THE COMPLETE
MENTAL
HEALTH
RESOURCE GUIDE

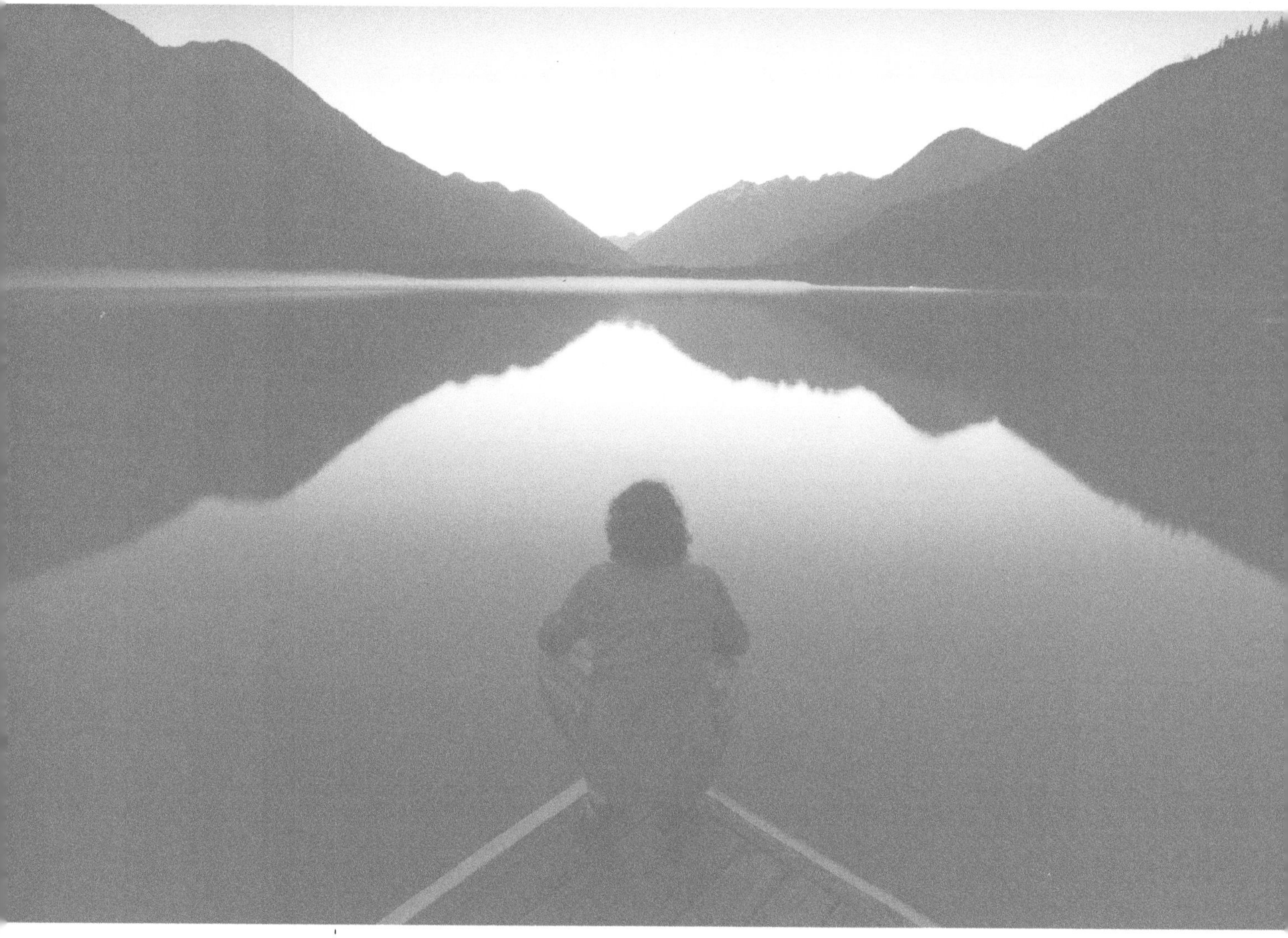

2018/2019
ELEVENTH EDITION

THE COMPLETE
MENTAL
HEALTH
RESOURCE GUIDE

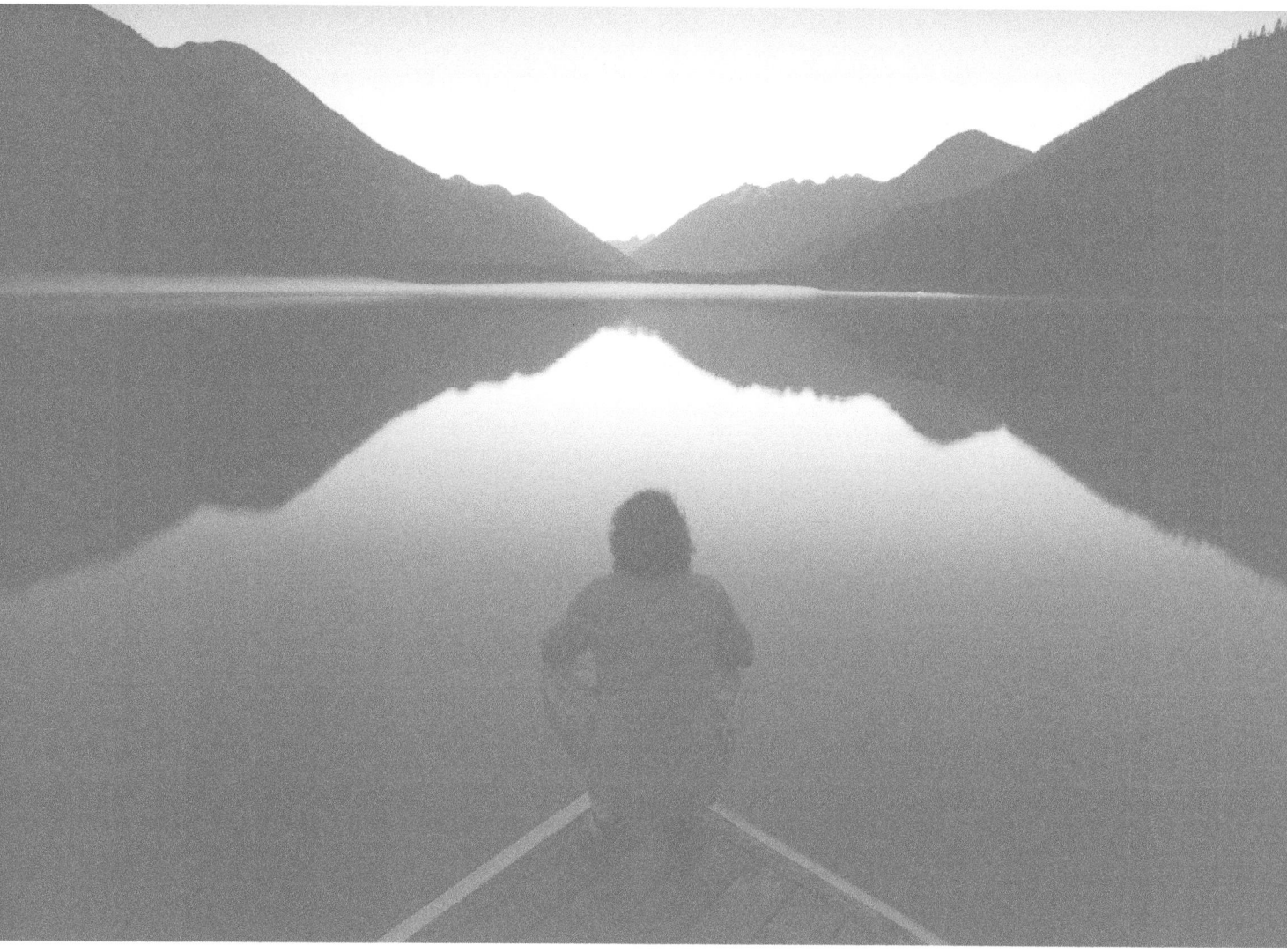

A SEDGWICK PRESS BOOK
GREY HOUSE PUBLISHING

PRESIDENT:	Richard Gottlieb
PUBLISHER:	Leslie Mackenzie
EDITORIAL DIRECTOR:	Laura Mars
PRODUCTION MANAGER:	Kristen Hayes
MARKETING DIRECTOR:	Jessica Moody

Grey House Publishing, Inc.
4919 Route 22
Amenia, NY 12501
518.789.8700
Fax: 518.789.0545
www.greyhouse.com
books@greyhouse.com

Publisher's Cataloging-In-Publication Data
(Prepared by The Donohue Group, Inc.)

Names: Gottlieb, Richard (Richard Harris), editor. | Grey House Publishing, Inc., publisher.
Title: The complete mental health resource guide : a comprehensive source book for professionals and
    individuals / [editor: Richard Gottlieb].
Description: Amenia, NY : Grey House Publishing, 2018- | "A Sedgwick Press Book." | Includes indexes.
Subjects: LCSH: Mental health services--United States--Directories. | LCGFT: Directories.
Classification: LCC RA790.6 .C625 | DDC 362.20973--dc23

ISBN: 978-1-68217-733-4

Table of Contents

Introduction

This eleventh edition of *The Complete Mental Health Resource Guide* (formerly *The Complete Mental Health Directory*) provides comprehensive coverage of 22 major mental health disorder categories, from ADHD to Trauma and Stressor-Related Disorders, with over 100 subcategories and specific disorders.

The major categories have been reorganized and, in some cases, renamed, to better reflect current, professional thought and changes regarding mental health. These changes include:

- Bipolar and Related Disorders, Depressive Disorders, Obsessive Compulsive Disorders, and Trauma and Stressor-Related Disorders now have their own sections;

- Neurocognitive Disorders, Neurodevelopmental Disorders, Feeding and Eating Disorders, and Sleep-Wake Disorders have been renamed to reflect current scholarship;

- Paraphilias are now part of Sexual Disorders;

- Impulse Disorders and Conduct Disorders have been combined under the new name—Disruptive, Impulse-Control and Conduct Disorders.

A repeat winner of the *National Health Information Awards* by the Health Information Resource Center for "the Nation's best consumer health programs and materials," this edition provides information on a subject that continues to grab headlines and fracture families and communities.

Praise for previous edition:

"... useful to libraries providing consumer health information and [to] medical libraries...valuable to professionals and patients..."

Cheryl A. Capitani, Chief Librarian, Harrisburg Hospital

"...the introductory essay's...thoughtful...comments...open many topics to discussion and searches for further information. Recommended. All levels."

Choice Magazine

"...array of materials...helpful addition to public, academic, medical libraries."

4-Star, Doody's Review Service

Coverage of more than 100 disorder categories include clear, concise descriptions, all updated with the most current diagnoses and treatment methods. Users will find a variety of disorder-specific resources, including Associations, Books, Periodicals, Research Centers, and Support Groups. In addition, *The Complete Mental Health Resource Guide* includes Professional Services, Publishers, Facilities, Clinical Management and Pharmaceutical Companies.

In addition to more than 4,500 listings, *The Complete Mental Health Resource Guide* includes several valuable elements:

- The State of Mental Health in America 2018 is a colorful report that combines narrative and charts for a complete look at this topic;

- NAMI - National Alliance on Mental Illness—reports on: Student Guide to Mental Health; Taking Charge of Your Mental Health; How to Help a Friend; and The Doctor is Out;

- Mental Disorders by Diagnostic Category educates patient and professional about categorical diagnoses, symptoms and treatments.

Section One: Disorders

This section consists of 22 chapters dealing with broad categories of mental health issues from Adjustment Disorders to Trauma and Stressor-Related Disorders. Each chapter begins with a description, written in clear, accessible language and includes symptoms, prevalence and treatment options.

These descriptions include information on specific syndromes within a general category, such as Agoraphobia, Social Anxiety, Selective Mutism and Separation Anxiety within the Anxiety Disorders chapter, and Delirium, Dementia and Anmestic Disorders within the Neurocognitive Disorders chapter.

Following the descriptions are specific resources relevant to the disorder, including Associations, Books, Government Agencies, Periodicals, Pamphlets, Support Groups, Hot Lines, Resource Centers, Audio & Video Tapes, and Web Sites.

Sections Two & Three: Associations, Organizations, Government Agencies

More than 1,000 National Associations, and Federal and State Agencies are profiled in these sections that offer general mental health services and support for patients and their families.

Section Four: Professional Support & Services

This section provides resources that support the many different professionals in the mental heath field. Included are specific chapters on Accreditation and Quality Assurance, Associations, Books, Conferences and Meetings, Periodicals, Training and Recruitment, Audio & Video Tapes, Web Sties, and Workbooks and Manuals.

Section Five: Publishers

This section lists major publishers of books and magazines that focus on health care or mental health issues. This material is suitable for both professionals in the mental health industry as well as patients and their network community.

Section Six: Facilities

This section lists major facilities and hospitals, arranged by state, which provide treatment for persons with mental health disorders.

Section Seven: Clinical Management

Here you will find products and services that support the Clinical Management aspect of the mental health industry, including Directories and Databases, Management Companies, and Information Services, which provide patient and medical data, as well as marketing information.

Section Eight: Pharmaceutical Companies

This section offers current information on the pharmaceutical companies that manufacture drugs to treat mental health disorders. This data is presented alphabetically by company name, including address, phone, fax, and web site.

PLUS an Appendix of Mental Health Drugs

This information is presented alphabetically by brand name of drug, with its generic name, the disorder/s it is typically prescribed for, and its manufacturers.

Three Indexes

- Disorder Index lists entries by disorders and disorder categories.

- Entry Index is an alphabetical list of all entries.

- Geographic Index lists entries by state.

For even easier access, *The Complete Mental Health Resource Guide* is available on our online database platform, http://gold.greyhouse.com. Subscribers have access to all of this health information, and can search by geographic area, disorder, contacts, keyword and so much more. With this online database, locating mental health resources has never been faster or easier.

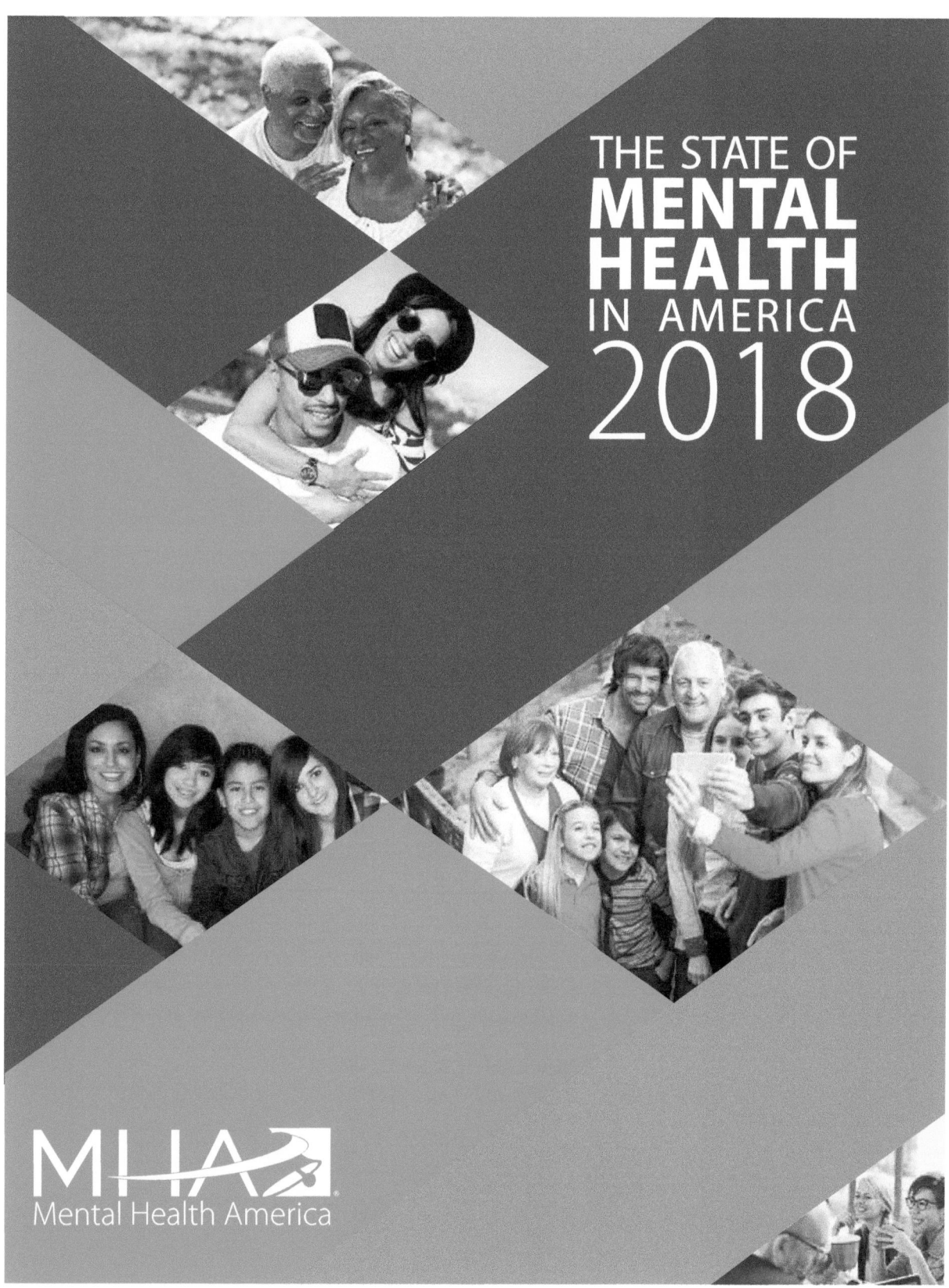

THE STATE OF
**MENTAL
HEALTH**
IN AMERICA
2018

MHA
Mental Health America

Key Facts and Findings

MENTAL HEALTH AND SUBSTANCE USE CONDITIONS ARE COMMON

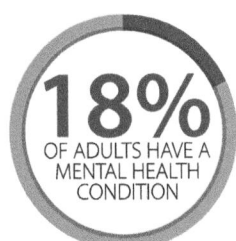

18% OF ADULTS HAVE A MENTAL HEALTH CONDITION

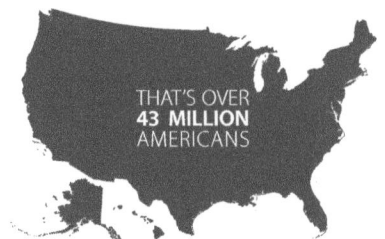

THAT'S OVER **43 MILLION** AMERICANS

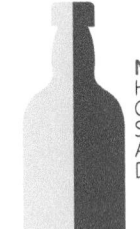

NEARLY HALF HAVE A CO-OCCURRING SUBSTANCE ABUSE DISORDER

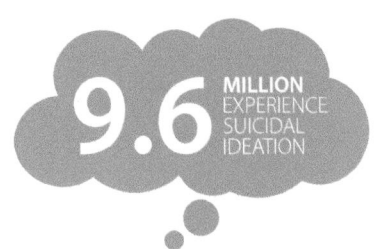

9.6 MILLION EXPERIENCE SUICIDAL IDEATION

MOST AMERICANS LACK ACCESS TO CARE

56% OF AMERICAN ADULTS WITH A MENTAL ILLNESS **DID NOT** RECEIVE TREATMENT

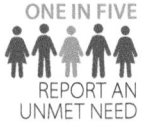

ONE IN FIVE REPORT AN UNMET NEED

7.7% OF YOUTH HAD **NO ACCESS** TO MENTAL HEALTH SERVICES THROUGH THEIR PRIVATE INSURANCE

YOUTH MENTAL HEALTH IS WORSENING AND ACCESS TO CARE IS LIMITED

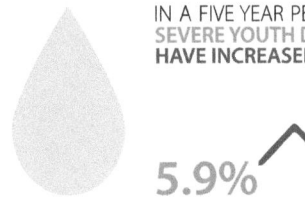

IN A FIVE YEAR PERIOD, RATES OF SEVERE YOUTH DEPRESSION **HAVE INCREASED**

5.9% → 8.2%

OVER 1.7 MILLION YOUTH WITH MAJOR DEPRESSIVE EPISODES **DID NOT** RECEIVE TREATMENT

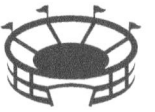

THAT'S ENOUGH TO FILL EVERY MAJOR LEAGUE BASEBALL STADIUM ON THE EAST COAST **TWICE**

THERE IS A SHORTAGE OF PROVIDERS

IN ALABAMA, THERE'S ONLY **ONE MENTAL HEALTH PROFESSIONAL PER 1,260 PEOPLE**

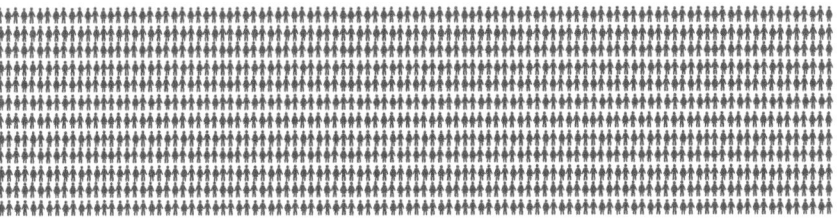

TO MEET THE NEED FOR MENTAL HEALTH CARE, PROVIDERS IN THE LOWEST RANKED STATES WOULD HAVE TO TREAT SIX TIMES AS MANY PEOPLE THAN PROVIDERS IN THE HIGHEST RANKED STATES

HEALTHCARE REFORM IS HELPING

RATES OF UNINSURED ADULTS WITH A MENTAL ILLNESS **DECREASED** BY

5%

STATES THAT **INCREASED** MEDICAID EXPANSION...

...SAW GREATER IMPROVEMENT IN YOUTH COVERAGE

...HAD FEWER UNINSURED ADULTS WITH MENTAL ILLNESS

Ranking Overview and Guidelines

This chart book presents a collection of data that provides a baseline for answering some questions about how many people in America need and have access to mental health services. This report is a companion to the online interactive data on the MHA website (http://www.mentalhealthamerica.net/issues/state-mental-health-america). The data and table include state and national data and sharable infographics.

MHA Guidelines

Given the variability of data, MHA developed guidelines to identify mental health measures that are most appropriate for inclusion in our ranking. Indicators were chosen that met the following guidelines:

- Data that are publicly available and as current as possible to provide up-to-date results.
- Data that are available for all 50 states and the District of Columbia.
- Data for both adults and youth.
- Data that captured information regardless of varying utilization of the private and public mental health system.
- Data that could be collected over time to allow for analysis of future changes and trends.

Our 2018 Measures

1. Adults with Any Mental Illness (AMI)
2. Adults with Alcohol Dependence and Illicit Drug Use (Marijuana, Heroin, and Cocaine)
3. Adults with Serious Thoughts of Suicide
4. Youth with At Least One Major Depressive Episode (MDE) in the Past Year
5. Youth with Alcohol Dependence and Illicit Drug Use (Marijuana, Heroin, and Cocaine)
6. Youth with Severe MDE
7. Adults with AMI who Did Not Receive Treatment
8. Adults with AMI Reporting Unmet Need
9. Adults with AMI who are Uninsured
10. Adults with Disability who Could Not See a Doctor Due to Costs
11. Youth with MDE who Did Not Receive Mental Health Services
12. Youth with Severe MDE who Received Some Consistent Treatment
13. Children with Private Insurance that Did Not Cover Mental or Emotional Problems
14. Students Identified with Emotional Disturbance for an Individualized Education Program
15. Mental Health Workforce Availability

A Complete Picture

While the above fifteen measures are not a complete picture of the mental health system, they do provide a strong foundation for understanding the prevalence of mental health concerns, as well as issues of access to insurance and treatment, particularly as that access varies among the states. MHA will continue to explore new measures that allow us to more accurately and comprehensively capture the needs of those with mental illness and their access to care.

Ranking

To better understand the rankings, it's important to compare similar states.

Factors to consider include geography, size, and political affiliation. For example, California and New York are similar. Both are large states with densely populated cities and tend to be Democratic leaning. They are less comparable to less populous or Republican leaning states like South Dakota North Dakota, Alabama, or Wyoming. Keep in mind that size of states and populations matter, both New York City and Los Angeles alone have more residents than North Dakota, South Dakota, Alabama, and Wyoming combined.

The rankings are based on the percentages, or rates, for each state collected from the most recently available data. For most indicators, the data represent data collected up to 2015. States with positive outcomes are ranked higher than states with poorer outcomes. The overall, adult, youth, prevalence and access rankings were analyzed by calculating a standardized score (Z score) for each measure, and ranking the sum of the standardized scores. For most measures, lower percentages equated to more positive outcomes (e.g. lower rates of substance use or those who are uninsured). There are two measures where high percentages equate to better outcomes. These include Youth with Severe MDE (Major Depressive Episode) who Received Some Consistent Treatment, and Students Identified with Emotional Disturbance for an Individualized Education Program. Here, the calculated standardized score was multiplied by -1 to obtain a Reverse Z Score that was used in the sum. All measures were considered equally important, and no weights were given to any measure in the rankings.

Along with calculated rankings, each measure is ranked individually with an accompanying chart and table. The table provides the percentage and estimated population for each ranking. The estimated population number is weighted and calculated by the agency conducting the applicable federal survey. The ranking is based on the percentage or rate. Data are presented with 2 decimal places when available.

Due to limitations in sample size for youth, measures for Youth with MDE who Did Not Receive Mental Health Services and Youth with Severe MDE who Received Some Consistent Treatment include data from various annual averages. Youth with MDE who Did Not Receive Mental Health Services includes data from years 2013 – 2015 and from 2010 – 2015. Those data from 2010 – 2015 are denoted noted by an (*). Data for Youth with Severe MDE who Received Some Consistent Treatment include annual averages from 2013 – 2015, 2010 – 2015 (*), and 2010-2013(**).

This year the measures Adults with Alcohol Dependence and Illicit Drug Use (Marijuana, Heroin, and Cocaine) and Youth with Alcohol Dependence and Illicit Drug Use (Marijuana, Heroin, and Cocaine) were determined by calculating the a weighted (.25) Z scores for measures Alcohol Dependence in the Past Year, Marijuana Use in the Past Year, Cocaine Use in the Past Year, and Heroin Use in the Past Year. The final measure is the sum of the weighted z scores.

Survey Limitations

Each survey has its own strengths and limitations. For example, strengths of both SAMHSA's *National Survey of Drug Use and Health* (NSDUH) and the CDC's Behavioral Risk Factor Surveillance System (BRFSS) are that they include national survey data with large sample sizes and utilized statistical modeling to provide weighted estimates of each state population. This means that the data is more representative of the general population. An example limitation of particular importance to the mental health community is that the NSDUH does not collect information from persons who are homeless and who do not stay at shelters, are active duty military personnel, or are institutionalized (i.e., in jails or hospitals). This limitation means that those individuals who have a mental illness who are also homeless or

incarcerated are not represented in the data presented by the NSDUH. If the data did include individuals who were homeless and/or incarcerated, we would possibly see prevalence of behavioral health issues increase and access to treatment rates worsen. It is MHA's goal to continue to search for the best possible data in future reports. Additional information on the methodology and limitations of the surveys can be found online as outlined in the glossary.

Overall Ranking

A high overall ranking indicates lower prevalence of mental illness and higher rates of access to care. A low overall ranking indicates higher prevalence of mental illness and lower rates of access to care. The combined scores of all 15 measures make up the overall ranking. The overall ranking includes both adult and youth measures as well as prevalence and access to care measures.

The 15 measures that make up the overall ranking include:

1. Adults with Any Mental Illness (AMI)
2. Adults with Alcohol Dependence and Illicit Drugs Use (Marijuana, Heroin, and Cocaine)
3. Adults with Serious Thoughts of Suicide
4. Youth with At Least One Major Depressive Episode (MDE) in the Past Year
5. Youth with Alcohol Dependence and Illicit Drugs Use (Marijuana, Heroin, and Cocaine)
6. Youth with Severe MDE
7. Adults with AMI who Did Not Receive Treatment
8. Adults with AMI Reporting Unmet Need
9. Adults with AMI who are Uninsured
10. Adults with Disability who Could Not See a Doctor Due to Costs
11. Youth with MDE who Did Not Receive Mental Health Services
12. Youth with Severe MDE who Received Some Consistent Treatment
13. Children with Private Insurance that Did Not Cover Mental or Emotional Problems
14. Students Identified with Emotional Disturbance for an Individualized Education Program
15. Mental Health Workforce Availability

The chart is a visual representation of the sum of the scores for each state. It provides an opportunity to see the difference between ranked states. For example, Massachusetts (ranked 1) has a score that is higher than Maryland (ranked 12). Rhode Island (ranked 23) has a score that is closest to the average.

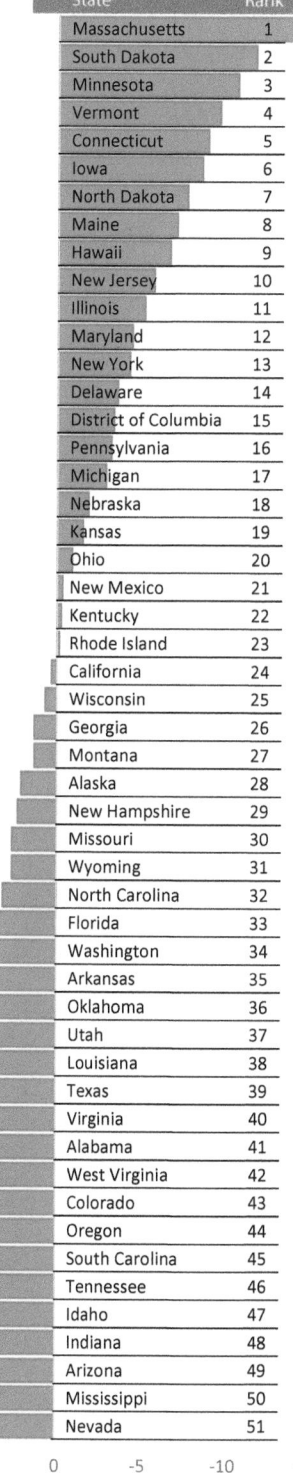

State	Rank
Massachusetts	1
South Dakota	2
Minnesota	3
Vermont	4
Connecticut	5
Iowa	6
North Dakota	7
Maine	8
Hawaii	9
New Jersey	10
Illinois	11
Maryland	12
New York	13
Delaware	14
District of Columbia	15
Pennsylvania	16
Michigan	17
Nebraska	18
Kansas	19
Ohio	20
New Mexico	21
Kentucky	22
Rhode Island	23
California	24
Wisconsin	25
Georgia	26
Montana	27
Alaska	28
New Hampshire	29
Missouri	30
Wyoming	31
North Carolina	32
Florida	33
Washington	34
Arkansas	35
Oklahoma	36
Utah	37
Louisiana	38
Texas	39
Virginia	40
Alabama	41
West Virginia	42
Colorado	43
Oregon	44
South Carolina	45
Tennessee	46
Idaho	47
Indiana	48
Arizona	49
Mississippi	50
Nevada	51

Adult Rankings

States with high rankings have lower prevalence of mental illness and higher rates of access to care for adults. Lower rankings indicate that adults have higher prevalence of mental illness and lower rates of access to care.

The 7 measures that make up the Adult Ranking include:

1. Adults with Any Mental Illness (AMI).
2. Adults with Alcohol Dependence and Illicit Drugs Use (Marijuana, Heroin, and Cocaine).
3. Adults with Serious Thoughts of Suicide.
4. Adults with AMI who Did Not Receive Treatment.
5. Adults with AMI Reporting Unmet Need.
6. Adults with AMI who are Uninsured.
7. Adults with Disability who Could Not See a Doctor Due to Costs.

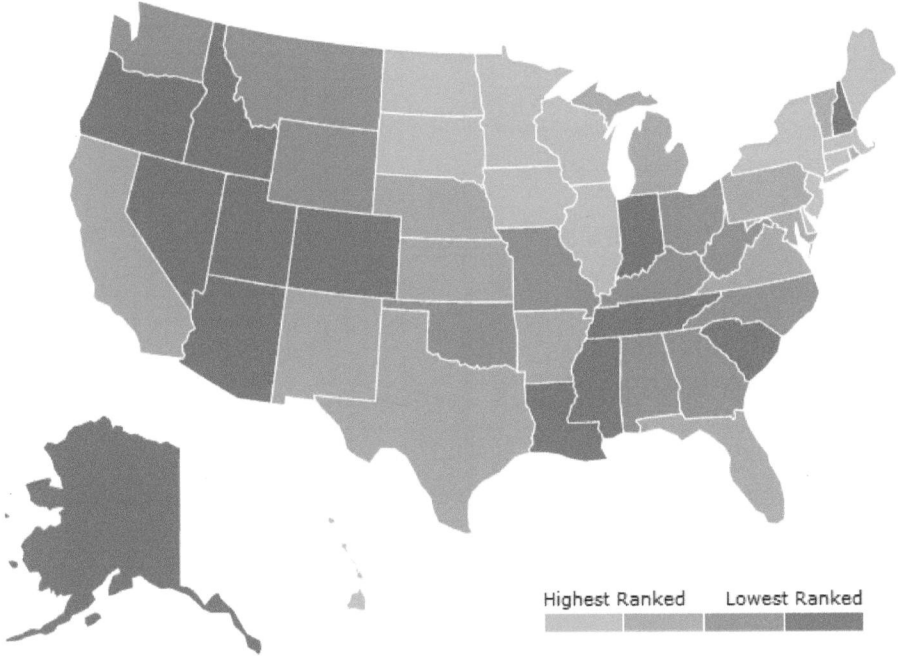

Highest Ranked   Lowest Ranked

Rank	State
1	Massachusetts
2	Iowa
3	Hawaii
4	North Dakota
5	South Dakota
6	Maine
7	Minnesota
8	Illinois
9	New Jersey
10	Connecticut
11	Wisconsin
12	Delaware
13	New York
14	Maryland
15	California
16	Pennsylvania
17	Vermont
18	Texas
19	Michigan
20	Rhode Island
21	Nebraska
22	Kansas
23	Virginia
24	Florida
25	New Mexico
26	Arkansas
27	Alabama
28	Ohio
29	Georgia
30	Wyoming
31	West Virginia
32	Kentucky
33	District of Columbia
34	Montana
35	Oklahoma
36	Missouri
37	North Carolina
38	Washington
39	South Carolina
40	Colorado
41	Louisiana
42	Arizona
43	Mississippi
44	Tennessee
45	Idaho
46	New Hampshire
47	Indiana
48	Oregon
49	Alaska
50	Nevada
51	Utah

Youth Rankings

States with high rankings have lower prevalence of mental illness and higher rates of access to care for youth. Lower rankings indicate that youth have
higher prevalence of mental illness and lower rates of access to care.

The 7 measures that make up the Youth Ranking include:

1. Youth with At Least One Major Depressive Episode (MDE) in the Past Year.
2. Youth with Alcohol Dependence and Illicit Drugs Use (Marijuana, Heroin, and Cocaine).
3. Youth with Severe MDE.
4. Youth with MDE who Did Not Receive Mental Health Services.
5. Youth with Severe MDE who Received Some Consistent Treatment.
6. Children with Private Insurance that Did Not Cover Mental or Emotional Problems.
7. Students Identified with Emotional Disturbance for an Individualized Education Program.

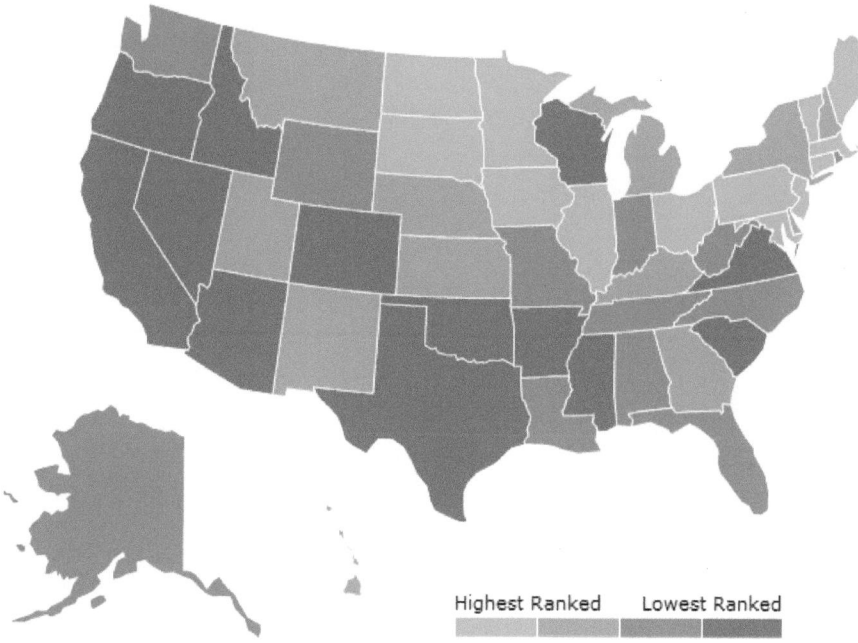

Highest Ranked   Lowest Ranked

Rank	State
1	South Dakota
2	Vermont
3	Minnesota
4	Massachusetts
5	Connecticut
6	North Dakota
7	District of Columbia
8	Iowa
9	New Jersey
10	Pennsylvania
11	Ohio
12	Maine
13	Illinois
14	Maryland
15	Kentucky
16	Alaska
17	Michigan
18	New York
19	Kansas
20	Georgia
21	Nebraska
22	New Hampshire
23	Delaware
24	Utah
25	New Mexico
26	Montana
27	Hawaii
28	Alabama
29	North Carolina
30	Missouri
31	Louisiana
32	Tennessee
33	Rhode Island
34	West Virginia
35	Washington
36	Wyoming
37	Florida
38	Indiana
39	California
40	Idaho
41	Oregon
42	South Carolina
43	Wisconsin
44	Texas
45	Oklahoma
46	Arkansas
47	Virginia
48	Colorado
49	Mississippi
50	Arizona
51	Nevada

Prevalence of Mental Illness

The scores for the six prevalence make up the Prevalence Ranking.

The 6 measures that make up the Prevalence Ranking include:

1. Adults with Any Mental Illness (AMI).
2. Adults with Alcohol Dependence and Illicit Drugs Use (Marijuana, Heroin, and Cocaine).
3. Adults with Serious Thoughts of Suicide.
4. Youth with At Least One Major Depressive Episode (MDE) in the Past Year.
5. Youth with Alcohol Dependence and Illicit Drugs Use.
6. Youth with Severe MDE.

A high ranking on the Prevalence Ranking indicates a lower prevalence of mental health and substance use issues. States that rank 1-10 have lower rates of mental health and substance use problems compared to states that ranked 42-51.

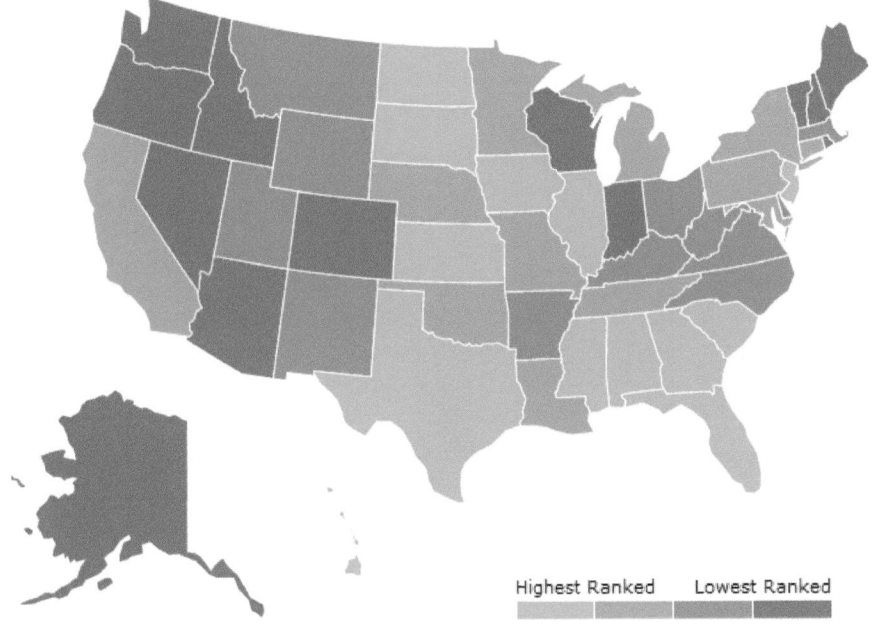

Rank	State
1	South Dakota
2	Hawaii
3	Georgia
4	North Dakota
5	Texas
6	New Jersey
7	South Carolina
8	Alabama
9	Illinois
10	Florida
11	Mississippi
12	Iowa
13	Kansas
14	Louisiana
15	Maryland
16	Tennessee
17	Missouri
18	Connecticut
19	District of Columbia
20	Nebraska
21	Pennsylvania
22	New York
23	Michigan
24	California
25	Oklahoma
26	Minnesota
27	Arkansas
28	Virginia
29	Delaware
30	North Carolina
31	New Mexico
32	Kentucky
33	Massachusetts
34	Montana
35	Wyoming
36	Ohio
37	Utah
38	West Virginia
39	Idaho
40	Maine
41	Washington
42	Wisconsin
43	Nevada
44	Alaska
45	Arizona
46	Vermont
47	Indiana
48	Rhode Island
49	Colorado
50	New Hampshire
51	Oregon

Access to Care Rankings

The Access Ranking indicates how much access to mental health care exists within a state. The access measures include access to insurance, access to treatment, quality and cost of insurance, access to special education, and workforce availability. A high Access Ranking indicates that a state provides relatively more access to insurance and mental health treatment.

The 9 measures that make up the Access Ranking include:

1. Adults with AMI who Did Not Receive Treatment.
2. Adults with AMI Reporting Unmet Need.
3. Adults with AMI who are Uninsured.
4. Adults with Disability who Could Not See a Doctor Due to Costs.
5. Youth with MDE who Did Not Receive Mental Health Services.
6. Youth with Severe MDE who Received Some Consistent Treatment.
7. Children with Private Insurance that Did Not Cover Mental or Emotional Problems.
8. Students Identified with Emotional Disturbance for an Individualized Education Program.
9. Mental Health Workforce Availability.

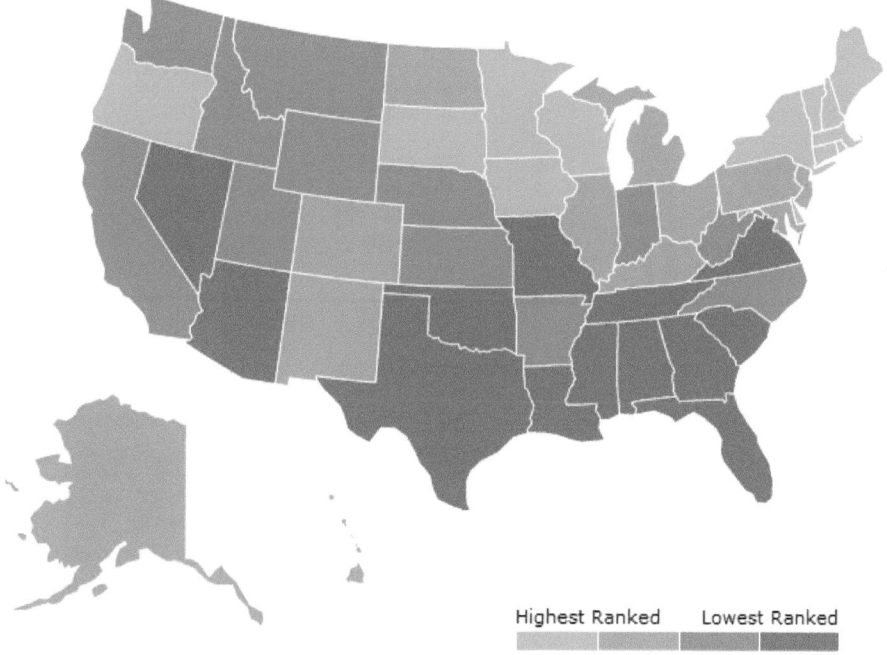

Highest Ranked   Lowest Ranked

Rank	State
1	Vermont
2	Massachusetts
3	Minnesota
4	Maine
5	Connecticut
6	Rhode Island
7	New Hampshire
8	South Dakota
9	Iowa
10	Delaware
11	New York
12	Oregon
13	Wisconsin
14	Ohio
15	North Dakota
16	Michigan
17	Colorado
18	Pennsylvania
19	Maryland
20	Alaska
21	District of Columbia
22	Illinois
23	New Mexico
24	Hawaii
25	Kentucky
26	New Jersey
27	Nebraska
28	Washington
29	Montana
30	California
31	Wyoming
32	Kansas
33	Indiana
34	Utah
35	West Virginia
36	North Carolina
37	Idaho
38	Arkansas
39	Arizona
40	Missouri
41	Oklahoma
42	Virginia
43	Georgia
44	Florida
45	Louisiana
46	Tennessee
47	Nevada
48	Alabama
49	Texas
50	South Carolina
51	Mississippi

Adult Prevalence of Mental Illness - Adults with Any Mental Illness (AMI)

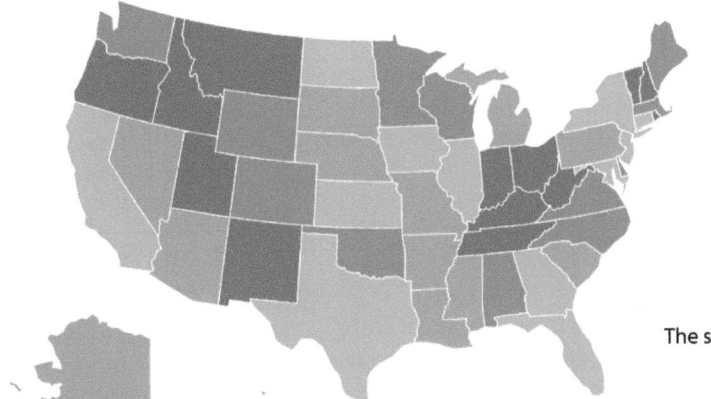

18.01% of adults struggle with mental health problems annually.

Equivalent to over 43.4 million Americans.

4.2 million live with an Anxiety Disorder

16 million live with Major Depression

The state prevalence of mental illness ranges from:

15.91% (Hawaii)	21.67 % (New Hampshire)
Highest Ranked	Lowest Ranked

Rank	State	%	#
1	Hawaii	15.91	168,000
2	Texas	15.98	3,127,000
3	Illinois	16.16	1,570,000
4	New Jersey	16.19	1,107,000
5	Maryland	16.62	756,000
6	Florida	16.77	2,630,000
7	North Dakota	16.78	94,000
8	California	17.04	4,997,000
9	Iowa	17.10	402,000
10	New York	17.22	2,638,000
11	Connecticut	17.42	483,000
12	Georgia	17.42	1,299,000
13	Kansas	17.52	372,000
14	South Carolina	17.52	644,000
15	South Dakota	17.57	110,000
16	Nevada	17.91	387,000
17	District of Columbia	17.95	97,000
18	Mississippi	17.95	394,000
19	Missouri	17.99	823,000
20	Arkansas	18.01	438,000
21	Michigan	18.07	1,373,000
22	Alaska	18.11	94,000
23	Nebraska	18.19	253,000
24	Pennsylvania	18.21	1,803,000
25	Arizona	18.32	925,000
26	Louisiana	18.42	634,000

Rank	State	%	#
27	Delaware	18.51	133,000
28	Wisconsin	18.75	824,000
29	Minnesota	18.78	777,000
30	Alabama	18.85	691,000
31	Massachusetts	18.99	1,008,000
32	Maine	19.16	203,000
33	Oklahoma	19.18	548,000
34	Virginia	19.18	1,203,000
35	North Carolina	19.48	1,459,000
36	Wyoming	19.51	85,000
37	Colorado	19.55	794,000
38	Washington	19.68	1,062,000
39	Tennessee	19.85	988,000
40	New Mexico	19.93	309,000
41	Montana	19.97	157,000
42	Ohio	20.20	1,778,000
43	Vermont	20.27	101,000
44	Idaho	20.41	243,000
45	Utah	20.48	417,000
46	Rhode Island	20.50	170,000
47	Indiana	20.56	1,014,000
48	West Virginia	20.89	301,000
49	Kentucky	21.30	707,000
50	Oregon	21.47	666,000
51	New Hampshire	21.67	227,000
	National	18.01	43,486,000

According to SAMHSA, "Any Mental Illness (AMI) is defined as having a diagnosable mental, behavioral, or emotional disorder, other than a developmental or substance use disorder. Any mental illness includes persons who have mild mental illness, moderate mental illness, and serious mental illness.

Adult Alcohol Dependence and Illicit Drug Use (Marijuana, Heroin, and Cocaine)

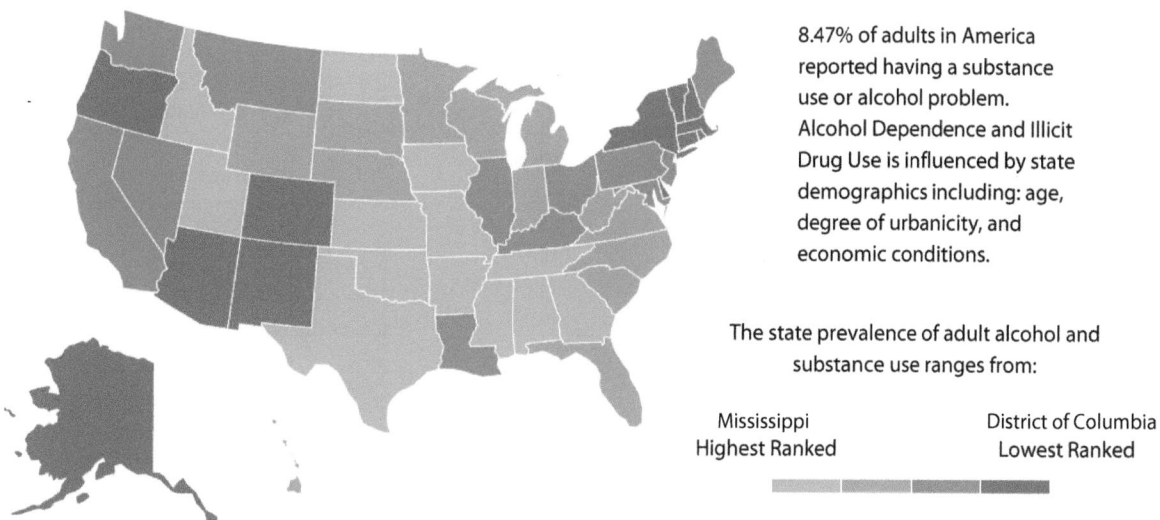

8.47% of adults in America reported having a substance use or alcohol problem. Alcohol Dependence and Illicit Drug Use is influenced by state demographics including: age, degree of urbanicity, and economic conditions.

The state prevalence of adult alcohol and substance use ranges from:

Mississippi
Highest Ranked

District of Columbia
Lowest Ranked

Rank	State	Weighted Sum of Z scores Adult Alcohol Dependence and Marijuana, Heroin, Cocaine Use
1	Mississippi	-1.1162
2	Utah	-1.1066
3	Iowa	-1.0318
4	Arkansas	-0.9161
5	Alabama	-0.9030
6	Kansas	-0.7833
7	Texas	-0.7578
8	North Dakota	-0.6849
9	Tennessee	-0.6252
10	Oklahoma	-0.6117
11	Idaho	-0.4811
12	Missouri	-0.4429
13	Georgia	-0.4228
14	West Virginia	-0.4071
15	South Dakota	-0.3809
16	Virginia	-0.3696
17	Nebraska	-0.3372
18	Florida	-0.3270
19	North Carolina	-0.2984
20	Hawaii	-0.2833
21	Michigan	-0.2612
22	Wyoming	-0.2548
23	Wisconsin	-0.2512
24	Minnesota	-0.2459
25	South Carolina	-0.2053
26	Indiana	-0.1411

Rank	State	Weighted Sum of Z scores Adult Alcohol Dependence and Marijuana, Heroin, Cocaine Use
27	Illinois	-0.1061
28	Nevada	-0.0763
29	Ohio	-0.0591
30	New Jersey	-0.0340
31	Kentucky	0.0091
32	Louisiana	0.0463
33	Montana	0.0756
34	Pennsylvania	0.1539
35	Washington	0.1952
36	Maine	0.2919
37	California	0.4569
38	Maryland	0.5607
39	New Mexico	0.5993
40	Massachusetts	0.6031
41	Delaware	0.7823
42	Arizona	0.8091
43	New York	0.8547
44	Oregon	0.8998
45	Rhode Island	1.0956
46	Connecticut	1.1272
47	New Hampshire	1.4512
48	Colorado	1.5944
49	Vermont	1.7503
50	Alaska	2.0697
51	District of Columbia	2.0943
	National	0.000

Adults with Serious Thoughts of Suicide

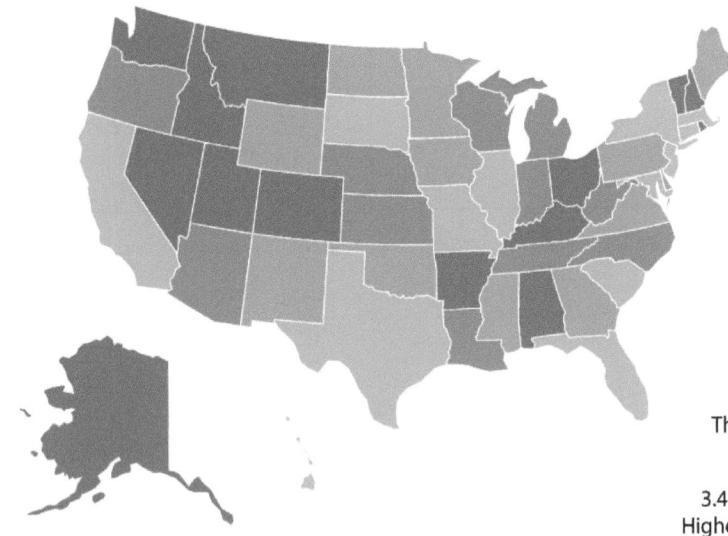

The percentage of adults reporting serious thoughts of suicide is 3.99%. The estimated number of adults with serious suicidal thoughts is over 9.6 million.

The percentage of adults who made a suicide plan in the past year was higher among adults aged 18 to 25.

The state prevalence of adult with serious thoughts of suicide range from:

3.46% (Texas)
Highest Ranked

5.25% (Utah)
Lowest Ranked

Rank	State	%	#
1	Texas	3.46	678,000
2	Connecticut	3.49	97,000
3	Florida	3.59	563,000
4	Maryland	3.65	166,000
5	South Dakota	3.66	23,000
6	South Carolina	3.73	137,000
7	New Jersey	3.78	259,000
8	California	3.80	1,115,000
9	New York	3.85	591,000
10	Hawaii	3.88	41,000
11	Massachusetts	3.88	206,000
12	Illinois	3.89	378,000
13	Missouri	3.92	179,000
14	Iowa	3.93	92,000
15	Virginia	3.94	247,000
16	North Dakota	3.95	22,000
17	Oklahoma	3.97	114,000
18	Alabama	4.02	148,000
19	Delaware	4.03	29,000
20	Georgia	4.03	301,000
21	Minnesota	4.07	168,000
22	New Mexico	4.08	63,000
23	Maine	4.10	43,000
24	Pennsylvania	4.10	407,000
25	Mississippi	4.13	91,000
26	Wyoming	4.14	18,000

Rank	State	%	#
27	Kansas	4.14	88,000
28	Michigan	4.14	314,000
29	Indiana	4.17	206,000
30	District of Columbia	4.18	23,000
31	Nebraska	4.18	58,000
32	Wisconsin	4.18	184,000
33	Louisiana	4.19	144,000
34	North Carolina	4.20	315,000
35	West Virginia	4.23	61,000
36	Tennessee	4.26	212,000
37	Arizona	4.34	219,000
38	Oregon	4.37	136,000
39	Idaho	4.39	52,000
40	Arkansas	4.41	98,000
41	Rhode Island	4.42	37,000
42	Nevada	4.45	96,000
43	Colorado	4.47	182,000
44	Washington	4.54	245,000
45	Vermont	4.59	23,000
46	Ohio	4.64	408,000
47	Kentucky	4.66	155,000
48	Alaska	4.68	24,000
49	New Hampshire	4.94	52,000
50	Montana	4.95	39,000
51	Utah	5.25	107,000
	National	3.99	9,653,000

Youth Prevalence of Mental Illness

Youth with At Least One Major Depressive Episode (MDE) in the Past Year

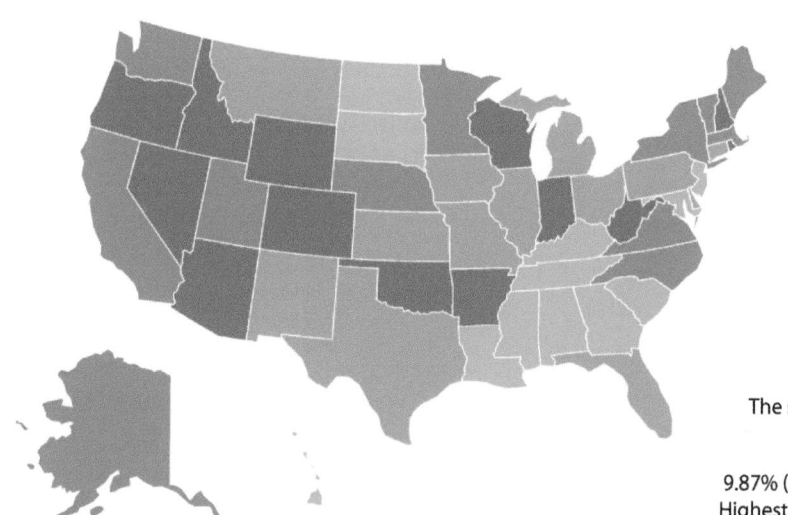

11.93% of youth (age 12-17) report suffering from at least one major depressive episode (MDE) in the past year. Major Depression is marked by significant and pervasive feelings of sadness that are associated with suicidal thoughts and impair a young person's ability to concentrate or engage in normal activities.

The number of youth experiencing MDE continues to rise, annually.

The state prevalence of youth with MDE ranges from:

9.87% (Hawaii)
Highest Ranked

14.64% (Indiana)
Lowest Ranked

Rank	State	%	#
1	Hawaii	9.87	10,000
2	South Dakota	9.90	7,000
3	District of Columbia	9.96	3,000
4	Georgia	10.08	85,000
5	New Jersey	10.32	72,000
6	North Dakota	10.47	5,000
7	Tennessee	10.92	55,000
8	South Carolina	10.96	40,000
9	Alabama	10.97	42,000
10	Louisiana	11.00	40,000
11	Maryland	11.03	50,000
12	Kentucky	11.05	38,000
13	Mississippi	11.08	27,000
14	Kansas	11.18	27,000
15	Illinois	11.20	115,000
16	Montana	11.42	8,000
17	Delaware	11.47	8,000
18	Connecticut	11.49	33,000
19	Missouri	11.49	54,000
20	New Mexico	11.50	19,000
21	Texas	11.53	272,000
22	Pennsylvania	11.64	109,000
23	Michigan	11.80	93,000
24	Ohio	11.85	109,000
25	Iowa	11.87	29,000
26	Florida	11.88	166,000

Rank	State	%	#
27	New York	11.92	170,000
28	Utah	11.97	35,000
29	Vermont	12.06	5,000
30	Nebraska	12.25	19,000
31	California	12.28	375,000
32	North Carolina	12.35	96,000
33	Massachusetts	12.37	60,000
34	Alaska	12.40	7,000
35	Virginia	12.47	78,000
36	Maine	12.51	12,000
37	Washington	12.54	67,000
38	Minnesota	12.55	53,000
39	Oklahoma	12.57	39,000
40	Arkansas	12.72	30,000
41	Idaho	13.03	19,000
42	Rhode Island	13.03	10,000
43	Arizona	13.20	72,000
44	West Virginia	13.26	17,000
45	Wyoming	13.31	6,000
46	New Hampshire	13.43	13,000
47	Wisconsin	13.64	61,000
48	Colorado	13.73	57,000
49	Nevada	13.94	31,000
50	Oregon	14.33	42,000
51	Indiana	14.64	79,000
	National	11.93	2,969,000

Youth with Alcohol Dependence and Illicit Drug Use

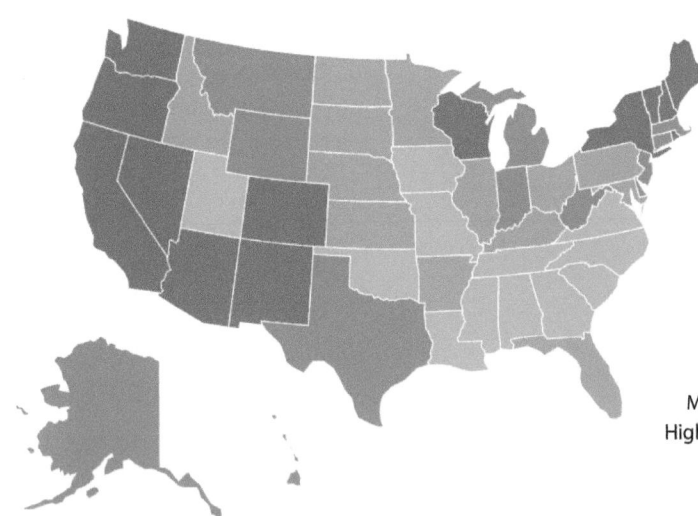

5.13% of youth in America report having a substance use or alcohol problem.

3.3 million youth reported the use of marijuana, cocaine, and/or heroin

National youth rates have decreased over time, but higher rates remain among special populations, such LGBTQ, Service members and American and Alaskan Natives.[1]

The state prevalence of youth alcohol and substance use ranges from:

Mississippi	Colorado
Highest Ranked	Lowest Ranked

Rank	State	Weighted Sum of Z scores
1	Mississippi	-1.3899
2	Alabama	-1.2295
3	Louisiana	-1.2050
4	North Carolina	-0.9268
5	Utah	-0.8959
6	Georgia	-0.8945
7	Iowa	-0.8936
8	Tennessee	-0.8374
9	South Carolina	-0.8049
10	District of Columbia	-0.7956
11	Oklahoma	-0.7809
12	Virginia	-0.7308
13	Missouri	-0.6696
14	Nebraska	-0.6455
15	South Dakota	-0.5813
16	Arkansas	-0.5321
17	Minnesota	-0.4994
18	Florida	-0.3702
19	North Dakota	-0.3618
20	Ohio	-0.3270
21	Kansas	-0.3114
22	Illinois	-0.2895
23	Maryland	-0.2096
24	Pennsylvania	-0.1863
25	Kentucky	-0.1861
26	Idaho	-0.1618

Rank	State	Weighted Sum of Z scores
27	Wyoming	-0.1383
28	Michigan	-0.1232
29	Montana	-0.0500
30	West Virginia	-0.0422
31	Indiana	-0.0020
32	Hawaii	0.0278
33	Delaware	0.0537
34	New Jersey	0.1256
35	Massachusetts	0.1732
36	Texas	0.2067
37	Connecticut	0.2392
38	Alaska	0.2928
39	New York	0.4384
40	Wisconsin	0.4389
41	Washington	0.5629
42	Maine	0.6482
43	Nevada	0.6500
44	Rhode Island	0.7792
45	California	0.9050
46	New Mexico	1.1088
47	Oregon	1.2007
48	New Hampshire	1.2217
49	Vermont	1.2473
50	Arizona	1.4244
51	Colorado	1.7503
	National	0.00

---

[1] Center for Substance Abuse Treatment. Substance Abuse Treatment and Family Therapy. Rockville (MD): Substance Abuse and Mental Health Services Administration (US); 2004. (Treatment Improvement Protocol (TIP) Series, No. 39.) Chapter 5 Specific Populations. Available from: https://www.ncbi.nlm.nih.gov/books/NBK64253/

Youth with Severe Major Depressive Episode

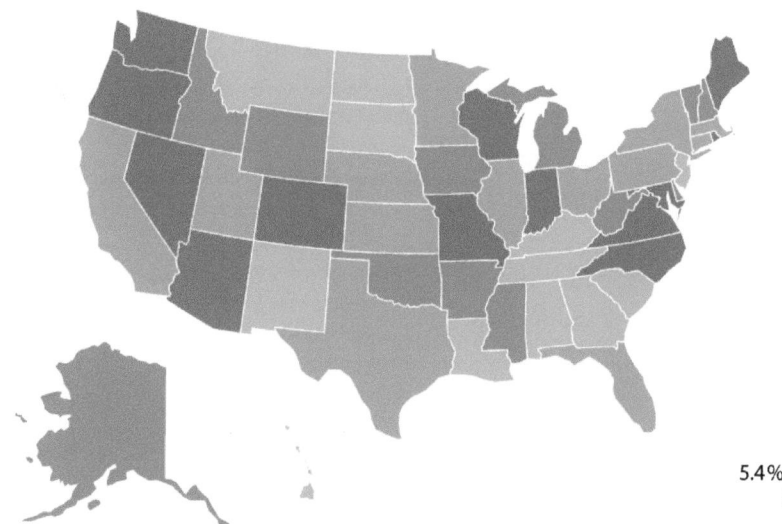

8.2% of youth (over 1.9 million youth) cope with severe major depression. Depressive symptoms result in significant interference in school, home and in relationships.

States with the highest rates (bottom 13 states) have almost **TWICE as many** severely depressed youth than states with the lowest rates (top 13 states).

The state prevalence of youth with severe MDE ranges from:

5.4% (South Dakota)
Highest Ranked

13.1% (Oregon)
Lowest Ranked

Rank	State	%	#
1	South Dakota	5.4	4,000
2	Kentucky	5.5	18,000
3	Georgia	5.6	46,000
4	New Mexico	5.8	9,000
5	Montana	5.9	4,000
6	North Dakota	6.0	3,000
7	Hawaii	6.2	6,000
8	Tennessee	6.5	32,000
9	New Jersey	6.6	45,000
10	District of Columbia	6.7	2,000
11	Alabama	6.8	25,000
12	Louisiana	6.9	25,000
13	South Carolina	7.1	25,000
14	New York	7.5	104,000
15	Pennsylvania	7.5	68,000
16	Texas	7.6	175,000
17	Nebraska	7.6	11,000
18	Utah	7.7	22,000
19	Kansas	7.7	18,000
20	California	7.8	232,000
21	Illinois	7.9	79,000
22	Ohio	8.0	72,000
23	Connecticut	8.0	22,000
24	Florida	8.1	111,000
25	Minnesota	8.2	34,000
26	Massachusetts	8.3	39,000

Rank	State	%	#
27	West Virginia	8.5	11,000
28	Vermont	8.5	4,000
29	Alaska	8.7	5,000
30	Michigan	8.7	67,000
31	New Hampshire	8.7	8,000
32	Wyoming	8.8	4,000
33	Mississippi	8.8	21,000
34	Iowa	8.8	21,000
35	Delaware	8.9	6,000
36	Arkansas	9.0	21,000
37	Oklahoma	9.1	28,000
38	Washington	9.3	48,000
39	Idaho	9.3	13,000
40	Maryland	9.4	42,000
41	Missouri	9.5	43,000
42	North Carolina	9.6	72,000
43	Virginia	9.9	60,000
44	Maine	10.3	9,000
45	Nevada	10.6	23,000
46	Arizona	10.6	56,000
47	Colorado	10.8	43,000
48	Wisconsin	11.5	51,000
49	Rhode Island	12.1	9,000
50	Indiana	12.1	63,000
51	Oregon	13.1	37,000
	National	8.2	1,996,000

According to SAMHSA, youth who experience a major depressive episode in the last year with severe role impairment (Youth with Severe MDE) reported the maximum level of interference over four role domains including: chores at home, school or work, family relationships, and social life.

Adult Access to Care
Adults with AMI who Did Not Receive Treatment

55.8% of adults with a mental illness received no treatment. Lack of access to treatment is slowly improving. In 2011, 59% of adults with a mental health problem did not receive any mental health treatment.

Reasons for not receiving treatment can be individual or systemic.

Making screening tools accessible would allow individuals to learn about, and address mental health concerns. Additionally, establishing contact with a healthcare provider at onset is critical.

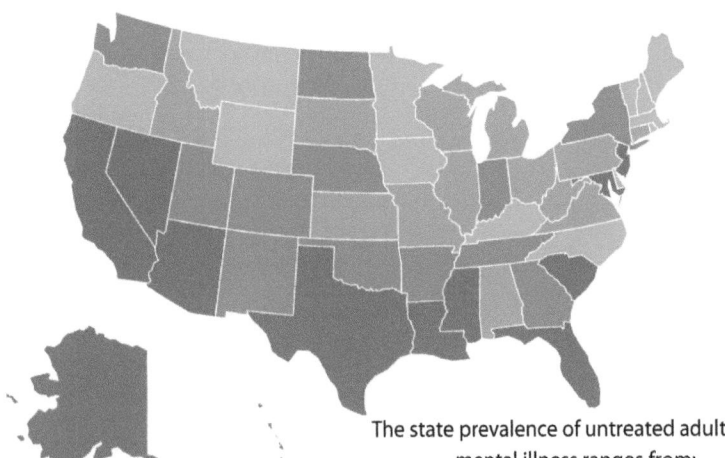

The state prevalence of untreated adults with mental illness ranges from:

41.4% (Maine)	66.0% (Nevada)
Highest Ranked	Lowest Ranked

Rank	State	%	#
1	Maine	41.4	87,000
2	Vermont	43.7	47,000
3	Minnesota	44.3	356,000
4	Iowa	45.6	170,000
5	Massachusetts	45.9	502,000
6	Montana	48.1	79,000
7	New Hampshire	49.0	111,000
8	Rhode Island	49.3	92,000
9	North Carolina	50.2	743,00
10	Delaware	50.6	69,000
11	Kentucky	50.6	363,000
12	Oregon	51.2	373,000
13	Wyoming	52.0	44,000
14	Idaho	52.2	129,000
15	Missouri	52.3	424,000
16	Wisconsin	52.4	436,000
17	Connecticut	52.5	247,000
18	Ohio	52.9	946,000
19	Virginia	53.0	630,000
20	Pennsylvania	53.2	933,000
21	Illinois	53.3	807,000
22	Kansas	53.7	193,000
23	Michigan	53.7	743,000
24	West Virginia	53.8	167,000
25	Alabama	54.0	382,000
26	South Dakota	54.3	56,000

Rank	State	%	#
27	Arkansas	54.8	251,000
28	Indiana	55.4	571,000
29	North Dakota	55.6	45,000
30	Washington	55.6	593,000
31	Utah	56.2	246,000
32	Oklahoma	56.3	298,000
33	New York	56.4	1,468,000
34	New Mexico	57.2	188,000
35	Colorado	57.3	433,000
36	Georgia	57.3	757,000
37	Nebraska	57.5	143,000
38	Tennessee	57.7	599,000
39	Mississippi	57.8	222,000
40	Louisiana	58.1	388,000
41	New Jersey	58.2	587,000
42	South Carolina	58.3	357,000
43	Arizona	58.5	539,000
44	District of Columbia	58.7	61,000
45	Maryland	59.5	417,000
46	Texas	60.4	1,890,000
47	California	61.2	3,104,000
48	Florida	61.7	1,557,000
49	Hawaii	63.5	114,000
50	Alaska	63.9	60,000
51	Nevada	66.0	268,000
	National	55.8	24,280,000

Adults with AMI Reporting Unmet Need

One out of five (20.1%) adults with a mental illness reported that were not able to receive the treatment they needed.

Individuals who are reporting unmet need are seeking treatment and facing barriers to getting the help they need.

Where you live could determine whether you receive timely treatment: individuals living in states with the highest levels of unmet need (bottom 13) were 1.6 times more likely to have people report unmet need.

Across the country, several systemic barriers to accessing care exclude and marginalize individuals with a great need. These include the following:

1) Lack of insurance or inadequate insurance
2) Lack of available treatment providers
3) Lack of available treatment types (inpatient treatment, individual therapy, intensive community services)
4) Insufficient finances to cover costs – including, copays, uncovered treatment types, or when providers do not take insurance.

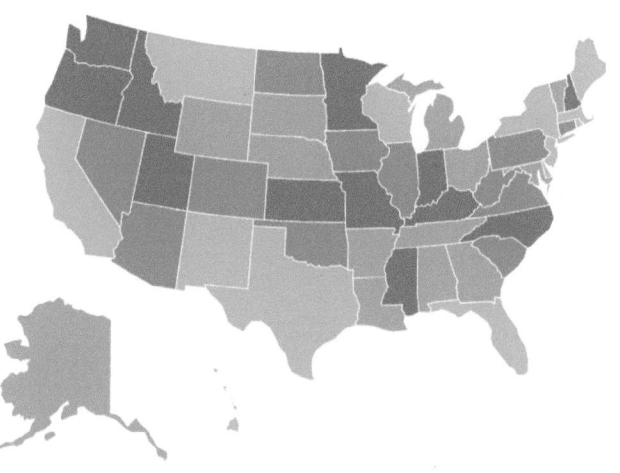

The state prevalence of adults with AMI reporting unmet treatment needs ranges from:

14.4% (Hawaii)	25.2% (District of Columbia)
Highest Ranked	Lowest Ranked

Rank	State	%	#
1	Hawaii	14.4	26,000
2	Massachusetts	15.6	169,000
3	Texas	16.9	530,000
4	Delaware	17.0	23,000
5	New Jersey	17.4	177,000
6	Rhode Island	17.9	33,000
7	New Mexico	18.2	60,000
8	California	18.2	922,000
9	Florida	18.3	464,000
10	Montana	18.4	30,000
11	New York	18.6	483,000
12	Wisconsin	19.0	158,000
13	Maine	19.1	40,000
14	Nebraska	19.2	48,000
15	Alaska	19.2	18,000
16	Georgia	19.3	255,000
17	Arkansas	19.4	89,000
18	South Dakota	19.6	20,000
19	Louisiana	19.6	131,000
20	Alabama	19.8	140,000
21	Tennessee	19.8	206,000
22	Maryland	20.0	140,000
23	Ohio	20.1	360,000
24	Michigan	20.1	279,000
25	Vermont	20.6	22,000
26	Iowa	20.6	77,000

Rank	State	%	#
27	Wyoming	20.6	18,000
28	Pennsylvania	20.6	362,000
29	Arizona	20.8	193,000
30	North Dakota	20.9	17,000
31	Illinois	21.3	324,000
32	South Carolina	21.3	130,000
33	Connecticut	21.6	102,000
34	Oklahoma	21.7	114,000
35	Colorado	21.8	163,000
36	Virginia	22.0	262,000
37	West Virginia	22.1	69,000
38	Nevada	22.4	91,000
39	Kansas	22.5	81,000
40	Utah	22.7	100,000
41	Mississippi	22.9	88,000
42	Kentucky	23.3	168,000
43	Washington	23.5	249,000
44	New Hampshire	23.8	54,000
45	Minnesota	24.0	194,000
46	North Carolina	24.3	362,000
47	Oregon	24.5	177,000
48	Indiana	24.5	247,000
49	Idaho	24.7	61,000
50	Missouri	25.1	203,000
51	District of Columbia	25.2	26,000
	National	20.1	8,752,000

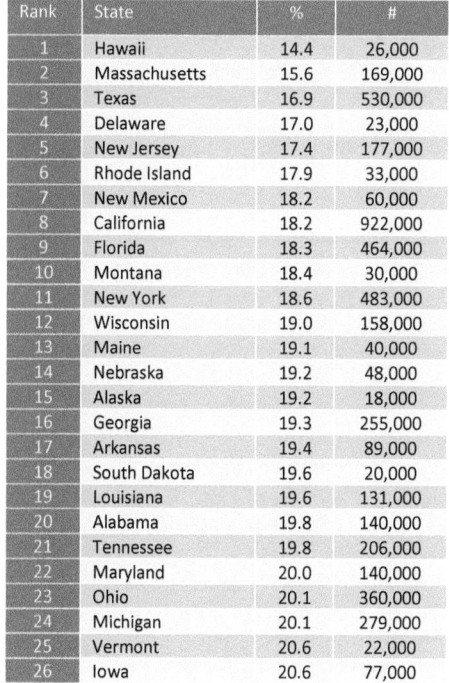

Adults with AMI who are Uninsured

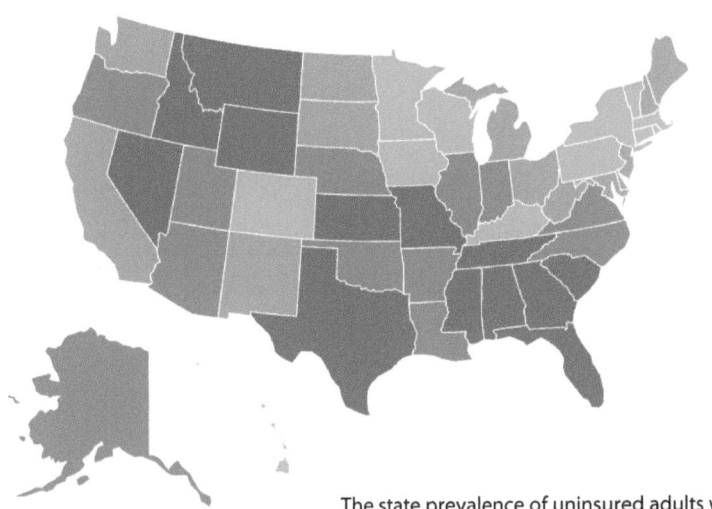

14.7% (over 6.3 million) of adults with a mental illness remain uninsured.

Missouri (7.7%), South Carolina (2.7%), and Kansas (2.4%) had the largest increase in Adults with AMI who Uninsured –three states that have not adopted Medicaid expansion.

With a national focus on health care access, the uninsured rate is improving (3% reduction).

Unfortunately, having insurance coverage does not mean access to needed treatment.

55.8% of adults with mental illness received no treatment in the past year. For those seeking treatment, 20.1% continue to report unmet treatment needs.

The state prevalence of uninsured adults with mental illness ranges from:

3.3% (Massachusetts)
Highest Ranked

23.8% (South Carolina)
Lowest Ranked

Rank	State	%	#
1	Massachusetts	3.3	36,000
2	District of Columbia	4.9	5,000
3	Hawaii	5.3	10,000
4	Vermont	5.6	6,000
5	Minnesota	6.8	55,000
6	Kentucky	8.1	58,000
7	Rhode Island	8.2	15,000
8	Colorado	8.7	66,000
9	Wisconsin	9.0	75,000
10	Connecticut	9.3	44,000
11	Iowa	9.3	35,000
12	Pennsylvania	9.6	170,000
13	New York	10.3	268,000
14	North Dakota	10.7	9,000
15	New Mexico	10.8	36,000
16	New Hampshire	10.9	25,000
17	Delaware	11.1	15,000
18	New Jersey	11.3	115,000
19	Maryland	11.3	79,000
20	South Dakota	11.8	12,000
21	Ohio	11.9	214,000
22	Washington	11.9	127,000
23	West Virginia	11.9	37,000
24	Michigan	12.5	174,000
25	California	13.3	675,000
26	Maine	13.3	28,000

Rank	State	%	#
27	Illinois	13.9	211,000
28	Oregon	14.5	106,000
29	Virginia	14.6	174,000
30	Alaska	14.9	14,000
31	North Carolina	15.0	224,000
32	Nebraska	15.3	38,000
33	Arizona	15.9	147,000
34	Indiana	16.1	165,000
35	Louisiana	17.7	119,000
36	Utah	17.7	78,000
37	Oklahoma	17.7	94,000
38	Arkansas	18.1	83,000
39	Kansas	18.5	66,000
40	Montana	18.6	31,000
41	Nevada*	19.0	77,000
42	Georgia	19.2	254,000
43	Alabama	19.3	136,000
44	Idaho	19.3	48,000
45	Mississippi	20.4	79,000
46	Wyoming	20.7	18,000
47	Florida	21.0	533,000
48	Missouri	22.5	183,000
49	Texas	23.3	731,000
50	Tennessee	23.6	247,000
51	South Carolina	23.8	145,000
	National	14.7	6,389,000

Adults with Disability who Could Not See a Doctor Due to Costs

21.62% of adults with a disability were not able to see a doctor due to costs.

An estimated 47% of adults are not receiving treatment because of costs.

People with mental health problems are more likely to have no insurance or to be on public insurance (43%).[1]

The inability to pay for treatment, due to high treatment costs and/or inadequate insurance coverage remains a barrier for those individuals despite being insured.

In recent years, there has also been a decline in employer-sponsored insurance, which has contributed to even greater disparities in mental healthcare.

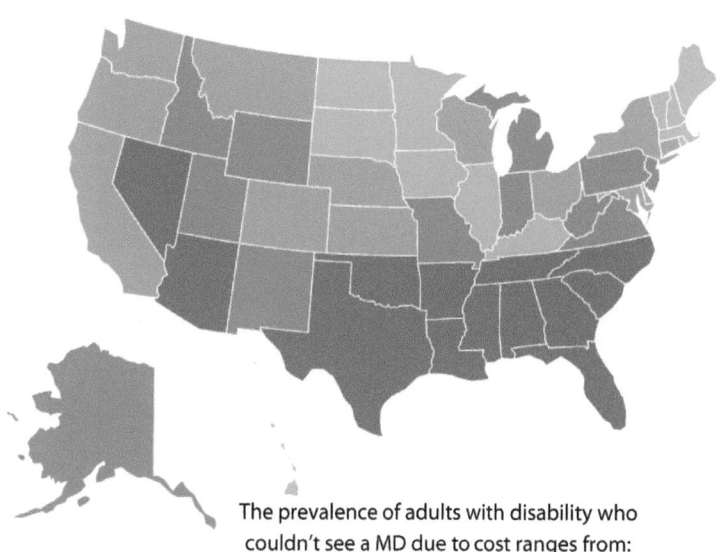

The prevalence of adults with disability who couldn't see a MD due to cost ranges from:

12.45% (Hawaii)
Highest Ranked

30.91% (Mississippi)
Lowest Ranked

Rank	State	%	#
1	Hawaii	12.45	22,097
2	Iowa	12.64	54,455
3	Vermont	12.66	13,144
4	North Dakota	13.26	12,981
5	New Hampshire	13.47	28,019
6	Massachusetts	13.64	141,320
7	District of Columbia	14.19	13,597
8	Minnesota	14.38	104,523
9	Illinois	15.38	262,507
10	Kentucky	15.38	188,778
11	Maine	15.89	40,150
12	South Dakota	16.11	21,437
13	Rhode Island	16.18	27,887
14	Colorado	17.30	133,762
15	Connecticut	17.53	93,597
16	Washington	17.53	219,597
17	Wisconsin	17.53	146,005
18	Ohio	17.59	319,279
19	Montana	18.21	34,492
20	Maryland	18.27	143,733
21	California	18.46	1,006,308
22	New York	18.79	531,331
23	Kansas	19.02	79,714
24	Oregon	19.23	152,156
25	Nebraska	19.39	48,379
26	Delaware	19.48	28,943

Rank	State	%	#
27	West Virginia	20.03	82,178
28	Pennsylvania	20.17	392,965
29	Idaho	20.74	56,031
30	Alaska	20.98	23,610
31	New Mexico	21.09	72,475
32	Wyoming	21.30	20,759
33	Michigan	21.43	363,203
34	Virginia	21.65	243,521
35	Utah	22.06	77,733
36	New Jersey	22.35	258,348
37	Indiana	22.86	237,916
38	Missouri	23.54	272,719
39	Arkansas	24.11	146,714
40	Arizona	24.14	249,660
41	Nevada	24.75	109,424
42	Tennessee	25.21	309,380
43	North Carolina	25.40	418,833
44	Oklahoma	25.45	188,785
45	Alabama	25.65	261,471
46	Georgia	26.96	407,162
47	Florida	27.11	875,479
48	South Carolina	28.12	244,082
49	Louisiana	28.73	225,771
50	Texas	29.19	956,390
51	Mississippi	30.91	170,133
	National	21.62	10,663,174

[7] Bradford, Kim, Braxton, and others, "Access to medical care among persons with psychotic and major affective disorders," Psychiatric Services 59(8), pp. 847-852, 2008 (AHRQ grant HS13353).

Youth Access to Care
Youth with MDE who Did Not Receive Mental Health Services

63.1% of youth with major depression do not receive any mental health treatment.

That means that **6 out of 10** young people who have depression and who are most at risk of suicidal thoughts, difficulty in school, and difficulty in relationships with others do not get the treatment needed to support them.

State-level budget cuts and coverage contraction has presented a challenge for federal programs, such as Medicaid, which is reported to have the greatest influence over mental health trends among children. [1]

The state prevalence of untreated youth with depression ranges from:

48.6% (Connecticut)
Highest Ranked

72.2% (Tennessee)
Lowest Ranked

Rank	State	%	#
1*	Connecticut	48.6	12,000
2	Maine	50.1	5,000
3	Vermont	50.6	2,000
4	Minnesota	51.9	21,000
5	Alaska	53.1	3,000
6	Oregon	54.9	26,000
7	Massachusetts	55.5	26,000
8	Maryland	55.6	24,000
9	Wyoming	55.7	3,000
10	Iowa	56.4	13,000
11	Ohio	58.0	56,000
12	New Hampshire	58.0	7,000
13	South Dakota	58.1	3,000
14	Delaware	58.8	4,000
15	West Virginia	59.9	8,000
16	Idaho	59.9	9,000
17	New York	60.3	91,000
18	Rhode Island	61.6	7,000
19	Illinois	61.8	66,000
20	Michigan	62.0	55,000
21	Colorado	62.1	36,000
22	Nebraska	62.1	8,000
23	Arizona	62.1	47,000
24	North Carolina	62.3	58,000
25	Washington	62.5	36,000
26	North Dakota	62.5	2,000

Rank	State	%	#
27	Indiana	62.7	50,000
28	Oklahoma	63.1	18,000
29	Kansas	63.3	14,000
30	New Jersey	63.5	34,000
31	Nevada	64.0	20,000
32	District of Columbia	64.1	1,000
33	Montana	64.6	4,000
34	Utah	64.7	19,000
35	Kentucky	64.9	20,000
36	California	65.0	233,000
37	Louisiana	65.0	19,000
38	Georgia	65.5	46,000
39	Missouri	66.3	30,000
40	Pennsylvania	66.4	65,000
41	Arkansas	66.6	17,000
42	Hawaii	66.7	6,000
43	Florida	66.8	106,000
44	Alabama	67.1	24,000
45	New Mexico	69.2	12,000
46	Texas	69.5	183,000
47	Mississippi	70.0	15,000
48	South Carolina	70.6	23,000
49	Virginia	70.8	55,000
50	Wisconsin	71.8	51,000
51	Tennessee	72.2	31,000
	National	63.0	1,548,000

* Due to data limitations, figures were taken from two sets of data: annual averages from 2013-2015 and 2010-2015. Data set denoted for each state in the Appendix- Table 1

[3] Waxman HA. Improving the Care of Children with Mental Illness: A Challenge for Public Health and the Federal Government. *Public Health Reports.* 2006;121(3):299-302.

Youth with Severe MDE who Received Some Consistent Treatment

Nationally, only 23.4% of youth with severe depression receive some consistent treatment (7-25+ visits in a year).

These numbers speak on the need for increased funding for community-based treatments proven to work for high needs children. Treatments must be made accessible to children with mental health conditions and their family—regardless of income.

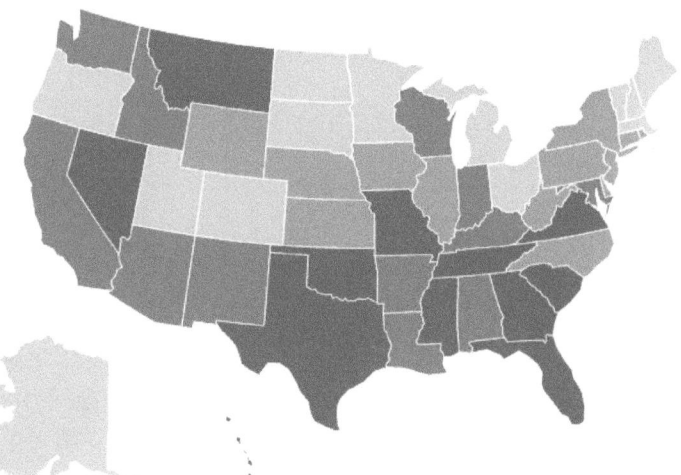

The state prevalence of youth with severe depression who received some outpatient treatment ranges from:

39.9 %(Minnesota)
Highest Ranked

11.30% (Mississippi)
Lowest ranked

High percentages are associated with positive outcomes and low percentages are associated with poorer outcomes.

Rank	State	%	#
1	Minnesota	39.90	11,000
2	South Dakota	39.50	2,000
3	Vermont	38.00	1,000
4	Alaska	35.10	1,000
5	Massachusetts	34.10	11,000
6	Maine	34.00	3,000
7	New Hampshire	31.80	2,000
8	North Dakota	31.60	1,000
9	Colorado	30.30	9,000
10	Ohio	29.80	21,000
11	Oregon	29.40	8,000
12	Michigan	29.00	19,000
13	Utah	29.00	4,000
14	New York	28.10	28,000
15	Kansas	27.90	4,000
16	West Virginia	27.90	2,000
17	Nebraska	27.60	2,000
18	Iowa	27.40	5,000
19	Wyoming	26.70	1,000
20	Delaware	26.50	1,000
21	Rhode Island	26.50	2,000
22	New Jersey	26.40	9,000
23	Illinois	26.20	20,000
24	Connecticut	25.60	5,000
25	North Carolina	25.50	14,000
26	Pennsylvania	25.20	16,000

Rank	State	%	#
27	Arkansas	25.10	4,000
28	Maryland	24.40	8,000
29	Washington	24.20	10,000
30	Louisiana	22.50	5,000
31	Indiana	22.00	9,000
32	New Mexico	21.90	2,000
33	California	21.50	47,000
34	Arizona	21.40	9,000
35	Wisconsin	21.40	8,000
36	Alabama	20.80	4,000
37	Idaho	19.50	2,000
38	Kentucky	19.50	4,000
39	Texas	18.90	32,000
40	Hawaii	18.70	1,000
41	Missouri	18.60	7,000
42	Florida	18.20	19,000
43	Oklahoma	16.80	3,000
44	District of Columbia	15.90	< 1,000
45	Virginia	15.50	8,000
46	South Carolina	14.60	3,000
47	Nevada	14.20	2,000
48	Montana	12.80	< 1,000
49	Tennessee	12.30	3,000
50	Georgia	11.30	5,000
51	Mississippi	11.30	2,000
	National	23.40	447,000

* Due to data limitations, figures were taken from three sets of data: annual averages from 2013-2015, 2010-2015, and 2010-2013 Data set denoted for each state in the Appendix-Table 2

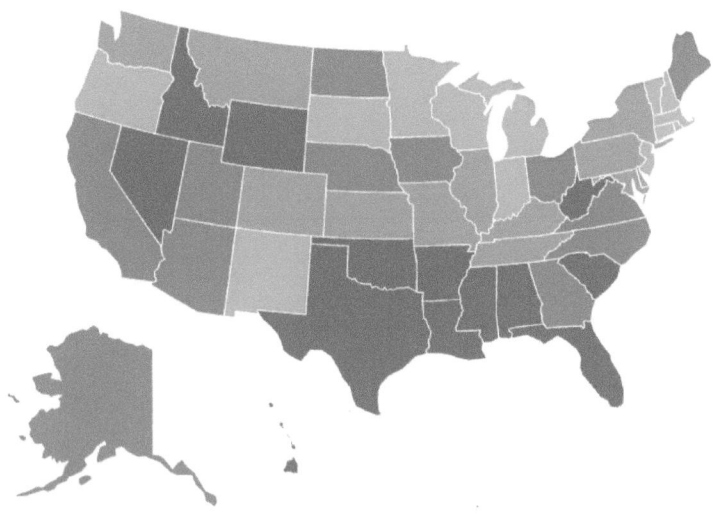

Children with Private Insurance that Did Not Cover Mental or Emotional Problems

The state prevalence of children lacking mental health coverage ranges from:

2.4 % (Massachusetts)   18.4 % (Mississippi)
Highest Ranked   Lowest Ranked

Rank	State	%	#
1	Massachusetts	2.4	7,000
2	Connecticut	2.7	4,000
3	South Dakota	4.2	1,000
4	Wisconsin	4.2	10,000
5	Indiana	4.3	12,000
6	New Hampshire	4.5	3,000
7	Michigan	4.7	20,000
8	New Mexico	4.7	3,000
9	Vermont	4.7	1,000
10	Oregon	5.0	7,000
11	New Jersey	5.1	21,000
12	Minnesota	5.4	13,000
13	Rhode Island	5.4	2,000
14	Pennsylvania	5.7	28,000
15	Kentucky	5.8	10,000
16	Maryland	6.0	16,000
17	Kansas	6.1	7,000
18	Washington	6.1	17,000
19	Montana	6.6	2,000
20	New York	6.6	47,000
21	District of Columbia	6.7	1,000
22	Colorado	6.9	15,000
23	Delaware	6.9	3,000
24	Tennessee	7.4	17,000
25	Illinois	7.5	36,000
26	Missouri	7.5	17,000
27	Utah	7.5	14,000
28	Alaska	7.6	2,000
29	North Carolina	7.9	23,000
30	Iowa	8.0	11,000
31	California	8.1	107,000
32	Maine	8.1	4,000
33	North Dakota	8.1	3,000
34	Ohio	8.1	39,000
35	Nebraska	8.3	6,000
36	Georgia	8.6	28,000
37	Virginia	8.7	26,000
38	Arizona	9.1	21,000
39	Idaho	9.7	6,000
40	Florida	10.1	52,000
41	Arkansas	10.5	9,000
42	West Virginia	10.6	6,000
43	Nevada	10.8	12,000
44	Alabama	11.5	17,000
45	Hawaii	11.6	5,000
46	Texas	11.6	103,000
47	South Carolina	12.5	18,000
48	Oklahoma	12.6	14,000
49	Wyoming	13.5	3,000
50	Louisiana	14.4	22,000
51	Mississippi	18.4	12,000
	National	7.7	884,000

Children and youth are more likely to have insurance coverage compared to adults.

Nationally, 7.7% of youth had private health insurance that did not cover mental or emotional problems.

Montana, Hawaii, New Jersey, and Ohio saw the largest increase in mental health coverage among children. These states have also had a significant increase in monthly Medicaid/Chip enrollment from Pre-ACA enrollment numbers.

- Montana: 75% increase in monthly enrollment
- Hawaii: 20% increase in monthly enrollment
- New Jersey: 36% increase in monthly enrollment
- Ohio: 29% increase in monthly enrollment[4]

Medicaid is the "largest single payer for mental health services", often providing more comprehensive mental healthcare than most private insurances. Private insurance remains costly for many people. Market autonomy, also allows private insurers to determine coverage based on levels of mental health conditions

[4] https://www.kff.org/health-reform/state-indicator/total-monthly-medicaid-and-chip-enrollment/?currentTimeframe=0&sortModel=%7B%22colId%22:%22Location%22,%22sort%22:%22asc%22%7D

Students Identified with Emotional Disturbance for an Individualized Education Program

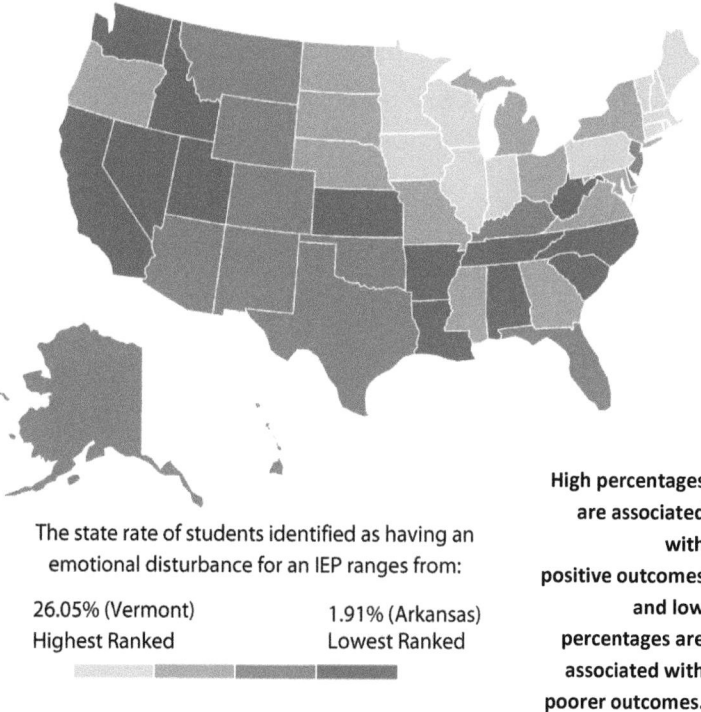

The state rate of students identified as having an emotional disturbance for an IEP ranges from:

26.05% (Vermont)
Highest Ranked

1.91% (Arkansas)
Lowest Ranked

High percentages are associated with positive outcomes and low percentages are associated with poorer outcomes.

Only .763% of students are identified as having an Emotional Disturbance (ED) for an Individualized Education Program (IEP).

For purposes of an IEP, the term "Emotional Disturbance" is used to define youth with a mental illness that is affecting their ability to succeed in school. Often youth with emotional or mental health problems are identified as having behavioral issues rather than an emotional or mental health problem.

Mental illness under the guise of a "behavioral issue", along with lower expectations for certain populations, and a lack of education in parents concerning the effects of trauma, prevent many high-risk students from receiving IEPs (Sarah Ozment, M Ed. Early Childhood Special Education, Interview, September 2017).

The rate for this measure is shown as a rate per 1,000 students. The calculation was made this way for ease of reading. Unfortunately, doing so hides the fact that the percentages are significantly lower. If states were doing a better job of identifying whether youth had emotional difficulties that could be better supported through an IEP – the rates would be closer to 8% instead of .8 percent.

Rank	State	%	#
1	Vermont	26.05	1,968
2	Minnesota	18.95	14,736
3	Massachusetts	17.61	15,137
4	Wisconsin	16.18	12,217
5	Pennsylvania	14.51	23,322
6	District of Columbia	14.36	885
7	Maine	13.61	2,234
8	Indiana	13.29	12,642
9	Iowa	12.85	5,610
10	Rhode Island	12.56	1,629
11	New Hampshire	12.44	2,107
12	Connecticut	11.08	5,395
13	Illinois	10.48	19,198
14	New York	9.82	24,377
15	Ohio	9.57	14,979
16	South Dakota	9.28	1,099
17	North Dakota	9.19	878
18	Oregon	8.89	4,704
19	Nebraska	8.46	2,313
20	Michigan	8.16	11,325
21	Virginia	8.15	9,398
22	Maryland	7.97	6,203
23	Mississippi	7.95	3,544
24	Missouri	7.87	6,439
25	Georgia	7.38	11,546
26	Arizona	7.31	7,456
27	Kentucky	7.26	4,422
28	Colorado	7.11	5,624
29	Oklahoma	6.90	4,078
30	Delaware	6.71	821
31	Wyoming	6.58	563
32	Florida	6.55	16,333
33	New Mexico	6.41	1,959
34	New Jersey	6.35	7,955
35	Montana	5.78	761
36	Texas	5.77	26,558
37	Hawaii	5.74	972
38	Alaska	5.66	665
39	Idaho	5.33	1,422
40	West Virginia	5.26	1,284
41	Kansas	5.20	2,290
42	Washington	4.70	4,601
43	Nevada	4.35	1,826
44	California	4.23	24,199
45	North Carolina	3.91	5,462
46	Tennessee	3.62	3,237
47	South Carolina	3.59	2,418
48	Utah	3.26	1,871
49	Louisiana	2.79	1,763
50	Alabama	2.00	1,348
51	Arkansas	1.91	836
	National	7.63	344,609

Mental Health Workforce Availability

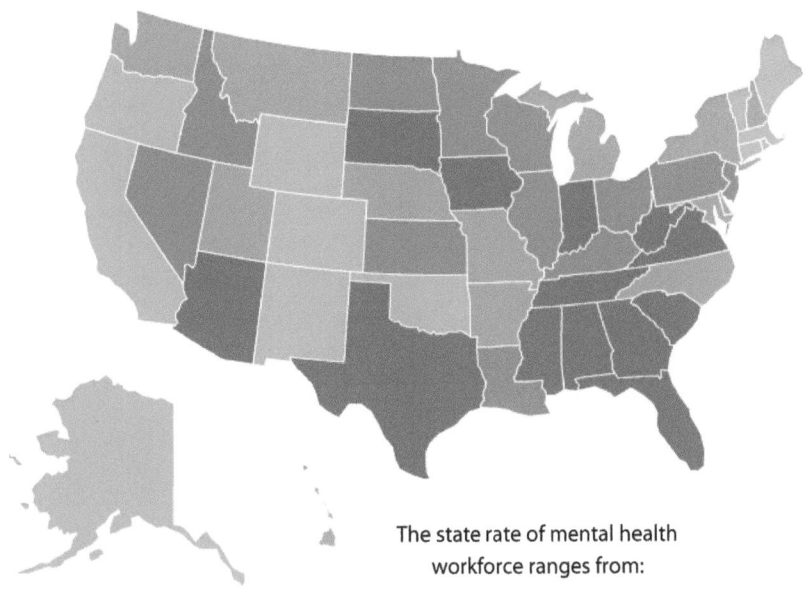

The state rate of mental health
workforce ranges from:

200:1 (Massachusetts)   1260:1 (Alabama)
Highest Ranked   Lowest Ranked

The term "mental health provider" includes: psychiatrists, psychologists, licensed clinical social workers, counselors, marriage and family therapists, and advanced practice nurses specializing in mental health care.

Over 4,000 areas across the US, containing more than 110,000,000 million people, are considered mental health professional shortage areas. These are individuals that are left to travel hours or across state lines to access services.[5] **Areas that are rural, and have low- income per capita are most affected.**

Although the ACA gave millions of individuals with mental health conditions the chance to seek treatment, these individuals now face a shortage of mental health providers. The demand, along with high turnover rates amongst mental health professionals (mainly due to a lack of social support and compensation) has created a "workforce crisis." [6]

To make matters worse, low reimbursement rates combined with a limited number of providers and high demand for help means that many providers do not accept insurance, forcing families and individuals to pay high out-of-pocket fees or go without care.

Peer support specialists, workforce development programs, telehealth, or primary care models like Collaborative Care are possible solutions to the significant mental health workforce gap in the states.

[5] Health Resources & Services Administration, Shortage Designation: Health http://www.hrsa.gov/shortage
[6] United States. (2013). Report to Congress on the nation's substance abuse and mental health workforce issues.

Rank	State	%
1	Massachusetts	200:1
2	District of Columbia	230:1
3	Maine	240:1
4	Oregon	250:1
5	Vermont	260:1
6	Oklahoma	270:1
7	New Mexico	280:1
8	Rhode Island	290:1
9	Alaska	300:1
10	Connecticut	310:1
11	California	350:1
12	Colorado	350:1
13	Wyoming	350:1
14	Missouri	360:1
15	Washington	360:1
16	Utah	380:1
17	New Hampshire	390:1
18	Montana	410:1
19	New York	420:1
20	Nebraska	440:1
21	Delaware	460:1
22	Michigan	460:1
23	Hawaii	470:1
24	Maryland	490:1
25	North Carolina	490:1
26	Arkansas	510:1
27	Minnesota	510:1
28	Idaho	550:1
29	Kentucky	560:1
30	Illinois	580:1
31	Kansas	580:1
32	Nevada	580:1
33	New Jersey	580:1
34	Louisiana	600:1
35	Pennsylvania	600:1
36	Wisconsin	600:1
37	Ohio	630:1
38	North Dakota	640:1
39	South Dakota	660:1
40	South Carolina	680:1
41	Indiana	730:1
42	Virginia	730:1
43	Florida	750:1
44	Tennessee	780:1
45	Iowa	820:1
46	Mississippi	820:1
47	Arizona	850:1
48	Georgia	900:1
49	West Virginia	950:1
50	Texas	1070:1
51	Alabama	1260:1
	National	536:1

Getting the Right Start
STUDENT GUIDE TO MENTAL HEALTH

KNOW THE 10 COMMON WARNING SIGNS

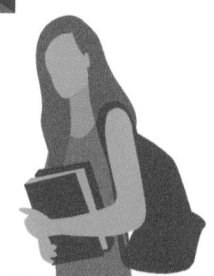

1. Feeling very sad or withdrawn for more than two weeks
2. Seriously trying to harm or kill oneself or making plans to do so
3. Severe out-of-control, risk-taking behaviors
4. Sudden, overwhelming fear for no reason
5. Not eating, throwing up or using laxatives to lose weight; significant weight loss or weight gain
6. Seeing, hearing or believing things that are not real
7. Repeatedly using drugs or alcohol
8. Drastic changes in mood, behavior, personality or sleeping habits
9. Extreme difficulty in concentrating or staying still
10. Intense worries or fears that get in the way of daily activities

WORRIED? TELL SOMEONE

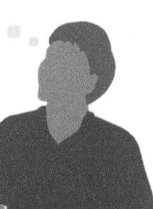

- ✓ A FAMILY MEMBER
- ✓ CLOSE FRIEND
- ✓ TEACHER OR PROFESSOR
- ✓ COUNSELOR OR COACH
- ✓ FAITH LEADER

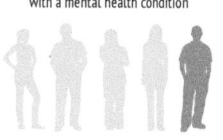

YOU ARE NOT ALONE
1 in 5 youth and young adults lives with a mental health condition

WHAT TO SAY

I haven't felt right lately and I don't know what to do. Can I talk to you about it?

I'm having a really hard time lately, will you go with me to see someone?

I'm worried about stuff that's going on right now, do you have time to talk?

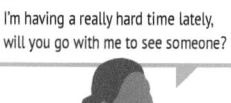

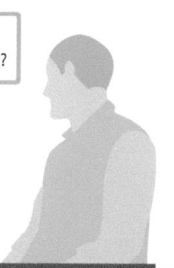

WHAT TO DO

Getting help early for mental health matters in keeping your life on track.

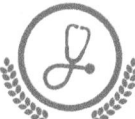

Your first stop is your primary care doctor, to rule out other physical health conditions

Be honest about what you're feeling and be clear about what you want

Ask for help finding a therapist or mental health specialist that works for you

KEEP IN MIND

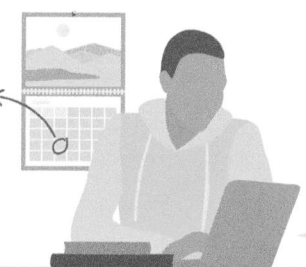

It can take a while to get an appointment with a specialist.

If you need to see a specialist right away, speak up to get an appointment sooner.

CONNECT WITH OTHERS

Lots of youth and young adults live with a mental health condition. You can connect with them at OK2Talk.org. Also, look in your community for peer and support groups and you will discover that you are not alone.

Follow Us!
- NAMI
- NAMIcommunicate
- NAMIcommunicate
- www.nami.org

nami
National Alliance on Mental Illness

Taking Charge of Your Mental Health

FIND THE RIGHT SPECIALIST

 Ask your doctor or nurse to help you find a specialist and make your first appointment

 There may be a long wait for your first visit, so speak up if you need to see someone right away

 If the first mental health specialist you see isn't a good fit, keep looking for one who works for you

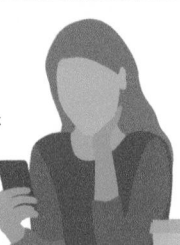

DON'T FORGET!

> Surround yourself with family and friends

> Talk to a counselor, social worker, nurse or trusted adult

> Continue doing what you love: reading, sports, writing, nature walks, creating art

MAKE YOUR FIRST APPOINTMENT COUNT

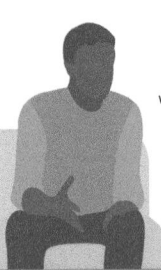

 Be ready to talk about your health history and what you're experiencing

You may be asked to fill out a questionnaire describing your mental health experience

 Be clear about what you want and need to get better

 Ask the mental health specialist to explain treatment options so you understand the plan and what you need to do

NAVIGATING YOUR INSURANCE

○ Involve someone with experience to help you

○ Call your insurance company to ask what mental health benefits are covered

○ To find a provider, visit your insurer's website or call the number on your insurance card

ASK QUESTIONS

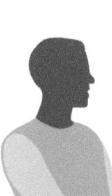

If I have thoughts that scare me what should I do?

Do I have to take medication? What does it help with? What are the side effects?

How often should we meet? What can I do between appointments if I need help?

How long will it take for me to feel better, a few days, weeks or months?

STAY INVOLVED

 Keep a wellness log and monitor your progress

 Ask for changes if your treatment plan is not working for you

 Stick with it; most therapies and medications take time to work

 Your treatment plan may change, so be an active partner in this process

LIVE WELL

☼ Remember that you have control over living well

☼ Find a routine that works for you that includes a healthy diet, exercise and regular sleep patterns

☼ Stay close to your support network. Engage family, friends, teammates and your faith community. Think about joining an online community

☼ Be realistic and mindful of your needs and know your limits

GETTING THROUGH IT

> Try staying away from drugs and alcohol. This is not always easy, so find strategies that work. Using drugs or alcohol to feel better is harmful to you.

> If you use alcohol or drugs, be honest and tell your therapist or doctor because it affects your care plan.

> Stay positive. Surround yourself with positive messages, people and activities. This will help you to feel better.

Follow Us!
f NAMI   🐦 NAMIcommunicate   NAMIcommunicate   🌐 www.nami.org

nami
National Alliance on Mental Illness

Want to Know How to Help a Friend?

STUDENT GUIDE TO MENTAL HEALTH

KNOW THE 10 COMMON WARNING SIGNS

1. Feeling very sad or withdrawn for more than two weeks
2. Seriously trying to harm or kill oneself or making plans to do so
3. Severe out-of-control, risk-taking behaviors
4. Sudden overwhelming fear for no reason
5. Not eating, throwing up or using laxatives to lose weight; significant weight loss or weight gain
6. Seeing, hearing or believing things that are not real
7. Repeatedly using drugs or alcohol
8. Drastic changes in mood, behavior, personality or sleeping habits
9. Extreme difficulty in concentrating or staying still
10. Intense worries or fears that get in the way of daily activities

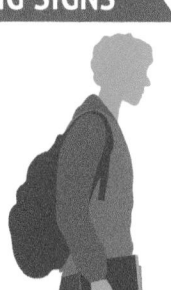

START THE CONVERSATION

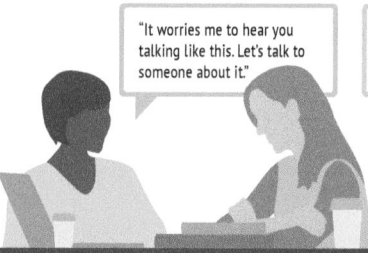

"It worries me to hear you talking like this. Let's talk to someone about it."

"I've noticed that you haven't been acting like yourself lately. Is something going on?"

"I've noticed you're [sleeping more, eating less, etc.], is everything ok today?"

OFFER SUPPORT

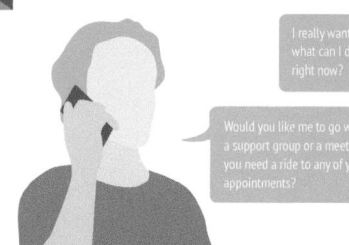

BE PATIENT, UNDERSTANDING AND PROVIDE HOPE.

I really want to help, what can I do to help you right now?

Would you like me to go with you to a support group or a meeting? Do you need a ride to any of your appointments?

Let's sit down together and look for places to get help. I can go with you too.

BE A FRIEND

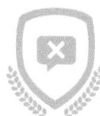

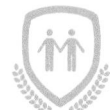

Your friend may feel alone; check in regularly and include your friend in your plans

Learn more about mental health conditions

Avoid saying things like "you'll get over it," "toughen up" or you're fine"

Tell your friend that having a mental health condition does not change the way you feel about them

Tell your friend it gets better; help and support are out there

GET ADVICE

You may want to reach out to someone to talk to about how you're feeling or to get advice on how to help your friend. Consider talking to a:

FAMILY MEMBER	TRUSTED FRIEND	SCHOOL COUNSELOR OR ADVISOR	TEACHER OR COACH	FAITH LEADER
★	★	★	★	★

Follow Us!
 NAMI   NAMIcommunicate   NAMIcommunicate   www.nami.org

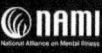

National Alliance on Mental Illness

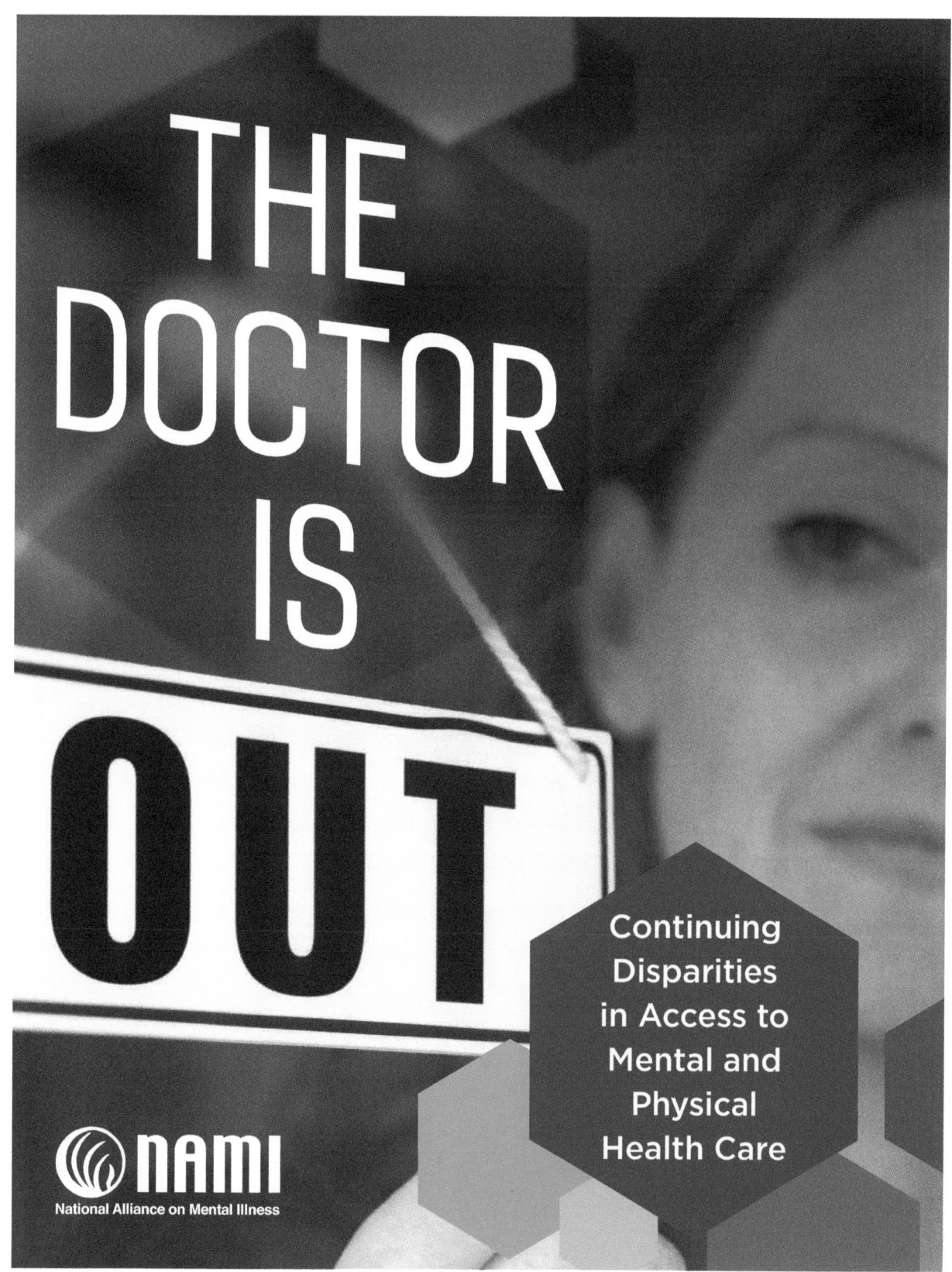

THE
DOCTOR
IS
OUT

Continuing
Disparities
in Access to
Mental and
Physical
Health Care

NAMI
National Alliance on Mental Illness

INTRODUCTION

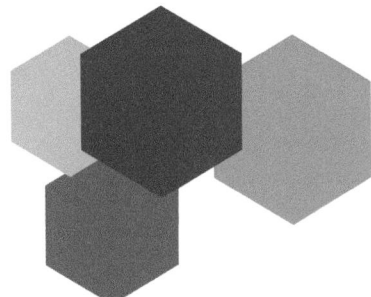

Each year, millions of Americans with mental illness struggle to find care. Nearly half of the 60 million adults and children living with mental health conditions in the United States go without any treatment. People who do seek treatment must navigate a fragmented and costly system full of obstacles.

Many people cannot access mental health care when they most need it. Despite passage of a federal mental health and addictions parity law in 2008, significant barriers exist in accessing mental health treatment and support. Barriers include high rates of denials of care by insurers, high out-of-pocket costs for mental health care, difficulties accessing psychiatric medications and problems finding psychiatrists and other mental health providers in health insurance networks.[1-3]

In 2016, NAMI, the National Alliance on Mental Illness, conducted its third nationwide survey to explore the relationship between health coverage and access to mental health care. The survey found that people with mental illness continue to experience significant barriers to finding affordable, accessible mental health care. These barriers exist whether the person is covered by private insurance or by a public plan such as Medicaid. This report identifies possible reasons for these barriers to finding mental health care in health insurance networks and suggests steps to remedy them.

SURVEY DESCRIPTION

NAMI conducted an online survey in 2016 to assess the experiences of health insurance beneficiaries when they seek mental health care. The survey drew responses from 3,177 individuals. To be eligible, respondents could have either private health insurance or public health coverage such as Medicaid or Medicare. The survey explored access to mental health and substance use care compared to primary and specialty medical care. Respondents could answer for themselves or for a relative for whom they could provide reliable information. Most respondents answered for themselves (63.1%) or their child (27.5%).

Participants were typically female (62%) and White/Caucasian (86%), and 50.3% were aged 26–49. Most respondents (59.6%) earned less than $25,000 per year, although 45% worked full- or part-time.

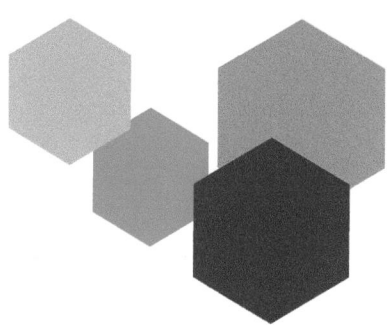

SURVEY RESULTS

The Paul Wellstone and Pete Domenici Mental Health Parity and Addictions Equity Act of 2008 (MHPAEA) requires parity in health insurance coverage of mental health and physical health benefits. These requirements apply both to quantifiable treatment limitations (co-pays, deductibles, annual and lifetime caps, etc.) and non-quantifiable treatment limitations, such as criteria for providers to participate in plan networks and the design of health plan networks. Despite these requirements, people are encountering mental health provider networks in health plans that are significantly narrower than those for primary care or specialty care. In addition, respondents incurred higher out-of-pocket costs for mental health services than for other types of medical care. These disparities in accessing mental health care relative to primary care and specialty care exist whether the care is outpatient, inpatient or residential.

Outpatient Mental Health Care

For the purposes of this study, outpatient mental health questions focused on two types of providers: (1) mental health prescribers (psychiatrists and other licensed providers who prescribe mental health medications) and (2) mental health therapists (licensed psychotherapists or counselors).

Of the respondents who received psychotherapy, 28% used an out-of-network provider. By contrast, only 7% of respondents used an out-of-network medical specialist and only 3% used an out-of-network primary care provider.

Thirty-four percent of respondents with private insurance reported difficulties finding *any* mental health therapist who would accept their insurance compared to other types of medical specialists (13%) or primary care providers (9%). This problem was present both in less populous rural regions and in urban or suburban regions with a greater supply of psychiatrists and other mental health professionals.

Searching for a New Provider

Obtaining a new provider is particularly challenging because the mental health workforce is in short supply. Nearly a third of the respondents reported that they had looked for a

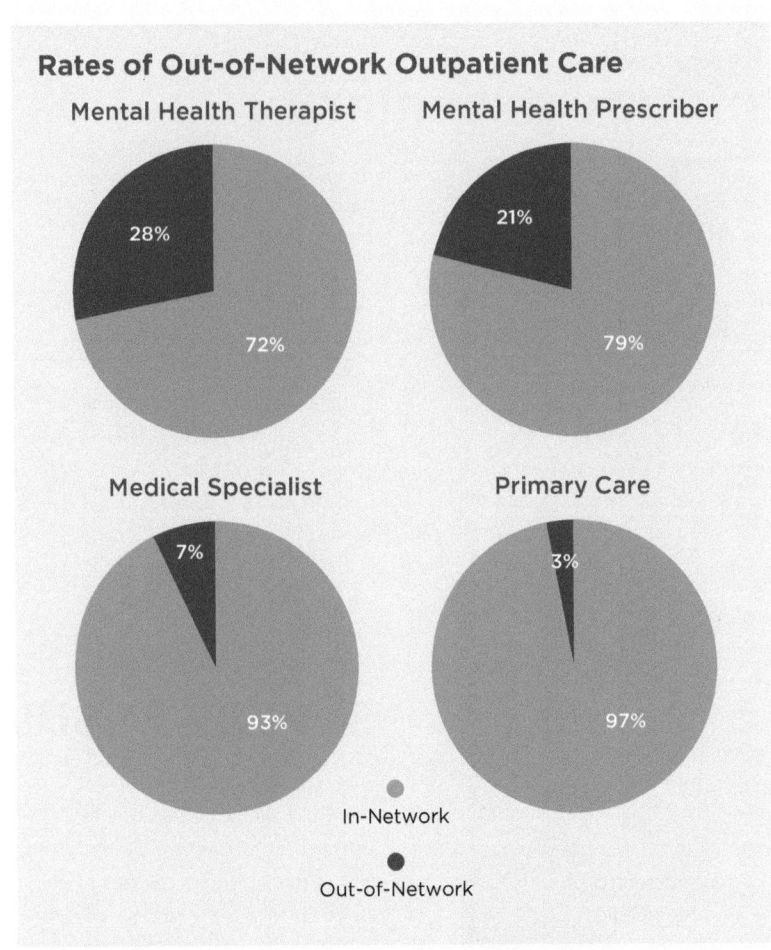

Rates of Out-of-Network Outpatient Care

Mental Health Therapist — 28% / 72%

Mental Health Prescriber — 21% / 79%

Medical Specialist — 7% / 93%

Primary Care — 3% / 97%

● In-Network

● Out-of-Network

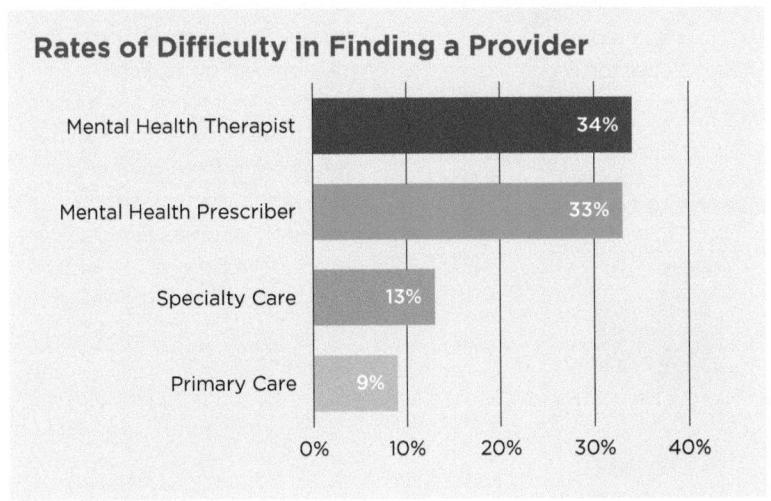

Rates of Difficulty in Finding a Provider

Mental Health Therapist — 34%

Mental Health Prescriber — 33%

Specialty Care — 13%

Primary Care — 9%

0% 10% 20% 30% 40%

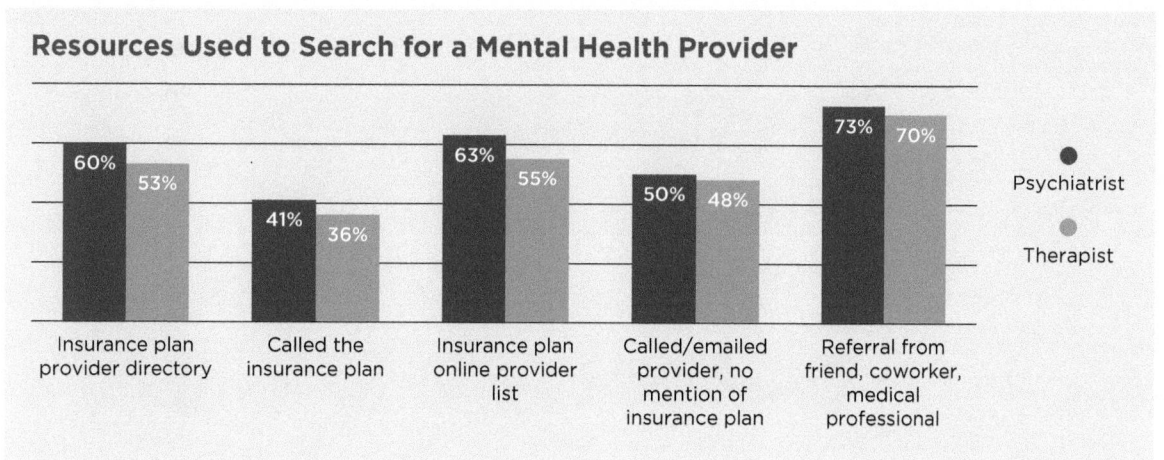

Resources Used to Search for a Mental Health Provider

new mental health provider in the last year—28% looked for a prescriber and 30% for a therapist. With respect to selecting resources used to locate a provider, the results were very similar whether the person had sought a psychiatrist or a therapist. The most common approach was to get a referral from a friend, coworker or medical professional (73% psychiatrist, 70% therapist). The next most common approach was to consult a provider list either in a directory or online (63% psychiatrist, 55% therapist).

Two in five called the health plan (41% psychiatrist, 36% therapist) and half called a provider directly without mentioning their health plan (50% psychiatrist, 48% therapist).

When trying to find a provider, respondents reported the most severe problems as follows:

1. Providers were not accepting new patients (55% psychiatrist, 45% therapist); or
2. Providers were not accepting their health plan (56% psychiatrist, 11% therapist).

The data shows that finding a new psychiatrist was more difficult than finding a therapist. About one-third of respondents had a severe problem with finding a provider close to home or work (36% psychiatrist, 33% therapist). Respondents remarked that many providers did not respond to telephone or email inquiries (29% psychiatrist, 22% therapist), while incorrect information in provider directories presented barriers for some respondents (16% psychiatrist, 15% therapist).

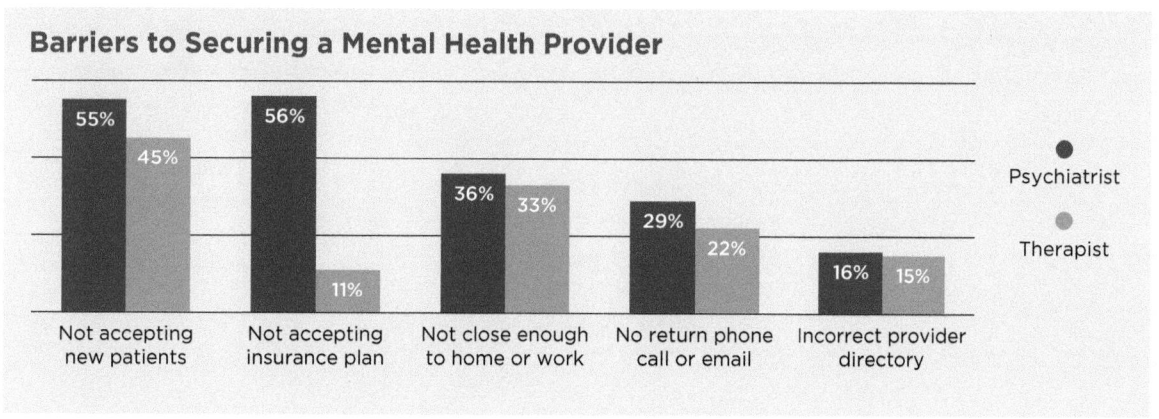

Barriers to Securing a Mental Health Provider

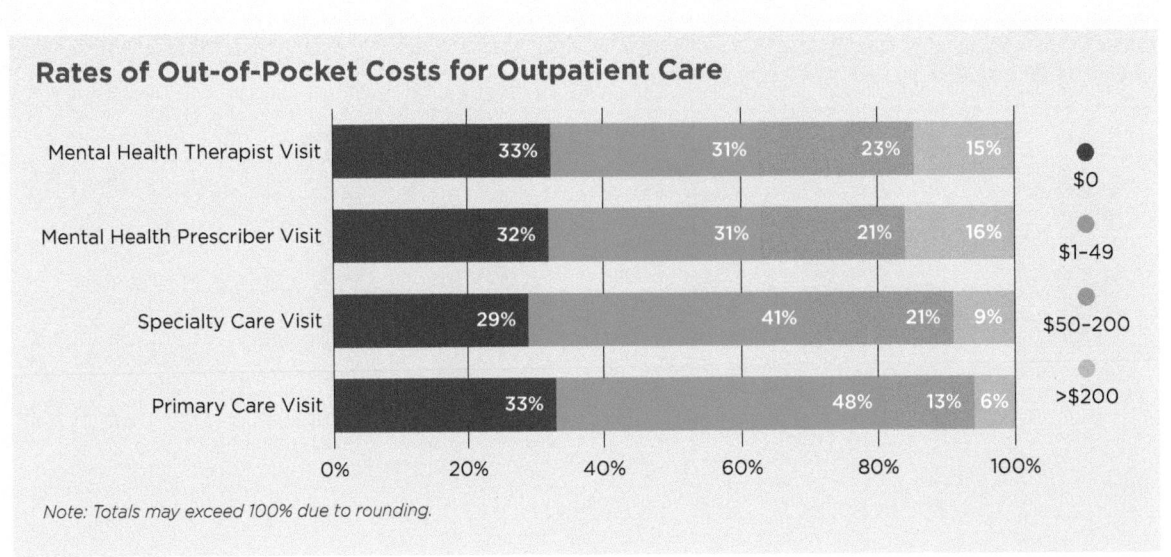

Rates of Out-of-Pocket Costs for Outpatient Care

	$0	$1–49	$50–200	>$200
Mental Health Therapist Visit	33%	31%	23%	15%
Mental Health Prescriber Visit	32%	31%	21%	16%
Specialty Care Visit	29%	41%	21%	9%
Primary Care Visit	33%	48%	13%	6%

Note: Totals may exceed 100% due to rounding.

Outpatient Service Costs

Respondents reported higher out-of-pocket costs, such as co-pays, for outpatient mental health services than for other types of medical care. Out-of-pocket costs exceeding $200 were more frequent for visits to mental health therapists (15%) and psychiatric prescribers (16%) compared to medical specialty care (9%). These results are concerning because higher out-of-pocket costs can lead people to get less care—or to go without any mental health treatment at all.

Inpatient Mental Health Care

Respondents also reported challenges locating inpatient mental health care. Respondents were far more likely to use an out-of-network hospital or residential facility for mental health care than for other medical needs. Psychiatric hospital care includes care received in state-operated psychiatric hospitals, private free-standing psychiatric hospitals and psychiatric units within general hospitals. Residential care refers to inpatient mental health services received in a longer-term residential setting.

Psychiatric Hospital Care

More than twice as many respondents (12%) who received psychiatric hospital care used an out-of-network hospital compared to those who used out-of-network medical hospital care (5%). In addition, twice as many (20%) had difficulty locating any inpatient psychiatric hospital, whether in- or out-of-network, compared to the 10% who reported difficulty finding any inpatient medical care.

Difficulties in finding inpatient psychiatric care are consistent with recent reports documenting significant shortages in psychiatric hospital beds. These shortages are particularly problematic for acute and emergency inpatient care and contribute to problems such as psychiatric emergency room boarding (keeping a person in the emergency room to wait for an available inpatient bed) and disproportionate numbers of people with mental illness who are inappropriately incarcerated in jails.[4-5]

Shortages of inpatient psychiatric beds are not attributable solely to inadequate insurance coverage. Other factors have contributed, including limitations in Medicaid and Medicare on paying for inpatient psychiatric care for adults, cuts in public funding for inpatient care and private hospitals' closing of psychiatric units in favor of more lucrative medical-surgical units.

Residential Mental Health Care

Of respondents who received residential mental health care, nearly one-quarter (24%) had to go out-of-network. Further, 27% of respondents reported difficulties finding any appropriate residential facility, either in- or out-of-network.

Medicaid In-Network Care More Likely

In many states, Medicaid provides a comprehensive array of well-researched, clinically-proven interventions that private insurance does not cover. Although Medicaid recipients who participated in the survey reported some difficulties locating mental health services, they were far more likely to use in-network services than were people with private insurance.

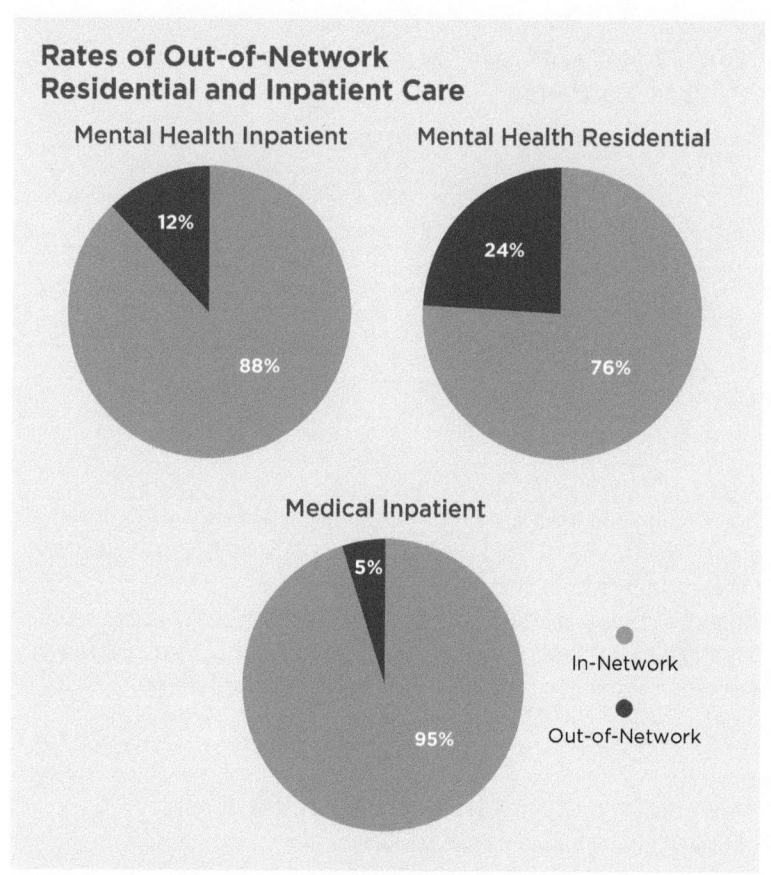

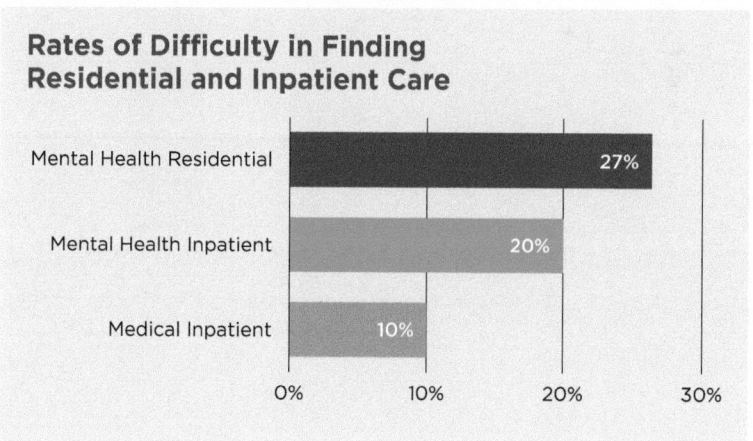

Out-of-Network Use by Medicaid vs. Private Insurance

Type of Service	Medicaid Out-of-Network	Private Insurance Out-of-Network
Mental Health Prescriber	13%	29%
Mental Health Therapist	14%	32%
Mental Health Hospital	8%	16%
Mental Health Residential	16%	38%

This is a significant advantage for people covered by Medicaid. However, this distinction may not apply to people in states that contract with managed care organizations to run their Medicaid behavioral health services, as these organizations may not have the same provider networks as are available under Medicaid fee-for-service programs.

Medicaid Outpatient Out-of-Pocket Costs Reported as a Barrier to Care

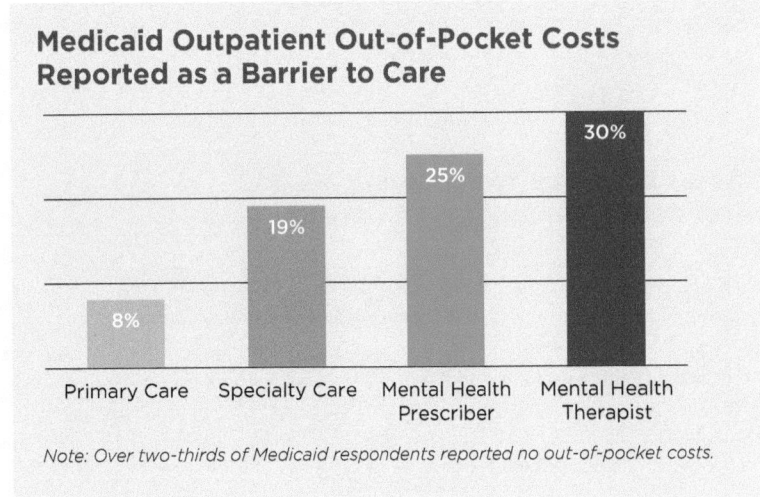

Note: Over two-thirds of Medicaid respondents reported no out-of-pocket costs.

Medicaid Out-of-Pocket Costs

Medicaid Outpatient Costs

Over two-thirds of the Medicaid enrollees who responded to the survey reported no out-of-pocket costs. Most state Medicaid programs do not impose cost-sharing on enrollees because even relatively minor out-of-pocket costs are shown to impede care for people with very low incomes.[6] Medicaid enrollees who did incur out-of-pocket costs reported these expenses as more of an impediment to accessing mental health care than other medical specialty care or primary care.

Of Medicaid recipients responding to the survey, 25% reported that out-of-pocket costs deterred them from seeking a mental health prescriber, and 30% reported being deterred from seeking a therapist. By contrast, 19% of respondents reported that out-of-pocket costs deterred them from seeking other medical specialty care and 8% from seeking primary care. These findings are important because a number of states have considered or are considering imposing out-of-pocket costs on Medicaid recipients—even on those Medicaid recipients who are most impoverished.

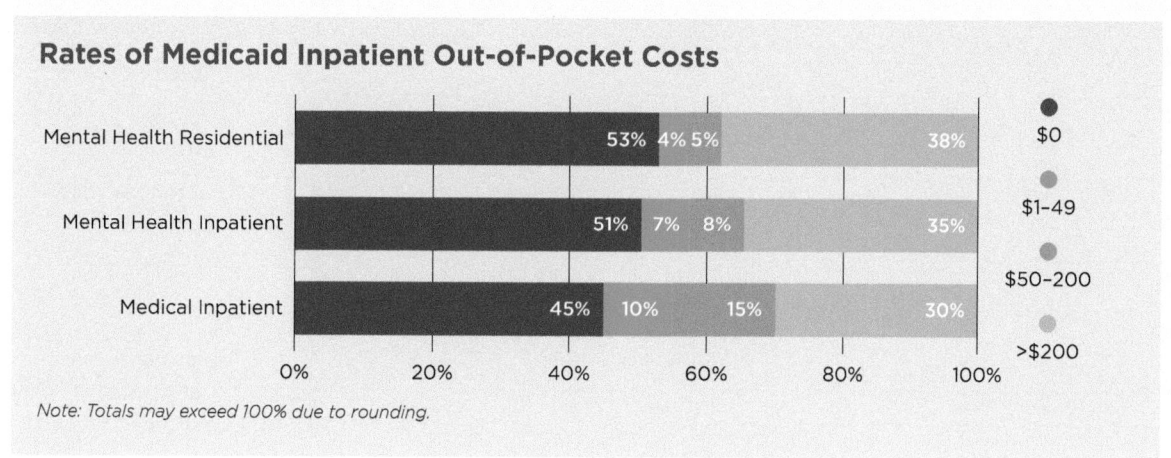

Rates of Medicaid Inpatient Out-of-Pocket Costs

Category	$0	$1-49	$50-200	>$200
Mental Health Residential	53%	4%	5%	38%
Mental Health Inpatient	51%	7%	8%	35%
Medical Inpatient	45%	10%	15%	30%

Note: Totals may exceed 100% due to rounding.

Medicaid Inpatient Costs

Out-of-pocket costs for mental health inpatient and residential care were more likely to be at the extremes than for medical inpatient care. Respondents were more likely to have no co-pay for mental health residential care (53%) or mental health hospital care (51%) compared to medical inpatient care (45%). However, when out-of-pocket costs were imposed, they were more likely to be more than $200 for mental health residential (38%) or mental health hospital care (35%) than for other inpatient medical care (30%).

Out-of-pocket costs were far lower for Medicaid enrollees than for people with private insurance. Three-quarters of those with Medicaid (74% for mental health residential to 78% for mental health inpatient care) had no out-of-pocket expenses, while those with private insurance were more likely to owe more than $200 in out-of-pocket costs.

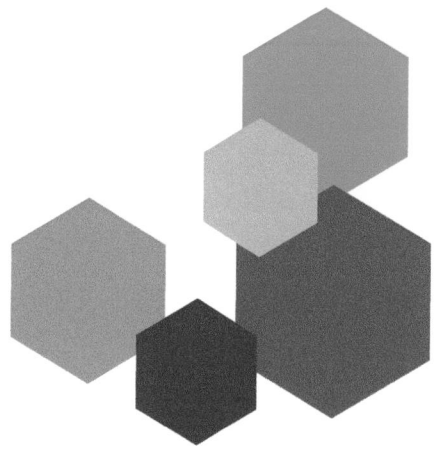

Disorders by Diagnostic Category

ADHD
    Adjustment Disorders

Anxiety Disorders
    Agoraphobia
    General Anxiety Disorder
    Panic Disorder
    Phobias
    Selective Mutism
    Separation Anxiety Disorder
    Social Anxiety Disorder

Autism Spectrum Disorders
    Autism
    Asperger's Syndrome

Bipolar and Related Disorders
    Depressive Disorders
    Depression
    Dysthymic Disorder
    Major Depression
    Postpartum Depression
    Premenstrual Dysphoric Disorder

Disruptive, Impulse-Control and Conduct Disorders
    Conduct Disorder
    Intermittent Explosive Disorder
    Kleptomania
    Pathological Gambling
    Pyromania
    Trichotillomania

Dissociative Disorders
    Depersonalization Disorder
    Dissociative Amnesia
    Dissociative Fugue
    Dissociative Identity Disorder

Feeding and Eating Disorders
    Anorexia Nervosa
    Bulimia Nervosa

Gender Dysphoria

Neurocognitive Disorders
    Delirium
    Dementias
    Amnestic Disorders

Neurodevelopmental Disorders
    Attention Deficit/Hyperactivity Disorder (ADHD)
    Autism Spectrum Disorder
    Asperger's Syndrome
    Autistic Disorder
    Conduct Disorder
    Tic Disorders
    Chronic Motor or Vocal Tic Disorder
    Transient Tic Disorder
    Tourette's Syndrome

Obsessive Compulsive Disorder

Personality Disorders
    Paranoid Personality Disorder
    Schizoid Personality Disorder
    Schizotypal Personality Disorder
    Antisocial Personality Disorder
    Borderline Personality Disorder
    Narcissistic Personality Disorder
    Avoidant Personality Disorder
    Dependent Personality Disorder
    Obsessive-Compulsive Disorder

Schizophrenia Spectrum and Other Psychotic Disorders
    Brief Psychotic Disorder
    Delusional Disorders
    Schizoaffective Disorder
    Schizophrenia

Sexual Disorders
    Sexual Desire Disorders
        Hypoactive Sexual Desire Disorder (HASSD)
        Sexual Aversion Disorder (SAD)
    Sexual Arousal Disorders
        Female Sexual Arousal Disorder (FSAD)
        Male Erectile Disorder (MED)
    Orgasmic Disorders
        Female and Male Orgasmic Disorders
        Premature Ejaculation
        Delayed Ejaculation
        Erectile Dysfunction
    Sexual Pain Disorders
        Dyspareunia
        Vaginismus
    Paraphilias
        Exhibitionism
        Fetishism
        Frotteurism
        Sexual Masochism
        Sexual Sadism
        Transvestic Fetishism
        Voyeurism

Sleep-Wake Disorders
    Breathing-related Sleep Disorder
    Circadian Rhythm Sleep Disorder
    Hypersomnolence
    Insomnia
    Narcolepsy
    Nightmare Disorder
    Parasomnias
    Restless Legs Syndrome
    Substance Abuse Induced Sleep Disorder
    Sleep Apnea
    Sleep Terror Disorder

Somatic Symptom and Related Disorders
    Hypochondria
    Factitious Disorder
    Malingering Disorder
    Somatization Disorder

Substance-Related and Addictive Disorders
    Substance-Related Abuse
    Substance-Related Dependence

Suicide

Tic Disorders

Trauma and Stressor-Related Disorders
    Post Traumatic Stress Syndrome (PTSD)
    Obsessive Compulsive Disorder (OCD)

User's Guide

Below is a sample listing illustrating the kind of information that is or might be included in an Association entry, with additional fields that apply to publication and trade show listings. Each numbered item of information is described in the paragraphs on the User's Key.

1. **12345**

    2. **Association for People with Mental Illness**
    3. 29 Simmons Street
        Philadelphia, PA 15201

    4. 234-555-1111
    5. 234-555-1112
    6. 800-555-1113
    7. TDD: 234-555-1114
    8. info@association-mh.com
    9. www.association-mh.com

10. William Lancaster, Executive Director
    Monty Spitz, Marketing Manager
    Kathleen Morrison, Medical Consultant

11. Association for Mental Health is funded by the Mental Health Community Support Program. The purpose of the association is to share information about services, providers, and ways to cope with mental illnesses. Available services include referrals, professional seminars, support gourps, and a variety of publications.

12. 1 M *Members*

13. *Founded*: 1984

14. Bi-monthly

15. $59.00

16. 110,000

User's Key

1. **Record Number:** Entries are listed alphabetically within each category and numbered sequentially. The entry numbers, rather than the page numbers, are used in the indexes to refer to listings.

2. **Title:** Formal name of association or publication. Where names are completely capitalized, the listing will appear at the beginning of the section. If listing is a publication or trade show, the publisher or sponsoring organization will appear below the title.

3. **Address:** Location or permanent address of the association.

4. **Phone Number:** The listed phone number is usually for the main office of the association, but may also be for the sales, marketing, or public relations office as provided.

5. **Fax Number:** This is listed when provided by the association.

6. **Toll-Free Number:** This is listed when provided by the association.

7. **TDD:** This is listed when provided by the association. It refers to Telephone Device for the Deaf.

8. **E-mail:** This is listed when provided by the association.

9. **Web Site:** This is listed when provided by the association and is also referred to as a URL address.

10. **Key Executives:** Lists key contacts of the association, publication or sponsoring organization.

11. **Description:** This paragraph contains a brief description of the association, their purpose and services.

12. **Members:** Total number of association members.

13. **Founded:** Year association was founded.

14. **Frequency:** If listing is a publication.

15. **Subscription Price:** If listing is a publication.

16. **Circulation:** If listing is a publication.

ADHD

Introduction

Attention Deficit Hyperactivity Disorder (ADHD) is characterized by three main symptoms: distractibility, impulsivity, and hyperactivity. ADHD primarily affects children. Since many children are inattentive, impulsive, and rambunctious at times, it is important to note that the diagnosis is not made unless these behaviors are more severe than is typical for a person at a comparable developmental level. At least some of the symptoms must appear before the age of seven.

The problems caused by hyperactivity show themselves in constant movement, especially among younger children. Preschool children with hyperactivity cannot sit still, even for quiet activities that usually absorb children of the same age. They are always on the move and run rather than walk. In older children the intensity of the hyperactivity is reduced but fidgeting, getting up during meals or homework, and excessive talking continue.

People with Attention Deficit Hyperactivity Disorder have great difficulty controlling all their impulses, not just the craving for movement and stimulation. They have little sense of time (five minutes seems like hours), and waiting for something is intolerable. Thus, they are impatient, interrupt, make comments out of turn, grab objects from others, clown around, and cause trouble at home, in school, at work, and in social settings.

The consequences of ADHD can be severe. From a young age, people with Attention Deficit Hyperactivity Disorder tend to experience failure repeatedly, including rejection by peers, resulting in low self-esteem and sometimes more serious problems.

SYMPTOMS

1. Inattention, as compared with others at the same developmental level
• Often fails to attend to details, or makes careless mistakes in schoolwork, work or other activities;
• Often finds it difficult to maintain attention in tasks or play activities;
• Often does not seem to listen when spoken to;
• Often does not follow through on instructions and does not finish schoolwork, chores, or tasks;
• Often has difficulty organizing tasks or activities;
• Often avoids tasks that demand sustained mental effort, such as schoolwork or homework;
• Often loses things needed for tasks or activities, such as toys and school assignments;
• Often is easily distracted;
• Often is forgetful in daily activities.

2. Hyperactivity, as compared with others at the same developmental level
• Often fidgets with hands or feet, or squirms in chair;
• Often leaves seat in classroom or other situations where remaining seated is expected;
• Often runs or climbs about in situations in which it is inappropriate (among adolescents or adults, this may be a feeling of restlessness);
• Often has difficulty playing or handling leisure activities quietly;
• Often is on the go, moving excessively.

3. Impulsivity, as compared with others at the same developmental level
• Often talks excessively;
• Often blurts out answers impulsively before questions are finished;
• Often has difficulty waiting in turn;
• Often intrudes impulsively on others' games, activities or conversations.

Parts of this description may apply to all or most children at times, but behaving in this way nearly all the time wreaks havoc on the child and family. Three distinctions are made in the diagnosis:

Attention Deficit Hyperactivity Disorder, Combined Type if symptoms of inattention, hyperactivity and impulsivity (Lists 1, 2, and 3) are exhibited;

Attention Deficit Hyperactivity Disorder, Predominantly Inattentive Type if six or more inattention symptoms (List 1 only) are displayed;

Attention Deficit Hyperactivity Disorder, Predominantly Hyperactive-Impulse Type if six or more hyperactivity and impulsivity symptoms (Lists 2 and 3 only) are applicable.

ASSOCIATED FEATURES

Certain behaviors often go along with Attention Deficit Hyperactivity Disorder. The person is often frustrated and angry, exhibiting outbursts of temper and bossiness. To others, the lack of application and inability to finish tasks may look like laziness or irresponsibility. Other conditions may also be associated with the disorder, including Hyperthyroidism (an overactive thyroid). There may be a higher prevalence of anxiety, depression, and learning disorders among people with ADHD.

A careful assessment and diagnosis by a professional familiar with ADHD are essential, especially since some of the typical ADHD behaviors may resemble those of other disorders. Family, school, and other possible problems must be taken into account and addressed. This is a lifelong disorder, though sometimes attenuated in adulthood.

The diagnosis is especially difficult to establish in young children, e.g., at the toddler and preschool level, because behavior that is typical at that age is similar to the symptoms of ADHD. Children at that age may be extremely active but not develop the disorder.

PREVALENCE

ADHD occurs in various cultures. It is much more frequent in males than females, with male to female ratios at 4:1 in the general population, and 9:1 in clinic populations. The prevalence among school-age children is from five percent to twelve percent.

ADHD can exist throughout a lifetime and, in fact, may be diagnosed in teen or adult years. There is emerging literature concerning adult ADHD, and evidence that some adults can benefit from the same treatments used for children.

TREATMENT OPTIONS

ADHD is treated using a three-tiered approach consisting of education programs (including resources and tutorial help), psychological programs (individual, group and family counseling) to help with self-esteem and stress, and medical therapy.

The person with ADHD has great need for external motivation, consistency, and structure. This should be provided by a professional who is familiar with the disorder. For a school-aged child, it is important to enlist the help of the school in designing a treatment plan which should include concrete steps aimed at developing specific compentencies (e.g., handling time, sequencing, problem-solving, and social interaction).

Medication is often prescribed but should not be the only treatment. Newer preparations of medications, such as Concerta and Biphentin, offer once or twice a day dosing, so that children do not need to take medication during the school day.

Since this condition affects all members of the family, the family needs help in providing consistency and structure, and in not defining the role of the person with ADHD as the one who always gets into trouble. Treatment should be based on an understanding that ADHD is not intentional, and that punishment is not a cure.

Current treatments can have a positive impact and, in some cases, transform behaviors so that a formerly chaotic life becomes more in control.

Associations & Agencies

2   **Attention Deficit Disorder Association**
PO Box 7557
Wilmington, DE 19803-9997
800-939-1019; *Fax:* 800-939-1019
www.add.org

Duane Gordon, President
Michelle Frank, PsyD, Vice President
Jeffrey Druce, Treasurer
Melinda Whetstone, PhD, Workplace Issues Chair

Provides information, support groups, publications, workshops, and networking opportunities for people with Attention Deficit Hyperactivity Disorder. Strives to improve the lives of those with ADHD.

3   **Center for Mental Health Services (CMHS)**
Substance Abuse and Mental Health Services
Administration
5600 Fishers Lane
Rockville, MD 20857
240-276-1310
877-726-4727
TTY: 800-487-4889
www.samhsa.gov/about-us/who-we-are/offices-centers

Paolo del Vecchio, MSW, Director
Anne Mathews-Younes, Acting Deputy Director
Keris Myrick, Director, Consumer Affairs
Patricia Gratton, Director, Program Analysis

Promotes the treatment of mental illness and emotional disorders by increasing accessibility to mental health programs; supporting outreach, treatment, rehabilitation, and support programs and networks; and encouraging the use of scientifically-based information when treating mental disorders. CMHS provides information about mental health via a toll-free number and numerous publications. Devel-

oped for users of mental health services and their families, the general public, policy makers, providers, and the media.
Year Founded: 1992

4   **Children and Adults with AD/HD (CHADD)**
4601 Presidents Drive
Suite 300
Lanham, MD 20706
301-306-7070
800-233-4050; *Fax:* 301-306-7090
www.chadd.org

Michael McKay, President
Belynda L. Gauthier, President Elect
Eugene M. Bell, Secretary
Harvey Parker, Founder

National nonprofit organization serving individuals with Attention Deficit Hyperactivity Disorder (ADHD) and their families. Offers support and information for individuals, parents, teachers, professionals, and others, and advocates for the rights of people with ADHD. Available on Facebook and Twitter.
Year Founded: 1987

5   **Learning Disabilities Association of America**
4156 Library Road
Pittsburgh, PA 15234-1349
412-341-1515; *Fax:* 412-344-0224
info@ldaamerica.org
www.ldaamerica.org

Beth McGaw, President
Mary-Clare Reynolds, Executive Director
Jonathan Jones, First Vice President
Jennifer Harkins, Secretary

Educates individuals with learning disabilities and their families through conferences, workshops, and symposiums; advocates for the rights of individuals with learning disabilities; provides support for parents; and promotes research in the assessment and prevention of learning disabilities.
Year Founded: 1964

6   **National Alliance on Mental Illness**
3803 North Fairfax Drive
Suite 100
Arlington, VA 22203
703-524-7600
800-950-6264
info@nami.org
www.nami.org

Steve Pitman, JD, President
Lacey Berumen, PhD, MNM, First Vice President
Mary Giliberti, Chief Executive Officer
David Levy, Chief Financial Officer

NAMI is an organization dedicated to raising awareness on mental health and providing support and education for Americans affected by mental illness. NAMI advocates for access to services and treatment and fosters an environment of awareness and understanding for those concerned with mental health.
Year Founded: 1979

7   National Association for the Dually Diagnosed (NADD)
132 Fair Street
Kingston, NY 12401
845-331-4336
info@thenadd.org
www.thenadd.org

Jeanne M. Farr, MA, Chief Executive Officer
Daniel Baker, PhD., President
Peggie Webb, MA, Vice President
George Zukotynski, PhD., Secretary

NADD is a nonprofit organization designed to increase awareness of, and provide services for, individuals with developmental disabilities and mental illness. NADD emphasizes the importance of quality mental healthcare for people with mental health needs and offers conferences, information resources, educational programs, and training materials to professionals, parents, and organizations.

Year Founded: 1983

8   National Center for Learning Disabilities
32 Laight Street
2nd Floor
New York, NY 10013
212-545-7510
888-575-7373; *Fax:* 212-545-9665
ncld@ncld.org
www.ncld.org

Frederic M. Poses, Chairman of the Board
Mimi Corcoran, President and CEO
Mary Kalikow, Vice Chairman
John R. Langeler, Treasurer

The National Center for Learning Disabilities (NCLD) aims to help individuals with learning disabilities succeed in school, work, and social settings. NCLD provides parents and educators with resources and promotes policies focused on enhancing the educational rights of those with learning disabilities.

Year Founded: 1977

9   National Federation of Families for Children's Mental Health
12320 Parklawn Drive
Rockville, MD 20852
240-403-1901
ffcmh@ffcmh.org
www.ffcmh.org

Lynda Gargan, PhD, Executive Director
Barbara Huff, Technical Assistance Provider
Sherri Luthe, President
Terry Stevens, Vice President

The National Federation of Families for Children's Mental Health is a national organization focused on advocating for the rights of children affected by mental health challenges, assisting family-run organizations across the nation, and ensuring that children and families concerned with mental health have access to services.

Year Founded: 1989

10   National Mental Health Consumers' Self-Help Clearinghouse
1211 Chestnut Street
Suite 1100
Philadelphia, PA 19107

267-507-3810
800-553-4539; *Fax:* 215-636-6312
info@mhselfhelp.org
www.mhselfhelp.org

Joseph Rogers, Founder and Executive Director
Susan Rogers, Director

The Clearinghouse is a peer-run national technical assistance center focused on achieving respect and equality of opportunity for those with mental illnesses. The Clearinghouse helps with the growth of the mental health consumer movement by evaluating mental health services, advocating for mental health reform, and providing consumers with news, information, publications, and consultation services.

Year Founded: 1986

11   National Resource Center on ADHD
Children and Adults with AD/HD
4601 PresidentsDrive
Suite 300
Lanham, MD 20706
800-233-4050
www.chadd.org/about-chadd/national-resource-center

Dr L. Eugene Arnold, MD, MEd, Resident Expert
Sarah Brown, NRC Program Manager
Ara Rich, Health Information Specialist

The National Resource Center, a program of CHADD, is a resource platform focused on disseminating the latest science-based information on ADHD. The NRC provides comprehensive information and program activities for children and adults with ADHD, parents, caregivers, professionals, and other members of the public.

12   PACER Center
8161 Normandale Boulevard
Bloomington, MN 55437
952-838-9000
800-537-2237; *Fax:* 952-838-0199
www.pacer.org

Paula F. Goldberg, Co-Founder & Executive Director
Matthew Woods, President
Tammy Pust, Vice President
Dan Levinson, Treasurer

PACER provides information, training, and assistance to parents of children and young adults with all disabilities (physical, learning, cognitive, emotional, and health). Its mission is to help improve the quality of life for young people with disabilities and their families.

Year Founded: 1977

13   The Center for Family Support
2811 Zulette Avenue
Bronx, NY 10461
718-518-1500; *Fax:* 718-518-8200
www.www.cfsny.org/

Steven Vernikoff, Executive Director
Lloyd Stabiner, President
Amy Bittinger, Vice President
Barbara Greenwald, Associate Executive Director

The Center for Family Support offers assistance to individuals with developmental and related disabilities, as well as their families, and provides support services and programs that are designed to accommodate individual needs. Offers services throughout New York City, Westchester County, Long Island, and New Jersey.

Year Founded: 1954

Books

14   A Birds-Eye View of Life with ADD and ADHD: Advice from Young Survivors
Cherish the Children
PO Box 189
Cedar Bluff, AL 35959-189
Fax: 256-779-5203
chirs@chrisdendy.com
www.www.chrisdendy.com/bev.htm

Chris A Zeigler Dendy, Author
Alex Zeigler, Author

Written expressly for teenagers, preteens, and young adults, by teenagers and a young adult who are struggling with ADD or ADHD. This survival guide offers factual information and practical advice in words and examples that young people can easily understand and put into practice. Written with humor and compassion, A Bird's Eye View offers down-to-earth tips for coping with a variety of issues: disorganization, forgetfulness, always being late, sleep problems, memorization, procrastination, restlessness, medication, writing essays, and algebra. This book is meant to be helpful yet still interesting to read.

15   ADD & Learning Disabilities: Reality, Myths, & Controversial Treatments
Bantam Doubleday Dell Publishing
1745 Broadway
New York, NY 10019-4343
212-782-9000

Barbara Ingersoll, Author
Sam Goldstein, PhD., Author

For parents of children with learning disabilities and attention deficit disorder - and for educational and medical professionals who encounter these children - two experts in the field have devised a handbook to help identify the very best treatments. *$10.36*

256 pages ISBN 0-385469-31-4

16   ADD & Romance: Finding Fulfillment in Love, Sex, & Relationships
ADD WareHouse
300 NW 70th Avenue
Suite 102
Plantation, FL 33317-2360
954-792-8100
800-233-9273; *Fax:* 954-792-8545
sales@addwarehouse.com
www.addwarehouse.com

Jonathan Halverstadt, Author
Daniel Amen, Author

Licensed therapist Jonathan Scott Halverstadt looks at how attention deficit disorder can damage romantic relationships when partners do not take time, or do not know how, to address this unique problem. The book aims to give people with A.D.D. and their partners the tools they need to build and sustain a more satisfying and fulfilling relationship. *$12.95*

230 pages Year Founded: 1998 ISBN 0-878332-09-X

17   ADD Kaleidoscope: The Many Faces of Adult Attention Deficit Disorder
Hope Press 91009-188
Fax: 818-358-3520
dcomings@earthlink.net
www.hopepress.com

Joan Andrews, Author
Denise E. Davis, Author

A comprehensive presentation of all aspects of attention deficit disorder in adults. While often thought of as a childhood disorder, ADD symptoms usually continue into adulthood where they can cause a wide range of problems with personal interactions, work performance, attitude towards one's employer, and interactions with spouses and children. *$24.95*

293 pages ISBN 1-878267-03-5

18   ADD Success Stories: Guide to Fulfillment for Families with Attention Deficit Disorder
ADD WareHouse
300 NorthWest 70th Avenue
Suite 102
Plantation, FL 33317-2360
954-792-8944
800-233-9273; *Fax:* 954-792-8545
websales@addwarehouse.com
www.addwarehouse.com

Thom Hartmann, Author
John J. Ratey, Author

Real-life stories of people with ADD who achieved success in school, at work, in marriages and relationships. Thousands of interviews and histories as well as new research show children and adults from all walks of life how to reach the next-step, a fulfilling, successful life with ADD. Discover which occupations are best for people with ADD. *$12.00*

288 pages Year Founded: 1995 ISBN 1-887424-03-2

19   ADD in the Workplace: Choices, Changes and Challenges
ADD WareHouse
300 NW 70th Avenue
Suite 102
Plantation, FL 33317-2360
954-792-8944
800-233-9273; *Fax:* 954-792-8545
sales@addwarehouse.com
www.addwarehouse.com

Kathleen Nadeau, Author

This book contains information that seeks to help adults move from resignation to determination in forging a path to success. Whether this means finding an ADD-friendly environment, requesting reasonable workplace accommodations, or creating a freelance nich, this book will point out the right directions. *$24.00*

256 pages Year Founded: 1997 ISBN 0-876308-47-7

20   ADD/ADHD Checklist: an Easy Reference for Parents & Teachers
ADD WareHouse
300 NorthWest 70th Avenue
Suite 102
Plantation, FL 33317-2360
954-792-8944
800-233-9273; *Fax:* 954-792-8545

websales@addwarehouse.com
www.addwarehouse.com

Harvey C Parker, Owner

Written by a nationally known educator with two decades of experience in working with ADD/ADHD students. For fast, reliable information about attention deficit disorder, parents and teachers need only to refer to The ADD/ADHD Checklist. *$12.00*

272 pages Year Founded: 2002

21   ADHD Monitoring System
ADD WareHouse
300 NorthWest 70th Avenue
Suite 102
Plantation, FL 33317-2360
954-792-8944
800-233-9273; *Fax: 954-792-8545*
websales@addwarehouse.com
www.addwarehouse.com

Harvey C Parker, Owner

Provides a simple, cost effective way to carefully monitor how well a student with ADHD is doing at school. Parents and teachers will be able to easily track behavior, academic performance, quality of student classwork and homework. Contains monitoring forms along with instructions for use. *$8.95*

22   ADHD Parenting Handbook: Practical Advice for Parents
Taylor Trade Publishing
5360 Manhattan Circle
Suite 100
Boulder, CO 80303-4249
303-543-7835; *Fax: 303-543-0043*
rrinehart@rowman.com
www.rowman.com/taylortrade

Colleen Alexander Roberts, Author

Practical advice for parents from parents, and proven techniques for raising hyperactive children without losing your temper.

224 pages Year Founded: 1994 ISBN 0-878338-62-4

23   ADHD Survival Guide for Parents and Teachers
Hope Press
PO Box 188
Duarte, CA 91009-188
818-303-0644
800-321-4039; *Fax: 626-358-3520*
dcomings@earthlink.net
www.hopepress.com

Richard A. Lougy,MFT, Author
David K. Rosenthal,MD, Author

Fills an important need expressed by parents, teachers, and other caretakers of ADHD children who have asked for clear, practical, and easily understood strategies to deal with ADHD children.

Year Founded: 2002 ISBN 1-878267-43-4

24   ADHD and Teens: Parent's Guide to Making it Through the Tough Years
ADD WareHouse
300 NorthWest 70th Avenue
Suite 102
Plantation, FL 33317-2360
954-792-8944
800-233-9273; *Fax: 954-792-8545*
websales@addwarehouse.com
www.addwarehouse.com

Colleen Alexander Roberts, Author

A manual of practical advice to help parents cope with the problems that can arise during these years. A crash course is offered on parenting styles that really work with teens with ADHD and how these styles allow the teen to safely move from dependence to independence. *$13.00*

199 pages Year Founded: 1995 ISBN 0-878338-99-3

25   ADHD and the Nature of Self-Control
Guilford Press
72 Spring Street
New York, NY 10012
212-431-9800
800-365-7006; *Fax: 212-966-6708*
info@guilford.com
www.guilford.com

Russell A. Barkley, PhD, Author

Provides a radical shift of perspective on ADHD, arguing that the disorder is a developmental problem of self control and that an attention deficit is a secondary characteristic. Combines neuropsychological research and the theory on the executive functions, illustrating how normally functioning individuals are able to bring behavior under the control of time and orient their actions toward the future. *$46.00*

410 pages Year Founded: 1973 ISBN 1-572302-50-X

26   ADHD in the Young Child: Driven to Redirection: A Guide for Parents and Teachers of Young Children with ADHD
ADD WareHouse
300 NW 70th Avenue
Suite 102
Plantation, FL 33317-2360
954-792-8944
800-233-9273; *Fax: 954-792-8545*
sales@addwarehouse.com
www.addwarehouse.com

Cathy Reimers PhD, Author
Bruce A. Brunger, Author

The authors sensitively and effectively describe what life is like living with a young child with ADHD. With the help of over 75 cartoon illustrations they provide practical solutions to common problems found at home, in school and elsewhere. *$18.95*

202 pages Year Founded: 1999 ISBN 1-886941-32-7

27   ADHD: A Complete and Authoritative Guide
American Academy Of Pediatrics
141 Northwest Point Boulevard
Elk Grove Village, IL 60007-1098
847-434-4000
800-433-9016; *Fax: 847-434-8000*
www.aap.org

Sherill Tippins, Editor
Michael I. Reiff MD, FAAP, Editor-in-Chief

Based on the American Academy of Pediatrics' own clinical practice guidelines for ADHD and written in clear, accessible language, ths book answers the common question: How is ADHD diagnosed? What are today's best treatment options? and Will my child outgrow ADHD?

355 pages Year Founded: 2004 ISBN 1-581101-21-X

28   Adventures in Fast Forward: Life, Love and Work for the ADD Adult
ADD WareHouse
300 NW 70th Avenue
Suite 102
Plantation, FL 33317-2360
954-792-8944
800-233-9273; *Fax:* 954-792-8545
sales@addwarehouse.com
www.addwarehouse.com

Kathleen G. Nadeu, Author

For all adults with ADD, this book is designed to be a practical guide for day-to-day life. No matter where you are in the scenario - curious about ADD, just diagnosed or experiencing particular problems, this book will give you effective strategies to help anticipate and negotiate the challenges that come with the condition. Filled with important tools and tactics for self-care and success. *$23.00*

224 pages Year Founded: 1996 ISBN 0-876308-00-0

29   All About Attention Deficit Disorder: Revised Edition
ADD WareHouse
300 NW 70th Avenue
Suite 102
Plantation, FL 33317-2360
954-792-8944
800-233-9273; *Fax:* 954-792-8545
sales@addwarehouse.com
www.addwarehouse.com

Harvey C Parker, Owner

A practical and comprehensive manual for parents and teachers interested in understanding the facts about ADD. Chapters on home management, the 1-2-3 Magic discipline method, facts about medication management and practical ideas for teachers to use in managing learning and classroom behavior. *$13.00*

165 pages

30   All Kinds of Minds
ADD WareHouse
300 NW 70th Avenue
Suite 102
Plantation, FL 33317-2360
954-792-8944
800-233-9273; *Fax:* 954-792-8545
sales@addwarehouse.com
www.addwarehouse.com

Dr. Mel Levine, Author

Young students with learning disorders- children in primary and elementary grades -can now gain insight into the difficulties they face in school. This book helps all children understand and respect all kinds of minds and can encourage children with learning disorders to maintain their motivation and keep from developing behavior problems stemming from their learning disorders. *$38.00*

283 pages

31   Answers to Distraction
ADD WareHouse
300 NorthWest 70th Avenue
Suite 102
Plantation, FL 33317-2360
954-792-8944
800-233-9273; *Fax:* 954-792-8545
websales@addwarehouse.com
www.addwarehouse.com

Edward M. Hallowell, Author
John J. Ratey, Author

A user's guide to ADD presented in a question and answer format ideal for parents of children and adolescents with ADD, adults with ADD and teachers who work with students who have ADD. *$13.00*

334 pages Year Founded: 1996 ISBN 0-553378-21-X

32   Attention Deficit Disorder and Learning Disabilities: Reality, Myths, and Controversial Treatments
Bantam Doubleday Dell Publishing
1745 Broadway
10th Floor
New York, NY 10019-4343
E-mail: ddaypub@randomhouse.com
www.www.randomhouse.com

Barbara D. Ingersoll, Author
Sam Goldstein, Author

Discusses ADHD and learning disabilities as well as their effective treatments. Warns against nutritional and other alternative treatments. *$12.95*

256 pages Year Founded: 1993 ISBN 0-385469-31-4

33   Attention Deficit Hyperactivity Disorder in Children: A Medication Guide
Madison Institute of Medicine
7617 Mineral Point Road
Suite 300
Madison, WI 53717-1623
608-827-2470
mim@miminc.org
www.factsforhealth.org

Hugh F. Johnston, Author
J. Jay Fruehling, Author

Written for parents, this explains the various medications used commonly to treat ADHD/ADD. It includes a review of the symptoms of ADHD, medication therapy, commonly asked questions, and side effects of medications. *$5.95*

41 pages

34   Attention Deficits and Hyperactivity in Children: Developmental Clinical Psychology and Psychiatry
Sage Publications
2455 Teller Road
Thousand Oaks, CA 91320-2234
800-818-7243; *Fax:* 800-583-2665
info@sagepub.com
www.sagepub.com

Stephen P. Hinshaw, Author

Provides background information and evaluates key debates and questions that remain unanswered about ADHD.

Includes what tools can be used to gain optimal information about this disorder and which factors predict subsequent functioning in adolescence and adulthood. Advances, challenges and unresolved problems in diverse but relevant areas are analyzed and placed in context. Paperback also available. *$43.95*

161 pages Year Founded: 1993 ISBN 0-803951-96-5

35 Attention-Deficit Hyperactivity Disorder in Adults: A Guide
Madison Institute of Medicine
6515 Grand Teton Plaza
Suite 100
Madison, WI 53719
608-827-2470; *Fax:* 608-827-2444
mim@miminc.org
www.factsforhealth.org

Hugh F. Johnston, MD, Author

This guide provides an overview of adult ADHD and how it is treated with medications and other treatment approaches. *$5.95*

58 pages Year Founded: 2002

36 Beyond Ritalin
ADD WareHouse
300 NorthWest 70th Avenue
Suite 102
Plantation, FL 33317-2360
954-792-8944
800-233-9273; *Fax:* 954-792-8545
websales@addwarehouse.com
www.addwarehouse.com

Stephen W. Garber, PhD, Author

Beyond Ritalin: Facts About Medication and Other Strategies for Helping Children, Adolescents and Adults with Attention Deficit Disorders. The authors respond to concerns all parents and individuals have about using medication to treat disorders such as ADHD, explain the importance of a treatment program for those with this condition and discuss fads and fallacies in current treatments. *$13.50*

272 pages Year Founded: 1996 ISBN 0-060977-25-6

37 Conduct Disorders in Children and Adolescents
American Psychiatric Publishing, Inc.
1000 Wilson Boulevard
Suite 1825
Arlington, VA 22209-3901
703-907-7322
800-368-5777; *Fax:* 703-907-1091
appi@psych.org
www.appi.org

G Pirooz Sholevar, M.D., Editor
Ron McMillen, Chief Executive Officer
John McDuffie, Editorial Director

Examines the phenomenology, etiology, and diagnosis of conduct disorders, and describes therapeutic and preventive interventions. Includes the range of treatments now availaable, including individual, family, group, and behavior therapy; hospitalization; and residential treatment. *$52.00*

414 pages Year Founded: 1995 ISBN 0-880485-17-5

38 Consumer's Guide to Psychiatric Drugs
NewHarbinger Publications
5674 Shattuck Avenue
Oakland, CA 94609-1662
510-652-0215
800-748-6273; *Fax:* 800-652-1613
customerservice@newharbinger.com
www.newharbinger.com

Mary C. Talaga, Author
John D. Preston, Author
John H. O'Neal, Author

The authors explain how each drug works, tell readers what to expect in terms of side-effects, interaction with other drugs and medical condition, and other concerns, and offer detailed information about treatments for depression, bipolar disorder, anxiety and sleep disorders, and a comprehensive range of other conditions. *$16.95*

340 pages Year Founded: 1973 ISBN 1-572241-11-X

39 Daredevils and Daydreamers: New Perspectives on Attention Deficit/Hyperactivity Disorder
ADD WareHouse
300 NW 70th Avenue
Suite 102
Plantation, FL 33317-2360
954-792-8100
800-233-9273; *Fax:* 954-792-8545
sales@addwarehouse.com
www.addwarehouse.com

Barbara Ingersoll, Author

From obtaining a good diagnosis through the most recent, cutting edge medical and psychological solutions offered, Ingersoll's examples and research have an immediacy missing from the other books in the field. In addition, the othor tackles a number of peripheral issues other books ignore such as the problem of the ADHD child in adoptive families, divorced families and step-families, and she handles real-world issues (like soiling and bed-wetting) that others disregard. *$11.00*

256 pages Year Founded: 1997 ISBN 0-385487-57-6

40 Distant Drums, Different Drummers: A Guide for Young People with ADHD
ADD WareHouse
300 NorthWest 70th Avenue
Suite 102
Plantation, FL 33317-2360
954-792-8944
800-233-9273; *Fax:* 954-792-8545
websales@addwarehouse.com
www.addwarehouse.com

Barbara D. Ingersoll, Author

This book presents a positive perspective of ADHD - one that stresses the value of individual differences. Written for children and adolescents struggling with ADHD, it offers young readers the opportunity to see themselves in a positive light and motivates them to face challenging problems. Ages 8-14. *$16.00*

48 pages Year Founded: 1995 ISBN 0-964854-80-6

41 Don't Give Up Kid
ADD WareHouse
300 NW 70th Avenue
Suite 102
Plantation, FL 33317-2360

954-792-8944
800-233-9273; *Fax:* 954-792-8545
sales@addwarehouse.com
www.addwarehouse.com

Jeanne Gehret, Author
M.A. Gehret, Author
Sandra A. Depauw, Illustrator

Alex, the hero of this book, is one of two million children in the US who have learning disabilities. This book gives children with reading problems and learning disabilities a clear understanding of their difficulties and the necessary courage to learn to live with them. Ages 5-12. *$13.00*

40 pages Year Founded: 1996 ISBN 1-884281-10-9

42   Down and Dirty Guide to Adult Attention Deficit Disorder
ADD WareHouse
300 NorthWest 70th Avenue
Suite 102
Plantation, FL 33317-2360
954-792-8944
800-233-9273; *Fax:* 954-792-8545
websales@addwarehouse.com
www.addwarehouse.com

Harvey C Parker, Owner

A book about ADD that is immensely entertaining, informative and uncomplicated. Describes concepts essential to understanding how this disorder is best identified and treated. You'll find a refreshing absence of jargon and an abundance of common sense, practical advice and healthy skepticism. *$17.00*

194 pages

43   Driven to Distraction: Recognizing and Coping with Attention Deficit Disorder from Childhood through Adulthood
ADD WareHouse
300 NorthWest 70th Avenue
Suite 102
Plantation, FL 33317-2360
954-792-8944
800-233-9273; *Fax:* 954-792-8545
websales@addwarehouse.com
www.addwarehouse.com

Harvey C Parker, Owner
John J Ratey MD

Through vivid stories of the experiences of their patients (both adults and children), this books shows the varied forms ADD takes - from the hyperactive search for high stimulation to the floating inattention of daydreaming - and the transforming impact of precise diagnosis and treatment. The authors explain when and how medication can be helpful, and since both authors have ADD, their advice on effective behavior-modification techniques is enriched by their own experience. Also available on audiotape for $16.00. *$13.00*

319 pages Year Founded: 1995

44   Drug Therapy and Childhood & Adolescent Disorders
Mason Crest Publishers
450 Parkway Drive
Suite D
Broomall, PA 19008-4017

610-543-6200
866-627-2665; *Fax:* 610-543-3878
dtaylor@masoncrest.com
www.masoncrest.com

Shirley Brinkerhoff, Author
Dan Hilferty, President
Michelle Luke, Director, Marketing
Michael Toglia, Special Sales

This book provides readers with an easy-to-understand introduction to this topic. Numerous case studies and examples give insight in the four disorders first diagnosed in childhood and adolescence that can be treated with psychiatric drugs, and helps readers understand the symptoms and treatments of these disorders.

128 pages ISBN 1-590845-63-3

45   Eagle Eyes: A Child's View of Attention Deficit Disorder
ADD WareHouse
300 NorthWest 70th Avenue
Suite 102
Plantation, FL 33317-2360
954-792-8944
800-233-9273; *Fax:* 954-792-8545
websales@addwarehouse.com
www.addwarehouse.com

Harvey C Parker, Owner

This book helps readers of all ages understand ADD and gives practical suggestions for organization, social cues and self calming. Expressive illustrations enhance the book and encourage reluctant readers. Ages 5-12. *$13.00*

30 pages

46   Eukee the Jumpy, Jumpy Elephant
ADD WareHouse
300 NorthWest 70th Avenue
Suite 102
Plantation, FL 33317-2360
954-792-8944
800-233-9273; *Fax:* 954-792-8545
websales@addwarehouse.com
www.addwarehouse.com

Harvey C Parker, Owner
Esther Trevino

A story about a bright young elephant who is not like all the other elephants. Eukee moves through the jungle like a tornado, unable to pay attention to the other elephants. He begins to feel sad, but gets help after a visit to the doctor who explains why Eukee is so jumpy and hyperactive. With love, support and help, Eukee learns ways to help himself and gain renewed self-esteem. Ideal for ages 3-8. *$15.00*

22 pages Year Founded: 1995

47   Facing AD/HD: A Survival Guide for Parents
Research Press
Dept 24 W
PO Box 9177
Champaign, IL 61826-9177
217-352-3273
800-519-2707; *Fax:* 217-352-1221
rp@researchpress.com
www.researchpress.com

Janet Morris, Author
Robert W Parkinson, Founder

Provides parents with the skills they need to help minimize the everyday struggles and frustrations associated with AD/HD. The book addresses structure, routines, setting goals, using charts, persistency with consistency, teamwork, treatment options, medication and more. *$ 14.95*

232 pages ISBN 0-878223-81-9

48 First Star I See
ADD WareHouse
300 NW 70th Avenue
Suite 102
Plantation, FL 33317-2360
954-792-8944
800-233-9273; *Fax:* 954-792-8545
sales@addwarehouse.com
www.addwarehouse.com

Harvey C Parker, Owner

This entertaining and funny look at ADD without hyperactivity is a must-read for middle grade girls with ADD, their teachers and parents. *$11.00*

150 pages

49 Gene Bomb
Hope Press
PO Box 188
Duarte, CA 91009-188
818-303-0644
800-321-4039; *Fax:* 626-358-3520
dcomings@earthlink.net
www.hopepress.com

David E Comings, Author

Gene Bomb: Does Higher Education and Advanced Technology Accelerate the Selection of Genes for Learning Disorders, Addictive and Disruptive Behaviors? Explores the hypothesis that autism, learning disorders, alcoholism, drug abuse, depression, attention deficit disorder, and other disruptive behavioral disorders are increaseing in frequency because of an increasing selection, in the 20th century, for the genes associated with these conditions. *$29.95*

304 pages ISBN 1-878267-38-8

50 Give Your ADD Teen a Chance: A Guide for Parents of Teenagers with Attention Deficit Disorder
ADD WareHouse
300 NorthWest 70th Avenue
Suite 102
Plantation, FL 33317-2360
954-792-8944
800-233-9273; *Fax:* 954-792-8545
websales@addwarehouse.com
www.addwarehouse.com

Harvey C Parker, Owner

Parenting teenagers is never easy, especially if your teen suffers from ADD. This book provides parents with expert help by showing them how to determine which issues are caused by 'normal' teenager development and which are caused by ADD. *$15.00*

299 pages

51 Grandma's Pet Wildebeest Ate My Homework
ADD WareHouse
300 NW 70th Avenue
Suite 102
Plantation, FL 33317-2360

954-792-8944
800-233-9273; *Fax:* 954-792-8545
sales@addwarehouse.com
www.addwarehouse.com

Harvey C Parker, Owner

Parents and teachers dealing with hyperactive or daydreaming kids will find this book outstanding. As an ADHD adult himself, Quinn draws upon his own experience, making use of straightforward, creative behavioral management techniques, along with a keen sense of humor. A highly informative and enlightened book. *$16.95*

272 pages

52 Healing ADD: Simple Exercises That Will Change Your Daily Life
ADD WareHouse
300 NW 70th Avenue
Suite 102
Plantation, FL 33317-2360
954-792-8944
800-233-9273; *Fax:* 954-792-8545
sales@addwarehouse.com
www.addwarehouse.com

Harvey C Parker, Owner

Presents simple methods involving visualization and positive thinking that can be readily picked up by adults and taught to children with ADD. *$10.00*

178 pages

53 Help 4 ADD@High School
ADD WareHouse
300 NorthWest 70th Avenue
Suite 102
Plantation, FL 33317-2360
954-792-8944
800-233-9273; *Fax:* 954-792-8545
websales@addwarehouse.com
www.addwarehouse.com

Harvey C Parker, Owner

This new book was written for teenagers with ADHD. Designed like a web site, it has short, easy-to-read information packed sections which tell you what you need to know about how to get your life together - for yourself, not for your parents or your teachers. Includes tips on studying, ways your high school can help you succeed, tips on getting along better at home, on dating, exercise and much more. *$19.95*

119 pages

54 HomeTOVA: Attention Screening Test
ADD WareHouse
300 NW 70th Avenue
Suite 102
Plantation, FL 33317-2360
954-792-8944
800-233-9273; *Fax:* 954-792-8545
sales@addwarehouse.com
www.addwarehouse.com

Harvey C Parker, Owner

Screen yourself or your child (ages 4 to 80 plus) for attention problems. After a simple installation on your home computer (Windows 95/98 OS only), the Home TOVA program runs with use of a mouse. Takes 21.6 minutes and measures how fast, accurate and consistent a person is in responding to squares flashing on a screen. Each program is limited to two administrators. *$29.95*

55   How to Do Homework without Throwing Up
ADD WareHouse
300 NorthWest 70th Avenue
Suite 102
Plantation, FL 33317-2360
954-792-8944
800-233-9273; *Fax:* 954-792-8545
websales@addwarehouse.com
www.addwarehouse.com

Harvey C Parker, Owner

Cartoons and witty insights teach important truths about homework and strategies for getting it done. Learn how to make a homework schedule, when to do the hardest homework, where to do homework, the benefits of homework and more. Useful in motivating students with ADD. For ages 8-13. *$9.00*

67 pages

56   Hyperactive Child, Adolescent, and Adult
Oxford University Press
198 Madison Avenue
New York, NY 10016-4341
212-726-6400
800-451-7556

Michael Cunningham, Manager

Discusses symptoms and treatment of ADD/ADHD in children and adults with practical suggestions for the management of children. *$27.00*

172 pages   ISBN 0-195042-91-3

57   Hyperactive Children Grown Up: ADHD in Children, Adolescents, and Adults
Guilford Press
72 Spring Street
New York, NY 10012-4068
212-431-9800
800-365-7006; *Fax:* 212-966-6708
info@guilford.com

Bob Matloff, President
Seymour Weingarten, Editor-in-Chief

Explores what happens to hyperactive children when they grow to adulthood. Based on the McGill prospective studies, which spans more than 30 years, the volume reports findings on the etiology, treatment and outcome of attention deficits and hyperactivity at all stages of development. Paperback also available. *$44.95*

473 pages   ISBN 0-898620-39-2

58   I'm Somebody, Too!
ADD WareHouse
300 NorthWest 70th Avenue
Suite 102
Plantation, FL 33317-2360
954-792-8944
800-233-9273; *Fax:* 954-792-8545
websales@addwarehouse.com
www.addwarehouse.com

Harvey C Parker, Owner

Because it is written for an older, non-ADD audience, this book explains ADD in depth and explains methods to han-

dle the feelings that often result from having a family member with ADD. For children ages 9 and older. *$13.00*

159 pages

59   Is Your Child Hyperactive? Inattentive? Impulsive? Distractible?
ADD WareHouse
300 NorthWest 70th Avenue
Suite 102
Plantation, FL 33317-2360
954-792-8944
800-233-9273; *Fax:* 954-792-8545
websales@addwarehouse.com
www.addwarehouse.com

Harvey C Parker, Owner

Written with compassion and hope, this parent guide prepares you for the process of determining if your child has ADD and guides you in your dealings with educators, doctors and other professionals. *$13.00*

256 pages   Year Founded: 1995

60   Learning to Slow Down and Pay Attention
ADD WareHouse
300 NorthWest 70th Avenue
Suite 102
Plantation, FL 33317-2360
954-792-8944
800-233-9273; *Fax:* 954-792-8545
websales@addwarehouse.com
www.addwarehouse.com

Harvey C Parker, Owner

Written for children to read, and illustrated with charming cartoons and activity pages, the book helps children identify problems and explains how their parents, teachers and doctors can help. For children 6-14. *$10.00*

96 pages

61   Living with Attention Deficit Disorder: Workbook for Adults with ADD
NewHarbinger Publications
5674 Shattuck Avenue
Oakland, CA 94609-1662
510-652-0215
800-748-6273; *Fax:* 800-652-1613
customerservice@newharbinger.com
www.newharbinger.com

M Susan Roberts, Author
Gerald J Jansen, Author

Includes strategies for handling common problems at work and school, dealing with intimate relationships, and finding support. *$17.95*

165 pages   Year Founded: 1973 ISBN 1-572240-63-6

62   Medications for Attention Disorders and Related Medical Problems: Comprehensive Handbook
ADD WareHouse
300 NW 70th Avenue
Suite 102
Plantation, FL 33317-2360
954-792-8944
800-233-9273; *Fax:* 954-792-8545
sales@addwarehouse.com
www.addwarehouse.com

Harvey C Parker, Owner

ADHD and ADD are medical conditions and often medical intervention is regarded by most experts as an essential component of the multimodal program for the treatment of these disorders. This text presents a comprehensive look at medications and their use in attention disorders. *$37.00*

420 pages

63 **Meeting the ADD Challenge: A Practical Guide for Teachers**
Research Press
PO Box-7886
Champaign, IL 61826
217-352-3273
800-519-2707; *Fax: 217-352-1221*
rp@researchpress.com
www.researchpress.com

Dr Michael J Asher, Author
Dr. Steven B Gordon, Author

Information on the needs and treatment of children and adolescents with ADD. The book addresses the defining characteristics of ADD, common treatment approaches, myths about ADD, matching intervention to student, use of behavior rating scales and checklists, evaluating interventions, regular versus special class placement, helping students regulate their own behavior and more. Includes case examples. *$21.95*

196 pages Year Founded: 1968 ISBN 0-878223-45-2

64 **Misunderstood Child: Understanding and Coping with Your Child's Learning Disabilities**
ADD WareHouse
300 NW 70th Avenue
Suite 102
Plantation, FL 33317-2360
954-792-8944
800-233-9273; *Fax: 954-792-8545*
sales@addwarehouse.com
www.addwarehouse.com

Harvey C Parker, Owner

In this revised and updated edition you will find promising treatment options for children, adolescents and adults with learning disabilities, discussion of ADHD, pros and cons of using medication, revision to federal and state laws covering discrimination and educational rights, new approaches for those of college age and older. *$15.00*

403 pages

65 **My Brother's a World Class Pain: Sibling's Guide to ADHD**
ADD WareHouse
300 NorthWest 70th Avenue
Suite 102
Plantation, FL 33317-2360
954-792-8944
800-233-9273; *Fax: 954-792-8545*
websales@addwarehouse.com
www.addwarehouse.com

Harvey C Parker, Owner

While they frequently bear the brunt of the ADHD child's impulsiveness and distractibility, siblings usually are not afforded opportunities to understand the nature of the problem and to have their own feelings and thoughts addressed.

This story shows brothers and sisters how they can play an important role in the family's quest for change. *$12.00*

34 pages Year Founded: 1992

66 **Put Yourself in Their Shoes: Understanding Teenagers with Attention Deficit Hyperactivity Disorder**
ADD WareHouse
300 NorthWest 70th Avenue
Suite 102
Plantation, FL 33317-2360
954-792-8944
800-233-9273; *Fax: 954-792-8545*
websales@addwarehouse.com
www.addwarehouse.com

Harvey C Parker, Owner

Contains up-to-date information on how ADHD affects the lives of adolescents at home, in school, in the workplace and in social relationships. Chapters discuss how to get a good assessment, controversial treatments and medications for ADHD, building positive communication at home, problem-solving strategies to resolve family conflict, ADHD and the military, study strategies to improve learning, ADHD and delinquency, two hundred educational accommodations for ADHD teens and more. *$19.00*

229 pages Year Founded: 1999

67 **RYAN: A Mother's Story of Her Hyperactive/ Tourette Syndrome Child**
Hope Press
PO Box 188
Duarte, CA 91009-188
818-303-0644
800-321-4039; *Fax: 626-358-3520*
dcomings@earthlink.net
www.hopepress.com

Susan Hughes, Author

A moving and informative story of how a mother struggled with the many behavioral problems presented by her son with Tourette syndrome, ADHD and oppositional defiant disorder. *$9.95*

153 pages ISBN 1-878267-25-6

68 **Shelley, The Hyperative Turtle**
ADD WareHouse
300 NorthWest 70th Avenue
Suite 102
Plantation, FL 33317-2360
954-792-8944
800-233-9273; *Fax: 954-792-8545*
websales@addwarehouse.com
www.addwarehouse.com

Harvey C Parker, Owner

The story of a bright young turtle who's not like all the other turtles. Shelley moves like a rocket and is unable to sit still for even the shortest periods of time. Because he and the other turtles are unable to understand why he is so wiggly and squirmy, Shelley begins to feel naughty and out of place. But after a visit to the doctor, Shelley learns what 'hyperactive' means and that it is necessary to take special medicine to control that wiggly feeling. Ideal for ages 3-7. *$14.00*

20 pages Year Founded: 1990

69 Sometimes I Drive My Mom Crazy, But I Know She's Crazy About Me
ADD WareHouse
300 NorthWest 70th Avenue
Suite 102
Plantation, FL 33317-2360
954-792-8944
800-233-9273; *Fax:* 954-792-8545
websales@addwarehouse.com
www.addwarehouse.com

Harvey C Parker, Owner

This warm and humorous story of a young boy with ADHD addresses the many difficult and frustrating issues kids like him confront every day - from sitting still in the classroom, to remaining calm, to feeling 'different' from other children. This book is an amusing look at how a youngster with ADHD can develop a sense of self-worth through better understanding of this disorder. Ages 6-12. *$16.00*

124 pages   Year Founded: 1990

70 Stuck on Fast Forward: Youth with Attention Deficit/Hyperactivity Disorder
Mason Crest Publishers
450 Parkway Drive
Suite D
Broomall, PA 19008-4017
610-543-6200
866-627-2665; *Fax:* 610-543-3878
dtaylor@masoncrest.com
www.masoncrest.com

Shirley Brinkerhoff, Author
Dan Hilferty, President
Michelle Luke, Director, Marketing
Michael Toglia, Special Sales

Provides a comprehensive, yet easy to understand, overview of attention deficit/hyperactivity disorder. ADHD is an increasingly common diagnosis for school-aged and preschool children today, as parents, educators, and medical professionals struggle to deal with children who often don't sit still, don't pay attention, or act impulsively and even inappropriately. The debate over diagnosis and treatment of such symptoms is intense, and Stuck on Fast Forward explores all sides of the issue.

128 pages   ISBN 1-590847-28-8

71 Succeeding in College with Attention Deficit Disorders: Issues and Strategies for Students, Counselors and Educators
ADD WareHouse
300 NorthWest 70th Avenue
Suite 102
Plantation, FL 33317-2360
954-792-8944
800-233-9273; *Fax:* 954-792-8545
websales@addwarehouse.com
www.addwarehouse.com

Harvey C Parker, Owner

Written for college students, their couselors and educators. Based on the real life experiances of adults who were interviewed as part of a research study, this book offers a vivid picture of how college students with ADD can cope and find success in school. *$18.00*

189 pages   Year Founded: 1990

72 Survival Guide for College Students with ADD or LD
ADD WareHouse
300 NorthWest 70th Avenue
Suite 102
Plantation, FL 33317-2360
954-792-8944
800-233-9273; *Fax:* 954-792-8545
websales@addwarehouse.com
www.addwarehouse.com

Harvey C Parker, Owner

A useful guide for high school or college students diagnosed with attention deficit disorder or learning disabilities. Provides the information needed to survive and thrive in a college setting. Full of practical suggestions and tips from an experienced specialist in the field and from college students who also suffer from these difficulties. *$10.00*

56 pages   Year Founded: 1990

73 Survival Strategies for Parenting Your ADD Child
Underwood Books
PO Box 1919
Nevada City, CA 95959
Fax: 530-274-7179
contact@underwoodbooks.com
www.underwoodbooks.com

George T Lynn, Author

Survival Strategies for Parenting Your ADD Child: Dealing with Obsessions, Compulsions, Depression, Explosive Behavior and Rage. Provides parents with methods which can heal the fractures and pain that occur in families with troubled children. *$12.95*

240 pages   ISBN 1-887424-19-9

74 Taking Charge of ADHD: Complete, Authoritative Guide for Parents
ADD WareHouse
300 NorthWest 70th Avenue
Suite 102
Plantation, FL 33317-2360
954-792-8944
800-233-9273; *Fax:* 954-792-8545
websales@addwarehouse.com
www.addwarehouse.com

Harvey C Parker, Owner

Written for parents who are ready to take charge of their child's life. Strong on advocacy and parental empowerment, this book provides step-by-step methods for managing a child with ADHD in a variety of everyday situations, gives information on medications and discusses numerous techniques for enhancing a child's school performance. *$18.00*

294 pages   Year Founded: 1990

75 Teenagers with ADD and ADHD: A Guide for Parents and Professionals
Woodbine House
6510 Bells Mill Road
Bethesda, MD 20817-1636
301-897-3570
800-843-7323; *Fax:* 301-897-5838
info@woodbinehouse.com
www.woodbinehouse.com

Chris A Zeigler Dendy,MS, Author

The newly updated and expanded guide to raising a teenager with an attention deficit disorder is more comprehensive than ever. Thousands more parents can rely on Dendy's compassionately presented expertise based on the latest research and decades of her experience as a parent, teacher, school psychologist, and mental health counselor.

418 pages   Year Founded: 1985

76   Teenagers with ADD: A Parent's Guide
Woodbine House
6510 Bells Mill Road
Bethesda, MD 20817-1636
301-897-3570
800-843-7323; *Fax:* 301-897-5838
info@woodbinehouse.com
www.woodbinehouse.com

Chris A Zeigler Dendy,MS, Author

Double-column book full of information, suggestions and case studies. Lively, upbeat, comprehensive and well targeted to the problems parents face with ADD teenagers. *$18.95*

370 pages   Year Founded: 1985 ISBN 0-933149-69-7

77   The AD/HD Forms Book: Identification, Measurement, and Intervention
Research Press
PO Box-7886
Champaign, IL 61826
217-352-3273
800-519-2707; *Fax:* 217-352-1221
rp@researchpress.com
www.researchpress.com

Dr Michael J Asher, Author
Dr. Steven B Gordon, Author

A collection of intervention procedures and over 30 reproducible forms and checklists for use with any AD/HD program for children or adolescents. Each item is prefaced by a brief description of its purpose and use. The AD/HD Forms Book helps educators, mental health professionals and parents translate their knowledge into action. *$ 25.95*

117 pages   Year Founded: 1968 ISBN 0-878223-78-9

78   The ADD Hyperactivity Handbook for Schools: Effective Strategies for Identifying and Teaching ADD Students in Elementary and Secondary Schools
ADD WareHouse
300 NorthWest 70th Avenue
Suite 102
Plantation, FL 33317-2360
954-792-8944
800-233-9273; *Fax:* 954-792-8545
websales@addwarehouse.com
www.addwarehouse.com

Harvey C. Parker, Author

Written in a practical, easy-to-read style, this handbook for educators who need to effectively assist children with ADD offers proven techniques teachers can use in elementary and secondary school classrooms to help students and families overcome the challenges of ADD. This text is also useful for school psychologists, guidance personnel, student education specialists, and administrators. *$29.00*

330 pages   Year Founded: 1990 ISBN 0-962162-92-2

79   Understanding Girls with Attention Deficit Hyperactivity Disorder
ADD WareHouse
300 NorthWest 70th Avenue
Suite 102
Plantation, FL 33317-2360
954-792-8944
800-233-9273; *Fax:* 954-792-8545
websales@addwarehouse.com
www.addwarehouse.com

Harvey C Parker, Owner

Symptoms of ADHD are often overlooked or misunderstood in girls who are often diagnosed much later, and their ADHD symptoms may go untreated. This groundbreaking book reveals how ADHD affects girls from preschool through high school years. Gender differences are discussed along with issues related to school success, medication treatment, family relationships and susceptibility to other disorders such as anxiety, depression and learning problems. *$19.95*

291 pages   Year Founded: 1990

80   Voices From Fatherhood: Fathers, Sons and ADHD
ADD WareHouse
300 NorthWest 70th Avenue
Suite 102
Plantation, FL 33317-2360
954-792-8944
800-233-9273; *Fax:* 954-792-8545
websales@addwarehouse.com
www.addwarehouse.com

Harvey C Parker, Owner
Patricia O Quinn MD

Written to specifically help fathers navigate the complex world of parenting and ADHD, this book helps fathers enhance and deepen their relationships with their sons while providing them with strategies for guiding their sons. *$20.00*

184 pages   Year Founded: 1990

81   What Makes Ryan Tick?
Hope Press
PO Box 188
Duarte, CA 91009-188
818-303-0644
800-321-4039; *Fax:* 626-358-3520
dcomings@earthlink.net
www.hopepress.com

Susan Hughes, Author

What Makes Ryan Tick? A Family's Triumph over Tourette's Syndrome and Attention Deficit Hyperactivity Disorder. A moving and informative story how a mother struggled with the many behavioral problems presented by her son with Tourettes syndrome, ADHD and oppositional defiant disorder. *$15.95*

303 pages   ISBN 1-878267-35-3

82   Women with Attention Deficit Disorder
ADD WareHouse
300 NorthWest 70th Avenue
Suite 102
Plantation, FL 33317-2360
954-792-8944
800-233-9273; *Fax:* 954-792-8545

websales@addwarehouse.com
www.addwarehouse.com

Harvey C Parker, Owner

Combines real-life histories, treatment experiences and recent clinical research to highlight the special challenges facing women with Attention Deficit Disorder. After describing what to look for and what to look out for in treatment and counseling, this book outlines empowering steps that women living with ADD may use to change their lives. Also available on audiotape. 3 hours on 2 cassettes for $20.00. *$12.00*

354 pages Year Founded: 1990

83   You Mean I'm Not Lazy, Stupid or Crazy?
ADD WareHouse
300 NorthWest 70th Avenue
Suite 102
Plantation, FL 33317-2360
954-792-8944
800-233-9273; *Fax:* 954-792-8545
websales@addwarehouse.com
www.addwarehouse.com

Harvey C Parker, Owner
Peggy Ramundo

This book is the first written by ADD adults for ADD adults. A comprehensive guide, it provides accurate information, practical how-to's and moral support. Readers will also get information on unique differences in ADD adults, the impact on their lives, treatment options available for adults, up-to-date research findings and much more. Also available on audiotape. *$14.00*

460 pages Year Founded: 1990

Periodicals & Pamphlets

84   ADDitude Magazine
ADD Warehouse
300 NW 70th Avenue
Suite 102
Plantation, FL 33317-2360
954-792-8944
800-233-9273; *Fax:* 954-792-8545
sales@addwarehouse.com
www.addwarehouse.com

Harvey C Parker, Owner

Provides valuable resource information for professionals-teachers, healthcare providers, employers and others-who interact with AD/HD people everyday. *$19.97*

85   Attention Magazine
Children and Adults with AD/HD (CHADD)
4601 Presidents Drive
Suite 300
Lanham, MD 20706
301-306-7070
800-233-4050; *Fax:* 301-306-7090
www.chadd.org

A bi-monthly magazine for members of CHADD that offers practical information, clinical insights, and strategies for managing ADHD. Attention manazine also offers a digital edition subscription. *$24.00*

6 per year

86   Attention-Deficit/Hyperactivity Disorder in Children and Adolescents
Center for Mental Health Services: Knowledge Exchange Network
PO Box 42557
Washington, DC 20015-557
800-789-2647; *Fax:* 301-984-8796
TDD: 866-889-2647
ken@mentalhealth.org
www.mentalhealth.samhsa.gov/publications/

This fact sheet defines attention-deficit/hyperactivity disorder, describes the warning signs, discusses types of help available, and suggests what parents or other caregivers can do.

3 pages Year Founded: 1997

87   Learning Disabilities: A Multidisciplinary Journal
Learning Disabilities Association of America
4156 Library Road
Pittsburgh, PA 15234-1349
412-341-1515; *Fax:* 412-344-0224
info@LDAAmerica.org
www.ldaamerica.org

Steven C Russell,PhD, Editor
Heather Nicklow, Accounting Manager
Sharon Tanner, Membership and Development
Maureen Swanson, Healthy Children Project

The most current research designed for professionals in the field of LD. *$60.00*

Year Founded: 1964

88   Treatment of Children with Mental Disorders
National Institute of Mental Health
6001 Executive Boulevard
Room 8184
Bethesda, MD 20892-9663
301-443-4513
866-615-6464
TTY: 301-443-8431
nimhinfo@nih.gov
www.www.nimh.nih.gov/

Francis S Collins MD, PhD, Director
James M Anderson, MD, PhD, Director
Robin L Kawazoe, Deputy Director

A short booklet that contains questions and answers about therapy for children with mental disorders. Includes a chart of mental disorders and medications used.

Support Groups & Hot Lines

89   Children and Adults with AD/HD (CHADD)
4601 Presidents Drive
Suite 300
Lanham, MD 20706
301-306-7070
800-233-4050; *Fax:* 301-306-7090
www.chadd.org

Michael McKay, President
Belynda L. Gauthier, President Elect
Eugene M. Bell, Secretary
Harvey Parker, Founder

Nonprofit organization serving individuals with AD/HD and their families. Over 16,000 members in 200 local chapters throughout the United States. Chapters offer support for individuals, parents, teachers, professionals, and others. Available on Facebook and Twitter.

Video & Audio

90   ADHD & LD: Powerful Teaching Strategies & Accomodations
ADD Warehouse
300 NW 70the Avenue
Suite 102
Plantation, FL 33317-2360
954-792-8100
800-233-9273; *Fax:* 954-792-8545
websales@addwarehouse.com
www.addwarehouse.com

Sandra Rief, Author

Provides instructional strategies for engaging attention and active participation, classroom management and behavioral interventions, gives academic strategies and accomodations, and collaborates teaming for success. 45 minutes. *$129.00*

Year Founded: 1990

91   ADHD-Inclusive Instruction & Collaborative Practices
ADD Warehouse
300 NW 70th Avenue
Suite 102
Plantation, FL 33317-2360
954-792-8100
800-233-9273; *Fax:* 954-792-8545
websales@addwarehouse.com
www.addwarehouse.com

Sandra Rief, Author

Describes classroom modifications, teaching strategies, and interventions that can be used to maximize learning and ensure that all students achieve success. 38 minutes. *$99.00*

Year Founded: 1990 ISBN 1-887943-04-8

92   ADHD: What Can We Do?
ADD WareHouse
300 NW 70th Avenue
Suite 102
Plantation, FL 33317-2360
954-792-8100
800-233-9273; *Fax:* 954-792-8545
websales@addwarehouse.com
www.addwarehouse.com

Russell A. Barkley, Author

Can serve as a companion to ADHD: What Do We Know?, this video focuses on the most effective ways to manage ADHD, both in the home and in the classroom. Scenes depict the use of behavior management at home and accommodations and interventions in the classroom which have proven to be effective in the treatment of ADHD. Thirty five minutes. *$95.00*

Year Founded: 1990 ISBN 0-898629-72-1

93   ADHD: What Do We Know?
ADD WareHouse
300 NW 70th Avenue
Suite 102
Plantation, FL 33317-2360

954-792-8100
800-233-9273; *Fax:* 954-792-8545
websales@addwarehouse.com
www.addwarehouse.com

Russell A. Barkley, Author

This video provides an overview of the disorder and introduces the viewer to three young people who have ADHD. Discusses how ADHD affects the lives of the children and adults, causes of the disorder, associated problems, outcome in adulthood and provides vivid illustrations of how individuals with ADHD function at home, at school and on the job. Thirty five minutes. *$95.00*

Year Founded: 1990 ISBN 0-898629-71-3

94   Adults with Attention Deficit Disorder: ADD Isn't Just Kids Stuff
ADD WareHouse
300 NW 70th Avenue
Suite 102
Plantation, FL 33317-2360
954-792-8100
800-233-9273; *Fax:* 954-792-8545
websales@addwarehouse.com
www.addwarehouse.com

Harvey C Parker, Owner

Explains this often misunderstood condition and the effects it has on one's work, home and social life. With the help of a panel of six adults, four ADD adults and two of their spouses, the book addresses the most common concerns of adults with ADD and provides information that will help families who are experiencing difficulties. 86 minutes. *$ 47.00*

Year Founded: 1990

95   Educating Inattentive Children
ADD WareHouse
300 NW 70th Avenue
Suite 102
Plantation, FL 33317-2360
954-792-8100
800-233-9273; *Fax:* 954-792-8545
websales@addwarehouse.com
www.addwarehouse.com

Samuel Goldstein, Ph.D., Author
Michael Goldstein, M.D., Author

This two-hour video is ideal for in-service to regular and special educators concerning problems experienced by inattentive elementary and secondary students. Provides educators with information necessary to indentify and evaluate classroom problems caused by inattention and a well-defined set of practical guidelines to help educate children with ADD. *$49.00*

Year Founded: 1990

96   Medication for ADHD
ADD WareHouse
300 NW 70th Avenue
Suite 102
Plantation, FL 33317-2360
954-792-8100
800-233-9273; *Fax:* 954-792-8545
websales@addwarehouse.com
www.addwarehouse.com

Dr. Andrew Adesman, Author

This comprehensive DVD addresses the critical questions regarding the use of medication in the treatment of ADD or ADHD. Allows those involved with ADHD to make well-informed and constructive decisions that may deeply change someone's life. *$39.95*

Year Founded: 1990 ISBN 1-889140-18-X

97 New Look at ADHD: Inhibition, Time and Self Control
Guilford Press
72 Spring Street
New York, NY 10012-4068
212-431-9800
800-365-7006; *Fax:* 212-966-6708
info@guilford.com

Bob Matloff, President
Seymour Weingarten, Editor-in-Chief

This video provides an accessible introduction to Russell A Barkley's influential theory of the nature and origins of ADHD. The program brings to life the conceptual framework delineated in Barkley's other books. Discusses concrete ways that our new understanding of the disorder might facilitate more effective clinical interventions. This lucid, state of the art program is ideal viewing for clinicians, students and inservice trainees, parents of children with ADHD and adults with the disorder. 30 minutes. *$95.00*

Year Founded: 2000 ISBN 1-572304-97-9

98 Outside In: A Look at Adults with Attention Deficit Disorder
ADD Warehouse
300 NW 70th Avenue
Suite 102
Plantation, FL 33317-2360
954-792-8100
800-233-9273; *Fax:* 954-792-8545
websales@addwarehouse.com
www.addwarehouse.com

Ted Kay, Director

Documentary film about adults with ADD and their journeys and the strategies they used to succeed. 29 minutes *$27.95*

Year Founded: 1990

99 Understanding Mental Illness
Educational Video Network
1401 19th Street
Huntsville, TX 77340
936-295-5767
800-762-0060; *Fax:* 936-294-0233
info at evn.org
www.www.evndirect.com

A video to learn and understand mental illness and how it affects you. *$79.95*

Year Founded: 2004 ISBN 1-589501-48-9

100 Understanding and Treating the Hereditary Psychiatric Spectrum Disorders
Hope Press
10 Mill Road
Duarte, CA 91010
626-622-4978
800-209-9182; *Fax:* 626-358-3520

dcomings@earthlink.net
www.hopepress.com

Books cover: ADHD, Tourette Syndrome, Obsessive-Compulsive Disorder, Conduct Disorder, Oppositional Defiant Disorder, Autism and other Hereditary Psychiatric Spectrum Disorders. *$75.00*

Year Founded: 1997

101 Understanding the Defiant Child
Guilford Press
72 Spring Street
New York, NY 10012-4068
212-431-9800
800-365-7006; *Fax:* 212-966-6708
info@guilford.com

Bob Matloff, President
Seymour Weingarten, Editor-in-Chief

Presents information on Oppositional Defiant Disorder and Conduct Disorder with scenes of family interactions, showing the nature and causes of these disorders and what can and should be done about it. Thirty five minutes with a manual that contains more information. 30 minutes. *$95.00*

Year Founded: 1997 ISBN 1-572301-66-X

102 Why Won't My Child Pay Attention?
ADD WareHouse
300 NW 70th Avenue
Suite 102
Plantation, FL 33317-2360
954-792-8100
800-233-9273; *Fax:* 954-792-8545
websales@addwarehouse.com
www.addwarehouse.com

Sam Goldstein, PhD, Author

Provides an easy-to-follow explanation concerning the effect ADD has on children at school, home and in the community. Provides guidelines to help parents and professionals successfully and happily manage the problems these behaviors can cause. 76 minutes. *$38.00*

Year Founded: 1990

Web Sites

103 www.CHADD.org
Children/Adults with Attention Deficit/Hyperactivity Disorder

104 www.LD-ADD.com
Attention Deficit Disorder and Parenting Site

105 www.aap.org
American Academy of Pediatrics Practice Guidelines on ADHD

Site serves the purpose of giving the public guidelines for diagnosing and evaluating children with possible ADHD.

106 www.add.about.com
Attention Deficit Disorder

Hundreds of sites.

107 **www.add.org**
Attention Deficit Disorder Association

Provides information, resources and networking to adults with ADHD and to the professionals who work with them.

108 **www.additudemag.com**
Happy Healthy Lifestyle Magazine for People with ADD

109 **www.addvance.com**
Answers to Your Questions About ADD

provides answers to questions about ADD, ADHD for families and individuals at every stage of life from preschool through retirement years.

110 **www.adhdnews.com/Advocate.htm**
Advocating for Your Child

111 **www.adhdnews.com/sped.htm**
Special Education Rights and Responsibilities

Writing IEP's and TIEPS. Pursuing special education services.

112 **www.babycenter.com/rcindex.html**
BabyCenter

113 **www.cfsny.org**
Center for Family Support (CFS)

Devoted to providing support and assistance to individuals with developmental and related disabilities, and to the family members who care for them.

114 **www.cyberpsych.org**
CyberPsych

Hosts the American Psychoanalyists Foundation, American Association of Suicideology, Society for the Exploration of Psychotherapy Intergration, and Anxiety Disorders Association of America. Also subcategories of the anxiety disorders, as well as general information, including panic disorder, phobias, obsessive compulsive disorder (OCD), social phobia, generalized anxiety disorder, post traumatic stress disorder, and phobias of childhood. Book reviews and links to web pages sharing the topics.

115 **www.nami.org**
National Alliance on Mental Illness

From its inception in 1979, NAMI has been dedicated to improving the lives of individuals and families affected by mental illness.

116 **www.nichcy.org**
National Information Center for Children and Youth with Disabilities

Excellent information in English and Spanish.

117 **www.nimh.nih.gov/publicat/adhd.cfm**
Attention Deficit Hyperactivity Disorder

Thirty page booklet.

118 **www.oneaddplace.com**
One ADD Place

119 **www.planetpsych.com**
Planetpsych.com

Learn about disorders, their treatments and other topics in psychology. Articles are listed under the related topic areas. Ask a therapist a question for free, or view the directory of professionals in your area. If you are a therapist sign up for the directory. Current features, self-help, interactive, and newsletter archives.

120 **www.psychcentral.com**
Psych Central

Personalized one-stop index for psychology, support, and mental health issues, resources, and people on the Internet.

121 **www.store.samhsa.gov**
Substance Abuse and Mental Health Services Administration

Resources on mental disorders as well as treatment and recovery.

122 **www.thenadd.org**
National Association for the Dually Diagnosed (NADD)

An association for persons with developmental disabilities and mental health needs.

Adjustment Disorders

Introduction

The experience of stress in life is inevitable. When we are faced with significant life changes, we do our best to cope, get through it, and move on. How we cope and how long it takes to get through it vary according to the stressful situation and the resources the individual brings to it. In most situations, we respond appropriately to the stressful event or situation and show an adaptive response.

Adjustment Disorders are maladaptive reactions to a stressful event or situation. The adjustment is to a real event or situation (e.g., the end of a relationship or job loss), and the disorder signifies that the reaction is more extreme than would be warranted considering the stressor, and/or keeps the individual from functioning as usual.

SYMPTOMS

• The development of emotional or behavioral symptoms is in response to an identifiable stressor, except bereavement, within three months of the appearance of the stressor;
• The emotions or behaviors are significant either because the distress is more extreme than would normally be caused by the stressor, or because the emotions or behaviors are clearly impairing the person's social, school, or work functioning;
• If the symptoms persist for less than six months after the stressor ends, the disorder is considered acute; if symptoms persist for longer than six months, the disorder is considered to be chronic.

Adjustment Disorders are divided into several subtypes:

• **Depressed Mood** - predominant mood is depression, with symptoms such as tearfulness, hopelessness, sadness, sleep disturbances;
• **Anxiety** - predominant symptoms are edginess, nervousness, worry, or in children, fears of separation from important attachment figures;
• **Anxiety and Depressed Mood** - chief manifestations are a combination of depression and anxiety;
• **Disturbance of Conduct** - predominant symptoms are conduct which involves either a violation of other people's rights (e.g., reckless driving, fighting), or the violation of social norms and rules;
• **Disturbance of Emotions and Conduct** - predominant manifestations are a combination of anxiety, depression, and behavioral symptoms;
• **Unspecified** - symptoms that differ fro those associated with other Adjustment Disorder subtypes, such as physical problems or issues related to home, work, or social life.

ASSOCIATED FEATURES

Many commonplace events can be stressful (e.g., first day of school, changing jobs). If the stressor is an acute event (like an impending surgical procedure), the onset of the disturbance is usually immediate but may not last more than six months after the stressor ends. If the stressor or its consequences continue (such as a long-term illness), the Adjustment Disorder may also continue. Whatever the nature of the event, it caused the person to feel overwhelmed. A person may be reacting to one or many stressors; the stressor may affect one person or the whole family. The more severe the stressor, the more likely that an Adjust-

ment Disorder will develop. If a person is already vulnerable, e.g., is suffering from a disability including a mental disorder, an Adjustment Disorder is more likely.

The diagnosis of an Adjustment Disorder is called a residual category, meaning that other possible diagnoses must be ruled out first. For example, symptoms that are part of a personality disorder and become worse under stress are not usually considered to be Adjustment Disorders unless they are new types of symptoms for the individual.

There are three questions to consider in diagnosing Adjustment Disorder: How out-of-proportion is the response to the stressor? How long does it go on? To what extent does it impair the person's ability to function in social, workplace, and school settings?

The emotional response may show itself in excessive worry and edginess, excessive sadness and hopelessness or a combination of these. There may also be changes in behavior in response to the stressful event or situation, with the person violating other people's rights or breaking agreed-upon rules and regulations. The emotional response and the changes in behavior persist, even after the stressful event or circumstances have ended. Finally, the response significantly affects the person's normal functioning in social, school or work settings.

Adjustment Disorders increase the risk of suicidal behavior and completed suicide, and they also complicate the course of other medical conditions (for example, patients may not take their medication, eat properly, etc).

PREVALENCE

Men and women of all ages, as well as children, can suffer from this disorder. Women are twice as likely as men to have an Adjustment Disorder, while chances are similar for boys and girls. In outpatient mental health centers, the diagnosis of Adjustment Disorder is made in five to twenty percent of patients. Adjustment Disorder is one of the most common mental disorders diagnosed in workers.

TREATMENT OPTIONS

Anyone who is experiencing one or more stressful events or circumstances, and feels overwhelmed or markedly distressed and cannot function normally, should seek help. A psychiatrist or other mental health professional should make an evaluation including a referral for physical examination if necessary. Treatment prescribed is often psychotherapy, and, depending on the circumstances, can include individual, couple, or family therapy. Medication is sometimes prescribed for a few weeks or months. In most instances long-term therapy will not be necessary, and the person can expect marked improvement within 8 to 12 sessions.

Associations & Agencies

124 **Alive Alone**
PO Box 182
Van Wert, OH 45891
419-238-7879
alivalon@bright.net
www.alivealone.org

Kay Bevington, Founder
Rodney Bevington, Founder
Sam Brewster, Webmaster

Alive Alone is a nonprofit organization dedicated to educating and supporting bereaved parents whose children are deceased. Alive Alone provides a self-help network and publishes bimonthly newsletters to help parents with no surviving children to find friendship and healing, resolve their grief, and work towards a positive future.

Year Founded: 1988

125 Center for Loss in Multiple Birth (CLIMB), Inc.
PO Box 190401
Anchorage, AK 99519
907-222-5321
climb@climb-support.org
www.climb-support.org

Jean Kollantai, Founder
Berney Richert, Webmaster

A nonprofit organization focused on educating the public on the risks of multiple births and the importance of preventing the losses associated with them. CLIMB provides support for parents who are coping with the loss of one or more of their multiple birth children from conception through early childhood, and also extends assistance to twins, caregivers, families, and multiples organizations.

Year Founded: 1987

126 Center for Mental Health Services (CMHS) Substance Abuse and Mental Health Services Administration
5600 Fishers Lane
Rockville, MD 20857
240-276-1310
877-726-4727
TTY: 800-487-4889
www.samhsa.gov/about-us/who-we-are/offices-centers

Paolo del Vecchio, MSW, Director
Anne Mathews-Younes, Acting Deputy Director
Keris Myrick, Director, Consumer Affairs
Patricia Gratton, Director, Program Analysis

Promotes the treatment of mental illness and emotional disorders by increasing accessibility to mental health programs; supporting outreach, treatment, rehabilitation, and support programs and networks; and encouraging the use of scientifically-based information when treating mental disorders. CMHS provides information about mental health via a toll-free number and numerous publications. Developed for users of mental health services and their families, the general public, policy makers, providers, and the media.

Year Founded: 1992

127 Empty Cradle
9880 N. Magnolia Avenue
#154
Santee, CA 92071
619-595-3887
Info@EmptyCradle.org
www.emptycradle.org

Rachel Redhouse, Director
Suzanne Wells, Assistant Director

A nonprofit peer support group for parents who have experienced the death of a baby. Focusing on parents in the San Diego and Riverside County area, Empty Cradle supports grieving families through educational resources, monthly meetings, and a network of volunteer parents seeking to offer friendship and emotional support.

Year Founded: 1982

128 First Candle
49 Locust Avenue
Suite 104
New Canaan, CT 06840
203-966-1300
800-221-7437
info@firstcandle.org
www.firstcandle.org

Alison Jacobson, Chief Executive Officer
David Cunningham, Chairman

First Candle is a nonprofit organization dedicated to preventing infant death from Sudden Infant Death Syndrome (SIDS), stillbirth, miscarriage, and other Sudden Unexpected Infant Deaths (SUID). First Candle offers support for bereaved families and promotes research, education, and advocacy programs focused on helping all babies to survive.

Year Founded: 1987

129 Grief Recovery After a Substance Passing (GRASP)
40569 Calle Balderas
Indio, CA 92203
302-492-7717
administrator@grasphelp.org
www.grasphelp.org

Denise Cullen, Executive Director

GRASP provides information resources, offers support, and organizes meetings and events for families or individuals who have experienced the death of a loved one as a result of substance abuse or addiction.

Year Founded: 2002

130 M.I.S.S. Foundation/Center for Loss & Trauma
PO Box 9195
Austin, TX 78766
602-279-6477
888-455-6477
info@missfoundation.org
www.missfoundation.org

Dr. Joanne Cacciatore, PhD., Founder and Chairman
Kelli Montgomery, Executive Director
Cindy Cunningham, Executive Assistant

M.I.S.S. Foundation is committed to supporting those who have experienced the death of a child and using research and education to limit the number of child deaths. The Foundation offers ongoing support for families coping with the loss of a child; provides information, newsletters, referrals, support groups, and online chat room support; and participates in legislative issues, advocacy movements, and community events.

Year Founded: 1996

131 National Association for the Dually Diagnosed (NADD)
132 Fair Street
Kingston, NY 12401
845-331-4336
info@thenadd.org
www.thenadd.org

Jeanne M. Farr, MA, Chief Executive Officer
Daniel Baker, PhD., President

Peggie Webb, MA, Vice President
George Zukotynski, PhD., Secretary

NADD is a nonprofit organization designed to increase awareness of, and provide services for, individuals with developmental disabilities and mental illness. NADD emphasizes the importance of quality mental healthcare for people with mental health needs and offers conferences, information resources, educational programs, and training materials to professionals, parents, and organizations.

Year Founded: 1983

132 National Mental Health Consumers' Self-Help Clearinghouse
1211 Chestnut Street
Suite 1100
Philadelphia, PA 19107
267-507-3810
800-553-4539; *Fax:* 215-636-6312
info@mhselfhelp.org
www.mhselfhelp.org

Joseph Rogers, Founder and Executive Director
Susan Rogers, Director

The Clearinghouse is a peer-run national technical assistance center focused on achieving respect and equality of opportunity for those with mental illnesses. The Clearinghouse helps with the growth of the mental health consumer movement by evaluating mental health services, advocating for mental health reform, and providing consumers with news, information, publications, and consultation services.

Year Founded: 1986

133 National Organization of Parents of Murdered Children
635 West 7th Street
Suite 104
Cincinnati, OH 45203
513-721-5683
888-818-7662; *Fax:* 513-345-4489
natlpomc@aol.com
www.pomc.com

Howard S. Klerk, Jr., President
Bev Warnock, National Executive Director
Terrie Jacoby, Vice President
Martha Lasher-Warner, Secretary

The organization provides ongoing support services for parents of children who were murdered, as well as other survivors, with the goal of helping them to work towards a healthy future. Monthly meetings, newsletters, and court accompaniment are also offered in many areas. This organization offers guidelines for starting local chapters. Parole Block Program and Second Opinion Services are also available.

Year Founded: 1978

134 National Youth Network
42165 Turqueries Avenue
Palm Desert, CA 92211
866-458-5441
www.nationalyouth.com

The National Youth Network, formerly known as the Western Youth Network, provides parents and professionals with information on programs and services for underachieving youth experiencing emotional and behavioral problems.

Year Founded: 1990

135 Survivors of Loved Ones' Suicides (SOLOS)
8310 Ewing Halsell Drive
San Antonio, TX 78229
210-885-7069
solossanantonio@gmail.com
www.solossa.org

Tony Mata, SOLOS Facilitator
Angie Navarette, SOLOS Facilitator

Located in San Antonio, Texas, SOLOS organizes ongoing support group meetings for persons affected by the loss of loved ones from suicide.

Year Founded: 1987

136 The Center for Family Support
2811 Zulette Avenue
Bronx, NY 10461
718-518-1500; *Fax:* 718-518-8200
www.www.cfsny.org/

Steven Vernikoff, Executive Director
Lloyd Stabiner, President
Amy Bittinger, Vice President
Barbara Greenwald, Associate Executive Director

The Center for Family Support offers assistance to individuals with developmental and related disabilities, as well as their families, and provides support services and programs that are designed to accommodate individual needs. Offers services throughout New York City, Westchester County, Long Island, and New Jersey.

Year Founded: 1954

137 UNITE, Inc.
1068 West Baltimore Pike
C/o Riddle Hospital
Media, PA 19063
610-296-2411
888-488-6483
administrator@unitegriefsupport.org
www.unitegriefsupport.org

Barbara Bond-Moury, Board Chairperson
Danielle Kennedy, President
Karen Powers, Vice President of Fundraising
John Flanagan, Treasurer

A nonprofit organization committed to providing support services for those who have lost a baby from miscarriage, stillbirth, ectopic pregnancy or early infant death. UNITE, Inc. organizes grief support groups for parents and offers educational programs, training workshops, literature, referrals, and group development assistance.

Year Founded: 1975

138 Zur Institute
321 S. Main Street
#29
Sebastopol, CA 95472
707-935-0655; *Fax:* 707-736-7045
info@zurinstitute.com
www.www.zurinstitute.com

Dr. Ofer Zur, Director

Provides quality online continuing education, tools, and services that enhance the ability of psychotherapists, couselors, therapists, social workers, and other health care professionals to meet the needs of those concerned with mental health.

Year Founded: 1995

Books

139 Don't Despair on Thursdays: the Children's Grief-Management Book
ADD WareHouse
300 NorthWest 70th Avenue
Suite 102
Plantation, FL 33317
954-792-8100
800-233-9273; *Fax:* 954-792-8545
websales@addwarehouse.com
www.addwarehouse.com

David Melton, Illustrator
Nancy R. Thatch, Editor
Adolph Moser, Author

Children are sure to be comforted by the friendly manner and sensitivity that this book imparts as it explains the grief process to children and helps them understand that grieving is a normal response. For children ages 4-10.

61 pages Year Founded: 1996 ISBN 0-933849-60-5

140 Don't Feed the Monster on Tuesdays: The Children's Self-Esteem Book
ADD WareHouse
300 NorthWest 70th Avenue
Suite 102
Plantation, FL 33317
954-792-8100
800-233-9273; *Fax:* 954-792-8545
websales@addwarehouse.com
www.addwarehouse.com

Adolph Moser, Author
Nancy R. Thatch, Editor
David Melton, Illustrator

Helps kids understand negative self-talk by picturing a nasty green monster who lives in your head and says mean things. With colorful cartoons and kid-friendly language, the book offers explanations for those bad feelings and ways to overcome them. *$18.95*

55 pages Year Founded: 1991 ISBN 0-933849-38-9

141 Drug Therapy and Adjustment Disorders
Mason Crest Publishers
450 Parkway Drive
Suite D
Broomall, PA 19008-4017
610-543-6200
866-627-2665; *Fax:* 610-543-3878
www.masoncrest.com

Sherry Bonice, Author
Michelle Luke, Mktg Dir & Public Relations
Louis Cohen, Principal & Creative Director
Sherry Bonnice, Author

Part of the Series: Psychiatric Disorders: Drugs & Psychology for the Mind and Body. Learn about the antidepressants and antianxiety drugs available to treat adjustment disorders. *$24.95*

128 pages Year Founded: 2004 ISBN 1-590845-60-8

142 Preventing Maladjustment from Infancy Through Adolescence
Sage Publications
2455 Teller Road
Thousand Oaks, CA 91320-2234
805-499-0721
800-818-7243; *Fax:* 800-583-2665
info@sagepub.com
www.sagepub.com

Annette U Rickel, Author
Larue Allen, Author
Tracey A Ozmina, EVP, Chief Opersting Officer
Chris Hickok, SVP, Chief Financial Officer

The book begins with a historical overview of prevention research, essential concepts and research practices for identifying populations at risk, and other types of intervention programs. *$83.22*

160 pages Year Founded: 1987 ISBN 0-803928-68-8

143 Stress Response Syndromes: Personality Styles and Interventions
The Rowman & Littlefield Publishing Group
4501 Forbes Blvd
Suite 200
Lanham, MD 20706
301-459-3366; *Fax:* 301-429-5746
customercare@rowman.com
www.rowman.com/RLPublishers

Mardi J Horowitz, Author
George Franzak, Chief Financial Officer
Karin Cholak, Senior Marketing Manager
Kimberly Lyons, Senior Marketing Manager

Incorporation of the most recent advances in the understanding and treatment of stress response syndromes to date. Describes the general characteristics, including signs and symptoms, and elaborates on treatment techniques that integrate cognitive and dynamic approaches. Fourth Edition *$61.00*

451 pages Year Founded: 2001 ISBN 0-765703-13-0

144 Transition from School to Post-School Life for Individuals with Disabilities: Assessment from an Educational and School Psychological Perspective
Charles C Thomas Publisher Ltd.
2600 South First Street
Springfield, IL 62704
217-789-8980
800-258-8980; *Fax:* 217-789-9130
books@ccthomas.com
www.ccthomas.com

Edward M. Levinson, Editor

Designed to assist professionals in developing and implementing transition services for students with disabilities. Specifically, this book focuses on the importance of assessment in transition planning and targets the various domains that should be included in any achool-to-work transition assessment. advocates a transdisciplinary school-based approach to transition assessment that involves not only school-based professionals in the assessment process but community agency representatives as well. Available in paperback for $41.95. *$131.47*

285 pages Year Founded: 1927 ISBN 0-398074-80-1

145 Treatment of Stress Response Syndromes
American Psychiatric Publishing, Inc.
1000 Wilson Boulevard
Suite 1825
Arlington, VA 22209-3901

703-907-7322
800-368-5777; *Fax:* 703-907-1091
appi@psych.org
www.appi.org

Mardi J Horowitz, M.D., Author
Ron McMillen, Chief Executive Officer
John McDuffie, Editorial Director

A comprehensive clinical guide to treating patients with disorders related to loss, trauma and terror. Author Mardi J Horowitz, MD, is the clinical researcher who is largely responsible for modern concepts of posttraumatic stress disorder (PTSD). In this book he reveals the latest strategies for treating PTSD and expands the coverage to include several related diagnoses. *$37.95*

136 pages Year Founded: 2003 ISBN 1-585621-07-1

146 When A Friend Dies: A Book for Teens About Grieving & Healing
Free Spirit Publishing Inc.
217 Fifth Avenue North
Suite 200
Minneapolis, MN 55401-1299
612-338-2068
800-737-7323; *Fax:* 866-419-5199
www.freespirit.com

Marilyn E Gootman Ed.D, Author
Marilyn E Gootman, Author

The death of a friend is a wrenching event for anyone at any age. Teenagers especially need help coping. This compassionate book answers questions grieving teens often have, like 'How should I be acting?''Is it wrong to go to parties and have fun?' and 'What if I can't handle my grief on my own?' The author has seen her children suffer from the death of a friend, and she knows what teens go through. Also recommended for parents and teachers of teens who have experienced a painful loss. *$4.77*

128 pages Year Founded: 1983 ISBN 0-915793-66-0

Periodicals & Pamphlets

147 A Journey Together
Bereaved Parents of the USA
PO Box 622
St Peters, MO 63376
443-865-9666
800-273-8255
jbgoodrich@sbcglobal.net
www.bereavedparentsusa.org

Richard Berman, Editor
Lee Ann Hutson, Vice President, Web Liason
Linda Fehrman, Secretary
John Goodrich, National Contact

The newsletter contains articles of interest to the bereaved about grief. It also has book reviews and information about upcoming Grief Gatherings and other support groups.

4 per year

148 Alive Alone Newsletter
PO Box 182
Van Wert, OH 45891
419-238-7879
alivalon@bright.net
www.alivealone.org

Kay Bevington, Founder
Rodney Bevington, Founder

The Alive Alone newsletter is published quarterly and contains articles on the topic of the loss of a child. The newsletter features articles, poems, and letters written by bereaved parents.

4 per year

149 Journal of Mental Health Research
NADD Press
132 Fair Street
Kingston, NY 12401-4802
845-331-4336
800-331-5362; *Fax:* 845-334-4569
info@thenadd.org
www.thenadd.org

Donna McNELIS,PhD, President
Robert J Fletcher DSW, Chief Executive Officer
Dan Baker,PhD, Vice President
Julia Pearce, Secretary

Bi-monthly publication designed to promote interest of professional and parent development with resources for individuals who have the coexistence of mental illness and developmental disabilities.

4 per year Year Founded: 1983

150 The NADD Bulletin
NADD Press
132 Fair Street
Kingston, NY 12401-4802
845-331-4336
800-331-5362; *Fax:* 845-334-4569
info@thenadd.org
www.thenadd.org

Donna McNELIS,PhD, President
Robert J Fletcher DSW, Chief Executive Officer
Dan Baker,PhD, Vice President
Julia Pearce, Secretary

Bi-monthly publication designed to promote interest of professional and parent development with resources for individuals who have the coexistence of mental illness and developmental disabilities.

6 per year Year Founded: 1983

Support Groups & Hot Lines

151 Bereaved Parents of the USA
PO Box 622
St Peters, MO 63376
708-748-7866
800-273-8255
jbgoodrich@sbcglobal.net
www.bereavedparentsusa.org

Lee Ann Hutson, President
Jodi Norman, Vice President
Delain Johnson, Secretary
Bill Lagemann, Treasurer

BP/USA is a national nonprofit self-help group that offers support, understanding, compassion and hope especially to the newly bereaved, whether they are granparents, parents or siblings.

152 Compassionate Friends, Inc
1000 Jorie Boulevard
Suite 140
Oak Brook, IL 60523
630-990-0010
877-969-0010; *Fax:* 630-990-0246
nationaloffice@compassionatefriends.org
www.compassionatefriends.org

Patrick O'Donnell, President
Lisa Corrao, Chief Operating Officer
Georgia Cockerham, Vice President
Alan Pederson, Interim Executive Director

Bereavement support for families grieving the death of a child of any age regardless of cause.

Year Founded: 1978

153 Friends for Survival, Inc.
PO Box 214463
Sacramento, CA 95821
916-392-0664
800-646-7322
ffs@truevine.net
www.friendsforsurvival.org

A national nonprofit outreach organization open to those who have lost family or friends by suicide, and also to professionals who work with those who have been touched by a suicide tragedy. Dedicated to providing a variety of peer support services that comfort those in grief, encourage healing and growth, foster the development of skills to cope with a loss and educate the entire community regarding the impact of suicide.

154 National Share Office
42 Jackson Street
Saint Charles, MO 63301-3468
636-947-6164
800-821-6819; *Fax:* 636-947-7486
info@nationalshare.org
www.www.nationalshare.org

Michael Margherio, President
Gary Wellman, Vice President
Matthew Hans, Secretary
Megan Rowekamp, CPA, Treasurer

Pregnancy and infant loss support.

Year Founded: 1977

155 Parents of Murdered Children, Inc.
4960 Ridge Avenue
Suite 2
Cincinnati, OH 45209
513-721-5683
888-818-7662; *Fax:* 513-345-4489
natlpomc@aol.com
www.pomc.com

Howard S Klerk Jr, President
Dan Levey, National Executive Director
Terrie Jacoby, Vice President
Carole DiAddezio, Treasurer

For the families and friends of those who have died by violence. Provides the on-going emotional support needed to help parents and other survivors facilitate the reconstruction of a new life and to promote a healthy resolution. Not only does POMC help survivors deal with their acute grief but also helps with the criminal justice system.

Year Founded: 1978

156 Rainbows
1007 Church Street
Suite 408
Evanston, IL 60201
847-952-1770
800-266-3206; *Fax:* 847-952-1774
info@rainbows.org
www.rainbows.org

Anthony Taglia, Chairman
Bob Thomas, Executive Director and CEO
Burt Heatherly, CFO
Bill Olbrisch, National Community Outreach Dir.

Rainbows is an international, nonprofit organization that fosters emotional healing among children grieving a loss from a life-altering crisis. Rainbows believes that grieving youth deserve supporting, loving listeners as they struggle with their feelings. Available to participants of all races and religions. Serves as an advocate for youth who face life-altering crises.

Year Founded: 1983

157 Survivors of Loved Ones' Suicides (SOLOS)
8310 Ewing Halsell Drive
San Antonio, TX 78229
210-885-7069
solossanantonio@gmail.com
www.solossa.org

Tony Mata, SOLOS Facilitator
Angie Navarette, SOLOS Facilitator

Located in San Antonio, Texas, SOLOS organizes ongoing support group meetings for persons affected by the loss of loved ones from suicide.

Year Founded: 1987

Video & Audio

158 Effective Learning Systems, Inc.
5108 W 74th
St #390160
Minneapolis, MN 55439
239-948-1660
800-966-0443; *Fax:* 239-948-1664
info@efflearn.com
www.effectivelearning.com

Robert E Griswold, President/ Founder
Deirdre M Griswold, VP

The mission of Effective Learning Systems is to develop and distribute the most effective programs- incorporating the most powerful, scientifically sound techniques- to help as many people as possible learn to use the power of their mind to achieve their goals and realize significant, positive changes in their lives. Audio tapes for self-help.

Year Founded: 1972

Web Sites

159 AtHealth.Com
At Health

Providing trustworthy online information, tools, and training that enhance the ability of practitioners to furnish high quality, personalized care to those they serve. For mental health consumers, find practitioners, treatment centers, learn about disorders and medications, news and resources.

160 forums.grieving.com
Death and Dying Grief Support

Information on grief and loss.

161 www.alivealone.org
Alive Alone

An organization for the education and charitable purposes to benefit bereaved parents, whose only child or all children are deceased, by providing a self-help network and publications to promote communication and healing, to assist in resolving their grief, and a means to reinvest their lives for a positive future.

162 www.bereavedparentsusa.org
Bereaved Parents of the USA (BP/USA)

Self-help group that offers support, understanding, compassion and hope especially to the newly bereaved be they bereaved parents, grandparents or siblings struggling to rebuild their lives after the death of their children, grandchildren or siblings.

163 www.cfsny.org
Center for Family Support (CFS)

Devoted to providing support and assistance to individuals with developmental and related disabilities, and to the family members who care for them.

164 www.climb-support.org
Center for Loss in Multiple Birth (CLIMB), Inc.

Support by and for parents who have experienced the death of one or more of their twins or higher multiples during pregnance, birth, in infancy, or childhood. Newsletter, information on specialized topics, pen pals, phone support.

165 www.compassionatefriends.org
The Compassionate Friends

Organization for those having lost a child.

166 www.counselingforloss.com
Counseling for Loss and Life Changes, Inc.

Offers individual and family counseling services for grieving people.

167 www.cyberpsych.org
CyberPsych

CyberPsych presents information about psychoanalysis, psychotherapy and topics like anxiety disorders, substance abuse, homophobia, and traumas. It hosts mental health organizations and individuals with content of interest to the public and professional communities. There is also a free therapist finder service.

168 www.divorceasfriends.com
Bill Ferguson's How to Divorce as Friends

Articles, Resources, and Support to help minimize conflict in divorce situations.

169 www.divorcecentral.com
Divorce Central

Offers helpful advice and suggestions on what to expect emotionally, and how to deal with the emotional effects of divorce.

170 www.divorceinfo.com
Divorce Information

Simply written and covers all the issues.

171 www.divorcemag.com
Divorce Magazine

The printed magazine's commercial site.

172 www.divorcesupport.com
Divorce Support

Covers all aspects of divorce.

173 www.emptycradle.org
Empty Cradle

A peer support group for parents who have experienced the loss of baby due to early pregnancy loss, stillbirth or infant death.

174 www.firstcandle.org
First Candle

For those who have suffered the loss of an infant through SIDS.

175 www.friendsforsurvival.org
Friends for Survival

Assisting anyone who has suffered the loss of a loved one through suicide death.

176 www.grasphelp.org
Grief Recovery After A Substance Passing

Support and advocacy group for parents who have suffered the death of a child due to substance abuse. Provides opportunity for parents to share theri greif and experiences without shame or recrimination. They will provide information and suggestions for those wanting to start a similar group elsewhere.

177 www.griefnet.org
GriefNet

Internet community of persons dealing with grief, death, and major loss.

178 www.mhselfhelp.org
National Mental Health Consumers' Self-Help Clearinghouse

Encouraging the development and growth of consumer self-help groups.

179 www.misschildren.org
Mothers in Sympathy and Support (MISS) Foundation

Provides immediate and ongoing support to grieving families, empowerment through community volunteerism opportunities, public policy and legislative education, and programs to reduce infant and toddler death through research and education.

180 www.nationalshare.org
National SHARE Office

Pregnancy and infant loss support.

181 www.planetpsych.com
PlanetPsych

Learn about disorders, their treatments and other topics in psychology. Articles are listed under the related topic areas. Ask a therapist a question for free, or view the directory of professionals in your area. If you are a therapist sign up for the directory. Current features, self-help, interactive, and newsletter archives.

182 www.pomc.com
National Organization of Parents Of Murdered Children, Inc.

Help for anyone who has suffered the loss of a murdered child.

183 www.psychcentral.com
Psych Central

Personalized one-stop index for psychology, support, and mental health issues, resources, and people on the Internet.

184 www.psycom.net/depression.central.grief.html
Grief and Bereavement

Helpful information for those grieving from the loss of a loved one.

185 www.rainbows.org
Rainbows

Group for grieving parents and children.

186 www.relationshipjourney.com
The Relationship Learning Center

Marriage and relationship counseling and information.

187 www.safecrossingsfoundation.org
Safe Crossings Foundation

For children facing a loved one's death.

188 www.spig.clara.net/guidline.htm
Shared Parenting Information Group (SPIG)

Useful information that helps to decrease the stress associated with separation.

189 www.store.samhsa.gov
Substance Abuse and Mental Health Services Administration

Resources on mental disorders as well as treatment and recovery.

190 www.thenadd.org
National Association for The Dually Diagnosed (NADD)

An association for persons with developmental disabilities and mental health needs.

191 www.unitegriefsupport.org
UNITE, Inc.

Grief support after miscarriage, stillbirth and infant death.

192 www.widownet.org
WidowNet

Online information and self-help resource for, and by, widows and widowers. Topics covered include grief, bereavement, recovery, and other information helpful to people who have suffered the death of a spouse or life partner.

Directories & Databases

193 After School and More
Resources for Children with Special Needs
116 E 16th Street
5th Floor
New York, NY 10003-2164
212-677-4650; *Fax:* 212-254-4070
info@resourcenyc.org
www.resourcesnyc.org

Rachel Howard, Executive Director
Stephen Stern, Director , Finance and Administr
Todd Dorman, Director, Communications and Out
Helen Murphy, Director, Program and Fund Devel

The most complete directory of after school programs for children with disabilities and special needs in the metropolitan New York area focusing on weekend and holiday programs. *$25.00*

ISBN 0-967836-57-3

Anxiety Disorders

Introduction

It is perfectly normal to feel worried or nervous sometimes, especially if there is an obvious reason: a loved one is late coming home; a pending yearly evaluation meeting at work; an important social event is looming. Even when you are nervous or anxious with good cause, you continue performing life's functions adequately. Indeed, some anxiety is not only normal, it is necessary, helping us to avoid trouble and danger - like preparing for a test in school, or making sure your child is safely buckled into a car. But if you cannot rid yourself of your worry, you worry all the time, and about everything, if people close to you comment that you seem bothered and unlike yourself, or if your nervousness is affecting your relationships and your work, it is time to seek help. Without treatment, anxiety disorders can worsen. Sometimes a person who suffers from persistent anxiety turns to alcohol or other drugs in an effort to seek relief.

Different kinds of Anxiety Disorders have been identified. Several of the most prevalent are discussed in detail below. Treatment is tailored to the particular disorder and has become more effective as a result.

SYMPTOMS

Agoraphobia
• Usually involves fears connected with being outside the home and alone;
• Anxiety about being in places or situations from which it is difficult or embarrassing to escape (e.g., in the middle seat of a row in a theatre) or in which help may not be immediately available (as in an airplane);
• Such situations are avoided or endured with distress and fear of having a panic attack;
• The anxiety significantly interferes with the individual's ability to participate normally in work, domestic, and/or recreational activities.

Social Anxiety Disorder
• Fear of being humiliated or embarrassed in a social situation with strangers or where other people are watching;
• Being in the situation causes intense anxiety, sometimes with panic attacks;
• Realizing that the fear is irrational;
• Unlike simple shyness, the fear leads to avoidance of important or uncomplicated social situations and interferes with the ability to function at work or with friends.

General Anxiety Disorder
• Excessive worry and anxiety on most days for at least six months about several events or activities such as work or school performance;
• Difficulty in controlling the worry;
• The anxiety is connected with at least three of the following: restlessness/feeling on edge; being easily tired; difficulty concentrating; irritability; muscle tension; difficulty falling/staying asleep or restless sleep;
• The anxiety or physical symptoms seriously affect the person's social life, work life, or other important areas.

Phobias
• Persistent, unreasonable, and exaggerated fear of the presence or anticipated presence of a particular object or situation (e.g., snake, flying in an airplane, blood);
• The presence of such an object or situation triggers immediate anxiety which may result in a panic attack;
• Knowledge that the fear is exaggerated and unreasonable;
• The phobic situation is either avoided or experienced with extreme distress;
• The avoidance, fearful anticipation, and distress seriously affects the person's normal routine, work and social activities, and relationships.

Panic Disorder
A panic attack is a period of intense fear in which four or more of the following symptoms escalate suddenly, reaching a peak within ten minutes, after which they diminish:
• Palpitations and pounding;
• Rapid heart beat;
• Sweating;
• Trembling or shaking;
• Shortness of breath;
• Feeling of choking;
• Chest pain;
• Nausea;
• Feeling dizzy or faint;
• Feelings of unreality or detachment;
• Fear of losing control or going crazy;
• Fear of dying;
• Numbness or tingling;
• Chills or hot flashes.

Selective Mutism
Those with Selective Mutism are full capable of speech and understanding language but do not speak in certain situations. This may be perceived as shyness or rudeness by others. A child with selective mutism my be silent at school, but speak quite freely at home.

Selective Mutism is characterized by the following:
• Consistent failure to speak in specific social situations, in which speaking is expected, despite speaking in other situations;
• The disturbance interferes with educational or occupational achievement or with social communication;
• The duration is at least one month;
• Failure to speak is not due to lack of knowledge or, or comfort with, the spoken language required in the social situation;
• The disturbance is not better accounted for by a communication disorder and does not occur exclusively during the course of autism spectrum disorder, schizophrenia, or other psychotic disorder.

Separation Anxiety Disorder
Separation Anxiety Disorder (SAD) is an anxiety disorder in which an individual experiences excessive anxiety regarding separation from home or from people to whom the indiviudal has a strong emotional attachment. To be diagnosed with SAD, one must display at least three of the following:

• Recurrent excessive distress when anticipating or experiencing separation from home or from major attachment figures;
• Persistent and excessive worry about losing major attachment figures or about possible harm to them;
• Persistent and excessive worry about experiencing an untoward event that causes separation from a major attachment figure;
• Persistent reluctance or refusal to go out, away from home, to school, to work, or elsewhere because of fear of separation;

• Persistent and excessive fear of or reluctance about being along or without major attachment figures at home or in other settings;
• Persistent reluctance or refusal to sleep away from home or to go to sleep without being near a major attachment figure;
• Repeated nightmares involving the theme of separation;
• Repeated complaints of physical symptoms when separation from major attachment figures occurs or is anticipated.

ASSOCIATED FEATURES

Anxiety can be acute and intense such as the fear of imminent death in a panic attack or it can be experienced as the state of chronic nagging worry in Generalized Anxiety Disorder. Whatever its intensity or frequency, it persists over time. One of the hallmarks of Anxiety Disorders is that the person is unable to control the anxiety, even when he or she knows it is exaggerated and unreasonable. To other people, the person may seem edgy, irritable, to have unexpected outbursts of anger, or to be consumed by an unreasonable fear. For the anxious person, the problem takes up time and effort and becomes a major preoccupation.

In addition to the psychological effects (and entangled with them) are the physical effects, that is, a frequent or constant state of physical arousal and tension. This can lead to gastrointestinal upset, headaches, and cardiovascular disease. Using alcohol or drugs to resolve the problem is common but ineffective and dangerous. Anxiety Disorders negatively affect all aspects of life—family, work, and friends.

PREVALENCE

Anxiety Disorders are the most common psychiatric disorders in the U.S. Anxiety Disorders are approximately twice as common in women as in men.

TREATMENT OPTIONS

It is very important to have a full evaluation so that a proper diagnosis can be made. In general, people should have a primary care evaluation as part of the diagnostic process for all disorders, so as to rule out a general medical condition that could be causing the signs and symptoms. For example, hyperthyroidism can cause anxiety problems and can look like depression. Self medication with alcohol, tranquilizers, or other drugs is dangerous and can lead to serious drug abuse. Many people who abuse drugs are likely suffering from an underlying Anxiety Disorder. Treatment will vary depending on which of the Anxiety Disorders is diagnosed. Medications, psychotherapy or both will be prescribed. Some psychotherapies which have proven helpful in certain cases are cognitive-behavioral therapies, including exposure therapy, and eye movement desensitisation reprogramming (EMDR). Benzodiazepines, or minor tranquillizers, can be useful for the acute treatment of anxiety symptoms; care must be taken, because these medications have addictive potential. Selective Serotonin Reuptake Inhibitors, or SSRIs, which were originally developed as antidepressants, have proven to be effective in several Anxiety Disorders and are now the mainstays of treatment. Since new drugs are frequently introduced, and already approved medications given new therapeutic indications by the USDA, it is wise to consult an expert or recent expert reference before making a treatment decision.

It is important to note that suddenly stopping an SSRI can cause rebound symptoms including sleeplessness, headaches, and irritability. Medications should be tapered under the care of a physician.

Associations & Agencies

195 A.I.M. Agoraphobics in Motion
PO Box 725363
Berkley, MI 48072
248-547-0400
boardofdirectors@aimforrecovery.com
www.aimforrecovery.com

Mary Ann Gogoleski, SWT, Director
James Fortune, President
Robert Diedrich, Vice President
Jaclyn Rymal White, Secretary

AIM is a nonprofit support group organization committed to the support and recovery of people with anxiety disorders, as well as their families.

Year Founded: 1983

196 Adventure Camp
Advanced Therapeutic Solutions
600 W 22nd Street
Suite 250
Oak Brook, IL 60523
630-230-6505; *Fax: 630-230-3362*
www.www.selectivemutismtreatment.net

Kelly Amrhein, PhD, Clinical Team
Theresa Gabby, LSCW, School Social Worker
Carmen M. Tumialan Lynas, PhD, Clinical Psychologist

A summer camp designed to help children with selective mutism. This exposure therapy program is designed to simulate a classroom environment, and each child is assigned a counselor for one-on-one therapy.

197 Anxiety and Depression Association of America
8701 Georgia Avenue
Suite 412
Silver Spring, MD 20910
240-485-1001; *Fax: 240-485-1035*
information@adaa.org
www.adaa.org

Mary E. Salcedo, MD, President
Susan K. Gurley, JD, Executive Director
Risa B. Weisberg, PhD, Treasurer
Cindy J. Aaronson, MSW, PhD, Secretary

An international nonprofit organization committed to the use of education and research to promote the prevention, treatment, and cure of anxiety, depressive, obssesive compulsive, and other trauma related disorders. ADAA's mission is to improve the lives of all people with anxiety and mood disorders.

Year Founded: 1979

198 Anxiety and Phobia Treatment Center
41 East Post Road
White Plains, NY 10601
914-681-1038
jchessa@wphospital.org
www.www.phobia-anxiety.org

John Gregory, PhD, Group Leader
Donna Pappalardo, LCSW, Group Leader
Judy Lake Chessa, LMSW, Coordinator

Treatment for individuals suffering from phobias and other anxiety disorders. Specializes in the use of cognitive-behavioral therapy and exposure therapy.

Year Founded: 1971

199   Center for Mental Health Services (CMHS)
Substance Abuse and Mental Health Services
Administration
5600 Fishers Lane
Rockville, MD 20857
240-276-1310
877-726-4727
TTY: 800-487-4889
www.samhsa.gov/about-us/who-we-are/offices-centers

Paolo del Vecchio, MSW, Director
Anne Mathews-Younes, Acting Deputy Director
Keris Myrick, Director, Consumer Affairs
Patricia Gratton, Director, Program Analysis

Promotes the treatment of mental illness and emotional disorders by increasing accessibility to mental health programs; supporting outreach, treatment, rehabilitation, and support programs and networks; and encouraging the use of scientifically-based information when treating mental disorders. CMHS provides information about mental health via a toll-free number and numerous publications. Developed for users of mental health services and their families, the general public, policy makers, providers, and the media.

Year Founded: 1992

200   Freedom From Fear
308 Seaview Avenue
Staten Island, NY 10305
718-351-1717
help@freedomfromfear.org
www.freedomfromfear.org

Daniel Deutsch. PhD, Board Member
Mary Guardino, Founder and Executive Director
Steve Jenkins, PhD, Board Member
Theresa Mazzeo, Board Member

A national nonprofit organization, the mission of Freedom From Fear is to aid and counsel individuals suffering from anxiety and depressive disorders through advocacy, education, research, and community support.

Year Founded: 1984

201   Goodwill's Community Employment Services
Goodwill Industries-Suncoast, Inc.
10596 Gandy Blvd.
St. Petersburg, FL 33702
727-523-1512
888-279-1988
TDD: 727-579-1068
www.goodwill-suncoast.org

Heather Ceresoli, CPA, Chair
Deborah A. Passerini, President
Martin W. Gladysz, Senior Vice Chair
Louise R. Lopez, Vice Chair

Program providing job coaching and community job placements for people with disabilities.

Year Founded: 1954

202   Mental Health America
500 Montgomery Street
Suite 820
Alexandria, VA 22314

703-684-7722
800-969-6642; *Fax:* 703-684-5968
www.mentalhealthamerica.net

Reginald Williams, Chair of the Board
Paul Gionfriddo, President and CEO
Jessica Kennedy, Chief of Staff/VP of Finance
Theresa Nguyen, VP of Policy and Programs

Mental Health America is a community-based nonprofit organization committed to enabling the mental wellness of all Americans. MHA advocates for greater access to quality health services and seeks to educate individuals on identifying symptoms, as well as intervention and prevention.

Year Founded: 1909

203   NAPCSE National Association of Parents with
Children in Special Education
3642 East Sunnydale Drive
Chandler Heights, AZ 85142
800-754-4421; *Fax:* 800-424-0371
contact@napcse.org
www.napcse.org

Dr. George Giuliani, President

The NAPCSE is dedicated to ensuring quality education for all children and adolescents with special needs. NAPCSE provides resources, support, and assistance to parents with children in special education.

204   National Alliance on Mental Illness
3803 North Fairfax Drive
Suite 100
Arlington, VA 22203
703-524-7600
800-950-6264
info@nami.org
www.nami.org

Steve Pitman, JD, President
Lacey Berumen, PhD, MNM, First Vice President
Mary Giliberti, Chief Executive Officer
David Levy, Chief Financial Officer

NAMI is an organization dedicated to raising awareness on mental health and providing support and education for Americans affected by mental illness. NAMI advocates for access to services and treatment and fosters an environment of awareness and understanding for those concerned with mental health.

Year Founded: 1979

205   National Anxiety Foundation
3135 Custer Drive
Lexington, KY 40517
859-272-7166
www.www.nationalanxietyfoundation.org/

Stephen Cox, MD, President
Linda Vernon Blair, Vice President
C. Todd Strecker, Secretary and Treasurer

Organization that seeks to alleviate suffering and save lives by educating the public about anxiety disorders.

206   National Association for the Dually Diagnosed
(NADD)
132 Fair Street
Kingston, NY 12401
845-331-4336
info@thenadd.org
www.thenadd.org

Jeanne M. Farr, MA, Chief Executive Officer
Daniel Baker, PhD., President
Peggie Webb, MA, Vice President
George Zukotynski, PhD., Secretary

NADD is a nonprofit organization designed to increase awareness of, and provide services for, individuals with developmental disabilities and mental illness. NADD emphasizes the importance of quality mental healthcare for people with mental health needs and offers conferences, information resources, educational programs, and training materials to professionals, parents, and organizations.

Year Founded: 1983

207 National Council for Behavioral Health

1400 K Street Northwest
Suite 400
Washington, DC 20005
202-684-7457
communications@thenationalcouncil.org
www.thenationalcouncil.org

Jeff Richardson, Chair
Linda Rosenberg, President and CEO
Jeannie Campbell, Executive VP and COO
Tim Swinfard, First Vice Chair

The National Council for Behavioral Health serves to unify America's behavioral health organizations. The council is dedicated to ensuring that quality mental health and addictions care is readily accessible to all Americans.

208 National Mental Health Consumers' Self-Help Clearinghouse

1211 Chestnut Street
Suite 1100
Philadelphia, PA 19107
267-507-3810
800-553-4539; *Fax:* 215-636-6312
info@mhselfhelp.org
www.mhselfhelp.org

Joseph Rogers, Founder and Executive Director
Susan Rogers, Director

The Clearinghouse is a peer-run national technical assistance center focused on achieving respect and equality of opportunity for those with mental illnesses. The Clearinghouse helps with the growth of the mental health consumer movement by evaluating mental health services, advocating for mental health reform, and providing consumers with news, information, publications, and consultation services.

Year Founded: 1986

209 Selective Mutism Association (SMA)

E-mail: info@selectivemutism.org
www.www.selectivemutism.org/

Rachel Busman, PsyD, President
Pamela Martis Zambriski, Treasurer
Nicole Caporino, PhD, Secretary
Lisa Kovac, Executive Director

An organization that increases awareness and education about selective mutism. SMA supports families and professionals through an annual conference, expert chat sessions, professional training, online resources, and providing connections with research institutions.

210 Selective Mutism Network

407-534-3500
forms@selectivemutismnetwork.org
www.www.selectivemutismnetwork.org/

A nonprofit organization that spreads awareness to the public about Selective Mutism. The Network offers resources for parents to provide to teachers and school administrators in order to help children with Selective Mutism while at school.

211 Selective Mutism Research Institute

505 North Old York Road
Jenkintown, PA 19046
215-887-5748
info@SelectiveMutismResearch.org
www.selectivemutismresearchinstitute.org/

Dr. Elisa Shipon Blum, Director
Rosemarie Manfredi, PsyD, Director of Clinical Research

A nonprofit organization dedicated to raising better awareness, treatment, and resources for children dealing with selective mutism and other social communication anxiety.

212 Sutcliffe Developmental & Behavioral Pediatrics

851 Fremont Avenue
Suite 110
Los Altos, CA 94024
650-941-1698; *Fax:* 650-434-3953
info@sutcliffedbp.com
www.www.sutcliffedbp.com/

Trenna Sutcliffe, MD, Medical Director
Jen Aronowitz, PhD, Neuropsychologist
Christy Tadros, Clinical Counselor
Hedva Redlich, Practice Manager

Sutcliffe Developmental & Behavioral Pediatrics is an organization that specializes in the treatment of ADHD, autism spectrum disorder, anxiety disorders, conduct disorders, learning disabilities, and more. Sutcliffe works with community services, school districs, and primary physicians, as well as provides family counseling.

213 Territorial Apprehensiveness (TERRAP) Anxiety & Stress Program

755 Park Avenue
Suite 140
Huntington, NY 11743
631-549-8867; *Fax:* 631-423-8446
www.anxietyandpanic.com

Julian Herskowitz, PhD, Director

Helps to treat anxiety and stress disorders through Territorial Apprehensiveness Programs, developed by Dr. Arthur Hardy in the 1960's. The program systematically addresses the behavioral and thought processes of those suffering from stress and anxiety.

Year Founded: 1975

214 The Center for Family Support

2811 Zulette Avenue
Bronx, NY 10461
718-518-1500; *Fax:* 718-518-8200
www.www.cfsny.org/

Steven Vernikoff, Executive Director
Lloyd Stabiner, President
Amy Bittinger, Vice President
Barbara Greenwald, Associate Executive Director

The Center for Family Support offers assistance to individuals with developmental and related disabilities, as well as their families, and provides support services and programs that are designed to accommodate individual needs. Offers services throughout New York City, Westchester County, Long Island, and New Jersey.

Year Founded: 1954

215   The Children's and Adult Center for OCD and Anxiety
3138 Butler Pike
Suite 200
Plymouth Meeting, PA 19462
www.childrenscenterocdanxiety.blogspot.ca/

Tamar Chansky, PhD, Founder

A center composed of six private practice psychologists delivering treatment and therapy to children and adults with OCD, Separation Anxiety, and other mental health disorders. They also offer parent workshops on skills and strategies to help their child cope with anxiety.

Year Founded: 1988

216   The SMart Center: Selective Mutism, Anxiety, & Related Disorders Treatment Center
505 Old York Road
Jenkintown, PA 19046
215-887-5748
www.selectivemutismcenter.org

Dr. Elisa Shipon-Blum, President and Director
Irina Khrapatina, PsyD, Director of Clinical Research
Jennifer Brittingham, MA, Lead Consultant
Laura Bansemer, Lead Clinical Coordinator

A center that provides treatment and support to children and young adults with selective mutism and other social communication issues. The SMart Center uses the evidence-based Social Communication Anxiety Treatment (S-CAT) program, and also offers products, services, and events for parents, professionals, researchers, and educators.

217   The Selective Mutism Foundation Inc.
PO Box 25972
Tamarac, FL 33320
E-mail: sue@selectivemutismfoundation.org
www.selectivemutismfoundation.org

Sue Newman, Co-Founder and Director
Carolyn Miller, Co-Founder and Director

An organization that promotes ongoing research and provides information on selective mutism. Seeks to help those with selective mutism achieve productivity, social interaction, and inclusion within the community.

Year Founded: 1991

218   Thriving Minds
10524 E Grand River Avenue
Suite 100
Brighton, MI 48116
810-225-3417
office@thrivingmindsbehavioralhealth.com
www.www.thrivingmindsbehavioralhealth.com/

Sheri Mehlhorn, Office Manager
Amanda Kay Espinoza, Registered Behavioral Technician
Dr. Aimee Kotrba, Clinical Psychologist
Dr. Brice Hella, Clinical Psychologist

Thriving Minds is an organization that offers therapy to people with anxiety, behavioral issues, and depression. With locations in Brighton and Chelsea, Thriving Minds uses a mix of research-based interventions, such as Cognitive Behavioral Therapy; parent coaching; and school interventions in order to help children, teens, and adults deal with their anxiety.

Books

219   100 Q&A About Panic Disorder
Jones and Bartlett Publishers
5 Wall Street
Burlington, MA 01803
978-443-5000
800-832-0034; *Fax: 978-443-8000*
info@jblearning.com
www.jblearning.com

Carol Berman,MD, Author
Ty Field, Chief Executive Officer
James Homer, President
Alison Pendergast, Chief Marketing Officer

$22.95

136 pages Year Founded: 1983 ISBN 9-780763-77-6

220   Acceptance and Commitment Therapy for Anxiety Disorders
NewHarbinger Publications
5674 Shattuck Avenue
Oakland, CA 94609-1662
510-652-0215
800-748-6273; *Fax: 800-652-1613*
customerservice@newharbinger.com
www.newharbinger.com

Georg H Eifert,PhD, Author
John P Forsyth,PhD, Author
Steven C Hayes,PhD, Author

The first step-by-step professional book that teaches how to apply and integrate acceptance and mindfulness for treatment with anxiety disorders. $59.95

304 pages Year Founded: 1973 ISBN 1-572244-27-5

221   An End to Panic: Breakthrough Techniques for Overcoming Panic Disorder
NewHarbinger Publications
5674 Shattuck Avenue
Oakland, CA 94609-1662
510-652-0215
800-748-6273; *Fax: 800-652-1613*
customerservice@newharbinger.com
www.newharbinger.com

Elke Zuercher-White,PhD, Author
Elke Zuercher-White, Author

A state of the art treatment program covers breathing retraining, taking charge of fear fueling thoughts, overcoming the fear of physical symptoms, coping with phobic situations, avoiding relapse, and living in the here and now. $24.95

232 pages Year Founded: 1973 ISBN 1-572241-13-8

222   Anxiety & Phobia Workbook
NewHarbinger Publications
5674 Shattuck Avenue
Oakland, CA 94609-1662

510-652-0215
800-748-6273; *Fax:* 800-652-1613
customerservice@newharbinger.com
www.newharbinger.com

Edmund J. Bourne,PhD, Author

This comprehensive guide is recommended to those struggling with anxiety disorders. Includes step by step instructions for the crucial cognitive - behavioral techniques that have given real help to hundreds of thousands of readers struggling with anxiety disorders. *$24.95*

496 pages Year Founded: 1973 ISBN 1-572248-91-5

223 Anxiety Cure: Eight Step-Program for Getting Well
John Wiley & Sons
605 3rd Avenue
New York, NY 10158-180
212-850-6301
info@wiley.com

Stephen M Smith, Pres., Chief Executive Officer
Ellis E Cousens, EVP, CFO, Operations Officer
William J Arlington, Senior Vice President of HR
Edward J Melando, VP, Corporate Controller

Anxiety disorders are the most common type of emotional trouble and among the most treatable. Dupont provides a practical guide featuring a step-by-step program for curing the six kinds of anxiety. *$14.95*

256 pages ISBN 0-471247-01-4

224 Anxiety Disorders
Cambridge University Press
40 W 20th Street
New York, NY 10011-4211
212-924-3900
800-872-7423; *Fax:* 212-691-3239
marketing@cup.org
www.cup.org

Stephen Bourne, Chief Press Executive / Director

This comprehensive text covers all the anxiety disorders found in the latest DSM and ICD classifications. Provides detailed information about seven principal disorders, including anxiety in the medically ill. For each disorder, the book covers diagnosis criteria, epidemiology, etiology and pathogenesis, clinical features, natural history and different diagnosis. Describes treatment approaches, both psychological and pharmacological. *$105.00*

394 pages ISBN 0-521515-57-3

225 Anxiety and Its Disorders
Guilford Press
72 Spring Street
New York, NY 10012-4068
212-431-9800
800-365-7006; *Fax:* 212-966-6708
info@guilford.com

Bob Matloff, President
David H Barlow, Author

Incorporating recent advances from cognitive science and neurobiology on the mechanisms of anxiety and using emotion theory as basic theoretical framework. Ties theory and research of emerging clinical knowledge to create a new model of anxiety with profound implications for treatment. *$76.50*

704 pages ISBN 1-572304-30-8

226 Anxiety, Phobias, and Panic
Grand Central Publishing
322 South Enterprise Blvd
Lebanon, IN 46052
800-759-0190
www.www.hachettebookgroup.com

Reneau Z Peurifoy, Author
Kenneth Michaels, EVP, Chief Operating Officer
Chris Barba, EVP, Sales and Marketing
Sophie Cottrell, VP, Communications Director

Congratulations! You are about to start a journey along the path to freedom.

400 pages Year Founded: 1837 ISBN 0-446692-77-9

227 Anxiety, Phobias, and Panic: Step-By-Step Program for Regaining Control of Your Life
Time Warner Books
3 Center Plaza
Boston, MA 02108-2084
800-759-0190; *Fax:* 800-331-1664

Reneau Z Peurifoy, Author

Helps you identify stress and reduce stress anxiety, recognize and change distorted mental habits, stop thinking and acting like a victim, eliminate the excessive need for approval, make anger your friend and ally, stand up for yourself and feel good about yourself, and conquer your fears and take charge of your life. *$11.00*

384 pages ISBN 0-446670-53-7

228 Beyond Anxiety and Phobia
NewHarbinger Publications
5674 Shattuck Avenue
Oakland, CA 94609-1662
510-652-0215
800-748-6273; *Fax:* 800-652-1613
customerservice@newharbinger.com
www.newharbinger.com

Edmund J. Bourne,PhD, Author

Helping people try to get beyond anxiety and their phobia. *$24.95*

264 pages Year Founded: 1973 ISBN 1-572242-29-9

229 Biology of Anxiety Disorders
American Psychiatric Publishing, Inc.
1000 Wilson Boulevard
Suite 1825
Arlington, VA 22209-3901
703-907-7322
800-368-5777; *Fax:* 703-907-1091
appi@psych.org
www.appi.org

Rudolf Hoehn-Saric, M.D, Editor
Daniel R McLeod, Ph.D, Editor
John McDuffie, Editorial Director

Provides the most recent data on the neurobiology and pathophysiology af anxiety from a variety of perspectives. *$32.00*

280 pages Year Founded: 1993 ISBN 0-880484-76-4

230 Comorbidity of Mood and Anxiety Disorders
American Psychiatric Publishing, Inc.
1000 Wilson Boulevard
Suite 1825
Arlington, VA 22209-3901

703-907-7322
800-368-5777; *Fax:* 703-907-1091
appi@psych.org
www.appi.org

Jack D Maser, Ph.D., Editor
C. Robert Cloninger, M.D., Editor
John McDuffie, Editorial Director
Jack Maser PhD, Author

Presents a systematic examination of the concurrence of different symptoms and syndromes in patients with anxiety or mood disorders. *$147.00*

888 pages Year Founded: 1990 ISBN 0-880483-24-5

231 Concise Guide to Anxiety Disorders
American Psychiatric Publishing, Inc.
1000 Wilson Boulevard
Suite 1825
Arlington, VA 22209-3901
703-907-7322
800-368-5777; *Fax:* 703-907-1091
appi@psych.org
www.appi.org

Eric Hollander, M.D., Author
Daphne Simeon, M.D, Author
John McDuffie, Editorial Director
Eric Hollander, MD, Author

Concise Guide to Anxiety Disorders summarizes the latest research and translates it into practical treatment strategies for the best clinical outcomes. Designed for daily use in the clinical setting, it serves as an instant library of current information, quick to access and easy to understand. Every clinician who diagnoses and treats patients with anxiety disorders-including psychiatrists, residents and medical students, psychologists, and mental health professionals-will find this book invaluable for making informed treatment decisions. *$53.00*

272 pages Year Founded: 2003 ISBN 1-585620-80-7

232 Consumer's Guide to Psychiatric Drugs
NewHarbinger Publications
5674 Shattuck Avenue
Oakland, CA 94609-1662
510-652-0215
800-748-6273; *Fax:* 800-652-1613
customerservice@newharbinger.com
www.newharbinger.com

Mary C. Talaga, Author
John D. Preston, Author
John H. O'Neal, Author

Helps consumers understand what treatment options are available and what side effects to expect. Covers possible interactions with other drugs, medical conditions and other concerns. Explains how each drug works, and offers detailed information about treatments for depression, bipolar disorder, anxiety and sleep disorders, as well as other conditions. *$16.95*

340 pages Year Founded: 1973 ISBN 1-572241-11-X

233 Coping with Anxiety
NewHarbinger Publications
5674 Shattuck Avenue
Oakland, CA 94609-1662
510-652-0215
800-748-6273; *Fax:* 800-652-1613

customerservice@newharbinger.com
www.newharbinger.com

Edmund J. Bourne,PhD, Author
Lorna Garano, Author

Ten simple steps, proven to help relieve anxiety. *$ 14.95*

176 pages Year Founded: 1973 ISBN 1-572243-20-1

234 Coping with Social Anxiety: The Definitive Guide to Effective Treatment Options
Holt Paperbacks
175 Fifth Avenue
New York, NY 10010-7703
646-307-5151; *Fax:* 212-633-0748
customerservice@mpsvirginia.com
www.us.macmillan.com

Eric Hollander, Author
Nickolas Bakalar, Author

An essential guide for the 5.3 million American sufferers of social anxiety from a leading psychiatrist and researcher. *$17.00*

256 pages Year Founded: 2005 ISBN 0-805075-82-8

235 Don't Panic: Taking Control of Anxiety Attacks
Anxiety Disorders Association of America
8701 Georgia Avenue
Suite 412
Silver Spring, MD 20910-3643
240-485-1001; *Fax:* 240-485-1035
AnxDis@adaa.org
www.adaa.org

Mark H Pollack,MD, President
Alies Muskin, Executive Director
Murray Stein,MD,MPH, Treasurer
Cindy J Aaronson,MSW,PhD, Secretary

Book on overcoming panic and anxiety.

Year Founded: 2009

236 Drug Therapy and Anxiety Disorders
Mason Crest Publishers
450 Parkway Drive
Suite D
Broomall, PA 19008-4017
610-543-6200
866-627-2665; *Fax:* 610-543-3878
dtaylor@masoncrest.com
www.masoncrest.com

Shirley Brinkerhoff, Author
Dan Hilferty, President
Michelle Luke, Director of Marketing
Michael Toglia, Special Sales

This volume provides readers with a clear introduction to anxiety disorders. Numerous case studies give insight into the world of mental disorders and helps readers understand the symptoms and treatments of this disorder, which includes: generalized anxiety disorder, social phobia, specific phobia, obsessive-compulsive disorder (covered more extensively in a separate column), post-traumatic stress disorder, and panic disorder.

128 pages ISBN 1-590845-61-7

237 Dying of Embarrassment: Help for Social Anxiety and Social Phobia
NewHarbinger Publications
5674 Shattuck Avenue
Oakland, CA 94609-1662
510-652-0215
800-748-6273; *Fax: 800-652-1613*
customerservice@newharbinger.com
www.newharbinger.com

Barbara G Markway, Author
C Alec Pollard, Author
Teresa Flynn, Author
Cheryl N Carmin, Author

Clear, supportive instructions for assessing your fears, improving or developing new social skills, and changing self defeating thinking patterns. *$13.95*

208 pages Year Founded: 1973 ISBN 1-879237-23-7

238 Emotions Anonymous Book
Emotions Anonymous International Service Center
PO Box 4245
Saint Paul, MN 55104-0245
651-647-9712; *Fax: 651-647-1593*
info@EmotionsAnonymous.org
www.EmotionsAnonymous.org

Karen Mead, Executive Director

The Big Book of EA: A fellowship of men and women who share their experience, strength and hope with each other, that they may solve their common problem and help others recover from emotional illness. *$15.00*

261 pages ISBN 0-960735-65-5

239 Encyclopedia of Phobias, Fears, and Anxieties
Facts on File
132 West 31st Street
17th Floor
New York, NY 10001-3406
212-613-2800
800-322-8755
custserv@factsonfile.com

Ronald M Doctor, PhD, Author
Ada Kahn, PhD, Author
Christine Adame, Author

Providing the basic information on common phobias and anxieties, some 2000 entries explain the nature of anxiety disorders, panic attacks, specific phobias, and obsessive-compulsive disorders. *$75.00*

592 pages Year Founded: 2000 ISBN 0-816039-89-5

240 Flying Without Fear
NewHarbinger Publications
5674 Shattuck Avenue
Oakland, CA 94609-1662
510-652-0215
800-748-6273; *Fax: 800-652-1613*
customerservice@newharbinger.com
www.newharbinger.com

Duane Brown, Author
Duane Brown, Author

Program to confront fears of flying and guides you through first takeoff and later flights. *$16.95*

184 pages Year Founded: 1973 ISBN 1-572240-42-3

241 Free from Fears: New Help for Anxiety, Panic and Agoraphobia
Anxiety Disorders Association of America
8730 Georgia Avenue
Suite 600
Silver Spring, MD 20910-3643
240-485-1001
AnxDis@adaa.org
www.adaa.org

Alies Muskin, Manager
Michelle Alonso, Communications/Membership

Book shows you how to recognize the avoidance trap, combat fears, and modify your behavior for a lasting cure.

242 Freeing Your Child from Anxiety: Powerful, Practical Solutions to Overcome Your Child's Fears, Worries, and Phobias
Broadway Books
1745 Broadway
New York, NY 10019-4368
212-662-0231
bwaypub@randomhouse.com

Sherif Isak, Owner
Tamar E Chansky, PhD, Author

From the children: When I was little my mom worked the graveyard shift at the hospital. *$13.99*

320 pages Year Founded: 2008 ISBN 0-307485-11-3

243 Healing Fear: New Approaches to Overcoming Anxiety
NewHarbinger Publications
5674 Shattuck Avenue
Oakland, CA 94609-1662
510-652-0215
800-748-6273; *Fax: 800-652-1613*
customerservice@newharbinger.com
www.newharbinger.com

Edmund Bourne,PhD, Author

Covers a wide range of healing strategies that help you learn how to relinquish control, discover a unique purpose that is bigger than your particular fears, and find ways to restructure your work and home environments to make them more congruent with the real you. *$ 16.95*

398 pages Year Founded: 1973 ISBN 1-572241-16-0

244 How to Help Your Loved One Recover from Agoraphobia
Anxiety Disorders Association of America
8730 Georgia Avenue
Suite 600
Silver Spring, MD 20910-3643
240-485-1001
AnxDis@adaa.org
www.adaa.org

Alies Muskin, Manager
Michelle Alonso, Communications/Membership

Book is helpful for sufferer and family members to understand what a sufferer is going through. *$45.00*

256 pages

245 Integrative Treatment of Anxiety Disorders
American Psychiatric Publishing, Inc.
1000 Wilson Boulevard
Suite 1825
Arlington, VA 22209-3901
703-907-7322
800-368-5777; *Fax:* 703-907-1091
appi@psych.org
www.appi.org

James M Ellison, M.D., M.P.H., Editor
Ron McMillen, Chief Executive Officer
John McDuffie, Editorial Director

An overview of the spectrum of anxiety disorders, and reviews the treatment alternatives. *$67.00*

349 pages Year Founded: 1996 ISBN 0-880487-15-1

246 It's Not All In Your Head: Now Women Can Discover the Real Causes of their Most Misdiagnosed Health Problems
Anxiety Disorders Association of America
8730 Georgia Avenue
Suite 600
Silver Spring, MD 20910-3643
240-485-1001
AnxDis@adaa.org
www.adaa.org

Susan Swedo,MD, Author
Henreitta Leonard,MD, Author

This book will present you with information about when, how and from whom to seek treatment.

336 pages

247 Managing Social Anxiety: A Cognitive Behavioral Therapy Approach Client Workbook
Oxford University Press
2001 Evans Road
Carry, NC 27513-2010
919-677-0977
800-445-9714; *Fax:* 919-677-2673
custserv.us@oup.com

Debra Hope, Author
Richard Heimberg, Author
Cynthia Turk, Author

This is a client workbook for those in treatment or considering treatment for social anxiety. *$39.95*

Year Founded: 2010 ISBN 0-195336-68-2

248 Master Your Panic and Take Back Your Life: Twelve Treatment Sessions to Overcome High Anxiety
Impact Publishers
PO Box 6016
Atascadero, CA 93423-6016
805-466-5917
800-246-7228; *Fax:* 805-466-5919
info@impactpublishers.com
www.impactpublishers.com

Denise F Beckfield, PhD, Author

Practical, self empowering book on overcoming agoraphobia and debilitating panic attacks is now completely revised and expanded to include the latest information and research findings on relaxation, breathing, medication and other treatments. *$17.95*

304 pages Year Founded: 1970 ISBN 1-886230-47-7

249 Mastery of Your Anxiety and Panic: Workbook
Oxford University Press
2001 Evans Road
Cary, NC 27513-2010
919-677-0977
800-445-9714; *Fax:* 919-677-2673
custserv.us@oup.com

David H Barlow, Author
Michelle G Craske, Author

If you are prone to panic attacks and constantly worry about when the next attack may come, you may suffer from panic disorder and/or agoraphobia. Though panic disorder seems irrational and uncontrollable, it has been proven that a treatment like the one outlined in this book can help you take control of your life. *$31.95*

Year Founded: 2006 ISBN 0-195311-35-3

250 Overcoming Anxiety, Depression, and Other Mental Health Disorders in Children and Adults
Interdesciplinary Council on Development and Learning Disorders
4938 Hampden Lane
Suite 800
Bethesda, MD 20814
301-656-2667
info@icdl.com
www.icdl.com

Dr Stanley I Greenspan, Author

Reveals strategies for family members as well as professionals from different disciplines to help both children and adults. The most common mental health disorders, including anxiety, depression, obsessive-compulsive patterns, ADD/ADHD, borderline states, and others, are discussed literally with a new set of eyeglasses

168 pages ISBN 0-976775-88-3

251 Panic Disorder and Agoraphobia: A Guide
Madison Institute of Medicine
7617 Mineral Point Road
Suite 300
Madison, WI 53717-1623
608-827-2470
mim@miminc.org
www.factsforhealth.org

John H. Greist, Author
James W Jefferson, MD, Author

Learn about the causes of panic disorder and agoraphobia and how patients can overcome these disabling disorders with medications and behavior therapy in this booklet written by leading experts on the subject. *$5.95*

69 pages Year Founded: 2004

252 Panic Disorder: Critical Analysis
Guilford Press
72 Spring Street
New York, NY 10012-4068
212-431-9800
800-365-7006; *Fax:* 212-966-6708
info@guilford.com

Bob Matloff, President
Richard McNally, Author

Provides a comprehensive, integrative exploration of panic disorder. Discusses the phenomenology of the disorder, with extensive reviews of the epidemiology, biological aspects and psychopharmacalogic treatments, followed by detailed explorations of psychological aspects, including predictability and controllability and psychological treatments including cognitive behavioral techniques. *$38.00*

276 pages Year Founded: 1994 ISBN 0-898622-63-8

253 Pharmacotherapy for Mood, Anxiety and Cognitive Disorders
American Psychiatric Publishing, Inc.
1000 Wilson Boulevard
Suite 1825
Arlington, VA 22209-3901
703-907-7322
800-368-5777; *Fax:* 703-907-1091
appi@psych.org
www.appi.org

Uriel Halbreich, M.D., Editor
Stuart A Montgomery, M.D., Editor
John McDuffie, Editorial Director

Takes a critical look at the different medications available for treating mood, anxiety and cognitive disorders. Also, it takes a look at their relevance to pathobiology and the underlying mechanisms, and the limitations. *$99.00*

832 pages Year Founded: 2000 ISBN 0-880488-85-9

254 Phobic and Obsessive-Compulsive Disorders: Theory, Research, and Practice
Kluwer Academic/Plenum Publishers
233 Spring Street
New York, NY 10013-1522
212-242-1490
www.kluweracademicpublishers.com

Paul M.G. Emmelkamp, Author

$24.95

366 pages Year Founded: 1992 ISBN 0-306410-44-3

255 Relaxation & Stress Reduction Workbook
NewHarbinger Publications
5674 Shattuck Avenue
Oakland, CA 94609-1662
510-652-0215
800-748-6273; *Fax:* 800-652-1613
customerservice@newharbinger.com
www.newharbinger.com

Martha Davis, Author
Elizabeth Robbins Eshelman, Author
Matthew McKay, Author

Step by step instructions cover progressive muscle relaxation, meditation, autogenics, visualization, thought stopping, refuting irrational ideas, coping skills training, job stress management, and much more. *$17.95*

392 pages Year Founded: 1973 ISBN 1-879237-82-2

256 Shy Children, Phobic Adults: Nature and Treatment of Social Phobia
American Psychological Association
750 First Street,NorthEast
Washington, DC 20002-4242
202-336-5500
800-374-2721; *Fax:* 202-336-5518
TDD: 202-336-6123

TTY: 202-336-6123
www.www.apa.org

Deborah C. Beidel,PhD,ABPP, Author
Sameuel M. Turner,PhD, Author

Recent advances in the understanding of social phobia. Isolates the controversies that have yet to be resolved. Provides a clear description of effective treatments now available.

398 pages Year Founded: 1998 ISBN 1-557984-61-1

257 Social Anxiety Disorder: A Guide
Madison Institute of Medicine
7617 Mineral Point Road
Suite 300
Madison, WI 53717-1623
608-827-2470
mim@miminc.org
www.factsforhealth.org

John H. Greist, Author
James W Jefferson, MD, Author
David J. Katzelnick, MD, Author

Do you fear public speaking or do you avoid social situations because you worry you may do something embarassing or humiliating? Learn how social anxiety disorder, also known as social phobia, is diagnosed and treated in this thorough publication written by leading experts on the subject. *$5.95*

67 pages Year Founded: 2007

258 Ten Simple Solutions To Panic
NewHarbinger Publications
5674 Shattuck Avenue
Oakland, CA 94609-1662
510-652-0215
800-748-6273; *Fax:* 800-652-1613
customerservice@newharbinger.com
www.newharbinger.com

Randi E McCabe, PhD., Author
Martin Antony, PhD., Author

Provides readers who have at one time or another experienced unexplainable, intense mental and physical attacks over time. *$11.95*

152 pages Year Founded: 1973 ISBN 1-572243-25-2

259 Textbook of Anxiety Disorders
American Psychiatric Publishing, Inc.
1000 Wilson Boulevard
Suite 1825
Arlington, VA 22209-3901
703-907-7322
800-368-5777; *Fax:* 703-907-1091
appi@psych.org
www.appi.org

Dan J Stein, M.D., Ph.D., Editor
Eric Hollander, M.D., Editor
Barbara O Rothbaum, Ph.D., A.B.P, Editor

US and international experts cover every major anxiety disorder, compare it with animal behavior and the similarities in the brain that exist, how disorders can relate to age specific groups, and covers the latest developments in understanding and treating these disorders. *$77.00*

822 pages Year Founded: 2010 ISBN 0-880488-29-8

260 The 10 Best-Ever Anxiety Management Techniques: Understanding How Your Brain Makes You Anxious and What You Can Do to Change It
W.W. Norton & Company, Inc.
500 Fifth Avenue
New York, NY 10110
212-354-5500
800-233-4830; *Fax:* 212-869-0856
www.books.wwnorton.com

Margaret Wehrenberg, Author

A strategy-filled handbook to understand, manage, and conquer your own your own stress. *$18.95*

256 pages Year Founded: 1923 ISBN 0-393705-56-0

261 The Agoraphobia Workbook
NewHarbinger Publications
5674 Shattuck Avenue
Oakland, CA 94609-1662
510-652-0215
800-748-6273; *Fax:* 800-652-1613
customerservice@newharbinger.com
www.newharbinger.com

C Allen Pollard,PhD, Author
Elke Zuercher-White, Author

Self-help resource to help readers overcome the disorder in all its forms *$19.95*

192 pages Year Founded: 1973 ISBN 1-572243-23-6

262 The American Psychiatric Publishing Textbook of Anxiety Disorders
American Psychiatric Publishing, Inc.
1000 Wilson Boulevard
Suite 1825
Arlington, VA 22209-3901
703-907-7322
800-368-5777; *Fax:* 703-907-1091
appi@psych.org
www.appi.org

Dan J Stein, M.D., Ph.D., Editor
Eric Hollander, M.D., Editor
Barbara O Rothbaum, Ph.D., A.B.P, Editor

Gives a detailed look at the history, classification, preclinical models, concepts and combined treatment of anxiety disorders. *$92.00*

822 pages Year Founded: 2010 ISBN 0-880488-29-8

263 The Anxiety & Phobia Workbook, 5th Edition
NewHarbinger Publications
5674 Shattuck Avenue
Oakland, CA 94609-1662
510-652-0215
800-748-6273; *Fax:* 800-652-1613
customerservice@newharbinger.com
www.newharbinger.com

Edmund J. Bourne, PhD, Author

Research conducted by the National Institute of Mental Health has shown that anxiety disorders are the number one mental health problem among American women and. *$24.95*

496 pages Year Founded: 1973 ISBN 1-572244-13-5

264 The Imp of the Mind: Exploring the Silent Epidemic of Obsessive Bad Thoughts
Plume
375 Hudson Street
New York, NY 10014-3657
212-366-2372; *Fax:* 212-366-2933

Lee Baer, PhD, Author

Dr. Lee Baer combines the latest research with his own extensive experience in treating this widespread syndrome. Drawing on information ranging from new advances in brain technology to pervasive social taboos, Dr. Baer explores the root causes of bad thoughts, why they can spiral out of control, and how to recognize the crucial difference between harmless and dangerous bad thoughts. *$12.99*

176 pages Year Founded: 1936 ISSN 978-0452283077ISSN 0-452283-07-8

265 The Worry Control Workbook
NewHarbinger Publications
5674 Shattuck Avenue
Oakland, CA 94609-1662
510-652-0215
800-748-6273; *Fax:* 800-652-1613
customerservice@newharbinger.com
www.newharbinger.com

Mary Ellen Copeland, Author

Self help program that shares experiences of people who have developed ways to overcome chronic worry. Step by step format helps identify areas likely to reoccur and develop new skills. *$15.95*

266 pages ISBN 1-572241-20-9

266 Traumatic Stress: Effects of Overwhelming Experience on Mind, Body and Society
Guilford Press
72 Spring Street
New York, NY 10012-4068
212-431-9800
800-365-7006; *Fax:* 212-966-6708
info@guilford.com

Besell van der Kolk, Author
Alexander McFarlane, Author

The current state of research and clinical knowledge on traumatic stress and its treatment. Contributions from leading authorities summarize knowledge emerging. Addresses the uncertainties and controversies that confront the field of traumatic stress, including the complexity of posttraumatic adaptations and the unproven effectiveness of some approaches to prevention and treatment. *$42.50*

596 pages Year Founded: 2006 ISBN 1-572300-88-4

267 Triumph Over Fear: A Book of Help and Hope for People with Anxiety, Panic Attacks, and Phobias
Bantam Dell Publishing Group
1745 Broadway
New York, NY 10019
212-782-9000
ecustomerservice@randomhouse.com
www.randomhouse.com

Jerilynn Ross, Author

Resource and guide for both lay and professional readers. *$16.00*

320 pages Year Founded: 1995 ISSN 9780553081329ISBN 0-553081-32-2

268 What to Do When You Worry Too Much: A Kid's Guide to Overcoming Anxiety
American Psychological Association
750 First Street,NorthEast
Washington, DC 20002-4242
202-336-5500
800-374-2721; *Fax: 202-336-5518*
TTY: 202-336-6123
www.apa.org

Dawn Huebner,PhD, Author
Bonnie Matthews, Illustrator

Interactive self-help book designed to guide 6-12 year olds and thier parents through the techniques most often used in the treatments of generalized anxiety. *$9.38*

88 pages Year Founded: 1892 ISBN 1-591473-14-4

269 What to Do When You're Scared and Worried: A Guide for Kids
Free Spirit Publishing
217 Fifth Avenue North
Suite 200
Minneapolis, MN 55401-1299
612-338-2068
800-735-7323; *Fax: 866-419-5199*
www.freespirit.com

James J Christ, Author

This book is all about fears and worries: things that everyone deals with at some point in thier lives.

128 pages Year Founded: 1983

270 When Perfect Isn't Good Enough: Strategies for Coping with Perfectionism
NewHarbinger Publications
5674 Shattuck Avenue
Oakland, CA 94609-1662
510-652-0215
800-748-6273; *Fax: 800-652-1613*
customerservice@newharbinger.com
www.newharbinger.com

Martin Antony,PhD, Author
Richard P Swinson,MD,FRCPC,FRCP, Author

This step by step guide explores the nature of perfectionism and offers a series of exercises to help you challenge unrealistic expectations and work on the specific situations in your life where perfectionism is a problem. *$14.95*

312 pages Year Founded: 1973 ISBN 1-572241-24-1

Periodicals & Pamphlets

271 Anxiety Disorders
National Institute of Mental Health
6001 Executive Boulevard
Rockville, MD 20852
301-443-4513
866-615-6464
TTY: 301-443-8431
nimhinfo@nih.gov
www.www.nimh.nih.gov/

Thomas Insel MD, Director
Phillip Sun Wang, Deputy Director

Marlene Guzman, Senior Advisor to the Director
Mayada Akil, Senior Advisor

A detailed booklet that describes the symptoms, causes, and treatments of the major anxiety disorders, with information on getting help and coping.

22 pages

272 Anxiety Disorders Fact Sheet
Center for Mental Health Services: Knowledge Exchange Network
3803 North Fairfax Drive
Suite 100
Arlington, VA 22203
703-524-7600
800-950-6264; *Fax: 703-524-9094*
TDD: 866-889-2647
ken@mentalhealth.org
www.www.nami.org

This fact sheet presents basic information on the symptoms, formal diagnosis, and treatment for generalized anxiety disorder, panic disorders, phobias, and post-traumatic stress disorder.

3 pages Year Founded: 1979

273 Anxiety Disorders in Children and Adolescents
Center for Mental Health Services: Knowledge Exchange Network
1 Choke Cherry Road
Rockville, MD 20015
800-789-2647; *Fax: 240-747-5470*
TDD: 866-889-2647
ken@mentalhealth.org
www.mentalhealth.samhsa.gov/

Tracy L Morris, Editor
John S March, Editor

This fact sheet defines anxiety disorders, identifies warning signs, discusses risk factors, describes types of help available, and suggests what parents or other caregivers can do.

395 pages

274 Facts About Anxiety Disorders
National Institute of Mental Health
6001 Executive Boulevard
Rockville, MD 20852
301-443-4513
866-615-6464
TTY: 301-443-8431
nimhinfo@nih.gov
www.www.nimh.nih.gov/

Series of fact sheets that provide overviews and descriptions of generalized anxiety disorder, obsessive-compulsive disorder, panic disorder, post-traumatic stress disorder, social phobia, and the Anxiety Disorders Education Program.

275 Families Can Help Children Cope with Fear, Anxiety
PO Box 42490
Washington, DC 20015
800-789-2647; *Fax: 301-984-8796*
TDD: 866-889-2647
www.mentalhealth.org

2 pages

276 Journal of Anxiety Disorders
Elsevier Publishing
1600 John F Kennedy Boulevard
Suite 1800
Philadelphia, PA 19103-2879
212-989-5800
800-325-4177; *Fax:* 212-633-3820
custserv.ehs@elsevier.com

Deborah Beidel, Author

Interdisciplinary journal that publishes research papers
dealing with all aspects of anxiety disorders for all age
groups (child, adolescent, adult and geriatrics). *$195.00*

8 per year Year Founded: 2012 ISSN 0887-6185

277 Let's Talk Facts About Panic Disorder
American Psychiatric Publishing, Inc.
1000 Wilson Boulevard
Suite 1825
Arlington, VA 22209-3901
703-907-7322
800-368-5777; *Fax:* 703-907-1091
appi@psych.org
www.appi.org

Robert E Hales MD, Editor-in-Chief
Ron McMillen, Chief Executive Officer
John McDuffie, Editorial Director

Contains an overview of the illness, its symptoms, and the
illness's effect on family and friends. A biliography and list
of resources make them ideal for libraries or patient education. *$29.95*

6 pages Year Founded: 2006 ISBN 0-890423-57-1

278 Panic Attacks
ETR Associates
4 Carbonero Way
Scotts Valley, CA 95066-4200
831-438-4060
800-321-4407; *Fax:* 831-438-3618
support@etr.freshdesk.com
www.etr.org

David Kitchen,MBA, Chief Financial Officer
Talita Sanders,BS, Director,Human Resources
Coleen Cantwell,MPH, Director,Business Development Pl
Matt McDowell,BS, Director,Marketing

Describes causes of panic attacks, including genetics,
stress, and drug use; prevention and treatment, and how to
stop a panic attack in its tracks. *$16.00*

279 Real Illness: Panic Disorder
National Institute of Mental Health
6001 Executive Boulevard
Room 8184
Bethesda, MD 20892
301-443-4513
866-615-6464
TTY: 301-443-8431
nimhinfo@nih.gov

Do you often have feelings of sudden fear that don't make
sense? If so, you may have panic disorder. Read this
pamplet of simple information about getting help.

9 pages

Research Centers

280 Columbia University Pediatric Anxiety and
Mood Research Clinic
1051 Riverside Drive
New York, NY 10032
646-774-5793
www.childadolescentpsych.cumc.columbia.edu

Laura Mufson, PhD, Unit Chief, Children's Day Unit
Pablo Goldberg, MD, Medical Director
Anthony C. Puliafico, PhD, Consulting Psychologist
Mara Eilenberg, MSW, LCSW, Clinician

A research clinic desinged to help children with anxiety,
depression, and OCD. The clinic provides evaluations, evidence-based therapy and medications, and a day-treatment
program. All evaluation and treatment services are free of
charge.

281 UAMS Psychiatric Research Institute
4224 Shuffield Drive
Little Rock, AR 72205
501-526-8100; *Fax:* 501-660-7542
kramerteresal@uams.edu
www.www.psychiatry.uams.edu

John Fortney PhD, Director
Geoff Curran PhD, Associate Director
Keith Berner MD, Clinical Faculty

Combining research, education and clinical services into
one facility, PRI offers inpatiend and outpatient services,
with 40 psychiatric beds, therapy options, and specialized
treatment for specific disorders, including: addictive eating,
anxiety, deppressive and post-traumatic stress disorders.
Research focuses on evidence-based care takes into consideration the education of future medical personnel while relying on research scientists to provide innovative forms of
treatment. PRI includes the Center for Addiction Research
as well as a methadone clinic.

Support Groups & Hot Lines

282 Agoraphobics Building Independent Lives
2008 Bremo Road
Suite #101
Richmond, VA 23226
804-257-5591
866-400-6428; *Fax:* 804-447-7786
info@mhav.org
www.mhav.org

Joanne Whitley, President
Ali Faruk, Vice President & Public Policy C
Anne Edgerton, Executive Director
Sarah Rudden, Project Coordinator

A nonprofit organization for people dealing with anxiety
and panic disorders, incorporated in the State of Virginia. It
has support groups nationwide.

283 Emotions Anonymous International Service
Center
PO Box 4245
St. Paul, MN 55104-0245
651-647-9712
director@emotionsanonymous.org
www.emotionsanonymous.org/

Elaine Weber Nelson, Executive Director
Gus S., President

Scott J., Vice President and Treasurer
John W., Secretary

Fellowship of men and women who share their experience, strength, and hope with each other, that they may solve their common problem and help others recover from emotional illness. Members come together in weekly meetings.

284 Recovery International
1415 W. 22nd Street
Tower Floor
Oak Brook, IL 60523
312-337-5661
866-221-0302; *Fax:* 312-726-4446
www.www.recoveryinternational.org

Sandra K. Wilcoxon, Chief Executive Officer
Joanne Lampey, President
Joan Nobiling, Vice President
Nicole Cilento, 2nd Vice President

Recovery International is an organization that uses a peer-to-peer,self-help training system developed by Abraham Low in order to help individuals with mental health issues lead more productive lives.

Year Founded: 1937

Video & Audio

285 Anxiety Disorders
American Counseling Association
5999 Stevenson Avenue
Alexandria, VA 22304-3304
703-823-9800
800-347-6647; *Fax:* 703-823-0252
TDD: 703-823-6862
webmaster@counseling.org
www.counseling.org

Cirecie A. West-Olatunji, President
Richard Yep, Executive Director
Thelma Daley, Treasurer

Increase your awareness of anxiety disorders, their symptoms, and effective treatments. Learn the effect these disorders can have on life and how treatment can change the quality of life for people presently suffering from these disorders. Includes 6 audiotapes and a study guide. *$140.00*

Year Founded: 1952

286 DSM-IV-TR
American Psychiatric Publishing, Inc.
1000 Wilson Boulevard
Suite 1825
Arlington, VA 22209-3901
703-907-7322
800-368-5777; *Fax:* 703-907-1091
appi@psych.org
www.appi.org

Cathryn A Galanter, M.D, Editor
Peter S Jensen, M.D, Editor
John McDuffie, Editorial Director

Series of three clinical programs that reveals additions and changes for mood, psychotic and anxiety disorders. Each video focuses on a different level of disorder as well as giving three 10 minute interviews. Approximately 60 minutes. *$57.00*

744 pages Year Founded: 2009 ISBN 0-880488-98-0

287 Dealing With Social Anxiety
Educational Video Network
1401 19th Street
Huntsville, TX 77340
936-295-5767
800-762-0060; *Fax:* 936-294-0233
info at evn.org
www.www.evndirect.com

A video to learn and understand social anxiety. *$89.95*

Year Founded: 2002 ISBN 1-589501-48-9

288 Driving Far from Home
NewHarbinger Publications
5674 Shattuck Avenue
Oakland, CA 94609-1662
510-652-0215
800-748-6273; *Fax:* 800-652-1613
customerservice@newharbinger.com
www.newharbinger.com

Edmund J. Bourne, Author

120 minute videotape that reduces fear associated with leaving the safety of your home base. *$15.95*

Year Founded: 1973 ISBN 1-572240-14-8

289 Effective Learning Systems, Inc.
5108 W 74th Street
#390160
Minneapolis, MN 55439
952-943-1660
800-966-0443
info@efflearn.com
www.www.effectivelearning.com

Bob Griswold, Founder
Deirdre M Griswold, VP

Audio tapes for stress management, deep relaxation, anger control, peace of mind, insomnia, weight and smoking, self-image and self-esteem, positive thinking, health and healing. Since 1972, Effective Learning Systems has helped millions of people take charge of their lives and make positive changes.

Year Founded: 1972

290 Understanding Mental Illness
Educational Video Network
1401 19th Street
Huntsville, TX 77340
936-295-5767
800-762-0060; *Fax:* 936-294-0233
info at evn.org
www.www.evndirect.com

A video to learn and understand mental illness and how it affects you. *$79.95*

Year Founded: 2004 ISBN 1-589501-48-9

291 Understanding and Treating the Hereditary Psychiatric Spectrum Disorders
Hope Press
PO Box 188
Duarte, CA 91009-188
818-303-0644
800-209-9182; *Fax:* 818-358-3520
dcomings@earthlink.net
www.hopepress.com

David E Comings MD, Presenter

Learn with ten hours of audio tapes from a two day seminar given in May 1997 by David E Comings MD. Tapes cover: ADHD, Tourette Syndrome, Obsessive-Compulsive Disorder, Conduct Disorder, Oppositional Defiant Disorder, Autism and other Hereditary Psychiatric Spectrum Disorders. Eight audio tapes. *$75.00*

Year Founded: 1997

Web Sites

292 www.bcm.tmc.edu/civitas/caregivers.htm
Caregivers Series

Sophisticated articles describing the effects of childhood trauma on brain development and relationships.

293 www.cyberpsych.org
CyberPsych

Presents information about psychoanalysis, psychotherapy and special topics such as anxiety disorders, the problematic use of alcohol, homophobia, and the traumatic effects of racism. Explains in detail what anxiety it is how it is treated and the symptoms associated with anxiety.

294 www.goodwill-suncoast.org
Career Assessment & Planning Services

A comprehensive assessment for the developmentally disabled persons who may be unemployed or underemployed.

295 www.guidetopsychology.com
A Guide To Psychlogy & Its Practice

Free information on various types of psychology.

296 www.healthanxiety.org
Anxiety and Phobia Treatment Center

Treatment groups for individuals suffering from phobias.

297 www.healthyminds.org
Anxiety Disorders

American Psychiatric Association publication diagnostic criteria and treatment.

298 www.lexington-on-line.com
Panic Disorder

Explains development and treatment of panic disorder.

299 www.mayoclinic.com
Mayo Clinic

Provides information on obsessive-compulsive disorder and anxiety.

300 www.mentalhealth.Samhsa.Gov
Center for Mental Health Services Knowledge Exchange Network

Information about resources, technical assistance, research, training, networks and other federal clearinghouses.

301 www.mentalhealth.com
Internet Mental Health

On-line information and a virtual encyclopedia related to mental disorders, possible causes and treatments. News, articles, on-line diagnostic programs and related links. Designed to improve understanding, diagnosis and treatment of mental illness throughout the world. Awarded the Top Site Award and the NetPsych Cutting Edge Site Award.

302 www.nami.org
National Alliance on Mental Illness

From its inception in 1979, NAMI has been dedicated to improving the lives of individuals and families affected by mental illness.

303 www.nimh.nih.gov/anxiety/anxiety/ocd
National Institute of Health

Information on anxiety disorders and OCD.

304 www.npadnews.com
National Panic/Anxiety Disorder Newsletter

This resource was founded by Phil Darren who collects and collates information of recovered anxiety disorder sufferers who want to distribute some of the lessons that they learned with a view to helping others.

305 www.panicattacks.com.au
Anxiety Panic Hub

Information, resources and support.

306 www.panicdisorder.about.com
Agoraphobia: For Friends/Family

307 www.planetpsych.com
Planetpsych.com

Learn about disorders, their treatments and other topics in psychology. Articles are listed under the related topic areas. Ask a therapist a question for free, or view the directory of professionals in your area. If you are a therapist sign up for the directory. Current features, self-help, interactive, and newsletter archives.

308 www.psychcentral.com
Psych Central

Personalized one-stop index for psychology, support, and mental health issues, resources, and people on the Internet.

309 www.selectivemutismfoundation.org
Selective Mutism Foundation

Promotes awareness and understanding for individuals and families affected by mutism.

310 www.selfhelpmagazine.com/articles/stress
Meditation, Guided Fantasies, and Other Stress Reducers

Meditative and stress reduction resources for eyes, ears, minds, and hearts.

311 www.terraphouston.com
Territorial Apprehensiveness Programs (TERRAP)

Shirley Riff, Director

Formed to disseminate information concerning the recognition, causes and treatment of anxieties, fears and phobias.

312 www.thenadd.org
National Association for the Dually Diagnosed (NADD)

An association for persons with developmental disabilities and mental health needs.

Autism Spectrum Disorders

Introduction

Autism Spectrum Disorders are a distinct group of neurological conditions characterized by impairment in language and communication skills; two of the most common are Autistic Disorder and Asperger's Syndrome. Other ASDs include Pervasive Development Disorder (not otherwise specified), Childhood Disintegrative Disorder, and Rett Syndrome.

Autistic Disorder is a pervasive developmental disorder whose main symptoms are a marked lack of interest in connecting, interacting, or communicating with others. People with this disorder cannot share something of interest with other people, rarely make eye contact with others, avoid physical contact, show little facial expression, and do not make friends. Autistic Disorder is a profound, lifelong condition associated with wide ranging and severe disabilities, including behavior problems, such as hyperactivity, obsessive compulsive behavior, self injury, and tics. Although present before age three, the disorder may not be apparent until later, although parents often sense that there is something wrong because of their child's marked lack of interest in social interaction. Very young children with autism not only show no desire for affection and cuddling, but show actual aversion to it. There is no socially directed smiling or facial responsiveness, and no responsiveness to the voices of parents and siblings. As a result, parents may sometimes worry that their child is deaf. Later, the child may be more willing to interact socially, but the quality of interaction is unusual, usually inappropriately intrusive with little understanding of social rules and boundaries. The autistic child seems not to have the abilities and desires that would make it possible for him or her to become a social being. Instead, the child seems locked up in an interior world which is both incomprehensible and inaccessible to parents, siblings, and others.

Asperger's Syndrome (AS) is named for Austrian pediatrician Hans Asperger, who in 1944, observed four children who had normal intelligence, but lacked nonverbal communication skills; additionally they did not demonstrate empathy with their peers, and were physically clumsy. Dr. Asperger called the condition 'Autistic psychopathy' and described it as a personality disorder marked by social isolation.

Twin and family studies have shown a genetic predisposition to AS and other ADs. Several genes, but not one specific gene, have recently been identified as associated with autism. Some researchers have proposed that the disorder may stem from abnormalities during critical stages of fetal development, including defects in the genes that control and regulate normal brain growth and growth patterns.

There is no standardized screening tool available to diagnose Asperger's Syndrome. Most doctors rely on the presence of a core group of behaviors to diagnose the syndrome.

SYMPTOMS

Autism: Impairment in the Quality of Social Interaction
• Gross lack of nonverbal behavior (e.g., eye contact, facial expression, body postures, and gestures), which gives meaning to social interaction and social behavior;
• Failure to make friends in age-appropriate ways;
• Lack of spontaneously seeking to share interests or achievements with others (e.g., not showing things to others, not pointing to, or bringing interesting objects to others);
• Lack of social or emotional give and take (e.g., not joining in social play or simple games with others);
• Notable lack of awareness of others. Oblivious of other children (including siblings), of their excitement, distress, or needs.

Autism: Marked Impairment in the Quality of Communication
• Delay in, or lack of, spoken language development. Those who speak cannot initiate or sustain communication with others;
• Lack of spontaneous make-believe or imitative play common among young children;
• When speech does develop, it may be abnormal and monotonous;
• Repetitive use of language.

Autism: Restricted Repetitive Patterns or Behavior
• Restricted range of interests often fixed on one subject and its facts (e.g., baseball);
• A great deal of exact repetition in play, (e.g., lining up play objects in the same way again and again);
• Resistance and distress if anything in the environment is changed, (e.g., a chair moved to a different place);
• Insistence on following certain rules and routines (e.g., walking to school by the same route each day);
• Repeated body movements (e.g., body rocking, hand clapping);
• Persistent preoccupation with details or parts of objects (e.g., buttons).

Asperger's Syndrome in Contrast to Autism:
Asperger's Syndrome causes two types of symptoms: problems with social interactions and stereotyped, repetitive patterns of behavior. Individuals with AS have limited interests and are preoccupied with a particular subject to the exclusion of other activities. Some other characteristics are:
• Repetitive routines or rituals;
• Peculiarities in speech and language, such as speaking in an overly formal manner or in a monotone, or taking figures of speech literally;
• Socially and emotionally inappropriate behavior and the inability to interact successfully with peers;
• Problems with non-verbal communication, including the restricted use of gestures, limited or inappropriate facial expressions, or a peculiar, stiff gaze;
• Clumsy and uncoordinated motor movements.

ASSOCIATED FEATURES

Autism seems to bring with it an increased risk of other disorders. Seventy-five percent of autistic children have cognitive deficits, and twenty-five percent have cognitive abilities at or above average. Twenty-five percent of individuals with autism also have seizure disorders. The development of intellectual skills is usually uneven. An autistic child may be able to read extremely early, but not be able to comprehend what he or she reads. Other symptoms include hyperactivity, short attention span, impulsivity, aggressiveness, and self injury, such as head banging, hair pulling, and arm biting (particularly in young children). There may be unusual responses to stimuli: less than normal sensitivity to pain but extreme sensitivity to sounds or to being touched. There may be abnormalities in emotional expression, giggling or weeping for no apparent reason, and little or no emotional reaction when one would be expected. Similar abnormal responses may be shown in relation to fear; an absence of fear in response to real danger, but great fearfulness in the presence of harmless objects.

In adolescence or adulthood, people with Autistic Disorder who have the capacity for insight may become depressed when they realize how seriously impaired they are. Autistic Disorder sometimes follows medical and obstetrical problems, such as encephalitis, anoxia (absence of oxygen) during birth, and prenatal infections (such as maternal rubella). There is some evidence of genetic transmission. The disorder is not caused by inappropriate parenting or by routine immunizations.

The person with Asperger's may not develop age-appropriate relationships or attempt to share interests or pleasures with others. He or she may be unable to reciprocate others' feelings, have difficulty using gestures or facial expressions, be extremely preoccupied with a very narrow area of interest, insist upon very rigid routines, make repetitive movements, and focus on parts of objects rather than the objects as a whole.

Asperger's Syndrome does not interfere with the development of language or thinking. However, its symptoms interfere with the individual's social or occupational functioning.

PREVALENCE

By definition, Autistic Disorder is present before age three. There are two to five cases of the disorder per 10,000 births. Rates of autism are four to five times greater among males than females. Females with Autistic Disorder are more likely to be severely affected by the disorder than males. Follow-up studies suggest that only a small percentage of people with Autistic Disorder live independent adult lives. Even the highest functioning adults continue to have problems in social interaction and communication, together with greatly restricted interests and activities. The siblings of people with the disorder are at increased risk.

After years of controversy, there is a growing consensus that the incidence and prevalence of autism spectrum disorders has increased significantly in recent years. The reason(s) for the increase are not clear.

The incidence of Asperger's Syndrome is estimated to be two out of every 10,000 children. Boys are three to four times more likely than girls to have the disorder. Although diagnosed mainly in children, it is being increasingly diagnosed in adults with other mental health conditions such as depression, obsessive-compulsive disorder, and attention-deficit/hyperactivity disorder.

TREATMENT OPTIONS

It is difficult or unusual to be able to eradicate all the symptoms of Autistic Disorder, but there are many intervention and education programs which help to improve functioning. It is extremely important, however, that a proper assessment and diagnosis be made. Since the disturbance in behavior is so wide ranging, this can require an array of professional skills - psychological, language development, neuropsychological, and medical. Such a multiple assessment establishes the presence or absence of other disorders, the level of intellectual functioning, together with individual strengths and weaknesses, and the child's capacity for social and personal self-sufficiency. Since the symptoms of Autistic Disorder vary widely, a proper assessment is the foundation for designing and planning an individually tailored intervention program.

The autistic person may benefit from a combination of educational and behavioral interventions, which may reduce many of the behavioral disturbances, and improve the quality of life for the person and his or her family. One treatment method is applied behavior analysis (ABA), which builds on social interaction, imitation and language skills, as well as attention to social stimuli. Other treatments include speech and language therapy, occupational therapy, life skills training and psychological counseling. In some cases, medication may also be prescribed for the symptoms that sometimes co-exist with Autistic Disorder (e.g., stimulant drugs for hyperactivity, antidepressants for anxiety). There is no drug that specifically treats the neurological problems associated with AD.

The diagnosis of Autistic Disorder can be a shattering experience for any family. The outcome of the diagnosis is open-ended and uncertain and includes a lifetime of care. Every member of the family is affected and it is vital to work with and support them.

Treatment for Asperger's Syndrome address the core symptoms of the disorder: poor communication skills; obsessive or repetitive routines; and physical clumsiness. No single treatment works best, but the program would include social skills training, cognitive behavioral therapy, medication, occupational/physical therapy, and parent training and support.

Associations & Agencies

314 Achieve Beyond
7000 Austin Street
Suite 200
Forest Hills, NY 11375
718-762-7633; *Fax:* 212-679-7867
info@achievebeyondusa.com
www.achievebeyondusa.com

Dr. Trudy Font Padron, PhD, Founder and Executive Director
Robert Padron, Executive Director

Achieve Beyond provides therapeutic and educational services to children with developmental disabilities and their families, with particular focus on children with bilingual needs. Services include special education, speech language therapy, occupational therapy, physical therapy, and behavioral management.
Year Founded: 1995

315 Asperger Autism Spectrum Education Network
9 Aspen Circle
Edison, NJ 08820
732-321-0880
info@aspennj.org
www.aspennj.org

Lori Shery, President and Executive Director
Rich Meleo, Vice President
Elizabeth Yamashita, Vice President
Ann Hiller, Secretary

A nonprofit organization seeking to assist individuals with Autism Spectrum Disorders and Nonverbal Learning Disabilities and their families. Provides educational resources on the disorders and issues surrounding them, supports individuals with ASDs and NLD in realizing their full potential, and advocates for public awareness, educational programs, and medical research funding.

316   Asperger/Autism Network (AANE)
51 Water Street
Suite 206
Watertown, MA 02472
617-393-3824
info@aane.org
www.aane.org

Dania Jekel, MSW, Executive Director
Brenda Dater, MSW, MPH, Associate Director
Ilia Walsh, MEd, MBA, Director, Adult Services
Nancy Parker, MSW, LICSW, Director, Child & Teen Services

An organization that helps people with Asperger Syndrome and related conditions live meaningful and productive lives. Provides information, offers support, and engages in advocacy while fostering awareness, respect, and acceptance for individuals with AS and their families.

Year Founded: 1996

317   Autism Network International
PO Box 35448
Syracuse, NY 13235-5448
www.autismnetworkinternational.org

Jim Sinclair, Coordinator
James Bordner, List Owner

Autism Network International is an organization run by autistic people and for autistic people. Advocates for awareness, acceptance of autistic people, and accessibility to support services.

318   Autism Research Foundation
72 East Concord Street
Room 1010
Boston, MA 02118
617-414-7012; *Fax:* 617-414-7207
www.theautismresearchfoundation.org

Dr. Margaret L. Bauman, Founding Director

A nonprofit, tax-exempt organization dedicated to researching autism and related developmental disorders. Supports changing developments in the field of autism through education, social inclusion programs, and family life resources.

Year Founded: 1990

319   Autism Research Institute
4182 Adams Avenue
San Diego, CA 92116
833-281-7165
www.autism.com

Stephen M. Edelson, PhD, Executive Director
Melanie Glock, Communcations Specialist
Kimberly Taylor, JD, Chairwoman
Christopher Flynn, Treasurer

A nonprofit organization that provides information and supports research on Autism and Asperger's Syndrome.
Year Founded: 1967

320   Autism Services Inc.
40 Hazelwood Drive
Amherst, NY 14228
716-631-5777
888-288-4764; *Fax:* 716-565-0671
vfedericoni@autism-services-inc.org
www.friendsofasi.org

Dr. Edmund Egan, President
Veronica Federiconi, Chief Executive Officer
John Lordi, PhD, Vice President
Matthew Shriver, Treasurer

An agency exclusively dedicated to providing educational programs, quality of life programs, and support services for children and adults with autism and their families.

321   Autism Society
4340 East-West Highway
Suite 350
Bethesda, MD 20814
301-657-0881
800-328-8476
info@autism-society.org
www.autism-society.org

Joseph P. Joyce, CPCU, CWCA, Executive Chair
Scott Badesch, President and CEO
John Dabrowski, Chief Financial Officer
Lori A. Ireland, Vice Chair

Promotes inclusivity for individuals on the autism spectrum and their families and works towards ensuring their full participation in the community through advocacy, public awareness, education, and research related to autism. Hosts a national conference, publishes a magazine, engages in public policy activities at local, state, and federal levels, and provides information and referral services via phone and email. The Autism Society consists of a nationwide network of local chapters.

Year Founded: 1965

322   Autism Speaks
1 East 33rd Street
4th Floor
New York, NY 10016
646-385-8500; *Fax:* 212-252-8676
familyservices@autismspeaks.org
www.autismspeaks.org

Angela Geiger, President and CEO
Anne Marie Forbes, Chief Field Officerrs
Thomas Frazer, PhD, Chief Science Officer
Kevin Roy, Executive VP of Advocacy

Autism Speaks was founded in 2005 and serves as an organization for autism science and advocacy. Autism Speaks funds biomedical research focused on the causes, treatments, and prevention of autism; educates the public and raises awareness about autism as well as its effects on people and society; and advocates for the needs of individuals and families concerned with autism.

Year Founded: 2005

323 Brain Resources and Information Network (BRAIN)
National Institute of Neurological Disorders and Stroke
PO Box 5801
Bethesda, MD 20824-5801
301-496-5751
800-352-9424
braininfo@ninds.nih.gov
www.ninds.nih.gov

Denise Dorsey, Chief Administrative Officer
Peter Soltys, Chief Information Officer
Walter J. Koroshetz, MD, Director, NINDS
Margo Warren, Deputy Director, Communications

Federal agency focused on supporting neuroscience research and working towards reducing the burdens associated with neurological disease.

Year Founded: 1950

324 Center for Mental Health Services (CMHS)
Substance Abuse and Mental Health Services Administration
5600 Fishers Lane
Rockville, MD 20857
240-276-1310
877-726-4727
TTY: 800-487-4889
www.samhsa.gov/about-us/who-we-are/offices-centers

Paolo del Vecchio, MSW, Director
Anne Mathews-Younes, Acting Deputy Director
Keris Myrick, Director, Consumer Affairs
Patricia Gratton, Director, Program Analysis

Promotes the treatment of mental illness and emotional disorders by increasing accessibility to mental health programs; supporting outreach, treatment, rehabilitation, and support programs and networks; and encouraging the use of scientifically-based information when treating mental disorders. CMHS provides information about mental health via a toll-free number and numerous publications. Developed for users of mental health services and their families, the general public, policy makers, providers, and the media.

Year Founded: 1992

325 Community Services for Autistic Adults and Children
8615 East Village Avenue
Montgomery Village, MD 20886
240-912-2220; *Fax:* 301-926-9384
csaac@csaac.org
www.csaac.org

Eric Salzano, Executive Director
Sakshi Gadoo, Director, Human Resources
Peter Donaghy, Director of Finance
Eva Muiruri, Assistant Executive Director

CSAAC provides quality services for people with autism, offers employment and early intervention programs, and operates community living residences in Montgomery County. CSAAC seeks to help individuals with autism to realize their highest potential and to become active participants in their community.

Year Founded: 1979

326 FACES Autism Services
220 D Twin Dolphin Drive
Redwood City, CA 94065

650-622-9601
info@facesforkids.org
www.pacificautism.org

Kurt Ohlfs, Executive Director, Paces
Karen Kennan, Assistant Executive Director
Maureen McNeil, Administrator
Meredith Loscialpo, Faces Clinical Manager

FACES is a behavioral program serving children with autism. The program implements teaching methods based upon Applied Behavior Analysis, including behavior assessment, behavior consultation, ABA therapy services, and parent and community training.

Year Founded: 1995

327 Families for Early Autism Treatment
PO Box 255722
Sacramento, CA 95865-5722
916-303-7405
feat@feat.org
www.feat.org

A nonprofit organization offering a support network for families with children who have an Autism Spectrum Disorder. Organizes meetings where families can meet and discuss autism, treatment options, and other issues surrounding the disorder.

Year Founded: 1993

328 Generation Rescue
13636 Ventura Boulevard
Suite 259
Sherman Oaks, CA 91423
877-982-8847
www.generationrescue.org

Candace McDonald, Executive Director
JB Handley, Co-Founder
Lisa Handley, Co-Founder
Zack Peter, Associate Director

Generation Rescue is an organization focused on providing assistance and medical treatment support for families with children affected by autism spectrum disorders. Generation Rescue is committed to the recovery of children with autism.

Year Founded: 2005

329 Indiana Resource Center for Autism (IRCA)
1905 North Range Road
Bloomington, IN 47408-9801
812-855-6508
800-825-4733; *Fax:* 812-855-9630
TTY: 812-855-9396
prattc@indiana.edu
www.iidc.indiana.edu/pages/irca

Cathy Pratt, PhD, BCBA, Center Director
Pamela Anderson, Outreach/Resource Specialist
Catherine Davies, MEd, MSC, LMHC, Educational Consultant

The Indiana Resource Center for Autism focuses on improving the quality of life for people with autism spectrum disorders, and promotes early diagnosis of autism and effective childhood programs, employment and living options, family support and other opportunities. The Center also conducts research on the most effective methods for supporting individuals with autism, and provides consultations and disseminates information on autism for families and professionals.

330 **National Alliance on Mental Illness**
3803 North Fairfax Drive
Suite 100
Arlington, VA 22203
703-524-7600
800-950-6264
info@nami.org
www.nami.org

Steve Pitman, JD, President
Lacey Berumen, PhD, MNM, First Vice President
Mary Giliberti, Chief Executive Officer
David Levy, Chief Financial Officer

NAMI is an organization dedicated to raising awareness on mental health and providing support and education for Americans affected by mental illness. NAMI advocates for access to services and treatment and fosters an environment of awareness and understanding for those concerned with mental health.

Year Founded: 1979

331 **National Association for the Dually Diagnosed (NADD)**
132 Fair Street
Kingston, NY 12401
845-331-4336
info@thenadd.org
www.thenadd.org

Jeanne M. Farr, MA, Chief Executive Officer
Daniel Bakers, PhD., President
Peggie Webb, MA, Vice President
George Zukotynski, PhD., Secretary

NADD is a nonprofit organization designed to increase awareness of, and provide services for, individuals with developmental disabilities and mental illness. NADD emphasizes the importance of quality mental healthcare for people with mental health needs and offers conferences, information resources, educational programs, and training materials to professionals, parents, and organizations.

Year Founded: 1983

332 **National Autism Center**
41 Pacella Park Drive
Door 2
Randolph, MA 02368
877-313-3833
www.nationalautismcenter.org

Lauren C. Solotar, PhD, ABPP, President
Cynthia M. Anderson, PhD, BCBA-D, Director
Ralph B. Sperry, PhD, ABPP, Chief Operating Officer
Debra Blair, MBA, CMA, CPA, Chief Financial Officer

The National Autism Center is committed to promoting evidence-based information and practices surrounding the treatment of autism spectrum disorder, and providing trustworthy resources for families and professionals.

333 **National Institute of Mental Health**
National Institutes of Health
6001 Executive Boulevard
Room 6200, MSC 9663
Bethesda, MD 20892-9663
301-443-4513
866-615-6464; *Fax:* 301-443-4279
TTY: 301-443-8431
nimhinfo@nih.gov
www.nimh.nih.gov

Joshua Gordon, MD, PhD, Director
Shelli Avenevoli, PhD, Deputy Director
Ann D. Huston, Associate Director, Management
Meredith A. Fox, PhD, Director of Communications

The National Institute of Mental Health conducts clinical research on mental disorders and seeks to expand knowledge on mental health treatments.

334 **National Institute on Deafness and Other Communication Disorders**
31 Center Drive
MSC 2320
Bethesda, MD 20892-2320
301-827-8183
800-241-1044; *Fax:* 301-402-0018
TTY: 800-241-1055
www.www.nidcd.nih.gov/

James F. Battey, MD, PhD, Director
Judith A. Cooper, PhD, Deputy Director
Timothy J. Wheeles, Executive Officer
Lisa Portnoy, Chief Administrative Officer

NIDCD is one of the institutes that comprise the National Institutes of Health, and is dedicated to conducting research on communication disorders through biomedical and behavioral research on hearing, balance, taste, speech, language, smell, and voice. The institute also addresses problems associated with communication impairments.

Year Founded: 1988

335 **National Mental Health Consumers' Self-Help Clearinghouse**
1211 Chestnut Street
Suite 1100
Philadelphia, PA 19107
267-507-3810
800-553-4539; *Fax:* 215-636-6312
info@mhselfhelp.org
www.mhselfhelp.org

Joseph Rogers, Founder and Executive Director
Susan Rogers, Director

The Clearinghouse is a peer-run national technical assistance center focused on achieving respect and equality of opportunity for those with mental illnesses. The Clearinghouse helps with the growth of the mental health consumer movement by evaluating mental health services, advocating for mental health reform, and providing consumers with news, information, publications, and consultation services.

Year Founded: 1986

336 **New England Center for Children**
33 Turnpike Road
Southborough, MA 01772-2108
508-481-1015; *Fax:* 508-485-3421
www.necc.org

John Y. Kim, Chair of the Board
Vincent Strully, Jr., President and CEO
Lisa Macenka, Vice Chair of the Board
Michael S. Downey, Chief Financial Officer

A nonprofit research organization dedicated to using education and technology to make a positive impact on the lives of children with autism around the world. Provides evidence-based educational services for parents and teachers and assists autistic children and their families.

Year Founded: 1975

337 The Center for Family Support
2811 Zulette Avenue
Bronx, NY 10461
718-518-1500; *Fax:* 718-518-8200
www.www.cfsny.org/

Steven Vernikoff, Executive Director
Lloyd Stabiner, President
Amy Bittinger, Vice President
Barbara Greenwald, Associate Executive Director

The Center for Family Support offers assistance to individuals with developmental and related disabilities, as well as their families, and provides support services and programs that are designed to accommodate individual needs. Offers services throughout New York City, Westchester County, Long Island, and New Jersey.

Year Founded: 1954

Books

338 A Book: A Collection of Writings from the Advocate
Autism Society of North Carolina Bookstore
4182 Adams Avenue
San Diego, CA 92116
919-743-0204
866-366-3361; *Fax:* 919-743-0208
www.www.autism.com

Beth Sposato, Author
Paul Wendler, Chief Financial Officer
David Laxton, Director, Communications
Kay Walker, Director, Development

A collection of articles and writings from the Advocate, the national newsletter of the Autism Society of America. *$12.00*

93 pages Year Founded: 1967

339 A Parent's Guide to Asperger Syndrome and High-Functioning Autism
Guilford Press
72 Spring Street
New York, NY 10012
212-431-9800
800-365-7006; *Fax:* 212-966-6708
info@guilford.com
www.guilford.com

Sally Ozonoff, Author
Geraldine Dawson, Author
James McPartland, Author

How to Meet the Challenges and Help Your Child Thrive. Covers definitions, diagnsosis, causes and treatments as well as living with AS-HFA, channeling a child's strengths, and dealing with home and social world and life as an adult. *$18.95*

278 pages Year Founded: 1973 ISBN 1-572305-31-2

340 Activities for Developing Pre-Skill Concepts in Children with Autism
Autism Society of North Carolina Bookstore
505 Oberlin Road
Suite 230
Raleigh, NC 27605-1345
919-743-0204
800-442-2762; *Fax:* 919-743-0208
www.www.autismsociety-nc.org

Toni Flowers, Author
Paul Wendler, Chief Financial Officer
David Laxton, Director, Communications
Kay Walker, Director, Development

Chapters include auditory development, concept development, social development and visual-motor integration. *$34.00*

217 pages

341 Adults with Autism
Cambridge University Press
32 Avenue of the Americas
New York, NY 10013-2473
212-337-5000
newyork@cambrigde.org
www.www.cambridge.org

Hugh Morgan, Author
Andrew Chandler, Chief Financial Officer
Richard Fisher, Managing Director
Andrew Gilfilan, Managing Director, Europe

Provides pratical help and guidance specifically for those caring for the growing recognized population of adults with autism. *$ 50.00*

312 pages Year Founded: 1534 ISBN 0-521456-83-5

342 Are You Alone on Purpose?
Autism Society of North Carolina Bookstore
505 Oberlin Road
Suite 230
Raleigh, NC 27605-1345
919-743-0204
800-442-2762; *Fax:* 919-743-0208
www.www.autismsociety-nc.org

Nancy Werlin, Author
Paul Wendler, Chief Financial Officer
David Laxton, Director, Communications
Kay Walker, Director, Development

This is the story of Alison, the twin sister of an autistic boy, who develops a friendship with a boy who has become paralyzed. Alison's feelings of isolation from her family and brother are discussed as she develops a true friendship. *$14.95*

211 pages

343 Aspects of Autism: Biological Research
Autism Society of North Carolina Bookstore
505 Oberlin Road
Suite 230
Raleigh, NC 27605-1345
919-743-0204
800-442-2762; *Fax:* 919-743-0208
www.www.autismsociety-nc.org

Lorba Wing, Author
Paul Wendler, Chief Financial Officer
David Laxton, Director, Communications
Kay Walker, Director, Development

Reviews the evidence for a physical cause of autism and the roles of genetics, magnesium and vitamin B6. *$15.00*

120 pages

344 Asperger Syndrome: A Practical Guide for Teachers
ADD WareHouse
300 NorthWest 70th Avenue
Suite 102
Plantation, FL 33317-2360
954-792-8944
800-233-9273; *Fax: 954-792-8545*
websales@addwarehouse.com
www.addwarehouse.com

Harvey C Parker, Owner

A clear and concise guide to effective classroom practice for teachers and support assistants working with children with Asperger Syndrome in school. The authors explain characteristics of children with Asperger Syndrome, discusses methods of assessment and offers practical strategies for effective classroom interventions. *$24.95*

90 pages Year Founded: 1990

345 Asperger's Syndrome: A Guide for Parents and Professionals
ADD WareHouse
300 NorthWest 70th Avenue
Suite 102
Plantation, FL 33317-2360
954-792-8944
800-233-9273; *Fax: 954-792-8545*
websales@addwarehouse.com
www.addwarehouse.com

Harvey C Parker, Owner

Providing a description and analysis of the unusual characteristics of Asperger's syndrome, with strategies to reduce those that are most conspicuous or debilitating. This guide brings together the most relevant and useful information on all aspects of the syndrome, from language and social behavior to motor clumsiness. *$18.95*

223 pages Year Founded: 1990

346 Autism
Autism Society of North Carolina Bookstore
505 Oberlin Road
Suite 230
Raleigh, NC 27605-1345
919-743-0204
800-442-2762; *Fax: 919-743-0208*
www.www.autismsociety-nc.org

Heather Bargett Veague,PhD, Author
Christine Collins,PhD, Editor
David Laxton, Director, Communications
Kay Walker, Directord, Development

In a question-and-answer format, the authors respond to questions about autism asked by countless parents and family members of children and youths with autism. *$26.00*

347 Autism & Asperger Syndrome
Cambridge University Press
32 Avenue of the Americas
New York, NY 10013-2473
212-337-5000
800-872-7423; *Fax: 212-691-3239*
newyork@cambrigde.org
www.www.cambridge.org

Uta Frith, Editor
Andrew Chandler, Chief Financial Officer

Richard Fisher, Managing Director
Andrew Gilfillan, Managidn Director, Europe

Six clinician-researchers present aspects of Asperger Syndrome, one form of autism. Research summaries are enlivened by case studies. *$24.00*

257 pages Year Founded: 1534

348 Autism & Sensing: The Unlost Instinct
Jessica Kingsley Publishers
400 Market Street
Suite 400
Philadelphia, PA 19106-2614
215-922-1161
866-416-1078; *Fax: 215-922-1474*
hello.usa@jkp.com
www.jkp.com

Donna Williams, Author
Dee Brigham, Company Secretary, Director
Jemima Kingsley, Director
Octavia Kingsley, Production Director

Available in paperback. *$26.95*

200 pages Year Founded: 1987 ISBN 1-853026-12-3

349 Autism Bibliography
TASH
29 W Susquehanna Avenue
Suite 210
Baltimore, MD 21204-5218
410-828-8274; *Fax: 410-828-6706*
info@tash.org
www.tash.org

Sobfey , Author
Jean Trainor, Vice President
Barbara Loescher, Treasurer

Three hundred recent references to publications on autism along with brief abstracts. *$9.00*

350 Autism Spectrum
Autism Society of North Carolina Bookstore
505 Oberlin Road
Suite 230
Raleigh, NC 27605-1345
919-743-0204
800-442-2762; *Fax: 919-743-0208*
www.www.autismsociety-nc.org

Chantal Sicile-Kira, Author
Paul Wendler, Chief Financial Officer
David Laxton, Director, Communications
Kay Walker, Director, Development

An excellent publication for new parents and professionals. *$28.95*

360 pages

351 Autism Spectrum Disorders: The Complete Guid to Understanding Autism, Asperger's Syndrome, Pervasive Developmental Disorder, and Other ASDs
Penguin Group (USA)
375 Hudson Street
New York, NY 10014-3672
212-366-2000; *Fax: 212-366-2933*
www.www.penguin.com

John Makinson, Chief Executive Officer
Coram Willimas, Chief Financial Officer
David Shanks, Chief Executive Officer

Twelve years ago, we were in the local doctor's office in a small village in England, where we had just moved.

352 Autism Treatment Guide
Autism Society of North Carolina Bookstore
505 Oberlin Road
Suite 230
Raleigh, NC 27605-1345
919-743-0204
800-442-2762; *Fax:* 919-743-0208
www.www.autismsociety-nc.org

Elizabeth K Gerlach, Author
Paul Wendler, Chief Financial Officer
David Laxton, Director, Communications
Kay Walker, Director, Development

A comprehensive book covering treatments and methods used to help individuals with autism. *$12.75*

157 pages

353 Autism and Pervasive Developmental Disorders
Cambridge University Press
32 Avenue of the Americas
New York, NY 10013-2473
212-337-5000; *Fax:* 212-691-3239
newyork@cambrigde.org
www.www.cambridge.org

Fred R Volkmar, Editor
Andrew Chandler, Chief Financial Officer
Richard Fisher, Managing Director
Andrew Gilfillan, Managing Director, Europe

Featuring contributions from leading authorities in the clinical and social sciences, this volume reflects recent progress in the understanding of autism and related conditions, and offers an international perspective on the present state of the discipline. Chapters cover current approaches to definition and diagnosis; prevalence and planning for service delivery; cognitive, genetic and neurobiological features and pathophysiological mechanisms. *$75.00*

356 pages Year Founded: 1534 ISBN 0-521553-86-5

354 Autism: An Inside-Out Approach An Innovative Look at the Mechanics of Autism and its Developmental Cousins
Jessica Kingsley Publishers
400 Market Street
Suite 400
Philadelphia, PA 19106-2614
215-922-1161
866-416-1078; *Fax:* 215-922-1474
hello.usa@jkp.com
www.jkp.com

Donna Williams, Author
Dee Brigham, Company Secretary, Director
Jemima Kingsley, Director
Octavia Kingsley, Production Director

Written by an autistic person for people with autism and related disorders, carers, and the professionals who work with them, is a practical handbook to understanding, living with and working with autism. *$23.95*

336 pages Year Founded: 1987 ISBN 1-853023-87-6

355 Autism: An Introduction to Psychological Theory
Harvard University Press
79 Garden Street
Cambridge, MA 02138-1400
617-495-2600; *Fax:* 617-495-5898
CONTACT_HUP@harvard.edu
www.www.hup.harvard.edu

Francesca Happe, Author

Provides a concise overview of current psychological theory and research that synthesizes the established work on the biological foundations, cognitive characteristics, and behavioral manifestations of this disorder. *$32.00*

160 pages Year Founded: 1913 ISBN 0-674053-12-5

356 Autism: Explaining the Enigma
Autism Society of North Carolina Bookstore
505 Oberlin Road
Suite 230
Raleigh, NC 27605-1345
919-743-0204
800-442-2762; *Fax:* 919-743-0208
www.www.autismsociety-nc.org

Uta Frith, Author
Paul Wendler, Chief Financial Officer
David Laxton, Director, Communications
Kay Walker, Director, Development

Explains the nature of autism. *$27.95*

264 pages

357 Autism: From Tragedy to Triumph
Branden Publishing Company
PO Box 812094
Wellesley, MA 02482-13
Fax: 781-790-1056
www.www.brandenbooks.com

Julia Crowder, Author
Carol Johnson, Author

A new book that deals with the Lovaas method and includes a foreward by Dr. Ivar Lovaas. The book is broken down into two parts, the long road to diagnosis and then treatment. *$12.95*

187 pages Year Founded: 1998 ISBN 0-828319-65-0

358 Autism: Identification, Education and Treatment
Autism Society of North Carolina Bookstore
505 Oberlin Road
Suite 230
Raleigh, NC 27605-1345
919-743-0204
800-442-2762; *Fax:* 919-743-0208
www.www.autismsociety-nc.org

Dianne Zager, Author
Psul Wendler, Chief Financial Officer
David Laxton, Director, Communications
Kay Walker, Director, Development

Chapters include medical treatments, early intervention and communication and development in autism. *$36.00*

392 pages

359 Autism: Nature, Diagnosis and Treatment
Guilford Press
72 Spring Street
Department 4E
New York, NY 10012-4019
212-431-9800
800-365-7006; *Fax:* 212-966-6708
exam@guilford.com

Geraldine Dawson, Author

Foremost experts explore new perspectives on the nature and treatment of autism. Covering theory, research and the development of hypotheses and models, this book provides a balance between depth and breadth by focusing on questions most central to the field. For each question, an expert examines theoretical issues as well as empirical findings to offer new directions and testable hypotheses for future research. *$51.00*

417 pages ISBN 0-898627-24-9

360 Autism: Strategies for Change
Groden Center
86 Mount Hope Avenue
Providence, RI 02906-1648
401-274-6310; *Fax:* 401-421-3280
grodencenter@grodencenter.org
www.grodencenter.org

Gerald Groden, Editor
M Grace Baron, Editor

A comprehensive approach to the education and treatment of children with autism and related disorders. Clinicians, parents, and students of autism who are, or want to be advocates for change will find in this book a blueprint, and much detail, on how to bring change about. This applies at the level of program planning and management as well as of clinical or education practice. *$21.95*

350 pages Year Founded: 1976

361 Autistic Adults at Bittersweet Farms
Haworth Press
10 Alice Street
Binghamton, NY 13904-1503
607-722-5857
800-429-6784; *Fax:* 607-722-1424
getinfo@haworthpressinc.com
www.haworthpress.com

Norman Giddan, Author
Jane J Giddan, Author

A touching view of an inspirational residential care program for autistic adolescents and adults. *$17.95*

226 pages ISBN 1-560240-57-1

362 Avoiding Unfortunate Situations
Autism Society of North Carolina Bookstore
505 Oberlin Road
Suite 230
Raleigh, NC 27605-1345
919-743-0204
800-442-2762; *Fax:* 919-743-0208
info@autismsociety-nc.org
www.www.autismsociety-nc.org

Dennis Debbaudt, Author
Ellen Kerfoot, Editor
David Laxton, Director, Communications
Kay Walker, Director, Development

A collection of tips and information from and about people with autism and other developmental disabilities. *$5.00*

18 pages Year Founded: 1970

363 Beyond Gentle Teaching
Autism Society of North Carolina Bookstore
505 Oberlin Road
Suite 230
Raleigh, NC 27605-1345
919-743-0204
800-442-2762; *Fax:* 919-743-0208
www.www.autismsociety-nc.org

John J McGee, Author
Frank J Menolascino, Author
David Laxton, Director, Communications
Kay Walker, Director, Development

A nonaversive approach to helping those in need. *$35.00*

233 pages

364 Biology of the Autistic Syndromes
Autism Society of North Carolina Bookstore
505 Oberlin Road
Suite 230
Raleigh, NC 27605-1345
919-743-0204
800-442-2762; *Fax:* 919-743-0208
www.www.autismsociety-nc.org

Christopher Gillberg, Author
Mary Coleman, Author
David Laxton, Director, Communications
Kay Walker, Director, Development

A revision of the original, classic text in the light of new developments and current knowledge. This book covers the epidemiological, genetic, biochemical, immunological and neuropsychological literature on autism. *$74.95*

300 pages

365 Camps 2009-2010
Resources for Children with Special Needs
116 E 16th Street
5th Floor
New York, NY 10003-2164
212-677-4650; *Fax:* 212-254-4070
info@resourcenyc.org
www.resourcesnyc.org

Rachel Howard, Executive Director
Vicky Garwood Burton, Executive, Development Assistant
Hilda Melendez, Family, Community Educator

The guide includes a dozen new camps and updates on more than 300 camps and programs that provide a wide range of summer activities for children with emotional, developmental, learning and physical disabilities, health issues and other special needs. Day camps in the New York metro area are included as well as sleepaway camps in the Northeast. *$25.00*

133 pages Year Founded: 2009 ISBN 0-967836-57-3

366 Children with Autism: A Developmental Perspective
Harvard University Press
79 Garden Street
Cambridge, MA 02138-1400
617-495-2600; *Fax:* 617-495-5898
CONTACT_HUP@harvard.edu
www.www.hup.harvard.edu

Marian Sigman, Author
Lisa Capps, Author

Views autism through the lens of developmental psychpathology, a discipline grounded in the belief that studies of normal and abnormal development can inform and enhance one another.

284 pages Year Founded: 1913

367 Children with Autism: Parents' Guide
Woodbine House
6510 Bells Mill Road
Bethesda, MD 20817-1636
301-897-3570
800-843-7323; *Fax:* 301-897-5838
info@woodbinehouse.com
www.woodbinehouse.com

Michael D. Powers, Editor

Recommended as the first book parents should read, this completely revised volume offers information and a complete introduction to autism, while easing the family's fears and concerns as they adjust and cope with their child's disorder. *$14.95*

456 pages ISBN 1-890627-04-6

368 Communication Unbound: How Facilitated Communication Is Challenging Views
Baker & Taylor International
2709 Water Ridge Parkway
Charlotte, NC 28217-4596
704-357-3500
800-775-1800
www.btol.com

Tom Morgan, Chairman, CEO
Arnie Wright, President, COO
Jeff Leonard, Chief Financial Officer
George Coe, Pres of Library Education

Addresses the ways in which we receive persons with autism in our society, our community and our lives. *$18.95*

240 pages

369 Diagnosis and Treatment of Autism
Autism Society of North Carolina Bookstore
505 Oberlin Road
Suite 230
Raleigh, NC 27605-1345
919-743-0204
800-442-2762; *Fax:* 919-743-0208
www.www.autismsociety-nc.org

Christopher Gillberg, Editor
Paul Wendler, Chief Financial Officer
David Laxton, Director, Communications
Kay Walker, Director, Development

Various chapters written by professionals working with autistic children and adults. *$110.00*

370 Facilitated Communication and Technology Guide
Autism Society of North Carolina Bookstore
505 Oberlin Road
Suite 230
Raleigh, NC 27605-1345
919-743-0204
800-442-2762; *Fax:* 919-743-0208
www.www.autismsociety-nc.org

Carol Lee Berger, Author
Paul Wendler, Chief Financial Officer
David Laxton, Director, Communications
Kay Walker, Director, Development

Chapters include technology and facilitated communication, augmentative and alternative communication, spelling boards, speech synthesizers and software. *$20.00*

371 Fighting for Darla: Challenges for Family Care & Professional Responsibility
Baker & Taylor International
2709 Water Ridge Parkway
Charlotte, NC 28217-4596
704-357-3500
800-775-1800
www.btol.com

Follows the story of Darla, a pregnant adolescent with autism. *$18.95*

176 pages ISBN 0-807733-56-3

372 Fragile Success - Ten Autistic Children, Childhood to Adulthood
Autism Society of North Carolina Bookstore
505 Oberlin Road
Suite 230
Raleigh, NC 27605-1345
919-743-0204
800-442-2762; *Fax:* 919-743-0208
www.www.autismsociety-nc.org

Virgina Walker Sperry, Author
Paul Wendler, Chief Financial Officer
David Laxton, Director, Communications
Kay Walker, Director, Development

A book about the lives of autistic children, whom the author has followed from their early years at the Elizabeth Ives School in New Haven, CT, through to adulthood. *$24.95*

304 pages

373 Handbook of Autism and Pervasive Developmental Disorders
ADD WareHouse
300 NW 70th Avenue
Suite 102
Plantation, FL 33317-2360
954-792-8944
800-233-9273; *Fax:* 954-792-8545
sales@addwarehouse.com
www.addwarehouse.com

Harvey C Parker, Owner

A comprehensive view of all information presently available about autism and other pervasive developmental disorders, drawing on findings and clinical experience from a number of related disciplines psychiatry, psychology, neurobiology and pediatrics. *$95.00*

1092 pages

374 Helping People with Autism Manage Their Behavior
Autism Society of North Carolina Bookstore
505 Oberlin Road
Suite 230
Raleigh, NC 27605-1345

919-743-0204
800-442-2762; *Fax:* 919-743-0208
www.www.autismsociety-nc.org

Nancy J Darylmple, Author
Paul Wendler, Chief Financial Officer
David Laxton, Director, Communications
Kay Walker, Director, Development

Covers the broad topic of helping people with autism manage their behavior. *$7.00*

375 Hidden Child: The Linwood Method for Reaching the Autistic Child
Woodbine House
6510 Bells Mill Road
Bethesda, MD 20817-1636
301-897-3570
800-843-7323; *Fax:* 301-897-5838
info@woodbinehouse.com
www.woodbinehouse.com

Jeanne Simons, Author
Sabine Oishi, Author

Chronicle of the Linwood Children's Center's successful treatment program for autistic children. *$14.95*

251 pages Year Founded: 1985 ISBN 0-933149-06-9

376 How to Teach Autistic & Severely Handicapped Children
Autism Society of North Carolina Bookstore
505 Oberlin Road
Suite 230
Raleigh, NC 27605-1345
919-743-0204
800-442-2762; *Fax:* 919-743-0208

Laura Schreibman, Author
Robert L Koegel, Author
David Laxton, Director, Communications
Kay Walker, Director, Development

Book provides procedures for effectively assessing and teaching autistic and other severely handicapped children. *$9.00*

377 I'm Not Autistic on the Typewriter
TASH
2013 H Street NW
Suite 715
Washington, D. 20006
202-540-9020; *Fax:* 202-540-9019
info@tash.org
www.tash.org

Barbara Trader, Executive Director
Jonathan Riethmaier, Advocacy Communications Manager
Edwin Canizalez, Events and Training Manager
Jenny Stonemeier, Education Policy Director

An introduction to the facilitated communication training method. *$25.00*

378 Inner Life of Children with Special Needs
Taylor & Francis
325 Chestnut Street
Philadelphia, PA 19106-2614
215-625-8900; *Fax:* 215-625-2940
www.taylorandfrancis.com

Ved Prakash Varma, Editor

210 pages

379 Joey and Sam
Autism Society of North Carolina Bookstore
505 Oberlin Road
Suite 230
Raleigh, NC 27605-1345
919-743-0204
800-442-2762; *Fax:* 919-743-0208
www.www.autismsociety-nc.org

IIlana Katz, Author
M.D.Ritvo Edward, Author
David Laxton, Director, Communications
Kay Walker, Director, Development

A beautifully illustrated storybook for children, focusing on a family with two sons, one of whom suffers from autism. *$16.95*

1 pages

380 Keys to Parenting the Child with Autism
Autism Society of North Carolina Bookstore
505 Oberlin Road
Suite 230
Raleigh, NC 27605-1345
919-743-0204
800-442-2762; *Fax:* 919-743-0208
www.www.autismsociety-nc.org

Marlene Targ Brill,Med, Author
Paul Wendler, Chief Financial Officer
David Laxton, Director, Communications
Kay Walker, Director, Development

This book explains what autism is and how it is diagnosed. *$7.95*

224 pages

381 Kristy and the Secret of Susan
Autism Society of North Carolina Bookstore
505 Oberlin Road
Suite 230
Raleigh, NC 27605-1345
919-743-0204
800-442-2762; *Fax:* 919-743-0208
www.www.autismsociety-nc.org

Tracey Sheriff, Chief Executive Officer
Paul Wendler, Chief Financial Officer
David Laxton, Director, Communications
Kay Walker, Director, Development

This book discusses Kristy and her new baby-sitting charge, Susan. Susan can't speak but sings beautifully. Susan is autistic. *$ 3.50*

382 Learning and Cognition in Autism
Kluwer Academic/Plenum Publishers
233 Spring Street
New York, NY 10013-1522
212-242-1490

Mads Soegaard, Editor-in-Chief

Collection of papers written by experts in the field of autism. Describes the cognitive and educational characteristics of people with autism and explains intervention techniques and strategies. Topics include motivating communication in children with autism and a chapter by a high-functioning woman with autism who discusses special learning problems and unique learning strengths that characterize their development and offers specific suggestions for working with people like herself. *$59.00*

368 pages ISBN 0-306448-71-8

383 Let Community Employment Be the Goal For Individuals with Autism
Autism Society of North Carolina Bookstore
505 Oberlin Road
Suite 230
Raleigh, NC 27605-1345
919-743-0204
800-442-2762; *Fax:* 919-743-0208
www.www.autismsociety-nc.org

Joanne Suomi, Author
Paul Wendler, Chief Financial Officer
David Laxton, Director, Communications
Kay Walker, Director, Development

A guide designed for people who are responsible for preparing individuals with autism to enter the work force. *$7.00*

60 pages

384 Let Me Hear Your Voice
Autism Society of North Carolina Bookstore
505 Oberlin Road
Suite 230
Raleigh, NC 27605-1345
919-743-0204
800-442-2762; *Fax:* 919-743-0208
www.www.autismsociety-nc.org

Catherine Maurice, Author
Paul Wendler, Chief Financial Officer
David Laxton, Director, Communications
Kay Walker, Director, Development

The Maruice family's second and third children were diagnosed with autism. This book recounts their experience with a home program using behavior therapy. *$13.95*

400 pages

385 Letting Go
Autism Society of North Carolina Bookstore
505 Oberlin Road
Suite 230
Raleigh, NC 27605-1345
919-743-0204
800-442-2762; *Fax:* 919-743-0208
www.www.autismsociety-nc.org

Philip Roth, Author
Paul Wendler, Chief Financial Officer
David Laxton, Director, Communications
Kay Walker, Director, Development

A book of poems about a journey, an emotional road of placing a child in a residential group home for children with autism. *$7.50*

640 pages

386 Management of Autistic Behavior
Pro-Ed Publications
8700 Shoal Creek Boulevard
Austin, TX 78757-6897
512-451-3246
800-897-3202; *Fax:* 512-451-8542
info@proedinc.com

Donald D Hammill, Owner

Comprehensive and practical book that tells what works best with specific problems. *$41.00*

450 pages ISBN 0-890791-96-1

387 Mindblindness: An Essay on Autism and Theory of Mind
Autism Society of North Carolina Bookstore
505 Oberlin Road
Suite 230
Raleigh, NC 27605-1345
919-743-0204
800-442-2762; *Fax:* 919-743-0208
www.www.autismsociety-nc.org

Simon Baron-Cohen, Author
David Laxton, Director, Communications
Kay Walker, Director, Development

Interpretations and research into the theory of mindblindness in children with autism. *$19.95*

200 pages ISBN 0-262023-84-9

388 Mixed Blessings
Autism Society of North Carolina Bookstore
505 Oberlin Road
Suite 230
Raleigh, NC 27605-1345
919-743-0204
800-442-2762; *Fax:* 919-743-0208
www.autismsociety-nc.org

Danielle Steel, Author
Paul Wendler, Chief Financial Officer
David Laxton, Director, Communications
Kay Walker, Director, Development

A real-life family discusses the raising of their autistic son. *$19.95*

432 pages

389 More Laughing and Loving with Autism
Autism Society of North Carolina Bookstore
505 Oberlin Road
Suite 230
Raleigh, NC 27605-1345
919-743-0204
800-442-2762; *Fax:* 919-743-0208
www.autismsociety-nc.org

R Wayne Gilpin, Author
Paul Wendler, Chief Financial Officer
David Laxton, Director, Communications
Kay Walker, Director, Development

A collection of warm and humorous parent stories about raising a child with autism. *$9.95*

108 pages

390 Neurobiology of Autism
Johns Hopkins University Press
2715 N Charles Street
Baltimore, MD 21218-4319
410-516-6900
800-537-5487; *Fax:* 410-516-6998
www.www.press.jhu.edu

Kathleen Keane, Director
Stacey Armstead, Info Systems Manager
Kelly Rogers, Rights Manager
Jack Holmes, Director, Development

This 2nd edition discusses recent advances in scientific research that point to a neurobiological basis for autism and examines the clinical implications of this research. *$44.95*

272 pages Year Founded: 2005 ISBN 0-801856-80-9

391 News from the Border: a Mother's Memoir of Her Autistic Son
Houghton Mifflin Company
222 Berkeley Street
Boston, MA 02116-3760
617-351-5000; *Fax:* 617-351-1105
www.www.hmhco.com/

Barry O'Callaghan, CEO

A searingly honest account of the author's family experiences with autism. Raising an autistic child is the central, ongoing drama of her married life in this riveting account of acceptance and coping. *$22.95*

384 pages

392 Nobody Nowhere
Autism Society of North Carolina Bookstore
505 Oberlin Road
Suite 230
Raleigh, NC 27605-1345
919-743-0204
800-442-2762; *Fax:* 919-743-0208
www.www.autismsociety-nc.org

Donna Williams, Author
Paul Wendler, Chief Finacial Officer
David Laxton, Director, Communications
Kay Walker, Director, Development

An autobiography giving readers a tour of the author's life with autism. *$14.00*

219 pages

393 Parent Survival Manual
Autism Society of North Carolina Bookstore
505 Oberlin Road
Suite 230
Raleigh, NC 27605-1345
919-743-0204
800-442-2762; *Fax:* 919-743-0208
www.autismsociety-nc.org

Eric Schopler, Editor
Paul Wendler, Chief Financial Officer
David Laxton, Director, Communications
Kay Walker, Director, Development

Compiled from three hundred fifty anecdotes told by parents of autistic and developmentally disabled children. *$38.50*

224 pages

394 Parent's Guide to Autism
Autism Society of North Carolina Bookstore
505 Oberlin Road
Suite 230
Raleigh, NC 27605-1345
919-743-0204
800-442-2762; *Fax:* 919-743-0208
www.www.autismsociety-nc.org

Charles A Hart, Author
Paul Wendler, Chief Financial Officer
David Laxton, Director, Communications
Kay Walker, Director, Development

An essential handbook for anyone facing autism. *$14.00*

256 pages

395 Please Don't Say Hello
Human Sciences Press
233 Spring Street
New York, NY 10013-1522
212-620-8000; *Fax:* 212-807-1047

A nine-year-old autistic boy is able to emerge from his shell with the support and love of his family and neighborhood children. *$10.95*

47 pages ISBN 0-898851-99-8

396 Preschool Issues in Autism
Kluwer Academic/Plenum Publishers
233 Spring Street
New York, NY 10013-1522
212-242-1490
www.www.springer.com

Derk Haank, Chief Executive Officer
Martin Mos, Chief Operating Officer
Dr Ulrich Vest, Chief Financial Officer
Ralf Birkelbach, Executive Vice President

Combines some of the most important theory and data related to the early identification and intervention in autism and related disorders. Addresses clinical aspects, parental concerns and legal issues. Helps professionals understand and implement state-of-the-art services for young children and their families. *$54.00*

276 pages ISBN 0-306444-40-2

397 Psychoeducational Profile
Autism Society of North Carolina Bookstore
505 Oberlin Road
Suite 230
Raleigh, NC 27605-1345
919-743-0204
800-442-2762; *Fax:* 919-743-0208
www.www.autismsociety-nc.org

Tracey Sheriff, Chief Executive Officer
Paul Wendler, Chief Financial Officer
David Laxton, Director, Communications
Kay Walker, Director, Development

The PEP-R is a revision of the popular instrument that has been used for over twenty years to assess skills and behavior of autistic and communication-handicapped children who function between the ages of 6 months and 7 years. *$74.00*

398 Reaching the Autistic Child: a Parent Training Program
Brookline Books/Lumen Editions
8 Trumbell Road
Suite B-001
Northampton, MA 01060
413-584-0184
800-666-2665; *Fax:* 413-584-6184
www.brooklinebooks.com

Detailed case studies of social and behavioral change in autistic children and their families show parents how to implement the principles for improved socialization and behavior. Revised and updated 1998. *$15.95*

ISBN 1-571290-56-7

399 Record Books for Individuals with Autism
Indiana Institute on Disability and Community
Indiana University
2853 E Tenth Street
Bloomington, IN 47408-2601
812-855-9396
800-280-7010; *Fax:* 812-855-9630
TTY: 812-855-9396
uap@indiana.edu
www.www.iidc.indiana.edu

Cathy Pratt, Center Director
Pamela Anderson, Outreach/Resource Specialist
Scott Bellini, PhD, Assistant Center Director
Donna Beasley, Adminstrative Program Secretary

This book was developed with parent information about an autistic child so that it is organized, easily accessible and can be copied as needed. *$5.00*

37 pages

400 Russell Is Extra Special
Autism Society of North Carolina Bookstore
505 Oberlin Road
Suite 230
Raleigh, NC 27605-1345
919-743-0204
800-442-2762; *Fax:* 919-743-0208
www.www.autismsociety-nc.org

Charles A Amenta, Author
Paul Wendler, Chief Financial Officer
David Laxton, Director, Communications
Kay Walker, Director, Development

A sensitive portrayal of an autistic boy written by his father. *$8.95*

32 pages

401 Schools for Students with Special Needs
Resources for Children with Special Needs
116 E 16th Street
Fifth Floor
New York City, NY 10003-2112
212-677-4650; *Fax:* 212-254-4070
info@resourcesnyc.org
www.resourcesnyc.org

Rachel Howard, Executive Director
Vicky Garwood Burton, Executive Development Asst
Hilda Melendez, Family and Community Educator

The first complete book listing private day and residential schools for parents, caregivers and professionals seeking schools for students 5 and up with developmental, emotional, physical and learning disabilities in the NYC metro area. More than 400 schools and residential programs that serve children in the elementary through high school grades are listed with contact information, ages and populations served, class sizes and student-teacher ratios, special services and diplomas offered. Includes a 46-page section of Schools for Children with Autism Spectrum Disorders, as well as a guide with a list of websites on autism spectrum disorders. *$25.00*

342 pages

402 Sex Education: Issues for the Person with Autism
Indiana Institute on Disability and Community
Indiana University
2853 E Tenth Street
Bloomington, IN 47408-2601
812-855-9396
800-280-7010; *Fax:* 812-855-9630
TTY: 812-855-9396
uap@indiana.edu

Michael McRobbie, President
Karen Adams, Chief of Staff
Kelly Kish, Deputy Chief of Staff

Discusses issues of sexuality and provides some methods of instruction for persons with autism. *$3.00*

18 pages

403 Siblings of Children with Autism: A Guide for Families
Autism Society of North Carolina Bookstore
505 Oberlin Road
Suite 230
Raleigh, NC 27605-1345
919-743-0204
800-442-2762; *Fax:* 919-743-0208
www.www.autismsociety-nc.org

Sandra L Harris, Author
Beth A Glasberg, Author
David Laxton, Director, Communications
Kay Walker, Director, Development

Offers information on the needs of a child with autism. *$16.95*

164 pages

404 Somebody Somewhere
Autism Society of North Carolina Bookstore
505 Oberlin Road
Suite 230
Raleigh, NC 27605-1345
919-743-0204
800-442-2762; *Fax:* 919-743-0208
www.autismsociety-nc.org

Donna Williams, Author
Paul Wendler, Chief Financial Officer
David Laxton, Director, Communications
Kay Walker, Director, Development

Offers a revealing account of the author's battle with autism. *$15.00*

256 pages

405 Soon Will Come the Light
Autism Society of North Carolina Bookstore
505 Oberlin Road
Suite 230
Raleigh, NC 27605-1345
919-743-0204
800-442-2762; *Fax:* 919-743-0208
www.autismsociety-nc.org

Thomas A McKean, Author
R Wayne Gilpin, Editor
David Laxton, Director, Communications
Kay Walker, Director, Development

Offers new perspectives on the perplexing disability of autism. *$19.95*

156 pages

406 Teaching Children with Autism: Strategies to Enhance Communication
Autism Society of North Carolina Bookstore
505 Oberlin Road
Suite 230
Raleigh, NC 27605-1345
919-743-0204
800-442-2762; *Fax:* 919-743-0208
www.autismsociety-nc.org

Kathleen Ann Quill, Editor
Paul Wendler, Chief Financial Officer
David Laxton, Director, Communications
Kay Walker, Director, Development

This valuable new book describes teaching strategies and instructional adaptations which promote communication and socialization in children with autism. *$34.95*

315 pages

407 Teaching and Mainstreaming Autistic Children
Love Publishing Company
9101 East Kenyon Avenue
Suite 2200
Denver, CO 80237-1854
303-221-7333; *Fax:* 303-221-7444
lpc@lovepublishing.com
www.lovepublishing.com

Peter Knoblock, Author

Dr Knoblock advocates a highly organized, structured environment for autistic children, with teachers and parents working together. His premise is that the learning and social needs of autistic children must be analyzed and a daily program be designed with interventions that respond to this functional analysis of their behavior. *$39.95*

360 pages Year Founded: 1968 ISBN 0-891081-11-9

408 Ten Things Every Child with Autism Wishes You Knew
Future Horizons
721 West Abram Street
Arlington, TX 76013-6995
817-277-0727
800-489-0727; *Fax:* 817-277-2270
www.fhautism.com

Ellen Notbohm, Author
Jennifer Gilpin, Vice President
Kelly Gilpin, Editorial Director

Framed in both humor and compassion, the book defines the top ten characteristics that illuminate the minds and hearts of cildren with autism. Ellen's personal experiences.

200 pages

409 The Comprehensive Directory
Resources For Children with Special Needs
116 East 16th Street
5th Floor
New York, NY 10003-2164
212-677-4650; *Fax:* 212-254-4070
info@resourcesnyc.org
www.resourcesnyc.org

Ellen Miller-Wachtel, Chair
Shon E Glusky, President
Rachel Howard, Executive Director
Stephen Stern, Director of Finance and Administ

The directory for everyone who needs to find services for children with disabilities and special needs. Designed for parents, caregivers and professionals, it includes more than 2,500 agencies providing more than 4,000 services and programs. *$30.00*

1096 pages Year Founded: 1983 ISBN 0-967836-51-4

410 The Hidden Child: Youth with Autism
Mason Crest Publishers
450 Parkway Drive
Suite D
Broomall, PA 19008-4017
610-543-6200
866-627-2665; *Fax:* 610-543-3878
dtaylor@masoncrest.com
www.masoncrest.com

Sherry Bonice, Author
Dan Hilferty, President
Michelle Luke, Dir of Marketing, PR
Michael Toglia, Special Sales

Hope is the keyword for the autistic child's future. Through education, early intervention, and continued research, children with autism can live normal lives. Factual information about autism, the Autism Society of America, sibshops, and different educational treatments will expand the reader's knowledge of this condition. A fictional story told from a sibling's point of view helps the reader understand the effects autism has on individuals and family members.

128 pages ISBN 1-590847-38-9

411 Thinking In Pictures, Expanded Edition: My Life with Autism
Vintage
1745 Broadway
New York, NY 10019
212-782-9000
800-733-3000; *Fax:* 212-572-6043
ecustomerservice@randomhouse.com
www.randomhouse.com

Temple Grandin, Author

304 pages ISBN 0-307275-65-5

412 Transition Matters from School to Independence
Resources for Children with Special Needs
116 East 16th Street
5th Floor
New York, NY 10003-2164
212-677-4650; *Fax:* 212-254-4070
info@resourcesnyc.org
www.resourcesnyc.org

Ellen Miller-Wachtel, Chair
Shon E Glusky, President
Rachel Howard, Executive Director
Stephen Stern, Director of Finance and Administ

Youth with disabilities need special guidance when moving from school to adult life. Transition Matters covers every aspect of moving from high school to the world of postsecondary education, job training, employment and idependent living. This guide for parents, caregivers and educators presents a wealth of information about the transition process, and lists 1,000 agencies and organizations that provide services for youth 14 and up. It explains entitlements and options and helps families navigate systems and procedures. *$15.00*

512 pages Year Founded: 1983 ISBN 0-967836-56-5

413 Ultimate Stranger: The Autistic Child
Autism Society of North Carolina Bookstore
505 Oberlin Road
Suite 230
Raleigh, NC 27605-1345
919-743-0204
800-442-2762; *Fax:* 919-743-0208
www.www.autismsociety-nc.org

Carl H Delacato, Author
Paul Wendler, Chief Financial Officer
David Laxton, Director, Communications
Kay Walker, Director, Development

Delacato's thesis is that autism is neuro-genic and not psy-cho-genic in origin. *$10.00*

240 pages

414 Understanding Autism
Fanlight Productions
32 Court Street
21st Floor
Brooklyn, NY 11201
718-488-8900
800-937-4113; *Fax:* 718-488-8642
info@fanlight.com
www.fanlight.com

Suzanne Newman, Director

Parents of children with autism discuss the nature and symptoms of this lifelong disability, and outline a treatment program based on behavior modification principles. *$195.00*

ISBN 1-572951-00-1

415 Until Tomorrow: A Family Lives with Autism
Autism Society of North Carolina Bookstore
505 Oberlin Road
Suite 230
Raleigh, NC 27605-1345
919-743-0204
800-442-2762; *Fax:* 919-743-0208
www.autismsociety-nc.org

Dorothy Zeitz, Author
Paul Wendler, Chief Financial Officer
David Laxton, Director, Communications
Kay Walker, Director, Development

The central theme of this book is an effort to show what it is like to live with a child who cannot communicate. *$10.00*

416 When Snow Turns to Rain
Woodbine House
6510 Bells Mill Road
Bethesda, MD 20817-1636
301-897-3570
800-843-7323; *Fax:* 301-897-5838
info@woodbinehouse.com
www.woodbinehouse.com

Craig B Schulze, Author

A gripping personal account of one family's experiences with autism. Chronicles a family's journey from parental bliss to devastation, as they learn that their son has autism. This book delves into diagnosis, treatments, and attitudes toward persons with autism. *$14.95*

216 pages Year Founded: 1985 ISBN 0-933149-63-8

417 Winter's Flower
Autism Society of North Carolina Bookstore
505 Oberlin Road
Suite 230
Raleigh, NC 27605-1345
919-743-0204
800-442-2762; *Fax:* 919-743-0208
www.autismsociety-nc.org

Ranae Johnson, Author
Paul Wendler, Chief Financial Officer
David Laxton, Director, Communications
Kay Walker, Director, Development

The story of Ranae Johnson's quest to rescue her son from a world of silence. A story of love, patience and dedication. *$12.95*

418 Without Reason
Autism Society of North Carolina Bookstore
505 Oberlin Road
Suite 230
Raleigh, NC 27605-1345
919-743-0204
800-442-2762; *Fax:* 919-743-0208
www.autismsociety-nc.org

Charles A Hart, Author
Paul Wendler, Chief Financial Officer
David Laxton, Director, Communications
Kay Walker, Director, Development

A story of a family coping with two generations of autism. *$19.95*

292 pages

Periodicals & Pamphlets

419 Autism Matters
Autism Society Ontario
1179 King Street West
Suite 004
Toronto, ON M6K 3-5
416-246-9592
800-472-7789; *Fax:* 416-246-9417
mail@autismsociety.on.ca
www.autismsociety.on.ca

Covers society activities and contains information on autism. Recurring features include news of research, a calendar of events, reports of meetings, and book reviews. *$25.00*

10 pages 4 per year

420 Autism Research Review International
Autism Research Institute
4182 Adams Avenue
San Diego, CA 92116-2599
619-281-7165; *Fax:* 619-563-6840
www.autism.com

Stephen M Edelson, PhD, Executive Director
Jane Johnson, Managing Director
Valerie Paradiz ,PhD, Director,ARI Autistic Global Ins
Rebecca McKenney, Office Manager

Discusses current research and provides information about the causes, diagnosis, and treatment of autism and related disorders. *$18.00*

8 pages 4 per year Year Founded: 1976 ISSN 0893-8474

421 Autism Society News
Utah Parent Center
230 West 200 South
Suite 1101
Salt Lake City, UT 84117-4428
801-272-1067
800-468-1160; *Fax:* 801-272-8907
www.utahparentcenter.org

Helen Post, Executive Director

Presents news, research information, and legislative updates regarding autism. Recurring features include a calendar of events and columns titled Parent Meetings, What's On in the News, Research News, Parent Corner, Legislative Summary, and A Big Thank You!

8 pages

422 Autism Spectrum Disorders in Children and Adolescents
Center for Mental Health Services: Knowledge Exchange Network
PO Box 42490
Washington, DC 20015
800-789-2647; *Fax:* 301-984-8796
TDD: 866-889-2647
ken@mentalhealth.org
www.mentalhealth.org

Lee A Wilkinson, Author

This fact sheet defines autism, describes the signs and causes, discusses types of help available, and suggests what parents or other caregivers can do.

264 pages

423 Autism in Children and Adolescents
Center for Mental Health Services: Knowledge Exchange Network
PO Box 42557
Washington, DC 20015-557
800-789-2647; *Fax:* 301-984-8796
TDD: 866-889-2647
ken@mentalhealth.org

This fact sheet defines autism, describes the signs and causes, discusses types of help available, and suggests what parents or other caregivers can do.

2 pages Year Founded: 1997

424 Facts About Autism
Indiana Institute on Disability and Community
1 East 33rd Street
4th Floor
New York, NY 10016
212-252-8584
800-280-7010; *Fax:* 212-252-8676
TTY: 812-855-9396
uap@indiana.edu
www.www.autismspeaks.org/

Liz Feld, President
Jennifer Bizub, Chief Human Resources Officer
Alec M Elbert, Chief Strategy and Development O
Jamitha Fields, Vice President - Community Affai

Provides concise information describing autism, diagnosis, needs of the person with autism from diagnosis through adulthood. Information on the Autism Society of America chapters in Indiana are listed in the back, along with a de-

scription of the Indiana Resource Center for Autism and suggested books to look for in the local library. Also available in Spanish. *$1.00*

425 Journal of Autism and Developmental Disorders
Springer Science & Business Media
Heidelberger Plate 3
14197 Berlin
Germany,
www.springer.com

Fred R. Volkmar, Editor-in-Chief

Features research and case studies involving the entire spectrum of interventions and advances in the diagnosis and classification of disorders.

6 per year Year Founded: 1842 ISSN 0162-3257

426 Sex Education: Issues for the Person with Autism
Autism Society of North Carolina Bookstore
955 Woodland Street
Nashville, TN 37206
615-385-2077
866-508-4987; *Fax:* 615-383-1176
support@autismtn.org
www.www.autismtn.org

Nancy Dalrympale, Author
Susan Gray, Author
Lisa Ruble, Author
Kay Walker, Director, Development

Discusses issues of sexuality and provides methods of instruction for people with autism. *$4.00*

18 pages

427 The Source Newsletter
MAAP
PO Box 524
Crown Point, IN 46308-524
219-662-1311; *Fax:* 219-662-0638
chart@netnitco.net

Story C Landis, Director
Wlater J Koroshetz, MD, Deputy Director
Caroline Lewis, Executive Officer

Newsletter from the Global Information and Support Network for More Advanced Persons with Austism and Asperger's Syndrome.

4 per year

428 Treatment of Children with Mental Disorders
National Institute of Mental Health
6001 Executive Boulevard
Room 8184,MSC 9663
Bethesda, MD 20892-9663
301-443-4513
866-615-6464
TTY: 301-443-8431
nimhinfo@nih.gov
www.www.nimh.nih.gov/

Francis S Collins, MD, PhD, Director

A short booklet that contains questions and answers about therapy for children with mental disorders. Includes a chart of mental disorders and medications used.

Research Centers

429   Indiana Resource Center for Autism (IRCA)
1905 North Range Road
Bloomington, IN 47408-9801
812-855-6508
800-825-4733; *Fax:* 812-855-9630
TTY: 812-855-9396
prattc@indiana.edu
www.iidc.indiana.edu/pages/irca

Cathy Pratt, PhD, BCBA, Center Director
Pamela Anderson, Outreach/Resource Specialist
Catherine Davies, MEd, MSC, LMHC, Educational
Consultant

The Indiana Resource Center for Autism focuses on improving the quality of life for people with autism spectrum disorders, and promotes early diagnosis of autism and effective childhood programs, employment and living options, family support and other opportunities. The Center also conducts research on the most effective methods for supporting individuals with autism, and provides consultations and disseminates information on autism for families and professionals.

430   TEACCH
CB# 6305
University of NC at Chapel Hill
Chapel Hill, NC 27599
919-966-2174; *Fax:* 919-966-4127
teacch@unc.edu
www.teacch.com

Dr Laura Klinger, Director
Rebecca Mabe, Assistant Director of Business a
Walter Kelly, Business Officer
Mark Klinger, Director, Research

This organization is the division for the treatment and education of autistic and related communication handicapped children.

Video & Audio

431   Asperger's Unplugged, an Interview with Jerry Newport
Program Development Associates
32 Court St
21st Floor
Brooklyn, NY 11201
315-452-0643
800-876-1710; *Fax:* 718-488-8642
info@disabilitytraining.com
www.disabilitytraining.com

Meet the man who answered a question in the film 'Rain Man' - How much is 4,343 x 1,234? - before the autistic savant character played by Dustin Hoffman answered it. Jerry Newport discovered Asperger's Syndrome while watching 'Rain Man' and has since become an engaging speaker and self-help organizer. This inspiring interview, available on VHS or DVD, supports teachers, staff developers and people with high functioning autism. 40 minutes. *$79.95*

432   Autism Spectrum Disorders and the SCERTS
Program Development Associates
32 Court St
21st Floor
Brooklyn, NY 11201
315-452-0643
800-876-1710; *Fax:* 718-488-8642
info@disabilitytraining.com
www.disabilitytraining.com

Early intervention for children with Autism Spectrum Disorders. Shows a model in action with higher-functioning children who require less support. 105 minutes between three tapes. *$279.00*

Year Founded: 2004

433   Autism in the Classroom
Program Development Associates
32 Court St
21st Floor
Brooklyn, NY 11201
315-452-0643
800-876-1710; *Fax:* 718-488-8642
info@disabilitytraining.com
www.disabilitytraining.com

Overviews symptoms, behaviors and treatments, and interviews children with autism, along with their parents and their teachers. 16 minutes. *$69.95*

Year Founded: 2004

434   Autism is a World
Program Development Associates
32 Court St
21st Floor
Brooklyn, NY 11201
315-452-0643
800-876-1710; *Fax:* 718-488-8642
info@disabilitytraining.com
www.disabilitytraining.com

Takes a look inside the life of a woman who lives with the disorder. She explains how she feels, how she relates to others, her obsession and why her behavior can be so very different. Gives teachers and professionals striving to understand Autism Spectrum Disorder a glimpse from the inside out of this developmental disability. 40 minutes & can also be ordered as a DVD with special features. *$99.95*

Year Founded: 2004

435   Autism: A Strange, Silent World
Filmakers Library
3212 Duke Street
Alexandria, VA 22314
212-808-4980
sales@alexanderstreet.com

Sue Oscar, Manager

British educators and medical personnel offer insight into autism's characteristics and treatment approaches through the cameos of three children. 52 minutes. *$295.00*

436   Autism: A World Apart
Fanlight Productions
32 Court Street
21st Floor
Brooklyn, NY 11201
718-488-8900
800-876-1710; *Fax:* 718-488-8642
fanlight@fanlight.com
www.fanlight.com

Karen Cunninghame, Author

In this documentary, three families show us what the textbooks and studies cannot; what it's like to live with autism day after day, raise and love children who may be withdrawn and violent and unable to make personal connections with their families. Video cassette. 29 minutes. *$199.00*

ISBN 1-572950-39-0

437 Autism: Being Friends
Indiana Institute on Disability and Community
Indiana University
2853 E Tenth Street
Bloomington, IN 47408-2601
812-855-9396
800-280-7010; *Fax:* 812-855-9630
TTY: 812-855-9396

David Mank, Executive Director

This autism awareness videotape was produced specifically for use with young children. The program portrays the abilities of the child with autism and describes ways in which peers can help the child to be a part of the everyday world. *$10.00*

Year Founded: 1991

438 Avoiding The Turbulance: Guiding Families of Children Diagnosed with Autism
Program Development Associates
32 Court St
21st Floor
Brooklyn, NY 11201
315-452-0643
800-876-1710; *Fax:* 718-488-8642
info@disabilitytraining.com
www.disabilitytraining.com

Focuses primarily on the best strategies of early intervention. Good resources for primary care medical providers and agency professionals involved in early intervention autism programs. 12 minutes. *$79.95*

Year Founded: 2005

439 Breakthroughs: How to Reach Students with Autism
ADD WareHouse
300 NW 70th Avenue
Suite 102
Plantation, FL 33317-2360
954-792-8100
800-233-9273; *Fax:* 954-792-8545
websales@addwarehouse.com
www.addwarehouse.com

Karen Sewell, Author

This video is designed for instructors of children with autism, K-12. The program provides a fully-loaded teacher's manual with reproducible lesson plans that will take you through an entire school year as well as an award-winning video that demonstrates the instructional and behavioral techniques recommended in the manual. Covers math, reading, fine motor, self-help, vocational, social and life skills. Features a veteran instructor who was named 'Teacher of the Year' by the Autism Society of America. *$89.00*

243 pages Year Founded: 1990

440 Children and Autism: Time is Brain
Program Development Associates
PO Box 2038
Syracuse, NY 13220-2038

315-452-0643
800-543-2119; *Fax:* 315-452-0710
info@disabilitytraining.com
www.disabilitytraining.com/autism

Video features Applied Behavior Analysis (ABA) as an autism treatment technique by focusing on two families raising a child with autism. Gives documentation on their interaction with therapists and behavior analysts. 28 minutes. *$99.95*

Year Founded: 2004

441 Dr. Tony Attwood: Asperger's Syndrome Volume 2 DVD
Program Development Associates
32 Court St
21st Floor
Brooklyn, NY 11201
315-452-0643
800-876-1710; *Fax:* 718-488-8642
info@disabilitytraining.com
www.disabilitytraining.com

Following rave national reviews that autism expert Dr. Tony Attwood received for his Volume 1 introduction to Asperger's Syndrome, here's the new DVD of his latest conference presentations. Volume 2 leaps off the DVD screen with Dr. Attwood's interactive, in-depth, theory-of-mind approach to Asperger's. 180 minutes. *$109.95*

442 Going to School with Facilitated Communication
Syracuse University, Facilitated Communication Institute
370 Huntington Hall
Syracuse, NY 13244-1
315-443-9657; *Fax:* 315-443-2274
fcstaff@sued.syr.edu
www.soeweb.syr.edu/thefci

Douglas Biklen, Author

A video in which students with autism and/or severe disabilities illustrate the use of facilitated communication focusing on basic principles fostering facilitated communication.

443 I'm Not Autistic on the Typewriter
Syracuse University, Facilitated Communication Institute
370 Huntington Hall
Syracuse, NY 13244-1
315-443-9657; *Fax:* 315-443-2274
www.soeweb.syr.edu/thefci

A video introducing facilitated communication, a method by which persons with autism express themselves.

11 pages

444 Interview with Dr. Pauline Filipek
Program Development Associates
PO Box 2038
Syracuse, NY 13220-2038
315-452-0643
800-543-2119; *Fax:* 315-452-0710
info@disabilitytraining.com
www.disabilitytraining.com/autism

An interview that presents early stage developmental autism, with diagnosis and age-level comparisons, research, interventions and myths and false and future treatments. 14 minutes. *$79.95*

Year Founded: 2005

445 Matthew: Guidance for Parents with Autistic Children
Program Development Associates
PO Box 2038
Syracuse, NY 13220-2038
315-452-0643
800-543-2119; *Fax:* 315-452-0710
info@disabilitytraining.com
www.disabilitytraining.com/autism

A resource video guide for parents of autistic children. Shows parents where they should go, who to consult and what did or did not work for Matthew and his parents. 28 minutes. *$79.95*

Year Founded: 2004

446 Rising Above a Diagnosis of Autism
Program Development Associates
32 Court St
21st Floor
Brooklyn, NY 11201
315-452-0643
800-876-1710; *Fax:* 718-488-8642
info@disabilitytraining.com

Focuses primarily on the period when a child receives a diagnosis of Autism. Meet with others who are involved somehow with autistic children, and hear recommendations from professionals and meet children that have Autism, PDD, Asperger's Syndrome or any other forms of Austism Spectrum Disorder. 30 minutes. *$99.95*

Year Founded: 2005

447 Rylee's Gift - Asperger Syndrome
Program Development Associates
PO Box 2038
Syracuse, NY 13220-2038
315-452-0643; *Fax:* 315-452-0710
info@disabilitytraining.com
www.disabilitytraining.com

Martha Rylee, Author

This video or DVD spotlights Rylee - through his mother, grandparents, doctor, teacher - and adults with Asperger's Syndrome. Balances views of difficult transitions and meltdown behaviors, with sensory therapy, socialization and the amazing capabilities of people with this syndrome/gift. 56 minutes. *$89.95*

448 Straight Talk About Autism with Parents and Kids
ADD WareHouse
300 NW 70th Avenue
Suite 102
Plantation, FL 33317-2360
954-792-8100
800-233-9273; *Fax:* 954-792-8545
websales@addwarehouse.com
www.addwarehouse.com

Jeff Schultz, Author

These revealing videos contain intimate interviews with parents of kids with autism and the young people themselves. Topics discussed include friends and social isolation, communication difficulties, hypersensitivities, teasing, splinter skills, parent support groups and more. One video focuses on childhood issues, while the second covers adolescent issues. Two 40 minute videos. *$99.00*

Year Founded: 1990

449 Struggling with Life: Asperger's Syndrome
Program Development Associates
PO Box 2038
Syracuse, NY 13220-2038
315-452-0643; *Fax:* 315-452-0710
info@disabilitytraining.com
www.disabilitytraining.com

ABC News correspondent Jay Schadler's report on the neurological disorder called Asperger's focuses on the telling line between intense interests and obsessions. The latter may be an early symptom of the syndrome. This closed caption video is grounded on studies by Fred Voklmar at Yale that explore compulsive fixations and unreadable facial expressions, both of which are typical of Asperger's and inhibit normal peer interactions among children. VHS or DVD. 14 minutes. *$ 69.95*

Web Sites

450 www.aane.org
Asperger's Association of New England

Working advocacy group of Massachusetts parents of adults and teens with AS who have come together with the goal of getting state funding for residential supports for adults with AS. At the present time no state agency will provide these needed supports. Interested parents and AS adults are welcome to join this working group.

451 www.ani.ac
Autism Network International

This organization is run by and for the autistic people. The best advocates for autistic people are autistic people themselves. Provides a forum for autistic people to share information, peer support, tips for coping and problem solving, as well as providing a social outlet for autistic people to explore and participate in autistic social experiences. In addition to promoting self advocacy for high-functioning autistic adults, ANI also works to improve the lives of autistic people who, whether they are too young or because they do not have the communication skills, are not able to advocate for themselves. Helps autistic people by providing information and referrals for parenting and teachers. Also strives to educate the public about autism.

452 www.aspennj.org
Asperger Syndrome Education Network (ASPEN)

Regionally-based non-profit organization headquarted in New Jersey, with 11 local chapters, providing families and those individuals affected with Asperger Syndrome, PDD-NOS, High Function Autism, and related disorders. Provides education about the issues surrounding Asperger Syndrome and other related disorders. Support in knowing that they are not alone and in helping individuals with AS achieve their maximum potential. Advocacy in areas of appropriate educational programs and placement, medical research funding, and increased public awareness and understanding.

453 www.aspergerinfo.com
Aspergers Resource Links

AspergerInfo.com offers a safe place to ask questions, share experiences, and discuss treatments relating to Asperger Syndrome.

454 www.aspergers.com
Aspergers Resource Links

Asperger's Disorder Homepage

455 www.aspergersyndrome.org
Aspergers Resource Links

Barbara Kirby, Founder

A collection of web resources on Asperger's Syndrome and related topics. Hosted by the University of Delaware.

456 www.aspiesforfreedom.com
Aspies for Freedom

Aspies for Freedom (AFF) is a web site with chat rooms, forums and information relating to Austism and Asperger's Syndrome.

457 www.autism-society.org
Autism Society of America

Promotes lifelong access and opportunities for persons within the autism spectrum and their families, to be fully included, participating members of their communities through advocacy, public awareness, education and research related to autism.

458 www.autism.org
Center for the Study of Autism (CSA)

Located in the Salem/Portland, Oregon area. Provides information about autism to parents and professionals, and conducts research on the efficacy of various therapeutic interventions. Much of our research is in collaboration with the Autism Research Institute in San Diego, California.

459 www.autismresearchinstitute.org
Autism Research Institute

Devoted to conducting research on the causes of autism and on the methods of preventing, diagnosing and treating autism and other severe behavioral disorders of childhood.

460 www.autismservicescenter.org
Autism Services Center

Makes available technical assistance in designing programs. Provides supervised apartments, group homes, respite services, independent living programs and job-coached employment.

461 www.autismspeaks.org
National Alliance for Autism Research (NAAR)

National non-profit, tax-exempt organization dedicated to finding the causes, preventions, effective treatments and, ultimately, a cure for the autism spectrum disorders. NAAR's mission is to fund, promote and support biomedical research into autism. Aims to have an aggressive and far-reaching research program. Seeks to encourage scientists outside the field of autism to apply their insights and experience to autism. Publishes a newsletter that focuses on developments in autism research. Supports brain banks and tissue consortium development.

462 www.autisticservices.com
Autistic Services

Dedicated to serving the unique lifelong needs of autistic individuals.

463 www.cfsny.org
Center for Family Support (CFS)

Devoted to providing support and assistance to individuals with developmental and related disabilities, and to the family members who care for them.

464 www.csaac.org
Community Services for Autistic Adults & Children

Enables individuals to achieve their highest potential and contribute as confident members in their community, instead of living in institutions.

465 www.cyberpsych.org
CyberPsych

Hosts the American Psychoanlyists Foundation, American Association of Suicideology, Society for the Exploration of Psychotherapy Intergration, and Anxiety Disorders Association of America. Also subcategories of the anxiety disorders, as well as general information, including panic disorder, phobias, obsessive compulsive disorder (OCD), social phobia, generalized anxiety disorder, post traumatic stress disorder, and phobias of childhood. Book reviews and links to web pages sharing the topics.

466 www.feat.org
Families for Early Autism Treatment

A non-profit organization of parents and professionals, designed to help families with children who are diagnosised with autism or pervasive developmental disorder. It offers a network of support for families. FEAT has a Lending Library, with information on autism and also offers Support Meetings on the third Wednesday of each month.

467 www.iidc.indiana.edu
Indiana Resource Center for Autism (IRCA)

Conducts outreach training and consultations, engage in research and develop and disseminate info on behalf of individuals across the autism spectrum.

468 www.ladders.org
The Autism Research Foundation

A non-profit, tax-exempt organization dedicated to researching the neurological underpinnings of autism and other related developmental brain disorders. Seeking to rapidly expand and accelerate research into the pervasive developmental disorders. To do this, time and efforts goes into investigating the neuropathology of autism in their laboratories, collecting and redistributing brain tissue to promising research groups for use by projects approved by the Tissue Resource Committee, studies frozen autistic brain tissue collected by TARF. They believe that only aggressive scientific and medical research will reveal the cure for this lifelong disorder.

469 www.maapservices.org
MAAP Services

Provides information and advice to people with Asperger Syndrome, Autism and Pervasive Developmental Disorders. Provides parents and professionals a chance to network with others to learn more within the autism spectrum.

470 www.mentalhealth.Samhsa.Gov
Center for Mental Health Services Knowledge Exchange Network

Information about resources, technical assistance, research, training, networks and other federal clearinghouses and fact sheets and materials.

471 www.mhselfhelp.org
National Mental Health Consumer's Self-Help Clearinghouse

Encourages the development and growth of consumer self-help groups.

472 www.nami.org
National Alliance on Mental Illness

From its inception in 1979, NAMI has been dedicated to improving the lives of individuals and families affected by mental illness.

473 www.necc.org
New England Center for Children

Serves students diagnosed with autism, learning disabilities, language delays, behavior disorders and related disabilities.

474 www.planetpsych.com
Planetpsych.com

Learn about disorders, their treatments and other topics in psychology. Articles are listed under the related topic areas. Ask a therapist a question for free, or view the directory of professionals in your area. If you are a therapist sign up for the directory. Current features, self-help, interactive, and newsletter archives.

475 www.resourcesnyc.org
Resources for Children with Special Needs

Gives a general introduction on autism, educational approaches, available resources, supplementary services, definitions and other related services are included.

476 www.son-rise.org
Son-Rise Autism Treatment Center of America

Training center for autism professionals and parents of autistic children. Programs focus on the design and implementation of home-based/child-centered alternatives.

477 www.thenadd.org
National Association for the Dually Diagnosed (NADD)

An association for persons with developmental disabilities and mental health needs.

478 www.wrongplanet.net
Wrong Planet

WrongPlanet.net is a web community designed for individuals with Asperger's Syndrome and other PDDs. They provide a forum where members can communicate with each other, may read or submit essays or how-to guides about various subjects, and a chatroom for communication with other Aspies.

Conferences & Meetings

479 Asperger Syndrome Education Network (ASPEN) Conference
9 Aspen Circle
Edison, NJ 08820-2832
732-321-0880
info@aspennj.org
www.www.aspennj.org

Lori Shery, President
Rich Meleo, Vice President
Elizabeth Yamashita, Vice President
Ann Hiller, Secretary

Annual conference.

Directories & Databases

480 After School and More
Resources for Children with Special Needs
116 E 16th Street
5th Floor
New York, NY 10003-2164
212-677-4650; *Fax:* 212-254-4070
info@resourcenyc.org
www.resourcesnyc.org

Rachel Howard, Executive Director
Stephen Stern, Director , Finance and Administr
Todd Dorman, Director, Communications and Out
Helen Murphy, Director, Program and Fund Devel

The most complete directory of after school programs for children with disabilities and special needs in the metropolitan New York area focusing on weekend and holiday programs. *$15.00*

252 pages ISBN 0-967836-57-3

Bipolar and Related Disorders

Introduction

Bipolar and Related Disorders discuss a group of severe mental illnesses characterized by alterations between depression and manic euphoria or irritability.

The two states are not independent of each other, but part of the same illness. Individuals in the manic phase of Bipolar Disorder may feel exuberant, invincible, or even immortal. They may be awake for days at a time, and be able to work tirelessly; they may rush from one idea to the next carried by a nearly uncontrollable burst of energy that leaves others bewildered and unable to keep up. (Some extraordinarily creative people, Vincent Van Gogh, for example, have had Bipolar Disorder. Whether or not the disorder makes a positive contribution to creativity is a controversial question.)

In the depressed phase which follows a manic high, the patient may be suicidal. The depressed phase of the illness mirrors a major depressive episode. There are three forms of Bipolar Disorders: Bipolar I Disorder, Bipolar II Disorder, and Cyclothymic Disorder. Bipolar II Disorder consists of repeated depressive episodes interspersed with hypomanic (not full blown mania) episodes. The individual with Cyclothymic Disorder has a history of at least two years of repeated episodes of elevated and depressed mood which don't meet all the criteria for mania or depression but which cause distress and/or decreased ability to function.

A number of researchers are closing in on genetic links to the illness. Like all mental disorders, however, the relationship between genetic physiologic, psychological, and environmental causes is complex. Lithium was the first medication found to be effective; several other medications are now available and effective. Many patients with Bipolar Disorders need a combination of medications to address both the manic and depressive aspects. While medication is quite effective, patients need psychotherapy as well, in order to address issues like compliance with medication, noting early signs of relapse, dealing with friends and family and environmental life stressors.

SYMPTOMS

A **manic episode** consists of the following:

• A distinct period of abnormally and persistently elevated, expansive, or irritable mood, lasting at least one week;
• Inflated self-esteem or grandiosity; decreased need for sleep;
• More talkative than usual;
• Flight of ideas (a succession of topics with little relationship to one another) or a subjective experience that thoughts are racing;
• Distractibility;
• Increase in goal-directed activity;
• Excessive involvement in activities that have a high potential for painful consequences;
• The mood disturbances are severe enough to cause impairment in social or occupational functioning;
• The symptoms are not due to the direct physiological effects of a substance.

The **depressive phase** of Bipolar Disorder consists of the following:

• Depressed mood most of the day, nearly every day, as indicated by either subjective report or observation;
• Markedly diminished interest or pleasure in almost all activities most of the day;
• Significant weight loss when not dieting, or weight gain, or decrease or increase in appetite nearly every day;
• Insomnia or hypersomnia nearly every night;
• Psychomotor agitation or retardation nearly every day;
• Fatigue or loss of energy nearly every day;
• Feelings of worthlessness or excessive or inappropriate guilt nearly every day.

ASSOCIATED FEATURES

Bipolar Disorder is a severe mental illness that can cause extreme disruption to individual lives and careers, and to whole families. While manic, patients may spend all of a family's money, borrow great sums, engage in indiscriminate sexual activity, and behave in other ways that leave lasting negative effects. Suicide is a risk factor in the illness, and an estimated ten percent to fifteen percent of individuals with Bipolar I Disorder commit suicide. Abuse of children, spouses or other family members, or other types of violence, may occur during the manic phase of the illness. Untreated mania, during which the individual gets no sleep, little or no nutrition, and expends great quantities of energy, can result in death as well.

It is important for patients with depression to be carefully screened for any manic or hypomanic symptoms so that Bipolar Disorder can be diagnosed and the appropriate treatment prescribed. Most people with Bipolar Disorder present, or are referred, for care while in the depressive state; it is essential that any individual diagnosed with depression be carefully evaluated to rule out bipolar disorder before antidepressant medication is prescribed. Antidepressant medication alone can precipitate a manic episode in an individual with Bipolar Disorder. The cycles of mood changes tend to become more frequent, shorter, and more intense as the patient gets older.

Disturbances in work, school or social functioning are common, resulting in frequent school truancy or failure, occupational failure, divorce, or episodic antisocial behavior. A variety of other mental disorders may accompany Bipolar Disorder; these include Feeding and Eating Disorders, ADHD, Panic Disorder, Social Phobia, and Substance-Related and Addictive Disorders.

PREVALENCE

The prevalence of Bipolar Disorder varies from 0.4 percent to 0.6 percent in the community. The average onset for Bipolar Disorder is usually between 18 and 24 years, but it can develop in childhood, or as late as the forties and fifties.

TREATMENT OPTIONS

Lithium is the most commonly prescribed drug for Bipolar Disorder and is effective for stabilizing patients in the manic phase of the illness and preventing mood swings. However, compliance is a problem among patients both because of the nature of the condition (some patients may actually miss the high of their mood swings and other people often envy their enthusiasm, energy, and confidence) and because of the side effects associated with the drug. These include weight gain, excessive thirst, tremors and muscle weakness. Lithium is also very toxic in overdose. Blood levels of lithium must be measured daily or weekly to begin with, and in at least six-month intervals thereafter. The distruptive nature of the condition also necessitates the use of psychotherapy and family therapy to help patients rebuild relationships, to maintain compliance with treatment and a positive attitude toward living with chronic illness, and to restore confidence and self-esteem.

Anticonvulsants/mood stabilizers, such as Valproate, Carbamazepine, Lamotrigine, Gabapentin, and Topiramate have also become first-line treatments, as have several antipsychotic medications.

Education of the family is crucial for successful treatment, as is education of patients about the disorder and treatment.

Associations & Agencies

482 Brain & Behavior Research Foundation
90 Park Avenue
16th Floor
New York, NY 10016
646-681-4888
800-829-8289
info@bbrfoundation.org
www.www.bbrfoundation.org/

Steve Lieber, Chairman of the Board
Jeffrey Borenstein, MD, President and CEO
Louis Innamorato, CPA, VP and Chief Financial Officer
Anne Abramson, Vice President

The Brain and Behavior Research Foundation awards grants aimed at advancing scientific understandings of mental health treatments and mental disorders such as depression and schizophrenia. The Brain and Behavior Research Foundation's mission is to eliminate the suffering caused by mental illness.

Year Founded: 1987

483 Center for Mental Health Services (CMHS)
Substance Abuse and Mental Health Services Administration
5600 Fishers Lane
Rockville, MD 20857
240-276-1310
877-726-4727
TTY: 800-487-4889
www.samhsa.gov/about-us/who-we-are/offices-centers

Paolo del Vecchio, MSW, Director
Anne Mathews-Younes, Acting Deputy Director
Keris Myrick, Director, Consumer Affairs
Patricia Gratton, Director, Program Analysis

Promotes the treatment of mental illness and emotional disorders by increasing accessibility to mental health programs; supporting outreach, treatment, rehabilitation, and support programs and networks; and encouraging the use of scientifically-based information when treating mental disorders. CMHS provides information about mental health via a toll-free number and numerous publications. Developed for users of mental health services and their families, the general public, policy makers, providers, and the media.

Year Founded: 1992

484 Depression & Bipolar Support Alliance
55 East Jackson Boulevard
Suite 490
Chicago, IL 60604
800-826-3632; *Fax:* 312-642-7243
info@dbsalliance.org
www.dbsalliance.org

Michael Kuhl, Chair
Allen Doederlein, EVP, External Affairs
Catherine Fields, JD, Vice Chair
Christy B. Beckmann, Treasurer

The Depression and Bipolar Support Alliance is a national organization focused on improving the lives of individuals with depression, bipolar disorder, and other mood disorders. DBSA organizes peer-led support groups; educates patients, families, professionals, and the public on mental health; and works to ensure the availability of quality care for all people.

485 Mood Disorders Center
Department of Psychiatry and Behavioral Sciences at Johns Hopkins
600 North Wolfe Street
Baltimore, MD 21218-7413
410-955-5212
877-666-3754
www.www.hopkinsmedicine.org/psychiatry/specialty_areas

J. Raymond DePaulo, MD, Co-Director
Kay Redfield Jamison, PhD, Co-Director
Mehdi Pirooznia, MD, Research Team
Peter Zandi, PhD, Research Team

The Mood Disorders Center at Johns Hopkins Medicine provides specialized clinical services to patients with mood disorders; conducts research on the causes of mood disorders, treatment responses, and brain function and structure; and educates patients, caregivers, and the public on mood disorders through symposia, publications, community presentations, and the Adolescent Depression Awareness Program.

486 National Alliance on Mental Illness
3803 North Fairfax Drive
Suite 100
Arlington, VA 22203
703-524-7600
800-950-6264
info@nami.org
www.nami.org

Steve Pitman, JD, President
Lacey Berumen, PhD, MNM, First Vice President
Mary Giliberti, Chief Executive Officer
David Levy, Chief Financial Officer

NAMI is an organization dedicated to raising awareness on mental health and providing support and education for Americans affected by mental illness. NAMI advocates for access to services and treatment and fosters an environment of awareness and understanding for those concerned with mental health.

Year Founded: 1979

487 National Association for the Dually Diagnosed (NADD)
132 Fair Street
Kingston, NY 12401

845-331-4336
info@thenadd.org
www.thenadd.org

Jeanne M. Farr, MA, Chief Executive Officer
Daniel Baker, PhD., President
Peggie Webb, MA, Vice President
George Zukotynski, PhD., Secretary

NADD is a nonprofit organization designed to increase awareness of, and provide services for, individuals with developmental disabilities and mental illness. NADD emphasizes the importance of quality mental healthcare for people with mental health needs and offers conferences, information resources, educational programs, and training materials to professionals, parents, and organizations.

Year Founded: 1983

488 National Institute of Mental Health
National Institutes of Health
6001 Executive Boulevard
Room 6200, MSC 9663
Bethesda, MD 20892-9663
301-443-4513
866-615-6464; *Fax:* 301-443-4279
TTY: 301-443-8431
nimhinfo@nih.gov
www.nimh.nih.gov

Joshua Gordon, PhD, Director
Shelli Avenevoli, PhD, Deputy Director
Ann D. Huston, Associate Director, Management
Meredith A. Fox, PhD, Director of Communications

The National Institute of Mental Health conducts clinical research on mental disorders and seeks to expand knowledge on mental health treatments.

489 National Mental Health Consumers' Self-Help Clearinghouse
1211 Chestnut Street
Suite 1100
Philadelphia, PA 19107
267-507-3810
800-553-4539; *Fax:* 215-636-6312
info@mhselfhelp.org
www.mhselfhelp.org

Joseph Rogers, Founder and Executive Director
Susan Rogers, Director

The Clearinghouse is a peer-run national technical assistance center focused on achieving respect and equality of opportunity for those with mental illnesses. The Clearinghouse helps with the growth of the mental health consumer movement by evaluating mental health services, advocating for mental health reform, and providing consumers with news, information, publications, and consultation services.

Year Founded: 1986

490 The Balanced Mind Parent Network
Depression and Bipolar Support Alliance
55 East Jackson Boulevard
Suite 490
Chicago, IL 60604
800-826-3632; *Fax:* 312-642-7243
support@thebalancedmind.org

Julia Small, Parent Volunteer Coordinator
Karen Cruise, Family Helpline Leader
Kathy Karle, Support Network Coordinator
Janice Cox, Support Network Coordinator

The Balanced Mind provides support, information, and assistance to families raising children with mood disorders and related conditions.

491 The Center for Family Support
2811 Zulette Avenue
Bronx, NY 10461
718-518-1500; *Fax:* 718-518-8200
www.www.cfsny.org/

Steven Vernikoff, Executive Director
Lloyd Stabiner, President
Amy Bittinger, Vice President
Barbara Greenwald, Associate Executive Director

The Center for Family Support offers assistance to individuals with developmental and related disabilities, as well as their families, and provides support services and programs that are designed to accommodate individual needs. Offers services throughout New York City, Westchester County, Long Island, and New Jersey.

Year Founded: 1954

Books

492 An Unquiet Mind: A Memoir of Moods and Madness
Random House
1745 Broadway
New York, NY 10019
212-782-9000
ecustomerservice@randomhouse.com
www.randomhouse.com

Kay Redfield Jamison, Author

The author examines bipolar illness from the dual perspectives of the healer and the healed, revealing both its terrors and the cruel allure that at times prompted her to resist taking medication. An Unquiet Mind is a memoir of enormous candor, vividness, and wisdom- a deeply powerful book that has both transformed and saved lives. *$15.00*

224 pages ISBN 0-679763-30-9

493 Bipolar Disorder Survival Guide: What You and Your Family Need to Know
The Guilford Press
72 Spring Street
New York, NY 10012-4019
212-431-9800
800-365-7006; *Fax:* 212-966-6708
info@guilford.com
www.www.guilford.com

David J. Miklowitz, PhD, Author

Gives ideas to the person diagnosed with the disorder how to come to terms with the diagnosis. Also shows who you should confide in and how to recognize mood swings. *$19.95*

342 pages Year Founded: 1973 ISBN 1-572305-25-8

494 Bipolar Disorder for Dummies
John Wiley and Sons
111 River Street
Hoboken, NJ 07030-5774
201-748-6000
877-762-2974; *Fax:* 201-748-6088
info@wiley.com
www.wiley.com

Candida Fink,MD, Author
Joe Kraynak, Author

Guide explains the brain chemistry behind the disease, and covers the latest medications and therapies. Sound advice and self-help techniques that everyone can use including children to ease and eliminate syptoms, function in a crisis, and plan ahead for manic or depressive episodes. *$19.99*

384 pages Year Founded: 2005 ISBN 0-764584-51-0

495 Bipolar Disorders: A Guide to Helping Children & Adolescents
ADD WareHouse
300 NW 70th Avenue
Suite 102
Plantation, FL 33317-2360
954-792-8100
800-233-9273; *Fax:* 954-792-8545
sales@addwarehouse.com
www.addwarehouse.com

Mitzi Waltz, Author

A million children and adolescents in the US may have childhood-onset bipolar disorder-including a significant number with ADHD. This new book helps parents and professionals recognize, treat and cope with bipolar disorders. It covers diagnosis, family life, medications, talk therapies, school issues, and other interventions. *$24.95*

442 pages Year Founded: 2000 ISBN 1-565926-56-0

496 Bipolar Disorders: Clinical Course and Outcome
American Psychiatric Publishing, Inc.
1000 Wilson Boulevard
Suite 1825
Arlington, VA 22209-3901
703-907-7322
800-368-5777; *Fax:* 703-907-1091
appi@psych.org
www.appi.org

Joseph F. Goldberg, Editor
Martin Harrow, Editor

An important and much-needed resource, this book related empirical data on outcome with practical information on the prognosis, course, and potential complications of bipolar disorders in the modern era. Pulling together current knowledge from leading investigators in the field, it provides a concise, up-to-date summary of affective relapse, comorbid psychopathology, functional disability, and psychosocial outcome in contemporary bipolar disorders. *$49.95*

344 pages Year Founded: 1999 ISBN 0-880487-68-2

497 Bipolar Puzzle Solution
Taylor and Francis
7625 Empire Drive
Florence, KY 41042-2919
800-634-7064; *Fax:* 800-248-4724
TDD: 703-516-7227
www.nami.org

Bryan L. Court, Author
Gerald E. Nelson, Author

An informative book on bipolar illness in a 187 question-and-answer format. *$18.50*

160 pages Year Founded: 1996

498 Consumer's Guide to Psychiatric Drugs
NewHarbinger Publications
5674 Shattuck Avenue
Oakland, CA 94609-1662
510-652-0215
800-748-6273; *Fax:* 800-652-1613
customerservice@newharbinger.com
www.newharbinger.com

Mary C. Talaga, Author
John D. Preston, Author
John H. O'Neal, Author

Helps consumers understand what treatment options are available and what side effects to expect. Covers possible interactions with other drugs, medical conditions and other concerns. Explains how each drug works, and offers detailed information about treatments for depression, bipolar disorder, anxiety and sleep disorders, as well as other conditions. *$16.95*

340 pages Year Founded: 1973 ISBN 1-572241-11-X

499 Divalproex and Bipolar Disorder: A Guide
Madison Institute of Medicine
6515 Grand Teton Plaza
Suite 100
Madison, WI 53719
608-827-2470
mim@miminc.org
www.www.miminc.org

James W. Jefferson, MD, Author
John H. Greist, MD, Author

A concise, up-to-date booklet that provides the reader with an overview of bipolar disorder and its treatment with the medication, divalproex (sometimes referred to as valproate). Information an administration and dosage, patient monitoring, and possible side effects is included in the guide, as well as other information important to anyone taking divalproex for bipolar disorder. *$5.95*

32 pages

500 Guildeline for Treatment of Patients with Bipolar Disorder
American Psychiatric Publishing, Inc.
1000 Wilson Boulevard
Suite 1825
Arlington, VA 22209-3901
703-907-7322
800-368-5777; *Fax:* 703-907-1091
appi@psych.org
www.appi.org

Provides guidance to psychiatrists who treat patients with bipolar I disorder. Summarizes the pharmacologic, somatic, and psychotherapeutic treatments used for patients. *$22.50*

96 pages ISBN 0-890423-02-4

501 Management of Bipolar Disorder: Pocketbook
American Psychiatric Publishing, Inc.
1000 Wilson Boulevard
Suite 1825
Arlington, VA 22209-3901
703-907-7322
800-368-5777; *Fax:* 703-907-1091
appi@psych.org
www.appi.org

Robert E Hales MD, Editor-in-Chief
Ron McMillen, Chief Executive Officer
John McDuffie, Editorial Director

Contains the need for treatment, what defines bipolar disorders, spectrum of the disorder, getting the best out of treatment, treatment of mania and bipolar depression, preventing new episodes, special problems in treatment, mood stabilizers and case studies. *$ 14.95*

96 pages ISBN 1-853172-74-X

502 Manic-Depressive Illness: Bipolar Disorders and Recurrent Depression, 2nd Edition
Oxford University Press
198 Madison Avenue
New York, NY 10016
212-726-6000
custserv.us@oup.com
www.www.oup.com/us/

Frederick K Goodwin, Author

The authors review the biological and genetic literature that has dominated the field in recent years and incorporate cutting-edge research conducted since publication of the first edition. They also update their surveys of psychological and epidemiological evidence, as well as that pertaining to diagnostice issues, course, and outcome, and they offer practical guidelines for differential diagnosis and clinical management.

503 Physician's Guide to Depression and Bipolar Disorders
McGraw-Hill Companies
PO Box 182604
Columbus, OH 43218-2604
877-833-5524; *Fax:* 614-759-3749
customer.service@mcgraw-hill.com
www.mcgraw-hill.com

Dwight L Evans,MD, Author
Dennis S Charney,MD, Author
Lydia Lewis, Author

Offers a clear definitive instruction on drug treatments for bipolar disorders with the exact dosages needed. Crucial to a diagnosis and treatment is the ability to identify a patients symptoms. *$59.00*

400 pages Year Founded: 2005 ISBN 0-071441-75-1

15

504 Taming Bipolar Disorders
Alpha
677 Elm Street, Ste 112
PO Box 255
Royersford, PA 19468
800-992-9124
www.alphapub.com

Contains cutting-edge research and straightforward advice from the most respectable names on bipolar disorder, along with the most up-to-date information on mental health organizations, support and advocacy groups. *$17.95*

400 pages Year Founded: 2004 ISBN 1-592572-85-5

Periodicals & Pamphlets

505 Bipolar Disorder
National Institute of Mental Health
6001 Executive Boulevard
Room 6200,MSC 9663
Bethesda, MD 20892-9663
301-443-4513
866-615-6464; *Fax:* 301-443-4279
TTY: 301-443-8431
nimhinfo@nih.gov
www.www.nimh.nih.gov

Tom Insel,MD, NIHM Director
William G Coleman, Scientific Director,NIMHD
Grace E O Ajao, Administrative Officer
Dionne D Draper, Administrative Officer

A detailed booklet that describes Bipolar Disorder symptons, causes, and treatments, with information on getting help and coping.

24 pages

506 DBSA Support Groups: An Important Step on the Road to Wellness
Depression and Bipolar Support Alliance
730 North Franklin Street
Suite 501
Chicago, IL 60654-7225
312-642-0049
800-826-3632; *Fax:* 312-642-7243
www.dbsalliance.org

Cheryl T Magrini,MS.Ed,MTS,PhD, Chair
Allen Doederlein, President
Cindy Specht, ExecutiveVice president
Gregory E Ostfeld, Treasurer

Support groups for people with depression or bipolar disorder to discuss the experiences, and helpful treatments.

10 pages Year Founded: 2003

507 Finding Peace of Mind: Treatment Strategies for Depression and Bipolar Disorder
Depression and Bipolar Support Alliance
730 North Franklin Street
Suite 501
Chicago, IL 60654-7225
312-642-0049
800-826-3632; *Fax:* 312-642-7243
www.dbsalliance.org

Helps to build a good, cooperative relationship with your doctor by explaining some of the treatments for mood disorders and how they work. Also includes a guide for medication that has been frequently prescribed and new treatments that are being investigated.

20 pages Year Founded: 2003

508 Getting Better Sleep: What You Need to Know
Depression and Bipolar Support Alliance
730 North Franklin Street
Suite 501
Chicago, IL 60654-7225
312-642-0049
800-826-3632; *Fax:* 312-642-7243
www.dbsalliance.org

Sue Bergeson, President

Describes some causes of sleep loss, and how sleep loss relates to bipolar disorder and depression. Also provides information on how to get better sleep.

509 Introduction to Depression and Bipolar Disorder
Depression and Bipolar Support Alliance
730 North Franklin Street
Suite 501
Chicago, IL 60654-7225
312-642-0049
800-826-3632; *Fax:* 312-642-7243
www.dbsalliance.org

Sue Bergeson, President

Quick and easy-to-read brochure describing syptoms and treatments for mood disorders.

510 McMan's Depression and Bipolar Weekly
McMan's Depression and Bipolar Web
PO Box 5093
Kendall Park, NJ 08824-5093
E-mail: mcman@mcmanweb.com
www.mcmanweb.com

John McManamy, Editor/Publisher

Online newsletter devoted to the issues of bipolar and depression disorders. There is no charge, just for you to understand different things about the disorders.

511 Mood Disorders
Center for Mental Health Services: Knowledge Exchange Network
PO Box 42490
Washington, DC 20015
800-789-2647; *Fax:* 301-984-8796
TDD: 866-889-2647
ken@mentalhealth.org
www.store.samhsa.gov

This fact sheet provides basic information on the symptoms, formal diagnosis, and treatment for bipolar disorder.

3 pages

512 Myths and Facts about Depression and Bipolar Disorders
Depression and Bipolar Support Alliance
730 North Franklin Street
Suite 501
Chicago, IL 60654-7225
312-642-0049
800-826-3632; *Fax:* 312-642-7243
www.dbsalliance.org

Gives some myths about depression and bipolar disorder and the truths that combat them.

513 Oxcarbazepine and Bipolar Disorder: A Guide
Madison Institute of Medicine
6515 Grand Teton Plaza
Suite 100
Madison, WI 53719
608-827-2470; *Fax:* 608-827-2444
mim@miminc.org
www.factsforhealth.org

W Jefferson James, Author
John H Greist, Author
David J Katzelnick, MD, Author

This 31 page booklet provides patients with the information they need to know about the use of oxcarbazepine in the treatment of bipolar disorder, including information about proper dosing, medication management, and possible side effects. *$5.95*

31 pages

514 Recovering Your Mental Health: a Self-Help Guide
SAMHSA'S National Mental Health Informantion Center
1 Choke Cherry Road
Rockville, MD 20857
877-726-4727
ken@mentalhealth.org
www.mentalhealth.samhsa.gov

Mary Ellen Copeland, Author
Edward B Searle, Deputy Director

This booklet offers tips for understanding symptoms of depression and other conditions and getting help. Also details the advantages of counseling, medications available, options for professional help, relaxation techniques and paths to positive thinking.

32 pages

515 Storm In My Brain
Depression & Bi-Polar Support Alliance
730 North Franklin Street
Suite 501
Chicago, IL 60654-7225
312-642-0049
800-826-3632; *Fax:* 312-642-7243
www.dbsalliance.org

Sue Bergeson, President
Ingrid Deetz, Program Director

Pamphlet free on the Internet or by mail. Discusses child or adolesent Bi-Polar symptoms.

516 You've Just Been Diagnosed...What Now?
Depression and Bipolar Support Alliance
730 North Franklin Street
Suite 501
Chicago, IL 60654-7225
312-642-0049
800-826-3632; *Fax:* 312-642-7243
www.dbsalliance.org

Sue Bergeson, President

Pamphlet to help you understand about the disorder you have just been diagnosed with. Tells you basic facts about mood disorders and will help you work towards a diagnosis.

19 pages Year Founded: 2002

Research Centers

517 Bipolar Clinic and Research Program
The Massachusetts General Hospital Bipolar Clinic & Research Program
50 Staniford Street
Suite 580
Boston, MA 02114-2540
617-726-5855; *Fax:* 617-726-6768
www.www.massgeneral.org

Michael Jellinek,MD, President
Laurie Ansorge Ball, Executive Director,MGH Departmen
Jerrold F Rosenbaum,MD, Chief of Psychiatry,MGH

Dedicated to providing quality clinical care, conducting clinically informative research, and educating our colleagues, patients, as well as the community.

518 Bipolar Disorders Clinic
Standford School of Medicine
401 Quarry Road
Stanford, CA 94305-5723
650-723-3305
www.bipolar.stanford.edu

Terrence A Ketter,MD, Chief,Bipolar Disorders Clinic
Shelley Hill,MS, Clinical Research Coordinator

Offers an on-going clinical treatment, manage clinical trials and neuroimaging studies, lecture and teach seminar courses at Stanford University and train residents in the School of Medicine.

519 Bipolar Research Program at University of Pennsylvania
3535 Market Street
6th Floor
Philadelphia, PA 19104-3413
215-898-4301; *Fax:* 215-898-0509
balthrop@mail.med.upenn.edu
www.www.med.upenn.edu/psych/bipolar_research.html

Laszlo Gyulai, MD, Program Director
Chang-Gyu Hahn, MD, Ph.D., Clinical Team Member

Offers and conducts research on treatments for bipolar disorders. The program provides comprehensive care for persons with bipolar affective disorder (manic depressive illness), seasonal affective disorder, and rapid cycling bipolar disorder. Services offered for individuals who are in the ages of 18 or older include evaluations, consultations, and ongoing treatment options.

520 Epidemiology-Genetics Program in Psychiatry
John Hopkins University School of Medicine
PO Box 1997
Baltimore, MD 21203
888-289-4095
www.www.hopkinsmedicine.org

The research program is to help characterize the genetic (biochemical) developmental, and environmental components of bipolar disorder. The hope is that once scientists understand the biological causes of this disorder new medications and treatments can be developed.

521 Yale Mood Disorders Research Program
Department of Psychiatry
300 George Street
Suite 901
New Haven, CT 06511-6624
203-785-2090; *Fax:* 203-785-2028
www.psychiatry.yale.edu

John H Krystal, Chair
Rajita Sinha, Chief,Psychology Section

MDRP is dedicated to understanding the science of mood disorders, including bipolar disorder and depression. The MDRP brings together a multi-disciplinary group of scientists from across the Yale campus in a highly collaborative research effort. Goals of the MDRP include the identifica-

tion of biological markers for mood disorders and discovery of new treatment strategies.

Support Groups & Hot Lines

522 Recovery International
1415 W. 22nd Street
Tower Floor
Oak Brook, IL 60523
312-337-5661
866-221-0302; *Fax:* 312-726-4446
www.www.recoveryinternational.org

Sandra K. Wilcoxon, Chief Executive Officer
Joanne Lampey, President
Joan Nobiling, Vice President
Nicole Cilento, 2nd Vice President

Recovery International is an organization that uses a peer-to-peer, self-help training system developed by Abraham Low in order to help individuals with mental health issues lead more productive lives.

Year Founded: 1937

Video & Audio

523 Anger Management-Enhanced Edition
Educational Video Network, Inc.
1401 19th Street
Huntsville, TX 77340
936-295-5767
800-762-0060; *Fax:* 936-294-0233
www.www.evndirect.com

Learn what causes anger and understand why our bodies react as they do when we're angry. Effective techniques for assuaging anger are discussed.

524 Bipolar Disorder: Shifting Mood Swings
Educational Training Videos
136 Granville St
Suite 200
Gahanna, OH 43230
Fax: 888-775-3919
www.educationaltrainingvideos.com

Different from the routine ups and downs of life, the symptoms of bipolar disorder are severe - even to the point of being life-threatening. In this insightful program, patients speak from their own experience about the complexities of diagnosis and the very real danger of suicide, while family members and close friends address the strain of the condition's cyclic behavior.

525 Clinical Impressions: Identifying Mental Illness
Educational Training Videos
136 Granville St
Suite 200
Gahanna, OH 43230
Fax: 888-775-3919
www.educationaltrainingvideos.com

How long can mental illness stay hidden, especially from the eyes of trained experts? This program rejoins a group of ten adults- five of them healthy and five of them with histories of mental illness- as psychiatric specialists try to spot and correctly diagnose the latter. Administering a series of collaborative and one-on-one tests, including assessments of personality type, physical self-image, and rational thinking, the panel gradually makes decisions about who suffers from depression, bipolar disorder, bulimia, and social anxiety.

526 Families Coping with Mental Illness
Mental Illness Education Project
25 West Street
Brookline Village, MA 01581
617-562-1111
800-343-5540; *Fax:* 617-779-0061
info@miepvideos.org
www.miepvideos.org

Ten family members share their experiences of having a family member with schizophrenia or bipolar disorder. Designed to provide insights and support to other families, the tape also profoundly conveys to professionals the needs of families when mental illness strikes. In two versions: a 22-minute version ideal for short classes and workshops, and a richer 43-minute version with more examples and details. Discounted price for families/consumers. *$99.95*

527 Kay Redfield Jamison: Surviving Bipolar Disorder
Educational Training Videos
136 Granville St
Suite 200
Gahanna, OH 43230
Fax: 888-775-3919
www.educationaltrainingvideos.com

Psychiatry professor and clinical psychologist Kay Redfield Jamison knows all about bipolar disorder- from the inside out. She talks frankly about her experiences with a mental illness that almost claimed her life.

528 Understanding Mental Illness
Educational Video Network, Inc.
1401 19th Street
Huntsville, TX 77340
936-295-5767
800-762-0060; *Fax:* 936-294-0233
www.www.evndirect.com

Contains information and classifications of mental illness. Mental illness can strike anyone, at any age. Learn about various organic and functional mental disorders as discussed and their causes and symptoms, and learn where to seek help for a variety of mental health concerns.

Web Sites

529 www.befrienders.org
Samaritans International

Support, helplines, and advice.

530 www.bpso.org
BPSO-Bipolar Significant Others

Informational site intended to provide information and support to the spouses, families, friends and other loved ones of those who suffer from bi-polar.

531 www.cfsny.org
Center for Family Support (CFS)

Devoted to providing support and assistance to individuals with developmental and related disabilities, and to the family members who care for them.

532 www.dbsalliance.org
Depression & Bi-Polar Support Alliance

Mental health news updates and local support group information.

533 www.goodwill-suncoast.org
Suncoast Residential Training Center

Group home that serves individuals diagnosed as developmentally disabled, with a secondary diagnosis of psychiatric difficulties as evidenced by problem behavior.

534 www.med.yale.edu
Yale University School of Medicine

Research center dedicated to understanding the science of mood disorders.

535 www.mentalhealth.Samhsa.Gov
Center for Mental Health Services Knowledge Exchange Network

Information about resources, technical assistance, research, training, networks, and other federal clearinghouses, fact sheets and materials.

536 www.mhselfhelp.org
National Mental Health Consumer's Self-Help Clearinghouse

Encourages the development and growth of consumer self-help groups.

537 www.miminc.org
Bipolar Disorders Treatment Information Center

Provides information on mood stabilizers other than lithium for bipolar disorders.

538 www.nami.org
National Alliance on Mental Illness

From its inception in 1979, NAMI has been dedicated to improving the lives of individuals and families affected by mental illness.

539 www.planetpsych.com
Planetpsych.com

Learn about disorders, their treatments and other topics in psychology. Articles are listed under the related topic areas. Ask a therapist a question for free, or view the directory of professionals in your area. If you are a therapist sign up for the directory. Current features, self-help, interactive, and newsletter archives.

540 www.psychcentral.com
Psych Central

Personalized one-stop index for psychology, support, and mental health issues, resources, and people on the Internet.

541 www.shpm.com
Self Help Magazine

Articles and discussion forums, resource links.

542 www.store.samhsa.gov
Substance Abuse and Mental Health Services Administration

Resources on mental disorders as well as treatment and recovery.

543 **www.thenadd.org**
National Association for the Dually Diagnosed
(NADD)

An association for persons with developmental disabilities
and mental health needs.

Depressive Disorders

Introduction

Feelings of sadness are common to everyone, and quite natural in response to unfortunate circumstances. The death of a loved one, the end of a relationshio, or other traumatic life experiences are bound to bring on the blues. But when feelings of sadness and despair persist beyond a reasonable period, arise for no particular reason, or begin to affect a person's ability to function, help is needed. Depression is a diagnosis made by a psychiatrist or other mental health professional to describe serious and prolonged symptoms of sadness or despair. While is is quite common, it is also a disease that should not be taken lightly; depression can be deadly. Many people who are deeply depressed think about or actually try to commit suicide; some commit suicide. Even a relatively mild depression, if untreated, can disrupt marriages and relationships or impeded careers.

Symptoms

Depression is diagnosed when an individual experiences 1) persistent feelings of sadness or 2) loss of interest or pleasure in usual activities, in addition to five of the following symptoms for at least two weeks:
• Significant weight gain or loss unrelated to dieting;
• Inability to sleep or, conversely, sleeping too much;
• Restlessness and agitation;
• Fatigue or loss of energy;
• Feelings of worthlessness or guilt;
• Diminished ability to think or concentrate;
• Recurrent thoughts of death or suicide;
• Distress not caused by a medication or the symtoms of a medical illness.

Associated Features

Because depression can range from mild to severe, people who are depressed may exhibit a variety of behaviors. Often, people who are depressed are tearful, irritable, or brooding. Problems sleeping (either insomnia or sleeping too much) are common. People with depression may worry uneccessarily about being sick or having a disease, or they may report physical symtoms such as headaches or other pains. Depression can seriously affect people's friendships and intimate relationships.

Depression can make people worry about having a disease, but this is not a central symptom. Depression very frequently coexists with anxiety disorder. There is a genetic predisposition in some people.

Within days to a year after giving birth, women may experience a spectrum of psychological symptoms related to both the abrupt hormonal changes and the psychological and social demands of motherhood. The mildest of these symptoms, 'baby blues,' is not a psychiatric condition. It consists of a few days of heightened emotionality starting within days after birth and resolving spontaneously. Women may become concerned when the emotionality leads to tears, but women with 'baby blues,' and their families, need only reassurance.

Postpartum depression is often a continuation of depression starting during or even before pregnancy. The symptoms, which are listed below, are much the same as those of depression occurring at any other time of life. The fact that the postpartum period is almost always associated with problems with sleep, appetite, libido, energy, and con-

centration makes those symptoms less useful for diagnosis at this time. Two cardinal questions are: 'Are you feeling sad most of the time?' and 'Are you unable to enjoy things that you usually enjoy?' Women with postpartum depression are preoccupied with concerns about their ability to be good mothers. Unlike an average, tired new mother, the depressed woman cannot enjoy her baby. She is often guilty and reluctant to tell her family about it because she knows she is supposed to appreciate her good fortune and be happy. Severe Postpartum Depression, or Postpartum Psychosis, that causes confusion, disorientation,delusions, and hallucinations, and can cause suicide or infanticide, is a serious medical condition demanding immediate professional attention. Fortunately, there is increasing awareness and understanding of postpartum depression among the general population.

Symptoms

In addition to the symptoms of Depression:
• Preoccupation with concerns of being a good mother;
• Inability to rest while the baby is sleeping;
• Inability to enjoy her baby accompanied with feelings of guilt.

Prevalence

Very mild depression after delivery, or 'baby blues,' affects over half, perhaps up to 90% of postpartum women. Baby blues is actually not depression at all; rather it is a common condition characterized by sensitivity and emotionality, both happy and sad. Postpartum Depression affects approximately 10% of new mothers. Much of postpartum depression is a continuation of depression that was already present during pregnancy. Postpartum Psychosis is estimated to affect one in 1,000 women after they give birth.

Treatment Options

Treatment for Postpartum Depression is similar to treatment for depression in general. Possible risks of medications taken during pregnancy and breastfeeding have to be weighed against the risks of leaving the depression untreated. Women who discontinue antidepressant medication because they wish to become or have become pregnant are at a very high risk of relapse.

Dysthymic Disorder is more low-level than chronic, with depressed mood consistently for at least two years, than major depressive episodes, which last about nine months. Dysthymia can be treated with medication and psychotherapy as well.

Psychotherapy, or talk therapy, may be used to help the patient improve the way he or she thinks about things and deals with specific life problems. Individual, family, or couples therapy may be recommended, depending on the patient's life experiences. If the Depression is not severe, treatment can take a few weeks; if the Depression has been a longstanding problem, it may take much longer, but in many cases, a patient will experience improvement in 10-15 sessions. Self-help groups and patient and family education may also be of benefit to people with depression.

Associations & Agencies

545 **Brain & Behavior Research Foundation**
90 Park Avenue
16th Floor
New York, NY 10016

646-681-4888
800-829-8289
info@bbrfoundation.org
www.www.bbrfoundation.org/

Steve Lieber, Chairman of the Board
Jeffrey Borenstein, MD, President and CEO
Louis Innamorato, CPA, VP and Chief Financial Officer
Anne Abramson, Vice President

The Brain and Behavior Research Foundation awards grants aimed at advancing scientific understandings of mental health treatments and mental disorders such as depression and schizophrenia. The Brain and Behavior Research Foundation's mission is to eliminate the suffering caused by mental illness.

Year Founded: 1987

546 Center for Mental Health Services (CMHS)
Substance Abuse and Mental Health Services
Administration
5600 Fishers Lane
Rockville, MD 20857
240-276-1310
877-726-4727
TTY: 800-487-4889
www.samhsa.gov/about-us/who-we-are/offices-centers

Paolo del Vecchio, MSW, Director
Anne Mathews-Younes, Acting Deputy Director
Keris Myrick, Director, Consumer Affairs
Patricia Gratton, Director, Program Analysis

Promotes the treatment of mental illness and emotional disorders by increasing accessibility to mental health programs; supporting outreach, treatment, rehabilitation, and support programs and networks; and encouraging the use of scientifically-based information when treating mental disorders. CMHS provides information about mental health via a toll-free number and numerous publications. Developed for users of mental health services and their families, the general public, policy makers, providers, and the media.

Year Founded: 1992

547 Depression & Bipolar Support Alliance
55 East Jackson Boulevard
Suite 490
Chicago, IL 60604
800-826-3632; *Fax:* 312-642-7243
info@dbsalliance.org
www.dbsalliance.org

Michael Kuhl, Chair
Allen Doederlein, EVP, External Affairs
Catherine Fields, JD, Vice Chair
Christy B. Beckmann, Treasurer

The Depression and Bipolar Support Alliance is a national organization focused on improving the lives of individuals with depression, bipolar disorder, and other mood disorders. DBSA organizes peer-led support groups; educates patients, families, professionals, and the public on mental health; and works to ensure the availability of quality care for all people.

548 Freedom From Fear
308 Seaview Avenue
Staten Island, NY 10305
718-351-1717
help@freedomfromfear.org
www.freedomfromfear.org

Daniel Deutsch, PhD, Board Member
Mary Guardino, Founder and Executive Director
Steve Jenkins, PhD, Board Member
Theresa Mazzeo, Board Member

A national nonprofit organization, the mission of Freedom From Fear is to aid and counsel individuals suffering from anxiety and depressive disorders through advocacy, education, research, and community support.

Year Founded: 1984

549 Mood Disorders Center
Department of Psychiatry and Behavioral Sciences
at Johns Hopkins
600 North Wolfe Street
Baltimore, MD 21218-7413
410-955-5212
877-666-3754
www.www.hopkinsmedicine.org/psychiatry/specialty_areas

J. Raymond DePaulo, MD, Co-Director
Kay Redfield Jamison, PhD, Co-Director
Mehdi Pirooznia, MD, Research Team
Peter Zandi, PhD, Research Team

The Mood Disorders Center at Johns Hopkins Medicine provides specialized clinical services to patients with mood disorders; conducts research on the causes of mood disorders, treatment responses, and brain function and structure; and educates patients, caregivers, and the public on mood disorders through symposia, publications, community presentations, and the Adolescent Depression Awareness Program.

550 National Alliance on Mental Illness
3803 North Fairfax Drive
Suite 100
Arlington, VA 22203
703-524-7600
800-950-6264
info@nami.org
www.nami.org

Steve Pitman, JD, President
Lacey Berumen, PhD, MNM, First Vice President
Mary Giliberti, Chief Executive Officer
David Levy, Chief Financial Officer

NAMI is an organization dedicated to raising awareness on mental health and providing support and education for Americans affected by mental illness. NAMI advocates for access to services and treatment and fosters an environment of awareness and understanding for those concerned with mental health.

Year Founded: 1979

551 National Association for the Dually Diagnosed
(NADD)
132 Fair Street
Kingston, NY 12401
845-331-4336
info@thenadd.org
www.thenadd.org

Jeanne M. Farr, MA, Chief Executive Officer
Daniel Baker, PhD., President
Peggie Webb, MA, Vice President
George Zukotynski, PhD., Secretary

NADD is a nonprofit organization designed to increase awareness of, and provide services for, individuals with developmental disabilities and mental illness. NADD emphasizes the importance of quality mental healthcare for people with mental health needs and offers conferences, information resources, educational programs, and training materials to professionals, parents, and organizations.

Year Founded: 1983

552 National Institute of Mental Health
National Institutes of Health
6001 Executive Boulevard
Room 6200, MSC 9663
Bethesda, MD 20892-9663
301-443-4513
866-615-6464; *Fax:* 301-443-4279
TTY: 301-443-8431
nimhinfo@nih.gov
www.nimh.nih.gov

Joshua Gordon, PhD, Director
Shelli Avenevoli, PhD, Deputy Director
Ann D. Huston, Associate Director, Management
Meredith A. Fox, PhD, Director of Communications

The National Institute of Mental Health conducts clinical research on mental disorders and seeks to expand knowledge on mental health treatments.

553 National Mental Health Consumers' Self-Help
Clearinghouse
1211 Chestnut Street
Suite 1100
Philadelphia, PA 19107
267-507-3810
800-553-4539; *Fax:* 215-636-6312
info@mhselfhelp.org
www.mhselfhelp.org

Joseph Rogers, Founder and Executive Director
Susan Rogers, Director

The Clearinghouse is a peer-run national technical assistance center focused on achieving respect and equality of opportunity for those with mental illnesses. The Clearinghouse helps with the growth of the mental health consumer movement by evaluating mental health services, advocating for mental health reform, and providing consumers with news, information, publications, and consultation services.

Year Founded: 1986

554 Postpartum Support International
6706 Southwest 54th Avenue
Portland, OR 97219
503-894-9453
800-944-4773; *Fax:* 503-894-9452
support@postpartum.net
www.postpartum.net

Ann Smith, CNM, President
Wendy N. Davis, PhD, Executive Director
Lianne Swanson, PSI Office Administrator
Lita Simanis, LCSW, Secretary

A nonprofit organization focused on providing support for pregnant, post-loss and postpartum women across the world. Postpartum Support International seeks to raise awareness about the emotional and mental health issues that women face during pregnancy and postpartum.

Year Founded: 1987

555 The Balanced Mind Parent Network
Depression and Bipolar Support Alliance
55 East Jackson Boulevard
Suite 490
Chicago, IL 60604
800-826-3632; *Fax:* 312-642-7243
support@thebalancedmind.org

Julia Small, Parent Volunteer Coordinator
Karen Cruise, Family Helpline Leader
Kathy Karle, Support Network Coordinator
Janice Cox, Support Network Coordinator

The Balanced Mind provides support, information, and assistance to families raising children with mood disorders and related conditions.

556 The Center for Family Support
2811 Zulette Avenue
Bronx, NY 10461
718-518-1500; *Fax:* 718-518-8200
www.www.cfsny.org/

Steven Vernikoff, Executive Director
Lloyd Stabiner, President
Amy Bittinger, Vice President
Barbara Greenwald, Associate Executive Director

The Center for Family Support offers assistance to individuals with developmental and related disabilities, as well as their families, and provides support services and programs that are designed to accommodate individual needs. Offers services throughout New York City, Westchester County, Long Island, and New Jersey.

Year Founded: 1954

Books

557 Against Depression
Viking Adult
375 Hudson Street
New York, NY 10014-3657
212-366-2372; *Fax:* 212-366-2933
ecommerce@us.penguingroup.com
www.www.us.penguingroup.com

Peter D. Kramer, Author

A deeply felt, deeply moving book, grounded in time spent with the depressed. As his argument unfolds, Kramer becomes a crusader, the author of a compassionate polemic that is fiercely against depression and the devastation it causes. This book will offer hope to millions who suffer from depression, and radically alter the debate on its treatment.

368 pages Year Founded: 1936 ISBN 0-670034-05-3

558 Anxiety and Depression in Adults and Children,
Banff International Behavioral Science Series
Sage Publications, Inc.
2455 Teller Road
Thousand Oaks, CA 91320-2234
805-499-0721
800-818-7243; *Fax:* 800-583-2665
info@sagepub.com
www.sagepub.com

Kenneth D. Craig, Author
Keith S. Dobson, Author

Collection of papers by well respected researchers in the field of anxiety and depression. Brings together desparate areas of research and integrates them in an informative and interesting way. Focuses on recent advances in treating anxiety and depression in adults and children. Topics include self-management therapy, assessing and treating sexually abused children and unipolar depression. Integrates empirical research with clinical applications. Paperback also available. *$46.95*

296 pages Year Founded: 1994 ISBN 0-803970-20-X

559 Breaking the Patterns of Depression
Random House
1745 Broadway
New York, NY 10019-4343
212-782-9000
800-733-3000; *Fax:* 212-782-9052
ecustomerservice@randomhouse.com
www.randomhouse.com

Michael D. Yapko,PhD, Author

Presents skills that enable readers to understand and ultimately avert depression's recurring cycles. Focusing on future prevention as well as initial treatment, the book includes over one hundred structured activities to help sufferers learn the skills necessary to become and remain depression-free. Translates the clinical literature on psychotherapy and antidepressant medication into understandable language. Defines what causes depression and clarifies what can be done about it. With this knowledge in hand, readers can control their depression, rather than having depression control them. *$13.95*

360 pages Year Founded: 1998 ISBN 0-385483-70-8

560 Brilliant Madness: Living with Manic-Depressive Illness
Bantam Books
1745 Broadway
3rd Floor
New York, NY 10019-4368
212-782-9000
bdpublicity@randomhouse.com

Patty Duke, Author
Gloria Hochman, Author

From what it's like to live with manic-depressive disorder to the latest findings on its most effective treatments, this compassionate and eloquent book provides profound insight into the challenge of mental illness. It offers hope for all those who suffer from mood disorders and for the family, friends, and physicians who love and care for them.

368 pages Year Founded: 1997 ISBN 0-553560-72-7

561 Broken Connection: On Death and the Continuity of Life
American Psychiatric Publishing, Inc.
1000 Wilson Boulevard
Suite 1825
Arlington, VA 22209-3901
703-907-7322
800-368-5777; *Fax:* 703-907-1091
appi@psych.org
www.appi.org

Robert Jay Lifton, Author

Exploration of the inescapable connections between death and life, the psychiatric disorders that arise from these connections, and the advent of the nuclear age which has jeopardized any attempts to ensure the perpetuation of the self beyond death. *$38.00*

512 pages Year Founded: 1996 ISBN 0-880488-74-3

562 Carbamazepine and Manic Depression: A Guide
Madison Institute of Medicine
6515 Grand Teton Plaza
Suite 100
Madison, WI 53719
608-827-2470; *Fax:* 608-827-2444
mim@miminc.org
www.www.miminc.org

James W. Jefferson, Author
Janet R. Medenwald, MD, Author
John H. Greist, Author

A concise guide to the use of carbamazepine for the treatment of manic depression with information about dosing, monitoring and side effects. *$5.95*

32 pages Year Founded: 1996 ISBN 1-890802-05-0

563 Clinical Guide to Depression in Children and Adolescents
American Psychiatric Publishing, Inc.
1000 Wilson Boulevard
Suite 1825
Arlington, VA 22209-3901
703-907-7322
800-368-5777; *Fax:* 703-907-1091
appi@psych.org
www.appi.org

Mohammad Shafii, Editor
Sharon Lee Shafii, Editor

The book begins with a discussion of depression's clinical manifestations, including epidemiology, neurobiology, and chronobiology of seasonal mood disorders. A section on diagnostic assessment and treatment addresses standardizes approaches to assessment and such treatment modalities as dynamic psychotherapy, group therapy, the latest advances in pharmacological treatment and inpatient treatment. A concluding section examines bipolar disorders clinical manifestations, natural history, genetics, and treatment. *$39.50*

320 pages Year Founded: 1991 ISBN 0-880483-56-3

564 Consumer's Guide to Psychiatric Drugs
NewHarbinger Publications
5674 Shattuck Avenue
Oakland, CA 94609-1662
510-652-0215
800-748-6273; *Fax:* 800-652-1613
customerservice@newharbinger.com
www.newharbinger.com

Mary C. Talaga, Author
John D. Preston, Author
John H. O'Neal, Author

Helps consumers understand what treatment options are available and what side effects to expect. Covers possible interactions with other drugs, medical conditions and other concerns. Explains how each drug works, and offers detailed information about treatments for depression, bipolar disorder, anxiety and sleep disorders, as well as other conditions. *$16.95*

340 pages Year Founded: 1973 ISBN 1-572241-11-X

565 Depression Workbook: a Guide for Living with Depression
NewHarbinger Publications
5674 Shattuck Avenue
Oakland, CA 94609-1662
510-652-0215
800-748-6273; *Fax:* 800-652-1613
customerservice@newharbinger.com
www.newharbinger.com

Mary Ellen Copeland, MS, MA, Author

Based on responses of participants sharing their insights, experiences, and strategies for living with extreme mood swings. *$ 19.95*

352 pages Year Founded: 1973 ISBN 1-572242-68-X

566 Depression and Its Treatment
Grand Central Publishing

John H. Greist, MD, Author
James W. Jefferson, MD, Author

Depression is the most common psychological disorder, and at least ten percent of Americans will experience a major depression at some point in their lives. This clearly-written, straightforward guide explains depression and its causes and discusses treatments from drugs to psychotherapy. Developed by the American Psychiatric Press. *$19.95*

157 pages Year Founded: 1994

567 Depression, the Mood Disease
Johns Hopkins University Press
2715 N Charles Street
Baltimore, MD 21218-4319
410-516-6900
800-537-5487; *Fax:* 410-516-6998

Francis Mark Mondimore, MD, Author

Explores the many faces of an illness that will affect as many as 36 million Americans at some point in their lives. Updated to reflect state-of-the-art treatment. *$12.76*

240 pages ISBN 0-801851-84-X

568 Diagnosis and Treatment of Depression in Late Life: Results of the NIH Consensus Development Conference
American Psychiatric Publishing, Inc.
1000 Wilson Boulevard
Suite 1825
Arlington, VA 22209-3901
703-907-7322
800-368-5777; *Fax:* 703-907-1091
appi@psych.org
www.appi.org

Lon S Schneider, M.D., Editor
Charles F Reynolds III, M.D, Editor
Barry D Lebowitz, Ph.D, Editor
Arnold Friedhoff, M.D, Editor

Provides comprehensive studies in early life depression versus late life depression, the prevalence of depression in the elderly and the risk factors involved. *$21.95*

550 pages Year Founded: 1993 ISBN 0-880485-56-6

569 Drug Therapy and Postpartum Disorders (Psychiatric Disorders: Drugs & Psychology for the Mind & Body)
Mason Crest Publishers
450 Parkway Drive
Suite D
Broomall, PA 19008-4017
610-543-6200
866-627-2665; *Fax:* 610-543-3878
dtaylor@masoncrest.com
www.masoncrest.com

Autumn Libal, Author

Pregnancy, childbirth and early motherhood are supposed to be times filled with the joy and wonder of bringing a new life into the world. Unfortunately, many women find that the struggles of early motherhood are accompanied by multiple sorrows that clash with the sentimental ideal. New mothers may feel alone in their struggles, but depression after childbirth is far more common than most people realize. This book provides information about the psychiatric conditions that can accompany new motherhood and the treatments that can help.

128 pages ISBN 1-590846-70-6

570 Emotions Anonymous Book
Emotions Anonymous International Service Center
PO Box 4245
Saint Paul, MN 55104-0245
651-647-9712; *Fax:* 651-647-1593
www.EmotionsAnonymous.org

The Big Book of EA: A fellowship of men and women who share their experience, strength and hope with each other, that they may solve their common problem and help others recover from emotional illness. *$15.00*

261 pages ISBN 0-960735-65-5

571 Encyclopedia of Depression (Facts on File Library of Health & Living)
Facts on File
132 W 31st Street
17th Floor
New York, NY 10001-3406
800-322-8755; *Fax:* 800-678-3633
custserv@factsonfile.com
www.www.infobasepublishing.com

This volume defines and explains all terms and topics relating to depression. *$58.50*

170 pages

572 Growing Up Sad: Childhood Depression and Its Treatment
WW Norton & Company
500 5th Avenue
New York, NY 10110-54
212-354-2907
800-233-4830; *Fax:* 212-869-0856
npb@wwnorton.com

Leon Cytryn, Author
Donald H. McKnew Jr., Author

The authors have updated their classic study, Why Isn't Johnny Crying? that looks at the symptoms and treatment of childhood - onset depression. The authors give an authoritative summary of research, counsel prompt diagnosis, and assert that the disorder is treatable. *$25.00*

216 pages Year Founded: 1998 ISBN 0-393317-88-9

573 Help Me, I'm Sad: Recognizing, Treating, and Preventing Childhood and Adolescent Depression
Penguin Publishers
375 Hudson Street
New York, NY 10014-3657
212-366-2372
800-847-5515; *Fax:* 212-366-2933
ecommerce@us.penguingroup.com
www.www.us.penguingroup.com

David G. Fassler, Author
Lynne Dumas, Author

Discusses how to tell if your child is at risk; how to spot symptoms; depressions link with other problems and its impact on the family; teen suicide; finiding the right diagnosis, therapist, and treatment; and what you can do to help.

224 pages Year Founded: 1936 ISBN 0-140267-63-1

574 Helping Someone with Mental Illness: A Compassionate Guide for Family, Friends, and Caregivers
Three Rivers Press
1745 Broadway
New York, NY 10019
212-782-9000
ecustomerservice@randomhouse.com
www.randomhouse.com

Rosalynn Carter, Author
Susan Golant MA, Author

The authors address the latest breakthroughs in understanding, research, and treatment of schizophrenia, depression, manic depression, panic attacks, obsessive-compulsive disorder, and other mental disorders. *$19.00*

368 pages Year Founded: 1999 ISSN 9780812928983ISBN 0-812928-98-9

575 Helping Your Depressed Teenager: a Guide for Parents and Caregivers
John Wiley & Sons
111 River Street
Hoboken, NJ 07030-5774
201-748-6000
800-225-5945; *Fax:* 201-748-6088
info@wiley.com
www.wiley.com

Gerald D. Oster, Author
Sarah S. Montgomery, Author

A practical guide offering family solutions to a family problem. This book will sensitize you to the hidden struggles of adolescents and assist in understanding their multifaceted problems. The authors are experts in this field and have help countless youngsters confront and overcome their depressed mood. *$19.95*

208 pages Year Founded: 1994 ISBN 0-471621-84-6

576 Lithium and Manic Depression: A Guide
Madison Institute of Medicine
6515 Grand Teton Plaza
Suite 100
Madison, WI 53719
608-827-2470; *Fax:* 608-827-2444
mim@miminc.org
www.www.miminc.org

John Bohn, MD, Author
James W. Jefferson, MD, Author

A concise, up-to-date guide written by a leading expert on manic depression (bipolar disorder) and its treatment. This publication includes the most important information every patient taking lithium needs to know about lithium dosing, monitoring and side effects. *$5.95*

31 pages Year Founded: 1996 ISBN 1-890802-04-2

577 Living Without Depression & Manic Depression: a Workbook for Maintaining Mood Stability
NewHarbinger Publications
5674 Shattuck Avenue
Oakland, CA 94609-1662
510-652-0215
800-748-6273; *Fax:* 800-652-1613
customerservice@newharbinger.com
www.newharbinger.com

Mary Ellen Copeland,MS,MA, Author

Outlines a program that helps people achieve breakthroughs in coping and healing. Contents include: self advocacy, building a network of support, wellness lifestyle, symptom prevention strategies, self-esteem, mood stability, a career that works, trauma resolution, dealing with sleep problems, diet, vitamin and herbal therapies, dealing with stigma, medication side effects, psychotherapy, and counseling alternatives. *$18.95*

288 pages Year Founded: 1973 ISBN 1-879237-74-1

578 Lonely, Sad, and Angry: a Parent's Guide to Depression in Children and Adolescents
ADD Warehouse
300 NorthWest 70th Avenue
Suite 102
Plantation, FL 33317-2360
954-792-8944
800-233-9273; *Fax:* 954-792-8545
websales@addwarehouse.com
www.addwarehouse.com

Richard R. Morrissey, PhD, Author

Covers the symptoms of depression, its diagnosis, causes, treatment (including medication), suicide, and management strategies at home and at school. For parents and teenagers. *$14.95*

225 pages Year Founded: 1990

579 Management of Depression
American Psychiatric Publishing, Inc.
1000 Wilson Boulevard
Suite 1825
Arlington, VA 22209-3901
703-907-7322
800-368-5777; *Fax:* 703-907-1091
appi@psych.org
www.appi.org

Robert E Hales MD, Editor-in-Chief
Ron McMillen, Chief Executive Officer
John McDuffie, Editorial Director

Comprehensive text covers all the important issues in the management of depression. *$39.95*

136 pages ISBN 1-853175-47-1

580 Mania: Clinical and Research Perspectives
American Psychiatric Publishing, Inc.
1000 Wilson Boulevard
Suite 1825
Arlington, VA 22209-3901
703-907-7322
800-368-5777; *Fax:* 703-907-1091
appi@psych.org
www.appi.org

Paul J Goodnick, M.D., Editor
Ron McMillen, Chief Executive Officer
John McDuffie, Editorial Director

Diagnostic considerations, biological aspects, and treatment
of mania. *$59.95*

440 pages Year Founded: 1998 ISBN 0-880487-28-3

581 Manic-Depressive Illness: Bipolar Disorders
and Recurrent Depression, 2nd Edition
Oxford University Press
198 Madison Avenue
New York, NY 10016
212-726-6000
custserv.us@oup.com
www.www.oup.com/us/

Frederick K Goodwin, Author

The authors review the biological and genetic literature that
has dominated the field in recent years and incorporate cutting-edge research conducted since publication of the first
edition. They also update their surveys of psychological
and epidemiological evidence, as well as that pertaining to
diagnostice issues, course, and outcome, and they offer
practical guidelines for differential diagnosis and clinical
management.

582 Mayo Clinic on Depression: Answers to Help
You Understand, Recognize and Manage
Depression
Mason Crest Publishers
370 Reed Road
Suite 302
Broomall, PA 19008-4017
866-627-2665; *Fax:* 610-543-3878
www.masoncrest.com

Keith G Kramlinger,MD, Author

Discusses factors that increase risk, indications of depression, what happens inside the brain, effective forms of psychotherapy, electroconvulsive therapy, new trends in
treatment, self-care strategies for staying healthy, and more.

194 pages

583 Mood Apart: The Thinker's Guide to Emotion
and Its Disorders
William Morrow Paperbacks, Harper Collins
Imprint
30 Bond Street
New York, NY 10012
212-253-1074; *Fax:* 212-253-1075
www.www.peterwhybrow.com/

Peter C. Whybrow, Author

An overview of depression and manic depression and the
available treatments for them. *$24.00*

384 pages Year Founded: 1998 ISBN 0-060977-40-X

584 Mood Apart: Thinker's Guide to Emotion & Its
Disorders
Harper Collins
30 Bond Street
New York, NY 10012
212-253-1074; *Fax:* 212-253-1075
sales@harpercollins.com
www.www.peterwhybrow.com/

Peter C. Whybrow, Author

Discussion of depression and mania includes symptoms,
human costs, biological underpinnings, and therapies. Au-
thoritatively written, it uses case histories, appendices, and
historical references. *$15.00*

ISBN 0-060977-40-X

585 Natural History of Mania, Depression and
Schizophrenia
American Psychiatric Publishing, Inc.
1000 Wilson Boulevard
Suite 1825
Arlington, VA 22209-3901
703-907-7322
800-368-5777; *Fax:* 703-907-1091
appi@psych.org
www.appi.org

George Winokur, M.D., Author
Ming T Tsuang, M.D., Ph.D., D, Author
John McDuffie, Editorial Director

An unusual look at the course of mental illness, based on
data from the Iowa 500 Research Project. *$42.50*

384 pages Year Founded: 1996 ISBN 0-880487-26-7

586 Overcoming Anxiety, Depression, and Other
Mental Health Disorders in Children and
Adults
Interdisciplinary Council on Development &
Learning Disorders
4938 Hampden Lane
Suite 800
Bethesda, MD 20814
301-656-2667
info@icdl.com
www.icdl.com

Dr Stanley I Greenspan, Author

Reveals strategies for family members as well as professionals from different disciplines to help both children and
adults. The most common mental health disorders, including anxiety, depression, obsessive-compulsive patterns,
ADD/ADHD, borderline states, and others, are discussed
literally with a new set of eyeglasses.

168 pages ISBN 0-976775-88-3

587 Overcoming Depression: The Definitive
Resource for Patients and Families Who Live
with Depression and Manic-Depression
Harper Collins
10 E 53rd Street
New York, NY 10022-5299
212-207-7000
www.harpercollins.com

Demitri Papolos, Author

Has become the book most often recommended by doctors
to their depressed patients because it clearly and sympa-
thetically presents state-of-the-art medical information and

the solid, practical advice that patients and their families need to participate actively in diagnosis and treatment. Now featuring all-new data on the latest drugs, research, treatment, and medical insurance, it also includes a frank discussion of psychiatric therapy in the era of managed care. *$15.00*

432 pages Year Founded: 1997 ISBN 0-060927-82-8

588 Pain Behind the Mask: Overcoming Masculine Depression
Haworth Press
711 Third Avenue
New York, NY 10017
212-216-7800
800-429-6784; *Fax:* 212-244-1563
getinfo@haworthpress.com
www.haworthpress.com

John R Lynch, PhD, Author
Christopher Kilmartin, PhD, Author

Presents a model of masculinity based on the premise that men express depression through behaviors that distort the feelings and human conflicts they experience. *$22.95*

210 pages Year Founded: 1999 ISBN 0-789005-58-1

589 Pastoral Care of Depression
Haworth Press
711 Third Avenue
New York, NY 10017
212-216-7800
800-429-6784; *Fax:* 212-244-1563
getinfo@haworthpressinc.com
www.haworthpress.com

Binford W Gilbert, PhD, Author
Harold G Koenig, Author

Helps caregivers by overcoming the simplistic myths about depressive disorders and probing the real issues. *$17.95*

136 pages Year Founded: 1997 ISBN 0-789002-65-5

590 Physician's Guide to Depression and Bipolar Disorders
McGraw-Hill Companies
PO Box 182604
Columbus, OH 43218-2604
877-833-5524; *Fax:* 614-759-3749
customer.service@mcgraw-hill.com
www.mcgraw-hill.com

Dwight L Evans,MD, Author
Dennis S Charney,MD, Author
Lydia Lewis, Author

Offers a clear definitive instruction on drug treatments for bipolar disorders with the exact dosages needed. Crucial to a diagnosis and treatment is the ability to identify a patients symptoms. *$59.00*

400 pages Year Founded: 2005 ISBN 0-071441-75-1

591 Post-Natal Depression: Psychology, Science and the Transition to Motherhood
Routledge
711 3rd Avenue
8th Floor
New York, NY 10017
212-216-7800; *Fax:* 212-563-2269
www.www.routledge.com

Paula Nicolson, Author

Challenges the expectation that it is normal to be a happy mother. It provides a radical critique of the traditional medical and social science explanations of post natal depression by supplying a systematic feminist psychological analysis of women's experiences following childbirth. This book makes an important contribution to the psychology of women and feminist research and will be of interest to psychologists, nurses, and doctors. *$23.95*

ISBN 0-415163-62-5

592 Postpartum Mood Disorders
American Psychiatric Publishing, Inc.
1000 Wilson Boulevard
Suite 1825
Arlington, VA 22209-3901
703-907-7322
800-368-5777; *Fax:* 703-907-1091
www.appi.org

Lee S Cohen, M.D., Editor
Ruta M Nonacs, M.D., Ph.D., Editor
John McDuffie, Editorial Director

Provides thorough coverage of a highly prevalent, but often misunderstood subject. *$38.50*

164 pages Year Founded: 2005 ISBN 0-880489-29-4

593 Practice Guideline for Major Depressive Disorders in Adults
American Psychiatric Publishing, Inc.
1000 Wilson Boulevard
Suite 1825
Arlington, VA 22209-3901
703-907-7322
800-368-5777; *Fax:* 703-907-1091
appi@psych.org
www.appi.org

Robert E Hales MD, Editor-in-Chief
Ron McMillen, Chief Executive Officer
John McDuffie, Editorial Director

Summarizes the specific forms of somatic, psychotherapeutic, psychosocial, and educational treatments developed to deal with major depressive order and its various subtypes. *$22.50*

1,612 pages Year Founded: 2006 ISBN 0-890423-01-6

594 Predictors of Treatment Response in Mood Disorders
American Psychiatric Publishing, Inc.
1000 Wilson Boulevard
Suite 1825
Arlington, VA 22209-3901
703-907-7322
800-368-5777; *Fax:* 703-907-1091
appi@psych.org
www.appi.org

Paul J Goodnick, M.D., Editor
Ron McMillen, Chief Executive Officer
John McDuffie, Editorial Director

Helps clinicians and managed care administrators assign the correct somatic therapy. *$29.00*

260 pages Year Founded: 1995 ISBN 0-880484-94-2

595 Prozac Nation: Young & Depressed in America, a Memoir
Houghton Mifflin Company
222 Berkeley Street
Boston, MA 02116-3760
617-351-5000; *Fax:* 617-351-1105

Elizabeth Wurtzel, Author

Struck with depression at 11, Wurtzel, now 27, chronicles her struggle with the illness. Witty, terrifying and sometimes funny, it tells the story of a young life almost destroyed by depression. *$19.95*

317 pages

596 Questions & Answers About Depression & Its Treatment
Charles Press Publishers
230 North 21st Street
Suite 202
Philadelphia, PA 19103
215-561-2786; *Fax:* 215-600-1248
mailbox@charlespresspub.com
www.charlespresspub.com

Ivan k Goldberg,MD, Author

All the questions you'd like to ask, with answers.

139 pages

597 Seasonal Affective Disorder and Beyond: Light Treatment for SAD and Non-SAD Conditions
American Psychiatric Publishing, Inc.
1000 Wilson Boulevard
Suite 1825
Arlington, VA 22209-3901
703-907-7322
800-368-5777; *Fax:* 703-907-1091
appi@psych.org
www.appi.org

Raymond W Lam, M.D., Editor
Ron McMillen, Chief Executive Officer
John McDuffie, Editorial Director

Summarizes issues around the therapeutic uses of light treatment. *$45.00*

344 pages Year Founded: 1998 ISBN 0-880488-67-0

598 Talking to Depression: Simple Ways to Connect When Someone In Your Life Is Depressed
Penguin Group
375 Hudson Street
New York, NY 10014-3657
212-366-2372
800-847-5515; *Fax:* 212-366-2933
ecommerce@us.penguingroup.com
www.www.us.penguingroup.com

Claudia J Strauss, Author
Martha Manning, Foreward

What to say and what not to say when a friend or family member is struggling with depression. *$14.00*

224 pages Year Founded: 1936 ISBN 0-451209-86-3

599 The Cognitive Behavorial Workbook for Depression: A Step-by-Step Program
NewHarbinger Publications
5674 Shattuck Avenue
Oakland, CA 94609-1662

510-652-0215
800-748-6273; *Fax:* 800-652-1613
customerservice@newharbinger.com
www.newharbinger.com

Dr William J Knaus, Ed.D., Author
Albert Ellis, Ph.D., Author

This type of cognitive behavioral therapy, called rational emotive behavior therapy (REBT) by Ellis, proved especially effective at relieving problems like anger, anxiety, and depression.

336 pages Year Founded: 1973

600 Touched with Fire: Manic-Depressive Illness and the Artistic Temperament
Free Press
40 Main Street
Suite 301
Florence, MA 01062-3100
877-888-1533; *Fax:* 413-585-8904
www.freepress.net

Kay Redfield Jamison, Author

'We of the craft are all crazy.' -remarked Lord Byron about himself and his fellow poets.

325 pages Year Founded: 1996 ISBN 0-684831-83-X

601 Treatment Plans and Interventions for Depression and Anxiety Disorders
Guilford Press
72 Spring Street
New York, NY 10012-4068
800-365-7006; *Fax:* 212-966-6708
info@guilford.com
www.www.guilford.com

Robert L Leahy, Author
Stephen J.F Holland, Author
Lata K McGinn, Author

Provides information on treatments for seven frequently encountered disorders: major depression, generalized anxiety, panic, agoraphobia, PTSD, social phobia, specific phobia and OCD. Serving as ready to use treatment packages, chapters describe basic cognitive behavioral therapy techniques and how to tailor them to each disorder. Also featured are diagnostic decision trees, therapist forms for assessment and record keeping, client handouts and homework sheets. *$ 49.50*

490 pages Year Founded: 1973 ISBN 1-572305-14-2

602 Treatment for Chronic Depression: Cognitive Behavioral Analysis System of Psychotherapy (CBASP)
Guilford Press
512 Glendale Drive
Richmond, VA 23229
804-740-7646
800-365-7006; *Fax:* 804-740-0305
jmccull@vcu.edu
www.www.cbasp.org/

James P. McCullough Jr, PhD, Author

This book describes CBASP, a research based psychotherapeutic approach designed to motivate chronically depressed patients to change and help them develop needed problem solving and relationship skills. Filled with illustrative case material that brings challenging clinical situations to life, this book now puts the power of CBASP in the hands of the clinician. Readers are provided with two essential assets: an innovative framework for understanding the patient's psychopathology and a disciplined plan for helping the individual overthrow depression. *$35.00*

326 pages ISBN 1-572305-27-4

603 When Nothing Matters Anymore: A Survival Guide for Depressed Teens
Free Spirit Publishing
217 Fifth Avenue North
Suite 200
Minneapolis, MN 55401-1299
612-338-2068
866-735-7323; *Fax:* 866-419-5199
help4kids@freespirit.com
www.freespirit.com

Bev Cobain,R.N.C, Author

Written for teens with depression and those who feel despondent, dejected or alone. This powerful book offers help, hope, and potentially lifesaving facts and advice. *$13.95*

160 pages Year Founded: 1983 ISBN 1-575420-36-8

604 Winter Blues: Seasonal Affective Disorder: What It Is and How to Overcome It
Guilford Press
72 Spring Street
New York, NY 10012-4068
212-431-9800
800-365-7006; *Fax:* 212-966-6708
info@guilford.com

Norman Rosenthal, Author

Complete information about Seasonal Affective Disorder and its treatment. *$14.95*

355 pages Year Founded: 1998 ISBN 1-572303-95-6

605 Yesterday's Tomorrow
Hazelden
PO Box 11
Center City, MN 55012-0176
651-213-4000
800-822-0080
www.www.hazelden.org

Barry Longyear, Author

At last, a meditation book that shows why and, more importantly, how recovery works written in no-nonsense language by a hard case who's been there, and been there, and been there. *$12.00*

384 pages ISBN 1-568381-60-3

606 You Can Beat Depression: Guide to Prevention and Recovery
Impact Publishers
PO Box 6016
Atascadero, CA 93423-6016
805-466-5917
800-246-7228; *Fax:* 805-466-5919
info@impactpublishers.com
www.impactpublishers.com

John Preston,Psy.D, Author

Includes material on prevention of depression, prevention of relapse after treatment, brief therapy interventions, exercise, other non medical approaches and the Prozac controversy. Helps readers recognize when and how to help

themsevles, and when to turn to professional treatment. *$14.95*

176 pages Year Founded: 1970 ISBN 1-886230-40-4

Periodicals & Pamphlets

607 Coping With Unexpected Events: Depression & Trauma
Depression & BiPolar Support Alliance
730 North Franklin Street
Suite 501
Chicago, IL 60654-7225
312-642-0049
800-826-3632; *Fax:* 312-642-7243
programs@dbsalliance.org
www.dbsalliance.org

Cheryl T Magrini,MS.Ed,MTS,PhD, Chair
Allen Doederlein, President
Cindy Specht, ExecutiveVice president
Gregory E Ostfeld, Treasurer

The mission of DBSA is to provide hope, help, and support to improve the lives of people living with mood disorders. DBSA pursues and accomplishes this mission through peer-based, recovery-oriented, empowering services and resources when people want them, where they want them, and how they want to receive them.

608 Coping with Mood Changes Later in Life
Depression & Bipolar Support Alliance
730 North Franklin Street
Suite 501
Chicago, IL 60654-7225
312-642-0049
800-826-3632; *Fax:* 312-642-7243
www.dbsalliance.org

Sue Bergeson, President

14 pages Year Founded: 2003

609 Depression
National Institute of Mental Health
6001 Executive Boulevard
Room 8184
Bethesda, MD 20892-1
301-443-4513
866-615-6464
TTY: 301-443-8431
nimhinfo@nih.gov

This brochure gives descriptions of major depression, dysthymia and bipolar disorder (manic depression). It lists symptoms, gives possible causes, tells how depression is diagnosed and discusses available treatments. This brochure provides help and hope for the depressed person, family and friends.

23 pages

610 Depression: Help On the Way
ETR Associates
4 Carbonero Way
Scotts Valley, CA 95066-4200
831-438-4060
800-321-4407; *Fax:* 831-438-3618
support@etr.freshdesk.com
www.etr.org

David Kitchen,MBA, Chief Financial Officer
Talita Sanders,BS, Director,Human Resources

Coleen Cantwell,MPH, Director,Business Development Pl
Matt McDowell,BS, Director,Marketing

Includes symptoms of minor depression, major depression, and seasonal affective depression; treatment options and medication, and the importance of exercise and laughter. Sold in lots of 50.

611   Depression: What Every Woman Should Know
National Institute of Mental Health
6001 Executive Boulevard
Room 8184,MSC 9663
Bethesda, MD 20892-9663
301-443-4513
866-615-6464
TTY: 301-443-8431
nimhinfo@nih.gov
www.www.nimh.nih.gov/

This booklet discusses the symptoms of depression and some of the reasons that make women so vulnerable. It also discusses the types of therapy and where to go for help.

24 pages

612   Finding Peace of Mind: Treatment Strategies
for Depression and Bipolar Disorder
Depression and Bipolar Support Alliance
730 North Franklin Street
Suite 501
Chicago, IL 60654-7225
312-642-0049
800-826-3632; *Fax:* 312-642-7243
www.dbsalliance.org

Helps to build a good, cooperative relationship with your doctor by explaining some of the treatments for mood disorders and how they work. Also includes a guide for medication that has been frequently prescribed and new treatments that are being investigated.

20 pages Year Founded: 2003

613   Getting Better Sleep: What You Need to Know
Depression and Bipolar Support Alliance
730 North Franklin Street
Suite 501
Chicago, IL 60654-7225
312-642-0049
800-826-3632; *Fax:* 312-642-7243
www.dbsalliance.org

Sue Bergeson, President

Describes some causes of sleep loss, and how sleep loss relates to bipolar disorder and depression. Also provides information on how to get better sleep.

614   Introduction to Depression and Bipolar
Disorder
Depression and Bipolar Support Alliance
730 North Franklin Street
Suite 501
Chicago, IL 60654-7225
312-642-0049
800-826-3632; *Fax:* 312-642-7243
www.dbsalliance.org

Sue Bergeson, President

Quick and easy-to-read brochure describing syptoms and treatments for mood disorders.

615   Let's Talk About Depression
National Institute of Mental Health
6001 Executive Boulevard
Room 8184,MSC 9663
Bethesda, MD 20892-9663
301-443-4513
866-615-6464
TTY: 301-443-8431
nimhinfo@nih.gov
www.www.nimh.nih.gov/

Facts about depression, and ways to get help. Target audience is teenaged youth.

616   Major Depression in Children and Adolescents
PO Box 42557
Washington, DC 20015-557
800-789-2647; *Fax:* 240-747-5470
TDD: 866-889-2647
ken@mentalhealth.org
www.mentalhealth.samhsa.gov

A Kathryn Power, MEd, Director
Edward B Searle, Deputy Director

2 pages

617   McMan's Depression and Bipolar Weekly
McMan's Depression and Bipolar Web
PO Box 5093
Kendall Park, NJ 08824-5093
E-mail: mcman@mcmanweb.com
www.mcmanweb.com

John McManamy, Editor/Publisher

Online newsletter devoted to the issues of bipolar and depression disorders. There is no charge, just for you to understand different things about the disorders.

618   Men and Depression
National Institute of Mental Health
6001 Executive Boulevard
Room 8184,MSC 9663
Bethesda, MD 20892-9663
301-443-4513
866-615-6464
TTY: 301-443-8431
nimhinfo@nih.gov
www.www.nimh.nih.gov/

Have you known a man who is grumpy, irritable, and has no sense of humor? Maybe he drinks too much or abuses drugs. Maybe he physically or verbally abuses his wife and his kids. Maybe he works all the time, or compulsively seeks thrills in high-risk behavior. Or maybe he seems isolated, withdrawn, and no longer interested in the people or activities he used to enjoy. Perhaps this man is you. Talk to a healthcare provider about how you are feeling, and ask for help.

36 pages

619   Myths and Facts about Depression and Bipolar
Disorders
Depression and Bipolar Support Alliance
730 North Franklin Street
Suite 501
Chicago, IL 60654-7225
312-642-0049
800-826-3632; *Fax:* 312-642-7243
www.dbsalliance.org

Gives some myths about depression and bipolar disorder and the truths that combat them.

620   New Message
Emotions Anonymous
PO Box 4245
Saint Paul, MN 55104-0245
651-647-9712; *Fax:* 651-647-1593
info@EmotionsAnonymous.org
www.EmotionsAnonymous.org

Features stories and articles of recovery, plus the latest news from EA International. *$8.00*

4 per year

621   Recovering Your Mental Health: a Self-Help Guide
SAMHSA'S National Mental Health Informantion Center
1 Choke Cherry Road
Rockville, MD 20857
877-726-4727
ken@mentalhealth.org
www.mentalhealth.samhsa.gov

Mary Ellen Copeland, Author
Edward B Searle, Deputy Director

This booklet offers tips for understanding symptoms of depression and other conditions and getting help. Also details the advantages of counseling, medications available, options for professional help, relaxation techniques and paths to positive thinking.

32 pages

622   What to do When a Friend is Depressed: Guide for Students
National Institute of Mental Health
6001 Executive Boulevard
Room 8184
Bethesda, MD 20892-1
301-443-4513
866-615-6464
TTY: 301-443-8431
nimhinfo@nih.gov
www.www.vamh.org

This brochure offers information on depression and its symptoms and suggests things a young person can do to guide a depressed friend in finding help. It is especially good for health fairs, health clinics, and school health units.

3 pages

623   You've Just Been Diagnosed...What Now?
Depression and Bipolar Support Alliance
730 North Franklin Street
Suite 501
Chicago, IL 60654-7225
312-642-0049
800-826-3632; *Fax:* 312-642-7243
www.dbsalliance.org

Sue Bergeson, President

Pamphlet to help you understand about the disorder you have just been diagnosed with. Tells you basic facts about mood disorders and will help you work towards a diagnosis.

19 pages Year Founded: 2002

Research Centers

624   Brain & Behavior Research Foundation
90 Park Avenue
16th Floor
New York, NY 10016
646-681-4888
800-829-8289
info@bbrfoundation.org
www.www.bbrfoundation.org/

Steve Lieber, Chairman of the Board
Jeffrey Borenstein, MD, President and CEO
Louis Innamorato, CPA, VP and Chief Financial Officer
Anne Abramson, Vice President

The Brain and Behavior Research Foundation awards grants aimed at advancing scientific understandings of mental health treatments and mental disorders such as depression and schizophrenia. The Brain and Behavior Research Foundation's mission is to eliminate the suffering caused by mental illness.

Year Founded: 1987

625   UAMS Psychiatric Research Institute
University of Arkansas for Medical Sciences
4224 Shuffield Drive
Little Rock, AR 72205
501-526-8100; *Fax:* 501-660-7542
www.psychiatry.uams.edu

Donald R Bobbitt, President
William Bowes,MS, Vice Chancellor,Finance And CFO
Roxane A Townsend,MD, Chief Executive Officer
Christina L Clark,BA, Chief of Staff

Combining research, education and clinical services into one facility, PRI offers inpatiend and outpatient services, with 40 psychiatric beds, therapy options, and specialized treatment for specific disorders, including: addictive eating, anxiety, deppressive and post-traumatic stress disorders. Research focuses on evidence-based care takes into consideration the education of future medical personnel while relying on research scientists to provide innovative forms of treatment. PRI includes the Center for Addiction Research as well as a methadone clinic.

626   University of Texas: Mental Health Clinical Research Center
6363 Forest Park Road
7th Floor, Suite 749
Dallas, TX 75390-9121
214-648-3111
www.utsouthwestern.edu

Research activity of major and atypical depression.

627   Yale Mood Disorders Research Program
Department of Psychiatry
300 George Street
Suite 901
New Haven, CT 06511-6624
203-785-2090; *Fax:* 203-785-2028
www.psychiatry.yale.edu

John H Krystal, Chair
Rajita Sinha, Chief,Psychology Section

MDRP is dedicated to understanding the science of mood disorders, including bipolar disorder and depression. The MDRP brings together a multi-disciplinary group of scientists from across the Yale campus in a highly collaborative research effort. Goals of the MDRP include the identification of biological markers for mood disorders and discovery of new treatment strategies.

Support Groups & Hot Lines

628 Depressed Anonymous
PO Box 17414
Louisville, KY 40217
502-569-1989
info@depressedanon.com
www.depressedanon.com

Formed to provide therapeutic resources for depressed individuals of all ages. Works with the chronically depressed and those recently discharged from health facilities who were treated for depression.

629 Emotions Anonymous International Service Center
PO Box 4245
St. Paul, MN 55104-0245
651-647-9712
director@emotionsanonymous.org
www.emotionsanonymous.org/

Gus S., President
Scott J., Vice President and Treasurer
John W., Secretary
Elaine Weber Nelson, Executive Director

Fellowship of men and women who share their experience, strength, and hope with each other, that they may solve their common problem and help others recover from emotional illness. Members come together in weekly meetings.

630 Recovery International
1415 W. 22nd Street
Tower Floor
Oak Brook, IL 60523
312-337-5661
866-221-0302; *Fax:* 312-726-4446
www.www.recoveryinternational.org

Sandra K. Wilcoxon, Chief Executive Officer
Joanne Lampey, President
Joan Nobiling, Vice President
Nicole Cilento, 2nd Vice President

Recovery International is an organization that uses a peer-to-peer, self-help training system developed by Abraham Low in order to help individuals with mental health issues lead more productive lives.

Year Founded: 1937

Video & Audio

631 A Madman's Journal
Educational Training Videos
136 Granville St
Suite 200
Gahanna, OH 43230
Fax: 888-775-3919
www.educationaltrainingvideos.com

For two years, the narrator of this program went through a nightmare, feeling a self-hatred and worthlessness beyond love and redemption that he described as the concentration camp of the mind. This video presents one man's attempt to convey the ordeal of severe depression by writing a memoir about the experience.

632 Beating Depression
Educational Training Videos
136 Granville St
Suite 200
Gahanna, OH 43230
Fax: 888-775-3919
www.educationaltrainingvideos.com

This program comes to grips with depression through the experiences of five patients whose backgrounds span the socioeconomic spectrum. Three cases of chronic depression, one of which is complicated by borderline personality disorder and another by alcohol abuse, and two cases of bipolar disorder, one of which is extreme, are presented.

633 Bundle of Blues
Fanlight Productions
32 Court Street
21st Floor
Brooklyn, NY 11201
718-488-8900
800-876-1710; *Fax:* 718-488-8642
info@fanlight.com
www.fanlight.com

Serena Down, Author

The stories in this thoughtful documentary represent a range of experiences from minor postpartum depression through postpartum psychosis. It stresses that PDD can happen to any new mother, but that it can be managed. 13 minutes.

634 Clinical Impressions: Identifying Mental Illness
Educational Training Videos
136 Granville St
Suite 200
Gahanna, OH 43230
Fax: 888-775-3919
www.educationaltrainingvideos.com

How long can mental illness stay hidden, especially from the eyes of trained experts? This program rejoins a group of ten adults- five of them healthy and five of them with histories of mental illness- as psychiatric specialists try to spot and correctly diagnose the latter. Administering a series of collaborative and one-on-one tests, including assessments of personality type, physical self-image, and rational thinking, the panel gradually makes decisions about who suffers from depression, bipolar disorder, bulimia, and social anxiety.

635 Coping with Depression
NewHarbinger Publications
5674 Shattuck Avenue
Oakland, CA 94609-1662
510-652-0215
800-748-6273; *Fax:* 800-652-1613
customerservice@newharbinger.com
www.newharbinger.com

Matthew McKay, Owner

60 minute videotape that offers a powerful message of hope for anyone struggling with depression. *$39.95*

Year Founded: 1973 ISBN 1-879237-62-8

636 Coping with Stress
Educational Video Network, Inc.
1401 19th Street
Huntsville, TX 77340

936-295-5767
800-762-0060; *Fax:* 936-294-0233
www.www.evndirect.com

Stress affects everyone, both emotionally and physically. For some, mismanaged stress can result in substance abuse, violence, or even suicide. This program answers the question, How can a person cope with stress?

637 Covert Modeling & Covert Reinforcement
NewHarbinger Publications
5674 Shattuck Avenue
Oakland, CA 94609-1662
510-652-0215
800-748-6273; *Fax:* 800-652-1613
customerservice@newharbinger.com
www.newharbinger.com

Matthew McKay, Owner

Based on the essential book of cognitive behavioral techniques for effecting change in your life, Thoughts & Feelings. Learn step-by-step protocols for controlling destructive behaviors such as anxiety, obsessional thinking, uncontrolled anger, and depression. *$ 11.95*

Year Founded: 1973 ISBN 0-934986-29-0

638 Dark Glasses and Kaleidoscopes: Living with Manic Depression
Depression and Bipolar Support Alliance
730 N Franklin Street
Suite 501
Chicago, IL 60654-7225
312-642-0049
800-826-3632; *Fax:* 312-642-7243
www.dbsalliance.org

Allen Doederlein, President
Cindy Specht, Executive Vice President
Lisa Goodale, Vice President, Peer Support Ser
Nancy Heffernan, Vice President, Finance and Admi

Dr. Kowatch speaks about the prevalence, diagnosis, comorbidity, medication treatment, and outcome of child/adolescent bipolar disorder. He addresses some of the unique traits of cild bipolar, as well as some factors that make it difficult to diagnose. He covers treatment options for both the manic and depressive phases in detail, using clinical studies as evidence. *$5.00*

639 Day for Night: Recognizing Teenage Depression
DRADA-Depression and Related Affective Disorders Association
2330 W Joppa Road
Suite 100
Lutherville, MD 21093-4614
410-583-2919; *Fax:* 410-583-2964
www.drada.org

Catherine Pollock, Executive Director
Sallie Mink, Director Education
Vice Preside

In an effort to help teens gain a better understanding of depression, this video was created to build awareness of the illness and, in the process, save lives. Offering an in-depth look at the signs, symptoms and treatment of teenage depression, this video includes interviews with young people who are dealing with clinical depression and bipolar disorder. Featuring their families and friends, as well as interviews with health professionals, the video's goal is to

provide education, support and hope to those suffering from this debilitating yet treatable disease. *$22.50*

640 Dealing with Depression
Educational Video Network, Inc.
1401 19th Street
Huntsville, TX 77340
936-295-5767
800-762-0060; *Fax:* 936-294-0233
www.www.evndirect.com

As more and more young people are falling victim to depression, it is important to understand what causes it and to know how to get the help that can rid a person of this life-wrecking affliction.

641 Depression & Anxiety Management
NewHarbinger Publications
5674 Shattuck Avenue
Oakland, CA 94609-1662
510-652-0215
800-748-6273; *Fax:* 800-652-1613
customerservice@newharbinger.com
www.newharbinger.com

Matthew McKay, Owner

Offers step-by-step help for identifying the thoughts that make one anxious and depressed, confronting unrealistic and distorted thinking, and replacing negative mental patterns with healthy, realistic thinking. *$11.95*

Year Founded: 1973 ISBN 1-879237-46-6

642 Depression: Fighting the Dragon
Fanlight Productions
32 Court Street
21st Floor
Brooklyn, NY 11201
718-488-8900
800-876-1710; *Fax:* 718-488-8642
info@fanlight.com
www.fanlight.com

Sue Ridout, Author

Follows five people who have struggled for years to overcome this debilitating condition. Two of the five have family histories of the disease. Their moving personal stories are enriched by the perspectives of leading researchers, and by glimpses of the sophisticated brain-imaging technologies which now enable us to see what is happening in the human brain during depression and its treatment. *$149.00*

643 FRONTLINE: The Released
PBS
2100 Crystal Drive
Arlington, VA 22202
www.pbs.org

Will Lyman, Actor
Narrator
Miri Navasky, Director
Karen O'Connor, Director

The documentary states that of the 700,000 inmates released from American prisons each year, half of them have mental disabilities. This work focused on those with severe problems who keep entering and exiting prison. Full of good information on the challenges they face with mental illnesses; housing, employment, stigmatization, and socialization.

Year Founded: 2009

644 Living with Depression and Manic Depression
NewHarbinger Publications
5674 Shattuck Avenue
Oakland, CA 94609-1662
510-652-0215
800-748-6273; *Fax:* 800-652-1613
customerservice@newharbinger.com
www.newharbinger.com

Matthew McKay, Owner

Describes a program based on years of research and hundreds of interviews with depressed persons. Warm, helpful, and engaging, this tape validates the feelings of people with depression while it encourages positive change. *$11.95*

Year Founded: 1973 ISBN 1-879237-63-6

645 Mental Disorder
Educational Training Videos
136 Granville St
Suite 200
Gahanna, OH 43230
Fax: 888-775-3919
www.educationaltrainingvideos.com

What is abnormality? Using the case studies of two young women; one who has depression, one who has an anxiety disorder; as a springboard, this program presents three psychological perspective on mental disorder.

646 No More Shame: Understanding Schizophrenia, Depression, and Addiction
Educational Training Videos
136 Granville St
Suite 200
Gahanna, OH 43230
Fax: 888-775-3919
www.educationaltrainingvideos.com

These programs examine research about the physiological, psychological, sociological, and cultural aspects of these disorders and their treatments. The goal of these programs is to explain what we do and do not know about each of these conditions, as well as to destigmatize the disorders by presenting them in the context of the same research process that is applied to all medical disorders.

647 Understanding Mental Illness
Educational Video Network, Inc.
1401 19th Street
Huntsville, TX 77340
936-295-5767
800-762-0060; *Fax:* 936-294-0233
www.www.evndirect.com

Contains information and classifications of mental illness. Mental illness can strike anyone, at any age. Learn about various organic and functional mental disorders as discussed and their causes and symptoms, and learn where to seek help for a variety of mental health concerns.

648 Why Isn't My Child Happy? Video Guide About Childhood Depression
ADD WareHouse
300 NW 70th Avenue
Suite 102
Plantation, FL 33317-2360
954-792-8100
800-233-9273; *Fax:* 954-792-8545
websales@addwarehouse.com
www.addwarehouse.com

Sam Goldstein, PhD, Author

The first of its kind, this new video deals with childhood depression. Informative and frank about this common problem, this book offers helpful guidance for parents and professionals trying to better understand childhood depression. 110 minutes. *$55.00*

Year Founded: 1990

Web Sites

649 www.befrienders.org
Samaritans International

Support, helplines, and advice.

650 www.blarg.net/~charlatn/voices
Voices of Depression

Compilation of writings by people suffering from depression.

651 www.cfsny.org
Center for Family Support (CFS)

Devoted to providing support and assistance to individuals with developmental and related disabilities, and to the family members who care for them.

652 www.cyberpsych.org
CyberPsych

Hosts the American Psychoanalyists Foundation, American Association of Suicideology, Society for the Exploration of Psychotherapy Intergration, and Anxiety Disorders Association of America. Also subcategories of the anxiety disorders, as well as general information, including panic disorder, phobias, obsessive compulsive disorder (OCD), social phobia, generalized anxiety disorder, post traumatic stress disorder, and phobias of childhood. Book reviews and links to web pages sharing the topics.

653 www.dbsalliance.org
Depression & Bi-Polar Support Alliance

Mental health news updates and local support group information.

654 www.emdr.com
EMDR Institute, Inc.

Discusses EMDR-Eye Movement Desensitization and Reprocessing-as an innovative clinical treatment for trauma, including sexual abuse, domestic violence, combat, crime, and those suffering from a number of other disorders including depressions, addictions, phobias and a variety of self-esteem issues.

655 www.goodwill-suncoast.org
Suncoast Residential Training Center

Group home that serves individuals diagnosed as developmentally disabled, with a secondary diagnosis of psychiatric difficulties as evidenced by problem behavior.

656 www.ifred.org
National Foundation for Depressive Illness

Support, helplines, and advice.

657 www.klis.com/chandler/pamphlet/dep/
Jim Chandler MD

White paper on depression in children and adolesents.

658 **www.manicdepressive.org**
The Massachusetts General Hospital Bipolar Clinic/Research Program

Dedicated to providing quality clinical care, conducting clinically informative research, and educating colleagues, patients and the community.

659 **www.med.yale.edu**
Yale University School of Medicine

Research center dedicated to understanding the science of mood disorders.

660 **www.mentalhealth.Samhsa.Gov**
Center for Mental Health Services Knowledge Exchange Network

Information about resources, technical assistance, research, training, networks, and other federal clearinghouses, fact sheets and materials.

661 **www.mhselfhelp.org**
National Mental Health Consumer's Self-Help Clearinghouse

Encourages the development and growth of consumer self-help groups.

662 **www.nami.org**
National Alliance on Mental Illness

From its inception in 1979, NAMI has been dedicated to improving the lives of individuals and families affected by mental illness.

663 **www.nimh.nih.gov/publicat/depressionmenu.cfm**
National Institute of Mental Health

National Institute of Mental Health offers brochures organized by topic. Depression discusses symptoms, diagnosis, and treatment options.

664 **www.nimh.nih.gov/publist/964033.htm**
National Institute of Mental Health

Discusses depression in older years, symptoms, treatment, going for help.

665 **www.planetpsych.com**
Planetpsych.com

Learn about disorders, their treatments and other topics in psychology. Articles are listed under the related topic areas. Ask a therapist a question for free, or view the directory of professionals in your area. If you are a therapist sign up for the directory. Current features, self-help, interactive, and newsletter archives.

666 **www.psychcentral.com**
Psych Central

Personalized one-stop index for psychology, support, and mental health issues, resources, and people on the Internet.

667 **www.psychologyinfo.com/depression**
Psychology Information On-line: Depression

Information on diagnosis, therapy, and medication.

668 **www.psycom.net/depression.central.html**
Dr. Ivan's Depression Central

Medication-oriented site. Clearinghouse on all types of depressive disorders.

669 **www.queendom.com/selfhelp/depression/depression.html**
Queendom

Articles, information on medication and support groups.

670 **www.shpm.com**
Self Help Magazine

Articles and discussion forums, resource links.

671 **www.store.samhsa.gov**
Substance Abuse and Mental Health Services Administration

Resources on mental disorders as well as treatment and recovery.

672 **www.thebalancedmind.org/flipswitch**
Flipswitch

Educational site dedicated to helping teens, parents and teachers understand symptoms of teenage depression. Provides resources for those ready to seek help.

673 **www.thenadd.org**
National Association for the Dually Diagnosed (NADD)

An association for persons with developmental disabilities and mental health needs.

674 **www.utsouthwestern.edu**
UT Southwestern Medical Center

Research to find the corticosteroid effects on the human brain, dual-diagnosed patients, and depression in asthma patients.

675 **www.wingofmadness.com**
Wing of Madness: A Depression Guide

Accurate information, advice, support, and personal experiences.

Disruptive, Impulse-Control and Conduct Disorders

Introduction

Everyone has experienced a situation in which they are tempted to do something that is harmful to themselves or others. This kind of behavior only becomes a disorder when the person is repeatedly and persistently unable to resist such temptations. Usually, the person feels a rising tension before acting on the need, feels pleasure and relief when giving into the impulse and, sometimes, feels remorse and guilt afterwards. Conduct disorder is characterized by a repetitive and persistent pattern of behavior in which societal norms and the basic rights of others are violated. These behaviors can include physical harm to people or animals, damage to property, deceitfulness or theft, and extreme violations of rules. It is important to note that troublesome behavior can also result from adverse circumstances; the circumstances need to be fully investigated, and attempts to rectify adversity made, before Conduct Disorder is diagnosed. The diagnosis can be divided into two types, depending on the age of diagnosis: childhood-onset type and adolescent-onset type. Early diagnosis and intensive, individualized therapy is necessary to help children and adolescents with conduct disorder make a successful transition to adulthood.

SYMPTOMS

Disruptive and Impulse-Control Disorders

Kleptomania
• Recurrent failure to resist the impulse to steal objects, often objects that the individual could have paid for or does not particularly want;
• Increased sense of tension immediately before the theft;
• Pleasure and relief during the theft;
• Theft is not due to anger, delusions, or hallucinations;
• Awareness that stealing is sensless and wrong;
• Feelings of depression and guilt after stealing.

Kleptomania should not be confused with thefts which are deliberate or for personal gain. Kleptomania is strongly associated with depression, anxiety disorders, and feeding and eating disorders.

Kleptomania is very rare, but is it usually kept secret, and is more common among females than males.

Behavior therapy, which focuses on changing the behavior, has had some success, as has anti-depressant medication.

Pyromania
• Purposefully setting fires more than once;
• Increased tension before the deed;
• Fascination with and curiosity about fire;
• Pleasure or relief when setting or watching fires;
• The fire is not set for financial gain or revenge.

Pyromaniacs make complicated preparations for setting a fire, seem not to care about consequenses, and may get pleaure from the destruction. Many who set fires often have symptoms of ADHD or Adjustment Disorders. It is more common among males with alcohol, learning and societal problems. Treatment is difficult, and may include anger management, problem solving, and behavior therapy. Psychotherapy and anti-depressants have been effective.

Pathological Gambling
• Recurrent gambling;
• Gambling disrupts family, work, and personal activities;
• Preoccupation with gambling;
• Excitement is more important than money. Greater bets and risks needed to produce desired excitement;
• Gambling continues despite repeated efforts to stop, accompanied by restlessness and irritability;
• Gambler lies to conceal gambling to family and others;
• May turn to criminal behavior to get money for gambling;
• May lose job, relationship, and career opportunities.

Compulsive gamblers are distorted in their thinking, are superstitious, deny their problem, and may be over confident, believing that money is the cause and solution to all their problems. They are often competitive, easily bored, extravagently generous, and concerned with other's approval. Compulsive gamblers are prone to medical issues dealing with stress and may suffer from ADHD, depression, bipolar disorder, and alcohol abuse. Both males and females can be compulsive gamblers. Men usually start gambling in adolescence, women somewhat later, often as an escape from depression. It is a difficult disorder to treat, but psychotherapy and Gambler's Anonymous, a 12-step program, has had some success.

Trichotillomania
• Repeated hair pulling so that hair loss is noticeable;
• Increasing tension just before the behavior or when trying to resist it;
• Pleasure or relief when pulling;
• Causes clear distress and problems in personal work or social functioning.

Examining the hair root, pulling the hair between the teeth, or eating hairs (Trichophagia) may accompany Trichotillomania. Hair pulling is usually done in private or in the presence of close family members. Pain is not usually reported. The hair pulling is mostly denied and concealed by wigs, hairstyling, and cosmetics. People with this disorder may also have Major Depressive Disorder, General Anxiety Disorder, Eating Disorder, or Mental Retardation. Among children, both males and females can have the disorder, but among adults, it is far more frequent in females. Symptoms usually emerge around the age of 13, but the condition may also affect children as young as five.

There is no agreement about the cause of this disorder, making treatment more difficult. Variable treatments that have been proposed include behavior therapy, hypnosis, and stress reduction. Cognitive behavior therapy (in which the patient learns to replace negative thoughts and behaviors with positive ones) is considered to be an effective treatment for trichotillomania. Medications such as serotonin reuptake inhibitors (SSRIs) are sometimes prescribed if cognitive behavior therapy is not successful.

Intermittent Explosive Disorder
• Recurrent instances of impulsive, aggressive behavior;
• Feelings of guilt and remorse after aggressive behavior;
• May lose job and relationships;
• Injuries as a result of fighting or accidents;
• Explosive outbursts likely among people with paranoid or obsessive characteristics.

Intermittent Explosive Disorder is associated with substance abuse disorders and certain neurological disorders, but should not be confused with the aggression seen in other forms of psychiatric and organic brain disorders, such as head trauma, substance withdrawal, and borderline personality disorder. Intermittent Explosive Disorder is a rare disorder, that is more common in men than women. Symptoms usually begin to emerge between late childhood and the early 20s.

Treatment for Intermittent Explosive Disorder may include cognitive behavior therapy and medications such as carbamazepine, propranolol, and lithium.

Conduct Disorder
• Aggression to people and animals, including bullying, fighting, using weapons, physical cruelty to people and animals, stealing, or forcing someone into sexual activity;
• Destruction of property;
• Deceitfulness and theft, including breaking and entering, lying to obtain goods/favors, or shoplifting;
• Violations of rules, including staying out past curfews, running away from home, and truancy from school.

ASSOCIATED FEATURES

Conduct disorder is often associated with early onset of sexual activity, drinking and smoking. The disorder leads to school disruption, problems with the police, sexually transmitted diseases, unplanned pregnancy, and injury from accidents and fights. Suicide and suicidal attempts are more common among adolescents with Conduct Disorder, probably both because they have a history of abuse and neglect and because their behavior results in adverse consequences. Individuals with Conduct Disorder appear to have little remorse for their acts, though they may learn that expressing guilt can diminish punishment; and they often show little or no empathy for the feelings, wishes, and well-being of others.

PREVALENCE

Prevalence of Conduct Disorder appears to have increased in recent years. The disorder seems to be more common in males than females. For males under 18 years of age, rates range from six percent to sixteen percent; for females, rates range from two percent to nine percent. Onset can be before the age of ten, or in adolescence.

TREATMENT OPTIONS

There is no agreement on the best way to treat conduct disorder. Approaches range from incarceration and 'tough love,' to psychotherapy (usually cognitive behavioral therapy with an emphasis on anger management techniques) and medication. This condition is stressful for family members of the affected child or adolescent; it is crucial that they are supported and involved in the treatment.

Associations & Agencies

677 American Association of Children's Residential Centers
648 North Plankinton Avenue
Suite 425
Milwaukee, WI 53203
877-332-2272
www.togetherthevoice.org

Laurah Currey, President
Kerry Ann Goldsmith, Secretary

Joe Ford, Vice President
Kari Sisson, Executive Director

The American Association of Children's Residential Centers is a national organization focused on providing residential therapeutic treatment for children and adolescents with behavioral health disorders.

Year Founded: 1956

678 Association for Behavioral and Cognitive Therapies
305 Seventh Avenue
16th Floor
New York, NY 10001
212-647-1890; *Fax:* 212-647-1865
www.abct.org

Sabine Wilhelm, PhD, President
Mary Jane Eimer, Executive Director
Mary Larimer, PhD, Secretary-Treasurer
David Teisler, Director of Communications

A multidisciplinary organization dedicated to utilizing and advancing scientific approaches in the understanding and prevention of human behavioral and cognitive problems.

Year Founded: 1966

679 Center for Mental Health Services (CMHS)
Substance Abuse and Mental Health Services Administration
5600 Fishers Lane
Rockville, MD 20857
240-276-1310
877-726-4727
TTY: 800-487-4889
www.samhsa.gov/about-us/who-we-are/offices-centers

Paolo del Vecchio, MSW, Director
Anne Mathews-Younes, Acting Deputy Director
Keris Myrick, Director, Consumer Affairs
Patricia Gratton, Director, Program Analysis

Promotes the treatment of mental illness and emotional disorders by increasing accessibility to mental health programs; supporting outreach, treatment, rehabilitation, and support programs and networks; and encouraging the use of scientifically-based information when treating mental disorders. CMHS provides information about mental health via a toll-free number and numerous publications. Developed for users of mental health services and their families, the general public, policy makers, providers, and the media.

Year Founded: 1992

680 Goodwill's Community Employment Services
Goodwill Industries-Suncoast, Inc.
10596 Gandy Blvd.
St. Petersburg, FL 33702
727-523-1512
888-279-1988
TDD: 727-579-1068
www.goodwill-suncoast.org

Heather Ceresoli, CPA, Chair
Deborah A. Passerini, President
Martin W. Gladysz, Senior Vice Chair
Louise R. Lopez, Vice Chair

Program providing job coaching and community job placements for people with disabilities.

Year Founded: 1954

681 Mental Health America
500 Montgomery Street
Suite 820
Alexandria, VA 22314
703-684-7722
800-969-6642; *Fax: 703-684-5968*
www.mentalhealthamerica.net

Reginald Williams, Chair of the Board
Paul Gionfriddo, President and CEO
Jessica Kennedy, Chief of Staff/VP of Finance
Theresa Nguyen, VP of Policy and Programs

Mental Health America is a community-based nonprofit organization committed to enabling the mental wellness of all Americans. MHA advocates for greater access to quality health services and seeks to educate individuals on identifying symptoms, as well as intervention and prevention.

Year Founded: 1909

682 Mental Health Matters
Carron Consulting
19206 65th Pl NE
Kenmore, WA 98028
425-402-6934
www.mental-health-matters.com

Sean Bennick, Operations Officer

Mental Health Matters serves as a source of information about mental health issues. Provides mental health consumers, professionals, and students with resources on disorders, symptoms, treatment, and medications.

683 National Association for the Dually Diagnosed (NADD)
132 Fair Street
Kingston, NY 12401
845-331-4336
info@thenadd.org
www.thenadd.org

Jeanne M. Farr, MA, Chief Executive Officer
Daniel Baker, PhD., President
Peggie Webb, MA, Vice President
George Zukotynski, PhD., Secretary

NADD is a nonprofit organization designed to increase awareness of, and provide services for, individuals with developmental disabilities and mental illness. NADD emphasizes the importance of quality mental healthcare for people with mental health needs and offers conferences, information resources, educational programs, and training materials to professionals, parents, and organizations.

Year Founded: 1983

684 National Mental Health Consumers' Self-Help Clearinghouse
1211 Chestnut Street
Suite 1100
Philadelphia, PA 19107
267-507-3810
800-553-4539; *Fax: 215-636-6312*
info@mhselfhelp.org
www.mhselfhelp.org

Joseph Rogers, Founder and Executive Director
Susan Rogers, Director

The Clearinghouse is a peer-run national technical assistance center focused on achieving respect and equality of opportunity for those with mental illnesses. The Clearinghouse helps with the growth of the mental health consumer movement by evaluating mental health services, advocating for mental health reform, and providing consumers with news, information, publications, and consultation services.

Year Founded: 1986

685 The Balanced Mind Parent Network
Depression and Bipolar Support Alliance
55 East Jackson Boulevard
Suite 490
Chicago, IL 60604
800-826-3632; *Fax: 312-642-7243*

Julia Small, Parent Volunteer Coordinator
Karen Cruise, Family Helpline Leader
Kathy Karle, Support Network Coordinator
Janice Cox, Support Network Coordinator

The Balanced Mind provides support, information, and assistance to families raising children with mood disorders and related conditions.

686 The Center for Family Support
2811 Zulette Avenue
Bronx, NY 10461
718-518-1500; *Fax: 718-518-8200*
www.www.cfsny.org/

Steven Vernikoff, Executive Director
Lloyd Stabiner, President
Amy Bittinger, Vice President
Barbara Greenwald, Associate Executive Director

The Center for Family Support offers assistance to individuals with developmental and related disabilities, as well as their families, and provides support services and programs that are designed to accommodate individual needs. Offers services throughout New York City, Westchester County, Long Island, and New Jersey.

Year Founded: 1954

687 The Shulman Center for Compulsive Theft, Spending & Hoarding
PO Box 250008
Franklin, MI 48025
248-358-8508
terrenceshulman@theshulmancenter.com
www.theshulmancenter.com

Terrence Shulman, JD, LMSW, CPC, Founder and Director

The Shulman Center provides counseling and professional services designed to help individuals with compulsive stealing, spending, and hoarding disorders. The Shulman Center supports individuals, families, companies, and communities through education, assessment, and treatment.

Year Founded: 1992

688 The TLC Foundation for Body-Focused Repetiti ve Behaviors
716 Soquel Avenue
Suite A
Santa Cruz, CA 95062
831-457-1004; *Fax: 831-427-5541*
info@bfrb.org
www.www.bfrb.org/

Brian Haslam, President
Jennifer Raikes, Executive Director
Rahel Y. Smith, Treasurer
Josie Sanctis, Secretary

The TLC Foundation, formerly The Trichotillomania Learning Center, serves to raise awareness on trichotillomania and related body-focused repetitive disorders, support research, and disseminate scientifically-based information about trichotillomania, and offer support services for individuals and families affected by the disorders. The TLC Foundation aims to eliminate the suffering caused by trichotillomania and body-focused repetitive behaviors.

Year Founded: 1991

Books

689 Angry All the Time: An Emergency Guide to Anger Control
NewHarbinger Publications
5674 Shattuck Avenue
Oakland, CA 94609-1662
510-652-0215
800-748-6273; *Fax:* 800-652-1613
www.newharbinger.com

Ronald T Potter-Efron MSW, PhD, Author

The book is organized to move readers along the shortest path to recovery. This edition includes tips for problem solving and directing anger in positive ways, new strategies for encouraging change, and a discussion of anger styles and the effects of jealousy on problem anger are just some of the engaging new concepts. *$16.95*

160 pages Year Founded: 1973 ISBN 1-572243-92-7

690 Antisocial Behavior by Young People
Cambridge University Press
32 Avenue of the Americas
New York, NY 10013-2473
212-337-5000; *Fax:* 212-691-3239
newyork@cambrigde.org
www.www.cambridge.org

Michael Rutter, Author
Henri Giller, Author
Ann Hagell, Author

Written by a child psychiatrist, a criminologist and a social psychologist, this book is a major international review of research evidence on anti-social behavior. Covers all aspects of the field, including descriptions of different types of delinquency and time trends, the state of knowledge on the individuals, social-psychological and cultural factors involved and recent advances in prevention and intervention. *$53.00*

492 pages Year Founded: 1534 ISBN 0-521646-08-6

691 Bad Men Do What Good Men Dream: a Forensic Psychiatrist Illuminates the Darker Side of Human Behavior
American Psychiatric Publishing, Inc.
1000 Wilson Boulevard
Suite 1825
Arlington, VA 22209-3901
703-907-7322
800-368-5777; *Fax:* 703-907-1091
appi@psych.org
www.appi.org

Robert I Simon, MD, Author

Provides insights into the minds of rapists, stalkers, serial killers, psychopaths, professional exploiters, and other individuals whose behavior both frightens and fascinates us. *$53.00*

339 pages Year Founded: 2008 ISBN 1-585622-94-8

692 Clinical Manual of Impulse-Control Disorders
American Psychiatric Publishing, Inc.
1000 Wilson Boulevard
Suite 1825
Arlington, VA 22209-3901
703-907-7322
800-368-5777; *Fax:* 703-907-1091
appi@psych.org
www.appi.org

Eric Hollander, Author
Dan J. Stein, Author

Focuses on all of the different impulse-control disorders as a group.

368 pages Year Founded: 2006 ISBN 1-585621-36-1

693 Conduct Disorders in Childhood and Adolescence, Developmental Clinical Psychology and Psychiatry
Sage Publications
2455 Teller Road
Thousand Oaks, CA 91320-2234
805-499-0721
800-818-7243; *Fax:* 800-583-2665
info@sagepub.com
www.sagepub.com

Alan E. Kazdin, Author

Conduct disorder is a clinical problem among children and adolescents that includes aggressive acts, theft, vandalism, firesetting, running away, truancy, defying authority and other antisocial behaviors. This book describes the nature of conduct disorder and what is currently known from research and clinical work. Topics include psychiatric diagnosis, parent psychopathology and child-rearing processes. Paperback also available. *$71.00*

191 pages Year Founded: 1995 ISBN 0-803971-81-8

694 Difficult Child
Bantam Doubleday Dell Publishing
1745 Broadway
New York, NY 10019-4343
212-782-9000
ecustomerservice@randomhouse.com
www.randomhouse.com

Stanley Turecki,MD, Author
Leslie Tonner, Author

Help for parents dealing with behavioral problems. *$ 17.00*

320 pages Year Founded: 2000 ISBN 0-553380-36-2

695 Drug Therapy and Impulse Control Disorders: Drugs & Psychology for the Mind & Body)
Mason Crest Publishers
450 Parkway Drive
Suite D
Broomall, PA 19008-4017
610-543-6200
866-627-2665; *Fax:* 610-543-3878
www.masoncrest.com

Autumn Libal, Author

The stories and information in this book will tell you more about impulse-control disorders, how they affect people's lives, and how they can be treated. *$24.95*

124 pages ISBN 1-590845-66-0

696 Dysinhibition Syndrome How to Handle Anger and Rage in Your Child or Spouse
Hope Press
PO Box 188
Duarte, CA 91009-188
818-303-0644
800-321-4039; *Fax:* 626-358-3520
dcomings@earthlink.net
www.hopepress.com

Rose Wood, Author

How to understand and handle rage and anger in your children or spouse. The book presents behavioral approaches that can be very effective and an understanding that can be family saving. *$18.96*

271 pages Year Founded: 1999 ISBN 1-878267-08-6

697 Helping Parents, Youth, and Teachers Understand Medications for Behavioral and Emotional Problems
American Psychiatric Publishing, Inc.
1000 Wilson Boulevard
Suite 1825
Arlington, VA 22209-3901
703-907-7322
800-368-5777; *Fax:* 703-907-1091
appi@psych.org
www.appi.org

Mina K. Dulcan, MD, Editor

Resource Book of Medication Information Handouts, Second Edition. Valuable resource for anyone involved in evaluating psychiatric disturbances in children and adolescents. Provides a compilation of information sheets to help promote the dialogue between the patient's family, caregivers and the treating physician. *$101.00*

759 pages Year Founded: 2007 ISBN 1-585622-53-5

698 Impulse Control Disorders: A Clinician's Guide to Understanding and Treating Behavioral Addictions
W.W. Norton & Company
500 Fifth Avenue
New York, NY 10110
212-354-5500; *Fax:* 212-869-0856
www.www.wwnorton.com

Jon E. Grant, Author

A comprehensive book on impulse control disorders topic for clinicians provides a screening instrument and a detailed method for assessing and treating them. *$26.95*

288 pages Year Founded: 2008

699 Impulsivity and Compulsivity
American Psychiatric Publishing, Inc.
1000 Wilson Boulevard
Suite 1825
Arlington, VA 22209-3901
703-907-7322
800-368-5777; *Fax:* 703-907-1091
appi@psych.org
www.appi.org

John M. Oldham, M.D., M.S., Editor
Eric Hollander, M.D., Editor
Andrew E. Skodol, M.D., Editor

Leading researchers and clinicians share their expertise on the phenomenological, biological, psychodynamic, and treatment aspects of these disorders. *$40.00*

312 pages Year Founded: 1996 ISBN 0-880486-76-7

700 One Hundred Four Activities That Build
Sunburst Media
2 Skyline Drive
Suite 101
Hawthorne, NY 10532-2142
888-367-6368; *Fax:* 914-347-1805
info@Childswork.com
www.Childswork.com

Full of interactive and fun games that can be used to encourage, modification of behavior, increase interaction with others, start discussions and build other life and social skills. *$23.95*

71 pages

701 Out of Control: Gambling and Other Impulse Control Disorders
Chelsea House Publishers
132 West 31st Street
17th Floor
New York, NY 10001-3406
800-322-8755; *Fax:* 800-678-3633
custserv@factsonfile.com
www.chelseahouse.infobasepublishing.com

Linda N. Bayer, Author

A ground-breaking series that provides up-to-date information on the history, causes and effects of, and treatment and therapies for problems affecting the human mind. *$35.00*

95 pages Year Founded: 2001 ISBN 0-791053-13-X

702 Preventing Antisocial Behavior Interventions from Birth through Adolescence
Guilford Press
72 Spring Street
New York, NY 10012-4068
212-431-9800
800-365-7006; *Fax:* 212-966-6708
info@guilford.com

Bob Matloff, President
Seymour Weingarten, Editor-in-Chief

Establishes the crucial link between theory, measurement, and intervention. Brings together a collection of studies that utilize experimental approaches for evaluating intervention programs for preventing deviant behavior. Demonstrates both the feasibility and necessity of independent evaluation. Also shows how the information obtained in such studies can be used to test and refine prevailing theories about human behavior in general and behavior changes in particular. *$55.00*

391 pages Year Founded: 1992 ISBN 0-898628-82-2

703 Pyromania, Kleptomania, and Other Impulse Control Disorders
Enslow Publishers, Inc.
40 Industrial Road
Box 398,Department F61
Berkeley Heights, NJ 07922-0398

908-771-9400
800-398-2504; *Fax:* 908-771-0925
customerservice@enslow.com
www.www.enslow.com

Julie Williams, Author

Describes the characterisitics of impulsive control disorders, from their early diagnoses and methods of treatment to today's available medications. *$26.60*

128 pages Year Founded: 1976 ISBN 0-766018-99-7

704 Skills Training for Children with Behavior Disorders
Courage to Change
PO Box 486
Wilkes-Barre, PA 18703-486
800-440-4003; *Fax:* 800-772-6499
customerservice@guidance-group.com
www.couragetochange.com

Michael L. Boomquist, Author

Written for both parents and therapists, this book provides backround, instructions, and many reproducible worksheets. Academic success, anger management, emotional well being and compliance/following rules are covered. *$36.00*

242 pages Year Founded: 1996 ISBN 1-572300-80-9

705 Stop Me Because I Can't Stop Myself: Taking Control of Impulsive Behavior
McGraw-Hill Companies
PO Box 182604
Columbus, OH 43272
877-833-5524; *Fax:* 614-759-3749
www.mcgraw-hill.com

S.W. Kim, Author
Jon E Grant, Author
Gregory Fricchione, Author

Offers the latest research and practical help for those who engage in all types of impulse-related behaviors.

224 pages Year Founded: 2004 ISBN 0-071433-68-6

706 When Anger Hurts: Quieting The Storm Within
NewHarbinger Publications
5674 Shattuck Avenue
Oakland, CA 94609-1662
510-652-0215
800-748-6273; *Fax:* 800-652-1613
customerservice@newharbinger.com
www.newharbinger.com

Matthew McKay,PhD, Author
Peter D Rogers, Author
Judith McKay, Author

Step-by-step guide to changing habitual, anger-generating thoughts while developing healthier, more effective ways of getting needs met. It is ideal for therapists who work with families or teach anger control and helpful for health professionals who treat the effects of Type A personality. *$16.95*

320 pages Year Founded: 1973 ISBN 1-572243-44-9

707 Youth with Impulse-Control Disorders: On the Spur of the Moment
Mason Crest Publishers
450 Parkway Drive
Suite D
Broomall, PA 19008-4017
610-543-6200
866-621-2665; *Fax:* 610-543-3878
www.masoncrest.com

Kenneth McIntosh, Author
Phyllis Livingston, Author

128 pages Year Founded: 2008 ISBN 1-422204-47-2

Periodicals & Pamphlets

708 Conduct Disorder in Children and Adolescents
PO Box 42557
Washington, DC 20015-557
800-789-2647; *Fax:* 240-747-5470
TDD: 866-889-2647
ken@mentalhealth.org
www.mentalhealth.samhsa.gov

G Pirooz Shovelar, Editor
Edward B Searle, Deputy Director

414 pages

709 Mental, Emotional, and Behavior Disorders in Children and Adolescents
SAMHSA'S National Mental Health Information Center
PO Box 42557
Washington, DC 20015-557
800-789-2647; *Fax:* 240-747-5470
TDD: 866-889-2647
ken@mentalhealth.org

A Kathryn Power, MEd, Director
Edward B Searle, Deputy Director

This fact sheet describes mental, emotional, and behavioral problems that can occur during childhood and adolescence and discusses related treatment, support services, and research.

4 pages

710 Treatment of Children with Mental Disorders
National Institute of Mental Health
6001 Executive Boulevard
Room 8184,MSC 9663
Bethesda, MD 20892-9663
301-443-4513
866-615-6464
TTY: 301-443-8431
nimhinfo@nih.gov
www.www.nimh.nih.gov/

Francis S Collins, MD, PhD

A short booklet that contains questions and answers about therapy for children with mental disorders. Includes a chart of mental disorders and medications used.

Year Founded: 2004

Research Centers

711 Child & Family Center
Menninger Clinic
21545 Centre Pointe Parkway
Santa Clarita, CA 91350
661-259-9439
800-351-9058; *Fax:* 661-255-6853
webmaster@menninger.edu
www.www.childfamilycenter.org/

Steven Zimmer, Board Chair
Darrell Paulk, CEO
Bill Cooper, Vice Chair
Joan Aschoff, Executive Vice President of Prog

The Center's goals: to further develop emerging understanding of the impact of childhood maltreatment and abuse; to chart primary prevention strategies that will foster healthy patterns of caregiving and attachment and reduce the prevalence of maltreatment and abuse; to develop secondary prevention strategies that will promote early detection of attachment-related problems and effective interventions to avert the development of chronic and severe disorders; and to develop more effective treatment approaches for those individuals whose early attachment problems have eventuated in severe psychopathology.

Year Founded: 1976

712 Impulse Control Disorders Clinic
University of Minnesota
231 Pillsbury Drive,South East.
240 Williamson Hall
Minneapolis, MN 55455-0213
612-625-2008
800-752-1000; *Fax:* 612-626-1693
TTY: 612-625-9051

A group of doctors and trainees engaged in research in Impulse-Control Disorders (ICD) and Obsessive-Compulsive Disorder (OCD) and treating patients in a specialty clinic. Conducts research to elucidate pathophysiological links to the ICD and OCD and conducts clinical trials to come up with better and improved treatments for patients.

Support Groups & Hot Lines

713 Gam-Anon Family Groups International
Service Office, Inc.
PO Box 307
Massapequa Park, NY 11762
718-352-1671
gamanonoffice@gam-anon.org
www.gam-anon.org

A 12 step self-help fellowship of men and women who have been affected by the gambling problems of a loved one. Their program works through literature and meetings. At meetings individuals learn how other members applied the Gam-Anon program to find serenity and a more normal way of thinking and living.

714 Gamblers Anonymous
PO Box 17173
Los Angeles, CA 90017
626-960-3500; *Fax:* 626-960-350
isomain@gamblersanonymous.org
www.gamblersanonymous.org

Fellowship of men and women who share their experience, strength and hope with each other so that they may solve their common problem and help others recover from a gambling problem.

Year Founded: 1957

715 Kleptomaniacs Anonymous
The Shulman Center for Compulsive Theft,
Spending & Hoarding
PO Box 250008
Franklin, MI 48025
248-358-8508
www.kleptomaniacsanonymous.com

Terrence Shulman,JD,LMSW, Founder/Director

Kleptomaniacs And Shoplifters Anonymous (CASA) is a unique, independent and secular weekly self-help group.

Year Founded: 1992

716 The TLC Foundation for Body-Focused
Repetiti ve Behaviors
716 Soquel Avenue
Suite A
Santa Cruz, CA 95062
831-457-1004; *Fax:* 831-427-5541
www.www.bfrb.org/

Brian Haslam, President
Josie Sanctis, Secretary
Rahel Y. Smith, Treasurer
Jennifer Raikes, Executive Director

The TLC Foundation, formerly The Trichotillomania Learning Center, serves to raise awareness on trichotillomania and related body-focused repetitive disorders, support research, and disseminate scientifically-based information about trichotillomania. The Foundation also offers support services for individuals and families affected by the disorders.

Year Founded: 1991

Video & Audio

717 A Desperate Act
Trichotillomania Learning Center
207 McPherson Street
Suite H
Santa Cruz, CA 95060-5863
831-457-1004; *Fax:* 831-427-5541
info@trich.org
www.trich.org

Joanna Heitz, President
Brenda Cameron, Secretary
Deborah M. Kleinman, Treasurer
Jennifer Raikes, Executive Director

A performance artist with TTM discusses her experiences in front of a live audience.

Year Founded: 1991

718 Active Parenting Now
Active Parenting Publishers
1220 Kennestone Circle
Suite 130
Marietta, GA 30066
770-429-0565
800-825-0060; *Fax:* 770-429-0334
cservice@activeparenting.com

Michael Popkin, PhD, Author

A complete video-based parenting education program curriculum. Helps parents of children ages two to twelve raise responsible, courageous children. Emphasizes nonviolent discipline, conflict resolution and improved communication. With Leader's Guide, videotapes, Parent's Guide and more. Also available in Spanish. *$ 349.00*

Year Founded: 2002 ISBN 1-880283-89-1

719 Addictive Behavior: Drugs, Food and Relationships
Educational Video Network, Inc.
1401 19th Street
Huntsville, TX 77340
936-295-5767
800-762-0060; *Fax:* 936-294-0233
www.www.evndirect.com

Addiction is a serious and very real problem for many people. It can come in the forms of caffeine, heroin, food or love. Find out what makes one person more likely to develop an addiction than someone else, learn about the different types of addiction, the signs and the consequences.

720 Aggression Replacement Training Video: A Comprehensive Intervention for Aggressive Youth
Research Press
PO Box 7886
PO Box 9177
Champaign, IL 61826
217-352-3273
800-519-2707; *Fax:* 217-352-1221
rp@researchpress.com
www.researchpress.com

Dr. Barry Glick, Author
Dr. John C. Gibbs, Author

This staff training video illustrates the training procedures in the Aggression Replacement Training (ART) book.It features scenes of adolescents participating in group sessions for each of ART's three interventions: Prosocial Skills, Anger Control, and Moral Reasoning. A free copy of the book accompanies the video program. *$35.95*

426 pages ISBN 0-878226-37-5

721 Anger Management-Enhanced Edition
Educational Video Network, Inc.
1401 19th Street
Huntsville, TX 77340
936-295-5767
800-762-0060; *Fax:* 936-294-0233
www.www.evndirect.com

Learn what causes anger and understand why our bodies react as they do when we're angry. Effective techniques for assuaging anger are discussed.

722 Clinical Impressions: Identifying Mental Illness
Educational Training Videos
136 Granville St
Suite 200
Gahanna, OH 43230
Fax: 888-775-3919
www.educationaltrainingvideos.com

How long can mental illness stay hidden, especially from the eyes of trained experts? This program rejoins a group of ten adults- five of them healthy and five of them with histories of mental illness- as psychiatric specialists try to spot

and correctly diagnose the latter. Administering a series of collaborative and one-on-one tests, including assessments of personality type, physical self-image, and rational thinking, the panel gradually makes decisions about who suffers from depression, bipolar disorder, bulimia, and social anxiety.

723 Coping with Stress
Educational Video Network, Inc.
1401 19th Street
Huntsville, TX 77340
936-295-5767
800-762-0060; *Fax:* 936-294-0233
www.www.evndirect.com

Stress affects everyone, both emotionally and physically. For some, mismanaged stress can result in substance abuse, violence, or even suicide. This program answers the question, How can a person cope with stress?

724 Dealing with ADHD: Attention Deficit/ Hyperactivity
Educational Video Network, Inc.
1401 19th Street
Huntsville, TX 77340
936-295-5767
800-762-0060; *Fax:* 936-294-0233
www.www.evndirect.com

Learn about attention deficit/hyperactivity disorder and learn what factors are thought to contribute to the development of this disorder. Other disorders that commonly co-exist with ADHD will be identified. The impulsivity and risk-taking behaviors of ADHD teens will be focused upon and tips that ADHD students can use to succeed academically will be provided. Laws that require schools to make special accommodations for ADHD students will be reviewed, and viewers will learn how to contact organizations that exist to help people who are dealing with ADHD.

725 FRONTLINE: The Released
PBS
2100 Crystal Drive
Arlington, VA 22202
www.pbs.org

Will Lyman, Actor
Narrator
Miri Navasky, Director
Karen O'Connor, Director

The documentary states that of the 700,000 inmates released from American prisons each year, half of them have mental disabilities. This work focused on those with severe problems who keep entering and exiting prison. Full of good information on the challenges they face with mental illnesses; housing, employment, stigmatization, and socialization.

Year Founded: 2009

726 Mental Disorder
Educational Training Videos
136 Granville St
Suite 200
Gahanna, OH 43230
Fax: 888-775-3919
www.educationaltrainingvideos.com

What is abnormality? Using the case studies of two young women; one who has depression, one who has an anxiety disorder; as a springboard, this program presents three psychological perspective on mental disorder.

727 No More Shame: Understanding Schizophrenia, Depression, and Addiction
Educational Training Videos
136 Granville St
Suite 200
Gahanna, OH 43230
Fax: 888-775-3919
www.educationaltrainingvideos.com

These programs examine research about the physiological, psychological, sociological, and cultural aspects of these disorders and their treatments. The goal of these programs is to explain what we do and do not know about each of these conditions, as well as to destigmatize the disorders by presenting them in the context of the same research process that is applied to all medical disorders.

728 Obsessions: Understanding OCD
Educational Training Videos
136 Granville St
Suite 200
Gahanna, OH 43230
Fax: 888-775-3919
www.educationaltrainingvideos.com

Are compulsive hair-pulling, hand-washing, and even gambling learned behaviors or inherited diseases? Where do obsessions come from and how can they be managed so they do not dominate a person's life? This two-part series attempts to understand the roots of obsessive-compulsive disorder, or OCD, and looks at both standard and experimental treatment options.

729 Our Personal Stories
Trichotillomania Learning Center
207 McPherson Street
Suite H
Santa Cruz, CA 95060-5863
831-457-1004; *Fax:* 831-427-5541
info@trich.org
www.trich.org

Joanna Heitz, President
Brenda Cameron, Secretary
Deborah M. Kleinman, Treasurer
Jennifer Raikes, Executive Director

Documentary detailing 8 womens' personal experiences with TTM. *$28.00*

Year Founded: 1991

730 Trichotillomania: Overview and Introduction to HRT
Trichotillomania Learning Center
207 McPherson Street
Suite H
Santa Cruz, CA 95060-5863
831-457-1004; *Fax:* 831-427-5541
info@trich.org
www.trich.org

Joanna Heitz, President
Brenda Cameron, Secretary
Deborah M. Kleinman, Treasurer
Jennifer Raikes, Executive Director

A lecture on Behavior Therapy and Habit Reversal Training for TTM. *$30.00*

Year Founded: 1991

731 Understanding & Managing the Defiant Child
Courage to Change
1 Huntington Quadrangle
Suite: 1N03
Melville, NY 11747
800-962-1141; *Fax:* 800-262-1886
www.couragetochange.com

Russell A Barkley, PhD, Presenter

Understanding and Managing the Defiant Child provides a proven approach to behavior management. *$205.95*

732 Understanding Mental Illness
Educational Video Network
1401 19th Street
Huntsville, TX 77340
936-295-5767
800-762-0060; *Fax:* 936-294-0233
info at evn.org
www.www.evndirect.com

Contains information and classifications of mental illness. Learn about various organic and functional mental disorders as discussed and their causes and symptoms, and learn where to seek help for a variety of mental health concerns. *$79.95*

Year Founded: 2004 ISBN 1-589501-48-9

733 Understanding and Treating the Hereditary Psychiatric Spectrum Disorders
Hope Press
PO Box 188
Duarte, CA 91009-188
818-303-0644
800-209-9182; *Fax:* 818-358-3520
dcomings@earthlink.net
www.hopepress.com

David E Comings MD, Presenter

Learn with ten hours of audio tapes from a two day seminar given in May 1997 by David E Comings, MD. Tapes cover: ADHD, Tourette Syndrome, Obsessive-Compulsive Disorder, Conduct Disorder, Oppositional Defiant Disorder, Autism and other Hereditary Psychiatric Spectrum Disorders. Eight audio tapes. *$75.00*

Year Founded: 1997

Web Sites

734 www.apa.org/pubinfo/anger.html
Controlling Anger-Before It Controls You

From the American Psychological Association.

735 www.cfsny.org
Center for Family Support (CFS)

Devoted to providing support and assistance to individuals with developmental and related disabilities, and to the family members who care for them.

736 www.cyberpsych.org
CyberPsych

Presents information about psychoanalysis, psychotherapy and special topics such as anxiety disorders, the problematic use of alcohol, homophobia, and the traumatic effects of racism. Includes an archive of older site content.

737 **www.members.aol.com/AngriesOut**
Get Your Angries Out

Guidelines for kids, teachers, and parents.

738 **www.mentalhelp.net/psyhelp/chap7**
Anger and Aggression

Therapeutic approaches.

739 **www.mhselfhelp.org**
National Mental Health Consumer's Self-Help Clearinghouse

A national consumer technical assistance center, has played a major role in the development of the mental health consumer movement.

740 **www.ncwd-youth.info/node/245**
Center for Mental Health Services Knowledge Exchange Network

Information about resources, technical assistance, research, training, networks and other federal clearinghouses, fact sheets and materials.

741 **www.planetpsych.com**
PlanetPsych.com

Learn about disorders, their treatments and other topics in psychology. Articles are listed under the related topic areas. Ask a therapist a question for free, or view the directory of professionals in your area. If you are a therapist sign up for the directory. Current features, self-help, interactive, and newsletter archives.

742 **www.psychcentral.com**
Psych Central

Personalized one-stop index for psychology, support, and mental health issues, resources, and people on the Internet.

743 **www.stopbitingnails.com**
Stop Biting Nails

Online organization created for those who bite their nails. Created a product which is used to prevent nailbiting.

744 **www.store.samhsa.gov**
Substance Abuse and Mental Health Services Administration

Resources on mental disorders as well as treatment and recovery.

745 **www.thenadd.org**
National Association for the Dually Diagnosed (NADD)

An association for persons with developmental disabilities and mental health needs.

Dissociative Disorders

Introduction

Dissociative Disorders are a cluster of mental disorders, characterized by a profound change in consciousness or a disruption in continuity of consciousness. People with a Dissociative Disorder may abruptly take on different personalities, or undergo long periods in which they do not remember anything that happened; in some cases, individuals may embark on lengthy international travels, returning home with no recollection of where they have been or why they had gone.

Dissociative Disorders are uncommon, mysterious and somewhat controversial; reports of Dissociative Disorders have grown more frequent in recent years and a degree of debate surrounds the validity of these reports. Some professionals say the disorders are far more rare than is reported, and that these individuals are highly vulnerable to the suggestions of others.

Dissociative Disorders are believed to be related in many cases to severe trauma, although the historical validity of these cases is difficult to determine. There are five types of Dissociative Disorders: Dissociative Amnesia; Dissociative Fugue; Dissociative Identity Disorder; Depersonalization Disorder; and Dissociative Disorder Not Otherwise Specified.

SYMPTOMS

Dissociative Amnesia
• One or more episodes of inability to recall important personal information, usually of a traumatic or stressful nature, that is too extensive to be explained by ordinary forgetfulness;
• The disturbance does not occur exclusively during the course of any other Dissociative Disorder and is not due to the direct physiological effects of a substance abuse or general medical condition;
• The symptoms cause clinically significant distress or impairment in social, occupational, or other important areas of functioning.

Dissociative Fugue
• A sudden, unexpected travel away from home or work, with inability to recall one's past;
• Confusion about personal identity or assumption of a new identity;
• The disturbance does not occur exclusively during the course of any other Dissociative Disorder and is not due to the direct physiological effects of a substance or a general medical condition;
• The symptoms cause clinically significant distress or impairment in social, occupational, or other important areas of functioning.

Dissociative Identity Disorder
• The presence of two or more distinct identities or personality states that take control of the person's behavior;
• Inability to recall important personal information;
• The disturbance is not due to the direct physiological effects of a substance or a general medical condition.

Depersonalization Disorder
• Persistent or reurrent experiences of feeling detached from one's body and mental processes;

• During the depersonalization experience, reality testing remains intact;
• The depersonalization causes clinically significant distress or impairment in social, occupational, or other important areas of functioning;
• The depersonalization does not occur during the course of another Dissociative Disorder or as a direct physiological effect of a substance or general medical condition;
• Akin to depersonalization (feeling one is not real) is derealization, which is feeling that one's environment and/or perceptions are not real.

ASSOCIATED FEATURES

Patients with any of the Dissociative Disorders may be depressed, and may experience depersonalization, or a feeling of not being in their own bodies. They often experience impairment in work or interpersonal relationships, and they may practice self-mutilation or have aggressive and suicidal impulses. They may also have symptoms typical of a Mood or Personality Disorder. Individuals with Dissociative Amnesia and Dissociative Identity Disorder (sometimes known as multiple personality disorder) often report severe physical and/or sexual abuse in childhood. Controversy surrounds the accuracy of these reports, in part because of the unreliability of some childhood memories. Individuals with Dissociative Identity Disorder may have symptoms typical of Post-Traumatic Stress Disorder, as well as BiPolar, Substance Abuse Related, Sexual, Eating, or Wake-Sleep Disorders.

PREVALENCE

The prevalence of Dissociative Disorders is difficult to ascertain, and subject to controversy. The recent rise in the US in reports of Dissociative Amnesia and Dissociative Identity Disorder related to traumatic childhood abuse has been very controversial. Some say these disorders are overreported, the result of suggestibility in individuals and the unreliability of childhood memories. Others say the disorders are underreported, given the propensity for children and adults to dismiss or forget abusive memories and the tendency of perpetrators to deny or obscure their abusive actions. For Dissociative Fugue, a prevalence rate of 0.2 percent of the population has been reported. Dissociative Identity Disorder is diagnosed three to nine times more frequently in females than in males, and Depersonalization Disorder is twice as likely to occur in women than men.

TREATMENT OPTIONS

Treatment for Dissociative Amnesia may involve supportive psychotherapy or hypnosis to help the patient recover traumatic memories. Another stage of psychotherapy may then be initiated to enable the patient to deal with the uncovered memories. For Dissociative Fugue, psychotherapy is often the principal treatment.

Treatment for Dissociative Identity Disorder may include hypnosis, psychotherapy, family therapy, and group therapy. Medications such as antidepressants and anti-anxiety agents may also be prescribed.

In some cases, Depersonalization Disorder can resolve on its own without therapy. In other cases, treatment such as hypnosis, psychodynamic psychotherapy (in which the focus is on unconscious thoughts and how they are revealed in a patient's behavior), or cognitive behavioral therapy (in which the patient learns to replace negative thoughts and behaviors with positive ones) may be used. Medications such as benzodiazepine tranquilizers, tricyclic antidepressants, and selective serotonin reuptake inhibitors (SSRIs) may also be prescribed.

Associations & Agencies

747 Center for Mental Health Services (CMHS)
Substance Abuse and Mental Health Services
Administration
5600 Fishers Lane
Rockville, MD 20857
240-276-1310
877-726-4727
TTY: 800-487-4889
www.samhsa.gov/about-us/who-we-are/offices-centers

Paolo del Vecchio, MSW, Director
Anne Mathews-Younes, Acting Deputy Director
Keris Myrick, Director, Consumer Affairs
Patricia Gratton, Director, Program Analysis

Promotes the treatment of mental illness and emotional disorders by increasing accessibility to mental health programs; supporting outreach, treatment, rehabilitation, and support programs and networks; and encouraging the use of scientifically-based information when treating mental disorders. CMHS provides information about mental health via a toll-free number and numerous publications. Developed for users of mental health services and their families, the general public, policy makers, providers, and the media.

Year Founded: 1992

748 International Society for the Study of Trauma and Dissociation
8400 Westpark Drive
Second Floor
McLean, VA 22102
703-610-9037; *Fax:* 703-610-0234
info@isst-d.org
www.isst-d.org

Kevin J. Connores, MS, MFT, President
D. Michael Coy, MA, LICSW, Treasurer
Robert B. Slater, MSW, LCSW-R, Secretary
Lisa Danylchuk, EdM, MFT, Director

ISSTD seeks to provide educational resources, programs, conferences, and publications on the prevalence and consequences of chronic trauma and dissociation.

749 National Association for the Dually Diagnosed (NADD)
132 Fair Street
Kingston, NY 12401
845-331-4336
info@thenadd.org
www.thenadd.org

Jeanne M. Farr, MA, Chief Executive Officer
Daniel Baker, PhD., President
Peggie Webb, MA, Vice President
George Zukotynski, PhD., Secretary

NADD is a nonprofit organization designed to increase awareness of, and provide services for, individuals with developmental disabilities and mental illness. NADD emphasizes the importance of quality mental healthcare for people with mental health needs and offers conferences, informa-

tion resources, educational programs, and training materials to professionals, parents, and organizations.

Year Founded: 1983

750 National Mental Health Consumers' Self-Help Clearinghouse
1211 Chestnut Street
Suite 1100
Philadelphia, PA 19107
267-507-3810
800-553-4539; *Fax:* 215-636-6312
info@mhselfhelp.org
www.mhselfhelp.org

Joseph Rogers, Founder and Executive Director
Susan Rogers, Director

The Clearinghouse is a peer-run national technical assistance center focused on achieving respect and equality of opportunity for those with mental illnesses. The Clearinghouse helps with the growth of the mental health consumer movement by evaluating mental health services, advocating for mental health reform, and providing consumers with news, information, publications, and consultation services.

Year Founded: 1986

751 Sidran Traumatic Stress Institute
PO Box 436
Brooklandville, MD 21022-0436
410-825-8888; *Fax:* 410-825-8888
info@sidran.org
www.sidran.org

Esther Giller, President and Director
Sheila Giller, Secretary and Treasurer
Stephanie Muszelik, Accountant
Ruta Mazelis, Editor, The Cutting Edge/Trainer

Sidran Institute assists with the recovery and treatment of sufferers of traumatic stress and dissociative disorders, and provides educational programming, publications, and other resources designed to help people understand trauma and recovery.

Year Founded: 1986

752 TARA Association for Personality Disorders
23 Greene Street
New York, NY 10013
212-966-6514
tara4bpd@gmail.com
www.tara4bpd.org

Valerie Porr, MA, Founder and President

A not-for-profit organization promoting educational programs and research on the causes and treatment of personality disorders. TARA seeks to raise awareness on personality disorder and to eliminate the stigma attached to it.

Year Founded: 1994

753 The Center for Family Support
2811 Zulette Avenue
Bronx, NY 10461
718-518-1500; *Fax:* 718-518-8200
www.www.cfsny.org/

Steven Vernikoff, Executive Director
Lloyd Stabiner, President
Amy Bittinger, Vice President
Barbara Greenwald, Associate Executive Director

The Center for Family Support offers assistance to individuals with developmental and related disabilities, as well as their families, and provides support services and programs that are designed to accommodate individual needs. Offers services throughout New York City, Westchester County, Long Island, and New Jersey.

Year Founded: 1954

Books

754 Amongst Ourselves: A Self-Help Guide to Living with Dissociative Identity Disorder
NewHarbinger Publications
5674 Shattuck Avenue
Oakland, CA 94609-1662
510-652-0215
800-748-6273; *Fax:* 800-652-1613
customerservice@newharbinger.com
www.newharbinger.com

Tracy Alderman, Author
Karen Marshall, Author

First person perspective of Dissociative Identity Disorder and practical suggestions to come to terms with and improve their lives. *$19.95*

240 pages Year Founded: 1973 ISBN 1-562241-22-5

755 Dialectical Behavior Therapy in Clinical Practice: Applications Across Disorders and Settings
Guilford Press
72 Spring Street
New York, NY 10012
800-365-7006
800-365-7006; *Fax:* 212-966-6708
info@guilford.com
www.www.guilford.com

Linda A Dimeff, Editor
Kelly Koerner, Editor

This book presents applications for depression, substance dependence, eating disorders, psychosis, assaultive behaviors and other problems. *$42.50*

363 pages Year Founded: 1973 ISBN 1-572309-74-6

756 Dialectical Behavior Therapy with Suicidal Adolescents
Guilford Press
72 Spring Street
New York, NY 10012
800-365-7006
800-365-7006; *Fax:* 212-966-6708
info@guilford.com
www.www.guilford.com

Alec L. Miller, Author
Jill H. Rathus, Author
Marsha M Linehan, Author

This book adapts the proven techniques of Dialectical Behavior Therapy among Dissociative Disorder sufferers to treatment. The authors take you step by step through understanding and assessing severe emotional dysregulation in teens and implementing individual family, family and group based interventions. *$42.50*

346 pages Year Founded: 1973 ISBN 1-593853-83-9

757 Dissociation Culture, Mind, and Body
American Psychiatric Publishing, Inc.
1000 Wilson Boulevard
Suite 1825
Arlington, VA 22209-3901
703-907-7322
800-368-5777; *Fax:* 703-907-1091
appi@psych.org
www.appi.org

David Spiegel, MD, Editor

Combines cultural anthropology, congitive psychology, neurophysiology, and the study of psychosomatic illness to present the latest information on the dissociative process. Designed for professionals in cross cultural psychiatry and the influence of the mind on the body. *$83.00*

246 pages Year Founded: 1994 ISBN 0-880485-57-9

758 Dissociation and the Dissociative Disorders: DSM-V and Beyond
Routledge
270 Madison Avenue
New York, NY 10016-601
212-695-6599
www.routledgementalhealth.com

Paul F. Dell, Author
John A. O'Neil, Author

This book draws together and integrates the most recent scientific and conceptual foundations of dissociation and the dissociative disorders field. *$93.56*

898 pages Year Founded: 2009 ISBN 0-415957-85-4

759 Dissociative Child: Diagnosis, Treatment and Management
Sidran Institute
PO Box 436
Brooklandville, MD 21022-0436
410-825-8888
888-825-8249; *Fax:* 410-560-0134
sidran@sidran.org
www.sidran.org

Joyanna L Silberg, PhD, Editor

This second groundbreaking edition addresses all aspects of caring for the dissociative child and adolescents. Contributors include experienced and eminent practitioners in the field of childhood DID. The section on diagnosis offers comprehensive coverage of various aspects of diagnosis, including diagnosis taxonomy, differential diagnosis, interviewing, testing and the special problems of male children and adolescents with DID. The section on treatment covers factors associated with positive theraputic outcome, therapeutic phases, the five-domain crisis model, promoting intergration in dissociative children, art therapy and group therapy. Includes ways school personnel can act to help the dissociative child, multiculturalism and other important information. *$37.00*

343 pages Year Founded: 1986

760 Drug Therapy and Dissociative Disorders
Mason Crest Publishers
450 Parkway Drive
Suite D
Broomall, PA 19008-4017
610-543-6200
866-627-2665; *Fax:* 610-543-3878

dtaylor@masoncrest.com
www.masoncrest.com

Autumn Libal, Author
Dan Hilferty, President
Michelle Luke, Director, Marketing, PR
Michael Toglia, Special Sales

Dissociative disorders are some of the most controversial disorders in psychiatry today. Despite newfound recognition and numerous diagnosis the very existence of these disorders is still hotly debated in some academic circles. these disorders make us question our assumptions about memory, self, and personality, and shed unique light on the mysterious complexities of the human mind. From amnesia to multiple personalities, dissociative disorders present treatment challenges to psychotherapy and psychopharmacology alike. Through stories of individuals' struggles with dissociative disorders, this book provides both historical overview of treatment and reviews the most up-to-date treatments available today.

128 pages ISBN 1-590845-64-1

761 Got Parts? An Insider's Guide to Managing Life Successfully with Dissociative Identity Disorder
Loving Healing Press
5145 Pontiac Trail
Ann Arbor, MI 48105-9627
734-929-0881
888-761-6268; *Fax:* 734-663-6861
info@lovinghealing.com
www.lovinghealing.com

A.T.W.

This book is directed towards people treating Dissociative Identity Disorder. It is a book for survivors written by a survivor. This book is filled with successful coping techniques and strategies to enhance the day to day functioning of a dult survivors of DID in relationships, work, and parenting.

132 pages Year Founded: 2003 ISBN 1-932690-03-4

762 Handbook for the Assessment of Dissociation: a Clinical Guide
American Psychiatric Publishing, Inc.
1000 Wilson Boulevard
Suite 1825
Arlington, VA 22209-3901
703-907-7322
800-368-5777; *Fax:* 703-907-1091
appi@psych.org
www.appi.org

Marlene Steinberg, M.D., Author
Ron McMillen, Chief Executive Officer
John McDuffie, Editorial Director

Offers guidelines for the systematic assessment of dissociation and posttraumatic syndromes for clinicians and researchers. Provides a comprehensive overview of dissociative symptoms and disorders and an introduction to the use of the SCID-D, a diagnostic interview for the dissociative disorders. *$54.00*

450 pages Year Founded: 1995 ISBN 0-880486-82-1

763 Lost in the Mirror: An Inside Look at Borderline Personality Disorder
Sidran Institute
200 E Joppa Road
Suite 207
Baltimore, MD 21286-3107
410-825-8888
888-825-8249; *Fax:* 410-337-0747
sidran@sidran.org
www.sidran.org

Richard A. Moskovitz,MD, Author
J G Goellner, Director Emertius
Stanley Platman, MD, Medical Advisor

Dr. Moskovitz considers BPD to be part of the dissociative continuum, as it has many causes, symptoms and behaviors in common with Dissociative Disorder. This book is intended for people diagnosed with BPD, their families and therapists. Outlines the features of BPD, including abuse histories, dissociation, mood swings, self harm, impulse control problems and many more. Includes an extensive resource section. *$13.95*

190 pages

764 New Hope for People with Borderline Personality Disorder
Three Rivers Press

Neil R. Bocklan, Author
Rob Viehman, Publisher
Amy England, Staff Writer
$18.95

Year Founded: 2004 ISBN 0-761527-18-4

765 Overcoming Borderline Personality Disorder: A Family Guide for Healing and Change
Oxford University Press

Valerie Porr, Author

a book for professional, families, and people suffering with Dissociative Disorders. *$24.95*

Year Founded: 2010 ISBN 0-195379-58-6

766 Rebuilding Shattered Lives: Responsible Treatment of Complex Post-Traumatic and Dissociative Disorders
John Wiley & Sons
111 River Street
Hoboken, NJ 07030-5774
201-748-6000
800-225-5945; *Fax:* 201-748-6088
info@wiley.com
www.wiley.com

James A Chu, Author

Essential for anyone working in the field of trauma therapy. Part I discusses recent findings about child abuse, the changes in attitudes toward child abuse over the last two decades and the nature of traumatic memory. Part II is an overview of principles of trauma treatment, including symptom control, establishment of boundaries and therapist self-care. Part III covers special topics, such as dissociative identity disorder, controversies, hospitalization and acute care. *$ 73.95*

271 pages Year Founded: 1998 ISBN 0-471247-32-4

767 Skills Training Manual for Treating Borderline Personality Disorder
Guilford Press
72 Spring Street
New York, NY 10012
800-365-7006
800-365-7006; *Fax:* 212-966-6708
info@guilford.com
www.www.guilford.com

Marsha M. Linehan, Author

This book is a step by step guide to teach clients four sets of skills: interpersonal effectiveness, emotion regulation, distress tolerance, and mindfulness. *$38.25*

180 pages Year Founded: 1973 ISBN 0-898620-34-4

768 The Abused Child Psychodynamic Understanding and Treatment
Guilford Press
72 Spring Street
New York, NY 10012
800-365-7006
800-365-7006; *Fax:* 212-966-6708
info@guilford.com
www.www.guilford.com

Toni Vaughn Heineman, Author

The book traces the interplay of neurobiological and psychological facats of behavior to show how abuse derails normal development and how psychodynamic psychotherapy can reestablish emotional connections. *$34.00*

243 pages Year Founded: 1973 ISBN 1-572303-75-1

769 Traumatic Stress The Effects of Overwhelming Experience on Mind, Body, And Society
Guilford Press
72 Spring Street
New York, NY 10012
800-365-7006
800-365-7006; *Fax:* 212-966-6708
info@guilford.com
www.www.guilford.com

Bessel A Van Der Kolk, Editor
Alexander C McFarlane, Editor
Lars Weisaeth, Editor

This best selling classic presents seminal theory and research on dissociation disorders. These leading editors and contributors comprehensively examine how trauma affects an individual's biology, conception of the world, and psychological functioning. *$42.50*

596 pages Year Founded: 1973 ISBN 1-572304-57-4

770 Treatment of Multiple Personality Disorder
American Psychiatric Publishing, Inc.
1000 Wilson Boulevard
Suite 1825
Arlington, VA 22209-3901
703-907-7322
800-368-5777; *Fax:* 703-907-1091
appi@psych.org
www.appi.org

Bennett G Braun, M.D., Editor
Ron McMillen, Chief Executive Officer
John McDuffie, Editorial Director

Authorities in the Multiple Personality Disorder field merge clinical understanding and research into therapeutic approaches that can be employed in clinical practice. *$22.50*

228 pages Year Founded: 1986 ISBN 0-880480-96-3

771 Understanding Dissociative Disorders and Addiction
Sidran Institute
200 E Joppa Road
Suite 207
Townson, MD 21286-3107
410-825-8888
888-825-8249; *Fax:* 410-337-0747
sidran@sidran.org
www.sidran.org

A Scott Winter, Author
J Gila Goellner, Director Emertius
Stanley Plantman, MD, Medical Advisor

This booklet discusses the origins and symptoms of dissociation, explains the links between dissociative disorder and chemical dependency. Addresses treatment options available to help in your recovery. The work book includes exercises and activities that help you acknowledge, accept and manage both your chemical dependency and your disociative disorder. *$7.20*

48 pages

772 Understanding Dissociative Disorders: A Guide for Family Physicians and Healthcare Workers
Crown House Publishing
6 Trowbridge Drive
Suite 5
Bethel, CT 06801-2882
203-778-1300

Marlene E. Hunter, Author

This volume outlines common presentations in the family physicians' practice, and offers realistic, practical answers to a multitude of questions. *$20.00*

Year Founded: 2009

Video & Audio

773 Different From You
Fanlight Publications
32 Court Street
21st Floor
Brooklyn, NY 11201
718-488-8900
800-876-1710; *Fax:* 718-488-8642
fanlight@fanlight.com
www.fanlight.com

Milt L. Kogan, MD, MPH, Author
Demetrio Cuzzocrea, Author

As a result of the 'deinstituionalization' of mental patients, people with mental illnesses now make up a majority of the homeless in many areas. This video explores the problem through the work of a compassionate physician who cares for mentally ill people living on the streets and in inadequate 'board and care' facilities in Los Angeles.

774 Understanding Mental Illness
Educational Video Network
1401 19th Street
Huntsville, TX 77340

936-295-5767
800-762-0060; *Fax:* 936-294-0233
info at evn.org
www.www.evndirect.com

A video to learn and understand mental illness and how it affects you. *$79.95*

Year Founded: 2004 ISBN 1-589501-48-9

775 Understanding Personality Disorders DVD
Educational Video Network
1401 19th Street
Huntsville, TX 77340
936-295-5767
800-762-0060; *Fax:* 936-294-0233

Defines to adolescents what a personality disorder really is. *$89.95*

Year Founded: 2006

776 Understanding Self Destructive Behavior
Educational Video Network
1401 19th Street
Huntsville, TX 77340
936-295-5767
800-762-0060; *Fax:* 936-294-0233

helps adolescents learn how to deal with their destructive behavior due to their mental illness. *$129.95*

Year Founded: 2004

Web Sites

777 www.cyberpsych.org
CyberPsych

Hosts the American Psychoanalyists Foundation, American Association of Suicideology, Society for the Exploration of Psychotherapy Intergration, and Anxiety Disorders Association of America. Also subcategories of the anxiety disorders, as well as general information, including panic disorder, phobias, obsessive compulsive disorder (OCD), social phobia, generalized anxiety disorder, post traumatic stress disorder, and phobias of childhood. Book reviews and links to web pages sharing the topics.

778 www.fmsf.com
False Memory Syndrome Facts

Access to literature.

779 www.isst-D.Org
International Society for the Study of Dissociation

A non-profit, professional society that promotes research and training in the identification and treatment of dissociative disorders, provides professional and public education about dissociative states, and serves as a catalyst for international communication and cooperation among clinicians and researchers working in this field.

780 www.planetpsych.com
Planetpsych.com

Learn about disorders, their treatments and other topics in psychology. Articles are listed under the related topic areas. Ask a therapist a question for free, or view the directory of professionals in your area. If you are a therapist sign up for the directory. Current features, self-help, interactive, and newsletter archives.

781 www.psychcentral.com
Psych Central

Personalized one-stop index for psychology, support, and mental health issues, resources, and people on the Internet.

782 www.sidran.org
Trauma Resource Area

Resources and Articles on Dissociative Experiences Scale and Dissociative Identity Disorder, PsychTrauma Glossary and Traumatic Memories.

783 www.store.samhsa.gov
Substance Abuse and Mental Health Services Administration

Resources on mental disorders as well as treatment and recovery.

Feeding and Eating Disorders

Introduction

Eating is integral to human health, and for many people food is a pleasure that can be enjoyed without too much thought. But an increasing number of people (mostly, but not exclusively, women) have eating disorders, which cause them to use food and dieting in ways that are extremely unhealthy, even life-threatening. The two principal feeding and eating disorders are Anorexia Nervosa and Bulimia Nervosa; though different in the symptoms they manifest, the two disorders are quite similar in their underlying pathology: an obsessive concern with food, body image, and body weight.

The enormous increase in the incidence of obesity may lead to a formal classification of overeating as a disorder. However, recent research reveals that the cause of obesity is not simply a lack of self-control, or too much self-indulgence, leading to the ingestion of too many calories. It appears that human beings are hard-wired, so to speak, to eat whenever food is available, and food is ever more available and more caloric. In addition, the eating patterns and weight of pregnant women seems to result in physiologic changes in their unborn babies, who are predisposed to become obese after birth regardless of diet.

Many people believe that feeding and eating disorders are, in part, culturally determined: in the Western world, and particularly the US, a pervasive cultural preference for slimness causes many people to spend extraordinary amounts of time, money, and energy dieting and exercisingin order to stay slim. At the same time, people are flooded with media; celebrations of anorexia, and suggested strategies for remaining thin, can be easily found on the Internet, on television, and in magazines. Cultural preference is likely to exert pressure on people, especially young women, who may be genetically or psychologically predisposed to the illness. It is important to be wary of media, including the Internet, which can expose young people to counterproductive influences. Overeating is another type of eating disorder, as it reflects the paradox that, as society values thinness more and more, more and more people are obese. Feeding and Eating Disorders may do lasting physical damage; because of this, treatment must first restore a patient to a safe and healthy body weight. Treatment of the disorder is a long-term process, involving psychotherapy, family interventions and, for depressed or obsessional patients, antidepressant medication. Fortunately, most people who are appropriately treated can and do recover.

SYMPTOMS

Anorexia Nervosa:
• Refusal to maintain body weight at or above eighty-five percent of a minimally normal weight for age and height;
• Intense fear of gaining weight or becoming fat, even though underweight;
• Disturbance in the way one's body weight or shape is experienced, undue influence of body weight or shape on self-evaluation, or denial of the seriousness of the current low body weight;
• In menstruating females, the absence of at least three consecutive menstrual cycles;
• Physical damage often occurs, such as imbalances in body chemicals, which if severe can cause cardiac arrest; purging often erodes tooth enamel, in which case a dentist might

make the diagnosis. Anorexia Nervosa is associated with amenorrhea and infertility, which may lead patients to seek help from a gynecologist, who must then make the diagnosis.

Bulimia Nervosa:
• Recurrent episodes of binge eating characterized by eating more food than most people would eat during a similar period of time and under similar circumstances;
• A sense of loss of control over eating;
• Recurrent inappropriate behavior in order to prevent weight gain, such as self-induced vomiting or misuse of laxatives, and excessive fasting or exercise;
• The binge-eating and inappropriate behaviors both occur, on average, at least twice a week for three months;
• Self-evaluation is unduly influenced by body shape and weight;
• The disturbance does not occur exclus ively during episodes of Anorexia Nervosa.

ASSOCIATED FEATURES

Patients with Anorexia Nervosa may be severely depressed, and may experience insomnia, irritability, and diminished interest in sex. These features may be exacerbated if the patient is severely underweight. People with Feeding and Eating Disorders also share many of the features of Obsessive Compulsive Disorder. For instance, someone with an Eating Disorder may have an excessive interest in food; they may hoard food, or spend unusual amounts of time reading and researching about foods, recipes, and nutrition. People with Anorexia Nervosa may also exhibit a strong need to control their environment, and may be socially and emotionally withdrawn. Approximately twenty to thirty percent of patients attempt suicide.

Individuals with Bulimia Nervosa are often within the normal weight range, but prior to the development of the disorder they may be overweight. Depression, Bipolar and other related disorders are common among people with bulimia. Substance abuse occurs in about one-third of individuals with bulimia.

Anxiety Disorders are common, and fear of social situations can be a precipitating factor in binging episodes.

PREVALENCE

Prevalence studies in females have found rates of 0.5 to one percent for Anorexia Nervosa. The prevalence of Anorexia Nervosa in males is approximately 0.3 percent. The prevalence of Bulimia Nervosa among adolescent females is approximately one to three percent. The rate of the disorder among males is approximately 0.5 percent.

TREATMENT OPTIONS

Medications, especially the newest SSRIs (Selective Serotonin Reuptake Inhibitors, which were originally developed as antidepressants), have been found to be very effective in the treatment of Feeding and Eating Disorders. They can help restore and build self-esteem, and thereby help the patient maintain a positive attitude as well as a safe and healthy body image and body weight.

Because of the physical damage these disorders can do to a patient, nutritional counseling and monitoring is often vital to restore and maintain proper body weight.

It is critical to recognize that Feeding and Eating Disorders are, in addition to being life-threatening, extremely complex: simply restoring the patient to an acceptable body weight is not enough. Many patients have complex and conflicting psychological issues that trigger the compulsion to binge, or the morbid fear of gaining weight. These issues need to be addressed by psychotherapy. Forms of psychotherapy that may be useful include psychodynamic psychotherapy (in which longstanding and sometimes unconscious emotional issues related to the feeding and eating disorders are explored) and cognitive behavior therapy, which aims to identify the thought patterns that trigger the disorder and to establish healthy eating habits. Recent literature suggests that psychotherapeutic approaches are often more effective than medications in the treatment of Anorexia. Family involvement in treatment is critical, and peer pressure can be used to compel patients to maintain adequate nutrition. Feeding and Eating Disorders are serious — untreated Anorexia can kill a patient — and treatment may be required over a course of many years. Treatment for Bulimia is similar to treatment for Anorexia.

Associations & Agencies

785 Alliance for Eating Disorders Awareness

1649 Forum Place
Suite 2
West Palm Beach, FL 33401
561-841-0900
866-662-1235
info@allianceforeatingdisorders.com
www.allianceforeatingdisorders.com

Leah Wypych, MPA, Board Chair
Johanna Kandel, Founder and CEO
Sharon Glynn, Director of Operations
Joann Hendelman,PhD,RN,FAED, Clinical Director

The Alliance for Eating Disorders Awareness is a nonprofit organization that serves to provide educational programs, information and referrals, and support and mentoring services focused on eating disorders, body image, and self-esteem. The Alliance advocates for health promotion and positive body image, and seeks to reduce size prejudice.

Year Founded: 2000

786 Center for Mental Health Services (CMHS)
Substance Abuse and Mental Health Services Administration

5600 Fishers Lane
Rockville, MD 20857
240-276-1310
877-726-4727
TTY: 800-487-4889
www.samhsa.gov/about-us/who-we-are/offices-centers

Paolo del Vecchio, MSW, Director
Anne Mathews-Younes, Acting Deputy Director
Keris Myrick, Director, Consumer Affairs
Patricia Gratton, Director, Program Analysis

Promotes the treatment of mental illness and emotional disorders by increasing accessibility to mental health programs; supporting outreach, treatment, rehabilitation, and support programs and networks; and encouraging the use of scientifically-based information when treating mental disorders. CMHS provides information about mental health via a toll-free number and numerous publications. Developed for users of mental health services and their families, the general public, policy makers, providers, and the media.

Year Founded: 1992

787 Council on Size and Weight Discrimination (CSWD)

PO Box 305
Mount Marion, NY 12456-305
845-679-1209; *Fax:* 845-679-1206
info@cswd.org
www.cswd.org

Miriam Berg, President
Lynn McAfee, Director of Medical Advocacy
William J. Fabrey, Media Project
Ragen Chastain, Media Spokesperson

The Council on Size and Weight Discrimination is a not-for-profit group aiming to change dominant perceptions about weight. CSWD advocates for the rights of larger people, particularly in the areas of media image, job discrimination, and medical treatment.

Year Founded: 1991

788 International Association of Eating Disorders Professionals Foundation

PO Box 1295
Pekin, IL 61555-1295
800-800-8126; *Fax:* 800-800-8126
iaedpmembers@earthlink.net
www.iaedp.com

Bonnie Harken, Managing Director
Blanche Williams, Media Relations Director
Holly Finlay, MA, LPCC, CEDS, President
Dena Cabrera, PsyD, CEDS, Secretary

IAEDP Foundation seeks to strengthen the level of quality among professionals who treat individuals with eating disorders. The Foundation provides training, education, and certifications; encourages professional and ethical standards; raises awareness on eating disorders; and participates in prevention efforts.

Year Founded: 1985

789 Multiservice Eating Disorders Association

288 Walnut Street
Suite 130
Newton, MA 02460
617-558-1881
866-343-6332
www.medainc.org

Rebecca Manley, MS, Founder
Mitchel Appelbaum, Chair
Beth Mayer, LICSW, Executive Director
Rachel Benson Monroe, Director, Clinical Programming

New England-based nonprofit organization dedicated to educating the public about eating disorders, as well as the causes, prevention, and treatment of eating disorders. Provides services and support designed to assist clients and families, as well as clinicians, educators, professionals, and the general public.

Year Founded: 1994

790 National Alliance on Mental Illness

3803 North Fairfax Drive
Suite 100
Arlington, VA 22203
703-524-7600
800-950-6264
info@nami.org
www.nami.org

Steve Pitman, JD, President
Lacey Berumen, PhD, MNM, First Vice President
Mary Giliberti, Chief Executive Officer
David Levy, Chief Financial Officer

NAMI is an organization dedicated to raising awareness on mental health and providing support and education for Americans affected by mental illness. NAMI advocates for access to services and treatment and fosters an environment of awareness and understanding for those concerned with mental health.

Year Founded: 1979

791 National Association for the Dually Diagnosed (NADD)

132 Fair Street
Kingston, NY 12401
845-331-4336
info@thenadd.org
www.thenadd.org

Jeanne M. Farr, MA, Chief Executive Officer
Daniel Baker, PhD., President
Peggie Webb, MA, Vice President
George Zukotynski, PhD., Secretary

NADD is a nonprofit organization designed to increase awareness of, and provide services for, individuals with developmental disabilities and mental illness. NADD emphasizes the importance of quality mental healthcare for people with mental health needs and offers conferences, information resources, educational programs, and training materials to professionals, parents, and organizations.

Year Founded: 1983

792 National Association of Anorexia Nervosa and Associated Disorders (ANAD)

220 North Green Street
Chicago, IL 60607
630-577-1333
630-577-1330
hello@anad.org
www.anad.org

Maria Rago, President
Warren Denardo, Treasurer
Lynn Slawsky, MPA, PMP, Executive Director
Kristen Portland, Coordinator, Volunteer/Support

A nonprofit organization dedicated to preventing anorexia nervosa, bulimia nervosa, binge eating disorder, and other eating disorders. ANAD serves as a clearinghouse of information with the goal of raising awareness and supports research and educational programs focused on understanding and preventing eating disorders.

Year Founded: 1976

793 National Association to Advance Fat Acceptance (NAAFA)

PO Box 4662
Foster City, CA 94404-0662
916-558-6880
www.naafaonline.com

Darliene Howell, Board Chair and Secretary
Peggy Howell, Public Relations Director
Tigress Osborn, Social Media Director

A nonprofit organization committed to defending the rights of fat people and improving their quality of life. NAAFA opposes discrimination against fat people, including discrimination in advertising, employment, fashion, medicine, insurance, social acceptance, the media, schooling, and public accommodations. Monitors legislative activity and litigation affecting fat people. Publications: NAAFA Newsletter, monthly.

Year Founded: 1969

794 National Eating Disorders Association

200 West 41st Street
Suite 1203
New York, NY 10036
212-575-6200
800-931-2237; *Fax:* 212-575-1650
info@nationaleatingdisorders.org
www.nationaleatingdisorders.org

Geoffrey Craddock, Chair
Claire Mysko, MA, Chief Executive Officer
Jessica Scheer, Chief Operationg Officer
Caitlin Hamilton, Director of Communications

NEDA offers a national information phone line, an international treatment referral directory, and a support group directory. The organization sponsors an annual conference; provides resources on eating disorders for individuals, parents, and educators; funds research; and raises awareness of eating disorders.

Year Founded: 2001

795 National Institute of Mental Health Eating Disorders Research Program

6001 Executive Boulevard
Room 7126, MSC 9632
Bethesda, MD 20892-9663
301-443-8942
866-615-6464; *Fax:* 301-443-4279
TTY: 301-443-8431
nimhinfo@nih.gov
www.www.nimh.nih.gov/

Mark Chavez, PhD, Program Chief

The program supports studies and research on eating disorders in areas including assessment, risk factors, and intervention development.

796 National Mental Health Consumers' Self-Help Clearinghouse

1211 Chestnut Street
Suite 1100
Philadelphia, PA 19107
267-507-3810
800-553-4539; *Fax:* 215-636-6312
info@mhselfhelp.org
www.mhselfhelp.org

Joseph Rogers, Founder and Executive Director
Susan Rogers, Director

The Clearinghouse is a peer-run national technical assistance center focused on achieving respect and equality of opportunity for those with mental illnesses. The Clearinghouse helps with the growth of the mental health consumer movement by evaluating mental health services, advocating for mental health reform, and providing consumers with news, information, publications, and consultation services.

Year Founded: 1986

797 TOPS Take Off Pounds Sensibly

4575 South 5th Street
PO Box 070360
Milwaukee, WI 53207-360

414-482-4620
wondering@tops.org
www.tops.org

Robert Dischinger, Jr., Chairman
Rick Danforth, President
Karen Tinlin, First Vice President
Sandra Seidlitz, Treasurer

TOPS is a nonprofit network of weight loss support groups and wellness education organizations. Promotes healthy lifestyles and sensible approaches to weight management. Provides meetings, educational tools and programs based on positive reinforcement and motivation. Supports people of all ages, sizes, and shapes.

Year Founded: 1948

798 The Center for Family Support

2811 Zulette Avenue
Bronx, NY 10461
718-518-1500; *Fax:* 718-518-8200
www.www.cfsny.org/

Steven Vernikoff, Executive Director
Lloyd Stabiner, President
Amy Bittinger, Vice President
Barbara Greenwald, Associate Executive Director

The Center for Family Support offers assistance to individuals with developmental and related disabilities, as well as their families, and provides support services and programs that are designed to accommodate individual needs. Offers services throughout New York City, Westchester County, Long Island, and New Jersey.

Year Founded: 1954

799 The National Association for Males with Eating Disorders, Inc.

2840 Southwest 3rd Avenue
Miami, FL 33129
www.namedinc.org

Scott Griffiths, Secretary
Andrew Walen, LCSW-C, President
Tiffany Ashton Brown, MS, Vice President

An organization dedicated to providing support for males with eating disorders. Provides information for males with eating disorders, families, treatment providers, and researchers.

Year Founded: 2006

Books

800 Anorexia Nervosa & Recovery: a Hunger for Meaning

Haworth Press
10 Alice Street
Binghamton, NY 13904-1503
607-722-5857
800-429-6784; *Fax:* 607-721-0012
getinfo@haworthpress.com
www.haworthpress.com

Ellen Cole, Author
Karen Way, MA, Author
Esther D Rothblum, Author
Karly Way Schramm, Author

Presents the most objective, complete, and compassionate picture of what anorexia nervosa is about. *$19.95*

142 pages Year Founded: 1993 ISBN 0-918393-95-7

801 Beyond Anorexia

Cambridge University Press
32 Avenue of the Americas
New York, NY 10013-2473
212-337-5000
newyork@cambrigde.org
www.www.cambridge.org

Catherine Garrett, Author

Beyond Anorexia is a sociological exploration of how people recover from what medicince lables 'eating disorders'. *$41.00*

260 pages Year Founded: 1534 ISBN 0-521629-83-6

802 Binge Eating: Nature, Assessment and Treatment

Guilford Press
72 Spring Street
New York, NY 10012-4068
212-431-9800
800-365-7006; *Fax:* 212-966-6708
info@guilford.com

Bob Matloff, President

Informative and practical text brings together original and significant contributions from leading experts from a wide variety of fields. Detailed manual covers all those who binge eat, including those who are overweight. *$21.95*

419 pages ISBN 0-898628-58-X

803 Body Image Workbook: An 8 Step Program for Learning to Like Your Looks

NewHarbinger Publications
5674 Shattuck Avenue
Oakland, CA 94609-1662
510-652-0215
800-748-6273; *Fax:* 800-652-1613
customerservice@newharbinger.com
www.newharbinger.com

Thomas Cash, PhD, Author

Workbook offering a program to help transform your relationship with your body. *$19.95*

240 pages Year Founded: 1973 ISBN 1-572240-62-8

804 Body Image, Eating Disorders, and Obesity in Youth

APA Books
750 First Street,NorthEast
Washington, DC 20002-4241
202-336-5500
800-374-2721; *Fax:* 202-336-5500
TDD: 202-336-6123
order@apa.org
www.apa.org

Linda Smolak, PhD, Editor
J. Kevin Thompson, PhD, Editor

Provides for clinicians including research, assessment and treatment suggestions on body image disturbances and eating disorders in children and adolescents. *$49.95*

389 pages Year Founded: 1892 ISBN 1-433804-05-2

805 Brief Therapy and Eating Disorders

John Wiley & Sons
111 River Street
Hoboken, NJ 07030-5774

201-748-6000; *Fax:* 201-748-6088
www.wiley.com

Barbara McFarland, Author

Demonstrates how solution-focused brief therapy is one of the more efficient approaches in treating eating disorders. *$36.95*

284 pages ISBN 0-787900-53-2

806 Bulimia
Jossey-Bass Publishers
989 Martket Street
San Francisco, CA 94103-1708
415-433-1740; *Fax:* 415-433-0499
www.leadertoleader.org

Barbara G Baeur,PhD, Author
Wayne P Anderson,PhD, Author
Robert W Hyatt,MD, Author

A step-by-step guide to this complex disease. Filled with practical information and advice, this essential resource offers hope to millions of bulimics and their loved ones. *$17.95*

167 pages ISBN 0-787903-61-2

807 Bulimia Nervosa
University of Minnesota Press
111 Third Avenue South
Suite 290
Minneapolis, MN 55401-2520
612-627-1970; *Fax:* 612-627-1980
ump@umn.edu
www.upress.umn.edu

James E. Mitchell, Author

A practical guide for health-care professionals to the diagnosis, treatment and management of bulimia by a leading expert in the field of eating disorders. Hardcover. *$27.95*

192 pages Year Founded: 1925 ISBN 0-816616-26-4

808 Bulimia Nervosa & Binge Eating: A Guide To Recovery
New York University Press
838 Broadway
3rd Floor
New York, NY 10003-4812
212-998-2575; *Fax:* 212-995-3833
www.nyupress.nyu.edu

Peter J Cooper, Author
Margie Guerra, Assistant Director
Monica McCormick, Program Officer

A self-help book designed to guide bilimics and binge-eaters to recovery. *$35.00*

170 pages ISBN 0-814715-22-2

809 Bulimia: a Guide to Recovery
Gurze Books
5145 B Avenida Encinas
Carlsbad, CA 92008
760-434-7533
800-756-7533; *Fax:* 760-434-5476
info@gurze.net
www.www.gurzebooks.com

Lindsey Hall, Author
Leigh Cohn,M.A.T, Author

Guidebook offers a complete understanding of bulimia and a plan for recovery. Includes a two-week program to stop binging, things-to-do instead of binging, a two-week guide for support groups, specific advice for loved ones, and Eating Without Fear - Hall's story of self-cure which has inspired thousands of other bulimics. *$14.95*

280 pages Year Founded: 1980 ISBN 0-936077-31-X

810 Clinical Handbook of Eating Disorders: An Integrated Approach
Informa Healthcare
52 Vanderbilt Avenue
New York, NY 10017-3808
646-443-3976; *Fax:* 646-661-5054
healthcare.enquiries@informa.com
www.informaworld.com

Timothy D Brewerton, Editor

Reviews the most current research on the assessment, epidemiology, etiology, risk factors, neurodevelopment, course of illness, and various empirically-based evaluation and treatment approaches relating to eating disorders-studying disordered eating in atypical patient populations, such as men, infants, and the elderly and highlighting gender, cultural, and age-related differences that have appeared in the study of these conditions.

740 pages

811 Controlling Eating Disorders with Facts, Advice and Resources
Oryx Press
88 Post Road W
Westport, CT 06880-4208
203-226-3571; *Fax:* 603-431-2214
info@oryxpress.com
www.oryxpress.com

Raymond Lemberg, Editor

256 pages

812 Coping with Eating Disorders
Rosen Publishing Group
29 East 21st Street
New York, NY 10010-6209
212-777-3017
800-237-9932; *Fax:* 888-436-4643
info@rosenpub.com
www.rosenpublishing.com

Barbara Moe, Author

Offers practical suggestions on coping with eating disorders. *$33.25*

149 pages Year Founded: 1950 ISBN 0-823921-33-6

813 Cult of Thinness
Oxford University Press
198 Madison Avenue
New York, NY 10016-4341
212-726-6400
800-445-9714
TTY: 800-445-9714
custserv.us@oup.com
www.www.oup.com

Sharlene Nagy Hesse-Biber, Author

Discusses eating patterns and disorders and their relationship to emotional states and self-esteem. *$29.95*

288 pages Year Founded: 2006 ISBN 0-195178-78-4

814 Developmental Psychopathology of Eating Disorders: Implications for Research, Prevention and Treatment
Lawrence Erlbaum Associates
10 Industrial Avenue
Mahwah, NJ 07430-2253
201-825-3200
800-926-6577; *Fax:* 201-236-0072
orders@erlbaum.com
www.erlbaum.com

Linda Smolak, Editor
Ruth H Striegel-Moore, Editor
Michael P Levine, Editor

This text provides backround material from developmental psychology and psychopathology - following the theory that eating problems and disorders are typically rooted in childhood. Applications are then outlined, including research, treatment, protective factors and primary prevention. *$79.95*

464 pages ISBN 0-805817-46-8

815 Disordered Eating Among Athletes
Human Kinetics Publishers
1607 North Market Street
PO Box 5076
Champaign, IL 61825-5076
800-747-4457; *Fax:* 217-351-1549
orders@hkusa.com

Katherine Beals, Author

Gives readers the information they need to identify and address major eating disorders such as: anorexia, bulimia nervosa, and eating disorders not otherwise specified. *$50.00*

264 pages Year Founded: 2004 ISBN 0-736042-19-2

816 Eating Disorder Hope
5112 Golden Lane
Fort Worth, TX 76123
817-231-5184
800-986-4160; *Fax:* 817-887-4025
info@eatingdisorderhope.com
www.www.eatingdisorderhope.com

Jaquelyn Ekern, MS, LPC, Founder and Director
Baxter Ekern,MBA, Vice President
Crystal Karges,MS,RDN,IBCLC, Special Projects Manager

Eating Disorder Hope was founded in January 2005. Their mission is to offer hope, information, and resources to individual eating disorder sufferers, their family members, and treatment providers.

Year Founded: 2005

817 Eating Disorders & Obesity: a Comprehensive Handbook
Guilford Press
72 Spring Street
New York, NY 10012-4068
212-431-9800
800-365-7006; *Fax:* 212-966-6708
info@guilford.com

Bob Matloff, President

Presents and integrates virtually all that is currently known about eating disorders and obesity in one authorative, accessible and eminently practical volume. *$57.95*

583 pages ISBN 0-898628-50-4

818 Eating Disorders Sourcebook
Omnigraphics
155 West Congress
Suite 200
Detroit, MI 48226
313-961-1340
800-234-1340; *Fax:* 313-961-1383
contact@omnigraphics.com
www.omnigraphics.com

Sandra J Judd, Author/Editor

Omnigraphics is the publisher of the Health Reference Series, a growing consumer health information resource with more than 100 volumes in print. Each title in the series features an easy to understand format, nontechnical language, comprehensive indexing and resources for further information. Material in each book has been collected from a wide range of government agencies, professional associations, periodicals and other sources. *$78.00*

583 pages Year Founded: 1985 ISBN 0-780803-35-3

819 Eating Disorders and Obesity, Second Edition : A Comprehensive Handbook
The Guilford Press
72 Spring Street
New York, NY 10012-4019
212-431-9800
800-365-7006; *Fax:* 212-966-6708
info@guilford.com

Bob Matloff, President

This unique handbook presents and integrates virtually all that is currently known about eating disorders and obesity in one authoritative, accessible, and eminently practical volume.

820 Eating Disorders: Reference Sourcebook
Oryx Press
88 Post Road W
Westport, CT 06880-4208
203-226-3571; *Fax:* 603-431-2214
www.oryxpress.com

Raymond Lemberg, Author
Leigh Cohn, Author

Listings of 200 centers and groups for care and treatment of eating disorders, such as anorexia nervosa, bulimia nervosa, and compulsive overeating. *$49.95*

272 pages

821 Emotional Eating: A Practical Guide to Taking Control
Lexington Books
4501 Forbes Boulevard
Suite 200
Lanham, MD 20706-4346
301-459-3366
800-426-6420; *Fax:* 301-429-5748

Edward Abramson, Author

Using case histories he explores some of the causes of emotional eating (childhood programming, family life, sexual abuse) and the manifestos of emotional eating ('sneaky snaking',grazing, and binging). Of particular interest is the last chaper, which helps the reader determine whether or not it is a good or bad time to diet. While not a diet book or a 12-step primer, this is a tool for developing healthier ways of handling emotions and food. *$19.95*

208 pages ISBN 0-029002-15-X

822 Encyclopedia of Obesity and Eating Disorders
Facts on File
11 Penn Plaza
New York, NY 10001-2006
212-290-8090
800-322-8755; *Fax:* 212-678-3633

From abdominoplasty to Zung Rating Scale, this volume defines and explains these disorders, along with medical and other problems associated with them. *$50.00*

272 pages

823 Feminist Perspectives on Eating Disorders
Guilford Press
72 Spring Street
New York, NY 10012-4068
212-431-9800
800-365-7006; *Fax:* 212-966-6708
info@guilford.com

Bob Matloff, President

Explores the relationship between the anguish of eating disorder sufferers and the problems of ordinary women. Examines the sociocultural pressure on women to conform to culturally ideal body types and how this affects individual self concept. Controversial topics include the relationship between sexual abuse and eating disorders, the use of medications and the role of hospitalization and 12-step programs. *$ 25.95*

465 pages ISBN 1-572301-82-1

824 Food for Recovery: The Next Step
Crown Publishing Group
201 E 50th Street
New York, NY 10022-7703
212-751-2600
www.randomhouse.com

Joseph D Beasley, Author
Susan Knightly, Author

A very practicle guide on every aspect needed by the patient and counselor to utilize nutrition as a therapeutic tool. *$ 14.00*

156 pages ISBN 0-517586-94-0

825 Golden Cage, The Enigma of Anorexia Nervosa
Random House
1745 Broadway 15-3
New York, NY 10019-4368
212-572-4985; *Fax:* 212-782-9052
www.randomhouse.com

Hilde Bruch, Author

One of the world's leading authorities offers a vivid and moving account of the causes, effects and treatment of this devastating disease. *$9.00*

174 pages ISBN 0-394726-88-X

826 Group Psychotherapy for Eating Disorders
American Psychiatric Publishing, Inc.
1000 Wilson Boulevard
Suite 1825
Arlington, VA 22209-3901
703-907-7322
800-368-5777; *Fax:* 703-907-1091

appi@psych.org
www.appi.org

Heather Harper-Giuffre, Author
K. Roy MacKenzie, Author

The first book to fully explore the use of group therapy in the treatment of eating disorders. *$101.00*

374 pages Year Founded: 1992 ISBN 0-880484-19-0

827 Hunger So Wide and Deep
University of Minnesota Press
111 Third Avenue South
Suite 290
Minneapolis, MN 55401-2520
612-627-1970; *Fax:* 612-627-1980
ump@umn.edu
www.upress.umn.edu

Becky W. Thompson, Author

$19.50

176 pages Year Founded: 1925 ISBN 0-816624-35-6

828 Hungry Self; Women, Eating and Identity
Harper Collins
10 East 53rd Street
New York, NY 10022-5299
212-207-7000
feedback2@harpercollins.com
www.harpercollins.com

Kim Chernin, Author

Answers the need for help among the five million American women who suffer from eating disorders. Paperback. *$13.00*

240 pages Year Founded: 1817 ISBN 0-060925-04-3

829 Insights in the Dynamic Psychotherapy of Anorexia and Bulimia
Jason Aronson
506 Clemant Street
San Francisco, CA 94118-2324
415-387-2272; *Fax:* 415-387-2377
www.greenapplebooks.com

Joyce Kraus Aronson, Author

The clinical insights that guide the dynamic psychotheray of anorexic and bulimic patients. *$45.00*

288 pages ISBN 0-876685-68-8

830 Making Peace with Food
Harper Collins
10 East 53rd Street
New York, NY 10022-5299
212-207-7000
800-242-7737
feedback2@harpercollins.com
www.www.harpercollins.com

Susan Kano, Author

For millions of diet-conscious Americans, the scientifically proven, step-by-step guide to overcoming repeated weight loss and gain, binge eating, guilt and anxieties about food and body image. *$15.00*

272 pages Year Founded: 1989 ISBN 0-060963-28-X

831 Obesity: Mechanisms & Clinical Management
Lippincott Williams &Wilkins
I 185 Avenue of the Americas
New York, NY 10013-1209
212-930-9500
800-638-3030; *Fax:* 212-869-3495
www.lww.com

Robert H. Eckel, MD, Author

A classic reference for clinicians dealing with obesity, this
volume provides the most up-to-date research, preclinical
and clinical information. *$139.00*

566 pages Year Founded: 2003 ISBN 0-781728-44-7

832 Overeaters Anonymous
Overeaters Anonymous
6075 Zenith Court NE
Rio Rancho, NM 87144-6424
505-891-2664; *Fax:* 505-891-4320
NYOAMentroOffice@yahoo.com
www.www.oa.org/

Personal stories demonstrating the struggles overcome and
accomplishments made. *$7.50*

204 pages Year Founded: 1958

**833 Psychobiology and Treatment of Anorexia
Nervosa and Bulimia Nervosa**
American Psychiatric Publishing, Inc.
1000 Wilson Boulevard
Suite 1825
Arlington, VA 22209-3901
703-907-7322
800-368-5777; *Fax:* 703-907-1091
appi@psych.org
www.appi.org

Katherine A. Halmi, MD, Editor

Combines clinical research concerning these distinct disorders and provides an overview of the psychobiology and
treatment. *$101.00*

376 pages Year Founded: 1992 ISBN 0-880485-06-7

**834 Psychosomatic Families: Anorexia Nervosa in
Context**
Harvard University Press
79 Garden Street
Cambridge, MA 02138-1400
617-495-2600; *Fax:* 617-495-5898
contact_hup@harvard.edu
www.www.hup.harvard.edu

Salvador Minuchin, Author
Bernice L Rosman, Author
Lester Baker, Author

Hardcover. *$76.50*

351 pages Year Founded: 1913 ISBN 0-674722-20-0

835 Shame and Anger: The Criticism Connection
Change for Good Coaching and Counseling
3801 Connecticut Avenue NorthWest
Washington, DC 20008-4530
202-362-3009; *Fax:* 202-204-6100
brockhansenlcsw@aol.com
www.change-for-good.org

Brock Hansen LCSW, Author

Coaching on learnable emotional skills to see goals clearly,
harness resources and get moving toward a successful outcome. *$16.98*

226 pages ISBN 0-615135-81-6

**836 Surviving an Eating Disorder: Perspectives and
Strategies**
Harper Collins
10 East 53rd Street
New York, NY 10022-5299
212-207-7000
feedback2@harpercollins.com
www.www.harpercollins.com

Michele Siegel, Author
Judith Brisman, PhD, Author
Margot Weinshel,MSW, Author

Addresses the cutting-edge advances made in the field of
eating disorders, discusses how the changes in health care
have affected treatment and provides additional strategies
for dealing with anorexia, bulimia and binge eating disorder. It also includes updated readings and a list of support
organizations. A terrrific resource for those suffering from
eating disorders, their families and professionals. Paperback. *$ 35.00*

288 pages Year Founded: 1817 ISBN 0-060952-33-4

837 Treating Eating Disorders
Jossey-Bass Publishers
10475 Crosspoint Boulevard
Indianapolis, IN 46256-3386
877-762-2974; *Fax:* 800-597-3299
consumers@wiley.com
www.josseybass.com

Joellen Werne, Author

Details how some of the most eminent clinicians in the
field combine and intergrate a wide variety of contemporary therapies — ranging from psychodynamic to systematic to cognitive behavioral—to successfully treat clients
with anorexia nervosa, bulimia nervosa, and binge eating
diorders. Filled with up to date information and important
approaches to assessment and treatment, the book offers a
hands-on approach that cogently illustrates both theory and
technique. *$29.95*

377 pages ISBN 0-787903-30-2

838 When Food Is Love
Geneen Roth and Associates
PO Box 682
Aptos, CA 95001
703-401-0871
877-243-6336; *Fax:* 703-852-3956
info@geneenroth.com
www.geneenroth.com

Geneen Roth, Author

Shows how dieting and compulsive eating often become a
subsititue for intimacy. Drawing on painful personal
experiece as well as the candid stories of those she has
helped in her seminars, Roth claims the crucial issues that
surrounds compulsive eating: need for control, dependency
on melodrama, desire for what is forbidden, and the belief
that the wrong move can mean catastrophe. She shows why
many people overeat in an attempt to satisfy their emotional hunger, and why weight loss frequently just uncovers
a new set of problems. This book will help readers break
destructive, self-perpetuating patterns and learn to satisfy

all the hungers - physical and emotional - that makes us human. *$13.98*

205 pages Year Founded: 1992

Periodicals & Pamphlets

839 Anorexia: Am I at Risk?
ETR Associates
4 Carbonero Way
Scotts Valley, CA 95066-4200
831-438-4060
800-321-4407; *Fax:* 831-438-3618
customerservice@etr.org
www.etr.org

David Kitchen, MBA, Chief Operations Officer
Laurie Searson, Publisher
Sarah Stevens, Director, Product Development
Yvonne Collins, Sales Director

Offers a clear overview of anorexia; Lists symptoms; Explains helath problems.

840 Body Image
ETR Associates
4 Carbonero Way
Scotts Valley, CA 95066-4200
831-438-4060
800-321-4407; *Fax:* 831-438-3618
support@etr.freshdesk.com
www.etr.org

David Kitchen,MBA, Chief Financial Officer
Talita Sanders,BS, Director,Human Resources
Coleen Cantwell,MPH, Director,Business Development Pl
Matt McDowell,BS, Director,Marketing

Discusses the difference between healthy and distorted body image; the link between poor body image and low self esteem; five point list to help people check out their own body image.

841 Bulimia
ETR Associates
4 Carbonero Way
Scotts Valley, CA 95066-4200
831-438-4060
800-321-4407; *Fax:* 831-438-3618
customerservice@etr.org
www.etr.org

Bonnie Graves, Author
Laurie Searson, Publisher
Sarah Stevens, Director, Product Development
Yvonne Collins, Sales Director

Includes warning signs that someone's bulimic, health consequesnces of bulimia, and how to help a friend.

842 Eating Disorder Sourcebook
Gurze Books
PO Box 2238
Carlsbad, CA 92018-2238
760-434-7533
800-756-7533; *Fax:* 760-434-5476
info@gurze.net
www.gurze.net

Carolyn Costin, Author
Lindsay Cohn, Co-Owner

Includes 125 books and tapes on eating disorders and related subjects for both lay and professional audiences, basic facts about eating disorders, a list of national organizations and treatment facilities. Also publishes a bimonthly newsletter for clinicians and are executive editors of Eating Disorders the Journal of Treatment and Prevention.

336 pages 1 per year

843 Eating Disorders
ETR Associates
4 Carbonero Way
Scotts Valley, CA 95066-4200
831-438-4060
800-321-4407; *Fax:* 831-438-3618
support@etr.freshdesk.com
www.etr.org

David Kitchen,MBA, Chief Financial Officer
Talita Sanders,BS, Director,Human Resources
Coleen Cantwell,MPH, Director,Business Development Pl
Matt McDowell,BS, Director,Marketing

Includes anorexia and bulimia, eating patterns versus eating disorders, treatment and getting help.

844 Eating Disorders: Facts About Eating Disorders and the Search for Solutions
National Institute of Mental Health
6001 Executive Boulevard
Room 8184,MSC 9663
Bethesda, MD 20892-9663
301-443-4513
866-615-6464
TTY: 301-443-8431
nimhinfo@nih.gov
www.www.nimh.nih.gov/

Francis S Collins PhD, Director

Eating is controlled by many factors, including appetite, food availability, family, peer, and cultural practices, and attempts at voluntary control. Dieting to a body weight leaner than needed for health is highly promoted by current fashion trends, sales campaigns for special foods, and in some activities and professions. Eating disorders involve serious disturbances in eating behavior, such as extreme and unhealthy reduction of food intake or severe overeating, as well as feelings of distress or extreme concern about body shape or weight. There is help, and there is every hope for recovery.

8 pages

845 Fats of Life
ETR Associates
4 Carbonero Way
Scotts Valley, CA 95066-4200
831-438-4060
800-321-4407; *Fax:* 831-438-3618
customerservice@etr.org
www.etr.org

Caroline M Pond, Author
Laurei Searson, Publisher
Sarah Stevens, Director, Product Development
Yvonne Collins, Sales Director

Stresses that health, not body weight, is what's important; dispels myths about dieting; includes chart to help people determine their body mass index.

344 pages

846 Food and Feelings
ETR Associates
4 Carbonero Way
Scotts Valley, CA 95066-4200
831-438-4060
800-321-4407; *Fax:* 831-438-3618
customerservice@etr.org
www.etr.org

David Kitchen, Chief Operations Officer
Laurie Searson, Publisher
Sarah Stevens, Director, Product Development
Yvonne Collins, Sales Director

Helps students recognize eating disorders; emphasizes the seriousness of eating disorders; encourages the sufferers to seek treatment.

847 Getting What You Want from Your Body Image
ETR Associates
4 Carbonero Way
Scotts Valley, CA 95066-4200
831-438-4060
800-321-4407; *Fax:* 831-438-3618
support@etr.freshdesk.com
www.etr.org

Melinda M Mueller, Author
Laurie Searson, Publisher
Sarah Stevens, Director, Product Development
Yvonne Collins, Sales Director

Discusses topics such as the influence of the media, the truth about dieting, and body image survival tips.

8 pages

848 Restrictive Eating
ETR Associates
4 Carbonero Way
Scotts Valley, CA 95066-4200
831-438-4060
800-321-4407; *Fax:* 831-438-3618
customerservice@etr.org
www.etr.org

David Kitchen, MBA, Chief Operations Officer
Laurie Searson, Publisher

Discusses the spectrum of eating patterns, signs of restrictive eating and why it is a problem, how to help a friend, and where to go for help.

849 Teen Image
ETR Associates
4 Carbonero Way
Scotts Valley, CA 95066-4200
831-438-4060
800-321-4407; *Fax:* 831-438-3618
customerservice@etr.org
www.etr.org

Mary Nelson, President

Dispels unrealistic media images; offers ways to boost body image and self esteem; includes tips to maintain a good body image.

850 Working Together
National Association of Anorexia Nervosa and Associated Disorders
750 East Diehl Road
Suite 127
Naperville, IL 60563
630-577-1333
630-577-1330; *Fax:* 847-433-4632
anadhelp@anad.org
www.anad.org

Laura Discipio, LCSW, Executive Director
Donna Rostamian, Community Organisational Manager
Melanie Zumm, Support Group Coordinator
Kyron Johnson-Brana, Administrative Assistant

Designed for individuals, families, group leaders and professionals concerned with eating disorders. Provides updates on treatments, resources, conferences, programs, articles by therapists, recovered victims, group members and leaders.

2 pages 4 per year Year Founded: 1976

Research Centers

851 Center for the Study of Anorexia and Bulimia
1841 Broadway 4th Floor
New York, NY 10023-7603
212-333-3444; *Fax:* 212-333-5444
www.www.icpnyc.org/csab/

Jill M Pollack, Director
Jill E Daino, Co-Director
Tracy McClair, CSAB Program Administrator

Established as a division of the Institute for Contemporary Psychotherapy in 1979 and is the oldest non-profit eating disorders clinic in New York City. Using an eclectic approach, the professional staff and affiliates are on the cutting edge of treatment in their field. The treatment staff includes social workers, psychologists, registered nurses and nutritionists, all with special training in the treatment of eating disorders.

Year Founded: 1979

852 Obesity Research Center
St. Luke's-Roosevelt Hospital
1111 Amsterdam Ave., Babcock 10
New York, NY 10025
212-523-4161; *Fax:* 212-523-4830
www.www.nyorc.org/

Lee C Bollinger, President
John H Coatsworth, Provost
Robert Kasdin, Sr Executive Vice President
Nicholas B Dirks, EVP, Arts ans Sciences

Helps reduce the the incidence of obesity and related diseases through leadership in basic research, clinical research, epidemiology and public health, patient care, and public education.

853 UAMS Psychiatric Research Institute
4224 Shuffield Drive
Little Rock, AR 72205
501-526-8100; *Fax:* 501-660-7542
kramerteresal@uams.edu
www.www.psychiatry.uams.edu

Dan Rahn, MD, Chancellor

Combining research, education and clinical services into one facility, PRI offers inpatiend and outpatient services, with 40 psychiatric beds, therapy options, and specialized treatment for specific disorders, including: addictive eating, anxiety, deppressive and post-traumatic stress disorders. Research focuses on evidence-based care takes into consideration the education of future medical personnel while relying on research scientists to provide innovative forms of treatment. PRI includes the Center for Addiction Research as well as a methadone clinic.

854 University of Pennsylvania Weight and Eating Disorders Program
3535 Market Street
Suite 3108
Philadelphia, PA 19104-3313
215-898-7314; *Fax:* 215-898-2878
cwilson@mail.med.upenn.edu
www.www.med.upenn.edu/weight/

Dwight L. Evans, MD, Chair

Conducts a wide variety of studies on the causes and treatment of weight-related disorders.

Support Groups & Hot Lines

855 Food Addicts Anonymous
529 N W Prima Vista Blvd.
#301 A
Port St. Lucie, FL 34983
772-878-9657
faawso@bellsouth.net
www.foodaddictsanonymous.org

Linda Closy, Manager

The FAA program is based on the belief that food addiction is a bio-chemical disease. We share our experience, strength, and hope with others allows us to recover from this disease.

856 MEDA
92 Pearl Street
Newton, MA 02458-1529
617-558-1881
866-343-6332
info@medainc.org
www.medainc.org

Rachel Benson, Clinical Programs Coordinator
Beth Mayer, LICSW, Executive Director
Lindsay Brady, LICSW, Clinical Director
Susie Stockwell, Communications and Development D

MEDA ia a nonprofit organization dedicated to the prevention and treatment of eating disorders and disordered eating. MEDA'S mission is to prevent the continuing spread of eating disorders through educational awareness and early detection. MEDA serves as a support network and resource for clients, loved ones, clinicians, educators and the general public.

857 National Center for Overcoming Overeating
PO Box 1257
Old Chelsea Station
New York, NY 10113-1257
212-875-0442
webmaster@overcomingovereating.com
www.overcomingovereating.com

Is an educational and training organization working to end body hatred and dieting.

858 Overeaters Anonymous General Service Office
6075 Zenith Court,NorthEast
Rio Rancho, NM 87144-6424
505-891-2664; *Fax:* 505-891-4320
info@oa.org
www.oa.org

OA offers a program of recovery from compulsive eating using the Twelve Steps and Twelve Traditions of OA. It addresses physical, emotional and spiritual well-being.
Year Founded: 1960

Video & Audio

859 Eating Disorder Video
Active Parenting Publishers
1955 Vaughn Road NW
Suite 108
Kennesaw, GA 30144-7808
770-429-0565
800-825-0060; *Fax:* 770-429-0334
cservice@activeparenting.com

Features compelling interviews with several young people who have suffered from anorexia nervosa, bulimia and compulsive eating. Discusses the treatments, causes and techniques for prevention with field experts. *$39.95*
ISSN Q6456

Web Sites

860 www.anred.com
Anorexia Nervosa and Related Eating Disorders
Online resource providing information about eating disorders and how to recover from them.

861 www.bulimia.us.com
Bulimia: News & Discussion Forum
Eating disorders forum with news and information about bulimia, anorexia, male and teen eating disorders; treatment, help and resources information, events and inspirational stories.

862 www.closetoyou.org/eatingdisorders
Close to You
Information about eating disorders, anorexia, bulimia, binge eating disorder, and compulsive overeating.

863 www.cyberpsych.org
CyberPsych
Hosts the American Psychoanalyists Foundation, American Association of Suicideology, Society for the Exploration of Psychotherapy Intergration, and Anxiety Disorders Association of America. Also subcategories of the anxiety disorders, as well as general information, including panic disorder, phobias, obsessive compulsive disorder (OCD), social phobia, generalized anxiety disorder, post traumatic stress disorder, and phobias of childhood. Book reviews and links to web pages sharing the topics.

864 **www.edap.org**
Eating Disorders Awareness and Prevention

A source of educational brochures and curriculum materials.

865 **www.gurze.com**
Gurze Bookstore

Hundreds of books on eating disorders.

866 **www.healthyplace.com/Communities/**
Peace, Love, and Hope

Click on Body Views for information on body dysmorphic disorder.

867 **www.kidsource.com/nedo/**
National Eating Disorders Organization

Educational materials on dynamics, causative factors and evaluating treatment options.

868 **www.mentalhelp.net**
Anorexia Nervosa General Information

Introductory text on Anorexia Nervosa.

869 **www.mirror-mirror.org/eatdis.htm**
Mirror, Mirror

Relapse prevention for eating disorders.

870 **www.planetpsych.com**
Planetpsych.com

Learn about disorders, their treatments and other topics in psychology. Articles are listed under the related topic areas. Ask a therapist a question for free, or view the directory of professionals in your area. If you are a therapist sign up for the directory. Current features, self-help, interactive, and newsletter archives.

871 **www.psychcentral.com**
Psych Central

Personalized one-stop index for psychology, support, and mental health issues, resources, and people on the Internet.

872 **www.something-fishy.com**
Something Fishy Music and Publishing

Continuously educating the world on eating disorders to encourage every sufferer towards recovery.

873 **www.store.samhsa.gov**
Substance Abuse and Mental Health Services Administration

Resources on mental disorders as well as treatment and recovery.

Gender Dysphoria

Introduction

With a wide scope of questions and confusion surrounding human sexuality and gender-explicit roles in the modern era, many children, adolescents, and adults have been perplexed by the concepts of homosexuality and cross-gender identification. Homosexuality is a matter of sexual orientation: whether one is sexually attracted to men or women. The American Psychiatric Association ceased to classify homosexuality as an illness in 1973. Gender identity, in contrast, is a matter of what gender one feels oneself to be; people with Gender Dysphoria feel that their psychological experience conflicts with the physical body with which they were born. Gender Dysphoria can have serious social and occupational repercussions.

Diagnosis of Gender Dysphoria requires two sets of criteria: (1) a heavy and persistent insistence that the individual is, or has a strong desire to be, of the opposite sex, and (2) a constant discomfort about his/her designated sex, a feeling of inappropriateness towards his/her biological designation. Typically, boys meeting critera for the disorder are predisposed to dressing as girls, drawing explicit pictures of females, playing with pre-designated feminine toys, fantasizing and role playing as females, and interacting primarily with girls. Girls who exhibit Gender Dysphoria are often mistaken for boys due to attire and hair style, and may assert that they will develop into men. For adolescents and adults, ostracism in school and the workplace is likely to occur, as is a profound inability to associate with others and poor relationships with family members and members of either sex.

There is a sharp divide among persons whose biological gender feels wrong: some insist that this is not a psychiatric disorder but rather a biological variant; others feel strongly that they have a psychiatric disorder. Some of this conviction is driven by the need to demonstrate 'medical necessity' in order for health insurance to cover hormonal or surgical interventions to make the individual look like the gender he or she feels they are.

SYMPTOMS

In boys
• A marked preoccupation with traditionally feminine activites;
• A preference for dressing as a girl;
• Attraction to stereotypical female games and toys;
• Portraying female characters in role playing;
• Assertion he is a girl;
• Insistence on sitting to urinate;
• Displaying disgust for his genitals, wishing to remove them.

In girls
• Aversion to traditional female attire;
• Shared interest in contact games;
• A preference for associating with boys;
• Refusing to urinate sitting down;
• Show little interest in playing with stereotypical female toys such as dolls;
• Assertion that she will grow a penis, not breasts;
• Identification with strong male figures.

In adolescents
• Ostracism in school and social situations;
• Social isolation, peer rejection and peer teasing;
• Significant cross-gender identification and mannerisms;
• Similar symptoms as children.

In adults
• Adoption of social roles, physical appearance, and mannerisms of opposite sex;
• Surgical and/or hormonal manipulation of biological state;
• Discomfort in being regarded by others, or functioning, as his/her designated sex;
• Cross-dressing;
• Transvestic Fetishism.

ASSOCIATED FEATURES

Those who have Gender Dysphoria are at risk of mental and physical harm resulting, not from the condition itself, but from the reactions of other people to the condition. In children, a manifestation of separation anxiety disorder, generalized anxiety disorder, and symptoms of depression may result. For adolescents, depression and suicidal thoughts or ideas, as well as actual suicide attempts can result from prolonged feelings of ostracism by peers. Relationships with either one or both parents may weaken from resentment, lack of communication, and misunderstanding; many with this condition may drop out of or avoid school due to peer teasing. For many, lives are built around attempts to decrease gender distress. They are often preoccupied with appearance. In extreme cases, males with the condition perform their own castration. Prostitution has been linked with the condition because young people who are rejected by their families and ostracized by others may resort to prostitution as the only way to support themselves, a practice which increases the risk of acquiring sexually transmitted diseases. Some people with the condition resort to substance abuse and other forms of abuse in an attempt to deal with the associated stress.

PREVALENCE

In most cases, the age of onset for Gender Dysphoria is in the pre-school years. However, it should be noted that Gender Dysphoria in childhood does not always continue into adulthood.

TREATMENT OPTIONS

Therapists who attempt to pathologize and 'cure' sexual orientation have been generally unsuccessful. So-called conversion therapy can cause more harm than good. In contrast, some people with Gender Dysphoria decide to live as members of the opposite sex; some choose to undergo sex-change surgery.

There is some controversy about the diagnosis; some groups protest that their condition, like homosexuality, should not be classified as a mental illness.

Psychological assistance can help individuals to gain acceptance of themselves, and can teach methods of dealing with discrimination, prejudice, and violence. Supportive counseling may also help families accept the gender identity of the family member with Gender Dysphoria.

For youth with Gender Dysphoria, treatment may include hormone blockers, which suppress the physical changes of puberty, and cross-sex hormone therapy. Treatment for adults may include hormone replacement therapy and supportive counseling.

It is important that people with Gender Dysphoria receive the support and therapy that they need in order to reduce the risk of depression and emotional distress, and increase the chance of a happy, productive life.

Associations & Agencies

875 Center for Mental Health Services (CMHS)
Substance Abuse and Mental Health Services
Administration
5600 Fishers Lane
Rockville, MD 20857
240-276-1310
877-726-4727
TTY: 800-487-4889
www.samhsa.gov/about-us/who-we-are/offices-centers

Paolo del Vecchio, MSW, Director
Anne Mathew-Younes, Acting Deputy Director
Keris Myrick, Director, Consumer Affairs
Patricia Gratton, Director, Program Analysis

Promotes the treatment of mental illness, emotional disorders, and other mental health concerns by increasing accessibility to mental health programs; supporting outreach, treatment, rehabilitation, and support programs and networks; and encouraging the use of scientifically-based information in mental health treatments. CMHS provides information about mental health via a toll-free number and numerous publications. Developed for users of mental health services and their families, the general public, policy makers, providers, and the media.

Year Founded: 1992

876 CenterLink
PO Box 24490
Ft Lauderdale, FL 33307
954-765-6024; *Fax:* 954-210-9870
centerlink@lgbtcenters.org
www.lgbtcenters.org

Lora Tucker, CEO
Denise Spivak, Deputy Director
Adriana Orozco, Controller
Julia Landis, Executive Office Manager

Founded in 1994, CenterLink is a member-based coalition designed to support the growth and development of LGBT community centers across the world. The organization collaborates with other national organizations to provide key information to LGBT community centers and to advocate for the rights of the LGBT community.

Year Founded: 1994

877 Gender Diversity
6523 California Avenue SW
Suite 360
Seattle, WA 98136
855-443-6337
info@genderdiversity.org
www.www.genderdiversity.org/

Aidan Key, Founder and Executive Director
Nikki Neuen, Associate Director
Huddle Blakefield, Parent Support Coordinator

A nonprofit organization that aims to increase awareness and understanding of gender diversity in children, adoles-

cents, and adults. Gender Diversity provides support groups for youth, adults, and families; education and training for schools and workplaces; and conferences.

878 Gender Spectrum San Leandro, CA
510-788-4412
info@genderspectrum.org
www.www.genderspectrum.org/

Lisa Kenney, Executive Director
Stephanie Brill, Founder and Chair
Jenna Hackman, Project Coordinator
Kim Westheimer, Director, Strategic Initiatives

An organization that provides a variety of serivces to support families, schools, professionals, and youth who are dealing with gender identity issues.

Year Founded: 2006

879 Human Rights Campaign
1640 Rhode Island Avenue Northwest
Washington, DC 20036-3278
202-628-4160
800-777-4723; *Fax:* 202-347-5323
TTY: 202-216-1572
feedback@hrc.org
www.hrc.org

Chad Griffin, President
Joni Madison, Chief Operating Officer
Olivia Alair Dalton, Senior VP of Communications
John Baez, Vice Presient of Marketing

Founded in 1980, the Human Rights Campaign is a civil rights organization that advocates for the rights of lesbian, gay, bisexual, and transgender people in the United States. HRC organizes grassroots movements, educates the public about LGBT issues, and works towards achieving a world in which lesbian, gay, bisexual, and transgender people are respected as equal and full members of society.

Year Founded: 1980

880 National Association for the Dually Diagnosed
(NADD)
132 Fair Street
Kingston, NY 12401
845-331-4336
info@thenadd.org
www.thenadd.org

Jeanne M. Farr, MA, Chief Executive Officer
Daniel Baker, PhD., President
Peggie Webb, MA, Vice President
George Zukotynski, PhD., Secretary

NADD is a nonprofit organization designed to increase awareness of, and provide services for, individuals with developmental disabilities and mental illness. NADD emphasizes the importance of quality mental healthcare for people with mental health needs and offers conferences, information resources, educational programs, and training materials to professionals, parents, and organizations.

Year Founded: 1983

881 National Coalition for LGBT Health
2000 S Street Northwest
Washington, DC 20009
202-232-6749; *Fax:* 202-232-6750
info@healthlgbt.org
www.healthlgbt.org

Brian Hujdich, Executive Director
Michael Beyer, Advocacy Manager
Scott Brawley, Director of Development
Dana Cropper-Williams, Director of Education

The National Coalition for LGBT Health is a coalition of over 70 state and national organizational advocates and health services providers dedicated to using advocacy, education, and research to improve the health of lesbian, gay, bisexual, and transgender individuals.

882 National Commission on Correctional Heath Care

1145 West Diversey Parkway
Chicago, IL 60614
773-880-1460; *Fax:* 773-880-2424
info@ncchc.org
www.ncchc.org

Barbara A. Wakeen, Chair
Nancy B. White, Treasurer
Oscar Aviles, Secretary
Thomas J. Fagan, Chair-Elect

The National Commission on Correctional Health Care is committed to improving the standards of health care provided for individuals in prisons, jails, and juvenile confinement facilities. The organization seeks to ensure that the needs of all correctional health patients, including gender nonconforming people and individuals with gender dysphoria, are met.

Year Founded: 1983

883 National Institute of Mental Health
National Institutes of Health

6001 Executive Boulevard
Room 6200, MSC 9663
Bethesda, MD 20892-9663
301-443-4513
866-615-6464; *Fax:* 301-443-4279
TTY: 301-443-8431
nimhinfo@nih.gov
www.nimh.nih.gov

Joshua Gordon, MD, PhD, Director
Shelli Avenevoli, PhD, Deputy Director
Ann D. Huston, Associate Director, Management
Meredith A. Foxx, PhD, Director of Communications

The National Institute of Mental Health conducts clinical research on mental disorders and seeks to expand knowledge on mental health treatments.

884 National LGBTQ Task Force

1325 Massachusetts Avenue Northwest
Suite 600
Washington, DC 20005
202-393-5177; *Fax:* 202-393-2241
thetaskforce@thetaskforce.org
www.thetaskforce.org

Hez Norton, Co-Chair
Roger Thomson, Co-Chair
Rea Carey, Executive Director
Kierra Johnson, Deputy Executive Director

The National LGBTQ Task Force advocates for justice and equality for LGBTQ people and mobilizes activists throughout the nation to eliminate discrimination against the LGBTQ community.

Year Founded: 1973

885 National Mental Health Consumers' Self-Help Clearinghouse

1211 Chestnut Street
Suite 1100
Philadelphia, PA 19107
267-507-3810
800-553-4539; *Fax:* 215-636-6312
info@mhselfhelp.org
www.mhselfhelp.org

Joseph Rogers, Founder and Executive Director
Susan Rogers, Director

The Clearinghouse is a peer-run national technical assistance center focused on achieving respect and equality of opportunity for those with mental illnesses. The Clearinghouse helps with the growth of the mental health consumer movement by evaluating mental health services, advocating for mental health reform, and providing consumers with news, information, publications, and consultation services.

Year Founded: 1986

886 PFLAG

1828 L Street Northwest
Suite 660
Washington, DC 20036
202-467-8180; *Fax:* 202-467-8194
info@pflag.org
www.pflag.org

Jean Hodges, President
Joellen Shiffman, Executive Office Administrator
Liz Owen, Director of Communications
Dale Bernstein, Vice President

An organization of families and friends of LGBTQ individuals. Dedicated to offering support for people who are LGBTQ and educating the public about LGBTQ issues.

Year Founded: 1973

887 The Center for Family Support

2811 Zulette Avenue
Bronx, NY 10461
718-518-1500; *Fax:* 718-518-8200
www.www.cfsny.org/

Steven Vernikoff, Executive Director
Lloyd Stabiner, President
Amy Bittinger, Vice President
Barbara Greenwald, Associate Executive Director

The Center for Family Support is committed to serving individuals with developmental disabilities and mental health needs, as well as their families. Offers services throughout New York City, Westchester County, Long Island, and New Jersey.

Year Founded: 1954

888 The Lesbian, Gay, Bisexual & Transgender Community Center

208 W. 13th Street
New York, NY 10011
212-620-7310; *Fax:* 212-924-2657
www.gaycenter.org/

Glennda Testone, Executive Director
Rob Wheeler, MPA, PHR, Deputy Executive Director/COO
Brian Daniel, Acting Chief Financial Officer
Jeffrey Klein, Chief Strategy Officer

An organization that advocates for LGBT individuals to lead healthy and successful lives. The Center offers health and wellness programs, as well as recovery and family support services.

Year Founded: 1983

889 Trans Youth Equality Foundation
PO Box 7441
Portland, ME 04112-7441
207-478-4087
contact@transyouthequality.org
www.www.transyouthequality.org/

Susan Maasch, Director
Jack Montgomery, Director
Rebecca Oglesby, Director and Treasurer

A nonprofit organization that provides education, advocacy, and support for transgender, gender nonconforming, and intersex youth ages 2-18, as well as their families. TYEF runs annual youth reatreats, a podcast program, training for educational and medical professionals, and youth workshops.

890 World Professional Association for Transgend er Health (WPATH)
www.www.wpath.org/

Gail Knudson, MD, FRCPC, President
Vin Tangpricha, MD, PhD, President-Elect
Randi Ettner, PhD, Secretary
Walter Pierre Bouman, MD, Treasurer

Formerly known as the Harry Benjamin International Gender Dysphoria Association, WPATH is a nonprofit organization dedicated to transgender health. Members of WPATH engage in clinical and academic research in order to further the understanding of Gender Dysphoria and to create a high quality of care for transsexual, transgender, and gender-nonconforming individuals globally.

Books

891 Gender Disorders and the Paraphilias
Intl Universities Pr Inc
59 Boston Post Rd.
Madison, CT 06443
203-245-4000; *Fax:* 203-245-0775
info@iup.com
www.www.iup.com

William B. Arndt, Jr., Author

488 pages Year Founded: 1991 ISBN 0-823621-50-2

892 Gender Identity Disorder: A Medical Dictionary, Bibliography, and Annotated Research Guide to Internet References
ICON Health Publications
7404 Trade Street
San Diego, CA 92121-3414
858-635-9414

Icon Group

This book was created for medical professionals, students, and members of the general public who want to conduct medical research using the most advanced tools available and spending the least amount of time doing so. *$28.95*

64 pages Year Founded: 2004 ISBN 0-497004-51-8

893 Handbook of Sexual and Gender Identity Disorders
John Wiley & Sons
111 River Street
Hoboken, NJ 07030-5774
201-748-6000; *Fax:* 201-748-6088
info@wiley.com
www.wiley.com

David L. Rowland, Editor
Luca Incrocci, Editor

The Handbook of Sexual and Gender Identity Disorders provides mental health professionals a comprehensive yet practical guide to the understanding, diagnosis, and treatment of a variety of sexual problems. *$120.00*

696 pages Year Founded: 2008 ISBN 0-471767-38-1

894 Identity Without Selfhood
32 Avenue of the Americas
New York, NY 10013-2473
212-337-5000
newyork@cambrigde.org
www.www.cambridge.org

Mariam Fraser, Author

226 pages Year Founded: 1534

895 Sexual Signatures: On Being a Man or a Woman
John Wiley & Sons
111 River Street
Hoboken, NJ 07030-5790
201-748-6000; *Fax:* 201-748-6088
info@wiley.com
www.wiley.com

John Money, Author
Patricia Tucker, Author

Sexual differentiations begins before birth and extends through puberty, when the sexual hormones become active. Case histories of children born with sexual anomalies becoming satisfactorily 'masculine' or 'feminine.' This shows how strongly culture shapes gender-personalitites. *$19.95*

250 pages Year Founded: 1975 ISBN 0-471767-38-1

Periodicals & Pamphlets

896 Similarities and Differences Between Sexual Orientation and Gender Identity
PFLAG
PO Box 3313
San Luis Obispo, CA 93403
805-801-2186
pflag.slo@gmail.com
www.pflagcentralcoastchapter.net

Moises Torreblanca, President
John Sullivan, Vice President
Val Barboza, Treasurer
Barabara Adams, Secretary

An explanation of the simialrities and differences of both a person sexual orientation and how they relate to gender.

897 The United Nations Speaks Out: Tackling Discrimination on Grounds of Sexual Orientation and Gender Identity
Unesco-Globe NY
E-mail: unescoglobe@gmail.com
www.www.unescoglobe.wordpress.com

Irina Bokova, UNESCO Director-General
Engida Getachew, Deputy Director-General, UNESCO

Year Founded: 2010

Support Groups & Hot Lines

898 Gender Trust
76 The Ridgeway
Astwood Bank, B96 6LX, WO
527-894-838
www.gendertrust.org.uk

Gender Trust is a listening ear, a caring support and an information centre for anyone with any question or problem concerning their gender identity, or whose loved one is struggling with gender identity issues.

899 TransYouth Family Allies
PO Box 1471
Holland, MI 49422-1471
888-462-8932
info@imatyfa.org
www.imatyfa.org

Shannon Garcia, Founding Member, President
Lisa Gilinger, Vice President
Amy G., Founding Member, Treasurer
Kim Pearson, Founding Member, Training Direct

TYFA empowers children and families by partnering with educators, service providers and communities to develop supportive environments in which gender may be expressed and respected.

Year Founded: 2006

Web Sites

900 www.cyberpsych.org
CyberPsych

Presents information about psychoanalysis, psychotherapy and special topics such as anxiety disorders, the problematic use of alcohol, homophobia, and the traumatic effects of racism.

901 www.gidreform.wordpress.com
Gender Identity Disorder Reform Advocates

GID Reform Advocates is a group of medical professionals, researchers, scholars, members of the transgender, bisexual, lesbian and gay communities, and other individuals who are concerned with the psychiatric classification of gender diversity as mental disorder and who advocate for the reform of the diagnostic criteria surrounding gender nonconforming people. The GID Reform Weblog addresses the issues surrounding these diagnostic categories.

902 www.health.nih.gov
National Institutes of Health

Part of the U.S. Department of Health and Human Services that is the nation's medical research agency-making important medical discoveries that improve health and save lives.

903 www.healthfinder.gov
Healthfinder

Developed by the U.S. Department of Health and Human Services, a key resource for finding the best government and nonprofit health and human services information on the internet.

904 www.intelihealth.com
Aetna InteliHealth

Aetna InteliHealth's mission is to empower people with trusted solutions for healthier lives.

905 www.kidspeace.org
KidsPeace

KidsPeace is a private charity dedicated to serving the behavioral and mental health needs of children, preadolescents and teens.

906 www.mayohealth.com
Mayo Clinic Health Oasis

Their mission is to empower people to manage their health. They accomplish this by providing useful and up-to-date information and tools that reflect the expertise and standard of excellence of Mayo Clinic.

907 www.nlm.nih.gov
National Library of Medicine

The National Library of Medicine (NLM), on the campus of the National Institutes of Health in Bethesda, Maryland, is the world's largest medical library. The Library collects materials and provides information and research services in all areas of biomedicine and health care

908 www.planetpsych.com
Planet Psych

The online resource for mental health information

909 www.psychcentral.com
Psych Central

The Internet's largest and oldest independent mental health social network created and run by mental health professionals to guarantee reliable, trusted information and support communities.

910 www.store.samhsa.gov
Substance Abuse and Mental Health Services Administration

Resources on mental disorders as well as treatment and recovery.

911 www.xs4all.nl/~rosalind/cha-assr.html
Support and Information on Sex Reassignement

The purpose of this newsgroup is to provide a supportive and informative environment for people who are undergoing or who have undergone sex reassignment surgery (SRS) and for their relatives and significant others.

Conferences & Meetings

912 Religion and Gender: Identity, Conflict, and Power Conference
Feminist Studies in Religion
Harvard Divinity School
45 Francis Avenue
Cambridge, MA 02138
617-384-8046
fsr@fsrinc.org
www.www.fsrinc.org

Dr Pushpa Iyer, Conference Chair
Quinn Van Valler-Campbell, Conference Administrator
Judith Plaskow, Founding Editor
Elisabeth Sch□ssler Fiorenza, Founding Editor

The conference will highlight the complex relationships between religion and gender in a global context. It seeks to explore conflicts that arise at the nexus of gender and religion while simultaneously promoting spaces for empowerment that arise in these interactions.

Year Founded: 1983

Neurocognitive Disorders

Introduction

Neurocognitive disorders are a group of conditions characterized by impairments in the ability to think, reason, plan, and organize. There are three types of cognitive disorders; delirium, dementia (of which Alzheimer's Disease is the most common), and amnestic disorders.

Delirium is a relatively short-term condition in which the level of conciousness waxes and wanes. It is common in patients after surgery or during illness, as with high fever. It resolves when the underlying problem resolves. There are three categories of causes of delirium: a general medical condition, substance-induced, and multiple causes. An amnestic disorder, in contrast to delirium or dementia, is a condition in which only memory is impaired; for instance the person is unable to recall important facts or events, making it difficult to function normally. Dementia is a chronic impairment of multiple cognitive functions. Persons with dementia may have severe memory loss and also be unable to plan or prepare for events or to care for themselves.

Dementia, Alzheimer's type, is a progressive disorder that slowly kills nerve cells in the brain. While definitive treatments are lacking, there is a prodigious amount of research on the condition, some of which suggests that a vaccine may be developed to prevent the condition. Though such hopeful breakthroughs remain distant, there is much that families and patients can do when the condition is recognized and care and support are sought early in the disorder's progression. Since other, serious, treatable disorders can resemble Alzeimer's Disease, it is very important for individuals who are losing cognitive functions to be evaluated by a physician. Early detection of Alzheimer's Disease, with early treatment, may improve the chances for slowing the rate of decline.

The following discusses Alzheimer's dementia, the most prevalent Neurocognitive Disorder.

SYMPTOMS

• Langugage disorders;
• Impaired ability to carry out motor activities despite intact motor function;
• Failure to recognize or identify objects despite intact sensory perception;
• Disturbance in executive functioning (planning, organizing, sequencing, abstracting);
• The deficits cause impairment in social or occupational functioning and represent a decline from previous level of functioning;
• The course is gradual and continuous;
• The deficits are not due to central nervous system conditions such as Parkinson's Disease, other conditions known to cause dementia, and are not substance-induced;
• The deficits do not occur during the course of delirium and are not better accounted for by severe depression or schizophrenia.

ASSOCIATED FEATURES

Dementia, Alzheimer's type, generally begins gradually, not with deficits in cognition but with a marked change in personality. For instance, a person may suddenly become given to fits of anger for no apparent reason.

Soon, however, family and acquaintances may notice that the individual begins to mix up facts, or gets lost driving to a familiar place. In the early stages the afflicted individual may become aware of slipping cognitive functions, adding to confusion, fright and depression. After a period, lapses in memory grow more obvious; patients with Alzheimer's are apt to repeat themselves, and may forget the names of grandchildren or longtime friends. They may also be increasingly agitated and combative when family members or other caretakers try to correct them or help with accustomed tasks. The memory lapses in patients with Alzheimer's differ markedly from those in normal aging: a patient with Alzheimer's may often forget entire experiences and rarely remembers them later; the patient only grudgingly acknowledges lapses. In contrast, the individual with normal aging or depression is extremely concerned about, and may even exaggerate, the extent of memory loss. In Alzheimer's, skills deteriorate and a patient is increasingly unable to follow directions, or care for him/herself. Eventually the disease leads to death.

PREVALENCE

An estimated one in 10 people over age 65 has dementia, Alzheimer's type. Other types of dementia are believed to be much less common. Prevalence of the condition increases with age, particularly after age 75. Of people who have been diagnosed with Alzheimer's dementia, 81 percent are age 75 or older.

TREATMENT OPTIONS

There is no known cure or definitive treatment for dementia, Alzheimer's type. However, research has suggested avenues that involve drugs, such as THA, Donepezil, and Rivastigmine, for regulating acetylcholine, seratonin or norepinephrine in the brain. According to the American Psychiatric Association, some progress has been seen in slowing the death rate among nerve cells using a chemical known as Alcar (acetyl-l-carnitine). One drug, memantine, has been developed to slow down the progression of Alzheimer's disease. However, these drugs do not offer a cure for Alzheimer's and do not stop the progression of the disease. Psychiatrists treating patients with dementia, Alzheimer's type, may also be able to prescribe medications that can treat the depression and anxiety that accompanies the condition.

Researchers suggest that close to half of the cases of Alzheimer's are related to modifiable risk factors, such as smoking and cognitive and physical inactivity. A healthy lifestyle may reduce the risk of developing Alzheimer's disease.

Families are strongly encouraged to take advantage of adjunctive services including support groups, counseling and psychotherapy. There is a high incidence of depression among family members caring at home for persons with Alzheimer's Disease.

Associations & Agencies

914 Alzheimer's Association National Office
225 North Michigan Avenue
17th Floor
Chicago, IL 60601-7633
312-335-8700
800-272-3900; *Fax:* 866-699-1246

TDD: 312-335-5886
info@alz.org
www.alz.org

Christopher Binkley, Chair
Harry Johns, President and CEO
Richard Hovland, Chief Operations Officer
Maria Carrillo, Chief Science Officer

Headquarters for Alzheimer's Association, an organization dedicated to helping all those with Alzheimer's disease and dementia, and their families. Funds Alzheimer's research, engages in Alzheimer's advocacy, and offers referrals, support groups, educational sessions, safety services, and publications.

Year Founded: 1980

915 Alzheimer's Disease Education and Referral Center
National Institute on Aging
PO Box 8250
Silver Spring, MD 20907-8250
301-495-3311
800-438-4380; *Fax:* 301-495-3334
adear@nia.nih.gov
www.nia.nih.gov/alzheimers

Richard J. Hodes, MD, Director
Patrick Shirdon, Director of Management
Luigi Ferrucci, MD, PhD, Scientific Director
Marie A. Bernard, MD, Deputy Director

The ADEAR Center provides information about Alzheimer's Disease and related disorders to health professionals, patients and their families, and the public.

Year Founded: 1990

916 Brain Resources and Information Network (BRAIN)
National Institute of Neurological Disorders & Stroke
PO Box 5801
Bethesda, MD 20824-5801
301-496-5751
800-352-9424
braininfo@ninds.nih.gov
www.ninds.nih.gov

Denise Dorsey, Chief Administrative Officer
Peter Soltys, Chief Information Officer
Walter J. Koroshetz, MD, Director
Margo Warren, Deputy Director, Communications

Federal agency focused on supporting neuroscience research and working towards reducing the burdens associated with neurological disease.

Year Founded: 1950

917 BrightFocus Foundation
22512 Gateway Center Drive
Clarksburg, MD 20871
800-437-2423; *Fax:* 301-258-9454
info@brightfocus.org
www.brightfocus.org

Scott Rodgville, CPA, Chair
Stacy Pagos Haller, President and CEO
Diane I. Marcello, Vice Chair
Nicholas W. Raymond, Treasurer

Raises awareness of Alzheimer's disease, macular degeneration, and glaucoma and supports research and programs to cure brain and eye diseases.

Year Founded: 1973

918 Caregiver Action Network
1150 Connecticut Avenue Northwest
Suite 501
Washington, DC 20036-3904
202-454-3970
info@caregiveraction.org
www.caregiveraction.org

Wes Metheny, Chair
John Schall, Chief Executive Officer
Lisa Winstel, Chief Operating Officer
Michael Shaughnessy, Vice Chair

Caregiver Action Network is a nonprofit organization that acts as a support and an advocate for family caregivers of individuals with chronic conditions, diabilities, diseases, or old age. CAN provides education, peer support, and resources free of charge.

Year Founded: 1993

919 Center for Mental Health Services (CMHS)
Substance Abuse and Mental Health Services Administration
5600 Fishers Lane
Rockville, MD 20857
240-276-1310
877-726-4727
TTY: 800-487-4889
www.samhsa.gov/about-us/who-we-are/offices-centers

Paolo del Vecchio, MSW, Director
Anne Mathews-Younes, Acting Deputy Director
Keris Myrick, Director, Consumer Affairs
Patricia Gratton, Director, Program Analysis

Promotes the treatment of mental illness and emotional disorders by increasing accessibility to mental health programs; supporting outreach, treatment, rehabilitation, and support programs and networks; and encouraging the use of scientifically-based information when treating mental disorders. CMHS provides information about mental health via a toll-free number and numerous publications. Developed for users of mental health services and their families, the general public, policy makers, providers, and the media.

Year Founded: 1992

920 Federation of Associations in Behavioral and Brain Sciences
1001 Connecticut Avenue Northwest
Suite 1100
Washington, DC 20036
202-888-3949
info@fabbs.org
www.fabbs.org

Nora Newcombe, PhD, President
Paula Skedsvold, JD, PhD, Executive Director
Eugene Borgida, PhD, Vice President
Leaetta Hough, PhD, Treasurer

FABBS is a coalition of scientific societies focused on expanding scientific knowledge on the brain, mind, and behavior. FABBS educates the public and policymakers on the importance of brain, mind, and behavior sciences research; provides quality sources to federal agencies and the media; advocates for research-focused policy and legislation; and promotes exchange of information among scientific organizations.

Year Founded: 1980

921 National Association for the Dually Diagnosed (NADD)

132 Fair Street
Kingston, NY 12401
845-331-4336
info@thenadd.org
www.thenadd.org

Jeanne M. Farr, MA, Chief Executive Officer
Daniel Baker, PhD., President
Peggie Webb, MA, Vice President
George Zukotynski, PhD., Secretary

NADD is a nonprofit organization designed to increase awareness of, and provide services for, individuals with developmental disabilities and mental illness. NADD emphasizes the importance of quality mental healthcare for people with mental health needs and offers conferences, information resources, educational programs, and training materials to professionals, parents, and organizations.

Year Founded: 1983

922 National Association of Councils on Developmental Disabilities

1825 K Street Northwest
Suite 600
Washington, DC 20006
202-506-5813
info@nacdd.org
www.nacdd.org/

Donna A. Meltzer, Chief Executive Officer
Shannon Buller, President
Steve Gieber, Vice President
Dan Shannon, Treasurer

A national membership association representing the 56 State and Territorial Councils on Developmental Disabilities. An organization with the purpose of promoting the programs and policies that its member councils advocate, as well as ensuring inclusion for Americans with developmental disabilities.

923 National Mental Health Consumers' Self-Help Clearinghouse

1211 Chestnut Street
Suite 1100
Philadelphia, PA 19107
267-507-3810
800-553-4539; *Fax:* 215-636-6312
info@mhselfhelp.org
www.mhselfhelp.org

Joseph Rogers, Founder and Executive Director
Susan Rogers, Director

The Clearinghouse is a peer-run national technical assistance center focused on achieving respect and equality of opportunity for those with mental illnesses. The Clearinghouse helps with the growth of the mental health consumer movement by evaluating mental health services, advocating for mental health reform, and providing consumers with news, information, publications, and consultation services.

Year Founded: 1986

924 National Niemann-Pick Disease Foundation PO Box 49

Fort Atkinson, WI 53538-0049
920-563-0930
877-287-3672; *Fax:* 920-563-0931
nnpdf@nnpdf.org
www.nnpdf.org

Lisa Chavez, Board Chair
Justin Hopkin, Vice Chair
Missy Ward, Secretary
Jill Flinton, Treasurer

The Foundations promotes research and offers support and funding for individuals with Niemann-Pick Disease and their support network.

Year Founded: 1992

925 The Center for Family Support

2811 Zulette Avenue
Bronx, NY 10461
718-518-1500; *Fax:* 718-518-8200
www.www.cfsny.org/

Steven Vernikoff, Executive Director
Lloyd Stabiner, President
Amy Bittinger, Vice President
Barbara Greenwald, Associate Executive Director

The Center for Family Support offers assistance to individuals with developmental and related disabilities, as well as their families, and provides support services and programs that are designed to accommodate individual needs. Offers services throughout New York City, Westchester County, Long Island, and New Jersey.

Year Founded: 1954

Books

926 Agitation in Patients with Dementia: a Practical Guide to Diagnosis and Management

American Psychiatric Publishing, Inc.
1000 Wilson Boulevard
Suite 1825
Arlington, VA 22209-3901
703-907-7322
800-368-5777; *Fax:* 703-907-1091
appi@psych.org
www.appi.org

George T Grossberg, M.D, Editor
Donald P Hay, M.D, Editor
Linda K Hay, R.N., Ph.D, Editor
John S Kennedy, M.D., F.R.C.P, Editor

Appealing to a wide audience of geriatric psychiatrists, primary care physicians and internists, general practitioners, nurses, social workers, psychologists, pharmacists and mental health care workers and practitioners in hospitals, nursing homes and clinics, this remarkable monograph offers practical direction on assessing and managing agitation in patients with dementia. *$57.00*

272 pages Year Founded: 2003 ISBN 0-880488-43-3

927 Alzheimer's Disease Sourcebook

Omnigraphics
155 West Congress
Suite 200
Detroit, MI 48226

313-961-1340
800-234-1340; *Fax:* 313-961-1383
contact@omnigraphics.com
www.omnigraphics.com

Amy L. Sutton, Author

Omnigraphics is the publisher of the Health Reference Series, a growing consumer health information resource with more than 100 volumes in print. Each title in the series features an easy to understand format, nontechnical language, comprehensive indexing and resources for further information. Material in each book has been collected from a wide range of government agencies, professional associations, periodicals, and other sources. *$95.00*

637 pages Year Founded: 1985 ISBN 0-780811-50-8

928 Alzheimer's Disease: Activity-Focused Care, Second Edition
Therapeutic Resources
PO Box 16814
Cleveland, OH 44116-814
440-331-7114
888-331-7114; *Fax:* 440-331-7118
contactus@therapeuticresources.com
www.therapeuticresources.com

Carly R. Hellen, OTR/L, Author

Provides practical and innovative strategies for care of people with Alzheimer's disease, emphasizing the activities that make up daily living - dressing, toileting, eating, exercising, and communication. The text is written from the viewpoint that activity-focused care promotes the resident's cognitive, physical, psychosocial, and spiritual well-being. *$559.95*

536 pages ISBN 0-750699-08-6

929 American Psychiatric Association Practice Guideline for the Treatment of Patients with Delirium
American Psychiatric Publishing, Inc.
1000 Wilson Boulevard
Suite 1825
Arlington, VA 22209-3901
703-907-7322
800-368-5777; *Fax:* 703-907-1091
appi@psych.org
www.appi.org

Robert E Hales MD, Editor-in-Chief
Ron McMillen, Chief Executive Officer
John McDuffie, Editorial Director
Rebecca Rinehart, Publisher

Best practices examined from the group whose vision is a society that has available, accessible quality psychiatric diagnosis and treatment. *$47.95*

75 pages Year Founded: 1999 ISBN 0-890423-13-4

930 Behavioral Complications in Alzheimer's Disease
American Psychiatric Publishing, Inc.
1000 Wilson Boulevard
Suite 1825
Arlington, VA 22209-3901
703-907-7322
800-368-5777; *Fax:* 703-907-1091
appi@psych.org
www.appi.org

Brian A. Lawlor, MD, Author

Practical management strategies for the identification, measurement and treatment of behavioral symptoms in patient with Alzheimer's disease. *$67.00*

303 pages Year Founded: 1995 ISBN 0-880484-77-0

931 Care That Works: A Relationship Approach to Persons with Dementia
Johns Hopkins University Press
2715 N Charles Street
Baltimore, MD 21218-4319
410-516-6900
800-537-5487; *Fax:* 410-516-6998

Jitka M. Zgola, Author

Provides caregivers the information with which they can develop their own approaches, evaluate their effectiveness, and continue to grow in skill and insight. Real life strategies for a challenging task. *$24.00*

272 pages Year Founded: 1999 ISBN 0-801860-25-6

932 Cognitive Therapy in Practice
WW Norton & Company
500 5th Avenue
New York, NY 10110-54
212-354-2907
800-233-4830; *Fax:* 212-869-0856
npd@wwnorton.com

Jacqueline Persons, Author

Basic text for graduate studies in psychotherapy, psycholgy nursing social work and counseling. *$29.00*

256 pages Year Founded: 1989 ISBN 0-393700-77-0

933 Dementia: A Clinical Approach
Elsevier Health Sciences
11830 Westline Industrial Drive
St. Louis, MO 63146-3313
314-872-8370
800-568-5136; *Fax:* 314-432-1380
orders@bhusa.com or custserv@bhusa.com
www.elsevier.com

Jeffrey L. Cummings, Author
Jeffrey L Cummings, Author

Third Edition, this is both a scholarly review of the dementias and a practical guide to their diagnosis and treatment. *$99.00*

432 pages Year Founded: 2003 ISBN 0-750674-70-9

934 Disorders of Brain and Mind: Volume 1
Cambridge University Press
32 Avenue of the Americas
New York, NY 10013-2473
212-337-5000; *Fax:* 212-691-3239
newyork@cambrigde.org
www.www.cambridge.org

Maria A. Ron, Author
Anthony S. David, Author

Discusses various neuropsychiatry topics where the brain and mind come together. *$113.00*

388 pages Year Founded: 1534 ISBN 0-521778-51-0

935 Drug Therapy and Cognitive Disorders
Mason Crest Publishers
450 Parkway Drive
Suite D
Broomall, PA 19008-4017
610-543-6200
866-627-2665; *Fax:* 610-543-3878
dtaylor@masoncrest.com
www.masoncrest.com

Sherry Bonice, Author
Carolyn Hoard, Author
Michelle Luke, Director, Marketing, PR
Michael Toglia, Special Sales

Alzheimer's disease is one of the most common cognitive disorder, one that affects millions of people. Patients, caregivers and loved ones all suffer as they experience the devastation of this often misunderstood disease. Researchers are working hard to find a cure for the symptoms of Alzheimer's and other cognitive disorders, and this book describes the most recent research. Coauthored by someone who has experienced the early stages of Alzheimer's firsthand, this volume will give readers a new understanding and appreciation of the treatment options for those who experience a cognitive disorder.

128 pages ISBN 1-590845-62-5

936 Progress in Alzheimer's Disease and Similar Conditions
American Psychiatric Publishing, Inc.
1000 Wilson Boulevard
Suite 1825
Arlington, VA 22209-3901
703-907-7322
800-368-5777; *Fax:* 703-907-1091
appi@psych.org
www.appi.org

Leonard L Heston, M.D., Editor
Ron McMillen, Chief Executive Officer
John McDuffie, Editorial Director

Details advances in research on human genetics that is broadening our knowledge of Alzheimer's disease and other related afflictions. Describes disease mechanisms, including prisons, that provide insight into the role environment plays in the development of disease. Includes stories about the pain inflicted by this disease on the patients and their family and friends as well as current efforts in management and treatment. *$77.00*

318 pages Year Founded: 1997 ISBN 0-880487-60-7

937 Treating Complex Cases: The Cognitive Behavioral Therapy Approach
John Wiley & Sons
111 River Street
Hoboken, NJ 07030-5774
201-748-6000; *Fax:* 201-748-6088
info@wiley.com
www.wiley.com

Nicholas Tarrier, Author
Adrian Wells, Author
Gillian Haddock, Author

This book brings together some of the most experiences and expert cognitive behavioral therapists to share their specialist experience of formulation and treatment of complex problems such as co-morbidity, psychotic conditions, and chronic conditions. The experienced clinician will find:

evidence-based approaches to assessment and formulation of complex cases; a wide range of problems not restricted to disorder categories, including anger, low self-esteem, abuse and shame; a concern with the realities of clinical practice which involves complex cases that do not fit into simple case conceptualisations or diagnostic categories. Copyright 2000. *$89.95*

458 pages Year Founded: 2000 ISBN 0-471978-39-8

938 Victims of Dementia: Service, Support, and Care
Haworth Press
10 Alice Street
Binghamton, NY 13904-1503
607-722-5857
800-429-6784; *Fax:* 607-721-0012
getinfo@haworthpressinc.com
www.haworthpress.com

William Michael Clemmer, PhD, Editor

Provides an in depth look at the concept, construction and operation of Wesley Hall, a special living area at the Chelsea United Methodist retirement home in Michigan. *$27.95*

161 pages Year Founded: 1993 ISSN 978156024-265-9

Periodicals & Pamphlets

939 Alzheimer's Disease Research and the American Health Assistance Foundation
American Health Assistance Foundation
22512 Gateway Center Drive
Clarksburg, MD 20871-2005
301-948-3244
800-437-2423; *Fax:* 301-258-9454
info@brightfocus.org
www.www.brightfocus.org

Grace Frisone, Chairman
Stacy Pagos Haller, President and CEO
Michael H Barnett,Esq, Vice Chairman
Nicholas W Raymond, Treasurer

Provides information on treatment, medication, medical referrals.

Video & Audio

940 A Change of Character
Fanlight Productions
32 Court Street
21st Floor
Brooklyn, NY 11201
718-488-8900
800-876-1710; *Fax:* 718-488-8642
fanlight@fanlight.com
www.fanlight.com

Neal Goodman, Author

Truett Allen's personality changed drastically after a series of strokes resulted in damage to the frontal lobes of his brain. this captivating video features neuroscientist Dr. Elkhonon Goldberg, author of The Executive Brain, as well as neurologist and best-selling author Dr. Oliver Sacks.

941 Effective Learning Systems
5108 W 74th
St #390160
Minneapolis, MN 55439
239-948-1660
800-966-0443; *Fax:* 239-948-1664
info@efflearn.com
www.effectivelearning.com

Robert E Griswold, President
Deirdre M Griswold, VP

Audio tapes for stress management, deep relaxation, anger control, peace of mind, insomnia, weight and smoking, self-image and self-esteem, positive thinking, health and healing. Since 1972, Effective Learning Systems has helped millions of people take charge of their lives and make positive changes. Over 75 titles available, each with a money-back guarantee. Price range $12-$14.

Year Founded: 1972

942 Understanding Mental Illness
Educational Video Network
1401 19th Street
Huntsville, TX 77340
936-295-5767
800-762-0060; *Fax:* 936-294-0233
info at evn.org
www.www.evndirect.com

A video to learn and understand mental illness and how it affects you. *$79.95*

Year Founded: 2004 ISBN 1-589501-48-9

Web Sites

943 www.Nia.Nih.Gov/Alzheimers
Alzheimer's Disease Education and Referral
Fax: 301-495-3334

A division of the National Institute on Aging of the National Institute of Health. Solid information and a list of federally funded centers for evaluation, referral, treatment.

944 www.aan.com
American Academy of Neurology

Provides information for both professionals and the public on neurology subjects, covering Alzheimer's and Parkinson's diseases to stroke and migraine, includes comprehensive fact sheets.

945 www.agelessdesign.com
Ageless Design

Information on age related diseases such as Alzheimer's disease.

946 www.ahaf.org/alzdis/about/adabout.htm
American Health Assistance Foundation

Alzheimer's resource for patients and caregivers.

947 www.alz.co.uk
Alzheimer's Disease International

Umbrella organization of associations that support people with dementia.

948 www.alzforum.org
Alzheimer Research Forum

Information in layman's terms, plus many references and resources listed.

949 www.alzheimersbooks.com/
Alzheimer's Disease Bookstore

950 www.alzheimersupport.Com
AlzheimerSupport.com

Information and products for people dealing with Alzheimer's Disease.

951 www.biostat.wustl.edu
Washington University - Saint Louis

Page on Alzheimer's information, from basic care to friends and family networking experiences for support.

952 www.cyberpsych.org
CyberPsych

Hosts the American Psychoanalyists Foundation, American Association of Suicideology, Society for the Exploration of Psychotherapy Intergration, and Anxiety Disorders Association of America. Also subcategories of the anxiety disorders, as well as general information, including panic disorder, phobias, obsessive compulsive disorder (OCD), social phobia, generalized anxiety disorder, post traumatic stress disorder, and phobias of childhood. Book reviews and links to web pages sharing the topics.

953 www.mayohealth.org/mayo/common/htm/
MayoClinic.com

Information for dealing with Alzheimer's Disease.

954 www.mentalhealth.com
Internet Mental Health

On-line information and a virtual encyclopedia related to mental disorders, possible causes and treatments. News, articles, on-line diagnostic programs and related links. Designed to improve understanding, diagnosis and treatment of mental illness throughout the world. Awarded the Top Site Award and the NetPsych Cutting Edge Site Award.

955 www.mindstreet.com/training.html
Cognitive Therapy: A Multimedia Learning Program

The basics of cognitive therapy are presented.

956 www.ninds.nih.gov
National Institute of Neurological Disorders & Stroke

Neuroscience updates and articles.

957 www.noah-health.org/en/bns/disorders/
alzheimer.html
Ask NOAH About: Aging and Alzheimer's Disease

Links to brochures on medical problems of the elderly.

958 www.ohioalzcenter.org/facts.html
University Memory and Aging Center

Alzheimer's disease fact page.

959 **www.planetpsych.com**
Planetpsych.com

Learn about disorders, their treatments and other topics in psychology. Articles are listed under the related topic areas. Ask a therapist a question for free, or view the directory of professionals in your area. If you are a therapist sign up for the directory. Current features, self-help, interactive, and newsletter archives.

960 **www.psych.org/clin_res/pg_dementia.cfm**
American Psychiatric Association

Practice guidelines for the treatment of patients with Alzheimer's.

961 **www.psychcentral.com**
Psych Central

Personalized one-stop index for psychology, support, and mental health issues, resources, and people on the Internet.

962 **www.rcpsych.ac.uk/info/help/memory**
Royal College of Psychiatrists

Memory and Dementia

963 **www.store.samhsa.gov**
Substance Abuse and Mental Health Services Administration

Resources on mental disorders as well as treatment and recovery.

964 **www.zarcrom.com/users/alzheimers**
Alzheimer's Outreach

Detailed and practical information.

965 **www.zarcrom.com/users/yeartorem**
Year to Remember

A memorial site covering many aspects of Alzheimer's disease.

Neurodevelopmental Disorders

Introduction

Neurodevelopmental Disorders describe a range of brain function disorders that affect emotion, learning, ability, self control, and memory which unfold as the individual grows. Parents, other relatives, guardians, and teachers are concerned about not missing the signs of a treatable disorder while, at the same time, not subjecting a child to unnecessary and potentially stigmatizing diagnosis and treatment. When there is publicity about a medical disorder, however, the number of diagnoses goes up. In the case of Bipolar Disorder, cases that may have been overlooked before such public awareness are being accurately diagnosed. Still, many cases are diagnosed and treated without a full evaluation. As noted in the chapter on Autism Spectrum Disorders, while awareness of the diagnosis has brought more children to diagnosis and treatment, it also seems that the actual incidence of the condition is on the rise; the reasons are still unknown. The American Academy of Child and Adolescent Psychiatry (http://www.aacap.org/) provides accurate and useful information to help those responsible for children decide: whether a child's behavior is normal for his or her age; if a child is being adversely influenced by circumstances; what is a warning sign for mental disorder; and what constitutes a mental disorder. Warning signs of mental illness in children and youth may include self-harm, substance abuse, sudden and unexplained weight loss, difficulty focusing, drastic behavior changes, dangerous or out-of-control behavior, and drastic mood swings.

In general, a child or adolescent is evaluated not only on the basis of particular behaviors that cause concern, but also with respect to meeting the milestones expected at his or her age. A child should be increasingly able to relate to other people, both children and adults, and to learn. An untreated mental disorder can deprive a child of essential years of social and educational growth. Anyone concerned about a child should start with the child's pediatrician. A child should not be given a diagnosis or prescribed medication without a complete physical health evaluation, specialized observation, and interviews with parents, teachers, and others familiar with him or her. There is a shortage of fully qualified experts in child and adolescent mental health; it may require considerable persistence to ensure that a child receives the attention necessary, but it will be worthwhile. There should be no hesitation to obtain a second opinion. Health professionals should be able to explain why a child was or was not given a specific diagnosis, and the pros and cons of the treatment choices.

Note: Vaccinations do not cause autism, and going un-vaccinated exposes both a child to diseases that can be serious, even fatal, and all those the child comes in contact with, before the signs of the disease are evident.

Associations & Agencies

967 AHRC New York City
83 Maiden Lane
New York, NY 10038
212-780-2500
www.www.ahrcnyc.org/

Angelo Aponte, President
Amy West, Chief Financial Officer

Kathy Broderick, Acting Chief Operating Officer
Marco R. Damiani, Chief Executive Officer

AHRC New York City is an organization dedicated to helping people with intellectual and developmental disabilities build full lives. Provides support services, training programs, clinics, workshops, schools, and residential facilities to individuals with developmental and intellectual disabilities.

Year Founded: 1949

968 American Academy of Child and Adolescent Psychiatry
3615 Wisconsin Avenue Northwest
Washington, DC 20016-3007
202-966-7300; *Fax:* 202-464-0131
www.aacap.org

Karen Wagner, MD, PhD, President
Andres Martin, MD, MPH, Secretary
Bennett L. Leventhal, MD, Treasurer
Heidi B. Fordi, CAE, Executive Director

Nonprofit membership-based organization comprised of child and adolescent psychiatrists committed to serving the health care needs of children and their families. The AACAP disseminates information and research findings on mental illnesses, promotes accessibility to proper treatment and services, and advances efforts in mental illness prevention.

Year Founded: 1953

969 American Academy of Pediatrics
345 Park Boulevard
Itasca, IL 60143
800-433-9016; *Fax:* 847-434-8000
www.aap.org

Colleen A. Kraft, MD, MBA, FAAP, President
Karen Remley, MD, MBA, FAAP, Executive VP and CEO
Kyle Yasuda, MD, FAAP, President-Elect

The American Academy of Pediatrics is an organization consisting of 66,000 pediatricians committed to ensuring the well-being, health, and safety of all infants, children, adolescents, and young adults.

Year Founded: 1930

970 American Pediatric Society
9303 New Trails Drive
Suite 350
The Woodlands, TX 77381
346-980-9707
info@aps1888.org
www.www.aps1888.org/

Elena Fuentes-Afflick, President
Bruce D. Gelb, Vice President
Christine A. Gleason, Secretary and Treasurer

Society of professionals working on pediatric health care issues, through research, advocacy, and education. The society offers conferences and a variety of publications.

Year Founded: 1888

971 Association for Children's Mental Health
6017 West St Joseph Highway
Suite 200
Lansing, MI 48917
517-372-4016
888-226-4543; *Fax:* 517-372-4032
www.acmh-mi.org

Jane Shank, Executive Director
Mary Porter, Business Manager
Terri Henrizi, Education Coordinator
Al Way, President of the Board

A Michigan-based nonprofit organization serving families of children and youth with emotional, behavioral, or mental health needs. Provides information, support, resources, referrals, advocacy, and networking and leadership opportunities for youth.

Year Founded: 1989

972 Federation for Children with Special Needs (FCSN)
529 Main Street
Suite 1M3
Boston, MA 02129
617-236-7210
800-331-0688; *Fax:* 617-241-0330
fcsninfo@fcsn.org
www.fcsn.org

Anne Howard, PhD, President
Rich Robinson, Executive Director
Tom Hamel, Director, Business and Finance
Michael Weiner, Treasurer

The Federation for Children with Special Needs is an organization dedicated to supporting parents of children with disabilities. The Federation seeks to ensure the full participation of all people in community life, including persons with disabilities.

973 INCLUDEnyc
116 East 16th Street
5th Floor
New York, NY 10003
212-677-4650; *Fax:* 212-254-4070
info@includenyc.org
www.includenyc.org

Ellen Miller-Wachtel, Chair
Sarah Berman, Vice President
Barbara A. Glassman, Executive Director
Stephen Stern, Director of Finance

INCLUDEnyc, formerly Resources for Children with Special Needs, is an organization dedicated to providing assistance and support to families and young people with disabilities across all five boroughs in New York City. INCLUDEnyc offers programs and services to help children with disabilities develop their skills and reach their full potential.

Year Founded: 1983

974 Lifespire
1 Whitehall Street
9th Floor
New York, NY 10004
212-741-0100; *Fax:* 212-463-9814
info@lifespire.org
www.lifespire.org

Michael S. Gross, Chairman
Thomas Lydon, CEO and President
Keith Lee, Chief Financial Officer
Bonita Hinson, Chief Operating Officer

Lifespire seeks to provide support to individuals with disabilities and assist them with the development of the skills needed to become independent and contributing members of the community.

Year Founded: 1951

975 Mentally Ill Kids in Distress (MIKID)
7816 North 19th Avenue
Phoenix, AZ 85021
602-253-1240; *Fax:* 602-840-3409
phoenix@mikid.org
www.mikid.org

Ted Williams, President
Sue Gilbertson, Founder
Dick Geasland, LCSW, Chief Executive Officer
Bonnie Kolakowski, MBA, Chief Financial Officer

Mentally Ill Kids in Distress provides support and assistance to families in Arizona with children and youth who are struggling with behavioral problems. MIKID seeks to improve the behavioral health and wellness of youth across Arizona. Offers information centers, assistance by phone, email or in person, support groups, educational meetings, referrals to resources, and direct support services.

Year Founded: 1987

976 National Federation of Families for Children's Mental Health
12320 Parklawn Drice
Rockville, MD 20852
240-403-1901
ffcmh@ffcmh.org
www.ffcmh.org

Lynda Gargan, PhD, Executive Director
Barbara Huff, Technical Assistance Provider
Sherri Luthe, President
Terry Stevens, Vice President

The National Federation of Families for Children's Mental Health is a national organization focused on advocating for the rights of children affected by mental health challenges, assisting family-run organizations across the nation, and ensuring that children and families concerned with mental health have access to services.

Year Founded: 1989

977 National Technical Assistance Center for Children's Mental Health
Georgetown University Center for Child and Human Development
Box 571485
Washington, DC 20057-1485
202-687-5000
childrensmh@georgetown.edu
www.gucchdtacenter.georgetown.edu

James R. Wotring, Director
Bruno Anthony, Director, Research & Evaluation
Phyllis R. Magrab, Principal Investigator
Sybil Goldman, Senior Advisor

The National Technical Assistance Center for Children's Mental Health is committed to sustaining and expanding mental health systems across the nation and improving the quality of life for children affected by mental health challenges.

Year Founded: 1984

978 Parent to Parent of Omaha
Ollie Webb Center
1941 South 42nd Street
Suite 122
Omaha, NE 68105-2942

402-346-5220; *Fax:* 402-342-4857
www.olliewebbinc.org/parent-to-parent

Laurie Ackermann, Executive Director
Robin McArthur, Operations Director
Denise Gehringer, Program Coordinator
Lisa Dougherty, Human Resource Manager

Consists of parents, professionals, and others who are interested in providing emotional and peer support to parents of children with disabilities. Offers a parent-matching program which matches new parents with parents who have had sufficient experience and training.

Year Founded: 1971

979 Parents Helping Parents
Sobrato Center for Nonprofits
1400 Parkmoor Avenue
Suite 100
San Jose, CA 95126
408-727-5775
855-727-5775; *Fax:* 408-286-1116
info@php.com
www.php.com

Maria Daane, Executive Director
Mark Fishler, Development Director
Jane Floethe Ford, Director of Education Services
Trudy Marsh Grable, Director of Community Services

Parents Helping Parents is a community-based organization dedicated to helping individuals with special needs realize their full potential through the provision of support services, information, training, and resources for children and adults with special needs, their families, and professionals.

Year Founded: 1976

980 Research and Training Center for Pathways to Positive Futures
Portland State University
1600 Southwest 4th Avenue
Suite 900
Portland, OR 97201
503-725-4040; *Fax:* 503-725-4180
rtcpubs@pdx.edu
www.pathwaysrtc.pdx.edu

Janet Walker, Director
Nancy Koroloff, Coordinator of Research
Emily Taylor, Dissemination Manager
Donna Fleming, Center Manager

The Research and Training Center for Pathways to Positive Futures conducts research, training, and information dissemination with the goal of improving the lives of youth and young adults with mental health needs.

Year Founded: 2009

981 Society for Pediatric Research
9303 New Trails Drive
Suite 350
The Woodlands, TX 77381
346-980-9710
info@societyforpediatricresearch.org
www.www.societyforpediatricresearch.org/

Michelle Gill, MD, PhD, President
Joel N. Hirschhorn, MD, PhD, Vice President
David Hunstad, MD, Secretary/Treasurer
Constine Stratakis, MD, DSc, President-Elect

A society that aims to improve pediatric health by creating a network of multi-disciplinary researchers through meetings/conferences, career opportunities, and advocacy on medical system issues.

982 The Center for Family Support
2811 Zulette Avenue
Bronx, NY 10461
718-518-1500; *Fax:* 718-518-8200
www.www.cfsny.org/

Steven Vernikoff, Executive Director
Lloyd Stabiner, President
Amy Bittinger, Vice President
Barbara Greenwald, Associate Executive Director

The Center for Family Support offers assistance to individuals with developmental and related disabilities, as well as their families, and provides support services and programs that are designed to accommodate individual needs. Offers services throughout New York City, Westchester County, Long Island, and New Jersey.

Year Founded: 1954

983 Young Adult Institute and Workshop (YAI)
460 West 34th Street
11th Floor
New York, NY 10001-2382
212-273-6100
www.yai.org

George Contos, Chief Executive Officer
Jeffrey A. Mordos, Chairman
Lewis A. Lindenberg, Esq., Vice Chair
Kevin Hogan, Treasurer

The YAI Network is an organization that serves people with intellectual and developmental disabilities. The YAI Network seeks to enhance the lives of people with disabilities by creating new opportunities for them. Provides a range of family support, employment training and placement, clinical, and residential services.

Year Founded: 1957

984 ZERO TO THREE: National Center for Infants, Toddlers, and Families
1255 23rd Street Northwest
Suite 350
Washington, DC 20037
202-638-1144
800-899-4301
www.zerotothree.org

Brenda Jones Harden, President
Matthew Melmed, Executive Director
Paul Spicer, Vice President
Laura Shiflett, Chief Financial Officer

A national, nonprofit organization that provides information and resources on early development to parents, professionals, and policymakers. Zero To Three's mission is to improve the lives of infants and toddlers, and to promote their health and development.

Year Founded: 1977

Books

985 After School and More
Resources for Children with Special Needs
116 East 16th Street
5th Floor
New York, NY 10003-2164
212-677-4650; *Fax:* 212-254-4070
info@resourcenyc.org
www.resourcesnyc.org

Ellen Miller-Wachtel, Chair
Shon E Glusky, President
Rachel Howard, Executive Director
Stephen Stern, Director of Finance and Administ

The most complete directory of after school programs for children with disabilities and special needs in the metropolitan New York area focusing on weekend and holiday programs. *$15.00*

252 pages Year Founded: 1983 ISBN 0-967836-57-3

986 Aggression Replacement Training: A Comprehensive Intervention for Aggressive Youth
Research Press
PO Box-7886
Champaign, IL 61826
217-352-3273
800-519-2707; *Fax:* 217-352-1221
rp@researchpress.com
www.researchpress.com

Dr Barry Glick, Author
Dr John C Gibbs, Author

Aggression Replacement Training (ART) offers a comprehensive intervention program designed to teach adolescents to understand and replace aggression and antisocial behavior with positive alternatives. The book is designed to be user-friendly and teacher-oriented. It contains summaries of ART's outcome evaluations and it discusses recent applications in schools and other settings. *$24.95*

426 pages Year Founded: 1968 ISBN 0-878223-79-7

987 Bibliotherapy Starter Set
The Guidance Group
303 Crossways Park Dr
Woodbury, NY 11797-2099
800-962-1141; *Fax:* 800-262-1886
info@Childswork.com
www.Childswork.com

Beth Ann Marcozzi, Author

Eight popular books for helping children ages four - twelve. Titles include Self Esteem, Divorce, ADHD, Feelings, and Anger. *$105.00*

988 Book of Psychotherapeutic Homework
Childs Work/Childs Play
303 Crossways Park Dr
Woodbury, NY 11797-2099
800-962-1141; *Fax:* 800-262-1886
info@Childswork.com
www.Childswork.com

Lawrence E Shapiro, Author

More than 80 home activities to guarantee your therapy won't lose momentum. Appropriate for ages five - ten. *$20.95*

Year Founded: 2001 ISBN 1-882732-55-3

989 Breaking the Silence: Teaching the Next Generation About Mental Illness
NAMI Queens/Nassau
1981 Marcus Avenue
Suite C-117
Lake Success, NY 11042
516-326-0797; *Fax:* 516-437-5785
btslessonplans@aol.com
www.www.btslessonplans.org/

Janet Susin, Author
Lorraine Kaplan, Author
Louise Slater, Author

Breaking the Silence (BTS) is an innovative teaching package which includes lesson plans, games and posters on serious mental illness for three grade levels: upper elementary, middle and high school. It is designed to fight stigma by putting a human face on mental illness, replacing fear and ridicule with compassion. BTS meets national health standards.

990 CARE Child and Adolescent Risk Evaluation: A Measure of the Risk for Violent Behavior
Research Press
Dept 24 W
PO Box 9177
Champaign, IL 61826-9177
217-352-3273
800-519-2707; *Fax:* 217-352-1221
rp@researchpress.com
www.researchpress.com

Dr Kathryn Siefert, Author

The CARE was developed as a prevention tool to identify youth, as early as possible, who are at risk for committing acts of violence. Unlike other evaluation programs, CARE includes a case management planning form that provides the information needed to develop a risk management intervention plan. The CARE Kit includes 25 assessment forms, 25 case management planning forms and manual. *$75.00*

50 pages

991 Camps 2009-2010
Resources for Children with Special Needs
116 E 16th Street
5th Floor
New York, NY 10003-2164
212-677-4650; *Fax:* 212-254-4070
www.resourcesnyc.org

Rachel Howard, Executive Director

The guide includes a dozen new camps and updates on more than 300 camps and programs that provide a wide range of summer activities for children with emotional, developmental, learning and physical disabilities, health issues and other special needs. Day camps in the New York metro area are included as well as sleepaway camps in the Northeast. *$25.00*

133 pages Year Founded: 2009 ISBN 0-967836-57-3

992 Children and Trauma: A Guide for Parents and Professionals
Courage to Change
303 Crossways Park Drive
Woodbury, NY 11797
800-440-4003; *Fax:* 800-772-6499
www.couragetochange.com

Cynthia Monahon, Author

Teaches parents and professionals about the effects of such ordeals on children and offers a blueprint for restoring a child's sense of safety and balance. Offers hope and reassurance for parents. The author suggests straightforward ways to help kids through tough times, and also describes in detail the warning signs that indicate a child needs professional help. Monahon helps adults understand psychological trauma from a child's point of view and explores the ways both parents and professionals can help children heal. *$19.95*

240 pages Year Founded: 1997 ISBN 0-787910-71-6

993 Children in Therapy: Using the Family as a Resource
WW Norton & Company
500 5th Avenue
New York, NY 10110-54
212-354-2907
800-233-4830; *Fax:* 212-869-0856
npb@wwnorton.com
www.wwnorton.com

Drake McFeely, CEO

This anthology presents theoretical perspectives of five different competency-based approaches: solution-oriented brief therapy, narrative therapy, collaborative language systems therapy, internal family systems therapy, and emotionally focused family therapy.

ISBN 0-393704-85-8

994 Childs Work/Childs Play
303 Crossways Park Dr
Woodbury, NY 11797-2099
800-962-1141; *Fax:* 800-262-1886
info@Childswork.com
www.Childswork.com

Catalog of books, games, toys and workbooks relating to child development issues such as recognizing emotions, handling uncertainty, bullies, ADD, shyness, conflicts and other things that children may need some help navigating.

995 Creative Therapy with Children & Adolescents
Impact Publishers
PO Box 6016
Atascadero, CA 93423-6016
805-466-5917
800-246-7228; *Fax:* 805-466-5919
info@impactpublishers.com
www.impactpublishers.com

Angela Hobday,M.Sc, Author
Kate Ollier,M.Psych, Author

Over 100 activities that can be used in working with children, adolescents, and families. Encourages creativity in therapy and assists therapists in talking with children to facilitate change. From simple ideas to fresh innovations, the activities are designed to be used as tools to supplement a variety of therapeutic approaches, and can be tailored to each child's needs. Therapists will find practical help in gaining rapport with clients who find it difficult to talk about feelings and experiences. Each activity is categorized according to the child's needs or the purpose of the activity, and cross-referenced by problem, activity, and by the features of each game/exercise. *$21.95*

192 pages Year Founded: 1970 ISBN 1-886230-19-6

996 Don't Feed the Monster on Tuesdays!: The Children's Self-Esteem Book
ADD WareHouse
300 NorthWest 70th Avenue
Suite 102
Plantation, FL 33317-2360
954-792-8944
800-233-9273; *Fax:* 954-792-8545
websales@addwarehouse.com
www.addwarehouse.com

Adolph J. Moser, Author
Nancy R. Thatch, Editor
David Melton, Illustrator

Strikes right at the heart of the basic elements of self-esteem. It presents valuable information to children that will help them understand the importance of their self worth. A friendly book that children ages 4 to 10 will love. *$18.95*

55 pages Year Founded: 1990 ISBN 0-933849-38-9

997 Don't Pop Your Cork on Mondays: The Children's Anti-Stress Book
ADD WareHouse
300 NorthWest 70th Avenue
Suite 102
Plantation, FL 33317-2360
954-792-8944
800-233-9273; *Fax:* 954-792-8545
websales@addwarehouse.com
www.addwarehouse.com

Adolph J. Moser, Author
Dav Pilkey, Illustrator

In this very informative and highly entertaining handbook for children, Dr. Adolph Moser offers practical approaches and effective techniques to help young people deal with stress. *$18.95*

48 pages Year Founded: 1990 ISBN 0-933849-18-4

998 Don't Rant and Rave on Wednesdays: The Children's Anger-Control Book
ADD WareHouse
300 NorthWest 70th Avenue
Suite 102
Plantation, FL 33317-2360
954-792-8944
800-233-9273; *Fax:* 954-792-8545
websales@addwarehouse.com
www.addwarehouse.com

Adolph Moser, Author
Nancy R. Thatch, Editor
David Melton, Illustrator

This book will delight both children and adults. It's informative and it's fun because Dr. Moser examines the complex feelings of human anger with the proper blend of sensitivity and humor. And David Melton's colorful illustrations are bright and witty. *$18.95*

61 pages Year Founded: 1990 ISBN 0-933849-54-0

999 Essentials of Lewis's Child and Adolescent Psychiatry
Lippincott Williams & Wilkins
333 Seventh Avenue
19th & 20th Floors
New York, NY 10001

301-223-2300
800-933-6525
www.lww.com

Fred R. Volkmar, Author
Andres Martin,MD MPH, Author

Companion guide to: Lewis's child and adolescent psychiatry.

432 pages Year Founded: 1998 ISBN 0-781775-02-7

1000 Forms for Behavior Analysis with Children
Research Press
Dept 12W
PO Box 9177
Champaign, IL 61826-9177
217-352-3273
800-519-2707; *Fax:* 217-352-1221
rp@researchpress.com
www.researchpress.com

Joseph R. Cautela, Author
Julie Cautela, Author
Sharon Esonis, Author

A unique collection of 42 reproducible assessment forms designed to aid counselors and therapists in making proper diagnoses and in developing treatment plans for children and adolescents. Different assessment formats are included, ranging from direct observations and interviews to informant ratings and self-reports. Certain forms are to be filled out by children and adolescents, while others are to be completed by parents, school personnel, significant others or the therapist. *$ 39.95*

208 pages ISBN 0-878222-67-7

1001 Forms-5 Book Set
Childs Work/Childs Play
303 Crossways Park Dr
Woodbury, NY 11797-2099
800-962-1141; *Fax:* 800-262-1886
info@Childswork.com
www.Childswork.com

Five-book pack with reproducible forms titled: Oppositional Child, Children with OCD, Counseling Children, ADHD Child and Socially Fearful Child. *$125.00*

1002 Handbook of Infant Mental Health 3rd Edition
The Guilford Press
72 Spring Street
New York, NY 10012
800-365-7006; *Fax:* 212-966-6708
info@guilford.com
www.guilford.com

Charles H. Zeanah Jr., MD, Editor

Widely regarded as the standard reference in the field, this state-of-the-art handbook offers a comprehensive analysis of developmental, clinical, and social aspects of mental health from birth to the preschool years. Leading authorities explore models of development; biological, family, and sociocultural risk and protective factors; and frequently encountered disorders and disabilities. Evidence-based approaches to assessment and treatment are presented, with an emphasis on ways to support strong parent-child relationships. The volume reviews the well-documented benefits of early intervention and prevention and describes applications in mental health, primary care, childcare, and child welfare settings.

622 pages Year Founded: 1973 ISBN 1-606233-15-7

1003 I Wish Daddy Didn't Drink So Much
Childs Work/Childs Play
303 Crossways Park Dr
Woodbury, NY 11797-2099
800-962-1141; *Fax:* 800-262-1886
info@Childswork.com
www.Childswork.com

Judith Vigna, Author

A young girl shares her feelings and frustrations about her alcoholic father's behavior. *$6.95*

32 pages ISBN 0-807535-26-5

1004 I'm Somebody, Too!
ADD WareHouse
300 NW 70th Avenue
Suite 102
Plantation, FL 33317-2360
954-792-8944
800-233-9273; *Fax:* 954-792-8545
sales@addwarehouse.com
www.addwarehouse.com

Harvey C Parker, Owner

When her brother responds to therapy for ADD, Emily no longer knows what her family role should be. *$13.00*

159 pages

1005 Kid Power Tactics for Dealing with Depression
Childswork/Childsplay
303 Crossways Park Drive
Woodbury, NY 11797
800-962-1141

Nicholas Dubuque, Author
Susan Dubuque, Author

Written by an 11 year-old boy with depression and his mother, inclues 15 strategies to deal with depression. *$12.95*

47 pages Year Founded: 1996 ISBN 1-882732-48-0

1006 Lewis's Child and Adolescent Psychiatry: A Comprehensive Textbook, 4th Edition
Lippincott Williams & Wilkins
333 Seventh Avenue
19th & 20th Floors
New York, NY 10001
301-223-2300
800-933-6525
www.lww.com

Fred R. Volkmar, Editor
Andres Martin, Editor

Established for fifteen years as the standard work in the field, this classic text emphasizes the relationship between basic science and clinical research and integrates scientific principles with the realities of drug interactions. Companion website provides instant access to the complete, fully searchable text.

1088 pages Year Founded: 1998 ISBN 0-781762-14-6

1007 My Body is Mine, My Feelings are Mine
Childs Work/Childs Play
303 Crossways Park Dr
Woodbury, NY 11797-2099
800-962-1141; *Fax:* 800-262-1886
info@Childswork.com
www.Childswork.com

Susan Hoke,LCSW,ACSW, Author
Bruce Van Patter, Illustrator
Charles Brenna, Designer

For ages 3 - 8. First part to be read to children, the second part teaches adults how to educate children about body safety. Sexual victimization can be prevented through explanation of how to identify inappropriate touching and what to do about it. *$20.95*

78 pages Year Founded: 1995 ISBN 1-882732-24-3

1008 My Listening Friend: A Story About the Benefits of Counseling
Childs Work/Childs Play
303 Crossways Park Dr
Woodbury, NY 11797-2099
800-962-1141; *Fax:* 800-262-1886
info@Childswork.com
www.Childswork.com

P J Michaels, Author
Anna Dewdney, Illustrator

For ages five - twelve, explores the feelings a child has the first time they see a counselor. Written from the point of view of the child. *$14.50*

57 pages Year Founded: 2001 ISBN 1-588150-43-7

1009 Neurodevelopmental Disabilities: Clinical Care for Children and Young Adults
Springer
11 West 42nd Street
15th Floor
New York, NY 10036
212-431-4370
877-687-7476; *Fax:* 212-941-7842
cs@springerpub.com
www.springerpub.com

Dilip R. Patel, Editor
Donald E. Greydanus, Editor
Hatim A. Omar, Editor
Joav Merrick, Editor

Increasingly more and more children with developmental disabilities survive into adulthood. Pediatricians and other clinicians are called upon to care for an increasing number of children with developmental disabilities in their practice and thus there is a need for a practical guide specifically written for pediatricians and primary care clinicians that addresses major concepts of neurodevelopmental pediatrics.

350 pages Year Founded: 1950 ISBN 9-400706-26-X

1010 Preventing Maladjustment from Infancy Through Adolescence
Sage Publications
2455 Teller Road
Thousand Oaks, CA 91320-2234
805-499-0721
800-818-7243; *Fax:* 800-583-2665
info@sagepub.com
www.sagepub.com

Annette U Rickel, Author
Larue Allen, Author

Authoritative and thoroughly researched, this book examines the theoretical and historical issues of prevention with children and youth, and delineates those factors which place the individual at risk. It will serve as an excellent text for advanced level undergraduate and graduate courses courses dealing with preventive interventions for infants, children, and adolescents.

160 pages Year Founded: 1987 ISBN 0-803928-68-8

1011 Psychotherapy with Infants and Young Children: Repairing the Effects of Stress and Trauma on Early Attachement
The Guilford Press
72 Spring Street
New York, NY 10012
800-365-7006; *Fax:* 212-966-6708
info@guilford.com
www.guilford.com

Alicia F. Lieberman, PhD, Author
Patricia Van Horn, PhD, Author

This eloquent book presents an empirically supported treatment that engages parents as the most powerful agents of their young children's healthy development. The book provides a comprehensive theoretical framework together with practical strategies for combining play, developmental guidance, trauma-focused interventions, and concrete assistance with problems of living. It is grounded in extensive clinical experience and important research on early development, attachment, neurobiology, and trauma.

366 pages Year Founded: 1973 ISBN 1-609182-40-5

1012 Saddest Time
Childs Work/Childs Play
303 Crossways Park Dr
Woodbury, NY 11797-2099
800-962-1141; *Fax:* 800-262-1886
info@Childswork.com
www.Childswork.com

Norma Simon, Author

Helps children ages 6 - 12 understand that death is sad and sometimes tragic, but it is also part of life. *$13.95*

Year Founded: 1999 ISBN 0-613141-80-6

1013 Schools for Students with Special Needs
Resources for Children with Special Needs
116 E 16th Street
Fifth Floor
New York City, NY 10003-2112
212-677-4650; *Fax:* 212-254-4070
info@resourcesnyc.org
www.resourcesnyc.org

Rachel Howard, Executive Director

The first complete book listing private day and residential schools for parents, caregivers and professionals seeking schools for students 5 and up with developmental, emotional, physical and learning disabilities in the NYC metro area. More than 400 schools and residential programs that serve children in the elementary through high school grades are listed with contact information, ages and populations served, class sizes and student-teacher ratios, special services and diplomas offered. Includes a 46-page section of Schools for Children with Autism Spectrum Disorders, as well as a guide with a list of websites on autism spectrum disorders. *$25.00*

342 pages

1014 Teen Relationship Workbook
Childs Work/Childs Play
303 Crossways Park Dr
Woodbury, NY 11797-2099
516-349-5520
800-962-1141; *Fax:* 800-262-1886
info@childswork.com
www.childswork.com

Kerry Moles, Author
Amy L Leutenberg-Brodsky, Illustrator

A reproducible workbook, this hands-on tool helps teens develop healthy relationships and prevent dating abuse and domestic violence. *$44.95*

135 pages

1015 Thirteen Steps to Help Families Stop Fighting Solve Problems Peacefully
Childs Work/Childs Play
303 Crossways Park Dr
Woodbury, NY 11797-2099
800-962-1141; *Fax:* 800-262-1886
info@Childswork.com
www.Childswork.com

Sharon Hernes Silverman, Author

Candid views on why families fight, and solutions to conflict. *$15.95*

Year Founded: 2001 ISBN 1-882732-77-4

1016 What Works When with Children and Adolescents: A Handbook of Individual Counseling Techniques
Research Press
PO Box-7886
Champaign, IL 61826
217-352-3273
800-519-2707; *Fax:* 217-352-1221
rp@researchpress.com
www.researchpress.com

Dr Ann Vernon, Author

This practical handbook is designed for counselors, social workers and psychologists in schools and mental health settings. It offers over 100 creative activities and effective interventions for individual counseling with children and adolescents (ages 6-18). Dr. Vernon provides strategies for establishing a therapeutic relationship with students who are sometimes apprehensive or opposed to counseling. Several case studies are included to help illustrate the counseling techniques and interventions. The book also includes a chapter on working with parents and teachers. *$39.95*

384 pages Year Founded: 1968 ISBN 0-878224-38-6

Periodicals & Pamphlets

1017 Helping Hand
Performance Resource Press
1270 Rankin Drive
Suite F
Troy, MI 48083-2843
248-588-7733
800-453-7733; *Fax:* 248-588-6633
www.store.amplifiedlifenetwork.com

Lyle Labardee,MS,LPC,NCC, President

A newsletter on child and adult behavioral health.

4 pages 9 per year

1018 Treatment of Children with Mental Disorders
National Institute of Mental Health
6001 Executive Boulevard
Room 8184,MSC 9663
Bethesda, MD 20892-9663
301-443-4513
866-615-6464
TTY: 301-443-8431
nimhinfo@nih.gov
www.www.nimh.nih.gov/

Ruth Dubois, Assistant Chief

A booklet with answers to frequently asked questions about the treatment of mental disorders in children, includes a medications chart.

Research Centers

1019 Child Neurology and Developmental Center
1510 Jericho Turnpike
New Hyde Park, NY 11040
516-352-2500; *Fax:* 516-352-2573
www.childbrain.com

Rami Grossmann, M.D.

Pediatric neurology practice of Rami Grossmann, M.D. in New York. Neurologists are highly trained to treat disorders of the nervous system. This includes diseases of the brain, spinal cord, nerves, and muscles. Common problems that Dr. Grossmann diagnoses and treats include the following: AD/HD, Autism, a form of PDD, Developmental delays, Epilepsy, Headaches, Learning difficulties, and Tic Disorders.

1020 KidsHealth
The Nemours Foundation
10140 Centurion Parkway
Jacksonville, FL 32256
904-697-4100; *Fax:* 904-697-4220
comments@KidsHealth.org
www.kidshealth.org

Alfred I. duPont, Nemour's Foundation Creator
Neil Izenberg, MD, Editor-in-Chief & Founder

KidsHealth is more than just the facts about health. As part of The Nemours Foundation's Center for Children's Health Media, KidsHealth also provides families with perspective, advice, and comfort about a wide range of physical, emotional, and behavioral issues that affect children and teens. The Nemours Center for Children's Health Media is a part of The Nemours Foundation, a nonprofit organization created by philanthropist Alfred I. duPont in 1936 and devoted to improving the health of children.

Year Founded: 1936

Support Groups & Hot Lines

1021 Alateen and Al-Anon Family Groups
1600 Corporate Landing Parkway
Virginia Beach, VA 23454-5617
757-563-1600
888-425-2666; *Fax:* 757-563-1655
wso@al-anon.org
www.al-anon.alateen.org

Mary Ann Keller, Director Members Services

Strength and hope for friends and families of problem drinkers.

1022 Girls and Boys Town of New York
281 Park Avenue South
5th Floor
New York, NY 10010
212-725-4260
800-448-3000; *Fax:* 212-725-4385
www.www.boystown.org

Guy Cleveland, Chairman
John C. Scott, Ph.D., Board Secretary
Jennifer Armstrong, Senior Vice President of New Pro
Crystal Denunzio, Vice President of Business Devel

Crisis intervention and referrals.

Year Founded: 1990

1023 Kidspeace National Centers
4085 Independence Drive
Schnecksville, PA 18078
800-257-3223; *Fax:* 610-391-8280
www.kidspeace.org

Mary Jane Willis, Chairman
William R Isemann, President & CEO
James Horan, Executive VP,CFO,Treasurer
Michael Slack, EVP,Business Development

Mission is to give hope, help and healing to children, families and communities. Helping people in need overcome challenges and transform their lives by providing emotional and physical healthcare and educational services in an atmosphere of teamwork, compassion and creativity.

1024 National Youth Crisis Hotline
5331 Mount Alifan Drive
San Diego, CA 92111-2622
800-448-4663
www.1800hithome.com/

Information and referral for runaways, and for youth and parents with problems.

1025 One Place for Special Needs
One Place for Special Needs, Ltd.
PO Box 9701
Naperville, IL 60567
E-mail: info@oneplaceforspecialneeds.com
www.oneplaceforspecialneeds.com

Dawn Villarreal, Founder

An information network and social community that allows the disability community to share resources and make connections in their own neighborhood. And a place where those who actively work with those who have disabilities can let families learn about their products, program and services.

Year Founded: 2002

1026 Rainbows
1360 Hamilton Parkway
Itasca, IL 60143
847-952-1770
800-266-3206; *Fax:* 847-952-1774
info@rainbows.org
www.rainbows.org

Anthony Taglia, Chair
Bob Thomas, Executive Director and CEO
Burt Heatherly, CFO

The largest international children's charity dedicated solely to helping youth successfully navigate the very difficult grief process. Every day, children are touched by emotional suffering caused by a death, divorce, deployment of a family member, incarceration of a loved one, or any of a multitude of significant event traumas including natural or manmade disasters.

Year Founded: 1983

1027 SADD: Students Against Destructive Decisions
255 Main Street
Marlborough, MA 01752-5505
508-481-3568
877-723-3462; *Fax:* 508-481-5759
info@sadd.org
www.sadd.org

Danna Mauch,PhD, Chairman
Penny Wells, President and CEO
Susan Scarola, Treasurer
James E Champagne, Secretary/Clerk

Providing students with the best prevention tools possible to deal with the issues of underage drinking, other drug use, risky and impaired driving, and other destructive decisions.

Year Founded: 1981

Video & Audio

1028 Aggression Replacement Training Video: A Comprehensive Intervention for Aggressive Youth
Research Press
PO Box 7886
PO Box 9177
Champaign, IL 61826
217-352-3273
800-519-2707; *Fax:* 217-352-1221
rp@researchpress.com
www.researchpress.com

This staff training DVD features scenes of adolescents participating in group sessions for each of ART's three interventions. Viewers will see a prosocial skills training group, an anger management session, and a moral reasoning group. *$125.00*

ISBN 0-878225-91-0

1029 Anger Management-Enhanced Edition
Educational Video Network, Inc.
1401 19th Street
Huntsville, TX 77340
936-295-5767
800-762-0060; *Fax:* 936-294-0233
www.www.evndirect.com

Learn what causes anger and understand why our bodies react as they do when we're angry. Effective techniques for assuaging anger are discussed.

1030 Are the Kids Alright?
Fanlight Productions
32 Court Street
21st Floor
Brooklyn, NY 11201
718-488-8900
800-876-1710; *Fax:* 718-488-8642
orders@fanlight.com
www.fanlight.com

Karen Bernstein, Author
Ellen Spiro, Author

Filmed in courtrooms, correctional institutions, treatment centers, and family homes, this searing documentary documents the results of the tragic decline in mental health services for children and adolescents at risk.

1031 Bipolar Disorder: Shifting Mood Swings
Educational Training Videos
136 Granville St
Suite 200
Gahanna, OH 43230
Fax: 888-775-3919
www.educationaltrainingvideos.com

Different from the routine ups and downs of life, the symptoms of bipolar disorder are severe - even to the point of being life-threatening. In this insightful program, patients speak from their own experience about the complexities of diagnosis and the very real danger of suicide, while family members and close friends address the strain of the condition's cyclic behavior.

1032 Bipolar Focus, Bipolar Disorder Audio and Video Files: Bipolar and Children/Adolescents
Bipolar Focus
www.pendulum.org/video/videospecial.htm

Website with list of playable video and audio files on topics including: children and mental health, antipsychotics in special populations: pediatrics and adolescents, mental health in childre, parts I and II, mental health and illness in teenagers, adult minds- mental health in early adulthood, college students and mental health, and pregnancy and the mind.

1033 Case Studies in Childhood Obsessive-Compulsive Disorder
Educational Training Videos
136 Granville St
Suite 200
Gahanna, OH 43230
Fax: 888-775-3919
www.educationaltrainingvideos.com

This edition of Primetime tracks the treatment of Bridget, Rocco, and Michelle as they attempt to reclaim their lives and overcome the stigma associated with the disorder. Original ABC News broadcast title: Kids Battle Obsessive-Compulsive Disorder.

1034 Children: Experts on Divorce
Courage to Change
1 Huntington Quadrangle
Suite: 1N03
Melville, NY 11747
800-962-1141; *Fax:* 800-262-1886
www.couragetochange.com/

Dede L Pitts, CEO

This DVD should be played for divorcing parents in your waiting room or client library. Children, ages 5-17, speak of what they need from their parents, what helps and what hurts. Judges, mediators, therapists and Karl Malone also appear on camera. DVD makes parents more ready to collaborate and make agreements that will benefit their children. Have a box of tissues handy. *$34.95*

1035 Chill: Straight Talk About Stress
Childs Work/Childs Play
303 Crossways Park Dr
Woodbury, NY 11797-2099
800-962-1141; *Fax:* 800-262-1886
info@Childswork.com
www.Childswork.com

Encourages youth to recognize, analyze and handle the stresses in their lives. 22 minutes. *$96.95*

1036 Clinical Impressions: Identifying Mental Illness
Educational Training Videos
136 Granville St
Suite 200
Gahanna, OH 43230
Fax: 888-775-3919
www.educationaltrainingvideos.com

How long can mental illness stay hidden, especially from the eyes of trained experts? This program rejoins a group of ten adults- five of them healthy and five of them with histories of mental illness- as psychiatric specialists try to spot and correctly diagnose the latter. Administering a series of collaborative and one-on-one tests, including assessments of personality type, physical self-image, and rational thinking, the panel gradually makes decisions about who suffers from depression, bipolar disorder, bulimia, and social anxiety.

1037 Coping with Emotions
Educational Video Network, Inc.
1401 19th Street
Huntsville, TX 77340
936-295-5767
800-762-0060; *Fax:* 936-294-0233
www.www.evndirect.com

Anger, indifference, sadness, confusion and ecstatic happiness are emotions that manifest themselves frequently during the teen years. The hormones that change the body physically also have a great effect on a teenager's emotions. Discover the gamut of emotions that rule a teenager's life and what can be done to control them.

1038 Coping with Stress
Educational Video Network, Inc.
1401 19th Street
Huntsville, TX 77340
936-295-5767
800-762-0060; *Fax:* 936-294-0233
www.www.evndirect.com

Stress affects everyone, both emotionally and physically. For some, mismanaged stress can result in substance abuse, violence, or even suicide. This program answers the question, How can a person cope with stress?

1039 Dark Voices: Schizophrenia
Educational Training Videos
136 Granville St
Suite 200
Gahanna, OH 43230
Fax: 888-775-3919
www.educationaltrainingvideos.com

This program seeks to understand how schizophrenia touches the lives of patients and their family members while examining the disease's etiology and pathology. A Discovery Channel Production.

1040 Dealing with ADHD: Attention Deficit/Hyperactivity
Educational Video Network, Inc.
1401 19th Street
Huntsville, TX 77340
936-295-5767
800-762-0060; *Fax:* 936-294-0233
www.www.evndirect.com

Learn about attention deficit/hyperactivity disorder and learn what factors are thought to contribute to the development of this disorder. Other disorders that commonly co-exist with ADHD will be identified. The impulsivity and risk-taking behaviors of ADHD teens will be focused upon and tips that ADHD students can use to succeed academically will be provided. Laws that require schools to make special accommodations for ADHD students will be reviewed, and viewers will learn how to contact organizations that exist to help people who are dealing with ADHD.

1041 Dealing with Depression
Educational Video Network, Inc.
1401 19th Street
Huntsville, TX 77340
936-295-5767
800-762-0060; *Fax:* 936-294-0233
www.www.evndirect.com

As more and more young people are falling victim to depression, it is important to understand what causes it and to know how to get the help that can rid a person of this life-wrecking affliction.

1042 Dealing with Grief
Educational Video Network, Inc.
1401 19th Street
Huntsville, TX 77340
936-295-5767
800-762-0060; *Fax:* 936-294-0233
www.www.evndirect.com

Grief allows us to acknowledge and mourn our losses so we can reconcile our feelings and move forward in life. Learn how to deal with your grief and become a better person for having gone through it.

1043 Dealing with Social Anxiety
Educational Video Network, Inc.
1401 19th Street
Huntsville, TX 77340
936-295-5767
800-762-0060; *Fax:* 936-294-0233
www.www.evndirect.com

Social anxiety is America's third-largest psychiatric disorder. It generally develops during the mid-teen years, and almost always before the age of 25. Understand what may trigger the development of anxiety and learn how it sometimes evolves into full-blown panic disorder, which is characterized by recurrent attacks of terror or fear. The consequences of social anxiety are examined and effective treatments are discussed.

1044 Don't Kill Yourself: One Survivor's Message
Educational Training Videos
136 Granville St
Suite 200
Gahanna, OH 43230
Fax: 888-775-3919
www.educationaltrainingvideos.com

This is the story of a young man, David, who at 16 years of age survived a suicide attempt. Now 22, he shares the events of his life leading up to the attempt, including how low self-esteem led to drug addiction, and how the addiction encouraged the sense that life was no longer worth living.

1045 Fetal Alcohol Syndrome and Effect DVD
Hazelden
15251 Pleasant Valley Road
PO Box 11
Center City, MN 55012-0011
651-213-4200
800-328-9000; *Fax:* 651-213-4793
info@hazelden.org
www.hazelden.org

Mark Mishek, President and CEO
James A. Blaha, Vice President Finance and Admin
Ann Bray, General Counsel and Vice Preside
Sharon Birnbaum, Corporate Director of Human Reso

Excellent for women in treatment, addiction professionals, and community education programs, the video is centered on the work being done with children affected by fetal alcohol and their families. It provides a factual definition of Fetal Alcohol Syndrome and Effect, explains how children are diagnossed and, most importantly, vividly illustrates the positive prognosis possible for fetal alcohol children. Medical and educational professionals, biological and adoptive parents and siblings, and the children themselves speak in this video about FAS. *$225.00*

Year Founded: 1949

1046 Legacy of Childhood Trauma: Not Always Who They Seem
Research Press
Dept 24 W
PO Box 9177
Champaign, IL 61826-9177
217-352-3273
800-519-2707; *Fax:* 217-352-1221
rp@researchpress.com
www.researchpress.com

Russell Pense, VP Marketing

Focuses on the connection between so-called delinquent youth and the experience of childhood trauma such as emotional, sexual, or physical abuse. The video features the unique stories of four young adults who are survivors of childhood trauma. They candidly discuss their troubled childhood and teenage years and reveal how, with the help of caring adults, they were able to salvage their lives. The caregivers, who helped these young adults through their teenage years, are joined by other helping professionals who provide thorough discussions of diagnosis and treatment issues. They offer valuable guidelines and insights on working with adolescents who have experienced childhood trauma. *$195.00*

1047 Mental Disorder
Educational Training Videos
136 Granville St
Suite 200
Gahanna, OH 43230
Fax: 888-775-3919
www.educationaltrainingvideos.com

What is abnormality? Using the case studies of two young women; one who has depression, one who has an anxiety disorder; as a springboard, this program presents three psychological perspective on mental disorder.

1048 Overcoming Obstacles and Self-Doubt
Educational Video Network, Inc.
1401 19th Street
Huntsville, TX 77340
936-295-5767
800-762-0060; *Fax:* 936-294-0233
www.www.evndirect.com

When feelings of self-doubt are combined with the sudden appearance of an overwhelming obstacle, the situation can be emotionally crippling.

1049 Suicide among Teens
Educational Video Network, Inc.
1401 19th Street
Huntsville, TX 77340
936-295-5767
800-762-0060; *Fax:* 936-294-0233
www.www.evndirect.com

Suicide devastates surviving loved ones. Find out why it should never be considered as a solution and learn how to recognize warning signs in a suicidal person.

1050 Teenage Anxiety, Depression, and Suicide
Educational Video Network, Inc.
1401 19th Street
Huntsville, TX 77340
936-295-5767
800-762-0060; *Fax:* 936-294-0233
www.www.evndirect.com

This program can provide helpful insight to those in need of assistance.

1051 Understanding Mental Illness
Educational Video Network, Inc.
1401 19th Street
Huntsville, TX 77340
936-295-5767
800-762-0060; *Fax:* 936-294-0233
www.www.evndirect.com

Contains information and classifications of mental illness. Mental illness can strike anyone, at any age. Learn about various organic and functional mental disorders as discussed and their causes and symptoms, and learn where to seek help for a variety of mental health concerns.

1052 Understanding Personality Disorders
Educational Video Network, Inc.
1401 19th Street
Huntsville, TX 77340
936-295-5767
800-762-0060; *Fax:* 936-294-0233
www.www.evndirect.com

For many people, the onset of a psychological disorder goes undiagnosed and untreated, and, as a result, they face a constant, if not impossible, struggle to maintain good mental health. This can be especially true when individuals suffer from a personality disorder. However, with identification and understanding, crippling personality disorders can be brought out of the shadows of ignorance and into the light of treatment.

1053 Why Isn't My Child Happy? Video Guide About Childhood Depression
ADD WareHouse
300 NW 70th Avenue
Suite 102
Plantation, FL 33317-2360
954-792-8100
800-233-9273; *Fax:* 954-792-8545
sales@addwarehouse.com
www.addwarehouse.com

Sam Goldstein, PhD, Author

The first of its kind, this new video deals with childhood depression. Informative and frank about this common problem, this book offers helpful guidance for parents and professionals trying to better understand childhood depression. 110 minutes. *$55.00*

Year Founded: 1990

Web Sites

1054 www.Al-Anon-Alateen.org
Al-Anon and Alateen

AA literature may serve as an introduction.

1055 www.CHADD.org
CHADD: Children/Adults with Attention Deficit/Hyperactivity Disorder

Offers support for individuals, parents, teachers, professionals, and others.

1056 www.aacap.org
American Academy of Child and Adolescent Psychiatry

Represents over 6,000 child and adolescent psychiatrists, brochures availible online which provide concise and up-to-date material on issues ranging from children who suffer from depression and teen suicide to stepfamily problems and child sexual abuse.

1057 www.adhdnews.com/Advocate.htm
Advocating for Your Child

1058 www.adhdnews.com/sped.htm
Special Education Rights and Responsibilities

Writing IEP's and TIEPS. Pursuing special education services.

1059 www.couns.uiuc.edu
Self-Help Brochures

Address issues teens deal with.

1060 www.freedomvillageusa.com
Freedom Village USA

Faith-based home for troubled teens.

1061 www.kidshealth.org/kid/feeling/index.html
Dealing with Feelings

Ten readings. Examples are: Why Am I So Sad; Are You Shy; Am I Too Fat or Too Thin; and A Kid's Guide to Divorce.

1062 www.naturalchild.com/home
Natural Child Project

Articles by experts.

1063 www.nospank.net
Project NoSpank

Site for those against paddling in schools.

1064 www.oneplaceforspecialneeds.com
One Place for Special Needs, Ltd.

1065 www.parentcenterhub.org
National Dissemination Center for Children with Disabilities

The Center for Parent Information and Resources hosts many of the resources published by the National Dissemination Center for Children with Disabilities, including English and Spanish resources.

1066 www.parenthood.com
Parenthood.Com

A leading online destination for moms, mothers-to-be, and families.

1067 www.rtckids.fmhi.usf.edu
Research & Training Center for Children's Mental Health

The Research and Training Center for Children's Mental Health at the University of South Florida was formed to conduct research, provide training, and contribute to the improvement of services for children with emotional and behavioral disabilities and their families. The Research and Training Center was funded by the National Institute on Disability and Rehabilitation Research and the Substance Abuse and Mental Health Services Administration from 1984 to 2009. Resources available on website.

1068 www.wholefamily.com
About Teens Now

Addresses important issues in teens lives.

1069 www2.mc.duke.edu/pcaad
Duke University's Program in Child and Anxiety Disorders

Obsessive Compulsive Disorder

Introduction

Obssessive-Compulsive Disorder, commonly known as OCD, is characterized by uncontrollable, reoccurring thoughts and behaviours that an individual feels the urge to repeat over and over. Almost everyone will have obsessive thoughts/compulsive behaviors at some point in their lives, but for people with OCD the obsessions and compulsions become so extreme that it consumes a lot of time and can interfere with other aspects of life, such as work, school, and personal relationships.

SYMPTOMS

Individuals with OCD have overwhelming obsessions and/or compulsions. Obsessions are repeated, intrusive, un- wanted thoughts that cause distressing emotions such as anxiety or anguish; a compulsion is a ceaseless urge to do something to lessen the anxiety caused by the obsession.
• Recurrent and persistent thoughts, impulses, or images that are experienced as intrusive and inappropriate and that cause marked anxiety or distress;
• Thoughts and worries are not simply excessive worries about real-life probelms, but can be inflated misinterpreta- tions of actions and words of others;
• Repetitive behvaiors that the person feels driven to per- form in response to an obsession, or according to rules that must be applied rigidly;
• The person recognizes that the obsessions or compulsions are unreasonable;
• The obsessions or compulsions are time consuming or sig- nificantly interfere with the person's normal routine, occupational or academic functioning, or usual social activities.

ASSOCIATED FEATURES

In OCD, the person is unable to control the anxiety even when he or she knows it is exaggerated and unreasonable. To other people, the person may seem edgy, irritable, to have unexpected outbursts of anger, or to be consumed by an unreasonable fear. The problem takes up time and effort and becomes a major preoccupation. The OCD affected persona can further that time and expenditure of energy in creating a ritual to manage the obsession, such as perform- ing an action a specific number of times in a particular order.

PREVALENCE

Obssessive Compulsive Disorder usually begins in adolescence or early adulthood, but may begin in childhood. In males the onset is earlier (between 6 and 15 years old) than for women (between 20 and 29), though it is equally common in both males and females.

TREATMENT OPTIONS

It is very important to have a full evaluation so that a proper diagnosis can be made. In general, people should have a primary care evaluation as part of the diagnostic proccess, so as to rule out a general medical condition that could be causing the signs and symptoms. Patients with OCD may benefit from bevhavioral therapy and/or a variety of medications. Particularly effective is exposure and response prevention therapy, in which a therapist carefully exposes the patient to situations that cause anxiety and provoke the obsessive compulsive behavior. Slowly the patient learns to decrease and eventually end the ritualistic behaviors.

Associations & Agencies

1071 Anxiety and Depression Association of America
8701 Georgia Avenue
Suite 412
Silver Spring, MD 20910
240-485-1001; *Fax:* 240-485-1035
information@adaa.org
www.adaa.org

Mary E. Salcedo, MD, President
Susan K. Gurley, JD, Executive Director
Risa B. Weisberg, PhD, Treasurer
Cindy J. Aaronson, MSW, PhD, Secretary

An international nonprofit organization committed to the use of education and research to promote the prevention, treatment, and cure of anxiety, depressive, obssessive com- pulsive, and other trauma related disorders. ADAA's mis- sion is to improve the lives of all people with anxiety and mood disorders.

Year Founded: 1979

1072 Center for Mental Health Services (CMHS)
Substance Abuse and Mental Health Services
Administration
5600 Fishers Lane
Rockville, MD 20857
240-276-1310
877-726-4727
TTY: 800-487-4889
www.samhsa.gov/about-us/who-we-are/offices-centers

Paolo del Vecchio, MSW, Director
Anne Mathews-Younes, Acting Deputy Director
Keris Myrick, Director, Consumer Affairs
Patricia Gratton, Director, Program Analysis

Promotes the treatment of mental illness and emotional dis- orders by increasing accessibility to mental health pro- grams; supporting outreach, treatment, rehabilitation, and support programs and networks; and encouraging the use of scientifically-based information when treating mental dis- orders. CMHS provides information about mental health via a toll-free number and numerous publications. Devel- oped for users of mental health services and their families, the general public, policy makers, providers, and the media.

Year Founded: 1992

1073 Goodwill's Community Employment Services
Goodwill Industries-Suncoast, Inc.
10596 Gandy Blvd.
St. Petersburg, FL 33702
727-523-1512
888-279-1988
TDD: 727-579-1068
www.goodwill-suncoast.org

Heather Ceresoli, CPA, Chair
Deborah A. Passerini, President
Martin W. Gladysz, Senior Vice Chair
Louise R. Lopez, Vice Chair

Program providing job coaching and community job place- ments for people with disabilities.

Year Founded: 1954

1074 International Obsessive Compulsive Disorder Foundation
18 Tremont Street
Suite 903
Boston, MA 02108
617-973-5801; *Fax:* 617-973-5803
info@iocdf.org
www.iocdf.org

Denise Egan Stack, LMHC, Secretary
Jeff Szymanski, PhD, Executive Director
Susan Boaz, President
Denis Asselin, Vice President

An organization for people with obsessive-compulsive disorder, as well as their families and friends. The Foundation aims to educate the public and professional communities about OCD and related disorders, work towards achieving increased accessibility to effective treatment, and support research into the causes and treatment methods of OCD.

Year Founded: 1986

1075 Mental Health America
500 Montgomery Street
Suite 820
Alexandria, VA 22314
703-684-7722
800-969-6642; *Fax:* 703-684-5968
www.mentalhealthamerica.net

Reginald Williams, Chair of the Board
Paul Gionfriddo, President and CEO
Jessica Kennedy, Chief of Staff/VP of Finance
Theresa Nguyen, VP of Policy and Programs

Mental Health America is a community-based nonprofit organization committed to enabling the mental wellness of all Americans. MHA advocates for greater access to quality health services and seeks to educate individuals on identifying symptoms, as well as intervention and prevention.

Year Founded: 1909

1076 NAPCSE National Association of Parents with Children in Special Education
3642 East Sunnydale Drive
Chandler Heights, AZ 85142
800-754-4421; *Fax:* 800-424-0371
contact@napcse.org
www.napcse.org

Dr. George Giuliani, President

The NAPCSE is dedicated to ensuring quality education for all children and adolescents with special needs. NAPCSE provides resources, support, and assistance to parents with children in special education.

1077 National Alliance on Mental Illness
3803 North Fairfax Drive
Suite 100
Arlington, VA 22203
703-524-7600
800-950-6264
info@nami.org
www.nami.org

Steve Pitman, JD, President
Lacey Berumen, PhD, MNM, First Vice President
Mary Giliberti, Chief Executive Officer
David Levy, Chief Financial Officer

NAMI is an organization dedicated to raising awareness on mental health and providing support and education for Americans affected by mental illness. NAMI advocates for access to services and treatment and fosters an environment of awareness and understanding for those concerned with mental health.

Year Founded: 1979

1078 National Anxiety Foundation
3135 Custer Drive
Lexington, KY 40517
859-272-7166
www.www.nationalanxietyfoundation.org/

Stephen Cox, MD, President
Linda Vernon Blair, Vice President
C. Todd Strecker, Secretary and Treasurer

Organization that seeks to alleviate suffering and save lives by educating the public about anxiety disorders.

1079 National Association for the Dually Diagnosed (NADD)
132 Fair Street
Kingston, NY 12401
845-331-4336
info@thenadd.org
www.thenadd.org

Jeanne M. Farr, MA, Chief Executive Officer
Daniel Baker, PhD., President
Peggie Webb, MA, Vice President
George Zukotynski, PhD., Secretary

NADD is a nonprofit organization designed to increase awareness of, and provide services for, individuals with developmental disabilities and mental illness. NADD emphasizes the importance of quality mental healthcare for people with mental health needs and offers conferences, information resources, educational programs, and training materials to professionals, parents, and organizations.

Year Founded: 1983

1080 National Council for Behavioral Health
1400 K Street Northwest
Suite 400
Washington, DC 20005
202-684-7457
communications@thenationalcouncil.org
www.thenationalcouncil.org

Jeff Richardson, Chair
Linda Rosenberg, President and CEO
Jeannie Campbell, Executive VP and COO
Tim Swinfard, First Vice Chair

The National Council for Behavioral Health serves to unify America's behavioral health organizations. The council is dedicated to ensuring that quality mental health and addictions care is readily accessible to all Americans.

1081 Sutcliffe Developmental & Behavioral Pediatrics
851 Fremont Avenue
Suite 110
Los Altos, CA 94024
650-941-1698; *Fax:* 650-434-3953
info@sutcliffedbp.com
www.www.sutcliffedbp.com/

Trenna Sutcliffe, MD, Medical Director
Jen Aronowitz, PhD, Neuropsychologist
Christy Tadros, Clinical Counselor
Hedva Redlich, Practice Manager

Sutcliffe Developmental & Behavioral Pediatrics is an organization that specializes in the treatment of ADHD, autism spectrum disorder, anxiety disorders, conduct disorders, learning disabilities, and more. Sutcliffe works with community services, school districs, and primary physicians, as well as provides family counseling.

1082 The Center for Family Support

2811 Zulette Avenue
Bronx, NY 10461
718-518-1500; *Fax:* 718-518-8200
www.www.cfsny.org/

Steven Vernikoff, Executive Director
Lloyd Stabiner, President
Amy Bittinger, Vice President
Barbara Greenwald, Associate Executive Director

The Center for Family Support offers assistance to individuals with developmental and related disabilities, as well as their families, and provides support services and programs that are designed to accommodate individual needs. Offers services throughout New York City, Westchester County, Long Island, and New Jersey.

Year Founded: 1954

1083 The Children's and Adult Center for OCD and Anxiety

3138 Butler Pike
Suite 200
Plymouth Meeting, PA 19462
www.childrenscenterocdanxiety.blogspot.ca/

Tamar Chansky, PhD, Founder

A center composed of six private practice psychologists delivering treatment and therapy to children and adults with OCD, Separation Anxiety, and other mental health disorders. They also offer parent workshops on skills and strategies to help their child cope with anxiety.

Year Founded: 1988

Books

1084 Boy Who Couldn't Stop Washing
Penguin Group

375 Hudson Street
New York, NY 10014-3672
212-366-2000
800-631-8571; *Fax:* 212-366-2933
online@penguinputnam.com

John Makinson, Chairman, CEO
Coram Williams, Chief Financial Officer
David Shanks, CEO
Judith Rapoport, Author

The Boy Who Wouldn't Stop Washing: Experience and Treatment of Obsessive-Compulsive Disorder. A comprehensive treatment of obsessive-compulsive disorder that summarizes evidence that the disorder is neurobiological. It also describes the effect of medication combined with behavioral therapy. *$7.99*

304 pages Year Founded: 1991 ISBN 0-451172-02-7

1085 Brain Lock: Free Yourself from Obsessive Compulsive Behavior
Harper Collins

10 E 53rd Street
New York, NY 10022-5299
212-207-7000

Brian Murray, Group President
Jeffrey M Schwartz, Author

A simple four-step method for overcoming OCD that is so effective, it's now used in academic treatment centers throughout the world. Proved by brain-imaging tests to actually alter the brain's chemistry, this method dosen't rely on psychopharmaceuticals but cognitive self-therapy and behavior modification to develop new patterns of response. Offers real-life stories of actual patients. Paperback. *$14.99*

256 pages Year Founded: 1997 ISBN 0-060987-11-1

1086 Childhood Obsessive Compulsive Disorder
Sage Publications

2455 Teller Road
Thousand Oaks, CA 91320-2234
805-499-0721
800-818-7243; *Fax:* 800-583-2665
info@sagepub.com
www.sagepub.com

Greta Francis, Author
Rod A Gragg, Author
Stephen Bar, Managing Director
Ziyad Marar, Deputy Managing Director

Childhood Obsessive Compulsive Disorder: Developmental Clinical Psychology and Psychiatry. *$62.00*

120 pages Year Founded: 1996 ISBN 0-803959-22-2

1087 Compulsive Acts: A Psychiatrist's Tales of Rituals and Obsessions
University of California Press

2120 Berkeley Way
Berkeley, CA 94704-1012
510-642-4247; *Fax:* 510-643-7127
www.ucpress.edu

Elias Aboujaoude, Author
Alison Mudditt, Director
Elias Aboujaude, Author

The author tells stories inspired by memorable patients he has treated, taking readers from his initial contact through the stages of the doctor-patient relationship. Stories include a man who can't let anyone get within a certain distance of his nose, two kleptomaniacs, an Internet addict who chooses virtual life over real life, a professor with a dangerous gambling habit, and others with equally debilitating compulsive conditions. *$29.95*

192 pages Year Founded: 2008 ISSN 978-0520255678ISBN 0-520255-67-4

1088 Consumer's Guide to Psychiatric Drugs
NewHarbinger Publications

5674 Shattuck Avenue
Oakland, CA 94609-1662
510-652-0215
800-748-6273; *Fax:* 800-652-1613
customerservice@newharbinger.com
www.newharbinger.com

Mary C. Talaga, Author
John D. Preston, Author
John H. O'Neal, Author

Helps consumers understand what treatment options are available and what side effects to expect. Covers possible interactions with other drugs, medical conditions and other concerns. Explains how each drug works, and offers detailed information about treatments for depression, bipolar disorder, anxiety and sleep disorders, as well as other conditions. *$16.95*

340 pages Year Founded: 1973 ISBN 1-572241-11-X

1089 Drug Therapy and Anxiety Disorders
Mason Crest Publishers
450 Parkway Drive
Suite D
Broomall, PA 19008-4017
610-543-6200
866-627-2665; *Fax:* 610-543-3878
dtaylor@masoncrest.com
www.masoncrest.com

Shirley Brinkerhoff, Author
Dan Hilferty, President
Michelle Luke, Director of Marketing
Michael Toglia, Special Sales

This volume provides readers with a clear introduction to anxiety disorders. Numerous case studies give insight into the world of mental disorders and helps readers understand the symptoms and treatments of this disorder, which includes: generalized anxiety disorder, social phobia, specific phobia, obsessive-compulsive disorder (covered more extensively in a separate column), post-traumatic stress disorder, and panic disorder.

128 pages ISBN 1-590845-61-7

1090 Drug Therapy and Obsessive-Compulsive Disorder
Mason Crest Publishers
450 Parkway Drive
Suite D
Broomall, PA 19008-4017
610-543-6200
866-627-2665; *Fax:* 610-543-3878
dtaylor@masoncrest.com
www.masoncrest.com

Shirley Brinkerhoff, Author
Dan Hilferty, President
Michelle Luke, Director of Marketing
Michael Toglia, Special Sales

This volume provides readers with a clear and understandable introduction to obsessive-compulsive disorder (OCD). Numerous case studies are included, which give insight into the world of those who experience this disorder; these anecdotes also help readers understand the symptoms and treatments of this disease. Famous historical figures who suffered from OCD, such as Samuel Johnson (1709-1784) and Howard Hughes (1905-1975) are mentioned as well.

128 pages ISBN 1-590845-69-2

1091 Freeing Your Child from Obsessive-Compulsive Disorder: A Powerful, Practical Program for Parents of Children and Adolescents
Three Rivers Publishing
1745 Broadway
New York, NY 10019
212-782-9000; *Fax:* 212-940-7408
crownpublicity@randomhouse.com
www.crownpublishing.com

Tamar Chansky, PhD, Author

Creates a clear road map to understanding and overcoming OCD based on her successful practice treating hundreds of children and teenages with this disorder. *$11.99*

368 pages Year Founded: 2011 ISBN 0-307794-44-4

1092 Funny, You Don't Look Crazy: Life With Obsessive Compulsive Disorder
Dilligaf Publishing
64 Court Street
Ellsworth, ME 04605
207-667-5031

An honest look at people who live with Obsessive Compulsive Disorder and those who love them.

128 pages Year Founded: 1994 ISBN 0-963907-00-X

1093 Getting Control: Overcoming Your Obsessions and Compulsions
Penguin Putnam
375 Hudson Street
New York, NY 10014-3672
212-366-2000
800-227-9604; *Fax:* 212-366-2933

David Shanks, CEO
Lee Baer, Author

Updated guide to treating OCD based on clinically proven techniques of behavior therapy. Offers a step-by-step program including assessing symptoms, setting realistic goals and creating specific therapeutic exercises. *$16.00*

272 pages Year Founded: 2000 ISBN 0-452281-77-6

1094 Let's Talk Facts About Obsessive Compulsive Disorder
American Psychiatric Publishing, Inc.
1000 Wilson Boulevard
Suite 1825
Arlington, VA 22209-3901
703-907-7322
800-368-5777; *Fax:* 703-907-1091
appi@psych.org
www.appi.org

Robert E Hales MD, Editor-in-Chief
Ron McMillen, Chief Executive Officer
John McDuffie, Editorial Director

$49.00

6 pages Year Founded: 2006 ISBN 0-890423-87-5

1095 OCD Workbook: Your Guide to Breaking Free From Obsessive-Compulsive Disorder
NewHarbinger Publications
5674 Shattuck Avenue
Oakland, CA 94609-1662
510-652-0215
800-748-6273; *Fax:* 800-652-1613
customerservice@newharbinger.com
www.newharbinger.com

Bruce M Hyman, PhD, LCSW, Author
Cherlene Pedrick, RN, Author

Offers the latest information about the neurobiological causes of obsessive-compulsive disorder(OCD), new developments in medication and other treatment options for the disorder, and a new chapter outlining cutting-edge daily coping strategies for sufferers. *$24.95*

352 pages Year Founded: 1973 ISBN 1-572249-21-9

1096 OCD in Children and Adolescents: A Cognitive-Behavioral Treatment Manual
Guilford Press
72 Spring Street
New York, NY 10012-4068
212-431-9800
800-365-7006; *Fax:* 212-966-6708
info@guilford.com

Bob Matloff, President
John S March, Author
Karen Mulle, Author

Written for clinicians, the book includes tips for parents, and treatment guidelines. The cognitive - behavioral approach to OCD has been problematic for many to understand because patients with symptoms of increased anxiety are told that their treatment initially involves further increases in their anxiety levels. The authors provide this in a modified and developmentally appropriate approach.
$39.00

298 pages Year Founded: 1998 ISBN 1-572302-42-6

1097 Obsessive Compulsive Anonymous
Obsessive Compulsive Anonymous
PO Box 215
New Hyde Park, NY 11040-0910
516-739-0662
west24th@aol.com
www.obsessivecompulsiveanonymous.com

Literature for the OCA program. *$19.00*

ISBN 0-962806-62-5

1098 Obsessive-Compulsive Disorder Casebook
American Psychiatric Publishing, Inc.
1000 Wilson Boulevard
Suite 1825
Arlington, VA 22209-3901
703-907-7322
800-368-5777; *Fax:* 703-907-1091
appi@psych.org
www.appi.org

John H Greist, M.D., Editor
James W Jefferson, M.D., Editor
John McDuffie, Editorial Director

Presents 60 case histories of OCD with a discussion by the author and editors regarding their opinion on each diagnosis. *$39.95*

220 pages ISBN 0-880487-29-1

1099 Obsessive-Compulsive Disorder Spectrum
American Psychiatric Publishing, Inc.
1000 Wilson Boulevard
Suite 1825
Arlington, VA 22209-3901
703-907-7322
800-368-5777; *Fax:* 703-907-1091
appi@psych.org
www.appi.org

Jose A Yaryura-Tobias, M.D., Author
Fugen A Neziroglu, Ph.D., Author
John McDuffie, Editorial Director

Comprehensive examination of OCD, related disorders and treatment regimens. *$68.50*

344 pages ISBN 0-880487-07-0

1100 Obsessive-Compulsive Disorder in Children and Adolescents: A Guide
Madison Institute of Medicine
7617 Mineral Point Road
Suite 300
Madison, WI 53717-1623
608-827-2470
mim@miminc.org
www.factsforhealth.org

Hugh F Johnston, Author
J.Jay Fruehling, Author
J. Jay Frueling, MA, Author

The guide is a comprehensive introduction to obsessive-compulsive disorder for parents who are learning about the illness. Discusses treating symptoms by a combination of behavioral therapy and medication and describes various drugs that can be used with children and adolescents in terms of their effects on brain functioning, symptom control, and side-effects. The book is attuned to the difficulties families of OCD children face. *$5.95*

66 pages ISBN 1-890802-28-X

1101 Obsessive-Compulsive Disorder in Children and Adolescents
American Psychiatric Publishing, Inc.
1000 Wilson Boulevard
Suite 1825
Arlington, VA 22209-3901
703-907-7322
800-368-5777; *Fax:* 703-907-1091
appi@psych.org
www.appi.org

Judith L Rapoport, M.D., Editor
Ron McMillen, Chief Executive Officer
John McDuffie, Editorial Director

Examines the early development of obsessive - compulsive disorder and describes effective treatments. *$47.50*

368 pages ISBN 0-880482-82-6

1102 Obsessive-Compulsive Disorder: Theory, Research and Treatment
Guilford Press
72 Spring Street
New York, NY 10012-4068
212-431-9800
800-365-7006; *Fax:* 212-966-6708
info@guilford.com

Bob Matloff, President
Richard Swinson, Author
Martin Antony, Author
S Rachman, Author

Part I: Psychopathology and Theoretical Perspectives; Part II: Assessment and Treatment; Part III: Obsessive Compulsive Spectrum Disorders; Appendix: List of Resources.
$38.25

478 pages Year Founded: 2001 ISBN 1-572307-32-0

1103 Obsessive-Compulsive Disorders: A Complete Guide to Getting Well and Staying Well
Oxford University Press
2001 Evans Road
Cary, NC 27513-2010
919-677-0977
800-445-9714; *Fax:* 919-677-2673
custserv.us@oup.com

In defining obsessive-compulsive disorders (OCDs), our language creates problems, because it treats the terms 'obsessive' and 'compulsion' very loosely. *$39.95*

Year Founded: 2000 ISBN 0-195140-92-3

1104 Obsessive-Compulsive Disorders: Practical Management
Elsevier
PO Box 28430
Saint Louis, MO 63146-930
314-453-7010
800-460-3110; *Fax:* 314-453-7095
www.elsevier.com

Michael A Jenike, MD, Author
Lee Baer, PhD, Author
Wiliam E Minichiello, EdD, Author

Topics include the clinical picture, illnesses relation to obsessive-compulsive disorder, spectrum disorders, patient and clinical management and pathophysiology and assessment. *$73.00*

886 pages Year Founded: 1998 ISBN 0-815138-40-7

1105 Obsessive-Compulsive Disorders: The Latest Assessment and Treatment Strategies
Jones & Bartlett
5 Wall Street
Burlington, MA 01803
978-443-5000
800-832-0034; *Fax:* 978-443-8000
info@jblearning.com
www.jblearning.com

Gail Steketee, PhD, Author
Teresa Pigott, MD, Author

Previously considered a rare mental condition, obsessive compulsive disorder (OCD) now appears to be a hidden epidemic with over 6.5 million sufferers. *$40.95*

104 pages Year Founded: 1983 ISBN 1-887537-28-5

1106 Obsessive-Compulsive Related Disorders
American Psychiatric Publishing, Inc.
1000 Wilson Boulevard
Suite 1825
Arlington, VA 22209-3901
703-907-7322
800-368-5777; *Fax:* 703-907-1091
appi@psych.org
www.appi.org

Eric Hollander, M.D., Editor
Ron McMillen, Chief Executive Officer
John McDuffie, Editorial Director

Discusses the way compulsivity and impulsivity are understood, diagnosed and treated. *$22.50*

304 pages Year Founded: 1992 ISBN 0-880484-02-0

1107 Over and Over Again: Understanding Obsessive-Compulsive Disorder
Jossey-Bass/Wiley
111 River Street
Hoboken, NJ 07030-5773
201-748-6000; *Fax:* 201-748-6088
custserv@wiley.com
www.wiley.com

Fugen Neziroglu, Author
Jose A Yarvura-Tobias, Author

This sensitive and insightful book, the result of the author's years of research and experimentation, is a much needed survival manual for OCD sufferers and the families and friends who share their pain. *$35.00*

240 pages Year Founded: 1997 ISBN 0-787908-76-8

1108 Overcoming Obsessive-Compulsive Disorder: Client Manual: A Behavioral and Cognitive Protocol for the Treatment of OCD
NewHarbinger Publications
5674 Shattuck Avenue
Oakland, CA 94609
800-748-6273; *Fax:* 800-652-1613
customerservice@newharbinger.com
www.newharbinger.com

Matthew McKay PhD, Founder/Author
Gail Steketee PhD, Author

This protocol outlines a fourteen-session treatment for individual adults diagnosed with obsessive-compulsive disorder. This protocol is based on imagined exposure, in vivo exposure, response prevention and avoidance reduction. Copyright 1998 *$29.95*

104 pages Year Founded: 1973 ISBN 1-572241-29-9

1109 Phobic and Obsessive-Compulsive Disorders: Theory, Research, and Practice
Kluwer Academic/Plenum Publishers
233 Spring Street
New York, NY 10013-1522
212-242-1490

Paul M.G. Emmelkamp, Author
 $24.95

366 pages Year Founded: 1992 ISBN 0-306410-44-3

1110 Real Illness: Obsessive-Compulsive Disorder
National Institute of Mental Health
6001 Executive Boulevard
Room 8184
Bethesda, MD 20892-1
301-443-4513
866-615-6464
TTY: 301-443-8431
nimhinfo@nih.gov

Do you have disturbing thoughts and behaviors you know don't make sense but that you can't seem to control? This easy brochure explains how to get help.

9 pages

1111 Rewind, Replay, Repeat: A Memoir of Obsessive-Compulsive Disorder
Hazelden Publishing & Educational Services
PO Box 11
Center City, MN 55012-0011
651-213-4200
800-257-7810; *Fax:* 651-213-4793
info@hazelden.org
www.hazelden.org

Jeff Bell, Author

The revealing story of one man's struggle with obsessive-compulsive disorder (OCD) and his hard-won recovery. Readers will learn what OCD feels like from the inside, and how healing from such a devastating condition is possible through therapy, determination, and the support of loved ones.

368 pages Year Founded: 1949 ISBN 1-592853-71-4

1112 School Personnel
Obsessive-Compulsive Foundation
18 Tremont Street
Suite 903
Boston, MA 02196
617-973-5801; *Fax:* 617-973-5803
info@iocdf.org
www.ocfoundation.org

Denise Egan Stack LMHC, President
Jeff Szymanski,PhD, Executive Director
Susan B Dailey, Vice President
Michael J Stack,CFA, Treasurer

School Personnel: A Critical Link in the Identification, Treatment and Management of OCD in Children and Adolescents. Recognizing OCD in the school setting, current treatments, the role of school personnel in identification, assessment, and educational interventions, are thoroughly covered in this brief, but informative booklet especially targeted to educators and guidance counselors. *$4.00*

19 pages Year Founded: 1986 ISBN B-0006QK-6V-6

1113 Stop Obsessing: How to Overcome Your Obsessions and Compulsions
Anxiety Disorders Association of America
8701 Georgia Avenue
Suite 412
Silver Spring, MD 20910-3643
240-485-1001
AnxDis@adaa.org
www.adaa.org

Edna Foa, Author
Reid Wilson, Author

Book provides knowledgeable descriptions of the steps, the challenges, and the value of self - treatment.

Year Founded: 1980

1114 The Imp of the Mind: Exploring the Silent Epidemic of Obsessive Bad Thoughts
Plume
375 Hudson Street
New York, NY 10014-3657
212-366-2372; *Fax:* 212-366-2933

Lee Baer, PhD, Author

Dr. Lee Baer combines the latest research with his own extensive experience in treating this widespread syndrome. Drawing on information ranging from new advances in brain technology to pervasive social taboos, Dr. Baer explores the root causes of bad thoughts, why they can spiral out of control, and how to recognize the crucial difference between harmless and dangerous bad thoughts. *$12.99*

176 pages Year Founded: 1936 ISSN 978-0452283077ISBN 0-452283-07-8

1115 Tormenting Thoughts and Secret Rituals: The Hidden Epidemic of Obsessive-Compulsive Disorder
Random House
1745 Broadway
3rd Floor
New York, NY 10019-4343
212-782-9000; *Fax:* 212-302-7985
ecustomerservice@randomhouse.com
www.randomhouse.com

Ian Osborn,MD, Author

Discusses the various forms Obsessive-Compulsive Disorder (OCD) takes and, using the most common focuses of obsession, presents detailed cases whose objects are filth, harm, lust, and blasphemy. He explains how the disorder is currently diagnosed and how it differs from addiction, worrying, and preoccupation. He summarizes the recent findings in the areas of brain biology, neuroimaging and genetics that show OCD to be a distinct chemical disorder of the brain. *$14.95*

336 pages Year Founded: 1999 ISBN 0-440508-47-9

1116 When Once Is Not Enough: Help for Obsessive Compulsives
NewHarbinger Publications
5674 Shattuck Avenue
Oakland, CA 94609-1662
510-652-0215
800-748-6273; *Fax:* 800-652-1613
customerservice@newharbinger.com
www.newharbinger.com

Gail Steketee, Author
Kerrin White, Author

How to recognize and confront fears, using simple rituals, positive coping strategies and handling complications. *$14.95*

229 pages Year Founded: 1973 ISBN 0-934986-87-8

Periodicals & Pamphlets

1117 OCD Newsletter
18 Tremont Street
Suite 903
Boston, MA 02196
617-973-5801; *Fax:* 617-973-5803
info@iocdf.org
www.ocfoundation.org

Denise Egan Stack LMHC, President
Jeff Szymanski,PhD, Executive Director
Susan B Dailey, Vice President
Michael J Stack,CFA, Treasurer

A source of news, entertainment, and inspiration to individuals with OCD, their loved ones, and to OCD professionals and researchers.

8-12 pages Year Founded: 1986

Support Groups & Hot Lines

1118 International OCD Foundation
18 Tremont Street
Suite 903
Boston, MA 02108
617-973-5801; *Fax:* 617-973-5803
info@ocfoundation.org
www.ocfoundation.org

Denise Egan Stack LMHC, President
Susan B. Dailey, Vice President
Michael J. Stack CFA, Treasurer
Diane Davey RN, Secretary

An international not-for-profit organization made up of people with Obsessive Compulsive Disorder and related disorders, as well as their families, friends, professionals and others.

Year Founded: 1986

1119 Obsessive-Compulsive Anonymous
PO Box 215
New Hyde Park, NY 11040
516-739-0662; *Fax:* 212-768-4679
west24th@aol.com
www.obsessivecompulsiveanonymous.com

Is a fellowship of people who share their Experience, Strength, and Hope with each other that they may solve their common problem and help others to recover from OCD.

Video & Audio

1120 Hope and Solutions for OCD
International OCD Foundation
18 Tremont Street
Suite 903
Boston, MA 02108
617-973-5801; *Fax:* 617-973-5803
info@ocfoundation.org
www.ocfoundation.org

Denise Egan Stack LMHC, President
Susan B. Dailey, Vice President
Michael J. Stack CFA, Treasurer
Diane Davey RN, Secretary

Finally, a video series about obsessive compulsive disorder. With some straight forward solutions, answers, and advice for individuals who have OCD, their families, their doctors, and school personnel. The Awareness Foundation for OCD & Related Disorders had produced this highly useful, informative, and inspirational series to help guide those with OCD towards confidence, recovery, and hope. *$89.95*

Year Founded: 1986

1121 Touching Tree
Obsessive-Compulsive Foundation
18 Tremont Street
Suite 903
Boston, MA 02108
617-973-5801; *Fax:* 617-973-5803
info@ocfoundation.org
www.ocfoundation.org

Denise Egan Stack LMHC, President
Susan B. Dailey, Vice President
Michael J. Stack CFA, Treasurer
Diane Davey RN, Secretary

This video will foster awareness of early onset obsessive-compulsive disorder (OCD) and demonstrate the symptoms and current therapies that are most successful. Typical ritualistic compulsions of children and adolescents such as touching, hand washing, counting, etc. are explained. *$49.95*

Year Founded: 1986

Web Sites

1122 www.cyberpsych.org
CyberPsych

Presents information about psychoanalysis, psychotherapy and special topics such as anxiety disorders, the problematic use of alcohol, homophobia, and the traumatic effects of racism. Explains in detail what anxiety it is how it is treated and the symptoms associated with anxiety.

1123 www.guidetopsychology.com
A Guide To Psychlogy & Its Practice

Free information on various types of psychology.

1124 www.mayoclinic.com
Mayo Clinic

Provides information on obsessive-compulsive disorder and anxiety.

1125 www.mentalhealth.Samhsa.Gov
Center for Mental Health Services Knowledge Exchange Network

Information about resources, technical assistance, research, training, networks and other federal clearinghouses.

1126 www.nami.org
National Alliance on Mental Illness

From its inception in 1979, NAMI has been dedicated to improving the lives of individuals and families affected by mental illness.

1127 www.nimh.nih.gov/anxiety/anxiety/ocd
National Institute of Health

Information on anxiety disorders and OCD.

1128 www.nimh.nih.gov/publicat/ocdmenu.cfm
Obsessive-Compulsive Disorder

Introductory handout with treatment recommendations.

1129 www.ocdhope.com/gdlines.htm
Guidelines for Families Coping with OCD

1130 www.ocfoundation.org
Obsessive-Compulsive Foundation

An international not-for-profit organization composed of people with obsessive compulsive disorder and related disorders, their families, friends, professionals and other concerned individuals.

1131 www.thenadd.org
National Association for the Dually Diagnosed (NADD)

An association for persons with developmental disabilities and mental health needs.

Personality Disorders

Introduction

Personality is deeply rooted in our sense of ourselves and how others see us; it is formed from a complex intermingling of genetic factors and life experience. Everyone has personality characteristics that are likable and unlikable, attractive and unattractive, to others. By adulthood, most of us have personality traits that are difficult to change. Sometimes, these deeply rooted personality traits can get in the way of our happiness, hinder relationships, and even cause harm to ourselves or others.

For example, a person may have a tendency to be deeply suspicious of other people with no good reason. Another person may assume a haughty, arrogant manner that is difficult to be around. Personality Disorders, by definition, do not cause symptoms, which are experiences that are troublesome to the individual. They consist of whole sets of distorted experiences of the outside world that pervade every or nearly every aspect of a person's life, causing traits and behaviors leading to interpersonal problems which only secondarily cause distress to the individual. The problem is blamed on other people. For example, people with dependent personality disorder feel that they need more care and protection than others, not that they are inordinately demanding of care and protection. People with narcissistic personality disorder feel that others do not respect them, not that they demand more attention and admiration than others; people with paranoid personality disorder feel that others are out to trick and cheat them, not that they are inordinately suspicious; people with obsessive personality disorder feel that others are sloppy, not that they are overly preoccupied with order and tidiness.

A diagnosis of a Personality Disorder should be distinguished from labeling someone as a bad or disagreeable person and not be used to stigmatize people who are simply unpopular, rebellious, or otherwise unorthodox. A Personality Disorder is not simply a personality style, but a condition that interferes with successful living. A Personality Disorder refers to an enduring pattern or experience and behavior that is inflexible, long lasting (often beginning in adolescence or early childhood) and which leads to distress and impairment. Personality disorders frequently co-exist with substance abuse, eating disorders, suicidal thinking and behavior, depression, and other mental disorders.

There are three distinct groups of personality disorders:

A.
• Paranoid Personality Disorder;
• Schizoid Personality Disorder;
• Schizotypal Personality Disorder;

B.
• Antisocial Personality Disorder;
• Borderline Personality Disorder;
• Narcissistic Personality Disorder;

C.
• Avoidant Personality Disorder;
• Dependent Personality Disorder;
• Obsessive-Compulsive Personality Disorder.

SYMPTOMS

An enduring pattern of inner experience and behavior that deviates markedly from the expectations of the individual's culture:
• This pattern is manifested in two or more of the following areas: cognition, affectivity, interpersonal functioning, and impulse control;
• The enduring pattern is inflexible and pervasive across a broad range of personal and social situations;
• The enduring pattern leads to clinically significant distress or impairment in social, occupational, or other important areas of functioning;
• The pattern is stable and of long duration and its onset can be traced back at least to adolescence or early adulthood;
• The enduring pattern is not better accounted for as a manifestation or consequence of another mental disorder;
• The enduring pattern is not due to the direct physiological effects of a substance or a general medical condition.

Antisocial Personality Disorder
• Irresponsible behavior;
• Disregard for the law and the rights of others;
• Symptoms in childhood may include lying, stealing, and disrespect for authority;
• Symptoms in adults may include aggression, frustration, reckless behavior, substance abuse, making irresponsible decisions about money and criminal activity;
• Deception or manipulation of others;
• Lack of remorse.

Avoidant Personality Disorder
• Self-criticism;
• Social awkwardness;
• Social anxiety;
• Social inhibition;
• Hyp ersensitivity;
• Self-criticism;
• May miss school, work, or social events due to fear of rejection, despite desires for a social life.

Borderline Personality Disorder
• Unstable behavior (e.g. self-harm, suicide attempts, suicidal thoughts);
• Unstable emotions (e.g. extreme anger, intense boredom, severe anxiety or depression);
• Unstable relationships;
• Unstable sense of identity (e.g. feelings of emptiness, lack of self-knowledge);
• Awareness problems (e.g. delusions, hallucinations).

Dependent Personality Disorder
• Exhibits an excessive need to be taken care of;
• Feelings of inadequacy, helplessness and incompetence;
• Lack of decision-making or self-motivation skills.

Narcissistic Personality Disorder
• Seeks admiration of others;
• Lack of empathy;
• Sense of entitlement;
• May resort to illegal means or use other people for personal gain.

Obsessive Compulsive Personality Disorder
• Obsession with orderliness, details, and scheduling;
• Need to constantly recheck things to avoid making a mistake;

- Black-and-white thinking;
- Workaholic tendencies;
- Inflexibility;
- Perfectionism that disrupts ever yday living;
- Over-criticism of self and others.

Paranoid Personality Disorder
- Unjustified mistrust and suspicion of others;
- Social isolation;
- Aggressiveness;
- Hostility.

Schizoid Personality Disorder
- Inability to relate to other people;
- Lack of emotion;
- Mechanical behavior;
- Social isolation;
- Social awkwardness;
- Lack of desire for personal interaction.

Schizotypal Personality Disorder
- Discomfort with close relationships;
- Passivity;
- Indifference;
- Awkward or inappropriate social behavior;
- Lack of emotion;
- Peculiarities in appearance (e.g. poor personal hygiene, ill-fitting clothing).

TREATMENT OPTIONS

Most people who suffer from a Personality Disorder do not see themselves as having psychological problems, and therefore do not seek treatment. For those who do, the most effective treatment is long-term (at least one year) psychotherapy. People with Personality Disorders generally seek treatment only because they are distressed about the behavior of those around them. It is important for a patient to find a mental health professional with expert knowledge and experience in treating personality disorders. Some therapists specialize in treating Borderline Personality Disorder. Antisocial Personality Disorder is notably difficult to treat, especially in extreme cases, when the affected individual lacks all concern for others.

Psychotherapy encourages patients to talk about their suspicions, doubts, and other personality traits that have a negative impact on their lives, and therefore helps to improve social interactions.

Psychotherapeutic treatment should include attention to family members, stressing the importance of emotional support, reassurance, explanation of the disorder, and advice on how to manage and respond to the patient. Group therapy is helpful in many situations.

Antipsychotic medication can be useful in patients with certain Personality Disorders, specifically Schizotypal and Borderline Disorders.

Associations & Agencies

1133 Center for Mental Health Services (CMHS)
Substance Abuse and Mental Health Services Administration
5600 Fishers Lane
Rockville, MD 20857

240-276-1310
877-726-4727
TTY: 800-487-4889
www.samhsa.gov/about-us/who-we-are/offices-centers

Paolo del Vecchio, MSW, Director
Anne Mathews-Younes, Acting Deputy Director
Keris Myrick, Director, Consumer Affairs
Patricia Gratton, Director, Program Analysis

Promotes the treatment of mental illness and emotional disorders by increasing accessibility to mental health programs; supporting outreach, treatment, rehabilitation, and support programs and networks; and encouraging the use of scientifically-based information when treating mental disorders. CMHS provides information about mental health via a toll-free number and numerous publications. Developed for users of mental health services and their families, the general public, policy makers, providers, and the media.

Year Founded: 1992

1134 Goodwill's Community Employment Services
Goodwill Industries-Suncoast, Inc.
10596 Gandy Blvd.
St. Petersburg, FL 33702
727-523-1512
888-279-1988
TDD: 727-579-1068
www.goodwill-suncoast.org

Heather Ceresoli, CPA, Chair
Deborah A. Passerini, President
Martin W. Gladysz, Senior Vice Chair
Louise R. Lopez, Vice Chair

Program providing job coaching and community job placements for people with disabilities.

Year Founded: 1954

1135 National Alliance on Mental Illness
3803 North Fairfax Drive
Suite 100
Arlington, VA 22203
703-524-7600
800-950-6264
info@nami.org
www.nami.org

Steve Pitman, JD, President
Lacey Berumen, PhD, MNM, First Vice President
Mary Giliberti, Chief Executive Officer
David Levy, Chief Financial Officer

NAMI is an organization dedicated to raising awareness on mental health and providing support and education for Americans affected by mental illness. NAMI advocates for access to services and treatment and fosters an environment of awareness and understanding for those concerned with mental health.

Year Founded: 1979

1136 National Association for the Dually Diagnosed (NADD)
132 Fair Street
Kingston, NY 12401
845-331-4336
info@thenadd.org
www.thenadd.org

Jeanne M. Farr, MA, Chief Executive Officer
Daniel Baker, PhD., President

Peggie Webb, MA, Vice President
George Zukotynski, PhD., Secretary

NADD is a nonprofit organization designed to increase awareness of, and provide services for, individuals with developmental disabilities and mental illness. NADD emphasizes the importance of quality mental healthcare for people with mental health needs and offers conferences, information resources, educational programs, and training materials to professionals, parents, and organizations.

Year Founded: 1983

1137 National Mental Health Consumers' Self-Help Clearinghouse

1211 Chestnut Street
Suite 1100
Philadelphia, PA 19107
267-507-3810
800-553-4539; *Fax:* 215-636-6312
info@mhselfhelp.org
www.mhselfhelp.org

Joseph Rogers, Founder and Executive Director
Susan Rogers, Director

The Clearinghouse is a peer-run national technical assistance center focused on achieving respect and equality of opportunity for those with mental illnesses. The Clearinghouse helps with the growth of the mental health consumer movement by evaluating mental health services, advocating for mental health reform, and providing consumers with news, information, publications, and consultation services.

Year Founded: 1986

1138 The Center for Family Support

2811 Zulette Avenue
Bronx, NY 10461
718-518-1500; *Fax:* 718-518-8200
www.www.cfsny.org/

Steven Vernikoff, Executive Director
Lloyd Stabiner, President
Amy Bittinger, Vice President
Barbara Greenwald, Associate Executive Director

The Center for Family Support offers assistance to individuals with developmental and related disabilities, as well as their families, and provides support services and programs that are designed to accommodate individual needs. Offers services throughout New York City, Westchester County, Long Island, and New Jersey.

Year Founded: 1954

Books

1139 Biology of Personality Disorders, Review of Psychiatry

American Psychiatric Publishing, Inc.
1000 Wilson Boulevard
Suite 1825
Arlington, VA 22209-3901
703-907-7322
800-368-5777; *Fax:* 703-907-1091
appi@psych.org
www.appi.org

Kenneth R. Silk, Editor

An all-inclusive guide for the study of the etiology and the treatment of personality disorders. For the many patients who suffer from personality disorders and the physicians who have the challenge of successfully treating them, this book is a welcome reference. *$25.00*

176 pages Year Founded: 1998 ISBN 0-880488-35-2

1140 Borderline Personality Disorder

American Psychiatric Publishing, Inc.
1000 Wilson Boulevard
Suite 1825
Arlington, VA 22209-3901
703-907-7322
800-368-5777; *Fax:* 703-907-1091
appi@psych.org
www.appi.org

John G. Gunderson, M.D., Author
Paul S Links, M.D., F.R.C.P.C, Author
John McDuffie, Editorial Director

Guide to the diagnosis and treatment of borderline personality disorder. *$34.00*

366 pages Year Founded: 2008 ISBN 0-880486-89-9

1141 Borderline Personality Disorder: Multidimensional Approach

American Psychiatric Publishing, Inc.
1000 Wilson Boulevard
Suite 1825
Arlington, VA 22209-3901
703-907-7322
800-368-5777; *Fax:* 703-907-1091
appi@psych.org
www.appi.org

Joel Paris, M.D., Author
Ron McMillen, Chief Executive Officer
John McDuffie, Editorial Director

Practical approach to the management of patients with BPD. *$33.00*

232 pages Year Founded: 1994 ISBN 0-880486-55-4

1142 Borderline Personality Disorder: A Patient's Guide to Taking Control

W.W. Norton & Company, Inc.
500 Fifth Avenue
New York, NY 10110
212-354-2907
800-233-4830; *Fax:* 212-869-0856
npb@wwnorton.com
www.books.wwnorton.com/books/

The Patient's Guide is your clients' means to begin to take command of their lives by following the therapeutic course described in these books. Provides a step-by-step cognitive program wich in worksheets and exercises to facilitate your clients' personal process of self-examination and problem solving.

ISBN 0-393703-53-3

1143 Borderline Personality Disorder: Etiology and Treatment

American Psychiatric Publishing, Inc.
1000 Wilson Boulevard
Suite 1825
Arlington, VA 22209-3901
703-907-7322
800-368-5777; *Fax:* 703-907-1091
appi@psych.org
www.appi.org

Robert E Hales MD, Editor-in-Chief
Ron McMillen, Chief Executive Officer
John McDuffie, Editorial Director

Provides empirical data as the basis for progress in understanding and treating the borderline patient. *$50.00*

420 pages ISBN 0-880484-08-X

1144 Borderline Personality Disorder: Tailoring the Psychotherapy to the Patient
American Psychiatric Publishing, Inc.
1000 Wilson Boulevard
Suite 1825
Arlington, VA 22209-3901
703-907-7322
800-368-5777; *Fax:* 703-907-1091
appi@psych.org
www.appi.org

Leonard Horwitz, Ph.D, Author
Glen O Gabbard, M.D, Author
Jon G Allen, Ph.D, Author
Donald B Colson, Ph.D, Author

Emphasizes how the clinician should decide between the use of supportive as opposed to expressive techniques, depending upon the characteristics of the patient. *$34.00*

272 pages Year Founded: 1996 ISBN 0-880486-89-9

1145 Borderline Personality Disorder: The Latest Assessment and Treatment Strategies
Jones & Bartlett Learning
5 Wall Street
Burlington, MA 01803-4211
978-443-5000
800-832-0034; *Fax:* 978-443-8000
info@jblearning.com
www.jblearning.com

Melanie Dean,PhD, Author

7 typical characteristics of those with BPD, differential diagnostic concerns, treatment strategies for interpersonal, cognitive, dialectical behavior, and group therapy, 13 predisposing factors for suicide, 4 psychometric assessment tools, new self-report and interview instruments, treatment dialogue examples for vaious theoretical approaches, comparison table of 6 classes of medications used to treat BPD and 6 key relapse prevention treatment strategies.

88 pages Year Founded: 1983

1146 Challenging Behaviour, Third Edition
Cambridge University Press
32 Avenue of the Americas
New York, NY 10013-2473
212-337-5000
newyork@cambridge.org
www.www.cambridge.org

Eric Emerson, Author
Stewart L Einfield, Author

This edition contains significantly expanded sections on the emergence and development of challenging behaviour and strategies for prevention, at the level of both individuals and service systems. Essential reading for students undertaking professional training in health and related aspects of intellectual disabilities, including psychologists, psychiatrists, nurses, teachers and social workers. This book is a key text for professional staff delivering health, educational and social care services to people with intellectual disabilities.

224 pages Year Founded: 1534 ISBN 0-521728-93-5

1147 Clinical Assessment and Management of Severe Personality Disorders
American Psychiatric Publishing, Inc.
1000 Wilson Boulevard
Suite 1825
Arlington, VA 22209-3901
703-907-7322
800-368-5777; *Fax:* 703-907-1091
appi@psych.org
www.appi.org

Paul S Links, M.D., F.R.C.P.C, Editor
Ron McMillen, Chief Executive Officer
John McDuffie, Editorial Director

Focuses on issues relevant to the clinician in private practice, including the diagnosis of a wide range of personality disorders and alternative management approaches. *$33.00*

250 pages Year Founded: 1995 ISBN 0-880484-88-8

1148 Cognitive Analytic Therapy & Borderline Personality Disorder: Model and the Method
John Wiley & Sons
111 River Street
Hoboken, NJ 07030-5774
201-748-6000
877-762-2974; *Fax:* 201-748-6088
info@wiley.com
www.wiley.com

Anthony Ryle, Author

This book documents CAT's recent theoretical and practical developments is a must for anyone interested in CAT itself and in integrative approaches, for those interested in brief, psychodynamically informed therapy, or indeed for those interested in developments in psychology generally. *$70.00*

206 pages Year Founded: 1997 ISBN 0-471976-18-0

1149 Cognitive Therapy of Personality Disorders, Second Edition
The Guilford Press
72 Spring Street
New York, NY 10012
212-431-9800
800-365-7006; *Fax:* 212-966-6708
info@guilford.com
www.guilford.com

Aaron T. Beck, M.D., Author
Arthur Freeman, Author
Denise D. Davis Ph.D., Author

This landmark work was the first to present a cognitive framework for understanding and treating personality disorders.

412 pages Year Founded: 1973 ISBN 1-572308-56-7

1150 Developmental Model of Borderline Personality Disorder: Understanding Variations in Course and Outcome
American Psychiatric Publishing, Inc.
1000 Wilson Boulevard
Suite 1825
Arlington, VA 22209-3901
703-907-7322
800-368-5777; *Fax:* 703-907-1091

appi@psych.org
www.appi.org

Patricia Hoffman Judd, Ph.D, Author
Thomas H McGlashan, M.D., Author
John McDuffie, Editorial Director

Landmark work on this difficult condition. Emphasizes a developmental approach to BPD based on treatment of in-patients at Chestnut Lodge in Rockville, Maryland, during the years through 1975. Using information gleaned from the original clinical notes and follow-up studies, the authors present four intriguing case studies to chart the etiology, long-term course, and clinical manifestations of BPD. *$34.95*

248 pages Year Founded: 2003 ISBN 0-880485-15-9

1151 Disordered Personalities
Rapid Psychler Press
2014 Holland Avenue
Suite 374
Port Huron, MI 48060-1994
519-667-2335
888-779-2453; *Fax:* 888-779-2457
rapid@psychler.com
www.psychler.com

David J. Robinson, MD, Author

Provides a comprehensive, practical and entertaining over-view of the DSM-IV personality disorders. The diagnostic, theoretical and therapeutic principles relevant to under-standing character pathology are detailed in the introduc-tory chapters. *$39.95*

430 pages Year Founded: 2005 ISBN 1-894328-09-4

1152 Disorders of Narcissism: Diagnostic, Clinical, and Empirical Implications
American Psychiatric Publishing, Inc.
1000 Wilson Boulevard
Suite 1825
Arlington, VA 22209-3901
703-907-7322
800-368-5777; *Fax:* 703-907-1091
appi@psych.org
www.appi.org

Elsa Ronningstam, Ph.D., Editor
Ron McMillen, Chief Executive Officer
John McDuffie, Editorial Director

Addresses important subjects at the forefront of the study of narcissism, including cognitive treatment, normal narcis-sism, pathological narcissism and suicide, and the connec-tion between pathological narcissism, trauma, and alexithymia. *$42.50*

512 pages Year Founded: 1998 ISBN 0-880487-01-1

1153 Drug Therapy and Personality Disorders
Mason Crest Publishers
450 Parkway Drive
Suite D
Broomall, PA 19008-4017
610-543-6200
866-627-2665; *Fax:* 610-543-3878
dtaylor@masoncrest.com
www.masoncrest.com

Shirley Brinkerhoff, Author

What is a personality disorder? Can it be treated? If so, how? What can people do about their troublsome symp-toms? These are just a few of the questions Drug Therapy and Personality Disorders answers. Learn about these com-mon forms of mental illness and the treatments that bring new hope to those who suffer with them.

128 pages Year Founded: 2004 ISBN 1-590845-71-4

1154 Fatal Flaws: Navigating Destructive Relationships with People with Disorders of Personality and Character
American Psychiatric Publishing, Inc.
1000 Wilson Boulevard
Suite 1825
Arlington, VA 22209-3901
703-907-7322
800-368-5777; *Fax:* 703-907-1091
appi@psych.org
www.appi.org

Stuart C. Yudofsky, Author

Featuring case vignettes from nearly 30 years of Dr. Yudofsky's clinical practice and incorporating the knowl-edge of gifted clinicians, educators, and research scientists with whom he has collaborated throughout that time.

512 pages Year Founded: 2005

1155 Field Guide to Personality Disorders: A Companion to Disordered Personalities
Rapid Psychler Press
2014 Holland Avenue
Suite 374
Port Huron, MI 48060-1994
519-667-2335
888-779-2453; *Fax:* 888-779-2457
rapid@psychler.com
www.psychler.com

David J. Robinson, MD, Author

Practical introduction to the DSM-IV personality disorders. Covers diagnosis, theoretical and therapeutic principles. Each chapter covers a different personality Synopsis of the text Disordered Personalities. *$19.95*

212 pages Year Founded: 2005 ISBN 1-894328-10-8

1156 Get Me Out of Here: My Recovery from Borderline Personality Disorder
Hazelden
PO Box 11
Center City, MN 55012-0011
651-213-4200
800-257-7810; *Fax:* 651-213-4793
info@hazelden.org
www.hazelden.org

Rachel Reiland, Author

With astonishing honesty, Reiland's memoir reveals what mental illness feels like and looks like from the inside, and how healing from such a devastating disease is possible through intensive therapy and the support of loved ones.

464 pages Year Founded: 1949 ISBN 1-592850-99-5

1157 I Hate You, Don't Leave Me: Understanding the Borderline Personality
Avon, Imprint of Harper Collins Publishers
10 East 53rd Street
11th Floor
New York, NY 20706-1002

212-207-7528
800-242-7737
orders@harpercollins.com
www.harpercollins.com

Jerold J. Kreisman MD, Author
Hal Strauss, Author

For years BPD was difficult to describe, diagnose, and treat. But now, for the first time, Dr. Jerold J. Kreisman and health writer Hal Straus offer much-needed professional advice, helping victims and their families to understand and cope with this troubling, shockingly widespread affliction.

288 pages Year Founded: 1991 ISBN 0-380713-05-5

1158 Lost in the Mirror: An Inside Look at Borderline Personality Disorder
Sidran Institute
200 E Joppa Road
Suite 207
Baltimore, MD 21286-3107
410-825-8888
888-825-8249; *Fax: 410-337-0747*
sidran@sidran.org
www.sidran.org

Richard A. Moskovitz,MD, Author

Dr. Moskovitz considers BPD to be part of the dissociative continuum, as it has many causes, symptoms and behaviors in common with Dissociative Disorder. This book is intended for people diagnosed with BPD, their families and therapists. Outlines the features of BPD, including abuse histories, dissociation, mood swings, self harm, impulse control problems and many more. Includes an extensive resource section. *$13.95*

190 pages

1159 Management of Countertransference with Borderline Patients
American Psychiatric Publishing, Inc.
1000 Wilson Boulevard
Suite 1825
Arlington, VA 22209-3901
703-907-7322
800-368-5777; *Fax: 703-907-1091*
appi@psych.org
www.appi.org

Glen O Gabbard, M.D, Author
Sallye M. Wilkinson, Ph.D., Author
John McDuffie, Editorial Director

Open and detailed discussion of the emotional reactions that clinicians experience when treating borderline patients. *$34.50*

272 pages Year Founded: 1994 ISBN 0-880785-63-9

1160 Personality Disorders in Modern Life
John Wiley & Sons
111 River Street
Hoboken, NJ 07030-5774
201-748-6000
877-762-2974; *Fax: 201-748-6088*
info@wiley.com
www.wiley.com

Carrie M. Millon, Author
Sarah Meagher, Author
Seth Grossman, Author
Rowena Ramnath, Author

Exploring the continuum from normal personality tests to the diagnosis amd treatment of severe cases of personality disorders.

624 pages Year Founded: 2004 ISBN 0-471237-34-5

1161 Personality and Psychopathology
American Psychiatric Publishing, Inc.
1000 Wilson Boulevard
Suite 1825
Arlington, VA 22209-3901
703-907-7322
800-368-5777; *Fax: 703-907-1091*
appi@psych.org
www.appi.org

C. Robert Cloninger, Editor

Compiles the most recent findings from more than 30 internationally recognized experts. Analyzes the association between personality and psychopathology from several interlocking perspective, descriptive, developmental, etiological, and therapeutic. *$58.50*

544 pages Year Founded: 1999 ISBN 0-880489-23-5

1162 Role of Sexual Abuse in Etiology of Borderline Personality Disorder
American Psychiatric Publishing, Inc.
1000 Wilson Boulevard
Suite 1825
Arlington, VA 22209-3901
703-907-7322
800-368-5777; *Fax: 703-907-1091*
appi@psych.org
www.appi.org

Mary C. Zanarini, Editor

Presenting the latest generation of research findings about the impact of traumatic abuse on the development of BPD. This book focuses on the theoretical basis of BPD, including topics such as childhood factors associated with the development, the relationship of child sexual abuse to dissociation and self-mutilation, severity of childhood abuse, borderline symptoms and family environment. Twenty six contributors cover every aspect of BPD as it relates to childhood sexual abuse. *$65.00*

264 pages Year Founded: 1996 ISBN 0-880484-96-9

1163 Stop Walking on Eggshells: Taking Your Life Back When Someone You Care About Has Borderline Personality Disorder
NewHarbinger Publications
5674 Shattuck Avenue
Oakland, CA 94609-1662
510-652-0215
800-748-6273; *Fax: 800-652-1613*
customerservice@newharbinger.com
www.newharbinger.com

Paul T. Mason, MS, Author
Randi Kreger, Author

Stop Walking on Eggshells has helped nearly half a million people with friends and family members suffering from BPD understand this destructive disorder, set boundaries, and help their loved ones stop relying on dangerous BPD behaviors. This fully revised edition has been updated with the very latest BPD research and includes coping and communication skills you can use to stabilize your relationship with the BPD sufferer in your life. *$15.95*

288 pages Year Founded: 1973 ISBN 1-572241-08-X

1164 Structured Interview for DSM-IV Personality (SIDP-IV)
American Psychiatric Publishing, Inc.
1000 Wilson Boulevard
Suite 1825
Arlington, VA 22209-3901
703-907-7322
800-368-5777; *Fax:* 703-907-1091
appi@psych.org
www.appi.org
Bruce Pfohl, M.D, Author
Nancee Blum, M.S.W, Author
Mark Zimmerman, M.D, Author

Semistructured interview uses nonperorative questions to examine behavior and personality traits from the patient's perspective. *$21.95*

48 pages Year Founded: 1997 ISBN 0-880489-37-5

1165 The Angry Heart: Overcoming Borderline and Addictive Disorders: An Interactive Self-Help Guide
NewHarbinger Publications
5674 Shattuck Avenue
Oakland, CA 94609-1662
510-652-0215
800-748-6273; *Fax:* 800-652-1613
customerservice@newharbinger.com
www.newharbinger.com
Joseph Santoro, Author
Ronald Jay Cohen, Author

The emotional turmoil and impulsive behavior that characterize borderline personality disorder are so often accompanied by alcoholism or drug abuse that some estimates suggest that as many as half of the millions of people with substance abuse prolems may have a masked borderline personality disorder. This self-help guide offers a range of exercises and step-by-step techniques to help you come to terms with the destructive aspects of your lifestyle *$15.95*

272 pages Year Founded: 1973 ISBN 1-572240-80-6

1166 The Borderline Personality Disorder Survival Guide: Everything You Need to Know About Living with BPD
NewHarbinger Publications
5674 Shattuck Avenue
Oakland, CA 94609-1662
510-652-0215
800-748-6273; *Fax:* 800-652-1613
customerservice@newharbinger.com
www.newharbinger.com
Alex L Chapman, Author
Kim L Gratz, Author

This book provides answers to many questions one might have about BPD: what is it, how long does it last, what other problems co-occur with BPD?

256 pages Year Founded: 1973 ISBN 1-572245-07-7

1167 Understanding the Borderline Mother: Helping Her Children Transcend the Intense, Unpredictable, and Volatile Relationship
Jason Aronson
4501 Forbes Blvd
Suite 200
Lanham, MD 20706
301-459-3366; *Fax:* 301-429-5748
www.www.rowmanlittlefield.com
Christine Ann Lawson, Author

Vividly describes how mothers who suffer from borderline personality disorder produce children who may flounder in life even as adults, futilely struggling to reach the safety of a parental harbor, unable to recognize that their borderline parent lacks a pier, or even a discernible shore. Four character profiles describe different symptom clusters that include the waif mother, the hermit mother, the queen mother, and the witch. Addressing the adult children of borderlines and the therapists who work with them, Dr. Lawson shows how to care for the waif without rescuing her, to attend to the hermit without feeding her fear, to love the queen without becoming her subject, and to live with the witch without becoming her victim. *$37.50*

352 pages Year Founded: 2002

Support Groups & Hot Lines

1168 Out of the FOG
www.www.outofthefog.net

Providing information and support to the family members and loved-ones of individuals who suffer from a personality disorder. A supportive, close-knit community encouraging one another through the many challenges that come with having a family member or significant other who has a personality disorder. FOG stands for Fear, Obligation, and Guilt, feelings which often result from being in a relationship with a person who suffers from a Personality Disorder.

Year Founded: 2007

1169 Paranoid Personality Disorder Forum
Mental Health Matters
www.www.psychforums.com/paranoid-personality/

A helpful user to user forum for support and information about Paranoid Personality Disorders.

1170 S.A.F.E. Alternatives
7115 W North Avenue
PMB 319
Oak Park, IL 60302-1002
708-366-9066
800-366-8288; *Fax:* 708-366-9065
info@selfinjury.com
www.selfinjury.com
Karen Conterio, CEO & Founder
Wendy Lader, PhD, M.Ed, Clinical Director
Michelle Seliner MSW, LCSW, Chief Operating Officer
Joni Nowicki, BA, Admissions Coordinator

A world-renowned treatment program that in it's more than twenty years of operation has helped thousands of people successfully end self-injurious behavior. A treatment team of experts uses therapy, education, and support to empower clients to identify healthier ways to cope with emotional distress. The S.A.F.E. Alternatives philosophy and model of treatment focus on shifting control to the client, empowering them to make healthy choices, including the choice to not self-injure.

Year Founded: 1986

Video & Audio

1171 Anger Management-Enhanced Edition
Educational Video Network, Inc.
1401 19th Street
Huntsville, TX 77340
936-295-5767
800-762-0060; *Fax:* 936-294-0233
www.www.evndirect.com

Learn what causes anger and understand why our bodies react as they do when we're angry. Effective techniques for assuaging anger are discussed.

1172 Beating Depression
Educational Training Videos
136 Granville St
Suite 200
Gahanna, OH 43230
Fax: 888-775-3919
www.educationaltrainingvideos.com

This program comes to grips with depression through the experiences of five patients whose backgrounds span the socioeconomic spectrum. Three cases of chronic depression, one of which is complicated by borderline personality disorder and another by alcohol abuse, and two cases of bipolar disorder, one of which is extreme, are presented.

1173 Clinical Impressions: Identifying Mental Illness
Educational Training Videos
136 Granville St
Suite 200
Gahanna, OH 43230
Fax: 888-775-3919
www.educationaltrainingvideos.com

How long can mental illness stay hidden, especially from the eyes of trained experts? This program rejoins a group of ten adults- five of them healthy and five of them with histories of mental illness- as psychiatric specialists try to spot and correctly diagnose the latter. Administering a series of collaborative and one-on-one tests, including assessments of personality type, physical self-image, and rational thinking, the panel gradually makes decisions about who suffers from depression, bipolar disorder, bulimia, and social anxiety.

1174 Dealing with Social Anxiety
Educational Video Network, Inc.
1401 19th Street
Huntsville, TX 77340
936-295-5767
800-762-0060; *Fax:* 936-294-0233
www.www.evndirect.com

Social anxiety is America's third-largest psychiatric disorder. It generally develops during the mid-teen years, and almost always before the age of 25. Understand what may trigger the development of anxiety and learn how it sometimes evolves into full-blown panic disorder, which is characterized by recurrent attacks of terror or fear. The consequences of social anxiety are examined and effective treatments are discussed.

1175 FRONTLINE: The Released
PBS
2100 Crystal Drive
Arlington, VA 22202
www.pbs.org

Will Lyman, Actor
Narrator
Miri Navasky, Director
Karen O'Connor, Director

The documentary states that of the 700,000 inmates released from American prisons each year, half of them have mental disabilities. This work focused on those with severe problems who keep entering and exiting prison. Full of good information on the challenges they face with mental illnesses; housing, employment, stigmatization, and socialization.

Year Founded: 2009

1176 Lost in the Mirror: Women with Multiple Personalities
Educational Training Videos
136 Granville St
Suite 200
Gahanna, OH 43230
Fax: 888-775-3919
www.educationaltrainingvideos.com

In this program, ABC News anchors Diane Sawyer and Sam Donaldson study the causes and key signs of dissociative identity disorder and the fragmented lives of two people dealing with its effects.

1177 Mental Disorder
Educational Training Videos
136 Granville St
Suite 200
Gahanna, OH 43230
Fax: 888-775-3919
www.educationaltrainingvideos.com

What is abnormality? Using the case studies of two young women; one who has depression, one who has an anxiety disorder; as a springboard, this program presents three psychological perspective on mental disorder.

1178 Multiple Personality Disorder: In the Shadows
Educational Training Videos
136 Granville St
Suite 200
Gahanna, OH 43230
Fax: 888-775-3919
www.educationaltrainingvideos.com

This program shows how therapy can integrate the multiple personalities and make a patient whole again. Following two MPD patients and health care professionals, the program traces the struggles and triumphs in treating this disorder.

1179 Understanding Mental Illness
Educational Video Network, Inc.
1401 19th Street
Huntsville, TX 77340
936-295-5767
800-762-0060; *Fax:* 936-294-0233
www.www.evndirect.com

Contains information and classifications of mental illness. Mental illness can strike anyone, at any age. Learn about various organic and functional mental disorders as discussed and their causes and symptoms, and learn where to seek help for a variety of mental health concerns.

1180 Understanding Personality Disorders
Educational Video Network, Inc.
1401 19th Street
Huntsville, TX 77340
936-295-5767
800-762-0060; *Fax:* 936-294-0233
www.www.evndirect.com

For many people, the onset of a psychological disorder goes undiagnosed and untreated, and, as a result, they face a constant, if not impossible, struggle to maintain good mental health. This can be especially true when individuals suffer from a personality disorder. However, with identification and understanding, crippling personality disorders can be brought out of the shadows of ignorance and into the light of treatment.

Web Sites

1181 www.cyberpsych.org
CyberPsych

Presents information about psychoanalysis, psychotherapy and special topics such as anxiety disorders, the problematic use of alcohol, homophobia, and the traumatic effects of racism

1182 www.mentalhealth.com
Internet Mental Health

Offers online psychiatric diagnosis in the hope of reaching the two-thirds of individuals with mental illness who do not seek treatment.

1183 www.mhsanctuary.com/borderline
Borderline Personality Disorder Sanctuary

Borderline personality disorder education, communities, support, books, and resources.

1184 www.nimh.nih.gov/publicat/ocdmenu.cfm
Obsessive-Compulsive Disorder

Introductory handout with treatment recommendations.

1185 www.ocdhope.com/ocd-families.php
OCD Resource Center of Florida

1186 www.outofthefog.net
Out of the FOG

Information and support for those with a family member or loved one who suffers from a personality disorder.

1187 www.planetpsych.com
Planetpsych.com

The online resource for mental health information.

1188 www.psychcentral.com
Psych Central

The Internet's largest and oldest independent mental health social network created and run by mental health professionals to guarantee reliable, trusted information and support communities to you.

1189 www.store.samhsa.gov
Substance Abuse and Mental Health Services Administration

Resources on mental disorders as well as treatment and recovery.

Schizophrenia Spectrum and Other Psychotic Disorders

Introduction

Schizophrenia is an old term meaning, approximately, 'split personality.' While the name of the diagnosis survives, the concept of split personality is outdated.

Schizophrenia is a devastating disease of the brain that severely impairs an individual's ability to think, feel, and function normally. Though not a common disorder, it is one of the most destructive, disrupting the lives of sufferers, as well as of family members and loved ones. Long misunderstood, people with Schizophrenia and their families have also borne a burden of stigma in addition to the burden of their illness.

Although family and other environmental stressors can play a role in precipitating or exacerbating episodes of illness, theories that the disease is caused by poor parenting have been discredited. Much has been learned about the disease in recent years and treatments have improved markedly.

Schizophrenia is a largely genetically determined disorder of the brain. One theory is that it is a disorder of information processing resulting from a defect in the prefrontal cortex of the brain. Because this system is defective, an individual with Schizophrenia is easily overwhelmed by the amount of information and stimuli coming from the environment. Schizophrenia causes hallucinations, which are sensory experiences in the absence of actual stimuli (hearing voices when no one is speaking), and delusions, which are bizarre beliefs (that the individual is God, that the television is conveying messages specifically aimed at the individual, that some power is removing the individual's thoughts from his or her mind). Speech may be tangential or confused. These are called 'positive symptoms.' The individual also loses some normal behaviors and experiences, engaging in little behavior or social interaction and displaying catatonic behavior and a flat or grossly inappropriate emotional state. These are called 'negative symptoms.' Schizophrenia is a chronic disease and, once diagnosed, a person often needs treatment for the rest of his or her life. However, great strides have been made in treating the disease and many individuals with schizophrenia can hold jobs, marry, parent children, and have gratifying and productive lives.

SYMPTOMS

So-called 'positive' symptoms (experiences not shared by people in society):
• Delusions or false and bizarre beliefs;
• Hallucinations.

Negative symptoms (the loss of normal behaviors):
• Withdrawing from social contact;
• Speaking less;
• Losing interest in things and the ability to enjoy them;
• Disorganized speech;
• Grossly disorganized or catatonic behavior (extremely agitated or zombie-like);
• The symptoms cause social and occupational dysfunction;
• Signs of the disturbance persist for at least six months;
• The symptoms must not be related to mood or depressive disorders, substance abuse, or general medical conditions.

ASSOCIATED FEATURES

People with Schizophrenia, because their disease causes difficulty in perceiving their environment and responding to it normally, often act strange, and have odd beliefs. They sometimes react to stimuli (voices or images originating inside their brains) as though they were originating in their environment; hallucinations and delusions can make a person's behavior appear bizarre to others. Anhedonia, the inability to enjoy pleasurable activities, is common in Schizophrenia, as are sleep disturbances and abnormalities of psychomotor activity. The latter may take the form of pacing, rocking, or immobility. Negative symptoms can be more disabling than positive ones. Family members often become annoyed because they think the individual is just lazy. Schizophrenia takes many forms, and there are a number of subtypes of the illness, including paranoid schizophrenia.

Individuals with untreated Schizophrenia, under the influence of hallucinations and delusions, have a slightly greater propensity for violence than the general population, but only when there is co-existing alcohol or substance abuse, which is quite common. Schizophrenia is known as a heterogenous disease, meaning that the illness takes many forms, depending on a variety of individual characteristics and circumstances. Patients who receive appropriate treatment are not more violent than the general population.

The life expectancy of people with Schizophrenia is shorter than the general population for a variety of reasons: suicide is common among people with the disease (about ten percent die from suicide) and people with Schizophrenia often have both poor medical care and poor health.

PREVALENCE

The first episode of Schizophrenia usually occurs in teenage years, although some cases may occur in the late thirties or forties. Onset prior to puberty is rare, though cases in five year olds have been reported. Women have a later average of onset and a better prognosis. Estimates of the prevalence of Schizophrenia vary widely around the world, but probably about one percent of the world population has the disease.

TREATMENT OPTIONS

Medications can diminish or eliminate many of the positive symptoms of Schizophrenia. Older medications, such as Haldol, are effective and inexpensive, but cause more side effects than newer medications, such as Zyprexa and Geodon. Clozapine was the first and is still one of the most effective treatments, but it causes a low incidence of a life-threatening blood disorder; therefore, people who take it must have blood tests at regular intervals. The newer medications are more effective in treating the negative, as well as the positive, symptoms.

Often, patients report that antipsychotic medications make them feel foggy, or lethargic. Antipsychotic medications can have serious side effects, including Tardive Dyskinesia, which consists of involuntary muscular movements. The newer antipsychotic medications are less sedating and have a decreased risk of causing Tardive Dyskinesia, but are associated with significant weight gain and increased risk of diabetes. There is considerable public controversy as to whether the weight gain, and risk of diabetes associated with the newer medications, along with their cost, outweigh their advantages.

Having Schizophrenia interferes with taking care of oneself and getting proper medical care in several ways; Schizophrenia often depletes financial resources so that patients cannot afford medication, nutrition, and medical care. Untreated Schizophrenia can also interfere with an individual's ability to understand signs and symptoms of medical disorders. Compliance with medication is often a problem, and failure to continue taking medication is a major cause of relapse. For this reason, treatment should include supportive therapy, in which a psychiatrist or other mental health professional provides counseling aimed at helping the patient maintain a positive and optimistic attitude focused on staying healthy. Other forms of therapy, such as social skills training, have also found some success and may be useful in helping a person with Schizophrenia learn appropriate social and interpersonal behavior. Cognitive behavioral therapy may also be helpful in treating Schizophrenia.

Families of persons with Schizophrenia are often also affected by the disease and can be helped by support and advocacy groups.

It is important to note that psychotic illness does not necessarily affect all aspects of an individual's thinking. People with Schizophrenia may have bizarre beliefs or behavior in one sphere of life but be perfectly able to make decisions and function in other areas. In addition, it is crucial not to destroy an individual or family's hopes of a normal life by communicating the message that Schizophrenia is hopeless.

Paranoid Schizophrenia is especially difficult to treat. Paranoia, the irrational conviction that other people, institutions (e.g., the FBI), or alien beings are attempting to harm the individual, prevents the individual from forming trusting relationships with care providers and adhe

Associations & Agencies

1191 Brain & Behavior Research Foundation
90 Park Avenue
16th Floor
New York, NY 10016
646-681-4888
800-829-8289
info@bbrfoundation.org
www.www.bbrfoundation.org/

Steve Lieber, Chairman of the Board
Jeffrey Borenstein, MD, President and CEO
Louis Innamorato, CPA, VP and Chief Financial Officer
Anne Abramson, Vice President

The Brain and Behavior Research Foundation awards grants aimed at advancing scientific understandings of mental health treatments and mental disorders such as depression and schizophrenia. The Brain and Behavior Research Foundation's mission is to eliminate the suffering caused by mental illness.

Year Founded: 1987

1192 Center for Mental Health Services (CMHS)
Substance Abuse and Mental Health Services
Administration
5600 Fishers Lane
Rockville, MD 20857

240-276-1310
877-726-4727
TTY: 800-487-4889
www.samhsa.gov/about-us/who-we-are/offices-centers

Paolo del Vecchio, MSW, Director
Anne Mathews-Younes, Acting Deputy Director
Keris Myrick, Director, Consumer Affairs
Patricia Gratton, Director, Program Analysis

Promotes the treatment of mental illness and emotional disorders by increasing accessibility to mental health programs; supporting outreach, treatment, rehabilitation, and support programs and networks; and encouraging the use of scientifically-based information when treating mental disorders. CMHS provides information about mental health via a toll-free number and numerous publications. Developed for users of mental health services and their families, the general public, policy makers, providers, and the media.

Year Founded: 1992

1193 Goodwill's Community Employment Services
Goodwill Industries-Suncoast, Inc.
10596 Gandy Blvd.
St. Petersburg, FL 33702
727-523-1512
888-279-1988
TDD: 727-579-1068
www.goodwill-suncoast.org

Heather Ceresoli, CPA, Chair
Deborah A. Passerini, President
Martin W. Gladysz, Senior Vice Chair
Louise R. Lopez, Vice Chair

Program providing job coaching and community job placements for people with disabilities.

Year Founded: 1954

1194 Mental Health America
500 Montgomery Street
Suite 820
Alexandria, VA 22314
703-684-7722
800-969-6642; *Fax:* 703-684-5968
www.mentalhealthamerica.net

Reginald Williams, Chair of the Board
Paul Gionfriddo, President and CEO
Jessica Kennedy, Chief of Staff/VP of Finance
Theresa Nguyen, VP of Policy and Programs

Mental Health America is a community-based nonprofit organization committed to enabling the mental wellness of all Americans. MHA advocates for greater access to quality health services and seeks to educate individuals on identifying symptoms, as well as intervention and prevention.

Year Founded: 1909

1195 National Alliance on Mental Illness
3803 North Fairfax Drive
Suite 100
Arlington, VA 22203
703-524-7600
800-950-6264
info@nami.org
www.nami.org

Steve Pitman, JD, President
Lacey Berumen, PhD, MNM, First Vice President

Mary Giliberti, Chief Executive Officer
David Levy, Chief Financial Officer

NAMI is an organization dedicated to raising awareness on mental health and providing support and education for Americans affected by mental illness. NAMI advocates for access to services and treatment and fosters an environment of awareness and understanding for those concerned with mental health.

Year Founded: 1979

1196 National Association for the Dually Diagnosed (NADD)
132 Fair Street
Kingston, NY 12401
845-331-4336
info@thenadd.org
www.thenadd.org

Jeanne M. Farr, MA, Chief Executive Officer
Daniel Baker, PhD., President
Peggie Webb, MA, Vice President
George Zukotynski, PhD., Secretary

NADD is a nonprofit organization designed to increase awareness of, and provide services for, individuals with developmental disabilities and mental illness. NADD emphasizes the importance of quality mental healthcare for people with mental health needs and offers conferences, information resources, educational programs, and training materials to professionals, parents, and organizations.

Year Founded: 1983

1197 National Mental Health Consumers' Self-Help Clearinghouse
1211 Chestnut Street
Suite 1100
Philadelphia, PA 19107
267-507-3810
800-553-4539; *Fax: 215-636-6312*
info@mhselfhelp.org
www.mhselfhelp.org

Joseph Rogers, Founder and Executive Director
Susan Rogers, Director

The Clearinghouse is a peer-run national technical assistance center focused on achieving respect and equality of opportunity for those with mental illnesses. The Clearinghouse helps with the growth of the mental health consumer movement by evaluating mental health services, advocating for mental health reform, and providing consumers with news, information, publications, and consultation services.

Year Founded: 1986

1198 The Center for Family Support
2811 Zulette Avenue
Bronx, NY 10461
718-518-1500; *Fax: 718-518-8200*
www.www.cfsny.org/

Steven Vernikoff, Executive Director
Lloyd Stabiner, President
Amy Bittinger, Vice President
Barbara Greenwald, Associate Executive Director

The Center for Family Support offers assistance to individuals with developmental and related disabilities, as well as their families, and provides support services and programs that are designed to accommodate individual needs. Offers services throughout New York City, Westchester County, Long Island, and New Jersey.

Year Founded: 1954

Books

1199 Biology of Schizophrenia and Affective Disease
American Psychiatric Publishing, Inc.
1000 Wilson Boulevard
Suite 1825
Arlington, VA 22209-3901
703-907-7322
800-368-5777; *Fax: 703-907-1091*
appi@psych.org
www.appi.org

Stanley J. Watson, MD, PhD, Editor

Provides a state-of-the-art look at the biological basis of several mental illness from the perspective of the researchers making these discoveries. This outstanding reference tool explores the explosive progress in the fields of biochemistry, molecular genetics, neuroscience, and brain circuit anatomy and the resultant advances in nearly every aspect of the biology of the brain and mental illness. The book also discusses treatment issues, including the mechanisms of action of antidepressants and atypical antipsychotic drugs. *$58.50*

560 pages Year Founded: 1995 ISBN 0-880487-46-7

1200 Breakthroughs in Antipsychotic Medications: A Guide for Consumers, Families, and Clinicians
National Alliance on Mental Illness
2107 Wilson Boulevard
Suite 300
Arlington, VA 22201-3080
703-524-7600
800-950-6264; *Fax: 703-524-9094*
TDD: 703-516-7227
generalinquiry@center4si.com
www.homeless.samhsa.gov

Ronald J. Diamond, Author
Ruth Ross, Author
Patricia L. Scheifler, Author
Peter J. Weiden, Author

Helps consumers and their families weigh the pros and cons of switching from older antipsychotics to newer ones. Answers frequently asked questions about antipsychotics and guides readers through the process of switching. Includes fact sheets on the new medications and their side effects. *$22.95*

208 pages Year Founded: 1999 ISBN 0-393703-03-7

1201 Concept of Schizophrenia: Historical Perspectives
American Psychiatric Publishing, Inc.
1000 Wilson Boulevard
Suite 1825
Arlington, VA 22209-3901
703-907-7322
800-368-5777; *Fax: 703-907-1091*
appi@psych.org
www.appi.org

John G. Howells, Editor

The authors question whether there is a psychodynamics of schizophrenia and discuss the insights that spring from this field of inquiry. Presenting material on the concept of schizophrenia this work shows how historical research can be of value to contemporary clinical practice. *$65.00*

211 pages Year Founded: 1991 ISBN 0-880481-08-0

1202 Contemporary Issues in the Treatment of Schizophrenia
American Psychiatric Publishing, Inc.
1000 Wilson Boulevard
Suite 1825
Arlington, VA 22209-3901
703-907-7322
800-368-5777; *Fax:* 703-907-1091
appi@psych.org
www.appi.org

Christian L. Shriqui, MD, Editor
Henry A. Nasrallah, MD, Editor

Covers the spectrum of therapeutic approaches to the disorder- biological, pharmacologica, and psychosocial- as well as presenting a wealth of new research on the course and outcome of schizophrenia. This volume should be a welcome addition to the libraries of psychiatrists, psychiatric residents, psychologists, and other health professionals working with schizophrenia. *$99.95*

889 pages Year Founded: 1995 ISBN 0-880486-81-3

1203 Drug Therapy and Schizophrenia
Mason Crest Publishers
450 Parkway Drive
Suite D
Broomall, PA 19008-4017
610-543-6200
866-627-2665; *Fax:* 610-543-3878
gbaffa@nationalhighlights.com
www.masoncrest.com

Shirley Brinkerhoff, Author

This volume provides a concise description of this disease, which is considered the most severe of the mental disorders. The book also includes a brief account of the disease in history, as well as explanations of how the brain operates and how psychiatric drugs work within the brain. Many case studies are presented to help readers better understand the nature of this difficult and potentially devastating mental disorder.

128 pages ISBN 1-590845-74-9

1204 Encyclopedia of Schizophrenia and Other Psychotic Disorders
Facts on File
132 W 31st Street
17th Floor
New York, NY 10001-3406
212-613-2800
800-322-8755
custserv@factsonfile.com

Richard Noll, Author

Details recent theories and research findings on schizophrenia and psychotic disorders, together with a complete overview of the field's history. *$65.00*

368 pages Year Founded: 2000 ISBN 0-816040-70-2

1205 Family Care of Schizophrenia: a Problem-solving Approach to the Treatment of Mental Illness
Guilford Press
72 Spring Street
New York, NY 10012-4068

212-431-9800
800-365-7006; *Fax:* 212-966-6708
info@guilford.com
www.www.guilford.com

Jeffrey L. Boyd, Author
Ian R.H. Falloon, Author
Christine W McGill, Author

Falloon and his colleagues have developed a model for the broad-based community treatment of schizophrenia and other severe forms of mental illness that taps this underutilized potential. The goal of their program is not merely the reduction of stress that can trigger florid episodes, but also the restoration of the patient to a level of social functioning that permits employment and socialization with people outside the family. As the author demonstrates, families can, with proper guidance, be taught to modulate intrafamilial stress, whether it derives from family tensions or external life events. *$27.95*

451 pages Year Founded: 1973 ISBN 0-898629-23-3

1206 Family Work for Schizophrenia: a Practical Guide
American Psychiatric Publishing, Inc.
1000 Wilson Boulevard
Suite 1825
Arlington, VA 22209-3901
703-907-7322
800-368-5777; *Fax:* 703-907-1091
appi@psych.org
www.appi.org

Liz Kuipers, Author
J.P. Leff, Author
Dominic Lam, Author

The techniques and strategies included in the guide are clearly described for use by clinical practitioners and are illustrated by case examples. The guide has been further enriched with the authors' experience of working with families over the ten years since the first edition was published.

1207 First Episode Psychosis
American Psychiatric Publishing, Inc.
1000 Wilson Boulevard
Suite 1825
Arlington, VA 22209-3901
703-907-7322
800-368-5777; *Fax:* 703-907-1091
appi@psych.org
www.appi.org

Robert E Hales MD, Editor-in-Chief
Ron McMillen, Chief Executive Officer
John McDuffie, Editorial Director

Professional discussion of early Psychosis presentation. *$39.95*

160 pages ISBN 1-853174-35-1

1208 Group Therapy for Schizophrenic Patients
American Psychiatric Publishing, Inc.
1000 Wilson Boulevard
Suite 1825
Arlington, VA 22209-3901
703-907-7322
800-368-5777; *Fax:* 703-907-1091
appi@psych.org
www.appi.org

Nick Kanas, M.D., Author
Ron McMillen, Chief Executive Officer
John McDuffie, Editorial Director

Acquaints mental health practitioners with this cost-effective method of treatment. *$29.00*

184 pages Year Founded: 1996 ISBN 0-880481-72-2

1209 Guidelines for the Treatment of Patients with Schizophrenia
American Psychiatric Publishing, Inc.
1000 Wilson Boulevard
Suite 1825
Arlington, VA 22209-3901
703-907-7322
800-368-5777; *Fax:* 703-907-1091
appi@psych.org
www.appi.org

Robert E Hales MD, Editor-in-Chief
Ron McMillen, Chief Executive Officer
John McDuffie, Editorial Director

Provides therapists with a set of patient care strategies that will aid their clinical decison making. Describes the best and most appropriate treatments available to patients. *$22.50*

160 pages ISBN 0-890423-09-1

1210 How to Cope with Mental Illness In Your Family: A Guide for Siblings and Offspring
Health Source
1404 K Street, NW
Washington, DC 20005-2401
202-789-7303
800-713-7122; *Fax:* 202-789-7899
healthsourcebooks@psych.org
www.healthsourcebooks.org

Diane T Marsh, Author
Rex M Dickens, Author

This book explores the nature of illnesses such as schizophrenia, major depression, while providing the tools to overcome the devasting effects of growing up or living in a family where they exist. Readers are led through the essential stages of recovery, from revisiting their childhood to revising their family legacy, and ultimately, to reclaiming their life. *$14.00*

206 pages ISBN 0-874779-23-5

1211 Innovative Approaches for Difficult to Treat Populations
American Psychiatric Publishing, Inc.
1000 Wilson Boulevard
Suite 1825
Arlington, VA 22209-3901
703-907-7322
800-368-5777; *Fax:* 703-907-1091
appi@psych.org
www.appi.org

Scott W Henggeler, Ph.D, Editor
Alberto W Santos, M.D., Editor
John McDuffie, Editorial Director

Firsthand look at the future direction of clinical services. Focuses on services for individuals who use the highest proportion of mental health resources and for whom traditional services have not been effective. *$65.00*

552 pages Year Founded: 1997 ISBN 0-880486-80-5

1212 Me, Myself, and Them: A Firsthand Account of One Young Person's Experience with Schizophrenia
Oxford University Press
198 Madison Avenue
New York, NY 10016-4341
800-445-9714; *Fax:* 919-677-1303
custserv.us@oup.com
www.oup.com/us

Kurt Snyder, Author
Raquel E Gur,MD, Author
Linda Wasmer Andrews, Author

Offers hope to young people who are struggling with schizophrenia, helping them to understand and manage the challenges of this illness and go on to lead healthy lives.

192 pages Year Founded: 1896 ISBN 0-195311-22-1

1213 Natural History of Mania, Depression and Schizophrenia
American Psychiatric Publishing, Inc.
1000 Wilson Boulevard
Suite 1825
Arlington, VA 22209-3901
703-907-7322
800-368-5777; *Fax:* 703-907-1091
appi@psych.org
www.appi.org

George Winokur, M.D, Author
Ming T Tsuang, M.D., Ph.D, Author
John McDuffie, Editorial Director

An unusual look at the course of mental illness, based on data from the Iowa 500 Research Project. *$42.50*

384 pages Year Founded: 1996 ISBN 0-880487-26-7

1214 New Pharmacotherapy of Schizophrenia
American Psychiatric Publishing, Inc.
1000 Wilson Boulevard
Suite 1825
Arlington, VA 22209-3901
703-907-7322
800-368-5777; *Fax:* 703-907-1091
appi@psych.org
www.appi.org

Alan F Breier, M.D, Editor
Ron McMillen, Chief Executive Officer
John McDuffie, Editorial Director

Discusses the new class of antipsychotic agents that promise superior efficacy and more favorable side-effects; offers an improved understanding of how to employ existing pharmachotherapeutic agents. *$32.50*

264 pages Year Founded: 1996 ISBN 0-880484-91-8

1215 Office Treatment of Schizophrenia
American Psychiatric Publishing, Inc.
1000 Wilson Boulevard
Suite 1825
Arlington, VA 22209-3901
703-907-7322
800-368-5777; *Fax:* 703-907-1091
appi@psych.org
www.appi.org

Robert E Hales MD, Editor-in-Chief
Ron McMillen, Chief Executive Officer
John McDuffie, Editorial Director

Examines options in outpatient treatment of schizophrenic patients. *$31.00*

208 pages

1216 Practicing Psychiatry in the Community: a Manual
American Psychiatric Publishing, Inc.
1000 Wilson Boulevard
Suite 1825
Arlington, VA 22209-3901
703-907-7322
800-368-5777; *Fax: 703-907-1091*
appi@psych.org
www.appi.org

Jerome V Vaccaro, M.D, Editor
Gordon H Clark, Jr., M.D., M.Di, Editor
John McDuffie, Editorial Director

Addressess the major issues currently facing community psychiatrists. *$67.50*

534 pages Year Founded: 1996 ISBN 0-880486-63-5

1217 Prenatal Exposures in Schizophrenia
American Psychiatric Publishing, Inc.
1000 Wilson Boulevard
Suite 1825
Arlington, VA 22209-3901
703-907-7322
800-368-5777; *Fax: 703-907-1091*
appi@psych.org
www.appi.org

Ezra S Susser, M.D., Dr.P.H, Editor
Alan S Brown, M.D., Editor
Jack M Gorman, M.D, Editor

Considers a range of epigenetic elements thought to interact with abnormal genes to produce the onset of illness. Attention to the evidence implicating obstetric complications, prenatal infection, autoimmunity and prenatal malnutrition in brain disorders. *$36.50*

296 pages Year Founded: 1999 ISBN 0-880484-99-3

1218 Psychiatric Rehabilitation of Chronic Mental Patients
American Psychiatric Publishing, Inc.
1000 Wilson Boulevard
Suite 1825
Arlington, VA 22209-3901
703-907-7322
800-368-5777; *Fax: 703-907-1091*
appi@psych.org
www.appi.org

Robert P Liberman, M.D., Editor
Ron McMillen, Chief Executive Officer
John McDuffie, Editorial Director

Provides highly detailed prescriptions for assessment and treatment techniques with case examples and learning exercises. *$28.00*

319 pages Year Founded: 1987 ISBN 0-880482-01-X

1219 Psychoses and Pervasive Development Disorders in Childhood and Adolescence
American Psychiatric Publishing, Inc.
1000 Wilson Boulevard
Suite 1825
Arlington, VA 22209-3901
703-907-7322
800-368-5777; *Fax: 703-907-1091*
appi@psych.org
www.appi.org

Robert E Hales MD, Editor-in-Chief
Ron McMillen, Chief Executive Officer
John McDuffie, Editorial Director

Provides a concise summary of currently knowledge of psychoses and pervasive developmental disorders of childhood and adolescence. Discusses recent changes in aspects of diagnosis and definition of these disorders, advances in knowledge, and aspects of treatment. *$46.50*

368 pages ISBN 1-882103-01-7

1220 Return From Madness
Jason Aronson
200 Livingston Street
Northvale, NJ 07647
201-767-4093
800-782-1005; *Fax: 201-767-1576*
www.aronson.com

Kathleen Degen, Author
Ellen Nasper, Author

The authors describe group therapy that helps patients identify and cope with unexpected, intense feelings such as sadness or painful memories of childhood trauma, increase their interpersonal skills, and advance their sense of self beyond that of their label as mental patients. Degen and Nasper show how to build on the phenomenal changes that the new medications provide. *$50.00*

256 pages ISBN 1-568216-25-4

1221 Schizophrenia
1000 Wilson Boulevard
Suite 1825
Arlington, VA 22209-3901
703-907-7322
800-368-5777; *Fax: 703-907-1091*
appi@psych.org
www.appi.org

Robert E Hales MD, Editor-in-Chief
Ron McMillen, Chief Executive Officer
John McDuffie, Editorial Director

760 pages

1222 Schizophrenia Revealed: From Neurons to Social Interactions
W.W. Norton & Company
500 Fifth Avenue
New York, NY 10110
212-354-2907; *Fax: 212-869-0856*
www.books.wwnorton.com/books/

Drake McFeely, CEO

In this much-needed book, and expert in the neurocognition of schizophrenia, presents an integrated overview of schizophrenia covering a wide range of topics in lively, understandable proze. He outlines a neurodevelopmental model of schizophrenia, discusses neurocognitive indicators of genetic vulnerability, the introduction of a new generation of medications, recent findings from brain imaging, cognitive remediation, and the determinants of functional outcome. He presents a modern view of schizophrenia based on neuroscience that goes far beyond the symptoms of the illness.

224 pages Year Founded: 2003

1223 Schizophrenia and Genetic Risks
National Alliance on Mental Illness
2107 Wilson Boulevard
Suite 300
Arlington, VA 22201-3080
703-524-7600
800-950-6264; *Fax:* 703-524-9094
TDD: 703-516-7227
info@nami.org
www.nami.org

Irving I. Gottesman, Author
Steven O. Moldin, Author

Provides basic facts about schizophrenia and its familial distribution so consumers and mental health workers can become informed enough to initiate appropriate actions. Includes suggested resources.

17 pages Year Founded: 1999 ISBN 9-997725-94-8

1224 Schizophrenia and Manic Depressive Disorder
National Alliance for the Mentally Ill
2107 Wilson Boulevard
Suite 300
Arlington, VA 22201-3080
703-525-0686
800-950-6264
TDD: 703-516-7227
info@nami.org
www.nami.org

E Fuller Torrey, Author

Explores the biological roots of mental illness with a primary focus on schizophrenia. *$27.00*

312 pages ISBN 0-465072-85-2

1225 Schizophrenia and Primitive Mental States
Jason Aronson Publishing
276 Livingston Street
Northvale, NJ 07647
570-342-1320
800-782-0015; *Fax:* 201-767-1576
www.aronson.com

Peter L. Giovacchini, Author

In this volume, renowned therapist Peter Giovacchini shows readers how to do more for psychotic patients than rely on medication to reduce their florid symptoms. Instead, he demonstrates how schizophrenic patients can be offered true cure and the possibility of living a full and related life through intensive psychotherapeutic treatment. *$50.00*

288 pages ISBN 0-765700-27-1

1226 Schizophrenia in a Molecular Age
American Psychiatric Publishing, Inc.
1000 Wilson Boulevard
Suite 1825
Arlington, VA 22209-3901
703-907-7322
800-368-5777; *Fax:* 703-907-1091
appi@psych.org
www.appi.org

Carol A Tamminga, M.D, Editor
Ron McMillen, Chief Executive Officer
John McDuffie, Editorial Director

Explores the multidimensional phenotype of schizophrenia, and use of molecular biology and anti-psychotic medications. Reviews the implications of early sensory procesing and subcortical involvement of cognitive dysfuntion in schizophrenia. Functional neuroimaging applied to the syndrome of schizophrenia. *$26.50*

204 pages Year Founded: 1999 ISBN 0-880489-61-8

1227 Schizophrenia: From Mind to Molecule
American Psychiatric Publishing, Inc.
1000 Wilson Boulevard
Suite 1825
Arlington, VA 22209-3901
703-907-7322
800-368-5777; *Fax:* 703-907-1091
appi@psych.org
www.appi.org

Nancy C Andreasen, M.D., Ph.D, Editor
Ron McMillen, Chief Executive Officer
John McDuffie, Editorial Director

Provides a thorough look at schizophrenia that includes neurobehavioral studies, traditional and emerging technologies, psychosocial and medical treatments, and future research opportunities. *$34.00*

294 pages Year Founded: 1994 ISBN 0-800489-50-2

1228 Schizophrenia: Straight Talk for Family and Friends
William Morrow & Company
10 East 53rd Street
New York, NY 10022-5244
212-872-1133; *Fax:* 212-872-1199

Maryellen Walsh, Author

This compassionate survival manual explains the malady and its effects, treatments, and prospects, as well as widespread myths and actual experiences. *$17.95*

Year Founded: 1985

1229 Stigma and Mental Illness
American Psychiatric Publishing, Inc.
1000 Wilson Boulevard
Suite 1825
Arlington, VA 22209-3901
703-907-7322
800-368-5777; *Fax:* 703-907-1091
appi@psych.org
www.appi.org

Paul J Fink, M.D, Editor
Allan Tasman, M.D., Editor
John McDuffie, Editorial Director

Collection of firsthand accounts on how society has stigmatized mentally ill individuals, their families and their caregivers. *$36.00*

256 pages Year Founded: 1992 ISBN 0-880484-05-5

1230 Surviving Schizophrenia: A Manual for Families, Consumers and Providers
Harper Collins
10 E 53rd Street
New York, NY 10022-5299
212-207-7000
800-242-7737

Since its first publication nearly twenty years ago, this has become the standard reference book on this disease, helping thousands of patients, families and mental health professionals to better deal with the condition. Dr. Fuller Torrey explains the nature causes, symptoms, and treatment of this often misunderstood illness. This fully revised 4th edition of Surviving Schizophrenia is a must-have for the multitude of people affected both directly and indirectly by this serious, yet treatable, disorder. *$15.00*

544 pages ISBN 0-060959-19-3

1231 The Complete Family Guide to Schizophrenia: Helping Your Loved One Get the Most Out of Life

The Guilford Press
72 Spring Street
New York, NY 10012-4019
212-431-9800
800-365-7006; *Fax:* 212-966-6708
info@guilford.com

Bob Matloff, President
Kim T Mueser, Author
Susan Gingerich, Author

This book walks readers through a range of treatment and support options that can lead to a better life for the entire family. Individual chapters hightlight special issues for parents, siblings, and partners, while other sections provide tips for dealing with problems including cognitive difficulties, substance abuse, and psychosis.

1232 Treating Schizophrenia

Jossey-Bass / John Wiley & Sons
111 River Street
Hokoken, NJ 07030-5790
201-748-6000; *Fax:* 201-748-6088
custserv@wiley.com
www.wiley.com

Sophia Vinogradov, Author

Using case studies from their own practices, the contributors describe how to conduct a successful assessment of schizophrenia. They then explore in detail the major treatment methods, including inpatient treatment, individual therapy, family therapy, group therapy, and the crucial role of medication. Th authors also address the timely issue of treating schizophrenia in the era of managed care. *$ 121.60*

372 pages Year Founded: 1995

1233 Understanding Schizophrenia: Guide to the New Research on Causes & Treatment

Free Press
40 Main St.
Suite 301
Florence, MA 01062
877-888-1533; *Fax:* 413-585-8904
consumer.customerservice@simonandschuster.com
www.simonsays.com

Richard Keefe, Author
Philip D Harvey, Author

Two noted researchers provide an accessible, timely guide to schizophrenia, discussing the nature of the disease, recent advances in understanding brain structure and function, and the latest psychological and drug treatments. *$25.95*

283 pages Year Founded: 1994 ISBN 0-029172-47-0

1234 Water Balance in Schizophrenia

American Psychiatric Publishing, Inc.
1000 Wilson Boulevard
Suite 1825
Arlington, VA 22209-3901
703-907-7322
800-368-5777; *Fax:* 703-907-1091
appi@psych.org
www.appi.org

David B. Schnur, Editor
Darrell G. Kirch, Editor

Represents the first attempt to provide clinicians with a consolidated guide to polydipsia-hyponatremia, associated with schizophrenia. Here, some of the foremost experts in the field address a variety of issues pertinent to both researchers and clinicians. All clinicians who treat schizophrenic patients will find this book an indispensable reference. Whenever possible, the editors provide details regarding methodolody and explicit management guidelines. They even include a detailed description of an inpatient polydipsia unit, as well as a comprehensive review of drug treatment. *$54.95*

360 pages Year Founded: 1996 ISBN 0-880484-85-3

Periodicals & Pamphlets

1235 Schizophrenia

National Institute of Mental Health
6001 Executive Boulevard
Room 8184
Bethesda, MD 20892-1
301-443-4513
866-615-6464
TTY: 301-443-8431
nimhinfo@nih.gov

This booklet answers many common questions about schizophrenia, one of the most chronic, severe and disabling mental disorders. Current research-based information is provided for people with schizophrenia, their family members, friends and the general public about the symptoms and diagnosis of schizophrenia, possible causes, treatments and treatment resources.

28 pages Year Founded: 1999

1236 Schizophrenia Research

1600 John F Kennedy Boulevard
Suite 1800
Philadelphia, PA 19103-2879
212-633-3730
800-545-2522; *Fax:* 800-535-9935
usbkinfo@elsevier.com
www.elsevier.com

H.A Nasrallah, Editor-in-Chief
L.E DeLisi, Editor-in-Chief

The journal of choice for international researchers and clinicians to share their work with the global schizophrenia research community. Publishes novel papers that really contribute to understanding the biology and treatment of schizophrenic disorders; Schizophrenia Research brings together biological, clinical and psychological research in order to stimulate the synthesis of findings from all disciplines involved in improving patient outcomes in schizophrenia.

Year Founded: 1880 ISSN 0920-9964

Research Centers

1237 Brain & Behavior Research Foundation
90 Park Avenue
16th Floor
New York, NY 10016
646-681-4888
800-829-8289
info@bbrfoundation.org
www.www.bbrfoundation.org/

Steve Lieber, Chairman of the Board
Jeffrey Borenstein, MD, President and CEO
Louis Innamorato, CPA, VP and Chief Financial Officer
Anne Abramson, Vice President

The Brain and Behavior Research Foundation awards grants aimed at advancing scientific understandings of mental health treatments and mental disorders such as depression and schizophrenia. The Brain and Behavior Research Foundation's mission is to eliminate the suffering caused by mental illness.

Year Founded: 1981

1238 Schizophrenia Research Branch: Division of Clinical and Treatment Research
6001 Executive Boulevard
Room 7122, MSC 9625
Bethesda, MD 20892-1
301-443-9233
866-615-6464; *Fax:* 301-443-5158
TTY: 301-443-8431
sarah.morris@nih.gov
www.www.nimh.nih.gov

Sarah E Morris, PhD, Program Chief

Plans, supports, and conducts programs of research, research training, and resource development of schizophrenia and related disorders. Reviews and evaluates research developments in the field and recommends new program directors. Collaborates with organizations in and outside of the National Institute of Mental Health (NIMH) to stimulate work in the field through conferences and workshops.

Support Groups & Hot Lines

1239 Common Ground Sanctuary
1410 S. Telegraph
Bloomfield Hills, MI 48302
248-456-8150
800-231-1127; *Fax:* 248-456-8147
www.www.commongroundsanctuary.org

Tony Rothschild, President & CEO
Steve Mitchell, Board Chair
Gary Dembs, Secretary
Charles Schmidt, Treasurer

A 24-hour nonprofit agency dedicated to helping youths, adults and families in crisis. Through its crisis line and in person through various programs, Common Ground Sanctuary provides professional and compassionate service to more than 40,000 people a year, with most services provided free of charge. Mission is to provide a lifeline for individuals and families in crisis, victims of crime, persons with mental illness, people trying to cope with critical situations and runaway and homeless youth.

Year Founded: 1998

1240 Family-to-Family: National Alliance on Mental Illness
3803 N. Fairfax Drive
Suite 100
Arlington, VA 22203
703-524-7600
888-999-6264; *Fax:* 703-524-9094
info@nami.org
www.nami.org

The NAMI Family-to-Family Education Program is a free, 12-week course for family caregivers of individuals with severe mental illnesses. The course is taught by trained family members, all instruction and course materials are free to class participants, and over 300,000 family members have graduated from this national program.

Video & Audio

1241 Bonnie Tapes
Mental Illness Education Project, Inc.
25 West Street
Westborough, MA 01581
617-562-1111
info@miepvideos.org
www.miepvideos.org

Bonnie's account of coping with schizophrenia will be a revelation to people whose view of mental illness has been shaped by the popular media. She and her family provide an intimate view of a frequently feared, often misrepresented, and much stigmatized illness-and the human side of learning to live with a psychiatric disability.

Year Founded: 1997

1242 Clinical Impressions: Identifying Mental Illness
Educational Training Videos
136 Granville St
Suite 200
Gahanna, OH 43230
Fax: 888-775-3919
www.educationaltrainingvideos.com

How long can mental illness stay hidden, especially from the eyes of trained experts? This program rejoins a group of ten adults- five of them healthy and five of them with histories of mental illness- as psychiatric specialists try to spot and correctly diagnose the latter. Administering a series of collaborative and one-on-one tests, including assessments of personality type, physical self-image, and rational thinking, the panel gradually makes decisions about who suffers from depression, bipolar disorder, bulimia, and social anxiety.

1243 Dark Voices: Schizophrenia
Educational Training Videos
136 Granville St
Suite 200
Gahanna, OH 43230
Fax: 888-775-3919
www.educationaltrainingvideos.com

This program seeks to understand how schizophrenia touches the lives of patients and their family members while examining the disease's etiology and pathology. A Discovery Channel Production.

1244 FRONTLINE: The Released
PBS
2100 Crystal Drive
Arlington, VA 22202
www.pbs.org

Will Lyman, Actor
Narrator
Miri Navasky, Director
Karen O'Connor, Director

The documentary states that of the 700,000 inmates released from American prisons each year, half of them have
mental disabilities. This work focused on those with severe
problems who keep entering and exiting prison. Full of
good information on the challenges they face with mental
illnesses; housing, employment, stigmatization, and
socialization.

Year Founded: 2009

1245 Families Coping with Mental Illness
Mental Illness Education Project
PO Box 470813
Brookline Village, MA 02447-813
617-562-1111
800-343-5540; *Fax:* 617-779-0061
info@miepvideos.org
www.miepvideos.org

Christine Ledoux, Executive Director

Designed to provide insights and support to other families,
the tape also has profound messages for professionals about
the needs of families when mental illness strikes. *$68.95*

Year Founded: 1997

1246 Mental Disorder
Educational Training Videos
136 Granville St
Suite 200
Gahanna, OH 43230
Fax: 888-775-3919
www.educationaltrainingvideos.com

What is abnormality? Using the case studies of two young
women; one who has depression, one who has an anxiety
disorder; as a springboard, this program presents three psychological perspective on mental disorder.

1247 My Name is Walter James Cross: The Reality
of Schizophrenia
Educational Training Videos
136 Granville St
Suite 200
Gahanna, OH 43230
Fax: 888-775-3919
www.educationaltrainingvideos.com

Walter James Cross tried to kill himself and failed, so he
decided to tell his story instead. Created by a psychiatrist
who has worked for many years with schizophrenic patients, this compelling dramatic monologue presents an
acurate depiction of a devastating, costly, much maligned,
and misunderstood illness.

1248 No More Shame: Understanding Schizophrenia,
Depression, and Addiction
Educational Training Videos
136 Granville St
Suite 200
Gahanna, OH 43230

Fax: 888-775-3919
www.educationaltrainingvideos.com

These programs examine research about the physiological,
psychological, sociological, and cultural aspects of these
disorders and their treatments. The goal of these programs
is to explain what we do and do not know about each of
these conditions, as well as to destigmatize the disorders by
presenting them in the context of the same research process
that is applied to all medical disorders.

1249 To See What I See - The Stigma of Mental
Illness
Northern Lakes Community Mental Health

People served by Northern Lakes Community Mental
Health have come together as Stigma Busters - creating art-
work, photographs, recovery stories, media campaigns, personal testimonies, buttons, and other projects for the
purpose of eliminating the stigma associated with mental
illness and spreading the word that recovery is possible.
This is their story.

1250 Understanding Mental Illness
Educational Video Network, Inc.
1401 19th Street
Huntsville, TX 77340
936-295-5767
800-762-0060; *Fax:* 936-294-0233
www.www.evndirect.com

Contains information and classifications of mental illness.
Mental illness can strike anyone, at any age. Learn about
various organic and functional mental disorders as discussed and their causes and symptoms, and learn where to
seek help for a variety of mental health concerns.

Web Sites

1251 www.cyberpsych.org
CyberPsych

Presents information about psychoanalysis, psychotherapy
and special topics such as anxiety disorders, the problematic use of alcohol, homophobia, and the traumatic effects
of racism.

1252 www.hopkinsmedicine.org/epigen
Epidemology-Genetics Program in Psychiatry

Research program to help characterize the genetic, developmental and environmental componenets of bipolar disorder and schizophrenia.

1253 www.mentalhealth.com
Internet Mental Health

Offers online psychiatric diagnosis in the hope of reaching
the two-thirds of individuals with mental illness who do not
seek treatment.

1254 www.naminys.org
National Alliance on Mental Illness

From its inception in 1979, NAMI has been dedicated to
improving the lives of individuals and families affected by
mental illness.

1255 www.planetpsych.com
Planetpsych.com

The online resource for mental health information.

1256 www.psychcentral.com
Psych Central

The Internet's largest and oldest independent mental health social network created and run by mental health professionals to guarantee reliable, trusted information and support communities to you.

1257 www.schizophrenia.com
Schizophrenia

A non-profit community providing in-depth information, support and education related to schizophrenia, a disorder of the brain and mind.

1258 www.schizophrenia.com/discuss/
Schizophrenia

On-line support for patients and families.

1259 www.schizophrenia.com/newsletter/buckets/
success.html
Schizophrenia

Success stories including biographical accounts, links to stories of famous people who have schizophrenia, and personal web pages.

1260 www.store.samhsa.gov
Substance Abuse and Mental Health Services
Administration

Resources on mental disorders as well as treatment and recovery.

Sexual Disorders

Introduction

It is not possible to know what degree of sexual interest, desire, or activity is 'normal'; at best, we have averages, not indications of the optimal state. A Sexual Disorder is diagnosed when lack of desire or activity is repeated, persists over time, and causes distress or interferes with the person's functioning in other important areas of life. Sexual Disorders are divided into four groups: Disorders of Sexual Desire; Disorders of Sexual Arousal; Orgasmic Disorders; and Disorders involving Sexual Pain. It is essential to know whether the problem is lifelong or was precipitated by a recent event, and whether it occurs only with a particular partner or in a particular situation. It is also essential not to make assumptions about sexual activity based on age, socioeconomic status, or sexual orientation.

SEXUAL DESIRE DISORDERS SYMPTOMS

Hypoactive Sexual Desire Disorder (HSDD)
• Persistent or repeated lack of sexual fantasies and desire for sexual activities;
• The lack of sexual fantasies and desire cause marked distress or interpersonal problems.

Sexual Aversion Disorder (SAD)
• Persistent or repeated extreme aversion to, and avoidance of, all or almost all genital sexual contact with a sexual partner;
• The aversion causes marked distress or interpersonal problems.

The person with a Sexual Desire Disorder commonly has a poor body image and avoids nudity. In HSDD, a person does not initiate sexual activity, or respond to the partner's initiation attempts. The disorder is often associated with the inability to achieve orgasm in women, and in the inability to achieve an erection in men. It can also be associated with other psychiatric and medical problems, including a history of sexual trauma and abuse.

Prevalence
HADD is common in both men and women but twice as many women as men report it. It is estimated at twenty percent overall, and as high as sixty-five-percent among those seeking treatment for sexual disorders. The prevalence of SAD is unknown.

Treatment Options
Treatment of Sexual Desire Disorders may include psychotherapy (to treat any underlying psychological problems that might be causing the symptoms) and couples counseling. Testosterone is sometimes prescribed to improve sex drive in post-menopausal women with Sexual Desire Disorders; however, it can have serious side effects.

SEXUAL AROUSAL DISORDER

Female Sexual Arousal Disorder (FSAD)
• Persistent or repeated inability to attain or maintain adequate lubrication-swelling (sexual excitement) response throughout sexual activity;
• The disorder causes clear distress or interpersonal problems.

Male Erectile Disorder (MED)
• Persistent or repeated inability to maintain an adequate erection throughout sexual activity;
• The disorder causes clear distress or interpersonal problems.

Associated Features
While both these disorders are common, men tend to be more upset by it than women. Contributing issues include performance anxiety (especially in men), fear of failure, inadequate stimulation, and relationship conflicts. Other problems are also associated with FSAD and MED, such as childhood sexual trauma, sexual identity concerns, religious orthodoxy, depression, lack of intimacy or trust, and power conflicts. MED is frequently associated with diabetes, peripheral nerve disorders, and hypertension, and is a side effect of a variety of medications. In addition, the medications used to treat MED are contraindicated in some medical conditions, such as heart conditions.

Prevalence
Prevalence information varies for FSAD. Most studies report a prevalence of 13% and 24%, with a range of 6% to 28% of women. It appears that prevalence of FSAD increases with increasing age, but also that women become less distressed by the disorder. In a study of happily married couples, about one third of women complained of difficulty in achieving or maintaining sexual excitement.

Erectile difficulties in men are estimated to be very common, affecting 20-30 million men in the US. The frequency of erectile problems increases steeply with age. In one survey, fifty-two percent of men aged 40-70 reported erectile problems, with three times as many older men reporting difficulties. The disorder is common among married, single, heterosexual, and homosexual men.

Treatment Options
In FSAD, cognitive-behavioral psychotherapy is often recommended, including practical help such as the use of water-soluble lubricating products. Hormone treatment, such as testosterone-estrogen compounds, is sometimes helpful.

An array of treatments is available for Male Erectile Dysfunction, including prosthetic devices for physiological penile problems. In cases of hormonal problems, testosterone treatments have had some results. (However, the use of testosterone to treat sexual disorders in menopausal women is controversial and can have serious side effects.) Viagra has produced success for male erectile dysfunction, as have two newer medications for MED, vardenafil (Levitra) and tadalafil (Cialis).

When sexual problems are limited to a particular partner or situation, psychotherapy (individual or couple) is necessary to resolve the difficulty.

ORGASMIC DISORDER

Female and Male Orgasmic Disorders
• Persistent or repeated delay in, or absence of, orgasm despite a normal sexual excitement phase;
• The disorder causes clear distress or interpersonal problems.

Premature Ejaculation
• Persistent or recurring ejaculation with minimal sexual stimulation before, upon, or shortly after penetration and earlier than desired;
• The disorder causes clear distress or interpersonal problems.

Associated Features
When FOD or MOD occur only in certain situations, difficulty with desire and arousal are often also present. All of these disorders are associated with poor body image, self-esteem, or relationship problems. In FOD or MOD, medical or surgical conditions can also play a role, such as multiple sclerosis, spinal cord injury, surgical prostatectomy (males), and some medications. PE is likely to be very distruptive. Some males may have had the disorder all their lives, for others it may be situational. Few illnesses or drugs are associated with PE.

Prevalence
FOD is probably the most frequent sexual disorder among females. Among those who have sought sex therapy twenty-four percent to thirty-seven percent report the problem. In general population samples, 15.4 percent of premenopausal women report the disorder, and 34.7 percent of postmenopausal women do so. More single than married women report that they have never had an orgasm. There is no association between FOD and race, socioeconomic status, education, or religion. MOD is relatively rare; only three percent to eight percent of men seeking treatment report having the disorder, though there is a higher prevalence among homosexual males (ten to fifteen percent).

PE is very common: twenty-five to forty percent of adult males report having, or having had PE.

Treatment Options
Psychotherapeutic treatments are similar to those for Sexual Desire and Sexual Arousal Disorders. In both males and females with Orgasmic Disorders there may be a lack of desire, performance anxiety, and fear of impregnation or disease. Therapy should take into account contextual and historical information concerning the onset and course of the problem. Cognitive-behavioral methods to help change the assumptions and thinking of the person have sometimes been helpful.

SEXUAL PAIN DISORDER

Dyspareunia
• Recurring or persistent pain with sexual intercourse in a male or female;
• The disorder causes clear distress or interpersonal problems.

Vaginismus
• Persistent or recurrent involunatry spasm of the vagina that interferes with sexual intercourse;
• The disorder causes clear distress or interpersonal problems.

Associated Features
Both Dyspareunia and Vaginismus may be associated with lack of desire or arousal. Women with Vaginismus tend to avoid gynecological exams, and the disorder is most often associated with psychological and interpersonal issues. Various physical factors are associated with Dyspareunia, such as pelvic inflammatory disease, hymenal or child-birth-related scarring, and vulvar vestibulitis. Dyspareunia is not a clear symptom of any physical condition, and in women it is often combined with Depression and interpersonal conflicts. Other associated psychosocial factors include religious orthodoxy, low self-esteem, poor body image, poor couple communication, and history of sexual trauma.

Prevalence
Dyspareunia is frequent in females but occurs infrequently in males. Vaginismus is seen quite often in sex therapy clinics - in fifteen to seventeen percent of women coming for treatment.

Treatment Options
The most successful treatment for women with these disorders is the reinsertion of a graduated sequence of dilators in the vagina. This treatment should be done in conjunction with relaxation training, sensate focusing exercises (which help people focus on the pleasures of sex rather than the performance), and sex therapy.

General Treatment Options
It is important to know whether or not a medicalor medication issue is present. However, many with these disorders do not seek treatment. Their lack of desire for sex is often combined with a lack of desire for sex therapy. Even with therapy, relapse is commonly reported. Treatments that have had some success are ones that challenge the cognitive assumptions and distortions of client(s), e.g., that sex should be perfect, that without intercourse and without both partners having an orgasm it is not real sex.

Therapy often also includes sensate focusing in which the person is encouraged and trained to give up the role of agitated spectator to love-making in favor of participating in it. A sexual history should be part of every mental health evaluation, and patients receiving psychotropic medications should be asked about sexual side effects. Having information about sexual function before medication is prescribed will prevent pre-existing sexual problems from being confused with any that may result from medication.

PARAPHILIAS
Paraphilias are sexual disorders or perversions in which sexual intercourse is not the desired goal. Instead, the desire is to use non-human objects or non-sexual body parts for sexual activities sometimes involving the suffering of, or inflicting pain onto, non-consenting partners.

Symptoms
• Recurrent, intense, sexually arousing fantasies, urges, or behavior involving the particular perversion for at least six months;
• The fantasies, urges, or behavior cause distress and/or disruption in the person's functioning in social, work, and interpersonal areas.

There are seven Paraphilias, described below, categorized as either victimless, or as victimizing someone who has not consented to the sexual activity, with relevant associated features.

Exhibitionism
The exposure of the genitals to a stranger or group of strangers. Sometimes the paraphiliac masturbates during exposure. The onset of this disorder usually occurs before age 18 and becomes less severe after age 40.

Fetishism
Using non-living objects, known as fetishes, for sexual gratification. Objects commonly used by men with the disorder include women's underwear, shoes, or other articles of women's clothing. The person often masturbates while holding, rubbing, or smelling the fetish object. This disorder usually begins in adolescence; it is chronic.

Frotteurism
Sexual arousal, and sometimes masturbation to orgasm, while rubbing against a non-consenting person. The behavior is usually planned to occur in a crowded place, such as on a bus, subway, or in a swimming pool, where detection is less likely. Frotteurism usually begins in adolescence, is most frequent between the ages of 15 and 25, then gradually declines.

Sexual Masochism
Acts of being bound, beaten, humiliated, or made to suffer in some other way in order to become sexually aroused. The behaviors can be self-inflicated or performed with a partner, and include physical bondage, blindfolding, and humiliation. Masochistic sexual fantasies are likely to have been present since childhood. The activities themselves begin at different times but are common by early adulthood; they are usually chronic. The severity of the behaviors may increase over time.

Sexual Sadism
Acts in which the person become sexually excited through the physical or psychological suffering of someone else. Some Sexual Sadists may conjure up thesadistic fantasies during sexual activity without acting on them. Others act on their sadistic urges with a consenting partner (who may be a Sexual Masochist), or act on their urges with a non-consenting partner. The behavior may involve forcing the other person to crawl, be caged or tortured. Sadistic sexual fantasies are likely to have been present in childhood. The onset of the behavior varies but most commonly occurs by early adulthood. The disorder is usually chronic, and severity tends to increase over time. When the disorder is severe or coupled with Antisocial Personality Disorder, the person is likely to seriously injure or kill his victim.

Transvestic Fetishism
Consists of heterosexual males dressing in women's clothes and makeup then masturbating. When not cross dressed, the man looks like an ordinary man. It is important to note that there is considerable controversy over this diagnosis; some people who cross dress seem to have little distress and function normally. This condition typically begins in childhood or adolescence. Often the cross dressing is not done publicly until adulthood.

Voyeurism
Peeping Tom disorder, involving the act of observing one or more unsuspecting persons (usually strangers) who are naked, in the process of undressing, or engaged in sexual activity, in order for the voyeur to become sexually excited. Sexual activity with the people being observes is not usually sought. The voyeur may masturbate during the observation or later. The onset of this disorder is usually before age 15. It tends to be chronic.

Prevalence
Paraphiliacs are almost exclusively male. Very few volunteer to disclose their activities or to seek treatment. It is estimated that more have deficits in interpersonal or sexual relationships. In one study, two thirds were diagnosed with Mood Disorders and fifty percent had alcohol or drug abuse problems.

Recent studies provide evidence that the great majority of Paraphiliacs are active in more than one form of sexually perverse behavior; less than ten percent have only one form; and thirty-eight percent engage in five or more difference sexually deviant behaviors. In a survey of college students, it was found that young males often fantasize about forced sex, and almost half have engaged in some form of sexual misconduct or sexual behavior with someone younger than age 14.

At the same time, the incidence and prevalence of some sexual perversions are hard to estimate, or unknown, because they are rarely reported or the people involved do not come into contact with authorities. All the Paraphilias are difficult to treat. It is important for the professional making the diagnosis to take a very careful history, and to be sensitive to the presence of other, e.g., personality, disorders. Relapse is common.

Diagnostic techniques can be useful. Penile plethysmography measures the degree of penile erection while the individual is exposed to visual sexual stimulation. Some people are treated in a formal Sex Offenders Program, developed for individuals arrested for and convicted of paraphilias that are crimes. Sometimes treatment occurs within the context of individual therapy where trust can be established. Other have been treated by means of conditioning techniques, e.g., where a fetish object is paired with an aversive stimulus such as a mild electric shock.

Medication is also used. Pedophilia and other Paraphilias are sometimes treated through the use of female hormones or other medications, which diminishes sexual appetite. Other medications may include serotonin reuptake inhibitors (SSRIs) and anti-androgens (agents that reduce the level of testosterone in the blood). Behavior therapy may also be used.

Treatment can be difficult because it is associated with the risk of reporting and punishment; many individuals do not have any real interest in being treated. They may deliberately deceive the professional, or deny the problem. Sex offenders are also more likely to exaggerate treatment gains, resist treatment, or end treatment prematurely.

Associations & Agencies

1262 American Association of Sexuality Educators, Counselors and Therapists (AASECT)
35 E Wacker Drive
Suite 850
Chicago, IL 60601
202-449-1099; *Fax:* 202-216-9646
info@aasect.org
www.www.aasect.org/

Debby Herbenick, PhD, MPH, President
Susan E. Stiritz, PhD, MSW, MBA, President-Elect
Melissa Novak, LCSW, CST, Secretary
Douglas Braun-Harvey, LMFT, Treasurer

A nonprofit professional organization for sexuality educators, cousnelors, sex therapists, physicians, social workers, and psychologists. Members of the association advance the fields of sexual therapy, counseling, and education.

Year Founded: 1967

1263 American Sexual Health Association (ASHA)
PO Box 13827
Research Triangle Park, NC 27709
919-361-8400
info@ashasexualhealth.org
www.www.ashasexualhealth.org/

Lynn Barclay, President and CEO
Deborah Arrindell, Vice President, Health Policy
Keith Walsh, Chair
Debra Hauser, Vice Chair

A nonprofit organization that aims to foster healthy sexual behaviours. ASHA's objectives are to educate individuals with scientifially based information, collaborate with other organizations, and advocate for beneficial changes in sexual health policy.

Year Founded: 1914

1264 American Society for Reproductive Medicine
1209 Montgomery Highway
Birmingham, AL 35216-2809
205-978-5000; *Fax:* 205-978-5005
asrm@asrm.org
www.www.asrm.org/

Christos Coutifaris, MD, PhD, President
Catherine Racowsky, PhD, HCLD, Vice President
Michael Thomas, MD, Secretary
Richard H. Reindollar, MD, Chief Executive Officer

A nonprofit, multidisciplinary organization composed of urologists, obstetricians/gynecologists, embryologists, mental health professionals, nurses, reproductive endocrinologists, and other reproductive health professionals. The society aims to advance the science and practice of reproductive medicine through education, research, and advocacy.

Year Founded: 1944

1265 American Urological Association
1000 Corporate Boulevard
Linthicum, MD 21090
410-689-3700
866-746-4282; *Fax:* 410-689-3800
aua@AUAnet.org
www.www.auanet.org/

J. Brantley Thrasher, MD, FACS, President
Robert C. Flanagan, MD, FACS, President-Elect

Manoj Monga, MD, FACS, Secretary
Michael T. Sheppard, CPA, CAE, Chief Executive Officer

An association of professionals who promote high standards of urological care, including male infertility. The Association provides support for urologists through education, funding for research, and networking/information sharing opportunities.

Year Founded: 1902

1266 Association of Reproductive Health Professionals
1300 19th Street NW
Suite 200
Washington, DC 20036
202-466-3825; *Fax:* 202-266-3826
arhp@arhp.org
www.www.arhp.org

Shannon Darlington, Interim Executive Director
Rebecca Sager, Development Director
Rebecca Theim, MS, MA, Communications Director
Melissa Werner, MPH, MAT, Education Director

An association of sexual health professionals dedicated to improving sexual and reproductive health care.

Year Founded: 1963

1267 Center for Healthy Sex
10700 Santa Monica Boulevard
Suite 311
Los Angeles, CA 90025
310-843-9902
info@centerforhealthysex.com
www.centerforhealthysex.com/

Douglas Evans, Executive Director
Eve Curtis, Lead Intake Counselor
Gaalan Michaelson, Intake Counselor
Alexandra Katehakis, Clinical Director

A therapy center that specializes in the treatment of sexual dysfunction, sexual aversion/anorexia, sex addiction, and love addiction.

Year Founded: 2005

1268 Center for Mental Health Services (CMHS)
Substance Abuse and Mental Health Services Administration
5600 Fishers Lane
Rockville, MD 20857
240-276-1310
877-726-4727
TTY: 800-487-4889
www.samhsa.gov/about-us/who-we-are/offices-centers

Paolo del Vecchio, MSW, Director
Anne Mathews-Younes, Acting Deputy Director
Keris Myrick, Director, Consumer Affairs
Patricia Gratton, Director, Program Analysis

Promotes the treatment of mental illness and emotional disorders by increasing accessibility to mental health programs; supporting outreach, treatment, rehabilitation, and support programs and networks; and encouraging the use of scientifically-based information when treating mental disorders. CMHS provides information about mental health via a toll-free number and numerous publications. Developed for users of mental health services and their families, the general public, policy makers, providers, and the media.

Year Founded: 1992

1269 Center for Women's Health
Kohler Pavilion, 7th Floor
808 SW Campus Drive
Portland, OR 97239
503-418-4500
cwh@ohsu.edu
www.www.ohsu.edu/xd/health/services/women/

Sharon Anderson, MD, Leadership Council Member
Katherine Bradley, RN, PhD, Leadership Council Member
Aaron Caughey, MD, PhD, Leadership Council Member
Jennifer DeVoe, MD, Leadership Council Member

A center dedicated to providing services in many areas of women's health, including women's sexual health.

1270 International Society for the Study of Women's Sexual Health (ISSWSH)
14305 Southcross Dr.
Suite 100
Burnsville, MN 55306
952-683-9025
952-314-8212
www.www.isswsh.org

Noel N. Kim, President
Tessa Benitez, Associate Executive Director
Vivian Gies, Meeting Director

The ISSWSH promotes communication among scholars, researchers, and practitioners about women's sexual function and sexual experience; supports high standards of ethics and professionalism in research, education, and clinical practice of women's sexuality; and provides the public with accurate information about women's sexuality and sexual health.

1271 National Association for the Dually Diagnosed (NADD)
132 Fair Street
Kingston, NY 12401
845-331-4336
info@thenadd.org
www.thenadd.org

Jeanne M. Farr, MA, Chief Executive Officer
Daniel Baker, PhD., President
Peggie Webb, MA, Vice President
George Zukotynski, PhD., Secretary

NADD is a nonprofit organization designed to increase awareness of, and provide services for, individuals with developmental disabilities and mental illness. NADD emphasizes the importance of quality mental healthcare for people with mental health needs and offers conferences, information resources, educational programs, and training materials to professionals, parents, and organizations.

Year Founded: 1983

1272 National Mental Health Consumers' Self-Help Clearinghouse
1211 Chestnut Street
Suite 1100
Philadelphia, PA 19107
267-507-3810
800-553-4539; *Fax:* 215-636-6312
info@mhselfhelp.org
www.mhselfhelp.org

Joseph Rogers, Founder and Executive Director
Susan Rogers, Director

The Clearinghoue is a peer-run national technical assistance center focused on achieving respect and equality of opportunity for those with mental illnesses. The Clearinghouse helps with the growth of the mental health consumer movement by evaluating mental health services, advocating for mental health reform, and providing consumers with news, information, publications, and consultation services.

Year Founded: 1986

1273 Sexual Medicine Society of North America
14305 Southcross Drive
Suite 100
Burnsville, MN 55306
952-683-1917; *Fax:* 612-808-0491
info@smsna.org
www.www.sexhealthmatters.org

Run Wang, MD, FACS, President
Hossein Sadeghi-Nejad, MD, President-Elect
Mohit Khera, MD, Secretary
Nelson Bennet, Jr., MD, Treasurer

A nonprofit professional association of physicians, researchers, nurses, and assistants who are dedicated to treating human sexual function and dysfunction.

Year Founded: 1994

1274 The Center for Family Support
2811 Zulette Avenue
Bronx, NY 10461
718-518-1500; *Fax:* 718-518-8200
www.www.cfsny.org/

Steven Vernikoff, Executive Director
Lloyd Stabiner, President
Amy Bittinger, Vice President
Barbara Greenwald, Associate Executive Director

The Center for Family Support offers assistance to individuals with developmental and related disabilities, as well as their families, and provides support services and programs that are designed to accommodate individual needs. Offers services throughout New York City, Westchester County, Long Island, and New Jersey.

Year Founded: 1954

1275 Urology Care Foundation
1000 Corporate Boulevard
Linthicum, MB 21090
410-689-3700
800-828-7866; *Fax:* 410-689-3998
info@UrologyCareFoundation.org
www.www.urologyhealth.org/

Harris M. Nagler, MD, FACS, President
Gopal H. Badlani, MD, Secretary
David F. Green, MD, FACS, Treasurer

Associated with the American Urological Association, the Urology Care Foundation is a nonprofit organization that partners with urological health professionals, reserchers, patients, caregivers, and families to support the treatment of urological diseases such as male erectile dysfunction.

Year Founded: 1987

Books

1276 Back on Track: Boys Dealing with Sexual Abuse
Sidran Institute
PO Box 436
Brooklandville, MD 21022-0436
410-825-8888
888-825-8249; *Fax:* 410-560-0134
sidran@sidran.org
www.sidran.org

Leslie Bailey Wright, Author
Mindy B Loiselle, Author

Written for boys age ten and up, this wookbook addresses adolescent boys directly, answering commonly asked questions, offering concrete suggestions for getting help and dealing with unspoken concerns such as homosexuality. Contains descriptions of what therapy may be like and brief explanations of social services and courts, as well as sections on family and friends. Exercises and interesting graphics break up the text. The book's important message is TELL: Just keep telling until someone listens who STOPS the abuse. *$14.00*

126 pages Year Founded: 1986 ISBN 1-884444-43-1

1277 Coping with Erectile Dysfunction: How to Regain Confidence and Enjoy Great Sex
New Harbinger Publications
5674 Shattuck Avenue
Oakland, CA 94609
800-748-6273; *Fax:* 800-652-1613
customerservice@newharbinger.com
www.www.newharbinger.com

Barry W. McCarthy, PhD, Co-Author
Michael E. Metz, PhD, Co-Author

A book on erectile dysfunction that includes facts and myths about ED, medicine and medical treatments, and an individualized relapse prevention plan. This book takes a comprehensive biological, psychological, and social approach to ED. *$18.95*

184 pages Year Founded: 2004 ISSN 9781572243866

1278 Coping with Premature Ejaculation: How to Overcome PE, Please Your Partner, and Have Great Sex
New Harbinger Publications
5674 Shattuck Avenue
Oakland, CA 94609
800-748-6273
customerservice@newharbinger.com
www.www.newharbinger.com

Barry W. McCarthy, PhD, Co-Author
Michael E. Metz, PhD, Co-Author

A book containing scientifally based methods for overcoming premature ejaculation. The book takes a bio-psychological approach, and includes assessment exercises, treatment strategies, and information about myths of male sexual performance. *$18.95*

184 pages Year Founded: 2003 ISSN 9781572243408

1279 Dangerous Sex Offenders: a Task Force Report of the American Psychiatric Association
American Psychiatric Publishing, Inc.
1000 Wilson Boulevard
Suite 1825
Arlington, VA 22209-3901
703-907-7322
800-368-5777; *Fax:* 703-907-1091
appi@psych.org
www.appi.org

Robert E Hales MD, Editor-in-Chief
Ron McMillen, Chief Executive Officer
John McDuffie, Editorial Director

Topics in this volume on sexually dangerous offenders include: epidemiology of sex offenders; sexual predator commitment laws; juvenile sex offenders; and pharmacological treatment of sexual offenders. *$40.95*

210 pages Year Founded: 1999 ISBN 0-890422-80-X

1280 Emonics: A Systemic Analysis of Emotional Identity in the Etiology of Sexual Paraphilias
CreateSpace
7290 B. Investment Drive
Charleston, SC 29418
E-mail: Info@CreateSpace.com

Dr. Pierre F. Walter, Author

A daring new approach to grasping the reality of emosexual attraction, from not a sexological but a bioenergetic perspective. It is especially geared toward understanding the true nature and etiology of sexual paraphilias and pedoemotions.

232 pages Year Founded: 2012 ISBN 1-475031-24-6

1281 Gender Disorders and the Paraphilias
Intl Universities Pr Inc
59 Boston Post Rd.
Madison, CT 06443
203-245-4000; *Fax:* 203-245-0775
www.www.iup.com

William B. Arndt, Jr., Author

488 pages Year Founded: 1991 ISBN 0-823621-50-2

1282 Interviewing the Sexually Abused Child
American Psychiatric Publishing, Inc.
1000 Wilson Boulevard
Suite 1825
Arlington, VA 22209-3901
703-907-7322
800-368-5777; *Fax:* 703-907-1091
appi@psych.org
www.appi.org

Robert E Hales MD, Editor-in-Chief
Ron McMillen, Chief Executive Officer
John McDuffie, Editorial Director

Guide for mental health professionals who need to know if a child has been sexually abused. Presents guidelines on the structure of the interview and covers the use of free play, toys, and play materials by focusing on the investigate interview of the suspected victim. *$27.95*

80 pages ISBN 0-880486-12-0

1283 Masculinity and Sexuality: Selected Topics
American Psychiatric Publishing, Inc.
1000 Wilson Boulevard
Suite 1825
Arlington, VA 22209-3901
703-907-7322
800-368-5777; *Fax:* 703-907-1091
appi@psych.org
www.appi.org

Jennifer Downey, Author/Editor
Richard C. Friedman, Editor

Sheds light on clinical issues important in the treatment of all male patients. Sexual experiences and related attitudes of patients and therapists influence symptoms, treatment, and outcome across diverse diagnostic categories. Chapters cover clinical issues related sexual thoughts, impulses, and desires and the way they are organized into erotic fantasies including the differences that exist in the way ment and women experience sexual fantasy. *$37.50*

172 pages Year Founded: 1999 ISBN 0-880489-62-6

1284 Perversion (Ideas in Psychoanalysis)
National Book Network
4501 Forbes Boulevard
Suite 200
Lanham, MD 20706-4346
301-459-3366
800-462-6420; *Fax:* 301-429-5746
customercare@nbnbooks.com
www.www.nbnbooks.com

Ivan Ward, Editor
Claire Pajaczkowska, Author

The concept of perversion is used to understand the unconscious dynamics of addiction, sexual abuse, delinquency, murder, sexual assault & even burglary. The concepts of narcissism, fetishism, voyeurism & sadomasochism are also useful as tools to analyze our culture, particularly in relation to film. *$7.24*

80 pages Year Founded: 1996 ISBN 1-840461-88-8

1285 Principles and Practice of Sex Therapy
The Guilford Press
72 Spring Street
New York, NY 10012-4019
212-431-9800
800-365-7006; *Fax:* 212-966-6708
info@guilford.com

Sandra R. Leiblum, Ph.D., Editor/Author

Provides a comprehensive guide to assessment and treatment of all of the major female and male sexual dysfunctions. Leading authorities demonstrate effective ways to integrate psychological, interpersonal, and medical interventions. Every chapter includes detailed clinical examples illustrating the process of therapy and the factors that influence treatment outcomes. *$95.00*

Year Founded: 2006 ISBN 1-593853-49-1

1286 Quickies: The Handbook of Brief Sex Therapy
W.W. Norton & Company
500 Fifth Avenue
New York, NY 10110
212-354-2907; *Fax:* 212-869-0856
www.wwnorton.com

Shelley K. Green, Author
Douglas Flemons, Author

The authors gather a wonderful array of approaches to brief sex therapy, each presented by a well known therapist in the field. Pleasure and humor are highlighted, the office and the bed, as readers are reminded that the point of sex therapy is a sexual change.

ISBN 0-393705-27-7

1287 Sex Crimes and Paraphilia
Prentice Hall Upper Saddle River, NJ
800-922-0579
www.pearsonhighered.com

Eric W. Hickey, Author

Offers a comprehensive examination of sex crimes, sex offenders, victims of sex crimes as well as intervention and treatment strategies. Examining a wide range of sex crimes ranging from non-violent offenses such as exhibitionism, voyeurism and obscene telephone calls to serial rapes and lust murders, this book looks to uncover the roots and causes of these behaviors to aid in the understanding of sex offenders and their crimes. *$60.98*

560 pages Year Founded: 2005 ISBN 0-131703-50-1

1288 Sexual Aggression
American Psychiatric Publishing, Inc.
1000 Wilson Boulevard
Suite 1825
Arlington, VA 22209-3901
703-907-7322
800-368-5777; *Fax:* 703-907-1091
appi@psych.org
www.appi.org

Jon A Shaw, M.D., Editor

Appropriate diagnosis and treatment options are presented. *$64.00*

360 pages Year Founded: 1999 ISBN 0-880487-57-7

1289 Sexual Deviance, Second Edition: Theory, Assessment, and Treatment
The Guilford Press
72 Spring Street
New York, NY 10012
800-365-7006; *Fax:* 212-966-6708
info@guilford.com
www.guilford.com

D. Richard Laws, PhD, Editor
William T. O'Donohue, PhD, Editor

This important work provides authoritative scientific and applied perspectives on the full range of paraphilias and other sexual behavior problems. For each major clinical syndrome, a chapter of psychopathology and theory is followed by a chapter on assessment and treatment. Challenges in working with sex offenders are considered in depth. New topics include an integrated etiological model, sexual deviance across the lifespan, Internet offenders, multiple paraphilias, neurobiological processes, the clinician as expert witness, and public health approaches.

642 pages Year Founded: 1973 ISBN 1-593856-05-9

1290 The Psychology of Lust Murder: Paraphilia, Sexual Killing, and Serial Homicide
Academic Press
1600 John F Kennedy Boulevard
Suite 1800
Philadelphia, PA 19103-2879

800-545-2522; *Fax:* 800-568-5136
usbkinfo@elsevier.com
www.elsevier.com

Catherine Purcell, Author
Bruce Arrigo, Author

Systematically examines the phenomenon of paraphilia in relationship to the crime of lust murder. By synthesizing the relevant theories on sexual homicide and serial killing, the authors develop an original, timely, sensible model that accounts for the emergence and progression of paraphilias expressed through increasingly violent erotic fantasies. Going well beyond theoretical speculation, the authors apply their integrated model to the gruesome and chilling case of Jeffrey Dahmer. They convincingly demonstrate where and how their conceptual framework provides a more complete explanation of lust homicide than any other model available in the field today.

192 pages Year Founded: 1880 ISBN 0-123705-10-X

1291 Therapy for Adults Molested as Children: Beyond Survival
Springer Publishing Company
11 West 42nd Street
15th Floor
New York, NY 10036-8002
212-431-4370
877-687-7476; *Fax:* 212-941-7842
cs@springerpub.com
www.springerpub.com

John Briere, PhD, Author

Substantially expanded and updated, this classic volume provides therapists with detailed information on how to treat sexual abuse survivors more effectively. Dr. Briere offers an integrated theory of postabuse symptom development and suggests certain core phenomena that account for many of the psychosocial difficulties associated with childhood sexual abuse. *$39.95*

270 pages Year Founded: 1950 ISBN 0-826156-41-X

1292 Treating Intellectually Disabled Sex Offenders: A Model Residential Program
Safer Society Foundation
PO Box 340
Brandon, VT 05733-0340
802-247-3132; *Fax:* 802-247-4233
www.safersociety.org

James Haaven, Author
Roger Little, Author
Dan Petre-Miller, Author

Describes how the intensive residential specialized Social Skills Program at Oregon State Hospital combines the principles of respect, self-help, and experiential learning with traditional sex-offender treatment methods. *$24.00*

152 pages ISBN 1-884444-30-X

Video & Audio

1293 Understanding Mental Illness
Educational Video Network, Inc.
1401 19th Street
Huntsville, TX 77340
936-295-5767
800-762-0060; *Fax:* 936-294-0233
www.www.evndirect.com

Contains information and classifications of mental illness. Mental illness can strike anyone, at any age. Learn about various organic and functional mental disorders as discussed and their causes and symptoms, and learn where to seek help for a variety of mental health concerns.

Web Sites

1294 www.emdr.com
EMDR Institute

Eye Movement Desensitization and Reprocessing (EMDR) integrates elements of many effective psychotherapies in structured protocols that are designed to maximize treatment effects. These include psychodynamic, cognitive behavioral, interpersonal, experiential, and body-centered therapies.

1295 www.mentalhealth.com
Internet Mental Health

Offers online psychiatric diagnosis in the hope of reaching the two-thirds of individuals with mental illness who do not seek treatment.

1296 www.planetpsych.com
Planetpsych.com

Online resource for mental health information.

1297 www.priory.com/sex.htm
Sexual Disorders

Diagnoses and treatments.

1298 www.psychcentral.com
Psych Central

The Internet's largest and oldest independent mental health social network created and run by mental health professionals to guarantee reliable, trusted information and support communities to you.

1299 www.shrinktank.com
Shrinktank

Psychology-related programs, shareware and freeware.

1300 www.store.samhsa.gov
Substance Abuse and Mental Health Services Administration

Resources on mental disorders as well as treatment and recovery.

1301 www.vaginismus.com
Vaginismus.com

An online resource for individuals who suffer from sexual pain. Vaginismus.com offers products, materials in a variety of languages, and a forum for people with Vaginismus to connect with each other.

Sleep-Wake Disorders

Introduction

Sleep-Wake Disorders are a group of disorders characterized by extreme distruptions in normal sleeping patterns. These include Insomnia, Hypersomnonlence, Narcolepsy, Sleep Apnea, Circadian Rhythm Sleep Disorder, Substance Abuse Induced Sleep Disorder, Nightmare Disorder, Sleep Terror Disorder, Parasomnias, and Restless Legs Syndrome.

Insomnia consists of the inability to sleep, with excessive daytime sleepiness, for at least one month, as evidenced by either prolonged sleep episodes or daytime sleep episodes that occur almost daily.

Narcolepsy is characterized by chronic, involuntary and irresistible sleep attacks; a person with the disorder can suddenly fall asleep at any time of the day and during nearly any activity, including driving a car.

Sleep Apnea is diagnosed when sleep is distrupted by an obstruction of the breathing apparatus.

Circadian Rhythm Sleep Disorder is a disruption of normal sleep patterns leading to a mismatch between the schedule required by a person's environment and his or her sleeping patterns; i.e., the individual is irresistibly sleepy when he or she is required to be awake, and awake at those times that he or she should be sleeping.

Nightmare Disorder is diagnosed when there is a repeated occurrence of frightening dreams that lead to waking.

Sleep Terror Disorder is the repeated occurrence of sleep terrors, or abrupt awakenings from sleeping with a shriek or a cry.

SYMPTOMS

This discussion addresses the disorder with the greatest prevalence: Insomnia. A diagnosis of Insomnia is made if the following criteria are met:

• Difficulty initiating or maintaining sleep or nonrestorative sleep for at least one month;
• The impairment causes clinically significant distress or impairment in social, occupational, or other important areas of functioning;
• The disturbance does not occur exclusively during the course of other sleep-related disorders;
• The disturbance is not due to another general medical or psychiatric disorder, or the direct physiological effects of a substance.

ASSOCIATED FEATURES

Individuals with Insomnia have a history of light sleeping. Interpersonal or work-related problems typically arise because of lack of sleep. Accidents and injuries may result from lack of attentiveness during waking hours, and sleep inducing, tranquillizer, or other medications may be misused or abused by people with Insomnia. Once general medical problems are ruled out, a careful sleep history will often reveal that the individual has poor sleep habits or is reacting to an adverse life situation. These problems can then be addressed with advice or psychotherapy.

PREVALENCE

Surveys indicate a one-year prevalence of Insomnia complaints in thirty percent to forty percent of adults. Insomnia becomes more prevalent with increased age, and women are more likely than men to suffer from Insomnia.

TREATMENT OPTIONS

Treatment for Sleep-Wale Disorders includes an examination by a primary care physician to determine physical condition and sleeping habits, and a discussion with a somnologist, a professional trained in Sleep-Wake Disorders, or other mental health professional, to determine the individual's emotional state.

Referrals may be made to sleep clinics, which can be situated in hospitals, or sleep disorder centers in hospitals, universities or psychiatric institutions. To determine the cause of sleep disturbances, an individual in a sleep clinic or sleep disorder center may undergo interviews, psychological tests and laboratory observation. The patient will sleep in the sleep laboratory while an overnight polysomnography is conducted. In this procedure, the person is wired to electrodes that monitor the various sleep stages. Polysomnography can also determine if the individual is suffering from Sleep Apnea.

The main treatments for Insomnia are behavioral therapy and sleep medications. Behavioral methods used to help people with Insomnia may include relaxation exercises, planning a transition time for unwinding before bed, going to bed only when sleepy, getting out of bed if unable to sleep, getting up at the same time every morning, reserving the bedroom for sleeping only, avoiding daytime naps and limiting the amount of time in bed to actual sleep time. People with Insomnia are also encouraged to practise good sleep habits, such as exercising regularly, avoiding stimulants and alcohol before bedtime, and keeping the bedroom quiet and dark.

Medications that may be part of treatment for Sleep-Wake Disorders include drugs known as hypnotics, or sleeping pills, including temazepam, Ambien, Sonata, and Lunesta. Some medications are more helpful with falling, and others with staying, asleep; a new formulation of Ambien has been developed in an attempt to address both. Melatonin supplementation and over-the-counter medications that contain diphenhydramine may also help in treating Insomnia. Many cases of Insomnia will resolve with improved sleep hygiene, and treatment of pain and other remediable causes. The drug Provigil helps people with Narcolepsy to stay awake. Sleep medications can lose effectiveness if taken over extended periods; use should always be supervised by a physician.

Associations & Agencies

1303 American Academy of Dental Sleep Medicine
1001 Warrenville Road
Suite 175
Lisle, IL 60532
630-686-9875; *Fax:* 630-686-9876
info@aadsm.org
www.aadsm.org

Harold Smith, DDS, President
Leslie Dort, DDS, Director

Alan Blanton, DDS, Director
Rose Sheats, DMD, Secretary and Treasurer

The American Academy of Dental Sleep Medicine is a professional membership organization focused on raising awareness on the involvement of dentistry in sleep-related breathing disorders treatment and research. The AADSM seeks to expand research on the use of oral appliances and dental surgery in the diagnosis and treatment of sleep-related breathing disorders. The AADSM assists in the education of practitioner dentists through clinical meetings and establishes relationships with sleep centers and other professional medical groups to help drive research on sleep breathing disorders.

Year Founded: 1991

1304 American Academy of Sleep Medicine

2510 North Frontage Road
Darien, IL 60561
630-737-9700; *Fax:* 630-737-9790
contact@aasm.org
www.aasmnet.org

Ilene M. Rosen, MD, President
Steve Van Hout, Executive Director
Kelly A. Carden, MD, MBA, Secretary and Treasurer
Douglas Kirsch, MD, President-Elect

The American Academy of Sleep Medicine is a professional society committed to fostering health care, research, and education in the field of sleep medicine. Consisting of 10,000 accredited members specializing in the study, diagnosis, and treatment of sleep-related disorders, the AASM seeks to improve sleep health. The AASM also advocates for accessibility to quality sleep care, organizes educational events on sleep medicine, and produces publications on the latest research findings in the field.

Year Founded: 1975

1305 International Restless Legs Syndrome Study Group

3270 19th Street NW
Suite 110
Rochester, MN 55901
507-316-0084; *Fax:* 612-465-5357
secretary@irlssg.org
www.irlssg.org/

Allan O'Bryan, Executive Director

A nonprofit organization of professionals aiming to advance clinical research of Restless Legs Syndrome.

1306 Narcolepsy Network

PO Box 2178
Lynnwood, WA 98036
401-667-2523
888-292-6522; *Fax:* 401-633-6567
narnet@narcolepsynetwork.org
www.narcolepsynetwork.org

Mark Patterson, MD, PhD, President
Eveline Honig, MD, MPH, Executive Director
Keith Harper, Vice President
Louise O'Connell, Treasurer

A nonprofit organization dedicated to providing support for individuals with narcolepsy and related sleep disorders. Narcolepsy Network offers information and resources, raises public awareness of narcolepsy, and provides services to assist and advocate for all persons with the sleep disorder.

Year Founded: 1986

1307 National Alliance on Mental Illness

3803 North Fairfax Drive
Suite 100
Arlington, VA 22203
703-524-7600
800-950-6264
info@nami.org
www.nami.org

Steve Pitman, JD, President
Lacey Berumen, PhD, MNM, First Vice President
Mary Giliberti, Chief Executive Officer
David Levy, Chief Financial Officer

NAMI is an organization dedicated to raising awareness on mental health and providing support and education for Americans affected by mental illness. NAMI advocates for access to services and treatment and fosters an environment of awareness and understanding for those concerned with mental health.

Year Founded: 1979

1308 National Association for the Dually Diagnosed (NADD)

132 Fair Street
Kingston, NY 12401
845-331-4336
info@thenadd.org
www.thenadd.org

Jeanne M. Farr, MA, Chief Executive Officer
Daniel Baker, PhD., President
Peggie Webb, MA, Vice President
George Zukotynski, PhD., Secretary

NADD is a nonprofit organization designed to increase awareness of, and provide services for, individuals with developmental disabilities and mental illness. NADD emphasizes the importance of quality mental healthcare for people with mental health needs and offers conferences, information resources, educational programs, and training materials to professionals, parents, and organizations.

Year Founded: 1983

1309 National Mental Health Consumers' Self-Help Clearinghouse

1211 Chestnut Street
Suite 1100
Philadelphia, PA 19107
267-507-3810
800-553-4539; *Fax:* 215-636-6312
info@mhselfhelp.org
www.mhselfhelp.org

Joseph Rogers, Founder and Executive Director
Susan Rogers, Director

The Clearinghouse is a peer-run national technical assistance center focused on achieving respect and equality of opportunity for those with mental illnesses. The Clearinghouse helps with the growth of the mental health consumer movement by evaluating mental health services, advocating for mental health reform, and providing consumers with news, information, publications, and consultation services.

Year Founded: 1986

1310 National Sleep Foundation
1010 North Glebe Road
Suite 420
Arlington, VA 22201
703-243-1697
nsf@sleepfoundation.org
www.sleepfoundation.org

Joseph M. Ojile, Chairman
Helene Emsellem, Vice Chairman
David M. Cloud, MBA, Chief Executive Officer

The National Sleep Foundation is committed to improving the health of Americans suffering from sleep problems and disorders. Through sleep education and advocacy, NSF provides patients, medical professionals, and the public with resources on sleep medicine, sleep hygiene, and sleep disorders. NSF seeks to help the public better understand the benefits of healthy sleep habits and the importance of identifying the signs of sleep problems so that they can be properly treated.

Year Founded: 1990

1311 Restless Legs Syndrome Foundation, Inc.
3006 Bee Caves Road
Suite D206
Austin, TX 78746
512-366-9109; *Fax:* 512-366-9189
info@rls.org
www.www.rls.org/

Karla Dzienkowski, RN, BSN, Executive Director
Hillary Hurst, Program Coordinator
Lewis Phelps, Chair
Linda R. Secretan, Secretary

A nonprofit organization dedicated to increasing awareness, and improving treatments and research in order to find a cure for Restless Legs Syndrome.

Year Founded: 1992

1312 The Center for Family Support
2811 Zulette Avenue
Bronx, NY 10461
718-518-1500; *Fax:* 718-518-8200
www.www.cfsny.org/

Steven Vernikoff, Executive Director
Lloyd Stabiner, President
Amy Bittinger, Vice President
Barbara Greenwald, Associate Executive Director

The Center for Family Support offers assistance to individuals with developmental and related disabilities, as well as their families, and provides support services and programs that are designed to accommodate individual needs. Offers services throughout New York City, Westchester County, Long Island, and New Jersey.

Year Founded: 1954

1313 The Johns Hopkins Center for Restless Legs Syndrome
Johns Hopkins University School of Medicine
Johns Hopkins Asthma & Allergy Center
5501 Hopkins Bayview Circle
Baltimore, MD 21224-6801
410-550-0571
410-464-6713
www.www.hopkinsmedicine.org/neurology_neurosurgery/

Richard P. Allen, PhD, Professor of Neurology
Christopher J. Early, PhD, MBBCh, Professor of
Neurology
Charlene Edie Gamaldo, MD, Associate Professor,
Neurology
Rachel Marie E. Salas, MD, Associate Professor,
Neurology

A reseach center dedicated to the research of Restless Legs Syndrome. The center is part of the Johns Hopkins University of Medicine, and provides dissemination of health information as well as programs related to the cause, prevention, and treatmet of RLS. The center is located in the Asthma and Allergy Center at the Johns Hopkins Bayview Campus.

Books

1314 100 Q&A About Sleep and Sleep Disorders, Second Edition
Jones and Bartlett Publishers, Inc.
5 Wall Street
Burlington, MA 01803
978-443-5000
800-832-0034; *Fax:* 978-443-8000
info@jblearning.com
www.jblearning.com

Sudhansu Chokroverty,MD,FRCP,FA, Author

The only text available to provide both the doctor's and patient's views, giving you authoritative, practical answers to the common questions about sleep and sleep disorders. Written by an expert on the subject, with insider commentary from actual patients, this book is an invaluable resource for anyone struggling with the medical, psychological, or emotional turmoil of these conditions.

188 pages Year Founded: 1983 ISBN 0-763741-20-5

1315 A Woman's Guide to Sleep Disorders
McGraw-Hill
1221 Avenue of the Americas
New York, NY 10020-1095
212-904-2000
www.mcgraw-hill.com

Meir H. Kryger, MD, Author

The first comprehensive book written about sleep disorders in women by a leading medical expert in the field. Dr. Kryger provides a thorough overview of sleep disorders among women. He shows how to determine whether a sleep problem is a disorder, help pinpoint causes, and what can be done to help. A resource guide, sleep questionnaire, and worksheet are included to assist the reader, and her doctor, in evaluating her condition.

337 pages Year Founded: 2004 ISBN 0-071425-27-6

1316 Concise Guide to Evaluation and Management of Sleep Disorders
American Psychiatric Publishing, Inc.
1000 Wilson Boulevard
Suite 1825
Arlington, VA 22209-3901
703-907-7322
800-368-5777; *Fax:* 703-907-1091
appi@psych.org
www.appi.org

Martin Reite, Author
Michael Weissberg, M.D., Author
John Ruddy, Author

Overview of sleep disorders medicine, sleep physiology and pathology, insomnia complaints, excessive sleepiness disorders, parasomnias, medical and psychiatric disorders and sleep, medications with sedative-hypnotic properties, special problems and populations. *$29.95*

395 pages Year Founded: 2009 ISBN 0-880489-06-5

1317 Drug Therapy and Sleep Disorders
Mason Crest Publishers
450 Parkway Drive
Suite D
Broomall, PA 19008-4017
610-543-6200
866-627-2665; *Fax:* 610-543-3878
dtaylor@masoncrest.com
www.masoncrest.com

Joan Esherick, Author

What are sleep disorders? Which drugs do doctors prescribe to treat them? What risks and benefits are involved? This book answers these and other questions by examining various sleep disorders, their symptoms and causes, common treatments, the drugs used to treat them, and how sleep drugs affect the brain.

128 pages ISBN 1-590845-76-5

1318 Getting a Good Night's Sleep A Cleveland Clinic Guide
Cleveland Clinic Press
9500 Euclid Avenue
Cleveland, OH 44195
216-444-2200
800-223-2273
TTY: 216-444-0261
www.cchealth.clevelandclinic.org/publications

Nancy Foldvary-Schaefer, Author

This book gives the sleepless what they need; real, substantive information from a source that is trusted by people all over the world. It provides a straightforward and clear examination of sleep problems and serves as a complete home reference for anyone.

228 pages Year Founded: 2006 ISBN 1-596240-14-8

1319 Parasomnias, An Issue of Sleep Medicine Clinics
Saunders: Elsevier, Health Sciences Division
1600 John F. Kennedy Blvd
Suite 1800
Philadelphia, PA 19103-2899
215-239-3900
800-523-1649; *Fax:* 215-239-3990
www.www.us.elsevierhealth.com

Mark Pressman, PhD, D.ABSM, Author

Articles examine disorders such as sleepwalking, sleep sex, sleep violence, sleep eating, and diagnostic methods of these. The issue also delves into forensic concerns, especially with regard to sleep violence. Other types of parasomnias discussed include sleep talking and sleep enuresis.

Year Founded: 2011 ISBN 1-455779-92-X

1320 Principles and Practice of Sleep Medicine
Elsevier, Inc.
1600 John F. Kennedy Boulevard.
Suite 1800
Philadelphia, PA 19103-2822

215-239-3900
800-523-1649; *Fax:* 215-239-3990
www.www.us.elsevierhealth.com

Meir H. Kryger, MD, Author/Editor
Thomas Roth, PhD, Author/Editor
William C. Dement, MD, PhD, Author/Editor

Delivers the comprehensive, dependable guidance you need to effectively diagnose and manage even the most challenging sleep disorders. Updates to genetics and circadian rhythms, occupational health, sleep in older people, memory and sleep, physical examination of the patient, comorbid insomnias, and much more keep physicians current on the newest areas of the field. A greater emphasis on evidence-based approaches helps you make the most well-informed clinical decisions. *$329.00*

1766 pages Year Founded: 2011 ISBN 1-437707-31-1

1321 Say Good Night to Insomnia: The Six-Week, Drug-Free Program Developed at Harvard Medical School
Henry Holt and Company
175 Fifth Avenue
New York, NY 10010
646-307-5151; *Fax:* 212-633-0748
customerservice@mpsvirginia.com
www.us.macmillan.com

Gregg D. Jacobs, PhD, Author
Dr. Herbert Benson, Introduction

The first clinician to offer proof that insomnia can be overcome without drugs, Dr. Jacob's program provides techniques for: eliminating sleeping pills, establishing sleep-promoting habits and lifestyle practices, changing negative stressful thoughts about sleep, implementing relaxation and stress-reduction techniques, enhancing peace of mind and reducing negative emotions.

256 pages Year Founded: 1999 ISBN 0-805055-48-7

1322 Sleep Apnea: Pathogenesis, Diagnosis, and Treatment
Informa Healthcare
52 Vanderbilt Ave.
New York, NY 10017
212-520-2777
866-861-0135
books@informa.com

Allan I. Pack, MBChB PhD, Author, Editor

Considers the relationship between obstructive sleep apnea (OSA) and cardiovascular disease, right and left ventricular dysfunction, and hypertension. A must-have, in-depth guide for pulmonologists; physiologists; chest, pulmonary, thoracic, and cardiovascular physicians and surgeons; cardiologists; respiratory therapists; clinical neurologists; sleep disorder specialists; and medical school students.

570 pages Year Founded: 2002 ISBN 0-824703-12-X

1323 Sleep Disorders Sourcebook
Omnigraphics
155 West Congress
Suite 200
Detroit, MI 48226
313-961-1340
800-234-1340; *Fax:* 313-961-1383
contact@omnigraphics.com
www.omnigraphics.com

Sandra J Judd, Author/Editor

Gathering information from government and relevant agency sources, this consumer reference addresses the biology of sleep, changing sleep needs throughout life, how to improve sleep quality and quantity, the diagnosis and treatment of specific sleep disorders in adults and children, and conditions that affect sleep. The volume includes a glossary, directory of resources, and suggested further reading. *$ 78.00*

561 pages Year Founded: 1985 ISBN 1-780807-43-X

1324 Sleep Medicine Essentials
Wiley-Blackwell
111 River Street
Hoboken, NJ 07030-5774
201-748-6000; *Fax:* 201-748-6088
info@wiley.com
www.wiley.com

Teofilo L. Lee-Chiong, Author

This is a concise, convenient, practical, and affordable handbook on sleep medicine. It consists of forty topic-focused chapters written by a panel of international experts covering a range of topics including insomnia, sleep apnea, narcolepsy, parasomnias, circadian sleep disorders, sleep in the elderly, sleep in children, sleep among women, and sleep in the medical, psychiatric, and neurological disorders.

280 pages Year Founded: 2009 ISBN 0-470195-66-5

1325 Sleep and Pain
Intl Association for the Study of Pain
1510 H Street,NorthWest
Suite 600
Washington, DC 20005-1020
202-524-5300; *Fax:* 202-524-5301
IASPdest@iasp-pain.org
www.iasp-pain.org

Gilles Lavigne, Editor
Barry J. Sessle, Editor
Manon Choiniere, Editor
Peter J. Soja, Editor

Many in the research and clinical communities are becoming increasingly aware of the interactions between sleep disorders and chronic pain syndromes. There are a number of obstacles on the path to better patient care, and there is considerable room for improvement in the way knowledge is shared between professionals in the sleep and pain communities. This book serves as the first step toward enhancing communication between the sleep and pain communities with the intent of improving patient care.

474 pages Year Founded: 1974 ISBN 0-931092-80-0

1326 The Dana Guide to Brain Health: A Practical Family Reference from Medical Experts
The Dana Foundation
505 Fifth Avenue
6th Floor
New York, NY 10017
212-223-4040; *Fax:* 212-317-8721
danainfo@dana.org
www.dana.org

Floyd E Bloom, MD, Editor
M. Flint Beal, MD, Editor
David J. Kupfer, MD, Editor

A milestone in health publishing, the first major home medical reference on the brain, the Dana Guide is based on the contributions of more than 100 of America's most distinguished scientists and clinicians. The most authoritative, comprehensive, and clearly written guide to the bodily organ that is the key to our everyday health. No home should be without it.

Year Founded: 2007

1327 The Parasomnias and Other Sleep-Related Movement Disorders
Cambridge University Press
32 Avenue of the Americas
New York, NY 10013-2473
212-337-5000
newyork@cambrigde.org
www.www.cambridge.org

Michael J. Thorpy, MD, Editor
Giuseppe Plazzi, MD, Editor

The first authoritative review on the parasomnias - disorders that cause abnormal behavior during sleep - this book contains many topics never before covered in detail. Appropriate behavioral and pharmacological treatments are addressed in detail. Sleep specialists, neurologists, psychiatrists, psychologists, and other healthcare professionals with an interest in sleep disorders will find this book essential reading.

356 pages Year Founded: 1534 ISBN 0-521111-57-9

Periodicals & Pamphlets

1328 Narcolepsy In the Classroom
Narcolepsy Network
129 Waterwheel Lane
North Kingstown, RI 02852
401-667-2523
888-292-6522; *Fax:* 401-633-6567
NarNet@narcolepsynetwork.org
www.narcolepsynetwork.org

Sara Kowalczyk, MA, MPH, President
Eveline Honig, MD, MPH, Executive Director
Mark Patterson,MD,PhD, Vice President
Louise O'Connell, Treasurer

Concerned about a sleepy student? Essential information for school nurses, administrators, special education teams, parents, teachers, and students.

Year Founded: 1986

1329 Narcolepsy Q&A
Narcolepsy Network
129 Waterwheel Lane
North Kingstown, RI 02852
401-667-2523
888-292-6522; *Fax:* 401-633-6567
NarNet@narcolepsynetwork.org
www.narcolepsynetwork.org

Sara Kowalczyk, MA, MPH, President
Eveline Honig, MD, MPH, Executive Director
Mark Patterson,MD,PhD, Vice President
Louise O'Connell, Treasurer

Common questions about narcolepsy for doctors' offices, public service buildings as well as psychiatrist offices and sleep study programs.

Year Founded: 1986

1330 Narcolepsy and You
Narcolepsy Network
129 Waterwheel Lane
North Kingstown, RI 02852
401-667-2523
888-292-6522; *Fax:* 401-633-6567
NarNet@narcolepsynetwork.org
www.narcolepsynetwork.org

Sara Kowalczyk, MA, MPH, President
Eveline Honig, MD, MPH, Executive Director
Mark Patterson, MD, PhD, Vice President
Louise O'Connell, Treasurer

This booklet provides information about narcolepsy and tips on how to live a healthy life with this often misunderstood condition.

16 pages Year Founded: 1986

1331 Sleep Health Journal
National Sleep Foundation
1010 North Glebe Road
Suite 420
Arlington, VA 22201
703-243-1697
sleephealthjournal@sleepfoundation.org
www.www.sleephealthjournal.org/

Lauren Hale, PhD, Editor-in-Chief
Orfeu Buxton, PhD, Associate Editor
Michael Grandner, PhD, Associate Editor
Amy Wolfson, PhD, Associate Editor

A peer-reviewed journal that advances the sleep health of all members of society. The journal covers the topic of sleep throughout a variety of disciplines, and includes articles, reports, letters to the editor, editorials, and commentaries.

ISSN 2352-7218

1332 Sleep and Breathing
American Academy of Dental Sleep Medicine
2510 North Frontage Road
Darien, IL 60561
630-737-9761; *Fax:* 630-737-9790
info@aadsm.org
www.www.aadsm.org

B. Gail Demko, DMD, President
Michael Simmons, DMD, Director
Todd Morgan, DMD, Director
Leslie C Dort, DDS, Secretary/Treasurer

The official peer-reviewed journal of the AADSM, features the most recent original research in dental sleep medicine. Timely and original studies on the management of the upper airway during sleep in addition to common sleep disorders and disruptions, including sleep apnea, insomnia and shiftwork. Coverage includes patient studies and studies that emphasize the principles of physiology and pathophysiology or illustrate novel approaches to diagnosis and treatment.

4x per year Year Founded: 1991

Research Centers

1333 Sleep Studies
eRiver Neurology of New York, LLC
21 Fox Street
Suite 102
Poughkeepsie, NY 12601-4723

845-452-9750; *Fax:* 845-452-9751
www.eriverneurology.com/Sleep%20Disorders%20Lab.htm

The all-night sleep study is frequently used by sleep physicians to evaluate adult patients when they are sleeping. This laboratory tet is extremely valuable for diagnosing and treating many sleep disorders, including neurologic disorders, movement disorders and breathing disorders at night. Sleep studies are generally easy to tolerate, comfortable for patients, and give sleep physicians the information they need to accurately diagnose and treat the sleep disorder.

1334 Standford Sleep Medicine Center
450 Broadway Street, Pavilion B
2nd Floor, MC 5730
Redwood City, CA 94063
650-723-6601
www.stanfordhealthcare.org/search-results.clinics.html

Fiona Barwick, PhD, Psychologist
Mark Buchfuhrer, MD, Sleep Specialist
Clete A. Kushida, MD, PhD, Sleep Specialist
Emmanuel Mignot, MD, PhD, Sleep Specialist

A research center that deals with sleep disorders in children and adults, including Restless Leg Syndrome, Sleep Apnea, Insomnia, Narcolepsy, Parasomnias, and more. The Sleep Medicine Center has three clinics specifically for Narcolepsy, Parasomnias, and Restless Legs Syndrome.

Support Groups & Hot Lines

1335 ASAA A.W.A.K.E. Network
American Sleep Apnea Association (ASAA)
6856 Eastern Avenue NW
Suite 203
Washington, DC 20012
202-293-3650; *Fax:* 202-293-3656
www.stanford.edu/~dement/sleeplinks.html#so

Plays a crucial role in the ASAA's educational and avocacy efforts. A.W.A.K.E. is an acronym for Alert, Well, And Keeping Energetic. A mutual-help support group for persons affected by sleep apnea, composed of more than 200 groups in 45 states. Meetings are held regularly and guest speakers are often invited to address the group. Topics may include advice on complying with CPAP therapy, legal issues affecting those with sleep apnea, weight loss, treatment options such as oral appliances, and new research findings. Baltimore, New York, California, Oakland California, and Western Pennsylvania are just a few of the many locations of A.W.A.K.E. groups.

1336 Night Terrors Forum
Night Terrors Resource Center
www.www.nightterrors.org/forum.htm

David W. Richards, Site Administrator

Helping people understand that there are medical solutions and reasons for Night Terrors. Information on causes, medications, personal stories, sleep stages, and frequently asked questions about night terrors.

Year Founded: 1996

1337 eHealthForum Sleep Disorder Support Forum
www.ehealthforum.com/health/sleep_disorders.html#b

A health community featuring member and doctor discussions ranging from a specific symptom to related conditions, treatment options, medication, side effects, diet, and emotional issues surrounding medical sleep conditions.

Video & Audio

1338 Clinical Impressions: Identifying Mental Illness
Educational Training Videos
136 Granville St
Suite 200
Gahanna, OH 43230
Fax: 888-775-3919
www.educationaltrainingvideos.com

How long can mental illness stay hidden, especially from the eyes of trained experts? This program rejoins a group of ten adults- five of them healthy and five of them with histories of mental illness- as psychiatric specialists try to spot and correctly diagnose the latter. Administering a series of collaborative and one-on-one tests, including assessments of personality type, physical self-image, and rational thinking, the panel gradually makes decisions about who suffers from depression, bipolar disorder, bulimia, and social anxiety.

1339 Coping with Stress
Educational Video Network, Inc.
1401 19th Street
Huntsville, TX 77340
936-295-5767
800-762-0060; *Fax:* 936-294-0233
www.www.evndirect.com

Stress affects everyone, both emotionally and physically. For some, mismanaged stress can result in substance abuse, violence, or even suicide. This program answers the question, How can a person cope with stress?

1340 Effective Learning Systems
5108 W 74th
St #390160
Minneapolis, MN 55439
952-943-1660
800-966-0443
www.effectivelearning.com

Audio tapes for stress management, deep relaxation, anger control, peace of mind, insomnia, weight and smoking, self-image and self-esteem, positive thinking, health and healing. Since 1972, Effective Learning Systems has helped millions of people take charge of their lives and make positive changes. Over 75 titles available.

Year Founded: 1972

1341 Insomnia
Educational Training Videos
136 Granville St
Suite 200
Gahanna, OH 43230
Fax: 888-775-3919
www.educationaltrainingvideos.com

An inability to sleep is far more than a nuisance- it's a genuine health problem. This program examines insomnia from a medical perspective, exploring the physical, emotional, and psychological aspects of the disorder. Interview with doctors who specialize in treating sleep difficulties provide historical background on the affliction, the personal and professional hazards it can present, and dietary and behavioral adjustments that can improve the quality of sleep.

1342 Mental Disorder
Educational Training Videos
136 Granville St
Suite 200
Gahanna, OH 43230
Fax: 888-775-3919
www.educationaltrainingvideos.com

What is abnormality? Using the case studies of two young women; one who has depression, one who has an anxiety disorder; as a springboard, this program presents three psychological perspective on mental disorder.

1343 Understanding Mental Illness
Educational Video Network, Inc.
1401 19th Street
Huntsville, TX 77340
936-295-5767
800-762-0060; *Fax:* 936-294-0233
www.www.evndirect.com

Contains information and classifications of mental illness. Mental illness can strike anyone, at any age. Learn about various organic and functional mental disorders as discussed and their causes and symptoms, and learn where to seek help for a variety of mental health concerns.

Web Sites

**1344 ehealthforum.com/health/sleep_disorders.
html#b**
eHealthForum Sleep Disorder Support Forum

A health community featuring member and doctor discussions ranging from a specific symptom to related conditions, treatment options, medication, side effects, diet, and emotional issues surrounding medical sleep conditions.

1345 www.aadsm.org
American Academy of Dental Sleep Medicine

Promotes research on the use of oral appliances and dental surgery for the treatment of sleep disordered breathing and provides training and resources for those who work directly with patients. The organization builds bridges and forms relationships with the medical community, especially in sleep centers, and other professional groups who play an integral part of the sleep disorders treatment and research team. The AADSM also reaches out to the community at large, working toward the creation of a positive public awareness of sleep disorders and the role of the dentist in recognition and treatment of sleep breathing disorders.

1346 www.aasmnet.org
American Academy of Sleep Medicine

A professional society that is dedicated exclusively to the medical subspecialty of sleep medicine.

1347 www.cyberpsych.org
CyberPsych

Presents information about psychoanalysis, psychotherapy and special topics such as anxiety disorders, the problematic use of alcohol, homophobia, and the traumatic effects of racism.

1348 www.mentalhealth.com
Internet Mental Health

Offers on-line psychiatric diagnosis in the hope of reaching the two-thirds of individuals with mental illness who do not seek treatment.

1349 www.narcolepsynetwork.org
Narcolepsy Network
www.narcolepsynetwork.org

A non profit organization dedicated to individuals with narcolepsy and related sleep disorders. Mission is to provide services to educate, advocate, support and improve awareness of this neurological sleep disorder.

1350 www.nhlbi.nih.gov/about/ncsdr
National Institute of Health National Center on Sleep Disorders

The Center seeks to fulfill its goal of improving the health of Americans by serving four key functions: research, training, technology transfer, and coordination.

1351 www.nightterrors.org/forum.htm
Night Terrors Resource Center, Night Terrors Forum

Helping people understand that there are medical solutions and reasons for Night Terrors. Information on causes, medications, personal stories, sleep stages, and frequently asked questions about night terrors.

1352 www.nlm.nih.gov/medlineplus/sleepdisorders.html
MEDLINEplus on Sleep Disorders

Compilation of links directs you to information on sleep disorders.

1353 www.planetpsych.com
Planetpsych.com

Online resource for mental health information.

1354 www.psychcentral.com
Psych Central

The Internet's largest and oldest independent mental health social network created and run by mental health professionals to guarantee reliable, trusted information and support communities to you.

1355 www.reggiewhitefoundation.org
Reggie White Sleep Disorders Research & Education Foundation, Inc.

Helping provide CPAP treatment equipment to those people who might otherwise be unable to secure the needed equipment. CPAP equipment is provided to patients who qualify for the foundation's assistance and who have a current prescription for it. Co-founded by Reggie White's wife, Sara, who recognized the role of her husbands sleep disorder in cutting his life short. Started the Foundation to help people of all economic backgrounds to understand the symptoms and risks of sleep disorders.

1356 www.sdrfoundation.org
Sleep Disorder Relief Foundation

A public non profit organization founded to: assist the underpriveleged suffering from sleep disorders by creating a network of relief, further the field of sleep medicine through organizing and funding sleep disorder researcch,

and spread domestic and international awareness about the importance of sleep and the prevalence of sleep disorders.

1357 www.sleepfoundation.org
National Sleep Foundation

Alerting the public, healthcare providers and policymakers to the live-and-death importance of adequate sleep is central to the mission of NSF. NSF is dedicated to improving the quality of life for Americans who suffer from sleep problems and disorders. This means helping the public better understand the importance of sleep and the benefits of good sleep habits, and recognizing the signs of sleep problems so that they can be properly diagnosed and treated.

1358 www.stanford.edu/~dement/sleeplinks.html#so
ASAA A.W.A.K.E. Network

Plays a crucial role in the ASAA's educational and avocacy efforts. A.W.A.K.E. is an acronym for Alert, Well, And Keeping Energetic. A mutual-help support group for persons affected by sleep apnea, composed of more than 200 groups in 45 states. Meetings are held regularly and guest speakers are often invited to address the group. Topics may include advice on complying with CPAP therapy, legal issues affecting those with sleep apnea, weight loss, treatment options such as oral appliances, and new research findings. Baltimore, New York, California, Oakland California, and Western Pennsylvania are just a few of the many locations of A.W.A.K.E. groups.

1359 www.store.samhsa.gov
Substance Abuse and Mental Health Services Administration

Resources on mental disorders as well as treatment and recovery.

1360 www.uic.edu/nursing/CNSHR/index.html
Center for Narcolepsy, Sleep & Health Research

Primary goal is to conduct important basic, clinical and bio-behavioral research for improving, preserving or promoting health through good sleep. The Center also aims to continue as an important source of sleep science and health expertise for colleagues, aspiring sleep researchers, clinicians, patients and families. Researching sleep and sleep-related disorders; educating young scientists for productive careers in sleep research; and transferring technologies and knowledge developed through research into practice or into the private sector.

Somatic Symptom and Related Disorders

Introduction

The disorders in this category are characterized by multiple physical symptoms or the conviction that one is ill despite negative medical examinations and laboratory tests. Those who have a somatizing disorder persist in believing they are ill, or experience physical symptoms over long periods, and their beliefs negatively affect all areas of their functioning.

Two main types of somatizing disorders are Hypochondriasis (also known as Hypochondria), which consists of being convinced that one is ill despite evidence to the contrary, and Somatization Disorder, consisting of experiencing physical symptoms without a discernible basis.

Factitious Disorder and Malingering are also conditions in which physical symptoms are not caused by an identifiable general medical condition, but in which symptoms are deliberately and consciously produced. A malingerer deliberately complains or mimics symptoms to achieve a specific goal, such as winning a medical malpractice suit or obtaining disability insurance.

Individuals with Factitious Disorder deliberately cause significant medical conditions in themselves, for example by introducing fecal contamination intravenously, or taking insulin to the point of severe hypoglycemia. The motivations for this behavior are unclear. Once the diagnosis is suspected, and the suspicion is conveyed to the patient, these individuals nearly always flee the medical care venue and are unwillingto undergo more definitive diagnostic examinations.

SYMPTOMS

HYPOCHONDRIASIS

• Pre occupation with fears of having a serious illness based on a misinterpretation of bodily symptoms or sensations;
• The preoccupation persists in spite of medical reassurance;
• The preoccupation is a source of distress and difficulty in social, work, and other areas;
• The duration of the preoccupation is at least six months.

SOMATIZATION DISORDER

• A history beginning before age 30 and continuing over years, resulting in a search for treatment or clear difficulties in social, work, or interpersonal areas;
• Four pain symptoms related to at least four anatomical areas or functions;
• Two gastrointestinal problems other than pain, e.g. nausea, diarrhea;
• One sexual symptom other than pain, e.g. irregular menstruation, sexual disinterest, erectile dysfunction;
• One pseudoneurological symptom other than pain, e.g., weakness, double vision;
• Symptoms cannot be explained by a medical condition;
• When a medical condition exists, physical complaints and social difficulties are greater than normal.

ASSOCIATED FEATURES

The person with either of these somatizing disorders visits many doctors, but physical examinations and negative lab results neither reassure them nor resolve their symptoms. They often believe they are not getting proper respect or attention, and, indeed, they may be viewed in medical settings as troublesome. Persons with these disorders often suffer from anxiety and depression as well. Physical symptoms appearing after the somatization diagnosis is made, however, should not be dismissed completely out of hand. Sufferers can have general medical disorders at the same time as Somatizing Disorders.

The person may be treated by several doctors at once, which can lead to unwitting and possibly dangerous combinations of treatments. There may be suicide threats and attempts, and deteriorating personal relationships. Individuals with these disorders often have associated Personality Disorders, such as Borderline or Antisocial Personality Disorder.

PREVALENCE

Hypochondriasis is equally common in both sexes. The age of onset is usually young adulthood. Its prevalence in the general population is estimated to be one to five percent. In general medical practice, two percent to seven percent of patients have the disorder. It is usually chronic.

Somatization Disorder was once thought to be mainly a disease of women, but occurs in both sexes. It is slightly less common among men in the general population of the US than in other countries, but not uncommon in general medical practice. It is more common among Puerto Rican and Greek men, which suggests that cultural factors influence the sex ratios. It is estimated that between 0.2 percent and two percent of the general population suffers from Somatization Disorder.

TREATMENT OPTIONS

These disorders are chronic by definition, and are difficult to manage. Repeated reassurance is not successful. The aim is to limit the extent to which the physical concerns and symptoms preoccupy an individual's thoughts and activities, and drain family, emotional, and financial resources. Individuals suffering from these disorders often resist mental health referral because they interpret it, sometimes correctly, as an indication that their symptoms are not being taken seriously. Treatment, whether by the primary care or mental health professional or both, should focus on maintaining function despite the symptoms. It is important that the psychological management and treatment is coordinated with medical treatment if possible by one physician only; one person should oversee all the medical treatment, including the psychological, so that care does not become fragmented and/or repetitive as the patient sees many different clinicians. Some individuals with Hypochondriasis respond to treatment which combines medication with intensive behavioral and cognitive techniques to manage anxiety and modify beliefs about the origin and course of physical symptoms.

People with Hypochondriasis and Somatization Disorders do not deliberately produce or falsely complain of physical symptoms; their beliefs and behaviors are engendered by psychological conflict, and often by modeling on someone who was important to them when they were growing up.

Treatment for Hypochondriasis may include psychological counseling and medication. Cognitive behavioral therapy, which gives patients techniques to manage anxiety and modify beliefs about the origin and course of physical symptoms, is considered helpful in treating Hypochondriasis. Other treatments may include stress management techniques and exposure therapy (in which patients practise confronting their anxieties until they are better able to manage them). Medications such as serotonin reuptake inhibitors (SSRIs) and tricyclic antidepressants are sometimes prescribed.

Treatment of Somatization Disorder may include cognitive behavioral therapy, as well as relaxation techniques and communication skills training. Patients are also encouraged to increase their activity level. Antidepressant medications may be prescribed to help treat symptoms.

Associations & Agencies

1362 Academy of Psychosomatic Medicine
5272 River Road
Suite 500
Bethesda, MD 20816
301-718-6520; *Fax:* 301-656-0989
info@apm.org
www.apm.org

James Rundell, MD, President
James Vrac, CAE, Executive Director
Michael Sharpe, MD, Vice President
Maria Tiamson-Kassab, MD, Treasurer

The Academy of Psychosomatic Medicine represents psychiatrists focused on improving education, medical science, and healthcare for individuals with comorbid psychiatric and general medical conditions. The Academy seeks to promote interdisciplinary education and drive research and public policy with the goal of achieving outstanding clinical care for patients with comorbid psychiatric and general medical conditions throughout the world. They also created the Foundation of the Academy of Psychosomatic Medicine, a scientific foundation supporting education and research programs.

1363 Center for Mental Health Services (CMHS)
Substance Abuse and Mental Health Services Administration
5600 Fishers Lane
Rockville, MD 20857
240-276-1310
877-726-4727
TTY: 800-487-4889
www.samhsa.gov/about-us/who-we-are/offices-centers

Paolo del Vecchio, MSW, Director
Anne Mathews-Younes, Acting Deputy Director
Keris Myrick, Director, Consumer Affairs
Patricia Gratton, Director, Program Analysis

Promotes the treatment of mental illness and emotional disorders by increasing accessibility to mental health programs; supporting outreach, treatment, rehabilitation, and support programs and networks; and encouraging the use of scientifically-based information when treating mental disorders. CMHS provides information about mental health via a toll-free number and numerous publications. Developed for users of mental health services and their families, the general public, policy makers, providers, and the media.

Year Founded: 1992

1364 Goodwill's Community Employment Services
Goodwill Industries-Suncoast, Inc.
10596 Gandy Blvd.
St. Petersburg, FL 33702
727-523-1512
888-279-1988
TDD: 727-579-1068
www.goodwill-suncoast.org

Heather Ceresoli, CPA, Chair
Deborah A. Passerini, President
Martin W. Gladysz, Senior Vice Chair
Louise R. Lopez, Vice Chair

Program providing job coaching and community job placements for people with disabilities.

Year Founded: 1954

1365 Institute for Contemporary Psychotherapy
1841 Broadway
4th Floor
New York, NY 10023
212-333-3444; *Fax:* 212-333-5444
www.icpnyc.org

Ron Taffel, PhD, Chairman
Andrea Green-Lewis, LCSW-R, Director of Operations
Fred Lipschitz, PhD, Treasurer and Co-Founder
Mary Labiento, Associate Director of Operations

The Institute for Contemporary Psychotherapy is a New York City-based mental health treatment and training facility. Consisting of a group of 150 licensed psychotherapists, the Institute focuses on educating the public about the issues surrounding mental health, providing post-graduate training for therapists, and offering therapy at moderate costs.

Year Founded: 1971

1366 National Association for the Dually Diagnosed (NADD)
132 Fair Street
Kingston, NY 12401
845-331-4336
info@thenadd.org
www.thenadd.org

Jeanne M. Farr. MA, Chief Executive Officer
Daniel Baker, PhD., President
Peggie Webb, MA, Vice President
George Zukotynski, PhD., Secretary

NADD is a nonprofit organization designed to increase awareness of, and provide services for, individuals with developmental disabilities and mental illness. NADD emphasizes the importance of quality mental healthcare for people with mental health needs and offers conferences, information resources, educational programs, and training materials to professionals, parents, and organizations.

Year Founded: 1983

1367 National Mental Health Consumers' Self-Help Clearinghouse
1211 Chestnut Street
Suite 1100
Philadelphia, PA 19107
267-507-3810
800-553-4539; *Fax:* 215-636-6312
info@mhselfhelp.org
www.mhselfhelp.org

Joseph Rogers, Founder and Executive Director
Susan Rogers, Director

The Clearinghouse is a peer-run national technical assistance center focused on achieving respect and equality of opportunity for those with mental illnesses. The Clearinghouse helps with the growth of the mental health consumer movement by evaluating mental health services, advocating for mental health reform, and providing consumers with news, information, publications, and consultation services.

Year Founded: 1986

1368 The Center for Family Support

2811 Zulette Avenue
Bronx, NY 10461
718-518-1500; *Fax:* 718-518-8200
www.www.cfsny.org/

Steven Vernikoff, Executive Director
Lloyd Stabiner, President
Amy Bittinger, Vice President
Barbara Greenwald, Associate Executive Director

The Center for Family Support offers assistance to individuals with developmental and related disabilities, as well as their families, and provides support services and programs that are designed to accommodate individual needs. Offers services throughout New York City, Westchester County, Long Island, and New Jersey.

Year Founded: 1954

Books

1369 Concise Guide to Psychopharmacology
American Psychiatric Publishing, Inc.
1000 Wilson Boulevard
Suite 1825
Arlington, VA 22209-3901
703-907-7322
800-368-5777; *Fax:* 703-907-1091
appi@psych.org
www.appi.org

Lauren B Marangell, M.D, Author
James M Martinez, M.D, Author
John McDuffie, Editorial Director
Lauren B Marangell MD, Author

The definitive pocket reference for convenient everyday use. This invaluable clinical companion begins with an overview of the general principles relevant to the safe and effective use of psychotropic medications. Subsequent chapters focus on the major classes of psychotropic medications and the disorders for which they are prescribed. *$47.95*

260 pages Year Founded: 2006 ISSN 9781585622559ISBN 1-585622-55-9

1370 Disorders of Simulation: Malingering, Factitious Disorders, and Compensation Neurosis
Psychosocial Press
59 Boston Post Road
Madison, CT 06443-2130
203-245-4000; *Fax:* 203-245-0775

Grant L. Hutchinson, Author

The book suggests that patients who suffer from disorders of simulation should be considered to have a bona fide

problem, one deserving of mental health attention, understanding, analysis, and treatment.

1371 Do No Harm? Munchhausen Syndrome by Proxy
Independent Publishers Group
814 North Franklin Street
Chicago, IL 60610-3813
312-337-0747
800-888-4741; *Fax:* 312-337-5985
frontdesk@ipgbook.com
www.ipgbook.com

Craig McGill, Author

The syndrome that causes parents and care workers to harm their children to get attention is separating many families. But has the fertile imagination of social workers and the publicc turned MSBP into the trendy disorder of our time? McGill traces the 25-year history of the disorder and examines high profile cases from six countries. He produces compelling stories from parents and care workers and asks what can be done to protect parents from being wrongly accused. *$16.95*

240 pages Year Founded: 1971 ISBN 1-901250-48-2

1372 Drug Therapy and Psychosomatic Disorders
Mason Crest Publishers
450 Parkway Drive
Suite D
Broomall, PA 19008-4017
610-543-6200
866-627-2665; *Fax:* 610-543-3878
dtaylor@masoncrest.com
www.masoncrest.com

Autumn Libal, Author

How can doctors treat pain and illness in the body that are caused by the mind? In this book, learn more about Kevin's story, what psychosomatic disorders are, and how these phantom disorders can be treated.

128 pages Year Founded: 2004 ISBN 1-590845-73-0

1373 Essentials of Psychosomatic Medicine
American Psychiatric Publishing, Inc.
1000 Wilson Boulevard
Suite 1825
Arlington, VA 22209-3901
703-907-7322
800-368-5777; *Fax:* 703-907-1091
appi@psych.org
www.appi.org

James L. Levenson, Author

This condensed version of The American Psychiatric Publishing Textbook of Psychosomatic Medicine focuses on psychiatric care for medically ill patients. Presents that portion of the larger work devoted to specific disorders, enabling the practitioner to assist patients with comorbid psychiatric and general medical illnesses complicating each other's management.

604 pages Year Founded: 2007

1374 Hypochondria: Woeful Imaginings
University of California Press
2120 Berkeley Way
Berkeley, CA 94704-5804

510-642-4247; *Fax:* 510-643-7127
askucp@ucpress.edu
www.ucpress.edu

Susan Baur, Author

Susan Baur illuminates the process by which hypochondri-
acs come to adopt and maintain illness as a way of life.
$25.00

260 pages Year Founded: 1989 ISBN 0-520067-51-7

**1375 Mind-Body Problems: Psychotherapy with
Psychosomatic Disorders**
Jason Aronson
230 Livingston Street
Northvale, NJ 07647-1726
570-342-1320
800-782-0015; *Fax:* 201-767-1576
www.aronson.com

Janet Schumacher Finell, Author

Animated case reports on specific disorders- anorexia, ar-
thritis, irritable bowel syndrome, even (speculatively) mis-
carriage- balance consideration of developmental questions
and treatment issues (transference/countertransference) and
techniques. *$70.00*

376 pages Year Founded: 1977 ISBN 1-568216-54-8

**1376 Munchausen by Proxy: Identification,
Intervention, and Case Management**
Routledge
270 Madison Avenue
New York, NY 10016-601
770-385-9799
louisalasher@mindspring.com
www.www.mbpexpert.com/

Louisa J. Lasher, Author
Louisa Lasher, Author

This step-by-step guide will help you identify and manage
cases of this unique form of child maltreatment. This
skills-base, practical book contains a thorough, up-to-date
overview of MBP and includes suggestions for identifying
and reporting to child protection agencies, investigating
and gathering evidence, and legal and court procedures. Its
easy readability and immediate applicability make this text
a valuable tool in identifying and preventing this form of
child abuse.

384 pages Year Founded: 2004 ISBN 0-789012-17-0

1377 Munchausen's Syndrome by Proxy
World Scientific Publishing Company
27 Warren Street
Suite 401-402
Hackensack, NJ 07601-5477
201-487-9655
800-227-7562; *Fax:* 201-487-9656
wspc@wspc.com
www.worldscibooks.com

Gwen Adshead, Editor
Deborah Brooke, Editor

This book reviews the current state of knowledge of
Munchausen's Syndrome by Proxy, a type of child abuse
which causes wide concern. Two main areas are covered:
new directions in research, and treatment of the perpetrator
in and outside the family. Unlike other books, this volume
provides a multidisciplinary perspective, with input from
social workers, pediatricians, child-psychiatrists and law-

yers, among others. It also offers an international perspective, with contributors from the USA, Canada and Austra-
lia. *$53.00*

252 pages Year Founded: 1981 ISBN 1-860941-34-6

**1378 Phantom Illness: Recognizing, Understanding,
and Overcoming Hypochondria**
Houghton Mifflin Company
222 Berkeley Street
Boston, MA 02116-3760
617-351-5000; *Fax:* 617-351-1105
www.houghtonmifflinbooks.com

Carla Cantor, Author

Offers hope to those who suffer from the debilitating disorder of hypochondria. Carla Cantor's long, dark road to hypochondria began when she crashed a car, killing a friend
of hers. She couldn't forgive herself, and a few years later
began imagining that she was suffering from Lupus. Many
years and two hospitalizations later, she wrote this book not
only about her experiences, but about hypochondria in general, now more politely referred to as a somatoform disorder. *$ 15.00*

351 pages ISBN 0-395859-92-1

**1379 Playing Sick?: Untangling the Web of
Munchausen Syndrome, Munchausen by
Proxy, Malingering, and Factitious Disorder**
Routledge
7625 Empire Drive
Florence, KY 41042-2919
800-634-7064; *Fax:* 800-248-4724
orders@taylorandfrancis.com
www.www.routledge.com

Maura May, Publisher

Based on years of research and clinical practice, this book
provides the clues that can help practitioners and family
members recognize these disorders, avoid invasive procedures, and sort out the motives that drive people to hurt
themselves and deceive others.

**1380 Somatoform and Factitious Disorders (Review
of Psychiatry)**
American Psychiatric Publishing, Inc.
1000 Wilson Boulevard
Suite 1825
Arlington, VA 22209-3901
703-907-7322
800-368-5777; *Fax:* 703-907-1091
appi@psych.org
www.appi.org

Katherine A Phillips, M.D., Editor
Ron McMillen, Chief Executive Officer
John McDuffie, Editorial Director

Offers clinicians a broad synthesis of the current knowledge about somatoform and factitious disorders.

216 pages Year Founded: 2001

**1381 The Divided Mind: The Epidemic of Mindbody
Disorders**
HarperCollins Publishers
10 East 53rd Street
New York, NY 10022-5299
212-207-7000; *Fax:* 212-207-6964
feedback2@harpercollins.com
www.harpercollins.com

John E. Sarno, Author

Traces the history of psychosomatic medicine, including Freud's crucial role as well as his failures. Most important, it describes the psychology of the human condition that is responsible for the broad range of psychosomatic illness. Dr. Sarno believes that the failure of medicine's practitioners to recognize and appropriately treat mindbody disorders had produced public health and economic problems of major proportions in the United States.

400 pages Year Founded: 1817 ISBN 0-060851-78-3

1382 What Your Patients Need to Know about Psychiatric Medications
American Psychiatric Publishing, Inc.
1000 Wilson Boulevard
Suite 1825
Arlington, VA 22209-3901
703-907-7322
800-368-5777; *Fax:* 703-907-1091
appi@psych.org
www.appi.org

Robert E Hales MD, Author
Robert H. Chew, Ph.D., Author
Stuart C. Yudofsky, MD, Author

This book includes all major classes of medications, along with detailed information on specific agents - information that's more in-depth and easier to understand than what can be obtained from pharmacies or found on the Internet.
$87.00

441 pages Year Founded: 2009 ISSN 9781585623563

Periodicals & Pamphlets

1383 Asher Meadow Newsletter
18209 Smoke House Court
Germantown, MD 20874-2425

Asher Meadow is a wholly-owned non-profit subsidiary of American Marvels, an Internet development company that provides a newsletter for survivors of MSBP.

Video & Audio

1384 Clinical Impressions: Identifying Mental Illness
Educational Training Videos
136 Granville St
Suite 200
Gahanna, OH 43230
Fax: 888-775-3919
www.educationaltrainingvideos.com

How long can mental illness stay hidden, especially from the eyes of trained experts? This program rejoins a group of ten adults- five of them healthy and five of them with histories of mental illness- as psychiatric specialists try to spot and correctly diagnose the latter. Administering a series of collaborative and one-on-one tests, including assessments of personality type, physical self-image, and rational thinking, the panel gradually makes decisions about who suffers from depression, bipolar disorder, bulimia, and social anxiety.

1385 Coping with Stress
Educational Video Network, Inc.
1401 19th Street
Huntsville, TX 77340

936-295-5767
800-762-0060; *Fax:* 936-294-0233
www.www.evndirect.com

Stress affects everyone, both emotionally and physically. For some, mismanaged stress can result in substance abuse, violence, or even suicide. This program answers the question, How can a person cope with stress?

1386 Dealing with Depression
Educational Video Network, Inc.
1401 19th Street
Huntsville, TX 77340
936-295-5767
800-762-0060; *Fax:* 936-294-0233
www.www.evndirect.com

As more and more young people are falling victim to depression, it is important to understand what causes it and to know how to get the help that can rid a person of this life-wrecking affliction.

1387 Dealing with Social Anxiety
Educational Video Network, Inc.
1401 19th Street
Huntsville, TX 77340
936-295-5767
800-762-0060; *Fax:* 936-294-0233
www.www.evndirect.com

Social anxiety is America's third-largest psychiatric disorder. It generally develops during the mid-teen years, and almost always before the age of 25. Understand what may trigger the development of anxiety and learn how it sometimes evolves into full-blown panic disorder, which is characterized by recurrent attacks of terror or fear. The consequences of social anxiety are examined and effective treatments are discussed.

1388 FRONTLINE: The Released
PBS
2100 Crystal Drive
Arlington, VA 22202
www.pbs.org

Will Lyman, Actor
Narrator
Miri Navasky, Director
Karen O'Connor, Director

The documentary states that of the 700,000 inmates released from American prisons each year, half of them have mental disabilities. This work focused on those with severe problems who keep entering and exiting prison. Full of good information on the challenges they face with mental illnesses; housing, employment, stigmatization, and socialization.

Year Founded: 2009

1389 Mental Disorder
Educational Training Videos
136 Granville St
Suite 200
Gahanna, OH 43230
Fax: 888-775-3919
www.educationaltrainingvideos.com

What is abnormality? Using the case studies of two young women; one who has depression, one who has an anxiety disorder; as a springboard, this program presents three psychological perspective on mental disorder.

1390 Mind-Body Problems: Psychotherapy with Psychosomatic Disorders
Jason Aronson, Inc.- Rowman Littlefield Imprint
4501 Forbes Blvd.
Suite 200
Lanham, MD 20706
301-459-3366; *Fax:* 301-429-5748
www.rowmanlittlefield.com

Janet Schumacher Finell, Author

The opening paper profitably links psychosomatic disorders to alexithymia, the absence or deadening of feeling, the inability to identify or express emotion.

376 pages Year Founded: 1977 ISBN 1-568216-54-8

1391 Neurotic, Stress-Related, and Somatoform Disorders
Educational Training Videos
136 Granville St
Suite 200
Gahanna, OH 43230
Fax: 888-775-3919
www.educationaltrainingvideos.com

This program, filmed in the UK, discusses the following disorders and their differential diagnoses; phobic anxiety; anxiety; obsessive-compulsive disorder, from minor to acute; stress reaction and adjustment; and dissociative disorders. Sub-disorders discussed include Korsakov's syndrome; agoraphobia and social phobia; generalized anxiety and mixed-anxiety-and-depressive disorder; panic disorder; and post-traumatic stress syndrome. Patients suffering from each disorder exhibit the various symptoms in interviews conducted by psychiatrists.

1392 Somatoform Disorders: A Medicolegal Guide
Cambridge University Press
32 Ave of the Americas
New York, NY 10013-2473
212-337-5000
newyork@cambridge.org
www.cambridge.org

Michael Trimble, Author

This book is an in-depth, clinically oriented review of the somatoform disorders and related clinical manifestations (such as chronic fatigue syndrome) and how they appear in a medico-legal setting. The volume is aimed at clinicians and lawyers who deal with injury claims where these disorders impact much more frequently than generally recognized.

268 pages Year Founded: 2011 ISBN 0-521169-25-9

1393 Understanding Mental Illness
Educational Video Network, Inc.
1401 19th Street
Huntsville, TX 77340
936-295-5767
800-762-0060; *Fax:* 936-294-0233
www.www.evndirect.com

Contains information and classifications of mental illness. Mental illness can strike anyone, at any age. Learn about various organic and functional mental disorders as discussed and their causes and symptoms, and learn where to seek help for a variety of mental health concerns.

Web Sites

1394 www.mbpexpert.com
MBP Expert Services

Expert services from Louisa J Lasher, MA, provides Munchausen by Proxy maltreatment training, case consultation, technical assistance, and expert witness services in an objective manner and in the best interest of the child or children involved.

1395 www.mentalhealth.com
Internet Mental Health

Offers online psychiatric diagnosis in the hope of reaching the two-thirds of individuals with mental illness who do not seek treatment.

1396 www.msbp.com
Mothers Against Munchausen Syndrome by Proxy Allegations

Begun in response to the fast growing number of false allegations of Munchausen Syndrome by Proxy.

1397 www.munchausen.com
Munchause Syndrome

Dr. Marc Feldman's Munchausen Syndrome, Malingering, Factitious Disorder, & Munchausen by Proxy page. Includes articles, related book list, personal stories and links.

1398 www.planetpsych.com
Planetpsych.com

Online resource for mental health information

1399 www.psychcentral.com
Psych Central

The Internet's largest and oldest independent mental health social network created and run by mental health professionals to guarantee reliable, trusted information and support communities to you.

1400 www.store.samhsa.gov
Substance Abuse and Mental Health Services Administration

Resources on mental disorders as well as treatment and recovery.

Substance-Related and Addictive Disorders

Introduction

Substance abuse and addictive disorders are among the most destructive mental disorders in America today, contributing to a host of medical and social problems and to widespread individual suffering. Alcohol, a drug that is widely available and socially approved, is the most abused of all substances, and alcohol addiction is a pervasive mental disorder. Like all addictive disorders, alcohol addiction is characterized by repeated use despite repeated adverse consequences, and by physical and psychological craving.

Alcohol addiction can be treated, but successful recovery is dependent on acceptance by the patient that he or she has an illness; lack of this acceptance is often the greatest stumbling block to treatment.

Relapse is common for several reasons: lack of acceptance of the diagnosis; genetic vulnerability; and social factors. Successful treatment very often requires involvement by the patient in some form of self-help group, such as Alcoholics Anonymous or another 12-step program. The great majority of motivated individuals with these disorders can recover, but it often requires three or more separate episodes of treatment to prevent relapse and lead to recovery.

Scientific understanding of how alcohol works on the body and the brain, and the underlying physiology of addiction, has advanced remarkably in recent years. With the help of brain imaging and other techniques, we can now see that these disorders are associated with structural changes in the brain.

The substances referred to in this section include: amphetamines; marijuana; cocaine (and its purer derivative, crack); hallucinogens, such as LSD; inhalants, such as butane gas or cleaning fluid; opioids, such as morphine, heroin, or codeine; and benzodiazepines like Valium and Xanax. Caffeine and nicotine, both of which have the potential for abuse and dependence, are not included. The United States Food and Drug Administration has proposed adding nicotine to the list of addictive substances they monitor.

SYMPTOMS

Substance-Related Abuse:
• Repeated use resulting in inability to fulfill fundamental obligations at work, school, or home, e.g., repeated absences, poor work performance, family neglect;
• Repeated use, resulting in dangerous situations, e.g., driving or operating a machine while impaired;
• Repeated alcohol and substance-related legal problems, e.g., arrests for disorderly conduct;
• Continued use despite persistent social or interpersonal problems worsened by the effects of substance abuse.

Substance-Related Dependence:
• Alcohol or substance is often taken in greater amounts or for a longer period than intended;
• Repeated wish or unsuccessful attempts to control use;
• A great deal of time is taken to get and use alcohol or substance or to recover from its effects;
• Important social, work, or recreational activities are missed because of use;

• Use continues in spite of the person knowing about the persistent psychological or physical problems it causes, e.g., depression induced by cocaine or continued drinking.

Tolerance:
• Need for increased amounts of alcohol or the substance to achieve desired effect;
• Diminished effects with continued use of the same amount of alcohol or substance;
• Alcohol abuse can occur without tolerance, as in binge drinking, a particular problem for young people on college campuses and elsewhere.

Withdrawal:
• Characteristic withdrawal syndrome, prolonged taking and then stopping/reducing alcohol or substance causing physical and mental symptoms, such as headaches, diarrhea, shaking, anxiety and depression;
• Same or a related substance is taken to avoid/alleviate the withdrawal symptoms.

ASSOCIATED FEATURES

Frequently, alcohol abuse and dependence occur together with dependence on other substances, and alcohol may be used to counteract the ill effects of these substances. Depression, anxiety, and sleep disorders are common in alcohol dependence.

Typically, accidents, injuries and suicide accompany alcohol dependence, and it is estimated that half of all traffic accidents involve alcoholic intoxication. Absenteeism, low work productivity and injuries on the job are often caused by alcohol dependence. Alcohol is also the most common cause of preventable birth defects, including fetal alcohol syndrome, according to the American Psychiatric Association.

Women and men tend to have different drinking patterns. Society is more tolerant of male drunkeness than of female; women tend to drink alone and in secret and are more susceptible to medical complications of alcoholism. Alcohol abuse severely damages organ systems including the brain, liver, heart, and digestive tract.

Genetics has a considerable influence on a person's propensity for substance abuse disorders, and such disorders are associated with significant changes in the brain. These changes underscore the fact that alcohol and substance abuse problems are medical diseases, not failure of character. At the same time, those suffering from these disorders have an obligation to seek and utilize treatment and to ensure that their disorders do not cause injury to others.

Many individuals with substance-relatedand addictive disorders take more than one substance and suffer from other mental symptoms and disorders as well. Individuals with a wide variety of mental disorders sometimes abuse drugs as an attempt to medicate themselves. People with Antisocial Personality Disorder often abuse substances, including amphetamines such as cocaine. Substance-related disorders can also lead to other mental disorders. Use of the synthetic hallucinogen Ecstasy is associated with acute and paranoid psychoses, and the prolonged use of cocaine (a stimulant) can lead to paranoid psychosis with violent behavior. Substance use and the effects on an individual's employment and relationships, as well as legal difficulties, can precipitate anxiety and mood disorders. Intravenous substance abuse is associated with a high risk of HIV infections and other medical complications.

Chronic drug and alcohol abuse can lead to difficulty in memory and problem solving, and impaired sexual functioning.

Childhood sexual abuse is strongly associated with substance dependence and with a number of other mental symptoms and disorders.

PREVALENCE

Alcohol dependence and abuse are among the most prevalent mental disorders in the general population. One community study in the US found that about eight percent of the adult population had alcohol dependence and about five percent had alcohol abuse at some time in their lives. Approximately six percent had alcohol dependence or abuse during the preceding year.

There are large cultural differences in attitudes toward the use of substances. In some cultures, mood altering drugs, including alcohol, are well accepted; in others they are strictly forbidden.

Those between the ages of 18 and 24 have a high prevalence for abuse of all substances. Early adolescent drug and alcohol use is associated with a slight but significant decline in intellectual abilities. Substance related disorders are more common among males than females. The lifetime prevalence of use of any drugs (aside from alcohol) in the US is 11.9 percent; in males it is twice as high as in females.

TREATMENT OPTIONS

Diagnosis and treatment of alcohol dependence has improved as understanding of the physiology of addiction has advanced. But successful treatment still relies on acceptance by the patient that he or she has an illness, as well as support from other people who have gone through the same process. For this reason, medical treatment is most often successful when it is accompanied by involvement in a support group, for both the patient and family members; these may include Alcoholics Anonymous (AA) and Al-Anon, 12-step spiritual programs that have gained popularity over the years. Local groups can be found in every community and are listed in the phone book and on the Internet. Recently, similar groups have formed that do not emphasize spirituality, as these do, but rely on group support for sobriety.

There is a growing controversy over the need for people who have had an alcohol problem to abstain completely from alcohol for the rest of their lives, one of the central beliefs of AA. Some researchers and clinicians argue that it is possible for some former alcoholics to resume controlled drinking. AA, in the past, has discouraged members from using psychotropic medications; this is often counterproductive. Many alcohol treatment programs have been developed with men's needs and personalities in mind. Successful programs for women are far less confrontational than men's programs and include arrangements for child care. There is a tendency for women's alcohol and substance abuse disorders to be addressed punitively rather than therapeutically. Women who are pregnant and/or are mothers may be disciplined to seek treatment if they risk imprisonment and loss of child

custody - outcomes that do not help them or their children.

Treatment for alcoholism has been hospital-based in the past, but has increasingly moved to the outpatient setting. New treatment protocols and medications allow for outpatient detoxification/withdrawal in many cases. There is a considerable dispute about the need for inpatient care, which may not be covered by health insurance. Much depends upon the nature of the individual's support system. Hospital treatment is necessary for withdrawal when alcohol use has been heavy and steady. Delirium tremens, a consequence of very heavy drinking, can be fatal.

Medical treatment of alcohol dependence may include Anabuse, a drug that makes an individual violently ill if alcohol is used. Group or hospital-based treatment may also be useful, and psychotherapy can help the patient more effectively deal with underlying conflicts and interpersonal problems.

Denial of illness and ambivalence about abstinence can make treatment difficult. A patient's cravings can be overwhelmingly intense, and the individual's social circle is often composed of other substance abusers, making it hard for the indvidual to maintain relationships while becoming or remaining abstinent - the goal of treatment. A wide range of intervention may be needed, including a general assessment of the drug abuse, and evaluation of medical, social, and psychological problems. It is best to involve partner, family and friends to help the person gain new understanding of the problem and to make the general assessment complete. An explicit treatment plan should be worked out with the person (and partner/family/friends if appropriate) with concrete goals for which the person takes responsibility, which should include not only stopping substance abuse, but also dealing with associated problems concerning health, personal relationships, and work.

Another option is maintenance therapy, in which a drug is prescribed that has a slower action and is less addictive than the street drug (e.g., methadone vs. heroin). Therapy is added to help with withdrawal and other problems associated with drug use. Cognitive behavioral therapy can help with increasing the substance abuser's personal skills, resulting in a reduced dependency on drugs. Relaxation techniques and prescription drugs can also help with withdrawal symptoms. Rehabilitation in a therapeutic community is another option.

Dropout during treatment and relapse after initial success are common, but many people do achieve lifelong cures with abstinence from further substance abuse.

Associations & Agencies

1402 **AMERSA The Association for Medical Education and Research in Substance Abuse**
135 Lyndon Road
Cranston, RI 02905
401-230-2165; *Fax:* 877-418-8769
doreen@amersa.org
www.amersa.org

Sharon Levy, MD. MPH, President
Doreen MacLane-Baeder, Executive Director
Victoria A. Osborne, PhD, MSW, Secretary
Kevin L. Kraemer, MD, MSc, Treasurer

AMERSA, founded in 1976, is a nonprofit organization of healthcare professionals dedicated to improving education and clinical care in the management of problems related to substance abuse.

Year Founded: 1976

1403 Adult Children of Alcoholics World Service Organization, Inc.
PO Box 811
Lakewood, CA 90714
310-534-1815
www.adultchildren.org

Adult Children of Alcoholics is a 12 Step, 12 Tradition program for adult women and men who grew up in alcoholic or otherwise dysfunctional homes, and for adults who have experienced abuse or neglect in the past. The program involves ACA members meeting with each other in a mutually respectful, safe environment and sharing their experiences, as well as applying the program's 12 Steps for recovery to their own lives.

Year Founded: 1978

1404 Alcoholics Anonymous (AA): Worldwide
475 Riverside Drive at West 120th Street
11th Floor
New York, NY 10115
212-870-3400
www.aa.org

Bill Wilson, Co-Founder
Dr. Bob Smith, Co-Founder

A fellowship of men and women around the world who share experiences, strength, and hope with each other with the goal of solving their drinking problem and helping others to recover from alcoholism.

Year Founded: 1935

1405 American Academy of Addiction Psychiatry (AAAP)
400 Massasoit Avenue
Suite 307, 2nd Floor
East Providence, RI 02914
401-524-3076; *Fax:* 401-272-0922
www.aaap.org

Shelly F. Greenfield, MD, MPH, President
Larissa Mooney, MD, Vice President
John J. Mariani, MD, Treasurer
Tim Fong, MD, Secretary

An organization of healthcare professionals dedicated to helping those with mental health disorders. Promotes the use of evidence-based research in the assessment and treatment of substance abuse and mental disorders, as well as in public policy and clinical practice. Provides education to healthcare professionals and the public on patient care, recovery, and the safe treatment of those suffering from substance abuse disorders.

1406 American Council on Alcoholism
1000 East Indian School Road
Suite B
Phoenix, AZ 85014
800-527-5344

Lloyd R. Vacovsky, Executive Director

ACA is a nonprofit organization committed to educating the public about alcoholism and the effects of alcohol abuse, and the necessity of having readily accessible, affordable, and effective alcoholism treatment.

1407 American Public Human Services Association
1133 19th Street Northwest
Suite 400
Washington, DC 20036
202-682-0100; *Fax:* 202-289-6555
memberservice@aphsa.org
www.aphsa.org

Tracy Wareing Evans, President/CEO
Nicole York, Human Resources Director
Jessica Garon, Communications Manager
Candy Hill, External Affairs Director

APHSA is a nonprofit organization dedicated to improving health and human services by supporting state and local agencies, and working with partners and policymakers to drive effective policies.

Year Founded: 1930

1408 American Society of Addiction Medicine
11400 Rockville Pike
Suite 200
Rockville, MD 20852
301-656-3920; *Fax:* 301-656-3815
email@asam.org
www.asam.org

Kelly J. Clark, MD, MBA, DFAPA, President
Penny S. Mills, MBA, Executive VP and CEO
Carolyn C. Lanham, CAE, Chief Operating Officer
Margaret A. Jarvis, MD, DFASAM, Vice President

ASAM's mission is to support the practice of Addiction Medicine and to improve the quality of care and treatment for people struggling with addiction.

Year Founded: 1954

1409 Center for Mental Health Services (CMHS) Substance Abuse and Mental Health Services Administration
5600 Fishers Lane
Rockville, MD 20857
240-276-1310
877-726-4727
TTY: 800-487-4727
www.samhsa.gov/about-us/who-we-are/offices-centers

Paolo del Vecchio, MSW, Director
Anne Mathews-Younes, Acting Deputy Director
Keris Myrick, Director, Consumer Affairs
Patricia Gratton, Director, Program Analysis

Promotes the treatment of mental illness and emotional disorders by increasing accessibility to mental health programs; supporting outreach, treatment, rehabilitation, and support programs and networks; and encouraging the use of scientifically-based information when treating mental disorders. CMHS provides information about mental health via a toll-free number and numerous publications. Developed for users of mental health services and their families, the general public, policy makers, providers, and the media.

Year Founded: 1992

1410 Centre for Addiction and Mental Health
1001 Queen Street West
30-60 White Squirrel Way
Toronto, ON M6J 1H4,

416-535-8501
800-463-2338
info@camh.ca
www.camh.ca

David Wilson, Board Chair
Dr Catherine Zahn, President and CEO
Tom Milroy, Chair, CAMH Foundation
Dr. Vicky Stergiopoulos, Physician-in-Chief

The Centre for Addiction and Mental Health is a mental health and addiction teaching hospital and research centre based in Canada. CAMH seeks to support people affected by mental health and addiction issues through research, education, policy development, clinical care, and the promotion of health.

1411 Community Anti-Drug Coalition of America
625 Slaters Lane
Suite 300
Alexandria, VA 22314
800-542-2322; *Fax:* 703-706-0565
www.cadca.org

Arthur T. Dean, Chairman and CEO
Jerilyn Simpson-Jordan, Vice Chairman
Gregory Puckett, Secretary
Donald K. Truslow, Treasurer

Community Anti-Drug Coalition of America is a national organization representing the interests of over 5,000 anti-drug coalitions across the United States. CADCA participates in public policy advocacy and provides community coalitions with marketing programs, technical assistance and training, and special events with the purpose of making communities safe and drug-free.

Year Founded: 1992

1412 Goodwill's Community Employment Services
Goodwill Industries-Suncoast, Inc.
10596 Gandy Blvd.
St. Petersburg, FL 33702
727-523-1512
888-279-1988
TDD: 727-579-1068
www.goodwill-suncoast.org

Heather Ceresoli, CPA, Chair
Deborah A. Passerini, President
Martin W. Gladysz, Senior Vice Chair
Louise R. Lopez, Vice Chair

Program providing job coaching and community job placements for people with disabilities.

Year Founded: 1954

1413 Grief Recovery After a Substance Passing (GRASP)
40569 Calle Balderas
Indio, CA 92203
302-492-7717
administrator@grasphelp.org
www.grasphelp.org

Denise Cullen, Executive Director

GRASP provides information resources, offers support, and organizes meetings and events for families or individuals who have experienced the death of a loved one as a result of substance abuse or addiction.

Year Founded: 2002

1414 Mental Health America
500 Montgomery Street
Suite 820
Alexandria, VA 22314
703-684-7722
800-969-6642; *Fax:* 703-684-5968
www.mentalhealthamerica.net

Reginald Williams, Chair of the Board
Paul Gionfriddo, President and CEO
Jessica Kennedy, Chief of Staff/VP of Finance
Theresa Nguyen, VP of Policy and Programs

Mental Health America is a community-based nonprofit organization committed to enabling the mental wellness of all Americans. MHA advocates for greater access to quality health services and seeks to educate individuals on identifying symptoms, as well as intervention and prevention.

Year Founded: 1909

1415 NAADAC, The Association for Addiction Professionals
44 Canal Center Plaza
Suite 301
Alexandria, VA 22314
703-741-7686
800-548-0497; *Fax:* 703-741-7698
naadac@naadac.org
www.naadac.org

Gerard J. Schmidt, MA, MAC, LPC, President
Diane Sevening, EdD, LAC, President Elect
John Lisy, LICDC, OCPS II, Secretary
Mita M. Johnson, EdD, LPC, Treasurer

The Association for Addiction Professionals is an organization representing the professional interests of over 85,000 healthcare professionals. Members consist of addiction counselors, healthcare professionals, and educators who specialize in addiction, including the areas of education, treatment, prevention, and recovery support. Dedicated to promoting and enabling healthier individuals, families, and communities.

Year Founded: 1972

1416 NAATP National Association of Addiction Treatment Providers
1120 Lincoln Street
Suite 1303
Denver, CO 80203
888-574-1008
info@naatp.org
www.naatp.org

Marvin Ventrell, JD, Executive Director
Katie Strand, CMP, Director of Operations
Jessica Scwan, NCAC, Outcomes Manager
Mark Dunn, Director of Policy

NAATP ensures the availability and accessibility of high quality addiction treatment across the country through leadership, advocacy, training, and other member support services.

Year Founded: 1978

1417 National Alliance on Mental Illness
3803 North Fairfax Drive
Suite 100
Arlington, VA 22203
703-524-7600
800-950-6264

info@nami.org
www.nami.org

Steve Pitman, JD, President
Lacey Berumen, PhD, MNM, First Vice President
Mary Giliberti, Chief Executive Officer
David Levy, Chief Financial Officer

NAMI is an organization dedicated to raising awareness on mental health and providing support and education for Americans affected by mental illness. NAMI advocates for access to services and treatment and fosters an environment of awareness and understanding for those concerned with mental health.

Year Founded: 1979

1418 National Association of State Alcohol/Drug Abuse Directors

1919 Pennsylvania Avenue NW
Suite M-250
Washington, DC 20006
202-293-0090; *Fax:* 202-293-1250
dcoffice@nasadad.org
www.nasadad.org

Cassandra Price, President
Robert Morrison, Executive Director
Hollis McMullen, Director of Finance
Rick Harwood, Deputy Executive Director

The National Association of State Alcohol and Drug Abuse Directors is a private, not-for-profit organization focused on the promotion of educational and scientific materials on alcohol, drug abuse, and related fields. NASADAD seeks to support and further the development of effective alcohol and other drug abuse treatment programs in the United States.

Year Founded: 1971

1419 National Coalition for the Homeless

2201 P Street Northwest
Washington, DC 20037
202-462-4822
info@nationalhomeless.org
www.nationalhomeless.org

Bob Erlenbusch, President
Megan Hastings, Interim Director
Barbara Anderson, Secretary
Annie Leomporra, Grassroots Analyst

The National Coalition for the Homeless is an organization serving to protect the needs of those experiencing homelessness, while striving to prevent and end homelessness. NCH promotes effective treatment, services, and programs for those struggling with homelessness as well as substance abuse problems.

Year Founded: 1982

1420 National Council for Behavioral Health

1400 K Street Northwest
Suite 400
Washington, DC 20005
202-684-7457
communications@thenationalcouncil.org
www.thenationalcouncil.org

Jeff Richardson, Chair
Linda Rosenberg, President and CEO
Jeannie Campbell, Executive VP and COO
Tim Swinfard, First Vice Chair

The National Council for Behavioral Health serves to unify America's behavioral health organizations. The council is dedicated to ensuring that quality mental health and addictions care is readily accessible to all Americans.

1421 National Council on Alcoholism and Drug Dependence

217 Broadway
Suite 712
New York, NY 10007
212-269-7797
800-622-2255
national@ncadd.org
www.ncadd.org

Andrew N. Pucher, President and CEO
Leah Brock, Director of Affiliate Relations
Jill Price, Director of Administration
Paul Warren, Executive Assistant

Founded in 1944 by Marty Mann, the National Council on Alcoholism and Drug Dependence is an advocacy organization focused on alcohol and drug dependence. NCADD raises awareness about addiction throughout the United States and provides education, information, and support services for those suffering from addiction and alcoholism.

Year Founded: 1944

1422 National Institute on Alcohol Abuse and Alcoholism
National Institute on Health

9000 Rockville Pike
Rockville, MD 20892
301-443-3860
niaaaweb-r@exchange.nih.gov
www.niaaa.nih.gov

Dr. George F. Koob, PhD, Director
Patricia Powell, Deputy Director
Kenneth Warren, Senior Advisor

NIAAA seeks to reduce alcohol-related problems by conducting scientific research in a range of areas, including neuroscience, treatment, prevention, and epidemiology; working with other research institutes, federal programs, and organizations focused on the issues surrounding alcohol abuse; and disseminating information to healthcare providers, researchers, policymakers, and the public.

1423 National Mental Health Consumers' Self-Help Clearinghouse

1211 Chestnut Street
Suite 1100
Philadelphia, PA 19107
267-507-3810
800-553-4539; *Fax:* 215-636-6312
info@mhselfhelp.org
www.mhselfhelp.org

Joseph Rogers, Founder and Executive Director
Susan Rogers, Director

The Clearinghouse is a peer-run national technical assistance center focused on achieving respect and equality of opportunity for those with mental illnesses. The Clearinghouse helps with the growth of the mental health consumer movement by evaluating mental health services, advocating for mental health reform, and providing consumers with news, information, publications, and consultation services.

Year Founded: 1986

1424 National Organization on Fetal Alcohol Syndrome
1200 Eton Court Northwest
3rd Floor
Washington, DC 20007
202-785-4585
800-666-6327; *Fax: 202-466-6456*
information@nofas.org
www.nofas.org

Kate Boyce, Chair
Tom Donaldson, President
Kathleen Tavenner Mitchell, MHS, Vice President
Andy Kachor, Communications Director

Educates the public about the risks associated with alcohol use during pregnancy, including Fetal Alcohol Spectrum Disorders, which causes birth defects and developmental disabilities in children. Dedicated to preventing alcohol consumption during pregnancy and reducing the number of birth defects. Provides support for individuals and families concerned with Fetal Alcohol Spectrum Disorders.

Year Founded: 1990

1425 Research Society on Alcoholism
7801 North Lamar Boulevard
Suite D-89
Austin, TX 78752-1038
512-454-0022; *Fax: 512-454-0812*
rsastaff@sbcglobal.net
www.rsoa.org

Cristine Czachowski, PhD, President
Mary Larimer, PhD, Vice President
Carol Casey, PhD, Secretary
Pranoti Mandrekar, PhD, Treasurer

The Research Society on Alcoholism, founded in 1976, serves as a forum for scientists and researchers focused on the fields of alcoholism and alcohol-related problems. The Society promotes research with the purpose of advancing treatment of alcoholism and finding potential cures.

Year Founded: 1976

1426 Section for Psychiatric and Substance Abuse Services (SPSPAS)
155 North Wacker Drive
Chicago, IL 60606
312-422-3000
800-424-4301
www.www.aha.org

Mary Lou Mastro, FACHE, Chair
John A. Miller, PhD, Chair-Elect
Michelle Hood, PhD, Board-Liaison

A membership section that represents over 1,660 behavioral health providers and professionals who are members of the American Hospital Association (AHA). The Section applies AHA policy, advocacy, and service efforts to advance understandings of behavioral health care and to emphasize its importance.

1427 Substance Abuse and Mental Health Services Administration (SAMHSA)
5600 Fishers Lane
Rockville, MD 20857
877-726-4727
TTY: 800-487-4889
www.www.samhsa.gov

Elinore F. McCance-Katz, MD, PhD, Assistant Secretary
Deepa Avula, MPH, Director, Financial Resources
Mirtha Beadle, Acting Director, Policy
Marla Hendriksson, MPM, Director, Communications

SAMHSA is a public agency within the US Department of Health and Human Services focused on expanding the accessibility of information, services, and research on mental health and substance abuse. SAMHSA's mission is to reduce the impact of mental illness and substance abuse on communities across America.

Year Founded: 1992

1428 The Center for Family Support
2811 Zulette Avenue
Bronx, NY 10461
718-518-1500; *Fax: 718-518-8200*
www.www.cfsny.org/

Steven Vernikoff, Executive Director
Lloyd Stabiner, President
Amy Bittinger, Vice President
Barbara Greenwald, Associate Executive Director

The Center for Family Support offers assistance to individuals with developmental and related disabilities, as well as their families, and provides support services and programs that are designed to accommodate individual needs. Offers services throughout New York City, Westchester County, Long Island, and New Jersey.

Year Founded: 1954

Books

1429 Woman's Journal: Helping Women Recover - Special Edition for Use in the Criminal Justice
Jossey-Bass / Wiley & Sons
111 River Street
Hoboken, NJ 07030-5774
201-748-6000; *Fax: 201-748-6088*
info@wiley.com
www.wiley.com

Stephanie S Covington, Author
Elias E Cousens, EVP, Chief Financial Officer
William J Arlington, Sr. Vice President HR
Gary M Rinck, SVP, General Counsel

Includes important new evidence-based data and new proven techniques for her unique and exclusive program, as well as new ways to treat trauma and substance abuse, new principles for gender responsive strategies with women offenders, and a new module on sexuality and women's recovery. The latest, and most up-to-date theory and practice for this very focused but substantial field of treatment. It contains exercises for use in group sessions, summaries of information presented from the facilitator's guide, and reflection questions and activities for use after group sessions. *$30.00*

156 pages Year Founded: 2008 ISBN 0-787988-71-5

1430 A Woman's Journal: Helping Women Recover - Special Edition for Use in the Criminal Justice System, Revised
Jossey-Bass / Wiley & Sons
111 River Street
Hoboken, NJ 07030-5774
201-748-6000; *Fax: 201-748-6088*
info@wiley.com
www.wiley.com

Stephanie S Covington, Author
Ellis E Cousens, EVP, Chief Financial Officer
William J Arlington, Sr Vice President HR
Gary M Rinck, SVP, General Counsel

Designed to meet the unique needs of substance-abusing women. Created for use with women's groups in a variety of correctional settings. Offers mental health professionals, corrections personnel, and program administrators the tools they need to implement this highly effective program. *$30.00*

156 pages Year Founded: 2008 ISBN 0-787988-71-5

1431 Addiction Workbook: A Step by Step Guide to Quitting Alcohol and Drugs
NewHarbinger Publications
5674 Shattuck Avenue
Oakland, CA 94609-1662
510-652-0215
800-748-6273; *Fax:* 800-652-1613
customerservice@newharbinger.com
www.newharbinger.com

Patrick Fanning, Author

This comprehensive workbook explains the facts about addiction and provides simple, step by step directions for working through the stages of the quitting process. *$18.95*

160 pages Year Founded: 1973 ISBN 1-572240-43-1

1432 Addiction: Why Can't They Just Stop?
Rodale Books
733 Third Avenue
New York, NY 10017-3293
212-697-2040; *Fax:* 212-682-2237
www.rodale.com

John Hoffman, Editor
Susan Froemke, Editor

Addiction offers a comprehensive and provocative look at the impact of chemical dependency on addicts, their loved ones, society, and the economy.

256 pages ISBN 1-594867-15-1

1433 Alcohol & Other Drugs: Health Facts
ETR Associates
4 Carbonero Way
Scotts Valley, CA 95066-4200
831-438-4060
800-321-4407; *Fax:* 800-435-8433
www.pub.etr.org

Lucas Stang, Author
Nora J Krantzler, Author
William M Kane, Author
Maria Quackenbush, Author

Offers clear, concise background information on alcohol and other drugs, and provides assessment of the impact on youth. Also, discusses risk and protective factors, current trends, and prevention strategies. *$17.00*

151 pages Year Founded: 1981

1434 Alcohol and the Community
Cambridge University Press
32 Avenue of the Americas
New York, NY 10013-2473
212-337-5000
800-872-7423

newyork@cambrigde.org
www.www.cambridge.org

Harold H Holder, Author

The authors challenge the current implicit models used in alcohol problem prevention and demonstrate an ecological perspective of the community as a complex adaptive system composed of interacting subsystems. This volume represents a new and sensible approach to the prevention of alcohol dependence and alcohol-related problems. *$110.00*

200 pages Year Founded: 1584 ISBN 0-521591-87-2

1435 Alcoholism Sourcebook
Omnigraphics
155 West Congress
Suite 200
Detroit, MI 48226
313-961-1340
800-234-1340; *Fax:* 313-961-1383
contact@omnigraphics.com
www.omnigraphics.com

Joyce Brennfleck Shannon, Author
Peter Ruffner, Co-Founder

Omnigraphics is the publisher of the Health Reference Series, a growing consumer health information resource with more than 100 volumes in print. Each title in the series features an easy to understand format, nontechnical language, comprehensive indexing, and resources for further information. Material in each book has been collected from a wide range of government agencies, professional associations, periodicals, and other sources. *$78.00*

610 pages Year Founded: 1985 ISBN 0-780803-25-6

1436 American Psychiatric Association Practice Guideline for the Treatment of Patients With Substance Use Disorders
American Psychiatric Publishing, Inc.
1000 Wilson Boulevard
Suite 1825
Arlington, VA 22209-3901
703-907-7322
800-368-5777; *Fax:* 703-907-1091
appi@psych.org
www.appi.org

Robert E Hales MD, Editor-in-Chief
Saul Levin, M.D., M.P.A., CEO and Medical Director
John McDuffie, Editorial Director
Laura W Roberts, M.D., Deputy Editor

Offers guidance to psychiatrists caring for patients with substance use disorders. Includes treatment for alcohol, cocaine and opioids addiction. *$29.50*

126 pages ISBN 0-890423-03-2

1437 Broken: My Story of Addiction and Redemption
The Viking Press, Penguin Publishers
375 Hudson Street
New York, NY 10014-3657
212-366-2372; *Fax:* 212-366-2933
ecommerce@us.penguingroup.com

William Cope Moyers, Author
Coram Williams, Chief Financial Officer
David Shanks, Chief Executive Officer

Broken tells the story of what happened between then and now-from growing up the privileged son of Bill Moyers to his descent into alcholism and drug addiction, his numerous stabs at getting clean, his many relapses, and how he managed to survive. *$5.43*

384 pages Year Founded: 1936 ISBN 0-143112-45-7

1438 Clinical Supervision in Alcohol and Drug Abuse Counseling: Principles, Models, Methods
Jossey-Bass
111 River Street
Hoboken, NJ 07030-5774
201-748-6000; *Fax:* 201-748-6088
info@wiley.com
www.as.wiley.com/WileyCDA/

David J. Powell, Author
Archie Brodsky, Author
William J Arlington, Sr Vice President HR
Edward Melando, VP, Corporate Controller

Firmly grounded in both theory and practice, this book offers methods of supervisory contracting, observation, case presentation, modeling, intervention, and evaluation. Ethical and legal concerns are also addressed. *$25.95*

448 pages Year Founded: 1998 ISBN 0-787973-77-7

1439 Concerned Intervention: When Your Loved One Won't Quit Alcohol or Drugs
NewHarbinger Publications
5674 Shattuck Avenue
Oakland, CA 94609-1662
510-652-0215
800-748-6273; *Fax:* 800-652-1613
customerservice@newharbinger.com
www.newharbinger.com

John O'Neill, Author
Pat O'Neill, Author

Practical guide to group intervention techniques with lessons from experiences of families seeking counseling and treatment. *$13.95*

190 pages Year Founded: 1973 ISBN 1-879237-37-7

1440 Concise Guide to Treatment of Alcoholism and Addictions
American Psychiatric Publishing, Inc.
1000 Wilson Boulevard
Suite 1825
Arlington, VA 22209-3901
703-907-7322
800-368-5777; *Fax:* 703-907-1091
appi@psych.org
www.appi.org

Avram H Mack, M.D, Author
Amy L Harrington, M.D, Author
Richard J Frances, M.D, Author
Rebecca D Rinehart, Publisher

Presents information on available treatment options for alcoholism and addictions, substance abuse in the workplace and laboratory testing. *$29.95*

172 pages ISBN 0-880483-26-1

1441 Drug Abuse Sourcebook
Omnigraphics
155 West Congress
Suite 200
Detroit, MI 48226

313-961-1340
800-234-1340; *Fax:* 313-961-1383
contact@omnigraphics.com
www.omnigraphics.com

Laura Larsen, Author
Peter Ruffner, Co-Founder

Basic consumer health information about the abuse of cocaine, club drugs, hallucinogens, heroin, inhalents, marijuana, and other illicit substances, prescription medications, and over-the-counter medicines: along with facts about addiction and related health effects, drug abuse treatment and recover, drug testing, prevention programs, glossaries of drug-related terms, and directories of resources for more information. *$95.00*

640 pages Year Founded: 1985 ISBN 0-780810-79-2

1442 Dynamics of Addiction
Hazelden
15251 Pleasant Valley Road
PO Box 11
Center City, MN 55012-0176
651-213-4200
800-328-9000
info@hazelden.org
www.www.hazelden.org

George A Mann, Author
Marvin Sappala MD, Chief Medical Officer
Nick Motu, Publisher, VP of Marketing
Mark Sheets, Executive Director

Offers practical advice on how to raise balanced kids who can stand on their own feet, resist unhealthy peer pressures, and still be accepted by others. *$2.50*

16 pages Year Founded: 1987 ISBN 0-935908-38-2

1443 Eye Opener
Hazelden
PO Box 11
Center City, MN 55012-0011
651-213-4200
800-328-9000; *Fax:* 651-213-4793
info@hazelden.org
www.hazelden.org

Mark Mishek, President and CEO,Hazeldon Betty
James A Blaha, VP Finance,Administration/CFO
Marvin D Seppala,MD, Chief Medical Officer
Mark Sheets, Execurive Director,Regional serv

Popular meditations on A.A. philosophy, written for every day of the year. This effective tool has been a recovery-basic for over 30 years. *$13.95*

384 pages Year Founded: 1949 ISBN 0-894860-23-2

1444 Fetal Alcohol Syndrome, Fetal Alcohol Effects: Strategies for Professionals
Hazelden
15251 Pleasant Valley Road
PO Box 176
Center City, MN 55012-176
651-213-4000
800-328-9000; *Fax:* 651-213-4590
customersupport@hazelden.org
www.hazelden.org

Diane Malbin, Author
Mark Sheets, Executive Director
Marvin Seppala MD, Chief Medical Officer
Nick Motu, Publisher, VP of Marketing

If you're a chemical dependency counselor or work with women in pregnancy planning or self-care, this resource is filled with facts to help you better meet your clients needs. *$5.25*

43 pages Year Founded: 1996 ISBN 0-894869-51-5

1445 Getting Beyond Sobriety: Clinical Approaches to Long-Term Recovery
Jossey-Bass / Wiley & Sons
111 River Street
Hoboken, NJ 07030-5790
201-748-5774; *Fax:* 201-748-6088
custserv@wiley.com
www.wiley.com

Michael Craig Clemmens, Author
Ellis E Cousens, EVP, Chief Financial Officer
William J Arlington, Sr Vice President HR
Edward J Melando, VP, Corporate Controller

This method will lead to a change in behavior within the individual, while developing and expanding connection with others. *$ 42.50*

198 pages Year Founded: 1997 ISBN 0-787908-40-1

1446 Getting Hooked: Rationality and Addiction
Cambridge University Press
32 Avenue of the Americas
New York, NY 10013-2473
212-337-5000
newyork@cambrigde.org
www.www.cambridge.org

John Elster, Editor
Ole Jorgen Skog, Editor
Richard Fisher, Managing Director
Andrew Gilfillan, Managing Director

The essays in this volume offer thorough and up-to-date discussion on the relationship between addiction and rationality. Includes contributions from philosophers, psychiatrists, neurobiologists, sociologists and economists. Offers the neurophysiology of addiction, examination of the Becker theory of rational addiction, an argument for a visceral theory of addiction, a discussion of compulsive gambling as a form of addiction, discussions of George Ainslie's theory of hyperbolic discounting, analyses of social causes and policy implications and an investigation into relapse. *$75.00*

300 pages Year Founded: 1584 ISBN 0-521640-08-3

1447 Handbook of the Medical Consequences of Alcohol and Drug Abuse (Contemporary Issues in Neuropharmacology)
Routledge, Taylor & Francis Group
8th Floor, 711 3rd Avenue
New York, NY 10017
212-563-7800
800-634-7064; *Fax:* 212-563-2269
orders@taylorandfrancis.com
www.www.routledge.com

Dr William Francis, Founder
Richard Taylor, Founder
John Brick, Author

Describes the most current research on the acute and chronic effects of alcohol, stimulants, inhalants, marijuana, and opiates on human organ systems and behavior. Also provides in-depth explanations of the mechanisms by which these psychoactive drugs exert their biobehavioral

effects as well as current thinking about- and definitions of-abuse, dependence, and alcohol/drug use.

354 pages Year Founded: 2003 ISBN 0-789018-63-2

1448 Inside Recovery: How the Twelve Step Program Can Work for You
The Rosen Publishing Group
29 East 21st Street
New York, NY 10010-6209
212-777-3017
800-237-9932; *Fax:* 888-436-4643
www.rosenpublishing.com

Susan Banfield, Author

Describes the practices and principles of twelve-step programs, how they can be used in dealing with such problems as alcoholism and drug addiction, and how to get involved in them. *$25.25*

64 pages Year Founded: 1950 ISBN 0-823926-34-6

1449 Inside a Support Group: Help for Teenage Children of Alcoholics
Rosen Publishing Group
29 East 21st Street
New York, NY 10010-6209
212-777-3017
800-237-9932; *Fax:* 888-436-4643
info@rosenpub.com
www.rosenpublishing.com

Margi Trapani, Author

Gives teens an inside look at Alateen, an organization designed to help teens cope with a loved one's addiction to alcohol. *$25.25*

64 pages Year Founded: 1950 ISBN 0-823925-08-7

1450 Kicking Addictive Habits Once & for All: A Relapse Prevention Guide, Revised
Jossey-Bass / Wiley & Sons
111 River Street
Hoboken, NJ 07030-5774
201-748-6000
800-956-7739; *Fax:* 201-748-6088
info@wiley.com
www.wiley.com

Dennis C Daley, Author
Ellis E Cousens, EVP, Chief Financial Officer
William J Arlington, Sr Vice President HR
Edward J Melando, VP, Corporate Controller

All aspects of changing bad habits and developing a balanced lifestyle are addressed in the book. *$26.00*

224 pages Year Founded: 1997 ISBN 0-787940-68-3

1451 LSD: Still With Us After All These Years: Based on the National Institute of Drug Abuse Studies on the Resurgence of Contemporary LSD Use
Jossey-Bass / Wiley & Sons
111 River Street
Hoboken, NJ 07030-5774
201-748-6000; *Fax:* 201-748-6088
info@wiley.com
www.wiley.com

Leigh A Henderson, Author
William J Glass, Author

William J Arlington, Sr Vice President HR
Edward J Melando, VP, Corporate Controller

Offers an insightful look at LSD use and provides an essential resource for parents, counselors, and educators. The book examines why young people are using LSD- its appeal, experience, and where kids are getting. Solidly researched and dispassionately written, this book weaves current studies and anecdotes with recent statistics to create a vivid, complete, and credible picture of contemporary LSD use. *$ 24.00*

176 pages Year Founded: 1998 ISBN 0-787943-79-7

1452 Let's Talk Facts About Substance Abuse & Addiction
American Psychiatric Publishing, Inc.
1000 Wilson Boulevard
Suite 1825
Arlington, VA 22209-3901
703-907-7322
800-368-5777; *Fax:* 703-907-1091
appi@psych.org
www.appi.org

Robert E Hales MD, Editor-in-Chief
Saul Levin, M.D., M.P.A., CEO and Medical Director
John McDuffie, Editorial Director
Laura W Roberts, M.D., Deputy Editor

Straight talk about a difficult subject. *$26.95*

1453 Living Skills Recovery Workbook
Elsevier Science, Health Science Division
10900 Euclid Avenue
Cleveland, OH 44106-7169
212-368-0808; *Fax:* 212-268-2295
custserv@elsevier.com
www.www.centerforebp.case.edu

Pat Precin,MS OTR/L, Author
Bill Godfrey, Chief Information Officer
Michael Hansen, Chief Executive Officer
Gavin Howe, Executive Vice President

Provides clinicians with the tools necessary to help patients with dual diagnoses acquire basic living skills. Focusing on stress management, time management, activities of daily living, and social skills training, each living skill is taught in relation to how it aids in recovery and relapse prevention for each patient's individual lifestyle and pattern of addiction. Book is now printed as ordered. *$39.95*

197 pages Year Founded: 1999 ISBN 0-750671-18-7

1454 Living Sober I
Jossey-Bass / Wiley & Sons
111 River Street
Hoboken, NJ 07030-5790
201-748-8677; *Fax:* 201-748-2665
www.wiley.com

Dr Dennis Daley, Presenter
Ellis E Cousens, EVP, Chief Financial Officer
William J Arlington, Sr Vice President, HR
Edward J Melando, VP, Corporate Controller

Emphasizes the specific coping skills essential to a client's recovery. *$495.00*

87 pages Year Founded: 1999

1455 Living Sober II
Jossey-Bass / Wiley & Sons
111 River Street
Hoboken, NJ 07030-5774
201-748-6000; *Fax:* 201-748-6088
info@wiley.com
www.wiley.com

Dennis C Daley, Author
Ellis E Cousens, EVP, Chief Financial Officer
William J Arlington, Sr Vice President HR
Edward J Melando, VP, Corporate Controller

Emphasizes the specific coping skills essential to a client's recovery.

27 pages

1456 Motivating Behavior Changes Among Illicit-Drug Abusers: Research on Contingency Management Interventions
American Psychological Association
750 First Street,NorthEast
Washington, DC 20002-4242
202-336-5500
800-374-2721; *Fax:* 202-336-5518
TDD: 202-336-6123
TTY: 202-336-6123
www.www.apa.org

Stephen T Higgins, Editor
Kenneth Silverman, Editor
Stephen T Higgins, Author
Kenneth Silverman, Author

Scientifically based method focused on the use of incentives to change behavior. Research in multiple applications of contingency management techniques. Test case of effective utilization of the method in treating illicit-drug abusers. *$39.95*

399 pages Year Founded: 1999 ISBN 1-557985-70-7

1457 Motivational Interviewing: Preparing People to Change Addictive Behavior
Guilford Press
72 Spring Street
New York, NY 10012-4068
800-365-7006; *Fax:* 212-966-6708
info@guilford.com
www.www.guilford.com

William R. Miller, Ph.D., Author
Stephen Rollnick, Ph.D., Author

Explains how to work through ambivalence to facilitate change, presents detailed guidelines for using the authors' approach with a variety of clinical populations, and reflect on the process of learning MI. Chapters contributed by other leading experts address such special topics as MI and the stages-of-change model; using the approach with groups, couples, and adolescents; and applications to general medical care, health promotion, and criminal justice settings. *$42.00*

348 pages Year Founded: 1973 ISBN 0-898624-69-X

1458 New Treaments for Chemical Addictions
American Psychiatric Publishing, Inc.
1000 Wilson Boulevard
Suite 1825
Arlington, VA 22209-3901
703-907-7322
800-368-5777; *Fax:* 703-907-1091

appi@psych.org
www.appi.org

Robert E Hales MD, Editor-in-Chief
Ron McMillen, Chief Executive Officer
John McDuffie, Editorial Director
Rebecca Rinehart, Publisher

Examines new approaches for an old problem. *$37.50*

248 pages ISBN 0-880488-38-7

1459 Points for Parents Perplexed about Drugs
Hazelden
PO Box 11
Center City, MN 55012-0011
651-213-4000
800-257-7810; *Fax:* 651-213-4793
info@hazelden.org
www.hazelden.org

David C Hancock, Author
Mark Sheets, Executive Director
Marvin Seppala MD, Chief Medical Officer
Nick Motu, Publisher, VP of Marketing

Clear guidelines help teachers, parents, family members
and others recognize, evaluate, and deal with adolescent
drug abuse. Excellent support for family counseling programs. *$3.25*

15 pages Year Founded: 1949 ISBN 0-894861-40-9

1460 Relapse Prevention for Addictive Behaviours: A
Manual for Therapists
Blackwell Publishing
Commerce Place
350 Main Street
Malden, MA 02148-5020
781-388-8200; *Fax:* 781-388-8210
www.www.blackwellpublishing.com

Wendy Wallace, Co-Author
Jane Pullin, Co-Author
F. Keaney, Co-Author
Richard D. T. Farmer, Co-Author

Applies cognitive-behavioral strategies and lifestyle procedures to treat people with addiction problems. *$43.95*

224 pages Year Founded: 1991 ISBN 0-632024-84-4

1461 Rethinking Substance Abuse: What the Science
Shows, and What We Should Do about It
The Guilford Press
72 Spring Street
New York, NY 10012-4019
800-365-7006; *Fax:* 212-966-6708
info@guilford.com
www.www.guilford.com

William R. Miller Ph.D., Editor
Kathleen M. Carroll Ph.D., Editor

This state-of-the-art book brings together leading experts to
describe what treatment and prevention would look like if it
were based on the best science available. The volume incorporates developmental, neurobiological, genetic, behavioral, and social-environmental perspectives. Tightly edited
chapters summarize current thinking on the nature and
causes of alcohol and other drug problems; discuss what
works at the individual, family, and societal levels; and offer robust principles for developing more effective
treatments and services.

320 pages Year Founded: 1973 ISBN 1-572302-31-3

1462 Sex, Drugs, Gambling & Chocolate: A
Workbook for Overcoming Addictions
Impact Publishers
PO Box 6016
Atascadero, CA 93423-6016
805-466-5917
800-246-7228; *Fax:* 805-466-5919
info@impactpublishers.com
www.impactpublishers.com

Robert Dr A.Thomas, Horvath
Author Emmons PhD, Founder

This workbook is loaded with practical suggestions and
will appeal to anyone who has unsuccessfully sought to
overcome a serious addiction or habit using more traditional (i.e. 12 step) treatment approaches. The workbook
approach is straightforward and adaptable to a variety of
addictive behaviors. The information presented is not hos-
tile towards, or totally incompatible with other approaches
to addiction, but is primarily intended for those who want a
scientifically proven, rational approach to behavior change.
$15.95

240 pages Year Founded: 1970 ISBN 1-886230-55-2

1463 Sober Siblings: How to Help Your Alcoholic
Brother or Sister-and Not Lose Yourself
Da Capo Press
250 West 57th Street
15th Floor
New York, NY 10107
212-340-8100
www.www.perseusbooksgroup.com/perseus/home.jsp

Patricia Olsen, Author
Petros Levounis, Author

An empowering, practical guide to help the brothers and
sisters of alcoholics-by a journalist and sibling of two alcoholics, and an addiction specialist *$16.00*

243 pages Year Founded: 2008 ISBN 1-600940-55-2

1464 Substance Abuse Treatment and the Stages of
Change: Selecting and Planning Interventions
The Guilford Press
72 Spring Street
New York, NY 10012-4019
800-365-7006; *Fax:* 212-966-6708
info@guilford.com

Gerard J. Connors, Co-Author
Dennis M. Donovan, Co-Author
Carlo C. DiClemente, Co-Author

Synthesizes the latest theory and research on the process of
addictive behavior change, helping the clinician more effectively conceptualize and address the needs of particular
clients. It offers concrete guidance for tailoring interventions to clients with varying levels of motivation or readi-
ness to change, describing what works- and what doesn't-
at different points in the recovery process. Ideal for practicing clinicians, the book is also an invaluable text for
graduate-level courses.

274 pages Year Founded: 2004 ISBN 1-593850-97-2

1465 Substance Abuse: Information for School
Counselors, Social Workers, Therapists, and
Counselors
Allyn & Bacon
800-922-0579
www.www.pearsoned.co.uk/Imprints/AllynBacon/

Gary L. Fisher, Author
Thomas C. Harrison, Author

This text provides updated coverage and practical clinical examples to reflect the rapid changes in the field of addiction. In a reader-friendly style, the authors present balanced coverage of various treatment models as well as objective discussions dealing with the controversies in this field. The text covers topics spanning the entire field- pharmacology, assessment and diagnosis, treatment, recovery, prevention, children, families, and other addictions- providing students with a broad view of the AOD field aswell as the pervasiveness of the problem in all areas of behavioral health and general fields.

384 pages Year Founded: 2004 ISBN 0-205403-36-0

1466 Teach & Reach: Tobacco, Alcohol & Other Drug Prevention
ETR Associates
4 Carbonero Way
Scotts Valley, CA 95066-4200
831-438-4060; *Fax:* 831-438-4284
www.www.etr.org

Peggy Flynn, Project Director
Nicole Ellen Jones, Board Member
Dr. Douglas Kirby, Advisory Board
Marcia Quackenbush, Author

Empowers students to build commitment to stay tobacco, alcohol and drug free; look to peer norms to support healthy, responsible choices; enhance protective factors that prevent tobacco, alcohol and other drug use; and learn skills that can keep them free of tobacco, alcohol and other drug use. For youth in grades 7-12. *$22.00*

Year Founded: 2004 ISBN 1-560716-98-3

1467 Teen Guide to Staying Sober (Drug Abuse Prevention Library)
Rosen Publishing
29 East 21st Street
New York, NY 10010-6209
212-777-3017
800-237-9932; *Fax:* 888-436-4643
info@rosenpub.com
www.rosenpublishing.com

Christina Chiu, Author

Discusses the social and physical effects of alcohol, the reasons teenagers drink, the problems caused by teenage alcoholism, and possible preventive measures and treatments. *$25.25*

64 pages Year Founded: 1950 ISBN 0-823927-65-2

1468 The Meaning of Addiction: An Unconventional View
Jossey-Bass / Wiley & Sons
111 River Street
Hoboken, NJ 07030-5774
201-748-6000; *Fax:* 201-748-6088
info@wiley.com
www.wiley.com

Stanton Peele, Author
Ellis E Cousens, EVP, Chief Financial Officer
William J Arlington, Sr Vice President HR
Edward J Melando, VP, Corporate Controller

A controversial and persuasive analysis of addiction. This compelling and controversial book challenges the widely accepted belief that alcohol and drug addiction have a genetic or biological basis. The so-called disease theory suggests that a substance or activity can cause the addict to lose control of his behavior. Stanton Peele demonstrates how this notion fails to make sense of scientific observations. *$34.00*

224 pages Year Founded: 1998 ISBN 0-787943-82-0

1469 The Mother's Survival Guide to Recovery: All About Alcohol, Drugs & Babies
NewHarbinger Publications
5674 Shattuck Avenue
Oakland, CA 94609-1662
510-652-0215
800-748-6273; *Fax:* 800-652-1613
customerservice@newharbinger.com
www.newharbinger.com

Laurie L Tanner, Author

Seeking to help women surmount the grief of using whilst pregnant, and tap into the strength that their addictions have buried, this text is aimed at women of all backgrounds. It explains what addiction is, helps to decide whether they are addicts, and where to get help. For women in addiction, this offers an alternative to the loneliness, desolation and rejection of their lives. *$12.95*

138 pages Year Founded: 1973 ISBN 1-572240-49-0

1470 The Science of Addiction: From Neurobiology to Treatment
W.W. Norton
500 Fifth Avenue
New York, NY 10110
212-354-5500
800-233-4830; *Fax:* 212-869-0856
www.books.wwnorton.com

Carlton K Erickson, Author

Presents a comprehensive overview of the rolse that brain function and genetics play in addiction.

312 pages Year Founded: 1923 ISBN 0-393704-63-7

1471 The Science of Prevention: Methodological Advances from Alcohol and Substance Research
American Psychological Association
750 First Street,NorthEast
Washington, DC 20002-4242
202-336-5500
800-374-2721; *Fax:* 202-336-5518
TDD: 202-336-6123
TTY: 202-336-6123
www.www.apa.org

Kendel J Bryant, Editor
Michael Windle, Editor
Stephen G West, Editor

The editors and contributors explore the implications of prospective longitudinal research that measures risk and protective factors, and illustrates developmental trajectories and the sequence of abuse. They look at intervention research with an eye toward how certain components may interact with individual and environmental factors and offer many concrete suggestions for improving methodological quality. *$39.95*

458 pages Year Founded: 1997 ISBN 1-557984-39-5

1472 The Selfish Brain: Learning from Addiction
Hazelden
PO Box 11
Center City, MN 55012-0011
651-213-4200
800-328-9000; *Fax:* 651-213-4793
info@hazelden.org
www.hazelden.org

Robert L Dupont,MD, Author
Mark Sheets, Executive Director
Marvin Seppala MD, Chief Medical Officer
Nick Motu, Publisher, VP Of Marketing

Helps clients or loved ones face addiction and recovery by exploring the biological, historical and cultural aspects of addiction and its destructiveness. *$18.95*

544 pages Year Founded: 1949 ISBN 1-568383-63-0

1473 The Seven Points of Alcoholics Anonymous
Hazelden
PO Box 11
Center City, MN 55012-0011
651-213-4200
800-328-9000; *Fax:* 651-213-4793
info@hazelden.org
www.hazelden.org

Richmond Walker, Author
Mark Sheets, Executive Director
Marvin Seppala MD, Chief Medical Director
Nick Motu, Publisher, VP of Marketing

This book is the summation of Walker's knowledge on the practice and fundamentals of 12 Step recovery. Topics include an overview and history of A.A., the nature of alcoholism and recovery, the 12 Step way and fellowship, surrender, character defects, amends, living One Day at a Time, and sharing. *$9.85*

112 pages Year Founded: 1949 ISBN 1-592850-50-2

1474 The Twelve-Step Facilitation Handbook: A Systematic Approach to Early Recovery from Alcoholism and Addiction
Hazelden Publishing
PO Box 11
Center City, MN 55012-0011
651-213-4200
800-257-7810
customersupport@hazelden.org
www.www.hazelden.org

Joseph Nowinski, Author
Stuart Baker, Author
Marvin Seppala MD, Chief Medical Director
Nick Motu, Publisher, VP of Marketing

This book provides clinicians with the tools they need to encourage chemically dependent clients to take advantage of the healing power of twelve-step programs. *$24.95*

248 pages Year Founded: 2003 ISBN 1-592850-96-0

1475 Treating Alcoholism (Jossey-Bass Library of Current Clinical Technique)
Jossey-Bass Publishers
111 River Street
Hoboken, NJ 07030-5774
201-748-6000; *Fax:* 201-748-6088
info@wiley.com
www.as.wiley.com/WileyCDA/

Stephanie Brown, Editor
Irvin D Yalom, General Editor
William J Arlington, Sr Vice President HR
Edward J Melando, VP, Corporate Controller

In this comprehensive book, editor Stephanie Brown presents a model of alcoholism treatment to help readers guide alcoholics and their families on the path to long-term recovery. Experts in the field give skills to address the myriad problems associated with alcoholism by providing up-to-date information and illustrative case examples. This book, filled with a wealth of information, will help set specific therapeutic techniques for working with alcoholics and the families of alcoholics in a clinical setting. *$40.00*

448 pages Year Founded: 1997 ISBN 0-787938-76-9

1476 Twenty-Four Hours a Day
Hazelden
PO Box 11
Center City, MN 55012-0011
651-213-4200
800-257-7810; *Fax:* 651-213-4793
info@hazelden.org
www.hazelden.org

Mark Mishek, President and CEO,Hazeldon Betty
James A Blaha, VP Finance,Administration/CFO
Marvin D Seppala,MD, Chief Medical Officer
Mark Sheets, Execurive Director,Regional serv

Daily meditation in this classic book helps clients develop a solid foundation in a spiritual program, learn to relate the Twelve Steps to their everyday lives and accomplish their treatment and aftercare goals. Includes 366 daily meditations with special consideration and extra encouragement given during holidays. Helps clients find the power to stay sober each day and not to take that first drink. *$14.95*

400 pages Year Founded: 1949 ISBN 0-894868-34-9

1477 When Parents Have Problems: A Book for Teens and Older Children Who Have a Disturbed or Difficult Parent
Charles C Thomas Publisher Ltd.
2600 South First Street
Springfield, IL 62704
217-789-8980
800-258-8980; *Fax:* 217-789-9130
books@ccthomas.com
www.ccthomas.com

Susan B Miller, Author
PhD Miller, Author

Numerous books have been written for adults who grew up coping with troubled and difficult parents. This newly revised second edition expands the information in the previous edition by updating current knowledge that provides a thorough overview for children who are coping with difficult and/or troubled parents. Two chapters have been added. The first addresses parents who have difficult personalities. The second new chapter addresses parents in poverty. Additional topics discuss mistreatment, selfishness, when parents are in pain, when parents cause pain, powerhouse feelings, troubled parents and ordinary teen life. An excellent resource for therapists, counselor, and others who work with children and teenagers. *$19.95*

105 pages Year Founded: 1927 ISBN 0-398087-13-5

1478 You Can Free Yourself from Alcohol and Drugs; How to Work a Program That Keeps You in Charge
NewHarbinger Publications
5674 Shattuck Avenue
Oakland, CA 94609-1662
510-652-0215
800-748-6273; *Fax:* 800-652-1613
customerservice@newharbinger.com
www.newharbinger.com

Doug Althauser, Author

An alternative approach that removes the traditional reliance on a higher power. This ten-goal programme respects the individual beliefs of addicts and alcoholics while still requiring them to change their lifestyle from one of dependence to recovery. *$13.95*

192 pages Year Founded: 1973 ISBN 1-572241-18-7

Periodicals & Pamphlets

1479 About Alcohol
ETR Associates
4 Carbonero Way
Scotts Valley, CA 95066-4200
831-438-4060
800-321-4407; *Fax:* 831-438-4284
support@etr.freshdesk.com
www.etr.org

David Kitchen,MBA, Chief Financial Officer
Talita Sanders,BS, Director,Human Resources
Coleen Cantwell,MPH, Director,Business Development Pl
Matt McDowell,BS, Director,Marketing

What it is, why it's dangerous, and its negative effects on the body and in prenatal development. Title #079.

1480 About Crack Cocaine
ETR Associates
4 Carbonero Way
Scotts Valley, CA 95066-4200
831-438-4060
800-321-4407; *Fax:* 831-438-4284
customerservice@etr.org
www.etr.org

Mary Nelson, President

Describes what crack cocaine is and why it's dangerous and lists the effects on the body. *$16.00*

1481 About Drug Addiction
ETR Associates
4 Carbonero Way
Scotts Valley, CA 95066-4200
831-438-4060
800-321-4407; *Fax:* 831-438-4284
support@etr.freshdesk.com
www.etr.org

David Kitchen,MBA, Chief Financial Officer
Talita Sanders,BS, Director,Human Resources
Coleen Cantwell,MPH, Director,Business Development Pl
Matt McDowell,BS, Director,Marketing

Includes answers to commonly asked questions about drug addiction, a 13'x 17' wall chart presents the stages of addiction and recovery, covers denial, withdrawal and relapse. *$18.00*

1482 Alateen Talk
Al-Anon Family Group Headquarters
1600 Corporate Landing Parkway
Virginia Beach, VA 23454-5617
757-563-1600
888-425-2666; *Fax:* 757-563-1655
wso@al-anon.org
www.al-anon.alateen.org

Alateen members from all over the world share their experience, strength, and hope through the written words of Alateen Talk. Their sharings relate to their personal lives, how their Alateen group is functioning, and ways in which to carry the Alateen message to young people who are still suffering from someone else's drinking. *$7.50*

4 pages 4 per year ISSN 1054-1411

1483 Alcohol ABC's
ETR Associates
4 Carbonero Way
Scotts Valley, CA 95066-4200
831-438-4060
800-321-4407; *Fax:* 831-438-4284
customerservice@etr.org
www.etr.org

PALS , Author

Presents the consequenes of drinking and explains the difference between use and abuse in a straightforward, matter-of-fact way. Title #R712.

1484 Alcohol Issues Insights
Beer Marketer's Insights
49 East Maple Avenue
Suffern, NY 10901-5507
845-507-0040; *Fax:* 845-507-0041
eric@beerinsights.com
www.beerinsights.com

Eric Shepard, Editor

Newsletter that provides information on the use and misuses of alcohol. Covers such topics as misrepresentation in the media, minimum age requirements, advertising bans, deterrence of drunk driving, and the effects of tax increases on alcoholic beverage consumption. *$375.00*

4 pages 12 per year ISSN 1067-3105

1485 Alcohol Self-Test
ETR Associates
4 Carbonero Way
Scotts Valley, CA 95066-4200
831-438-4060
800-321-4407; *Fax:* 831-438-4284
support@etr.freshdesk.com
www.etr.org

David Kitchen,MBA, Chief Financial Officer
Talita Sanders,BS, Director,Human Resources
Coleen Cantwell,MPH, Director,Business Development Pl
Matt McDowell,BS, Director,Marketing

Thought provoking questions include: What do I know about alcohol? How safely do I drink? When and why do I drink? Title #H259.

1486 Alcohol: Incredible Facts
ETR Associates
4 Carbonero Way
Scotts Valley, CA 95066-4200

831-438-4060
800-321-4407; *Fax:* 831-438-4284
support@etr.freshdesk.com
www.etr.org

David Kitchen,MBA, Chief Financial Officer
Talita Sanders,BS, Director,Human Resources
Coleen Cantwell,MPH, Director,Business Development Pl
Matt McDowell,BS, Director,Marketing

Strange but true facts to trigger discussion about alcohol use, social consequences, and risks involved. Title #R719.

1487 Alcoholism: A Merry-Go-Round Named Denial
Hazelden
PO Box 11
Center City, MN 55012-0011
651-213-4200
800-257-7810; *Fax:* 651-213-4793
info@hazelden.org
www.hazelden.org

Joseph L Kellerman, Author

Revised and expanded for today's recovering person, family, and concerned others, this classic piece defines the roles of the alcoholic and those who are close to the alcoholic. This new version includes easier-to-understand, more accessible language and expanded descriptions of The Enabler, The Victim, and The Provoker roles. Also includes a section on the disease in adolescents and seniors- increasing its value to everyone touched by substance abuse. *$3.50*

20 pages Year Founded: 1949 ISBN 0-894860-22-4

1488 Alcoholism: A Treatable Disease
Hazelden
PO Box 11
Center City, MN 55012-0011
651-213-4200
800-257-7810
info@hazelden.org
www.hazelden.org

A hard look at the disease of chemical dependence, the confusion and delusion that go with it, intervention and a hopeful conclusion - alcoholism is treatable. *$2.95*

20 pages Year Founded: 1978 ISBN 0-935908-37-4

1489 American Journal on Addictions
American Academy of Addiction Psychiatry
400 Massasoit Avenue
Suite 307,2nd Floor
Easy Providence, RI 02914
401-524-3076; *Fax:* 401-272-0922
aja@aaap.org
www.www.aaap.org

Ismene L Petrakis,MD, Chair,Area Director
Laurence M Westreich MD, President
Thomas R Kosten,MD, Editor-in-Chief,AJA
Shelly F Greenfield,MD,MPH, Vice President

Covers a wide variety of topics ranging from codependence to genetics, epidemiology to dual diagnostics, etiology to neuroscience, and much more. Features of the journal, all written by experts in the field, include special overview articles, clinical or basic research papers, clinical updates, and book reviews within the area of addictions.

ISSN 1055-0496

1490 Binge Drinking: Am I At Risk?
ETR Associates
4 Carbonero Way
Scotts Valley, CA 95066-4200
831-438-4060
800-321-4407; *Fax:* 831-438-4284
support@etr.freshdesk.com
www.etr.org

David Kitchen,MBA, Chief Financial Officer
Talita Sanders,BS, Director,Human Resources
Coleen Cantwell,MPH, Director,Business Development Pl
Matt McDowell,BS, Director,Marketing

Easy-to-follow checklists help students decide if they have a problem with binge drinking, make a plan, and get help. Title #R018.

1491 Crossing the Thin Line: Between Social Drinking and Alcoholism
Hazelden
PO Box 11
Center City, MN 55012-0011
651-213-4200
800-257-7810; *Fax:* 651-213-4793
info@hazelden.org
www.hazelden.org

Terence Williams, Author
Mark Sheets, Executive Director
Marvin Seppala MD, Chief Medical Officer
Nick Motu, Publisher, VP of Marketing

This pamphlet encourages people to look at their own drinking habits to decide if they are crossing the very thin line between social drinking and alcoholism. An excellent resource for anyone who has wondered about his or her own drinking habits. *$2.95*

20 pages Year Founded: 1949 ISBN 0-894860-77-1

1492 Designer Drugs
ETR Associates
4 Carbonero Way
Scotts Valley, CA 95066-4200
831-438-4060
800-321-4407; *Fax:* 831-438-4284
customerservice@etr.org
www.etr.org

M Foster Olive, Author

Traces the evolution of designer drugs like China White and MDMA, explains how addiction works and suggests why designer drugs are so addictive. *$16.00*

112 pages

1493 Drinking Facts
ETR Associates
4 Carbonero Way
Scotts Valley, CA 95066-4200
831-438-4060
800-321-4407; *Fax:* 831-438-4284
support@etr.freshdesk.com
www.etr.org

David Kitchen,MBA, Chief Financial Officer
Talita Sanders,BS, Director,Human Resources
Coleen Cantwell,MPH, Director,Business Development Pl
Matt McDowell,BS, Director,Marketing

Addresses changing attitudes about drinking, and examines the basic facts of alcohol. Shows how to avoid risky situations, explains about the blood alcohol levels, and offers tips for curbing consumption. Title #R843

1494 Drug Dependence, Alcohol Abuse and Alcoholism
Elsevier Publishing
1600 John F Kennedy Boulevard
Suite 1800
Philadelphia, PA 19103-2879
314-872-8370
800-542-2522; *Fax:* 314-432-1380
usbkinfo@elsevier.com
www.elsevier.com

Erik Engstrom, CEO

This journal aims to provide its readers with a swift, yet complete, current awareness service. Careful selection of relevent abstracts (and other bibliographic data) from the latest issues of 4,000 leading international biomedical journals. The journal covers all aspects of the abuse of drugs, alcohol and organic solvents and includes material relating to experimental pharmacology of addiction, although, in general, experimental pharmacology of narcotics is not covered.

Year Founded: 1880 ISSN 0925-5958

1495 Drug Facts Pamphlet
ETR Associates
4 Carbonero Way
Scotts Valley, CA 95066-4200
831-438-4060
800-321-4407; *Fax:* 831-435-8433
support@etr.freshdesk.com
www.etr.org

David Kitchen,MBA, Chief Financial Officer
Talita Sanders,BS, Director,Human Resources
Coleen Cantwell,MPH, Director,Business Development Pl
Matt McDowell,BS, Director,Marketing

Overview of 11 of the most commonly abused drugs includes: Description of drug, short-term effects and long-term effects. *$18.00*

1496 Drug and Alcohol Dependence An International Journal on Biomedical an Psychosocial Approaches
Customer Support Services
1600 John F Kennedy Boulevard
Suite 1800
Philadelphia, PA 19103-2879
212-633-3730
800-654-2452; *Fax:* 212-633-3680
www.elsevier.com

Eric C. Strain, Editor-in-Chief
Andraya Dolbee, Editorial Office Manager

An international journal devoted to publishing original research, scholarly reviews, commentaries, and policy analyses in the area of drug, alcohol and tobacco use and dependence. Articles range from studies of the chemistry of substances of abuse, their actions at molecular and cellular sites, in vitro and in vivo investigations of their biochemical, pharacological and behavioural actions, laboratory-based and clinical research in humans, substance abuse treatment and prevention research, and studies employing methods from epidemiology, sociology, and economics.

15 per year Year Founded: 1880 ISSN 0376-8716

1497 DrugLink
Facts and Comparisons
Red Lion Lane
Trefoil House
Hemel Hempstead, UK HP3 9-E
192-326-0733
800-223-0554; *Fax:* 192-327-1781
www.www.druglink.co.uk

Rosemary Farmer, Chairman
John Pins, VP of Finance
Denise Basow MD, VP, General Manager, Editor
David Del Toro, VP, General Manager

DrugLink is an eight-page newsletter that provides abstracts of drug-related articles from various journals. DrugLink allows health care professionals to stay up-to-date on hot topics without having to subscribe to multiple publications. *$52.95*

8 pages Year Founded: 1984 ISBN 1-089559-0 -

1498 Drugs: Talking With Your Teen
ETR Associates
4 Carbonero Way
Scotts Valley, CA 95066-4200
831-438-4060
800-321-4407; *Fax:* 831-435-8433
support@etr.freshdesk.com
www.etr.org

David Kitchen,MBA, Chief Financial Officer
Talita Sanders,BS, Director,Human Resources
Coleen Cantwell,MPH, Director,Business Development Pl
Matt McDowell,BS, Director,Marketing

Suggestions for effective communication include: avoid scare tatics, clarify family rules, other alternative for drug use. *$ 16.00*

1499 Getting Involved in AA
Hazelden
PO Box 11
Center City, MN 55012-0011
651-213-4200
800-328-9000; *Fax:* 651-213-4793
info@hazelden.org
www.hazelden.org

Bob W, Author
Mark Sheets, Executive Director
Marvin Seppala MD, Chief Medical Officer
Nick Motu, Publisher, VP of Marketing

Shares the experiences of many members in joining AA and answers questions readers may have. The author's message is that your entry to AA can go smoothly. *$3.50*

32 pages Year Founded: 1949 ISBN 0-894861-36-0

1500 Getting Started in AA
Hazelden
PO Box 11
Center City, MN 55012-0011
651-213-4200
800-328-9000; *Fax:* 651-213-4793
info@hazelden.org
www.hazelden.org

Hamilton B, Author

The tradition and wisdom associated with the Twelve Step AA program has been captured in this comprehensive guide. Practical suggestions for staying sober; summaries of AA principles, concepts, and slogans; and a historical overview help the reader understand the spirit of the program. *$13.95*

232 pages Year Founded: 1949 ISBN 1-568380-91-7

1501 Getting What You Want From Drinking
ETR Associates
4 Carbonero Way
Scotts Valley, CA 95066-4200
831-438-4060
800-321-4407; *Fax: 831-438-3618*
support@etr.freshdesk.com
www.etr.org

David Kitchen,MBA, Chief Financial Officer
Talita Sanders,BS, Director,Human Resources
Coleen Cantwell,MPH, Director,Business Development Pl
Matt McDowell,BS, Director,Marketing

Practical ideas for drinking more safely, preventing hangovers, weight gain, and injuries; blood alcohol chart shows the effect of alcohol on the mind and body. Title #H220.

1502 Hazelden Voice
Hazelden Foundation
PO Box 11
Center City, MN 55012-0011
612-213-4200
800-257-7810; *Fax: 651-213-4793*
info@hazelden.org
www.hazelden.org

Mark Mishek, President and CEO,Hazeldon Betty
James A Blaha, VP Finance,Administration/CFO
Marvin D Seppala,MD, Chief Medical Officer
Mark Sheets, Execurive Director,Regional serv

Reports on Hazelden activities and programs, and discusses developments and issues in chemical dependency treatment and prevention. Carries notices of professional education opportunities, reviews of resources in the field, and a calendar of events.

Year Founded: 1949

1503 I Can't Be an Alcoholic Because...
Hazelden
PO Box 11
Center City, MN 55012-0011
651-213-4200
800-328-9000; *Fax: 651-213-4793*
info@hazelden.org
www.hazelden.org

David C Hancock, Author
Mark Sheets, Executive Director
Marvin Seppala MD, Chief Medical Officer
Nick Motu, Publisher, VP of Marketing

This pamphlet describes fallacies and misconceptions about alcoholism and includes facts and figures about alcohol, its use, and its abuse. Available in Spanish. *$1.95*

20 pages Year Founded: 1949 ISBN 0-894861-58-1

1504 ICPA Reporter
ICPADD
12501 Old Columbia Pike
Silver Spring, MD 20904-6601
301-680-6719; *Fax: 301-680-6707*
www.www.icpa.ca

Ed Wozniak, Executive Director
Tineke De Waele, Executive Director Designee

Cassandra Johnson, Business Manager
Koert Swierstra, Office of the President

Reports on activities of the Commission worldwide, which seeks to prevent alcoholism and drug dependency. Recurring features include a calendar of events and notices of publications available.

4 pages 4 per year

1505 Journal of Substance Abuse Treatment
Elsevier Publishing
1600 John F Kennedy Boulevard
Suite 1800
Philadelphia, PA 19103-2879
314-872-8370
800-545-2522; *Fax: 314-432-1380*
custserv@elsevier.com
www.elsevier.com

Mark P. McGovern, Editor-in-Chief

Features original research, systematic reviews and reports on meta-analyses and, with editorial approval, special articles on the assessment and treatment of substance use and addictive disorders, including alcohol, illicit and prescription drugs, and nicotine.

Year Founded: 1880 ISSN 0740-5472

1506 NIDA Notes
National Institute of Drug Abuse (NIDA)
6001 Executive Boulevard
Room 5213,MSC 9561
Bethesda, MD 20892-9561
301-443-1124; *Fax: 301-443-7397*
www.drugabuse.gov

Beverly Jackson, Manager
Beverly Jackson, Public Information Director

Covers the areas of drug abuse treatment and prevention research, epidemiology, neuroscience and behavioral research, health services research and AIDS. Seeks to report on advances in the field, identify resources, promote an exchange of information, and improve communications among clinicians, researchers, administrators, and policymakers. Recurring features include synopses of research advances and projects, NIDA news, news of legislative and regulatory developments, and announcements.

1507 Real World Drinking
ETR Associates
4 Carbonero Way
Scotts Valley, CA 95066-4200
800-321-4407; *Fax: 831-438-3618*
customerservice@etr.org
www.etr.org

Mary Nelson, President

Credible young people talk about benefits of not drinking and risks of drinking. Title #R746.

1508 Teens and Drinking
ETR Associates
4 Carbonero Way
Scotts Valley, CA 95066-4200
800-321-4407; *Fax: 831-438-3618*
customerservice@etr.org
www.etr.org

Mary Nelson, President

Includes common sense messages about drinking, binge drinking, and important things to know about drinking. Title #R717.

1509 The Chalice
Calix Society
PO Box 9085
St Paul, MN 55109-9969
651-773-3117
800-398-0524
www.calixsociety.org

William J Montroy, Founder

Directed toward Catholic and non-Catholic alcoholics who are maintaining their sobriety through affiliation with and participation in Alcoholics Anonymous. Emphasizes the virtue of total abstinence, through contributed stories regarding spiritual and physical recovery. Recurring features include statistics, book announcements, and research. *$15.00*

4-6 pages   24 per year

1510 The Prevention Researcher
Integrated Research Services
66 Club Road
Suite 370
Eugene, OR 97401-2464
541-683-9278
800-929-2955; *Fax: 541-683-2621*
info@tpronline.org

Steven Ungerleider PhD, Advisory Board
Gerald Mader PhD, Advisory Board
Juan Jerry Lopez MSW, Advisory Board

A quarterly journal that provides professionals with practical, relevant research for their work with youth. Each issue features a single topic focused on successful adolescent development. Articles are written by authors who lead in their respective fields and whose research covers the latest findings on significant issues facing today's youth. *$20.00*

12-16 pages   4 per year   ISSN 1086-4385

1511 When Someone You Care About Abuses Drugs and Alcohol: When to Act, What to Say
Hazelden
PO Box 11
Center City, MN 55012-0011
651-213-4200
800-328-9000; *Fax: 651-213-4793*
info@hazelden.org
www.hazelden.org

Mark Mishek, President and CEO,Hazeldon Betty
James A Blaha, VP Finance,Administration/CFO
Marvin D Seppala,MD, Chief Medical Officer
Mark Sheets, Execurive Director,Regional serv

Assists concerned family members and friends in determining their options for helping someone abusing alcohol and/or drugs. Addictive behavior is described, with clear guidelines for how and when to respond to the abuser's behavior. Throughout, the personal responsibility of concerned family and friends is reinforced, with suggestions for examining our motives for intervening. *$2.95*

20 pages   Year Founded: 1949 ISBN 1-592855-29-6

1512 Why Haven't I Been Able to Help?
Hazelden
15251 Pleasant Valley Road
PO Box 176
Center City, MN 55012-176
651-213-4200
800-257-7810; *Fax: 651-213-4590*
customersupport@hazelden.org
www.hazelden.org

Mark Mishek, President, CEO
Mark Sheets, Executive Director
Marvin Seppala MD, Chief Medical Officer
Nick Motu, Publisher, VP of Marketing

Explains how the spouse also gets trapped by the disease, and discusses how the disease progresses within the alcoholic. Ends on a note of hope by briefly indicating how the alcoholic, the spouse, and other family members can escape the trap of alcoholism. *$2.50*

18 pages   ISBN 0-935908-40-4

1513 Your Brain on Drugs
Hazelden
PO Box 11
Center City, MN 55012-0011
651-213-4200
800-257-7810
info@hazelden.org
www.www.hazelden.org

John O'Neill, L.C.D.C., Author
Carlton Erickson, Author
Nick Motu, Publisher, VP of Marketing
Marvin Seppala MD, Chief Medical Officer

This pamphlet explains the effects of alcohol and other drugs on the brain. Illustrations, activities, and exercises help to reinforce easy-to-read text. *$3.50*

32 pages   Year Founded: 1996 ISBN 1-568389-04-3

Research Centers

1514 UAMS Psychiatric Research Institute
4224 Shuffield Drive
Little Rock, AR 72205
501-526-8100; *Fax: 501-660-7542*
kramerteresal@uams.edu
www.www.psychiatry.uams.edu

Combining research, education and clinical services into one facility, PRI offers inpatiend and outpatient services, with 40 psychiatric beds, therapy options, and specialized treatment for specific disorders, including: addictive eating, anxiety, deppressive and post-traumatic stress disorders. Research focuses on evidence-based care takes into consideration the education of future medical personnel while relying on research scientists to provide innovative forms of treatment. PRI includes the Center for Addiction Research as well as a methadone clinic.

Support Groups & Hot Lines

1515 Adult Children of Alcoholics
PO Box 3216
Torrance, CA 90510-3216
562-595-7831
info@adultchildren.org
www.adultchildren.org

An anonymous Twelve Step, Twelve Tradition program of women and men who grew up in an alcoholic or otherwise dysfunctional homes.

1516 Al-Anon Family Group National Referral Hotline
1600 Corporate Landing Parkway
Virginia Beach, VA 23454-5617
757-563-1600; *Fax:* 757-563-1655
wso@al-anon.org
www.al-anon.alateen.org

Al-Anon is a mutual support group of peers who share their experience in applying the Al-Anon principles to problems related to the effects of a problem drinker in their lives. It is not group therapy and is not led by a counselor or therapist; This support network complements and supports professional treatment.

1517 Alateen and Al-Anon Family Groups
1600 Corporate Landing Parkway
Virginia Beach, VA 23454-5617
757-563-1600
888-425-2666; *Fax:* 757-563-1655
wso@al-anon.org

Mary Ann Keller, Director Members Services

A fellowship of men, women, children and adult children affected by another persons drinking.

1518 Alcoholics Anonymous (AA): World Services
475 Riverside Drive at West 120th Street
11th Floor
New York, NY 10115
212-870-3400
www.aa.org

For men and women who share the common problems of alcoholism.

Year Founded: 1935

1519 Chemically Dependent Anonymous
PO Box 423
Severna Park, MD 21146
888-232-4673
www.www.cdaweb.org

A 12-step fellowship for anyone seeking freedom from drug and alcohol addiction. The basis of the program is abstinence from all mood-changing and mind-altering chemicals, including street-type drugs, alcohol and unnecessary medication.

1520 Cocaine Anonymous
21720 S. Wilmington Ave
Suite 304
Long Beach, CA 90810-1641
310-559-5833; *Fax:* 310-559-2554
cawso@ca.org
www.ca.org

Fellowship of men and women who share their experience, stength and hope with each other in hope that they may solve their common problem and help others recover from their addiction.

1521 Infoline
United Way of Connecticut
1344 Silas Deane Highway
Rocky Hill, CT 06067-1350

860-571-7500
800-203-1234; *Fax:* 860-571-7525
TTY: 800-671-0737
www.ctunitedway.org

Richard Porth, CEO

Infoline is a free, confidential, help-by-telephone service for information, referral, and crisis intervention. Trained professionals help callers find information, discover options or deal with a crisis by locating hundreds of services in their area on many different issues, from substance abuse to elder needs to suicide to volunteering in your community. Infoline is certified by the American Association of Suicidology. Operates 24 hours a day, everyday. Multilingual caseworkers are available. For Child Care Infoline, call 1-800-505-1000.

1522 Join Together Online
352 Park Avenue South
9th Floor
New York, NY 10010
212-922-1560
855-378-4373; *Fax:* 212-922-1570
www.www.drugfree.org/join-together

Patricia F Russo, Chairman
Stephen J Pasierb, President,CEO
Robert Caruso, CFO
Paul Healy, Chief Development Officer

Join Together is a collaboration of the Boston University School of Public Health and The Partnership at Drugfree.org, dedicated to advancing effective drug and alcohol policy, prevention and treatment.

1523 MADD-Mothers Against Drunk Drivers
511 E John Carpenter Freeway
Suite 700
Irving, TX 75062-8187
877-275-6233; *Fax:* 214-869-2206
www.www.madd.org

Jan Withers, National President
Debbie Weir, CEO

Mission is to stop drunk driving, support the victims of this violent crime and prevent underage drinking. MADD's work has saved nearly 300,000 lives and counting.

Year Founded: 1980

1524 Marijuana Anonymous
PO Box 7807
Torrance, CA 90504-9207
800-766-6779
office@marijuana-anonymous.org
www.marijuana-anonymous.org

A fellowship of men and women who share experience, strength and hope with each other to solve common problem and help others recover from marijuana addiction.

1525 Nar-Anon Family Groups
22527 Crenshaw Blvd
Suite 200B
Torrance, CA 90505
310-534-8188
800-477-6291; *Fax:* 310-534-8688
www.nar-anon.org

Cathy Khaledi, Executive Director

Twelve-step program for families and friends of addicts.

1526 Narcotics Anonymous
PO Box 9999
Van Nuys, CA 91409-9099
818-773-9999; *Fax:* 818-700-0700
www.na.org

For narcotic addicts: Peer support for recovered addicts.

1527 Pathways to Promise
5400 Arsenal Street
Saint Louis, MO 63139-1403
Fax: 314-516-8405
info@pathways2promise.org
www.pathways2promise.org

An interfaith cooperative of many faith groups, providing assistance and a resource center which offers liturgical and educational materials, program models, caring ministry with people experiencing a mental illness and their families.

1528 Rational Recovery
PO Box 800
Lotus, CA 95651-800
530-621-2667
www.rational.org

Jack Trimpey, President

Exclusive, worldwide source of counseling, guidance and direct instruction on self-recovery from addiction to alcohol and other drugs through planned, permanent abstinence.

Year Founded: 1986

1529 SADD: Students Against Destructive Decisions
255 Main Street
Marlborough, MA 01752-5505
508-481-3568
877-723-3462; *Fax:* 508-481-5759
info@sadd.org
www.sadd.org

Danna Mauch,PhD, Chairman
Penny Wells, President and CEO
Susan Scarola, Treasurer
James E Champagne, Secretary/Clerk

SADD's mission is to provide students with the best prevention tools possible to deal with the issues of underage drinking, other drug use, risky and impaired driving, and other destructive decisions.

Year Founded: 1981

1530 SMART-Self Management and Recovery Training
7304 Mentor Avenue
Suite F
Mentor, OH 44060-5463
440-951-5357
866-951-5357; *Fax:* 440-951-5358
info@smartrecovery.org
www.smartrecovery.org

Shari Allwood, Executive Director

The leading self-empowering addiction recovery support group. Participants learn tools for addiction recovery based on the latest scientific research and participate in a world-wide community which includes free, self-empowering, science-based mutual help groups.

Video & Audio

1531 Alcohol Abuse Dying For A Drink
Educational Video Network
1401 19th Street
Huntsville, TX 77340
936-295-5767
800-762-0060; *Fax:* 936-294-0233
info at evn.org
www.www.evndirect.com

A video explaining alcohol abuse and its consequenses.
$59.95

Year Founded: 2004 ISBN 1-589501-48-9

1532 Alcohol and Sex: Prescription for Poor Decision Making
ETR Associates
4 Carbonero Way
Scotts Valley, CA 95066-4200
831-438-4060
800-321-4407; *Fax:* 800-435-8433
customerservice@etr.org
www.etr.org

Pamela Anderson, PhD, Senior Research Associate
Eric Blanke, BS, Director, Solutions
Nancy Calvin, CES, Administrative Specialist
Shannon Campe, BA, Research Associate III

Explains how alcohol use can interfere with healthy decisions about sex and intimacy, as well as describing the effects of alcohol on the brain. Also, includes information about the date rape drug, how alcohol affects relationships, and includes a Teacher Resource Book. *$139.95*

1533 Alcohol and You
Educational Video Network
1401 19th Street
Huntsville, TX 77340
936-295-5767
800-762-0060; *Fax:* 936-294-0233
info at evn.org
www.www.evndirect.com

A video explaining alcohol abuse and its consequenses.
$49.95

Year Founded: 2001 ISBN 1-588451-32-7

1534 Alcohol and the Brain
Educational Video Network
1401 19th Street
Huntsville, TX 77340
936-295-5767
800-762-0060; *Fax:* 936-294-0233
www.www.evndirect.com

A video explaining alcohol abuse and its consequenses.
$79.95

Year Founded: 2004 ISBN 1-589501-32-7

1535 Alcohol: the Substance, the Addiction, the Solution
Hazelden
15251 Pleasant Valley Road
PO Box 11
Center City, MN 55012-0011
651-213-4200
800-328-9000; *Fax:* 651-213-4793

info@hazelden.org
www.hazelden.org

Mark Mishek, President and CEO
James A. Blaha, Vice President Finance and Admin
Ann Bray, General Counsel and Vice Preside
Sharon Birnbaum, Corporate Director of Human Reso

Weaves dramatic personal stories of recovery from alcoholism with essential facts about alcohol itself. Emphasizes the impact of using and abusing alcohol in conjunction with other drugs. Educates about the dangers of this legally sanctioned drug, including the myth of safer versions such as wine and beer. *$149.00*

Year Founded: 1949

1536 Binge Drinking
ETR Associates
4 Carbonero Way
Scotts Valley, CA 95066-4200
831-438-4060
800-321-4407; *Fax:* 831-438-3618
customerservice@etr.org
www.etr.org

Pamela Anderson, PhD, Senior Research Associate
Eric Blanke, BS, Director, Solutions
Nancy Calvin, CES, Administrative Specialist
Shannon Campe, BA, Research Associate III

Explains the physiological and psychological effects of alcohol, covers the warning signs for alcohol poisoning and procedures to take to save someone, and delivers a no-nonsense message about why binge drinking is dangerous. Describes the catastrophic realities that can result from party behavior, such as car crashes, falls, bad decisions and acquaintance rape. *$139.95*

1537 Cocaine & Crack: Back from the Abyss
Hazelden
15251 Pleasant Valley Road
PO Box 11
Center City, MN 55012-0011
651-213-4200
800-257-7810; *Fax:* 651-213-4793
info@hazelden.org
www.hazelden.org

Mark Mishek, President and CEO
James A. Blaha, Vice President Finance and Admin
Ann Bray, General Counsel and Vice Preside
Sharon Birnbaum, Corporate Director of Human Reso

Provides clients in correctional, educational, and treatment settings an understanding of the history, pharamacology, and medical impact of cocaine/crack use through personal stories of addiction and recovery. Reveals proven methods for overcoming addiction and discusses the best ways to maintain recovery. 46 minutes. *$149.00*

Year Founded: 1949 ISBN 1-592852-97-1

1538 Cross Addiction: The Back Door to Relapse
Hazelden
15251 Pleasant Valley Road
PO Box 11
Center City, MN 55012-0011
651-213-4200
800-328-9000; *Fax:* 651-213-4793
info@hazelden.org
www.hazelden.org

Mark Mishek, President and CEO
James A. Blaha, Vice President Finance and Admin
Ann Bray, General Counsel and Vice Preside
Sharon Birnbaum, Corporate Director of Human Reso

Firsthand testimony from recovering alcoholics and addicts, chemicl dependency professionals, and a medical doctor dispel the myth that there is any such thing as a safe substance for people in recovery. *$225.00*

Year Founded: 1949

1539 Disease of Alcoholism Video
Hazelden
15251 Pleasant Valley Road
PO Box 11
Center City, MN 55012-0011
651-213-4200
800-328-9000; *Fax:* 651-213-4793
info@hazelden.org
www.hazelden.org

Mark Mishek, President and CEO
James A. Blaha, Vice President Finance and Admin
Ann Bray, General Counsel and Vice Preside
Sharon Birnbaum, Corporate Director of Human Reso

This video is used daily in treatment, corporations, and schools. Dr. Ohlms discusses startling and convincing information on the genetic and physiological aspects of alcohol addiction. *$395.00*

Year Founded: 1949

1540 Effective Learning Systems, Inc.
5108 W 74th Street
#390160
Minneapolis, MN 55439
239-948-1660
800-966-0443
www.www.effectivelearning.com

Bob Griswold, Founder
Deirdre M Griswold, VP

Audio tapes for stress management, deep relaxation, anger control, peace of mind, insomnia, weight and smoking, self-image and self-esteem, positive thinking, health and healing. Since 1972, Effective Learning Systems has helped millions of people take charge of their lives and make positive changes. Over 75 titles available, each with a money-back guarantee. Price range $12-$14.

Year Founded: 1972

1541 Fetal Alcohol Syndrome and Effect
Hazelden
15251 Pleasant Valley Road
PO Box 11
Center City, MN 55012-0011
651-213-4200
800-328-9000; *Fax:* 651-213-4793
info@hazelden.org
www.hazelden.org

Mark Mishek, President and CEO
James A. Blaha, Vice President Finance and Admin
Ann Bray, General Counsel and Vice Preside
Sharon Birnbaum, Corporate Director of Human Reso

If you're a chemical dependency counselor or work with women in pregnancy planning or self-care, this resource is filled with facts to help you better meet your clients needs. *$225.00*

Year Founded: 1949

1542 Fetal Alcohol Syndrome and Effect, Stories of Help and Hope
Hazelden
15251 Pleasant Valley Road
PO Box 11
Center City, MN 55012-0011
651-213-4200
800-328-9000; *Fax:* 651-213-4793
info@hazelden.org
www.hazelden.org

Mark Mishek, President and CEO
James A. Blaha, Vice President Finance and Admin
Ann Bray, General Counsel and Vice Preside
Sharon Birnbaum, Corporate Director of Human Reso

Provides clients with a factual defintion of the medical diagonosis of fetal alcohol syndrome and its effects, including how children are diagnosed and the positive prognosis possible for these children. *$225.00*

Year Founded: 1949

1543 Heroin: What Am I Going To Do?
Hazelden
15251 Pleasant Valley Road
PO Box 11
Center City, MN 55012-0011
651-213-4200
800-328-9000; *Fax:* 651-213-4793
info@hazelden.org
www.hazelden.org

Mark Mishek, President and CEO
James A. Blaha, Vice President Finance and Admin
Ann Bray, General Counsel and Vice Preside
Sharon Birnbaum, Corporate Director of Human Reso

Shares powerful stories and keen insights from recovering heroin addicts and the rewards of clean living. Teaches clients how to use honesty, surrender and responsibility as the power tools for a successful recovery. Deglamorizes heroin use, with a portrait of drug's inevitable degration of the mind, body and spirit. 30 minutes. *$225.00*

Year Founded: 1949

1544 I'll Quit Tomorrow
Hazelden
15251 Pleasant Valley Road
PO Box 11
Center City, MN 55012-0011
651-213-4200
800-328-9000; *Fax:* 651-213-4793
info@hazelden.org
www.hazelden.org

Mark Mishek, President and CEO
James A. Blaha, Vice President Finance and Admin
Ann Bray, General Counsel and Vice Preside
Sharon Birnbaum, Corporate Director of Human Reso

Show clients the progressive nature of alcoholism through one of the most powerful films ever made about this disease. This three-part video series and facilitator's guide use a dramatic personal story to provide a clear and thorough introduction to the disease concept of alcoholism, enabling the intervention process, treatment and the hope of healing and recovery. *$300.00*

Year Founded: 1949

1545 Marijuana: Escape to Nowhere
Hazelden
15251 Pleasant Valley Road
PO Box 11
Center City, MN 55012-176
651-213-4200
800-328-9000; *Fax:* 651-213-4793
info@hazelden.org
www.hazelden.org

Mark Mishek, President and CEO
James A. Blaha, Vice President Finance and Admin
Ann Bray, General Counsel and Vice Preside
Sharon Birnbaum, Corporate Director of Human Reso

Challenges myths about marijuana by clearly stating that marijuana is addictive and use results in physical, emotional and spiritual consequences. Explains to clients in simple language the pharmacology of today's more potent marijuana and shares the hope and healing of recovery. 30 minutes. *$225.00*

Year Founded: 1949

1546 Medical Aspects of Chemical Dependency
Active Parenting Publishers
Hazelden
15251 Pleasant Valley Road
PO Box 11
Center City, MN 55012-0011
651-213-4200
800-328-9000; *Fax:* 651-213-4793
info@hazelden.org
www.hazelden.org

Mark Mishek, President and CEO
James A. Blaha, Vice President Finance and Admin
Ann Bray, General Counsel and Vice Preside
Sharon Birnbaum, Corporate Director of Human Reso

This curriculum helps professionals educate clients in treatment and other settings about medical effects of chemical use and abuse. The program includes a video that explains body and brain changes that can occur when using alcohol or other drugs, a workbook that helps clients apply the information from the video to their own situations, a handbook that provides in-depth information on addiction, brain chemistry and the physiological effects of chemical dependency and a pamphlet that answers critical questions clients have about the medical effects of chemical dependency. Available to purchase separately. Program value packages available. *$225.00*

Year Founded: 1949

1547 Methamphetamine: Decide to Live Prevention Video
Hazelden
15251 Pleasant Valley Road
PO Box 11
Center City, MN 55012-0011
651-213-4200
800-328-9000; *Fax:* 651-213-4793
info@hazelden.org
www.hazelden.org

Mark Mishek, President and CEO
James A. Blaha, Vice President Finance and Admin
Ann Bray, General Counsel and Vice Preside
Sharon Birnbaum, Corporate Director of Human Reso

Methamphetamine: Decide to Live presents the latest information on the devastating consequences of meth addiction and the struggles and rewards of recovery. Facts, medical aspects, personal stories, and insights on the recovery process illuminate the path to healing. The video is divided into two parts and is 38 minutes long. *$225.00*

Year Founded: 1949

1548 Prescription Drugs: Recovery from the Hidden Addiction
Hazelden
15251 Pleasant Valley Road
PO Box 11
Center City, MN 55012-0011
651-213-4200
800-328-9000; *Fax: 651-213-4793*
info@hazelden.org
www.hazelden.org

Mark Mishek, President and CEO
James A. Blaha, Vice President Finance and Admin
Ann Bray, General Counsel and Vice Preside
Sharon Birnbaum, Corporate Director of Human Reso

Combines essential facts about prescription drugs with vivid personal stories of addiction and recovery. Classifies prescription medications and gives the corresponding street forms. Offers solutions to problems unique to presciption drugs, addresses the particular needs of older adults and elaborates on the dangers of cross-addiction. 31 minutes. *$225.00*

Year Founded: 1949

1549 Reality Check: Marijuana Prevention Video
Hazelden
15251 Pleasant Valley Road
PO Box 11
Center City, MN 55012-0011
651-213-4200
800-328-9000; *Fax: 651-213-4793*
info@hazelden.org
www.hazelden.org

Mark Mishek, President and CEO
James A. Blaha, Vice President Finance and Admin
Ann Bray, General Counsel and Vice Preside
Sharon Birnbaum, Corporate Director of Human Reso

This video creates a strong message for kids about the dangers of marijuana use. A combination of humor, animated graphics, testimonials and music deliver the facts on the pharmacology of marijuana and both it's short and long use consequences. Suitable for kids grades 7-12.
15 minute video. *$225.00*

Year Founded: 1949

1550 SmokeFree TV: A Nicotine Prevention Video
Hazelden
15251 Pleasant Valley Road
PO Box 11
Center City, MN 55012-0011
651-213-4200
800-328-9000; *Fax: 651-213-4793*
info@hazelden.org
www.hazelden.org

Mark Mishek, President and CEO
James A. Blaha, Vice President Finance and Admin
Ann Bray, General Counsel and Vice Preside
Sharon Birnbaum, Corporate Director of Human Reso

Key facts, consequences of use and refusal skills guide children in understanding why they should avoid nicotine.

Animated graphics, stories, humor, and music appeal to young people. Pharmacology of nicotine, its consequences and ways to refuse it are also explored. 15 minute video. *$225.00*

Year Founded: 1949

1551 Straight Talk About Substance Use and Violence
ADD WareHouse
300 NW 70th Avenue
Suite 102
Plantation, FL 33317-2360
954-792-8100
800-233-9273; *Fax: 954-792-8545*
websales@addwarehouse.com
www.addwarehouse.com

Mark Mishek, President and CEO
James A. Blaha, Vice President Finance and Admin
Ann Bray, General Counsel and Vice Preside
Sharon Birnbaum, Corporate Director of Human Reso

Substance abuse and violence prevention begins with this three video program featuring the frank testimonials of 19 teens with significant chemical dependency issues who range in age from 13 to 22. In the starkest terms they discuss their most personal issues: substance abuse, sexual abuse, physical abuse, suicide attempts, violent acting out, depression, and abusive relationships. Includes 95 page discussion guide and three 30 minute videos. *$259.00*

Year Founded: 1990

1552 What Should I Tell My Child About Drinking?
NADD-National Council on Alcoholism and Drug Dependence, Inc.
217 Broadway
Suite 712
New York, NY 10007-3128
212-269-7797
800-622-2255; *Fax: 212-269-7510*
national@ncadd.org
www.www.ncadd.org

Greg Muth, Chairman
William H. Foster, PhD, President and Chief Executive Of
Leah Brock, Director of Affiliate Relations
Jayne Restivo, Director of Development

Offers a series of teachable moments for different age groups that provide parents a structured opportunity to discuss alcohol with their children *$59.99*

12 pages Year Founded: 1944

Web Sites

1553 www.aa.org
AA-Alcoholics Anonymous

Group sharing their experience, strength and hope with each other to recover from alcoholism.

1554 www.addictionresourceguide.com
Addiction Resource Guide

A comprehensive directory of addiction treatment facilities online.

1555 www.adultchildren.org
Adult Children of Alcoholics World Services Organization, Inc.

12 step and 12 tradition program for adults raised in an environment including alcohol or other dysfunctions.

1556 www.al-anon.alateen.org
Al-Anon/Alateen

Program for relatives and friends of persons with alcohol problems.

1557 www.alcoholism.about.com
The Alcoholism Home Page

Information about addictive drug use, behaviors, and alcoholism.

1558 www.cfsny.org
Center for Family Support (CFS)

Devoted to providing support and assistance to individuals with developmental and related disabilities, and to the family members who care for them.

1559 www.doitnow.org
The Do It Now Foundation

Copies of brochures on drugs, alcohol, smoking, drugs and kids, and street drugs.

1560 www.drugabuse.gov
National Institute on Drug Abuse

Many publications useful for patients. Research Reports, summaries about chemicals and treatments.

1561 www.drugabuse.gov/drugpages
Commonly Abused Drugs: Street Names for Drugs of Abuse

Current names, periods of detection, medical uses.

1562 www.drugfree.org/join-together
Join Together

Alcohol and substance abuse information, legislative alerts, new and updates.

1563 www.higheredcenter.org
National Clearinghouse for Alcohol & Drug Information

One-stop resource for information about abuse prevention and addiction treatment.

1564 www.jacsweb.org
Jewish Alcoholics Chemically Dependent Persons

Ten articles dealing with denial and ignorance.

1565 www.lifering.org
LifeRing

Offers nonreligious approach with links to groups.

1566 www.madd.org
MADD-Mothers Against Drunk Driving

A crusade to stop alcohol consumption, and underage drinking.

1567 www.mentalhealth.com
Internet Mental Health

On-line information and a virtual encyclopedia related to mental disorders, possible causes and treatments. News, articles, on-line diagnostic programs and related links. Designed to improve understanding, diagnosis and treatment of mental illness throughout the world. Awarded the Top Site Award and the NetPsych Cutting Edge Site Award.

1568 www.mhselfhelp.org
National Mental Health Consumers Self-Help Clearinghouse

Encourages the development and growth of consumer self-help groups.

1569 www.naadac.org
The Association for Addiction Professionals

NAADAC is the premier global organization of addiction focused professionals who enhance the health and recovery of individuals, families and communities. NAADAC's mission is to lead, unify and empower addiction focused professionals to achieve excellence through education, advocacy, knowledge, standards of practice, ethics, professional development and research.

1570 www.niaaa.nih.gov
National Institute on Alcohol Abuse & Alcoholism

Supports research nationwide on alcohol abuse and alcoholism.

1571 www.nofas.org
National Organization on Fetal Alcohol Syndrome

Develops and implements innovative prevention and education strategies assessing fetal alcohol syndrome.

1572 www.psychcentral.com
Psych Central

Personalized one-stop index for psychology, support, and mental health issues, resources, and people on the Internet.

1573 www.sadd.org
SADD-Students Against Destructive Decisions

Peer leadership organization dedicated to preventing destructive decisions.

1574 www.samhsa.gov
Substance Abuse and Mental Health Services Administration

Provides links to government resources related to substance abuse and mental health.

1575 www.sapacap.com
American Council on Alcohol Problems

Referrals to DWI classes and treatment centers.

1576 www.smartrecovery.org
Self Help for Substance Abuse & Addiction

Four-Point program includes maintaining motivation, coping with urges, managing feelings and behavior, balancing momentary/enduring satisfactions.

1577 **www.soulselfhelp.on.ca/coda.html**
Souls Self Help Central

Discusses self-help, mental health, issues of co-dependency.

1578 **www.store.samhsa.gov**
SAMHSA's National Mental Health Info Center

Information about resources, technical assistance, research, training, networks, and other federal clearing houses, and fact sheets and materials.

1579 **www.thenationalcouncil.org**
National Council for Commuity Behavioral Healthcare

A network for sharing information and provding assistance among those working in the healthcare management field.

1580 **www.well.com**
Web of Addictions

Links to fact sheets from trustworthy sources.

Directories & Databases

1581 **National Directory of Drug and Alcohol Abuse Treatment Programs**
SAMHSA
1 Choke Cherry Road
Rockville, MD 20857
877-SAM-SA 7
www.store.samhsa.gov

Directory of substance abuse treatment programs for use by persons seeking treatment and by professionals. Lists facility name, address, telephone number and services offered. Updated annually. Searchable on-line version on web site. CD-ROM

Suicide

Introduction

Suicide is an event, not a mental disorder, but it is the lethal consequence of some mental disorders. Suicide involves a complex interaction of psychological, neurological, medical, social, and family factors.

Most professionals distinguish at least two suicide groups: those who actually kill themselves, i.e. completed suicides; and those who attempt it, usually harming themselves, but survive. Those who succeed in killing themselves are nearly always suffering from one or more psychiatric disorders, most commonly depression, often along with alcohol or substance abuse. Some individuals plan suicide very carefully, taking steps to ensure that they will not be discovered and rescued, and they use lethal means (shooting themselves, or jumping from high places). Some act impulsively, such as reacting to a life disappointment by jumping off a nearby bridge. Some suicide attempts or gestures use means that make discovery and rescue probable, and are not likely to be lethal (e.g. taking insufficient pills). Some people make repeated suicide attempts. Unfortunately, recurrent suicidal gestures cannot be dismissed; each unsuccesful attempt increases the likelihood of a completed suicide.

ASSOCIATED FEATURES

Nine of ten suicides are associated with some form of mental disorder, especially Depression, Schizophrenia, Alcohol/Substance Abuse, Bipolar Disorder, and Anxiety Disorders. In addition, Personality Disorders have been diagnosed in one-third to one-half of people who kill themselves. These suicides often occur in younger people who live in an environment where drug and alcohol abuse, as well as violence, are common. The most common personality disorders associated with suicide are Borderline Personality Disorder, Antisocial Personality Disorder, and Narcissistic Personality Disorder. Among people with Schizophrenia, especially those suffering from Paranoid Schizophrenia, suicide is the main reason for premature death.

Drug and alcohol abuse is a risk factor for suicide. In a study among 113 young people who killed themselves in California, fifty-five percent had some kind of substance abuse problems, usually long-standing and including several different drugs. A history of trauma or abuse is also a risk factor for suicide, as is a family history of suicide, loss of a job, loss of a loved one, lack of social support, and barriers to accessible health care.

Some suicides result from insufficiently treated, severe, debilitating, or terminal physical illness. The pain, restricted function, and dread of dependence can all contribute to suicidal behavior, especially in illnesses such as Huntington's Disease, cancer, MS, spinal cord injuries and AIDS. Some or many of these risk factors are present in most completed suicides. Depression and suicide are not inevitable for people with severe general medical diagnoses. The recognition and treatment of depression, when it does occur, can prevent many suicides.

PREVALENCE

Suicide is the tenth leading cause of death in the United States and the second leading cause among 15-24 year-olds. It is estimated that over five million people have suicidal thoughts, though there are only 30,000 deaths from it each year. This may be a serious underestimate, however, since suicide is still stigmatized and often goes unreported. Boys are more likely to complete suicide than girls, largely because they use more lethal means, such as firearms. Compared to other countries, guns are particularly common in the U.S. as a means of suicide. Children who kill themselves often have a history of antisocial behavior, and depression and suicide is more common in their families than in families in general.

More males than females commit suicide, both among adults and adolescents. Among adults, the most likely suicides are among men who are widowed, divorced, or single, who lack social support, who are unemployed, who have a diagnosed mental disorder (especially Depression), who have a physical illness, a family history of suicide, who are in psychological turmoil, who have made previous attempts, who use or abuse alcohol, and/or who have easy access to firearms. Among adolescents, the most likely suicides are married males (or unwed and pregnant females), who have suffered from parental abuse or absence, who have academic problems, Bipolar Disorder, who are substance abusers, suffer from AD/HD or epilepsy, who have conduct disorder, problems with impulse control, a family history of suicide, and/or access to firearms. Keeping guns in the home is a suicide risk for both males and females.

Elderly people (those over age 65) are more likely than any other age group to commit suicide. As in other population groups, elderly men are more likely to kill themselves than elderly women but the difference between the sexes is much bigger in this age group than in other age groups. Among all ages, the rate of suicide for men is about 20 per 100,000 and for women five per 100,000. Among the elderly, the rate for men is about 42 per 100,000 and for women about six and one-half per 100,000. Thus the great overall gender differences become even bigger among the elderly and more so as the elderly get older. The highest rate of suicide is among elderly white men, probably because their economic and social status drops severely with age, and because they may lack good social support systems and be reluctant to ask for help.

Although all the factors discussed here are risk factors, it should be kept in mind that 99.9 percent of those at risk do not commit suicide.

TREATMENT OPTIONS

Considering the risk factors, a professional must first make a careful assessment, taking all the risk factors into account, including the availabilty of weapons, pill and other lethal means, as well as whether or not the person has conveyed the intention to commit suicide, and whether the method the patient plans to use is available (one can only jump off a bridge if there is a bridge, or drive into a wall if one has access to a vehicle). Every individual who feels that life is not worth living, or who is contemplating suicide, should be asked about guns in the home and should be encouraged to remove them. The same is true for medications that are dangerous in overdose.

Someone who has no thought of death or has thoughts of death that are not connected with suicide is at a lower risk than someone who is thinking about suicide. Among those who are thinking of it, those who have not worked out the means of committing suicide are at a lower risk than those who have thought of a specific method of carrying it out.

Treatment is partly based on the level of intervention that is believed to be required. If the person is seriously depressed and is also anxious, tense and angry, and in overwhelming psychological anguish, the risk is more acute. The first priority is to ensure the safety of the client. To that end, hospitalization may be necessary.

After safety is assured, treatment is aimed at the underlying disorder. It may include psychological support, medication, and other therapies: group, art, dance/movement, music. Professional treatment should involve working with the family when possible, and other medical staff, e.g. a physician, and should include regular reassessments.

In cases of Personality Disorders, there may be anger and aggression, and the suicidal thoughts and ideas may be chronic or repetitive. This is a particular strain on professionals, patients, and family. They all must work together to understand the chronicity of the condition, and the fact that suicide cannot always be prevented. It is essential to develop a working alliance between the therapist and client, based on trust, mutual respect, and on the client's belief that the therapist genuinely cares about him/her. At the same time, the therapist must set limits on patient demands to prevent burn out.

Reassessments include getting information from other professionals involved in treating the patient, including medication with the prescribing physician, and from family members or others significant in the life of the client who should participate in planning and following up. Assessment must also include assessment of the client's ability to understand and participate in the treatment, information about his/her psychological state (hopeless, despairing, depressed) and cognitive competence.

Associations & Agencies

1583 American Association of Suicidology
5221 Wisconsin Avenue Northwest
Washington, DC 20015
202-237-2280; *Fax:* 202-237-2282
www.suicidology.org

Julie Cerel, PhD, President
Colleen Creighton, Executive Director
Amy Boland, CPA, Treasurer
Jonathan Singer, PhD, Secretary

The American Association of Suicidology is a nonprofit membership organization for those affected by suicide, as well as those involved in suicide prevention and intervention. AAS aims to foster an environment of understanding and support for all those who have been affected by suicide. AAS works towards the advancement of suicide prevention programs and scientific efforts through research, education, and training, information dissemination, and support services for survivors.

Year Founded: 1968

1584 Byron Peter Foundation for Hope
31 Hartfort Pike
North Scituate, RI 02857
401-647-9295
www.byronpeterfoundation.org

Marilynn Hammond, President and Founder
Seth W. Harrington, Vice President
Phoebe M. Harrington, Secretary and Treasurer

A nonprofit foundation established to honor the life of Byron Peter Harrington II, a young man who took his own life in 2001. The Foundation seeks to inspire troubled young people to attain hope for the future. The Foundation provides opportunities for at risk youth, including those struggling with depression or drug use.

1585 National Alliance on Mental Illness
3803 North Fairfax Drive
Suite 100
Arlington, VA 22203
703-524-7600
800-950-6264
info@nami.org
www.nami.org

Steve Pitman, JD, President
Lacey Berumen, PhD, MNM, First Vice President
Mary Giliberti, Chief Executive Officer
David Levy, Chief Financial Officer

NAMI is an organization dedicated to raising awareness on mental health and providing support and education for Americans affected by mental illness. NAMI advocates for access to services and treatment and fosters an environment of awareness and understanding for those concerned with mental health.

Year Founded: 1979

1586 National Center for the Prevention of Youth Suicide
American Association of Suicidology
5221 Wisconsin Avenue Northwest
Washington, DC 20015
202-237-2280; *Fax:* 202-237-2282
ajkulp@suicidology.org
www.suicidology.org/ncpys

Julie Cerel, PhD, President
Amy Kulp, MS, Director, National Center
Amy Boland, CPA, Treasurer
Jonathan Singer, PhD, Secretary

The goal of the National Center for the Prevention of Youth Suicide is to reduce the rate of suicide attempts and deaths among youth. The National Center provides information on the warning signs of suicide, works with other organizations to help develop effective suicide prevention practices among youth caregivers, promotes better mental health and forms strategies to address suicide risk factors, and encourages youth to participate in grassroots suicide prevention movements.

Year Founded: 1968

1587 National Organization for People of Color Against Suicide
1006 Kennon Court
Rockville, MD 20851
301-523-7794
dbarnes@nopcas.org
www.nopcas.org/

Donna Barnes, PhD, Co-Founder and President
Doris Smith, Co-Founder, VP and Treasurer
Les Franklin, Co-Founder
Nicole Aandahl, Policy Advisor

NOPCAS is a national organization whose mission is to raise awareness on suicide and to promote suicide education, particularly within communities of color. NOPCAS works with minorities in suicide prevention through the production of education resources and publications for communities of color, the development of culturally appropriate training opportunities for professionals, and the promotion of community-based strategies that mobilize minority communities around suicide prevention efforts.

1588 National P.O.L.I.C.E. Suicide Foundation

7015 Clarke Road
Seaford, DE 19973
302-536-1214
866-276-4615; *Fax:* 302-536-1214
redoug2001@aol.com
www.psf.org

Robert E. Douglas, Jr., Founder and Executive Director
Carolyn Douglas, Administrative Assistant

A nonprofit educational foundation focused on the issue of police suicide. Provides support services and training programs on suicide awareness and prevention for police, emergency responders, and their families. Seeks to address the psychological, emotional, and spiritual needs of officers and law enforcement families affected by suicide.

Year Founded: 1997

1589 Screening for Mental Health, Inc. (SMH)

One Washington Street
Suite 304
Wellesley Hills, MA 02481
781-239-0071; *Fax:* 781-431-7447
smhinfo@mentalhealthscreening.org
www.mentalhealthscreening.org

Douglas Jacobs, MD, Founder and Medical Director
Norm Gorin, President and CEO
Jill Buchanan, Director of Marketing
Meghan Diamon, Director, Suicide Prevention

Screening For Mental Health Inc. is an organization focused on providing education, screening, and treatment resources to the public with the goal of improving mental health. Since 1991, SMH has led the development of large-scale mental health screening and education programs, which provide mental health education and screen individuals for depression, bipolar disorder, eating disorders, alcohol use disorders, generalized anxiety disorder, post traumatic stress disorder, and suicide.

Year Founded: 1991

1590 Suicide Awareness Voices of Education (SAVE)

8120 Penn Avenue South
Suite 470
Bloomington, MN 55431
952-946-7998
www.save.org

Joseph W. Stackhouse, Chair
Jennifer A. Facciani, Treasurer
Patrick M. Klinger, Vice President

Suicide Awareness Voices of Education's mission is to prevent suicide through the elimination of stigma and the organization of education programs designed to raise awareness on depression, mental illnesses, the importance of assessment, treatment and intervention, the warning signs of suicide, and community resources. SAVE also provides resources for those who have been affected by suicide.

Year Founded: 1989

1591 Survivors of Loved Ones' Suicides (SOLOS)

8310 Ewing Halsell Drive
San Antonio, TX 78229
210-885-7069
solossanantonio@gmail.com
www.solossa.org

Tony Mata, SOLOS Facilitator
Angie Navarette, SOLOS Facilitator

Located in San Antonio, Texas, SOLOS organizes ongoing support group meetings for persons affected by the loss of loved ones from suicide.

Year Founded: 1987

1592 The Jason Foundation, Inc.

18 Volunteer Drive
Hendersonville, TN 37075
615-264-2323
888-881-2323; *Fax:* 615-264-0188
contact@jasonfoundation.com
www.jasonfoundation.com

Clark Flatt, President
Michele Ray, Senior Vice President and CEO
Deanne Ray, Vice President and COO
Morgan Marks, National Director of Divisions

An educational organization dedicated to the awareness and prevention of youth suicide. Develops educational programs that provide young people, youth workers, educators, and parents with the knowledge and resources needed to help identify and support at-risk youth.

1593 Yellow Ribbon Suicide Prevention Program
Light for Life Foundation International

7300 Lowell Boulevard
Suite 35, PO Box 644
Westminster, CO 80036
303-429-3530
ask4help@yellowribbon.org
www.yellowribbon.org

Dale Emme, Co-Founder/Executive Director
Dar Emme, Co-Founder/Deputy Director

The Yellow Ribbon Suicide Prevention Program provides support services for survivors; promotes the participation of communities, families, and individuals in suicide prevention efforts; develops community-based programs; partners with local agencies to organize suicide prevention trainings; and gives motivational presentations to schools, youth, and adults.

Year Founded: 1994

Books

1594 Adolescent Suicide
American Psychiatric Publishing, Inc.

1000 Wilson Boulevard
Suite 1825
Arlington, VA 22209-3901
703-907-7322
800-368-5777; *Fax:* 703-907-1091
appi@psych.org
www.appi.org

Presents techniques that allow psychiatrists and other professionals to respond to signs of distress with timely therapeutic intervention. It also suggests measures of anticipatory prevention. Adolescent Suicide presents an overview of adolescent suicidal behavior. It explores risk factors, the identification and evaluation of the suicidal adolescent, and approaches to therapy. *$38.95*

210 pages Year Founded: 1996 ISBN 0-873182-08-9

1595 Adolescent Suicide: A School-Based Approach to Assessment and Intervention
Research Press
Dept 12 W
PO Box 9177
Champaign, IL 61826-9177
217-352-3273
800-519-2707; *Fax:* 217-352-1221
rp@researchpress.com
www.researchpress.com

Dr William G Kirk, Author

Presents the information required to accurately identify potentially suicidal adolescents and provides the skills necessary for effective intervention. The book includes many case examples derived from information provided by parents, mental health professionals and educators, as well as adolescents who have considered suicide or survived suicide attempts. An essential resource for school counseling staff, psychologists, teachers and administrators. *$16.95*

175 pages Year Founded: 1993 ISBN 0-878223-36-3

1596 After a Suicide: An Activity Book for Grieving Kids
The Dougy Center
PO Box 86852
Portland, OR 97286
503-775-5683
866-775-5683
help@dougy.org
www.dougy.org

In this hands-on, interactive workbook, children who have been exposed to a suicide can learn from other grieving kids. The workbook includes drawing activities, puzzles, stories, advice from other kids and helpful suggestions for how to navigate the grief process after a suicide death.

48 pages Year Founded: 2001 ISBN 1-890534-06-4

1597 Anatomy of Suicide: Silence of the Heart
Charles C Thomas Publisher Ltd.
2600 S First Street
Springfield, IL 62704-4730
217-789-8980
800-258-8980; *Fax:* 217-789-9130
books@ccthomas.com
www.ccthomas.com

Louis Everstine, Author

The author explores the scope of this problem which involves clinical and ethical issues; the myth of depression; the path to suicide; unfinished business; staying alive; early warnings; first interventions; the self-contract; cases in point; and the future of suicide. Written for psychologists, counselors, and mental health professionals, this book is an excellent resource that will further our understanding of suicide and seek new ways for prevention. *$42.95*

153 pages Year Founded: 1998 ISSN 0-398-06803-8ISBN 0-398068-02-X

1598 Exuberance: The Passion for Life
Knopf Publishing Group
1745 Broadway
New York, NY 10019-4343
212-782-9000; *Fax:* 212-940-7390
knopfpublicity@randomhouse.com
www.knopfdoubleday.com

Kay Redfield Jamison, Author

An exploration of exuberance and how it fuels our most important creative and scientific achievements. In a fascinating and intimate coda to the rest of the book, renowned scientists, writers, and politicians share their thoughts on the forms and role of exuberance in their own lives. Original, inspiring, authoritative, Exuberance brims with the very energy and passion that it celebrates.

416 pages Year Founded: 2004 ISBN 0-375401-44-X

1599 Harvard Medical School Guide to Suicide Assessment and Intervention
Jossey-Bass / Wiley & Sons
111 River Street
Hoboken, NJ 07030-5774
201-748-6000; *Fax:* 201-748-6088
info@wiley.com
www.wiley.com

Douglas G. Jacobs, Editor

This vital resource is the definitive guide for helping mental health professionals determine the risk for suicide and appropriate interventions for suicidal or at-risk patients. Created primarily for mental health clinicians, the book is a hands-on guide for those who are often the first line of defense for assessing if a patient or client is suicidal. *$59.95*

736 pages Year Founded: 1998 ISBN 0-787943-03-7

1600 In the Wake of Suicide: Stories of the People Left Behind
Jossey-Bass / Wiley & Sons
10475 Crosspoint Blvd.
Indianapolis, IN 46256
877-762-2974; *Fax:* 800-597-3299
consumers@wiley.com
www.wiley.com

Victoria Alexander, Author

Offers survivors the understanding, compassion, and hope they need to guide them on their own path in the wake of this most painful loss. Breathtaking stories of incredible power for anyone struggling to find the meaning in the suicidal death of a loved one and for all readers seeking writing that moves and inspires. *$27.00*

256 pages Year Founded: 1998 ISBN 0-787940-52-6

1601 Left Alive: After a Suicide Death in the Family
Charles C Thomas Publisher Ltd.
2600 S 1st Street
Springfield, IL 62704-4730
217-789-8980
800-258-8980; *Fax:* 217-789-9130
books@ccthomas.com
www.ccthomas.com

Linda Rosenfeld, Author
Marilynne Prupas, Author

$21.95

100 pages Year Founded: 1984 ISBN 0-398066-50-7

1602 My Son...My Son: A Guide to Healing After Death, Loss, or Suicide
Bolton Press Atlanta
1090 Crest Brook Lane
Roswell, GA 30075-3403
770-645-1886; *Fax:* 770-649-0999
contactus@boltonpress.com
www.boltonpress.com

Iris Bolton, Author
Curtis Mitchell, Collaborator

A moving story of love, loss and recovery that will grab your heart, nourish your soul and open your eyes. A must read for anyone who has experienced a great loss and is trying to find some path out of the darkness of their despair or to understand those that are.

120 pages Year Founded: 1983 ISBN 0-961632-60-7

1603 Night Falls Fast: Understanding Suicide
Vintage Books A Division Of Random House
1745 Broadway
20th Floor
New York, NY 10019
212-782-9000
800-733-3000; *Fax:* 212-302-7985
ecustomerservice@randomhouse.com
www.randomhouse.com

Kay Redfield Jamison, Author

Tragically timely: suicide has become one of the most common killers of Americans between the ages of fifteen and forty-five. Weaving together a historical and scientific exploration of the subject with personal essays on individual suicides, the author not only brings her remarkable conpassion and literary skill but also all of her knowledge and research to bear on this devastating problem. This is a book that helps us to understand the suicidal mind, to recognize and come to the aid of those at risk, and to comprehend the profound effects on those left behind. It is critical reading for parents, educators, and anyone wanting to understand this tragic epidemic.

448 pages ISBN 0-375701-47-8

1604 No Time to Say Goodbye: Surviving the Suicide of a Loved One
Three Rivers Press
1745 Broadway
New York, NY 10019
212-782-9000
ecustomerservice@randomhouse.com
www.randomhouse.com

Carla Fine, Author

With No Time to Say Goodbye, the author brings suicide survival from the darkness into light, speaking frankly about the overwhelming feelings of confusion, guilt, shame, anger, and loneliness that are shared by all survivors. Fine draws on her own experience and on conversations with many other survivors- as well as on the knowledge of counselors and mental health professionals.

272 pages Year Founded: 1999 ISBN 0-385485-51-4

1605 Someone I Love Died by Suicide: A Story for Child Survivors and Those Who Care for Them
Grief Guidance Inc.
PO Box 32789
Palm Beach Gardens, FL 33420-2789

561-625-6751; *Fax:* 561-625-6751
www.griefguidance.com

Doreen Cammarata, Author

This book is designed for adult caregivers to read to surviving youngsters following a suicidal death. Although the language used in the book is simplistic enough to be read along with children ultimately stimulating family discussion, it can be beneficial to all who have been tragically devastated by suicide. It is recommended for this book to be utilized in conjunction with therapy.

40 pages Year Founded: 2001 ISBN 0-970933-29-0

1606 Suicidal Patient: Principles of Assessment, Treatment, and Case Management
American Psychiatric Publishing, Inc.
1000 Wilson Boulevard
Suite 1825
Arlington, VA 22209-3901
703-907-7322
800-368-5777; *Fax:* 703-907-1091
appi@psych.org
www.appi.org

John A. Chiles, Author
Kirk D. Strosahl, Author

Presents a clinical approach and valuable assessment strategies and techniques. Demonstrates an easy to use innovative clinical model with specific stages of treatment and associated interventions outlined for inpatient and outpatient settings. *$45.50*

282 pages Year Founded: 1995 ISBN 0-800485-54-X

1607 Suicide Over the Life Cycle
American Psychiatric Publishing, Inc.
1000 Wilson Boulevard
Suite 1825
Arlington, VA 22209-3901
703-907-7322
800-368-5777; *Fax:* 703-907-1091
appi@psych.org
www.appi.org

Susan J. Blumenthal, Editor
David J. Kupfer, Editor

This book attempts to solve the mystery of suicide by filling in the gaps in our understanding about risk factors and treatment of suicidal patients, and by integrating and translating current knowledge about suicidal behavior into practical treatment considerations. This book brings together the research studies and clinical experience of more than 40 internationally recognized contributors who paint an insightful and thought-provoking portrait of the suicidal patient at various stages of the life span. A comprehensive guide, this superb text is a practical and encyclopedic compendium of assessment and intervention strategies that the clinician can use in day-to-day treatment of suicidal patients.

828 pages Year Founded: 1990 ISBN 0-880483-07-5

1608 Understanding and Preventing Suicide: New Perspectives
Charles C Thomas Publisher Ltd.
PO Box 19265
Springfield, IL 62794-9265
217-789-8980
800-258-8980; *Fax:* 217-789-9130

books@ccthomas.com
www.ccthomas.com

David Lester, Author

Seven perspectives for understanding and preventing suicidal behavior, illustrating their implications for prevention. This book discusses suicide from a crimnological perspective, and whether the theories in it have any applicability to suicidal behavior, both in furthering our understanding of suicide and in seeing new ways to prevent suicide. Armed with this information, we may move far toward understanding and preventing suicide in the twenty-first century. *$35.95*

121 pages Year Founded: 1990 ISSN 0-398-06235-8ISBN 0-398057-09-5

1609 Why Suicide? Answers to 200 of the Most Frequently Asked Questions about Suicide, Attempted Suicide, and Assisted Suicide
HarperOne
10 East 53rd Street
New York, NY 10022
212-207-7000
www.harpercollins.com

Eric Marcus, Author

$14.95

256 pages Year Founded: 1996 ISBN 0-062511-66-9

Periodicals & Pamphlets

1610 Suicide Talk: What To Do If You Hear It
ETR Associates
4 Carbonero Way
Scotts Valley, CA 95066-4200
831-438-4060
800-321-4407; *Fax:* 831-438-3618
support@etr.freshdesk.com
www.etr.org

David Kitchen,MBA, Chief Financial Officer
Talita Sanders,BS, Director,Human Resources
Coleen Cantwell,MPH, Director,Business Development Pl
Matt McDowell,BS, Director,Marketing

Includes suicide warning signs, how to help a friend, and ways to relieve stress. *$16.00*

1611 Suicide: Who Is at Risk?
ETR Associates
4 Carbonero Way
Scotts Valley, CA 95066-4200
831-438-4060
800-321-4407; *Fax:* 831-438-3618
customerservice@etr.org
www.etr.org

Infinite Mind, Author

Includes warning signs, symptoms, and what to do. *$ 16.00*

Research Centers

1612 American Foundation for Suicide Prevention
120 Wall Street
29th Floor
New York, NY 10005
212-363-3500
888-333-2377; *Fax:* 212-363-6237

info@afsp.org
www.afsp.org

Nancy Farrell,M.P.A, Chairman
Yeates Conwell,M.D, President
Maria Oquendo,M.D, Vice President
Robert Gebbia, Chief Executive Officer

AFSP has been at the forefront of a wide range of suicide prevention initiatives, each designed to reduce loss of life from suicide. AFSP is investing in groundbreaking research, new educational campaigns, innovative demonstration projects and critical policy work. Also expanding assistance to people whose lives have been affected by suicide, reaching out to offer support and offering opportunities to become involved in prevention.

Year Founded: 1987

Support Groups & Hot Lines

1613 Covenant House Nineline
461 Eighth Avenue
New York, NY 10001
212-613-0300
800-388-3888; *Fax:* 212-629-3756
www.nineline.org

Andrew P. Bustillo, Board Chair
Kevin Ryan, President and CEO

Nationwide crisis/suicide hotline.

Year Founded: 1972

Video & Audio

1614 A Madman's Journal
Educational Training Videos
136 Granville St
Suite 200
Gahanna, OH 43230
Fax: 888-775-3919
www.educationaltrainingvideos.com

For two years, the narrator of this program went through a nightmare, feeling a self-hatred and worthlessness beyond love and redemption that he described as the concentration camp of the mind. This video presents one man's attempt to convey the ordeal of severe depression by writing a memoir about the experience.

1615 Bipolar Disorder: Shifting Mood Swings
Educational Training Videos
136 Granville St
Suite 200
Gahanna, OH 43230
Fax: 888-775-3919
www.educationaltrainingvideos.com

Different from the routine ups and downs of life, the symptoms of bipolar disorder are severe - even to the point of being life-threatening. In this insightful program, patients speak from their own experience about the complexities of diagnosis and the very real danger of suicide, while family members and close friends address the strain of the condition's cyclic behavior.

1616 Clinical Impressions: Identifying Mental Illness
Educational Training Videos
136 Granville St
Suite 200
Gahanna, OH 43230

Fax: 888-775-3919
www.educationaltrainingvideos.com

How long can mental illness stay hidden, especially from the eyes of trained experts? This program rejoins a group of ten adults- five of them healthy and five of them with histories of mental illness- as psychiatric specialists try to spot and correctly diagnose the latter. Administering a series of collaborative and one-on-one tests, including assessments of personality type, physical self-image, and rational thinking, the panel gradually makes decisions about who suffers from depression, bipolar disorder, bulimia, and social anxiety.

1617 Coping with Stress
Educational Video Network, Inc.
1401 19th Street
Huntsville, TX 77340
936-295-5767
800-762-0060; *Fax:* 936-294-0233
www.www.evndirect.com

Stress affects everyone, both emotionally and physically. For some, mismanaged stress can result in substance abuse, violence, or even suicide. This program answers the question, How can a person cope with stress?

1618 Dealing with Depression
Educational Video Network, Inc.
1401 19th Street
Huntsville, TX 77340
936-295-5767
800-762-0060; *Fax:* 936-294-0233
www.www.evndirect.com

As more and more young people are falling victim to depression, it is important to understand what causes it and to know how to get the help that can rid a person of this life-wrecking affliction.

1619 Dealing with Grief
Educational Video Network, Inc.
1401 19th Street
Huntsville, TX 77340
936-295-5767
800-762-0060; *Fax:* 936-294-0233
www.www.evndirect.com

Grief allows us to acknowledge and mourn our losses so we can reconcile our feelings and move forward in life. Learn how to deal with your grief and become a better person for having gone through it.

1620 Don't Kill Yourself: One Survivor's Message
Educational Training Videos
136 Granville St
Suite 200
Gahanna, OH 43230
Fax: 888-775-3919
www.educationaltrainingvideos.com

This is the story of a young man, David, who at 16 years of age survived a suicide attempt. Now 22, he shares the events of his life leading up to the attempt, including how low self-esteem led to drug addiction, and how the addiction encouraged the sense that life was no longer worth living.

1621 FRONTLINE: The Released
PBS
2100 Crystal Drive
Arlington, VA 22202
www.pbs.org

Will Lyman, Actor
Narrator
Miri Navasky, Director
Karen O'Connor, Director

The documentary states that of the 700,000 inmates released from American prisons each year, half of them have mental disabilities. This work focused on those with severe problems who keep entering and exiting prison. Full of good information on the challenges they face with mental illnesses; housing, employment, stigmatization, and socialization.

Year Founded: 2009

1622 Suicide among Teens
Educational Video Network, Inc.
1401 19th Street
Huntsville, TX 77340
936-295-5767
800-762-0060; *Fax:* 936-294-0233
www.www.evndirect.com

Suicide devastates surviving loved ones. Find out why it should never be considered as a solution and learn how to recognize warning signs in a suicidal person.

1623 Teenage Anxiety, Depression, and Suicide
Educational Video Network, Inc.
1401 19th Street
Huntsville, TX 77340
936-295-5767
800-762-0060; *Fax:* 936-294-0233
www.www.evndirect.com

This program can provide helpful insight to those in need of assistance.

Web Sites

1624 www.afsp.org
American Foundation for Suicide Prevention

AFSP has been at the forefront of a wide range of suicide prevention initiatives, each designed to reduce loss of life from suicide. AFSP is investing in groundbreaking research, new educational campaigns, innovative demonstration projects and critical policy work. Also expanding assistance to people whose lives have been affected by suicide, reaching out to offer support and offering opportunities to become involved in prevention.

1625 www.break-the-silence.org
Break the Silence

A non profit organization whose basis and foundation came from first-hand knowledge and experience that inpatient safety is not always provided to those in need of protection, causing a desperate need for a watch-dog organization like Break the Silence.

1626 www.friendsforsurvival.org
Friends for Survival

Assisting anyone who has suffered the loss of a loved one through suicide death.

1627 www.griefguidance.com
Grief Guidance Inc.

A company created by Doreen Cammarata to promote intervention services for suicide survivors.

1628 www.jasonfoundation.com
The Jason Foundation, Inc.

An educational organization dedicated to the awareness and prevention of youth suicide. JFI believes that awareness and education are the first steps to prevention.

1629 www.mentalhealth.samhsa.gov
Substance Abuse & Mental Health Services Administration

Information about resources, technical assistance, research, training, networks, and other federal clearing houses, and fact sheets and materials. Information specialists refer callers to mental health resources in their communities as well as state, federal and nonprofit contacts.

1630 www.nami.org
National Alliance on Mental Illness

Nation's leading self-help organization for all those affected by severe brain disorders. Mission is to bring consumers and families with similar experiences together to share information about services, care providers, and ways to cope with the challenges of schizophrenia, manic depression, and other serious mental illnesses.

1631 www.nineline.org
Covenant House Nineline

Nationwide crisis/suicide hotline.

1632 www.nopcas.com
National Organization for People of Color Against Suicide

NOPCAS serves as the only national organization of its kind addressing the issue of suicide prevention and intervention, specifically in communities of color. Primary focus and mission is to increase suicide education and awareness. Offering unique opportunities for outreach partnerships and community education efforts directed at communities of color across the nation.

1633 www.psf.org
National P.O.L.I.C.E. Suicide Foundation

This foundation provides educational training seminars for emergency responders, primarily associated with law enforcement on the issue of police suicide. Providing police suicide awareness and prevention training programs and support services that will meet the psychological, emotional, and spiritual needs of law enforcement, on every level, and their families.

1634 www.save.org
Suicide Awareness Voices of Education (SAVE)

One of the nation's first organizations dedicated to the prevention of suicide and was a co-founding member of the National Council for Suicide Prevention. Leading national non profit organization with staff dedicated to prevent suicide. Based on the foundation and belief that suicide should no longer be considered a hidden or taboo topic and that through raising awareness and educating the public, we can SAVE lives.

1635 www.solossa.org
Survivors of Loved Ones' Suicides (SOLOS)

Organization to help provide support for the families and friends who have suffered the suicide loss of a loved one.

1636 www.store.samhsa.gov
Substance Abuse and Mental Health Services Administration

Resources on mental disorders as well as treatment and recovery.

1637 www.suicide.supportgroups.com
SupportGroups

An online support group community bringing people together around life's challenges by providing concise, up-to-date information and a meeting place for individuals, their friends and families, and professionals who offer pathways to help.

1638 www.suicidology.org
American Association of Suicidology

AAS is a membership organization for all those involved in suicide prevention and intervention, or touched by suicide. AAS is a leader in the advancement of scientific and programmatic efforts in suicide prevention through research, education and training, the development of standards and resources, and survivor support services.

1639 www.yellowribbon.org
Yellow Ribbon Suicide Prevention Program

Dedicated to preventing suicide and attempts by making suicide prevention accessible to everyone and removing barriers to help by empowering individuals and communities through leadership, awareness and education, and by collaborating and partnering with support networks to reduce stigma and help save lives.

Tic Disorders

Introduction

A tic is described as an involuntary, sudden, rapid, recurrent, non-rhythmic motor movement or vocalization. Four disorders are associated with tics: Chronic Motor or Vocal Tic Disorder, Transient Tic Disorder, Tic Disorder Not Otherwise Specified, and Tourette's Syndrome. Tourette's Syndrome is the most extreme case, consisting of multiple motor tics and one or more vocal tics, and will be the focus of this chapter. The most common initial symptom of Tourette's Syndrome is a facial tic, such as rapid eye blinking or mouth twitching. Sometimes, the first sign of the disorder is throat clearing or sniffling. The vocalizations of Tourette's Syndrome can consist of grunts, obscenities, or other words the individual otherwise would not make. They are disruptive and can be profoundly embarrassing.

SYMPTOMS

• Multiple motor, as well as one or more vocal tics have been present during the illness, not necessarily at the same time;
• The tics occur many times during a day (often in bouts) nearly every day or intermittently throughout for more than one year, and during this period there was never a tic-free period of more than three consecutive months;
• The disturbance causes clear distress or difficulties in social, work, or other areas;
• The onset is before age 18;
• The involuntary movements or vocalizations are not due to the direct effects of a substance (e.g., stimulants) or a general medication condition.

ASSOCIATED FEATURES

Between ten percent and forty percent of people with Tourette's Syndrome also have echolalia (automatically repeating words spoken by others) or echopraxia (imitating someone else's movements). Fewer than ten percent have coprolalia (the involuntary utterance of obscenities).

There seems to be a clear association between tic disorders, such as Tourette's Syndrome, and Obsessive Compulsive Disorder (OCD). As many as twenty percent to thirty percent of people with OCD report having or having had tics, and between five percent and seven percent of those with OCD also have Tourette's Syndrome. In studies of patients with Tourette's Syndrome it was found that thirty-six percent to fifty-two percent also meet the criteria for OCD. There is evidence that Tourette's Syndrome and Obsessive Compulsive Disorder share a genetic basis or some underlying pathological/physiological disturbance. The genetic evidence is further strengthened by the concordance rate in twins (i.e., the likelihood that if one member of the pair has the disorder, the other will also develop it): in identical twins, who have the same genes, the concordance is fifty-three percent, whereas in fraternal twins, who are no more closely related than other siblings, it is eight percent.

Other conditions commonly associated with Tourette's Syndrome are hyperactivity, distractibility, impulsivity, difficulty in learning, emotional disturbances, and social problems. The disorder causes social uneasiness, shame, self-consciousness, and depression. The person may be rejected by others and may develop anxiety about the tics, negatively affecting social, school, and work functioning.

In severe cases, the disorder may interfere with everyday activities like reading and writing.

PREVALENCE

Tourette's Syndrome is reported in a variety of ethnic and cultural groups. It is one and one-half to three times more common in males than females and about 10 times more prevalent in children and adolescents than in adults. Overall prevalence is estimated at between four and five people in 10,000.

While the age of onset can be as early as two years, it commonly begins during childhood or early adolescence. The median age for the development of tics is seven years. The disorder usually lasts for the life of the person, but there may be periods of remission of weeks, months, or years. The severity, frequency, and variability of the tics often diminish during adolescence and adulthood. In some cases, tics can disappear entirely by early adulthood.

TREATMENT OPTIONS

Many treatments have been tried. Children who are not bothered by their tics should not be treated with medications. Medications are reserved for those whose tics lead to symptoms which impair behavioral, physiologic, or social function. Haloperidol, an antipsychotic drug, may be used for more severe cases; it acts directly on the brain source of the tic, counteracting the overactivity, and can have a calming effect. However, it also can have unwanted side effects and can sometimes cause other movement disorders after prolonged use. SSRIs (Selective Serotonin Reuptake Inhibitors) have also been effective in some cases of Tic Disorders. Simple tics respond to benzodiazepines (tranquilizers).

Whether drug treatment is used or not, patients and their families may need counseling to deal with the disease's secondary effects (e.g., bullying at school, conflict within the family). During periods of high stress, relaxation techniques and biofeedback may be useful. Other alternative therapies like acupuncture and yoga may also be of some benefit. In many cases, comprehensive behavioral intervention for tics (CBIT) is an effective treatment. With this approach, patients are shown ways to prevent themselves from engaging in a tic so that the tic is diminished over time.

Symptoms of the disorder usually become less severe with increasing age, and many people learn to live with them.

Associations & Agencies

1641 **Centers for Disease Control & Prevention**
Division of Human Development and Disability
1600 Clifton Road
Atlanta, GA 30329-4027
800-232-4636
TTY: 888-232-6348
www.www.cdc.gov/ncbddd/

Georgina Peacock, MD, MPH, FAAP, Director

Centers for Disease Control and Prevention serves to provide health information and promote the use of science and advanced technology to protect America from disease, disability, and other health concerns. The Division of Human Development and Disability aims to improve the lives of individuals with disabilities through programs, surveillance, research, and policies that facilitate better healthcare. DHDD focuses on the best outcomes for infants and adults with ADHD, mental disorders, and Tourette Syndrome.

1642 National Alliance on Mental Illness

3803 North Fairfax Drive
Suite 100
Arlington, VA 22203
703-524-7600
800-950-6264
info@nami.org
www.nami.org

Steve Pitman, JD, President
Lacey Berumen, PhD, MNM, First Vice President
Mary Giliberti, Chief Executive Officer
David Levy, Chief Financial Officer

NAMI is an organization dedicated to raising awareness on mental health and providing support and education for Americans affected by mental illness. NAMI advocates for access to services and treatment and fosters an environment of awareness and understanding for those concerned with mental health.

Year Founded: 1979

1643 National Association for the Dually Diagnosed (NADD)

132 Fair Street
Kingston, NY 12401
845-331-4336
info@thenadd.org
www.thenadd.org

Jeanne M. Farr, MA, Chief Executive Officer
Daniel Baker, PhD., President
Peggie Webb, MA, Vice President
George Zukotynski, PhD., Secretary

NADD is a nonprofit organization designed to increase awareness of, and provide services for, individuals with developmental disabilities and mental illness. NADD emphasizes the importance of quality mental healthcare for people with mental health needs and offers conferences, information resources, educational programs, and training materials to professionals, parents, and organizations.

Year Founded: 1983

1644 National Mental Health Consumers' Self-Help Clearinghouse

1211 Chestnut Street
Suite 1100
Philadelphia, PA 19107
267-507-3810
800-553-4539; *Fax:* 215-636-6312
info@mhselfhelp.org
www.mhselfhelp.org

Joseph Rogers, Founder and Executive Director
Susan Rogers, Director

The Clearinghouse is a peer-run national technical assistance center focused on achieving respect and equality of opportunity for those with mental illnesses. The Clearinghouse helps with the growth of the mental health consumer movement by evaluating mental health services, advocating for mental health reform, and providing consumers with news, information, publications, and consultation services.

Year Founded: 1986

1645 The Center for Family Support

2811 Zulette Avenue
Bronx, NY 10461
718-518-1500; *Fax:* 718-518-8200
www.www.cfsny.org/

Steven Vernikoff, Executive Director
Lloyd Stabiner, President
Amy Bittinger, Vice President
Barbara Greenwald, Associate Executive Director

The Center for Family Support offers assistance to individuals with developmental and related disabilities, as well as their families, and provides support services and programs that are designed to accommodate individual needs. Offers services throughout New York City, Westchester County, Long Island, and New Jersey.

Year Founded: 1954

1646 Tourette Association of America

42-40 Bell Boulevard
Suite 205
Bayside, NY 11361-2874
888-486-8738
support@tourette.org
www.tourette.org

Amanda Talty, EVP and Interim CEO
Diana Shineman, VP, Research/Medical Programs
Sonja Mason-Vidal, VP, Finance/Administration
Diana Felner, VP, Public Policy

The Tourette Association of America is a nonprofit membership organization dedicated to raising awareness about Tourette Syndrome and tic disorders, educating professionals and the public, advancing scientific understandings about tic disorders as well as care and treatment options, and advocating for public policies and services that support the needs of those affected by tic disorders. The Tourette Association seeks to challenge stereotypes about tic disorders and promote social acceptance across the nation.

Year Founded: 1972

Books

1647 A Mind of Its Own: Tourette's Syndrome: a Story and a Guide

Oxford University Press
198 Madison Avenue
New York, NY 10016-4341
212-726-6000
800-445-9714; *Fax:* 919-677-1303
custserv.us@oup.com
www.www.oup.com/us/

Ruth Dowling Bruun, Author
Bertel Bruun, Author

In spite of the attention paid to Tourette's syndrome in recent years, there was still no book which explains the condition to patients and their families in an informative, comprehensive, and accessible manner. This book fills that need. It presents factual information on all important aspects of TS along with a composite case history. The story of Michael Lockman, who typifies the average child with TS, is woven into the factual text which contains information on symptomology, diagnosis, natural history, biochemistry, genetics, associated disorders, treatment and related topiccs.

174 pages Year Founded: 1994 ISBN 0-195065-87-5

1648 Adam and the Magic Marble
Hope Press
PO Box 188
Duarte, CA 91009-188
800-321-4039; *Fax:* 626-358-3520
dcomings@earthlink.net
www.hopepress.com

Adam Buehrens, Author
Carol Buehrens, Author

Exciting reading for all ages, and a must for those who have been diagnosed with Tourette syndrome or other disabilities. An up-beat story of three heros, two with Tourette syndrome, one with cerebal palsy. Constantly taunted by bullies, the boys find a marble full of magic power, they aim a spell at the bullies and the adventure begins. *$6.95*

108 pages

1649 Children with Tourette Syndrome: A Parent's Guide (Special Needs Collection)
ADD WareHouse
300 NorthWest 70th Avenue
Suite 102
Plantation, FL 33317-2360
954-792-8944
800-233-9273; *Fax:* 954-792-8545
websales@addwarehouse.com
www.addwarehouse.com

Tracy Haerle, Editor
Jim Eisenreich, Foreword

This handbook for parents of children and teenagers with Tourette Syndrome offers up-to-date informaion and compassionate advice for dealing with what is perhaps one of the most misunderstood and misdiagnosed neurological disorders. Written by a team of professionals and parents, this book covers medical, educational, legal, family life, daily care and emotional issues. *$17.00*

361 pages Year Founded: 1990 ISBN 0-933149-44-1

1650 Don't Think About Monkeys: Extraordinary Stories Written by People with Tourette Syndrome
Hope Press
Fax: 626-358-3520
dcomings@earthlink.net
www.hopepress.com

Adam Ward Seligman, Editor
John S Hilkevich, Editor

A remarkable collection of stories written by fourteen people who live with Tourette syndrome. Ranging from three teenagers learning to come to grips with treatment to adults encountering discrimination, the collection represents the incredible diversity of a disorder as diverse as life itself. The drama of living with a disability and the comedy of a Tourette syndrome conference show the range of a book that Oliver Sacks called, A fascinatingly varied book! *$12.95*

200 pages Year Founded: 1992 ISBN 1-878267-33-7

1651 Echolalia: an Adult's Story of Tourette Syndrome
Hope Press
Fax: 626-358-3520
dcomings@earthlink.net
www.hopepress.com

Adam Ward Seligman, Author

Echolalia is the story of best selling writer Jackson Evans, who is diagnosed as having Tourette syndrome, a complex genetic disorder characterized by tics and vocal noises (including obscenities), and obsessive-compulsive behavior. At first, he is grateful for the answers it brings him, but Jackson soon realizes that the real problems are just beginning. The story is told in a style that captures the rhythms that soothe the Tourette. It ends with the ultimate truth- the answer isn't in being diagnosed, the answer is in living with the diagnosis. *$11.95*

165 pages Year Founded: 1991 ISBN 1-878267-31-0

1652 Hi, I'm Adam: a Child's Book About Tourette Syndrome
Hope Press
Fax: 626-358-3520
dcomings@earthlink.net
www.hopepress.com

Adam Buehrens, Author

A child's story of how it feels to have Tourette syndrome and hyperactivity (attention deficit hyperactivity disorder). *$4.95*

35 pages Year Founded: 1990 ISBN 1-878267-29-9

1653 I Can't Stop!: A Story About Tourette Syndrome
Albert Whitman & Company
250 South Northwest Highway
Suite 320
Park Ridge, IL 60068-4272
847-581-2800
800-255-7675; *Fax:* 847-581-0039
mail@awhitmanco.com
www.albertwhitman.com

Holly L. Niner, Author
Meryl Treatner, Illustrator

Kindergarten-Grade 4 level, An introduction for parents and teachers gives more information about it an notes that tics are common among children. The plot and primarily one-dimensional characters are devices to educate readers about TS. There is a lot of dialogue, and the students in Nathan's class represent diverse cultures. Very few books are available for young audiences on this medical concern; what's out there tends to be nonfiction for older readers. Thus, this title does fill a void.

32 pages Year Founded: 1919 ISBN 0-807536-20-2

1654 Neurodevelopmental Disabilities: Clinical Care for Children and Young Adults
Springer
11 West 42nd Street
15th Floor
New York, NY 10036
212-431-4370
877-687-7476; *Fax:* 212-941-7842
cs@springerpub.com
www.springerpub.com

Dilip R. Patel, Editor
Donald E. Greydanus, Editor
Hatim A. Omar, Editor
Joav Merrick, Editor

Increasingly more and more children with developmental disabilities survive into adulthood. Pediatricians and other clinicians are called upon to care for an increasing number of children with developmental disabilities in their practice and thus there is a need for a practical guide specifically written for pediatricians and primary care clinicians that addresses major concepts of neurodevelopmental pediatrics.

350 pages Year Founded: 1950 ISBN 9-400706-26-X

1655 RYAN: A Mother's Story of Her Hyperactive/ Tourette Syndrome Child
Hope Press
Fax: 626-358-3520
dcomings@earthlink.net
www.hopepress.com

Susan Hughes, Author

A moving and informative story of how a mother struggled with the many behavioral problems presented by her son with Tourette syndrome, ADHD and oppositional defiant disorder. *$9.95*

153 pages Year Founded: 1990 ISBN 1-878267-25-6

1656 Raising Joshua: One Mother's Story of the Challenges of Parenting a Child With Tourette Syndrome
Hope Press
Fax: 626-358-3520
dcomings@earthlink.net
www.hopepress.com

Sheryl Johnson Hamer, RN, Author

The harrowing and heartwarming story of Josh, a boy caught in Tourette Syndrome, and Attention Deficit Hyperactivity Disorder, as told by his mother. The true story of two souls caught in a modern jungle of medical ignorance, powerful drugs, and the ravaging behavior of a mysterious condition. Their indomitable spirits of love and courage help them walk hand in hand through their special world. *$14.95*

150 pages Year Founded: 1997 ISBN 0-965750-16-7

1657 Tics and Tourette Syndrome: A Handbook for Parents and Professionals
Jessica Kingsley Publishers
400 Market Street
Suite 400
Philadelphia, PA 19106
215-922-1161
866-416-1078; *Fax:* 215-922-1474
hello.usa@jkp.com
www.jkp.com

Uttom Chowdhury, Author
Isobel Heyman, Foreword

This essential guide to tic disorders and Tourette Syndrome tackles problems faced both at home and at school, such as adjusting to the diagnosis, the effect on siblings and classroom difficulties. Dr. Chowdhury offers advice on how to manage symptoms, describing psychological techniques such as habit reversal and massed practice and reviewing available medical treatments. In clear, accessible language, this book explains the clinical signs and symptoms of Tourette and related conditions, and their possible causes. Presenting practical strategies for dealing with associated difficulties, including low self-esteem, anger management and bullying, this book will be invaluable to parents, teachers, social workers and other professionals.

160 pages Year Founded: 1987 ISBN 1-843102-03-X

1658 Tourette Syndrome and Human Behavior
Hope Press
110 Mill Run
Monrovia, CA 91016-1658
Fax: 626-358-3520
dcomings@earthlink.net
www.hopepress.com

David E. Comings, Author

The story of how Tourette syndrome provides insights into the cause and treatment of a wide range of human behavioral problems. It covers diagnosis, associated behaviors including ADHD, learning disorders, dyslexia, conduct disorder, OCD, alcoholism, drug abuse, obesity, depression, panic attacks, phobias, night terrors, bed wetting, sleep disturbances, lying, stealing, inappropriate sexual behavior, and others: brain structure and chemistry, treatment and implications for society, over 2,500 references, 30-page Tourette Syndrom-Human Behavior Questionnaire, and Extensive index. *$39.95*

850 pages Year Founded: 1990 ISBN 1-878267-28-0

1659 Tourette's Syndrome- Tics, Obsession, Compulsions: Developmental Psychopathology & Clinical Care
John Wiley & Sons
605 3rd Avenue
New York, NY 10158-180
212-850-6301
info@wiley.com

James F. Leckman, Author
Donald J. Cohen, Author

Edited by two of the leading international authorities on Tourette's Syndrome and tic-related, obsessive-compulsive disorders, this book is the most up-to-date edited reference covering this neuropsychiatric disorder and related disorders from a variety of perspectives. Featuring contributors from the world-renowned Yale Child Study Center, this volume introduces a groundbreaking developmental framework for understanding Tourette's-defined by persistent motor and vocal tics and frequently associated with obsessions, compulsions, and attentional difficulties- and maps out the diagnosis, genetics, manifestations, and treatment. This comprehensive resource describes the major categories of disorders. *$189.00*

584 pages Year Founded: 2001 ISBN 0-471160-37-7

1660 Tourette's Syndrome: The Facts, Second Edition
Oxford University Press
198 Madison Avenue
New York, NY 10016-4341
212-726-6400
800-451-7556

Mary Robertson, Editor
Andrea Cavanna, Editor

This text explains the causes of the syndrome, how it is diagnosed, and how to cope if you have been recently diagnosed. It provides information on the treatment and therapies that are available, and advice on how individuals can manage their symptoms. It clearly explains the different presentations that can affect individuals, covering a spectrum from very mild to more uncommon severe forms of TS, and also discusses disorders that can be mistaken for

TS. This edition contains new chapters focusing on education, employment and empowerment, and famous and successful people who acheived their goals despite their diagnosis. *$ 19.95*

110 pages Year Founded: 2008 ISBN 0-198523-98-X

1661 Treating Tourette Syndrome and Tic Disorders: A Guide for Practitioners
The Guilford Press
72 Spring Street
New York, NY 10012
800-365-7006; *Fax:* 212-966-6708
info@guilford.com
www.guilford.com

Douglas W. Woods, PhD, Editor
John C. Piacentini, PhD, Editor
John T. Walkup, MD, Editor
Peter Hollenbeck, PhD, Foreword

Grounded in a comprehensive model of Tourette syndrome (TS) and related disorders, this state-of-the-art volume provides a multidisciplinary framework for assessment and treatment. Leading authorities present the latest knowledge on the neurobehavioral underpinnings of TS, its clinical presentation, and how to distinguish it from frequently encountered co-occurring disorders, such as obsessive-compulsive disorder and attention-deficit/hyperactivity disorder. Strategies for managing symptoms and providing effective support to children and families are thoroughly detailed, with an emphasis on integrating medication and psychosocial therapies. Several chapters also address clinical work with adults with TS.

287 pages Year Founded: 1973 ISBN 1-593854-80-3

1662 What Makes Ryan Tick: A Family's Triumph over Tourette Syndrome and Attention Deficiency Hyperactivity Disorder
Hope Press
Fax: 626-358-3520
dcomings@earthlink.net
www.hopepress.com

Susan Hughes, Author

A follow-up to Susan Hughes best selling book RYAN - A Mother's Story of her Hyperactivity Tourette Syndrome Child, covering his particularly difficult teenage years.

303 pages Year Founded: 1996 ISBN 1-878267-35-3

Research Centers

1663 Child Neurology and Developmental Center
1510 Jericho Turnpike
New Hyde Park, NY 11040
516-352-2500; *Fax:* 516-352-2573
www.childbrain.com

Rami Grossmann, M.D.

Pediatric neurology practice of Rami Grossmann, M.D. in New York. Neurologists are highly trained to treat disorders of the nervous system. This includes diseases of the brain, spinal cord, nerves, and muscles. Common problems that Dr. Grossmann diagnoses and treats include the following: AD/HD, Autism, a form of PDD, Developmental delays, Epilepsy, Headaches, Learning difficulties, and Tic Disorders.

1664 KidsHealth
The Nemours Foundation
10140 Centurion Parkway
Jacksonville, FL 32256
904-697-4100; *Fax:* 904-697-4220
comments@KidsHealth.org
www.kidshealth.org

Alfred I. duPont, Nemour's Foundation Creator
Neil Izenberg, MD, Editor-in-Chief & Founder

KidsHealth is more than just the facts about health. As part of The Nemours Foundation's Center for Children's Health Media, KidsHealth also provides families with perspective, advice, and comfort about a wide range of physical, emotional, and behavioral issues that affect children and teens. The Nemours Center for Children's Health Media is a part of The Nemours Foundation, a nonprofit organization created by philanthropist Alfred I. duPont in 1936 and devoted to improving the health of children.

Year Founded: 1936

Support Groups & Hot Lines

1665 DailyStrength: Tourette Syndrome Support Forum
3280 Peachtree Rd
Suite 600
Atlanta, GA 30305
www.dailystrength.org

DailyStrength is a subsidiary of Sharecare, Inc., the first truly interactive healthcare ecosystem giving consumers the ability to ask, learn, and act on the questions of health. DailyStrength was created and operated by some very passionate and dedicated people that get great satisfaction knowing that this site can be a positive force for everyone who faces challenges in their lives.

Video & Audio

1666 After the Diagnosis...The Next Steps
Tourette Syndrome Association
42-40 Bell Boulevard
Suite 205
Bayside, NY 11361-2874
718-224-2999
888-486-8738; *Fax:* 718-279-9596
ts@tsa-usa.org
www.tsa-usa.org

Judit Ungar, President
Gary Frank, EVP
Mark Levine, VP Development
Richard Dreyfuss, Narrator

When the diagnosis is Tourette Syndrome, what do you do first? How do you sort out the complexities of the disorder? Whose advice do you follow? What steps do you take to lead a normal life? Six people with TS—as different as any six people can be—relate the sometimes difficult, but finally triumphant path each took to lead the rich, fulfilling life they now enjoy. Narrated by Academy Award-winning actor, Richard Dreyfuss, the stories are refreshing blends of poignancy, fact, and inspiration illustrating that a diagnosis of TS can be approached with confidence and hope. Includes comments by family and friends, teachers, counselors and leading medical authorities on Tourette Syndrome. A must-see for the newly diagnosed child, teen or adult. *$35.00*

Year Founded: 1972

1667 Clinical Counseling: Toward a Better Understanding of TS
Tourette Syndrome Association
42-40 Bell Boulevard
Suite 205
Bayside, NY 11361-2874
718-224-2999
888-486-8738; *Fax:* 718-279-9596
ts@tsa-usa.org
www.tsa-usa.org

Judit Ungar, President
Gary Frank, EVP
Mark Levine, VP Development
Dylan McDermott, Narrator

Certain key issues often surface during the counseling sessions of people wwith TS and their families. These important areas of concern are explored for counselors, social workers, educators, psychologists and other allied professionals. Expert clinical practitioners offer invaluable insights for those working with people affected by Tourette Syndrome. *$30.00*

Year Founded: 1972

1668 Clinical Impressions: Identifying Mental Illness
Educational Training Videos
136 Granville St
Suite 200
Gahanna, OH 43230
Fax: 888-775-3919
www.educationaltrainingvideos.com

How long can mental illness stay hidden, especially from the eyes of trained experts? This program rejoins a group of ten adults- five of them healthy and five of them with histories of mental illness- as psychiatric specialists try to spot and correctly diagnose the latter. Administering a series of collaborative and one-on-one tests, including assessments of personality type, physical self-image, and rational thinking, the panel gradually makes decisions about who suffers from depression, bipolar disorder, bulimia, and social anxiety.

1669 Complexities of TS Treatment: Physician's Roundtable
Tourette Syndrome Association
42-40 Bell Boulevard
Suite 205
Bayside, NY 11361-2874
718-224-2999
888-486-8738; *Fax:* 718-279-9596
ts@tsa-usa.org
www.tsa-usa.org

Judit Ungar, President
Gary Frank, EVP
Mark Levine, VP Development

Three of the most highly regarded experts in the diagnosis and treatment of Tourette Syndrome offer insight, advice and treatment strategies to fellow physicians and other healthcare professionals. *$ 30.00*

Year Founded: 1972

1670 Family Life with Tourette Syndrome... Personal Stories
Tourette Syndrome Association
42-40 Bell Boulevard
Suite 205
Bayside, NY 11361-2874
718-224-2999
888-486-8738; *Fax:* 718-279-9596
ts@tsa-usa.org
www.tsa-usa.org

Judit Ungar, President
Gary Frank, EVP
Mark Levine, VP Development

In extended, in-depth interviews, all the people engagingly profiled in After the Diagnosis. The Next Steps, reveal the individual ways they developed to deal with TS. Each shows us that the key to leading a successful life in spite of having TS, is having a loving, supportive network of family and friends. Available in its entirety or as separate vignettes. *$50.00*

Year Founded: 1972

1671 Understanding and Treating the Hereditary Psychiatric Spectrum Disorders
Hope Press
PO Box 188
Duarte, CA 91009-188
818-303-0644
800-209-9182; *Fax:* 818-358-3520
dcomings@earthlink.net
www.hopepress.com

David E Comings MD, Presenter

Learn with ten hours of audio tapes from a two day seminar given in May 1997 by David E Comings, MD. Tapes cover: ADHD, Tourette Syndrome, Obsessive-Compulsive Disorder, Conduct Disorder, Oppositional Defiant Disorder, Autism and other Hereditary Psychiatric Spectrum Disorders. Eight Audio tapes. *$75.00*

Year Founded: 1997

Web Sites

1672 www.mentalhealth.com
Internet Mental Health

Offers online psychiatric diagnosis in the hope of reaching the two-thirds of individuals with mental illness who do not seek treatment.

1673 www.planetpsych.com
Planetpsych.com

Online resource for mental health information.

1674 www.psychcentral.com
Psych Central

The Internet's largest and oldest independent mental health social network created and run by mental health professionals to guarantee reliable, trusted information and support communities to you.

1675 www.store.samhsa.gov
Substance Abuse and Mental Health Services Administration

Resources on mental disorders as well as treatment and recovery.

1676 www.tourette-syndrome.com
Tourette Syndrome

Online community devoted to children and adults with
Tourette Syndrome disorder and their families, friends,
teachers, and medical professionals. Provides an interactive
meeting place for those interested in Tourette Syndrome or
people wanting to help others who have TS.

1677 www.tourettesyndrome.net
Tourette Syndrome Plus

Parent and teacher friendly site on Tourette Syndrome, Attention Deficit Disorder, Executive Dysfunction, Obessive
Compulsive Disorder, and related conditions.

1678 www.tsa-usa.org
Tourette Syndrome Association

Web site of the association dedicated to identifying the
cause, finding the cure and controlling the effects of TS.

Information Services

1679 Tourette Syndrome Plus
Leslie E. Packer, PhD
940 Lincoln Place
North Bellmore, NY 11710-1016
516-785-2653
admin@tourettesyndrome.net
www.www.tourettesyndrome.net

Leslie E. Packer, PhD

Information on Tourette Syndrome PLUS the Associated
Disorders.

Trauma and Stressor-Related Disorders

Introduction

Post-traumatic stress disorder, or PTSD, consists of the psychological and physiological symptoms that arise from experiencing, witnessing, or participating in a traumatic event. PTSD affects a significant number of individuals returning from war zones, as well as those affected by terrorism and natural disasters. Post-traumatic stress disorder has been recognized for over a hundred years at least. During and after World War I, traumatized soldiers' symptoms of hypersensitivity, avoidance, and other characteristics of what we now call PTSD were called 'shell shock' in the past. PTSD continues to be identified with military service, but it is not limited to members of the military. It can affect adults and children exposed to terrifying and dangerous events in any circumstances: natural disasters, physical and/or sexual attacks, acts of terrorism, and accidents. By definition, the precipitating event must be outside the bounds of everyday human experience and the individual must feel helpless to protect him or herself from the event. Women appear to be somewhat more vulnerable to PTSD than men.

SYMPTOMS

PTSD symptoms occur in three categories: re-experiencing, heightened emotional arousal, and numbing.

Re-experiencing is the group of symptoms we hear most about; these include:
• Intense anxiety when the individual is exposed to a situation reminiscent of the event;
• Recurrent distressing flashbacks, nightmares, and/or dreams of the event;
• Acting or feeling as if the traumatic event were taking place immediately in the present. At these times, physiologic changes, such as a fast heartbeat, breathlessness, or gastrointestinal symptoms occur along with the anxiety.

Heightened emotional arousal includes:
• Jumpiness, where the individual responds to ordinary touch or noises as though they were a signal of mortal danger;
• Extreme avoidance of stimuli associated with the trauma;
• Bouts of anger out of proportion to a situation.

Numbing refers to:
• Diminished general responsiveness;
• Desensitization of emotional response whether the events affect them or those close to them.

The duration of the disturbance is more than one month, and it causes clinically significant distress or impairment. It is easy to see how any or all of these symptoms not only cause terrible distress for the individual, but also are incomprehensible and disturbing to members of the family.

ASSOCIATED FEATURES

The recognition of PTSD as a disorder has been a great relief to those current and past members of the military who had no explanation for symptoms that are extremely painful to them and disruptive to their families when they return from active duty. Instead of being grateful to have survived, and able to relax and enjoy the safety and affection at home, they are irritable and jumpy. Now that their symptoms have a name, they can seek treatment. Increasing knowledge about PTSD has also benefited other individuals with previously unexplained symptoms, including those who had been diagnosed as having a personality disorder, specifically borderline personality disorder. For example, women who developed symptoms as a result of domestic violence had been labeled 'borderline,' which made it seem that they, rather than their abusers, were responsible for their symptoms. Under these circumstances, a loving and capable, but symptomatic, mother might have lost custody of her children to the abusive partner who was the cause of her symptoms.

If a person survives a life-threatening event, they may experience feelings of guilt, particularly if others did not survive the event. People with PTSD often avoid situations that remind them of the traumatic event, which can seriously disrupt normal life (e.g. taking detours to go to work or run errands). People with PTSD may experience a dissociative state when in threatening situations, allowing them to have no recollection afterwards. They may also experience somatic physical problems with no discernible anatomic or physiological explanation. People with PTSD may also suffer from other mental illnesses brought on by the PTSD, such as depression, OCD, or substance abuse.

PREVALENCE

Most people exposed to a particular traumatic event do not develop PTSD. Some of the vulnerability is genetic. Because we might assume that people repeatedly exposed to trauma, for example those living in war zones or other dangerous areas, would develop resistance to the resulting anxiety, it is especially important to note that the opposite is true; people who have been traumatized in the past are more likely to develop PTSD after a future traumatic event.

TREATMENT OPTIONS

There is some controversy over the best way to treat PTSD. After 9/11, volunteer counselors of all sorts offered to work with survivors and those traumatized in the course of trying to rescue people or retrieve human remains. However, encouraging people to talk about a trauma right after it happens is generally not helpful. Many people exposed to trauma would rather go to a safe, and, if possible, familiar, place; take care of any immediate needs like food, clothing, or shelter, and do comforting things like take a bath and spend time with friends and loved ones.

Medications, including paroxetine and sertraline, can help with symptoms but are not a cure for PTSD. Non-pharmacologic treatments have been more successful. The underlying concept is the elimination of traumatic memories by gradual and controlled exposure of the patient to memories or reminders of the traumatic event or events, in a safe environment. One method is called Eye Movement Desensitization and Reprocessing, or EMDR. Therapists have a patient make specific eye movements or listen to beep tones, while bringing traumatic memories to mind, however,there is considerable controversy over this method. Patients have achieved better resolution of symptoms by recounting the memories and their feelings (not immediately after the event) to a therapist. Therapists may also help patients who are avoiding places or situations to gradually tolerate exposure to them.

Psychiatrists have discussed the problem with military leaders. While it is a relief to know that one's symptoms are part of a recognized illness that affects many others, and while access to treatment can require medical diagnosis, there is also stigma against having a mental illness. The President of the United States has agreed to give veterans afflicted with PTSD the same recognition of battle-related injuries, with medals of honor for example, that are given to those with more obvious bodily injuries. Members of the military continue to be concerned, sometimes with good reason, that having a psychiatric diagnosis will adversely affect their military careers. The ongoing discussions may enable us to develop a special descriptive term, other than 'disorder' for PTSD resulting from the trauma of war.

Associations & Agencies

1681 Association of Traumatic Stress Specialists
5000 Old Buncombe Road
Suite 27-11
Greenville, SC 29617
864-294-4337
admin@atss.info
www.atss.info

Linda Hood, BA, CTSS, President
John Robertson, CTSS, Vice President
Bonita S. Frazer, CTTS, Secretary and Treasurer
Diane Travers, LCSW, CTS, Chair of Certification Board

An international organization that helps those suffering from trauma by offering education, training, and professional development resources.

1682 Center for Mental Health Services (CMHS)
Substance Abuse and Mental Health Services Administration
5600 Fishers Lane
Rockville, MD 20857
240-276-1310
877-726-4727
TTY: 800-487-4889
www.samhsa.gov/about-us/who-we-are/offices-centers

Paolo del Vecchio, MSW, Director
Anne Mathews-Younes, Acting Deputy Director
Keris Myrick, Director, Consumer Affairs
Patricia Gratton, Director, Program Analysis

Promotes the treatment of mental illness and emotional disorders by increasing accessibility to mental health programs; supporting outreach, treatment, rehabilitation, and support programs and networks; and encouraging the use of scientifically-based information when treating mental disorders. CMHS provides information about mental health via a toll-free number and numerous publications. Developed for users of mental health services and their families, the general public, policy makers, providers, and the media.

Year Founded: 1992

1683 Goodwill's Community Employment Services
Goodwill Industries-Suncoast, Inc.
10596 Gandy Blvd.
St. Petersburg, FL 33702
727-523-1512
888-279-1988
TDD: 727-579-1068
www.goodwill-suncoast.org

Heather Ceresoli, CPA, Chair
Deborah A. Passerini, President
Martin W. Gladysz, Senior Vice Chair
Louise R. Lopez, Vice Chair

Program providing job coaching and community job placements for people with disabilities.

Year Founded: 1954

1684 International Critical Incident Stress Foundation
3290 Pine Orchard Lane
Suite 106
Ellicott City, MD 21042
410-750-9600; *Fax:* 410-750-9601
www.icisf.org

Dave Evans, CPA, Chair of the Board
Lisa Joubert, Recording Secretary/CFO
Richard Barton, Chief Executive Officer
Richard Bloch, Foundation Counsel

A nonprofit, open membership foundation committed to preventing disabling stress by providing education, training, support, and consultation services for emergency service professionals and organizations around the world.

1685 International Society for Traumatic Stress Studies
One Parkview Plaza
Suite 800
Oakbrook Terrace, IL 60181
847-686-2234; *Fax:* 847-686-2251
info@istss.org
www.istss.org

Diane Elmore Borbon, PhD, MPH, President
Amanda Amstadter, PhD, Vice President
Rick Koepke, Executive Director
Amy Street, PhD, Treasurer

An organization that serves as a forum for the sharing of research, clinical strategies, public policy concerns, and other information resources on trauma throughout the world. Dedicated to discovering information and circulating knowledge about policies, programs, and services that focus on reducing traumatic stressors and their consequences.

Year Founded: 1985

1686 Mental Health America
500 Montgomery Street
Suite 820
Alexandria, VA 22314
703-684-7722
800-969-6642; *Fax:* 703-684-5968
www.mentalhealthamerica.net

Reginald Williams, Chair of the Board
Paul Gionfriddo, President and CEO
Jessica Kennedy, Chief of Staff/VP of Finance
Theresa Nguyen, VP of Policy and Programs

Mental Health America is a community-based nonprofit organization committed to enabling the mental wellness of all Americans. MHA advocates for greater access to quality health services and seeks to educate individuals on identifying symptoms, as well as intervention and prevention.

Year Founded: 1909

1687 National Alliance on Mental Illness
3803 North Fairfax Drive
Suite 100
Arlington, VA 22203
703-524-7600
800-950-6264
info@nami.org
www.nami.org

Steve Pitman, JD, President
Lacey Berumen, PhD, MNM, First Vice President
Mary Giliberti, Chief Executive Officer
David Levy, Chief Financial Officer

NAMI is an organization dedicated to raising awareness on mental health and providing support and education for Americans affected by mental illness. NAMI advocates for access to services and treatment and fosters an environment of awareness and understanding for those concerned with mental health.

Year Founded: 1979

1688 National Association for the Dually Diagnosed (NADD)
132 Fair Street
Kingston, NY 12401
845-331-4336
info@thenadd.org
www.thenadd.org

Jeanne M. Farr, MA, Chief Executive Officer
Daniel Baker, PhD., President
Peggie Webb, MA, Vice President
George Zukotynski, PhD., Secretary

NADD is a nonprofit organization designed to increase awareness of, and provide services for, individuals with developmental disabilities and mental illness. NADD emphasizes the importance of quality mental healthcare for people with mental health needs and offers conferences, information resources, educational programs, and training materials to professionals, parents, and organizations.

Year Founded: 1983

1689 Territorial Apprehensiveness (TERRAP) Anxiety & Stress Program
755 Park Avenue
Suite 140
Huntington, NY 11743
631-549-8867; *Fax:* 631-423-8446
www.anxietyandpanic.com

Julian Herskowitz, PhD, Director

Helps to treat anxiety and stress disorders through Territorial Apprehensiveness Programs, developed by Dr. Arthur Hardy in the 1960's. The program systematically addresses the behavioral and thought processes of those suffering from stress and anxiety.

Year Founded: 1975

1690 The Center for Family Support
2811 Zulette Avenue
Bronx, NY 10461
718-518-1500; *Fax:* 718-518-8200
www.www.cfsny.org/

Steven Vernikoff, Executive Director
Lloyd Stabiner, President
Amy Bittinger, Vice President
Barbara Greenwald, Associate Executive Director

The Center for Family Support offers assistance to individuals with developmental and related disabilities, as well as their families, and provides support services and programs that are designed to accommodate individual needs. Offers services throughout New York City, Westchester County, Long Island, and New Jersey.

Year Founded: 1954

Books

1691 After the Crash: Assessment and Treatment of Motor Vehicle Accident Survivors
American Psychological Publishing
750 First Street,NorthEast
Washington, DC 20002-4242
202-336-5500
800-374-2721; *Fax:* 202-336-5518
TDD: 202-336-6123
TTY: 202-336-6123
www.apa.org

Edward B Blanchard,PhD,ABPP, Author
Edward J Hickling, PsyD, Author
Suzanne Bennett-Johnson, PhD, President

In this timely second edition, written in a clear and lucid style and illustrated by a wealth of charts, guides, case studies, and clinical advice, the authors report on new, international research and provide updates on their own long-standing research protocols within the groundbreaking Alabny MVA Project. *$29.95*

475 pages Year Founded: 1892 ISBN 1-591470-70-6

1692 Aging and Post Traumatic Stress Disorder
American Psychiatric Publishing, Inc.
1000 Wilson Boulevard
Suite 1825
Arlington, VA 22209-3901
703-907-7322
800-368-5777; *Fax:* 703-907-1091
appi@psych.org
www.appi.org

Robert E Hales MD, Editor-in-Chief
Rebecca D Rinehart, Publisher
John McDuffie, Editorial Director

Provides both literature reviews and data about animal and clinical studies and training for important current concepts of aging, the stress response and the interaction between them. *$85.00*

280 pages ISBN 0-880485-13-5

1693 Children and Trauma: A Guide for Parents and Professionals
Courage to Change
303 Crossways Park Drive
Woodbury, NY 11797
800-440-4003; *Fax:* 800-772-6499
www.couragetochange.com

Cynthia Monahon, Author

Teaches parents and professionals about the effects of such ordeals on children and offers a blueprint for restoring a child's sense of safety and balance. Offers hope and reassurance for parents. The author suggests straightforward ways to help kids through tough times, and also describes in detail the warning signs that indicate a child needs professional help. Monahon helps adults understand psychological trauma from a child's point of view and explores the ways both parents and professionals can help children heal. *$19.95*

240 pages Year Founded: 1997 ISBN 0-787910-71-6

1694 Coping with Post-Traumatic Stress Disorder
Rosen Publishing Group
29 East 21st Street
New York, NY 10010-6209
212-777-3017
800-237-9932; *Fax:* 888-436-4643
info@rosenpub.com
www.rosenpublishing.com

Carolyn Simpson, Author
Dwain Simpson, Author

$33.25

176 pages Year Founded: 1950 ISBN 0-823934-56-X

1695 Coping with Trauma: A Guide to Self
Understanding
8730 Georgia Avenue
Suite 600
Silver Spring, MD 20910-3643
240-485-1001
AnxDis@adaa.org
www.adaa.org

Jon G Allen, Author
Michelle Alonso, Communications/Membership

1696 Coping with Trauma: A Guide to Self
Understanding
1000 Wilson Boulevard
Suite 1825
Arlington, VA 22209-3901
703-907-7322
800-368-5777; *Fax:* 703-907-1091
appi@psych.org
www.appi.org

Robert E Hales MD, Editor-in-Chief
Ron McMillen, Chief Executive Officer
John McDuffie, Editorial Director
Jon G Allen, Author

385 pages

1697 Effecive Treatments for PTSD: Practice
Guidelines from the International Society for
Traumatic Stress Studies
The Guilford Press
72 Spring Street
New York, NY 10012-4019
212-431-9800
800-365-7006; *Fax:* 212-966-6708
info@guilford.com

Bob Matloff, President
Edna Foa, Author
Terence Keane, Author
Matthew Friedman, Author

The treatment guidelines presented in this book were developed under the auspices of the PTSD Treatment Guidelines Task Force established by the Board of Directors. *$38.25*

658 pages Year Founded: 2010 ISBN 1-609181-49-9

1698 Effective Treatments for PTSD
Guilford Press
72 Spring Street
New York, NY 10012-4068
212-431-9800
800-365-7006; *Fax:* 212-966-6708
info@guilford.com

Bob Matloff, President

Represents the collaborative work of experts across a range of theoretical orientations and professional backgrounds. Addresses general treatment considerations and methodological issues, reviews and evaluates the salient literature on treatment approaches for children, adolescents and adults. *$44.00*

379 pages ISBN 1-572305-84-3

1699 Handbook of PTSD: Science and Practice
The Guilford Press
72 Spring Street
New York, NY 10012-4019
212-431-9800
800-365-7006; *Fax:* 212-966-6708
info@guilford.com

Bob Matloff, President
Seymour Weingarten, Editor-in-Chief
Matthew Friedman, Author

Unparalleled in its breadth and depth, this state-of-the-art handbook reviews the latest scientific advances in understanding trauma and PTSD. *$42.50*

592 pages Year Founded: 2010 ISBN 1-609181-74-1

1700 Haunted by Combat: Understanding PTSD in
War Veterans
Rowman & Littlefield Publishers
4501 Forbes Boulevard
Suite 200
Lanham, MD 20706
301-459-3366
301-459-5748; *Fax:* 301-429-5748
www.rowman.com

Daryl S Paulson, Author
Stanley Krippner, Author
Jeff Harris, Vice President of Credit
Mike Cornell, Vice President of Operations

Across history, the condition has been called soldier's heart, shell shock, or combat fatigue. *$18.99*

226 pages Year Founded: 2010 ISBN 1-442203-91-4

1701 I Can't Get Over It: Handbook for Trauma
Survivors
NewHarbinger Publications
5674 Shattuck Avenue
Oakland, CA 94609
510-652-0215
800-748-6273; *Fax:* 800-652-1613
customerservice@newharbinger.com
www.newharbinger.com

Aphrodite T Matsakis, PhD, Author

Guides readers through the healing process of recovering from Post Traumatic Stress Disorder. From the emotional experience to the process of healing, this book is written for survivors of all types of trauma including war, sexual abuse, crime, family violence, rape and natural catastrophes. *$16.95*

416 pages Year Founded: 1973 ISBN 1-572240-58-X

1702 Managing Traumatic Stress Risk: A Proactive Approach
Charles C Thomas Publisher Ltd.
2600 South First Street
Springfield, IL 62794-9265
217-789-8980
800-258-8980; *Fax:* 217-789-9130
www.ccthomas.com

This volume represents the first systematic review of critical incident and disaster hazards, the contextual factors that influence risk, and their implications for traumatic stress risk management. It provides the hazard assessment and risk analysis information which, combined with information on resilience, facilitates the systematic analysis of traumatic stress risk and proactive and methodical development of mitigation and risk reduction strategies. This book is also available in paperback for $41.95. *$61.95*

258 pages Year Founded: 2004 ISBN 0-398075-17-4

1703 Post-Traumatic Stress Disorder: Assessment, Differential Diagnosis, and Forensic Evaluation
Professional Resource Press
PO Box 3197
Sarasota, FL 34230-3197
941-343-9601
800-443-3364; *Fax:* 941-343-9201
orders@prpress.com
www.prpress.com

Carroll L Meek, Author,Editor

A concise yet thorough examination of PTSD. An excellent resource for psychologists, psychiatrists, and lawyers involved in litigation concerning PTSD. *$26.95*

264 pages Year Founded: 1990 ISBN 0-943158-35-4

1704 Posttraumatic Stress Disorder in Litigation: Guidelines for Forensic Assessment
American Psychiatric Publishing, Inc.
1000 Wilson Boulevard
Suite 1825
Arlington, VA 22209-3901
703-907-7322
800-368-5777; *Fax:* 703-907-1091
appi@psych.org
www.appi.org

Robert I Simon, M.D., Editor
Ron McMillen, Chief Executive Officer
John McDuffie, Editorial Director

This essential collection by 13 leading US experts sheds important new light on forensic guidelines for effective assessment and diagnosis and determination of disability, serving both plaintiffs and defendants in litigation involving PTSD claims. Mental health and legal professionals, third-party payers, and interested laypersons will welcome this balanced approach to a complex and difficult field. *$44.95*

272 pages Year Founded: 2003 ISBN 1-585620-66-1

1705 Posttraumatic Stress Disorder: A Guide
6515 Grand Teton Plaza
Suite 100
Madison, WI 53719
608-827-2470; *Fax:* 608-827-2444
mim@miminc.org

John H. Greist, MD, Author
James W. Jefferson, MD, Author
David J. Katzelnick, MD, Author

68 pages Year Founded: 2007

1706 Psychiatric Treatment of Victims and Survivors of Sexual Trauma: A Neuro-Bio-Psychological Approach
Charles C Thomas Publisher Ltd.
2600 South First Street
Springfield, IL 62704
217-789-8980
800-258-8980; *Fax:* 217-789-9130
books@ccthomas.com
www.ccthomas.com

Jamshid A Marvasti, MD, Author

Psychological trauma is a multifaceted phenomenon with extensive involvement of biochemical and neurological changes. This book originated on the basis of clinical observations and the authors believe that trauma is the region in which psych and soma meet each other and integrate, becoming a single entity. The authors attempt to integrate the psychosocial and bio-neuro-endocrine aspects of human experience, including trauma. *$53.95*

234 pages Year Founded: 1927 ISBN 0-398074-60-7

1707 Psychological Trauma
American Psychiatric Publishing, Inc.
1000 Wilson Boulevard
Suite 1825
Arlington, VA 22209-3901
703-907-7322
800-368-5777; *Fax:* 703-907-1091
appi@psych.org
www.appi.org

Rachel Yehuda, Ph.D., Editor
Ron McMillen, Chief Executive Officer
John McDuffie, Editorial Director

Epidemiology of trauma and post-traumatic stress disorder. Evaluation, neuroimaging, neuroendocrinology and pharmacology. *$29.00*

236 pages Year Founded: 1998 ISBN 0-880488-37-9

1708 Rebuilding Shattered Lives: Responsible Treatment of Complex Post-Traumatic and Dissociative Disorders
John Wiley & Sons
111 River Street
Hoboken, NJ 07030-5774
201-748-6000
800-225-5945; *Fax:* 201-748-6088
info@wiley.com
www.wiley.com

James A Chu, Author

Essential for anyone working in the field of trauma therapy. Part I discusses recent findings about child abuse, the changes in attitudes toward child abuse over the last two decades and the nature of traumatic memory. Part II is an overview of principles of trauma treatment, including symptom control, establishment of boundaries and therapist self-care. Part III covers special topics, such as dissociative identity disorder, controversies, hospitalization and acute care. *$ 73.95*

271 pages Year Founded: 1998 ISBN 0-471247-32-4

1709 Relaxation & Stress Reduction Workbook
NewHarbinger Publications
5674 Shattuck Avenue
Oakland, CA 94609-1662
510-652-0215
800-748-6273; *Fax:* 800-652-1613
customerservice@newharbinger.com
www.newharbinger.com

Martha Davis, Author
Elizabeth Robbins Eshelman, Author
Matthew McKay, Author

Step by step instructions cover progressive muscle relaxation, meditation, autogenics, visualization, thought stopping, refuting irrational ideas, coping skills training, job stress management, and much more. *$17.95*

392 pages Year Founded: 1973 ISBN 1-879237-82-2

1710 Risk Factors for Posttraumatic Stress Disorder
1000 Wilson Boulevard
Suite 1825
Arlington, VA 22209-3901
703-907-7322
800-368-5777; *Fax:* 703-907-1091
appi@psych.org
www.appi.org

Robert E Hales MD, Editor-in-Chief
Ron McMillen, Chief Executive Officer
John McDuffie, Editorial Director

320 pages

1711 Stress Response Syndromes: Personality Styles and Interventions
Jason Aronson-Rowman & Littlefield Publishers
200 Park Avenue South
Suite 1109
New York, NY 10003-1512
212-529-3888
custerv@rowman.com
www.rowmanlittlefield.com

Mardi J Horowitz, Author

Incorporation of the most recent advances in the understanding and treatment of stress response syndromes to date. Describes the general characteristics, including signs and symptoms, and elaborates on treatment techniques that integrate cognitive and dynamic approaches. *$43.00*

451 pages ISBN 0-765703-13-0

1712 Stress-Related Disorders Sourcebook
Omnigraphics
155 West Congress
Suite 200
Detroit, MI 48226
313-961-1340
800-234-1340; *Fax:* 313-961-1383
contact@omnigraphics.com
www.omnigraphics.com

Amy L. Sutton, Author

Omnigraphics is the publisher of the Health Reference Series, a growing consumer health information resource with more than 100 volumes in print. Each title in the series features an easy to understand format, nontechnical language, comprehensive indexing and resources for further information. Material in each book has been collected from a wide range of government agencies, professional associations, periodicals, and other sources. *$85.00*

621 pages Year Founded: 1985 ISBN 0-780805-60-7

1713 Take Charge: Handling a Crisis and Moving Forward
American Institute for Preventive Medicine
30445 Northwestern Highway
Suite 350
Farmington Hills, MI 48334-3107
248-539-1800
800-345-2476; *Fax:* 248-539-1808
aipm@healthy.net
www.HealthyLife.com

Don R Powell, PhD, President/CEO
Elaine Frank,M.Ed,R.D, Vice President
Jeanette Karwan, Director,Product Development

Take Charge helps people effectively live their lives after September 11th. This full color booklet provides just the right amount of information to effectively address the many concerns people have today. It will help people to be prepared for any kind of disaster, be it a terrorist attack, fire or flood. *$4.25*

32 pages Year Founded: 1983

1714 Traumatic Stress: Effects of Overwhelming Experience on Mind, Body and Society
Guilford Press
72 Spring Street
New York, NY 10012-4068
212-431-9800
800-365-7006; *Fax:* 212-966-6708
info@guilford.com

Besell van der Kolk, Author
Alexander McFarlane, Author

The current state of research and clinical knowledge on traumatic stress and its treatment. Contributions from leading authorities summarize knowledge emerging. Addresses the uncertainties and controversies that confront the field of traumatic stress, including the complexity of posttraumatic adaptations and the unproven effectiveness of some approaches to prevention and treatment. *$42.50*

596 pages Year Founded: 2006 ISBN 1-572300-88-4

1715 Trust After Trauma: A Guide to Relationships for Survivors and Those Who Love Them
NewHarbinger Publications
5674 Shattuck Avenue
Oakland, CA 94609-1662
510-652-0215
800-748-6273; *Fax:* 800-652-1613
customerservice@newharbinger.com
www.newharbinger.com

Aphrodite T Matsakis, PhD, Author

Survivors guided through process of strengthening existing bonds, building new ones, and ending cycles of withdrawal and isolation. *$24.95*

352 pages Year Founded: 1973 ISBN 1-572241-01-2

1716 Understanding Post Traumatic Stress Disorder and Addiction
Sidran Institute
200 E Joppa Road
Suite 207
Baltimore, MD 21286-3107
410-825-8888
888-825-8249; *Fax:* 410-337-0747

sidran@sidran.org
www.sidran.org

Katie Evans, Author

This booklet discusses PTSD, how to recognize it and how to begin a dual recovery program from chemical dependency and PTSD. The workbook includes information to enhance your understanding of PTSD, activities to help identify the symptoms of dual disorders, a self evaluation of your recovery process and ways to handle situations that may trigger PTSD. *$7.20*

48 pages

1717 Who Gets PTSD? Issues of Posttraumatic Stress Vulnerability
Charles C Thomas Publisher Ltd.
2600 South First Street
Springfield, IL 62704
217-789-8980
800-258-8980; *Fax:* 217-789-9130
books@ccthomas.com
www.ccthomas.com

John M. Violanti, Author, Editor
Douglas Paton, Editor

Major topics in the text include: assessing psychological distress and physiological vulnerability in police officers, personal, organizational, and contextual influences in stress vulnerability; differences in vulnerability to posttraumatic deprivation: gender differences in police work , stress and trauma, trauma types, etc. *$ 46.95*

216 pages Year Founded: 1927 ISBN 3-980761-89-

Periodicals & Pamphlets

1718 101 Stress Busters
ETR Associates
4 Carbonero Way
Scotts Valley, CA 95066-4200
831-438-4060
800-321-4407; *Fax:* 831-438-3618
support@etr.freshdesk.com
www.etr.org

David Kitchen,MBA, Chief Financial Officer
Talita Sanders,BS, Director,Human Resources
Coleen Cantwell,MPH, Director,Business Development Pl
Matt McDowell,BS, Director,Marketing

These 101 stress busters were written by students to help fellow students relieve stress: tell a joke, laugh out loud, beat a pillow to smitherines. *$16.00*

1719 Five Smart Steps to Less Stress
ETR Associates
4 Carbonero Way
Scotts Valley, CA 95066-4200
831-438-4060
800-321-4407; *Fax:* 831-438-3618
support@etr.freshdesk.com
www.etr.org

David Kitchen,MBA, Chief Financial Officer
Talita Sanders,BS, Director,Human Resources
Coleen Cantwell,MPH, Director,Business Development Pl
Matt McDowell,BS, Director,Marketing

Steps to managing stress include: know what stresses you, manage your stress, take care of your body, take care of your feelings, ask for help. *$16.00*

1720 Five Ways to Stop Stress
ETR Associates
4 Carbonero Way
Scotts Valley, CA 95066-4200
831-438-4060
800-321-4407; *Fax:* 831-438-3618
support@etr.freshdesk.com
www.etr.org

David Kitchen,MBA, Chief Financial Officer
Talita Sanders,BS, Director,Human Resources
Coleen Cantwell,MPH, Director,Business Development Pl
Matt McDowell,BS, Director,Marketing

An easy to read pamphlet that discusses how to recognize the signs of stress, explains the big and little changes that can produce stress and the different causes of stress. *$18.00*

1721 Getting What You Want From Stress
ETR Associates
4 Carbonero Way
Scotts Valley, CA 95066-4200
831-438-4060
800-321-4407; *Fax:* 831-438-3618
customerservice@etr.org
www.etr.org

Mary Nelson, President

Includes signs of stress, some stress can be healthy, and when to change, when to adapt. *$18.00*

1722 Helping Children and Adolescents Cope with Violence and Disasters
National Institute of Mental Health
6001 Executive Boulevard
Room 8184,MSC 9663
Bethesda, MD 20892-9663
301-443-4513
866-615-6464
TTY: 301-443-8431
nimhinfo@nih.gov
www.www.nimh.nih.gov/

A booklet that describes what parents can do to help children and adolescents cope with violence and disasters.

1723 Let's Talk Facts About Post-Traumatic Stress Disorder
American Psychiatric Publishing, Inc.
1000 Wilson Boulevard
Suite 1825
Arlington, VA 22209-3901
703-907-7322
800-368-5777; *Fax:* 703-907-1091
appi@psych.org
www.appi.org

Robert E Hales MD, Editor-in-Chief
Ron McMillen, Chief Executive Officer
John McDuffie, Editorial Director

$12.50

8 pages Year Founded: 2005 ISBN 0-890423-63-6

1724 Real Illness: Post-Traumatic Stress Disorder
6001 Executive Boulevard
Room 8184
Bethesda, MD 20892
301-443-4513
866-615-6464

TTY: 301-443-8431
nimhinfo@nih.gov
9 pages

1725 Stress
ETR Associates
4 Carbonero Way
Scotts Valley, CA 95066-4200
831-438-4060
800-321-4407; *Fax:* 831-438-3618
customerservice@etr.org
www.etr.org

Mary Nelson, President

Includes common changes that cause stress, symptoms of stress, and effects on feelings, actions and physical health.

1726 Stress Incredible Facts
ETR Associates
4 Carbonero Way
Scotts Valley, CA 95066-4200
831-438-4060
800-321-4407; *Fax:* 831-438-3618
support@etr.freshdesk.com
www.etr.org

David Kitchen,MBA, Chief Financial Officer
Talita Sanders,BS, Director,Human Resources
Coleen Cantwell,MPH, Director,Business Development Pl
Matt McDowell,BS, Director,Marketing

Strange-but-true facts to trigger discussion about how stress affects the body, how to use it and long-term risks.

1727 Stress in Hard Times
ETR Associates
4 Carbonero Way
Scotts Valley, CA 95066-4200
831-438-4060
800-321-4407; *Fax:* 831-438-3618
customerservice@etr.org
www.etr.org

Mary Nelson, President

Discusses stress caused by troubling world events, describes short and long term symptoms, and suggests ways to cope. *$ 16.00*

1728 Teen Stress!
ETR Associates
4 Carbonero Way
Scotts Valley, CA 95066-4200
831-438-4060
800-321-4407; *Fax:* 831-438-3618
support@etr.freshdesk.com
www.etr.org

David Kitchen,MBA, Chief Financial Officer
Talita Sanders,BS, Director,Human Resources
Coleen Cantwell,MPH, Director,Business Development Pl
Matt McDowell,BS, Director,Marketing

Explains what stress is, outlines the causes and effects and offers ideas for handling stress. *$16.00*

Video & Audio

1729 Anxiety Disorders
American Counseling Association
5999 Stevenson Avenue
Alexandria, VA 22304-3304

703-823-9800
800-347-6647; *Fax:* 703-823-0252
TDD: 703-823-6862
webmaster@counseling.org
www.counseling.org

Cirecie A. West-Olatunji, President
Richard Yep, Executive Director
Thelma Daley, Treasurer

Increase your awareness of anxiety disorders, their symptoms, and effective treatments. Learn the effect these disorders can have on life and how treatment can change the quality of life for people presently suffering from these disorders. Includes 6 audiotapes and a study guide. *$140.00*

Year Founded: 1952

1730 Legacy of Childhood Trauma: Not Always Who They Seem
Research Press
Dept 12 W
PO Box 9177
Champaign, IL 61826-9177
217-352-3273
800-519-2707; *Fax:* 217-352-1221
rp@researchpress.com
www.researchpress.com

This powerful video focuses on the connection between so-called delinquent youth, and the experience of childhood trauma such as emotional, sexual, or physical abuse. Four young adults, survivors of childhood trauma, candidly discuss their troubled childhood and teenage years and reveal how, with the help of caring adults, they were able to salvage their lives. They offer valuable guidelines and insights on working with adolescents who have experienced childhood trauma. *$ 195.00*

1731 Treating Trauma Disorders Effectively
Colin A Ross Institute for Psychological Trauma
1701 Gateway
Suite 349
Richardson, TX 75080-3546
972-918-9588; *Fax:* 972-918-9069
rossinst@rossinst.com
www.rossinst.com

Dr Colin A Ross,MD, Founder,President
Melissa Caldwell, Manager

A training video that gives a comprehensive overview of clinical interventions with trauma patients. The video teaches advanced techniques for treating Dissociative Identity Disorder, Post Traumatic Stress Disorder, & trauma related Depression, Anxiety, Addictions, and Borderline Personality Disorder. The video's teaching modalities consist of case examples, with dramatic reenactments, and narrator discussion by Colin Ross, M.D. The teaching methods used clearly demonstrate effective therapeutic techniques that are backed by years of experience and research. *$85.00*

Year Founded: 1995

Web Sites

1732 www.apa.org/practice/traumaticstress.html
American Psychological Association

Provides tips for recovering from disasters and other traumatic events.

1733 **www.bcm.tmc.edu/civitas/caregivers.htm**
Caregivers Series

Sophisticated articles describing the effects of childhood trauma on brain development and relationships.

1734 **www.cyberpsych.org**
CyberPsych

CyberPsych presents information about psychoanalysis, psychotherapy and topics like anxiety disorders, substance abuse, homophobia, and traumas. It hosts mental health organizations and individuals with content of interest to the public and professional communities. There is also a free therapist finder service.

1735 **www.icisf.org**
International Critical Incident Stress Foundation

A nonprofit, open membership foundation dedicated to the prevention and mitigation of disabling stress by education, training and support services for all emergency service professionals. Continuing education and training in emergency mental health services for psychologists, psychiatrists, social workers and licensed professional counselors.

1736 **www.mentalhealth.com**
Internet Mental Health

On-line information and a virtual encyclopedia related to mental disorders, possible causes and treatments. News, articles, on-line diagnostic programs and related links. Designed to improve understanding, diagnosis and treatment of mental illness throughout the world. Awarded the Top Site Award and the NetPsych Cutting Edge Site Award.

1737 **www.ncptsd.org**
National Center for PTSD

Aims to advance the clinical care and social welfare of U.S. Veterans through research, education and training on PTSD and stress-related disorders

1738 **www.planetpsych.com**
PlanetPsych

Learn about disorders, their treatments and other topics in psychology. Articles are listed under the related topic areas. Ask a therapist a question for free, or view the directory of professionals in your area. If you are a therapist sign up for the directory. Current features, self-help, interactive, and newsletter archives.

1739 **www.psychcentral.com**
Psych Central

Personalized one-stop index for psychology, support, and mental health issues, resources, and people on the Internet.

1740 **www.ptsdalliance.org**
Post Traumatic Stress Disorder Alliance

Website of the Post Traumatic Stress Disorder Alliance.

1741 **www.sidran.org**
Sidran Institute, Traumatic Stress Education & Advocacy

Helps people understand, recover from, and treat traumatic stress (including PTSD), dissociative disorders, and co-occuring issues, such as addictions, self injury, and suicidality.

1742 **www.sidran.org/trauma.html**
Trauma Resource Area

Resources and Articles on Dissociative Experiences Scale and Dissociative Identity Disorder, PsychTrauma Glossary and Traumatic Memories.

1743 **www.store.samhsa.gov**
Substance Abuse and Mental Health Services Administration

Resources on mental disorders as well as treatment and recovery.

1744 **www.trauma-pages.com**
David Baldwin's Trauma Information Pages

Focus primarily on emotional trauma and traumatic stress, including PTSD (Post-traumatic Stress Disorder) and dissociation, whether following individual traumatic experience(s) or a large-scale disaster.

Associations & Organizations

National

1745 Advocates for Human Potential (AHP)
490-B Boston Post Road
Sudbury, MA 01776
978-443-0055; *Fax:* 978-443-4722
cgalland@ahpnet.com
www.ahpnet.com

Neal Shifman, MA, President and CEO
Charles R. Galland, MD, MBA, Chief Operating Officer
David Wetherbee, MBA, Chief Information Officer
Damien Newman, CPA, MBA, Chief Financial Officer

Excels in research and evaluation; technical assistance and training; system and program development, including strategic planning and information management; and resource development and dissemination. Staff are experts in content areas critical to addressing the behavioral health needs of vulnerable populations: mental health policy and services, addictions and substance abuse, criminal justice, health care reform, housing, homelessness, population health management, veterans, and workforce development.

Year Founded: 1980

1746 American Academy of Child and Adolescent Psychiatry
3615 Wisconsin Avenue Northwest
Washington, DC 20016-3007
202-966-7300; *Fax:* 202-464-0131
communications@aacap.org
www.aacap.org

Karen Wagner, MD, President
Andres Martin, MD, MPH, Secretary
Bennett L. Leventhal, MD, Treasurer
Heidi B. Fordi, CAE, Executive Director

The AACAP is the leading national professional medical association dedicated to treating and improving the quality of life for children, adolescents, and families affected by these disorders. Members actively research, evaluate, diagnose, and treat psychiatric disorders and pride themselves on giving direction to and responding quickly to new developments in addressing the health care needs of children and their families. Widely distributes information in an effort to promote an understanding of mental illnesses and remove the stigma associated with them; advance efforts in prevention of mental illnesses; and assure proper treatment and access to services for children and adolescents.

Year Founded: 1953

1747 American Academy of Pediatrics
345 Park Boulevard
Itasca, IL 60143
800-433-9016; *Fax:* 847-434-8000
www.aap.org

Colleen A. Kraft, MD, MBA, FAAP, President
Karen Remley, MD, MBA, FAAP, Executive VP and CEO
Kyle Yasuda, MD, FAAP, President-Elect

The mission of the AAP is to attain optimal physical, mental, and social health and well-being for all infants, children, adolescents, and young adults. A professional membership organization of 66,000 primary care pediatricians, pediatric medical sub-specialists, and pediatric surgical specialists.

Year Founded: 1930

1748 American Association for Geriatric Psychiatry
6728 Old McLean Village Drive
McLean, VA 22101
703-556-9222; *Fax:* 703-556-8729
main@aagponline.org
www.aagponline.org

Melinda Lantz, MD, President
Christopher N. Wood, Executive Director
Victoria LaLiberte, Executive Assistant
Carrie Stankiewicz, Consultant

The only national association that has products, activities, and publications which focus exclusively on the challenges of geriatric psychiatry. Practitioners, researchers, educations, students, and the public have relied on AAGP as the key driver for progress for elderly mental health care.

Year Founded: 1978

1749 American Association on Intellectual and Developmental Disabilities (AAIDD)
501 3rd Street NW
Suite 200
Washington, DC 20001
202-387-1968; *Fax:* 202-387-2193
www.aaidd.org

Susan Havercamp, PhD, President
Margaret Nygren, EdD, Executive Director and CEO
Paul D. Aitken, CPA, Director, Finance/Administration
Ajith Mathew, Contracts Manager

AAIDD provides worldwide leadership in the field of intellectual and developmental disabilities. The oldest and largest interdisciplinary organization of professionals and citizens concerned about intellectual and developmental disabilities. AAIDD promotes progressive policies, research, and universal human rights for people with intellectual and developmental disabilities.

Year Founded: 1876

1750 American Holistic Health Association
PO Box 17400
Anaheim, CA 92817-7400
714-779-6152
mail@ahha.org
www.ahha.org

Suzan V. Walter, MBA, President
Gena E. Kadar, DC, CNS, Secretary
Susan J. Negus, HHD, Treasurer

The leading national resource connecting people with vital solutions for reaching a higher level of wellness through a holistic approach to health and healthcare.

Year Founded: 1989

1751 American Network of Community Options and Resources (ANCOR)
1101 King Street
Suite 380
Alexandria, VA 22314
703-535-7850; *Fax:* 703-535-7860
ancor@ancor.org
www.ancor.org

Angela King, President
Barbara Merrill, Chief Executive Officer
Gabrielle Sedor, Chief Operations Officer
Sean Luechtefeld, Communications Director

A national trade association representing private providers of community living, employment supports, and services to individuals with disabilities. As a nonprofit organization, ANCOR continually advocates for the crucial role private providers play in enhancing and supporting the lives of people with disabilities and their families.

1752 American Pediatric Society

9303 New Trails Drive
Suite 350
The Woodlands, TX 77381
346-980-9707; *Fax: - - 2*
info@aps1888.org
www.www.aps1888.org/

Elena Fuentes-Afflick, President
Bruce D. Gelb, Vice President
Christine A. Gleason, Secretary and Treasurer

Society of professionals working on pediatric health care issues, through research, advocacy, and education. The society offers conferences and a variety of publications.

Year Founded: 1888

1753 American Psychiatric Association

800 Maine Avenue Southwest
Suite 900
Washington, DC 20024
202-559-3900
888-357-7924
apa@psych.org
www.psych.org

Anita Everett, MD, President
Altha J. Stewart, MD, President-Elect
Philip R. Muskin, MD, MA, Secretary
Bruce Schwartz, MD, Treasurer

The world's largest psychiatric organization. It is a medical specialty society representing more than 37,800 psychiatric physicians from the United States and around the world. Its member physicians work together to ensure humane care and effective treatment for all persons with mental disorders. Members are primarily medical specialists who are psychiatrists or in the process of becoming psychiatrists.

Year Founded: 1844

1754 American Psychological Association

750 First Street NE
Washington, DC 20002-4242
202-336-5500
800-374-2721
TDD: 202-336-6123
TTY: 202-336-6123
www.apa.org

Jessica Henderson Daniel, PhD, President
Arthur C. Evans, Jr., PhD, Chief Executive Officer and EVP
Jennifer F. Kelly, PhD, ABPP, Secretary
Jean A. Carter, PhD, Treasurer

The American Psychological Association seeks to advance psychology as a science, a profession, and as a means of promoting health, education, and human welfare. This organization of researchers, educators, clinicians, consultants, and students promotes research in psychology and the improvment of research methods; establishes high standards of ethics, conduct, and education; and disseminates psychological knowledge through professional and academic networks.

1755 American Speech-Language-Hearing Association

2200 Research Boulevard
Rockville, MD 20850-3289
301-269-5700
800-638-8255; *Fax: 301-296-8580*
TTY: 301-296-5650
www.asha.org

Elise Davis-McFarland, PhD, President
Janet Koehnke, PhD, CCC-A, Vice President Academic Affairs
Arlene Carney, CCC-A, Vice President, Standards/Ethics
Arlene A. Pietranton, PhD, CAE, Chief Executive Officer

The professional, scientific, and credentialing association for members and affiliates who are audiologists, speech-language pathologists, and speech, language, and hearing scientists in the United States and internationally. Supports audiologists and speech-language scientists in their research and practices.

Year Founded: 1925

1756 Association for Behavioral Health and Wellness

1325 G Street, NW
Suite 500
Washington, DC 20005
202-449-7660; *Fax: 202-449-7659*
info@abhw.org
www.www.abhw.org

Pamela Greenberg, MPP, President and CEO
Tiffany Huth, Director, Communications
Michael Golinkoff, PhD, MBA, Chair
Charles Gross, PhD, Treasurer

An association of the nation's leading behavioral health and wellness companies that manage behavioral health insurance. These companies provide an array of services related to mental health, substance use, employee assistance, disease management, and other health and wellness programs to over 175 million people in both the public and private sectors.

Year Founded: 1994

1757 Association of Mental Health Librarians (AMHL)

140 Old Orangeburg Road
Orangeburg, NY 10962
845-398-6576; *Fax: 845-398-5551*
moss@nki.rfmh.org
www.mhlib.org

Pam Hastings, President
Stuart Moss, Treasurer
Kate Elder, Secretary
Len Levin, President-Elect

A professional organization of individuals working in the field of mental health information delivery. The organization is open to libraries, library assistants, and library associates. AMHL hosts an annual conference, and provides opportunities for networking and enhancing professional skills.

1758 Attitudinal Healing International

3001 Bridgeway
Suite K-368
Sausalito, CA 94965-3100

877-244-3392
info@ahinternational.org
www.ahinternational.org

Gerald G. Jampolsky, MD, Founder
Diane V. Cirincione-Jampolsky, Executive Director and Founder
Paige Peterson, Chief Consult/Growth & Devel.
Lynne Law, International Liaison

Attitudinal Healing is based on the principle that it is not other people or situations that cause individuals distress. Rather, it is their own thoughts and attitudes that are responsible. AHInternational's mission is to create, develop, and support the official home portal for Attitudinal Healing and to help facilitate the organic creation and growth of independent centers, groups, and individuals worldwide.

Year Founded: 1975

1759 Bazelon Center for Mental Health Law

1101 15th Street NW
Suite 1212
Washington, DC 20005
202-467-5730
intakes@bazelon.org
www.www.bazelon.org/

Holly O'Donnell, President and CEO
Ira Burnim, Director
Jennifer Mathis, Deputy Director
Lewis Bossing, Senior Staff Attorney

National legal advocate for people with mental disabilities. Through precedent-setting litigation and in the public policy arena, the Bazelon Center works to advance and preserve the rights of people with mental illnesses and development disabilities.

Year Founded: 1972

1760 Bellefaire Jewish Children's Bureau

One Pollock Circle
22001 Fairmont Boulevard
Cleveland, OH 44118
216-932-2800
800-879-2522
www.bellefairejcb.org

Adam G. Jacobs, PhD, President
Jeffrey Lox, LISW-S, ACSW, Executive Director
Tom Browne, Chief Financial Officer
Leigh Johnson, General Counsel

Bellefaire JCB provides a variety of behavioral health, education, and prevention services for children, adolescents, and their families. Serves children, families, and young adults throughout the United States through its residential and autism treatment programs. Bellefaire JCB also meets the needs of children internationally through its Hague-accredited international adoption program.

Year Founded: 1868

1761 Best Buddies International (BBI)

100 Southeat Second Street
Suite 2200
Miami, FL 33131
305-374-2233; *Fax: 305-789-5577*
Info@BestBuddies.org
www.bestbuddies.org

Anthony K. Shriver, Founder and Chairman
John Carlin, Senior Director, Major Gifts

Jen Miller, SVP, Finance and Operations
Lisa Derx, VP, Government Relations

An international organization that has grown from one original chapter to almost 1,500 middle school, high school, and college chapters worldwide. Best Buddies programs engage participants in each of the 50 United States, and in 50 countries around the world, to help enhance the lives of people with intellectual and developmental disabilities.

Year Founded: 1989

1762 Bethesda Lutheran Communities

600 Hoffmann Drive
Watertown, WI 53094
920-261-3050
800-369-4636; *Fax: 920-261-8441*
www.bethesdalutherancommunities.org

Mike Thirtle, President and CEO
Jeff Kaczmarski, Executive Vice President
Lori Anderson, Chief Operating Officer
Dave Griebl, Chief Financial Officer

A Christian organization whose mission is to provide homes, support, and awareness for people with intellectual and developmental disabilities.

1763 Black Mental Health Alliance for Education & Consultation, Inc.

900 East Fayette Street
Suite 22111
Baltimore, MD 21203
410-338-2642; *Fax: 410-338-1771*
bhealthall@blackmentalhealth.com
www.blackmentalhealth.com

Jan A. Desper Peters, Executive Director
Cherly Maxwell, Program Manager

BMHA promotes appropriate mental health care, service delivery, and theoretical understanding of all the mental health programs. An organization that provides training, education, consultation, public information, support groups, and resource referrals regarding mental health and related issues. The primary mission of BMHA is to provide a forum and promote a holistic, culturally relevant approach to the development and maintenance of optimal mental health programs and services for African Americans and other people of color.

Year Founded: 1984

1764 Canadian Art Therapy Association

PO Box 658, Stn Main
Parksville, BC, ZZ
E-mail: admin@canadianarttherapy.org
www.www.canadianarttherapy.org/

Haley Toll, President
Michelle Winkel, Vice President
Sharona Bookbinder, Treasurer
Waqas Yousafzai, Director, Government Relations

A nonprofit organization promoting art therapy in Canada. Objectives are to encourage professional growth of art therapy through the exchange and collaboration of Art Therapists; to maintain national standards of training, practice, and professional registration; to foster research and publications in art therapy; and to increase awareness of art therapy as an important mental health discipline within the community Services.

Year Founded: 1977

1765 Canadian Federation of Mental Health Nurses
1 Concorde Gate
Suite 109
Toronto, ON, M3C 3N6, ZZ
416-426-7229
drosser@firststageinc.com
www.cfmhn.org

Florence Budden, President
Sergio Grice, Treasurer
Doug Rosser, General Manager
Marg Osborne, Advisor

The CFMHN is a membership organization that provides a
voice for pssychiatric and mental health nursing in Canada.
An associate group of the Canadian Nurses' Association
(CNA), CFMHN assures the development and application
of mental health and psychiatric nursing standards, addresses mental health issues, facilitates psychiatric and
mental health nursing through professional and networking
opportunities, and examines government policy.

Year Founded: 1988

1766 Canadian Mental Health Association
Canadian Mental Health Association
250 Dundas Street West
Suite 500
Toronto, ON M5T 2Z5,
416-646-5557
info@cmha.ca
www.cmha.ca

Dr. Patrick Smith, National CEO
Katherine Janson, National Director, Communication
Steven Presser, National VP/CDO
Cal Crocker, Chair

As a nation-wide, voluntary organization, the Canadian
Mental Health Association promotes the mental health of
all and supports the resilience and recovery of people experiencing mental illness. The CMHA accomplishes this mission through advocacy, education, research, and services.
CMHA has programs that assist with employment, housing,
early intervention for youth, peer support, recreation services for people with mental illness, stress reduction workshops, and public education campaigns for the community.
It also acts as a social advocate to encourage public action
and commitment to strengthening community mental health
services and legislation.

Year Founded: 1918

1767 Center for Mental Health Services (CMHS)
Substane Abuse and Mental Health Services
Administration
5600 Fishers Lane
Rockville, MD 20857
240-276-1310
877-726-4727
TTY: 800-487-4889
www.samhsa.gov/about-us/who-we-are/offices-centers

Paolo del Vecchio, MSW, Director
Anne Mathews-Younes, Acting Deputy Director
Keris Myrick, Director, Consumer Affairs
Patricia Gratton, Director, Program Analysis

Promotes the treatment of mental illness and emotional disorders by increasing accessibility to mental health programs; supporting outreach, treatment, rehabilitation, and
support programs and networks; and encouraging the use of
scientifically-based information when treating mental dis-

orders. CMHS provides information about mental health
via a toll-free number and numerous publications. Developed for users of mental health services and their families,
the general public, policy makers, providers, and the
media.

Year Founded: 1992

1768 Centre for Addiction and Mental Health
1001 Queen Street West
30-60 White Squirrel Way
Toronto, ON M6J 1H4,
416-535-8501
800-463-2338
info@camh.ca
www.camh.ca

Dr Catherine Zahn, President and CEO
David Wilson, Board Chair
Tom Milroy, Chair, CAMH Foundation

CAMH is Canada's leading addiction and mental health organization, integrating specialized clinical care with innovative research, education, health promotion and policy
development. CAMH is fully affiliated with the University
of Toronto, and is a Pan American Health Organiza-
tion/World Health Organization Collaborating Centre.
CAMH combines clinical care, research, education, policy
and health promotion to transform the lives of people
affected by mental health and addiction issues.

Year Founded: 1998

1769 Child & Parent Resource Institute (CPRI)
600 Sanatorium Road
London, ON N6H 3W7,
519-858-2774
877-494-2774; *Fax:* 519-858-3913
TTY: 519-858-0257
www.cpri.ca

A tertiary centre that provides highly specialized voluntary
services to children and youth with multi complex, severe
behavioural disturbances and/or developmental challenges
that impacts the child/youth in all areas i.e. home, school,
and/or community. 100% funded by the Ontario Ministry
of Children and Youth Services and services are offered at
no charge.

1770 Child Mind Institute
101 East 56th Street
New York, NY 10022
212-308-3118
www.childmind.org/

Brooke Garber Neidich, Co-Founder and Co-Chair
Ram Sundaram, Co-Chair
Debra G. Perelman, Co-Founder and Vice Chair

An independant, national nonprofpit organization that helps
children and their families struggling with mental health
disorders through free resources, access to effective treatments, and the advancement of pediatric research to improve diagnosis and treatment of mental health disorders in
children.

1771 Community Access
2 Washington Street
9th Floor
New York, NY 10004
212-780-1400
www.communityaccess.org

Stephen H. Chase, President
Catherine G. Patsos, Vice President
Cal Hedigan, Deputy CEO
Steve Coe, CEO

Community Access assists people with psychiatric disabilities in making the transition from shelters and institutions to independent living. Community Access provides safe, affordable housing and support services, and advocates for the rights of people to live without fear or stigma. They provide a range of housing, job skills, employment placement, and professional support services to help break the cycle of homelessness, institutionalization, and/or incarceration that often complicates the lives of people who have a history of mental illness. Community access creates pathways to meaningful and successful community life.

Year Founded: 1974

1772 Council for Learning Disabilities

11184 Antioch Road
Box 405
Overland Park, KS 66210
913-491-1011; *Fax:* 913-491-1011
CLDinfo@cldinternational.org
www.www.council-for-learning-disabilities.org

Deborah Reed, President
Lindy Crawford, Vice President
Brittany Hott, Secretary
Linda Nease, Executive Director

An international organization that promotes evidence-based teaching, collaboration, research, leadership, and advocacy. CLD is comprised of professionals who represent diverse disciplines and are committed to enhancing the education and quality of life for individuals with learning disabilities and others who experience challenges in learning.

1773 Council on Quality and Leadership (CQL)

100 West Road
Suite 300
Towson, MD 21204
410-583-0060
info@thecouncil.org
www.thecouncil.org

Mary Kay Rizzolo, President and CEO
Trina Douglas, VP, Finance and Administration
Jennifer Becher, Chair
Trina Sieling, Vice Chair

CQL offers consultation, accreditation, training, and certification services to organizations and systems that share the vision of dignity, opportunity, and community for all people. CQL provides leadership to improve the quality of life for people with disabilities, people with mental illness, and older adults.

Year Founded: 1969

1774 Emotions Anonymous International Service Center

PO Box 4245
St. Paul, MN 55104-0245
651-647-9712
director@emotionsanonymous.org
www.emotionsanonymous.org/

Gus S., President
Scott J., Vice President and Treasurer
John W., Secretary
Elaine Weber Nelson, Executive Director

Fellowship of men and women who share their experience, strength, and hope with each other, that they may solve their common problem and help others recover from emotional illness. Members come together in weekly meetings.

1775 Eye Movement Desensitization and Reprocessing International Association (EMDRIA)

5806 Mesa Drive
Suite 360
Austin, TX 78731-3785
512-451-5200; *Fax:* 512-451-5256
info@emdria.org
www.emdria.org

Michael Bowers, Executive Director
Gayla Turner, Deputy Executive Director
Evelyn Wright, LCSW, President
Mark Nickerson, LICSW, Secretary

A professional association for EMDR practitioners seeking high standars of practice in EDMR therapy.

Year Founded: 1995

1776 Families Anonymous, Inc.

701 Lee Street
Suite 670
Des Plaines, IL 60016
847-294-5877
800-736-9805; *Fax:* 847-294-5837
famanon@familiesanonymous.org
www.familiesanonymous.org

A 12 Step fellowship for families and friends of individuals who have dealt or are dealing with mental health issues, whether caused by drugs, alcohol, or related behavioral problems.

1777 Federation for Children with Special Needs (FCSN)

529 Main Street
Suite 1M3
Boston, MA 02129
617-236-7210
800-331-0688; *Fax:* 617-241-0330
fcsninfo@fcsn.org
www.fcsn.org

Anne . Howard, PhD, President
Rich Robison, Executive Director
Tom Hamel, Director, Business and Finance
Michael Weiner, Treasurer

The federation provides information, support, and assistance to parents of children with disabilities, their professional partners, and their communities. Promotes the active and informed participation of parents of children with disabilities in shaping, implementing, and evaluating public policy that affects them.

Year Founded: 1974

1778 Gam-Anon Family Groups International Service Office, Inc.

PO Box 307
Massapequa Park, NY 11762
718-352-1671
gamanonoffice@gam-anon.org
www.gam-anon.org

A 12 step self-help organization for close friends and family of compulsive gamblers.

1779 Genetic Alliance
4301 Connecticut Avenue NW
Suite 404
Washington, DC 20008-2369
202-966-5557; *Fax:* 202-966-8553
info@geneticalliance.org
www.geneticalliance.org

Sharon Terry, MA, CEO
Natasha Bonhomme, Chief Strategy Officer
Ruth Child, Chief Financial Officer
Tetyana Murza, MES, Managing Director

Genetic Alliance is the world's leading nonprofit health advocacy organization committed to transforming health through genetics and promoting an environment of openness centered on the health of individuals, families, and communities.

Year Founded: 1986

1780 Healing for Survivors
PO Box 8405
Fresno, CA 93747-8405
559-442-3600; *Fax:* 559-442-3600
jankister@email.com
www.healingforsurvivors.org

Jan Kister, Director/Founder

A community based non profit organization dedicated to provideing education, counseling, resources, and a safe place for individuals and families impacted by physical, emotional and/or sexual abuse to pursue wholeness and healing.

1781 Hong Fook Mental Health Association
3320 Midland Avenue
Suite 201
Scarborough, ON M1V 5E6,
416-493-4242; *Fax:* 416-493-2214
info@hongfook.ca
www.hongfook.ca

Dr. Lin Fang, President
Grace Kangmeehae Lee, Vice President
Eric Man, Vice President
Peter Lee, Treasurer

Hong Fook Mental Health Association aims to facilitate access to mental health services for people with linguistic and cultural barriers. Mental health services includes self-help programs; family initiatives; clinical services, including group psychotherapy, intake, and case management; youth programs; and prevention and promotion programs.

Year Founded: 1982

1782 Human Services Research Institute
7690 SW Mohawk St.
Bldg K.
Tualatin, OR 97062
503-924-3783
www.hsri.org

David Hughes, President
John Agosta, Executive Vice President
Julie Bershadsky, Dir., Aging and Disabilities
Teresita Camacho-Gonsalves, Co-Dir., Behavioral Health

Assists state and federal government to enhance services and support people with mental illness and people with developmental disabilities.

Year Founded: 1976

1783 Institute of Living-Anxiety Disorders Center; Center for Cognitive Behavioral Therapy
The Institute of Living/Hartford Hospital
200 Retreat Avenue
Hartford, CT 06106
860-545-7685
800-673-2411
ADC@hhchealth.org
www.harthosp.org/instituteofliving/

David Tolin, PhD, ABPP, Director

The Anxiety Disorders Center provides treatment, conducts research, and educates mental health professionals on anxiety disorders. Treatment options include group therapy, cognitive behavioral therapy, and virtual reality therapy, and are offered at no cost.

1784 Institute on Violence, Abuse and Trauma at Alliant International University
10065 Old Grove Road
Suite 101
San Diego, CA 92131
858-527-1860; *Fax:* 858-527-1743
ivat@ivatcenters.org
www.www.ivatcenters.org/

Robert Geffner, PhD, President
Sandi Capuano Morrison, MA, Chief Executive Officer
Morgan Shaw, PsyD, Clinical Director
Tiffany Robbins, Exec. Administrative Assistant

IVAT strives to be a comprehensive resource, training, and research center dealing with all aspects of violence, abuse, and trauma. IVAT interfaces with Alliant International University's academic schools and centers, which provide resource support and educational training. Through a focus on collaborations with various partnering organizations, IVAT desires to bridge gaps and help improve current systems of care on a local, national, and global level.

Year Founded: 2006

1785 International Society of Psychiatric-Mental Health Nurses
2424 American Lane
Madison, WI 53704-3102
608-443-2463; *Fax:* 608-443-2474
info@ispn-psych.org
www.ispn-psych.org

Steven Pryjmachuk, PhD, President
Vicki Hines-Martin, PhD, RN, President-Elect
Helen Teresa Buckland, PhD, MEd, Treasurer
Kathy Kuehn, ISPN Executive Director

The mission of ISPN is to unite and strengthen the presence and the voice of specialty psychiatric-mental health nursing while influencing health care policy to promote equitable, evidence-based and effective treatment and care for individuals, families, and communities.

Year Founded: 1999

1786 Judge Baker Children's Center
53 Parker Hill Avenue
Boston, MA 02120-3225
617-232-8390; *Fax:* 617-232-8399
info@jbcc.harvard.edu
www.jbcc.harvard.edu

Robert P. Franks, PhD, President and CEO
Elizabeth Fitzsimons, Director of Development

Christopher Bellonci, MD, Chief Medical Officer
Nina Rodriguez, Director of Facilities

A nonprofit organization dedicated to improving the lives of children whose emotional and behavioral problems threaten to limit their potential. Integrating education, service, research, and training, the Center is the oldest child mental health organization in New England and a national leader in the field of children's mental health. Promoting the best possible mental health of children through the integration of research, intervention, training, and advocacy.

Year Founded: 1917

1787 Learning Disabilities Association of America

4156 Library Road
Pittsburgh, PA 15234-1349
412-341-1515; *Fax:* 412-344-0224
info@ldaamerica.org
www.LDAAmerica.org

Beth McGaw, President
Mary-Clare Reynolds, Executive Director
Jonathan Jones, First Vice President
Jennifer Harkins, Secretary

LDA's mission is to create opportunities for success for all individuals affected by learning disabilities and to reduce the incidence of learning disabilities in future generations.

Year Founded: 1964

1788 Life Development Institute

18001 N 79th Avenue
Suite B-42
Glendale, AZ 85308
866-736-7811
www.lifedevelopmentinstitute.org

Rob Crawford, MEd, Chief Executive Officer
Veronica Lieb Crawford, MA, President
Justin Coller, BS, Director of Operations
Mia Coudret, BA, Resource Support Specialist

LDI is a special education school dedicated to motivating and inspiring its students to seek and experience success. Learning disability program staff and administrators are devoted to actively working with and supporting parents to help their child succeed and be independent for life.

1789 Lifespire

1 Whitehall Street
9th Floor
New York, NY 10004
212-741-0100; *Fax:* 212-463-9814
info@lifespire.org
www.lifespire.org

Michael S. Gross, Chairman
Thomas Lydon, CEO and President
Keith Lee, Chief Financial Officer
Bonita Hinson, Chief Operating Officer

Lifespire seeks to provide support to individuals with disabilities and assist them with the development of the skills needed to become independent and contributing members of the community.

Year Founded: 1951

1790 Menninger Clinic

12301 Main Street
Houston, TX 77035
713-275-5000
800-351-9058; *Fax:* 713-275-5107
www.www.menningerclinic.com

Tony Gaglio, CPA, MBA, Acting President and CEO
Tony Gaglio, CPA, MBA, Senior VP and CFO
Bella Schanzer, MD, MPH, Chief of Staff
Avni Cirpili, RN, DNP, Sr. VP and Chief Nursing Officer

Menninger is a leading psychiatric hospital dedicated to treating individuals with mood, personality, anxiety, and addictive disorders; teaching mental health professionals; and advancing mental healthcare through research.

Year Founded: 1925

1791 Mental Health America

500 Montgomery Street
Suite 820
Alexandria, VA 22314
703-684-7722
800-969-6642; *Fax:* 703-684-5968
TTY: 800-433-5959
www.mentalhealthamerica.net

Reginald Williams, Chair of the Board
Paul Gionfriddo, President and CEO
Jessica Kennedy, Chief of Staff/VP of Finance
Theresa Nguyen, VP of Policy and Programs

Mental Health America is a community-based nonprofit organization committed to enabling the mental wellness of all Americans and improving treatments and services for individuals with mental health needs. Provides information about a range of disorders, including panic disorder, obsessive-compulsive disorder, post traumatic stress, generalized anxiety disorder and phobias; advocates for policies focused on advancing early intervention and prevention; and organizes education and outreach initiatives.

Year Founded: 1909

1792 Mental Health Media

25 West Street
Westborough, MA 01581
617-562-1111
www.www.mentalhealth-media.org/

Mental Health Media, formerly The Mental Illness Education Project, is engaged in the production of video-based educational and support materials for the following specific populations: people with psychiatric disabilities, families, mental health professionals, special audiences, and the general public. The videos are designed to be used in hospital, clinical, and educational settings, and at home by individuals and families.

Year Founded: 1995

1793 Mental Health and Aging Network (MHAN) of the American Society on Aging (ASA)

American Society on Aging
575 Market Street
Suite 2100
San Francisco, CA 94105-2869
415-974-9600
800-537-9728; *Fax:* 415-974-0300
info@asaging.org
www.asaging.org

Robert Stein, President and CEO
Robert R. Lowe, Chief Operating Officer
Carole Anderson, Vice President of Education
Krista Brown, Director of Education

MHAN is dedicated to improving the supportive interventions for older adults with mental health problems and their caregivers by creating a network of professionals with expertise in geriatric mental health, improving systems of care for older adults with dementia, and advocating services and programs that help older adults with mental health issues.

Year Founded: 1954

1794 Nathan S. Kline Institute for Psychiatric Research
140 Old Orangeburg Road
Orangeburg, NY 10962
845-398-5500; *Fax:* 845-398-5510
webmaster@nki.rfmh.org
www.www.rfmh.org/nki

Donald C. Goff, MD, Director
Antonio Convit, MD, Deputy Director
Thomas O. O'Hara, MBA, Deputy Director Administration

A facility of the New York State Office of Mental Health that has earned a national and international reputation for its pioneering contributions in psychiatric research, especially in the areas of psychopharmacological treatments for schizophrenia and major mood disorders, and in the application of computer technology to mental health services. A broad range of studies are conducted at NKI, including basic, clinical, and services research. All work is intended to improve care for people suffering from these complex, psychobiologically-based, severely disabling mental disorders.

Year Founded: 1952

1795 National Alliance on Mental Illness
3803 North Fairfax Drive
Suite 100
Arlington, VA 22203
703-524-7600
800-950-6264
info@nami.org
www.nami.org

Steve Pitman, JD, President
Lacey Berumen, PhD, MNM, First Vice President
Mary Giliberti, Chief Executive Officer
David Levy, Chief Financial Officer

A grassroots mental health organization dedicated to improving the lives of all Americans affected by mental illness. NAMI provides education programs to communities across America; advocates for access to mental health services and treatment; offers support, information, referrals, and resources; and raises public awareness on mental illness through events, activities, and other efforts. NAMI seeks to eliminate stigma and to foster an environment of awareness and understanding for those concerned with mental health. Financial contributions allow NAMI to work towards fulfilling their mission.

Year Founded: 1979

1796 National Association for Rural Mental Health
660 North Capital Street
Suite 400
Washington, DC 20001
202-942-4276; *Fax:* 202-478-1659
info@narmh.org
www.narmh.org

Jennifer Christman, President
Virginia Shaw, PhD, Membership Chair, Secretary
Lori Irvine, LCSW, Secretary
Tammy Barnes, Treasurer

NARMH provides a forum for rural mental health professionals and advocates to identify and solve challenges, to work cooperatively toward improving the delivery of rural mental health services, and to promote the unique needs and concerns of rural mental health policy and practice issues. NARMH sponsors an annual conference where rural mental health professionals benefit from the sharing of knowledge and resources.

Year Founded: 1977

1797 National Association for the Dually Diagnosed (NADD)
132 Fair Street
Kingston, NY 12401
845-331-4336
info@thenadd.org
www.thenadd.org

Daniel Baker, PhD, President
Jeanne M. Farr, MA, Chief Executive Officer
Peggie Webb, MA, Vice President
George Zukotynski, PhD, Secretary

NADD is a nonprofit organization designed to increase awareness of, and provide services for, individuals with developmental disabilities and mental illness. NADD emphasizes the importance of quality mental healthcare for people with mental health needs and offers conferences, information resources, educational programs, and training materials to professionals, parents, and organizations.

Year Founded: 1983

1798 National Association of State Mental Health Program Directors (NASMHPD)
66 Canal Center Plaza
Suite 302
Alexandria, VA 22314
703-739-9333; *Fax:* 703-548-9517
brian.hepburn@nasmhpd.org
www.nasmhpd.org

Brian Hepburn, MD, Executive Director
Jay Meek, CPA, MBA, Chief Financial Officer
Raul Almazar, RN, MA, Senior Public Health Advisor
Meighan Haupt, MS, Chief of Staff

The only national association to represent state mental health commissioners/directors and their agencies. A private nonprofit membership organization, NASMHPD helps set the agenda and determine the direction of state mental health agency interests across the country, including state mental health planning, service delivery, and evaluation. The association provides members with the opportunity to exchange diverse views and experiences, learning from one another in areas vital to effective public policy development and implementation. Provides a broad array of services designed to identify and respond to critical policy issues, cutting-edge consultation, training, and technical assistance.

Year Founded: 1959

1799 National Center for Learning Disabilities
32 Laight Street
2nd Floor
New York, NY 10013

212-545-7510
888-575-7373; *Fax:* 212-545-9665
www.ncld.org

Frederic M. Poses, Chairman
Mimi Corcoran, President and CEO
Mary Kalikow, Vice Chairman
John R. Langeler, Treasurer

The NCLD's mission is to ensure success for all individuals with learning disabilities in school, at work, and in life. They connect parents with resources, guidance, and support to advocate effectively for their children; deliver evidence-based tools, resources, and professional development to educators to improve student outcomes; and develop policies and engage advocates to strengthen educational rights and opportunities.

Year Founded: 1977

1800 National Center on Addiction and Substance Abuse (CASA) at Columbia University

633 3rd Avenue
19th Floor
New York, NY 10017-6706
212-841-5200
contact@casacolumbia.org
www.casacolumbia.org

Joseph J. Plumeri, Executive Chair
Joseph A. Califano, Founder and Chairman Emeritus
James G. Niven, Co-Chair
Creighton Drury, President

The National Center on Addiction and Substance Abuse (CASA) at Columbia University is a science-based, multidisciplinary organization focused on transforming society's understanding of and responses to substance use and the disease of addiction. Founded by Former U.S. Secretary of Health, Education, and Welfare Joseph A. Califano, Jr., CASA remains the only national organization that assembles under one roof all of the professional skill needed to research and develop proven, effective ways to prevent and treat substance abuse and addiction to all substances - alcohol, nicotine as well as illegal, prescription, and performance enhancing drugs - in all sectors of society.

Year Founded: 1992

1801 National Council for Behavioral Health

1400 K Street NW
Suite 400
Washington, DC 20005
202-684-7457
communications@thenationalcouncil.org
www.TheNationalCouncil.org

Jeff Richardson, Chairman
Linda Rosenburg, President and CEO
Mohini Venkatesh, VP, Business and Strategy
Jeannie Campbell, Executive Vice President and COO

The unifying voice of America's behavioral health organizations. The National Council is committed to providing comprehensive, quality care that affords every opportunity for recovery and inclusion in all aspects of community life. The National Council advocates for public policies in mental and behavioral health that ensure that people who are ill can access comprehensive healthcare services, and also offer state-of-the-science education and practice improvement resources so that services are efficient and effective.

1802 National Disability Rights Network, Inc.

820 1st Street, NE
Suite 740
Washington, DC 20002
202-408-9514; *Fax:* 202-408-9520
TTY: 220-408-9521
info@ndrn.org
www.ndrn.org

Michael Kirkman, President
Tom Masseau, Vice President
Curtis L. Decker, JD, Executive Director
Zachary Martin, Director of Operations

NDRN is a nonprofit membership organization for the Protection and Advocacy Systems and the Client Assistance Programs. These programs work to guard against abuse, advocate for basic rights, and ensure acocunability throughout a variety of areas for people with disabilities and mental illnesses.

Year Founded: 1982

1803 National Empowerment Center

599 Canal Street
Lawrence, MA 01840
978-685-1494
800-769-3728; *Fax:* 978-681-6426
info4@power2u.org
www.power2u.org/

Daniel B. Fisher, MD, PhD, Chief Executive Officer
Oryx Cohen, MPA, Chief Operating Officer
Maria Ostheimer, Coordinator, Emotional CPR

A consumer/survivor/expatient-run organization that is dedicated to helping people with mental health issues, trauma, and/or extreme states. Their central message revolves around recovery, empowerment, and healing.

1804 National Federation of Families for Children's Mental Health

12320 Parklawn Drive
Rockville, MD 20852
240-403-1901
ffcmh@ffcmh.org
www.www.ffcmh.org

Lynda Gargan, PhD, Executive Director
Barbara Huff, Technical Assistance Provider
Sherri Luthe, President
Terry Stevens, Vice President

The National Federation of Families for Children's Mental Health is a national organization focused on advocating for the rights of children affected by mental health challenges, assisting family-run organizations across the nation, and ensuring that children and families concerned with mental health have access to services.

Year Founded: 1989

1805 National Institute of Drug Abuse (NIDA) Office of Science Policy & Communications, Public Information Branch

6001 Executive Boulevard
Room 5213, MSC 9561
Bethesda, MD 20892-9561
301-443-1124
www.drugabuse.gov

Dr. Nora Volkow, Director
Dr. Wilson Compton, Deputy Director

Joellen Austin, Associate Director, Management
Steven Gust, PhD, Director, International Program

NIDA is part of the National Institute of Health, and aims to advance research on the causes and consequences of drug use and addiction in order to improve public health.

1806 National Institute of Mental Health
Information Resource Center
6001 Executive Boulevard
Room 6200, MSC 9663
Bethesda, MD 20892-9663
301-443-4513
866-615-6464; *Fax:* 301-443-4279
TTY: 301-443-8431
nimhinfo@nih.gov
www.www.nimh.nih.gov/

Joshua A. Gordon, MD, PhD, Director
Shelli Avenevoli, PhD, Deputy Director

One of 27 components of the National Institutes of Health, the Federal government's principal biomedical and behavioral research agency. The National Institute of Mental Health is an expert in mental disorders and aims to improve the treatment and recovery of mental illness through clinical research.

1807 National Institutes of Health Clinical Center
9000 Rockville Pike
Building 10
Bethesda, MD 20892
301-496-2563; *Fax:* 301-402-2984
ccpressgroup@cc.nih.gov
www.cc.nih.gov

James K. Gilman, MD, Chief Executive Officer
Pius A. Aiyelawo, FACHE, Chief Operating Officer
Colleen A. McGowan, MHA, FACHE, Executive Officer
Gwenyth R. Wallen, PhD, RN, Chief Nurse Officer

The NIH Clinical Center is composed of the Warren Grant Magnuson Clinical Center and the later addition, The Mark O. Hatfield Clinical Research Center. The Center was designed with patient care facilities close to research laboratories so new findings of basic and clinical scientists can be quickly applied to the treatment of patients. Upon referral by physicians, patients are admitted to NIH clinical studies.

Year Founded: 1953

1808 National Mental Health Consumers' Self-Help
Clearinghouse
1211 Chestnut Street
Suite 1100
Philadelphia, PA 19107
267-507-3810
800-553-4539; *Fax:* 215-636-6312
info@mhselfhelp.org
www.mhselfhelp.org

Joseph Rogers, Founder and Executive Director
Susan Rogers, Director

The Clearinghouse is a peer-run national technical assistance center focused on achieving respect and equality of opportunity for those with mental illnesses. The Clearinghouse helps with the growth of the mental health consumer movement by evaluating mental health services, advocating for mental health reform, and providing consumers with news, information, publications, and consultation services.

Year Founded: 1986

1809 National Network for Mental Health
PO Box 1539
Station Main
St. Catharines, ON, ZZ
www.nnmh.ca

May Recollect, Indigenous Representative
Sarah Bell, Manitoba/Youth Representative
William Pringle, Saskatchewan Representative
Marilyn McGurran, NWT Representative

The purpose of the NNMH is to advocate, educate, and provide expertise and resources that benefit the Canadian consumer/survivor community. The focus of the organization is to network with Candian consumer/survivors and family and friends of consumer/survivors to provide opportunities for resource sharing, information distribution, and education on issues impacting persons living with mental health issues/illness/disability.

1810 National Organization on Disability
77 Water Street
Suite 204
New York, NY 10005
646-505-1191; *Fax:* 646-505-1184
info@nod.org
www.nod.org

Thomas Ridge, Chairman
Carol Glazer, President
Luke Visconti, Vice Chairman
Sue Meirs, Chief Operating Officer

NOD is a private, nonprofit organization that is dedicatd to helping people with disabilities live full, independent lives. NOD conducts research on disability employment issues, including the field's most widely used polls on employment trends and the quality of life for people with disabilities. They work in partnership with employers, schools, the military, service providers, researchers, and disability advocates. Current employment progrmas are benefiting high school students with disabilities, seriously injured service members returning from Iraq and Afghanistan, employers seeking to become more disability friendly, and state governments engaged in policy reform.

Year Founded: 1982

1811 National Rehabilitation Association
PO Box 150235
Alexandria, VA 22315
703-836-0850
888-258-4295; *Fax:* 703-836-0848
membership@nationalrehab.org
www.www.nationalrehab.org

Greg Mason, President
Dr. Frederic K. Schroeder, PhD, Executive Director
James Liin, Membership Coordinator
Veronica Hamilton, Office Manager

The National Rehabilitation Association is concerned with the rights of people with disabilities. Their mission is to provide advocacy, awareness, and career advancement for professionals in the fields of rehabilitation. Members include rehab counselors; physical, speech, and occupational therapists; job trainers; consultants; independent living instructors; and other professionals involved in the advocacy of programs and services for people with disabilities.

Year Founded: 1927

1812 New Hope Foundation
80 Conover Road
Marlboro, NJ 07746
723-946-3030
800-705-4673
www.newhopefoundation.org

Tony Comerford, PhD, President and CEO
David Roden, LCSW, LCADC, Vice President and COO

A nonprofit corporation serving those in need of treatment for alcoholism, drug addiction, and compulsive gambling. Over the years, New Hope has expanded its capacity and capabilities to include specialized programming for adolescents, women, and those with co-occuring disorders. New Hope constantly strives to advance the quality of addiction treatment through ongoing professional education and participation in select research projects.

1813 Parents Helping Parents
Sobrato Center for Nonprofits
1400 Parkmoor Avenue
Suite 100
San Jose, CA 95126
408-727-5775
855-727-5775; *Fax:* 408-286-1116
info@php.com
www.php.com

Maria Daane, Executive Director
Mark Fishler, Development Director
Jane Floethe Ford, Director of Education Services
Trudy Marsh Grable, Director of Community Services

PHP's mission is to help children and adults with special needs receive the support and services they need to reach their full potential by providing information, training, and resources to build strong families and improve systems of care.

Year Founded: 1976

1814 Recovery International
1415 W. 22nd Street
Tower Floor
Oak Brook, IL 60523
312-337-5661
866-221-0302; *Fax:* 312-726-4446
www.www.recoveryinternational.org

Sandra K. Wilcoxon, Chief Executive Officer
Joanne Lampey, President
Joan Nobiling, Vice President
Nicole Cilento, 2nd Vice President

Recovery International is an organization that uses a peer-to-peer, self-help training system developed by Abraham Low in order to help individuals with mental health issues lead more productive lives.

Year Founded: 1937

1815 Sidran Traumatic Stress Institute
PO Box 436
Brooklandville, MD 21022-0436
410-825-8888; *Fax:* 410-825-8888
info@sidran.org
www.sidran.org

Esther Giller, President and Director
Sheila Giller, Secretary and Treasurer
Stephanie Muszelik, Accountant
Ruta Mazelis, Editor, The Cutting Edge/Trainer

Sidran Institute provides useful, practical information for child and adult survivors of any type of trauma, for families/friends, and for the clinical and frontline service providers who assist in their recovery. Sidran's philosophy of education through collaboration brings together great minds (providers, survivors, and loved ones) to develop comprehensive programs to address the practical, emotional, spiritual, and medical needs of trauma survivors.

Year Founded: 1986

1816 The Arc New York
29 British American Boulevard
2nd Floor
Latham, NY 12110
518-439-8311
Info@TheArcNY.org
www.www.thearcny.org/

Laura J. Kennedy, President
Mark van Voorst, Executive Director
Tania F. Seaburg, Esq., Chief Policy/Operations Officer
Brian Cregin, Chief Financial Officer

Formerly known as NYSARC, The Arc's goal is to improve the quality of life for people with intellectual and other developmental disabilities by providing support, information, direction, and services; to have one of the best service delivery systems in the nation, including family members, self-advocates, and professionals in all matters; and to continually build training and educational opportunities into all aspects of The Arc New York.

Year Founded: 1949

1817 The Center for Family Support
2811 Zulette Avenue
Bronx, NY 10461
718-518-1500; *Fax:* 718-518-8200
www.www.cfsny.org/

Steven Vernikoff, Executive Director
Barbara Greenwald, Associate Executive Director
Lloyd Stabiner, President
Amy Bittinger, Vice President

The Center is committed to providing support and assistance to individuals with developmental and related disabilities, and to the family members who care for them. The Center supports individuals to live the lives they want; respects diversity, individual choice, and overall family needs; provides families with the support they need at all stages of life; involves individuals in the communities; and delivers excellent, individualized support to all.

Year Founded: 1954

1818 The Center for Workplace Mental Health
c/o American Psychiatric Foundation
800 Maine Avenue SW
Suite 900
Washington, DC 20024
202-559-3900
econnors@psych.org
www.workplacementalhealth.org

Darcy Gruttadaro, JD, Director
Ewuria Darley, MS, Associate Director

The Center works with businesses to ensure that employees and their families living with mental illness, including substance use disorders, receive effective care. It does so in recognition that employers purchase healthcare for millions of American workers and their families.

1819 The SickKids Centre for Community Mental Health
440 Jarvis Street
Toronto, ON M4Y 2H4,
416-924-1164
855-944-4673; *Fax:* 416-924-8208
info@sickkidscmh.ca
www.www.hincksdellcrest.org/

Dr. Michael Apkon, President and Chair
Christina Bartha, Executive Director
Dr. Diane Philipp, Acting Medical Director
Neil Carson, Clinical Director

A nonprofit children's mental health centre providing mental health services to infants, children, youth, and families. Formerly known as The Hincks-Dellcrest Centre, the SickKids Center provides prevention, intervention, outpatient, and residential treatment programs; assists with the education and training of mental health clinicians and managers; conducts research and develops and evaluates new methods for treatment; and increases awareness of the issues surrounding children's mental health. CCMH seeks to eradicate the stigma about mental illness and to promote social, emotional, and behavioral health in children and families.

Year Founded: 1998

1820 The World Bank Group
1818 H Street NW
Washington, DC 20433
202-473-1000
www.www.worldbank.org

Jim Yong Kim, President
Joaquim Levy, Chief Financial Officer
Kristalina Georgieva, Chief Executive Officer
Shaolin Yang, Chief Administrative Officer

The World Bank helps develop low and middle income countries to improve peoples health and to guard against the poverty that can result from sudden illness, including mental disorders.

Year Founded: 1944

1821 Thresholds
4101 N. Ravenswood Avenue
Chicago, IL 60613
773-572-5500
contact@thresholds.org
www.thresholds.org

Dan Klaff, President
Mark Ishaug, MA, Chief Executive Officer
Debbie Pavick, LCSW, Chief Clinical Officer
Mark Furlong, LCSW, Chief Operating Officer

Thresholds is an organization that serves people with severe and persistent mental illness with a range of programs designed with the individual's recovery as a goal. Strong leadership, an enduring vision, and a solid belief in the resilience and value of all individuals has made Thresholds one of the nation's most successful and respected provider of services for people with severe mental illness. Their goal is to help those with mental illness reclaim their lives through care, employment, advocacy, and housing.

Year Founded: 1959

1822 VOR
836 S. Arlington Heights Road
Suite 351
Elk Grove Village, IL 60007
Fax: 877-866-8377
info@vor.net
www.vor.net

Joanne St. Amand, President
Hugo Dwyer, Executive Director
Mary Vitale, Vice President
Larry Innis, Treasurer

Through national programs, VOR achieves its mission to unite advocates, as well as educate and assist families, organizations, public officials, and individuals concerned with the quality of life and choice for persons with intellectual disabilities within a full array of residential options, including community and facility-based care. VOR is the only national organization to advocate for a full range of quality residential options and services, including own home, family home, community-based service options. VOR advocates for the right of individuals with intellectual/developmental disabilities and their right to choose what is best for them.

Year Founded: 1983

1823 Willowglen Academy-Wisconsin, Inc.
5151 West Silver Spring Drive
Milwaukee, WI 53218
414-527-6940
contactWI@phoenixcaresystems.com
www.willowglen-academy.com/wisconsin

Julia Warzynski, Associate Executive Director
Jessica Zoch, Associate Executive Director

As a wholly owned subsidiary of Phoenix Care Systems, Inc., Willowglen Academy provides therapeutic residential treatment and educational services to children, adolescents, and young adults with mental health, emotional, cognitive, and developmental disabilities. Our accrediting bodies include COA, CARF, and JCAHO.

Year Founded: 1972

1824 World Federation for Mental Health
PO BOX 807
Occoquan, VA 22125
E-mail: info@wfmh.com

Alberto Trimboli, President
Prof. Abd Malak, VP, Program Development
Yoram Cohen, Corporate Secretary
Janet Paleo, Treasurer

An international organization to advance the prevention of mental and emotional disorders, the proper treatment and care of those with such disorders, and the promotion of mental health. The Federation has responded to international mental health crises through its role as the only worldwide grassroots advocacy and public education organization in the mental health field. The organization's broad and diverse membership makes possible collaboration among governments and non-governmental organizations to advance the cause of mental health services, research, and policy advocacy worldwide.

Year Founded: 1948

1825 Young Adult Institute and Workshop (YAI)
460 West 34th Street
11th Floor
New York, NY 10001-2382
212-273-6100
www.yai.org

George Contos, Chief Executive Officer
Jeffrey A. Lewis, Chairman
Lewis A. Lindenberg, Esq., Vice Chair
Kevin Hogan, Treasurer

Serves more than 20,000 people of all ages and levels of mental, developmental, and learning disabilities. Provides a full range of early intervention, preschool, family supports, employment training and placement, clinical and residential services, as well as recreation and camping services. YAI/National Intitute for People with Disabilities is also a professional organization, nationally renowned for its publications, conferences, training seminars, video training tapes, and innovative television programs.

Year Founded: 1957

1826 ZERO TO THREE: National Center for Infants, Toddlers, and Families
1255 23rd Street Northwest
Suite 350
Washington, DC 20037
202-638-1144
800-899-4301
www.zerotothree.org

Brenda Jones Harden, President
Matthew Melmed, Executive Director
Paul Spicer, Vice President
Laura Shiflett, Chief Financial Officer

A national, nonprofit organization that provides information and resources on early development to parents, professionals, and policymakers. Zero to Three's mission is to improve the lives of infants and toddlers, and to promote their health and development. Publishes books and pamphlets on the social and emotional development of infants, toddlers, and their families. Produces the Zero to Three journal, a professional publication. Sponsors the National Training Institute, an annual professional training conference in December, and offers a fellowship program.

Year Founded: 1977

State

Alabama

1827 Horizons School
2018 15th Avenue South
Birmingham, AL 35205
205-322-6606
800-822-6242; *Fax:* 205-322-6605
www.horizonsschool.org

Don Lutomski, President
Brian Geiger, EdD, Executive Director
Karen Dixon, PhD, Assistant Director
Anita Bosley, Manager of Development

The Horizons School provides a non-degree transition program designed to help students with specific learning disabilities and other mild learning problems develop the skills necessary to become independent, productive individuals. Classes teach life skills, social skills and career

training. The program aims to prepare students for successful transitions to the community.

Year Founded: 1991

1828 Mental Health Center of North Central Alabama
1316 Somerville Road Southeast
Suite 1
Decatur, AL 35601
256-355-5904
800-365-6008
www.mhcnca.org

William Hudson, President
John King, Vice President
Blythe Bowman, Secretary
Franklin Penn, Treasurer

Non-profit organization serving Lawrence, Limestone and Morgan counties. Provides treatment, education and assistance services and programs for people affected by mental health problems.

Year Founded: 1967

1829 NAMI Alabama (National Alliance on Mental Illness)
1401 I-85 Parkway
Suite A
Montgomery, AL 36106-2861
334-396-4797
800-626-4199; *Fax:* 334-396-4794
wlaird@namialabama.org
www.namialabama.org

James Walsh, President
Joan Elder, First Vice President
Shannon Weston, Second Vice President
Joel Willis, Treasurer

NAMI Alabama is a non-profit organization of local support and advocacy groups committed to improving the treatment and care available to persons diagnosed with a mental illness in Alabama. NAMI Alabama aims to enhance the quality of life for Alabamians with mental health needs.

Year Founded: 1979

Alaska

1830 Alaska Association for Infant and Early Childhood Mental Health
PO Box 81728
Fairbanks, AK 99708
E-mail: alaska.aimh@gmail.com
www.akaimh.org

Meghan Johnson, MS, President

Nonprofit organization of parents and professionals dedicated to supporting the healthy mental, emotional and social development of infants and young children.

Year Founded: 2009

1831 National Alliance on Mental Illness: Alaska
PO Box 201753
Anchorage, AK 99520-1753
907-277-1300
800-478-4462
alaskanami@gmail.com
www.nami.org/local-nami?state=AK

John Hartle, President
Pamela Robinson, Vice President
Avee M Evans, Secretary
Sheila Harris, Chapter Administrator

A nonprofit support, education and advocacy organization serving individuals with mental illnesses and their families and friends. Educates communities about mental illness and treatment, provides support groups, and advocates for people affected by mental illness.

Arizona

1832 Community Partners Inc.
4575 East Broadway
Tucson, AZ 85711-3509
520-325-4268
www.communitypartnersinc.org

Neal J Cash, President and CEO
Charles Andrade, BS, Chief Financial Officer
Bethanne Enoki, MA, SPHR, Chief Human Resources Officer
Edward M Gentile, DO, MBA, FAPA, Chief Medical Officer

Formerly Community Partnership of Southern Arizona, Community Partners Inc. is an organization that offers services in behavioral health care across Arizona.

Year Founded: 2013

1833 Devereux Arizona
11000 North Scottsdale Road
Scottsdale, AZ 85254
480-998-2920
800-345-1292; *Fax: 480-443-5587*
www.devereuxaz.org

Lane Barker, Executive Director
Yvette Jackson, Director of Operations
Donovan S Carman, MBA, Director of Finance
Janelle Westfall, Clinical Director

Nonprofit behavioral health organization providing clinical, educational and employment programs and services for individuals affected by learning, behavioral and emotional challenges.

Year Founded: 1967

1834 Mental Health America of Arizona
5110 North 40th Street
Suite 201
Phoenix, AZ 85018
480-982-5305
www.mhaarizona.org

Michael Shafer, Chair
Joshua Mozell, Vice Chair
Jason Bernstein, CPA, Treasurer
Kristina Sabetta, Secretary

An affiliate of Mental Health America, the organization promotes care and treatment for people with mental illness, educates Arizonans about mental health and participates in advocacy efforts, and strives for better mental health for people in Arizona.

Year Founded: 1954

1835 Mentally Ill Kids in Distress (MIKID)
7816 North 19th Avenue
Phoenix, AZ 85021

602-253-1240; *Fax: 602-840-3409*
phoenix@mikid.org
www.mikid.org

Ted Williams, President
Sue Gilbertson, Founder
Dick Geasland, LCSW, Chief Executive Officer
Bonnie Kolakowski, MBA, Chief Financial Officer

Mentally Ill Kids in Distress provides support and assistance to families in Arizona with children and youth who are struggling with behavioral problems. MIKID seeks to improve the behavioral health and wellness of youth across Arizona. Offers information centers, assistance by phone, email or in person, support groups, educational meetings, referrals to resources, and direct support services.

Year Founded: 1987

1836 National Alliance on Mental Illness: Arizona
5025 East Washington Street
Suite 112
Phoenix, AZ 85034
602-244-8166
800-626-5022; *Fax: 602-252-1349*
www.namiaz.org

Jim Dunn, Executive Director

NAMI Arizona serves as a state organization of the National Alliance on Mental Illness and is dedicated to improving the quality of life for individuals and families affected by mental illness.

Arkansas

1837 National Alliance on Mental Illness: Arkansas
1012 Autumn Road
Suite 1
Little Rock, AR 72211-3704
501-661-1548
800-844-0381; *Fax: 501-312-7540*
nami-ar@namiarkansas.org
www.namiarkansas.org

Kim Arnold, Executive Director

A non-profit organization dedicated to assisting individuals with mental illness, their families, and their communities. Formerly known as Arkansas Alliance for the Mentally Ill (AAMI), NAMI Arkansas operates across the state and provides support, education, and advocacy services through a network of local support groups.

California

1838 Assistance League of Los Angeles
826 Cole Avenue
Los Angeles, CA 90038
323-469-1973
www.assistanceleaguela.org

Andrea Goodman, President
Shelagh Callahan, Vice President
Flo Fowkes, Treasurer

Provides services to meet the physical and emotional needs of children and families. Focuses on helping children who live in poverty within Los Angeles communities through the development of programs designed to promote learning and improve self-esteem.

Year Founded: 1919

1839 California Association of Marriage and Family Therapists
7901 Raytheon Road
San Diego, CA 92111-1606
858-292-2638; *Fax:* 858-292-2666
www.camft.org

Laura Strom, LMFT, President
Jurgen Braungardt, LMFT, Chief Financial Officer
Jill Epstein, JD, Executive Director
Cathy Atkins, JD, Deputy Executive Director

Independent professional organization representing the interests of licensed marriage and family therapists. Dedicated to advancing marriage and family therapy as a mental health profession. Seeks to maintain standards of quality and ethics for the profession and to raise awareness of the profession.

88 pages 6 per year Year Founded: 2002 ISSN 1540-2770

1840 California Association of Social Rehabilitation Agencies
815 Marina Vista, Suite D
PO Box 388
Martinez, CA 94553
925-229-2300; *Fax:* 925-229-9088
casra@casra.org
www.casra.org

Betty Dahlquist, Executive Director
Debra Brasher, Director, Training and Education
Lucinda Dei Rossi, Public Policy Coordinator

Aims to improve the lives of people with psychiatric disabilities by developing mental health programs and services that promote growth and recovery, addressing legislative issues surrounding mental health services, and providing educational and training opportunities that address the importance of meeting mental health needs and social rehabilitation.

Year Founded: 1989

1841 California Health Information Association
1915 North Fine Avenue
Suite 104
Fresno, CA 93727-1565
559-251-5038; *Fax:* 559-251-5836
info@californiahia.org
www.californiahia.org

Sharon Lewis,MBA,RHIA,FAHIMA, CEO and Executive Director
Deborah Collier, RHIA, President
Debi Boynton, Finance Manager
Rissa Herman, Administrative Assistant

Nonprofit association that offers education, advocacy and resources for health information management professionals in California. Members contribute to the delivery of quality patient care through the management of personal health information.

1842 California Institute for Behavioral Health Solutions
2125 19th Street
2nd Floor
Sacramento, CA 95818
916-556-3480; *Fax:* 916-556-3483
www.cibhs.org

Al Rowlett, LCSW, MBA, Chair
Sandra Naylor Goodwin, PhD, President and CEO

Percy Howard III, LCSW, Chief Program Officer
Gail Leslie Zwier-Villanueva, PhD, Treasurer

Nonprofit agency that assists professionals and agencies with improving the lives of individuals struggling with mental illness and substance use problems through training, technical assistance, research and policy development.

1843 California Psychiatric Association (CPA)
921 11th Street
Suite 502
Sacramento, CA 95814
916-442-5196; *Fax:* 916-442-6515
calpsych@calpsych.org
www.calpsych.org

Lila Schmall, Executive Director
Randall Hagar, Director of Government Affairs

Non-profit organization representing psychiatrists who specialize in the care of patients with mental and emotional disorders. The California Psychiatric Association advocates for access to quality care, educates the public about psychiatry, and provides news and information on mental health issues. CPA is area six of the American Psychiatric Association, and is composed of members of APA's five district branches in California.

1844 California Psychological Association
1231 I Street
Suite 204
Sacramento, CA 95814-2933
916-286-7979; *Fax:* 916-286-7971
membership@cpapsych.org
www.cpapsych.org

Jo Linder-Crow, Chief Executive Officer
Jorge Wong, PhD, President
Patricia Van Woerkom, Director, Administration
Pat Jaspin, Director, Accounting

A non-profit professional association for licensed psychologists in California. Provides support for psychologists by educating the public about psychological services, engaging in legislative advocacy, and promoting training, education and research in the field of psychology.

Year Founded: 1948

1845 Calnet
3625 East Thousand Oaks Boulevard
Suite 128
Westlake Village, CA 91362
805-778-0055; *Fax:* 805-778-0054
www.calnetcare.com

Craig Lambdin, Chairman
Cary Quashen, Vice Chairman of the Board
Steven Wright, Secretary and Treasurer
Bill Redder, Director

A not-for-profit network serving to bring mental health and chemical dependency treatment providers together with managed care organizations for business opportunities.

Year Founded: 1983

1846 Filipino American Service Group
135 North Park View Street
Los Angeles, CA 90026-5215
213-487-9804
www.fasgi.org

Cris B Liban, PE, Chairman
Allison Aquino-Silva, Vice Chairman

Rafael Bernardino Jr, Secretary
Bruce Brown, Treasurer

Filipino American Service Group focuses on improving the physical and mental well-being of mentally ill, homeless, and/or low income individuals in Los Angeles. Provides independent health and social services. Aims to help enhance the quality of life for members of the community in Historic Filipinotown and the Greater Los Angeles area.

Year Founded: 1981

1847 Five Acres: Boys and Girls Aid Society of Los Angeles County

760 West Mountain View Street
Altadena, CA 91001-4925
626-798-6793
800-696-6793
wecanhelp@5acres.org
www.5acres.org

John Reith, Chairman
Rustin Mork, Vice Chair
Christianne Kerns, Vice Chair
Chanel Boutakidis, Chief Executive Officer

Serves to prevent child abuse and neglect, and connect children to safe and loving families. Develops support services and outreach programs to help treat and educate abused and neglected children, conducts research and promotes evidence-based treatment, engages in advocacy, and provides educational resources to family, professionals and the community on the prevention of child abuse and neglect.

Year Founded: 1888

1848 Health Services Agency: Behavioral Health

1080 Emeline Avenue
Santa Cruz, CA 95060-1966
831-454-4000; *Fax:* 831-454-4488
TDD: 831-454-4123
www.santacruzhealth.org

Giang Nguyen, RN, MSN, Agency Director

Serves to improve and protect the public health of Santa Cruz County and to ensure access to quality health care and treatment for residents. The Health Services Agency develops programs and services in mental health, as well as environmental health, public health, medical care, and substance abuse prevention and treatment. The HSA advocates for public health policy and seeks to eliminate the stigma associated with mental illness and other diseases.

1849 National Alliance on Mental Illness: California

1851 Heritage Lane
Suite 150
Sacramento, CA 95815
916-567-0163; *Fax:* 916-567-1757
nami.california@namica.org
www.namica.org

Sergio Aguilar-Gaxiola, President
Jessica Cruz, Executive Director
Steven Kite, Deputy Director
Frank Ruz, Accounts Manager

Grassroots organization providing support for individuals and families affected by mental illness through advocacy, legislation, education and policy development. Seeks to combat discrimination and stigma associated with mental illness and advocates for respect and equality for those with mental health needs.

1850 National Alliance on Mental Illness: Gold Country

PO Box 1088
Angels Camp, CA 95222-1088
209-736-4264; *Fax:* 209-736-4264
www.nami.org

Marilyn Ricci, MS, RD, President

Local chapter of the National Alliance on Mental Illness, an organization dedicated to raising awareness on mental health and providing support and education for Americans affected by mental illness. Mission is to help consumers and families share information about services, care providers, and ways to cope with the challenges of mental illness.

1851 National Health Foundation

515 South Figueroa Street
Suite 1300
Los Angeles, CA 90071
213-538-0700; *Fax:* 213-629-4272
www.nhfca.org

Kelly Bruno, MSW, President and CEO
Danielle Cameron, MPH, Chief Strategy Officer
Mia Arias, MPA, Director of Programs
Gwen Edwards, MBA, Secretary

Public charity whose mission is to improve the healthcare available to underserved groups through the development, support and provision of programs that address the systemic barriers in healthcare access and delivery.

1852 Orange County Psychiatric Society

17322 Murphy Avenue
Irvine, CA 92614
949-250-3157; *Fax:* 949-398-8120
www.ocps.org

Brenda Jensen, MD, President
Yujuan Choy, MD, Secretary
David Safani, MD, Treasurer

Works to promote public awareness of mental health and improve care for people affected by mental illness.

1853 UCLA Department of Psychiatry & Biobehavioral Sciences

760 Westwood Plaza
Los Angeles, CA 90095
310-825-0511
www.psychiatry.ucla.edu

Peter Whybrow, Director

Programs for clinical research on the causes of and treatments for psychiatric and behavioral disorders in adults and children.

1854 United Advocates for Children and Families

2035 Hurley Way
Suite 290
Sacramento, CA 95825
916-643-1530; *Fax:* 916-643-1592
TTY: 916-643-1532
www.uacf4hope.org

Dr Oscar Wright, Chief Executive Officer
Elisa Gonzalez, President
Mary Jane Gross, Treasurer
Errol Campbell, Secretary

A nonprofit organization that works on behalf of children and youth with mental, emotional, and behavioral challenges and their families.

Year Founded: 1993

Colorado

1855 CAFCA
1120 Lincoln Street
Suite 701
Denver, CO 80203-2137
720-570-8402; *Fax:* 720-570-8408
info@cafca.net
www.cafca.net

Bentley Smith, President
Skip Barber, Executive Director
Monica Mendoza, Executive Assistant Director

Provides agencies dedicated to helping Colorado's vulnerable children with research, education and training. The services provided by member agencies include: adoption, alcohol and drug treatment, day treatment, education, family support and preservation, foster care, group homes, independent living, kinship care, mental health treatment and counseling, pregnancy counseling, residential care at all levels, services for homeless and runaway youth, services for sexually reactive youth, sexual abuse services and transitional living.

1856 CHINS UP Youth and Family Services
Griffith Centers for Children
10 North Farragut Avenue
Colorado Springs, CO 80909
719-636-2122; *Fax:* 719-634-0482
info@griffithcenters.org
www.griffithcenters.org

Barbara B Ritchie, President and CEO
Ken Lingle, Chief Operating Officer
Sue Johnson, Director of Finance
Christina Murphy, Director of Business Development

A division of The Griffith Centers for Children, Chins Up is a nonprofit multi-service agency serving Colorado Springs children and adolescents with emotional or behavioral problems, as well as children who were victims of abuse. Chins Up provides community-based programs and services with the hope of healing the broken lives of children and families.

Year Founded: 1974

1857 Colorado Health Partnerships
9925 Federal Drive
Suite 100
Colorado Springs, CO 80921
800-804-5040
800-804-5008
www.coloradohealthpartnerships.com

Myron Unruh, Market President
Dr Lisa Clements, Vice President of Transformation

Comprised of partnerships between ValueOptions (now Beacon Health Options) and eight community mental health centers. Provides mental health services to Medicaid eligible individuals in southern and Western Colorado.

Year Founded: 1995

1858 Federation of Families for Children's Mental Health: Colorado Chapter
7475 West Fifth Avenue
Suite 307
Lakewood, CO 80226
303-893-7984
844-252-8202
www.coloradofederation.org

Sarah Davidon, President and Chair
Randy Garfield, Vice President
Jane Thomas, Secretary
Ian Andersen, Treasurer

Advocates for children, youth, and families affected by mental illness and aims to improve mental health programs, services, and policies in Colorado.

1859 Mental Health America of Colorado
1120 Lincoln Street
Suite 1606
Denver, CO 80203
720-208-2220
800-456-3249
www.mhacolorado.org

Andrew Romanoff, President and CEO
Laura Cordes, VP of External Affairs and COO
Moe Keller, VP of Public Policy
Jon Monteith, Communications Director

Nonprofit organization serving to address mental health issues in Colorado. Strives for the intervention, treatment, and prevention of mental illness and substance use disorders. Seeks to improve diagnosis, care, and quality of life for people with mental health needs.

Year Founded: 1953

1860 National Alliance on Mental Illness: Colorado
2280 South Albion Street
Denver, CO 80222
303-321-3104
888-566-6264; *Fax:* 303-321-0912
admin@namicolorado.org
www.namicolorado.org

Sherry Stevens, President
Scott Glaser, Executive Director
Cheri Bishop, Director of Education Programs
Elsa Erickson, Director of Communications

Grassroots organization providing support for individuals and families affected by mental illness through advocacy, legislation, education and policy development.

Connecticut

1861 Joshua Center Programs
Natchaug Hospital
189 Storrs Road
Mansfield Center, CT 06250-1683
860-456-1311
800-426-7792
www.natchaug.org

Brett Carra, Director

The Joshua Center Programs at Natchaug Hospital provide a range of services designed to treat children and adolescents who are struggling with emotional and behavioral problems, including mental illness, emotional trauma, and substance abuse. Intensive, structured treatment programs include group therapy, psycho-education, individual and family treatment, and medication management. Programs utilize a positive approach with the goal of maintaining recovery. Treatment programs offered with Joshua Centers include: Partial Hospital Program, Intensive Outpatient Program, and Extended Day Program. Natchaug Hospital provides Joshua Center programs at seven locations throughout Connecticut.

Year Founded: 1989

1862 National Alliance on Mental Illness: Connecticut
576 Farmington Avenue
Hartford, CT 06105
860-882-0236
800-215-3021; *Fax: 860-882-0240*
namicted@namict.org
www.namict.org

Marisa Walls, President
Kate Mattias, MPH, JD, Executive Director
Daniela Giordano, MSW, Public Policy Director
Paloma Bayona, Program Director

NAMI Connecticut is an affiliate of the National Alliance on Mental Illness, a grassroots organization providing support for individuals and families affected by mental illness. NAMI Connecticut serves all people impacted by mental health conditions through support, education, and advocacy.

1863 Women's Support Services
158 Gay Street
PO Box 341
Sharon, CT 06069
860-364-1080; *Fax: 860-364-5767*
info@wssdv.org
www.wssdv.org

Maria Horn, Chair
Louisa Yap, Vice Chair
Dr D Elizabeth Mauro, Executive Director

Support and advocacy for those affected by emotional, physical, psychological, or sexual trauma in the Northwest region of Connecticut and nearby areas in New York and Massachusetts. Raises awareness on domestic abuse and seeks to engage all members of the community in the movement to end domestic violence.

Delaware

1864 Mental Health Association of Delaware
100 West 10th Street
Suite 600
Wilmington, DE 19801-6604
302-654-6833
800-287-6423
information@mhainde.org
www.mhainde.org/wp/

Lawrence G Boyer, President
James Lafferty, Executive Director
Paul E Lakeman, Vice President
Cheryl Santaniello, Treasurer

Nonprofit organization focused on improving mental health for people in Delaware through education, support, and advocacy for mental health issues.

Year Founded: 1932

1865 National Alliance on Mental Illness: Delaware
2400 West 4th Street
Wilmington, DE 19805-3306
302-427-0787
888-427-2643; *Fax: 302-427-2075*

namide@namide.org
www.namidelaware.org

Mary Berger, President
Edward M McNally, Esq., Secretary
Julius Meisel, PhD, Treasurer

A statewide organization consisting of mental health consumers, families, friends, and professionals focused on improving the quality of life for individuals with mental illness. Provides support, promotes education on mental health, and advocates for access to adequate mental health services.

1866 National Association of Social Workers: Delaware Chapter
100 West 10th Street
Suite 608
Wilmington, DE 19801
302-288-0931
www.naswde.org

Norwood James Coleman, Jr, President
Vicki Root, Vice President
Shannon Baker, Treasurer
Silja Fiona Walter, Secretary

Member organization of professional social workers serving to help with the development of its members and the practice of social work, and to assist with improving the well-being of individuals and families through work and advocacy.

District of Columbia

1867 Department of Health and Human Services/OAS
200 Independence Avenue Southwest
Washington, DC 20201
202-619-0257
877-696-6775
www.hhs.gov

Sylva Mathews Burwell, HHS Secretary
Madhura Valverde, Executive Secretary
Susannah Fox, Chief Technology Officer
William B Schultz, General Counsel

The DHHS is the United States government's principal agency for protecting the health of all Americans, providing health and human services, and supporting initiatives in medicine, public health, and social services.

Florida

1868 Family Network on Disabilities
2196 Main Street
Suite L
Dunedin, FL 34698-5694
727-523-1130
800-825-5736; *Fax: 727-523-8687*
fnd@fndusa.org
www.fndusa.org

Rich La Belle, Executive Director
Jan La Belle, Director of Programs
Jane Soltys, Director of Finance
Laura Mattson, Trust and Operations Director

Family Network on Disabilities is a grassroots organization for individuals with disabilities or special needs and their families, as well as professionals and concerned citizens. FND seeks to assist families affected by disabilities through support services and the sharing of information. FND strives to eradicate systemic barriers and to work towards inclusion and equality of people with disabilities. FND organizes a number of programs in Florida, including the Parent Education Network, Family STAR (Support, Training, Assistance, Resources), and the Youth Advocacy and Action Project.

Year Founded: 1985

1869 Federation of Families of Central Florida
National Federation of Families for Children's Mental Health
237 Fernwood Boulevard
Suite 101
Fern Park, FL 32730
407-334-8049
info.ffcfl@gmail.com
www.ffcflinc.org

Muriel Jones, Executive Director

An affiliate of the National Federation of Families for Children's Mental Health, the Federation of Families of Central Florida serves children and youth with emotional, behavioral, and mental health challenges and their families through advocacy, support, and education.

1870 Florida Alcohol and Drug Abuse Association
2868 Mahan Drive
Suite 1
Tallahassee, FL 32308
850-878-2196; *Fax:* 850-878-6584
fadaa@fadaa.org
www.fadaa.org

Frank Rabbito, President
Mark Fontaine,MSW,CAP, Executive Director
Laureen Pagel, Vice President
Angie Durbin, Director of Finance and HR

Statewide membership organization that represents more than 100 community-based substance abuse treatment and prevention agencies throughout Florida. FADAA supports providers and programs dedicated to the advancement of substance abuse treatment, prevention, and research, and has provided advocacy for substance abuse policies and related practice improvement.

Year Founded: 1981

1871 Florida Health Care Association
307 West Park Avenue
PO Box 1459
Tallahassee, FL 32301-1457
850-224-3907; *Fax:* 850-681-2075
www.fhca.org

Joe Mitchell, President
J Emmett Reed, CAE, Executive Director
Kristen Knapp, APR, CAE, Director of Communications
Tom Parker, Director of Reimbursement

FHCA is dedicated to providing the highest quality care for elderly, chronically ill, and disabled individuals in Florida.

Year Founded: 1954

1872 Mental Health Association of West Florida
840 West Lakeview Avenue
Pensacola, FL 32501-1967
850-438-9879; *Fax:* 850-438-5901
www.mhawfl.org

Offers support services, advocacy, information and referrals for individuals and families affected by mental illness.

Year Founded: 1957

1873 National Alliance on Mental Illness: Florida
PO Box 961
Tallahassee, FL 32302
850-671-4445
877-626-4352; *Fax:* 850-671-5272
info@namiflorida.org
www.namiflorida.org

Dr. Rajiv Tandon, President
Carol Weber, Program Director
Diana Williams, Treasurer
Stephen Thompson, Consumer Council Chair

Contains thirty-six affiliates in communities throughout Florida that provide education, advocacy, and support groups for individuals and families affected by mental illness. Seeks to help persons with mental health needs become productive members of the community.

Year Founded: 1984

1874 National Association of Social Workers Florida Chapter
1931 Dellwood Drive
Tallahassee, FL 32303-4815
850-224-2400
800-352-6279; *Fax:* 850-561-6279
naswfl@naswfl.org
www.naswfl.org

Billy Spivey, LCSW, ACSW, President
Tara Moser, LCSW, RPT-S, Vice President
Paula Lupton, LCSW, Secretary
Tanya Fookes, LCSW, ACSW, Treasurer

NASW Florida is a membership organization for professional social workers in Florida. NASWFL provides: continuing education, information and resources, and advocacy for employment and legislation.

Georgia

1875 Georgia Parent Support Network
1381 Metropolitan Parkway
Atlanta, GA 30310-4455
404-758-4500
800-832-8645; *Fax:* 404-758-6833
info@gpsn.org
www.gpsn.org

Kathy Dennis, President
Sue L Smith, EdD, Chief Executive Officer
Brett Barton, LPC, Chief Operating Officer
Linda Seay, Treasurer

The Georgia Parent Support Network assists children with mental, emotional, and behavioral challenges and their families through support, education, and advocacy.

1876 Grady Health Systems: Behavioral Health Services
10 Park Place
Atlanta, GA 30303
404-616-4444
www.gradyhealth.org

John Haupert, CEO
Mark Meyer, EVP and CFO

Grady Behavioral Health Services focuses on the treatment of individuals with chronic and mental illnesses in Fulton and DeKalb counties and strives to offer quality, evidence-based mental health and substance abuse care for clients. Grady provides a full range of adult behavioral health services, including peer support, individual and group treatment, and medication clinics, and conducts research with the goal of advancing the treatment of clients with trauma and mental illness.

Year Founded: 1892

1877 National Alliance on Mental Illness: Georgia
3180 Presidential Drive
Suite A
Atlanta, GA 30340-3916
770-234-0855
800-728-1052; *Fax:* 770-234-0237
namigeorgia@namiga.org
www.namiga.org

Faye Taylor, President
Kim H Jones, Executive Director
Viktoria Varnado-Wooten, Interim Program Coordinator
Pat Strode, CIT Administrator

The mission of NAMI Georgia is to enhance the quality of life for Georgians with mental illness and their families through support, education, and the promotion of policies that work to improve the resources, services, and treatments available to mentally ill persons.

1878 Together Georgia
50 Hurt Plaza
Suite 1555
Atlanta, GA 30303
404-572-6170; *Fax:* 404-572-6171
www.togetherga.net

Ron Scroggy, Executive Director
Carolyn Fjeran, Deputy Director

Together Georgia, formerly the Georgia Association of Homes and Services for Children, is an organization consisting of child and family service providers dedicated to caring for children who have experienced risk and neglect. Together Georgia provides staff training and information, organizes regular meetings for members, and strives for a positive future for Georgia's children and families.

Hawaii

1879 Hawaii Families As Allies
99-209 Moanalua Road
Suite 305
Aiea, HI 96701
808-487-8785
866-361-8825; *Fax:* 808-487-0514
hfaa@hfaa.net

Shanelle Lum, Public Policy Specialist

Support and outreach group for parents with children who have mental disorders.

1880 National Alliance on Mental Illness: Hawaii
770 Kapiolani Boulevard
Suite 613
Honolulu, HI 96813-5212
808-591-1297; *Fax:* 808-591-2058
info@namihawaii.org
www.namihawaii.org

Mike Durant, President
Steven Katz, First Vice President
Robert Collesano, Second Vice President
Dana Anderson, Secretary

Organization providing support for individuals and families affected by mental illness through support, advocacy and education. Seeks to raise awareness on mental health issues and combat the stigmatization of mental illness.

Idaho

1881 National Alliance on Mental Illness: Idaho
PO Box 95
Hailey, ID 83333
208-242-7430
idahonami@gmail.com
www.idahonami.org

Mike Sandvig, President
Kathie Garrett, Vice President
Sharlisa Davis, Treasurer
Catherine Perusse, Secretary

Nationwide organization dedicated to serving people with mental illness and their families through support, advocacy, research and education.

Year Founded: 1991

Illinois

1882 Allendale Association
PO Box 1088
Lake Villa, IL 60046-1088
847-356-2351
888-255-3631; *Fax:* 847-356-0289
www.allendale4kids.org

Connie Borucki, Senior VP, Human Resources
Sue Gaddy, Associate VP, Communications
Dr. Sandra EJ Clavelli, Director of Clinical Training
Judy Griffeth, Placement Director

The Allendale Association is a private, non-profit organization committed to providing quality care, education, treatment, support, and advocacy for troubled children in need of intervention and their families.

Year Founded: 1897

1883 Baby Fold
108 East Willow Street
Normal, IL 61761
309-454-1770; *Fax:* 309-452-0115
www.thebabyfold.org

Julie Dobski, Chair
Dianne Schultz, President and CEO
Debi Armstrong, VP of Information Systems
Jennifer Keen, VP of Finance and Facility

The Baby Fold is an Illinois-based multi-service agency that provides residential, special education, child welfare, and family support services to children with emotional and behavioral disabilities and autism spectrum disorders, as well as at-risk children.

Year Founded: 1902

1884 Chaddock
205 South 24th Street
Quincy, IL 62301-4492

217-222-0034
888-242-3625; *Fax:* 217-222-3865
www.chaddock.org

Debbie Reed, President and CEO
Kristen Patton, Director of Finance
Amy Hyer, Director of Human Resources
Matt Obert, Director of Operations

A faith-based, not-for-profit organization dedicated to supporting children and families and providing hope and healing. Chaddock offers educational and treatment services for children who have experienced abuse, neglect, or trauma, including child and adolescent residential treatment, independent living and group home programs, special education school, in-home intensive program, and foster care and adoption services.

Year Founded: 1853

1885 Chicago Child Care Society

5467 South University Avenue
Chicago, IL 60615-5193
773-643-0452; *Fax:* 773-643-0620
www.cccsociety.org

Dara T Munson, MPA, Chief Executive Officer
Julia Beringer, President
Robert Lindstrom, Vice President
Curt Holderfield, LCSW, Associate Director

Chicago Child Care Society strives to meet the needs of vulnerable children and their families through the provision of community-based education and social service programs. CCCS provides vulnerable children with services and opportunities designed to help enable their physical, mental, and social development. CCCS programs focus on a range of issues, including teen pregnancy, poverty, and inadequate child healthcare. The Chicago Child Care Society was founded in 1849 and is the oldest child welfare agency in Illinois.

Year Founded: 1849

1886 Children's Home Association of Illinois

2130 North Knoxville Avenue
Peoria, IL 61603-2497
309-685-1047; *Fax:* 309-687-7299
www.chail.org

Matt George, Chief Executive Officer
Melissa Riddle, President and CFO
Cindy Hoffman, Executive Vice President
Tegan Camden, VP, Behavioral Health

Not-for-profit, multiple program and social service organization dedicated to providing community-based counseling, education and support programs for children and families in the Peoria area.

1887 Coalition of Illinois Counselor Organizations

PO Box 1086
Northbrook, IL 60065-1086
815-787-0515
myimhca@gmail.com
www.cico-il.org

Daniel Stasi, Executive Director

The Coalition of Illinois Counselor Organizations represents and advocates for counselors and psychologists and their clients in Illinois, with focus on government branches and agencies, relevant segments of the private sector, and mental health organizations.

1888 Family Service Association of Greater Elgin Area

1140 North McLean Boulevard
Suite 1
Elgin, IL 60123
847-695-3680; *Fax:* 847-695-4552
www.fsaelgin.org

Lisa La Forge, Executive Director
Amanda Rankin, Director of Crisis Services
Bernadette May, Associate Director
Martine Lyle, Supervisor of Crisis Services

A private, non-profit agency, Family Service Association has served children, adolescents, and adults in the Greater Elgin area since 1931. The Family Service Association provides a range of counseling services and programs, including family support, outpatient therapy, school-based therapy and screening assessments.

Year Founded: 1931

1889 Human Resources Development Institute

222 South Jefferson Street
Chicago, IL 60661-5603
312-441-9009
info@hrdi.org
www.hrdi.org

Joel K Johnson, President and CEO
Evelyn Willis, MBA, CPA, Chief Financial Officer
Kerri Brown, Esq., Chief Administrative Officer

Community-based behavioral healthcare organization. Human Resources Development Institute seeks to provide quality community and behavioral health care services and programs in the areas of mental health, disabilities, alcohol and substance abuse, family services, community health, and youth prevention.

Year Founded: 1974

1890 Illinois Alcoholism and Drug Dependence Association

937 South Second Street
Springfield, IL 62704-2701
217-528-7335; *Fax:* 217-528-7340
iadda@iadda.org
www.iadda.org

Mary Beth Sheets, Chair
Sara Moscato Howe, Chief Executive Officer
Eric Foster, Chief Operating Officer
Jessica Hayes, Treasurer

The Illinois Alcoholism and Drug Dependence Association represents over 50 substance abuse and mental health prevention and treatment agencies, as well as individual members who are interested in the field of substance abuse. IADDA advocates for sound public policies that address behavioral health issues. The goal of the IADDA is to work towards a healthier society with accessibility to mental health and addiction treatments, and reduced occurrences in substance use and mental disorders.

Year Founded: 1967

1891 Little City Foundation (LCF)

650 East Algonquin Road
Schaumburg, IL 60173
847-358-5510; *Fax:* 847-358-3291
www.littlecity.org

Shawn E Jeffers, Executive Director
Kim Tyler, Chief Financial Officer

Edward J Hockfield, Chief Development Officer
Larry Heisler, Chief Marketing Officer

The mission of Little City Foundation is to provide quality services for children and adults with intellectual and developmental disabilities and to offer opportunities that will enable them to lead productive and fulfilling lives.

1892 Mental Health America of Illinois
1103 Westgate
Suite 302
Oak Park, IL 60301
312-368-9070; *Fax:* 312-368-0283
www.mhai.org

Joyce Gallagher, President
Ray Connor, Co-Vice President
Joseph Troiani, PhD, CADC, Co-Vice President
Phillip Hall, Treasurer and CFO

Promotes mental health, works towards the prevention of mental illness and addictions, and seeks to improve access to high quality care for all persons with mental and emotional challenges. Mental Health America of Illinois focuses on providing education, advocacy, and services for those with mental health needs.

Year Founded: 1909

1893 Metropolitan Family Services
One North Dearborn
Suite 1000
Chicago, IL 60602
312-986-4000; *Fax:* 312-986-4289
contactus@metrofamily.org
www.metrofamily.org

John L MacCarthy, Chair
Ricardo Estrada, President and CEO
Colleen M Jones, Executive VP and COO
Denis Hurley, Chief Financial Officer

Metropolitan Family Services provides programs and services designed to help families across Chicago, DuPage County, Evanston/Skokie and the southwest suburbs achieve stability and self-sufficiency.

Year Founded: 1857

1894 National Alliance on Mental Illness: Illinois
218 West Lawrence
Springfield, IL 62704-2612
217-522-1403
800-346-4572; *Fax:* 217-522-3598
namiil@sbcglobal.net
www.namiillinois.org

John Schladweiler, President
Suzanne Spears, Vice President
Lisa Guardiola, Secretary
Bob Barger, Treasurer

A statewide, not-for-profit organization comprised of local Illinois affiliates dedicated to improving the lives of individuals and families affected by mental illness. NAMI Illinois provides education and support programs and raises awareness on the issues surrounding mental health.

Indiana

1895 Indiana Resource Center for Autism (IRCA)
1905 North Range Road
Bloomington, IN 47408-9801

812-855-6508
800-825-4733; *Fax:* 812-855-9630
TTY: 812-855-9396
prattc@indiana.edu
www.iidc.indiana.edu/pages/irca

Cathy Pratt, PhD, BCBA, Center Director
Pamela Anderson, Outreach/Resource Specialist
Catherine Davies, MEd, MSC, LMHC, Educational Consultant

The Indiana Resource Center for Autism focuses on providing communities, organizations, and families with the information and skills to support children and individuals with autism, Asperger's syndrome, and other pervasive developmental disorders. The IRCA conducts outreach training and research, disseminates information about autism spectrum disorders, and encourages communication among professionals and families concerned with autism.

1896 National Alliance on Mental Illness: Indiana
PO Box 22697
Indianapolis, IN 46222
317-925-9399
800-677-6442; *Fax:* 317-925-9398
info@namiindiana.org
www.namiindiana.org

Joshua G. Sprunger, MA, Executive Director
Joanne Abbott, ASN, Program Director
Marianne Halbert, JD, Criminal Justice Director
Linda Williams, Program Coordinator

Statewide grassroots public charity dedicated to improving the quality of life for individuals and families affected by mental illness.

Iowa

1897 Iowa Federation of Families for Children's Mental Health
106 South Booth
PO Box 362
Anamosa, IA 52205
319-462-2187
888-400-6302; *Fax:* 319-462-6789
www.iffcmh.org

Lori Reynolds, Executive Director
Heidi Reynolds, Program Director

Iowa Federation of Families for Children's Mental Health provides support and assistance to parents of children who have emotional or behavioral disorders, are receiving mental health or special education services, or are in the juvenile justice system. Mission is to work towards a system that will allow families to live in safe and stable environments.

1898 National Alliance on Mental Illness: Iowa
3839 Merle Hay Road
Suite 226
Des Moines, IA 50310
515-254-0417
800-417-0417; *Fax:* 515-254-0417
www.namiiowa.com

Jim Rixner, President
Nancy Hale, Executive Director
Ed Arnold, Treasurer
John Rowley, Administrative Assistant

Statewide grassroots organization providing support for individuals, families, and friends affected by mental illness. NAMI Iowa's mission is to promote public awareness and research about mental illness, improve treatment, and advance the system of care in Iowa.

Year Founded: 1984

Kansas

1899 Keys for Networking: Kansas Parent Information & Resource Center

900 South Kansas Avenue
Suite 301
Topeka, KS 66612
785-233-8732
800-499-8732; *Fax: 785-235-6659*

Mary Ellen Conlee, President
Greg Whittaker, Treasurer
Juan Perez, Secretary
Cheryl Renolds-Buckley, Secretary

A non-profit organization offering assistance to families in Kansas whose children have behavioral, educational, emotional, and substance abuse challenges. Mission is to provide parents and youth in Kansas with services, information, resources, support, education, and training.

1900 National Alliance on Mental Illness: Kansas

610 Southwest 10th Avenue
Suite 203
Topeka, KS 66612-1674
800-539-2660; *Fax: 785-233-4804*
info@namiKansas.org
www.namikansas.org

Rick Cagan, Executive Director
Lindsey Spooner-Gabaldon, Program Manager

Statewide organization of the National Alliance on Mental Illness, an organization providing support for individuals and families affected by mental illness. Mission is to provide peer support, education, advocacy, and research and to improve the quality of life for people with mental disorders and their families.

Kentucky

1901 Beacon Health Options

240 Corporate Boulevard
Norfolk, VA 23502
757-459-5100
www.beaconhealthoptions.com

Timothy Murphy, Chief Executive Officer
Bill Fandrich, Chief Operating Officer
Brian Wheelan, EVP and Chief Strategy Officer
Dr Hal Levine, EVP and Chief Medical Officer

Beacon Health Options combines two behavioral health companies, Beacon Health Strategies and ValueOptions. Seeks to improve the quality and delivery of behavioral health care for regional health plans, employers, and federal, state and local governments. Provides behavioral health care services and programs in employee assistance and work and life support.

1902 Children's Alliance

420 Capital Avenue
Frankfort, KY 40601
502-875-3399; *Fax: 502-223-4200*
www.childrensallianceky.org

Jeff Choate, Chair
Michelle Sanborn, President
Melissa Muse, Director of Member Services
Kathy Adams, Director of Public Policy

Mission is to enhance the well-being of at-risk children and families in Kentucky. Engages in public policy advocacy and promotes the provision of quality and effective services to children and families.

Year Founded: 1961

1903 KY-SPIN (Kentucky Special Parent Involvement Network)

10301-B Deering Road
Louisville, KY 40272-4000
502-937-6894
800-525-7746; *Fax: 502-937-6464*
spininc@kyspin.com
www.kyspin.com

Non-profit organization dedicated to helping individuals with disabilities and their families improve their quality of life through information, resources, programs, training opportunities, and support networks.

Year Founded: 1988

1904 Kentucky Partnership for Families and Children

207 Holmes Street
1st Floor
Frankfort, KY 40621
502-875-1320
800-369-0533; *Fax: 502-875-1399*
kpfc@kypartnership.org
www.kypartnership.org

Carol W Cecil, Executive Director
Brittany Roberts, Program Coordinator
Carmilla Ratliff, Youth Empowerment Specialist
Barbara Greene, Project Coordinator

Non-profit organization focused on the needs of children and youth with behavioral health challenges and their families. Works to enhance the quality of services, effect policy changes, and educate legislators about emotional disabilities in children.

1905 Kentucky Psychiatric Medical Association

649 Charity Court
Suite 13
Frankfort, KY 40601
502-695-4843; *Fax: 502-695-4441*
www.kypsych.org

Kathy M Vincent, MD, President
Bonnie Cook, Executive Director
Rebecca Tamas, MD, Treasurer
Todd R Cheever, MD, Secretary

A non-profit association of physicians specializing in the treatment of mental illnesses and substance use disorders.

1906 National Alliance on Mental Illness: Kentucky

808 Monticello Street
Building 103
Somerset, KY 42501
606-451-6935
800-257-5081; *Fax: 606-677-4050*
namiky@bellsouth.net
www.namikyadvocacy.com

Brenda Huntsman, Chair
Donia Shuhaiber, First Vice Chair
Larry Gregory, Second Vice Chair
Susan Faris, Secretary

NAMI Kentucky is a non-profit, self-help organization and the state chapter of the National Alliance on Mental Illness, an organization dedicated to improving the quality of life for mentally ill individuals and reducing the stigma associated with mental illness. NAMI Kentucky focuses on providing support, education, and advocacy for people with mental illnesses and their families.

1907 National Association of Social Workers: Kentucky Chapter
76 C Michael Davenport Boulevard
Suite 4
Frankfort, KY 40601-4390
502-352-2220
800-526-8098; *Fax:* 502-589-3602
www.naswky.com

Robyn Napier, LCSW, President
April Murphy, PhD, MSW, Treasurer
Jerry Grugin, MSW, Secretary

Membership organization representing professional social workers across Kentucky.

Louisiana

1908 Louisiana Federation of Families for Children's Mental Health
5627 Superior Drive
Suite A-2
Baton Rouge, LA 70816-6085
225-293-3508
800-224-4010; *Fax:* 225-293-3510
info@laffcmh.org
www.laffcmh.org

Anthony D Beasley, President
Megan Harrison, Vice President
Ashle Hayes, Secretary

A parent-run organization focused on addressing the needs of children and youth with emotional, behavioral or mental challenges and their families. Works with parents to provide resources and advocate for improved mental health care for children in Louisiana.

Year Founded: 1991

1909 National Alliance on Mental Illness: Louisiana
307 France Street
Suite A
Baton Rouge, LA 70802
225-291-6262
800-437-0303; *Fax:* 225-291-6244
info@namilouisiana.org
www.namilouisiana.org

Dr Juliana Fort, President
Karen Kovach Soileau, Vice President
Dr Holly Houk Cullen, Treasurer
Linda Kelly, Secretary

NAMI Louisiana is a non-profit organization dedicated to eliminating the stigma and misconceptions of mental illness and improving the quality of life for all persons with mental illnesses and their families.

Year Founded: 1984

Maine

1910 National Alliance on Mental Illness: Maine
1 Bangor Street
Augusta, ME 04330-4701
207-622-5767
800-464-5767; *Fax:* 207-621-8430
info@namimaine.org
www.namimaine.org

Jenna Mehnert, MSW, Executive Director
Christine Canty Brooks, Director, Peer/Family Programs
Sophie M Gabrion, MS, Director, Public Education
Shelley O'Brian, Director, Finance/Operations

Dedicated to improving the lives of all people affected by mental illness. Advocates for quality services, offers resources on mental health, and provides support for individuals with mental illnesses. NAMI Maine provides services across the entire state of Maine.

Year Founded: 1977

Maryland

1911 Analysis and Services Research Branch SAMHSA's Center for Behavioral Health Statistics and Quality
1 Choke Cherry Road
Room 2-1049
Rockville, MD 20857
240-276-1250
www.samhsa.gov/about-us/who-we-are/offices-centers

Albert Woodward, PhD, Branch Chief

Federally funded agency providing statistics on behavioral health.

1912 Community Behavioral Health Association of Maryland: CBH
18 Egges Lane
Catonsville, MD 21228-4511
410-788-1865; *Fax:* 410-788-1768
info@mdcbh.org
www.mdcbh.org

Shannon Hall, Executive Director
Lori Doyle, Public Policy Director
JoAnn Clarke, Director of Administration

Professional association representing the network of community behavioral health providers operating in the public and private sectors in Maryland. Strives to improve the quality of care for individuals and families with mental illness, addiction and substance use problems.

1913 Maryland Psychiatric Research Center
55 Wade Avenue
Catonsville, MD 21228-4663
410-402-7666

Robert W Buchanan, MD, Director

The Maryland Psychiatric Research Center is a research center within the University of Maryland School of Medicine. The MPRC studies the causes and treatments of schizophrenia and related disorders, and provides treatments for patients with schizophrenia.

Year Founded: 1807

1914 Mental Health Association of Maryland
1301 York Road
Suite 505
Lutherville, MD 21093
443-901-1550
800-572-6426; *Fax:* 443-901-0038
info@mhamd.org
www.mhamd.org

Oscar Morgan, President
Linda J Raines, Chief Executive Officer
Lea Ann Browning-McNee, Chief Program Officer
Adrienne Ellis, Director, Healthcare Reform

The Mental Health Association of Maryland is a nonprofit organization committed to promoting mental health and preventing mental illness. MHAMD provides mental health research, education and training through outreach, advocacy, education and services oversight programs.

1915 National Alliance on Mental Illness: Maryland
10630 Little Patuxent Parkway
Suite 475
Columbia, MD 21044-3264
410-884-8691
877-878-2371; *Fax:* 410-884-8695
info@namimd.org
www.namimd.org

Steve Gray, President
Kate Farinholt, Executive Director
Jessica Honke, Policy and Advocacy Director
Jessica Wong, Program and Training Coordinator

A grassroots organization dedicated to helping people with mental illnesses and their families build better lives through education, support, and advocacy.

1916 National Association of Social Workers: Maryland Chapter
5750 Executive Drive
Suite 100
Baltimore, MD 21228-1700
410-788-1066
800-867-6776; *Fax:* 410-747-0635
nasw.md@verizon.net
www.nasw-md.org

Christine Garland, President
Terry Morris, Vice President
Daphne McClellan, PhD, Executive Director
Jenny Williams, Director of Communications

The National Association of Social Workers, Maryland Chapter supports the social work profession and the professional development of social workers, and advocates for just social policies and professional social work standards.

1917 National Federation of Families for Children's Mental Health
12320 Parklawn Drive
Rockville, MD 20852
240-403-1901
ffcmh@ffcmh.org
www.ffcmh.org

Lynda Gargan, PhD, Executive Director
Barbara Huff, Technical Assistance Provider
Sherri Luthe, President
Terry Stevens, Vice President

The National Federation of Families for Children's Mental Health is a national family-run organization that works to develop policies and service systems that meet the needs of children and youth experiencing emotional, behavioral, and mental health challenges and their families. The mission of the National Federation is to advocate for the rights of children with mental health needs and to collaborate with other organizations to help improve mental health care in America. The National Federation seeks to provide support and services for children affected by emotional, behavioral and mental health challenges, and to assist them in realizing their full potential.

Year Founded: 1989

1918 Sheppard Pratt Health System
6501 N Charles Street
Baltimore, MD 21204-6893
410-938-3800
888-938-4207
info@sheppardpratt.org
www.www.sheppardpratt.org

Steven S Sharfstein, CEO
Dr Robert Roca, VP & Medical Director

Massachusetts

1919 Association for Behavioral Healthcare
251 West Central Street
Suite 21
Natick, MA 01760-3758
508-647-8385; *Fax:* 508-647-8311

Vic DiGravio, President and CEO
Constance Peters, VP, Addiction Services
Lydia Conley, VP, Mental Health
Amanda Gilman, Senior Director, Public Policy

The Association for Behavioral Healthcare, formerly Mental Health and Substance Abuse Corporations of Massachusetts, is dedicated to promoting community-based mental health and substance abuse services, advocating for public policy changes, and addressing issues surrounding mental health and addiction treatment services.

1920 Behavioral Health Clinics and Trauma Services
Justice Resource Institute
160 Gould Street
Suite 300
Needham, MA 02494-2300
781-559-4900; *Fax:* 978-263-3088
www.jri.org

Arden O'Connor, Chairperson
Andy Pond, MSW, MAT, President
Deborah Reuman, MBA, Chief Financial Officer
Joseph Spinazzola, PhD, Vice President

Provides outpatient mental health services for children and families with developmental disabilities, behavioral and emotional problems, and medical complications. Services include in-home and outpatient therapies, mentoring services, in-home behavioral support, parent and caregiver support, and education, and mental health evaluation and consultation services to juvenile courts.

1921 Bridgewell
471 Broadway
Lynnfield, MA 01940
781-593-1088; *Fax:* 781-593-5731
info@bridgewell.org
www.bridgewell.org

Robert S Stearns, MEd, President and CEO
Kimberley J Haley, LMHC, Director of Clinical Services
John Hyland, Director of IT
Kelly J Johnson, MBA, Chief Operations Officer

Private, non-profit corporation that provides services and support for persons with developmental and psychiatric disabilities. Services offered include residential services, behavioral health services, employment training, affordable housing, transitional homeless services, and substance abuse and addiction services.

Year Founded: 1958

1922 CASCAP

231 Somerville Avenue
Somerville, MA 02143
617-492-5559; *Fax:* 617-492-6928
info@cascap.org
www.cascap.org

Shawn Luther, Chair
Michael Haran, Chief Executive Officer
Ted McKie, MS, Vice Chair
Thomas M Sadtler, MSW, MBA, Treasurer

Cascap Inc. seeks to assist underserved and disadvantaged members of the community and improve their quality of life. Provides a range of clinical, residential, and educational services for disabled, impoverished, or elderly individuals.

Year Founded: 1973

1923 Depression and Bipolar Support Alliance of Boston

115 Mill Street
PO Box 102
Belmont, MA 02478
617-855-2795; *Fax:* 617-855-3666
info@dbsaboston.org
www.dbsaboston.netfirms.com

Chuck Weinstein, LMHC, CPRP, President
Lillian Cravotta-Crouch, Vice President
Barry Park, Treasurer
Susan Reynolds, Secretary

DBSA-BOSTON is a non-profit organization dedicated to helping people with psychiatric illnesses lead healthy lives.

1924 Jewish Family and Children's Service

1430 Main Street
Waltham, MA 02451
781-647-5327
info@jfcsboston.org
www.jfcsboston.org

Rimma Zelfand, Chief Executive Officer
David Schechter, President
Bruce Haskin, Chief Financial Officer
Alan Jacobson, Senior VP of Programs

The Jewish Family & Children's Service supports families and individuals through the provision of health care programs based upon Jewish traditions of social responsibility, compassion, and respect for all community members. JF&CS assists all persons in need of care, with particular focus on vulnerable populations such as children and adults with disabilities or mental illness, seniors, and people experiencing domestic abuse, hunger, or financial crisis.

1925 Massachusetts Behavioral Health Partnership

1000 Washington Street
Suite 310
Boston, MA 02118-5002
617-790-4000
800-495-0086; *Fax:* 617-790-4128
www.masspartnership.com

Carol Kress, LICSW, Chief Executive
James Thatcher, MD, Chief Medical Officer
Nancy E Norman, MD, MPH, Medical Director of Integration

The Massachusetts Behavioral Health Partnership provides medical and behavioral health care for MassHealth Members who select the Division's Primary Care Clinician Plan, as well as children in state custody.

Year Founded: 1996

1926 Massachusetts National Alliance on Mental Illness

529 Main Street
Suite 1M17
Boston, MA 02129
617-580-8541
800-370-9085; *Fax:* 617-580-8673
namimass@aol.com
www.namimass.org

Steve Rosenfeld, President
Laurie Martinelli, Executive Director
Marilyn DeSantis, Bookkeeper/Donor Relations
Karen Gromis, Events and Walk Manager

Nation's leading self-help organization for all those affected by severe brain disorders. Mission is to bring consumers and families with similar experiences together to share information about services, care providers, and ways to cope with the challenges of schizophrenia, manic depression, and other serious mental illnesses.

1927 Parent Professional Advocacy League

15 Court Square
Suite 660
Boston, MA 02108
617-542-7860
866-815-8122; *Fax:* 617-542-7832
info@ppal.net
www.ppal.net

William O'Brien, Chair
Lisa Lambert, Executive Director
Anne Silver, Director of Operations
Meri Viano, Associate Director

Grassroots family organization providing support, education, publications, and advocacy for children with mental health needs and their families.

Michigan

1928 Borgess Behavioral Health

1521 Gull Road
Kalamazoo, MI 49048-1640
269-226-7000

Joni Knapper, Vice Chair
Beth Brutsche, Secretary
Susan Pozo, PhD, Treasurer

Offers patients and families a wide array of services to address their mental health concerns.

1929 Holy Cross Children's Services
8759 Clinton-Macon Road
Clinton, MI 49236-9569
517-423-7455; *Fax:* 517-423-5442
info@hccsnet.org
www.holycrossservices.org

Timothy Patton, Chairperson
Francis Boylan, Executive Director
John Lynch, Chief Financial Officer
Sharon Berkobien, Chief Operations Officer

Holy Cross Children's Services is a private, not-for-profit child and family services provider based in Michigan. The mission of Holy Cross Children's Services is to assist children and adults in leading productive and healthy lives.

Year Founded: 1948

1930 Macomb County Community Mental Health
22550 Hall Road
Clint Township, MI 48036
586-469-5275
855-996-2264
www.mccmh.net

John Kinch, Executive Director
Jim Losey, Deputy Director
Norma Josef, MD, Medical Director
Herbert Wendt, Director, Finance

Offers a range of mental health treatment and support services for individuals affected by mental illness, developmental disabilities, and substance use disorders, and seeks to advance their recovery, independence, and self-sufficiency.

1931 Michigan Association for Children with Emotional Disorders: MACED
230233 Southfield Road
Suite 219
Southfield, MI 48076
248-433-2200; *Fax:* 248-433-2299
info@michkids.org
www.michkids.org

Samuel L Davis, Clinical Director

Ensures that children with serious emotional disorders receive appropriate mental health and educational services so that they reach their full potential. To provide support to families and to encourage community understanding of the need for specialized programs for their children.

1932 Michigan Association for Children's Mental Health
6017 West St Joseph Highway
Suite 200
Lansing, MI 48917
517-372-4016
888-226-4543; *Fax:* 517-372-4032
www.acmh-mi.org

Jane Shank, Executive Director
Mary Porter, Business Manager
Terri Henrizi, Education Coordinator
Kayle Roose, Family Resource Specialist

Michigan-based non-profit organization serving families of children and youth with emotional, behavioral, or mental health needs. Provides information, support, resources, referrals, advocacy, and networking and leadership opportunities for youth.

Year Founded: 1989

1933 National Alliance on Mental Illness: Michigan
401 South Washington
Lansing, MI 48933
517-485-4049
800-331-4264
info@namimi.org
www.namimi.org

Holly Rhode, President
Kevin Fischer, Executive Director

Grassroots mental health organization committed to improving the quality of life of individuals and families affected by mental illness. NAMI Michigan assists affiliates, provides support and education programs, engages in advocacy, organizes events to raise awareness, and promotes research on mental illness.

Year Founded: 1979

1934 Southwest Solutions
5716 Michigan Avenue
Suite 3000
Detroit, MI 48210
313-481-3102
www.swsol.org

Seth Lloyd, Chair
John Van Camp, President and CEO
Lenora Hardy-Foster, Executive Director
Ozzie Rivera, Director, Community Engagement

Southwest Solutions provides human development, economic development, and community engagement programs for individuals living with mental illness. Southwest seeks to help marginalized persons build meaningful futures.

1935 Woodlands Behavioral Healthcare Network
960 M-60 East
Cassopolis, MI 49031-9339
800-323-0335; *Fax:* 269-445-3216
www.woodlandsbhn.org

Kathy Emans, LMSW, Director

Provides community behavioral health services.

Minnesota

1936 NASW Minnesota Chapter
Iris Park Place, Suite 340
1885 University Avenue West
Saint Paul, MN 55104-3458
651-293-1935
888-293-6279; *Fax:* 651-293-0952
admin@naswmn.org
www.nasw-heartland.org

Deborah Tallen, MPA, MBA, Executive Director
Whitney Gladden, Program Coordinator

NASW-MN is the state chapter of the National Association of Social Workers, a membership organization representing the interests of professional social workers. The mission of NASW-MN is to advance and promote the profession of social work, support the professional growth of its members, and advocate for clients through the promotion of social policies.

1937 National Alliance on Mental Illness: Minnesota
800 Transfer Road
Suite 31
Saint Paul, MN 55114-1414

651-645-2948
888-626-4435; *Fax:* 651-645-7379
namihelps@namimn.org
www.namihelps.org

Deborah Erickson, President
Sue Abderholden, Executive Director
Morgan Caldwell, Peer Programming Coordinator
Donna Fox, Director of Adult Programming

A non-profit organization dedicated to helping individuals with mental illness and their families build better lives. NAMI Minnesota offers education, support, and advocacy and promotes the development of accessible mental health services and programs.

Year Founded: 1976

1938 North American Training Institute

314 West Superior Street
Suite 508
Duluth, MN 55802-1868
218-722-1503
888-989-9234; *Fax:* 218-722-0346
info@nati.org
www.nati.org

Elizabeth George, Chief Executive Officer

The North American Training Institute is a not-for-profit organization based in Minnesota. NATI's mission is to promote research and professional training about gambling addiction. NATI provides resources and services for individuals at risk of developing a gambling addiction, particularly adolescents.

Year Founded: 1988

1939 Pacer Center

8161 Normandale Boulevard
Bloomington, MN 55437
952-838-9000
800-537-2237; *Fax:* 952-838-0199
www.pacer.org

Paula F. Goldberg, Co-Founder & Executive Director
Dan Levinson, Treasurer
Tammy Pust, Vice President
Matthew Woods, President

PACER provides information, training, and assistance to parents of children and young adults with all disabilities (physical, learning, cognitive, emotional, and health). Its mission is to help improve the quality of life for young people with disabilities and their families.

Year Founded: 1977

Mississippi

1940 National Alliance on Mental Illness: Mississippi

2618 Southerland Street
Suite 100
Jackson, MS 39216
601-899-9058
803-357-0388; *Fax:* 601-899-9058
stateoffice@namims.org
www.namims.org

Debbie Waller, President
Tameka Tobias Smith, Executive Director
Carla McGowan, LCSW, Education Coordinator
Reagan Harvey, Community Outreach Coordinator

Nonprofit state organization of the National Alliance on Mental Illness. Dedicated to improving the lives of individuals with mental illnesses and their families through education, support, advocacy, and research.

Year Founded: 1989

Missouri

1941 Depressive and Bipolar Support Alliance (DBSA)

730 N Franklin Street
Suite 501
Chicago, IL 60654-7225
800-826-3632; *Fax:* 312-642-7243
info@dbsalliance.org
www.dbsalliance.org

Cheryl T. Magrini, MS.Ed, MTS, P, Chair
Allen Doederlein, President
Cindy Specht, Executive Vice President
Lisa Goodale, Vice President, Peer Support Ser

The Depression and Bipolar Support Alliance is the leading patient-directed national organization focusing on the most prevalent mental illnesses. The organization fosters an environment of understanding about the impact and management of these life threatening illnesses by providing up-to-date, scientifically based tools and information written in language the general public can understand.

Year Founded: 1985

1942 Missouri Coalition for Community Behavioral Healthcare

221 Metro Drive
Jefferson City, MO 65109
573-634-4626; *Fax:* 573-634-8858
admin@mocoalition.org
www.mocoalition.org

Brent McGinty, President and CEO
Rachelle Glavin, Director of Clinical Operations
Paula Stanley, MEd, Director of Administration
Misty Snodgrass, MPA, Director of Public Policy

The Missouri Coalition for Community Behavioral Healthcare seeks to improve access to mental health services for all residents of Missouri.

Year Founded: 1963

1943 Missouri Institute of Mental Health

4633 World Parkway Circle
Saint Louis, MO 63134-3115
314-516-8400; *Fax:* 314-516-8405
info@mimh.edu
www.mimh.edu

Robert Paul, Director
Rita E Adkins, Project Director
Rachel Kryah, Project Director
Edward G Riedel, Project Director

The Missouri Institute of Mental Health is a health services research organization providing professional training, research, program evaluation, policy development, and community outreach to the Missouri Department of Mental Health, as well as state agencies, service provider agencies, and other organizations and individuals pursuing information on mental health and related issues.

Year Founded: 1962

1944 National Alliance on Mental Illness: Missouri
3405 West Truman Boulevard
Suite 102
Jefferson City, MO 65109-5861
573-634-7727
800-374-2138; *Fax:* 573-761-5636
namimosb@yahoo.com
www.namimissouri.org

Leslie Joslyn, President and Chairman
Cindi R Keele, Executive Director
Diana Harper, Secretary
James Owen, Treasurer

Statewide nonprofit organization committed to the recovery and improved quality of life for individuals with mental illness and their families. NAMI Missouri educates the public about mental health and supports research on mental illness.

Montana

1945 Mental Health America of Montana
205 Haggerty Lane
Suite 170
Bozeman, MT 59771
406-587-7774
info@montanamentalhealth.org
www.montanamentalhealth.org

Dan Aune, MSW, Executive Director
Shellie Aune, Prevention Services Director
Julio Brionez, MS, Technical Assistance Consultant

A statewide education and advocacy organization working towards improved mental health for all people and advocating for quality services for individuals with mental illnesses.

1946 National Alliance on Mental Illness: Montana
555 Fuller Avenue
Suite 3
Helena, MT 59601
406-443-7871
info@namimt.org
www.namimt.org

Gary Popiel, President
Matthew Kuntz, Executive Director
Colleen Rahn, Education Director

NAMI Montana is the state chapter of the National Alliance on Mental Illness, a grassroots organization for persons affected by mental illness. NAMI Montana serves Montanans with mental illnesses and their families through support, education, and advocacy.

Nebraska

1947 Department of Health and Human Services Division of Public Health
Licensure Unit
Lincoln, NE 68508-4986
402-471-2115
www.dhhs.ne.gov

Joseph M. Acierno, MD, JD, Director
Helen Meeks, Administrator of Licensure Unit

The Licensure Unit's mission is to assure the public that health-related practices provided by individuals, facilities and programs are safe, of acceptable quality, and that the cost of expanded services is justified by the need.

1948 Mutual of Omaha's Health and Wellness Programs
Mutual of Omaha Plaza
Omaha, NE 68175-1
402-342-7600
800-238-9354; *Fax:* 402-351-2775
www.mutualofomaha.com

Daniel P Neary, CEO

Mutual of Omaha's Health and Wellness Programs provide assistance and professional support in a variety of areas including family concerns; depression/anxiety; gambling and other addictions; parenting issues; drug/alcohol abuse; grief issues and life changes.

1949 National Alliance on Mental Illness: Nebraska
415 South 25th Avenue
Building LH
Omaha, NE 68131
402-345-8101
877-463-6264; *Fax:* 402-346-4070
www.naminebraska.org

Nancy Kelley, PhD, President
Cheryl Willis, Vice President
Mary Thunker, Secretary
Lee Kortus, Treasurer

NAMI Nebraska is a non-profit grassroots organization dedicated to providing support and assistance for individuals with mental illness and their families and friends. NAMI Nebraska educates the public about mental illness, advocates for mental health reform, and aims to improve mental health services throughout the state.

1950 National Association of Social Workers: Nebraska Chapter
650 'J' Street
Suite 208
Lincoln, NE 68508
402-477-7344
877-816-6279; *Fax:* 402-477-0374
www.nasw-heartland.org

Konnie Kirchner, President
Sue Kloch, Vice President
Terry Werner, Executive Director
Amy West, Secretary

NASW-NE is an affiliate of the National Association of Social Workers, a membership organization representing professional social workers.

1951 Nebraska Family Support Network
3568 Dodge Street
Suite 2
Omaha, NE 68131-3851
402-345-0791
800-245-6081; *Fax:* 402-444-7722
info@nefamilysupport.org
www.nefamilysupportnetwork.org

Chinedu Igbokwe, Board President
Tim Flott, Vice President
Dan Jackson, Executive Director
Steven Bauer, Program Director

1952 Parent to Parent of Omaha
Ollie Webb Center
1941 South 42nd Street
Suite 122
Omaha, NE 68105-2942

402-346-5220; *Fax:* 402-342-4857
www.olliewebbinc.org/parent-to-parent

Laurie Ackermann, Executive Director
Robin McArthur, Operations Director
Denise Gehringer, Program Coordinator
Lisa Dougherty, Human Resource Manager

Consists of parents, professionals, and others who are interested in providing emotional and peer support to parents of children with disabilities. Offers a parent-matching program which matches new parents wih parents who have had sufficient experience and training. Publications: The Gazette, newsletter, published 6 times a year. Also has chapters in Arizona and limited other states.

Year Founded: 1971

Nevada

1953 National Alliance on Mental Illness: Western Nevada
PO Box 4633
Carson City, NV 89702-4633
775-440-1626
www.namiwesternnevada.org

Sarah Adler, President
Robin Reedy, Vice President
Rick Porzig, Treasurer
Sandie Draper, Secretary

Part of the National Alliance on Mental Illness, a self-help organization for all those with mental disorders. The mission of NAMI Western Nevada is to help individuals affected by mental illness and their families lead dignified lives, and to end the stigma associated with mental illness. NAMI Western Nevada educates the public about mental health and seeks to expand mental health services across rural Nevada.

1954 Nevada Principals' Executive Program
2101 South Jones Boulevard
Suite 120
Las Vegas, NV 89146-3106
702-388-8899
800-216-5188; *Fax:* 702-388-2966
pepinfo@nvpep.org
www.nvpep.org

Karen Taycher, Executive Director
Natalie Filipic, Director of Operations
Stephanie Vrsnik, Community Development Director
Robin Kincaid, Educational Services Director

To strengthen and renew the knowledge, skills, and beliefs of public school leaders so that they might help improve the conditions for teaching and learning in schools and school districts.

New Hampshire

1955 Monadnock Family Services
64 Main Street
Suite 201
Keene, NH 03431-3701
603-357-4400
www.mfs.org

Jane Larmon, Chair
Elizabeth Cleary, Vice Chair
Michael Chelstowski, Treasurer
Dr Robert Englund, Secretary

A nonprofit community mental health agency serving the mental health needs of children, youth and adults through counseling, support services, and programs in parent education, family support, youth development, and substance abuse prevention and treatment.

1956 National Alliance on Mental Illness: New Hampshire
85 North State Street
Concord, NH 03301
603-225-5359
800-242-6264; *Fax:* 603-228-8848
info@naminh.org
www.naminh.org

Michele Grennon, President
Ken Norton, LICSW, ACSW, Executive Director
Tammy Murray, Chief Financial Officer
Linda Paquette, Secretary

A statewide grassroots organization providing education, support, and advocacy for all individuals, families, and friends affected by mental illness or emotional disorders. NAMI New Hampshire works towards a quality, comprehensive mental health service system.

New Jersey

1957 Advocates for Children of New Jersey
35 Halsey Street
2nd Floor
Newark, NJ 07102-3000
973-643-3876; *Fax:* 973-643-9153
advocates@acnj.org
www.acnj.org

Cecilia Zalkind, Executive Director
Mary Coogan, Assistant Director
Carla Ross, Operations Manager
Diane Dellanno, Policy Analyst

Advocates for Children of New Jersey is a statewide non-profit organization focused on advocating for the rights of children. ACNJ operates on behalf of children and families by collaborating with local, state and federal leaders to enact law and policy changes that will benefit the children of New Jersey. The mission of ACNJ is to raise awareness and to serve the needs of children through research, policy and strategic communications. ACNJ seeks to help children lead healthy, safe and educated lives so that they can become productive members of New Jersey's communities. ACNJ operates a children's legal resource center that serves to provide information on children and legal issues for parents, children, service providers, educators, attorneys and others.

Year Founded: 1847

1958 Community Resource Council
PO Box 443
Hackensack, NJ 07601
201-343-4900
www.crchelpline.org

Non-profit alliance of agencies and individuals serving to promote the health of the residents of Bergen County, New Jersey. Provides assistance, information and referrals through The HELPLINE Service.

1959 Disability Rights New Jersey
210 S Broad Street
3rd Floor
Trenton, NJ 08608-2404
609-292-9742
800-922-7233; *Fax:* 609-777-0187
TTY: 609-633-7106
advocate@drnj.org
www.drnj.org

Joseph B Young, Executive Director
Maritza Williams, Intake Coordinator
Lillie Lowe-Reid, CAP, Coordinator/PABSS Project Direct
Rachel Parsio, Senior Staff Advocate

Legal and non legal advocacy, information and referral, technical assistance and training, outreach and education in support of the human, civil, and legal rights of people with disabilities in New Jersey.

Year Founded: 1994

1960 Jewish Family Service of Atlantic and Cape May Counties
607 North Jerome Avenue
Margate, NJ 08402-1527
609-822-1108; *Fax:* 609-882-1106
www.jfsatlantic.org

Andrea Steinberg, LCSW, Chief Executive Officer
Richard B Wise, MD, President
Johanna Perskie, Vice President
Jessica Goldstein, Vice President

Multi-service family counseling agency committed to strengthening and preserving individual, family, and community well-being while following Jewish philosophy and values.

Year Founded: 1930

1961 Mental Health Association in New Jersey
88 Pompton Avenue
Verona, NJ 07044
800-367-8850; *Fax:* 973-857-1777
njconnect@mhanj.org
www.mhanj.org

Bill Waldman, MSW, Chairman
Victoria Brown, MSW, LCSW, Vice Chairman
Harold B Garwin, Esq., Acting Treasurer

The Mental Health Association in New Jersey seeks to eliminate barriers to recovery and care and to improve mental health for all people through advocacy, education, training, and services.

1962 National Alliance on Mental Illness: New Jersey
1562 Route 130
North Brunswick, NJ 08902-3090
732-940-0991; *Fax:* 732-940-0355
info@naminj.org
www.naminj.org

Mark Perrin, President
Sylvia Axelrod, Executive Director
Phil Lubitz, Associate Director
Aruna Rao, Associate Director

A statewide non-profit organization dedicated to improving the quality of life for persons with mental illness and their families. Provides education, support, advocacy, and programs to raise awareness on mental illness, abolish stigma, and promote mental health research.

Year Founded: 1985

1963 New Jersey Association of Mental Health and Addiction Agencies
3575 Quakerbridge Road
Suite 102
Trenton, NJ 08619
609-838-5488; *Fax:* 609-838-5489
info@njamhaa.org
www.njamhaa.org

Debra Wentz, President and CEO
Julia Schneider, Chief Financial Officer
Shauna Moses, Vice President, Public Affairs
June Noto, Vice President, IT and HR

The New Jersey Association of Mental Health and Addiction Agencies represents mental healthcare and substance use treatment providers serving New Jersey residents affected by mental illness or addictions and their families.

Year Founded: 1951

1964 New Jersey Psychiatric Association
PO Box 428
Bedminster, NJ 07921
908-719-2222; *Fax:* 908-719-4747
info@njpsychiatry.org

Theresa M Miskimen MD, President
Carla A Ross, Executive Director

A professional organization of about 100 physicians qualified by training and experience in the treatment of mental illness.

Year Founded: 1935

New Mexico

1965 National Alliance on Mental Illness: New Mexico
2015 Wyoming Boulevard Northeast
Suite E
Albuquerque, NM 87112
505-260-0154
800-953-6745; *Fax:* 505-260-0342
naminm@aol.com
www.naminewmexico.org

Kimmie Jordan, President
Linda Givens, Treasurer
Kate Jackson, Secretary

NAMI New Mexico is an organization serving to enhance the quality of life for individuals affected by mental illness through advocacy, support services, and education programs.

New York

1966 Compeer
1600 South Avenue
Suite 230
Rochester, NY 14620-3924
585-445-5700
800-836-0475; *Fax:* 585-442-7573
www.compeer.org

J. Theodore Smith, Chair
Johanna Ambrose, CEO and President
Barb Mestler, Affiliate Program Specialist
Nancy Dhurjaty, Project Specialist

Nonprofit mental wellness organization. Develops a model program that matches volunteers and mentors with children and adults with mental health needs. Seeks to improve the quality of life for individuals and families with mental health challenges through support and inclusion.

Year Founded: 1973

1967 Families Together in New York State
737 Madison Avenue
Albany, NY 12208
518-432-0333
888-326-8644; *Fax:* 518-434-6478
info@ftnys.org
www.ftnys.org

Paige Pierce, Chief Executive Officer
Geraldine Burton, President
Daphnne Brown, Director of Family Involvement
Clare Graham, Director of Finance

Non-profit, parent-run organization that serves families of children and youth affected by social, emotional, and behavioral challenges through advocacy, information, referrals, public awareness, education, and training.

1968 Finger Lakes Parent Network, Inc.
25 W Steuben Street
Bath, NY 14810
607-776-2164
800-934-4244; *Fax:* 607-776-4327
flpninc25@flpn.org
www.flpn.org

Pamela Maglier, President
Sue M arosek, Vice President
Patti DiNardo, Executive Director
Jeannine Struble, Assistant Director

A parent-governed organization, focused on the needs of children and youth with emotional, behavioral, and /or mental disorders and their families. Supports and empowers families so that they can improve the quality of their lives and help their child to achieve his/her full potential within the community.

Year Founded: 1990

1969 Healthcare Association of New York State
1 Empire Drive
Rensselaer, NY 12144-5729
518-431-7600; *Fax:* 518-431-7915
www.hanys.org

Dennis Whalen, President
Valerie Grey, Executive Vice President
Richard Cook, Chief Operating Officer
William F Streck, MD, Chief Medical Officer

Statewide healthcare association serving as the primary advocate for more than 550 non-profit and public hospitals, health systems, long-term care, home care, hospice, and other health care organizations throughout New York State.

1970 Mental Health America of Dutchess County
253 Mansion Street
Poughkeepsie, NY 12601
845-473-2500; *Fax:* 845-473-4870
info@mhadutchess.org
www.mhadutchess.org

Andrew O'Grady, LCSW-R, Executive Director
Jennifer Nelson, Director of Finance and HR
Janet Caruso, MSLS, Director of Community Education

Mental Health America of Dutchess County is a not-for-profit organization committed to the promotion of mental health and improved, accessible care for persons with mental illnesses. Provides education, programs, advocacy, and community support.

1971 Mental Health Association in Orange County Inc
73 James P Kelly Way
Middletown, NY 10940
845-342-2400
800-832-1200; *Fax:* 845-343-9665
mha@mhaorangeny.com
www.mhaorangeny.com

David Goggins, President of the Board
Nadia Allen, Executive Director

Seeks to promote the positive mental health and emotional well-being of Orange County residents, working towards reducing the stigma of mental illness, developmental disabilities, and providing support to victims of sexual assault and other crimes.

1972 National Alliance on Mental Illness: Westchester
100 Clearbrook Road
Elmsford, NY 10523
914-592-5458; *Fax:* 914-592-2652
info@namiwestchester.org
www.namiwestchester.org

Jennifer Jacquet-Murray, President
Irwin Lubell, First Vice President
Sharon McCarthy, Program Director
Marie Considine, Director of Development

Grassroots organization providing support and assistance to individuals and families affected by mental illness. Provides support and education, advocates for access to services and treatment, and raises mental health awareness.

1973 National Association of Social Workers New York State Chapter
188 Washington Avenue
Albany, NY 12210-2394
518-463-4741
800-724-6279; *Fax:* 518-463-6446
www.naswnys.org

Peter Chernack, DSW, LCSW-R, President
Diane Bessel Matteson, PhD, Vice President
Ronald Bunce, LMSW, Executive Director
Karin Carreau, MSW, Director of Policy

The National Association of Social Workers is a membership association representing professional social workers. NASW New York State advocates for public policies that address health, welfare, and education issues involving individuals and families, continues the education of its members through workshops and seminars, and maintains professional standards within social work practice.

Year Founded: 1955

1974 New York Association of Psychiatric Rehabilitation Services
194 Washington Avenue
Suite 400
Albany, NY 12210
518-436-0008; *Fax:* 518-436-0044
www.nyaprs.org

Carla Rabinowitz, Co-President
Alison Carroll, Co-President

Harvey Rosenthal, Executive Director
Michelle Jensen, Vice President

New York Association of Psychiatric Rehabilitation Services (NYAPRS) is a statewide coalition of New Yorkers who receive or provide mental health services. NYAPRS is committed to improving the quality and availability of services for individuals with psychiatric disabilities. NYAPRS promotes mental health recovery and rehabilitation and works to fight the discrimination that persons with psychiatric disabilities face both within the mental health system and in the larger community.

Year Founded: 1981

1975 Northeast Business Group on Health

61 Broadway
Suite 2705
New York, NY 10006
212-252-7440; *Fax:* 212-252-7448
www.nebgh.org

Laurel Pickering, MPH, President and CEO
Janaera J Gaston, MPA, Director, Programs
Shawn Nowicki, MPH, Director, Health Policy
Kathy Sakraida, Director, Quality Initiatives

The Northeast Business Group on Health is a not-for-profit coalition of providers, insurers, and organizations in New York, New Jersey, Connecticut and Massachusetts. The mission of NEBGH is to promote a value-based health care system by improving health care delivery and contributing to health care decisions.

1976 State University of New York at Stony Brook Department of Psychiatry

101 Nicolls Road
Stony Brook, NY 11794
631-444-2990
registrar_office@stonybrook.edu
www.medicine.stonybrookmedicine.edu/psychiatry/

Ramin Parsey, MD, PhD, Chairman
Michael Talento, CPA, Administrator
Kevin Kelly, PhD, Director of Information Systems
Michael McClain, Director of Communications

Conducts clinical and translational psychiatry research and provides clinical services.

North Carolina

1977 Autism Society of North Carolina

5121 Kingdom Way
Suite 100
Raleigh, NC 27607
919-743-0204
800-442-2762
info@autismsociety-nc.org
www.autismsociety-nc.org

Elizabeth Phillippi, Chair
Tracey Sheriff, Chief Executive Officer
Paul Wendler, Chief Financial Officer
Ruth Hurst, Vice Chair

Committed to providing support for individuals within the autism spectrum and their families through advocacy, training and education, and residential, recreational, vocational, and community-based services.

1978 National Alliance on Mental Illness: North Carolina

309 West Millbrook Road
Suite 121
Raleigh, NC 27609-4394
919-788-0801
800-451-9682; *Fax:* 919-788-0906
mail@naminc.org
www.naminc.org

David Smith, President
Deby Dihoff, Acting Executive Director
Lori Matteson, Coordinator, Programs/Membership
Virginia Hamlet Rodillas, MS, Helpline Manager

The mission of NAMI North Carolina is to improve the lives of persons with mental health needs. NAMI North Carolina assists individuals and families affected by mental illness through the provision of support, education, advocacy, and public awareness efforts.

1979 National Association of Social Workers: North Carolina Chapter

412 Morson Street
PO Box 27582
Raleigh, NC 27601
919-828-9650
800-280-6207; *Fax:* 919-828-1341
www.naswnc.org

Kathy Boyd, MSW, ACSW, CMSW, Executive Director
Valerie Arendt, MSW, MPP, Associate Executive Director
Kay Castillo, BSW, Director of Advocacy and Policy
Debbie Conner, Finance Director

NASW North Carolina is a state chapter of the National Association of Social Workers, a membership organization serving to promote and protect social workers and the social work profession. NASW aims to help improve the well-being of families and individuals through work and advocacy.

Year Founded: 1955

1980 North Carolina Mental Health Consumers Organization

916 Richardson Drive
Raleigh, NC 27603
919-832-2285
800-326-3842; *Fax:* 919-828-6999

Roger Hyman, President
Sharon Campbell, Executive Administrator
Henry Jacobs, Senior Program Coordinator

The North Carolina Mental Health Consumers' Organization is a non-profit organization providing support for individuals in North Carolina with mental illness through advocacy, resources, and education.

North Dakota

1981 National Association of Social Workers: North Dakota Chapter

1120 College Drive, Suite 100
PO Box 1775
Bismarck, ND 58503
701-223-4161; *Fax:* 701-223-4161
www.nasw-heartland.org

Heidi Borstad, President

NASW North Dakota is the state chapter of the National Association of Social Workers, an organization representing professional social workers. NASWND promotes the profession of social work and advocates for access to services for all.

1982 North Dakota Federation of Families for Children's Mental Health

PO Box 3061
Bismarck, ND 58502-3061
701-222-3310
877-822-6287; *Fax:* 701-222-3310
www.ndffcmh.org

Carlotta McCleary, Executive Director
Jamie Becker, Executive Assistant

The North Dakota Federation of Families for Children's Mental Health is an advocacy organization working to meet the needs of children and youth with emotional, behavioral and mental challenges and their families.

Year Founded: 1994

Ohio

1983 National Alliance on Mental Illness: Ohio

1225 Dublin Road
Suite 125
Columbus, OH 43215
614-224-2700
800-686-2646; *Fax:* 614-224-5400
namiohio@namiohio.org
www.namiohio.org

Lee Dunham, President
Terry Russell, Executive Director
Stacey Smith, Director of Operations
Peg Morrison, Director of Programs

Grassroots mental health advocacy organization and affiliate of the National Alliance on Mental Illness. The mission of NAMI Ohio is to help individuals living with serious mental disorders lead dignified lives. NAMI Ohio provides support, education, and advocacy for persons and families affected by mental illness and promotes public policies that benefit those with mental health needs.

1984 National Association of Social Workers: Ohio Chapter

400 West Wilson Bridge Road
Suite 103
Worthington, OH 43085
614-461-4484; *Fax:* 614-461-9793
info@naswoh.org
www.naswoh.org

Danielle Smith, MSW, MA, LSW, Executive Director
Dorothy Martindale, BSSW, LSW, Membership Associate
Colleen Dempsey, MSW, LISW, Practice Associate

NASW Ohio represents the interests of professional social workers in Ohio. The mission of NASW Ohio is to strengthen the profession of social work, maintain social work professional standards, and advocate for equitable social policies.

1985 Ohio Association of Child Caring Agencies

1151 Bethel Road
Suite 104B
Columbus, OH 43220
614-461-0014; *Fax:* 614-228-7004
www.oacca.org

Tracey Izzard, President
Mark M Mecum, Executive Director
Nancy Harvey, Treasurer
Matt Kresic, Secretary

The Ohio Association of Child Caring Agencies is an association of child and family service providers in Ohio. The mission of the association is to strengthen the quality of services for children, young adults, and families in Ohio through efforts in policy advocacy, as well as support of member agencies.

Year Founded: 1973

1986 Ohio Council of Behavioral Health & Family Services Providers

35 East Gay Street
Suite 401
Columbus, OH 43215-3138
614-228-0747; *Fax:* 614-228-0740
www.theohiocouncil.org

Hubert Wirtz, Chief Executive Officer
Brenda Cornett, Associate Director, Membership
Lori Criss, Associate Director
Teresa Lampl, Associate Director

A trade association representing Ohio-based organizations that provide alcohol and drug addiction treatment, mental health, behavioral healthcare and family services to their communities.

1987 Ohio Department of Mental Health & Addiction Services

30 East Broad Street
36th Floor
Columbus, OH 43215-3430
614-466-2596
877-275-6364
TDD: 614-752-9696
TTY: 614-752-9696
questions@mha.ohio.gov
www.mha.ohio.gov

Tracy J Plouck, Director
Mark A Hurst, MD, Medical Director
Michaela J Peterson, Deputy Director, Legal Services
Missy Craddock, Deputy Director, Public Affairs

State agency responsible for the oversight and funding of public mental health programs and services.

1988 Planned Lifetime Assistance Network of Northeast Ohio
Jewish Family Service Association of Cleveland

5010 Mayfield Road
Lyndhurst, OH 44124
216-504-6483
www.jfsa-cleveland.org

Harvey Kotler, Board Chair
Susan Bichsel, PhD, President and CEO
David Hlavac, Vice President and CFO
Michael Weiner, Treasurer

PLAN is a membership organization that provides help and support for individuals living with mental illness, cognitive disabilities, and autism spectrum disorder and their families. PLAN seeks to help people achieve emotional and cognitive development through the provision of social and wellness programs, work and volunteer opportunities, and family advocacy.

Year Founded: 1989

1989 Positive Education Program
3100 Euclid Avenue
Cleveland, OH 44115-2508
216-361-4400; *Fax:* 216-361-8600
info@pepcleve.org
www.pepcleve.org

Frank A Fecser, PhD, Chief Executive Officer
Claudia Lann Valore, Chief Program Officer
Habeebah R Grimes, Chief Clinical Officer
Shadi W Roman, PhD, Chief Operating Officer

The Positive Education Program (PEP) is a non-profit
agency serving to help troubled children and youth develop
skills to learn and grow successfully.

Year Founded: 1971

1990 Six County
2845 Bell Street
Zanesville, OH 43701-1794
740-454-9766; *Fax:* 740-588-6452
www.sixcounty.org

James McDonald, President and CEO
Robert Santos, Chief Operating Officer
Sue Ellen Foraker, Chief Financial Officer
William Mason, Chief Information Officer

Six County Inc. is a private not-for-profit community mental health service provider operating in Coshocton, Guernsey, Morgan, Muskingum, Noble and Perry counties.
Provides traditional treatment services and specialized services. Counseling and support services include outpatient
counseling services, medication management, 24-hour crisis intervention, employee assistance, residential services,
and peer support.

Oklahoma

1991 National Alliance on Mental Illness: Oklahoma
3812 North Santa Fe Avenue
Suite 305
Oklahoma City, OK 73118
405-601-8283
800-583-1264; *Fax:* 405-602-8539
namiok@coxinet.net
www.namioklahoma.org

Cynthia Adair, President
Brandon Pettit, Executive Director
Andrea Michaels, Director of Operations/CFO

NAMI Oklahoma is devoted to improving the lives of individuals and families affected by mental illness. Provides
support, educates the public about mental health, and advocates for equal access to quality healthcare, housing, education and employment for people with mental disorders.

1992 Oklahoma Mental Health Consumer Council
3200 NW 48th
Suite 102
Oklahoma City, OK 73112-5911
405-604-6975
888-424-1305
www.omhcc.org

Becky Tallent, Executive Director

Oregon

1993 National Alliance on Mental Illness: Oregon
4701 Southeast 24th Avenue
Suite E
Portland, OR 97202-1552
503-230-8009
800-343-6264; *Fax:* 503-230-2751
namioregon@namior.org
www.namior.org

Chuck Martin, President
Chris Bouneff, Executive Director
Michelle Madison, Events and Outreach Manager
Peter Link, Education Programs Manager

A statewide grassroots organization serving Oregonians affected by mental illness. NAMI Oregon seeks to help improve the lives of individuals living with mental illness and
their families through support, education, and advocacy.

1994 Oregon Family Support Network
1300 Broadway Street Northeast
Suite 403
Salem, OR 97301
503-363-8068
800-323-8521; *Fax:* 503-390-3161
www.ofsn.org

David de Fiebre, President
Sandy Bumpus, Executive Director
Leah Skipworth, Operations Manager
Janelle Rasmussen, Bookkeeper

A non-profit organization working to help families with
children and youth affected by mental or behavioral disorders and to represent families and youth in local and state
policy making. Provides advocacy, support, education and
services.

Year Founded: 1991

1995 Oregon Psychiatric Physicians Association
PO Box 21571
Keizer, OR 97307
503-406-2526; *Fax:* 503-406-2526
info@oregonpsychiatric.org

Patrick Sieng, Executive Director
Amy Goodall, Government Affairs Director
Patti Legarda, Program Committee Coordinator
Jennifer Boverman, Membership Coordinator

The Oregon Psychiatric Physicians Association is an organization of medical doctors in Oregon specializing in psychiatry. The OPPA works to ensure the effective treatment
of individuals with mental disorders through public education, advocacy, and the provision of resources.

Pennsylvania

**1996 American Anorexia & Bulimia Association of
Philadelphia**
PO Box 27156
Philadelphia, PA 19118
215-221-1864
aabaphilly@gmail.com
www.aabaphila.org

The American Anorexia and Bulimia Association of Philadelphia is a non-profit organization serving individuals
with eating disorders and their families. Its purpose is to
aid in the education and prevention of eating disorders.

AABA provides support, resources, and advocacy to assist in the treatment and recovery process.

1997 Health Federation of Philadelphia
1211 Chestnut Street
Suite 801
Philadelphia, PA 19107-4120
215-567-8001; *Fax:* 215-567-7743
healthfederation@healthfederation.org
www.healthfederation.org

Patricia Deitch, Chair
Natalie Levkovich, Executive Director
Ronald Heigler, Vice Chair
Phyllis Cater, Secretary and Treasurer

A non-profit membership organization of community health centers in Southeastern Pennsylvania. The Health Federation of Philadelphia seeks to improve the availability and quality of health care services for underserved families and people.

Year Founded: 1983

1998 Mental Health Association of Southeastern Pennsylvania (MHASP)
1211 Chestnut Street
Suite 1100
Philadelphia, PA 19107-4103
215-751-1800
800-688-4226; *Fax:* 215-636-6300
www.mhasp.org

Stephen St. Vincent, Chair
Michael Brody, President and CEO
Joseph Rogers, Chief Advocacy Officer
Christopher Nasto, Chief Financial Officer

The Mental Health Association of Southeastern Pennsylvania (MHASP) is a nonprofit corporation that seeks to transform mental health services to better meet the needs of individuals with mental illnesses and their families. MHASP addresses mental health issues through advocacy, support, training and education, information and referral, and technical assistance. MHASP's mission is to create opportunities for recovery for individuals with mental health challenges. MHASP offers services in Bucks, Chester, Delaware, Montgomery and Philadelphia counties.

Year Founded: 1951

1999 National Alliance on Mental Illness: Southwestern Pennsylvania
105 Braunlich Drive
McKnight Plaza, Suite 200
Pittsburgh, PA 15237
412-366-3788
888-264-7972; *Fax:* 412-366-3935
info@namiswpa.org
www.namiswpa.org

Charma D Dudley, PhD, FPPR, President
Kathy Testoni, Vice President
Mim Schwartz, Secretary
Eileen Lovell, Treasurer

A grassroots, non-profit organization serving individuals and families affected by mental illness. Provides support, education, and advocacy and promotes improvements to the mental health system.

2000 Pennsylvania Alliance for the Mentally Ill
2149 North 2nd Street
Harrisburg, PA 17110-1005
717-238-1514
800-223-0500; *Fax:* 717-238-4390
nami-pa@nami.org
www.nami-pa.org

Richard H. Rugen, President
Gwen DeYoung, Vice President
Tim Grumbacher, Secretary
Bill Kennedy, Treasurer

The largest statewide non-profit organization dedicated to helping mental health consumers and their families rebuild their lives and conquer the challenges posed by severe and persistent mental illness.

2001 Pennsylvania Psychiatric Society
777 East Park Drive
PO Box 8820
Harrisburg, PA 17105-8820
800-422-2900; *Fax:* 717-558-7841
papsych@pamedsoc.org
www.papsych.org

Robert E Wilson, MD, PhD, President
Gail A Edelsohn, MD, MSPH, Vice President
M Ahmad Hameed, MD, Treasurer
Keith R Stowell, MD, MSPH, MBA, Secretary

A district branch of the American Psychiatric Association, the PPS is a non-profit association comprising of 1,800 physicians who specialize in psychiatry. The Pennsylvania Psychiatric Society represents the interests of the psychiatric profession and their patients, and seeks to ensure the provision of high quality psychiatric services through education, advocacy, and the maintenance of ethical standards.

2002 University of Pittsburgh Medical Center
200 Lothrop Street
Pittsburgh, PA 15213-2582
412-647-8762
800-533-8762
www.upmc.com

G Nicholas Beckwith III, Chairperson
Jeffrey A Romoff, President and CEO
Robert A DeMichiei, Chief Financial Officer
C Talbot Heppenstall Jr, Treasurer

The University of Pittsburgh Medical Center is a health care provider and insurer focused on developing new models of patient-centered care. Its mission is to engage in clinical research, education and innovation to ensure excellence in patient care.

Rhode Island

2003 National Alliance on Mental Illness: Rhode Island
154 Waterman Street
Suite 5B
Providence, RI 02906-3116
401-331-3060
800-749-3197; *Fax:* 401-274-3020
info@namirhodeisland.org
www.namirhodeisland.org

Dana Dillon, PhD, President
Dana Parker, Executive Director
Jeremiah S Rainville, CCSP/CPRS, Coordinator of Peer

Programs
Alex Nunnelly, Policy & Advocacy Coordinator

A non-profit organization serving Rhode Island families and individuals affected by mental illnesses. NAMI Rhode Island educates the public about mental health, provides resources and support services for those living with mental illness, advocates for the rights of people with mental illness, and promotes research into the causes and treatment of mental disorders.

2004 Parent Support Network of Rhode Island
535 Centerville Road
Suite 202
Warwick, RI 02886
401-467-6855
800-483-8844; *Fax:* 401-467-6903
www.psnri.org

Linda Winfield, Board President
George McDonough, Vice President
Lisa Conlan Lewis, Executive Director
Brenda Alejo, Peer Mentor Program Director

Non-profit organization of families providing support for families with children and youth who have, or are at risk for, behavioral, emotional, or mental health problems. Parent Support Network promotes mental health and well-being with the goal of strengthening families. Parent Support Network provides advocacy, training, support services, and education, and works to raise public awareness on children and behavioral health. Parent Support Network works on behalf of children and families and aims to ensure access to effective services for all.

South Carolina

2005 Federation of Families of South Carolina
810 Dutch Square Boulevard
Suite 205
Columbia, SC 29210
803-772-5210
866-779-0402; *Fax:* 803-772-5212
www.fedfamsc.org

Kathleen Scharer, President
Roxann McKinnon, Vice President
Diane Revels Flashnick, Executive Director
Pheobe S Malloy, EdS, CPSP, Outreach Coordinator

Nonprofit organization providing assistance and support for families of children with emotional, behavioral, or psychiatric disorders. The Federation offers support networks, educational materials, publications, conferences, workshops, and other activities. The goal of the Federation of Families of South Carolina is to meet the needs of children and youth with emotional, behavioral, and mental disorders and their families, and assist them in building productive lives.

2006 Mental Health America of South Carolina
1823 Gadsden Street
Columbia, SC 29201-2344
803-779-5363
800-375-9894; *Fax:* 803-467-3547
www.mha-sc.org

Joy Jay, Executive Director
Natasha M Scott, Director of Operations
Kayce Bragg, MA, LPC, CAC/P, Clinical Director
Jean Ann Lambert, Community Resource Director

Mental Health America of South Carolina is an affiliate of Mental Health America, a national mental health advocacy organization. MHASC focuses on educating the public about mental illness, advocating for adequate mental health care and sound mental health practices, and organizing conferences designed to address the issues surrounding mental health.

2007 National Alliance on Mental Illness: South Carolina
PO Box 1267
Columbia, SC 29202-1267
803-733-9592
800-788-5131; *Fax:* 803-733-9593
namisc@namisc.org
www.namisc.org

Jim Hayes, MD, President
Bill Lindsey, Executive Director
Corinne Matthews, Office Manager
Betsey O'Brien, Director of Education and Family

A state chapter of the National Alliance on Mental Illness. Mission is to improve the lives of individuals and families living with mental illnesses. Provides information on mental illnesses and offers educational programs, support groups, and treatment facilities across South Carolina.

Year Founded: 1986

South Dakota

2008 National Alliance on Mental Illness: Brookings
PO Box 88808
Sioux Falls, SD 57109
605-271-1871
800-551-2531
www.nami.org

Nancy Sonnenburg, President
Judy Karen, Vice President
Brenda Johnson, Vice President
Vicki Graves, Treasurer

Nation's leading self-help organization for all those affected by mental illness. Mission is to bring consumers and families with similar experiences together to share information about services, care providers, and ways to cope with the challenges of schizophrenia, manic depression, and other serious mental illnesses.

2009 National Alliance on Mental Illness: South Dakota
PO Box 88808
Sioux Falls, SD 57109-8808
605-271-1871
800-551-2531
namisd@midconetwork.com
www.namisouthdakota.org

Wendy Giebink, Executive Director
John Williams, Fund Development Consultant
Marilyn Charging, Education & Outreach Specialist

Provides education and support for individuals and families impacted by mental illnesses and advocates for the development of a comprehensive mental health service system. Seeks to improve the lives of people affected by mental illness and to reduce the stigma of mental illness among the general public.

Tennessee

2010 Memphis Business Group on Health
5050 Poplar Avenue
Suite 509
Memphis, TN 38157
901-767-9585; *Fax:* 901-767-6592
www.memphisbusinessgroup.org

Cristie Upshaw Travis, Chief Executive Officer
Janis M Slivinski, Administrative Assistant
Tara Hill, Project Coordinator

Memphis Business Group on Health is a coalition of member employers seeking to manage health benefits, implement wellness programs and promote a healthy workforce.

Year Founded: 1985

2011 National Alliance on Mental Illness: Tennessee
1101 Kermit Drive
Suite 605
Nashville, TN 37217-5110
615-361-6608
800-467-3589; *Fax:* 615-361-6698
info@namitn.org
www.namitn.org

Leslie El-Sayad, President
Jeff Fladen, Executive Director
Roger Stewart, Deputy Director
Susan Ezzell, Finance Coordinator

NAMI Tennessee is a grassroots, non-profit organization serving individuals and families affected by mental illness. Provides support for people with mental health needs, educates families and communities, and promotes public policies with the goal of improving the quality of life for those living with mental illness.

2012 Tennessee Association of Mental Health Organization
42 Rutledge Street
Nashville, TN 37210-2043
615-244-2220
800-568-2642; *Fax:* 615-254-8331
tamho@tamho.org
www.tamho.org

Ellyn Wilbur, Executive Director
Alysia Williams, Director of Policy and Advocacy
Teresa Fuqua, Director of Member Services
Laura Jean, Office Manager

State wide trade association representing primarily community mental health centers, community-owned corporations that have historically served the needs of the mentally ill and chemically dependent citizens of Tennessee regardless of their ability to pay.

2013 Tennessee Mental Health Consumers' Association
3931 Gallatin Pike
Nashville, TN 37216
615-250-1176
888-539-0393; *Fax:* 615-383-1176
info@tmhca-tn.org
www.tmhca-tn.org

Anthony Fox, President/Chief Executive Office
Stacey Murphy, Vice President of Administrative
Carolina George, Vice President of Clinical Servi
Lori Abbot Rash, Vice President of Support Servic

A not for profit organization whose members are mental health consumers and other individuals and groups who support our mission. TMHCA recognizes our members as individuals whose life experiences and dreams for the future are invaluable in the structuring of ourplans and policies.

Year Founded: 1988

2014 Tennessee Voices for Children
701 Bradford Avenue
Nashville, TN 37204
615-269-7751
800-670-9882; *Fax:* 615-269-8914
TVC@tnvoices.org
www.tnvoices.org

Dick Blackburn, President
Paula Sandidge, M.D., Board Secretary
Chad Poff, Board Treasurer

Speaks out as active advocates for the emotional and behavioral well-being of children and their families. A non-profit organization of families, professionals, business and community leaders, and government representatives committed to improving and expanding services related to the emotional and behavioral well-being of children. Available on FaceBook and LinkedIn.

Year Founded: 1990

2015 Vanderbilt University: John F Kennedy Center for Research on Human Development
110 Magnolia Circle
Peabody College
Nashville, TN 37203
615-322-8240; *Fax:* 615-322-8236
TDD: 615-343-2958
kc@vanderbilt.edu
www.kc.vanderbilt.edu

Pat Leavitt PhD, Center Acting Director
Jan Rosemergy PhD, Director Communications

Research and research training related to disorders of thinking, learning, perception, communication, mood and emotion caused by disruption of typical development. Available services include behavior analysis clinic, referrals, lectures and conferences, and a free quarterly newsletter.

Year Founded: 1963

Texas

2016 Children's Mental Health Partnership
1210 San Antonio Street
Suite 200
Austin, TX 78701
512-454-3706; *Fax:* 512-454-3725
mhainfo@mhatexas.org
www.mhatexas.org

A coalition of human services providers, parents, educators and juvenile court professionals who care about the special mental health needs of Austin area youth and families.

Year Founded: 1935

2017 Depression and Bipolar Support Alliance Greater Houston
3800 Buffalo Speedway
Suite 300
Houston, TX 77098

713-600-1131; *Fax:* 713-600-1137
dbsahouston@dbsahouston.org
www.www.dbsahouston.org

Mary Collins, President & CEO
Jennifer Strich, LPC-S, NCC, Vice President of Programs

Depression and Bipolar Support Alliance Greater Houston provides free and confidential peer support groups for individuals living with, and family and friends affected by, depression and bipolar disorders.

2018 Jewish Family Service of Dallas

5402 Arapaho Road
Dallas, TX 75248-6905
972-437-9950; *Fax:* 972-437-1988
info@jfsdallas.org
www.jfsdallas.org

Michael Fleisher, Chief Executive Officer
Cathy Barker, Chief Operating Officer
Beth Donahue, Director, Marketing Communicatio
Allison Harding, Director, Career and Employment

2019 Jewish Family Service of San Antonio

12500 NW Military Hwy
#250
San Antonio, TX 78231-1871
210-302-6808; *Fax:* 210-349-6952
johnsonb@jfs-sa.org
www.www.jfs-sa.org/

Ilene Kramer, President
M.H. Levine, Executive Director
Susan Gordon, Secretary
David Scotch, Treasurer

2020 Mental Health America of Greater Dallas

624 North Good-Latimer Expy
Suite 200
Dallas, TX 75204-5818
214-871-2420; *Fax:* 214-954-0611
www.mhadallas.org

Matt Roberts, President
Janie Metzinger, Public Policy Director
Ricardo Aguilar, Consumer Programs Director
Donna Ebow, Executive Administrator

Mental Health America of Greater Dallas is a non-profit organization serving to promote mental health and meet the needs of individuals with mental illness in the Greater Dallas area. Provides information, education, and advocacy on mental health issues and offers preventive programs that target high-risk populations.

2021 Mental Health America of Southeast Texas

505 Orleans
Suite 301
Beaumont, TX 77701
409-833-9657
www.mentalhealthamerica.net

Jayne Bordelon, Executive Director

Non-profit agency dedicated to improving the well-being of individuals with mental and substance use disorders in Southeast Texas. Provides information, referral services, educational programs, and advocacy.

2022 Mental Health America of Texas

1210 San Antonio Street
Suite 200
Austin, TX 78701

512-454-3706; *Fax:* 512-454-3725
www.mhatexas.org

Lynn Lasky Clark, President and CEO
Colette Duciaume-Wright, Vice President
Julie Burch, Communications Director
Gyl Switzer, Public Policy Director

Mental Health America of Texas promotes mental health, works towards the prevention of mental illness and addictions, and seeks to improve access to high quality care through education, advocacy, and the provision of services.

Year Founded: 1935

2023 National Alliance on Mental Illness: Texas

PO Box 300817
Austin, TX 78703
512-693-2000
800-633-3760; *Fax:* 512-693-8000
officemanager@namitexas.org
www.namitexas.org

John Dornheim, President
Holly Doggett, Executive Director
Greg Hansch, LMSW, Public Policy Director
Bill Matthews, Treasurer

Nonprofit organization and affiliate with the National Alliance on Mental Illness. NAMI Texas aims to improve the lives of all persons affected by mental illness. NAMI Texas raises awareness about mental illness through the dissemination of information, and seeks to address the mental health needs of Texans through education and support programs for persons with mental illness, families, friends, professionals, and communities.

2024 Texas Counseling Association (TCA)

1204 San Antonio
Suite 201
Austin, TX 78701-1870
512-472-3403
800-580-8144; *Fax:* 512-472-3756
jan@txca.org
www.txca.org

Jan Friese, Executive Director

The Texas Counseling Association is dedicated to providing leadership, advocacy and education to promote the growth and development of the counseling profession and those that are served.

2025 Texas Psychological Association

1464 E. Whitestone Blvd
Suite 410
Cedar Park, TX 78613
512-528-8400
888-872-3435; *Fax:* 888-511-1305
admin@texaspsyc.org
www.texaspsyc.org/

David White, Executive Director
Sherry Reisman, Assistant Executive Director
Brian Stagner, PhD, Director of Professional Affairs
Amanda McCoy, Office Manager/Communications Co

2026 Texas Society of Psychiatric Physicians

401 W 15th Street
Suite 675
Austin, TX 78701-1665
512-370-1533
TxPsychiatry@aol.com
www.tsge.org

Michael Guirl, MD, FACG, President
Ira Flax, Secretary
Stephen Utts, Treasurer

2027 University of Texas Southwestern Medical Center
5323 Harry Hines Boulevard
Dallas, TX 75390-7200
214-648-3111
www.www.utsouthwestern.edu/

Daniel K Podolsky, M.D., President
J. Gregory Fitz, M.D., Executive Vice President for Aca
Willis C Maddrey, M.D., Assistant to the President
Amanda Billings, Interim Vice President for Devel

Year Founded: 1943

Utah

2028 Healthwise of Utah
3110 State Office Building
Suite 30270
Salt Lake City, UT 84114
801-538-3800
800-439-3805
www.insurance.utah.gov

Todd E. Kiser, Insurance Commissioner

2029 National Alliance on Mental Illness: Utah
1600 West 2200 South
Suite 202
West Valley City, UT 84119
801-323-9900
877-230-6264; *Fax: 801-323-9799*
www.namiut.org

Brian Miller, President
Jamie Justice, Executive Director
Francisca Blanc, Development Director
Tracy Bunner, Account Manager

NAMI Utah's mission is to improve the quality of life for individuals and families affected by mental illness and to help them lead dignified lives. NAMI Utah provides support, education, and advocacy for those living with mental illnesses.

2030 Utah Parent Center
230 West 200 South
Suite 1101
Salt Lake City, UT 84117-4428
801-272-1051
800-468-1160; *Fax: 801-272-8907*
info@utahparentcenter.org
www.utahparentcenter.org

Helen Post, Executive Director
Jennie Gibson, Associate Director

The Utah Parent Center is a statewide nonprofit organization founded in 1984 to provide training, information, referral and assistance to parents of children and youth with all disabilities: physical, mental, learning and emotional. Staff at the center are primarily parents of children and youth with disabilities who carry out the philosophy of Parents Helping Parents.

2031 Utah Psychiatric Association
310 E 4500 Sth
Suite 500
Salt Lake City, UT 84107

801-747-3500; *Fax: 801-747-3501*
paige@utahmed.org
Paige De Mille, Executive Director
Year Founded: 1951

Vermont

2032 Fletcher Allen Health Care
111 Colchester Avenue
Burlington, VT 05401-1416
802-847-0000
800-358-1144
www.www.fletcherallen.org

Melinda L Estes, MD, President/CEO
Richarad Magnuson, CFO
Angeline Marano, COO
Theresa Alberghini Dipalma, VP/Government External Affairs

2033 National Alliance on Mental Illness: Vermont
600 Blair Park
Suite 301
Williston, VT 05495
802-876-7949
800-639-6480; *Fax: 802-244-1405*
info@namivt.org
www.namivt.org

Ann Moore, President and Chair
Laurie Emerson, Executive Director
Jana Beagley, Development Director
Carla Vecchione, Program Director

NAMI Vermont is a statewide volunteer organization of individuals, family members, and friends affected by mental illness. NAMI Vermont's mission is to help all persons with mental illness lead better lives through the provision of education programs, advocacy efforts, and support groups.

Year Founded: 1983

2034 Retreat Healthcare
Anna Marsh Lane
PO Box 803
Brattleboro, VT 05302-803
802-257-7755
800-738-7328; *Fax: 802-258-3791*
TDD: 802-258-8770
www.retreathealthcare.org/

Richard T Palmisano, President/CEO
Gregory A Miller, VP Medical Affairs
Robert Soucy, COO
John E Blaha, VP/CFO

2035 Vermont Federation of Families for Children's Mental Health
600 Blair Park Road
PO Box 1577
Williston, VT 05495
802-244-1955
800-639-6071; *Fax: 802-828-2135*
vffcmh@vffcmh.org
www.vffcmh.org

Ted Tighe, President
Sherry Schoenberg, Vice President
Kathy Holsopple, Executive Director
Matt Wolf, Young Adult Coordinator

Supports families and children where a child or youth, age 0-22, is experiencing or at risk to experience emotional, behavioral, or mental health challenges.

Virginia

2036 Garnett Day Treatment Center
University of Virginia Health System/UVHS
1 Garnet Center Drive
Charlottesville, VA 22911-8572
434-977-3425; *Fax:* 434-977-8529
www.healthsystem.virginia.edu/internet/homehealth/
Byrd S Leavell Jr, MD, President UVHS

2037 National Alliance on Mental Illness
3803 North Fairfax Drive
Suite 100
Arlington, VA 22203
703-524-7600
888-950-9264; *Fax:* 703-524-9094
info@nami.org
www.nami.org

Marilyn Ricci, MS, RD, President
Janet Edelman, MS, First Vice President
Mary Giliberti, JD, Chief Executive Officer
David Levy, Chief Financial Officer

Dedicated to the elimination of mental illnesses and to the improvement of the quality of life for all individuals and families affected by mental illness.
Year Founded: 1979

2038 National Alliance on Mental Illness: Virginia
PO Box 8260
Richmond, VA 23226-0260
804-285-8264
888-486-8264; *Fax:* 804-285-8464
namiva@verizon.net
www.namivirginia.org

Barbara Collins, President
Peter Nicewicz, JD, Second Vice President
Mira Signer, Executive Director
Danny Aldred, Administrative Assistant

NAMI Virginia was created in 1984 to serve individuals and families in Virginia affected by mental illness. The mission of NAMI Virginia is to encourage the recovery of Virginians living with mental illness and to improve their quality of life. NAMI Virginia provides support, education, and advocacy and seeks to fight the stigma surrounding mental illness.
Year Founded: 1984

2039 Parent Resource Center
Division of Special Education And Student Services
Virginia Department of Education
P O Box 2120
Richmond, VA 23218-2120
804-371-7421
800-422-2083; *Fax:* 804-559-6835
www.www.doe.virginia.gov/special_ed/parents/
Patricia I. Wright, Superintendent of Public Instruc

Washington

2040 A Common Voice
Hope Center, Lakewood Boys/Girls Club
10402 Kline Street SW
Lakewood, WA 98499
253-537-2145
acvsherry@msn.com
www.acommonvoice.org

Marge Critchlow, Director
Sharon Lyons, Assistant Director

A parent driven, nonprofit organization funded by Washington State Mental Health. Their goal is to provide support, technical assistance, and to bring Pierce County parents together who have experience raising children with complex needs, facilitaing partnership between communities, systems, familes, and schools.
Year Founded: 1995

2041 Children's Alliance
718 6th Avenue South
Seattle, WA 98104
206-324-0340; *Fax:* 206-325-6291
seattle@childrensalliance.org
www.childrensalliance.org

Tom Rembiesa, Chairman
Paola Maranan, Executive Director
Nancy Norman, Finance and Operations Director
Jon Gould, Deputy Director

Washington's statewide child advocacy organization. We champion public policies and practices that deliver the essentials that kids need to thrive — confidence, stability, health and safety.
Year Founded: 1983

2042 Mental Health & Spirituality Support Group
Nami Eastside-Family Resource Center
16315 NE 87th Street
Suite B-3
Redmond, WA 98052-3537
425-489-4084
info@nami-eastside.org
www.nami-eastside.org/

Paul Beatty, Co - President
Manka Dhingra, Co - President
Shari Shovlin, Vice President
Michael C.Maloney, Secretary

Nation's leading self-help organization for all those affected by severe brain disorders. Mission is to bring consumers and families with similar experiences together to share information about services, care providers, and ways to cope with the challenges of schizophrenia, manic depression, and other serious mental illnesses.

2043 National Alliance on Mental Illness Washington Coast
PO Box 153 Aberdeen, WA 98520
360-268-2385
nami@nami-wacoast.org
www.nami-wacoast.org

Clyde Lulham, President
Otis Leathers, Vice President

NAMI Washington Coast is an organization serving to improve the quality of life for those affected by mental illness. Provides support for individuals with mental illness and their families, offers education programs and meetings on mental health, and advocates for the wellness of all people with mental illness.

2044 National Alliance on Mental Illness: Washington
7500 Greenwood Avenue North
Seattle, WA 98103
206-783-4288
800-782-9264
office@namiwa.org
www.www.namiwa.org

Tim Osborne, President
Cheryl Strange, Vice President
Lauren Simonds, Executive Director

Grassroots organization dedicated to helping Americans with mental illness build better lives. NAMI Washington offers outreach programs and educational resources on mental health, organizes events, provides support, and engages in advocacy. The mission of NAMI Washington is to improve the lives of persons affected by mental illness.

Year Founded: 1979

2045 National Alliance on Mental Illness: Pierce County
PO Box 111923
Tacoma, WA 98411-1923
253-677-6629
info@namipierce.org
www.namipierce.org

Bob Winslow, President
Laura Grealish, Vice President
Dahni Kronschnabel, Secretary
Tami Haleva, Treasurer

NAMI Pierce County is a local chapter of the National Alliance on Mental Illness, an organization dedicated to providing support for individuals and families affected by mental illness. NAMI Pierce provides support groups, classes, public information, forums, and literature on mental health, as well as sponsors Recovery Education programs.

2046 North Sound Regional Support Network
North Sound Mental Health Administration
117 North First Street
Suite 8
Mount Vernon, WA 98273-2858
360-416-7013
800-684-3555; *Fax:* 360-419-7017
TTY: 360-419-9008
www.nsmha.org

Kurt Aemmer, Quality Specialist
Annette Calder, Executive Assistant
Julie de Losada, Quality Specialist Coordinator
Shari Downing, Accounting Specialist

It is the purpose of the North Sound Regional Support Network (NSRSN) to ensure the provision of quality and integrated mental health services for the five counties (San Juan, Skagit, Snohomish, Island, and Whatcom) served by the NSRSN Prepaid Health Plan (PHP). We join together to enhance our community's mental health and support recovery for people with mental illness served in the North Sound region, through high quality culturally competent services.

2047 Nueva Esperanza Counseling Center
720 W Court Street
Suite 8
Pasco, WA 99301-4178
509-545-6506

Maria A Morcuende

2048 Sharing & Caring for Consumers, Families Alliance for the Mentally Ill
NAMI-Eastside Family Resource Center
16315 NE 87th Street
Suite B-11
Redmond, WA 98052-3537
425-885-6264
info@nami-eastside.org
www.nami-eastside.org/

Paul Beatty, Co - President
Manka Dhingra, Co - President
Shari Shovlin, Vice President
Michael C.Maloney, Secretary

Nation's leading self-help organization for all those affected by severe brain disorders. Mission is to bring consumers and families with similar experiences together to share information about services, care providers, and ways to cope with the challenges of schizophrenia, manic depression, and other serious mental illnesses.

2049 South King County Alliance for the Mentally Ill
515 West Harrison Street
Suite 215
Kent, WA 98032-4403
253-854-6264
NAMIskc@qwestoffice.net
www.nami.org/sites/NAMISouthKingCounty

John Corr, President
Sandy Klungness

Nation's leading self-help organization for all those affected by severe brain disorders. Mission is to bring consumers and families with similar experiences together to share information about services, care providers, and ways to cope with the challenges of schizophrenia, manic depression, and other serious mental illnesses.

2050 Spanish Support Group Alliance for the Mentally Ill
NAMI-Eastside
2601 Elliott Avenue
Suite 4143
Seattle, WA 98121-1399
425-747-7892
www.nami-eastside.org/

Paul Beatty, Co - President
Manka Dhingra, Co - President
Shari Shovlin, Vice President
Michael C.Maloney, Secretary

Nation's leading self-help organization for all those affected by severe brain disorders. Mission is to bring consumers and families with similar experiences together to share information about services, care providers, and ways to cope with the challenges of schizophrenia, manic depression, and other serious mental illnesses.

2051 Spokane Mental Health
107 South Division Street
Spokane, WA 99202-1510

509-838-4651; *Fax:* 509-458-7456
www.fbhwa.org

David Panken, CEO
Jennifer Allen, UC Coordinator

Since 1970, Spokane Mental Health, a not-for-profit organization, has served children, families, adults and elders throughout Spokane County. Our professional staff provides quality treatment and rehabilitation for those with mental illness and co-occurring disorders. These services include crisis response services; individual, family and group therapy; case management and support; vocational rehabilitation; psychiatric and psychological services; medication management and consumer education. We tailor services to the unique needs and strengths of each person seeking care.

2052 Washington Advocates for the Mentally Ill
NAMI Eastside Family Resource Center
16315 NE 87th Street
Suite B-11
Redmond, WA 98052-3537
425-885-6264
800-782-9264
info@nami-eastside.org
www.nami-eastside.org/

Paul Beatty, Co - President
Manka Dhingra, Co - President
Shari Shovlin, Vice President
Michael C.Maloney, Secretary

Nation's leading self-help organization for all those affected by severe brain disorders. Mission is to bring consumers and families with similar experiences together to share information about services, care providers, and ways to cope with the challenges of schizophrenia, manic depression, and other serious mental illnesses.

2053 Washington Institute for Mental Illness Research and Training
Washington State University, Spokane
PO Box 1495
Spokane, WA 99210-1495
509-358-7514; *Fax:* 509-358-7619
www.spokane.wsu.edu/research&service/

Michael Hendrix, Director
Sandie Kruse, Training Coordinator

Governmental organization focusing on mental illness research.

2054 Washington State Psychological Association
PO Box 95168
Seattle, WA 98145-2168
206-547-4220; *Fax:* 206-547-6366
wspa@wapsych.org
www.wapsych.org

Kathleen Hosfeld, Interim Executive Director
Lucy Homans, EdD, Director of Professional Affairs
Kevand Topping, Member Services Coordinator

To support, promote and advance the science, education and practice of psychology in the public interest.

Year Founded: 1947

West Virginia

2055 CAMC Family Medicine Center of Charleston
PO Box 1547
Suite 108
Charleston, WV 25326
304-347-4600; *Fax:* 304-347-4621
www.www.camc.org

Robert M D'Alessandri, MD, Vice President Health Sciences

2056 Mountain State Parent Child and Adolescent Contacts
1201 Garfield Street
McMechen, WV 26003-9062
304-233-5399
800-244-5385; *Fax:* 304-233-3847
www.mspcan.org

Joyce Floyd, President
Hope Coleman, Vice President
Jackie Hensley, Secretary
Donna Moss, Treasurer

A private non-profit, family-run organization that improves outcomes for children with serious emotional disorders and their families.

Wisconsin

2057 National Alliance on Mental Illness: Wisconsin
4233 West Beltline Highway
Madison, WI 53711-3814
608-268-6000
800-236-2988; *Fax:* 608-268-6004
nami@namiwisconsin.org
www.namiwisconsin.org

Jim Connors, President
Thomas Christensen, Vice President
Julianne Carbin, Executive Director
Katherine Rybak, Secretary

The mission of NAMI Wisconsin is to help improve the lives of individuals with mental illness and to promote their recovery through public education, advocacy, and support.

Year Founded: 1977

2058 Wisconsin Association of Family and Child Agency
131 W Wilson Street
Suite 901
Madison, WI 53703-3259
608-257-5939; *Fax:* 608-257-6067
www.wafca.org

Linda A Hall, Executive Director
Kathy Markeland, Associate Director
Carla Shedivy, Projects Manager

2059 Wisconsin Family Ties
16 N Carroll Street
Suite 230
Madison, WI 53703-2783
608-267-6888
800-422-7145; *Fax:* 608-267-6801
info@wifamilyties.org
www.wifamilyties.org

Hugh Davis, Executive Director
Joan Maynard, Information Referral Coordinator

Wyoming

2060 Central Wyoming Behavioral Health at Lander Valley
1320 Bishop Randall Drive
Lander, WY 82520-3939
307-332-4420
800-788-9446; *Fax:* 307-332-3548
www.landerhospital.com/patientservices.htm

Rebecca K Smith

2061 National Alliance on Mental Illness: Wyoming
137 West 6th Street
Casper, WY 82601
307-265-2573
888-882-4968; *Fax:* 307-265-0968
info@namiwyoming.org
www.namiwyoming.org

Roy C Walworth, President
Victor Ashear, PhD, Vice President
Tammy Noel, Executive Director
Becky Spahn, Program Coordinator

NAMI Wyoming serves to help persons living with mental illness and their families. NAMI Wyoming provides educational and support services, organizes events, and offers resources for individuals, family members, and caregivers affected by mental illness.

2062 Uplift
4007 Greenway Street
Suite 201
Cheyenne, WY 82001-4434
307-778-8686
888-875-4383; *Fax:* 307-778-8681
www.upliftwy.org/

Brenden McKinney, President
Peggy Nikkel, Executive Director
Sandy Reoff-Elledge, Vice President

Wyoming Chapter of the Federation of Familes for Children's Mental Health. Providing support, education, advocacy, information and referral for parents and professionals focusing on emotional, behavioral and learning needs of children and youth.

Government Agencies

Federal

2063 Administration for Children and Families
330 C Street SW
Washington, DC 20201
www.www.acf.hhs.gov

Steven Wagner, Acting Assistant Secretary
Anna Pilato, Deputy Assistant Secretary
Ben Goldhaber, Deputy Asst. Secretary, Admin.
Stacey Ecoffey, Acting Deputy Asst. Secretary

The Administration for Children and Families is responsible for federal programs that promotes the economic and social well-being of families, children, individuals, and communities.

2064 Administration on Aging
Administration for Community Living
330 C Street SW
Washington, DC 20201
202-401-4634
www.www.acl.gov

Lance Robertson, Secretary for Aging
Edwin L. Walker, Deputy Assistant Secretary
Dr. Whitney Bailey, Deputy Administrator, Operations
Dan Berger, Dep. Admin, Management/Budget

One of the nation's largest providers of home and community-based care for older persons and their caregivers. The mission is to promote the dignity and independence of older people, and help society prepare for an aging population. The Administration on Aging is part of the Administration for Community Living.

2065 Administration on Intellectual and Developmental Disabilities
Administration for Community Living
330 C Street SW
Washington, DC 20201
202-401-4634
www.www.acl.gov

Mary Lazare, Acting Commissioner
Dr. Robert Jaeger, Director, NIDRR
Bob Williams, Director, Indepdendent Living

AIDD ensures that people with disabilities are able to live without abuse, neglect, or expoitation, as well as supports their efforts to live full, independent lives. AIDD forms networks throughout each state, made up of State Councils; State Protection and Advocacy Systems; and University Centers. AIDD is a part of the Administration for Community Living, and runs the President's Committee on Intellectual Disabilities.

2066 Agency for Healthcare Research and Quality
Office of Communications and Knowledge Transfer
5600 Fishers Lane
7th Floor
Rockville, MD 20857
301-427-1104
www.www.ahrq.gov/

Gopal Khanna, MBA, Director
Francis D. Chesley, Jr., MD, Acting Deputy Director
Howard E. Holland, Director of Communications
Jeffrey Tovven, Chief Operating Officer

The Agency provides policymakers and other health care leaders with information needed to make critical health care decisions.

2067 Association of Maternal and Child Health Programs (AMCHP)
1825 K Street
Suite 250
Washington, DC 20006-1202
202-775-0436; *Fax:* 202-478-5120
info@amchp.org
www.www.amchp.org/

Susan Chacon, MSW, LISW, President
Lori Tremmel Freeman, MBA, Chief Executive Office
Caroline Stampfel, MPH, Director of Programs
Susan Colburn, Secretary

A national nonprofit organization representing state public health workers. AMCHP provides leadership to assure the health and well-being of women of reproductive age, children, youth, including those with special health care needs, and their families.

2068 Center for Behavioral Health Statistics and Quality
Substance Abuse and Mental Health Services Administration
5600 Fishers Lane
Rockville, MD 20857
240-276-1250
www.samhsa.gov

Daryl Kade, MA, Director
Michael Corriere, PhD, Deputy Director

The Center for Behavioral Health Statistics Quality, formerly the Office of Applied Studies, provides the latest national data on behavioral health statistics. The center also collaborates with Federal agencies to develop national health statistics policy, and promotes research in behavioral health data systems.

2069 Center for Mental Health Services Homeless Programs Branch
Substance Abuse and Mental Health Services Administration
5600 Fishers Lane
Rockville, MD 20857
240-276-1310
877-726-4727
TTY: 800-487-4889
www.samhsa.gov/about-us/who-we-are/offices-centers

Paolo del Vecchio, MSW, Director
Anne Mathews-Younes, Acting Deputy Director
Keris Myrick, Director, Consumer Affairs
Patricia Gratton, Director, Program Analysis

A Federal agency concerned with the prevention and treatment of mental illness and the promotion of mental health. Homeless Programs Branch administers a variety of programs and activities. Provides professional leadership for collaborative intergovernmental initiatives designed to assist persons with mental illnesses who are homeless. Also supports a contract for the National Resource Center on Homelessness and Mental Illness.

Year Founded: 1992

2070 Center for Substance Abuse Treatment
Substance Abuse Mental Health Services
Administration
5600 Fishers Lane
Rockville, MD 20857
240-276-1660
www.samhsa.gov/about-us/who-we-are/offices-centers

Kathryn Power, Acting Director
Marla Hendriksson, MPM, Acting Director, Consumer
Affair
Audra Stock, LPC, MAC, Director, Systems Improvement
Gerlinda Somerville, Chief, Health Systems Branch

CSAT promotes the quality and availability of community based substance abuse treatment services for individuals and families who need them. CSAT works with State and community based groups to improve and expand existing subsance abuse treatment services under the Substance Abuse Prevention and Treatment Block Grant Program.

2071 Centers for Disease Control & Prevention
1600 Clifton Road
Atlanta, GA 30329
800-232-4636
TTY: 888-232-6348
cdcinfo@cdc.gov
www.cdc.gov

Robert R. Redfield, MD, Director, CDC
Anne Schuchat, MD, Principal Deputy Director

The CDC protects the health and safety of people at home and abroad, provides credible information to enhance health decisions, and promotes health through strong partnership. The CDC serves as the national focus for developing and applying disease prevention and control, environmental health, and health promotion in education activities designed to improve the health of the people of the United States.

2072 DC Department of Behavioral Health
Government of the District of Columbia
64 New York Avenue, NE
3rd Floor
Washington, DC 20002
202-673-2200; *Fax:* 202-673-3433
TTY: 202-673-7500
dbh@dc.gov
www.dbh.dc.gov/

Dr. Tanya A. Royster, Director

The goal of the Department of Behavioral Health is to develop, support, and oversee a comprehensive, community-based, consumer driven, culturally competent, quality mental health system. This system should be responsive and accessible to children, youths, adults, and their families. It should leverage continuous positive change through its ability to learn and to partner. It should also ensure that mental health providers are accountable to consumers and offer services that promote recovery from mental illness.

2073 Equal Employment Opportunity Commission
131 M Street NE
Washington, DC 20507
202-663-4900
800-669-4000
TTY: 800-663-4494
www.www.eeoc.gov

Victoria A. Lipnic, Acting Chair
Chai R. Feldblum, Commissioner
Charlotte A. Burrows, Commissioner

The EEOC is dedicated to eradicating workplace discrimination. They enforce federal laws that make it illegal to discriminate against an employee/job applicant based on race, religion, color, sex, age, or disability.

Year Founded: 1965

2074 Health Care For All (HCFA)
One Federal Street
Boston, MA 02110
617-350-7279; *Fax:* 617-451-5838
TTY: 617-350-0974
www.www.hcfama.org

Amy Rosenthal, Executive Director
Maria Gonzalez Albuixech, Director, Communications
Suzanne Curry, Associate Director, Policy
Glitza Crowley, Human Resources Coordinator

HCFA is dedicated to working with state, federal, and local administrations to improve the health care system so that everyone in Massachusstts has affordable and comprehensive health coverage.

2075 Health and Human Services Office of Assistant
Secretary for Planning & Evaluation
200 Independence Avenue SW
Room 415F
Washington, DC 20201
202-690-7858
osaspeinfo@hhs.gov
www.aspe.hhs.gov

John R. Graham, Acting Assistant Secretary
Kara Osborne Townsend, Deputy Assistant Secretary
Gavin Kennedy, Acting Dir., Behavioral Health
Bill Marton, Dir., Disability/Aging Policy

ASPE is the principal advisor to the Secretary of the U.S. Department of Health and Human Services on policy development, and is responsible for major activities in policy coordination, legislation development, strategic planning, policy research, evaluation, and economic analysis.

Year Founded: 1972

2076 National Institutes of Mental Health Division of
Intramural Research Programs (IRP)
Science Writing, Press, & Dissemination Branch
6001 Executive Boulevard
Bethesda, MD 20892
866-615-6464; *Fax:* 301-443-4279
IRPinfo@mail.nih.gov
www.intramural.nimh.nih.gov

Susan G. Amara, PhD, Scientific Director

The Division of Intramural Research Programs (IRP) at the National Institute of Mental Health (NIMH) is the internal research division of the NIMH. NIMH DIRP scientists conduct research ranging from studies into mechanisms of normal brain function, conducted at the behavioral, systems, cellular, and molecular levels, to clinical investigations into the diagnosis, treatment, and prevention of mental illness. Major disease entities studied throughout the lifespan include mood disorders and anxiety, schizophrenia, obsessive-compulsive disorder, attention deficit hyperactivity disorder, and pediatric autoimmune neuropsychiatric disorders.

2077 National Association of Community Health Centers
7501 Wisconsin Avenue
Suite 1100W
Bethesda, MD 20814
301-347-0400
www.nachc.com

James Luisi, Chair of the Board
Tom Van Coverden, President and CEO
Dave Taylor, Chief Operating Officer
Glenda White, Associate VP/Chief of Staff

NACHC, is a national advocacy organization for community-based health centers, as well as for persons who are uninsured. NACHC conducts research and informs public and private sectors on the value of community health centers on the health care system, and also provides training to health centers.

Year Founded: 1971

2078 National Center for HIV, STD and TB Prevention
Centers For Disease Control and Prevention
1600 Clifton Road
Atlanta, GA 30329-4027
800-232-4636
TTY: 888-232-6348
cdcinfo@cdc.gov
www.www.cdc.gov/nchhstp/default.htm

Jonathan Mermin, MD, MPH, Director

CDC's mission is to collaborate to create the expertise, information, and tools that people and communities need to protect their health - through health promotion, prevention of disease, injury and disability, and prepaedness for new health threats and diseases. The National Center aims to eradicate HIV/AIDS, STDs, and TB.

2079 National Institute of Alcohol Abuse & Alcoholism
National Institute Of Health
9000 Rockville Pike
Bethesda, MD 20892
301-443-3860
niaaaweb-r@exchange.nih.gov.
www.niaaa.nih.gov/

Dr. George F. Koob, Director
Dr. Patricia A. Powell, Deputy Director
Vicki Buckley, Executive Officer
Kenneth Warren, Senior Advisor

NIAAA provides leadership in the national effort to reduce alcohol-related problems by conducting and supporting research in a wide range of scientific areas including genetics, neuroscience, epidemiology, health risks and benefits of alcohol consumption, prevention, and treatment.

2080 National Institute of Drug Abuse (NIDA)
6001 Executive Boulevard
Room 5213, MSC 9561
Bethesda, MD 20892-9561
301-443-1124
www.drugabuse.gov

Nora D. Volkow, MD, Director
Wilson M. Compton, MD, MPE, Deputy Director
Joellen Austin, MPAff, MSM, Associate Director,
Management

NIDA covers the areas of drug abuse treatment and prevention research, epidemiology, neuroscience and behavioral research, health services research, and AIDS. NIDA seeks to report on advances in the field, identify resources, promote an exchange of information, and improve communications among clinicians, researchers, administrators, and policymakers. Recurring features include synopses of research advances and projects, NIDA news, news of legislative and regulatory developments, and announcements.

2081 National Institute of Mental Health: Schizophrenia Spectrum Disorders Research Program
6001 Executive Boulevard
Room 7122, MSC 9625
Bethesda, MD 20892-9625
301-443-9233
866-615-6464
TTY: 301-443-8431
nimhinfo@nih.gov
www.www.nimh.nih.gov

Sarah E. Morris, PhD, Program Chief

A program that supports research into Schizophrenia. The goals of the program are to uncover information on the origin, onset, causes, and outcome of Schizophrenia, so that there may be better prevention and treatment of the disorder put in place.

2082 National Institute of Mental Health: Geriatr ics and Aging Processes Research Branch
National Institutes of Health
6001 Executive Boulevard
Room 7131, MSC 9634
Bethesda, MD 20892
301-443-1369
866-615-6464
nimhinfo@nih.gov
www.www.nimh.nih.gov

George T. Neiderehe, PhD, Branch Chief

The Geriatrics and Aging Processes Research Branch supports programs and research into mental disorders that occur later in life, such as Alzheimer's. This branch also looks into the relationship between aging and mental disorders, as well as the treatment and prevention of aging-related disorders.

2083 National Institute of Mental Health: Office of Science Policy, Planning, and Communications
National Institutes of Health
6001 Executive Boulevard
Room 6196
Bethesda, MD 20892
301-443-4335
866-615-6464
TTY: 301-443-8431
nimhinfo@nih.gov
www.www.nimh.nih.gov

Meredith A. Fox, PhD, Director
Julie L. Mason, PhD, Deputy Director

The Office of Science Policy, Planning, and Communications plans and directs efforts for science program planning, research training and coordination, and technology and information transfer. The Office is also responsible for the Institute's information dissemination, media relations, and internal communications.

2084 National Institute on Alcohol Abuse and Alcoholism
National Institute on Health
9000 Rockville Pike
Rockville, MD 20892
301-443-3860
www.niaaa.nih.gov

Dr. George F. Koob, PhD, Director
Patricia Powell, Deputy Director
Kenneth Warren, Senior Advisor

NIAAA's vision is to increase the understanding of normal and abnormal biological functions and behavior relating to alcohol use; to improve the diagnosis, prevention, and treatment of alcohol use disorders; and to enhance the quality of health care.

2085 National Institute on Drug Abuse: Division of Neuroscience and Behavior
6001 Executive Boulevard
Room 4282, MSC 9555
Bethesda, MD 20892-9555
301-443-1887; *Fax:* 301-594-6043
www.drugabuse.gov

Rita Valentino, PhD, Director
Roger Little, PhD, Deputy Director
Steven Grant, PhD, Health Scientist Administrator

The Division of Neuroscience and Behavior addresses the problem on drug use and addiction by supporting clinical biomedical neuroscience and behavioral research.

2086 National Institute on Drug Abuse: Office of Science Policy and Communications
6001 Executive Boulevard
Room 5213, MSC 9561
Bethesda, MD 20892-9561
301-443-1124
www.drugabuse.gov

Jack Stein, PhD, Director
Carole Andrews, Lead Program Analyst
Holly Buchanan, Staff Assitant
Geoffrey Laredo, MPA, Program Analysis Officer

The Office of Science Policy and Communications (OSPC) carries out a wide variety of functions in support of the Director, NIDA, and on behalf of the Institute. OSPC is made up of the Office of the Director and three branches, the Digital Communications Branch, the Public Information and Liaison Branch, and the Science Policy Branch.

2087 National Institutes of Mental Health: Office on AIDS
National Institutes of Health
6001 Executive Boulevard
Room 6105, MSC 9615
Bethesda, MD 20892-9619
301-443-2781
www.www.nimh.nih.gov

Dianne M. Rausch, PhD, Director

The Office on AIDS supports biomedical and behvaioral research in order to develop a better understanding of HIV, which leads to better diagnosis, treatment, and prevention of HIV/AIDS. The Office also collaborates with other NIH components, Federal agencies, and health organizations to identify AIDS-related needs.

2088 National Library of Medicine
National Institutes of Health
8600 Rockville Pike
Bethesda, MD 20894
301-594-5983
888-346-3656
www.www.nlm.nih.gov/

Dr. Patricia Flatley Brennan, Director
Jerry Sheehan, Deputy Director
Dr. Milton Corn, Deputy Director, Research
Kathy Cravedi, Director, Communications

The National Library of Medicine (NLM), on the campus of the National Institutes of Health in Bethesda, Maryland, is the world's largest medical library. The Library collects materials and provides information and research services in all areas of biomedicine and health care.

Year Founded: 1836

2089 Office of Disease Prevention & Health Promotion
US Department of Health and Human Services
1101 Wootton Parkway
Suite LL100
Rockville, MD 20852
240-453-8281
odphpinfo@hhs.gov
www.health.gov

Don Wright, MD, MPH, Director

The Office of Disease Prevention and Health Promotion works to strengthen the disease prevention and health promotion priorities of the Department within the collaborative framework of the HHS agencies. ODPHP is part of the HHS, under the Office of the Assistant Secretary for Health.

Year Founded: 1976

2090 Office of National Drug Control Policy
Drug Policy Information Clearinghouse
PO Box 6000
Rockville, MD 20849-6000
Fax: 301-519-5212
www.whitehousedrugpolicy.gov/

Jim Carroll, Acting Director

The Office of National Drug Control Policy is a component of the Executive Office of the President. The director acts as the principal advisor to the president on drug control activities, and the ONDCP coordinates the activities of 16 federal departments and agencies. The ONDCP also produces an annual publication, the National Drug Control Strategy, which outlines the efforts to reduce drug abuse.

2091 Office of Science Policy OD/NIH
6705 Rockledge Drive
Rockledge 1, Suite 750
Bethesda, MD 20817
301-496-9838; *Fax:* 301-402-1759

Sarah Carr, Acting Director
Marina Volkov, PhD, Acting Director
Jacqueline Corrigan-Curay, JD, Acting Director
Marina Volkov, PhD, Acting Director

Advises the NIH Director on science policy issues affecting the medical research community; Participates in the development of new policy and program initiatives; Monitors and coordinates agency planning and evaluation activities; Plans and implements a comprehensive science education program and Develops and implements NIH policies and procedures for the safe conduct of recombinant DNA and other biotechnology activities.

2092 President's Committee for People with Intellectual Disabilities
US DHHS, Administration for Children & Families
330 C Street SW
Washington, DC 20201
202-401-4802; *Fax:* 202-401-5706
www.www.acf.hhs.gov

J. Janelle George, Acting Dir., Community Services
Yolanda J. Butler, Dir., Social Services
Lauren Christopher, Dir., Energy Assistance
Seth Hassett, Dir., Community Assistance

The Committee acts in an advisory capacity to the President and the Secretary of Health and Human Services on matters relating to programs and services for persons with intellectual disabilities. It has adopted several national goals in order to better recognize and uphold the right of all people with intellectual disabilities to enjoy a quality of life that promotes independence, self-determination and participation as productive members of society.

2093 Presidential Commission on Employment of the Disabled
Frances Perkins Building
200 Constitution Avenue, NW
Washington, DC 20210-1
866-633-7365; *Fax:* 202-693-7888
TTY: 866-633-2365
www.dol.gov/odep

Thomas E. Perez, Secretary of Labor
Rhonda Basha, Chief of Staff
Dylan Orr, Specail Assistant/Advisor
Elena Carr, Acting Executive Officer

The Office of Disability Employment Policy (ODEP) was authorized by Congress in the Department of Labor's FY 2001 appropriation. Recognizing the need for a national policy to ensure that people with disabilities are fully integrated into the 21 st Century workforce, the Secretary of Labor Elaine L. Chao delegated authority and assigned responsibility to the Assistant Secretary for Disability Employment Policy. ODEP is a sub-cabinet level policy agency in the Department of Labor.

2094 Protection and Advocacy Program for the Mentally Ill
US Department of Health and Human Services
1 Choke Cherry Road
Rockville, MD 20857-1
240-276-1310; *Fax:* 240-276-1320
www.samhsa.gov/index.aspx

Federal formula grant program to protect and advocate the rights of people with mental illnesses who are in residential facilities and to investigate abuse and neglect in such facilities.

2095 Public Health Foundation
1300 L Street NW
Suite 800
Washington, DC 20005-4208
202-218-4400; *Fax:* 202-218-4409
info@phf.org
www.phf.org

Rachel H. Stevens, EDd, RN, Chair
Sue Madden, Chief Operating Officer/Chief Fi
Lois Banks, Director, TRAIN
Margie Beaudry, Senior Associate, Performance Im

A high-performing public health system that protects and promotes health in every community by improving public health infrastructure and performance through innovative solutions and measurable results.

2096 Substance Abuse & Mental Health Services Administration of the US Dept of Health and Human Services
1 Choke Cherry Road
Rockville, MD 20857
240-276-2000
www.samhsa.gov

Pamela Hyde JD, Administrator
Eric Broderick DDS, MPH, Deputy Adminstrator
Kana Enomoto MA, Advisor to the Administrator
Elaine Parry MS, Director of Program Services

SAMHSA's mission is to reduce the impact of substance abuse and mental illness on America's communities. The Agency was established by Congress to target effectively substance abuse and mental health services to the people most in need and to translate research in these areas more effectively and more rapidly into the general health care system. SAMHSA has demonstrated that prevention works, treatment is effective, and people recover from mental and substance use disorders. Behavioral health services improve health statuse and reduce health care costs to society. The Agency's programs are carried out through: the Center for Mental Health Services (CMHS); The Centers for Substance Abuse Prevention and Treatment (CSAP/T); and the Office of Applied Studies.

Year Founded: 1992

2097 Substance Abuse and Mental Health Services Administration: Center for Mental Health Services
SAMHSA
1 Choke Cherry Road
Rockville, MD 20857
240-221-4022
800-487-4889; *Fax:* 240-221-4021
TDD: 866-889-2647
www.www.samhsa.gov

Pamela S. Hyde, J.D., Administrator
Kana Enomoto, M.A., Principal Deputy Administrator
Marla Hendriksson, M.P.M., Director, Communications
Daryl W. Kade, M.A., SAMHSA, Chief Financial Officer and Dire

Year Founded: 1992

2098 The Alcohol Policy Information System (APIS) National Institute Of Alcohol Abuse and Alcoholism
National Institute of Health
9000 Rockville Pike
Bethesda, MD 20892
301-443-3860
niaaaweb-r@exchange.nih.gov
www.alcoholpolicy.niaaa.nih.gov/

Dr. George F. Koob, Director, NIAAA
Dr. Patricia A. Powell, Deputy Director, NIAAA

Vicki Buckley, Executive Officer, NIAAA
Kenneth Warren, Senior Advisor, NIAAA

The Alcohol Policy Information System (APIS) is an online resource that provides detailed information on a wide variety of alcohol-related policies in the United States at both State and Federal levels. It features compilations and analyses of alcohol-related statutes and regulations. Designed primarily as a tool for researchers, APIS simplifies the process of ascertaining the state of the law for studies on the effects and effectiveness of alcohol-related policies.

2099 US Department of Health and Human Services: Office of Women's Health
200 Independence Avenue SW
SW Room 712E
Washington, DC 20201
202-690-7650; *Fax:* 202-205-2631
www.www.womenshealth.gov

Barbara F. James, M.P.H., Acting Director
Valerie Borden, M.P.A., Acting Director
Lisa Begg, Dr.P.H., R.N., Acting Director
Frances E. Ashe-Goins, R.N., M.P., Associate Director for Partnership

The Office on Women's Health (OWH) was established in 1991 within the U.S. Department of Health and Human Services. OWH coordinates the efforts of all the HHS agencies and offices involved in women's health. OWH works to improve the health and well-being of women and girls in the United States through its innovative programs, by educating health professionals, and motivating behavior change in consumers through the dissemination of health information.

State

Alabama

2100 Alabama Department of Human Resources
Center For Communications
Gordon Persons Building, Suite 2104
50 North Ripley Street
Montgomery, AL 36130-1001
334-242-1310; *Fax:* 334-353-1115
www.www.dhr.alabama.gov

Nancy Jinright, Director

Member of the National Leadership Council. The mission of the Alabama Department of Human Resources is to partner with communities to promote family stability and provide for the safety and self-sufficiency of vulnerable Alabamians.

Year Founded: 1935

2101 Alabama Department of Mental Health
100 North Union Street
PO Box 301410
Montgomery, AL 36130-1410
334-242-3454
800-367-0955; *Fax:* 334-242-0725
Alabama.DMH@mh.alabama.gov
www.mh.alabama.gov

Lynn T. Beshear, Commissioner
Kim Boswell, Associate Commissioner

State agency charged with providing services to citizens with mental illness, developmental disabilities and substance abuse disorders.

2102 Alabama Department of Public Health
201 Monroe Street
Montgomery, AL 36104-3735
334-206-5300
800-252-1818
www.adph.org

Donald E Williamson, MD, State Officer

Provides public health related information about the State of Alabama.

2103 Alabama Disabilities Advocacy Program
PO Box 870395
Tuscaloosa, AL 35487-395
205-348-4928
800-826-1675; *Fax:* 205-348-3909
adap@adap.ua.edu
www.adap.ua.edu/

Angie Allen, Case Advocate
Nancy Anderson, Sr. Staff Attorney
Patrick Hackney, Sr. Staff Attorney
James Tucker, Director

Federally mandated, statewide, Protection and Advocacy system serving eligible individuals with disabilities in Alabama. ADAP's five programs are: Protection and Advocacy for Persons with Developmental Disabilities, Protection and Advocacy for Individuals with Mental Illness, Protection and Advocacy of Individual Rights, Protection and Advocacy for Assistive Technology and Protection and Advocacy for Beneficiaries of Social Security.

Alaska

2104 Alaska Council on Emergency Medical Services
20321 Middle Road
Eagle River, AK 99577-7931
907-465-3028
www.dhss.alaska.gov

Shelley K Owens, Public Health Specialist

The mission of the Emergency Medical Services program in Alaska is to reduce both the human suffering and economic loss to society resulting from premature death and disability due to injuries and sudden illness.

2105 Alaska Department of Health & Social Services
350 Main Street, Room 404
PO Box 110601
Juneau, AK 99811-0601
907-465-3030; *Fax:* 907-465-3068
www.hss.state.ak.us

Tara Horton, Special Assistant
Ward Hurlburt, Chief Medical Officer
William Streve, Deputy Commissioner
Craig Christenson, Deputy Commissioner for Medicaid

The mission of the Alaska Department of Health and Social Services is to promote and protect the health and well being of Alaskans.

2106 Alaska Division of Mental Health and Developmental Disabilities
PO Box 110620
Juneau, AK 99811-620
907-465-3370; *Fax:* 907-465-2668
www.dhss.alaska.gov

Stacy Toner, Division Operations Manager

The mission of the Division of Behavioral Health is to manage an integrated and comprehensive behavioral health system based on sound policy, effective practices and partnerships.

2107 Alaska Health and Social Services Division of Behavioral Health

350 Main Street, Room 404
PO Box 110601
Juneau, AK 99811-0601
907-465-3030; *Fax:* 907-465-3068
www.dhss.alaska.gov

William J. Streur, Commissioner
Ward Hurlburt, Chief Medical Officer
Clay Butcher, Department Communications Manage
Jason Hooley, Special Assistant

The mission of the Division of Behavioral Health is to manage an integrated and comprehensive behavioral health system based on sound policy, effective practices and partnerships.

2108 Alaska Mental Health Board

431 N Franklin Street
Suite 200
Juneau, AK 99801-1186
907-465-8920; *Fax:* 907-465-4410
www.http://hss.state.ak.us/amhb

Brenda Moore, Chair
Ramona Duby, Vice Chair
J. Kate Burkhart, Executive Director
Teri Tibbett, Advocacy Coordinator

Planning and advocacy body for public mental health services. The board works to ensure that Alaska's mental health program is integrated and comprehensive. It recommends operating and capital budgets for the program. The Governor appoints twelve - sixteen members to the board. At least half the members must be consumers of mental health services or family members. Two members are mental health service providers and one an attorney.

2109 Mental Health Association in Alaska

4045 Lake Otis Parkway
Suite 209
Anchorage, AK 99508-5227
907-563-0880; *Fax:* 907-563-0881
www.alaska.net/~mhaa/

Virginia L. Hostman, M.S., Chairman
Janet McGillivary, M.Ed., President & CEO
William F. Hostman, B.A., Assistant to the CEO

The Mental Health Association in Alaska (MHAA) is a Division of the National Mental Health Association and is dedicated to the promotion of good mental health, the prevention of mental illness and ongoing improvement in the care and treatment of the mentally ill through advocacy, education, referral, research, legislative input and the monitoring of existing programs.

Arizona

2110 Arizona Department of Health Services

150 North 18th Avenue
Phoenix, AZ 85007
602-542-1025; *Fax:* 602-542-0883

Will Humble, Director

Promotes and protects the health of Arizona's children and adults. Its mission is to set the standard for personal and community health through direct care, science, public policy, and leadership

2111 Arizona Department of Health Services: Behavioral Health Services

150 N. 18th Avenue
#200
Phoenix, AZ 85007-3238
602-364-4558; *Fax:* 602-364-4570

Dr. Laura K Nelson, Deputy Director

Administers Arizona's publicly funded behavioral health service system for individuals, families and communities.

Year Founded: 1986

2112 Northern Arizona Regional Behavioral Health Authority

1300 South Yale Street
Flagstaff, AZ 86001-6328
928-774-7128
877-923-1400; *Fax:* 855-408-3400
info@narbha.org
www.narbha.org

Mary Jo Gregory, President and CEO
Lindsay Miller, CIO/Chief Business Officer
Teresa Bertsch, Chief Medical Officer
Michael Kuzmin, Chief Financial Officer

The Northern Arizona Regional Behavioral Health Authority's (NARBHA) mission is to provide solutions that improve the health and healthcare experience of diverse communities. We serve individuals and families across northern Arizona who are eligible for State and federally-funded behavioral health services.

Year Founded: 1967

Arkansas

2113 Arkansas Department of Human Services

Donaghey Plaza
PO Box 1437
Little Rock, AR 72203-1437
501-682-1001; *Fax:* 501-682-6836
TDD: 501-682-8820
www.humanservices.arkansas.gov

John Selig, DHS Director
Janie Huddleston, Deputy Director
Keesa Smith, Deputy Director
Amy Webb, Director, Communications

The Arkansas Department of Human Services provides Medicaid, mental health and substance abuse resources.

Year Founded: 1977

2114 Arkansas Division of Children & Family Service

700 Main Street
P O Box 1437 Slot S 560
Little Rock, AR 72203-1437
501-682-8770; *Fax:* 501-682-6968
TDD: 501-682-1442
www.humanservices.arkansas.gov/about-dhs/dcfs

John Selig, Director
Janie Huddleston, Deputy Director
Keesa Smith, Deputy Director
Amy Webb, Director, Communications

The Arkansas Division of Children's Services is a member of the National Leadership Council and provides information and resources on adoption, daycare and child abuse prevention.

2115 Arkansas Division on Youth Services
700 Main Street
Slot 450
Little Rock, AR 72203-1437
502-682-8654; *Fax:* 501-682-1351
www.humanservices.arkansas.gov/dys

Michael Sanders, Program Development Manager
Judy Miller, Interstate Compact Coordinator
Justin Rash, Program Administrator
Brett Smith, Education Director

The Division of Youth Services (DYS) provides in a manner consistent with public safety, a system of high quality programs to address the needs of the juveniles who come in contact with, or are at risk of coming into contact with the juvenile justice system.

2116 Mental Health Council of Arkansas
501 Woodlane Drive
Suite 136S
Little Rock, AR 72201-1058
501-372-7062; *Fax:* 501-372-8039
mhca@mhca.org
www.mhca.org

Pamela Christie, Executive Director
Janie Cotton, President

The Mental Health Council of Arkansas is a non-profit organization governed by a board of directors with a representative from each of the 13 participating community mental health centers and their affiliates. The MHCA assists its members to achieve the goal of community based treatment which focuses on the whole person with emphasis on physical, mental and emotional wellness and promotes the comprehensive diagnostic, treatment, and wrap around services provided by the private non-profit community mental health centers of Arkansas. The MHCA is dedicated to improving the overall health and well-being of the citizens and communities of Arkansas.

California

2117 California Department of Alcohol and Drug Programs
PO Box 997413
MS# 2603
Sacramento, CA 95899-7413
916-445-9338
800-879-2772
www.www.adp.ca.gov

Edmund G Brown, Governor
Michael Cunnigham, Acting Director

The California Department of Alcohol and Drug Program's mission is to lead California's strategy to reduce alcohol and other drug problems by developing, administering, and supporting prevention and treatment programs.

2118 California Department of Alcohol and Drug Programs: Resource Center
PO Box 997413
MS# 2603
Sacramento, CA 95899-7413
916-445-9338
800-444-3066

Edmund G Brown, Governor
Michael Cunnigham, Acting Director

The Resource Center at the California Department of Alcohol and Drug Programs maintains a comprehensive collection of alcohol, tobacco, and other drug prevention and treatment information. This information is provided to all California residents at no cost through a Clearinghouse, a full-service Library, Internet communication links, and a telephone information and referral system. These services can be accessed by letter, fax, Internet, e-mail, telephone, or in person during the business hours of 8:00 a.m. to 4:30 p.m., Monday through Friday, excluding state holidays.

2119 California Department of Corrections and Rehabilitation
1515 S Street
Suite 502
Sacramento, CA 95811-7243
916-445-1310; *Fax:* 916-322-2998
www.www.cdcr.ca.gov

Dr Grant Jordon, Chief Psychiatrist
Dr Rob Prentice, Sr Psychologist Supervisor
Kathie Moon, Supervising Psych Social Worker

Our mission is founded on delivering a balance of quality and cost-effective health care in a safe, secure correctional setting.

2120 California Department of Education: Healthy Kids, Healthy California
313 West Winston Avenue
Room 176
Hayward, CA 94544-2720
510-670-4581
888-318-8188; *Fax:* 510-670-4582
www.californiahealthykids.org

Deborah Wood, Executive Director
Angela Amarillas, Program Manager

The California Healthy Kids Resource Center was established to assist schools in promoting health literacy. Health literacy is the capacity of an individual to obtain, interpret, and understand basic health information and services and the competence to use such information and services in ways that are health enhancing.

2121 California Hispanic Commission on Alcohol Drug Abuse
2101 Capitol Avenue
Sacramento, CA 95816-5720
916-443-5473; *Fax:* 916-443-1732
www.chcada.org

James Hernandez, Executive Director

Services can consist of developing Latino-based agencies, program management, consultation related to proposal development, Board of Directors training, program planning, and information dissemination. Populations or groups served include Latino alcohol and drug service agencies, groups and/or individuals planning to initiate services to Latinos, other AOD agencies with a commitment to serve the Latino community, and County Alcohol and Drug Program offices.

Year Founded: 1975

2122 California Institute for Mental Health
2125 19th Street
2nd Floor
Sacramento, CA 95818-1673
916-556-3480; *Fax:* 916-556-3483
sgoodwin@cimh.org
www.cimh.org

Mark Refowitz, Chairman
Sandra Naylor Goodwin, PhD, M, President and CEO
Doretha Williams-Flournoy, MS, Deputy Director, Chief Operating
Michelle Elder, Chief Financial Officer

Promoting excellence in mental health services through training, technical asistances, research and policy development.

Colorado

2123 Colorado Department of Health Care Policy and Financing
1570 Grant Street
Denver, CO 80203-1818
303-866-2993
800-221-3943; *Fax:* 303-866-3552
Jane.Wilson@state.co.us
www.www.colorado.gov/hcpf?

Sue Birch, Executive Director
Kady Lanoha, Chief of Startegy

The Department of Health Care Policy and Financing manages the Colorado Medicaid Community Mental Health Services program. the program provides mental health care to medicaid clients in Colorado, through Behavioral Health Organization contracts.

2124 Colorado Department of Human Services (CDHS)
1575 Sherman Street
Denver, CO 80203-1702
303-866-5700; *Fax:* 303-866-4047
cdhs.communications@state.co.us
www.www.colorado.gov

Nikki Hatch, Deputy Exec Director, Co-Chair

CDHS oversees the state's 64 county departments of social/human services, the state's public mental health system, Colorado's system of services for people with developmental disabilities, the state's juvenile corrections system and all state and veterans' nursing homes, through more than 5,000 employees and thousands of community-based service providers. Colorado is a state-supervised, county-administered system for the traditional social services, including programs such as public assistance and child welfare services.

2125 Colorado Department of Human Services: Alcohol and Drug Abuse Division
4055 S. Lowell Blvd.
Denver, CO 80236-3120
303-866-7480; *Fax:* 303-866-7481
www.www.colorado.gov

Roxy Huber, Executive Director

The Alcohol and Drug Abuse Division (ADAD) of the Colorado Department of Human Services was established by state law in 1971 to: promote healthy, drug-free lifestyles; reduce alcohol and other drug abuse and to reduce abuse-associated illnesses and deaths.

2126 Colorado Medical Assistance Program Information Center
Department of Health Care Policy and Financing
1570 Grant Street
Denver, CO 80203-1818
303-866-2993
customerservice@hcpf.state.co.us
www.www.colorado.gov

Susan Birch, Executive Director
Laurel Karabatsos, Director, Medicaid Program
Christopher Underwood, Director, State Programs

Provides numerous resources for policymakers, health care consumers, providers, and all citizens of Colorado.

2127 Colorado Traumatic Brain Injury Trust Fund Program
1575 Sherman Street
4th Floor
Denver, CO 80203-1702
303-866-4085; *Fax:* 303-866-4905
www.www.colorado.gov

Nancy Smith, Board Chair
Holly Batal, MD, Board Member
Deborah Boyle, Board Member
Susan Charlifue, PhD, Board Member

The TBI Trust Fund will strive to support all people in Colorado with traumatic brain injury through services, research and education.

2128 El Paso County Human Services
1675 W. Garden of the Gods
Colorado Springs, CO 80907-1409
719-636-0000
www.dhs.elpasoco.com

Richard Bengtsson, Executive Director
Rebecca Jacobs, Employment & Family Support Dire
Shirley Rhodus, Child Welfare Administrator
Jennifer Brown, Media Contact

The mission of the El Paso County Department of Human Services is to strengthen families, assure safety, promote self-sufficiency, eliminate poverty, and improve the quality of life in our community. They aim to keep families together and help them to become self sufficient and enable them to work closely with community organizations to stretch the safety net they provide even further.

Connecticut

2129 Connecticut Department of Mental Health and Addiction Services
410 Capitol Avenue
P O Box 341431
Hartford, CT 06134-1431
860-418-7000
800-446-7348
TDD: 860-418-6707
www.www.ct.gov

Pat Rehmer, Commissioner
Paul Di Leo, Deputy Commissioner
William Quinn, Director, Audit Division
Sabrina Trocchi, Chief of Staff

The mission of the Department of Mental Health and Addiction Services is to improve the quality of life of the people of Connecticut by providing an integrated network of comprehensive, effective and efficient mental health and addiction services that foster self-sufficiency, dignity and respect.

2130 Connecticut Department of Children and Families

505 Hudson Street
Hartford, CT 06106-7107
860-550-6300
866-637-4737
commissioner.dcf@ct.gov
www.state.ct.us/dcf/

Joette Katz, Commissioner

The mission of the Department of Children and Families is to protect children, improve child and family well-being and support and preserve families. These efforts are accomplished by respecting and working within individual cultures and communities in Connecticut, and in partnership with others. Member of the National Leadership Council

Delaware

2131 Delaware Department of Health & Social Services

1901 North Dupont Highway
Main Building
New Castle, DE 19720
302-255-9040; *Fax:* 302-255-4429
www.dhss.delaware.gov

Rita M Landgraf, Secretary
Henry Smith III, Deputy Secretary

The mission of the Delaware Department of Health and Social Services is to improve the quality of life for Delaware's citizens by promoting health and well-being, fostering self-sufficiency, and protecting vulnerable populations.

2132 Delaware Division of Child Mental Health Services

1825 Faulkland Road
Wilmington, DE 19805-1121
302-633-2571; *Fax:* 302-633-5118
cmh.dscyf@state.de.us

Susan Cycyk, Executive Director

The Division of Child Mental Health Services (DCMHS) is part of the Delaware Department of Services for Children, Youth and Their Families. Its primary responsibility is to provide and manage a range of services for children who have experienced abandonment, abuse, adjudication, mental illness, neglect, or substance abuse. Its services include prevention, early intervention, assessment, treatment, permanency, and after care.

2133 Delaware Division of Family Services

1825 Faulkland Road
Wilmington, DE 19805-1195
302-663-2665
info.dscyf@state.de.us

Jennifer Ranji, Cabinet Secretary
Rodney Grittingham, Deputy Director

The Division of Family Services is mandated by law to investigate complaints about child abuse and neglect. Since 1875, state agencies have been balancing the children's right of safety and the parent's right to choose what is good for the family. The Adoption and Safe Families Act of 1997 clearly puts the focus on the protection, safety and perma-

nency plan of children as the first priority. Services provided are child oriented and family focused.

Year Founded: 1983

District of Columbia

2134 DC Commission on Mental Health Services

64 New York Avenue, NE
4th Floor
Washington, DC 20002-3329
202-673-7440
888-793-4357
www.dmh.dc.gov/dmh/site/default.asp

Stephen T Baron, Director, Mental Health

Regulates the District's mental health system for adults, children and youth, and their families, and provides mental health services directly through the Community Service Agency (for community-based consumers of mental health services) and St. Elizabeths Hospital.

2135 DC Department of Human Services

64 New York Avenue NE
6th Floor
Washington, DC 20032-2601
202-671-4200; *Fax:* 202-671-4326
dhs@dc.gov
www.dhs.dc.gov/dhs

David A Berns, Director

The Department of Human Services provides protection, intervention and social services to meet the needs of vulnerable adults and families to help reduce risk and promote self sufficiency.

2136 Health & Medicine Counsel of Washington DDNC Digestive Disease National Coalition

507 Capital Court NE
Suite 200
Washington, DC 20002-7705
202-544-7497; *Fax:* 202-546-7105
www.ddnc.org

Dale Dirks, Administrator
Linda Aukett, Chair

The Digestive Disease National Coalition (DDNC) is an advocacy organization comprised of the major national voluntary and professional societies concerned with digestive diseases. The DDNC focuses on improving public policy related to digestive diseases and increasing public awareness with respect to the many diseases of the digestive system. The DDNC was founded in 1978 and is based in Washington D.C.

Year Founded: 1978

Florida

2137 Florida Department Health and Human Services: Substance Abuse Program
Department of Children and Families

1317 Winewood Boulevard
Building 1 Suite 207
Tallahassee, FL 32399-6570
850-487-1111; *Fax:* 850-922-2993
www.www.myflfamilies.com

Paul Keith, President
David Wilkins, Secretary

Gerald Peter Digre, Deputy Secretary
Suzanne Vitale, Asst. Deputy Secretary

The Substance Abuse Program Office is dedicated to the development of a comprehensive system of prevention, emergency/detoxification, and treatment services for individuals and families at risk of or affected by substance abuse; to promote their safety, well-being, and self-sufficiency.

2138 Florida Department of Children and Families

1317 Winewood Boulevard
Building 1, Room 202
Tallahassee, FL 32399-6570
850-487-1111; *Fax:* 850-922-2993
www.www.myflfamilies.com

Esther Jacobo, Interim Secretary
Gerald Peter Dilge, Deputy Secretary
Suzanne Vitale, Asst Deputy Secretary
John Cooper, Asst Secretary for Operations

Provides rules, regulations, monitoring of fifteen district mental health program offices and mental health providers throughout the state.

2139 Florida Department of Health and Human Services

2585 Merchants Row Boulevard
Tallahassee, FL 32399-1
850-245-4444
www.www.floridahealth.gov

Dr Steve Harris, Interim State Surgeon General
Kimberly A Berfield, Deputy Secretary

The mission of the Florida Department of Health and Human Services is to promote and protect the health and safety of all people in Florida through the delivery of quality public health services and the promotion of health care standards.

Year Founded: 1996

2140 Florida Department of Mental Health and Rehabilitative Services
Department of Children and Families

1317 Winewood Boulevard
Building 6
Tallahassee, FL 32399-6570
850-487-1111; *Fax:* 850-922-2993
www.www.myflfamilies.com

Paul Keith, President

The Mental Health Program Office is committed to focusing its resources to meet the needs of people who cannot otherwise access mental health care.

2141 Florida Medicaid State Plan

2727 Mahan Drive
Tallahassee, FL 32308-5407
888-419-3456
www.ahca.myflorida.com

Elizabeth Dudek, Secretary
Jenn Ungru, Chief of Staff
Molly McKinstry, Deputy Secretary
Justin Senior, Deputy Secretary

Provides information about the Medicare plans, benefits and how to enroll in them. Medicaid is the state and federal partnership that provides health coverage for selected categories of people with low incomes. Its purpose is to improve the health of people who might otherwise go without medical care for themselves and their children. Florida implemented the Medicaid program on January 1, 1970, to provide medical services to indigent people. Over the years, the Florida Legislature has authorized Medicaid reimbursement for additional services. A major expansion occurred in 1989, when the United States Congress mandated that states provide all Medicaid services allowable under the Social Security Act to children under the age of 21.

Georgia

2142 Georgia Department of Behavioral Health and Developmental Disabilities (DBHDD)

2 Peachtree Street NW
24th Floor
Atlanta, GA 30303
404-657-2252
www.dbhdd.georgia.gov

Judy Fitzgerald, Commissioner

Provides treatment and support services to people with mental illnesses and addictive diseases, and support to people with developmental disabilities. DBHDD serves people of all ages with the most severe and likely to be long-term conditions. The division also funds evidenced-based prevention services aimed at reducing substance abuse and related problems.

2143 Georgia Department of Human Resources

60 Executive Park South, NE
Suite 3-130
Atlanta, GA 30329
404-679-4940
800-359-4663; *Fax:* 404-656-9655
TDD: 877-204-1194
www.dca.state.ga.us

Clyde L Reese III, Esq, Commissioner
Sharon King, Deputy Commissioner
Marsha Hopkins, Deputy Commissioner

Provides programs that control the spread of disease, enable older people to live at home longer, prevent children from developing lifelong disabilities, train single parents to find and hold jobs, and help people with mental or physical disabilities live and work in their communities.

2144 Georgia Department of Human Resources: Division of Public Health

60 Executive Park South, NE
Atlanta, GA 30329
404-679-4940
800-359-4663; *Fax:* 404-656-9655
TDD: 877-204-1194
www.dca.state.ga.us

C Wade Sellers, MD, Director, District I
David N Westfall, MD, Director, District II
John Kennedy, Director, District III
Michael Brackett, MD, Director, District IV

Our mission is to promote and protect the health of people in Georgia wherever they live, work, and play. We unite with individuals, families, and communities to improve their health and enhance their quality of life.

Hawaii

2145 Hawaii Department of Health

1250 Punchbowl Street
Honolulu, HI 96813-2416

808-586-4400
808-586-4444
www.hawaii.gov/health

Loretta Fuddy, Director
Keith Yamamoto, Deputy Director
Gary Gill, Environmental Health
Lynn Fallin, Behavioral Health

The mission of the Department of Health is to protect and improve the health and environment for all people in Hawaii.

Idaho

2146 Department of Health and Welfare: Medicaid Division
450 West State Street
PO Box 83720
Boise, ID 83720-1
208-334-5546
877-456-1233; *Fax:* 208-334-6558

Richard Armstrong, Director
Leslie Clement, Deputy Director, Medicaid
David Taylor, Deputy Director, Support Service
Drew Hall, Deputy Director, Family Services

Our mission is to promote and protect the health and safety of all Idahoans. From birth throughout life, we can help enrich and protect the lives of the people of our state.

2147 Idaho Bureau of Maternal and Child Health
PO Box 83720
Boise, ID 83720-3
208-332-6910
www.healthandwelfare.idaho.gov/

Zsolt H. B Koppanyi, Author

Our mission is to promote and protect the health and safety of all Idahoans. From birth throughout life, we can help enrich and protect the lives of the people of our state.

2148 Idaho Department of Health & Welfare
PO Box 83720
Boise, ID 83720-3
208-332-6910

Richard Armstrong, Director
Leslie Clement, Seputy Director

Our mission is to promote and protect the health and safety of all Idahoans. From birth throughout life, we can help enrich and protect the lives of the people of our state.

2149 Idaho Department of Health and Welfare: Family and Child Services
PO Box 83720
Boise, ID 83720-3
208-334-6800
www.healthandwelfare.idaho.gov/

Richard Armstrong, Director
Leslie Clement, Deputy Director

Our mission is to promote and protect the health and safety of all Idahoans. From birth throughout life, we can help enrich and protect the lives of the people of our state.

2150 Idaho Mental Health Center
PO Box 83720
Boise, ID 83720-3
208-332-6910
www.healthandwelfare.idaho.gov/

Richard Armstrong, Director
Leslie Clement, Deputy Director

The Idaho Department of Health and Welfare's programs and services are designed to help people live healthy and be productive, strengthening individuals, families and communities. From birth throughout life, we help people improve their lives.

Illinois

2151 Illinois Alcoholism and Drug Dependency Association
937 S 2nd Street
Springfield, IL 62704-2701
217-528-7335; *Fax:* 217-528-7340
iadda@iadda.org
www.iadda.org

Bruce Suardini, Chairman
Eric Foster, Chief Operating Officer
Pel Thomas, Business Manager
Mary Jo Davies, External Program Manager

The IADD Association works hard to educate the general public about the disease of addiction, sharing the message that addiction can be prevented. It can be treated and people can recover from it. It is done through comprehensive media campaigns, community forums, town hall meetings, and letter writing efforts.

2152 Illinois Department of Alcoholism and Substance Abuse
401 South Clinton Street
Chicago, IL 60607-3224
312-793-2354
800-843-6154; *Fax:* 312-814-1436
TTY: 312-793-2354
www.www.dhs.state.il.us

Michelle Saddler, Secretary
Grace Hong Duffin, Chief of Staff
Tom Green, Director
Mary Lisa Sullivan, General Counsel

DASA consists of three operational Bureau's designed to reflect our mission and planning goals and objectives. Primary responsibilities are to develop, maintain, monitor and evaluate a statewide treatment delivery system designed to provide screening, assessment, customer-treatment matching, referral, intervention, treatment and continuing care services for indigents alcohol and drug abuse and dependency problems. These services are provided by numerous community-based substance abuse treatment organizations contracted by DASA according to the needs of various communities and populations.

Year Founded: 1997

2153 Illinois Department of Children and Family Services
100 W Randolph Street
Suite 6-200
Chicago, IL 60601-3208
312-814-6800; *Fax:* 312-814-1436
TDD: 312-814-8783
www.www.state.il.us/dcfs

Richard H Calica, Acting Director

The Illinois Department of Children and Family Services provides child welfare services in Illinois. It is also the nation's largest state child welfare agency to earn accreditation from the Council on Accreditation for Children and Family Services (COA). The Department's organization includes the Divisions of Child Protection, Placement Permanency, Field Operations, Guardian & Advocacy, Clinical Practice & Professional Development, Service Intervention, Budget & Finance, Planning & Performance Management, and Communications.

2154 Illinois Department of Health and Human Services
401 South Clinton Street
Chicago, IL 60607-3800
800-843-6154
TTY: 312-793-2354
www.www.dhs.state.il.us/

Michelle R B Saddler, Secretary
Grace Hong Duffin, Chief Of Staff

DHS serves Illinois citizens through seven main programs: Welfare programs, including temporary assistance for needy families, Food Stamps, and child care; Alcoholism and substance abuse treatment and prevention services; Developmental disabilities; Health services for pregnant women and mothers, infants, children, and adolescents; Prevention services for domestic violence and at-risk youth; Mental health and Rehabilitation services.

Year Founded: 1997

2155 Illinois Department of Healthcare and Family Services
201 S Grand Avenue E
Springfield, IL 62763-1
217-782-1200; *Fax:* 217-782-5672
www.www2.illinois.gov/hfs

Julie Hamos, Director
Sharron Matthews, Assistant Director
Bradley Hart, Inspector General
Amy Delcomyn, Project Mangement Officer

The Illinois Department of Healthcare and Family Services, formerly the Department of Public Aid, is the state agency dedicated to improving the lives of Illinois' families through health care coverage, child support enforcement and energy assistance.

2156 Illinois Department of Human Services: Office of Mental Health
160 N LaSalle
10th Floor
Chicago, IL 60601-3124
312-793-2800
www.www.dhs.state.il.us

Michelle R B Saddler, Secretary
Grace Hong Duffin, Chief of Staff

Works to improve the lives of persons with mental illness by integrating state operated services, community based programs, and other support services to create an effective and responsive treatment and care network. Management office which plans, organizes, and controls the activities of the organization, but does not offer services to the public.

2157 Illinois Department of Mental Health and Developmental Disabilities
100 South Grand Avenue
2nd Floor
Springfield, IL 62765-1

217-524-7065
800-843-6154
TTY: 217-557-2134
www.dhs.state.il.us/mhdd/dd/

Michelle R B Saddler, Secretary
Grace Hong Duffin, Chief of Staff

Our mission is to provide a full array of quality, outcome-based, person- and community-centered services and supports for individuals with developmental disabilities and their families in Illinois.

2158 Illinois Department of Public Health: Division of Food, Drugs and Dairies/FDD
535 W Jefferson Street
Springfield, IL 62761-1
217-782-4977; *Fax:* 217-782-3987
TTY: 800-547-0466
www.www.idph.state.il.us

Julie Hamos, Director
Sharron Matthews, Assistant Director
Bradley Hart, Inspector General
Carolyn Williams-Meza, Chief Admin Officer

The mission of the Illinois Department of Public Health is to promote the health of the people of Illinois through the prevention and control of disease and injury.

Indiana

2159 Indiana Department of Public Welfare Division of Family Independence: Food Stamps/Medicaid/Training
Family and Social Services Administration
402 W Washington Street
PO Box 7083
Indianapolis, IN 46207-7083
317-232-4946
800-901-1133; *Fax:* 317-233-4693
www.in.gov/fssa

Michael A Gargano, Secretary
Susie Howard, Chief of Staff
Paul Bowling, Chief Financial Officer
Lisa Hughes, Executive Assistant

The mission of the Division of Family Independence is to strengthenfamilies and children through temporary assistance to needy families, food stamps, housing, child care, foster care, adoption, energy assistance, homeless services, and job programs.

2160 Indiana Family & Social Services Administration
402 W Washington Street
PO Box 7083
Indianapolis, IN 46207-7083
317-233-4454
800-901-1133; *Fax:* 317-233-4693
www.in.gov/fssa

Michael A Gargano, Secretary
Susie Howard, Chief of Staff
Paul Bowling, Chief Financial Officer
Lisa Hughes, Executive Assistant

The mission of the Indiana Department of Family and Social Services is to strengthen families and children through temporary assistance to needy families, food stamps, housing, child care, foster care, adoption, energy assistance, homeless services, and job programs.

2161 Indiana Family And Social Services Administration
402 W Washington Street
PO Box 7083
Indianapolis, IN 46207-7083
317-233-4454
800-901-1133; *Fax:* 317-233-4693
www.in.gov/fssa

Michael A Gargano, Secretary
Susie Howard, Chief of Staff
Paul Bowling, Chief Financial Officer
Lisa Hughes, Executive Assistant

The mission of the Indiana Bureau of Family Protection is to strengthen families and children through temporary assistance to needy families, food stamps, housing, child care, foster care, adoption, energy assistance, homeless services, and job programs.

2162 Indiana Family and Social Services Administration: Division of Mental Health
402 W Washington Street
Suite W-353
Indianapolis, IN 46204-2779
317-233-4319
800-901-1133; *Fax:* 317-233-3472
www.www.in.gov/fssa/dmha/2688.htm

Michael A Gargano, Secretary
Susie Howard, Chief of Staff
Paul Bowling, Chief Financial Officer
Lisa Hughes, Executive Assistant

The mission of the Indiana Family and Social Services Administration Division of Mental Health is to strengthening families and children through temporary assistance to needy families, food stamps, housing, child care, foster care, adoption, energy assistance, homeless services, and job programs.

2163 The Indiana Consortium for Mental Health Services Research (ICMHSR)
Institute for Social Research Indiana University
1022 East Third Street
Bloomington, IN 47401-3779
812-855-3841; *Fax:* 812-856-5713
acapshew@indiana.edu
www.indiana.edu/~icmhsr/

Bernice A Pescosolido Ph.D, Director, Indiana Consortium for
Alex Capshew, Administrative Operations Manage
Jack K. Martin, Director, Karl F. Schuessler Ins
Mary Hannah, Production & Dissemination Manag

The Indiana Consortium for Mental Health Services Research (ICMHSR) focuses on developing high quality scholarly and applied research projects on mental health and related services for people with severe mental disorders. A major commitment of the ICMHSR is to use research to foster public awareness and improve public policy and decision-making regarding these devastating illnesses.

Iowa

2164 Iowa Department of Human Services
1305 East Walnut
Des Moines, IA 50319-114
515-281-6899
contactdhs@dhs.state.ia.us
www.dhs.state.ia.us

Charles M Palmer, Director

The Mission of the Iowa Department of Human Services is to help individuals and families achieve safe, stable, self-sufficient, and healthy lives, thereby contributing to the economic growth of the state. We do this by keeping a customer focus, striving for excellence, sound stewardship of state resources, maximizing the use of federal funding and leveraging opportunities, and by working with our public and private partners to achieve results.

2165 Iowa Department of Public Health
321 E 12th Street
Des Moines, IA 50319-75
515-281-7689
866-227-9878

Marcia Spangler, Division Director

Under the direction of the director, the Iowa Department of Public Health exercises general supervision of the state's public health; promotes public hygiene and sanitation; does health promotion activities, prepares for and responds to bioemergency situations; and, unless otherwise provided, enforces laws on public health.

2166 Iowa Department of Public Health: Division of Substance Abuse
321 12th Street
Des Moines, IA 50319-1002
515-281-4417

Kathy Stone, Division Director

The Office of Substance Abuse Prevention/Staff of the Office of Substance Abuse Prevention provides the following services: technical assistance to individuals, groups, and contracted agencies and organizations; Coordinate and collaborate with multiple state agencies and organizations for assessment, planning, and implementation of statewide prevention initiatives; and Coordinate, train, and monitor funding to local community-based organizations for alcohol, tobacco, and other drug prevention services.

2167 Iowa Mental Health and Disability Services Commission (MHDS)
1305 E Walnut Street
Des Moines, IA 50319
515-281-3785; *Fax:* 515-242-6036
jmaas@dhs.state.ia.us
www.dhs.iowa.gov

Julie Maas, Contact

The Mental Health and Disability Services Commission is the state policy-making body for the provision of services to persons with mental illness, intellectual disabilities or other developmental disabilities, or brain injury.

Kansas

2168 Kansas Council on Developmental Disabilities
Kansas Department of Social and Rehabilitation Services
915 SW Harrison Street
Room 141
Topeka, KS 66612
785-296-2608
888-369-4777
TTY: 785-296-1491
www.www.dcf.ks.gov

Phyllis Gilmore, Secretary

The Kansas Department of Social and Rehabilitation Services was established in 1973 as an umbrella agency to over see social services and state institutions. With amission to protect children and promote adult self sufficiency, SRS serves over 500,000 Kansans today.

12 pages

Kentucky

2169 Kentucky Cabinet for Health and Family Services: Division of Behavioral Health (DBH)
275 East Main Street, 4WG
Frankfort, KY 40621
502-564-4456; *Fax:* 503-564-9010
www.dbhdid.ky.gov/dbh

Koleen Slusher, Director

Administers state and federally funded mental health and substance abuse treatment services throughout the commonwealth.

2170 Kentucky Cabinet for Health and Human Services
275 East Main Street
1e-B
Frankfort, KY 40621-1
502-564-5497; *Fax:* 502-564-9523
www.chfs.ky.gov/

Steve Beshear, Governor
Jerry Abramson, Lt Governor
Allison Lundergan-Grimes, Secretary of State
Adam Edelen, State Auditor

The goal of the Cabinet for Health and Family Services is to provide the finest health care possible for people in our state facilities; To provide the best preventative services through our public health programs; To provide the most outstanding service for our families and children; To protect and prevent the abuse of children, elders and people with disabilities and To build quality programs across-the-board; and by doing all of these things.

2171 Kentucky Justice Cabinet: Department of Juvenile Justice
1025 Capital Center Drive
Frankfort, KY 40601-8205
502-573-2738
www.djj.ky.gov/

Hasan Davis, Acting Commissioner
Sheree Smith Jones, Deputy Commissioner
Diana McGuire, Acting Deputy Commissioner

The Kentucky Department of Juvenile Justice's mission is to improve public safety by providing balanced and comprehensive services that hold youth accountable, and to provide the opportunity for youth to develop into productive, responsible citizens.

Louisiana

2172 Louisiana Commission on Law Enforcement and Administration (LCLE)
602 North Fifth Street
Room 1230
Baton Rouge, LA 70802
225-342-1500
www.cole.state.la.us/

Joey Watson, Executive Director
Robert Mehrtens, Deputy Director
Tyler Downing, Confidential Assistant
Hope Davis, Human Resources

Lastest news and information on LCLE programs, resources, job openings, and general agency information on a monthly basis and for an in-depth review of our criminal justice programs.

2173 Louisiana Department of Health and Hospitals: Office of Mental Health
Bienville Building
628 N 4th Street
Baton Rouge, LA 70802-5342
225-342-9500; *Fax:* 225-342-5568
www.www.dhh.louisiana.gov

Bruce D Greenstein, Secretary

The Mission of the Office of Mental Health (OMH) is to perform the functions of the state which provide or lead to treatment, rehabilitation and follow-up care for individuals in Louisiana with mental and emotional disorders. OMH administers and/or monitors community-based services, public or private, to assure active quality care in the most cost-effective manner in the least restrictive environment for all persons with mental and emotional disorders.

2174 Louisiana Department of Health and Hospitals: Louisiana Office for Addictive Disorders
628 N 4th Street
PO Box 2790, Bin 18
Baton Rouge, LA 70821-2790
225-342-9500; *Fax:* 225-342-5568
lelsie.deville@la.gov
www.new.dhh.louisiana.gov

Bruce D Greenstein, Secretary

It is the philosophy of this agency that treatment and prevention services should be of high quality and easily accessible to all citizens of the state. The Office for Addictive Disorders offers comprehensive treatment and prevention services through ten Regional/District Offices throughout the state.

Maine

2175 Maine Department Health and Human Services Children's Behavioral Health Services
2 Anthony Avenue
Augusta, ME 04333-11
207-624-7900
888-568-1112; *Fax:* 207-287-5282
TTY: 207-606-0215
www.www.maine.gov/dhhs/ocfs/cbhs/

Julia Cabral, Juvenile Program Manager
Rebecca Thompson-Greaves, Director, Collateral Services

Children's Behavioral Health Services (CBHS), a branch of the Department of Health and Human Services (DHHS) has a long tradition of advocacy for children with special needs. Once known as the Bureau of Children's with Special Needs (BCSN), this part of the Department became known as Children's Services in 1995. In a continuing effort to meet the diverse and growing needs of Maine families, Children's Behavioral Health Services (CBHS) is going through a further transition. Most services formerly provided directly through the Department are now delivered through contracted community agencies.

2176 Maine Office of Substance Abuse: Information and Resource Center
295 Water Street
Suite 200
Augusta, ME 04330
207-621-8118
800-499-0027; *Fax:* 207-621-8362
TTY: 800-606-0215
osa.ircosa@maine.gov
www.www.masap.org

Pat Kimball, President
Peter McCorison, Vice President
Ruth E. Blauer, Executive Director
Catherine Ryder, Secretary

Provides Maine's citizens with alcohol, tobacco and other drug information, resources and research for prevention, education and treatment.

Maryland

2177 Centers for Medicare and Medicaid Services: Office of Financial Management/OFM
7500 Security Boulevard
Baltimore, MD 21244-1849
410-786-3000
www.www.cms.gov

Deborah Taylor, Director and Chief Financial Off
George Mills, Jr, Deputy Director
Maria Montilla, Director and Deputy Chief Financ
Janet Loftus, Director, Division of Accounting

OFM has overall reponsibility for the fiscal integrity of CMS' programs.

2178 Maryland Alcohol and Drug Abuse Administration
201 West Preston Street
55 Wade Avenue, Room 216
Baltimore, MD 21201
410-767-6500
877-463-3464; *Fax:* 410-402-8601
www.adaa.dhmh.maryland.gov/

Joshua M Sharfstein, MD, Secretary

The Alcohol and Drug Abuse Administration (ADAA) is the single state agency responsible for the provision, coordination, and regulation of the statewide network of substance abuse prevention, intervention and treatment services. It serves as the initial point of contact for technical assistance and regulatory interpretation for all Maryland Department of Health and Mental Hygiene (DHMH) prevention and certified treatment programs.

2179 Maryland Department of Health and Mental Hygiene
201 West Preston Street
Baltimore, MD 21201-2301
410-767-6500
877-463-3464
www.dhmh.maryland.gov

Joshua M Sharfstein, MD, Secretary

Provides information on a variety of services including mental health and substance abuse, health plans and providers, nutrition and maternal care, environmental health and developmental disabilities.

Massachusetts

2180 Massachusetts Department of Mental Health
25 Staniford Street
11th Floor
Boston, MA 02114
617-626-8068
800-221-0053
TTY: 617-727-9842
dmhinfo@dmh.state.ma.us
www.www.mass.gov/dmh

Marcia Fowler, Commissioner
Clifford Robinson, Deputy Commissioner
Liam Seward, Chief of Staff
Stephen Cidlevich, Director, Constituent Affairs

The Massachusetts Department of Mental Health provides clinical, rehabilitative and supportive services for adults with serious mental illness, and children and adolescents with serious mental illness or serious emotional disturbance.

2181 Massachusetts Department of Public Health
1000 Washington Street
Suite 310
Boston, MA 02118-5002
617-790-4000
800-495-0086; *Fax:* 617-790-4128
TTY: 617-624-6001
www.masspartnership.com

John Auerbach, Commissioner, Public Health

Our mission, to serve all the people in the Commonwealth, particularly the under served, and to promote healthy people, healthy families, healthy communities and healthy environments through compassionate care, education and prevention. Your health is our concern.

2182 Massachusetts Department of Public Health: Bureau of Substance Abuse Services
1000 Washington Street
Suite 310
Boston, MA 02118-5002
617-790-4000
800-495-0086; *Fax:* 617-790-4128
TTY: 617-536-5872
www.masspartnership.com

John Auerbach, Commissioner, Public Health

The Bureau of Substance Abuse Services oversees the substance abuse prevention and treatment services in the Commonwealth. Responsibilities include: licensing programs and counselors; funding and monitoring prevention and treatment services; providing access to treatment for the indigent and uninsured; developing and implementing policies and programs; and, tracking substance abuse trends in the state.

2183 Massachusetts Department of Transitional Assistance
Massachusetts Department of Health and Human Services
600 Washington Street
Boston, MA 02111-1751
617-348-8500
www.mass.gov/dta/

Julia Kehoe, Commissioner, Transistional

The mission of the Department of Transitional Assistance is to serve the Commonwealth's most vulnerable families and individuals with dignity and respect, ensuring those eligible for our services have access to those services in an accurate, timely and culturally sensitive manner and in a way that promotes client's independence and long term self-sufficiency.

2184 Massachusetts Executive Office of Public Safety

1 Ashburton Place
Suite 2133
Boston, MA 02108-1504
617-727-7775; *Fax:* 617-727-4764
eopsinfo@state.ma.us
www.www.mass.gov/eopss/

Dr Jusy Ann Bigby, Secretary
Marilyn Chase, Assistant Secretary
Christine Griffin, Assistant Secretary
Stacey Monahan, Chief of Staff

Plans and manages public safety efforts by supporting, supervising and providing planning and guidance to a variety of state agencies.

Michigan

2185 Michigan Department of Community Health
Department of Mental Health

Capitol View Building
201 Townsend Street
Lansing, MI 48913-1
517-373-3740
800-649-3777
mccurtisj@michigan.gov
www.michigan.gov/mdch/

Nick Lyon, Deputy Director
Angela Minicuci, Public Information Officer
Matthew Davis, M.D., Chief Medical Executive
Melanie Brim, Public Health Administration, De

Provides information on drug control and substance abuse treatment policies.

2186 Michigan Department of Human Services

235 S Grand Ave
PO Box 30037
Lansing, MI 48909-7537
517-373-2305; *Fax:* 517-335-6101
TTY: 517-373-8071
www.michigan.gov/dhs/

The Department of Human Services (DHS) is Michigan's public assistance, child and family welfare agency. DHS directs the operations of public assistance and service programs through a network of over 100 county department of human service offices around the state.

2187 National Council on Alcoholism and Drug Dependence: Greater Detroit Area

2400 East McNichols
Detroit, MI 48212
313-868-1340; *Fax:* 313-865-8951
www.ncadd-detroit.org/

Benjamin Jones, President, CEO
Don Denault, Chief Financial Officer
Linda Woodward, Director of Treatment
James Boyce, Jr, Service Leader

The National Council on Alcoholism and Drug Dependence-Greater Detroit Area is a voluntary, non-profit agency committed to improving health through providing substance abuse prevention, education, training, treatment and advocacy for the metropolitan Detroit area.

Minnesota

2188 Department of Human Services: Chemical Health Division

PO Box 64977
Saint Paul, MN 55164-977
651-431-2460
800-366-5411; *Fax:* 651-431-7449
www.mn.gov/dhs/

Lucinda Jesson, Commissioner
Anne Barry, Deputy Commissioner
Charles Johnson, CFO, Chief Operating Officer
Loren Colman, Asst Commissioner

The Chemical Health Division is the state alcohol and drug authority responsible for defining a statewide response to drug and alcohol abuse. This includes providing basic information on chemical health. It also includes planning a broad-based community service system, evaluating the effectiveness of various chemical dependency services, and funding innovative programs to promote reduction of alcohol and other drug problems and their effects on individuals, families and society

2189 Lake Area Youth Services Bureau

244 North Lake Street
Forest Lake, MN 55025-2517
651-464-3685; *Fax:* 651-464-3687
Jeanne.Walz@ysblakesarea.org

Jeanne Walz, Executive Director
Matt Howard, Community Justice Program Mgr
Aaron Lynch, Community Justice Case Manager
Kari Lyn Wampler, Youth, Family Therapist

Provides enrichment programs and intervention support to youth and families. Available on FaceBook and Twitter
Year Founded: 1976

2190 Minnesota Department of Human Services

444 Lafayette Road
Saint Paul, MN 55155-3899
651-431-3515
800-366-5411; *Fax:* 651-431-7476
www.mn.gov/dhs/

Lucinda Jesson, Commissioner
Anne Barry, Deputy Commissioner
Charles Johnson, CFO, Chief Operating Officer
Loren Colman, Assistant Commissioner

The Minnesota Department of Human Services helps people meet their basic needs by providing or administering health care coverage, economic assistance, and a variety of services for children, people with disabilities and older Minnesotans.

Mississippi

2191 Mississippi Alcohol Safety Education Program

1 Research Blvd
Suite 103
Starkville, MS 39759
662-325-7127; *Fax:* 662-325-7966
www.www.ssrc.msstate.edu

Alicia Falls, Administrative Assistant I
Angela Robertson, SSRC Interim Director and Resear
Anne Buffington, Technical Writer
Jennifer Alberson, Service Leader

MASEP is the statewide program for first-time offenders convicted of driving under the influence of alcohol or another substance which has impaired one's ability to operate a motor vehicle.

2192 Mississippi Department of Human Services
750 North State Street
Jackson, MS 39202-3033
601-359-4500
800-345-6347
www.www.mdhs.state.ms.us

Cathy Sykes, Director

The mission of the Department of Human Services is to provide services for people in need by optimizing all available resources to sustain the family unit and to encourage traditional family values thereby promoting self-sufficiency and personal responsibility for all Mississippians.

2193 Mississippi Department of Mental Health: Division of Alcohol and Drug Abuse
239 N Lamar Street
1101 Robert F Lee Building
Jackson, MS 39201
601-359-1288
877-210-8513; *Fax:* 601-359-6295
TDD: 601-359-6230
www.www.dmh.ms.gov

Dr. Jim Herzog, Chair
Sampat Shivangi, M.D., Vice Chair

The Division of Alcohol and Drug Abuse Services is responsible for establishing, maintaining, monitoring and evaluating a statewide system of alcohol and drug abuse services, including prevention, treatment and rehabilitation. The division has designed a system of services for alcohol and drug abuse prevention and treatment reflecting its philosophy that alcohol and drug abuse is a treatable and preventable illness.

2194 Mississippi Department of Mental Health
1101 Robert E Lee Building
239 N. Lamar Street
Jackson, MS 39201-1328
601-359-1288
877-210-8513; *Fax:* 601-359-6295
TDD: 601-359-6230
www.www.dmh.ms.gov

Has the primary responsibility for the development and implementation of services to meet the needs of individuals with developmental disabilities.

2195 Mississippi Department of Mental Health: Division of Medicaid
239 N Lamar Street
1101 Robert F Lee Building
Jackson, MS 39201
601-359-1288
877-210-8513; *Fax:* 601-359-6295
TDD: 601-359-6230
www.www.dmh.ms.gov

Dr. Jim Herzog, Chair
Sampat Shivangi, M.D., Vice Chair

Medicaid is a national health care program. It helps pay for medical services for low-income people. For those eligible for full Medicaid services, Medicaid is paid to providers of health care. Providers are doctors, hospitals and pharmacists who take Medicaid. We strive to provide financial assistance for the provision of quality health services to our beneficiaries with professionalism, integrity, compassion and commitment. We are advocates for, and accountable to the people we serve.

2196 Mississippi Department of Rehabilitation Services: Office of Vocational Rehabilitation (OVR)
1281 Highway 51
PO Box 1698
Madison, MS 39110
601-853-5100
800-443-1000
www.www.mdrs.ms.gov

Jack Virden, Chairman
Anita Naik, Office Director???
Chris Howard, Deputy Director, Financial
Tommy Browning, Office Director???, Administrati

The Office of Vocational Rehabilitation (OVR) provides services designed to improve economic opportunities for individuals with physical and mental disabilities through employment. Work related services are individualized and may include but are not limited to: counseling, job development, job training, job placement, supported employment, transition services and employability skills training program. OVR has a network of 17 community rehabilitation centers (Allied Enterprises) located throughout the state, which provide vocational assessment, job training and actual work experience for individuals with disabilities. Thousands of Mississippians are successfully employed each year through the teamwork at OVR.

Missouri

2197 Missouri Department Health & Senior Services
912 Wildwood
PO Box 570
Jefferson City, MO 65102-570
573-751-6400; *Fax:* 573-751-6010
info@health.mo.gov
www.health.mo.gov/

Gail Vasterling, Director
Margaret T Donnelly, Director
Kathy Branson, Deputy Director
Jennifer Stilabower, General Counsel

The Missouri Department of Health and Senior Services provides information on a variety of topics including senior services and health, current news and public notices, laws and regulations, and statistical reports.

2198 Missouri Department of Mental Health
1706 E Elm Street
P O Box 687
Jefferson City, MO 65102-687
573-751-4122
800-364-9687; *Fax:* 573-751-8224
TTY: 573-526-1201
dbhmail@dmh.mo.gov
www.dmh.mo.gov/

Keith Schafer, Director
Jan Heckemeyer, Deputy Director

Bob Bax, Director, Finance
Rikki Wright, General Counsel

State law provides three principal missions for the department: (1) the prevention of mental disorders, developmental disabilities, substance abuse, and compulsive gambling; (2) the treatment, habilitation, and rehabilitation of Missourians who have those conditions; and (3) the improvement of public understanding and attitudes about mental disorders, developmental disabilities, substance abuse, and compulsive gambling.

2199 Missouri Department of Public Safety
301 W. High Street
PO Box 36
Jefferson City, MO 65102
573-751-2764; *Fax:* 573-526-3898
dpsinfo@dps.mo.gov
www.www.dps.mo.gov

Jerry Lee, Director
Andrea Spillars, Deputy Director, Gen Counsel
Tracy McGinnis, General Counsel
Chris Pickering, Homeland Security Coordinator

The Office of the Director is the Department of Public Safety's central administrative unit. Our office administers federal and state funds in grants for juvenile justice, victims' assistance, law enforcement, and narcotics control. Other programs in the Director's Office provide support services and resources to assist local law enforcement agencies and to promote crime prevention.

2200 Missouri Department of Social Services
221 West High Street
P O Box 1527
Jefferson City, MO 65102-1527
573-751-4815; *Fax:* 573-751-3203
TDD: 800-735-2966
www.dss.mo.gov/

Brian Kinkade, Interim Director

A true measure of a society is the extent of its concern for those less fortunate-its intent of keeping families together, preventing abuse and neglect, and encouraging self-sufficiency and independence. In Missouri, programs dealing with these concerns are administered by the state Department of Social Services.

2201 Missouri Department of Social Services:
Medical Services Division
615 Howerton Court
P O Box 6500
Jefferson City, MO 65102-6500
573-751-3425
800-735-2966; *Fax:* 573-751-6564
www.dss.mo.gov/mhd/

Brian Kinkade, Interim Director

The purpose of the Division of Medical Services is to purchase and monitor health care services for low income and vulnerable citizens of the State of Missouri. The agency assures quality health care through development of service delivery systems, standards setting and enforcement, and education of providers and recipients. We are fiscally accountable for maximum and appropriate utilization of resources

2202 Missouri Division of Alcohol and Drug Abuse
P O Box 687
1706 E Elm Street
Jefferson City, MO 65101-4130
573-751-4942
800-575-7480
dbhmail@dmh.mo.gov
www.dmh.mo.gov/mentalillness/

Brian Kinkade, Interim Director

The Division provides funding for prevention, outpatient, residential, and detoxification services to community-based programs that work with communities to develop and implement comprehensive coordinated plans. The Division provides technical assistance to these agencies and operates a certification program that sets standards for treatment programs, qualified professionals, and alcohol and drug related educational programs.

2203 Missouri Division of Comprehensive Psychiatric Service
PO Box 687
1706 E Elm Street
Jefferson City, MO 65101-4130
573-751-8017
cpsmail@dmh.mo.gov

Vicky Davidson, Executive Director
Sherrie Hanks, Office Manager
Bernard Simons, Division Director
Mary Luebbert, Administrative Assistant

The division is committed to serving four target populations: persons with serious and persistent mental illness (SMI); persons suffering from acute psychiatric conditions; children and youth with serious emotional disturbances (SED) and forensic clients. In addition, CPS has identified four priority groups within the target populations: (1) individuals in crisis, (2) people who are homeless, (3) those recently discharged from inpatient care and (4) substantial users of public funds. These target populations currently constitute the majority of clientele whom the Division serves both in inpatient and ambulatory settings.

2204 Missouri Division of Developmental Disabilities
1706 E Elm Street
Jefferson City, MO 65102
573-751-4054; *Fax:* 573-751-9207
ddmail@dmh.mo.gov
www.dmh.mo.gov/dd

Valerie Huhn, Division Director
Julia LePage, Director, Community Supports
April Maxwell, Director, State-Operated Program

The Division of Developmental Disabilities (DD), established in 1974, serves a population that has developmental disabilities such as intellectual disabilities, cerebral palsy, head injuries, autism, epilepsy, and certain learning disabilities. Its mission is to improve lives of individuals with developmental disabilities through supports and services that foster self-determination.

Montana

2205 Montana Department of Health and Human Services: Child & Family Services Division
Cogswell Building
1400 Broadway
Helena, MT 59601-5231

406-444-5900
www.dphhs.mt.gov/

The Child and Family Services Division (CFSD) is a part of the Montana Department of Public Health and Human Services. Its mission is to keep Montana's children safe and families strong. The division provides state and federally mandated protective services to children who are abused, neglected, or abandoned. This includes receiving and investigating reports of child abuse and neglect, working to prevent domestic violence, helping families to stay together or reunite, and finding placements in foster or adoptive homes.

2206 Montana Department of Human & Community Services

111 N Jackson Street, 5th Floor
PO Box 202925
Helena, MT 59601-4168
406-444-5902; *Fax:* 406-444-2547
TTY: 406-444-1421
www.dphhs.mt.gov/

Jamie Palagi, Division Adminstrator
Kathe Quittenton, Public Aid Bureau
Jim Nolan, Human Services Management
Vacant , Early Childhood Services

The mission of the Montana Department of Human & Community Services is to promote job preparation and work as a means to help needy families become self-sufficient.

2207 Montana Department of Public Health & Human Services: Addictive and Mental Disorders

555 Fuller Avenue
PO Box 202905
Helena, MT 59601-3394
406-444-3964
www.dphhs.mt.gov/

Lou Thompson, Administrator
Joan Cassidy, Chemical Dependency Chief
E Lee Simes, Medical Director
Deb Matteucci, Behavioral Health

The mission of the Addictive and Mental Disorders Division (AMDD) of the Montana Department of Public Health and Human Services is to implement and improve an appropriate statewide system of prevention, treatment, care, and rehabilitation for Montanans with mental disorders or addictions to drugs or alcohol.

2208 Montana Department of Public Health and Human Services: Montana Vocational Rehabilitation Programs
Disability Services Division
111 North Last Chance Gulch
Suite 4c
Helena, MT 59601-4520
406-444-2590
877-296-1197; *Fax:* 406-444-3632
www.dphhs.mt.gov/

Jim Marks, Program Director
Clay Calton, Budget Analyst
Barbara Kriskovich, Grant Project Director

The mission of the Disability Services Division (DSD) of the Montana Department of Public Health and Human Services is to provide services that help Montanans with dis-

abilities to live, work and fully participate in their communities.

Nebraska

2209 Nebraska Department of Health and Human Services (NHHS)

301 Centennial Mall South
PO Box 95026
Lincoln, NE 68509-5026
402-471-3121
dhhs.helpline@nebraska.gov
www.dhhs.ne.gov

Kerry Winterer, Chief Executive Officer
Eric Henrichsen, Information Systems
Kathle Osterman, Director, Communications
Matt Clough, Director, Operations

The mission of the NHHS is to help people live better lives through effective health and human services.

2210 Nebraska Health & Human Services: Medicaid and Managed Care Division

Department of Finance & Support
PO Box 95026
Lincoln, NE 68509-5026
402-471-3121
www.hhs.state.ne.us

Vivianne Chaumont, Director
Dr Alan Nissen, Medical Director
Ruth Vineyard, Medicaid Initiatives
Catherine Gekas-Steeby, Eligibility Administrator

The Finance and Support agency aligns human resources, financial resources, and information needs for the Nebraska Health and Human Services System and is the designated Title XIX (Medicaid) agency responsible for provider enrollment activities.

2211 Nebraska Health and Human Services Division: Department of Mental Health

P O Box 95026
Lincoln, NE 68509-5026
402-471-7824

Jim Harvey, Behavioral Health Housing Manage
Blaine Shaffer, PhD, Chief Clinical Officer

Mental health services are designed for individuals and their families who have a serious and persistent mental illness that can create lifetime disabilities, and in some cases make the individuals dangerous to themselves or others. Services are also designed for people experiencing acute, serious mental illnesses, which in some cases may cause a life threatening event such as suicide attempts. In addition, services are provided for children and to their families.

2212 Nebraska Mental Health Centers

4545 South 86th Street
Lincoln, NE 68526-9227
402-483-6990
888-210-8064; *Fax:* 402-483-7045
www.www.nmhc-clinics.com/?

Jill Zlome McPherson, Owner, Executive Director
Dr Lee Zlomke, Clinical Director
Lisa Logsden, Psy.D., Staff Psychologist

We are a primary mental health care center that is truly committed to being of service to the Lincoln/Lancaster community and Greater Nebraska.

Nevada

2213 Nevada Department of Health and Human Services
4126 Technology Way
Room 100
Carson City, NV 89706-2013
775-684-4000
www.dhhs.nv.gov

Mike Willden, Director
Ellen Crecelius, Fiscal Services, Deputy Director
Amber Joiner, Programs, Deputy Director
Kareen Masters, Administrative Services, Deputy

The Department of Health and Human Services (DHHS) promotes the health and well-being of Nevadans through the delivery or facilitation of essential services to ensure families are strengthened, public health is protected, and individuals achieve their highest level of self-sufficiency.

2214 Nevada Division of Mental Health & Developmental Services
4126 Technology Way
2nd Floor
Carson City, NV 89706-2027
775-684-5943; *Fax:* 775-684-5966
mhdswebmaster@mhds.nv.gov
www.mhds.state.nv.us

Richard Whitley, Acting Administrator
Jane Gruner, Deputy Adminstrator
Tracey Green, MD, Northen Medical Director
Karen Hayes, Office Manager

The Nevada Division of Mental Health provides a full array of clinical services to over 24,000 consumers each year. Services include: crisis intervention, hospital care, medication clinic, outpatient counseling, residential support and other mental health services targeted to individuals with serious mental illness.

2215 Nevada Employment Training & Rehabilitation Department
500 East Third Street
Carson City, NV 89713-1
775-684-3849; *Fax:* 775-684-3850
TTY: 775-687-5353
www.nvdetr.org/

Larry Mosley, Director

The Department of Employment, Training and Rehabilitation (DETR) is comprised of four divisions with numerous bureaus programs, and services housed in offices throughout Nevada to provide citizens the state's premier source of employment, training, and rehabilitative programs.

2216 Northern Nevada Adult Mental Health Services
480 Galletti Way
Sparks, NV 89431-5573
775-688-2001; *Fax:* 775-688-2192
www.mhds.state.nv.us

Richard Whitely, Acting Administrator
Jane Gruner, Deputy Administrator
Tracey Green, MD, Northern Medical Director

The mission of Northern Nevada Adult Mental Health Services is to provide psychiatric treatment and rehabilitation services in the least restrictive setting to support personal recovery and enhance quality of life.

2217 Southern Nevada Adult Mental Health Services
6161 W Charleston Boulevard
Las Vegas, NV 89146-1148
702-486-6000
www.mhds.state.nv.us

Richard Whitley, Acting Administrator
Jane Gruner, Deputy Administrator
Tracey Green, MD, Northern Medical Director

State operated community mental health center. Provides inpatient and outpatient psychiatric services.

New Hampshire

2218 New Hampshire Department of Health & Human Services: Bureau of Community Health Services
29 Hazen Drive
Concord, NH 03301-6503
603-271-4638
800-852-3345; *Fax:* 603-271-8705
TDD: 800-735-2964
www.www.dhhs.state.nh.us/dphs/bchs/index.htm

The Bureau of Community Health Services oversees grants to community-based agencies for medical and preventive health services, sets policy, provides technical assistance and education, and carries out quality assurance activities in its programmatic areas of expertise.

2219 New Hampshire Department of Health and Human Services: Bureau of Developmental Services
105 Pleasant Street
Concord, NH 03301-3852
603-271-5034
800-852-3345; *Fax:* 603-271-5166
TDD: 800-735-2964
www.www.dhhs.state.nh.us/dcbcs/bds/index.htm

The NH developmental services system offers its consumers with developmental disabilities and acquired brain disorders a wide range of supports and services within their own communities. BDS is comprised of a main office in Concord and 12 designated non-profit and specialized service agencies that represent specific geographic regions of NH; the community agencies are commonly referred to as Area Agencies. All direct services and supports to individuals and families are provided in accordance with contractual agreements between BDS and the Area Agencies.

2220 New Hampshire Department of Health and Human Services: Bureau of Behavioral Health
105 Pleasant Street
Concord, NH 03301-3852
603-271-5000
800-852-3345; *Fax:* 603-271-5058
TDD: 800-735-2964
www.www.dhhs.state.nh.us/dcbcs/bbh/index.htm

The Bureau of Behavioral Health (BBH) seeks to promote respect, recovery, and full community inclusion for adults, including older adults, who experience a mental illness and children with an emotional disturbance. By law and rule, BBH is mandated to ensure the provision of efficient and effective services to those citizens who are most severely and persistently disabled by mental, emotional, and behavioral dysfunction. To this end, BBH has apportioned the entire state into community mental health regions. Each of the ten regions has a BBH contracted Community Mental

Health Center and many regions have Peer Support Agencies.

New Jersey

2221 Juvenile Justice Commission

1001 Spruce Street
Suite 202
Trenton, NJ 08638-3957
609-292-1400; *Fax:* 609-943-4611
commission@njjjc.org
www.www.nj.gov/lps/jjc/index.html

Kevin M. Brown, Executive Director
Felix Mickens, Deputy Executive Director
Keith Poujol, Director, Administration
Robert Montalbano, Deputy Executive Dir., Programs

The Juvenile Justice Commission (JJC) has three primary responsibilities: the care and custody of juvenile offenders committed to the agency by the courts, the support of local efforts to plan for and provide services to at-risk and court-involved youth through County Youth Services Commissions and the state Incentive Program, and the supervision of youth on aftercare/parole.

2222 New Jersey Department of Human Services
Capital Place One

P O Box 700
222 S Warren Street
Trenton, NJ 08608-2306
609-292-3717; *Fax:* 609-292-3824
www.www.state.nj.us/humanservices/

Jennifer Velez, Esq, Commissioner

The New Jersey Department of Human Services (DHS) is the state's social services agency, serving more than one million of New Jersey 's most vulnerable citizens, or about one of every eight New Jersey residents. Through the work of DHS and its 13 major divisions, individuals and families in need are able to keep their lives on track, their families together, a roof over their heads, and their health protected. Human Services offers individuals and families the breathing room they need in order to find permanent solutions to otherwise daunting problems.

2223 New Jersey Division of Mental Health Services

PO Box 700
PO Box 727
Trenton, NJ 08625
800-382-6717
www.www.state.nj.us/humanservices/dmhs/

Jennifer Velez, Esq, Commissioner

The Division of Mental Health Services (DMHS) serves adults with serious and persistent mental illnesses. Central to the Division's mission is the fact that these individuals are entitled to dignified and meaningful lives. With an operating budget of $588,377,000 for FY 2005 and 5,700 employees, services are available to anyone in the state who feels they need help with a mental health problem.

New Mexico

2224 New Mexico Behavioral Health Collaborative

37 Plaza La Prensa
PO Box 2348
Santa Fe, NM 87507-2348

505-827-6250; *Fax:* 505-827-3185
deborah.fickling@state.nm.us
www.www.bhc.state.nm.us

Linda Roebuck, Chief Executive Officer

At the heart of the Collaborative's vision is the expectation that the lives of individuals with mental illness and substance use disorders (customers) will improve, that customers and family members will have an equal voice in the decisions that affect them and their loved ones, and that those most affected by mental illness and substance abuse can recover to lead full, meaningful lives within their communities. To achieve this will require a paradigm shift not only within the service delivery culture but also within the existing customer/family member networks.

2225 New Mexico Department of Health

1190 S St. Francis Drive
PO Box 26110
Santa Fe, NM 87505-4173
505-827-2613
www.nmhealth.org

Alfredo Vigil, Manager

The mission of the New Mexico Department of Health is to promote health and sound health policy, prevent disease and disability, improve health services systems and assure that essential public health functions and safety net services are available to New Mexicans.

2226 New Mexico Department of Human Services

PO Box 2348
Santa Fe, NM 87504-2348
505-827-7750; *Fax:* 505-827-6286
eckert@state.nm.us
www.state.nm.us/hsd/

Sidone Squier, Secretary
Lisa Medina Lujan, Constituent Services
Matt Kennicott, Communications Director
Betina McCracken, Public Records Custodian

The Department strives to provide New Mexicans access to support and services so that they may move toward self-sufficiency.

2227 New Mexico Health & Environment Department

1190 St. Francis Drive
Suite N4050
Santa Fe, NM 87505-4173
800-219-6157
www.nmenv.state.nm.us/

Elaine Olah, Administrative Services Division

Our mission is to provide the highest quality of life throughout the state by promoting a safe, clean and productive environment.

2228 New Mexico Kids, Parents and Families Office of Child Development: Children, Youth and Families Department

760 Motel Blvd
Suite C
Las Cruces, NM 88007-4169
505-827-7946; *Fax:* 505-476-0490
www.newmexicokids.org/Family/

Dan Haggard, Director

The Children, Youth and Families Department Office of Child Development (OCD) works collaboratively with the

State Department of Education, Department of Health, Department of Labor and higher education and community programs to establish a five-year plan for Early Care, Education and Family Support Professional Development. The New Mexico Professional Development Initiative supports OCD's legislative mandate to articulate and implement training and licensure requirements for individuals working in all recognized settings with children from birth to age eight.

New York

2229 New York State Office of Mental Health
44 Holland Avenue
Albany, NY 12229-1
518-474-5554
800-597-8481
www.www.omh.ny.gov

Michael Hogan, Director

Promoting the mental health of all New Yorkers with a particular focus on providing hope and recovery for adults with serious mental illness and children with serious emotional disturbances.

North Carolina

2230 North Carolina Division of Mental Health
325 North Salisbury Street
Raleigh, NC 27603-1388
919-733-7011; *Fax:* 919-508-0951
contactdmh@ncmail.net
www.www.ncdhhs.gov/mhddsas/

Courtney Cantrell, Acting Director
Jim Jarrard, Deputy Director
Diana Simmons, Human Resources Manager
Ureh N. Lekwauwa, Chief, Clinical Policy

North Carolina will provide people with, or at risk of, mental illness, developmental disabilities and substance problems and their families the necessary prevention, intervention, treatment, services and supports they need to live successfully in communities of their choice.

2231 North Carolina Division of Social Services
820 S. Boylan Avenue
Dorothea Dix Campus, McBryde Building
Raleigh, NC 27603
919-527-6335; *Fax:* 919-334-1018
www.www.ncdhhs.gov/dss/

Sherry S Bradsher, Director
Laketha Miller, Controller
Emery Edwards Miliken, General Counsel

The North Carolina Dept of Health and Human Services, in collaboration with its partners, protects the health and safety of all North Carolinians and provides essential human services.

2232 North Carolina Substance Abuse Professional Certification Board (NCSAPCB)
PO Box 10126
Raleigh, NC 27605-126
919-832-0975; *Fax:* 919-833-5743

Anna Misenheimer, Executive Director
Barden Culbreth, Associate Director
Katie Faulkner, Associate
Matt Musselwhite, Controller

Provides guidelines for the certification of professionals in the substance abuse field of human services.

North Dakota

2233 North Dakota Department of Human Services Division of Mental Health and Substance Abuse Services
1237 West Divide Avenue
Suite 1C
Bismarck, ND 58501-1208
701-328-8920
800-755-2719; *Fax:* 701-328-8969
www.nd.gov/dhs/services/mentalhealth

Steve Jordan, Director
Jim Jarrard, Deputy Director
Diana Simmons, Human Resources Manager
Jesse Sowa, Support, Clinical Policy

Provides leadership for the planning, development and oversight of a system of care for children, adults and families with severe emotional disorders, mental illness and/or substance abuse issues. Mental health and substance abuse services are delivered through eight Regional Human Services Centers and the North Dakota State Hospital in Jamestown.

Ohio

2234 Ohio Department of Mental Health
30 East Broad Street
8th Floor
Columbus, OH 43215-3430
614-466-2596
877-275-6364
TTY: 614-752-9696
questions@mha.ohio.gov
www.www.mha.ohio.gov

Tracy J Plouk, Director
Mark A Hurst, MD, Medical Director
James Lapczynski, Administration Assistant Directo
Angie Bergefurd, Community Assistant Director

Ensures high quality mental health care is available to all Ohioans, particularly individuals with severe mental illness.

Oklahoma

2235 Oklahoma Department of Human Services
2400 North Lincoln Blvd
Oklahoma City, OK 73105
405-521-3646
800-522-3511

Diane Haser-Bennett, Director

The mission of the Oklahoma Department of Human Services is to help individuals and families in need help themselves lead safer, healthier, more independent and productive lives.

2236 Oklahoma Department of Mental Health and Substance Abuse Service (ODMHSAS)
1200 NE 13th Street
PO Box 53277
Oklahoma City, OK 73152-3277
405-522-3908
800-522-9054; *Fax:* 405-522-3650

TDD: 405-522-3851
www.www.ok.gov

Vacant , Director

State agency responsible for mental health, substance abuse, and domestic violence and sexual assault services.

2237 Oklahoma Healthcare Authority

2401 N W 23rd Street
Suite 1A
Oklahoma City, OK 73107-3400
405-522-7300
www.www.okhca.org

Charles Ed McFall, Chairman
Tony Armstrong, Vice Chairman

Provides health and medical policy information to Medicaid consumers and providers, administers SoonerCare and other health related programs.

2238 Oklahoma Mental Health Consumer Council

3200 NW 48th
Suite 102
Oklahoma City, OK 73112-5911
405-604-6975
888-424-1305
www.omhcc.org

Becky Tallent, Executive Director

2239 Oklahoma Office of Juvenile Affairs

3812 North Santa Fe
Suite 400
Oklahoma City, OK 73118-8500
918-530-2800; *Fax:* 918-530-2890
www.ok.gov/oja/

T. Keith Wilson, Executive Director
James Adams, Chief of Staff
Jeff Gifford, Division Director, Support Servi
Jim Goble, Division Administrator, Juvenile

State agency charged with delivery of programs and services to delinquent youth. Services include delinquency prevention, diversion, counseling in both community and secure residential programs. OJA provides counseling services with counselors, social workers and psychologists, as well as contracted service providers.

Year Founded: 1995

Oregon

2240 Marion County Health Department

3180 Center Street North East
Suite 2100
Salem, OR 97301
503-588-5357; *Fax:* 503-364-6552
health@co.marion.or.us
www.co.marion.or.us

Jeff White, Chief Financial Officer
Laurie Steel, Treasurer

The Marion County Health Department fosters wellness, monitors health trends, and responds to community health needs.

2241 Oregon Department of Human Resources: Division of Health Services

800 NE Oregon Street
Portland, OR 97232-2162

971-673-1555; *Fax:* 971-673-1562
TTY: 971-673-0372
www.oregonindependentcontractors.com

Stephanie Hoskins, Chief Executive Officer
Jerry Waybrant, Deputy Asst Director
Sandy Dugan, Operations Support Manager

Health Services administers low-income medical programs, and mental health and substance abuse services. It provides public health services such as monitoring drinking-water quality and communicable-disease outbreaks, inspecting restaurants and promoting healthy behaviors.

2242 Oregon Health Policy and Research: Policy and Analysis Unit

1225 Ferry Street Se
1st Floor
Salem, OR 97301-4278
503-373-1824
www.oregon.gov/

Facilitates collaborative health services and research and policy analysis on issues affecting the Oregon Health Plan population and works to effectively communicate timely, quality results of health services research and analysis in the interest of informing health policy.

Pennsylvania

2243 Pennsylvania Department of Human Services: Office of Mental Health and Substance Abuse Services

PO Box 2675
Harrisburg, PA 17105-2675
717-787-6443
www.dhs.pa.gov

Lynn Kovich, Program Officer

The Office provides individuals with opportunities for growth, recovery and inclusion, and culturally competent services and supports.

Rhode Island

2244 Rhode Island Council on Alcoholism and Other Drug Dependence

500 Prospect Street
Suite 202
Pawtucket, RI 02860-6260
401-725-0410; *Fax:* 401-725-0768
info@ricaodd.org
www.www.ricaodd.org

Heather Cabral, Director of Community Housing
Athena Sirignano, Administrative Assistant
Stephanie Coolbaugh, Housing Coordinator
Nicholas Sousa, Case Manager - Veterans

The Rhode Island Council on Alcoholism and Other Drug Dependence is a private, non-profit corporation whose mission is to help individuals, youth and families who are troubled with alcohol, tobacco and other drug dependence.

Year Founded: 1969

2245 Rhode Island Department of Behavioral Healthcare, Developmental Disabilities and Hospitals

14 Harrington Road
Cranston, RI 02920-3080

401-462-3201; *Fax:* 401-462-3204
TDD: 401-462-6087
BHDDH.AskDD@bhddh.ri.gov
www.www.bhddh.ri.gov

Craig S Stenning, Executive Director

The department's mission is to serve individuals who live with mental illness, substance use disorder and/or a developmental disability by maintaining a system of high quality, safe, affordable and coordinated care across the spectrum of behavioral health care services.

2246 Rhode Island Division of Substance Abuse
14 Harrington Road
Cranston, RI 02920-3080
401-462-4680; *Fax:* 401-462-6078

Craig Stenning, Executive Director

Substance Abuse Treatment and Prevention Services (SATPS) is responsible for planning, coordinating and administering a comprehensive statewide system of substance abuse, treatment and prevention activities. SATPS develops, supports and advocates for high quality, accessible, comprehensive and clinically appropriate substance abuse prevention and treatment services in order to decrease the negative effects of alcohol, tobacco and other drug use in Rhode Island, and improve the overall behavioral health of Rhode Islanders.

South Carolina

2247 South Carolina Department of Alcohol and Other Drug Abuse Services
2414 Bull street
PO Box 8268
Columbia, SC 29201
803-896-5555; *Fax:* 803-896-5557
btooney@daodas.sc.gov
www.www.daodas.state.sc.us

Bob Toomey, Director
Kaitlin Blanco-Silva, Project manager
Lillian Roberson, Manager,Division of Operations
Lachelle Frederick, Administrative Coordinator

DAODAS is the cabinet-level department responsible for ensuring the availability of comprehensive alcohol and other drug abuse services for the citizens of South Carolina.

Year Founded: 1957

2248 South Carolina Department of Mental Health
2414 Bull Street
Columbia, SC 29202
803-898-8319
TTY: 864-297-5130
www.www.state.sc.us

John H Magill, Executive Director

The administrative offices of the South Carolina Department of Mental Health are located in Columbia and provide support services including long-range planning, performance and clinical standards, evaluation and quality assurance, personnel management, communications, information resource management, legal counsel, financial, and procurement. In addition, the central office administers services for the hearing impaired; children, adolescents and their families; people with developmental disabilities; those needing alcohol and drug treatment; the elderly; and patients who need long-term care.

2249 South Carolina Department of Social Services
1535 Confederate Avenue Extension
P O Box 1520
Columbia, SC 29202-1520
803-898-7601
www.dss.sc.gov

Kathleen Hayes, State Director

The mission of the South Carolina Department of Social Services is to ensure the safety and health of children and adults who cannot protect themselves, and to assist those in need of food assistance and temporary financial assistance while transitioning into employment.

South Dakota

2250 South Dakota Department of Social Services Office of Medical Services
700 Governors Drive
Pierre, SD 57501-2291
605-773-3165; *Fax:* 605-773-4950
Medical@STATE.SD.US
www.www.dss.sd.gov

Dan Siebersma, Director

The South Dakota Office of Medical Services covers medical care provided to low income people who meet eligibility standards either under Medicaid (Title XIX) or the Children's Health Insurance Program (CHIP). These programs are financed jointly by state and federal government and are managed by the SD Department of Social Services.

2251 South Dakota Human Services Center
3515 Broadway Avenue
PO Box 7600
Yankton, SD 57078-7600
605-668-3100
800-273-8255; *Fax:* 605-668-3460
www.dss.sd.gov/behavioralhealth/hsc/services.aspx

Ric Compton, Administator

To provide persons who are mentally ill or chemically dependent with effective, individualized professional treatment that enables them to achieve their highest level of personal independence in the most therapeutic environment.

Tennessee

2252 Bureau of TennCare: State of Tennessee
310 Great Circle Road
Nashville, TN 37243-1700
800-342-3145
Tenn.Care@tn.gov
www.state.tn.us/tenncare/

Darin Gordon, Deputy Commissioner

On January 1, 1994, Tennessee began a new health care reform program called TennCare. This program, which required no new taxes, essentially replaced the Medicaid program in Tennessee. TennCare was designed as a managed care model. It extended coverage to uninsured and uninsurable persons who were not eligible for Medicaid.

2253 Council for Alcohol & Drug Abuse Services (CADAS)
207 Spears Avenue
Chattanooga, TN 37405

423-756-7644
877-282-2327; *Fax:* 423-756-7646
TTY: 423-752-0352
info@cadas.org
www.cadas.org

Paul Fuchcar MEd, EdD, Executive Director

Welcome to CADAS, founded in 1964. The CADAS mission is to deliver the highest quality treatment, prevention, and educational services to the chemically dependent, their families, and the community at large.

Year Founded: 1964

2254 Memphis Alcohol and Drug Council
1430 Poplar Avenue
Memphis, TN 38104-2901
901-274-0056

Catherine Bailey, Director

Provides referrals, alcohol and other drug prevention, intervention and treatment services. Also, regional and county school prevention coordination, and a clearinghouse for Shelby County including national data search and materials distribution.

2255 Middle Tennessee Mental Health Institute
221 Stewarts Ferry Pike
Nashville, TN 37214-3325
615-902-7400; *Fax:* 615-902-7571
www.state.tn.us

Robert Micinski, CEO

TDMHDD operates 5 Regional Mental Health Institutes (RMHIs). Lakeshore Mental Health Institute (Knoxville), Moccasin Bend Mental Health Institute (Chattanooga) and Memphis Mental Health Institute provide in-patient psychiatric services for adults; Middle Tennessee Mental Health Institute (Nashville) and Western Mental Health Institute (Bolivar) provide in-patient psychiatric services for both adults and children/youth. Most RMHI admissions are on an emergency involuntary basis, with a variety of court-ordered inpatient evaluation and treatment services also provided. The RMHIs provide psychiatric services based upon the demonstrated and emerging best practices of each clinical discipline.

2256 Tennessee Commission on Children and Youth
502 Deaderick St., 9th Fl.
Andrew Jackson Bldg
Nashville, TN 37243-0800
615-741-2633
www.www.tennessee.gov/tccy/

Linda O'Neal, Executive Director
Pat Wade, Program Director

2257 Tennessee Department of Health
710 James Robertson Parkway
Andrew Johnson Tower
Nashville, TN 37243-3400
615-741-3111

Suzanne Hayes, Director

Provides information on a wide variety of topics including community services, health maintenance organizations, immunizations and alcohol and drug services.

2258 Tennessee Department of Human Services
400 Deaderick Street
15th Floor
Nashville, TN 37243-1403
615-313-4700; *Fax:* 615-741-1791
www.www.tn.gov

Gina Lodge, Commissioner

Provides information about available programs and services, such as family assistance and child support, community programs, and rehabilitation services.

Texas

2259 Texas Commission on Alcohol and Drug Abuse
Texas Department of State Health Services
909 West 45th Street
Austin, TX 78751-2803
512-206-5000
contact@tcada.state.tx.us
www.tcada.state.tx.us/

The Department of State Health Services promotes optimal health for individuals and communities while providing effective health, mental health and substance abuse services to Texans.

2260 Texas Department of Family and Protective Services
701 West 51st Street
PO Box 149030
Austin, TX 78714-9030
512-438-4800
800-720-7777
www.www.dfps.state.tx.us

Christina Martin, Chairman
Imogen Sherman Papadopoulos, Vice Chairman
Traci Henderson, Chief Financial Officer
Jennifer Sims, Chief Operating Officer(interim)

The mission of the Texas Department of Family and Protective Services (DFPS) is to protect the unprotected _ children, elderly, and people with disabilities _ from abuse, neglect, and exploitation.

2261 The Harris Center for Mental Health and IDD
9401 Southwest Freeway
Houston, TX 77074
713-970-7000
866-970-4770
www.mhmraharris.org

The center provides high quality, efficient, and cost effective services to persons with mental disabilities, so that they may live with dignity as fully functioning, participating and contributing members of the community, regardless of their ability to pay.

Utah

2262 Utah Department of Health
288 North 1460 West
Cannon Health Building
Salt Lake Cty, UT 84116-3231
801-538-6003
www.health.utah.gov

W David Patton,PhD, Executive Director
Robert T Rolfs,MD,MPH, Deputy Director
Michael Hales,MPA, Deputy Director,Medicaid Health
Wu Xu,PhD, Director,Center for Health Data

Oversees and regulates health care services for children, seniors, the mentally ill, substance abusers, and all residents of Utah.

2263 Utah Department of Health: Health Care Financing Box 143101
Salt Lake City, UT 84114-3101
801-538-6406
www.health.utah.gov/medicaid

Provides information and assistance on Utah Medicaid programs including eligibility and additional contact info and links for administrators of the program.

2264 Utah Department of Human Services
195 North 1950 West
Salt Lake City, UT 84116
801-538-4171
800-662-3722; *Fax:* 801-538-4016
www.dhs.utah.gov

Ann S Williamson, Executive Director
Jennifer Evans, Chief Financial Officer
Mark Brasher, Deputy Director
Lana Stohl, Deputy Director

Provides services for the elderly, substance abusers, people with disabilities,ed children, youthful offenders, mentally ill and others.ple with disabilities,

2265 Utah Department of Human Services: Division of Substance Abuse And Mental Health
195 North 1950 West
Salt Lake City, UT 84116
801-538-4171; *Fax:* 801-538-9892
dsamh@utah.gov
www.www.dsamh.utah.gov

Douglas P Thomas, Director
Paula Bell, Vice Chair

The Utah State Division of Substance Abuse and Mental Health Division is the agency responsible for ensuring that substance abuse and mental health prevention and treatment services are available statewide. The Division also acts as a resource by providing general information, research, and statistics to the public regarding substances of abuse and mental health services.

2266 Utah Division of Substance Abuse and Mental Health
195 North 1950 West
Salt Lake City, UT 84116
801-538-4171; *Fax:* 801-538-9892
dsamh@utah.gov

Douglas P Thomas, Director

The Utah Division of Mental Health is the State agency responsible for ensuring that prevention and treatment services for subsatnce abuse and mental health are available statewide.

Virginia

2267 Virginia Department of Behavioral Health and Developmental Services (DBHDS)
PO Box 1797
Richmond, VA 23218-1797
804-786-3921
800-451-5544; *Fax:* 804-371-6638

TDD: 804-371-8977
www.dbhds.virginia.gov

Jack Barber, Interim Commissioner
Chris Foca, Director,Administrative Services
Ken Gunn, Director, Financial Reporting
Dawn M Adams, Director, Health Services

The Virginia Department of Behavioral Health and Developmental Services is a mental health and substance abuse services system working to improve the quality of treatment and prevention services for individuals and families whose lives are affected by mental illness, intellectual disabilities, or substance abuse disorders.

2268 Virginia Department of Medical Assistance Services
600 East Broad Street
Richmond, VA 23219-1832
804-786-7933
TDD: 800-343-0634
www.www.dmas.virginia.gov

Patrick Finnerty, Director

DMAS is the agency that administers Medicaid and the State Childrens Health Insurance Program (CHIP) in the State of Virginia.

2269 Virginia Department of Social Services
801 East Main Street
Richmond, VA 23219-2901
804-726-7000
800-552-3431
TDD: 800-828-1120
TTY: 800-828-1120
citizen.services@dss.virginia.gov
www.dss.virginia.gov

Margaret Ross Schultze, Commissioner

Social services system providing programs, services and benefits designed to ensure the health and well-being of citizens, families and communities.

2270 Virginia Office of the Secretary of Health and Human Resources
1111 East Broad Street
Richmond, VA 23219
804-786-2211; *Fax:* 804-371-6351
healthandhumanresources@governor.virginia.gov
www.hhr.virginia.gov

William A Hazel Jr., MD, Secretary

The Secretary of Health and Human Resources oversees the state agencies that provide services to the people of Virginia, including individuals with disabilities, low-income working families, children, the aging community, and caregivers.

West Virginia

2271 West Virginia Bureau for Behavioral Health and Health Facilities
West Virginia Department of Health and Human Resources
350 Capitol Street
Room 350
Charleston, WV 25301-1757
304-356-4811; *Fax:* 304-558-1008
www.dhhr.wv.gov/bhhf/

Damon Iarossi, Deputy Commissioner

The mission of the Bureau for Behavioral Health and Health Facilities is to help individuals with mental illness, intellectual and developmental disabilities, and substance abuse disorders realize their full potential and build positive and meaningful futures. The Bureau provides support for families and communities, and assists with the improvement of services in West Virginia.

2272 West Virginia Department of Health & Human Resources (DHHR)
One Davis Square
Suite 100 East
Charleston, WV 25301
304-558-0684; *Fax:* 304-558-1130
www.dhhr.wv.gov

Karen L Bowling, Secretary

The DHHR consists of five bureaus that serve to promote the health and well-being of the citizens of West Virginia.

2273 West Virginia Department of Welfare Bureau for Children and Families
West Virginia Department of Health and Human Resources
350 Capitol Street
Room 730
Charleston, WV 25301-1757
304-558-0628; *Fax:* 304-558-4194
www.dhhr.wv.gov/bcf/

Nancy Exline, Commissioner

The Bureau for Children and Families works to provide a service system for individuals and families in West Virginia. The Bureau's mission is to ensure the well-being of West Virginia's children, families and adults, and to help them improve their quality of life.

Wisconsin

2274 Journey Mental Health Center
625 West Washington Avenue
Madison, WI 53703-2637
608-280-2700; *Fax:* 608-280-2707
www.journeymhc.org

James Christiansen, Chair
William Greer, President and CEO
Lynn Brady, MPA, Chief Operating Officer
Karen Milner, MD, Medical Director

The Journey Mental Health Center is a nonprofit agency and outpatient mental health and substance abuse treatment clinic serving to assist Southern Wisconsin residents with mental illnesses and substance use disorders. The Journey Mental Health Center seeks to improve the lives of the people of Southern Wisconsin through the provision of behavioral health programs and services.

2275 University of Wisconsin Population Health Institute
610 Walnut Street
575 WARF
Madison, WI 53726-2336
608-263-6294; *Fax:* 608-262-6404
uwphi@med.wisc.edu
www.uwphi.pophealth.wisc.edu/programs/

Karen Timberlake, JD, Director
Matthew Call, BS, Program Manager

Allison Espeseth, MA, Outreach Specialist
Alison Bergum, MPA, Associate Researcher

The University of Wisconsin Population Health Institute, within the University of Wisconsin-Madison School of Medicine and Public Health, works to improve health and well-being for all people. The Institute strives to address an array of problems related to health; build partnerships between researchers and private and public policy makers; and contribute to the development of programs and policies designed to advance the population's health and well-being.

2276 Wisconsin Department of Health and Family Services
1 West Wilson Street
Madison, WI 53703-3445
608-266-1865
TTY: 888-701-1251
www.dhs.wisconsin.gov

Kitty Rhoades, Secretary
Tom Engels, Deputy Secretary

The Wisconsin Department of Health and Family Services administers services to clients in the areas of public health, mental health, substance abuse, medical assistance, aging, and disability. The mission of the Department of Health Services is to advance the health and safety of the people of Wisconsin.

Wyoming

2277 Wyoming Department of Family Services
2300 Capitol Avenue
Hathaway Building, 3rd Floor
Cheyenne, WY 82002
307-777-7561; *Fax:* 307-777-7747
www.dfsweb.wyo.gov

Steve Corsi, Psy.D, Director
Tony Lewis, Deputy Director and CCO
Chris Smith, Human Resources Manager
Kristie Langley, Senior Policy Advisor

The Wyoming Department of Family Services is an agency dedicated to advancing the well-being and safety of families in Wyoming. The DFS serves to connect people in Wyoming with child and family resources, programs and services in order to help build healthy and self-sufficient families.

Professional & Support Services

Accreditation & Quality Assurance

2279 American Board of Examiners in Clinical Social Work
241 Humphrey Street
Shetland Park
Marblehead, MA 01945
781-639-5270
800-694-5285; *Fax:* 781-639-5278
abe@abecsw.org
www.www.abecsw.org

Bob Booth, CEO
Robert Booth, Executive Director
Michael Brooks MSW BCD, Business Development, Policy Dir

Clinical Social Work certifying and standard setting organization. ABE's no cost online and CD ROM directories (both searchable/sortable) are sources used by the healthcare industry nationwide for network development and referrals. They contain verified information about the education, training, experience and practice specialties of over 11,000 Board Certified Diplomates in Clinical Social Work (BCD). Visit our website for the directory, employment resources, continuing education and other services.

2280 American Board of Examiners of Clinical Social Work Regional Offices
645 Broadway
Suite C
Sonoma, CA 95476
707-938-5833
888-279-9378; *Fax:* 781-639-5278
abe@abecsw.org
www.abecsw.org

Yvette Colon,PhD,BCD, President
Robert Booth, Executive Director
Carolyn Messner,DSW,BCD, Vice President
Bob Booth, Chief Executive Officer

Sets national practice standards, issues an advance-practice credential, and publishes reference information about its board-certified clinicians.

Year Founded: 1987

2281 Brain Imaging Handbook
WW Norton & Company
500 5th Avenue
New York, NY 10110-54
212-354-5500
800-233-4830; *Fax:* 212-869-0856
npb@wwnorton.com
www.books.wwnorton.com/

J. Douglas Bremner, Author

The past 10 years have seen an explosion in the use of brain imaging technologies to aid treatment of medical as well as mental health conditions. MRI, CT scans, and PET scans are now common. This book is the first quick reference to these technologies, rich in illustrations and including discussions of which techniques are best used in particular instances of care.

224 pages

2282 CARF International
6951 East SouthPoint Road
Tucson, AZ 85756-9407
520-325-1044
888-281-6531; *Fax:* 520-318-1129
TTY: 888-281-6531
www.carf.org

Brian J Boon,PhD, President/CEO
Cindy L Johnson,CPA, Chief Resource and Strategic Dev
Leslie Ellis-Lang, Managing Director
Amanda Birch, Administrator of Operations

CARF assists organizations to improve the quality of their services, to demonstrate value, and to meet internationally recognized organizational and practice standards.

Year Founded: 1966

2283 Cenaps Corporation
13194 Spring Hill Drive
Spring Hill, FL 34609
352-596-8000; *Fax:* 352-596-8002
info@cenaps.com
www.cenaps.com

Tresa Watson, Business Manager

CENAPS is an acronym for the Center for Applied Sciences. They are a private training firm committed to providing advanced clinical skills training for the addiction and behavioral health fields.

2284 CompHealth Credentialing
6440 South Millrock Drive
Suite 175
Salt Lake City, UT 84121
801-930-3000
800-453-3030; *Fax:* 801-930-4517
info@comphealth.com
www.comphealth.com

Assists in analyzing the total costs involved in credentialing verifications, including some items frequently overlooked; assesses and/or develops a provider application to meet accreditation standards; can assess current credentialing files; can assist in developing policy and procedures for the verification process.

2285 Consumer Satisfaction Team
1210 Stanbridge Street
Suite 600
Norristown, PA 19401-5300
610-270-3685; *Fax:* 610-270-9155
www.cstmont.com

Sue Soriano, President
Tim Tunner, Vice President
Molly Frantz, Treasurer
Dr Romani George, Secretary

The central role of CST is to provide the Montgomery County Office of MH/MR/DD with information about satisfaction with the mental health services that adults are receiving and make recommendations for change.

2286 Council on Social Work Education
1701 Duke Street
Suite 200
Alexandria, VA 22314-3457
703-683-8080; *Fax:* 703-683-8099
info@cswe.org
www.cswe.org

Barbara W Shank, Chairman
Darla Spence Coffey,PhD,MSW, President and Chief
Executive Of
Alejandro Garcia, Vice Chair/Secretary
Armin H Leopold, Director,Finance and Administrat

A national association that preserves and enhances the quality of social work education for the purpose of promoting
the goals of individual and community well being and social justice. Pursues this mission through setting and maintaining policy and program standards, accrediting bachelors
and masters degree programs in social work, promoting research and faculty development, and advocating for social
work education.

Year Founded: 1952

2287 Healtheast Behavioral Care

559 Capitol Boulevard
Saint Paul, MN 55103-2101
651-232-2228
www.healtheast.org

Robert Beck, President/CEO
Robert D. Gill, VP Finance/CFO
Robert J. Beck, VP Medical Affairs

Assessment and referral for: Psychiatric, Inpatient, Chemical Dependancy.

2288 Joint Commission on Accreditation of Healthcare Organizations

1 Renaissance Boulevard
Oakbrook Terrace, IL 60181-4294
630-792-5000; *Fax:* 630-792-5617
customerservice@jcaho.org
www.jointcommission.org

Mark Chassin, President
Mark Angood, VP/Chief Patient Safety Officer

The Joint Commission evaluates and accredits nearly
20,000 health care organizations and programs in the
United States. An independent, not-for-profit organization,
the Joint Commission is the nation's predominant stan-
dards-setting and accrediting body in health care. The Joint
Commission has developed state-of-the-art, profession-
ally-based standards and evaluated the compliance of
health care organizations against these benchmarks.

Year Founded: 1951

2289 Lanstat Incorporated

4663 Mason Street
Port Townsend, WA 98368
425-334-3124
800-672-3166; *Fax:* 425-334-3124
info@lanstat.com
www.lanstat.com

Landon Kimbrough, President
Sherry Kimbrough, VP/Co-Founder

Provides quality technical assistance to behavioral health
treatment agencies nationwide, including tribal and
goverment agencies.

2290 Med Advantage

11301 Corporate Boulevard
Suite 300
Orlando, FL 32817-1445
407-282-5131; *Fax:* 407-282-9240
info@med-advantage.com
www.www.med-advantage.com

John Witty, Owner

Fully accredited by URAC and certified in all 11 elements
by NCQA, Med Advantage is one of the oldest credentials
verification organizations in the country. Over the past
eight years, they have developed sophisticated computer
systems and one of the largest data warehouses of medical
providers in the nation, containing information on over
900,000 healthcare providers. Their system is continually
updated from primary source data required to meet the
standards of the URAC, NCQA and JCAHO.

2291 Mertech

PO Box 787
Norwell, MA 02061-787
781-659-0701
888-794-7447; *Fax:* 781-659-2049
kwoodman@mertech.org
www.mertech.org

John Kopacz, Founder

A business development organization that specializes in
helping clients capitalize on business opportunities in an efficient and effective manner to meet their goals and objectives. They have three business units: Mertech Health
Care Consultants, Mertech Personal Health Improvement
Program and Managed Care Information Systems.

2292 National Board for Certified Counselors

3 Terrace Way
Greensboro, NC 27403-3670
336-547-0607; *Fax:* 336-547-0017
nbcc@nbcc.org
www.nbcc.org

Joseph D. Wehrman, Chairman
Thomas Clawson, President/CEO
Brandon Hunt, Vice Chair
Kylie P. Dotson-Blake, Secretary

National voluntary certification board for counselors. Certified counselors have met minimum criteria. Referral lists
can be provided to consumers.

Year Founded: 1982

2293 National Register of Health Service Providers in Psychology

1200 New York Ave NW
Ste 800
Washington, DC 20005
202-783-7663; *Fax:* 202-347-0550
www.nationalregister.org

Raymond A. Follen, President/Chairman
Glenace E. Edwall, Vice President/Vice-Chair
Erica H. Wise, Secretary
William A. Hancur, Treasurer

Nonprofit credentialing organization for psychologists;
evaluates education, training, and experience of licensed
psychologists. Committed to advancing psychology as a
profession and improving the delivery of health services to
the public.

Year Founded: 1974

2294 SUPRA Management

2424 Edenborn Avenue
Suite 660
Metairie, LA 70001-6465
504-837-5557

Associations

2295 Academy of Psychosomatic Medicine
5272 River Road
Suite 500
Bethesda, MD 20816
301-718-6520; *Fax:* 301-656-0989
apm@apm.org
www.apm.org

James Rundell, MD, President
James Vrac, CAE, Executive Director
Michael Sharpe, MD, Vice President
Maria Tiamson-Kassab, MD, Treasurer

Represents psychiatrists dedicated to the advancement of medical science, education, and healthcare for persons with comorbid psychiatric and general medical conditions and provides national and international leadership in the furtherance of those goals.

2296 Agency for Healthcare Research & Quality
Office of Communications and Knowledge Transfer
540 Gaither Road
Suite 2000
Rockville, MD 20850-6649
301-427-1364; *Fax:* 301-427-1364
info@ahrq.gov
www.www.ahrq.gov

Jeffrey Toven, Chief Operating Officer
Richard Kronick,PhD, Director
Boyce Ginieczki,PhD, Acting Deputy Director

The Agency for Healthcare Research and Quality's (AHRQ) mission is to improve the quality, safety, efficiency, and effectiveness of health care for all Americans. Information from AHRQ's research helps people make more informed decisions and improve the quality of healthcare services.

Year Founded: 1989

2297 Alliance for Children and Families
11700 W Lake Park Drive
Milwaukee, WI 53224-3021
414-359-1040
800-221-3726; *Fax:* 414-359-1074
pgoldberg@alliance1.org
www.www.alliance1.org

Dennis Richardson, Chair
Susan Dreyfus, President/CEO
Polina Makievsky, Senior Vice President of Knowled

National membership association representing more than three hundred forty private, nonprofit child and family-serving organizations. It's mission is to strengthen members' capacity to serve and advocate for children, families and communities.

2298 American Academy of Addiction Psychiatry (AAAP)
400 Massasoit Avenue
Suite 307, 2nd Floor
East Providence, RI 02914
401-524-3076; *Fax:* 401-272-0922
info@aaap.org
www.aaap.org

Kathryn Cates-Wessel, Executive Director
Miriam Giles, Director, Professional Dvlpmt
Joe Barboza, Director, Grants Administration
Christina Kettell, Executive Assistant

Professional membership organization with approximately 1,000 members in the United States and around the world. The membership consists of psychiatrists who work with addiction in their practices, faculty at various academic institutions.

2299 American Academy of Child & Adolescent Psychiatry
3615 Wisconsin Avenue NW
Washington, DC 20016-3007
202-966-7300; *Fax:* 202-966-2891
communications@aacap.org
www.www.aacap.org

Paramjit T. Joshi, M.D., President
Aradhana Sood, M.D., Secretary
David G. Fassler, M.D., Treasurer

Provides information on childhood psychiatric disorders.

2300 American Academy of Clinical Psychiatrists
PO Box 458
Glastonbury, CT 06033-458
860-633-6023; *Fax:* 866-668-9858
aacp@cox.net
www.aacp.com

Donald W Black MD, President
Richard Baton, Vice President
James Wilcox DO, PhD, Secretary/Treasurer

Practicing board-eligible or board-certified psychiatrists. Promotes the scientific practice of psychiatric medicine. Conducts educational and teaching research. Publications: Annals of Clinical Psychiatry, quarterly journal. Clinical Psychiatry Quarterly, newsletter. Annual conference and exhibits in fall.

Year Founded: 1975

2301 American Academy of Medical Administrators
330 N Wabash Avenue
Suite 2000
Chicago, IL 60611
312-321-6815; *Fax:* 312-673-6705
info@aameda.org
www.aameda.org

Eric Conde, MSA, CFAAMA, Chairman
Thomas Draper, MBA, FAACVPR,, Treasurer
Maj (Retired Bonds, MA, BS, CFAAMA, Vice Chair
Susan Eget, Director, Communications

Their mission is to advance Academy member and the field of healthcare management, and promote excellence and integrity in healthcare delivery and leadership.

Year Founded: 1957

2302 American Academy of Psychiatry and the Law (AAPL)
One Regency Drive
PO Box 30
Bloomfield, CT 06002-30
860-242-5450
800-331-1389; *Fax:* 860-286-0787
office@aapl.org
www.aapl.org

Robert Weinstock,MD, President
Jacquelyn T Coleman,C.A.E, Executive Director
Richard L Frierson,MD, Vice President
Emily A Keram,MD, Vice President

Seeks to exchange ideas and experience in areas where psychiatry and the law overlap and develop standards of practice in the relationship of psychiatry to the law and encourage the development of training programs for psychiatrists in this area. Publications: Journal of the American Academy of Psychiatry and the Law, quarterly. Scholarly articles on forensic psychiatry. Newsletter of the American Academy of Psychiatry and Law, quarterly. Membership Directory, annual.

Year Founded: 1969

2303 American Academy of Psychoanalysis and Dynamic Psychiatry

One Regency Drive
PO Box 30
Bloomfield, CT 06002-30
888-691-8281; *Fax: 860-286-0787*
info@aapdp.org
www.aapsa.org

Michael Blumenfield,MD, President
Jacquelyn T Coleman CAE, Executive Director
Eugenio M Rothe,MD, Treasurer
Eugene Della Badia,D.O, Secretary

Founded in 1956 to provide an open forum for psychoanalysts to discuss relevant and responsible views of human behavior and to exchange ideas with colleagues and other social behavioral scientists. Aims to develop better communication among psychoanalysts and psychodynamic psychiatrists in other disiplines in science and the humanities. Meetings of the Academy provide a forum for inquiry into the phenomena of individual and interpersonal behavior. Advocates an acceptance of all relevant and responsible psychoanalytic views of human behavior, rather than adherence to one particular doctrine.

Year Founded: 1956

2304 American Association for Marriage and Family Therapy

PO Box 2276
Bellingham, VA 98227
360-733-1753
888-553-1228; *Fax: 703-838-9805*
central@aamft.org
www.wamft.org

Kim Gilliland, President
Kirk Roberts, Executive Director
Robin Gray, Treasurer
Susan Arneson, Secretary

The professional association for the field of marriage and family therapy. They represent the professional interests of more than 23,000 marriage and family therapists throughout the United States, Canada and abroad. They facilitate research, theory development and education. They develop standards for graduate education and training, clinical supervision, professional ethics and the clinical practice of marriage and family therapy. They host an annual national training conference each fall as well as a week-long series of continuing education institutes in the summer.

2305 American Association of Community Psychiatrists (AACP)

PO Box 570218
Dallas, TX 75357-218
972-613-0985; *Fax: 972-613-5532*
frda1@airmail.net
www.www.communitypsychiatry.org/

Anita Everett MD, DFAFA, President
Annelle Primm, Vice President
Francis Bell, Administrative Director

The mission of AACP is to inspire, empower and equip Community Psychiatrists to promote and provide quality care and to integrate practice with policies that improve the well being of individuals and communities.

2306 American Association of Chairs of Departments of Psychiatry (AACDP)

AACDP C/O Lucille Meinsler #319
1594 Cumberland Street
Lebanon, PA 17042-4532
717-270-1673
aacdp@verizon.net
www.aacdp.org

Laura Roberts MD, MA, President
Stuart Munro MD, President-Elect
David Baron DO, Secretary/Treasurer
Leighton Huey MD, Advocacy Task Force

Represents the leaders of departments of psychiatry in all the medical schools in the United States and Canada. They are committed to promotion of excellence in psychiatric education, research and clinical care. They are also committed to advocating for health policy to create appropriate and affordable psychiatric care for all.

2307 American Association of Children's Residential Centers

648 North Plankinton Avenue
Suite 425
Milwaukee, WI 53203
877-332-2272
ksisson@togetherthevoice.org
www.aacrc-dc.org

Laurah Currey, President
Kery Ann Goldsmith, Secretary
Joe Ford, Vice President
Kari Sisson, Executive Director

The American Association of Children's Residential Centers is a national organization focused on providing residential therapeutic treatment for children and adolescents with behavioral health disorders.

Year Founded: 1956

2308 American Association of Directors of Psychiatric Residency Training

1594 Cumberland Street
Lebanon, PA 17042-4532
717-270-1673
aadprt@verizon.net
www.aadprt.org

Lucille Meinsler, Administrative Director
Lucille Meinsler, Administrative Manager

To better meet the nation's mental healthcare needs, the mission of the American Association of Directors of Psychiatric Residency Training is to promote excellence in education and training of future psychiatrists.

2309 American Association of Geriatric Psychiatry (AAGP)

7910 Woodmont Avenue
Suite 1050
Bethesda, MD 20814-3004

301-654-7850; *Fax:* 301-654-4137
main@aagponline.org
www.aagponline.org

Susan K. Schultz, MD, President
Christine deVries, Chief Executive Officer/Executiv
Denise Disque, Office Manager/Executive Assista
Kate McDuffie, Director, Communications & Marke

Members are psychiatrists interested in promoting better mental health care for the elderly. Maintains placement service and speakers' bureau. Publications: AAGP Membership Directory, annual. Geriatric Psychiatry News, bimonthly newsletter. Growing Older and Wiser, covers consumer and general public information. Annual meeting and exhibits in February or March.

Year Founded: 1978

2310 American Association of Healthcare Consultants

5938 N Drake Avenue
Chicago, IL 60659-3203
888-350-2242; *Fax:* 773-463-3552
www.www.consultprism.com/aahc.htm

Billy Adkisson, Chairman

Serve as the preeminent credentialing, professional, and practice development organization for the healthcare consulting profession; to advance the knowledge, quality, and standards of practice for consulting to management in the healthcare industry; and to enhance the understanding and image of the healthcare consulting profession and Member Firms among its various publics.

Year Founded: 1949

2311 American Association of Homes and Services for the Aging

2519 Connecticut Avenue NW
Washington, DC 20008-1520
202-783-2242; *Fax:* 202-783-2255
info@LeadingAge.org

William L Minnix Jr, President and Chief Executive Of
Katrinka Smith Sloan, COO/SVP Member Services
Bruce Rosenthal, Vice President, Corporate Partne
Lea Chambers-Johnson, Assistant to the Preside

An association committed to advancing the vision of healthy, affordable, ethical long term care for America. The association represents 5,600 million driven, not-for-profit nursing homes, continuing care facilities and community care retirement facilities and community service organizations.

2312 American Association of Pastoral Counselors

9504A Lee Highway
Fairfax, VA 22031-2303
703-385-6967; *Fax:* 703-352-7725
info@aapc.org
www.aapc.org

Alice M. Graham, Ph.D., President
Pamela Holliman, Ph.D., Vice President
Douglas M. Ronsheim, Executive Director
William Manseau, Secretary

Organized in 1963 to promote and support the ministry of pastoral counseling within religious communities and the field of mental health in the United States and Canada.

Year Founded: 1963

2313 American Association of Pharmaceutical Scientists

2107 Wilson Boulevard
Suite 700
Arlington, VA 22201-3042
703-243-2800; *Fax:* 703-243-9650
www.aaps.org

Karen Habucky, President
John Lisack, Executive Director

The American Association of Pharmaceutical Scientists will be the premier organization of all scientists dedicated to the discovery, development and manufacture of pharmaceutical products and therapies through advances in science and technology.

2314 American Association of Retired Persons

601 E Street NW
Washington, DC 20049-2
202-434-2277
888-687-2277; *Fax:* 202-434-7599
TTY: 877-434-7598
www.aarp.org

A Barry Rand, CEO
Erik Olsen, President

AARP is a non profit membership organization of persons 50 and older dedicated to addressing their needs and interests.

2315 American Association on Intellectual and Developmental Disabilities (AAIDD)

501 3rd Street NW
Suite 200
Washington, DC 20001
202-387-1968; *Fax:* 202-387-2193
www.aaidd.org

Susan Havercamp, PhD, President
Margaret Nygren, EdD, Executive Director and CEO
Paul D. Aitken, CPA, Director, Finance/Administration
Ajith Mathew, Contracts Manager

AAIDD provides worldwide leadership in the field of intellectual and developmental disabilities. The oldest and largest interdisciplinary organization of professionals and citizens concerned about intellectual and developmental disabilities. AAIDD promotes progressive policies, research, and universal human rights for people with intellectual and developmental diabilities.

Year Founded: 1876

2316 American Board of Professional Psychology (ABPP)

600 Market Street
Suite 300
Chapel Hill, NC 27516
919-537-8031; *Fax:* 919-537-8034
office@abpp.org
www.abpp.org

Randy K. Otto, PhD, ABPP, President
David R. Cox, PhD, ABPP, Executive Officer
Nancy O. McDonald, Assistant Executive Officer
Jerry Sweet, PhD, ABPP, Treasurer

The mission is to increase consumer protection through the examination and certification of psychologists who demonstrate competence in approved specialty areas in professional psychology

2317 American Board of Psychiatry and Neurology (ABPN)
2150 E Lake Cook Road
Suite 900
Buffalo Grove, IL 60089-1875
847-229-6500; *Fax:* 847-229-6600
www.abpn.com

Burton Reifler, President
Patricia Coyle, Vice President

ABPN is a nonprofit organization that promotes excellence in the practice of psychiatry and neurology through lifelong certification including compentency testing processes.

2318 American College Health Association
1362 Mellon Road
Suite 180
Hanover m, MD 21076
410-859-1500; *Fax:* 410-859-1510
www.acha.org

Pat Ketcham, PhD, CHES, FA, President
Keith Anderson, PhD, FACHA, Vice President
Charley Bradley, BPS, RNBC, FA, Treasurer

Principal advocate and leadership organization for college and university health. Provides advocacy, education, communications, products and services as well as promotes research and culturally competent practices to enhance its members' ability to advance the health of all students and the campus community.

Year Founded: 1920

2319 American College of Health Care Administrators (ACHCA)
1321 Duke Street
Suite 400
Alexandria, VA 22314
202-536-5120; *Fax:* 888-874-1585
wodonnell@achca.org
www.achca.org

Marianna Kern Grachek, MSN, CNH, President & CEO
Becky Reisinger, Director, Membership and Busines
Whitney O'Donnell, Coordinator, Member Services
Chelsea Whitman-Rush, Coordinator, Member and Chapter

A non-profit professional membership association which provides superior educataional programming, professional certification, and career development opportunities for its members. Available on Facebook.

Year Founded: 1962

2320 American College of Healthcare Executives
One N Franklin Street
Suite 1700
Chicago, IL 60606-3529
312-424-2800; *Fax:* 312-424-0023
contact@ache.org
www.ache.org

Christine M. Candio, Chairman
Deborah J. Bowen, FACHE, President and CEO
Thomas C Dolan, President, CEO

International professional society of nearly 30,000 healthcare executives. ACHE is known for its prestigious credentialing and educational programs. ACHE is also known for its journal, Journal of Healthcare Management, and magazine, Healthcare Executive, as well as groundbreaking research and career development programs. Through its efforts, ACHE works toward its goal of im-

proving the health status of society by advancing healthcare management excellence.

2321 American College of Mental Health Administration (ACMHA)
7804 Loma del Norte Road NE
Albuquerque, NM 87109-5419
505-822-5038
www.acmha.org

Colette Croze, MSW, President
Kris Ericson, PhD, Executive Director
Christopher Wilkins, Sr., MHA, Treasurer
Steve Scoggin, PsyD, LPC, Secretary

Advancing the field of mental health and substance abuse administration and to promote the continuing education of clinical professionals in the areas of administration and policy. Publication: ACMHA Newsletter, quarterly. Annual Santa Fe Summit, conference.

Year Founded: 1979

2322 American College of Osteopathic Neurologists & Psychiatrists
142 E. Ontario St.
Suite 200
Chicago, IL 60611-2864
312-202-8000
800-062- 177; *Fax:* 312-202-8200
acn-aconp@msn.com
www.osteopathic.org

Norman E. Vinn, DO, President
Adrienne White-Faines, MPA, Executive Director and CEO

Purpose is to promote the art and science of osteopathic medicine in the fields of neurology and psychiatry; to maintain and further elevate the highest standards of proficiency and training among osteopathic neurologists and psychiatrists; to stimulate original research and investigation in neurology and psychiatry; and to collect and disseminate the results of such work for the benefit of the members of the college, the public, the profession at large, and the ultimate benefit of all humanity.

2323 American College of Psychiatrists
122 S. Michigan Ave
Suite 1360
Chicago, IL 60603-6185
312-662-1020; *Fax:* 312-662-1025
angel@acpsych.org
www.acpsych.org

Maureen Shick, Executive Director
Angel Waszak, Administrative Assistant

Nonprofit honorary association of psychiatrists who, through excellence in their chosen fields, have been recognized for thier significant contributions to the profession. The society's goal is to promote and support the highest standards in psychiatry through education, research and clinical practice.

Year Founded: 1963

2324 American College of Psychoanalysts (ACPA)
PO Box 570218
Dallas, TX 75357-218
972-613-0985
www.acopsa.org

Ralph H. Beaumont, III, M.D., President
Barbara Young, M.D., Secretary, General Counsel
Mervin S. Stewart, M.D., Treasurer

Honorary, scientific and professional organization for physician psycholanalysts. Goal is to contribute to the leadership and support high standards in the practice of psychoanalysis, and understanding the relationship between mind and brain.

2325 American Counseling Association

5999 Stevenson Avenue
Alexandria, VA 22304-3304
703-823-9800
800-347-6647; *Fax:* 703-823-0252
webmaster@counseling.org
www.counseling.org

Richard Yep, CAE, Executive Director
Dr Don W Locke, President
Dr Bradley T Erford, President Elect

ACA serves professional counselors in the US and abroad. Provides a variety of programs and services that support the personal, professional and program development goals of its members. ACA works to provide quality services to the variety of clients who use their services in college, community agencies, in mental health, rehabilitation and related settings. Offers a large catalog of books, manuals and programs for the professional counselor.

Year Founded: 1952

2326 American Counseling Association (ACA)

5999 Stevenson Avenue
Alexandria, VA 22304-3304
703-823-9800
800-347-6647; *Fax:* 703-823-0252
webmaster@counseling.org
www.counseling.org

Richard Yep, Executive Director

A not-for-profit, professional and educational organization that is dedicated to the growth and enhancement of the counseling profession.

Year Founded: 1952

2327 American Geriatrics Society

40 Fulton Street
18th Floor
New York, NY 10038
212-308-1414; *Fax:* 212-832-8646
info@americangeriatrics.org

Cathy Alessi, MD, AGSF, President
Nancy Lundebjerg, Deputy EVP, COO
Marianna Drootin, Associate Director
Melissa Fisher, Director of Development

Nationwide, nonprofit association of geriatric health care professionals, research scientists and other concerned individuals dedicated to improving the health, independence and quality of life for all older people. Pivotal force in shaping attitudes, policies and practices regarding health care for older people.

Year Founded: 1942

2328 American Group Psychotherapy Association

25 E 21st Street
6th Floor
New York, NY 10010-6207

212-477-2677
877-668-2472
info@agpa.org
www.agpa.org

Les R. Greene, President
Marsha S. Block, CAE, CFRE, Chief Executive Officer
Angela Stephens, CAE, Professional Development Directo
Diane C. Feirman, CAE, Public Affairs Director

Interdisciplinary community that has been enhancing practice, theory and research of group therapy for over 50 years. Provides support to enhance your work as a mental health care professional, or your life as a member of a therapeutic group.

Year Founded: 1942

2329 American Health Care Association

1201 L Street NW
Washington, DC 20005-4046
202-842-4444; *Fax:* 202-842-3860
www.www.ahcancal.org

Bruse Yarwood, President

Nonprofit federation of affiliated state health organizations, together representing nearly 12,000 nonprofit and for profit assisted living, nursing facility, developmentally disabled and subacute care providers that care for more than 1.5 million elderly and disabled individuals nationally. AHCA represents the long term care community at large — to government, business leaders and the general public. It also serves as a force for change within the long term care field, providing information, education, and administrative tools that enhance quality at every level.

2330 American Health Information Management Association

233 N Michigan Avenue
21st Floor
Chicago, IL 60601-5809
312-233-1100; *Fax:* 312-233-1090
info@ahima.org
www.ahima.org

Linda Kloss, Executive Director
Linda L Kloss CAE, CEO

Dynamic professional association that represents more than 46,000 specially educated health information management professionals who work throughout the healthcare industry. Health information management professionals serve the health care industry and the public by managing, analyzing and utilizing data vital for patient care and making it accessible to healthcare providers when it is needed most.

2331 American Humane Association

1400 16th Street,NorthWest
Suite 360
Washington, DC 20036
303-792-9900
800-227-4645; *Fax:* 303-792-5333
info@americanhumane.org
www.americanhumane.org

John Payne, Chair
Robert R Ganzert,PhD, President and Chief Executive Of
Clifford Rose, Chief Financial Officer
Audrey Lang, Chief of Staff

Leader in developing programs, policies and services to prevent the abuse and neglect of children, while strengthening families and communities and enhancing social service systems.

Year Founded: 1877

2332 American Medical Association

330 N. Wabash Ave.
Chicago, IL 60611-5885
312-464-5000
800-621-8335; *Fax:* 312-464-4184
www.ama-assn.org

James L Madara, MD, CEO, Executive Vice President
Bernard L Hengesbaugh, Chief Operating Officer
Denise M. Hagerty, Senior Vice President & Chief Fi
Craig Ethridge, Group Vice President & Chief Inf

Speaks out in issues important to patients and the nation's health. AMA policy on such issues is decided through its democratic policy making process, in the AMA House of Delegates, which meets twice a year. The House is comprised of physician delegates representing every state; nearly 100 national medical specialty societies, federal service agents, including the Surgeon General of the US; and 6 sections representing hospital and clinic staffs, resident physicians, medical students, young physicians, medical schools and international medical graduates. The AMA's envisioned future is to be a part of the professional life of every physician and an essential force for progress in improving the nation's health.

Year Founded: 1847

2333 American Medical Directors Association

11000 Broken Land Parkway
Suite 400
Columbia, MD 21044-3532
410-740-9743
800-876-2632; *Fax:* 410-740-4572
webmaster@amda.com
www.www.amda.com

Matthew S Wayne, MD, President
Leonard Gelman. MD, Vice President
Milta O Little, Secretary

Professional association of medical directors and physicians practicing in the long-term care continuum, dedicated to excellence in patient care by providing education, advocacy and professional development.

2334 American Medical Group Association

One Prince Street
Alexandria, VA 22314
703-838-0033; *Fax:* 703-548-1890
roconnor@amga.org
www.amga.org

Donald W. Fisher, Ph.D., President/CEO

The American Medical Group Association (AMGA) is a 501(c)(6) trade association representing medical groups, health systems and other organized systems of care, including some of the nation's largest, most prestigious integrated delivery systems. AMGA is a leading voice in advocating for efficient, team-based, and accountable care. AMGA members encompass all models of organized systmes of care in the healthcare industry. MOre than 150,000 physicians practice in AMGA member organizations, providing healthcare services for 120 million patients (approximately 1 in 3 Americans). AMGA's mission is to support its members in enhancing population health and care for patients through integrated systems of care.

Year Founded: 1950

2335 American Medical Informatics Association

4720 Montgomery Lane
Suite 500
Bethesda, MD 20814-6052
301-657-1291; *Fax:* 301-657-1296
mail@amia.org
www.amia.org

Blackford Middleton, MD, MPH, MS, Chairman
Karen Greenwood, Executive Vice President & COO
Ross D. Martin, MD, MHA, Vice President of Policy and Dev
Susanna Aguirre, Policy and Development Specialis

Nonprofit membership organization of individuals, institutions and corporations dedicated to developing and using information technologies to improve health care. Our members include physicians, nurses, computer and information scientists, biomedical engineers, medical librarians, academic researchers and educators. Holds an annual syposium, 2 congresses, prints a journal and maintains a resource center.

Year Founded: 1988

2336 American Mental Health Counselors Association (AMHCA)

801 N Fairfax Street
Suite 304
Alexandria, VA 22314-1775
703-548-6002
800-326-2642; *Fax:* 703-548-4775
vmoore@amhca.org
www.amhca.org

Judith Bertenthal-Smith, President
Joel E. Miller, Executive Director & CEO
James K. Finley, Associate Executive Director & D
Linda Morano, Manager for Membership & Member

Professional counselors employed in mental health services and students. Aims to deliver quality mental health services to children, youth, adults, families and organizations and to improve the availability and quality of services through licensure and certification, training standards and consumer advocacy. Publishes an Advocate Newsletter, Journal of Mental Health Counseling, quarterly, Mental Health Brights, brochures. Annual National Conference.

2337 American Neuropsychiatric Association

700 Ackerman Road
Suite 625
Columbus, OH 43202-4505
614-447-2077; *Fax:* 614-263-4366
anpa@osu.edu
www.www.anpaonline.org

Sandy Bornstein, Executive Director
C. Edward Coffey, Treasurer

An association of professionals in neuropsychiatry and clinical neurosciences. Their mission is to promote neuroscience for the benefit of people. They work together in a collegial fashion to provide a forum for learning and provide excellent, scientific and compassionate care. They hold their annual scientific meeting in the early spring.

Year Founded: 1988

2338 American Nurses Association
8515 Georgia Avenue
Suite 400
Silver Spring, MD 20910-3492
301-628-5000
800-274-4262; *Fax:* 301-628-5001
webmaster@ana.org
www.nursingworld.org

Karen Daley, PhD, RN, FAAN, President
Marla J. Weston, PhD, RN, FAAN, Chief Executive Officer
Cindy R. Balkstra, MS, RN, CNS-, First Vice President
Jennifer S. Mensik, PhD, RN, NEA-B, Second Vice President

A full-service professional organization representing the nation's 2.7 million registered nurses through its 54 constituent members associations. The ANA advances the nursing profession by fostering high standards of nursing practice, promoting the economic and general welfare of nurses in the workplace, projecting a positive and realistic view of nursing, and by lobbying the Congress and regulatory agencies on health care issues affecting nurses and the public.

2339 American Pharmacists Association
2215 Constitution Avenue NW
Washington, DC 20037
202-628-4410
800-237-2742; *Fax:* 202-783-2351
feedback@pharmacist.com
www.pharmacist.com

Joseph J. Janela, Chief Financial Officer
Elizabeth K. Keyes, Chief Operating Officer
Stacie Maass, Senior Vice President, Pharmacy
Thomas E. Menighan, Chief Executive Officer

National professional society of pharmacists, formerly the American Pharmaceutical Association. Our members include practicing pharmacists, pharmaceutical students, pharmacy scientists, pharmacy technicians, and others interested in advancing the profession. Provides professional information and education for pharmacists and advocates for improved health of the American public through the provision of comprehensive pharmaceutical care.

Year Founded: 1852

2340 American Psychiatric Association (APA)
800 Maine Avenue Southwest
Suite 900
Washington, DC 20024
202-559-3900
888-357-7924
apa@psych.org
www.www.psychiatry.org

Anita Everett, MD, President
Altha J. Stewart, MD, President-Elect
Philip R. Muskin, MD, MA, Secretary
Bruce Schwartz, MD, Treasurer

The American Psychiatric Association is a medical specialty society comprised of over 37,800 members who work together to ensure appropriate care and effective treatment for all persons with mental disorders, including developmental disabilities and substance-related disorders.

Year Founded: 1844

2341 American Psychiatric Nurses Association
3141 Fairview Park Drive
Suite 625
Falls Church, VA 22042
571-533-1919
855-863-2762; *Fax:* 855-883-2762
clement.1@osu.edu
www.apna.org

Nick Croce, Executive Director
Karla Lewis, Director of Finance & Administra
Lisa Deffenbaugh Nguyen, MS, Director of Operations
Patricia Federinko, Membership Manager

Provides leadership to promote the psychiatric-mental health nursing profession, improve mental health care for culturally diverse individuals, families, groups and communities and shape health policy for the delivery of mental health services.

2342 American Psychiatric Publishing
1000 Wilson Boulevard
Suite 1825
Arlington, VA 22209-3924
703-907-7300
888-357-7924; *Fax:* 703-907-1085
apa@psych.org
www.psych.org

Tara L Burkholder, Marketing
Joan Lang, Treasurer

Year Founded: 1844

2343 American Psychoanalytic Association (APsaA)
309 E 49th Street
New York, NY 10017-1601
212-752-0450; *Fax:* 212-593-0571
info@apsa.com
www.apsa.org

Dean K. Stein, Executive Director
Tina Faison, Administrative Assistant to Exec
Carolyn Gatto, Scientific Program & Meetings Di
Michael Candela, Meetings & Exhibits Coordinator

Professional Membership Organization with approximately 3,500 members nationwide, with 43 Affiliate Societies and 29 Training Institutes. Seeks to establish and maintain standards for the training of psychoanalysts and for the practice of psychoanalysis, fosters the integration of psychoanalysis with other disciplines (psychiatry, psychology, social work), and encourages research. Publications include: Journal of the Psychoanalyst (JAPA), American Psychoanalyst, a quarterly newsletter; Ethics Case Book; and Roster. Twice a year the organization sponsors scientific meetings and exhibits.

2344 American Psychologial Association: Division of Family Psychology
750 1st Street NE
Washington, DC 20002-4242
202-336-5500
800-374-2721; *Fax:* 202-336-5518
TDD: 202-336-6123
TTY: 202-336-6123
webmaster@apa.org
www.apa.org

Nadine Kaslow, PhD, President
Norman B Anderson, Chief Executive Officer and Exec
Jennifer F Kelly, Secretary
Bonnie Markham, PhD, PsyD, Treasurer

A division of the American Psychological Association. Psychologists intersted in research, teaching, evaluation, and public interest initiatives in family psychology. Seeks to promote human welfare through the development, dissemination, and application of knowledge about the dynamics, structure, and functioning of the family. Conducts research and specialized education programs.

2345 American Psychological Association

750 First Street NE
Washington, DC 20002-4242
202-336-5500
800-374-2721
TDD: 202-336-6123
TTY: 202-336-6123
www.apa.org

Jessica Henderson Daniel, PhD, President
Arthur C. Evans, Jr., PhD, Chief Executive Officer and EVP
Jennifer F. Kelly, PhD, ABPP, Secretary
Jean A. Carter, PhD, Treasurer

The American Psychological Association seeks to advance psychology as a science, a profession, and as a means of promoting health, education, and human welfare. This organization of researchers, educators, clinicians, consultants, and students promotes research in psychology and the improvment of research methods; establishes high standards of ethics, conduct, and education; and disseminates psychological knowledge through professional and academic networks.

2346 American Psychological Association: Applied Experimental and Engineering Psychology

750 First Street NE
Washington, DC 20002-4242
202-336-6013; *Fax:* 202-336-5518
www.apa.org

Frank A Drews, President
Scott Shappell, Secretary-Treasurer

A division of the American Psychological Association. Individuals whose principal fields of study, research, or work are within the area of applied experimental and engineering psychology. Promotes research on psychological factors in the design and use of environments and systems within which human beings work and live.

2347 American Psychology- Law Society (AP-LS)
AP-LS Central Office

750 First St. NE
Washington, DC 20002-4242
202-336-5500
TDD: 202-336-6123
TTY: 202-336-6123
www.ap-ls.org

Jennifer Skeem, President
Eve Brank, Treasurer
Jeremy Blumenthal, Secretary

A division of the American Psychological Association. It is an interdisciplinary organization devoted to the scholarship, practice and public service in psychology and law. Their goals include advancing the contributions of psychology to the understanding of law and legal institutions through basic and applied research; promoting the education of psychologists in matters of law and education of legal personnel in matters of psychology.

2348 American Psychosomatic Society

6728 Old McLean Village Drive
McLean, VA 22101-3906
703-556-9222; *Fax:* 703-556-8729
info@psychosomatic.org
www.psychosomatic.org

Karen L. Weihs, MD, President
George K. Degnon, CAE, Executive Director
Laura E. Degnon, CAE, Associate Executive Director
Urs Markus Nater, PhD, Secretary-Treasurer

A worldwide community of scholars and clinicians dedicated to the scientific understanding of the interaction of mind, brain, body and social context in promoting health and contributing to the pathogenesis, course and treatment of disease. Holds an annual meeting in a different location each year.

Year Founded: 1942

2349 American Society for Adolescent Psychiatry (ASAP)

PO Box 570218
Dallas, TX 75357-218
972-613-0985; *Fax:* 972-613-5532
info@adolpsych.org
www.adolpsych.org

Frances Bell, Executive Director
Mohan Nair, President

Psychiatrists concerned with the behavior of adolescents. Provides for the exchange of psychiatric knowledge, encourages the development of adequate standards and training facilities and stimulates research in the psychopathology and treatment of adolescents. Publications: Adolescent Psychiatry, annual journal. American Society for Adolescent Psychiatry Newsletter, quarterly. ASAP Membership Directory, biennial. Journal of Youth and Adolescence, bimonthly. Annual conference. Workshops.

Year Founded: 1967

2350 American Society for Clinical Pharmacology & Therapeutics

528 N Washington Street
Alexandria, VA 22314-2314
703-836-6981; *Fax:* 703-836-5223
info@ascpt.org
www.ascpt.org

Sharon J. Swan, CAE, Chief Executive Officer
Judy E. Dalie, Director, Education and Meetings
Natalie Ngo, Publications Manager
Lisa Williamson, Director of Member Services

Over 1,900 professionals whose primary interest is to promote and advance the science of human pharmacology and theraputics. Most of the members are physicians or other doctoral scientists. Other members are pharmacists, nurses, research coordinators, fellows in training and other professionals.

Year Founded: 1900

2351 American Society of Addiction Medicine

11400 Rockville Pike
Suite 200
Rockville, MD 20852
301-656-3920; *Fax:* 301-656-3815
email@asam.org
www.asam.org

Kelly J. Clark, MD, MBA, DFAPA, President
Penny S. Mills, MBA, Executive VP/CEO
Margaret A. Jarvis, MD, DFASAM, Vice President
Carolyn C. Lanham, CAE, Chief Operating Officer

Increase access to and improve the quality of addictions treatment. Educate physicians, medical and osteopathic, and the public.

2352 American Society of Consultant Pharmacists
1321 Duke Street
Alexandria, VA 22314-3507
703-739-1300
800-355-2727; *Fax: 703-739-1321*
info@ascp.com
www.ascp.com

Sean M. Jeffery, Chairman of the Board
Jeffrey C. Delafuente, President
Jan Allen, Secretary/Treasurer
Jessilyn Dechevalier, Educational Affairs

International professional association that provides leadership, education, advocacy and resources to advance the practice of senior care pharmacy. Consultant pharmacists specializing in senior care pharmacy practice are essential participants in the health care system, ensuring that their patients medications are the most appropriate, effective, the safest possible and are used correctly. They identify, resolve and prevent medication related problems that may interfere with the goals of therapy.

Year Founded: 1969

2353 American Society of Group Psychotherapy & Psychodrama
301 N Harrison Street
Suite 508
Princeton, NJ 08540-3512
609-737-8500; *Fax: 609-737-8510*
asgpp@asgpp.org
www.asgpp.org

Dave Moran, ASGPP, President
Eduardo Garcia, Executive Director
Sue Barnum, Secretary

Fosters national and international cooperation among all concerned with the theory and practice of psychodrama, sociometry, and group psychotherapy. Promotes research and fruitful application and publication of the findings. Maintains a code of professional standards.

Year Founded: 1942

2354 American Society of Health System Pharmacists
7272 Wisconsin Avenue
Bethesda, MD 20814-4836
301-657-3000; *Fax: 301-664-8877*
Custserv@ashp.org
www.ashp.org

Gerald Meyer, Chairman of the Board
Paul W. Abramowitz, CEO

Thirty thousand member national professional association that represents pharmacists who practice in hospitals, health maintenance organizations, long-term care facilities, ambulatory care, home care and other components of health care systems. ASHP helps people make the best use of their medications, advances and supports the professional practice of pharmacists in hospitals and health sys-

tems and serves as their collective voice on issues related to medication use and public health.

2355 American Society of Psychoanalytic Physicians (ASPP)
13528 Wisteria Drive
Germantown, MD 20874-1049
301-540-3197
cfcotter@aspp.net
www.aspp.net

Christine Cotter, Executive Director

An organization of physicians established for non-profit education, scientific, and professional purposes. Its objective is to futher the study of psyhcoanalytic methods for the treatment and prevention of emotional disorders and mental illnesses. The Society provides scientific meetings to foster its aims and to share information, namely research, evaluation of treatment, dissemination of information, and to publish and recognize achievement and provide professional opportunities among its members.

Year Founded: 1985

2356 American Society on Aging
575 Market St.
Suite 2100
San Francisco, CA 94105-2869
415-974-9600
800-537-9728; *Fax: 415-974-0300*
info@asaging.org
www.asaging.org

Ken Dychtwald, President and CEO
Robert Lowe, Director Of Operations

Nonprofit organization committed to enhancing the knowledge and skills of those working with older adults and their families. They produce educational programs, publications, conferences and workshops.

Year Founded: 1954

2357 Annie E Casey Foundation
701 St. Paul Street
Baltimore, MD 21202-2311
410-547-6600; *Fax: 410-547-6624*
webmail@aecf.org
www.aecf.org

Patrick McCarthy, President and Chief Executive Of
Teresa Markowitz, Vice President, Center for Syste
Ryan Chao, Vice President, Civic Sites and
Debra Joy P,rez, Vice President, Research, Evalua

Working to build better futures for disadvantaged children and their families in the US. The primary mission of the Foundation is to foster policies, human service reforms and community supports that more effectively meet the needs of today's vulnerable children and families.

Year Founded: 1948

2358 Association for Academic Psychiatry (AAP)
562 S. Hillcrest Avenue
#147
Elmhurst, IL 60126
770-222-2265; *Fax: 866-884-6103*
lhedrick@academicpsychiatry.org
www.academicpsychiatry.org

Carole Berney MA, Administrative Director
Joan Anzia, President

Focuses on education in psychiatry at every level from beginning of medical school through lifelong learning for psychiatrists and other physicians. It seeks to help psychiatrists who are interested in careers in academic psychiatry develop the skills and knowledge in teaching, research and career development that they must have to succeed. The Association provides a forum for members to exchange ideas on teaching techniques, curriculum, and other issues to work together to solve problems. It works with other professional organizations on mutual interests and objectives through committee liaison and collaborative programs.

2359 Association for Ambulatory Behavioral Healthcare

247 Douglas Avenue
Portsmouth, VA 23707-1520
757-673-3741; *Fax:* 757-966-7734
mickey@aabh.org
www.www.aabh.org/?

Christopher McGowan, President

Powerful forum for people engaged in providing mental health services. Promoting the evolution of flexible models of responsive cost-effective ambulatory behavioral healthcare.

2360 Association for Applied Psychophysiology & Biofeedback

10200 W 44th Avenue
Suite 304
Wheat Ridge, CO 80033-2840
303-422-8436
800-477-8892; *Fax:* 303-422-8894
info@aapb.org
www.www.aapb.org/

David Stumph, Executive Director
Monta Greenfield, Associate Director

Their purpose is to advance the development, dissemination, and utilization of knowledge about applied psychophysiology and biofeedback to improve health and the quality of life through research, education and practice.

Year Founded: 1969

2361 Association for Behavior Analysis

550 W. Centre Avenue
Portage, MI 49024
269-492-9310; *Fax:* 269-492-9316
mail@abainternational.org
www.abainternational.org

Janet Twyman, President
Maria E Malott PhD, Executive Director

Their purpose is to develop, enhance and support the growth and vitality of behavior analysis through research, education and practice.

Year Founded: 1974

2362 Association for Behavioral and Cognitive Therapies

305 Seventh Avenue
16th Floor
New York, NY 10001
212-647-1890; *Fax:* 212-647-1865
www.www.abct.org

Mary Jane Eimer, Executive Director
Sabine Wilhelm, PhD, President

David Teisler, Director of Communications
Mary Larimer, PhD, Secretary-Treasurer

Professional, interdisciplinary organization that is concerned with the application of behavioral and cognitive sciences to understanding human behavior, developing interventions to enhance the human condition, and promoting the appropriate utilization of these interventions.

Year Founded: 1966

2363 Association for Birth Psychology

PO Box 150966
Lakewood, CO 80215
707-887-2838; *Fax:* 707-887-2838
consultant@birthpsychology.com
www.birthpsychology.com

Maureen Wolfe, Executive Director
David Chamberlain, Treasurer/Website Editor

Obstetricians, pediatricians, midwives, nurses, psychotherapists, psychologists, counselors, social workers, sociologists, and others interested in birth psychology, a developing discipline concerned with the experience of birth and the correlation between the birth process and personality development. Seeks to promote communication among professionals in the field; encourage commentary, research and theory from different points of view; establish birth psychology as an autonomous science of human behavior; develop guidelines and give direction to the field. Annual conference, regional meetings, workshops.

2364 Association for Child Psychoanalysis (ACP)

7820 Enchanted Hills Blvd
#A-233
Rio Rancho, NM 87144
505-771-0372
childanalysis@comcast.net
www.childanalysis.org

Anita Schmukler, D.O., President
Tricia Hall, Administrator

An international not-for-profit organization in which all members are highly trained child and adolescent psychoanalysts. Provides a forum for the interchange of ideas and clinical experience in order to advance the psychological treatment and understanding of children and adolescents and their families.

2365 Association for Hospital Medical Education

109 Brush Creek Road
Irwin, PA 15642-9504
724-864-7321
866-617-4780; *Fax:* 724-864-6153
info@ahme.org
www.ahme.org

Carrie Eckart, MBA, President and Board Chairman
Kimball Mohn, MD, Executive Director
Margie Kleppick, Association Staff Manager
Sandi Parsons, Director of Association and Meet

National, nonprofit professional association involved in the continuum of medical education — undergraduate, graduate, and continuing medical education. More than 600 members represent hundreds of teaching hospitals, academic medical centers and consortia nationwide. Promotes improvement in medical education to meet health care needs, serves as a forum and resource for medical education information, advocates the value of medical education in health care.

Year Founded: 1956

2366 Association for Humanistic Psychology

14B Beach Road
PO Box 1190
Tiburon, CA 94920
310-692-0495; *Fax:* 415-435-1654
ahpoffice@aol.com
www.ahpweb.org

Carroy U Ferguson, Co-President
Leland Bagget, Co-President
M.A. Bjarkman, Treasurer

Enhances the quality of human experience and to advance
the evolution of human consciousness.

Year Founded: 1962

2367 Association for Pre- & Perinatal Psychology and Health

PO Box 150966
Lakewood, CO 80215
707-887-2838; *Fax:* 707-887-2838
consultant@birthpsychology.com
www.birthpsychology.com

Maureen Wolfe, Executive Director
David Chamberlain, Treasurer/Website Editor

Forum for individuals from diverse backgrounds and disciplines interested in psychological dimensions of prenatal
and perinatal experiences. Typically, this includes childbirth educators, birth assistants, doulas, midwives, obstetricians, nurses, social workers, perinatologists, pediatricians,
psychologists, counselors researchers and teachers at all
levels. All who share these interests are welcome to join.
Quarterly journal published.

Year Founded: 1983

2368 Association for Psychoanalytic Medicine (APM)

41 Union Square West
Rm. 402
New York, NY 10003
718-548-6088; *Fax:* 212-866-4817
gsagi@mac.com
www.theapm.org

Marvin Wasserman, President
Juliette Meyer, Ph.D, Secretary
David Gutman, M.D., Treasurer

A non-profit organization that is a component society of
both the American Psychoanalytic Association and the International Psychoanalytic Association.

Year Founded: 1945

2369 Association for Psychological Science (APS)

1133 15th Street NW
Suite 1000
Washington, DC 20005
202-293-9300; *Fax:* 202-293-9350
akraut@psychologicalscience.org
www.psychologicalscience.org

Elizabeth A. Phelps, President
Alan G. Kraut, Executive Director
G☐n R. Semin, Secretary
Roberta L. Klatzky, Treasurer

The APS (previously the American Psychological Society)
is a nonprofit organization dedicated to the advancement of
scientific psychology and its representation at the national
and international levels. The Association's mission is to

promote, protect, and advance the interests of scientifically
oriented psychology in research, application, teaching and
the improvement of human welfare. Available on Facebook
and Twitter.

Year Founded: 1988

2370 Association for Psychological Type

2415 Westwood Ave.
Suite B
Richmond, VA 23230
804-523-2907
800-847-9943; *Fax:* 804-288-3551
www.aptinternational.org

Susan Nash, President
Jane Kise, President

Individuals involved in organizational development, religion, management, education and counseling, and who are
interested in psychological type, the Myers-Briggs Type Indicator, and the works of Carl G Jung. Purpose is to share
ideas related to the uses of MBTI and the application of
personality type theory in any area; promotes research, development, and education in the field. Sponsors seminars,
conferences, and training sessions on the use of
psychological type.

2371 Association for Women in Psychology
Florida International University

DM 212
University Park
Miami, FL 33199-1
305-348-2408; *Fax:* 305-348-3143
awp@fiu.edu
www.awpsych.org

Suzanna Rose PhD, Director

Nonprofit scientific and educational organization committed to encouraging feminist psychological research, theory
and activism. They are an organization with a history of af-
firming and celebrating differences, deepening challenges,
and experiencing growth as feminists.

Year Founded: 1969

2372 Association for the Advancement of Psychology

PO Box 38129
Colorado Springs, CO 80937-8129
800-869-6595; *Fax:* 719-520-0375
www.AAPNet.org

Stephen M Pfeiffer PhD, Executive Officer
Karen Rivard, Administrator

Promotes the interests of all psychologists before public
and governmental bodies. AAP's fundamental mission is
the support of candidates for the US Congress who are
sympathetic to psychology's concerns, through electioneer-
ing activities.

Year Founded: 1974

2373 Association of Black Psychologists

7119 Allentown Road
Suite 203
Ft. Washington, DC 20744
301-449-3082; *Fax:* 301-449-3084
www.abpsi.org

Taasogle Daryl Rowe, Ph.D., President
Satira Streeter, Ph.D., Secretary
Carolyn Moore, Ph.D, Treasurer

Members are professional psychologists and others in associated disciplines. Aims to: enhance the psychological well-being of black people in America; define mental health in consonance with newly established psychological concepts and standards, develop policies for local, state, and national decision making that have impact on the mental health of the black community; support established black sister organizations and aid in the development of new, independent black institutions to enhance the psychological educational, cultural, and economic situation. Offers training and information on AIDS. Conducts seminars, workshops and research. Periodic conference, annual convention.

Year Founded: 1968

2374 Association of State and Provincial Psychology Boards
PO Box 3079
Peachtree City, GA 30269
678-216-1175; *Fax: 678-216-1176*
aspbb@asppb.org
www.asppb.org

Fred Mill n, President
Stephen T. DeMers, Ed.D., Chief Executive Officer
Carol Webb, Ph.D., ABPP, Chief Operating Officer
Mark Russell, CPA, Financial Officer

ASPPB is the association of psychology licensing boards in the United States and Canada. They create the Examination for Professional Practice in Psychology which is used in licensing boards to assess candidates for licensure and certification. They also publish training materials for training programs and for students preparing to enter the profession

Year Founded: 1961

2375 Association of the Advancement of Gestalt Therapy
PO Box 42221
Portland, OR 97242
971-238-2248; *Fax: 212-202-3974*
www.aagt.org

Peter Philippson, President
Sylvie Falschlunger, Administrative Assistant

Dynamic, inclusive, energetic nonprofit organization committed to the advancement of theory, philosophy, practice and research in Gestalt Therapy and its various applications. This includes but is not limited to personal growth, mental health, education, organization and systems development, political and social development and change, and the fine and performing arts. Their international member base includes psychiatrists, psychologists, social workers, teachers, academics, artists, writers, organizational consultants, political and social analysts, activists and students.

2376 Bazelon Center for Mental Health Law
1101 15th Street NW
Suite 1212
Washington, DC 20005
202-467-5730
intakes@bazelon.org
www.bazelon.org

Holly O'Donnell, President and CEO
Ira Burnim, Director
Jennifer Mathis, Deputy Director
Lewis Bossing, Senior Staff Attorney

National legal advocate for people with mental disabilities. Through precedent-setting litigation and in the public policy arena, the Bazelon Center works to advance and preserve the rights of people with mental illnesses and development disabilities.

Year Founded: 1972

2377 Behavioral Health Systems
2 Metroplex Drive
Suite 500
Birmingham, AL 35209-6827
205-879-1150
800-245-1150; *Fax: 205-879-1178*
generalwebsite@bhs-inc.com
www.behavioralhealthsystems.com

Deborah L Stephens, Founder, Chairman & CEO
Kyle Strange, Executive Vice President & MCO
William M Patterson, M.D., Medical Director
Pat Friedley, Executive Vice President & CQO

Provides behavioral health services to business and industry which are high quality and state of the art, cost effective and accountable, uniformly accessible over a broad geographic area and care continuum, and managed within a least restrictive treatment approach.

2378 CG Jung Foundation for Analytical Psychology
28 E 39th Street
New York, NY 10016-2587
212-697-6430; *Fax: 212-953-3989*
info@cgjungny.org
www.www.cgjungny.org

David Rottman, President
Joenine Roberts, Vice President
Rollin Bush, Treasurer
Anne Ortelee, Secretary

Analysts who follow the precepts of Carl G Jung, a Swiss psychologist, and any other persons interested in analytical psychology. Sponsors public lectures, films, continuing education, courses and professional seminars. Operates book service which provides publications on analytical psychology and related topics, and lectures on audio cassettes. Publishes journal, Quadrant.

Year Founded: 1962

2379 California Psychological Association
1231 I Street
Suite 204
Sacramento, CA 95814-2933
916-286-7979; *Fax: 916-286-7971*
membership@cpapsych.org
www.cpapsych.org

Robert deMayo, Ph.D., ABPP, President
Jo Linder-Crow PhD, Chief Executive Officer
Patricia VanWoerkom, Director Administration & Direct
April Fernando, Ph.D., Secretary

A non-profit professional association for licensed psychologists and others affiliated with the delivery of psychological services.

Year Founded: 1948

2380 Center for Applications of Psychological Type
2815 NW 13th Street
Suite 401
Gainesville, FL 32609-2878

352-375-0160
800-777-2278; *Fax:* 352-378-0503
customerservice@capt.org
www.capt.org

Nonprofit organization founded to conduct research and develop applications of the Myers-Briggs Type Indicator for the constructive use of differences. The MBTI is based on CG Jung's theory of psychological types. CAPT provides training for users of the MBTI and the Murphy-Meisgeier Type Indicator for Children, publishes and distributes books and resource materials, and maintains the Isabel Briggs Myers memorial library and the MBTI Bibliography. The MBTI is used in counseling individuals and families, to understand differences in learning styles, and for improving leadership and teamwork in organizations.

Year Founded: 1975

2381 Children's Health Council

650 Clark Way
Palo Alto, CA 94304-2340
650-326-5530; *Fax:* 650-688-3676
info@chconline.org
www.chconline.org

Andrew P Valentine, Chair
James Otieno, Vice-Chair
Carol M Roccuzzo, MBA, CHC, Director of Operations & Human R
Chris Harris, MEd, Director of CHC Schools & Head o

Working to make a measurable difference in the lives of children who face severe or complex behavioral and developmental challenges by providing interdisciplinary educational, assessment and treatment services and professional training.

2382 Christian Association for Psychological Studies

PO Box 365
Batavia, IL 60510-0365
630-639-9478; *Fax:* 630-454-3799
info@caps.net
www.caps.net

Stephen P Greggo, Psy.D., Chair
Sally Schwer Canning, Ph.D., Vice Chair
Rod Marshall, Ed.S., Treasurer
Julia P Grimm, Ph.D., Secretary

Psychologists, marriage and family therapists, social workers, educators, physicians, nurses, ministers, researchers, pastoral counselors, and rehabilitation workers and others professionally engaged in the fields of psychology, counseling, psychiatry, pastoring and related areas. Association is based upon a genuine commitment to superior clinical, pastoral and scientific enterprise in the theoretical and applied social sciences and theology, assuming persons in helping professions will be guided to professional and personal growth and a greater contribution to others in this way.

Year Founded: 1956

2383 Clinical Social Work Federation

PO Box 10
Garrisonville, VA 22463
703-340-1456
855-279-2669; *Fax:* 703-269-0707
nfscswlo@aol.com
www.www.clinicalsocialworkassociation.org

Stephanie Hadley, LCSW, President
Michael Rose, Ph.D., LCSW, Treasurer
Angela Oddone, LCSW, Secretary

A confederation of 31 state societies for clinical social work. The state societies are formed as voluntary associations for the purpose of promoting the highest standards of professional education and clinical practice. Each society is active with legislative advocacy and lobbying efforts for adequate and appropriate mental health services and coverage at their state and national levels of government.

2384 Commission on Accreditation of Rehabilitation Facilities

6951East Southpoint Road
Tucson, AZ 85756-9407
520-325-1044
888-281-6531; *Fax:* 520-318-1129
TTY: 888-281-6531
www.carf.org

Brian J Boon PhD, President/CEO
Amanda E Birch, Administrator of Operations

Promotes the quality, value and optimal outcomes through a consultative accreditation process that centers on enhancing the lives of the people served.

Year Founded: 1966

2385 Commonwealth Fund

One E 75th Street
New York, NY 10021-2692
212-606-3800; *Fax:* 212-606-3500
cmwf@cmwf.org
www.www.commonwealthfund.org

James R. Tallon, Jr., Chairman
David Blumenthal, President
John E. Craig, Executive Vice President and Chi
Donald Moulds, Executive Vice President for Pro

Private foundation that supports independent research on health and social issues and make grants to improve health care practice and policy.

2386 Community Action Partnership

1140 Connecticut Avenue
Suite 1210
Washington, DC 20036
202-265-7546; *Fax:* 202-265-5048
info@communityactionpartnership.com
www.communityactionpartnership.com

Thomas Tenorio, CCAP, Chair
Joyce J Dorsey, 1st Vice Chair
Dalitso S Sulamoyo, CCAP, 2nd Vice Chair
Peter Kilde, 3rd Vice Chair

The national organization representing the interests of the 1,000 Community Action Agencies working to fight poverty at the local level.

Year Founded: 1971

2387 Community Anti-Drug Coalitions of America

625 Slaters Lane
Suite 300
Alexandria, VA 22314-1176
703-706-0560
800-542-2322; *Fax:* 703-706-0565
info@cadca.org
www.www.cadca.org

Arthur T. Dean, Chairman & CEO
Celeste Brown, Office Manager
Jasmine Carrasco, Youth Programs Associate
Na'Denna Colbert, Membership Manager

With more than five thousand members across the country, CADCA is working to build and strengthen the capacity of community coalitions to create safe, healthy, and drug free communities. CADCA supports its members with technical assistance and training, public policy, media and marketing, conferences and special events.

Year Founded: 1992

2388 Corporate Counseling Associates

475 Park Avenue South
Fifth Floor
New York, NY 10016-6901
212-686-6827
800-833-8707; *Fax:* 212-686-6511
info@corporatecounseling.com
www.www.ccainc.com

Robert Levy, President
Thomas Diamante, PhD, Principal
Georgia Critsimilios, LCSW, Senior Vice President
Russell Correa, EdM, Director

Customized, integrated workplace solutions designed to enhance business performance by enriching employee productivity.

Year Founded: 1984

2389 Council on Social Work Education

1701 Duke Street
Suite 200
Alexandria, VA 22314-3457
703-683-8080; *Fax:* 703-683-8099
info@cswe.org
www.cswe.org

Julia M. Watkins PhD, Executive Director
Nicole Demarco, Executive Assistant To Exec. Dir

A national association that preserves and enhances the quality of social work education for the purpose of promoting the goals of individual and community well being and social justice. Pursues this mission through setting and maintaining policy and program standards, accrediting bachelors and masters degree programs in social work, promoting research and faculty development, and advocating for social work education.

Year Founded: 1952

2390 Developmental Disabilities Nurses Association

PO Box 536489
Orlando, FL 32853-6489
407-835-0642
800-888-6733; *Fax:* 407-426-7440
www.ddna.org

Kathy Brown, President
Wendy Herbers, RN, CDDN, QDD, Vice-President
Richanne Cunningham, RN, QMRP,, Secretary
Karen Hill, RN, BSN, CDDN, Treasurer

National nonprofit professional association for nurses working with individuals with developmental disabilities. Publishes a quarterly newsletter.

Year Founded: 1992

2391 Division of Independent Practice of the American Psychological Association (APADIP)

919 W Marshall Avenue
Phoenix, AZ 85013-1734
602-246-6219; *Fax:* 602-246-6577
div42apa@cox.net
www.division42.org

Gordon I Herz PhD, President
Gerald Koocher PhD, Treasurer
June W J Ching PhD, President-Elect

Members of the American Psychological Association engaged in independent practice. Works to ensure that the needs and concerns of independent psychology practitioners are considered by the APA. Gathers and disseminates information on legislation affecting the practice of psychology, managed care, and other developments in the health care industries, office management, malpractice risk and insurance, hospital management. Offers continuing professional and educational programs. Semiannual convention, with board meeting.

2392 Employee Assistance Professionals Association
EAPA Exchange

4350 North Fairfax Drive
Suite 740
Arlington, VA 22203
703-387-1000; *Fax:* 703-522-4585
www.eapassn.org

Jill Royer, President
Linda Dismuke, Acting Secretary

International association of approximately 5,000 members who are primarily employee assistance professionals as well as individuals in related fields such as human resources, chemical dependency treatment, mental health treatment, managed behavioral health care, counseling and benefits administration. Hosts annual EAP conference.

Year Founded: 1971

2393 Employee Assistance Society of North America

2001 Jefferson Davis Highway
Suite 1004
Arlington, VA 22202-3617
703-416-0060; *Fax:* 703-416-0014
www.www.easna.org

George Martin, President
Judith Plotkin, MSW, Vice President
Bob Mc Lean, Executive Director
Patrick Gagne, Treasurer

International group of professional leaders with competencies in such specialties as workplace and family wellness, employee benefits and organizational development. Maintains accreditation program, membership services and professional training opportunities, promotes high standards of employee assistance programs.

Year Founded: 1985

2394 Gerontoligical Society of America

1220 L Street NW
Suite 901
Washington, DC 20005-1503
202-842-1275; *Fax:* 202-842-1150
geron@geron.org
www.geron.org

Patricia Walker, Executive Director
Linda Krogh Harootyan, Interim Executive Director

Nonprofit professional organization with more than 5000 members in the field of aging. GSA provides researchers, educators, practitioners and policy makers with opportunities to understand, advance, integrate and use basic and applied research on aging to improve the quality of life as one ages.

2395 Gorski-Cenaps Corporation Training & Consultation

13194 Spring Hill Drive
Spring Hill, FL 34609
352-596-8000; *Fax:* 352-596-8002
tresa@cenaps.com
www.cenaps.com

Tresa Watson, Manager
Tresa Watson, Business Manager

Cenaps provides advanced clinical skills training for the addiction behavioral health and mental health fields. Their focus is recovery and relapse prevention.

2396 Group for the Advancement of Psychiatry

PO Box 570218
Dallas, TX 75357-218
972-613-0985; *Fax:* 972-613-5532
www.ourgap.org

Frances Roton, Executive Director

An organization of nationally respected psychiatrists dedicated to shaping psychiatric thinking, public programs and clinical practice in mental health. Meets twice a year at the Renaissance Westchester Hotel in White Plains, NY.

Year Founded: 1946

2397 Institute of HeartMath

14700 W Park Avenue
Boulder Creek, CA 95006-9318
831-338-8700
800-711-6221; *Fax:* 831-338-8504
info@heartmath.org
www.heartmath.org

Katherine Floriano, Chairwoman
Sara Childre, President and CEO
Rollin McCraty, Ph.D., Executive Vice President and Dir
Brian Kabaker, Chief Financial Officer and Dire

Nonprofit research and education on stress, emotional physiology and heart-brain interactions. Purpose is to reduce stress, school violence, improve mental and emotional attitudes, promote harmony within facilities and communities, improve academic performance and improve workplace health and performance. Research facility provides psychometric assessments for both individual and organizational assessment as well as autonomic assessments for physiological assessment and diagnostic purposes. Education initiative currently developing curriculum for rehabilitation of incarcerated teen felons in drug and alcohol recovery program.

Year Founded: 1991

2398 Institute on Psychiatric Services: American Psychiatric Association

1000 Wilson Boulevard
Suite 1825
Arlington, VA 22209-3924
703-907-7300
888-35 -7924

apa@psych.org
www.psych.org

Carol Robinowitz, President

Open to employees of all psychiatric and related health and educational facilities. Includes lectures by experts in the field and workshops and accredited courses on problems, programs and trends. Offers on-site Job Bank, which lists opportunities for mental health professionals. Organized scientific exhibits. Publications: Psychiatric Services, monthly journal. Annual Institute on Psychiatric Services conference and exhibits in October, Chicago, IL.

2399 International Center for the Study of Psychiatry And Psychology (ISCPP)

1036 Park Avenue
Suite 1B
New York, NY 10028-971
212-861-7400
djriccio@aol.com
www.icspp.org

Peter Breggin, Founder/Director Emeritus
Dominick Riccio PhD, Executive Director

Nonprofit research and educational network whose focus is the critical study of the mental health movement. ICSPP is completely independent and their funding consists solely of individual membership dues. Fosters prevention and treatment of mental and emotional disorders. Promotes alternatives to administering psychiatric drugs to children.

2400 International Society for Developmental Psychobiology

8181 Tezel Road
#10269
San Antonio, TX 78250-3092
830-796-9393
866-377-4416; *Fax:* 830-796-9394
www.isdp.org

Pamela Hunt, President
Hawley Montgomery-Downs, Conference Coordinator
Susan Swithers, Program Director
Gale Kleven, Treasurer

Members are research scientists in the field of developmental psychobiology and biology and psychology students. Promotes research in the field of developmental psychobiology, the study of the brain and brain behavior throughout the life span and in relation to other biological proccesses. Stimulates communication and interaction among scientists in the field. Provides the editorship for the journal, Development Psychobiology. Bestows awards. Compiles statistics. Annual conference.

2401 International Society of Political Psychology
Moynihan Institute of Global Affairs

126 Ward Street
Suite 1213
Columbus, NC 28722
828-894-5422; *Fax:* 315-443-9085
ispp@maxwell.syr.edu
www.http://ispp.org

Stanley Feldman, President
Severine Bennett, Executive Director

Facilitates communication across disciplinary, geographic and political boundaries among scholars, concerned individuals in government and public posts, the communication media and elsewhere who have a scientific interest in the relationship between politics and psychological processes. ISPP seeks to advance the quality of scholarship in political psychology and to increase the usefulness of work in political psychology.

2402 International Transactional Analysis Association (ITAA)

2843 Hopyard Road
Suite 155
Pleasanton, CA 94588
925-600-8110; *Fax: 925-600-8112*
info@itaa-net.org
www.www.itaaworld.org

Ken Fogleman, Manager
Lee Beer, Webmaster

A non-profit educational organization with members in over 65 countries. Its purpose is to advance the theory, methods and principles of transactional analysis.

2403 Jean Piaget Society: Society for the Study of Knowledge and Development (JPSSSKD)
Department Of Psychology

Clark University
950 Main St
Worcester, MA 01610-1400
508-793-7250; *Fax: 508-793-7265*
webmaster@piaget.org
www.piaget.org

Nancy Budwig, President
Ashley Maynard, Treasurer

Scholars, teachers, and researchers interested in exploring the nature of the developmental construction of human knowledge. Purpose is to further research on knowledge and development, especially in relation to the work of Jean Piaget, a Swiss developmentalist noted for his work in child psychology, the study of human development, and the origin and growth of human knowledge. Conducts small meetings and programs.

2404 Med Advantage

11301 Corporate Boulevard
Suite 300
Orlando, FL 32817-1445
407-282-5131; *Fax: 407-282-9240*
info@med-advantage.com
www.www.med-advantage.com/

John Witty, Owner

Fully accredited by URAC and certified in all 11 elements by NCQA, Med Advantage is one of the oldest credentials verification organizations in the country. Over the past eight years, they have developed sophisticated computer systems and one of the largest data warehouses of medical providers in the nation, containing information on over 900,000 healthcare providers. Their system is continually updated from primary source data required to meet the standards of the URAC, NCQA and JCAHO.

2405 Medical Group Management Association

104 Inverness Terrace E
Englewood, CO 80112-5313
303-799-1111
877-275-6462; *Fax: 303-643-9599*
service@mgma.com
www.mgma.com

William Jessee, CEO
Steve Hellebush, COO

The national membership association providing information networking and professional development for the individuals who manage and lead medical group practices.

Year Founded: 1926

2406 Mental Health America

500 Montgomery Street
Suite 820
Alexandria, VA 22314
703-684-7722
800-969-6642; *Fax: 703-684-5968*
www.mentalhealthamerica.net

Reginald Williams, Chair of the Board
Paul Gionfriddo, President and CEO
Jessica Kennedy, Chief of Staff/VP of Finance
Theresa Nguyen, VP of Policy and Programs

Committed to enabling the mental wellness of all Americans and improving treatments and services for individuals with mental health needs. Provides information about a range of disorders; advocates for policies focused on advancing early intervention and prevention; and organizes education and outreach initiatives.

Year Founded: 1909

2407 Mental Health Corporations of America

1876-A Eider Court
Tallahassee, FL 32308-4537
850-942-4900; *Fax: 850-942-0560*
www.mhca.com

Chris Wyre MBA, Chairman
Dale Shreve, President & CEO
Tara Boyter, Director, Communications & Membe
Glenda Deal, Director, Conference Services &

Membership in MHCA is by invitation only. It is the organization's intent to include in its network only the highest quality behavioral healthcare organizations in the country. Their alliance is designed to strengthen members' competitive position, enhance their leadership capabilities and facilitate their strategic networking opportunities.

2408 Mental Health Materials Center (MHMC)

PO Box 304
Bronxville, NY 10708-304
914-337-6596; *Fax: 914-779-0161*

Alex Sareyan, President

Professionals of mental health and health education, seeking to stimulate the development of wider, more effective channels of communication between health educators and the public. Provides consulting services to nonprofit organizations on the implementation of their publishing operations in areas related to mental health and health. Publications: Study on Suicide Training Manual. Survival Manual for Medical Students. Books, booklets and pamphlets. Annual Meeting in New York City.

2409 National Academy of Neuropsychology (NAN)

7555 E Hampden Ave
Ste 525
Denver, CO 80231-4836
303-691-3694; *Fax: 303-691-5983*
office@nanonline.org
www.nanonline.org

Daniel Allen, Ph.D., President
Laurie Ryan, Ph.D., Treasurer
Donna Broshek, Ph.D., Secretary

Clinical neuropsychologists and others interested in brain-behavior relationships. Works to preserve and advance knowledge regarding the assessment and remediation of neuropsychological disorders. Promotes the development of neuropsychology as a science and profession; develops standard of practice and training guidelines for the field; fosters communication between members, represents the professional interests of members, serves as an information resource, facilitates the exchange of information among related organizations. Offers continuing education programs, conducts research.

Year Founded: 1975

2410 National Association For Children's Behavioral Health

1025 Connecticut Avenue NW
Suite 1012
Washington, DC 20036-5417
202-857-9735; *Fax:* 202-362-5145
www.www.nacbh.org

Beth Chadwick, President
Joy Midman, Executive Director

To promote the availability and delivery of appropriate and relevant services to children and adolescents with, or at risk of, serious emotional disturbances and their families. Advocate for the full array of mental health and related services necessary, the development and use of assessment and outcome tools based on functional as well as clinical indicators, and the elimination of categorial funding barriers.

2411 National Association for Advancement of Psychoanalysis

80 Eighth Avenue
Suite 1501
New York, NY 10011-5126
212-741-0515; *Fax:* 212-366-4347
NAAP@NAAP.org
www.naap.org

Doughlas F. Maxwell, President
Margery Quackenbush, Executive Director
Kirsty Cardinale, NAAP News Editor
Lucinda Antrim, Secretary

Year Founded: 1972

2412 National Association for the Advancement of Psychoanalysis

NAAP News, E-Bulletin

80 Eighth Avenue
Suite 1501
New York, NY 10011-5126
212-741-0515; *Fax:* 212-366-4347
NAAP@NAAP.org
www.naap.org

Margery Quackenbush, Executive Director
Douglas F. Maxwell, President
Kirsty Cardinale, NAAP News Editor

Certified psychoanalysts disseminating psychoanalytic principles to the medical-psychiatric profession and the general community. Conducts scientific meetings. Supports research programs, sponsors public educational lectures. Publications: NAAP News, Quarterly; Registry of Psychoanalysts, Annual, E-Bulletin, Online Publication

Year Founded: 1972

2413 National Association of Addiction Treatment Providers

11380 ProsperityFarms Road
Suite 209A
Palm BeachGardens, FL 33410
561-429-4527; *Fax:* 561-429-4650
rhunsicker@naatp.org
www.naatp.org

Michael E. Walsh, MS, CAP, BRI I, President/CEO

The mission of the National Association of Addiction Treatment Providers (NAATP) is to promote, assist and enhance the delivery of ethical, effective, research-based treatment for alcoholism and other drug addictions. Provides members and the public with accurate, responsible information and other resources related to the treatment of these diseases, advocates for increased access to and availability of quality treatment for those who suffer from alcoholism and other drug addictions; works in partnership with other organizations and individuals that share NAATP's mission and goals.

Year Founded: 1978

2414 National Association of Community Health Centers

7501 Wisconsin Avenue
Suite 1100W
Bethesda, MD 20814
301-347-0400
www.nachc.com

Tom Van Coverdan, President and CEO
Dave Taylor, Chief Operating Officer
Glenda White, Associent VP/Chief of Staff
James Luisi, Chair of the Board

A nonprofit organization whose mission is to enhance and expand access to quality, community-responsive health care for America's medically underserved and uninsured. A major source for information, data, research, and advocacy on key issues affecting community-based health centers and the delivery of health care. Provides education, training, technical assistance, and leadership development to health center staff, boards, and others to promote excellence and cost-effectiveness in health delivery practice and community board governance. Builds partnerships and linkages that stimulate public and private sector investment in the delivery of quality health care services to medically underserved communities.

Year Founded: 1971

2415 National Association of Nouthetic Counselors

2825 Lexington Road
Louisville, KY 40280
502-410-5526; *Fax:* 317-337-9199
info@nanc.org

Heath Lambert, Executive Director
Randy Patten, Director of Training & Advanceme
Jim Patten, Conference Director
Amber Komatsu, Membership Services Coordinator

NANC is a fellowship of Christian counselors and laymen who have banded together to promote excellence in biblical counseling. NANC was founded in 1975 in service to Christ to address several needs in the counseling community.

Year Founded: 1975

2416 National Association of Psychiatric Health Systems
900 17th Street NW
Suite 420
Washington, DC 20006-2507
202-393-6700; *Fax:* 202-783-6041
naphs@naphs.org
www.naphs.org

Mark Covall, CEO
Kathleen McCann, Director of Quality
Maria Merlie, Director of Administration
Caroline Scott, Administrative Assistant

Advocates for behavioral health and represents provider systems that are committed to the delivery of responsive, accountable, and clinically effective treatment and prevention programs for children, adolescents, adults and older adults with mental and substance abuse disorders.

Year Founded: 1933

2417 National Association of School Psychologists (NASP)
4340 East West Highway
Suite 402
Bethesda, MD 20814-4468
301-657-0270; *Fax:* 301-657-0275
sgorin@naspweb.org
www.nasponline.org

Sally Baas, President
Susan Gorin, Executive Director
Laura Benson, Chief Operating Officer
Katie Britton, Manager, Special Projects

School psychologists who serve the mental health and educational needs of all children and youth. Encourages and provides opportunites for professional growth of individual members. Informs the public on the services and practice of school psychology, and advances the standards of the profession. Operates national school psychologist certification system. Sponsers children's services.

2418 National Association of Social Workers
750 First Street NE
Suite 700
Washington, DC 20002-4241
202-408-8600
800-638-8799; *Fax:* 202-336-8313
www.socialworkers.org

Jeane W. Anastas, PhD, LMSW, President
E. Jane Middleton, DSW, MSW, Vice President
Jacqueline Durham, MSW, LCSW, Secretary
Mary L. McCarthy, PhD, LMSW, Treasurer

Works to enhance the professional growth and development of its members, to create and maintain professional standards, and to advance sound social policies.

2419 National Association of State Mental Health Program Directors (NASMHPD)
66 Canal Center Plaza
Suite 302
Alexandria, VA 22314
703-739-9333; *Fax:* 703-548-9517
brian.hepburn@nasmhpd.org
www.nasmhpd.org

Brian Hepburn, MD, Executive Director
Jay Meek, CPA, MBA, Chief Financial Officer

Raul Almazar, RN, MA, Senior Public Health Advisor
Meighan Haupt, MS, Chief of Staff

The only national association to represent state mental health commissioners/directors and their agencies. A private nonprofit membership organization, NASMHPD helps set the agenda and determine the direction of state mental health agency interests across the country, including state mental health planning, service delivery, and evaluation. The association provides members with the opportunity to exchange diverse views and experiences, learning from one another in areas vital to effective public policy development and implementation.

Year Founded: 1959

2420 National Business Coalition Forum on Health (NBCH)
1015 18th Street NW
Suite 730
Washington, DC 20036-5207
202-775-9300; *Fax:* 202-775-1569
awebber@nbch.org
www.www.nbch.org

Brian Klepper, Chief Executive Officer
Susan Dorsey, Vice President of Education
Sara Hanlon, Vice President of Member Support
Maria Cornejo, Director of Operations

A national, non-profit membership organization of employer-based coalitions. Dedicated to value-based purchasing of health care services through the collective action of public and private purchasers. NCBH seeks to accelerate the nations progress towards safe, efficient, high quality health care and the improved health status of the American population.

2421 National Coalition for the Homeless
2201 P Street Northwest
Washington, DC 20037
202-462-4822
info@nationalhomeless.org
www.www.nationalhomeless.org

Bob Erlenbusch, President
Megan Hastings, Interim Director
Barbara Anderson, Secretary
Annie Leomporra, Grassroots Analyst

The National Coalition for the Homeless is an organization serving to protect the needs of those experiencing homelessness, while striving to prevent and end homelessness. NCH promotes effective treatment, services, and programs for those struggling with homelessness as well as substance abuse problems.

Year Founded: 1982

2422 National Committee for Quality Assurance
1100 13th Street NW
Suite 1000
Washington, DC 20005-4285
202-955-3500; *Fax:* 202-955-3599
www.ncqa.org

Margaret E O'Kane, President
Tom Fluegel, Chief Operating Officer
Patricia Barrett, Vice President, Product Developm
Mary Barton, Vice President, Performance Meas

A non-profit organization whose mission is to improve health care quality everywhere and to transform health care quality through measurement, transparency and accountability.

2423 National Council of Juvenile and Family Court Judges

PO Box 8970
Reno, NV 89507-8970
775-784-6012; *Fax:* 775-784-6628
staff@ncjfcj.org
www.ncjfcj.org

David Stucki, President
Mari Kay Bickett, JD, Chief ExecutiveOfficer
Cheryl Dailey, CPA, CMA, CFE,, Chief Financial Officer
Cheryl Davidek, Chief Administrative Officer

Their mission is to improve courts and systems practice and raise awareness of the core issues that touch the lives of many of our nation's childrens and families.

Year Founded: 1937

2424 National Council on Aging

1901 L Street NW
4th Floor
Washington, DC 20036-3540
202-479-1200; *Fax:* 202-479-0735
info@ncoa.org
www.ncoa.org

Richard Browdie, Chair
James Firman, EdD, President and CEO
Andrew Greene, Secretary & Treasurer
Jay Greenberg, ScD, CEO, NCOA Services, LLC

NCOA is a nonprofit service and advocacy organization. NCOA is a ntional voice for millions of older adults, especially those that are vulnerable and disadvantaged and the community organizations that serve them. It brings together non profit organizations, businesses, and government to develop creative solutions that improve the lives of older adults.

Year Founded: 1950

2425 National Nurses Association

1767 Business Center Drive
Suite 150
Reston, VA 20190-5332
703-438-3000
877-662-6253
info@nationalnurses.org
www.nationalnurses.org

Laurie Campbell PhD, Executive Director

Purpose is to help enhance the personal development as well as economic well being of its members. They provide services and benefits meaningful to the unique demands of the nursing professional.

Year Founded: 1984

2426 National Pharmaceutical Council

1717 Pennsylvania Ave., NW
Suite 800
Washington, DC 20006
202-827-2100; *Fax:* 202-827-0314
info@npcnow.com
www.www.npcnow.org/?

Dan Leonard, MA, President
Patricia L. Adams, VP, Business Operations & Extern
Robert W. Dubois, MD, PhD, Chief Science Officer
Melissa Baulkwill, Director, Administration

NPC sponsors a variety of research and education projects aimed at demonstrating that the appropriate use of pharmaceuticals improves both patient treatment outcomes and the cost effective delivery of overall health care services.

2427 National Psychological Association for Psychoanalysis (NPAP)

40 West 13th Street
New York, NY 10011-7802
212-924-7440; *Fax:* 212-989-7543
info@npap.org
www.npap.org

Carl Weinberg, President
Rosaleen Horn, Vice President
Ann Rose Simon, Treasurer
Penny Rosen, Corresponding Secretary

Professional society for practicing psychoanalysts. Conducts training program leading to certification in psychoanalysis. Offers information and private referral service for the public. Operates speakers' bureau. Publications: National Psychological Association for Psychoanalysis-Bulletin, biennial. National Psychological Association for Psychoanalysis-News and Reviews, semiannual. Psychoanalytic Review, bimonthly journal.

Year Founded: 1948

2428 National Register of Health Service Providers in Psychology

1200 New York Avenue NW
Suite 800
Washington, DC 20005-3873
202-783-7663; *Fax:* 202-347-0550
www.nationalregister.org

Raymond A Folen, PhD, President/Chair
Andrew P Boucher, Assistant Director
Julia Bernstein, Membership Coordinator
Deanne Canieso, Communications Coordinator, MPH,

Psychologists who are licensed or certified by a state/provincial board of examiners of psychology and who have met council criteria as health service providers in psychology.

Year Founded: 1974

2429 National Treatment Alternative for Safe Communities

1500 N Halsted
Chicago, IL 60642-2517
312-376-0950; *Fax:* 312-376-5889
information@tasc-il.org
www.tasc-il.org

Marcia J. Lipetz, PhD, Chair
Cecil V. Curtwright, Vice Chair / Secretary
Andreason Brown, Chief Financial Officer
Lancert A. Foster, CPA, Treasurer

TASC is a not-for-profit organization that provides behavioral health recovery management services for individuals with substance abuse and mental health disorders. They provide direct services, design model programs and build collaborative networks between public systems and community-based human service providers. TASC's purpose is to see that under-served populations gain access to the services they need for health and self-sufficiency, while also ensuring that public and private resources are used most efficiently.

2430 North American Society of Adlerian Psychology (NASAP)
NASAP
429 E. Dupont Road
Suite 276
Fort Wayne, IN 46825
260-267-8807; *Fax:* 260-818-2098
www.alfredadler.org

Richard Watts, President
Susan Belangee, Vice President
Michele Frey, Secretary
Susan (Zsuzs Burak, Treasurer

NASAP is a professional organization for couselors, educators, psychologists, parent educators, business professionals, researchers and others who are interested in Adler's Individual Psychology. Membership includes journals, newsletters, conferences and training.

Year Founded: 1952

2431 Pharmaceutical Care Management Association
601 Pennsylvania Avenue NW
7th Floor
Washington, DC 20004-2601
202-756-7210; *Fax:* 202-207-3623
info@pcmanet.org
www.pcmanet.org

Dirk McMahon, Chairman
Mark Merritt, President & Chief Executive Offi
Kristin Bass, Senior Vice President, Federal A
Timothy Brogan, Assistant Vice President, Public

A national association representing Pharmacy Benefit Managers. They are dedicated to enhancing the proven tools and techniques that PBMs have pioneered in the marketplace and working to lower the cost of prescription drugs for more than 200 million Americans.

2432 Physicians for a National Health Program
29 E Madison
Suite 602
Chicago, IL 60602-4406
312-782-6006; *Fax:* 312-782-6007
info@pnhp.org
www.pnhp.org

Andrew D Coates, MD, FACP, President
Quentin D Young, MD, MACP, National Coordinator
Claudia M Fegan, MD, CHCQM, FACP, Treasurer
Gordon Schiff, MD, Secretary

A single issue organization advocating a universal, comprehensive Single-Payer National Health Program.

Year Founded: 1987

2433 Professional Risk Management Services
The Psychiatrists' Program
1401 Wilson Boulevard
Suite 700
Arlington, VA 22209-2434
800-245-3333
www.www.prms.com

Stephen Sills, CEO
Denny Rodriguez, JD, COO

PRMS, Inc. specializes in medical professional liability insurance programs and claims and risk management services - on a bundled and unbundled basis for individual healthcare providers, group practices, facilities, associations, and organizations.

2434 Psychiatric Society of Informatics American Association for Technology in Psychiatry
PO Box 11
Bronx, NY 10464-11
718-502-9469
aatp@techpsych.org
www.techpsych.org

Robert Kennedy, Executive Director
Carlyle Chan, Secretary
Naakesh Dewan, President

Year Founded: 1995

2435 Psychohistory Forum
627 Dakota Trail
Franklin Lakes, NJ 07417-1043
201-891-7486
pelovitz@aol.com
www.cliospsyche.org

Paul H Elovitz PhD, Editor

Psychologists, psychiatrists, psychotherapists, social workers, historians, psychohistorians and others having a scholarly interest in the integration of depth psychology and history. Aids individuals in psychohistorical research. Holds lecture series. Publications: Clio's Psyche: Understanding the Why of Current Events and History, quarterly journal. Immigrant Experience: Personal Narrative and Psychological Analysis, monograph. Periodic Meeting.

Year Founded: 1994

2436 Psychology of Religion
Doctoral Program in Clinical Psychology
750 First Street NE
Washington, DC 20002-4242
202-336-6013; *Fax:* 202-218-3599
division@apa.org
www.www.apa.org/about/division/div36.aspx

Elizabeth Hall, President
Gina Magyar-Russell, Secretary

A division of the American Psychologial Association. Seeks to encourage and accelerate research, theory, and practice in the psychology of religion and related areas. Facilitates the dissemination of data on religious and allied issues and on the integration of these data with current psychological research, theory and practice.

2437 Psychonomic Society
2785 E. Posse Court
Green Valley, AZ 85614
520-232-3117; *Fax:* 520-232-3117
secretary-treasurer@psychonomic.org
www.psychonomic.org

Gavin Wilson, Manager
Roger Mellgren, Convention Manager

Persons qualified to conduct and supervise scientific research in psychology or allied sciences; members must hold a PhD degree or its equivalent and must have published significant research other than doctoral dissertation. Promotes the communication of scientific research in psychology and allied sciences.

Year Founded: 1959

2438 Rapid Psychler Press
2014 Holland Ave
Suite 374
Port Huron, MI 48060-1994

519-667-2335
888-779-2453; *Fax:* 519-675-0610
rapid@psychler.com
www.psychler.com

David Robinson, Publisher

Produces books and presentation media for educating mental health professionals. Products cover a wide range of learning needs. Where possible, humor is incorporated as an educational aid to enhance learning and retention.

2439 Risk and Insurance Management Society

1065 Avenue Of The Americas
13th Floor
New York, NY 10018
212-286-9292; *Fax:* 212-986-9716
www.rims.org

Carolyn Snow, President
Mary Roth, Executive Director
Richard Roberts, Vice President
Aurea Hernando, Executive Assistant

2440 Screening for Mental Health

1 Washington Street
Suite 304
Wellesley Hills, MA 02481-1706
781-239-0071; *Fax:* 781-431-7447
smhinfo@mentalhealthscreening.org
www.mentalhealthscreening.org

Douglas George Jacobs, M.D., President & Medical Director

Nonprofit organization devoted to assisting people with undiagnosed, untreated mental illness connect with local treatment resources via national screening programs for depression, anxiety, eating disorders and alcohol problems.

2441 Sigmund Freud Archives (SFA)

16 Channing Place
c/o Harold P Blum, MD
Cambridge, MA 02138
516-621-6850
aok@kris.org
www.www.freudarchives.org

Deanna Holtzman, President
Anton O. Kris, Executive Director
John M. Ross, Secretary/Treasurer

Psychoanalysts interested in the preservation and collection of scientific and personal writings of Sigmund Freud. Assists in research on Freud's life and work and the evolution of psychoanalytic thought. Collects and classifies all documents, papers, publications, personal correspondence and historical data written by, to, and on Freud. Transmits all materials collected to the Library of Congress. Annual meeting in New York City.

Year Founded: 1951

2442 Society for Pediatric Psychology (SPP)
Citadel

PO Box 3968
Lawrence, KS 66046
785-856-0713; *Fax:* 785-856-0759
APAdiv54@gmail.com
www.www.apadivisions.org/division-54/index.aspx

Lori Stark, President
Christina Adams, Secretary

Dedicated to research and practice addressing the relationship between children's physical, cognitive, social, and emotional functioning and their physical well-being, including maintenance of health, promotion of positive health behaviors, and treatment of chronic and serious medical conditions. A division of the APA. Bimonthly Journal, Newletter three times a year.

2443 Society for Personality Assessment

6109H Arlington Boulevard
Falls Church, VA 22044-2708
703-534-4772; *Fax:* 703-564-6905
manager@spaonline.org
www.personality.org

Ronald J Ganellen, Ph.D., President
Giselle Hass, PsyD, Secretary
John McNulty, Ph.D., Treasurer
Robert Bornstein, PhD, President-Elect

International professional trade association for psychologists, behavioral scientists, anthropologists, and psychiatrists. Promotes the study, research development and application of personality assessment.

2444 Society for Psychophysiological Research

2424 American Lane
Madison, WI 53704-3102
608-443-2470; *Fax:* 608-443-2474
homeoffice@scmhr.org
www.scmhr.org

Lisa Nelson, Manager
Karen Quigley, Treasurer

Founded in 1960, the Society for Psychophysiological Research is an international scientific society. The purpose of the society is to foster research on the interrelationship between physiological and phychological aspects of behavior.

2445 Society for Women's Health Research (SWHR)

1025 Connecticut Avenue NW
Suite 601
Washington, DC 20036-5447
202-223-8224; *Fax:* 202-833-3472
info@swhr.org
www.www.womenshealthresearch.org

Susan Alpert, PhD, MD, Chair
Phyllis Greenberger, MSW, President & CEO
Mary V. Hornig, COO & CFO
Yonas G. Weldemariam, MBA, Director of Finance

The nation's only not-for-profit organization whose sole mission is to improve the health of women through research. Founded in 1990, The SWHR advocates increased funding for research on women's health, encourages the study of sex differences that may affect the prevention, diagnosis and treatment of disease, and promotes the inclusion of women in medical research studies.

Year Founded: 1990

2446 Society for the Advancement of Social
Psychology (SASP)

630 Convention Tower
Buffalo, NY 14202
301-405-5921; *Fax:* 301-314-9566
info@sesp.org
www.sesp.org

Garold Stasser, Secretary
Charles Stangor, Executive Officer

Social psychologists and students in social psychology. Advances social psychology as a profession by facilitating communication among social psychologists and improving dissemination and utilization of social psychological knowledge. Annual meeting every October.

2447 Society for the Psychological Study of Social Issues (SPSSI)
208 I Street NE
Washington, DC 20002-4340
202-675-6956
877-310-7778; *Fax:* 202-675-6902
spssi@spssi.org
www.www.spssi.org

Susan Dudley, Executive Director
Anila Balkissoon, Administrative & Awards Coordina
Brad Sickels, Administrative Assistant
Gabriel Twose, Policy Director

An international group of over 3,500 psychologists, allied scientists, students, and others who share a common interest in research on the psychological aspects of important social issues. The Society seeks to bring theory and practice into focus on human problems of the group, the community, and nations as well as the increasingly important problems that have no national boundaries.

2448 Society of Behavioral Medicine
555 East Wells Street
Suite 1100
Milwaukee, WI 53202-3823
414-918-3156; *Fax:* 414-276-3349
info@sbm.org
www.sbm.org

Dawn K Wilson, PhD, President
Michael A Diefenbach, PhD, Secretary/Treasurer
Lisa M Klesges, PhD, President-Elect

A non-profit organization is a scientific forum for over 3,000 behavioral and biomedical researchers and clinicians to study the interactions of behavior, physiological and biochemical states, and morbidity and mortality. SBM provides an interactive network for education and collaboration on common research, clinical and public policy concerns related to prevention, diagnosis and treatment, rehabilitation, and health promotion.

Year Founded: 1978

2449 Society of Multivariate Experimental Psychology (SMEP)
University of Virginia
102 Gilmer Hall
Department of Psychology
Charlottesville, VA 22903
804-924-0656
shrout@psych.nyu.edu
www.smep.org

Steve West, President
Wayne Velicer, President-Elect

An organization of researchers interested in multivariate quantitative methods and their application to substantive problems in psychology. Membership is limited to 65 regular active members. SMEP oversees the publication of a research journal which publishes research articles on multivariate methodology and its use in psychological research. Annual meeting held every October.

Year Founded: 1960

2450 Society of Teachers of Family Medicine
11400 Tomahawk Creek Parkway
Suite 540
Leawood, KS 66211-2681
913-906-6000
800-274-2237; *Fax:* 913-906-6096
www.stfm.org

Stacy Brungardt, Executive Director
Tom Vansaghi, PhD, Chief Development Officer
Dana Greco, CAE, Chief Financial Officer
Priscilla Noland, Senior Meeting Planner

Mulitdisciplinary, medical organization that offers numerous faculty development opportunities for individuals involved in family medicine education. STFM publishes a monthly journal, hosts a web site, distributes books, coordinates CME conferences devoted to family medicine teaching and research and other activities designed to improve teaching skills of family medicine educators.

2451 United States Psychiatric Rehabilitation Organization (USPRA)
1760 Old Meadow Road
Suite 500
McLean, VA 22102
703-442-2078; *Fax:* 703-506-3266
info@uspra.org
www.uspra.org

Lisa Razzano, PhD, CPRP, Chair
Tom Gibson, Interim Chief Executive Officer
Casey Goldberg, Chief Staff Officer, Certificati
Cherilyn Cepriano, CAE, JD,, Vice President, Public Policy

The USPRA, formerly IAPSRS, is an organization of psychosocial rehabilitation agencies, practitioners, and interested organizations and individuals dedicated to promoting, supporting and strengthening community-oriented rehabilitation services and resources for persons with psychiatric disabilities.

Year Founded: 1975

2452 Wellness Councils of America
17002 Marcy St.
Suite 140
Omaha, NE 68118
402-827-3590; *Fax:* 402-827-3594
wellworkplace@welcoa.org
www.welcoa.org

Stephen M. LaCagnin, Chairman
Ryan Picarella, MS, SPHR, President
David Hunnicutt, PhD, CEO
Brittanie Leffelman, MS, Vice President of Operations

A national non-profit membership organization dedicated to promoting healthier life styles for all Americans, especially through health promotion initiatives at the worksite. They publish a number of source books, a monthly newsletter, an extensive line of brochures and conducts numerous training seminars.

Year Founded: 1987

2453 WorldatWork
14040 N Northsight Boulevard
Scottsdale, AZ 85260-3627
877-951-9191
480-951-9191; *Fax:* 866-816-2962

customerrelations@worldatwork.org
www.worldatwork.org
Anne Ruddy, President
Marcia Rhodes, Media Relations

A not-for-profit professional association dedicated to knowledge leadership in compensation, benefits and total rewards. Focuses on human resources disciplines associated with attracting, retaining and motivating employees. Provides education programs, a monthly magazine, online information resources, surveys, publications, conferences, research and networking opportunities.

Year Founded: 1955

Books

2454 A Primer on Rational Emotive Behavior Therapy
Research Press
PO Box 7866
Champaign, IL 61826-9177
217-352-3273
800-519-2707; *Fax:* 217-352-1221
rp@researchpress.com
www.researchpress.com

Dr Windy Dryden, Author
Dr Raymond DiGiuseppe, Author
Michael Neenan, Author

This concise, systematic guide addresses recent developments in the theory and practice of Rational Emotive Behavior Therapy (REBT). The authors discuss rational versus irrational thinking, the ABC framework, the three basic musts that interfere wtih rational thinking and behavior, two basic biological tendencies, two fundamental human disturbances, and the theory of change in REBT. A detailed case example that includes verbatim dialogue between therapist and client illustrates the 18-step REBT treatment sequence. An appendix by Albert Ellis examines the special features of REBT. *$13.95*

136 pages ISBN 0-878224-78-5

2455 A Research Agenda for DSM-V
American Psychiatric Publishing, Inc.
1000 Wilson Boulevard
Suite 1825
Arlington, VA 22209-3901
703-907-7322
800-368-5777; *Fax:* 703-907-1091
appi@psych.org
www.appi.org

Michael B First, M.D, Editor
David J. Kupfer, M.D, Editor
Darrel Regier, M.D., M.P.H., Editor

In the ongoing quest to improve our psychiatric diagnostic system, we are now searching for new approaches to understanding the etiological and pathophysiological mechanisms that can improve the validity of our diagnoses and the consequent power of our preventative and treatment interventions-venturing beyond the current DSM paradigm and DSM-IV framework. This volume represents a far-reaching attempt to stimulate research and discussion in the field in preparation for the start of the DSM-V process, still several years away, and to integrate information from a wide variety of sources and technologies. Copyright 2002. *$38.95*

336 pages Year Founded: 2002 ISBN 0-890422-92-3

2456 Addressing the Specific needs of Women with Co-Occuring Disorders in the Criminal Justice System
Policy Research Associates
345 Delaware Avenue
Delmar, NY 12054-1905
518-439-7415
800-444-7415; *Fax:* 518-439-7612
pra@prainc.com
www.prainc.com

Henry Steadman, President

Brochure emphasizes the need for gender specific programs to meet the management needs of female offenders. For law enforcement and justice administrators.

2457 Advances in Projective Drawing Interpetation
Charles C Thomas Publisher Ltd.
2600 S 1st Street
Springfield, IL 62704-4730
217-789-8980
800-258-8980; *Fax:* 217-789-9130
books@ccthomas.com
www.ccthomas.com

Michael P Thomas, President

Exceptional contributors were chosen for their pertinence, range and inventiveness. This outstanding book assembles the progress in the science and in the clinical art of projective drawings as we enter the twenty-first century. Copyright 1997. *$80.95*

476 pages ISBN 0-398067-43-0

2458 Advancing DSM: Dilemmas in Psychiatric Diagnosis
American Psychiatric Publishing, Inc.
1000 Wilson Boulevard
Suite 1825
Arlington, VA 22209-3901
703-907-7322
800-368-5777; *Fax:* 703-907-1091
appi@psych.org
www.appi.org

Katharine A Phillips, M.D, Editor
Michael B First, M.D, Editor
Harold Alan Pincus, M.D, Editor

Presents case studies from leading clinicians and researchers that illuminate the need for a revamped system. Each chapter presents a diagnostic dilemma from clinical practice that is intriguing, controversial, unresolved and remarkable in its theoretical and scientific complexity. Chapter by chapter, Advancing DSM raises important questions about the nature of diagnosis under the current DSM system and recommends broad changes. Copyright 2002. *$41.95*

264 pages Year Founded: 2003 ISBN 0-890422-93-1

2459 Adverse Effects of Psychotropic Drugs
Gilford Press
72 Spring Street
New York, NY 10012-4019
212-431-9800; *Fax:* 212-966-6708

John M. Kane, Editor
Jeffrey A. Lieberman, Editor
$63.00

2460 Agility in Health Care
John Wiley & Sons
111 River Street
Hoboken, NJ 07030-5773
201-748-6000; *Fax: 210-748-6088*
www.wiley.com

$42.95

250 pages ISBN 0-787942-11-1

2461 American Psychiatric Glossary
American Psychiatric Publishing, Inc.
1000 Wilson Boulevard
Suite 1825
Arlington, VA 22209-3901
703-907-7322
800-368-5777; *Fax: 703-907-1091*
appi@psych.org
www.appi.org

Robert E Hales MD, Editor-in-Chief
Ron McMillen, Chief Executive Officer
John McDuffie, Editorial Director

Hardcover. Paperback also available. Copyright 1994.
$28.50

224 pages ISBN 0-880485-26-4

2462 American Psychiatric Publishing Textbook of
Clinical Psychiatry
American Psychiatric Publishing, Inc.
1000 Wilson Boulevard
Suite 1825
Arlington, VA 22209-3901
703-907-7322
800-368-5777; *Fax: 703-907-1091*
appi@psych.org
www.appi.org

Robert E Hales MD, Editor-in-Chief
Ron McMillen, Chief Executive Officer
John McDuffie, Editorial Director

This densely informative textbook comprises 40 scholarly,
authorative chapters by an astonishing 89 experts and combines junior and senior authors alike to enhance the rich diversity and quality of clinical perspectives. Copyright
2002. *$239.00*

1776 pages ISBN 1-585620-32-7

2463 Americans with Disabilities Act and the
Emerging Workforce
AAMR
444 N Capitol Street NW
Suite 846
Washington, DC 20001-1569
202-637-0475
800-424-3688; *Fax: 202-637-0585*
dcroser@aamr.org

David L. Braddock, Author
Peter David Blanck, Author

Presents an empirical investigation of ADA issues and their
effect on the employment of people with disabilities. Filled
with legal cases, court opinions, charts, and tables. *$39.95*

303 pages ISBN 0-940898-52-7

2464 Assesing Problem Behaviors
AAMR
444 N Capitol Street NW
Suite 846
Washington, DC 20001-1569
202-637-0475
800-424-3688; *Fax: 202-637-0585*
dcroser@aamr.org

Mary Ann Demchak, Author
Karen W. Bossert, Author

Shows how to conduct a functional assessment, to link assessment results to interventions, and gives an example of
completed fuctional analysis. *$21.95*

44 pages ISBN 0-940898-39-X

2465 Basic Personal Counseling: Training Manual
for Counslers
Charles C Thomas Publisher Ltd.
2600 S 1st Street
Springfield, IL 62704-4730
217-789-8980
800-258-8980; *Fax: 217-789-9130*
books@ccthomas.com
www.ccthomas.com

David Geldard, Author

Contents: Becoming a Counselor; The Counseling Rela-
tionship; An Overview of Skills Training; Attending to the
Client and the Use of Minimal Responses; Reflection of
Feeling; Reflection of Content and Feeling; The Seeing,
Hearing, and Feeling Modes; Asking Questions; Summa-
rizing; Exploring Options; Reframing; Confrontation;
Challenging Self-Destructive Beliefs; Termination; Proce-
dure of the Counseling Experience; The Immediacy of the
Counseling Experience; The Human Personality as it
Emerges in the Counseling Experience; The Angry Client;
Loss and Grief Counseling; The Suicidal Client; Arrange-
ment of the Counseling Room; Keeping Records of Coun-
seling Sessions; Confidentiality; Supervision and Ongoing
Training; and The Counselor's Own Well-Being. Copyright
1989. *$42.95*

214 pages Year Founded: 1989 ISBN 0-398055-40-8

2466 Boundaries and Boundary Violations in
Psychoanalysis
American Psychiatric Publishing, Inc.
1000 Wilson Boulevard
Suite 1825
Arlington, VA 22209-3901
703-907-7322
800-368-5777; *Fax: 703-907-1091*
appi@psych.org
www.appi.org

Glen O Gabbard, M.D, Author
Eva P Lester, M.D, Author
John McDuffie, Editorial Director

Copyright 2002.

240 pages Year Founded: 2003 ISBN 1-585620-98-X

2467 Brain Calipers: Descriptive Psychopathology
and the Mental Status Examination, Second
Edition
Rapid Psychler Press
2014 Holland Ave
Suite 374
Port Huron, MI 48060-1994

519-667-2335
888-779-2453; *Fax:* 519-675-0610
rapid@psychler.com
www.psychler.com

David Robinson, Publisher

$34.95

ISBN 1-894328-02-7

2468 Breakthroughs in Antipsychotic Medications: A Guide for Consumers, Families, and Clinicians
WW Norton & Company
500 5th Avenue
New York, NY 10110-54
212-354-5500
800-233-4830; *Fax:* 212-869-0856
admalmud@wwnorton.com
www.books.wwnorton.com/

Ronald J. Diamond, Author
Ruth Ross, Author
Patricia L. Scheifler, Author
Peter J. Weiden, Author

Gives patients and their families needed information about the pros and cons of switching medications, possible side effects. Copyright 1999. *$22.95*

208 pages ISBN 0-393703-03-7

2469 Brief Coaching for Lasting Solutions
WW Norton & Company
500 5th Avenue
New York, NY 10110-54
212-354-5500
800-233-4830; *Fax:* 212-869-0856
npb@wwnorton.com
www.books.wwnorton.com/

Insoo Kim Berg, Author
Peter Szab¢, Author

Successful coaching is about finding solutions and optimizing clients' lives. Insoo Kim Berg, one of the founders of solution-focused psychotherapy, collaborates with Peter Szabo in order to show how to help clients achieve their goals by applying their therapeutic approach to coaching.

264 pages ISBN 0-393704-72-6

2470 Brief Therapy and Managed Care
Joh Wiley & Sons
111 River Street
Hoboken, NJ 07030-5774
201-748-6000; *Fax:* 201-748-6088
www.wiley.com

Provides focused, time-sensitive treatment to your patients. Pratical guidelines on psychotherapy that are conscientiously managed, appropriate, and sensitive to a client's needs. *$40.95*

443 pages ISBN 0-787900-77-X

2471 Brief Therapy with Intimidating Cases
Jossey-Bass Publishers
111 River Street
Hoboken, NJ 07030-5774
201-748-6000
800-956-7739; *Fax:* 201-748-6088
info@wiley.com
www.as.wiley.com

Richard Fisch, Author
Karin Schlanger, Author

This hands-on guide shows you how to apply the proven principles of brief therapy to a range of complex psychological problems once thought to be treatable only through long-term therapy or with medication. Learn how to focus on your clients' primary complaint and understand how and in what context the undesired behavior is performed. *$34.95*

192 pages Year Founded: 1998 ISBN 0-787943-64-9

2472 CURRENT Diagnosis & Treatment: Psychiatry
McGraw-Hill Medical Publishing Group
2 Penn Plaza
New York, NY 10121
212-904-2000; *Fax:* 212-904-6030
www.mhprofessional.com/product/php?isbn=0071422927

Michael H Ebert, Co-Author
Peter T Loosen, Co-Author
Barry Nurcombe, Co-Author
James F Leckman, Co-Author

This second edition is a reference for quickly answering day-to-day questions on psychiatric illness in both adults and children. Comprehensive in scope, and streamlined in coverage, this is a time-saving clinical companion. It reviews essential psychopharmacologic and psychotherapeutic approaches to the full range of psychiatric disorders. Copyright 2008. *$72.95*

758 pages ISBN 0-071422-92-7

2473 Cambridge Handbook of Psychology, Health and Medicine
Cambridge University Press
32 Avenue of the Americas
New York, NY 10013-2473
212-337-5000; *Fax:* 212-691-3239
customer_service@cambridge.org
www.cambridge.org

Andrew Baum, Editor
Susan Ayers, Editor
Chris McManus, Editor
Stanton Newman, Editor

This important text collates international and interdisciplinary expertise to form a unique encyclopedic handbook to this field that will be valuable to medical practitioners as well as psychologists. Copyright 1997. *$85.00*

678 pages ISBN 0-521436-86-9

2474 Challenging Behavior of Persons with Mental Health Disorders and Severe Developmental Disabilities
AAMR
444 N Capitol Street NW
Suite 846
Washington, DC 20001-1569
202-637-0475
800-424-3688; *Fax:* 202-637-0585
dcroser@aamr.org

Ronald H. Hanson, Author
Norman A. Wiesler, Editor

Provides a valuable compendium of the current knowledge base and empirically tested treatments for individuals with severe developmental disabilities, especially when problematic patterns of behavior are evident. *$39.95*

278 pages ISBN 0-940898-66-7

2475 Changing Health Care Marketplace
John Wiley & Sons
111 River Street
Hoboken, NJ 07030-5774
201-748-6000; *Fax:* 201-748-6088
www.wiley.com

$35.95

366 pages ISBN 0-787902-52-7

2476 Clinical Dimensions of Anticipatory Mourning
Research Press
PO Box 7866
Champaign, IL 61826-9177
217-352-3273
800-519-2707; *Fax:* 217-352-1221
rp@researchpress.com
www.researchpress.com

Russell Pense, VP Marketing

Dr. Therese Rando is joined by 17 contributing authors to present the most comprehensive resource available on the perspectives, issues, interventions, and changing views associated with anticipatory mourning. *$29.95*

616 pages ISBN 0-878223-80-0

2477 Clinical Integration
Jossey-Bass Publishers
111 River Street
Hoboken, NJ 07030-5774
201-748-6000
800-956-7739; *Fax:* 201-748-6088
info@wiley.com
www.as.wiley.com

Mary Tonges, Editor

Learn how to create information systems that can support care coordination and management across delivery sites, develop a case management model program for multi-provider systems, and more. *$41.95*

239 pages Year Founded: 1998 ISBN 0-787940-39-9

2478 Cognitive Therapy in Practice
WW Norton & Company
500 5th Avenue
New York, NY 10110-54
212-354-5500
800-233-4830; *Fax:* 212-869-0856
npd@wwnorton.com
www.books.wwnorton.com/

Jacqueline B Persons, Author

Basic text for graduate studies in psychotherapy, psycholgy nursing social work and counseling. *$29.00*

224 pages Year Founded: 1989 ISBN 0-393700-77-1

2479 Collaborative Therapy with Multi-Stressed Families
Guilford Press
72 Spring Street
New York, NY 10012-4068
212-431-9800
800-365-7006; *Fax:* 212-966-6708
info@guilford.com

William C. Madsen, Author

Written with a clear and fresh style, this is a guide to working in collaboration with clients, therapists and agencies. Experienced and beginning clinicians will appreciate a progressive approach to intricate problems. Copyrigt 1999. *$31.50*

388 pages ISBN 1-572304-90-1

2480 Communicating in Relationships: A Guide for Couples and Professionals
Research Press
PO Box 7866
Champaign, IL 61826-9177
217-352-3273
800-519-2707; *Fax:* 217-352-1221
rp@researchpress.com
www.researchpress.com

Russell Pense, VP Marketing

Addresses the behavioral, affective and cognitive aspects of communicating in relationships. The book can be used by couples as a self-help guide, by professionals as an adjunct to therapy, or as a supplementary text for related college courses. Numerous readings are interspersed with 44 exercises that provide a hands-on approach to learning. The authors outline 18 steps for developing communication skills and describe procedures for integrating the skills into relationships. *$29.95*

280 pages ISBN 0-878223-42-8

2481 Community-Based Instructional Support
AAMR
444 N Capitol Street NW
Suite 846
Washington, DC 20001-1569
202-637-0475
800-424-3688; *Fax:* 202-637-0585
dcroser@aamr.org

David Wesley Test, Author
Fred Spooner, Author

Offers practical guidelines for applying instructional strategies for adults who are learning community-based tasks. *$12.95*

34 pages ISBN 0-940898-43-8

2482 Comprehensive Textbook of Geriatric Psychiatry
WW Norton & Company
500 5th Avenue
New York, NY 10110-54
212-354-5500
800-233-4830; *Fax:* 212-869-0856
npb@wwnorton.com
www.books.wwnorton.com/

George T. Grossberg, Editor
Lissy F. Jarvik, Editor
Barnett S. Meyers, Editor
Joel Sadavoy, Editor

Sponsored by the American Association for Geriatric Psychiatry (AAGP), this invaluable reference covers the entire range of geriatric psychiatry, including: the ageing process; psychiatric disorders of the elderly; princpiles of diagnosis and treatment; medical-legal, ethical, and financial issues.

1352 pages ISBN 0-393704-26-2

2483 Computerization of Behavioral Healthcare
Jossey-Bass Publishers
111 River Street
Hoboken, NJ 07030-5774
201-748-6000
800-956-7739; *Fax:* 201-748-6088
info@wiley.com
www.as.wiley.com

Tom Trabin, Author

How computers and networked interactive information systems can help to contain costs, improve clinical outcomes, make your organizations more competitive using practical guidelines. Copyright 1996. *$27.95*

284 pages Year Founded: 1996 ISBN 0-787902-21-7

2484 Concise Guide to Marriage and Family Therapy
American Psychiatric Publishing, Inc.
1000 Wilson Boulevard
Suite 1825
Arlington, VA 22209-3901
703-907-7322
800-368-5777; *Fax:* 703-907-1091
appi@psych.org
www.appi.org

Robert E Hales MD, Editor-in-Chief
Ron McMillen, Chief Executive Officer
John McDuffie, Editorial Director

Developed for use in the clinical setting, presents the core knowledge in the field in a single quick-reference volume. With brief, to-the-point guidance and step-by-step protocols, it's an invaluable resource for the busy clinician. Copyright 2002. *$29.95*

240 pages ISBN 1-585620-77-7

2485 Concise Guide to Psychiatry and Law for Clinicians
American Psychiatric Publishing, Inc.
1000 Wilson Boulevard
Suite 1825
Arlington, VA 22209-3901
703-907-7322
800-368-5777; *Fax:* 703-907-1091
appi@psych.org
www.appi.org

Robert E Hales MD, Editor-in-Chief
Ron McMillen, Chief Executive Officer
John McDuffie, Editorial Director

Practical information for psychiatrists in understanding legal regulations, legal decisions and present managed care applications. Copyright 1998. *$29.95*

296 pages ISBN 0-880483-29-6

2486 Concise Guide to Psychopharmacology
American Psychiatric Publishing, Inc.
1000 Wilson Boulevard
Suite 1825
Arlington, VA 22209-3901
703-907-7322
800-368-5777; *Fax:* 703-907-1091
appi@psych.org
www.appi.org

Lauren B Marangell, M.D, Author
James M Martinez, M.D, Author
John McDuffie, Editorial Director

Packed with practical information that is easy to access via detailed tables and charts, this pocket-sized volume (it literally fits into a lab coat or jacket pocket) is designed to be immediately useful for students, residents and clinicians working in a variety of treatment settings, such as inpatient psychiatry units, outpatient clinics, consultation-liaison services and private offices. Copyright 2002. *$29.95*

260 pages Year Founded: 2006 ISBN 1-585620-75-0

2487 Consent Handbook for Self-Advocates and Support Staff
AAMR
444 N Capitol Street NW
Suite 846
Washington, DC 20001-1569
202-637-0475
800-424-3688; *Fax:* 202-637-0585
dcroser@aamr.org

Cathy Ficker Terrill, Author, Editor

Offers options for self-advocates and those for people who cannot consent on their own. *$14.95*

36 pages ISBN 0-904898-69-1

2488 Countertransference Issues in Psychiatric Treatment
American Psychiatric Publishing, Inc.
1000 Wilson Boulevard
Suite 1825
Arlington, VA 22209-3901
703-907-7322
800-368-5777; *Fax:* 703-907-1091
appi@psych.org
www.appi.org

Glen O Gabbard, M.D, Editor
Ron McMillen, Chief Executive Officer
John McDuffie, Editorial Director

Overview of countertransference: theory and technique. Copyright 1999. *$37.50*

144 pages Year Founded: 1999 ISBN 0-880489-59-6

2489 Crisis: Prevention and Response in the Community
AAMR
444 N Capitol Street NW
Suite 846
Washington, DC 20001-1569
202-637-0475
800-424-3688; *Fax:* 202-637-0585
dcroser@aamr.org

Ronald Halton Hanson, Author
Norman Anthony Wieseler, Editor

Provides a look at crisis services for people with developmental disabilities and how they impact the surrounding community. *$49.95*

240 pages ISBN 0-940898-74-8

2490 Cross-Cultural Perspectives on Quality of Life
AAMR
444 N Capitol Street NW
Suite 846
Washington, DC 20001-1569
202-637-0475
800-424-3688; *Fax:* 202-637-0585
dcroser@aamr.org

Robert L. Schalock, Author
Kenneth D. Keith, Editor

Provides a global outlook on quality-of-life issues for people with developmental disabilities. *$47.95*

380 pages ISBN 0-940898-70-5

2491 Cruel Compassion: Psychiatric Control of Society's Unwanted
John Wiley & Sons
605 3rd Avenue
New York, NY 10158-180
212-850-6301
info@wiley.com

Thomas Szasz, Author

Demonstrates that the main problem that faces mental health policy makers today is adult dependency. A sobering look at some of our most cherished notions about our humane treatment of society's unwanted, and perhaps more importantly, about ourselves as a compassionate and democratic people. Copyright 1994. *$19.95*

184 pages ISBN 0-471010-12-X

2492 Culture & Psychotherapy: A Guide to Clinical Practice
American Psychiatric Publishing, Inc.
1000 Wilson Boulevard
Suite 1825
Arlington, VA 22209-3901
703-907-7322
800-368-5777; *Fax:* 703-907-1091
appi@psych.org
www.appi.org

Wen-Shing Tseng, M.D, Editor
Jon Streltzer, M.D, Editor
John McDuffie, Editorial Director

Case presentations, analysis, special issues and populations are covered. Copyright 2001. *$51.50*

320 pages Year Founded: 2001 ISBN 0-880489-55-3

2493 Cutting-Edge Medicine: What Psychiatrists Need to Know
American Psychiatric Publishing, Inc.
1000 Wilson Boulevard
Suite 1825
Arlington, VA 22209-3901
703-907-7322
800-368-5777; *Fax:* 703-907-1091
appi@psych.org
www.appi.org

Nada L Stotland, M.D., M.P.H, Editor
Ron McMillen, Chief Executive Officer
John McDuffie, Editorial Director

Offers a comprehensive overview of recent developments in cardiovascular illness, gastrointestinal disorders, transplant medicine, and premenstrual mood disorders. Copyright 2003. *$36.95*

164 pages Year Founded: 2002 ISBN 1-585620-72-6

2494 Cybermedicine
John Wiley & Sons
111 River Street
Hoboken, NJ 07030-5774
201-748-6000; *Fax:* 201-748-6088
www.wiley.com

A passionate plea for the use of computers for initial diagnosis and assessment, treatment decisions, and for self-care, research, prevention, and above all, patient empowerment. *$25.00*

235 pages ISBN 0-787903-43-4

2495 DRG Handbook
Dorland Health
1500 Walnut Street
Suite 1000
Philadelphia, PA 19102-3512
215-875-1212
800-784-2332; *Fax:* 215-735-3966
info@dorlandhealth.com
www.dorlandhealth.com

Diagnosis-related groups are the building blocks of hospital reimbursement under the Medicare Prospective Payment System. Also provides the ability to forecast and manage information at DRG-specific levels using comparison groups of like hospitals, a critical tool for both providers and payers. Copyright 1998. *$399.00*

1 per year ISBN 1-573721-39-5

2496 DSM: IV Diagnostic & Statistical Manual of Mental Disorders
American Psychiatric Publishing, Inc.
1000 Wilson Boulevard
Suite 1825
Arlington, VA 22209-3901
703-907-7322
800-368-5777; *Fax:* 703-907-1091
appi@psych.org
www.appi.org

Robert E Hales MD, Editor-in-Chief
Ron McMillen, Chief Executive Officer
John McDuffie, Editorial Director

Focuses on clinical, research and educational findings. Practical and useful for clinicians and researchers of many orientations. Leatherbound. Hardcover and paperback also available. Copyright 1994. *$75.00*

991 pages Year Founded: 2013 ISBN 0-890420-64-5

2497 DSM: IV Personality Disorders
Rapid Psychler Press
2014 Holland Ave
Suite 374
Port Huron, MI 48060-1994
519-667-2335
888-779-2453; *Fax:* 519-675-0610
rapid@psychler.com
www.psychler.com

David Robinson, Publisher
$9.95

ISBN 1-894328-23-x

2498 Designing Positive Behavior Support Plans
AAMR
444 N Capitol Street NW
Suite 846
Washington, DC 20001-1569
202-637-0475
800-424-3688; *Fax:* 202-637-0585
dcroser@aamr.org

Provides a conceptual framework for understanding, designing, and evaluating positive behavior support plans. *$21.95*

43 pages ISBN 0-940898-55-1

2499 Developing Mind: Toward a Neurobiology of Interpersonal Experience
Guilford Press
72 Spring Street
New York, NY 10012-4068
212-431-9800
800-365-7006; *Fax:* 212-966-6708
info@guilford.com

Daniel J. Siegel, MD, Author

Concise research results as to the origins of our behavior based on cognitive neuroscience.

2500 Disability at the Dawn of the 21st Century and the State of the States
AAMR
444 N Capitol Street NW
Suite 846
Washington, DC 20001-1569
202-637-0475
800-424-3688; *Fax:* 202-637-0585
dcroser@aamr.org

Consumate source book on the analysis of financing services and supports for people with developmental disabilities in the United States. A detailed state-by-state analysis of public financial support for persons with MR/DD, mental illness, and physical disabilities.

512 pages ISBN 0-940898-85-3

2501 Diversity in Psychotherapy: The Politics of Race, Ethnicity, and Gender
Praeger
2727 Palisade Avenue
Suite 4H
Bronx, NY 10463-1020
718-796-0971; *Fax:* 718-796-0971
www.vd6@columbia.edu

Victor De La De La Cancela, Author
Jean Lau Chin, Author
Yvonne M. Jenkins, Author

This challenging and insightful work wrestles with difficult treatment problems confronting both culturally and socially oppressed clients and psychotherapists. Case studies offer highly valuable resource material and insights into challenging perpsectives on behavioral health services. Copyright 1993. *$49.95*

224 pages ISBN 0-275941-80-9

2502 Doing What Comes Naturally: Dispelling Myths and Fallacies About Sexuality and People with Developmental Disabilities
High Tide Press
Ste 2n
2081 Calistoga Dr
New Lenox, IL 60451-4833
815-206-2054
888-487-7377
managing.editor@hightidepress.com

Orieda Horn Anderson, Author
Jennifer Luvert, Author

Uncovers misconceptions about adults whose sexual needs vary greatly, and yet are often treated as children or non-sexual people. Includes heartwarming success stories from adults Mrs. Anderson has supported, as well as suggestions for teaching and a guide to sexual incident reporting. *$19.95*

127 pages ISBN 1-892696-13-4

2503 Dynamic Psychotherapy: An Introductory Approach
American Psychiatric Publishing, Inc.
1000 Wilson Boulevard
Suite 1825
Arlington, VA 22209-3901
703-907-7322
800-368-5777; *Fax:* 703-907-1091
appi@psych.org
www.appi.org

Robert E Hales MD, Editor-in-Chief
Ron McMillen, Chief Executive Officer
John McDuffie, Editorial Director

Principles and techniques. Copyright 1990. *$33.50*

229 pages

2504 Electroconvulsive Therapy: A Guide
Madison Institute of Medicine
7617 Mineral Point Road
Suite 300
Madison, WI 53717-1623
608-827-2470
mim@miminc.org
www.factsforhealth.org

Margarett Baudhuin, Manager

ECT is an extremely effective method of treatment for severe depression that does not respond to medication. This guidebook explains what ECT is and how it is used today to help patients overcome depression and other serious, treatment resistant psychiatric disorders. *$5.95*

19 pages

2505 Emergencies in Mental Health Practice
Guilford Press
72 Spring Street
New York, NY 10012-4068
212-431-9800
800-365-7006; *Fax:* 212-966-6708
info@guilford.com

Phillip M. Kleespies PhD, Editor

Focusing on acute clinical situations in which there is an imminent risk of serious harm or death to self or others, this practical resource helps clinicians evaluate and manage a wide range of mental health emergencies. The volume provides guidelines for interviewing with suicidal patients, potentially violent patients, vulnerable victims of violence, as well as patients facing life-and-death medical decisions, with careful attention to risk management and forensic issues. *$24.95*

450 pages ISBN 1-572305-51-7

2506 Essential Guide to Psychiatric Drugs
St. Martin's Press
175 5th Avenue
New York, NY 10010-7848
212-674-5151; *Fax:* 212-674-3179

Jack M. Gorman, Author

Information not found in other drug references. Lists many common drugs and not so common side effects, including drug interaction and the individual's reaction, including sexual side effects. Expert but nontechnical narrative. Copyright 1998. *$6.99*

448 pages ISBN 0-312954-58-1

2507 Essentials of Clinical Psychiatry: Based on the American Psychiatric Press Textbook of Psychiatry
American Psychiatric Publishing, Inc.
1000 Wilson Boulevard
Suite 1825
Arlington, VA 22209-3901
703-907-7322
800-368-5777; *Fax:* 703-907-1091
appi@psych.org
www.appi.org

Robert E Hales MD, Editor-in-Chief
Ron McMillen, Chief Executive Officer
John McDuffie, Editorial Director

51 distinguished experts have created a compelling reference reflecting a biopsychosocial approach to patient treatment that is at once exciting and accessible. Copyright 1999. *$77.00*

1032 pages ISBN 0-880488-48-4

2508 Ethical Way
John Wiley & Sons
111 River Street
Hoboken, NJ 07030-5774
201-748-6000; *Fax:* 201-748-6088
www.wiley.com

Leads you through a maze of ethical principles and crucial issues confronting mental health professionals. *$38.95*

254 pages ISBN 0-787907-41-X

2509 Evidence-Based Mental Health Practice: A Textbook
WW Norton & Company
500 5th Avenue
New York, NY 10110-54
212-354-5500
800-233-4830; *Fax:* 212-869-0856
npb@wwnorton.com
www.books.wwnorton.com/

Robert E. Drake, Editor
David W. Lynde, Editor
Matthew R. Merrens, Editor

The specific term evidence-based medicine was introduced in 1990 to refer to a systematic approach to helping doctors to apply scientific evidence to decision-making at the point of contact with a specific consumer. As support for evidence-based medicine grows in mental health, the need to clarify its fundamental principles also increases. An essential primer for all practititioners and students who are grappling with the new age of evidence-based practice.

528 pages ISBN 0-393704-43-2

2510 Executive Guide to Case Management Strategies
John Wiley & Sons
111 River Street
Hoboken, NJ 07030-5774
201-748-6000; *Fax:* 201-748-6088
www.wiley.com

A guide to plan, organize, develop, improve and help case management programs reach their full potential in the clinical and financial management of care. *$58.00*

160 pages ISBN 1-556481-28-4

2511 Family Approach to Psychiatric Disorders
American Psychiatric Publishing, Inc.
1000 Wilson Boulevard
Suite 1825
Arlington, VA 22209-3901
703-907-7322
800-368-5777; *Fax:* 703-907-1091
appi@psych.org
www.appi.org

Richard A Perlmutter, M.D., Author
Ron McMillen, Chief Executive Officer
John McDuffie, Editorial Director

Examines how treatment can and should involve the family of the patient. Copyright 1996. *$67.50*

406 pages Year Founded: 1996

2512 Family Stress, Coping, and Social Support
Charles C Thomas Publisher Ltd.
2600 S 1st Street
Springfield, IL 62704-4730
217-789-8980
800-258-8980; *Fax:* 217-789-9130
books@ccthomas.com
www.ccthomas.com

Michael P Thomas, President

Copyright 1982. *$48.95*

294 pages ISSN 0-398-06275-7ISBN 0-398046-92-1

2513 Family Therapy Progress Notes Planner
John Wiley & Sons
10475 Crosspoint Boulevard
Indianapolis, IN 46256-3386
317-572-3000; *Fax:* 317-572-4000
consumers@wiley.com
www.wiley.com

Arthur E. Jongsma, Jr., Author
David J Berghuis, MA, LLP, Author

Extends the line into the growing field of family therapy. Included is critical information about HIPAA guidelines, which greatly impact the privacy status of patient progress notes. Helps mental health practitioners reduce the amount of time spent on paperwork by providing a full menu of pre-written progress notes that can be easily and quickly adapted to fit a particular patient need or treatment situation. *$ 49.95*

352 pages ISBN 0-471484-43-1

2514 Fifty Ways to Avoid Malpractice: A Guidebook for Mental Health Professionals
Professional Resource Press
PO Box 3197
Sarasota, FL 34230-3197

941-343-9601
800-443-3364; *Fax:* 941-343-9201
orders@prpress.com
www.prpress.com

Laurie Girsch, Managing Editor

Offers straightforward guidance on providing legally safe and ethically appropriate services to your clients. Copyright 1988. *$ 18.95*

158 pages ISBN 0-943158-54-0

2515 First Therapy Session
John Wiley & Sons
111 River Street
Hoboken, NJ 07030-5774
201-748-6000; *Fax:* 201-748-6088
www.wiley.com

Presents an effective, straightforward approach for conducting first therapy sessions, showing step-by-step, how to identify client problems and help solve them within families. *$27.95*

ISBN 1-555421-94-6

2516 Five-HTP: The Natural Way to Overcome Depression, Obesity, and Insomnia
Bantam Doubleday Dell Publishing
1745 Broadway
New York, NY 10019-4343
212-782-9000

Jeff Rechtzigel, Publisher

An authorative and comprehensive guide to realizing the health benefits of 5-HTP. Explains how this natural amino acid can safely and effectively regulate low serotonin levels, which have been linked to depression, obesity, insomnia, migraines, and anxiety. 5-HTP is also a powerful antioxidant that can protect the body from free-radical damage, reducing the risk of serious illnesses such as cancer. Copyright 1999. *$11.95*

304 pages ISBN 0-553379-46-1

2517 Flawless Consulting
Jossey-Bass Publishers
111 River Street
Hoboken, NJ 07030-5774
201-748-6000
800-956-7739; *Fax:* 201-748-6088
info@wiley.com
www.as.wiley.com

Peter Block, Author

This book offers advice on what to say and what to do in specific situations to see your recommendations through. *$39.95*

214 pages ISBN 0-893840-52-1

2518 Forgiveness: Theory, Research and Practice
Guilford Press
72 Spring Street
New York, NY 10012-4068
212-431-9800
800-365-7006; *Fax:* 212-966-6708
info@guilford.com

Michael E. McCullough Phd, Editor
Kenneth I. Pargament PhD, Editor
Carl E. Thoresen Phd, Editor

Scholarly, up-to-date examination of forgiveness ranges many disiplines for mental health professionals. Copyright 2000. *$ 35.00*

334 pages ISBN 1-572305-10-X

2519 Foundations of Mental Health Counseling 4th Edition
Charles C Thomas Publisher Ltd.
2600 S 1st Street
Springfield, IL 62704-4730
217-789-8980
800-258-8980; *Fax:* 217-789-9130
books@ccthomas.com
www.ccthomas.com

Artis J. Palmo, Author
William J. Weikel, Author
David P. Borsos, Author

The importance of mental health counseling has grown, including the array of mental health issues that arise in an uncertain and fragile world. This fourth edition expands the information in the previous editions by updating the positive changes in the field of mental health counseling including the recognition of licensed professional counselors by managed care organizations and insurance companies. This book continues to be the most up-to-date resource in the field of mental health counseling and is a must read for anyone working or aspiring to work as a mental health counselor. *$87.95*

508 pages Year Founded: 2011 ISBN 0-398086-35-0

2520 Fundamentals of Psychiatric Treatment Planning
American Psychiatric Publishing, Inc.
1000 Wilson Boulevard
Suite 1825
Arlington, VA 22209-3901
703-907-7322
800-368-5777; *Fax:* 703-907-1091
appi@psych.org
www.appi.org

James A Kennedy, M.D., Author
Ron McMillen, Chief Executive Officer
John McDuffie, Editorial Director

Professional discussion of important basics. Copyright 2002. *$49.00*

350 pages Year Founded: 2003 ISBN 1-585620-61-0

2521 Group Involvement Training
NewHarbinger Publications
5674 Shattuck Avenue
Oakland, CA 94609-1662
510-652-0215
800-748-6273; *Fax:* 510-652-5472
customerservice@newharbinger.com
www.newharbinger.com

Matthew McKay, Owner

This book shows how training chronically ill mental patients in a series of structured group tasks can be used to treat the symptoms of apathy, withdrawl, poor interpersonal skills, helplessness, and the inability to structure leisure time constructively. Copyright 1988. *$24.95*

160 pages ISBN 0-934986-65-7

2522 Guide to Possibility Land: Fifty One Methods for Doing Brief, Respectful Therapy
WW Norton & Company
500 5th Avenue
New York, NY 10110-54
212-354-5500; *Fax:* 212-869-0856
admalmud@wwnorton.com
www.books.wwnorton.com/

Sandy Beadle, Author
Bill O'Hanlon, Author

The creator of Possibility therapy, William O'Hanlon, outlines acknowledging patient's experience and opinions about their lives while seeing that possibilites for change are explored and underlined. Copyright 1999. *$13.00*

94 pages ISBN 0-393702-97-9

2523 Guide to Treatments That Work
Oxford University Press/Oxford Reference
198 Madison Avenue
New York, NY 10016-4308
212-726-6400
800-451-7556

Peter E. Nathan, Author
Jack M. Gorman, Author

A systematic review of various treatments currently in use for virtually all of the recognized mental disorders. Copyright 1997. *$75.00*

784 pages ISBN 0-195102-27-4

2524 Handbook on Quality of Life for Human Service Practitioners
AAMR
444 N Capitol Street NW
Suite 846
Washington, DC 20001-1569
202-637-0475
800-424-3688; *Fax:* 202-637-0585
dcroser@aamr.org

Robert L. Schalock, Author
Miguel Angel Verdugo, Author

Revolutionary generic model for quality of life that integrates core domains and indicators with a cross-cultural systems prespective that can be used in all human services. *$59.95*

430 pages ISBN 0-940898-77-2

2525 Health Insurance Answer Book
Garner Consulting
630 North Rosemead Blvd
Suite 300
Pasadena, CA 91107
626-351-2300; *Fax:* 626-351-2331
info@garnerconsulting.com
www.garnerconsulting.com

Gerti Reagan Garner, President
John C Garner, Chief Executive Officer
Carl Isaacs, Principal
Araceli Sandoval, Associate

This easy-to-use guide will help you manage a cost effective health insurance plan and ensure that your decisions are in compliance with constantly changing health care legislation. Offers instant access to information on everything from HMOs, PPOs, COBRA, HIPPA, OBRA anad flexible benefits to plan rating, funding, cost containment, and administration. *$290.00*

1100 pages ISBN 0-735582-18-7

2526 Helper's Journey: Working with People Facing Grief, Loss, and Life-Threatening Illness
Research Press
PO Box 7866
Champaign, IL 61826-9177
217-352-3273
800-519-2707; *Fax:* 217-352-1221
rp@researchpress.com
www.researchpress.com

Dr Dale G Larson, Author

Written for both professional and volunteer caregivers, this unique manual provides exercises, activities and specific strategies for more successful caregiving, increased personal growth and effective stress management. The author explores the theory and practice of helping. He includes numerous case examples and verbatim disclosures of fellow caregivers that powerfully convey the joys and sorrows of the helper's journey. Cited as a 'Book of the Year' by the American Journal of Nursing. *$21.95*

292 pages ISBN 0-878223-44-4

2527 High Impact Consulting
Jossey-Bass Publishers
111 River Street
Hoboken, NJ 07030-5774
201-748-6000
800-956-7739; *Fax:* 201-748-6088
info@wiley.com
www.as.wiley.com

Robert H Schaffer, Author

Offers a new model for consulting services that shows how to produce short-term successes and use them as a springboard to larger accomplishments and, ultimately, to organization-wide continuous improvement. Also includes specific guidance to assist clients in analyzing their situation, identifying their real needs, and choosing an appropriate consultant. *$26.00*

288 pages Year Founded: 2002 ISBN 0-787903-41-8

2528 Home Maintenance for Residential Service Providers
High Tide Press
Ste 2n
2081 Calistoga Dr
New Lenox, IL 60451-4833
815-206-2054
888-487-7377
managing.editor@hightidepress.com

Nathan Cohen, Author

What happens when a human service organization becomes a large, commercial landlord, not unlike a real estate firm or condominium management company? Property management for homes supporting persons with disabilities requires a unique blend of human services and physical plant expertise. Provides detailed checklists for all house systems, fixtures and furnishings. Includes a discussion of maintaining an attractive residence that blends with the neighborhood. *$10.95*

43 pages ISBN 0-965374-46-7

2529 How to Partner with Managed Care
John Wiley & Sons
605 3rd Avenue
New York, NY 10158-180
212-850-6301
info@wiley.com

Charles H. Browning, Author
Beverly J Browning, Author

A Do It Yourself Kit for Building Working Relationships &
Getting Steady Referrals. Copyright 1996.

358 pages

2530 Improving Clinical Practice
John Wiley & Sons
111 River Street
Hoboken, NJ 07030-5774
201-748-6000; *Fax:* 201-748-6088
www.wiley.com

Enhance your organization's clinical decision making, and
ultimately improve the quality of patient care. *$41.95*

342 pages ISBN 0-787900-93-1

2531 Improving Therapeutic Communication
Jossey-Bass Publishers
111 River Street
Hoboken, NJ 07030-5774
201-748-6000
800-956-7739; *Fax:* 201-748-6088
info@wiley.com
www.as.wiley.com

D. Corydon Hammond, Author
Dean H Hepworth, Author
Veon G Smith, Author

Improve your communication technique with this definitive
guide for counselors, therapists, and caseworkers. Focuses
on the four basic skills that facilitate communication in
therapy: empathy, respect, authenticity, and confrontation.
$62.95

400 pages Year Founded: 2002 ISBN 0-875893-08-2

**2532 In Search of Solutions: A New Direction in
Psychotherapy**
WW Norton & Company
500 5th Avenue
New York, NY 10110-54
212-354-5500
800-233-4830; *Fax:* 212-869-0856
npb@wwnorton.com
www.books.wwnorton.com/

Bill O'Hanlon, Author
Michele Weiner-Davis, Author

O'Hanlon and Weiner-Davis provide guidelines for clinicians in implementing solution-oriented language and explain how to aviod dead ends. New material bring the
reader up to date on advances in this field since the book's
original publication in 1989.

ISBN 0-393704-37-8

2533 Increasing Variety in Adult Life
AAMR
501 3rd Street
NW Suite 200
Washington, DC 20001

202-387-1968
800-424-3688; *Fax:* 202-387-2193
dcroser@aamr.org
www.www.aaidd.org

Step-by-step guidelines for implementing the general-case
instructional process and shows how the process can be
used across a variety of activities. *$12.95*

38 pages ISBN 0-940898-43-2

**2534 Independent Practice for the Mental Health
Professional**
Brunner/Routledge
325 Chestnut Street
Philadelphia, PA 19106-2614
800-821-8312; *Fax:* 215-269-0363

Ralph H Earle PhD, Author
Dorothy J Barnes MC, Author

An excellent resource for beginning therapists considering
private practice or for experienced therapists moving from
agency or institutional settings into private practice. Offers
practical, down-to-earth suggestions for practice settings,
marketing and working with clients. The authors provide
worksheets and examples of successful planning for the
growth of a practice. *$24.95*

192 pages ISBN 0-876308-38-8

**2535 Infanticide: Psychosocial and Legal
Perspectives on Mothers Who Kill**
American Psychiatric Publishing, Inc.
1000 Wilson Boulevard
Suite 1825
Arlington, VA 22209-3901
703-907-7322
800-368-5777; *Fax:* 703-907-1091
appi@psych.org
www.appi.org

Margaret C Spinelli, M.D., Editor
Ron McMillen, Chief Executive Officer
John McDuffie, Editorial Director

Written to help remedy today's dearth of up-to-date, research-based literature, this unique volume brings together
a multidisciplinary group of 17 experts who focus on the
psychiatric perspective of this tragic cause of infant death.
Balanced perspective on a highly emotional issue will find
a wide audience among psychiatric and medical professionals, legal professionals, public health professionals and interested laypersons. Copyright 2002. *$53.50*

296 pages Year Founded: 2003 ISBN 1-585620-97-1

**2536 Innovative Approaches for Difficult to Treat
Populations**
American Psychiatric Publishing, Inc.
1000 Wilson Boulevard
Suite 1825
Arlington, VA 22209-3901
703-907-7322
800-368-5777; *Fax:* 703-907-1091
appi@psych.org
www.appi.org

Scott W Henggeler, Ph.D, Editor
Alberto B Santos, M.D., Editor
John McDuffie, Editorial Director

Alternate methods when the usual approaches are not helpful. Copyright 1997. *$86.95*

552 pages Year Founded: 1997

2537 Insider's Guide to Mental Health Resources Online
Guilford Press
72 Spring Street
New York, NY 10012-4068
212-431-9800
800-365-7006; *Fax:* 212-966-6708
info@guilford.com

John M. Grohol PsyD, Author
John M. Grohol, Author

This guide helps readers take full advantage of Internet and world-wide-web resources in psychology, psychiatric, self-help and patient education. The book explains and evaluates the full range of search tools, newsgroups, databases and describes hundreds of specific disorders, find job listings and network with other professionals, obtain needed articles and books, conduct grant searches and much more. *$ 21.95*

338 pages ISBN 1-572305-49-5

2538 Instant Psychopharmacology
WW Norton & Company
500 5th Avenue
New York, NY 10110-54
212-354-5500
800-233-4830; *Fax:* 212-869-0856
admalmud@wwnorton.com
www.books.wwnorton.com/

Ronald J. Diamond, Author

Revision of the best selling guide to all the new medications. Straightforward book teaches non medical therapists, clients and their families how the five different classes of drugs work, advice on side effects, drug interaction warnings and much more practical information. Copyright 2002. *$18.95*

168 pages ISBN 0-393703-91-6

2539 Integrated Treatment of Psychiatric Disorders
American Psychiatric Publishing, Inc.
1000 Wilson Boulevard
Suite 1825
Arlington, VA 22209-3901
703-907-7322
800-368-5777; *Fax:* 703-907-1091
appi@psych.org
www.appi.org

Jerald Kay, M.D., Editor
Ron McMillen, Chief Executive Officer
John McDuffie, Editorial Director

Psychodynamic therapy and medication. Copyright 2001. *$34.95*

216 pages Year Founded: 2001 ISBN 1-585620-27-0

2540 Integrating Psychotherapy and Pharmacotherapy: Disolving the Mind-Brain Barrier
WW Norton & Company
500 5th Avenue
New York, NY 10110-54
212-354-5500
800-233-4830; *Fax:* 212-869-0856
npb@wwnorton.com
www.books.wwnorton.com/

Drake McFeely, CEO

Will help all mental health clinicians to dissolve their conceptual mind/brain barriers by recognizing the reciprocal influences of psychological and pharmacological interventions. The reader responds to thought-provoking questions and vignettes of problematic cases.

ISBN 0-393704-03-3

2541 Integrative Brief Therapy: Cognitive, Psychodynamic, Humanistic & Neurobehavioral Approaches
Impact Publishers, Inc.
PO Box 6016
Atascadero, CA 93423-6016
805-466-5917
800-246-7228; *Fax:* 805-466-5919
info@impactpublishers.com
www.impactpublishers.com

John Preston, Psy.D., Author

Thorough discussion of the factors that contribute to effectiveness in therapy carefully integrates key elements from diverse theoretical viewpoints. *$27.95*

272 pages Year Founded: 2006 ISBN 1-886230-09-5

2542 International Handbook on Mental Health Policy
Greenwood Publishing Group
88 Post Road W
PO Box 5007
Westport, CT 06881-5007
203-226-3571; *Fax:* 203-222-1502

Donna R. Kemp, Editor

Major reference book for academics and practitioners that provides a systematic survey and analysis of mental health policies in twenty representative countries. Copyright 1993. *$125.00*

512 pages ISBN 0-313275-67-X

2543 Interpersonal Psychotherapy
American Psychiatric Publishing, Inc.
1000 Wilson Boulevard
Suite 1825
Arlington, VA 22209-3901
703-907-7322
800-368-5777; *Fax:* 703-907-1091
appi@psych.org
www.appi.org

John C Markowitz, M.D, Editor
Ron McMillen, Chief Executive Officer
John McDuffie, Editorial Director

An overview of interpersonal psychotherapy for depression, preventative treatment for depression, bulimia nervosa and HIV positive men and women. Copyright 1998. *$37.50*

184 pages Year Founded: 1998 ISBN 0-880488-36-0

2544 Introduction to Time: Limited Group Psychotherapy
American Psychiatric Publishing, Inc.
1000 Wilson Boulevard
Suite 1825
Arlington, VA 22209-3901
703-907-7322
800-368-5777; *Fax:* 703-907-1091

appi@psych.org
www.appi.org

K Roy MacKenzie, M.D., F.R.C, Author
Ron McMillen, Chief Executive Officer
John McDuffie, Editorial Director

Do more with limited time and sessions. Copyright 1997.
$57.95

336 pages Year Founded: 1990

2545 Introduction to the Technique of Psychotherapy: Practice Guidelines for Psychotherapists
Charles C Thomas Publisher Ltd.
2600 S 1st Street
Springfield, IL 62704-4730
217-789-8980
800-258-8980; *Fax:* 217-789-9130
books@ccthomas.com
www.ccthomas.com

Samuel I Greenberg, Author

A basic, simply written book, with a minimum of theory, helpful to the beginning therapist. Discuss how to conduct psychotherapy: by having a format in mind, taking a comprehensive history, and a careful, observing examination of the patient. Copyright 1998. *$34.95*

122 pages Year Founded: 1998 ISSN 0-398-06905-0ISBN 0-398069-04-2

2546 Languages of Psychoanalysis
Analytic Press
7625 Empire Drive
Florence, KS 41042-2919
510-547-7860
800-634-7064; *Fax:* 800-248-4724
orders@taylorandfrancis.com
www.www.routledgementalhealth.com/

John E Gedo, Author
John Kerr PhD, Sr Editor

A guide to understanding the full range of human discourse, especially behavioral conflicts and communicational deficits as they impinge upon the transactions of the analytic dyad. Available in hardcover. Copyright 1996. *$39.95*

224 pages ISBN 0-881631-86-8

2547 Leadership and Organizational Excellence
AAMR
444 N Capitol Street NW
Suite 846
Washington, DC 20001-1569
202-637-0475
800-424-3688; *Fax:* 202-637-0585
dcroser@aamr.org

Examines key managerial and organizational strategies that can be used to help ensure high-quality work environments for both staff and service delivery for people with developmental disabilities. *$ 14.95*

33 pages ISBN 0-940898-78-0

2548 Making Money While Making a Difference: Achieving Outcomes for People with Disabilities
High Tide Press
Ste 2n
2081 Calistoga Dr
New Lenox, IL 60451-4833
815-206-2054
888-487-7377
managing.editor@hightidepress.com

Diane J Bell, Managing Editor

Unique handbook for corporations and nonprofits alike. The authors guide readers through a step-by-step process for implementing strategic alliances between nonprofit organizations and corporate partners. Learn the tenets of cause related marketing and much more. *$14.95*

231 pages ISBN 0-965374-49-1

2549 Managed Mental Health Care in the Public Sector: a Survival Manual
Brunner/Routledge
325 Chestnut Street
Philadelphia, PA 19106-2614
800-821-8312; *Fax:* 215-269-0363

Manual for administrators, planners, clinicians and consumers with concepts and strategies to maneuver in public sector managed mental healthcare system. Copyright 1996. *$35.00*

336 pages ISBN 9-057025-37-X

2550 Managing Client Anger: What to Do When a Client is Angry with You
NewHarbinger Publications
5674 Shattuck Avenue
Oakland, CA 94609-1662
510-652-0215
800-748-6273; *Fax:* 510-652-5472
customerservice@newharbinger.com
www.newharbinger.com

Matthew McKay, Owner

Guide to help therapists understand their reactions and make interventions when clients express anger toward them. Copyright 1998. *$49.95*

261 pages ISBN 1-572241-23-3

2551 Manual of Clinical Psychopharmacology
American Psychiatric Publishing, Inc.
1000 Wilson Boulevard
Suite 1825
Arlington, VA 22209-3901
703-907-7322
800-368-5777; *Fax:* 703-907-1091
appi@psych.org
www.appi.org

Alan F Schatzberg, M.D, Author
Jonathan O Cole, M.D., Author
Charles DeBattista, D.M.H., M., Author

Examines the recent changes and standard treatments in psychopharmacology. Copyright 2002. *$63.00*

744 pages Year Founded: 2010 ISBN 0-880488-65-4

2552 Mastering the Kennedy Axis V: New Psychiatric Assessment of Patient Functioning
American Psychiatric Publishing, Inc.
1000 Wilson Boulevard
Suite 1825
Arlington, VA 22209-3901
703-907-7322
800-368-5777; *Fax:* 703-907-1091
appi@psych.org
www.appi.org

James A Kennedy, M.D., Author
Ron McMillen, Chief Executive Officer
John McDuffie, Editorial Director

Professional evaluation methods. Copyright 2002. *$44.00*

294 pages Year Founded: 2003 ISBN 1-585620-62-9

2553 Meditative Therapy Facilitating Inner-Directed Healing
Impact Publishers
PO Box 6016
Atascadero, CA 93423-6016
805-466-5917
800-246-7228; *Fax:* 805-466-5919
info@impactpublishers.com
www.impactpublishers.com

Michael L Emmons, Ph.D., Author
Janet Emmons, M.S., Author

Offers to the professional therapist a full description of the therapeutic procedures that facilitate inner-directed healing and explains the therapist's role in guiding clients' growth psychologically, physiologically and spiritually. Copyright 1999. *$27.95*

230 pages ISBN 1-886230-11-0

2554 Mental Disability Law: Primer, a Comprehensive Introduction
Commission on the Mentally Disabled
1800 M Street NW
Washington, DC 20036-5802
202-331-2240

An updated and expanded version of the 1984 edition provides a comprehensive overview of mental disability law. Part I of the Primer examines the scope of mental disability law, defines the key terms and offers tips on how to provide effective representation for clients. Part II reviews major federal legislative initiatives including the Americans with Disabilities Act. *$15.00*

ISBN 0-897077-98-9

2555 Mental Health Rehabilitation: Disputing Irrational Beliefs
Charles C Thomas Publisher Ltd.
2600 S 1st Street
Springfield, IL 62704-4730
217-789-8980
800-258-8980; *Fax:* 217-789-9130
books@ccthomas.com
www.ccthomas.com

Michael P Thomas, President

Applicable to a wide variety of disciplines involved with therapeutic counseling of people with mental and/or physical disabilities such as rehabilitation counseling, mental health counseling, pastoral counseling, school counseling, clinical social work, clinical and counseling psychology,

and behavioral science oriented medical specialities and related health and therapeutic professionals. Copyright 1995. *$36.95*

106 pages ISBN 0-398065-31-4

2556 Mental Health Resources Catalog
Paul H Brookes Company
PO Box 10624
Baltimore, MD 21285-624
410-337-9580
800-638-3775; *Fax:* 410-337-8539
custserv@brookespublishing.com
www.brookespublishing.com

This catalog offers practical resources for mental health professionals serving young children and their families, including school psychologists, teachers and early intervention professionals. FREE.

2 per year

2557 Metaphor in Psychotherapy: Clinical Applications of Stories and Allegories
Impact Publishers
PO Box 6016
Atascadero, CA 93423-6016
805-466-5917
800-246-7228; *Fax:* 805-466-5919
info@impactpublishers.com
www.impactpublishers.com

Comprehensive resource aids therapists in helping clients change distorted views of the human experience. Dozens of practical therapeutic activities involving metaphor, drama, fantasy, and meditation. Copyright 1998. *$29.95*

320 pages ISBN 1-886230-10-2

2558 Microcounseling
Charles C Thomas Publisher Ltd.
2600 S 1st Street
Springfield, IL 62704-4730
217-789-8980
800-258-8980; *Fax:* 217-789-9130
books@ccthomas.com
www.ccthomas.com

Thomas Daniels, Author
Allen Ivey, Author

Innovations in Interviewing, Counseling, Psychotherapy, and Psychoeducation. Copyright 1978. *$91.95*

296 pages Year Founded: 2007 ISSN 0-398-06175-0ISBN 0-398037-12-4

2559 Natural Supports: A Foundation for Employment
AAMR
444 N Capitol Street NW
Suite 846
Washington, DC 20001-1569
202-637-0475
800-424-3688; *Fax:* 202-637-0585
dcroser@aamr.org

Step-by-step strategy for developing a network of natural supports aimed at promoting the goals and interests of all individuals in the work setting. *$12.95*

34 pages ISBN 0-940898-65-9

2560 Negotiating Managed Care: Manual for Clinicians
American Psychiatric Publishing, Inc.
1000 Wilson Boulevard
Suite 1825
Arlington, VA 22209-3901
703-907-7322
800-368-5777; *Fax:* 703-907-1091
appi@psych.org
www.appi.org

Michael A Fauman, Ph.D., M.D., Author
Ron McMillen, Chief Executive Officer
John McDuffie, Editorial Director

Help for professionals to successfully present a case during clinical review. Copyright 2002. *$26.95*

128 pages Year Founded: 2002 ISBN 1-585620-42-4

2561 Neurobiology of Violence
American Psychiatric Publishing, Inc.
1000 Wilson Boulevard
Suite 1825
Arlington, VA 22209-3901
703-907-7322
800-368-5777; *Fax:* 703-907-1091
appi@psych.org
www.appi.org

Jan Volavka, M.D., Ph.D., Author
Ron McMillen, Chief Executive Officer
John McDuffie, Editorial Director

Important information on the basic science of violence, including genetics, with topics of great practical value to today's clinician, including major mental disorders and violence; alcohol and substance abuse and violence; and psychopharmacological approaches to managing violent behavior. Copyright 2002. *$69.00*

410 pages Year Founded: 2002 ISBN 1-585620-81-5

2562 Neurodevelopment & Adult Psychopathology
Cambridge University Press
40 W 20th Street
New York, NY 10011-4211
212-924-3900; *Fax:* 212-691-3239
marketing@cup.org
www.cup.org

2563 Neurology for Clinical Social Work: Theory and Practice
WW Norton & Company
500 5th Avenue
New York, NY 10110-54
212-354-5500
800-233-4830; *Fax:* 212-869-0856
npb@wwnorton.com
www.books.wwnorton.com/

Bernard D. Beitman, Author
Barton J. Blinder, Author
Michael E. Thase, Author
Debra L. Safer, Author

Social work educators Jeffrey Applegate and Janet Shapiro demystify the explosion of recent research on neurobiology and present it anew with social workers specifically in mind. Abundant case examples show clinicians how to make use of neurobiological concepts in assessment as well as in designing treatment plans and interventions. Commu-

nity mental health, family service agencies, and child welfare settings are discussed.

ISBN 0-393704-20-3

2564 Neuropsychiatry and Mental Health Services
American Psychiatric Publishing, Inc.
1000 Wilson Boulevard
Arlington, VA 22209-3901
703-907-7322
800-368-5777; *Fax:* 703-907-1091
appi@psych.org
www.appi.org

Fred Ovsiew, M.D., Editor
Ron McMillen, Chief Executive Officer
John McDuffie, Editorial Director

Cognitive therapy practices in conjunction with mental health treatment. Copyright 1999. *$79.95*

420 pages Year Founded: 1999 ISBN 0-880487-30-5

2565 Neuropsychology of Mental Disorders: Practical Guide
Charles C Thomas Publisher Ltd.
2600 S 1st Street
Springfield, IL 62704-4730
217-789-8980
800-258-8980; *Fax:* 217-789-9130
books@ccthomas.com
www.ccthomas.com

Michael P Thomas, President

Discusses the advances in diverse areas such as biology, electrophysiology, genetics, neuroanatomy, pharmacology, psychology, and radiology which are increasingly important for a practical understanding of behavior and its pathology. Copyright 1994. *$70.95*

338 pages ISBN 0-398059-05-5

2566 New Roles for Psychiatrists in Organized Systems of Care
American Psychiatric Publishing, Inc.
1000 Wilson Boulevard
Suite 1825
Arlington, VA 22209-3901
703-907-7322
800-368-5777; *Fax:* 703-907-1091
appi@psych.org
www.appi.org

Jeremy A Lazarus, M.D, Editor
Steven S Sharfstein, M.D, Editor
John McDuffie, Editorial Director

Comprehensive view of opportunities, challenges and roles for psychiatrists who are working for or with new organized systems of care. Discusses the ethical dilemmas for psychiatrists in managed care settings and training and identity of the field as well as historical overviews of health care policy. Copyright 1998. *$50.00*

288 pages Year Founded: 1998 ISBN 0-880487-58-5

2567 Of One Mind: The Logic of Hypnosis, the Practice of Therapy
WW Norton & Company
500 5th Avenue
New York, NY 10110-54
212-354-5500
800-233-4830; *Fax:* 212-869-0856

admalmud@wwnorton.com
www.books.wwnorton.com/

Douglas Flemons, Author

A new approach to an old treatment, the author explains his ideas on connecting with patients in hypno and brief therapies. Copyright 2001. *$30.00*

240 pages ISBN 0-393703-82-7

2568 On Being a Therapist
John Wiley & Sons
111 River Street
Hoboken, NJ 07030-5774
201-748-6000; *Fax:* 201-748-6088
www.wiley.com

This thoroughly revised and updated edition shows you how to use the insights gained from your clients' experiences to solve your own problems, realize positive change in yourself, and become a better therapist. *$22.00*

320 pages ISBN 1-555425-55-0

2569 On the Counselor's Path: A Guide to Teaching Brief Solution Focused Therapy
NewHarbinger Publications
5674 Shattuck Avenue
Oakland, CA 94609-1662
510-652-0215
800-748-6273; *Fax:* 510-652-5472
customerservice@newharbinger.com
www.newharbinger.com

Matthew McKay, Owner

A teacher's guide for conducting training sessions on solution focused techniques. Copyright 1996. *$24.95*

92 pages ISBN 1-572240-48-2

2570 Opportunities for Daily Choice Making
AAMR
444 N Capitol Street NW
Suite 846
Washington, DC 20001-1569
202-637-0475
800-424-3688; *Fax:* 202-637-0585
dcroser@aamr.org

Provides strategies for increasing choice-making opportunities for people with developmental disabilities. It describes basic principles of choice-making, shows how to teach choice-making skills to the passive learner, describes how to build in multiple choice-making opportunities within daily routines, introduces self-scheduling, and addresses common questions. *$12.95*

48 pages ISBN 0-904898-44-6

2571 Participatory Evaluation for Special Education and Rehabilitation
AAMR
444 N Capitol Street NW
Suite 846
Washington, DC 20001-1569
202-637-0475
800-424-3688; *Fax:* 202-637-0585
dcroser@aamr.org

Nine-step method for identifying and weighing the importance of disparate goals and outcomes. *$31.95*

90 pages ISBN 0-940898-73-X

2572 Person-Centered Foundation for Counseling and Psychotherapy
Charles C Thomas Publisher Ltd.
2600 S 1st Street
Springfield, IL 62704-4730
217-789-8980
800-258-8980; *Fax:* 217-789-9130
books@ccthomas.com
www.ccthomas.com

Angelo V Boy, Author
Gerald J Pine, Author

Focusing on counseling and psychotherapy, its goals are to renew interest in the person-centered approach in the US, make a signigicant contribution to extending person-centered theory and practice, and promote fruitful dialogue and futher development of person-centered theory. Presents: the rationale for an eclectic application of person-centered counseling; the rationale and process for reflecting clients' feelings; the importance of the theory as the foundation for the counseling process; the importance of values and their influence on the counseling relationship; the modern person-centered counselor's role; and the essential characteristics of a person-centered counseling relationship. Copyright 1999.

274 pages Year Founded: 1999 ISSN 0-398-06966-2ISBN 0-398069-64-6

2573 PharmaCoKinetics and Therapeutic Monitering of Psychiatric Drugs
Charles C Thomas Publisher Ltd.
2600 S 1st Street
Springfield, IL 62704-4730
217-789-8980
800-258-8980; *Fax:* 217-789-9130
books@ccthomas.com
www.ccthomas.com

Michael P Thomas, President

$52.95

226 pages ISBN 0-398058-41-5

2574 Positive Bahavior Support for People with Developmental Disabilities: A Research Synthesis
AAMR
444 N Capitol Street NW
Suite 846
Washington, DC 20001-1569
202-637-0475
800-424-3688; *Fax:* 202-637-0585
dcroser@aamr.org

Offers a careful analysis documenting that positive behavioral procedures can produce important change in the behavior and lives of people with disabilities. *$31.95*

128 pages ISBN 0-940898-60-8

2575 Positive Behavior Support Training Curriculum
AAMR
501 3rd Street
NW Suite 200
Washington, DC 20001
202-387-1968
800-424-3688; *Fax:* 202-387-2193
dcroser@aamr.org
www.www.aaidd.org

Dennis H. Reid, Author
Marsha B. Parsons, Author

Designed for training supervisors of direct support staff, as well as direct support professionals themselves in the values and practices of positive behavior support.

2576 Practical Guide to Cognitive Therapy
WW Norton & Company
500 5th Avenue
New York, NY 10110-54
212-354-5500; *Fax:* 212-869-0856
admalmud@wwnorton.com
www.books.wwnorton.com/

Dean Schuyler, Author

Based on highly successful workshops by the author, this book provides a framework to apply cognitive therapy model to office practices. Copyright 1991. *$22.95*

200 pages ISBN 0-393701-05-0

2577 Practical Psychiatric Practice Forms and Protocols for Clinical Use
American Psychological Publishing
1400 K Street NW
Washington, DC 20005-2403
202-682-6262
800-368-5777; *Fax:* 202-789-2648
appi@psych.org
www.appi.org

Katie Duffy, Marketing Assistant

Designed to aid psychiatrists in organizing their work. Provides rating scales, model letters, medication tracking forms, clinical pathology requests and sample invoices. Handouts on disorders and medication are provided for patients and their families. Spiralbound. Copyright 1998. *$47.50*

312 pages ISBN 0-880489-43-X

2578 Practice Guidelines for Extended Psychiatric Residential Care: From Chaos to Collaboration
Charles C Thomas Publisher Ltd.
2600 S 1st Street
Springfield, IL 62704-4730
217-789-8980
800-258-8980; *Fax:* 217-789-9130
books@ccthomas.com
www.ccthomas.com

Michael P Thomas, President
Stanley McCracken, Author/Editor
Joseph Mehr, Author/Editor

Presents a set of practice guidelines that represent state-of-the-art treatments for consumers of extended residential care. Written for line-level staff charged with the day-to-day services: psychiatrists, psychologists, social workers, activity therapists, nurses, and psychiatric technicians who work closely with consumers in residential programs and program administrators who have immediate responsibility for supervising treatment teams. Copyright 1995. *$47.95*

176 pages ISSN 0-398-06536-5ISBN 0-398065-35-7

2579 Primer of Brief Psychotherapy
WW Norton & Company
500 5th Avenue
New York, NY 10110-54

212-354-5500; *Fax:* 212-869-0856
admalmud@wwnorton.com
www.books.wwnorton.com/

John F. Cooper, Author

Positive guide to brief therapy is a task oriented aid with emphasis on the first session and details of procedures afterward. Copyright 1995. *$19.55*

348 pages ISBN 0-393701-89-1

2580 Primer of Supportive Psychotherapy
Analytic Press
7625 Empire Drive
Florence, KS 41042-2919
201-358-9477
800-634-7064; *Fax:* 800-248-4724
orders@taylorandfrancis.com
www.www.routledgementalhealth.com/

Henry Pinsker, Author
John Kerr PhD, Sr Editor

Focuses on the rationale for and techniques of supportive psychotherapy as a form of dyadic intervention distinct from expressive psychotherapies. The realities, ironies, conundrums and opportunities of the therapeutic encounter are vividly portrayed in scores of illustrative dialogues drawn from actual treatments. Among the topics covered are how to provide reassurance in the realistic way, how to handle requests for advice, the role of praise and reinforcement, the appropriate use of reframing techniques and of modeling, negotiating patients' concerns about medication and other collateral forms of treatment. *$45.00*

296 pages Year Founded: 1997 ISBN 0-881632-74-0

2581 Psychiatry in the New Millennium
American Psychiatric Publishing, Inc.
1000 Wilson Boulevard
Suite 1825
 22209-3901
703-907-7322
800-368-5777; *Fax:* 703-907-1091
appi@psych.org
www.appi.org

Sidney Weissman, M.D, Editor
Melvin Sabshin, M.D, Editor
Harold Eist, M.D, Editor

Keeping the standards and utilizing advances in diagnosis and treatment. *$66.50*

392 pages Year Founded: 1999 ISBN 0-880489-38-3

2582 Psychoanalysis, Behavior Therapy & the Relational World
American Psychological Association
750 1st St NE
Washington, DC 20002-4242
202-336-5500; *Fax:* 202-336-5518
www.apa.org

Paul L Wachtel, Author

484 pages

2583 Psychoanalytic Therapy as Health Care Effectiveness and Economics in the 21st Century
Analytic Press
7625 Empire Drive
Florence, KS 41042-2919

201-358-9477
800-634-7064; *Fax:* 800-248-4724
orders@taylorandfrancis.com
www.www.routledgementalhealth.com/

Harriette Kaley, PhD, Editor
Morris Eagle, Ph.D, Editor
David L Wolitzky, Ph.D, Editor

Drawing on a wide range of clinical and empirical evidence, authors argue that contemporary psychoanalytic approaches are applicable to seriously distressed persons in a variety of treatment contexts. Failure to include such long term therapies within health care delivery systems, they conclude, will deprive many patients of help they need, and help from which they can benefit in enduring ways that far transcend the limited treatment goals of managed care. Available in hardcover. *$ 49.95*

312 pages Year Founded: 1999 ISBN 0-881632-02-3

2584 Psychodynamic, Affective, and Behavioral Theories to Psychotherapy
Charles C Thomas Publisher Ltd.

2600 South First Street
Springfield, IL 62704
800-258-8980; *Fax:* 217-789-9130
books@ccthomas.com

Marty Sapp, Author

The goal of this book is to examine three major theories and their approach to psychotherapy psychodynamic, affective, and behavioral which are defined as specific skills that a clinician or student can readily understand. Experiential exercises, glossaries, and examination questions are included in each chapter. This unique and comprehensive book will be of interest to mentalhealth workers, educational therapists, counselors, psychologists, psychiatrists, and students. *$59.95*

242 pages Year Founded: 2010 ISBN 0-398078-95-9

2585 Psychological Aspects of Women's Health Care
American Psychiatric Publishing, Inc.

1000 Wilson Boulevard
Suite 1825
Arlington, VA 22209-3901
703-907-7322
800-368-5777; *Fax:* 703-907-1091
appi@psych.org
www.appi.org

Nada L Stotland, M.D., M.P.H, Editor
Donna E Stewart, M.D., D.Psych, Editor
John McDuffie, Editorial Director

The Interface Between Psychiatry and Obstetrics and Gynecology, Second Edition. Discussion from major leaders in the specialties of psychiatry and obstetrics/gynecology covering every major area of contemporary concern. Issues in pregnancy, gynecology, and general issues such as reproductive choices, breast disorders, violence, lesbian health care, and the male perspective are included. *$77.00*

672 pages Year Founded: 2001 ISBN 0-880488-31-X

2586 Psychologists' Desk Reference
Oxford University Press/Oxford Reference Book Society

198 Madison Avenue
New York, NY 10016-4308
212-726-6400
800-451-7556

Gerald P. Koocher, Editor
John C. Norcross, Editor
Beverly A. Greene, Editor

For the practicing psychologist; easily accessible, current information on almost any topic by some of the leading thinkers and innovators in the field. *$65.00*

840 pages Year Founded: 1998 ISBN 0-195111-86-9

2587 Psychoneuroendocrinology: The Scientific Basis of Clinical Practice
American Psychiatric Publishing, Inc.

1000 Wilson Boulevard
Suite 1825
Arlington, VA 22209-3901
703-907-7322
800-368-5777; *Fax:* 703-907-1091
appi@psych.org
www.appi.org

Owen M Wolkowitz, M.D., Editor
Anthony J Rothschild, M.D, Editor
John McDuffie, Editorial Director

Applications of scientific research.

606 pages Year Founded: 2003 ISBN 0-880488-57-3

2588 Psychopharmacology Desktop Reference
Manisses Communications Group

208 Governor Street
Providence, RI 02906-3246
401-831-6020
800-333-7771; *Fax:* 401-861-6370
manissescs@manisses.com
www.manisses.com

Karienne Stovell, Editor

Covers medications for all types of mental disorders. Provides detailed information on all the latest drugs as well as colored photographs of the different kinds of drugs. Helps you spot side effects and avoid drug interactions. Includes revealing case studies and outcomes data. *$159.00*

ISBN 1-864937-69-1

2589 Psychopharmacology Update
Manisses Communications Group

208 Governor Street
Providence, RI 02906-3246
401-831-6020
800-333-7771; *Fax:* 401-861-6370
manissescs@manisses.com
www.manisses.com

Karienne Stovell, Editor

Offers psychopharmacology advice for general practitioners and nonprescribing professionals in the mental health field. Covers child psychopharmacology and street drugs. Contains case reports. Recurring features include news of research and book reviews. *$147.00*

12 per year   ISSN 1068-5308

2590 Psychosocial Aspects of Disability
Charles C Thomas Publisher Ltd.

PO Box 19265
Springfield, IL 62794-9265
217-789-8980
800-258-8980; *Fax:* 217-789-9130
www.ccthomas.com

George Henderson, Author
Willie V Bryan, Author

This expanded and updated new edition continues the theme of the first and second editions of emphasizing that attitudinal barriers create environmental barriers for persons with disabilities. The new edition is improved as a primary introductory text or a supplemental text for student helping professionals with the addition of chapters on employment, understanding ethnic groups, concepts, theories, therapies, and issues for the twenty-first century. Available in paperback for $55.95. *$75.95*

274 pages Year Founded: 2011 ISBN 0-398074-86-0

2591 Psychotherapist's Duty to Warn or Protect
Charles C Thomas Publisher Ltd.
2600 S 1st Street
Springfield, IL 62704-4730
217-789-8980
800-258-8980; *Fax:* 217-789-9130
books@ccthomas.com
www.ccthomas.com

Michael P Thomas, President

$47.95

194 pages Year Founded: 1989 ISBN 0-398055-46-7

2592 Psychotherapist's Guide to Cost Containment: How to Survive and Thrive in an Age of Managed Care
Sage Publications
2455 Teller Road
Thousand Oaks, CA 91320-2234
805-499-0721
800-818-7243; *Fax:* 805-499-0871
info@sagepub.com
www.sagepub.com

Bernard D Beitman, Author

$23.50

176 pages Year Founded: 1998 ISBN 0-803973-81-0

2593 Psychotherapy Indications and Outcomes
American Psychiatric Publishing, Inc.
1000 Wilson Boulevard
Suite 1825
Arlington, VA 22209-3901
703-907-7322
800-368-5777; *Fax:* 703-907-1091
appi@psych.org
www.appi.org

David S Janowsky, M.D., Editor
Ron McMillen, Chief Executive Officer
John McDuffie, Editorial Director

Clinical approaches to different symptoms. *$66.50*

432 pages Year Founded: 1999 ISBN 0-880487-61-5

2594 Psychotropic Drug Information Handbook
Lexicomp Inc.
1100 Terex Road
Hudson, OH 44236-4438
330-650-6506
800-837-5394; *Fax:* 330-650-6506
www.lexi.com

Steven Kerscher, Owner

Concise handbook, designed to fit into your lab coat, is a current and portable psychotropic drug reference with 150

drugs and 35 herbal monographs. Perfect companion to Drug Information Handbook for Psychiatry. *$38.75*

1 per year ISBN 1-591951-15-1

2595 Psychotropic Drugs: Fast Facts
WW Norton & Company
500 5th Avenue
New York, NY 10110-54
212-354-5500
800-233-4830; *Fax:* 212-869-0856
npb@wwnorton.com
www.books.wwnorton.com/

Sidney H. Kennedy, Author
Jerrold S. Maxmen, Author
Roger S. McIntyre, Author

Now in its third edition, Psychotropic Drugs: Fast Facts continues to present valuable information in a clear and accessible format. The book organizaes and presents data clinicians need to choose the right treatment for common psychiatric problems and to anticipate and deal with problems that arise in treatment.

ISBN 0-393703-01-0

2596 Quality of Life: Volume II
AAMR
444 N Capitol Street NW
Suite 846
Washington, DC 20001-1569
202-637-0475
800-424-3688; *Fax:* 202-637-0585
dcroser@aamr.org

Focuses on how the concepts and research on quality of life can be applied to people with developmental disabilities. *$19.95*

267 pages ISBN 0-940898-41-1

2597 Questions of Competence
Cambridge University Press
40 W 20th Street
New York, NY 10011-4211
212-924-3900; *Fax:* 212-691-3239
marketing@cup.org
www.cup.org

2598 Reaching Out in Family Therapy: Home Based, School, and Community Interventions
Guilford Press
72 Spring Street
New York, NY 10012-4068
212-431-9800
800-365-7006; *Fax:* 212-966-6708
info@guilford.com

Brenna Hafer Bry, Author
Nancy Boyd-Franklin, Author

Practical framework for clinicians using multisystems intervention. *$27.00*

244 pages Year Founded: 2000 ISBN 1-572305-19-3

2599 Recognition and Treatment of Psychiatric Disorders: Psychopharmacology Handbook for Primary Care
American Psychiatric Publishing, Inc.
1000 Wilson Boulevard
Suite 1825
Arlington, VA 22209-3901

703-907-7322
800-368-5777; *Fax:* 703-907-1091
appi@psych.org
www.appi.org

Robert E Hales MD, Editor-in-Chief
Ron McMillen, Chief Executive Officer
John McDuffie, Editorial Director

Provides the primary care physician with practical and timely strategies for screening and treating patients who have psychiatric disorders. Includes an overview of the epidemiology, pathophysiology, presentation, diagnostic criteria and screening tests for common psychiatric disorders including anxiety, mood, substance abuse, somatization and eating disorders, as well as insomnia, dementia and schizophrenia. *$35.00*

324 pages

2600 Recognition of Early Psychosis
Cambridge University Press
40 W 20th Street
New York, NY 10011-4211
212-924-3900; *Fax:* 212-691-3239
marketing@cup.org
www.cup.org

2601 Review of Psychiatry
American Psychiatric Publishing, Inc.
1000 Wilson Boulevard
Suite 1825
Arlington, VA 22209-3901
703-907-7322
800-368-5777; *Fax:* 703-907-1091
appi@psych.org
www.appi.org

Robert E Hales MD, Editor-in-Chief
Ron McMillen, Chief Executive Officer
John McDuffie, Editorial Director

Cognitive therapy, repressed memories and obsessive-compulsive disorder across the life cycle. *$59.95*

928 pages Year Founded: 1997 ISBN 0-880484-43-8

2602 Schools for Students with Special Needs
Resources for Children with Special Needs
116 E 16th Street
Fifth Floor
New York City, NY 10003-2112
212-677-4650; *Fax:* 212-254-4070
info@resourcesnyc.org
www.resourcesnyc.org

Rachel Howard, Executive Director

The first complete book listing private day and residential schools for parents, caregivers and professionals seeking schools for students 5 and up with developmental, emotional, physical and learning disabilities in the NYC metro area. More than 400 schools and residential programs that serve children in the elementary through high school grades are listed with contact information, ages and populations served, class sizes and student-teacher ratios, special services and diplomas offered. Includes a 46-page section of Schools for Children with Autism Spectrum Disorders, as well as a guide with a list of websites on autism spectrum disorders. *$25.00*

342 pages

2603 Selecting Effective Treatments: a
Comprehensive, Systematic, Guide for Treating
Mental Disorders
Jossey-Bass Publishers
111 River Street
Hoboken, NJ 07030-5774
201-748-6000
800-956-7739; *Fax:* 201-748-6088
info@wiley.com
www.as.wiley.com

Linda Seligman, Author
Lourie W Reichenberg, Author

$39.95

609 pages Year Founded: 2014 ISBN 0-787943-07-X

2604 Social Work Dictionary
National Association of Social Workers
750 1st Street NE
Suite 700
Washington, DC 20002-4241
202-408-8600
800-227-3590; *Fax:* 202-336-8313
press@naswdc.org
www.naswpress.org

Robert L Barker, Author

More than 8,000 terms are defined in this essential tool for understanding the language of social work and related disciplines. The resulting reference is a must for every human services professional. *$34.95*

620 pages Year Founded: 1999 ISBN 0-871012-98-7

2605 Strategic Marketing: How to Achieve
Independence and Prosperity in Your Mental
Health Practice
Professional Resource Press
PO Box 3197
Sarasota, FL 34230-3197
941-343-9601
800-443-3364; *Fax:* 941-343-9201
orders@prpress.com
www.prpress.com

Laurie Girsch, Managing Editor

Presents ways to reshape your practice to capitalize on new opportunities for success in today's healthcare marketplace. *$21.95*

152 pages Year Founded: 1997 ISBN 1-568870-31-0

2606 Surviving & Prospering in the Managed Mental
Health Care Marketplace
Professional Resource Press
PO Box 3197
Sarasota, FL 34230-3197
941-343-9601
800-443-3364; *Fax:* 941-343-9201
orders@prpress.com
www.prpress.com

Laurie Girsch, Managing Editor

Includes examples of different managed care models, extensive references, and checklists. Offers examples of the typical steps in providing outpatient treatment in a managed care milieu, and other extremely useful resources. *$14.95*

106 pages Year Founded: 1994 ISBN 1-568870-04-3

2607 Suzie Brown Intervention Maze
High Tide Press
Ste 2n
2081 Calistoga Dr
New Lenox, IL 60451-4833
815-206-2054
888-487-7377
managing.editor@hightidepress.com

John Shephard, Author

Suzie Brown, age 25, has severe developmental disabilities. She lives in a staffed house for six adults, where you work as a team. She has major communication difficulties, is prone to self-injurious behavior, and no longer responds to all the usual calming methods. What can you do? This workbook offers a practical blueprint for group decision making. Each option page presents a new scenario and ideas for moving forward. Decision logs keep track of decisions as they are made. The binder format allows for easy photocopying. *$69.99*

72 pages ISBN 1-892696-09-6

2608 Teaching Goal Setting and Decision-Making to Students with Developmental Disabilities
AAMR
444 N Capitol Street NW
Suite 846
Washington, DC 20001-1569
202-637-0475
800-424-3688; *Fax:* 202-637-0585
dcroser@aamr.org

Link four basic steps of goal setting and decision making to twelve instructional principles that engage students in activities. *$12.95*

34 pages ISBN 0-940898-97-7

2609 Teaching Practical Communication Skills
AAMR
444 N Capitol Street NW
Suite 846
Washington, DC 20001-1569
202-637-0475
800-424-3688; *Fax:* 202-637-0585
dcroser@aamr.org

Discusses strategies for teaching students to request their preferences, protest non-preferred activities, and clarify misunderstandings. *$12.95*

30 pages ISBN 0-940898-42-X

2610 Teaching Students with Severe Disabilities in Inclusive Settings
AAMR
501 3rd Street
NW Suite 200
Washington, DC 20001
202-387-1968
800-424-3688; *Fax:* 202-387-2193
dcroser@aamr.org
www.www.aaidd.org

MaryAnn Demchak, Author

Presents student-specific strategies for teaching students with severe disabilities in inclusive settings. Strategies include how to write IEPs in inclusive settings; effective scheduling; planning for adaptations of objectives; materials, responses, and settings; and anticipating the need for support. *$12.95*

50 pages ISBN 0-940898-49-7

2611 Textbook of Family and Couples Therapy: Clinical Applications
American Psychiatric Publishing, Inc.
1000 Wilson Boulevard
Suite 1825
Arlington, VA 22209-3901
703-907-7322
800-368-5777; *Fax:* 703-907-1091
appi@psych.org
www.appi.org

G Pirooz Sholevar, M.D, Editor
Linda D Schwoeri, Ph.D, Editor
John McDuffie, Editorial Director

Blending theoretical training and up-to-date clinical strategies. It's a must for clinicians who are currently treating couples and families, a major resource for training future clinicians in these highly effective therapeutic techniques. *$63.00*

968 pages Year Founded: 2003 ISBN 0-880485-18-3

2612 The Annals of Clinical Psychiatry
American Academy of Clinical Psychiatrists
PO Box 458
Glastonbury, CT 06033-458
860-633-6023; *Fax:* 866-668-9858
aacp@cox.net
www.aacp.com

Sanjay Gupta MD, President
John B Reichman MD, Vice President
James Wilcox DO, PhD, Secretary/Treasurer
Donald W Black MD, President-Elect/Author

The journal of the American Academy of Clinical Psychiatrists. The Annals publishes high-quality articles that focus on the advancement of patient care. Contributions furnish professionals and students with a continuing medical perspective on their discipline, addressing problems and concerns that arise in clinical practice as well as their potential solutions. Covers ongoing research and the theories and techniques used by leading authorities in the field.

2613 The Pathology of Man: A Study of Human Evil
Charles C Thomas Publisher Ltd.
PO Box 19265
Springfield, IL 62794-9265
217-789-8980
800-258-8980; *Fax:* 217-789-9130
www.ccthomas.com

Charles C Thomas, Publisher

Deals with a topic that is both timely and of enduring importance. Expected to be a unique and important contribution that responds to the concerns of students and professionals in a wide range of diciplines. A comprehensive and solid study of the multi-casual nature of phonomenon that, until now, has been treated almost exclusively in terms of religion, myth, symbolism, moral philosophy, and ethics. Available in paperback for $53.95. *$73.95*

376 pages Year Founded: 1927 ISBN 0-398075-57-3

2614 The Role of Companion Animals in Counseling and Psychology, Discovering Their Use in the Therapeutic Process
Charles C Thomas Publisher Ltd.
2600 South First Street
Springfield, IL 62704
800-258-8980; *Fax:* 217-789-9130
books@ccthomas.com

Jane K. Wilkes, Author

The human health benefits derived from relationships with companion animals has attracted an abundance of scientific interest and research. However, there is a need for theoretical conceptualizations in order to understand the healinig benefits of human-animal interactions. The goal of this book is to seek these answers and the how and why companion animals play a role in counseling and psychology. In-depth semi-structured interviews were conducted with three psychologists who use animals in their therapy settings. Replete with informative appendices that will serve as valuable knowledge, this book is a significant resource on the subject of animal-assisted therapy for mental health professionals such as counselors, clinical social workers, and therapists. *$32.95*

168 pages Year Founded: 2009 ISBN 0-398078-63-8

2615 Theory and Technique of Family Therapy
Charles C Thomas Publisher Ltd.
2600 S 1st Street
Springfield, IL 62704-4730
217-789-8980
800-258-8980; *Fax:* 217-789-9130
books@ccthomas.com
www.ccthomas.com

Michael P Thomas, President
Ramon Garrido Corrales, Author

Contents: The Family as an Interactional System; The Family as an Intergenerational System; A Model for the Therapeutic Relationship in Family Theory, The Therapeutic Process and Related Concerns; Therapeutic Intervention Techniques and Adjuncts; Marital Group and Multiple Family Therapy; Counseling at Two Critical Stages of Family Development, Formation and Termination of Marriage. Useful information for students and practitioners of family therapy, social workers, the clergy, psychiatrists, psychologists, counselors, and related professionals. *$55.95*

352 pages Year Founded: 1981 ISBN 0-398038-59-7

2616 Thesaurus of Psychological Index Terms
American Psychological Association Database Department/PsycINFO
750 1st Street NE
Washington, DC 20002-4242
202-336-5500
800-374-2722; *Fax:* 202-336-5518
TDD: 202-336-6123
psycinfo@apa.org
www.apa.org

Norman B Anderson, CEO

Reference to the PsycINFO database vocabulary of over 5,400 descriptors. Provides standardized working to represent each concept for complete, efficient and precise retrieval of psychological information and is updated regularly. 9th edition published 2001. *$60.00*

379 pages ISBN 1-557987-75-0

2617 Three Spheres: Psychiatric Interviewing Primer
Rapid Psychler Press
2014 Holland Ave
Suite 374
Port Huron, MI 48060-1994
519-667-2335
888-779-2453; *Fax:* 519-675-0610
rapid@psychler.com
www.psychler.com

David Robinson, Publisher

$16.95

ISBN 0-968032-49-4

2618 Through the Patient's Eyes
Jossey-Bass Publishers
111 River Street
Hoboken, NJ 07030-5774
201-748-6000
800-956-7739; *Fax:* 201-748-6088
info@wiley.com
www.as.wiley.com

Margaret Gerteis, Editor
Thomas Delbanco, Editor
Susan Edgman-Levitan, Editor
Jennifer Daley, Editor

Learn how providers can improve their ability to meet patient's needs and enhance the quality of care by bringing the patient's perspective to the design and delivery of health services. *$36.95*

360 pages Year Founded: 2002 ISBN 7-555425-44-5

2619 Tools of the Trade: A Therapist's Guide to Art Therapy Assessments
Charles C Thomas Publisher Ltd.
PO Box 19265
Springfield, IL 62794-9265
217-789-8980
800-258-8980; *Fax:* 217-789-9130
www.ccthomas.com

Stephanie L. Brooke, Author

Provides critical reviews of art therapy tests along with some new reviews of assessments and updated research in the field. Comprehensive in the approach to consider reliability and validity evidence provided by test authors. Available in paperback for $35.95. *$53.95*

256 pages Year Founded: 2004 ISBN 0-398075-21-2

2620 Training Behavioral Healthcare Professionals
Jossey-Bass Publishers
350 Sansome Street
5th Floor
San Francisco, CA 94104-1310
800-956-7739

James M. Schuster, Editor
Mark R. Lovell, Editor
Anthony M. Trachta, Editor

Provides text on strategies for training mental health professionals in the skills necessary for providing services in a framework of limited resources. *$46.00*

180 pages Year Founded: 1997 ISBN 0-787907-95-2

2621 Training Families to do a Successful Intervention: A Professional's Guide
Hazelden
15251 Pleasant Valley Road
PO Box 176
Center City, MN 55012-176
651-213-2121
800-328-9000; *Fax:* 651-213-4590
customersupport@hazelden.org
www.hazelden.org

Helps professionals explain basic intervention concepts and give clients step-by-step instructions. *$15.95*

152 pages ISBN 1-562461-16-8

2622 Treatment of Complicated Mourning
Research Press
PO Box 7866
Champaign, IL 61826-9177
217-352-3273
800-519-2707; *Fax:* 217-352-1221
rp@researchpress.com
www.researchpress.com

Dr. Therese Rando, Author

This is the first book to focus specifically on complicated mourning, often referred to as pathological, unresolved or abnormal grief. It provides caregivers with practical therapeutic strategies and specific interventions that are necessary when traditional grief counseling is unsufficient. The author provides critically important information on the prediction, identification, assessment, classification and treatment of complicated mourning. *$39.95*

768 pages ISBN 0-878223-29-0

2623 Treatments of Psychiatric Disorders
American Psychiatric Publishing, Inc.
1000 Wilson Boulevard
Suite 1825
Arlington, VA 22209-3901
703-907-7322
800-368-5777; *Fax:* 703-907-1091
appi@psych.org
www.appi.org

Robert E Hales MD, Editor-in-Chief
Ron McMillen, Chief Executive Officer
John McDuffie, Editorial Director

Examines customary approaches to the major psychiatric disorders. Diagnostic, etiologic and therapeutic issues are clearly addressed by experts on each topic. *$307.00*

2800 pages Year Founded: 1995 ISBN 0-880487-00-3

2624 Using Computers In Educational and Psychological Research
Charles C Thomas Publisher Ltd.
PO Box 19265
Springfield, IL 62794-9265
217-789-8980
800-258-8980; *Fax:* 217-789-9130
www.ccthomas.com

This book has been designed to assist researchers in the social sciences and education fields who are interested in learning how information technologies can help them successfully navigate the research process. Most researchers are familiar with the use of programs like SPSS to analyze data, but many are not aware of other ways informaiton

technologies can support the research process. This book is available in paperback for $44.95. *$69.95*

274 pages Year Founded: 2006 ISBN 0-398076-16-2

2625 Values Clarification for Counselors
harles C Thomas Publisher Ltd.
2600 S 1st Street
Springfield, IL 62704-4730
217-789-8980
800-258-8980; *Fax:* 217-789-9130
books@ccthomas.com
www.ccthomas.com

Michael P Thomas, President

How Counselors, Social Workers, Psychologists, and Other Human Service Workers Can Use Available Techniques. *$24.95*

104 pages Year Founded: 1978 ISBN 0-398038-47-3

2626 What Psychotherapists Should Know About Disability
Guilford Press
72 Spring Street
New York, NY 10012-4068
212-431-9800
800-365-7006; *Fax:* 212-966-6708
info@guilford.com

Rhoda Olkin Phd, Author

Available in alternate formats for people with disabilities, this guide confronts biases and relates the human dimesions of disability. Stereotypes and discomfort can get in the way of even a well intentioned therapist, this helps achieve a clearer professional relationship with clients of special need. *$35.00*

368 pages Year Founded: 1999 ISBN 1-572302-27-5

2627 Where to Start and What to Ask: An Assessment Handbook
WW Norton & Company
500 5th Avenue
New York, NY 10110-54
212-354-5500
800-233-4830; *Fax:* 212-869-0856
npb@wwnorton.com
www.books.wwnorton.com/

Susan Lukas, Author

As a life raft for beginners and their supervisors, provides all the necessary tools for garnering information from clients. Offers a framework for thinking about that information and formulating a thorough assessment, helps neophytes organize their approach to the initial phase of treatment. Copyright 1993.

ISBN 0-393701-52-2

2628 Women's Mental Health Services: Public Health Perspecitive
Sage Publications
2455 Teller Road
Thousand Oaks, CA 91320-2234
805-499-0721
800-818-7243; *Fax:* 805-499-0871
info@sagepub.com
www.sagepub.com

Bruce Lubotsky Levin, Author
Andrea K Blanch, Author
Ann Jennings, Author

Paperback, hardcover also available. *$29.95*

448 pages Year Founded: 1998 ISBN 0-761905-09-X

2629 Working with the Core Relationship Problem in Psychotherapy
Jossey-Bass Publishers
111 River Street
Hoboken, NJ 07030-5774
201-748-6000
800-956-7739; *Fax:* 201-748-6088
info@wiley.com
www.as.wiley.com

Althea J Horner, Author

Learn to reveal, understand, and use the core relationship problem, which is formed from earliest childhood and creates an image of the self in relation to others so it can aid in understanding the underlying conflict that repeatedly plays out in a client's behavior. *$39.95*

185 pages Year Founded: 1998 ISBN 0-787943-01-0

2630 Writing Behavioral Contracts: A Case Simulation Practice Manual
Research Press
PO Box 7866
Champaign, IL 61826-9177
217-352-3273
800-519-2707; *Fax:* 217-352-1221
rp@researchpress.com
www.researchpress.com

Dr William J DeRiski, Author
Dennis Wiziecki, Marketing

The most difficult aspect of using contingency contracting is designing a contract acceptable to and appropriate for all involved parties. This unusually versatile book improves contract-writing skills through practice with typical cases. Valuable for social workers, mental health professionals and educators. *$11.95*

94 pages ISBN 0-878221-23-9

2631 Writing Psychological Reports: A Guide for Clinicians
Professional Resource Press
PO Box 3197
Sarasota, FL 34230-3197
941-343-9601
800-443-3364; *Fax:* 941-343-9201
orders@prpress.com
www.prpress.com

Greg J Wolber, Author
William F Carne, Author

Presents widely accepted structured format for writing psychological reports. Numerous useful suggestions for experienced clinicians, and qualifies as essential reading for all clinical psychology students. *$21.95*

158 pages Year Founded: 2002 ISBN 1-568870-76-0

ADHD

2632 ADHD in Adolesents: Diagnosis and Treatment
Guilford Press
72 Spring Street
New York, NY 10012-4068
212-431-9800
800-365-7006; *Fax:* 212-966-6708
info@guilford.com
www.www.guilford.com

Bob Matloff, President
Seymour Weingarten, Editor-in-Chief

Practical reference with a down to earth approach to diagnosing and treatment of ADHD in adolesents. A structured intervention program with guidelines to using educational, psycholgical and medical components to help patients. Many reproducible handouts, checklists and rating scales. *$24.95*

461 pages Year Founded: 1973 ISBN 1-572305-45-2

2633 ADHD in Adulthood: Guide to Current Theory, Diagnosis and Treatment
Johns Hopkins University Press
2715 North Charles Street
Baltimore, MD 21218-4363
410-516-6900
800-537-5487; *Fax:* 410-516-6998
webmaster@jhupress.jhu.edu
www.www.press.jhu.edu

William Brody, President

Discusses how ADHD manifests itself in adult life and answers popular questions posed by physicians and by adults with ADHD. Provides health professionals with a practical approach for treatment and diagnosis in adult ADHD patients. *$49.95*

392 pages Year Founded: 1878 ISBN 0-801861-41-1

2634 All About ADHD: Complete Practical Guide for Classroom Teachers
ADD WareHouse
300 NW 70th Avenue
Suite 102
Plantation, FL 33317-2360
954-792-8100
800-233-9273; *Fax:* 954-792-8545
websales@addwarehouse.com
www.addwarehouse.com

Harvey C Parker, Owner

Brings together both the art and science of effective teaching for students with ADHD using the Parallel Teaching Model as the base for blending behavior management and teaching, particularly in regular classroom settings. Real-life examples are used throughout the book and are intended to help you design strategies for you own classrooms to help your students be the best they can be. *$17.00*

175 pages Year Founded: 1990

2635 Attention Deficit Disorder ADHD and ADD Syndromes
Pro-Ed Publications
8700 Shoal Creek Boulevard
Austin, TX 78757-6897

512-451-3246
800-897-3202; *Fax:* 512-451-8542
info@proedinc.com
www.www.proedinc.com

Donald D Hammill, Owner

This book enters its third edition with even more complete explanations of how ADHD and ADD interfere with: classroom learning, behavior at home, job performance, and social skills development. *$ 19.00*

216 pages Year Founded: 1998 ISBN 0-890797-42-0

2636 Attention Deficit Disorder and Learning Disabilities: Realities, Myths and Controversial Treatments
ADD WareHouse
300 NW 70th Avenue
Suite 102
Plantation, FL 33317-2360
954-792-8100
800-233-9273; *Fax:* 954-792-8545
websales@addwarehouse.com
www.addwarehouse.com

Harvey C Parker, Owner

Designed to help parents and professionals recognize symptoms of learning disabilities and attentional disorders. Covers in detail conventional treatments that have been scientifically validated plus more controversial methods of treatment such as orthomolecular therapies, amino acid supplementation, dietary interventions, EEG biofeedback, cognitive therapy and visual training. *$13.00*

240 pages Year Founded: 1990

2637 Attention Deficit/Hyperactivity Disorder
American Psychiatric Publishing, Inc.
1000 Wilson Boulevard
Suite 1825
Arlington, VA 22209-3901
703-907-7322
800-368-5777; *Fax:* 703-907-1091
appi@psych.org
www.appi.org

Robert E Hales, M.D., M.B.A., Editor-in-Chief
Ron McMillen, Chief Executive Officer
John McDuffie, Editorial Director
RebeccaD. Rinehart, Publisher

Clinical Guide to Diagnosis and Treatment for Health and Mental Health Professionals making the proper diagnosis, and treatment strategies. *$29.95*

298 pages Year Founded: 1999 ISBN 0-880489-40-5

2638 Attention-Deficit Hyperactivity Disorder: A Handbook for Diagnosis and Treatment
Guilford Press
72 Spring Street
New York, NY 10012-4068
212-431-9800
800-365-7006; *Fax:* 212-966-6708
info@guilford.com
www.www.guilford.com

Bob Matloff, President
Seymour Weingarten, Editor-in-Chief

This second edition incorporates the latest finding on the nature, diagnosis, assessment and treatment of ADHD. Includes select chapters by seasoned colleagues covering

their respective areas of expertise and providing clear guidelines for practice in clinical, school and community settings. *$56.95*

602 pages Year Founded: 1973 ISBN 1-572302-75-5

2639 Attention-Deficit/Hyperactivity Disorder in the Classroom
Pro-Ed Publications
8700 Shoal Creek Boulevard
Austin, TX 78757-6897
512-451-3246
800-897-3202; *Fax:* 512-451-8542
info@proedinc.com
www.www.proedinc.com

Donald D Hammill, Owner

Provides educators with a complete guide on how to deal effectively with students with attention deficits in their classroom. Emphasizes practical applications for teachers to use that will facilitate the success of students, both academically and socially, in a school setting. *$29.00*

291 pages Year Founded: 1998 ISBN 0-890796-65-3

2640 Family Therapy for ADHD: Treating Children, Adolesents and Adults
Guilford Press
72 Spring Street
New York, NY 10012-4068
212-431-9800
800-365-7006; *Fax:* 212-966-6708
info@guilford.com
www.www.guilford.com

Bob Matloff, President
Seymour Weingarten, Editor-in-Chief

ADHD affects the entire family. This book helps the clinician evaluate its impact on marital dynamics, parent/sibling/child relationships and the complex treatment of ADHD in a larger context. Includes session by session plans and clinical material. *$32.95*

270 pages Year Founded: 1973 ISBN 1-572304-38-3

2641 How to Operate an ADHD Clinic or Subspecialty Practice
ADD WareHouse
300 NW 70th Avenue
Suite 102
Plantation, FL 33317-2360
954-792-8100
800-233-9273; *Fax:* 954-792-8545
websales@addwarehouse.com
www.addwarehouse.com

Harvey C Parker, Owner

This book goes beyond academic discussions of ADHD and gets down to how to establish and manage an ADHD practice. In addition to practice guidelines and suggestions, this guide presents a compendium of clinic forms and letters, interview formats, sample reports, tricks of the trade and resource listings, all of which will help you develop or refine your clinic/counseling operation. *$65.00*

325 pages Year Founded: 1990

2642 Medications for Attention Disorders and Related Medical Problems: A Comprehensive Handbook
ADD WareHouse
300 NW 70th Avenue
Suite 102
Plantation, FL 33317-2360
954-792-8100
800-233-9273; *Fax:* 954-792-8545
websales@addwarehouse.com
www.addwarehouse.com

Harvey C Parker, Owner

ADHD and ADD are medical conditions and often medical intervention is regarded by most experts as an essential component of the multimodal program for the treatment of these disorders. This text presents a comprehensive look at medications and their use in attention disorders. *$37.00*

420 pages Year Founded: 1990

2643 Parenting a Child With Attention Deficit/Hyperactivity Disorder
Pro-Ed Publications
8700 Shoal Creek Boulevard
Austin, TX 78757-6897
512-451-3246
800-897-3202; *Fax:* 512-451-8542
info@proedinc.com
www.www.proedinc.com

Donald D Hammill, Owner

Offers proven parenting approaches for helping children between the ages of 5-11 years improve their behavior. *$29.00*

150 pages Year Founded: 1999 ISBN 0-890797-91-9

2644 Pretenders: Gifted People Who Have Difficulty Learning
High Tide Press
2081 Calistoga Dr
Suite 2N
New Lenox, IL 60451-4833
815-717-3780
888-487-7377; *Fax:* 815-717-3783
www.www.hightidepress.com

Monica Regan, Managing Editor

Profiles of 8 adults with dyslexia and/or ADD with whom the author has worked. Informative, fascinating, at times heartbreaking, but ultimately inspiring. *$24.50*

177 pages ISBN 1-892696-06-1

Adjustment Disorders

2645 Ambiguous Loss: Learning to Live with Unresolved Grief
Harvard University Press
79 Garden Street
Cambridge, MA 02138-1400
617-495-1000; *Fax:* 617-495-5898
CONTACT_HUP@harvard.edu

William Sisler, President

$22.00

192 pages Year Founded: 1999 ISBN 0-674017-38-2

2646 Attachment and Interaction
Jessica Kingsley
711 3rd Avenue
8th Floor
New York, NY 10017
212-216-7800; *Fax:* 212-564-7854
www.taylorandfrancis.com

Available in paperback. *$29.95*

238 pages Year Founded: 1998 ISBN 1-853025-86-0

2647 Body Image: Understanding Body Dissatisfaction in Men, Women and Children
Routledge
2727 Palisade Avenue
Suite 4H
Bronx, NY 10463-1020
718-796-0971; *Fax:* 718-796-0971

Sarah Grogan, Author

$75.00

264 pages Year Founded: 1998 ISBN 0-415147-84-0

2648 Cognitive Therapy in Practice
WW Norton & Company
500 5th Avenue
New York, NY 10110-54
212-354-5500
800-233-4830; *Fax:* 212-869-0856
npd@wwnorton.com
www.books.wwnorton.com/

Jacqueline B Persons, Author

Basic text for graduate studies in psychotherapy, psycholgy nursing social work and counseling. *$29.00*

224 pages Year Founded: 1989 ISBN 0-393700-77-1

Anxiety Disorders

2649 Anxiety Disorders: A Scientific Approach for Selecting the Most Effective Treatment
Professional Resource Press
PO Box 3197
Sarasota, FL 34230-3197
941-343-9601
800-443-3364; *Fax:* 941-343-9201
orders@prpress.com
www.prpress.com

Laurie Girsch, Managing Editor

Presents descriptive and empirical information on the differential diagnosis of DSM-IV and DSM-III-R categories of anxiety disorders. Explicit decision rules are provided for developing treatment plans based on both scientific research and clinical judgement. *$14.95*

114 pages Year Founded: 1994 ISBN 1-568870-00-0

2650 Applied Relaxation Training in the Treatment of PTSD and Other Anxiety Disorders
NewHarbinger Publications
5674 Shattuck Avenue
Oakland, CA 94609-1662
510-652-0215
800-748-6273; *Fax:* 510-652-5472
customerservice@newharbinger.com
www.newharbinger.com

Matthew McKay, Owner

Comes with a one hundred five minute video tape and a 52 page paperback manual. *$100.00*

Year Founded: 1998 ISBN 1-889287-08-3

2651 Assimilation, Rational Thinking, and Suppression in the Treatment of PTSD and Other Anxiety Disorders
New Harbinger Publications
5674 Shattuck Avenue
Oakland, CA 94609-1662
510-652-0215
800-748-6273; *Fax:* 510-652-5472
customerservice@newharbinger.com
www.newharbinger.com

Matthew McKay, Owner

Comes with two videotapes and a ninety four page paperback manual. *$150.00*

Year Founded: 1998 ISBN 1-889287-06-7

2652 Client's Manual for the Cognitive Behavioral Treatment of Anxiety Disorders
New Harbinger Publications
5674 Shattuck Avenue
Oakland, CA 94609-1662
510-652-0215
800-748-6273; *Fax:* 510-652-5472
customerservice@newharbinger.com
www.newharbinger.com

Matthew McKay, Owner

$10.00

106 pages Year Founded: 1994 ISBN 1-889287-99-7

2653 Cognitive Therapy
American Psychiatric Publishing, Inc.
1000 Wilson Boulevard
Suite 1825
Arlington, VA 22209-3901
703-907-7322
800-368-5777; *Fax:* 703-907-1091
appi@psych.org
www.appi.org

Jesse H Wright, M.D., Ph.D, Editor
Michael E Thase, M.D., Editor
John McDuffie, Editorial Director

Cognitive therapy for anxiety, substance abuse, personality, eating and mental disorders. *$37.50*

174 pages Year Founded: 1997 ISBN 0-880484-45-4

2654 Cognitive Therapy in Practice
WW Norton & Company
500 5th Avenue
New York, NY 10110-54
212-354-5500
800-233-4830; *Fax:* 212-869-0856
npd@wwnorton.com
www.books.wwnorton.com

Drake McFeely, CEO

Basic text for graduate studies in psychotherapy, psychology nursing social work and counseling. *$29.00*

224 pages Year Founded: 1923 ISBN 0-393700-77-1

2655 Gender Differences in Mood and Anxiety Disorders: From Bench to Bedside
American Psychiatric Publishing, Inc.
1000 Wilson Boulevard
Suite 1825
Arlington, VA 22209-3901
703-907-7322
800-368-5777; *Fax:* 703-907-1091
appi@psych.org
www.appi.org

Robert E Hales, M.D., M.B.A., Editor-in-Chief
Ron McMillen, Chief Executive Officer
John McDuffie, Editorial Director
RebeccaD. Rinehart, Publisher

Gender differences in neuroimaging. Discusses women, stress and depression, sex differences in hypothalamic-pituitary-adrenal axis regulation, modulation of anxiety by reproductive hormones. Questions if hormone replacement and oral contraceptive therapy induce or treat mood symptoms. *$37.50*

224 pages Year Founded: 1999 ISBN 0-880489-58-8

2656 Generalized Anxiety Disorder: Diagnosis, Treatment and Its Relationship to Other Anxiety Disorders
American Psychiatric Publishing, Inc.
1000 Wilson Boulevard
Suite 1825
Arlington, VA 22209-3901
703-907-7322
800-368-5777; *Fax:* 703-907-1091
appi@psych.org
www.appi.org

Robert E Hales, M.D., M.B.A., Editor-in-Chief
Ron McMillen, Chief Executive Officer
John McDuffie, Editorial Director
RebeccaD. Rinehart, Publisher

Historical introduction, diagnosis, classification and differential diagnosis. Relationship with depression, panic and OCD. Treatments. *$74.95*

96 pages Year Founded: 1998 ISBN 1-853176-59-1

2657 Integrative Treatment of Anxiety Disorders
American Psychiatric Publishing, Inc.
1000 Wilson Boulevard
Suite 1825
Arlington, VA 22209-3901
703-907-7322
800-368-5777; *Fax:* 703-907-1091
appi@psych.org
www.appi.org

Robert E Hales, M.D., M.B.A., Editor-in-Chief
Ron McMillen, Chief Executive Officer
John McDuffie, Editorial Director
RebeccaD. Rinehart, Publisher

Up-to-date look at combined pharmacotherapy and cognitive behavioral therapy in the treatment of anxiety disorders. *$41.50*

320 pages Year Founded: 1995 ISBN 0-880487-15-1

2658 Long-Term Treatments of Anxiety Disorders
American Psychiatric Publishing, Inc.
1000 Wilson Boulevard
Suite 1825
Arlington, VA 22209-3901

703-907-7322
800-368-5777; *Fax:* 703-907-1091
appi@psych.org
www.appi.org

Robert E Hales, M.D., M.B.A., Editor-in-Chief
Ron McMillen, Chief Executive Officer
John McDuffie, Editorial Director
RebeccaD. Rinehart, Publisher

Treatment of anxiety disorders encapsulating important advances made over the past two decades. *$56.00*

464 pages Year Founded: 1996 ISBN 0-880486-56-2

2659 Overcoming Agoraphobia and Panic Disorder
New Harbinger Publications
5674 Shattuck Avenue
Oakland, CA 94609-1662
510-652-0215
800-748-6273; *Fax:* 510-652-5472
customerservice@newharbinger.com
www.newharbinger.com

Matthew McKay, Owner
Patrick Fanning, Co-Founder

A twelve to sixteen session treatment. *$11.95*

88 pages Year Founded: 1973 ISBN 1-572241-46-2

2660 Overcoming Specific Phobia
New Harbinger Publications
5674 Shattuck Avenue
Oakland, CA 94609-1662
510-652-0215
800-748-6273; *Fax:* 510-652-5472
customerservice@newharbinger.com
www.newharbinger.com

Matthew McKay, Owner
Patrick Fanning, Co-Founder

$9.95

72 pages Year Founded: 1973 ISBN 1-572241-15-2

2661 Panic Disorder: Clinical Diagnosis,
Management and Mechanisms
American Psychiatric Publishing, Inc.
1000 Wilson Boulevard
Suite 1825
Arlington, VA 22209-3901
703-907-7322
800-368-5777; *Fax:* 703-907-1091
appi@psych.org
www.appi.org

Robert E Hales, M.D., M.B.A., Editor-in-Chief
Ron McMillen, Chief Executive Officer
John McDuffie, Editorial Director
RebeccaD. Rinehart, Publisher

Novel and important new discoveries for biological research together with up to date information for the diagnosis and treatment for the practicing clinician. *$75.00*

264 pages Year Founded: 1998 ISBN 1-853175-18-8

2662 Panic Disorder: Theory, Research and Therapy
John Wiley & Sons
111 River Street
Hoboken, NJ 07030-5774
201-748-6000; *Fax:* 201-748-6088
info@wiley.com
www.www.wiley.com

Stephen M. Smith, President and Chief Executive Of
Ellis E. Cousens, Executive Vice President, Chief
John Kritzmacher, Executive Vice President, Chief
MJ O'Leary, Senior Vice President, Human Res

364 pages Year Founded: 1807

2663 Phobias: Handbook of Theory, Reseach and
Treatment
John Wiley & Sons
111 River Street
Hoboken, NJ 07030-5774
201-748-6000; *Fax:* 201-748-6088
info@wiley.com
www.www.wiley.com

Stephen M. Smith, President and Chief Executive Of
Ellis E. Cousens, Executive Vice President, Chief
John Kritzmacher, Executive Vice President, Chief
MJ O'Leary, Senior Vice President, Human Res

Provides an up-to-date summary of current knowledge of phobias. Psychological treatments available for specific phobias have been refined considerably in recent years. This extensive handbook acknowledges these treatments and includes the description and nature of prevalent phobias, details of symptoms, prevalence rates, individual case histories, and a brief review of of our knowledge of the etiology of phobias.

364 pages Year Founded: 1807

2664 Practice Guideline for the Treatment of
Patients with Panic Disorder
American Psychiatric Publishing, Inc.
1000 Wilson Boulevard
Suite 1825
Arlington, VA 22209-3901
703-907-7322
800-368-5777; *Fax:* 703-907-1091
appi@psych.org
www.appi.org

Robert E Hales, M.D., M.B.A., Editor-in-Chief
Ron McMillen, Chief Executive Officer
John McDuffie, Editorial Director
RebeccaD. Rinehart, Publisher

Summarizes data, evaluation of the patient for coexisting mental disorders and issues specific to the treatment of panic disorders in children and adolescents. *$22.50*

160 pages Year Founded: 1998 ISBN 0-890423-11-3

2665 Shy Children, Phobic Adults: Nature and
Treatment of Social Phobia
American Psychiatric Publishing, Inc.
1000 Wilson Boulevard
Suite 1825
Arlington, VA 22209-3901
703-907-7322
800-368-5777; *Fax:* 703-907-1091
appi@psych.org
www.appi.org

Robert E Hales, M.D., M.B.A., Editor-in-Chief
Ron McMillen, Chief Executive Officer
John McDuffie, Editorial Director
RebeccaD. Rinehart, Publisher

Describes the similiarities and differences in the syndrome across all ages. Draws from the clinical, social and developmental literatures, as well as from extensive clinical experience. Illustrates the impact of developmental stage on phenomenology, diagnoses and assessment and treatment of social phobia. *$39.95*

321 pages Year Founded: 1998 ISBN 1-557984-61-1

2666 Social Phobia: Clinical and Research Perspectives
American Psychiatric Publishing, Inc.
1000 Wilson Boulevard
Suite 1825
Arlington, VA 22209-3901
703-907-7322
800-368-5777; *Fax:* 703-907-1091
appi@psych.org
www.appi.org

Robert E Hales, M.D., M.B.A., Editor-in-Chief
Ron McMillen, Chief Executive Officer
John McDuffie, Editorial Director
RebeccaD. Rinehart, Publisher

Comprehensive and practice guide for mental health professionals who encounter individuals with social phobia. *$48.00*

384 pages Year Founded: 1995 ISBN 0-880486-53-8

2667 Standing in the Spaces: Essays on Clinical Process, Trauma, and Dissociation
Analytic Press
7625 Empire Drive
Florence, KY 41042-2919
800-634-7064; *Fax:* 215-269-0363
orders@taylorandfrancis.com
www.www.routledgementalhealth.com

Paul E Stepansky PhD, Managing Director
John Kerr PhD, Sr Editor

Bromberg's essays are delightfully unpredictable, as they strive to keep the reader continually abreast of how words can and cannot capture the subtle shifts in relatedness that characterize the clinical process. Radiating clinical wisdom infused with compassion and wit, Standing in the Spaces, is a classic destined to be read and reread by anlysts and therapists for decades to come. *$55.00*

376 pages Year Founded: 1998 ISBN 0-881632-46-5

2668 Treating Anxiety Disorders
Jossey-Bass Publishers
111 River Street
Hoboken, NJ 07030-5774
201-748-6000; *Fax:* 201-748-6088
www.www.wiley.com

Stephen M. Smith, President and Chief Executive Of
Ellis E. Cousens, Executive Vice President, Chief
John Kritzmacher, Executive Vice President, Chief
MJ O'Leary, Senior Vice President, Human Res

$30.95

288 pages Year Founded: 1999 ISBN 0-787903-16-7

2669 Treating Anxiety Disorders with a Cognitive Cognitive-behavioral Exposure Based Approach and the Eye-movement Technique: A Viewer's Guide for Video Tape
New Harbinger Publications
5674 Shattuck Avenue
Oakland, CA 94609-1662
510-652-0215
800-748-6273; *Fax:* 510-652-5472

customerservice@newharbinger.com
www.newharbinger.com

Matthew McKay, Owner
Patrick Fanning, Co-Founder

Fifty eight-minute videotape and a fifty one page paperback manual. *$100.00*

Year Founded: 1973 ISBN 1-889287-02-4

2670 Treating Panic Disorder and Agoraphobia: A Step by Step Clinical Guide
New Harbinger Publications
5674 Shattuck Avenue
Oakland, CA 94609-1662
510-652-0215
800-748-6273; *Fax:* 510-652-5472
customerservice@newharbinger.com
www.newharbinger.com

Matthew McKay, Owner
Patrick Fanning, Co-Founder

Treatment program covering breath control training, changing automatic thoughts and underlying beliefs. *$49.95*

296 pages Year Founded: 1973 ISBN 1-572240-84-9

Autism Spectrum Disorders

2671 Asperger Syndrome Diagnostic Scale (ASDS)
Pro-Ed
8700 Shoal Creek Boulevard
Austin, TX 78757-6897
512-451-3246
800-897-3202; *Fax:* 512-451-8542
feedback@proedinc.com
www.www.proedinc.com

Donald D Hammill, Owner
Stacey Bock
Richard Simpson

The ASDS is a quick, easy-to-use rating scale that helps determine whether a child has Asperger Syndrome. Anyone who knows the child or youth well can complete the scale. Parents, teachers, siblings, paraeducators, speech-language pathologists, psychologists, psyciatrists and other professionals can answer the 50 yes/no items in 10 to 15 minutes. *$100.00*

2672 Asperger Syndrome: a Practical Guide for Teachers
ADD WareHouse
300 NW 70th Avenue
Suite 102
Plantation, FL 33317-2360
954-792-8100
800-233-9273; *Fax:* 954-792-8545
websales@addwarehouse.com
www.addwarehouse.com

Harvey C Parker, Owner

A clear and concise guide to effective classroom practice for teachers and support assistants working with children with Asperger Syndrome in school. The authors explain characteristics of children with Asperger Syndrome, discuss methods of assessment and offer practical strategies for effective classroom interventions. *$24.95*

90 pages Year Founded: 1990

2673 Children and Youth with Asperger Syndrome
Program Development Associates
32 Court St
21st Floor
Brooklyn, NY 11201
315-452-0643
800-876-1710; *Fax:* 718-488-8642
info@disabilitytraining.com
www.disabilitytraining.com

Classroom teachers now get special information to accommodate students with Asperger Syndrome, who display symptoms similar to, but milder than, autism. Strategies include research-based instructional, behavioral and environmental modifications. *$35.95*

200 pages Year Founded: 1997

Bipolar and Related Disorders

2674 Bipolar Disorder Survival Guide: What You and Your Family Need to Know
The Guilford Press
72 Spring Street
New York, NY 10012-4019
212-431-9800
800-365-7006; *Fax:* 212-966-6708
info@guilford.com
www.www.guilford.com

David J. Miklowitz, PhD, Author

Gives ideas to the person diagnosed with the disorder how to come to terms with the diagnosis. Also shows who you should confide in and how to recognize mood swings. *$19.95*

342 pages Year Founded: 1973 ISBN 1-572305-25-8

2675 Bipolar Disorders: A Guide to Helping Children & Adolescents
ADD WareHouse
300 NW 70th Avenue
Suite 102
Plantation, FL 33317-2360
954-792-8100
800-233-9273; *Fax:* 954-792-8545
sales@addwarehouse.com
www.addwarehouse.com

Mitzi Waltz, Author

A million children and adolescents in the US may have childhood-onset bipolar disorder-including a significant number with ADHD. This new book helps parents and professionals recognize, treat and cope with bipolar disorders. It covers diagnosis, family life, medications, talk therapies, school issues, and other interventions. *$24.95*

442 pages Year Founded: 2000 ISBN 1-565926-56-0

2676 Bipolar Disorders: Clinical Course and Outcome
American Psychiatric Publishing, Inc.
1000 Wilson Boulevard
Suite 1825
Arlington, VA 22209-3901
703-907-7322
800-368-5777; *Fax:* 703-907-1091
appi@psych.org
www.appi.org

Joseph F. Goldberg, Editor
Martin Harrow, Editor

An important and much-needed resource, this book related empirical data on outcome with practical information on the prognosis, course, and potential complications of bipolar disorders in the modern era. Pulling together current knowledge from leading investigators in the field, it provides a concise, up-to-date summary of affective relapse, comorbid psychopathology, functional disability, and psychosocial outcome in contemporary bipolar disorders. *$49.95*

344 pages Year Founded: 1999 ISBN 0-880487-68-2

2677 Bipolar Puzzle Solution
Taylor and Francis
7625 Empire Drive
Florence, KY 41042-2919
800-634-7064; *Fax:* 800-248-4724
TDD: 703-516-7227
www.nami.org

Bryan L. Court, Author
Gerald E. Nelson, Author

An informative book on bipolar illness in a 187 question-and-answer format. *$18.50*

160 pages Year Founded: 1996

2678 Concise Guide to Mood Disorders
American Psychiatric Publishing, Inc.
1000 Wilson Boulevard
Suite 1825
Arlington, VA 22209-3901
703-907-7322
800-368-5777; *Fax:* 703-907-1091
appi@psych.org
www.appi.org

Robert E Hales, M.D., M.B.A., Editor-in-Chief
Ron McMillen, Chief Executive Officer
John McDuffie, Editorial Director
RebeccaD. Rinehart, Publisher

Designed for daily use in the clinical setting, the Concise Guide to Mood Disorders is a fingertip library of the latest information, easy to understand and quick to access. This practical reference summarizes everything a clinician needs to know to diagnose and treat unipolar and bipolar mood disorders. *$29.95*

320 pages Year Founded: 2002 ISBN 1-585620-56-4

2679 Guildeline for Treatment of Patients with Bipolar Disorder
American Psychiatric Publishing, Inc.
1000 Wilson Boulevard
Suite 1825
Arlington, VA 22209-3901
703-907-7322
800-368-5777; *Fax:* 703-907-1091
appi@psych.org
www.appi.org

Provides guidance to psychiatrists who treat patients with bipolar I disorder. Summarizes the pharmacologic, somatic, and psychotherapeutic treatments used for patients. *$22.50*

96 pages ISBN 0-890423-02-4

2680 Manic-Depressive Illness: Bipolar Disorders and Recurrent Depression, 2nd Edition
Oxford University Press
198 Madison Avenue
New York, NY 10016

212-726-6000
custserv.us@oup.com
www.www.oup.com/us/

Frederick K Goodwin, Author

The authors review the biological and genetic literature that has dominated the field in recent years and incorporate cutting-edge research conducted since publication of the first edition. They also update their surveys of psychological and epidemiological evidence, as well as that pertaining to diagnostice issues, course, and outcome, and they offer practical guidelines for differential diagnosis and clinical management.

Depressive Disorders

2681 Active Treatment of Depression
WW Norton & Company
500 5th Avenue
New York, NY 10110-54
212-354-5500; *Fax:* 212-869-0856
admalmud@wwnorton.com
www.books.wwnorton.com

Drake McFeely, CEO

A candid discussion on depression and effective, hopeful therapy strategies. *$35.00*

272 pages   Year Founded: 1923   ISSN 70322-3

2682 Antidepressant Fact Book: What Your Doctor Won't Tell You About Prozac, Zoloft, Paxil, Celexa and Luvox
Perseus Books Group
2465 Central Avenue
Boulder, CO 80301
303-444-3541
800-386-5656; *Fax:* 720-406-7336
westview.orders@perseusbooks.com
www.perseusbooksgroup.com

David Steinberger, President & CEO

What antidepressants will and won't treat, documented side and withdrawl effects, plus what parents need to know about teenagers and antidepressants. The author has been a medical expert in many court cases invloving the use and misuse of psychoactive drugs. *$13.00*

240 pages   Year Founded: 2001   ISBN 0-738204-51-X

2683 Cognitive Therapy of Depression
Guilford Press
72 Spring Street
New York, NY 10012-4068
212-431-9800
800-365-7006; *Fax:* 212-966-6708
info@guilford.com
www.www.guilford.com

Bob Matloff, President
Seymour Weingarten, Editor-in-Chief

Shows how psychotherapists can effectively treat depressive disorders. Case examples illustrate a wide range of strategies and techniques. Chapter topics include the role of emotions in cognitive therapy, application of behavioral techniques and cognitive therapy and antidepressant medications. Hardcover. Paperback also available. *$ 46.95*

425 pages   Year Founded: 1973   ISBN 0-898620-00-7

2684 Concise Guide to Women's Mental Health
American Psychiatric Publishing, Inc.
1000 Wilson Boulevard
Suite 1825
Arlington, VA 22209-3901
703-907-7322
800-368-5777; *Fax:* 703-907-1091
appi@psych.org
www.appi.org

Robert E Hales, M.D., M.B.A., Editor-in-Chief
Ron McMillen, Chief Executive Officer
John McDuffie, Editorial Director
RebeccaD. Rinehart, Publisher

Examines the biological, psychological, and sociocultural factors that influence a woman's mental health and often contribute to psychiatric disorders. Supplies clinicians with important information on gender related differences on differential diagnosis, case formulation and treatment planning. Topics include premenstrual dysphoric disorder, hormonal contraception and effects on mood, psychiatric disorders in pregnancy, postpartum psychiatric disorders and perimenopause and menopause. *$21.95*

187 pages   Year Founded: 1997   ISBN 0-880483-43-1

2685 Depression in Context: Strategies for Guided Action
WW Norton & Company
500 5th Avenue
New York, NY 10110-54
212-354-5500; *Fax:* 212-869-0856
admalmud@wwnorton.com
www.books.wwnorton.com

Drake McFeely, CEO

Description of Behavioral Activation, a new treatment for Depression. *$32.00*

224 pages   Year Founded: 1923   ISSN 70350-9

2686 Evaluation and Treatment of Postpartum Emotional Disorders
Professional Resource Press
PO Box 3197
Sarasota, FL 34230-3197
941-343-9601
800-443-3364; *Fax:* 941-343-9201
cs.prpress@gmail.com
www.prpress.com

Laurie Girsch, Managing Editor

Teaches how to recognize and treat postpartum emotional disorders. Procedures for clinical assessment, psychotherapeutic interventions, and medical - psychiatric treatments are described. *$ 13.95*

110 pages   Year Founded: 1980   ISBN 1-568870-24-8

2687 Handbook of Depression
Guilford Press
72 Spring Street
New York, NY 10012-4068
212-431-9800
800-365-7006; *Fax:* 212-966-6708
info@guilford.com
www.www.guilford.com

Bob Matloff, President
Seymour Weingarten, Editor-in-Chief

Brings together well-known authorities who address the need for a comprehensive review of the most current information available on depression. Surveys current theories and treatment models, covering both what the MD and non-MD needs to know. *$65.00*

628 pages Year Founded: 1973 ISBN 0-898628-41-5

2688 Postpartum Mood Disorders
American Psychiatric Publishing, Inc.
1000 Wilson Boulevard
Suite 1825
Arlington, VA 22209-3901
703-907-7322
800-368-5777; *Fax:* 703-907-1091
appi@psych.org
www.appi.org

Robert E Hales, M.D., M.B.A., Editor-in-Chief
Ron McMillen, Chief Executive Officer
John McDuffie, Editorial Director
RebeccaD. Rinehart, Publisher

$38.50

280 pages Year Founded: 1999 ISBN 0-880489-29-4

2689 Scientific Foundations of Cognitive Theory and Therapy of Depression
John Wiley & Sons
111 River Street
Hoboken, NJ 07030-5774
201-748-6000; *Fax:* 201-748-6088
info@wiley.com
www.www.wiley.com

Stephen M. Smith, President and Chief Executive Of
Ellis E. Cousens, Executive Vice President, Chief
John Kritzmacher, Executive Vice President, Chief
MJ O'Leary, Senior Vice President, Human Res

A synthesis of decades of research and practice, this semminal book presents and critically evaluates this scientific and emprical status of co author Aaron Beck's revised cognitive theory and therapy of depression. The authors explore the evolution of cognitive theory and therapy of depression and discuss the future directions for the treatment of depression.

364 pages Year Founded: 1807

2690 Symptoms of Depression
John Wiley & Sons
111 River Street
Hoboken, NJ 07030-5774
201-748-6000; *Fax:* 201-748-6088
info@wiley.com
www.www.wiley.com

Stephen M. Smith, President and Chief Executive Of
Ellis E. Cousens, Executive Vice President, Chief
John Kritzmacher, Executive Vice President, Chief
MJ O'Leary, Senior Vice President, Human Res

364 pages Year Founded: 1807

2691 Treating Depressed Children: A Therapeutic Manual of Proven Cognitive Behavioral Techniques
New Harbinger Publications
5674 Shattuck Avenue
Oakland, CA 94609-1662
510-652-0215
800-748-6273; *Fax:* 510-652-5472

customerservice@newharbinger.com
www.newharbinger.com

Matthew McKay, Owner
Patrick Fanning, Co-Founder

A full twelve session treatment program incorporates cartoons and role playing games to help children recognize emotions, change negative thoughts, gain confidence and learn crucial interpersonal skills. *$49.95*

160 pages Year Founded: 1973 ISBN 1-572240-61-X

2692 Treating Depression
Jossey-Bass Publishers
111 River Street
Hoboken, NJ 07030-5774
201-748-6000; *Fax:* 201-748-6088
info@wiley.com
www.www.wiley.com

Stephen M. Smith, President and Chief Executive Of
Ellis E. Cousens, Executive Vice President, Chief
John Kritzmacher, Executive Vice President, Chief
MJ O'Leary, Senior Vice President, Human Res

$27.95

364 pages Year Founded: 1807 ISBN 0-787915-85-8

2693 Treatment of Recurrent Depression
American Psychiatric Publishing, Inc.
1000 Wilson Boulevard
Suite 1825
Arlington, VA 22209-3901
703-907-7322
800-368-5777; *Fax:* 703-907-1091
appi@psych.org
www.appi.org

Robert E Hales, M.D., M.B.A., Editor-in-Chief
Ron McMillen, Chief Executive Officer
John McDuffie, Editorial Director
RebeccaD. Rinehart, Publisher

Five topics covered are, Lifetime Impact of Gender on Recurrent Major Depressive Disorder in Women, Treatment Stategies, Prevention of Recurrences in Bipolar Patients, Potential Applications and Updated Recommondations. *$29.95*

208 pages Year Founded: 2001 ISBN 1-585620-25-4

Disruptive, Impulse-Control and Conduct Disorders

2694 Abusive Personality: Violence and Control in Intimate Relationships
Guilford Press
72 Spring Street
New York, NY 10012-4068
212-431-9800
800-365-7006; *Fax:* 212-966-6708
info@guilford.com
www.www.guilford.com

Bob Matloff, President
Seymour Weingarten, Editor-in-Chief

A study of domestic violence, especially male perpetrators. *$26.95*

214 pages Year Founded: 1973 ISBN 1-572303-70-0

2695 Behavioral Risk Management
Jossey-Bass Publishers
111 River Street
Hoboken, NJ 07030-5774
201-748-6000; *Fax:* 201-748-6088
info@wiley.com
www.www.wiley.com

Stephen M. Smith, President and Chief Executive Of
Ellis E. Cousens, Executive Vice President, Chief
John Kritzmacher, Executive Vice President, Chief
MJ O'Leary, Senior Vice President, Human Res

Learn to identify potential mental health and behavioral problems on the job and apply effective intervention strategies for behavioral risk. *$41.95*

364 pages Year Founded: 1807 ISBN 0-787902-20-9

2696 Beyond Behavior Modification:
Cognitive-Behavioral Approach to Behavior
Management in the School
Pro-Ed Publications
8700 Shoal Creek Boulevard
Austin, TX 78757-6897
512-451-3246
800-897-3202; *Fax:* 512-451-8542
info@proedinc.com
www.www.proedinc.com

Donald D Hammill, Owner

Focuses on traditional behavior modification, and presents a social learning theory approach. *$39.00*

643 pages Year Founded: 1995 ISBN 0-890796-63-7

2697 Coping With Self-Mutilation: a Helping Book
for Teens Who Hurt Themselves
Rosen Publishing Group
29 E 21st Street
New York, NY 10010-6209
212-777-3017
800-237-9932; *Fax:* 888-436-4643
info@rosenpub.com
www.rosenpublishing.com

Roger Rosen, President

Examines the reasons for this phenomenon, and ways one might seek help. *$17.95*

Year Founded: 1950 ISBN 0-823925-59-5

2698 Dealing with Anger Problems:
Rational-Emotive Therapeutic Interventions
Professional Resource Press
PO Box 3197
Sarasota, FL 34230-3197
941-343-9601
800-443-3364; *Fax:* 941-343-9201
cs.prpress@gmail.com
www.prpress.com

Laurie Girsch, Managing Editor

Demonstrates ways to apply rational-emotive therapy techniques to help your clients control their anger. Offers step-by-step anger control treatment program that includes a variety of cognitive, emotive, and behavioral homework assignments, and procedures for modifying behaviors and facilitating change. *$11.95*

68 pages Year Founded: 1980 ISBN 0-943158-59-1

2699 Domestic Violence 2000: Integrated Skills
Program for Men
WW Norton & Company
500 5th Avenue
New York, NY 10110-54
212-354-5500; *Fax:* 212-869-0856
admalmud@wwnorton.com
www.books.wwnorton.com

Drake McFeely, CEO

Various theories are examined to deal with this difficult social problem. For group classes. *$23.20*

224 pages Year Founded: 1923 ISSN 70314-2

2700 Inclusion Strategies for Students with Learning
and Behavior Problems
Pro-Ed Publications
8700 Shoal Creek Boulevard
Austin, TX 78757-6897
512-451-3246
800-897-3202; *Fax:* 512-451-8542
info@proedinc.com
www.www.proedinc.com

Donald D Hammill, Owner

Provides the components necessary to implement successful inclusion by presenting the experience of those directly impacted by inclusion: an individual with a disability; parents of a student with a disbility; teachers who implement inclusion; and researchers of best practices. Integrates theory and practice in an easy, how-to manner. *$36.00*

416 pages Year Founded: 1997 ISBN 0-890796-98-X

2701 Outrageous Behavior Mood: Handbook of
Strategic Interventions for Managing
Impossible Students
Pro-Ed Publications
8700 Shoal Creek Boulevard
Austin, TX 78757-6897
512-451-3246
800-897-3202; *Fax:* 512-451-8542
info@proedinc.com
www.www.proedinc.com

Donald D Hammill, Owner

This handbook is for educators who have had success in managing difficult students. Introduces such methods as planned confusion, disruptive word pictures, unconscious suggestion, double-bind predictions, off the wall interpretations, and even some straight faced paradoxical assignments. *$26.00*

154 pages Year Founded: 1999 ISBN 0-890798-17-6

2702 Sex Murder and Sex Aggression:
Phenomenology Psychopathology,
Psychodynamics and Prognosis
Charles C Thomas Publisher Ltd.
2600 S 1st Street
Springfield, IL 62704-4730
217-789-8980
800-258-8980; *Fax:* 217-789-9130
books@ccthomas.com
www.ccthomas.com

Michael P Thomas, President
Charles C Thomas, Publisher

By Eugene Revitch, Robert Wood Johnson School of Medicine, Piscataway, New Jersey, and Louis B Schlesinger,

New Jersey Medical School, Newark. With a foreword by Robert R Hazelwood. Contents: The Place of Gynocide and Sexual Aggression in the Classification of Crime; Catathymic Gynocide; Compulsive Gynocide; Psychodynamics, Psychopathology and Differential Diagnosis; Prognostic Considerations. *$43.95*

152 pages Year Founded: 1927 ISSN 0-398-06346-XISBN 0-398055-56-4

2703 Teaching Behavioral Self Control to Students
Pro-Ed Publications
8700 Shoal Creek Boulevard
Austin, TX 78757-6897
512-451-3246
800-897-3202; *Fax:* 512-451-8542
info@proedinc.com
www.www.proedinc.com

Donald D Hammill, Owner

Demonstrates how teachers, counselors and parents can help children of all ages and ability levels to modify their own behavior. Clear step-by-step methods describe how common childhood problems can be solved by helping children become more responsible and independent. *$ 21.00*

122 pages Year Founded: 1995 ISBN 0-890796-17-3

Dissociative Disorders

2704 Dissociative Identity Disorder: Diagnosis, Clinical Features, and Treatment of Multiple Personality
John Wiley & Sons
111 River Street
Hoboken, NJ 07030-5774
201-748-6000; *Fax:* 201-748-6088
info@wiley.com
www.www.wiley.com

Stephen M. Smith, President and Chief Executive Of
Ellis E. Cousens, Executive Vice President, Chief
John Kritzmacher, Executive Vice President, Chief
MJ O'Leary, Senior Vice President, Human Res

Comprehensive and interesting, this account of the history of MPD dispells many myths and presents new insight into the treatment of MPD. Perfect for sexual abuse clinics, child abuse agencies, correctional facilities and clinicians of all fields. *$64.50*

364 pages Year Founded: 1807 ISBN 0-471132-65-9

2705 Rebuilding Shattered Lives: Responsible Treatment of Complex Post-Traumatic and Dissociative Disorders
John Wiley & Sons
111 River Street
Hoboken, NJ 07030-5774
201-748-6000; *Fax:* 201-748-6088
info@wiley.com
www.www.wiley.com

Stephen M. Smith, President and Chief Executive Of
Ellis E. Cousens, Executive Vice President, Chief
John Kritzmacher, Executive Vice President, Chief
MJ O'Leary, Senior Vice President, Human Res

The most up-to-date, integrative and emperically sound account of trauma theory and practice availible. Based on more than a decade of clinical research and treatment experience at the Harvard Medical School, this comprehensive and nontechnical text offers a stage oriented approach to

understanding and treating complex and difficult traumatized patients, integrating modern trauma theory with traditional theraputic interventions. *$47.50*

364 pages Year Founded: 1807 ISBN 0-471247-32-4

Feeding and Eating Disorders

2706 Biting The Hand That Starves You: Inspiring Resistance to Anorexia/Bulimia
WW Norton & Company
500 5th Avenue
New York, NY 10110-54
212-354-5500
800-233-4830; *Fax:* 212-869-0856
npb@wwnorton.com
www.books.wwnorton.com

Drake McFeely, CEO

Details a unique way of thinking and speaking about anorexia/bulimia (a/b), by having conversations with insiders in which the problem is viewed as an external influence rather than a part of the person. Coercion is sidestepped in favor of practices that are collaborative, accountable, and spirit-nurturing.

Year Founded: 1923 ISBN 0-393703-37-1

2707 Drug Therpay and Eating Disorders
Mason Crest Publishers
370 Reed Road
Suite 302
Broomall, PA 19008-4017
610-543-6200
866-627-2665; *Fax:* 610-543-3878
dtaylor@masoncrest.com
www.masoncrest.com

Provides a clear, concise account of the history, symptoms, and current treatment of anorexia nervosa and bulimia nervosa. It is estimated the eating disorders affect five million Americans each year, and many more millions among other nations.

ISBN 1-590845-65-X

2708 Handbook of Treatment for Eating Disorders
Guilford Press
72 Spring Street
New York, NY 10012-4068
212-431-9800
800-365-7006; *Fax:* 212-966-6708
info@guilford.com
www.www.guilford.com

Bob Matloff, President
Seymour Weingarten, Editor-in-Chief

Includes coverage of binge eating and examines pharmacological as well as therapeutic approaches to eating disorders. Presents cognitive behavioral, psychoeducational, interpersonal, family, feminist, group and psychodynamic approaches, as well as the basics of pharmacological management. Features strategies for handling sexual abuse, substance abuse, concurrent medical conditions, personality disorder, prepubertal eating disorders and patients who refuse therapy. *$56.95*

540 pages Year Founded: 1973 ISBN 1-572301-86-4

2709 Interpersonal Psychotherapy
American Psychiatric Publishing, Inc.
1000 Wilson Boulevard
Suite 1825
Arlington, VA 22209-3901
703-907-7322
800-368-5777; *Fax:* 703-907-1091
appi@psych.org
www.appi.org

Robert E Hales, M.D., M.B.A., Editor-in-Chief
Ron McMillen, Chief Executive Officer
John McDuffie, Editorial Director
RebeccaD. Rinehart, Publisher

An overview of interpersonal psychotherapy for depression, preventative treatment for depression, bulimia nervosa and HIV positive men and women. *$26.00*

156 pages Year Founded: 1998 ISBN 0-880488-36-0

2710 Sexual Abuse and Eating Disorders
200 E Joppa Road
PO Box 436
Brooklandville, MD 21022-0436
410-825-8888
888-825-8249; *Fax:* 410-560-0134
sidran@sidran.org
www.sidran.org

Esther Giller, President and Director
Sheila Sidran Giller, Secretary/Treasurer
J. G. Goellner, Director Emeritus
Tracy Howard, Book Sales/Office Manager

This is the first book to explore the complex relationship between sexual abuse and eating disorders. Sexual abuse is both an extreme boundary violation and a disruption of attachment and bonding; victims of such abuse are likely to exhibit symptoms of self injury, including eating disorders. This volume is a discussion of the many ways that sexual abuse and eating disorders are related, also has accounts by a survivor of both. Investigates the prevalence of sexual abuse among individuals with eating disorders. Also examines how a history of sexual violence can serve as a predictor of subsequent problems with food. Looks at related social factors, reviews trauma based theories, more controversial territory and discusses delayed memory versus false memory. *$34.95*

345 pages Year Founded: 1986

Gender Dysphoria

2711 Gender Loving Care
WW Norton & Company
500 5th Avenue
New York, NY 10110-54
212-354-5500; *Fax:* 212-869-0856
admalmud@wwnorton.com
www.books.wwnorton.com

Drake McFeely, CEO

Understanding and treating gender identity disorder, especially transexuals, who may feel stuck in the wrong-sexed body. *$ 25.00*

196 pages Year Founded: 1923 ISBN 0-393703-40-5

2712 Homosexuality and American Psychiatry: The Politics of Diagnosis
Princeton University Press
41 William Street
Princeton, NJ 08540
609-258-4900
800-777-4726; *Fax:* 609-258-6305
www.www.press.princeton.edu

Fred Appel, Executive Editor
Al Bertrand, Assistant Director
Eric Crahan, Senior Editor
Seth Ditchik, Executive Editor

$18.00

249 pages Year Founded: 1905 ISBN 0-691028-37-0

2713 Principles and Practice of Sex Therapy
Guilford Press
72 Spring Street
New York, NY 10012-4068
212-431-9800
800-365-7006; *Fax:* 212-966-6708
info@guilford.com
www.www.guilford.com

Bob Matloff, President
Seymour Weingarten, Editor-in-Chief

Many new developments in theory, diagnosis and treatment of sexual disorders have occured in the past decade. The authors set clear guidlines for assessment and treatment with fresh clinical material. A text for professionals and students in a wide range of mental health fields; sexual disorders, male and female, paraphilias, gender identity disorders, vasoactive drugs and more are covered. *$50.00*

518 pages Year Founded: 1973 ISBN 1-572305-74-6

2714 Psychoanalytic Therapy & the Gay Man
Analytic Press
7625 Empire Drive
Florence, KY 41042-2919
800-634-7064; *Fax:* 215-269-0363
orders@taylorandfrancis.com
www.www.routledgementalhealth.com

Paul E Stepansky PhD, Managing Director
John Kerr PhD, Sr Editor

Explores of the subjectivities of gay men in psychoanalytic psychotherapy. It is a vitally human testament to the richly varied inner experiences of gay men. Offers that sexual identity, which encompass a spectrum of possibilities for any gay man, must be addressed in an atmosphere of honest encounter that allows not only for exploration of conflict and dissasociation but also for restitutive conformation of the patient's right to be himself. Available in hardcover. *$55.00*

384 pages Year Founded: 1998 ISBN 0-881632-08-2

Neurocognitive Disorders

2715 Cognitive Therapy in Practice
WW Norton & Company
500 5th Avenue
New York, NY 10110-54
212-354-5500
800-233-4830; *Fax:* 212-869-0856
npd@wwnorton.com
www.books.wwnorton.com

Drake McFeely, CEO

Basic text for graduate studies in psychotherapy, psycholgy nursing social work and counseling. *$29.00*

224 pages Year Founded: 1923 ISBN 0-393700-77-1

2716 Geriatric Mental Health Care: A Treatment Guide for Health Professionals
Guilford Press
72 Spring Street
New York, NY 10012-4068
212-431-9800
800-365-7006; *Fax:* 212-966-6708
info@guilford.com
www.www.guilford.com

Bob Matloff, President
Seymour Weingarten, Editor-in-Chief

Designed for mental health practitioners and primary care providers without advanced training in geriatric psychiatry. Covers depression, anxiety, the dementias, psychosis, mania, sleep disturbances, personality and pain disorders, adapting principles, sexuality, elder issues, alcohol and substance abuse, suicide risk, consultation, legal and ethic issues, exercise and much more. *$39.00*

347 pages Year Founded: 1973 ISBN 1-572305-92-4

2717 Guidelines for the Treatment of Patients with Alzheimer's Disease and Other Dementias of Late Life
American Psychiatric Publishing, Inc.
1000 Wilson Boulevard
Suite 1825
Arlington, VA 22209-3901
703-907-7322
800-368-5777; *Fax:* 703-907-1091
appi@psych.org
www.appi.org

Robert E Hales, M.D., M.B.A., Editor-in-Chief
Ron McMillen, Chief Executive Officer
John McDuffie, Editorial Director
RebeccaD. Rinehart, Publisher

Diagnosis and treatment strategies. *$22.50*

40 pages Year Founded: 1995 ISBN 0-890423-04-0

2718 Loss of Self: Family Resource for the Care of Alzheimer's Disease and Related Disorders
WW Norton & Company
500 5th Avenue
New York, NY 10110-54
212-354-2907; *Fax:* 212-869-0856
admalmud@wwnorton.com
www.books.wwnorton.com

Drake McFeely, CEO

How to help a relative and also meet a family's own needs during the long and tragic period of care involved with Alzheimer's Disease. Challenges are more than medical and can be emotional, involve family conflict, sexuality, abuse, and eventually, dealing with death. As well as the emotional challenges, the latest treatments, drugs and diagnosis information, plus causes and preventative measures are included. *$27.95*

432 pages Year Founded: 1923 ISBN 0-393050-16-5

2719 Neurobiology of Primary Dementia
American Psychiatric Publishing, Inc.
1000 Wilson Boulevard
Suite 1825
Arlington, VA 22209-3901
703-907-7322
800-368-5777; *Fax:* 703-907-1091
appi@psych.org
www.appi.org

Robert E Hales, M.D., M.B.A., Editor-in-Chief
Ron McMillen, Chief Executive Officer
John McDuffie, Editorial Director
RebeccaD. Rinehart, Publisher

Study of aging and Alzheimer's. Contains investigations of the basic neurobiologic aspects of the etiology of dementia, clear discussions of the diagnostic process with regard to imaging and other laboratory tests, psychopharmacologic treatment and genetic counseling. *$61.50*

440 pages Year Founded: 1998 ISBN 0-880489-15-4

2720 Strange Behavior Tales of Evolutionary Neurology
WW Norton & Company
500 5th Avenue
New York, NY 10110-54
212-354-5500
800-233-4830; *Fax:* 212-869-0856
webmaster@wwnorton.com
www.books.wwnorton.com

Drake McFeely, CEO

Both educational and entertaining, the author presents an array of people with unusual problems who have one thing in common, brain disorder. Carefully constructed, this book outlines the functioning of the brain and evolution of language skills. *$13.95*

256 pages Year Founded: 1923 ISBN 0-393321-84-3

2721 The New Handbook of Cognitive Therapy Techniques
WW Norton & Company
500 5th Avenue
New York, NY 10110-54
212-354-5500
800-233-4830; *Fax:* 212-869-0856
npb@wwnorton.com
www.books.wwnorton.com

Drake McFeely, CEO

Describes, explains, and demonstrates over a hundred cognitive therapy techniques, offering for each the theorretical basis, a thumbnail description of the method, case examples, and resources for further information.

Year Founded: 1923 ISBN 0-393703-13-4

2722 Treating Complex Cases: The Cognitive Behavioral Therapy Approach
John Wiley & Sons
111 River Street
Hoboken, NJ 07030-5774
201-748-6000; *Fax:* 201-748-6088
info@wiley.com
www.www.wiley.com

Stephen M. Smith, President and Chief Executive Of
Ellis E. Cousens, Executive Vice President, Chief

John Kritzmacher, Executive Vice President, Chief
MJ O'Leary, Senior Vice President, Human Res

This book brings together some of the most experiences and expert cognitive behavioral therapists to share their specialist experience of formulation and treatment of complex problems such as co-morbidity, psychotic conditions, and chronic conditions. The experienced clinician will find: evidence-based approaches to assessment and formulation of complex cases; a wide range of problems not restricted to disorder categories, including anger, low self-esteem, abuse and shame; a concern with the realities of clinical practice which involves complex cases that do not fit into simple case conceptualisations or diagnostic categories. Copyright 2000. *$80.00*

364 pages Year Founded: 1807 ISBN 0-471978-39-8

Neurodevelopmental Disorders

2723 Adolescents in Psychiatric Hospitals: A Psychodynamic Approach to Evaluation and Treatment
harles C Thomas Publisher Ltd.
2600 S 1st Street
Springfield, IL 62704-4730
217-789-8980
800-258-8980; *Fax:* 217-789-9130
books@ccthomas.com
www.ccthomas.com

Michael P Thomas, President
Charles C Thomas, Publisher

A short history of adolescent inpatient psychiatry and its clinical methods, and a month-long, running account of the morning meetings of a typical inpatient ward. For trainees in child and adolescent psychiatry, nurses, social workers, administrators, and psychologists working in the field of adolescent inpatient psychiatry. *$32.95*

208 pages Year Founded: 1927 ISBN 0-398068-60-7

2724 Adolescents, Alcohol and Drugs: A Practical Guide for Those Who Work With Young People
Charles C Thomas Publisher Ltd.
2600 S 1st Street
Springfield, IL 62704-4730
217-789-8980
800-258-8980; *Fax:* 217-789-9130
books@ccthomas.com
www.ccthomas.com

Michael P Thomas, President
Charles C Thomas, Publisher

   $41.95

210 pages Year Founded: 1927 ISBN 0-398053-93-6

2725 Adolescents, Alcohol and Substance Abuse: Reaching Teens through Brief Interventions
Guilford Press
72 Spring Street
New York, NY 10012-4019
212-431-9800
800-365-7006; *Fax:* 212-966-6708
info@guilford.com
www.www.guilford.com

Bob Matloff, President
Seymour Weingarten, Editor-in-Chief

Reviews a range of empirically supported approachs to dealing with the growing problems of substance use and abuse among young people. While admission to specialized treatment programs is relatively rare in today's health care climate, there are many opportunities for brief interventions. Brief interventions also allow the clinician to work with the teen on his or her home turf, emphasize autonomy and personal responsibility, and can be used across the full range of teens who are engaging in health risk-behavior.

350 pages Year Founded: 1973 ISBN 1-572306-58-0

2726 Adolesent in Family Therapy: Breaking the Cycle of Conflict and Control
Guilford Press
72 Spring Street
New York, NY 10012-4068
212-431-9800
800-365-7006; *Fax:* 212-966-6708
info@guilford.com
www.www.guilford.com

Bob Matloff, President
Seymour Weingarten, Editor-in-Chief

Family relationships that are troubled can be catalysts for change. A guide to treating a wide range of parent/adolesent problems with straightforward advice. *$19.95*

336 pages Year Founded: 1973 ISBN 1-572305-88-6

2727 At-Risk Youth in Crises
Pro-Ed Publications
8700 Shoal Creek Boulevard
Austin, TX 78757-6897
512-451-3246
800-897-3202; *Fax:* 512-451-8542
info@proedinc.com
www.www.proedinc.com

Donald D Hammill, Owner

This edition has updated material in the chapters covering divorce, loss, abuse, severe depression and suicide. *$31.00*

268 pages Year Founded: 1994 ISBN 0-890795-74-6

2728 Attachment, Trauma and Healing: Understanding and Treating Attachment Disorder in Children and Families
200 E Joppa Road
PO Box 436
Brooklandville, MD 21022-0436
410-825-8888
888-825-8249; *Fax:* 410-560-0134
sidran@sidran.org
www.sidran.org

Esther Giller, President and Director
Sheila Sidran Giller, Secretary/Treasurer
J. G. Goellner, Director Emeritus
Tracy Howard, Book Sales/Office Manager

An in depth look at the causes of attachment disorder, explains the normal development of attachment, examines the research in this area and present treatment plans. Numerous appendices include a sample intake packet, two brief day in the life accounts of children with attachment disorder, assessment guides, treatment plans and references. *$34.95*

345 pages Year Founded: 1986

2729 Basic Child Psychiatry
American Psychiatric Publishing, Inc.
1000 Wilson Boulevard
Suite 1825
Arlington, VA 22209-3901
703-907-7322
800-368-5777; *Fax:* 703-907-1091
appi@psych.org
www.appi.org

Robert E Hales, M.D., M.B.A., Editor-in-Chief
Ron McMillen, Chief Executive Officer
John McDuffie, Editorial Director
RebeccaD. Rinehart, Publisher

$46.95

416 pages   Year Founded: 1995 ISBN 0-632037-72-5

2730 Behavior Modification for Exceptional Children and Youth
Pro-Ed Publications
8700 Shoal Creek Boulevard
Austin, TX 78757-6897
512-451-3246
800-897-3202; *Fax:* 512-451-8542
info@proedinc.com
www.www.proedinc.com

Donald D Hammill, Owner

An authoritative textbook for courses in behavior modification. Serves as a practical, comprehensive reference work for clinicians working with people with disabilities and behavior problems. $37.00

296 pages   Year Founded: 1993 ISBN 1-563720-42-6

2731 Behavior Rating Profile
Pro-Ed Publications
8700 Shoal Creek Boulevard
Austin, TX 78757-6897
512-451-3246
800-897-3202; *Fax:* 512-451-8542
info@proedinc.com
www.www.proedinc.com

Donald D Hammill, Owner

Provides different evaluations of a student's behavior at home, at school, and in interpersonal relationships from the varied perpsectives of parents, teachers, peers, and the target students themselves. Identifies students whose behavior is perceived to be deviant, the settings in which behavior problems are prominent, and the persons whose perceptions of student's behavior are different from those of other respondents. $194.00

Year Founded: 1990

2732 Behavioral Approach to Assessment of Youth with Emotional/Behavioral Disorders
Pro-Ed Publications
8700 Shoal Creek Boulevard
Austin, TX 78757-6897
512-451-3246
800-897-3202; *Fax:* 512-451-8542
info@proedinc.com
www.www.proedinc.com

Donald D Hammill, Owner

This new book addresses one of the most challenging aspects of special education: evaluating students referred for suspected emotional/behavioral disorders. Geared to the practical needs and concerns of school-based practitioners, including special education teachers, school psychologists and social workers. $44.00

729 pages   Year Founded: 1996 ISBN 0-890796-25-4

2733 Brief Therapy for Adolescent Depression
Professional Resource Press
PO Box 3197
Sarasota, FL 34230-3197
941-343-9601
800-443-3364; *Fax:* 941-343-9201
cs.prpress@gmail.com
www.prpress.com

Laurie Girsch, Managing Editor

Useful book for practicing clinicians and advanced students interested in building new skills for working with depressed young people. Written from the perspective that adaptations of cognitive therapy are necessary when working with adolescents both because of the difference in thinking (relative verses absolute) between adults and adolescents, and because adolescents are deeply embedded in their families of origin and effective treatment rarely can be conducted without intervening with the family. Includes detailed clinical vignettes to illustrate key principles and techniques of this treatment model. $13.95

112 pages   Year Founded: 1980 ISBN 1-568870-28-0

2734 Candor, Connection and Enterprise in Adolesent Therapy
WW Norton & Company
500 5th Avenue
New York, NY 10110-54
212-354-5500; *Fax:* 212-869-0856
admalmud@wwnorton.com
www.books.wwnorton.com

Drake McFeely, CEO

Suggestions and troubleshooting for therapists dealing with uncooperative adolesent patients. Avoiding the appearence of trying too hard, dialouges that seem to go nowhere, and gaining the faith of a child who may not appreciate efforts on their behalf. $35.00

208 pages   Year Founded: 1923 ISSN 70356-8

2735 Child Friendly Therapy: Biophysical Innovations for Children and Families
WW Norton & Company
500 5th Avenue
New York, NY 10110-54
212-354-5500; *Fax:* 212-869-0856
admalmud@wwnorton.com
www.books.wwnorton.com

Drake McFeely, CEO

Family centered treatment for children. Suggestions and case studies, therapy room set up and session structure, multi sensory skill building leading to a fresh understanding of often misunderstood children. Family members can be incorporated to work as a team to help with therapy. $32.00

256 pages   Year Founded: 1923 ISSN 70355-X

2736 Child Psychiatry
American Psychiatric Publishing, Inc.
1000 Wilson Boulevard
Suite 1825
Arlington, VA 22209-3901

703-907-7322
800-368-5777; *Fax:* 703-907-1091
appi@psych.org
www.appi.org

Robert E Hales, M.D., M.B.A., Editor-in-Chief
Ron McMillen, Chief Executive Officer
John McDuffie, Editorial Director
RebeccaD. Rinehart, Publisher

Provides the essential facts and concepts for everyone involved in child psychiatry, the book includes 200 questions
and answers for trainees approaching professional examinations. *$46.95*

336 pages Year Founded: 1987 ISBN 0-632038-85-3

2737 Child Psychopharmacology
American Psychiatric Publishing, Inc.
1000 Wilson Boulevard
Suite 1825
Arlington, VA 22209-3901
703-907-7322
800-368-5777; *Fax:* 703-907-1091
appi@psych.org
www.appi.org

Robert E Hales, M.D., M.B.A., Editor-in-Chief
Ron McMillen, Chief Executive Officer
John McDuffie, Editorial Director
RebeccaD. Rinehart, Publisher

Includes: Tic disorders and obsessive-compulsive disorder;
Attention-deficit/hyperactivity disorder; Children and adolescents with psychotic disorders; Affective disorders in
children and adolescents; Anxiety disorders; Eating disorders. *$26.00*

200 pages ISBN 0-880488-33-6

2738 Child and Adolescent Mental Health
Consultation in Hospitals, Schools and Courts
American Psychiatric Publishing, Inc.
1000 Wilson Boulevard
Suite 1825
Arlington, VA 22209-3901
703-907-7322
800-368-5777; *Fax:* 703-907-1091
appi@psych.org
www.appi.org

Robert E Hales, M.D., M.B.A., Editor-in-Chief
Ron McMillen, Chief Executive Officer
John McDuffie, Editorial Director
RebeccaD. Rinehart, Publisher

Leading experts present a practical guide for mental health
professionals. *$38.50*

316 pages Year Founded: 1993 ISBN 0-880484-18-7

2739 Child and Adolescent Psychiatry: Modern
Approaches
American Psychiatric Publishing, Inc.
1000 Wilson Boulevard
Suite 1825
Arlington, VA 22209-3901
703-907-7322
800-368-5777; *Fax:* 703-907-1091
appi@psych.org
www.appi.org

Robert E Hales, M.D., M.B.A., Editor-in-Chief
Ron McMillen, Chief Executive Officer

John McDuffie, Editorial Director
RebeccaD. Rinehart, Publisher
ISBN 0-632028-21-1

2740 Child-Centered Counseling and Psychotherapy
Charles C Thomas Publisher Ltd.
2600 S 1st Street
Springfield, IL 62704-4730
217-789-8980
800-258-8980; *Fax:* 217-789-9130
books@ccthomas.com
www.ccthomas.com

Michael P Thomas, President
Charles C Thomas, Publisher

Topics include an introduction to child-centered counseling, counseling as a three-phase process, applying the re-
flective process, phase three alternatives, counseling
through play, consultation, and professional issues. It represents the status of child-centered counseling which also
indentifies ideas which can influence its future. *$62.95*

262 pages Year Founded: 1927 ISSN 0-398-06522-5ISBN
0-398065-21-7

2741 Childhood Behavior Disorders: Applied
Research and Educational Practice
Pro-Ed Publications
8700 Shoal Creek Boulevard
Austin, TX 78757-6897
512-451-3246
800-897-3202; *Fax:* 512-451-8542
info@proedinc.com
www.www.proedinc.com

Donald D Hammill, Owner

Provides the balance of theory, research and practical relevance needed by students in graduate and undergraduate introductory courses, as well as practicing teachers and other
professionals. *$ 39.00*

550 pages Year Founded: 1998 ISBN 0-890797-19-6

2742 Childhood Disorders
Brunner/Routledge
7625 Empire Drive
Florence, KY 41042-2919
800-634-7064; *Fax:* 215-269-0363
orders@taylorandfrancis.com
www.www.routledgementalhealth.com

Provides an up-to-date summary of the current information
about the psychological disorders of childhood as well as
their causes, nature and course. Together with discussion
and evaluation of the major models that guide psychological thinking about the disorders. Gives detailed consideration of the criteria used to make the diagnoses, a
presentation of the latest research findings on the nature of
the disorder and an overview of the methods used and evaluations conducted for the treatment of the disorders.
$26.95

240 pages ISBN 0-863776-09-4

2743 Children in Therapy: Using the Family as a
Resource
WW Norton & Company
500 5th Avenue
New York, NY 10110-54
212-354-5500
800-233-4830; *Fax:* 212-869-0856

npb@wwnorton.com
www.books.wwnorton.com

Drake McFeely, CEO

This anthology presents theoretical perspectives of five different competency-based approaches: solution-oriented brief therapy, narrative therapy, collaborative language systems therapy, internal family systems therapy, and emotionally focused family therapy.

Year Founded: 1923 ISBN 0-393704-85-8

2744 Childs Work/Childs Play
303 Crossways Park Dr
Woodbury, NY 11797-2099
800-962-1141; *Fax: 800-262-1886*
info@childswork.com
www.childswork.com

Catalog of books, games, toys and workbooks relating to child development issues such as recognizing emotions, handling uncertainty, bullies, ADD, shyness, conflicts and other things that children may need some help navigating.

2745 Clinical & Forensic Interviewing of Children & Families
Jerome M Sattler
PO Box 3557
La Mesa, CA 91944-1060
619-460-3667; *Fax: 619-460-2489*
www.sattlerpublisher.com

2746 Clinical Application of Projective Drawings
Charles C Thomas Publisher Ltd.
2600 S 1st Street
Springfield, IL 62704-4730
217-789-8980
800-258-8980; *Fax: 217-789-9130*
books@ccthomas.com
www.ccthomas.com

Michael P Thomas, President
Charles C Thomas, Publisher

On its way to becoming the classic in the field of projective drawings, this book provides a grounding in fundamentals and goes on to consider differential diagnosis, appraisal of psychological resources as treatment potentials and projective drawing usage in therapy. *$65.95*

688 pages Year Founded: 1927 ISBN 0-398007-68-3

2747 Clinical Child Documentation Sourcebook
John Wiley & Sons
111 River Street
Hoboken, NJ 07030-5774
201-748-6000; *Fax: 201-748-6088*
info@wiley.com
www.www.wiley.com

Stephen M. Smith, President and Chief Executive Of
Ellis E. Cousens, Executive Vice President, Chief
John Kritzmacher, Executive Vice President, Chief
MJ O'Leary, Senior Vice President, Human Res

This easy to use resource offers child psychologists and therapists a full array of forms, inventories, checklists, client handouts, and clinical records essential to a successful practice in either and organizational or clinical setting. *$49.95*

364 pages Year Founded: 1807 ISBN 0-471291-11-0

2748 Concise Guide to Child and Adolescent Psychiatry
American Psychiatric Publishing, Inc.
1000 Wilson Boulevard
Suite 1825
Arlington, VA 22209-3901
703-907-7322
800-368-5777; *Fax: 703-907-1091*
appi@psych.org
www.appi.org

Robert E Hales, M.D., M.B.A., Editor-in-Chief
Ron McMillen, Chief Executive Officer
John McDuffie, Editorial Director
RebeccaD. Rinehart, Publisher

Topics include evaluation and treatment planning, axis I disorders usually first diagnosed in infancy, childhood or adolescence, attention deficit and disruptive behavior disorders, developmental disorders, special clinical circumstances, psychopharmacology, and psychosocial treatments. *$21.95*

400 pages Year Founded: 1998 ISBN 0-880489-05-7

2749 Counseling Children with Special Needs
American Psychiatric Publishing, Inc.
1000 Wilson Boulevard
Suite 1825
Arlington, VA 22209-3901
703-907-7322
800-368-5777; *Fax: 703-907-1091*
appi@psych.org
www.appi.org

Robert E Hales, M.D., M.B.A., Editor-in-Chief
Ron McMillen, Chief Executive Officer
John McDuffie, Editorial Director
RebeccaD. Rinehart, Publisher

$29.95

224 pages Year Founded: 1997 ISBN 0-632041-51-

2750 Creative Therapy with Children and Adolescents
Impact Publishers
PO Box 6016
Atascadero, CA 93423-6016
805-466-5917
800-246-7228; *Fax: 805-466-5919*
info@impactpublishers.com
www.impactpublishers.com

Encourages creativity in therapy, assists therapists in talking with children to facilitate change. From simple ideas to fresh innovations, the activities are to be used as tools to supplement a variety of therapeutic approaches, and can be tailored to each child's needs. *$21.95*

192 pages Year Founded: 1999 ISBN 1-886230-19-6

2751 Defiant Teens
Guilford Press
72 Spring Street
New York, NY 10012-4068
212-431-9800
800-365-7006; *Fax: 212-966-6708*
info@guilford.com
www.www.guilford.com

Bob Matloff, President
Seymour Weingarten, Editor-in-Chief

Guidelines for best practices in working with families and their teenaged children.

250 pages Year Founded: 1973 ISBN 1-572304-40-5

2752 Developmental Therapy/Developmental Teaching
Pro-Ed Publications
8700 Shoal Creek Boulevard
Austin, TX 78757-6897
512-451-3246
800-897-3202; *Fax:* 512-451-8542
info@proedinc.com
www.www.proedinc.com

Donald D Hammill, Owner

Provides extensive applications for teachers, counselors, parents and other adults concerned about the behavior and emotional stability of children and teens. The focus is on helping children and youth to cope effectively with the stresses of comtemporary life, with an emphasis on the positive effects adults can have on students when they adjust strategies to the social emotional needs of children. *$41.00*

398 pages Year Founded: 1996 ISBN 0-890796-64-5

2753 Drug Information for Teens: Health Tips About the Physical and Mental Effects of Substance Abuse
Omnigraphics
615 Giswold
Detroit, MI 48226-3900
313-961-1340; *Fax:* 313-961-1383
info@omnigraphics.com
www.omnigraphics.com

Provides students with facts about drug use, abuse, and addiction. It describes the physical and mental effects of alcohol, tobacco, marijuana, ecstasy, inhalants and many other drugs and chemicals that are often abused. It includes information about the process that leads from casual use to addiction and offers suggestions for resisting peer pressure and helping friends stay drug free.

452 pages ISBN 0-780804-44-9

2754 Effective Discipline
Pro-Ed Publications
8700 Shoal Creek Boulevard
Austin, TX 78757-6897
512-451-3246
800-897-3202; *Fax:* 512-451-8542
info@proedinc.com
www.www.proedinc.com

Donald D Hammill, Owner

Designed to provide principals, counselors, teachers, and college students preparing to become educators with information about research-based techniques that reduce or eliminate school behavior problems. Provides the knowledge to prevent discipline problems, identify specific behaviors that disrupt the environment, match interventions with behavioral infractions, implement a variety of intervention tactics, and evaluate the effectiveness of the intervention program. *$28.00*

220 pages Year Founded: 1993 ISBN 0-890795-79-7

2755 Empowering Adolesent Girls
WW Norton & Company
500 5th Avenue
New York, NY 10110-54

212-354-5500; *Fax:* 212-869-0856
admalmud@wwnorton.com
www.books.wwnorton.com

Drake McFeely, CEO

Strategies and activities for professionals who work with adolesent girls (teachers, counselors, therapists) to offer support and encouagement through the Go Girls program. *$32.00*

256 pages Year Founded: 1923 ISSN 70347-9

2756 Enhancing Social Competence in Young Students
Pro-Ed Publications
8700 Shoal Creek Boulevard
Austin, TX 78757-6897
512-451-3246
800-897-3202; *Fax:* 512-451-8542
info@proedinc.com
www.www.proedinc.com

Donald D Hammill, Owner

Addresses conceptual and practical issues of providing social competence-enhancing interventions for young students in schools, based on research findings. Summarizes recent advances in social skills programming for at-risk students and prevention interventions for all students. Discussions of developmental issues of childhood maladjustment, intervention strategies, implementation issues and assessment/evaluation issues are provided. *$28.00*

281 pages Year Founded: 1995 ISBN 0-890796-20-3

2757 Group Therapy With Children and Adolescents
American Psychiatric Publishing, Inc.
1000 Wilson Boulevard
Suite 1825
Arlington, VA 22209-3901
703-907-7322
800-368-5777; *Fax:* 703-907-1091
appi@psych.org
www.appi.org

Robert E Hales, M.D., M.B.A., Editor-in-Chief
Ron McMillen, Chief Executive Officer
John McDuffie, Editorial Director
RebeccaD. Rinehart, Publisher

Explores a major treatment modality often used with adult populations and rarely considered for child and adolescent treatments. With contributions from international experts, this book looks at the effectiveness of treatment and cost of group therapy as it applies to this particular age group. *$52.00*

400 pages ISBN 0-880484-06-3

2758 Handbook of Child Behavior in Therapy and in the Psychiatric Setting
John Wiley & Sons
111 River Street
Hoboken, NJ 07030-5774
201-748-6000; *Fax:* 201-748-6088
info@wiley.com
www.www.wiley.com

Stephen M. Smith, President and Chief Executive Of
Ellis E. Cousens, Executive Vice President, Chief
John Kritzmacher, Executive Vice President, Chief
MJ O'Leary, Senior Vice President, Human Res

364 pages Year Founded: 1807

2759 Handbook of Infant Mental Health
Guilford Press
72 Spring Street
New York, NY 10012-4068
212-431-9800
800-365-7006; *Fax:* 212-966-6708
info@guilford.com
www.www.guilford.com

Bob Matloff, President
Seymour Weingarten, Editor-in-Chief

Included are chapters on neurobiology, diagnostic issues, parental mental health issues and family dynamics. *$60.00*

588 pages Year Founded: 1973 ISBN 1-572305-15-0

2760 Handbook of Parent Training: Parents as Co-Therapists for Children's Behavior Problems
John Wiley & Sons
111 River Street
Hoboken, NJ 07030-5774
201-748-6000; *Fax:* 201-748-6088
info@wiley.com
www.www.wiley.com

Stephen M. Smith, President and Chief Executive Of
Ellis E. Cousens, Executive Vice President, Chief
John Kritzmacher, Executive Vice President, Chief
MJ O'Leary, Senior Vice President, Human Res

This completely revised handbook shows professionals who work with troubled children how to teach parents to become co-therapists. It presents various techniques and behavior modification skills that will help parents to better relate, communicate, and respond to their child. Updates are provided on such problems as noncompliance, ADHD, and conduct disorder, and a new section on special needs parents which includes adolescent mothers, aggressive parents, substance abusing parents, and more.

364 pages Year Founded: 1807

2761 Handbook of Psychiatric Practice in the Juvenile Court
American Psychiatric Publishing, Inc.
1000 Wilson Boulevard
Suite 1825
Arlington, VA 22209-3901
703-907-7322
800-368-5777; *Fax:* 703-907-1091
appi@psych.org
www.appi.org

Robert E Hales, M.D., M.B.A., Editor-in-Chief
Ron McMillen, Chief Executive Officer
John McDuffie, Editorial Director
RebeccaD. Rinehart, Publisher

Examines the role that psychiatrists and other mental health professionals are asked to play when children, adolescents, and their families end up in court. *$12.95*

198 pages ISBN 0-890422-33-8

2762 Helping Parents, Youth, and Teachers Understand Medications for Behavioral and Emotional Problems
American Psychiatric Publishing, Inc.
1000 Wilson Boulevard
Suite 1825
Arlington, VA 22209-3901

703-907-7322
800-368-5777; *Fax:* 703-907-1091
appi@psych.org
www.appi.org

Robert E Hales, M.D., M.B.A., Editor-in-Chief
Ron McMillen, Chief Executive Officer
John McDuffie, Editorial Director
RebeccaD. Rinehart, Publisher

Valuable resource for anyone involved in evaluating psychiatric disturbances in children and adolescents. Provides a compilation of information sheets to help promote the dialogue between the patient's family, caregivers, and the treating physician. *$39.95*

196 pages Year Founded: 1999 ISBN 0-880487-94-1

2763 How to Teach Social Skills
Pro-Ed Publications
8700 Shoal Creek Boulevard
Austin, TX 78757-6897
512-451-3246
800-897-3202; *Fax:* 512-451-8542
info@proedinc.com
www.www.proedinc.com

Donald D Hammill, Owner

$8.00

ISBN 0-890797-61-7

2764 In the Long Run... Longitudinal Studies of Psychopathology in Children
American Psychiatric Publishing, Inc.
1000 Wilson Boulevard
Suite 1825
Arlington, VA 22209-3901
703-907-7322
800-368-5777; *Fax:* 703-907-1091
appi@psych.org
www.appi.org

Robert E Hales, M.D., M.B.A., Editor-in-Chief
Ron McMillen, Chief Executive Officer
John McDuffie, Editorial Director
RebeccaD. Rinehart, Publisher

$29.95

224 pages Year Founded: 1999 ISBN 0-873182-11-1

2765 Infants, Toddlers and Families: Framework for Support and Intervention
Guilford Press
72 Spring Street
Department 4E
New York, NY 10012-4019
212-431-9800; *Fax:* 212-966-6708
www.www.guilford.com

Bob Matloff, President
Seymour Weingarten, Editor-in-Chief

Examines the complex development in a child's first 3 years of life. Instead of preaching or judging, this book acknowledges the challenges facing all families, especially vulnerable ones, and offers straightforward advice. *$28.95*

204 pages Year Founded: 1973 ISBN 1-572304-87-1

2766 Interventions for Students with Emotional Disorders
Pro-Ed Publications
8700 Shoal Creek Boulevard
Austin, TX 78757-6897
512-451-3246
800-897-3202; *Fax:* 512-451-8542
info@proedinc.com
www.www.proedinc.com

Donald D Hammill, Owner

This graduate textbook for special education students advocates an eclectic approach toward teaching children with social adjustment problems. Provides how-to information for implementing various techniques to successfully enhance positive sociobehavioral development in children with emotional disorders. *$36.00*

212 pages Year Founded: 1991 ISBN 0-890792-96-8

2767 Interviewing Children and Adolescents: Skills and Strategies for Effective DSM-IV Diagnosis
Guilford Press
72 Spring Street
New York, NY 10012-4068
212-431-9800
800-365-7006; *Fax:* 212-966-6708
info@guilford.com
www.www.guilford.com

Bob Matloff, President
Seymour Weingarten, Editor-in-Chief

Guide to developmentally appropriate interviewing. *$ 45.00*

482 pages Year Founded: 1973 ISBN 1-572305-01-0

2768 Interviewing the Sexually Abused Child
American Psychiatric Publishing, Inc.
1000 Wilson Boulevard
Suite 1825
Arlington, VA 22209-3901
703-907-7322
800-368-5777; *Fax:* 703-907-1091
appi@psych.org
www.appi.org

Robert E Hales, M.D., M.B.A., Editor-in-Chief
Ron McMillen, Chief Executive Officer
John McDuffie, Editorial Director
RebeccaD. Rinehart, Publisher

A guide for mental health professionals who need to know if a child has been sexually abused. Presents guidelines on the structure of the interview and covers the use of free play, toys, and play materials by focusing on the investigate interview of the suspected victim. *$15.00*

80 pages Year Founded: 1993 ISBN 0-880486-12-0

2769 Learning Disorders and Disorders of the Self in Children and Adolesents
WW Norton & Company
500 5th Avenue
New York, NY 10110-54
212-354-5500; *Fax:* 212-869-0856
admalmud@wwnorton.com
www.books.wwnorton.com

Drake McFeely, CEO

Clinicians who work with learning disabled children need to understand the complex, integrated framework of learn-

ing and self image problems. Specific problems and treatments are discussed. *$32.00*

332 pages Year Founded: 1923 ISSN 70377-0

2770 Living on the Razor's Edge: Solution-Oriented Brief Family Therapy with Self-Harming Adolesents
WW Norton & Company
500 5th Avenue
New York, NY 10110-54
212-354-5500; *Fax:* 212-869-0856
admalmud@wwnorton.com
www.books.wwnorton.com

Drake McFeely, CEO

Research supported stategies and a therapy model for self harming adolesents and their families to devlop a closer and more meaningful relationships. *$25.60*

320 pages Year Founded: 1923 ISSN 70335-5

2771 Making the Grade: Guide to School Drug Prevention Programs
Drug Strategies
1616 P Street NW
Washington, DC 20036-1434
202-289-9070; *Fax:* 202-414-6199
dspoilcy@aol.com

Mathea Falco, President

Updated and expanded from the 1996 original, this guide to drug prevention programs in America helps parents and educators make informed decisions with often limited budgets. *$14.95*

2772 Manual of Clinical Child and Adolescent Psychiatry
American Psychiatric Publishing, Inc.
1000 Wilson Boulevard
Suite 1825
Arlington, VA 22209-3901
703-907-7322
800-368-5777; *Fax:* 703-907-1091
appi@psych.org
www.appi.org

Robert E Hales, M.D., M.B.A., Editor-in-Chief
Ron McMillen, Chief Executive Officer
John McDuffie, Editorial Director
RebeccaD. Rinehart, Publisher

Addresses current issues such as cost containment, insurance complications, and legal and ethical issues, as well as neuropsychology, alcohol, and substance abuse, and developmental disabilities and genetics. *$42.50*

528 pages ISBN 0-880485-28-0

2773 Myth of Maturity: What Teenagers Need from Parents to Become Adults
WW Norton & Company
500 5th Avenue
New York, NY 10110-54
212-354-5500; *Fax:* 212-869-0856
admalmud@wwnorton.com
www.books.wwnorton.com

Drake McFeely, CEO

Debunking outdated and misguided ideas about maturity, the author discusses the amount of support teens need from their parents, what is too much for independence, or not enough. *$24.95*

256 pages Year Founded: 1923 ISBN 0-393049-42-6

2774 Narrative Therapies with Children and Adolescents
Guilford Press
72 Spring Street
New York, NY 10012-4068
212-431-9800
800-365-7006; *Fax:* 212-966-6708
info@guilford.com
www.www.guilford.com

Bob Matloff, President
Seymour Weingarten, Editor-in-Chief

Many renowned, creative contributors collaborate to bring this professional resource to the shelf. Transcripts of case examples, using many different methods and mediums are shown to engage children of different perspectives and ages. This book can serve as a text for child/adolesent psychotherapy, or is a useful guide for mental health professionals. *$39.95*

469 pages Year Founded: 1973 ISBN 1-572302-53-4

2775 National Survey of American Attitudes on Substance Abuse VI: Teens
Center on Addiction at Columbia University
633 3rd Avenue
19th Floor
New York, NY 10017-6706
212-841-5200
800-662-4357; *Fax:* 212-956-8020
www.casacolumbia.org

Jeffrey B. Lane, Chairman
Joseph A. Califano, Jr., Founder and Chairman Emeritus
Samuel A. Ball, Ph.D., President and Chief Executive Of
Susan P. Brown, Vice President and Director of F

Results of the sixth annual CASA National Survey of teens 12 - 17 years old reveals that parents that are more involved with their children's activities and have house rules and expectations can greatly influence teen behavior choices. Other statistics about availability of illegal substances and who may use them. *$22.00*

Year Founded: 1992

2776 No-Talk Therapy for Children and Adolescents
WW Norton & Company
500 5th Avenue
New York, NY 10110-54
212-354-5500; *Fax:* 212-869-0856
admalmud@wwnorton.com
www.books.wwnorton.com

Drake McFeely, CEO

Creative approach to treatment of young people who cannot respond to conversation based therapy. Seemingly sullen patients can be helped to find a voice of their own. *$.27*

288 pages Year Founded: 1923 ISSN 70286-3

2777 Ordinary Families, Special Children: Systems Approach to Childhood Disability
Guilford Press
72 Spring Street
New York, NY 10012-4068

212-431-9800
800-365-7006; *Fax:* 212-966-6708
info@guilford.com
www.www.guilford.com

Bob Matloff, President
Seymour Weingarten, Editor-in-Chief

Families, including siblings and grandparents are impacted by the special needs of a child's disability. The authors explore personal accounts that shape a family's response to childhood disability and how they come to adapt these unique needs to a satisfactory lifestyle. Available in hardcover and paperback. *$35.00*

324 pages Year Founded: 1973 ISBN 1-572301-55-4

2778 Outcomes for Children and Youth with Emotional and Behavioral Disorders and their Families
Pro-Ed Publications
8700 Shoal Creek Boulevard
Austin, TX 78757-6897
512-451-3246
800-897-3202; *Fax:* 512-451-8542
info@proedinc.com
www.www.proedinc.com

Donald D Hammill, Owner

This new book addresses one of the most challenging aspects of serving children and youth with emotional and behavioral disorders-evaluating the outcomes of the services you've provided. Also includes information on such topics as: child and family outcomes, system level anaylsis, case study analysis, cost analysis, cultural diversity, managed care, and consumer satisfaction. *$44.00*

730 pages Year Founded: 1998 ISBN 0-890797-50-1

2779 PTSD in Children and Adolescents
American Psychiatric Publishing, Inc.
1000 Wilson Boulevard
Suite 1825
Arlington, VA 22209-3901
703-907-7322
800-368-5777; *Fax:* 703-907-1091
appi@psych.org
www.appi.org

Robert E Hales, M.D., M.B.A., Editor-in-Chief
Ron McMillen, Chief Executive Officer
John McDuffie, Editorial Director
RebeccaD. Rinehart, Publisher

Mental health and other professionals who work with Post Traumatic Stress Disorder and the young people who suffer from it will find discussions of evaluation, biological treatment strategies, the need for an integrated approach to juvenille offenders who suffer from PTSD and more. *$29.95*

208 pages Year Founded: 2001

2780 Pediatric Psychopharmacology: Fast Facts
WW Norton & Company
500 5th Avenue
New York, NY 10110-54
212-354-2907
800-233-4830; *Fax:* 212-869-0856
npb@wwnorton.com
www.books.wwnorton.com

Drake McFeely, CEO

This new title in the Fast Facts series, full of up-to-date and authoritative infomration, is a critical resource for all health care professionals, including psychiatrists, prescribing psychologists, psychotherapists, pediatricians, family practice physicians, pediatric neurologists, nurse practitioners, and allied mental health professionals. Clear explanations of clinical directions for the prescriber and nonprescriber alike.

Year Founded: 1923 ISBN 0-393704-61-0

2781 Play Therapy with Children in Crisis: Individual, Group and Family Treatment
Guilford Press
72 Spring Street
New York, NY 10012-4068
212-431-9800
800-365-7006; *Fax:* 212-966-6708
info@guilford.com
www.www.guilford.com

Bob Matloff, President
Seymour Weingarten, Editor-in-Chief

  $45.00

506 pages Year Founded: 1973 ISBN 1-572304-85-5

2782 Post Traumatic Stress Disorders in Children and Adolescents Handbook
WW Norton & Company
500 5th Avenue
New York, NY 10110-54
212-354-2907
800-233-4830; *Fax:* 212-869-0856
npb@wwnorton.com
www.books.wwnorton.com

Drake McFeely, CEO

The 15 chapters gathered here address different aspects of childhood and adolescent trauma-some consider a distinct therapeutic situation (abuse and neglect), others pertain to standard clinical procedure (assessment), and still others focus on complex research issues (neurobiology and genetics of PSTD).

Year Founded: 1923 ISBN 0-393704-12-2

2783 Power and Compassion: Working with Difficult Adolesents and Abused Parents
Guilford Press
72 Spring Street
New York, NY 10012-4068
212-431-9800
800-365-7006; *Fax:* 212-966-6708
info@guilford.com
www.www.guilford.com

Bob Matloff, President
Seymour Weingarten, Editor-in-Chief

Useful as a supplemental text, or for mental health professionals dealing with aggressive teenagers and their parents. Pragmatic guide to help demoralized parents be more understanding, but more decisive. *$16.95*

196 pages Year Founded: 1973 ISBN 1-572304-70-7

2784 Practical Charts for Managing Behavior
Pro-Ed Publications
8700 Shoal Creek Boulevard
Austin, TX 78757-6897

512-451-3246
800-897-3202; *Fax:* 512-451-8542
info@proedinc.com
www.www.proedinc.com

Donald D Hammill, Owner

  $29.00

160 pages Year Founded: 1998 ISBN 0-890797-36-6

2785 Proven Youth Development Model that Prevents Substance Abuse and Builds Communities
Center on Addiction at Columbia University
633 3rd Avenue
19th Floor
New York, NY 10017-6706
212-841-5200
800-662-4357; *Fax:* 212-956-8020
www.casacolumbia.org

Jeffrey B. Lane, Chairman
Joseph A. Califano, Jr., Founder and Chairman Emeritus
Samuel A. Ball, Ph.D., President and Chief Executive Of
Susan P. Brown, Vice President and Director of F

How-to manual developed with nine years of research. The program is a collaboration of local school, law enforcement, social service and health teams to help high risk youth between the ages of 8 - 13 years old and their families prevent substance abuse and violent behavior. Used in 23 urban and rural communities in 11 states and the District of Columbia. *$50.00*

79 pages Year Founded: 1992

2786 Psychological Examination of the Child
John Wiley & Sons
111 River Street
Hoboken, NJ 07030-5774
201-748-6000; *Fax:* 201-748-6088
info@wiley.com
www.www.wiley.com

279 pages Year Founded: 1991

2787 Psychotherapies with Children and Adolescents
American Psychiatric Publishing, Inc.
1000 Wilson Boulevard
Suite 1825
Arlington, VA 22209-3901
703-907-7322
800-368-5777; *Fax:* 703-907-1091
appi@psych.org
www.appi.org

Robert E Hales, M.D., M.B.A., Editor-in-Chief
Ron McMillen, Chief Executive Officer
John McDuffie, Editorial Director
RebeccaD. Rinehart, Publisher

Illustrated with case histories and demonstrates how psychoanalytic techniques can be modified to meet the therapeutic needs of children and adolescents in specific clinical situations. *$47.50*

346 pages ISBN 0-880484-06-3

2788 Safe Schools/Safe Students: Guide to Violence Prevention Stategies
Drug Strategies
770 Broadway
New York, NY 10003

212-206-4400; *Fax:* 202-414-6199
dspoilcy@aol.com
www.www.aol.com

Tim Armstrong, Chairman and Chief Executive Off
Curtis Brown, Executive Vice President and Chi
Karen Dykstra, Executive Vice President and Chi

Practical assistance in rating over 84 violence prevention programs for classroom use, helps examine school policies and possible changes for student protection. *$14.95*

Year Founded: 1985

2789 Severe Stress and Mental Disturbance in Children
American Psychiatric Publishing, Inc.
1000 Wilson Boulevard
Suite 1825
Arlington, VA 22209-3901
703-907-7322
800-368-5777; *Fax:* 703-907-1091
appi@psych.org
www.appi.org

Robert E Hales, M.D., M.B.A., Editor-in-Chief
Ron McMillen, Chief Executive Officer
John McDuffie, Editorial Director
RebeccaD. Rinehart, Publisher

Uniquely blends current research and clinical data on the effects of severe stress on children. Each chapter is written by international experts in their field. *$69.95*

708 pages ISBN 0-880486-57-0

2790 Structured Adolescent Pscyhotherapy Groups
Professional Resource Press
PO Box 3197
Sarasota, FL 34230-3197
941-343-9601
800-443-3364; *Fax:* 941-343-9201
cs.prpress@gmail.com
www.prpress.com

Laurie Girsch, Managing Editor

Provides specific techniques for use in the beginning, middle, and end phase of time-limited structured psychotherapy groups. Offers concrete suggestions for working with hard to reach and difficult adolescents, providing feedback to parents, and dealing with administrative, legal, and ethical issues. Examples of pre/post evaluation forms, therapy contracts, evaluation feedback letters, parent response forms, therapist rating scales, co-therapist rating forms, problem identification forms, supervision and session records, client and patient handouts, and specific group exercises. Solidly anchored to research on the curative factors in group therapy, this book includes empirical data, references, theoretical formulations and examples of group sessions. *$19.95*

164 pages Year Founded: 1980 ISBN 0-943158-74-5

2791 Teaching Buddy Skills to Preschoolers
AAIDD
501 3rd Street NW
Suite 200
Washington, DC 20001
202-387-1968
800-424-3688; *Fax:* 202-387-2193
anam@aaidd.org
www.aaidd.org

Margaret A. Nygren, EdD, Executive Director & CEO
Danielle Webber, MSW, Manager
Kathleen McLane, Director
Paul D. Aitken,CPA, Director

Shows how the rewards of social interactions must outweigh the costs to encouraging friendships between pre-schoolers with and without disabilities. *$12.95*

40 pages ISBN 0-940898-45-4

2792 Textbook of Child and Adolescent Psychiatry
American Psychiatric Publishing, Inc.
1000 Wilson Boulevard
Suite 1825
Arlington, VA 22209-3901
703-907-7322
800-368-5777; *Fax:* 703-907-1091
appi@psych.org
www.appi.org

Robert E Hales, M.D., M.B.A., Editor-in-Chief
Ron McMillen, Chief Executive Officer
John McDuffie, Editorial Director
RebeccaD. Rinehart, Publisher

Includes chapter on changes in DSM-IV classification and discusses the latest research and treatment advances in the areas of epidemiology, fenetics, developmental neurobiology, and combined treatments. A special section covers essential issues such as HIV and AIDS, gender identity disorders, physical and sexual abuse, and substance abuse, for the child and adolescent psychiatrist. *$140.00*

960 pages ISBN 1-882103-03-3

2793 Textbook of Pediatric Neuropsychiatry
American Psychiatric Publishing, Inc.
1000 Wilson Boulevard
Suite 1825
Arlington, VA 22209-3901
703-907-7322
800-368-5777; *Fax:* 703-907-1091
appi@psych.org
www.appi.org

Robert E Hales, M.D., M.B.A., Editor-in-Chief
Ron McMillen, Chief Executive Officer
John McDuffie, Editorial Director
RebeccaD. Rinehart, Publisher

Comprehensive textbook on pediatric medicine. *$175.00*

1632 pages Year Founded: 1998 ISBN 0-880487-66-6

2794 The Special Education Consultant Teacher
Charles C Thomas Publisher Ltd.
PO Box 19265
Springfield, IL 62794-9265
217-789-8980
800-258-8980; *Fax:* 217-789-9130
www.ccthomas.com

Michael P Thomas, President
Charles C Thomas, Publisher

This book is intended for special education teachers and other professionals providing special education services with information, guidelines and suggestions relating to the role and responsibilities of the special education consultant teacher. Available in paperback for $ 45.95. *$67.95*

330 pages Year Founded: 1927 ISBN 0-398075-10-7

2795 Through the Eyes of a Child
WW Norton & Company
500 5th Avenue
New York, NY 10110-54
212-354-2907
800-233-4830; *Fax:* 212-869-0856
npb@wwnorton.com
www.books.wwnorton.com

Drake McFeely, CEO

Comprehensive and helpful, this book helps therapists
work with children and parents in the application of EMDR
with children. *$ 37.00*

*288 pages Year Founded: 1923 ISSN 70287-1ISBN
0-393702-87-1*

**2796 Transition Matters From School to
Independence: a Guide & Directory of Services
for Children & Youth with Disabilities &
Special Needs in the Metro New York Area**
Resources for Children with Special Needs
116 E 16th Street
5th Floor
New York, NY 10003-2164
212-677-4650; *Fax:* 212-254-4070
info@resourcesnyc.org
www.resourcesnyc.org

Ellen Miller-Wachtel, Chairman
Shon E. Glusky, President
Rachel Howard, Executive Director
Stephen Stern, Director

Youth with disabilities need special guidance when moving
from school to adult life. Transition Matters covers every
aspect of moving from high school to the world of
postsecondary education, job training, employment and
idependent living. This guide for parents, caregivers and
educators presents a wealth of information about the transition process, and lists 1,000 agencies and organizations that
provide services for youth 14 and up. It explains
entitlements and options and helps families navigate systems and procedures. *$15.00*

500 pages Year Founded: 1983 ISBN 0-967836-56-5

**2797 Treating Depressed Children: A Therapeutic
Manual of Proven Cognitive Behavior
Techniques**
NewHarbinger Publications
5674 Shattuck Avenue
Oakland, CA 94609-1662
510-652-0215
800-748-6273; *Fax:* 510-652-5472
customerservice@newharbinger.com
www.newharbinger.com

Matthew McKay, Owner
Patrick Fanning, Co-Founder

Program incorporating cartoons and role playing games to
help children recognize emotions, change negative
thoughts, gain confidence, and learn interpersonal skills.
$49.94

160 pages Year Founded: 1973 ISBN 1-572240-61-

**2798 Treating the Aftermath of Sexual Abuse: a
Handbook for Working with Children in Care**
Child Welfare League of America
440 First Street NW
Third Floor
Washington, DC 20001-2028
202-638-2952; *Fax:* 202-638-4004
www.cwla.org

A handbook for working with children in care who have
been sexually abused. The authors review the impact of
sexual abuse on a child's physical and emotional development and describe the effect of abuse on basic life experiences. Paperback. *$18.95*

176 pages Year Founded: 1998 ISBN 0-878686-93-2

**2799 Treating the Tough Adolesent: Family Based
Step by Step Guide**
Guilford Press
72 Spring Street
New York, NY 10012-4068
212-431-9800
800-365-7006; *Fax:* 212-966-6708
info@guilford.com
www.www.guilford.com

Bob Matloff, President
Seymour Weingarten, Editor-in-Chief

Model for effective family therapy, with reproducible handouts. *$35.00*

320 pages Year Founded: 1973 ISBN 1-572304-22-7

**2800 Troubled Teens: Multidimensional Family
Therapy**
WW Norton & Company
500 5th Avenue
New York, NY 10110-54
212-354-2907; *Fax:* 212-869-0856
admalmud@wwnorton.com
www.books.wwnorton.com

Drake McFeely, CEO

Based on 17 years of research, this treatment manual is for
therapists who work with youth referred for substance
abuse and behavior counseling. Treatment involves drug
counseling, family and individual sessions and interventions. People or systems of influence outside the family are
also considered. *$35.00*

320 pages Year Founded: 1923 ISBN 0-393703-40-1

**2801 Understanding and Teaching Emotionally
Disturbed Children and Adolescents**
Pro-Ed Publications
8700 Shoal Creek Boulevard
Austin, TX 78757-6897
512-451-3246
800-897-3202; *Fax:* 512-451-8542
info@proedinc.com
www.www.proedinc.com

Donald D Hammill, Owner

Shows how diverse theoretical perspectives translate into
practice by exploring forms of therapy and types of interventions currently employed with children and adolescents.
$41.00

620 pages Year Founded: 1993 ISBN 0-890795-75-4

2802 Ups & Downs: How to Beat the Blues and Teen Depression
Price Stern Sloan Publishing
375 Hudson Street
New York, NY 10014-3657
212-366-2000; *Fax:* 212-366-2933
www.penguingroup.com

John Makinson, Chairman and Chief Executive Off
Coram Williams, Chief Financial Officer
David Shanks, Chief Executive Officer
Susan Peterson Kennedy, President

This book discusses how to recognize depression in teens and what to do about it. Informal, yet informative, using quotes and case studies representing typical young people who are dealing with mood swings, eating disorders and problems at school or at home. The book also demystifies therapy and advises readers on how to seek help, particularly if they, or their friends, have suicidal thoughts. Reading level ages nine to twelve. *$4.99*

90 pages Year Founded: 1938 ISBN 0-843174-50-1

2803 Working with Self-Harming Adolescents: A Collaborative, Strengths-Based Therapy Approach
WW Norton & Company
500 5th Avenue
New York, NY 10110-54
212-354-2907
800-233-4830; *Fax:* 212-869-0856
npb@wwnorton.com
www.books.wwnorton.com

Drake McFeely, CEO

A unique approach to this illness combines flexability, compassion, and candor. His integration of the family in these treatments demonstrates the complex interplay between self-harming teens and their parents, peers, communities, and culture. Originally published in hardcover as Living on the Razor's Edge.

Year Founded: 1923 ISBN 0-393704-99-8

2804 Youth Violence: Prevention, Intervention, and Social Policy
American Psychiatric Publishing, Inc.
1000 Wilson Boulevard
Suite 1825
Arlington, VA 22209-3901
703-907-7322
800-368-5777; *Fax:* 703-907-1091
appi@psych.org
www.appi.org

Robert E Hales, M.D., M.B.A., Editor-in-Chief
Ron McMillen, Chief Executive Officer
John McDuffie, Editorial Director
RebeccaD. Rinehart, Publisher

Based on more than a decade of clinical research and treatment experience, this comprehensive and non-technical book offers a stage-oriented approach to understanding and treating complex and difficult traumatized patients, integrating modern trauma theory with traditional therapeutic interventions. *$48.50*

336 pages Year Founded: 1998 ISBN 0-880488-09-3

Obsessive Compulsive Disorder

2805 Current Treatments of Obsessive-Compulsive Disorder
American Psychiatric Publishing, Inc.
1000 Wilson Boulevard
Suite 1825
Arlington, VA 22209-3901
703-907-7322
800-368-5777; *Fax:* 703-907-1091
appi@psych.org
www.appi.org

Robert E Hales, M.D., M.B.A., Editor-in-Chief
Ron McMillen, Chief Executive Officer
John McDuffie, Editorial Director
RebeccaD. Rinehart, Publisher

Helps clinicians better match treatment approaches with each patients unique needs.

Year Founded: 01 ISBN 0-880487-79-8

2806 Obsessive-Compulsive Disorder: Contemporary Issues in Treatment
Lawrence Erlbaum Associates
10 Industrial Avenue
Mahwah, NJ 07430-2253
201-825-3200
800-926-6577; *Fax:* 201-236-0072
www.erlbaum.com

Hardcover.

Year Founded: 00 ISBN 0-805828-37-0

2807 Obsessive-Compulsive and Related Disorders in Adults: a Comprehensive Clinical Guide
Cambridge University Press
100 Gold Street
2nd Floor
New York, NY 10038
212-924-3900; *Fax:* 212-691-3239
marketing@cup.org
www.www.nyc.gov

The author challenges the current implicit models used in alcohol problem prevention and demonstrates an ecological perspective of the community as a complex adaptive systems composed of interacting subsystems. This volume represents a new and sensible approach to the prevention of alcohol dependence and alcohol-related problems. *$65.00*

380 pages Year Founded: 1999 ISBN 0-521559-75-8

2808 Overcoming Obsessive-Compulsive Disorder
New Harbinger Publications
5674 Shattuck Avenue
Oakland, CA 94609-1662
510-652-0215
800-748-6273; *Fax:* 510-652-5472
customerservice@newharbinger.com
www.newharbinger.com

Matthew McKay, Owner
Patrick Fanning, Co-Founder

A fourteen session treatment. *$11.95*

72 pages Year Founded: 1973 ISBN 1-572241-29-2

2809 Treatment of Obsessive Compulsive Disorder
Guilford Press
72 Spring Street
New York, NY 10012-4068
212-431-9800
800-365-7006; *Fax:* 212-966-6708
info@guilford.com
www.www.guilford.com

Bob Matloff, President
Seymour Weingarten, Editor-in-Chief

Provides everything the mental health professional needs
for working with clients who suffer from obsessions and
compulsions. Supplies background by describing in detail
up-to-date clinically relevant information and a
step-by-step guide for conducting behavioral treatment.
$39.95

224 pages Year Founded: 1973 ISBN 0-898621-84-4

Personality Disorders

2810 Biological Basis of Personality
Charles C Thomas Publisher Ltd.
2600 S 1st Street
Springfield, IL 62704-4730
217-789-8980
800-258-8980; *Fax:* 217-789-9130
books@ccthomas.com
www.ccthomas.com

Michael P Thomas, President
Charles C Thomas, Publisher

 $70.95

420 pages Year Founded: 1927 ISBN 0-398005-38-9

2811 Biology of Personality Disorders
American Psychiatric Publishing, Inc.
1000 Wilson Boulevard
Suite 1825
Arlington, VA 22209-3901
703-907-7322
800-368-5777; *Fax:* 703-907-1091
appi@psych.org
www.appi.org

Robert E Hales, M.D., M.B.A., Editor-in-Chief
Ron McMillen, Chief Executive Officer
John McDuffie, Editorial Director
RebeccaD. Rinehart, Publisher

Content topics include neurotransmitter function in personality disorders, new biological researcher strategies for personality disorders, the genetics psychobiology of the seven
- factor model of personality disorders, and significance of
biological research for a biopsychosocial model of personality disorders. *$25.00*

166 pages Year Founded: 1998 ISBN 0-880488-35-2

2812 Borderline Personality Disorder: A Therapist
Guide to Taking Control
WW Norton & Company
500 5th Avenue
New York, NY 10110-54
212-354-5500
800-233-4830; *Fax:* 212-869-0856
npb@wwnorton.com
www.books.wwnorton.com

Drake McFeely, CEO

From identification to relapse prevention, this guide helps
therapists manage a patient's treatment for the rather complex problem of Borderline Personality Disorder, an often
difficult and sometimes life threatening condition. *$27.50*

224 pages Year Founded: 1923 ISBN 0-393703-52-5

2813 Borderline Personality Disorder: Tailoring the
Psychotherapy to the Patient
American Psychiatric Publishing, Inc.
1000 Wilson Boulevard
Suite 1825
Arlington, VA 22209-3901
703-907-7322
800-368-5777; *Fax:* 703-907-1091
appi@psych.org
www.appi.org

Robert E Hales, M.D., M.B.A., Editor-in-Chief
Ron McMillen, Chief Executive Officer
John McDuffie, Editorial Director
RebeccaD. Rinehart, Publisher

 $34.00

256 pages Year Founded: 1996 ISBN 0-880486-89-9

2814 Cognitive Therapy for Personality Disorders: a
Schema-Focused Approach
Professional Resource Press
PO Box 3197
Sarasota, FL 34230-3197
941-343-9601
800-443-3364; *Fax:* 941-343-9201
cs.prpress@gmail.com
www.prpress.com

Laurie Girsch, Managing Editor

A guide to treating the most difficult cases in your practice:
personality disorders and other chronic, self - defeating
problems. Contains rationale, theory, practical applications,
and active cognitive behavioral techniques. *$13.95*

96 pages Year Founded: 1980 ISBN 1-568870-47-7

2815 Cognitive Therapy of Personality Disorders
Guilford Press
72 Spring Street
New York, NY 10012-4068
212-431-9800
800-365-7006; *Fax:* 212-966-6708
info@guilford.com
www.www.guilford.com

Bob Matloff, President
Seymour Weingarten, Editor-in-Chief

Focuses on the use of cognitive therapy to treat people with
personality disorders who do not usually engage in therapy.
Emanates the research and practical experience of Beck
and his associates and is the first to focus specifically on
this diverse and clinically demanding population. Case vignettes are used throughout. *$43.00*

396 pages Year Founded: 1973 ISBN 0-989624-34-7

2816 Dealing With the Problem of Low Self-Esteem:
Common Characteristics and Treatment
Charles C Thomas Publisher Ltd.
2600 S 1st Street
Springfield, IL 62704-4730
217-789-8980
800-258-8980; *Fax:* 217-789-9130

books@ccthomas.com
www.ccthomas.com

Michael P Thomas, President
Charles C Thomas, Publisher

Considers the practice of psychotherapy from the self-esteem perspective. Describes the common characteristics of low self-esteem that are manifested in clients with diverse problems; focuses on the functions the therapist performs in addressing these characteristics. The third is to consider the modalities of treatment through which the therapist delivers these therapeutic functions. *$ 48.95*

228 pages Year Founded: 1927 ISSN 0-398-05951-9ISBN 0-398059-36-5

2817 Disorders of Personality: DSM-IV and Beyond
John Wiley & Sons
111 River Street
Hoboken, NJ 07030-5774
201-748-6000; *Fax:* 201-748-6088
info@wiley.com
www.www.wiley.com

Stephen M. Smith, President and Chief Executive Of
Ellis E. Cousens, Executive Vice President, Chief
John Kritzmacher, Executive Vice President, Chief
MJ O'Leary, Senior Vice President, Human Res

Clarifies the distinctions between the vast array of personality disorders and helps clinicians make accurate diagnoses; thoroughly updated to incorporate the recent change in the DSM - IV. Guides the clinicians throught the intricate maze of personality disorders, with special attention on changes in their conceptualization over the last decade. DSM-V due out in 2013 *$85.00*

364 pages Year Founded: 1807 ISBN 0-471011-86-X

2818 Group Exercises for Enhancing Social Skills & Self-Esteem
Professional Resource Press
PO Box 3197
Sarasota, FL 34230-3197
941-343-9601
800-443-3364; *Fax:* 941-343-9201
cs.prpress@gmail.com
www.prpress.com

Laurie Girsch, Managing Editor

Includes exercises for enhancing self-esteem utilizing proven social, emotional, and cognitive skill-building techniques. These exercises are useful in therapeutic, psychoeducational, and recreational settings. *$24.95*

150 pages Year Founded: 1980 ISBN 1-568870-20-5

2819 Personality Characteristics of the Personality Disordered
John Wiley & Sons
111 River Street
Hoboken, NJ 07030-5774
201-748-6000; *Fax:* 201-748-6088
info@wiley.com
www.www.wiley.com

Stephen M. Smith, President and Chief Executive Of
Ellis E. Cousens, Executive Vice President, Chief
John Kritzmacher, Executive Vice President, Chief
MJ O'Leary, Senior Vice President, Human Res

364 pages Year Founded: 1807

2820 Personality Disorders and Culture: Clinical and Conceptual Interactions
John Wiley & Sons
111 River Street
Hoboken, NJ 07030-5774
201-748-6000; *Fax:* 201-748-6088
info@wiley.com
www.www.wiley.com

Stephen M. Smith, President and Chief Executive Of
Ellis E. Cousens, Executive Vice President, Chief
John Kritzmacher, Executive Vice President, Chief
MJ O'Leary, Senior Vice President, Human Res

Discusses two of the most timely and complex areas in mental health, personality disorders and the impact of cultural variables. Treading on the timeless nature - nurture debate, it suggests that social variables have a dramatic impact on the definition, development, and manifestation of personality disorders.

364 pages Year Founded: 1807

2821 Personality and Stress: Individual Differences in the Stress Process
John Wiley & Sons
111 River Street
Hoboken, NJ 07030-5774
201-748-6000; *Fax:* 201-748-6088
info@wiley.com
www.www.wiley.com

Stephen M. Smith, President and Chief Executive Of
Ellis E. Cousens, Executive Vice President, Chief
John Kritzmacher, Executive Vice President, Chief
MJ O'Leary, Senior Vice President, Human Res

364 pages Year Founded: 1807

2822 Psychotherapy for Borderline Personality
John Wiley & Sons
111 River Street
Hoboken, NJ 07030-5774
201-748-6000; *Fax:* 201-748-6088
info@wiley.com
www.www.wiley.com

Stephen M. Smith, President and Chief Executive Of
Ellis E. Cousens, Executive Vice President, Chief
John Kritzmacher, Executive Vice President, Chief
MJ O'Leary, Senior Vice President, Human Res

Based on the work of a research team, this manual offers techniques and strategies for treating patients with Borderline Personality Disorder using Transference Focused Psychology. Provides therapists with an overall strategy for treating BPD patients and helpful tactics for working with individual patients on a session by session basis.

364 pages Year Founded: 1807

2823 Role of Sexual Abuse in the Etiology of Borderline Personality Disorder
200 E Joppa Road
PO Box 436
Brooklandville, MD 21022-0436
410-825-8888
888-825-8249; *Fax:* 410-560-0134
sidran@sidran.org
www.sidran.org

Esther Giller, President and Director
Sheila Sidran Giller, Secretary/Treasurer

J. G. Goellner, Director Emeritus
Tracy Howard, Book Sales/Office Manager

Presenting the latest generation of research findings about the impact of traumatic abuse on the development of BPD. This book focuses on the theoretical basis of BPD, including topics such as childhood factors associated with the development, the relationship of child sexual abuse to dissociation and self mutilation, severity of childhood abuse, borderline symptoms and family environment. Twenty six contributors cover every aspect of BPD as it relates to childhood sexual abuse. *$42.00*

345 pages Year Founded: 1986

2824 Shorter Term Treatments for Borderline Personality Disorders
NewHarbinger Publications
5674 Shattuck Avenue
Oakland, CA 94609-1662
510-652-0215
800-748-6273; *Fax:* 510-652-5472
customerservice@newharbinger.com
www.newharbinger.com

Matthew McKay, Owner
Patrick Fanning, Co-Founder

This guide offers approaches designed to help clients stabilize emotions, decrease vulnerability and work toward a more adaptive day to day functioning. *$49.95*

184 pages Year Founded: 1973 ISBN 1-572240-92-X

Schizophrenia Spectrum and Other Psychotic Disorders

2825 Behavioral High-Risk Paradigm in Psychopathology
Springer-Verlag New York
175 5th Avenue
New York, NY 10010-7703
212-477-8200
800-777-4643; *Fax:* 212-473-6272
custserv@springer-ny.com
www.www.springer.com

Derk Haank, CEO
Martin Moss, COO
Ulrich Vest, CFO

Examines both traditional clinical research on psychopathology and psychophysiological research on psychopathology, with an emphasis on risk for schizophrenia and for mood disorders. Complementing treatments of risk for psychopathology in other sources which emphasize either genetic factors or large-scale psychosocial factors, chapters focus on research in specific areas of each disorder. Hardcover. *$98.00*

304 pages Year Founded: 1842 ISBN 0-387945-04-0

2826 Cognitive Therapy for Delusions, Voices, and Paranoia
John Wiley & Sons
111 River Street
Hoboken, NJ 07030-5774
201-748-6000; *Fax:* 201-748-6088
info@wiley.com
www.www.wiley.com

Stephen M. Smith, President and Chief Executive Of
Ellis E. Cousens, Executive Vice President, Chief

John Kritzmacher, Executive Vice President, Chief
MJ O'Leary, Senior Vice President, Human Res

A cognitive view of delusions and voices. The practice of therapy and the problem of engagement.

364 pages Year Founded: 1807

2827 Delusional Beliefs
John Wiley & Sons
111 River Street
Hoboken, NJ 07030-5774
201-748-6000; *Fax:* 201-748-6088
info@wiley.com
www.www.wiley.com

Stephen M. Smith, President and Chief Executive Of
Ellis E. Cousens, Executive Vice President, Chief
John Kritzmacher, Executive Vice President, Chief
MJ O'Leary, Senior Vice President, Human Res

Unique collection of ideas and empirical data provided by leading experts in a variety of disciplines. Each offers perspectives on questions such as: What criteria should be used to identify, describe and classify delusions? How can delusional individuals be identified? What distinguishes delusions from normal beliefs? *$95.00*

364 pages Year Founded: 1807 ISBN 0-471836-35-4

2828 Families Coping with Schizophrenia: Practitioner's Guide to Family Groups
John Wiley & Sons
111 River Street
Hoboken, NJ 07030-5774
201-748-6000; *Fax:* 201-748-6088
info@wiley.com
www.www.wiley.com

Stephen M. Smith, President and Chief Executive Of
Ellis E. Cousens, Executive Vice President, Chief
John Kritzmacher, Executive Vice President, Chief
MJ O'Leary, Senior Vice President, Human Res

364 pages Year Founded: 1807

2829 Practice Guideline for the Treatment of Patients with Schizophrenia
American Psychiatric Publishing, Inc.
1000 Wilson Boulevard
Suite 1825
Arlington, VA 22209-3901
703-907-7322
800-368-5777; *Fax:* 703-907-1091
appi@psych.org
www.appi.org

Robert E Hales, M.D., M.B.A., Editor-in-Chief
Ron McMillen, Chief Executive Officer
John McDuffie, Editorial Director
RebeccaD. Rinehart, Publisher

$22.00

146 pages Year Founded: 1997

2830 Schizophrenia Revealed: From Nuerons to Social Interactions
WW Norton & Company
500 5th Avenue
New York, NY 10110-54
212-354-5500
800-233-4830; *Fax:* 212-869-0856

admalmud@wwnorton.com
www.books.wwnorton.com

Drake McFeely, CEO

Helps explain some of the former mysteries of Schizophrenia that are now possible to study through advances in neuroscience. *$ 10.80*

Year Founded: 1923 ISBN 0-398704-48-1

Sexual Disorders

2831 Assessing Sex Offenders: Problems and Pitfalls
Charles C Thomas Publisher Ltd.
PO Box 19265
Springfield, IL 62794-9265
217-789-8980
800-258-8980; *Fax:* 217-789-9130
www.ccthomas.com

Charles C Thomas, Publisher

This book reviews the scientific evidence relevant to assessing the recidivism risk of sex offenders. Too often, the issues detailed in these chapters have been overlooked and/or misinterpreted. As a result, the likelihood of psychologists misusing and abusing scientific data when assessing sex offenders whould not be underestimated. The text identifies numerous instances of such misuse and abuse. Paperback is available for $41.95. *$61.95*

266 pages Year Founded: 1927 ISBN 0-398075-02-6

2832 Cognitive Therapy in Practice
WW Norton & Company
500 5th Avenue
New York, NY 10110-54
212-354-5500
800-233-4830; *Fax:* 212-869-0856
npd@wwnorton.com
www.books.wwnorton.com

Drake McFeely, CEO

Basic text for graduate studies in psychotherapy, psycholgy nursing social work and counseling. *$29.00*

224 pages Year Founded: 1923 ISBN 0-393700-77-1

2833 Erectile Dysfunction: Integrating Couple
Therapy, Sex Therapy and Medical Treatment
WW Norton & Company
500 5th Avenue
New York, NY 10110-54
212-354-5500; *Fax:* 212-869-0856
admalmud@wwnorton.com
www.books.wwnorton.com

Drake McFeely, CEO

Helpful to marriage and couple therapists, very up to date and encompassing, with simple and professional writing. *$30.00*

208 pages Year Founded: 1923 ISSN 70330-4

2834 Hypoactive Sexual Desire: Integrating Sex and
Couple Therapy
WW Norton & Company
500 5th Avenue
New York, NY 10110-54
212-354-5500; *Fax:* 212-869-0856
admalmud@wwnorton.com
www.books.wwnorton.com

Drake McFeely, CEO

Discussion of treating the couple, not the individual with lack of desire, the authors include distinguishing between organic and psychogenic problems plus how to combine relational and sex therapy. Although lack of desire is one of the most common problems couples face, it is one of the most challenging to treat. *$30.00*

288 pages Year Founded: 1923 ISSN 70344-4

Somatic Symptom and Related Disorders

2835 Anatomy of a Psychiatric Illness: Healing the
Mind and the Brain
American Psychiatric Publishing, Inc.
1000 Wilson Boulevard
Suite 1825
Arlington, VA 22209-3901
703-907-7322
800-368-5777; *Fax:* 703-907-1091
appi@psych.org
www.appi.org

Robert E Hales, M.D., M.B.A., Editor-in-Chief
Ron McMillen, Chief Executive Officer
John McDuffie, Editorial Director
RebeccaD. Rinehart, Publisher

 $22.95

232 pages Year Founded: 1993

2836 Concise Guide to Neuropsychiatry and
Behavioral Neurology
American Psychiatric Publishing, Inc.
1000 Wilson Boulevard
Suite 1825
Arlington, VA 22209-3901
703-907-7322
800-368-5777; *Fax:* 703-907-1091
appi@psych.org
www.appi.org

Robert E Hales, M.D., M.B.A., Editor-in-Chief
Ron McMillen, Chief Executive Officer
John McDuffie, Editorial Director
RebeccaD. Rinehart, Publisher

Provides brief synopsis of the major neuropsychiatric and neurobehavioral syndromes, discusses their clinical assessment, and provides guidelines for management. *$21.00*

368 pages Year Founded: 1995 ISBN 0-880483-43-1

2837 Concise Guide to Psychodynamic
Psychotherapy: Principles and Techniques in
the Era of Managed Care
American Psychiatric Publishing, Inc.
1000 Wilson Boulevard
Suite 1825
Arlington, VA 22209-3901
703-907-7322
800-368-5777; *Fax:* 703-907-1091
appi@psych.org
www.appi.org

Robert E Hales, M.D., M.B.A., Editor-in-Chief
Ron McMillen, Chief Executive Officer
John McDuffie, Editorial Director
RebeccaD. Rinehart, Publisher

Thoroughly updated coverage of all the major principles and important issues in psychodynamic psychotherapy and issues not commonly addressed in the standard training curriculum, including the office setting, suicidal and dangerous patients, and what to do when the therapist makes an error. *$21.00*

272 pages Year Founded: 1998 ISBN 0-880483-47-4

2838 Manual of Panic: Focused Psychodynamic Psychotherapy
American Psychiatric Publishing, Inc.
1000 Wilson Boulevard
Suite 1825
Arlington, VA 22209-3901
703-907-7322
800-368-5777; *Fax:* 703-907-1091
appi@psych.org
www.appi.org

Robert E Hales, M.D., M.B.A., Editor-in-Chief
Ron McMillen, Chief Executive Officer
John McDuffie, Editorial Director
RebeccaD. Rinehart, Publisher

A psychodynamic formulation applicable to many or most patients with Axis 1 panic disorders. *$28.00*

112 pages Year Founded: 1997 ISBN 0-880488-71-9

2839 Munchausen Syndrome by Proxy: Issues in Diagnosis and Treatment
Lexington Books
4501 Forbes Boulevard
Suite 200
Lanham, MD 20706-4346
301-459-3365

AV Levin, Editor
MS Sheridan, Editor

Reference/Resource material for professionals.

Year Founded: 1995

2840 Somatization, Physical Symptoms and Psychological Illness
American Psychiatric Publishing, Inc.
1000 Wilson Boulevard
Suite 1825
Arlington, VA 22209-3901
703-907-7322
800-368-5777; *Fax:* 703-907-1091
appi@psych.org
www.appi.org

Robert E Hales, M.D., M.B.A., Editor-in-Chief
Ron McMillen, Chief Executive Officer
John McDuffie, Editorial Director
RebeccaD. Rinehart, Publisher

$99.95

351 pages Year Founded: 1990 ISBN 0-632028-39-4

2841 Somatoform Dissociation: Phenomena, Measurement, and Theoretical Issues
WW Norton & Company
500 5th Avenue
New York, NY 10110-54
212-354-5500
800-233-4830; *Fax:* 212-869-0856
npb@wwnorton.com
www.books.wwnorton.com

Drake McFeely, CEO

In this first North Americacn edition of his work, Nijenhuis expands upon his theory of somatoform dissociation by providing two new chapters-one on dissociation and the re-

call of sexual abuse and a second on the phycometric characteristics of the Traumatic Experiences Checklist (TEC).

Year Founded: 1923 ISBN 0-393704-60-2

2842 Somatoform and Factitious Disorders
American Psychiatric Publishing, Inc.
1000 Wilson Boulevard
Suite 1825
Arlington, VA 22209-3901
703-907-7322
800-368-5777; *Fax:* 703-907-1091
appi@psych.org
www.appi.org

Robert E Hales, M.D., M.B.A., Editor-in-Chief
Ron McMillen, Chief Executive Officer
John McDuffie, Editorial Director
RebeccaD. Rinehart, Publisher

Consise yet thorough, this book covers Factitious disorders, Somatization disorder, Conversion disorder, Hypochondriasis and Body dysmorphic disorder. Explores the latest on these conditions and emphasises the need for further research to improve patient treament and understanding. *$29.95*

208 pages Year Founded: 2001 ISBN 1-585620-29-7

Substance-Related and Addictive Disorders

2843 Addiction Treatment Homework Planner
John Wiley & Sons
10475 Crosspoint Boulevard
Indianapolis, IN 46256-3386
317-572-3000; *Fax:* 317-572-4000
consumers@wiley.com
www.wiley.com

James R Finley, Author
Brenda S Lenz, Author

Helps clients suffering from chemical and nonchemical addictions develop the skills they need to work through problems. *$ 49.95*

384 pages ISBN 0-471274-59-3

2844 Addiction Treatment Planner
John Wiley & Sons
10475 Crosspoint Boulevard
Indianapolis, IN 46256-3386
317-572-3000; *Fax:* 317-572-4000
www.wiley.com

Robert R Perkinson, Editor
Arthur E. Jongsma, Jr., Editor

Provides all the elements necessary to quickly and easily develop formal treatment plans that satisfy the demands of HMOs, managed care companies, third-party payers, and state and federal review agencies. *$49.95*

384 pages ISBN 0-471418-14-5

2845 Addictive Behaviors Across the Life Span
Sage Publications
2455 Teller Road
Thousand Oaks, CA 91320-2234
805-499-0721
800-818-7243; *Fax:* 805-499-0871

info@sagepub.com
www.sagepub.com

John S Baer, Author
G Alan Marlatt, Author
Robert J McMahon, Author

Leading scholars, researchers and clinicians in the field of addictive behavior provide and examination of drug dependency from a life span perspective in this authoritative volume. Four general topic areas include: etiology; early intervention; integrated treatment; and policy issues across the life span. Other topics include biopsychosocial perspectives on the intergenerational transmission of alcoholism to children and reducing the risks of addictive behaviors. *$59.95*

358 pages Year Founded: 1993 ISBN 0-803950-78-0

2846 Addictive Thinking: Understanding Self-Deception
Health Communications
292 Fernwood Avenue
Edison, NJ 08837-3839
732-346-0027; *Fax:* 732-346-0442
www.hcomm.com

Exposes the irrational and contradictory patterns of addictive thinking, and shows how to overcome them and barriers they create; low self-esteem and relapse.

140 pages ISBN 1-568381-38-7

2847 Adolescents, Alcohol and Drugs: A Practical Guide for Those Who Work With Young People
Charles C Thomas Publisher Ltd.
2600 S 1st Street
Springfield, IL 62704-4730
217-789-8980
800-258-8980; *Fax:* 217-789-9130
books@ccthomas.com
www.ccthomas.com

Michael P Thomas, President

 $41.95

210 pages Year Founded: 1988 ISBN 0-398053-93-6

2848 American Psychiatric Press Textbook of Substance Abuse Treatment
American Psychiatric Publishing, Inc.
1000 Wilson Boulevard
Suite 1825
Arlington, VA 22209-3901
703-907-7322
800-368-5777; *Fax:* 703-907-1091
appi@psych.org
www.appi.org

Marc Galanter, M.D, Editor
Herbert D. Kleber, M.D, Editor
John McDuffie, Editorial Director

Comprehensive view of basic science and psychology underlying addiction and coverage of all treatment modalities. New topics include the neurobiology of alcoholism, stimulants, marijuana, opiates and hallucinogens, club drugs, and addiction in women. *$95.00*

770 pages Year Founded: 2008 ISBN 0-880488-20-4

2849 An Elephant in the Living Room: Leader's Guide for Helping Children of Alcoholics
Hazelden
15251 Pleasant Valley Road
PO Box 176
Center City, MN 55012-176
651-213-2121
800-328-9000; *Fax:* 651-213-4590
www.hazelden.org

Marion H Typpo PhD, Co-Author
Jill M Hastings PhD, Co-Author

Practical guidance for education and health professionals who help young people cope with a family member's chemical dependency. *$9.95*

144 pages ISBN 1-568380-34-8

2850 Assessing Substance Abusers with the Million Clinical Multiaxial Inventory
Charles C Thomas Publisher Ltd.
PO Box 19265
Springfield, IL 62794-9265
217-789-8980
800-258-8980; *Fax:* 217-789-9130
www.ccthomas.com

The construct validity of a psychological test is assessed by a multitrai-multimethod nomothetic matrix, which means that the psychometric properties of an assessment instrument are studied with a variety of populations and in a variety of settings and weighed against a variety of other measures that purportedly assess the same construct.This concept implies that a test might have strong validity with some populations and weak validity with others, and this is the central theme of this book. Also, the book comes in paperback for only $26.95. *$ 46.95*

164 pages Year Founded: 2005 ISBN 0-398075-91-3

2851 Before It's Too Late: Working with Substance Abuse in the Family
WW Norton & Company
500 5th Avenue
New York, NY 10110-54
212-354-5500; *Fax:* 212-869-0856
admalmud@wwnorton.com
www.books.wwnorton.com/

David C. Treadway, Author

Sometimes, the problem a patient or the family of the patient's root cause to the problem they seek help for, is actually substance abuse. How to present the problem, and step-by-step models for working with families dealing with substance abuse are examined. *$ 23.95*

224 pages Year Founded: 1989 ISBN 0-393700-68-2

2852 Behind Bars: Substance Abuse and America's Prison Population
Center on Addiction at Columbia University
633 3rd Avenue
19th Floor
New York, NY 10017-8155
212-841-5200; *Fax:* 212-956-8020
www.casacolumbia.org

William H Foster, CEO

Results of a three year study of American prisons and the reason drugs are responsible for the booming prison population and escalating costs. *$25.00*

Year Founded: 1998

2853 Blaming the Brain: The Truth About Drugs and Mental Health
Free Press
866 3rd Avenue
New York, NY 10022-6221
212-744-0379
800-323-7445
www.freepeople.com

Erin Legg, Manager

Exposes weaknesses inherent in the scientific arguments supporting the theory that biochemical imbalances are the main cause of mental illness. It discusses how the accidental discovery of mood-altering drugs stimulated an interest in psychopharmacology. *$25.00*

320 pages Year Founded: 1998 ISBN 0-684849-64-X

2854 Building Bridges: States Respond to Substance Abuse and Welfare Reform
Center on Addiction at Columbia University
633 3rd Avenue
19th Floor
New York, NY 10017-8155
212-841-5200; *Fax:* 212-956-8020
www.casacolumbia.org

William H Foster, CEO

Prepared in partnership with the American Public Human Services Association, this two year study among the front line workers in the nation's welfare offices, job training programs and substance abuse agencies reveals what they find works and does not work in helping clients. *$15.00*

Year Founded: 1999

2855 CASAWORKS for Families: Promising Approach to Welfare Reform and Substance-Abusing Women
Center on Addiction at Columbia University
633 3rd Avenue
19th Floor
New York, NY 10017-8155
212-841-5200; *Fax:* 212-956-8020
www.casacolumbia.org

William H Foster, CEO

Designed for TANF recipients, this promising approach to welfare reform is used in 11 cities and nine states. *$5.00*

Year Founded: 2001

2856 Clinician's Guide to the Personality Profiles of Alcohol and Drug Abusers: Typological Descriptions Using the MMPI
Charles C Thomas Publisher Ltd.
2600 S 1st Street
Springfield, IL 62704-4730
217-789-8980
800-258-8980; *Fax:* 217-789-9130
books@ccthomas.com
www.ccthomas.com

Michael P Thomas, President
Dennis M Eshbaugh, Author
Michael A Murphy, Author

$39.95

156 pages Year Founded: 1993 ISSN 0-399-06463-6ISBN 0-398058-85-7

2857 Critical Incidents: Ethical Issues in Substance Abuse Prevention and Treatment
Hazelden
15251 Pleasant Valley Road
PO Box 176
Center City, MN 55012-176
651-213-2121
800-328-9000; *Fax:* 651-213-4590
www.hazelden.org

Two hundred critical situations for health care professionals to sharpen their decision-making skills about everyday ethical dilemmas that arise in their field. *$17.95*

276 pages ISBN 0-938475-03-7

2858 Dangerous Liaisons: Substance Abuse and Sex
Center on Addiction at Columbia University
633 3rd Avenue
19th Floor
New York, NY 10017-8155
212-841-5200; *Fax:* 212-956-8020
www.casacolumbia.org

William H Foster, CEO

An intensive report on the dangerous and sometimes life-threatening connection between alcohol, drug abuse and sexual activity. Parents, guidance professionals and others will find this useful. *$22.00*

170 pages Year Founded: 1999

2859 Determinants of Substance Abuse: Biological, Psychological, and Environmental Factors
Kluwer Academic/Plenum Publishers
233 Spring Street
New York, NY 10013-1522
212-242-1490

Mark Galizio, Editor
Stephen A. Maisto, Editor

Hardcover. *$90.00*

443 pages Year Founded: 1985 ISBN 0-306418-73-8

2860 Drug Information for Teens: Health Tips About the Physical and Mental Effects of Substance Abuse
Omnigraphics
615 Giswold
Detroit, MI 48226-3900
313-961-1340; *Fax:* 313-961-1383
info@omnigraphics.com
www.omnigraphics.com

Provides students with facts about drug use, abuse, and addiction. It describes the physical and mental effects of alcohol, tobacco, marijuana, ecstasy, inhalants and many other drugs and chemicals that are often abused. It includes information about the process that leads from casual use to addiction and offers suggestions for resisting peer pressure and helping friends stay drug free.

452 pages ISBN 0-780804-44-9

2861 Ethics for Addiction Professionals
Hazelden
15251 Pleasant Valley Road
PO Box 176
Center City, MN 55012-176

651-213-2121
800-328-9000; *Fax:* 651-213-4590
www.hazelden.org

The first on ethics written by and for addiction professionals that addresses complex issues such as patient confidentiality versus mandatory reporting, clinician relapse, personal and social relationships with clients and other important related issues. *$14.95*

60 pages ISBN 0-894864-54-8

2862 Hispanic Substance Abuse
Charles C Thomas Publisher Ltd.
2600 S 1st Street
Springfield, IL 62704-4730
217-789-8980
800-258-8980; *Fax:* 217-789-9130
books@ccthomas.com
www.ccthomas.com

Michael P Thomas, President

Addresses the concerns of students and professionals who work with Hispanics. Brings together current research on this problem by well-known experts in the fields of alcohol and drug abuse. Useful for scholars and researchers, practitioners in the human services, and the general public. There is shown the extent of substance abuse problems in Hispanic communities, the differences between the Hispanic subgroups and the casual factors that are involved. There are detailed strategies for prevention and the necessary approaches to treatment. *$57.95*

258 pages Year Founded: 1993 ISSN 0-398-06274-9ISBN 0-398058-49-0

2863 Jail Detainees with Co-Occurring Mental Health and Substance Use Disorders
Policy Research Associates
345 Delaware Avenue
Delmar, NY 12054-1905
518-439-7415
800-444-7415; *Fax:* 518-439-7612
pra@prainc.com
www.prainc.com

Henry Steadman, President

Brief report that discusses the issue of keeping federal benefits for jail detainees.

2864 Love First: A New Approach to Intervention for Alcoholism and Drug Addiction
Hazelden
15245 Pleasant Valley Road
PO Box 11-CO 3
Center City, MN 55012-9640
651-257-4010
800-257-7810; *Fax:* 651-213-4394
www.hazelden.org

Mark Mishek, CEO

A straightforward, simple and practical resource written specifically for families seeking to help a loved one struggling with substance addiction.

280 pages ISBN 1-568385-21-8

2865 Malignant Neglect: Substance Abuse and America's Schools
Center on Addiction at Columbia University
633 3rd Avenue
19th Floor
New York, NY 10017-8155
212-841-5200; *Fax:* 212-956-8020
www.casacolumbia.org

William H Foster, CEO

Six years of exhaustive research of focus groups, schools, parents and professionals. Findings of the costs of drug abuse in dollars, student behavior, truancy and more. *$22.00*

117 pages Year Founded: 2001

2866 Missed Opportunity: National Survey of Primary Care Physicians and Patients on Substance Abuse
Center on Addiction at Columbia University
633 3rd Avenue
19th Floor
New York, NY 10017-8155
212-841-5200; *Fax:* 212-956-8020
www.casacolumbia.org

William H Foster, CEO

Findings and recomendations based on a CASA report that revealed 94% of primary care physicians fail to diagnose symptoms of alcohol abuse in adult patients, and 41% of pediatricians missed a diagnosis of drug abuse when presented with a classic description of a teenage patient with these symptoms. The report also sheds light on the fact that many physicians feel unprepared to diagnose substance abuse and have little confidence in the effectiveness of treatments available. *$22.00*

Year Founded: 2000

2867 Motivational Interviewing: Prepare People to Change Addictive Behavior
Hazelden
15251 Pleasant Valley Road
PO Box 176
Center City, MN 55012-176
651-213-2121
800-328-9000; *Fax:* 651-213-4590
www.hazelden.org

William K Miller, Co-Author
Stephen Rollnick, Co-Author

A key resource for clinical psychologists, social workers and chemical dependency counselors for mastering interviewing skills and working with resistant clients. *$21.95*

348 pages ISBN 0-898624-69-X

2868 Narrative Means to Sober Ends: Treating Addiction and Its Aftermath
Guilford Press
72 Spring Street
New York, NY 10012-4068
212-431-9800
800-365-7006; *Fax:* 212-966-6708
info@guilford.com

Jonathan Diamond, Author

This eloquently written volume illuminates the devastating power of addiction and describes an array of innovative approaches to facilitating clients' recovery. Demonstrated are creative ways to help clients explore their relationship to drugs and alcohol, take the first steps toward sobriety and develop meaningful ways of living without addiction. *$37.95*

386 pages ISBN 1-572305-66-5

2869 No Place to Hide: Substance Abuse in Mid-Size Cities and Rural America
Center on Addiction at Columbia University
633 3rd Avenue
19th Floor
New York, NY 10017-8155
212-841-5200; *Fax:* 212-956-8020
www.casacolumbia.org

William H Foster, CEO

Surprisingly to some, young people in smaller cities and rural areas are more likely to use many forms of illegal substances. Tobacco use is also higher away from the major cities. The findings on other statistics of drugs and rural adolescent and teenager use are included. *$10.00*

Year Founded: 2000

2870 No Safe Haven: Children of Substance-Abusing Parents
Center on Addiction at Columbia University
633 3rd Avenue
19th Floor
New York, NY 10017-8155
212-841-5200; *Fax:* 212-956-8020
www.casacolumbia.org

William H Foster, CEO
Peggy Macchetto, Author
Susan Foster, Author

Comprehensive report with shattering facts and figures reveals the impact of substance abuse on parenting skills and child neglect. The number of children affected by their parent's substance abuse driven behavior has more than doubled in the last ten years, greater than the rise in children's overall population. This report calls for a reworking of the child welfare system, and provides guidelines to when the child should be permanently remove from the home. *$22.00*

Year Founded: 1999

2871 Non Medical Marijuana: Rite of Passage or Russian Roulette?
Center on Addiction at Columbia University
633 3rd Avenue
19th Floor
New York, NY 10017-8155
212-841-5200; *Fax:* 212-956-8020
www.casacolumbia.org

William H Foster, CEO

The most recent numbers available find that more teens from 19 years old and younger enter treatment for marijuana abuse than for any other drug, including alcohol. Many teens also have a problem with secondary drugs. This report released by CASA at Columbia University, concludes that non medical marijuana is indeed a dangerous substance. *$20.00*

Year Founded: 1999

2872 Perfect Daughters
Health Communications
292 Fernwood Avenue
Edison, NJ 08837-3839
732-346-0027; *Fax:* 732-346-0442

Identifies what differentiates the adult daughters of alcoholics from other women. Adult daughters of alcoholics operate from a base of harsh and limiting views of themselves and the world. Having learned that they must function perfectly in order to avoid unpleasant situations, these women often assume responsibility for the failures of others. They are drawn to chemically dependent men and are more likely to become addicted themselves. This book collects the thoughts, feelings and experience of twelve hundred perfect daughters, offering readers an opportunity to explore their own life's dynamics and thereby heal and grow.

350 pages ISBN 1-558749-52-7

2873 Principles of Addiction Medicine
American Society of Addiction Medicine
4601 N Park Avenue
Suite 101, Upper Arcade
Chevy Chase, MD 20815-4519
301-656-3920
800-844-8948; *Fax:* 301-656-3815
www.asam.org

Eileen McGrath, Executive VP

Textbook on the basic and clinical science of prevention and treatment of alcohol, nicotine, and other drug dependencies and addictions. *$155.00*

1338 pages ISBN 1-880425-04-0

2874 Proven Youth Development Model that Prevents Substance Abuse and Builds Communities
Center on Addiction at Columbia University
633 3rd Avenue
19th Floor
New York, NY 10017-8155
212-841-5200; *Fax:* 212-956-8020
www.casacolumbia.org

William H Foster, CEO

How-to manual developed with nine years of research. The program is a collaboration of local school, law enforcement, social service and health teams to help high risk youth between the ages of 8 - 13 years old and their families prevent substance abuse and violent behavior. Used in 23 urban and rural communities in 11 states and the District of Columbia. *$50.00*

79 pages Year Founded: 2001

2875 Psychological Theories of Drinking and Alcoholism
Guilford Press
72 Spring Street
New York, NY 10012-4068
212-431-9800
800-365-7006; *Fax:* 212-966-6708
info@guilford.com

Howard T. Blane, Editor
Kenneth E. Leonard, Editor

Multidisciplinary approach discusses biological, pharmacological and social factors that influence drinking and alcoholism. Contributors review established and emerging approaches that guide research into the psychological processes influencing drinking and alcoholism. *$47.95*

467 pages Year Founded: 1999 ISBN 1-572304-10-3

2876 Relapse Prevention Maintenance: Strategies in the Treatment of Addictive Behaviors
Guilford Press
72 Spring Street
New York, NY 10012-4068
212-431-9800
800-365-7006; *Fax:* 212-966-6708
info@guilford.com

G. Alan Marlatt PhD, Editor
Dennis M. Donovan PhD, Editor

Research on relapse prevention to problem drinking, smoking, substance abuse, eating disorders and compulsive gambling. Analyzes factors that may lead to relapse and offers practical techniques for maintaining treatment gains. *$55.00*

416 pages Year Founded: 1985 ISBN 0-898620-09-0

2877 Relapse Prevention Maintenance: Strategies in the Treatment of Addictive Behaviors
Guilford Press
72 Spring Street
New York, NY 10012-4068
212-431-9800
800-365-7006; *Fax:* 212-966-6708
info@guilford.com

G. Alan Marlatt PhD, Editor
Dennis M. Donovan PhD, Editor

Research on relapse prevention to problem drinking, smoking, substance abuse, eating disorders and compulsive gambling. Analyzes factors that may lead to relapse and offers practical techniques for maintaining treatment gains. *$55.00*

416 pages Year Founded: 1985 ISBN 0-898620-09-0

2878 So Help Me God: Substance Abuse, Religion and Spirituality
Center on Addiction at Columbia University
633 3rd Avenue
19th Floor
New York, NY 10017-8155
212-841-5200; *Fax:* 212-956-8020
www.casacolumbia.org

William H Foster, CEO

Results of a 2 year study, finding that spirituality has enormous power to potentially lower the risks of substance abuse. When this is combined with professional treatment, an individual's religion helps greatly with recovery. *$10.00*

Year Founded: 2001

2879 Solutions Step by Step: Substance Abuse Treatment Manual
WW Norton & Company
500 5th Avenue
New York, NY 10110-54
212-354-5500; *Fax:* 212-869-0856
admalmud@wwnorton.com
www.books.wwnorton.com/

Insoo Kim Berg, Author
Norman H. Reuss, Author

Quick tips, questions and examples focusing on successes that can be experienced helping substance abusers help themselves. *$ 25.00*

192 pages Year Founded: 1997 ISSN 70251-0

2880 Substance Abuse and Learning Disabilities: Peas in a Pod or Apples and Oranges?
Center on Addiction at Columbia University
633 3rd Avenue
19th Floor
New York, NY 10017-8155
212-841-5200; *Fax:* 212-956-8020
www.casacolumbia.org

William H Foster, CEO

Report originating from a conference in 1999 sponsored by CASA, the relationship between learning disabilities that are not addressed, and possible substance abuse by these same children is examined. Attention Deficit/Hyperactivity Disorder and Conduct Disorder and the link to substance abuse is also considered. *$10.00*

00 pages

2881 Substance Abuse: A Comprehensive Textbook
Lippincott Williams & Wilkins
PO Box 1600
Hagerstown, MD 21741-1600
301-714-2300
800-638-3030; *Fax:* 301-824-7390
www.lww.com

$162.00

956 pages Year Founded: 1997 ISBN 0-683181-79-3

2882 Teens and Alcohol: Gallup Youth Survey Major Issues and Trends
Mason Crest Publishers
450 Parkway Drive
Suite D
Broomall, PA 19008-4017
866-627-2665; *Fax:* 610-543-3878
gbrffr@masoncrest.com
www.masoncrest.com

Eighty-seven percent of high school seniors have tried alcohol and, according to a Gallup Youth Survey, 27 percent of teenagers say it is very easy for them to get alcoholic beverages. Alcohol is a contributor to the three leading causes of death for teens and young adults: automobile crashes, homicide and suicides.

112 pages ISBN 1-590847-23-7

2883 Therapeutic Communities for Addictions: Reading in Theory, Research, and Practice
Charles C Thomas Publisher Ltd.
2600 S 1st Street
Springfield, IL 62704-4730
217-789-8980
800-258-8980; *Fax:* 217-789-9130
books@ccthomas.com
www.ccthomas.com

Michael P Thomas, President
James T Ziegenfuss Jr, Author

Contents: The Therapeutic Community (TC) for Substance Abuse; Democratic TCs or Programmatic TCs or Both?; Motivational Aspects of Heroin Addicts in TCs; A Sociological View of the TC; Psychodynamics of TCs for Treatment of Heroin Addicts; Britain and the Psychoanalytic Tradition in TCs; TC Research; Outcomes of Drug Abuse Treatment; 12-Year Follow-up Outcomes, College Training in a TC; Client Evaluations of TCs and Retention; Side Bets and Secondary Adjustments; Measuring Program Implementation; The TC Looking Ahead; TCs within Prisons; Uses and Abuses of Power and Authority. *$51.95*

282 pages Year Founded: 1986 ISBN 0-398052-06-9

2884 Treating Substance Abuse: Part 1
American Counseling Association
5999 Stevenson Avenue
Alexandria, VA 22304-3304
703-823-9800
800-422-2648; *Fax:* 703-823-0252
TDD: 703-823-6862
webmaster@counseling.org
www.counseling.org

Richard Yep, Executive Director

The first of a two-volume set presents up-to-date findings on the treatment of alcoholism and addiction to cocaine, caffeine, hallucinogens, and marijuana. Techniques and case examples are offered from a variety of approaches, including motivational enhancement therapy, marriage and family therapy as well as cognitive-behavioral. *$26.95*

280 pages ISBN 1-886330-48-4

2885 Treating Substance Abuse: Part 2
American Counseling Association
5999 Stevenson Avenue
Alexandria, VA 22304-3304
703-823-9800
800-422-2648; *Fax:* 703-823-0252
webmaster@counseling.org
www.counseling.org

Richard Yep, Executive Director

For treating select populations of substance-abusing clients, including those with disabilities, psychiatric disorders, schizophrenia and major depression. Also serves adolescents, older adults, pregnant women and clients whose addictions affect their ability to function in the workplace. *$29.95*

311 pages ISBN 1-886330-49-2

2886 Treating the Alcoholic: Developmental Model of Recovery
John Wiley & Sons
605 3rd Avenue
New York, NY 10158-180
212-850-6301
info@wiley.com

376 pages Year Founded: 1985

2887 Under the Rug: Substance Abuse and the Mature Woman
Center on Addiction at Columbia University
633 3rd Avenue
19th Floor
New York, NY 10017-8155
212-841-5200; *Fax:* 212-956-8020
www.casacolumbia.org

William H Foster, CEO

Discusses the fact that millions of mature women are robbed of a healthy and longer lifespan due to a substance abuse problem that they discreetly hide. Their reluctance to get help costs them and the health systems billions. *$25.00*

Year Founded: 1998

2888 Understanding Psychiatric Medications in the Treatment of Chemical Dependency and Dual Diagnoses
Charles C Thomas Publisher Ltd.
2600 S 1st Street
Springfield, IL 62704-4730
217-789-8980
800-258-8980; *Fax:* 217-789-9130
books@ccthomas.com
www.ccthomas.com

Michael P Thomas, President

Designed to address coexisting chemical dependency and psychiatric disorder (dual diagnoses) and specifically to focus on the appropriate role of psychotropic medications in the treatment of dual diagnonsis patients. The text presents a comprehensive overview of psychiatric medication treatment for dual diagnoses that speaks to a broad professional audience while being sensitive to the values and beliefs of the chemical dependents. *$39.95*

134 pages Year Founded: 1995 ISSN 0-398-05964-0ISBN 0-398059-63-2

2889 Your Drug May Be Your Problem: How and Why to Stop Taking Pyschiatric Medications
Perseus Books Group
550 Central Avenue
Boulder, CO 80301
800-386-5656; *Fax:* 720-406-7336
westview.orders@perseusbooks.com
www.perseusbooksgroup.com

In a very short time, a doctor may prescribe a drug which an individual may take for months, years, even the rest of their lives. This book provides up-to-date, descriptions of the pros and cons of taking psychiatric medication, dangers involved, and explains a safe method of withdrawl if needed. *$17.00*

288 pages Year Founded: 2000 ISBN 0-738203-48-3

Suicide

2890 A Woman Doctor's Guide to Depression
Hyperion
237 Park Avenue
New York, NY 10017
www.hyperionbooks.com

Mitch Albom, Author
Lauren Groff, Author
Caroline Kennedy, Author
Jamie Oliver, Author

Includes information on what depression feels like and how it affects daily life, women's unique risks of developing depression throughout the life cycle from puberty to menopause and current treatment strategies and their risks and benefits, preventive measures and warning signs. *$9.95*

176 pages Year Founded: 1997 ISBN 0-786881-46-1

2891 Antidepressant Fact Book: What Your Doctor Won't Tell You About Prozac, Zoloft, Paxil, Celexa and Luvox
Perseus Books Group
2465 Central Avenue
Boulder, CO 80301
303-444-3541
800-386-5656; *Fax: 720-406-7336*
www.perseusbooksgroup.com

David Steinberger, President & CEO

What antidepressants will and won't treat, documented side and withdrawl effects, plus what parents need to know about teenagers and antidepressants. The author has been a medical expert in many court cases invloving the use and misuse of psychoactive drugs. *$13.00*

240 pages Year Founded: 2001 ISBN 0-738204-51-X

2892 Assessment and Prediction of Suicide
Guilford Press
72 Spring Street
New York, NY 10012-4068
212-431-9800
800-365-7006; *Fax: 212-966-6708*
info@guilford.com
www.www.guilford.com

Bob Matloff, President
Seymour Weingarten, Editor-in-Chief

Comprehensive reference volume that includes contributions from top suicide experts of the current knowledge in the field of suicide. Covers concepts and theories, methods and quantification, in-depth case histories, specific single predictors applied to the case histories and comorbidity. *$90.00*

697 pages Year Founded: 1973 ISBN 0-898627-91-5

2893 Comprehensive Textbook of Suicidology
Guilford Press
72 Spring Street
New York, NY 10012-4068
212-431-9800
800-365-7006; *Fax: 212-966-6708*
info@guilford.com
www.www.guilford.com

Bob Matloff, President
Seymour Weingarten, Editor-in-Chief

This volume presents an authoritative overview of current scientific knowledge about suicide and suicide prevention. Multidisciplinary and comprehesive in scope, the book provides a solid foundation in theory, research and clinical applications. Topics covered include the classification and prevalence of suicidal behaviors, psychiatric and medical factors, ethical and legal issues in intervention as well as the social, cultural and gender context of suicide. *$70.00*

650 pages Year Founded: 1973 ISBN 1-572305-41-X

2894 Interpersonal Psychotherapy
American Psychiatric Publishing, Inc.
1000 Wilson Boulevard
Suite 1825
Arlington, VA 22209-3901
703-907-7322
800-368-5777; *Fax: 703-907-1091*
appi@psych.org
www.appi.org

Robert E Hales, M.D., M.B.A., Editor-in-Chief
Ron McMillen, Chief Executive Officer
John McDuffie, Editorial Director
RebeccaD. Rinehart, Publisher

An overview of interpersonal psychotherapy for depression, preventative treatment for depression, bulimia nervosa and HIV positive men and women. *$26.00*

156 pages Year Founded: 1998 ISBN 0-880488-36-0

2895 Practical Art of Suicide Assessment: A Guide for Mental Health Professionals and Substance Abuse Counselors
John Wiley & Sons
111 River Street
Hoboken, NJ 07030-5774
201-748-6000; *Fax: 201-748-6088*
info@wiley.com
www.www.wiley.com

Lou Peragallo, Manager

Covers the critical elements of suicide assessment, from risk factor analysis to evaluating clients with borderline personality disorders or psychotic process.

316 pages ISBN 0-471237-61-2

2896 Suicide From a Psychological Prespective
Charles C Thomas Publisher Ltd.
2600 S 1st Street
Springfield, IL 62704-4730
217-789-8980
800-258-8980; *Fax: 217-789-9130*
books@ccthomas.com
www.ccthomas.com

Michael P Thomas, President
Charles C Thomas, Publisher

$39.95

142 pages Year Founded: 1927 ISBN 0-398057-09-5

2897 Teens and Suicide
Mason Crest Publishers
370 Reed Road
Suite 302
Broomall, PA 19008-4017
866-627-2665; *Fax: 610-543-3878*
www.masoncrest.com

Suicide is the third-leading cause of death among adolescents in the United States; in a recent study by The Gallup Organization, 47 percent of teenagers between the ages of 13 and 17 said they know someone who has tried to take their own lives. This volume examines the cause of teen-age suicide and explores such issues as teens and guns as well as suicide rates among minorities.

2898 Treatment of Suicidal Patients in Managed Care
American Psychiatric Publishing, Inc.
1000 Wilson Boulevard
Suite 1825
Arlington, VA 22209-3901
703-907-7322
800-368-5777; *Fax: 703-907-1091*
appi@psych.org
www.appi.org

Robert E Hales, M.D., M.B.A., Editor-in-Chief
Ron McMillen, Chief Executive Officer

John McDuffie, Editorial Director
RebeccaD. Rinehart, Publisher

Suicide is an all too common cause of death and preventable, but the managed care concerns of cost control with rapid diagnosis and treatment of depression puts the clinician in a dilemma. This book guides the professional with advice on knowing who to contact, and getting more of what is needed from the patient's managed care provider. *$39.00*

240 pages Year Founded: 2001 ISBN 0-880488-28-x

Trauma and Stressor-Related Disorders

2899 Applied Relaxation Training in the Treatment of PTSD and Other Anxiety Disorders
NewHarbinger Publications
5674 Shattuck Avenue
Oakland, CA 94609-1662
510-652-0215
800-748-6273; *Fax:* 510-652-5472
customerservice@newharbinger.com
www.newharbinger.com

Matthew McKay, Owner

Comes with a one hundred five minute video tape and a 52 page paperback manual. *$100.00*

Year Founded: 1998 ISBN 1-889287-08-3

2900 Assimilation, Rational Thinking, and Suppression in the Treatment of PTSD and Other Anxiety Disorders
New Harbinger Publications
5674 Shattuck Avenue
Oakland, CA 94609-1662
510-652-0215
800-748-6273; *Fax:* 510-652-5472
customerservice@newharbinger.com
www.newharbinger.com

Matthew McKay, Owner

Comes with two videotapes and a ninety four page paperback manual. *$150.00*

Year Founded: 1998 ISBN 1-889287-06-7

2901 Body Remembers: Psychophysiology of Trauma and Trauma Treatment
WW Norton & Company
500 5th Avenue
New York, NY 10110-54
212-354-5500; *Fax:* 212-869-0856
admalmud@wwnorton.com
www.books.wwnorton.com/

Babette Rothschild, Author

Unites traditional verbal therapy and body oriented therapies for Post Traumatic Stress Disorder patients, as memories sometimes present in a physical disorder. *$30.00*

224 pages Year Founded: 2000 ISSN 70327-4

2902 Brief Therapy for Post Traumatic Stress Disorder
John Wiley & Sons
605 3rd Avenue
New York, NY 10158-180
212-850-6301
info@wiley.com

Stephen Bisbey, Author
Lori Beth Bisbey, Author

Discusses a new and exciting treatment technique that has proven to be more effective than the widely used direct theraputic exposure technique. Fills the growing need for a step by step practical treatment manual for PTSD using Traumatic Incident Reduction. It is an ideal companion to training workshops.

192 pages Year Founded: 1998

2903 Cognitive Processing Therapy for Rape Victims
Sage Publications
2455 Teller Road
Thousand Oaks, CA 91320-2234
805-499-0721
800-818-7243; *Fax:* 805-499-0871
info@sagepub.com
www.sagepub.com

Blaise R Simqu, CEO

Information regarding the assessment and treatment of rape victims. Discusses disorders that result from rape and add to a victim's suffering such as post traumatic stress, depression, poor self-esteem, interpersonal difficulties and sexual dysfunction. *$46.00*

192 pages Year Founded: 1993 ISBN 0-803949-01-4

2904 Concise Guide to Brief Dynamic Psychotherapy
American Psychiatric Publishing, Inc.
1000 Wilson Boulevard
Suite 1825
Arlington, VA 22209-3901
703-907-7322
800-368-5777; *Fax:* 703-907-1091
appi@psych.org
www.appi.org

Robert E Hales, M.D., M.B.A., Editor-in-Chief
Ron McMillen, Chief Executive Officer
John McDuffie, Editorial Director
RebeccaD. Rinehart, Publisher

Seven brief psychodynamic therapy models including supportive, time - limited, interpersonal, time - limited dynamic, short term dynamic for post traumatic stress disorder and brief dynamic for substance abuse. *$21.00*

224 pages Year Founded: 1997 ISBN 0-880483-46-6

2905 Does Stress Damage the Brain? Understanding Trauma-Related Disorders from a Mind-Body Perspective
WW Norton & Company
500 5th Avenue
New York, NY 10110-54
212-354-5500
800-233-4830; *Fax:* 212-869-0856
npb@wwnorton.com
www.books.wwnorton.com

Drake McFeely, CEO

Shows that extreme stress may result in lasting damage to the brain, especially a part of the brain involved in memory. This new neurobiological understanding of the relation between cognitive problems and trauma has many important implications for both self-understanding of trauma survivors and for the treatment of the effects of trauma.

Year Founded: 1923 ISBN 0-393704-74-2

2906 Effective Treatments for PTSD: Practice Guidelines from the International Society for Traumatic Stress Studies
Guilford Press
72 Spring Street
New York, NY 10012-4068
212-431-9800
800-365-7006; *Fax:* 212-966-6708
info@guilford.com
www.www.guilford.com

Bob Matloff, President
Seymour Weingarten, Editor-in-Chief

Developed under the auspices of the PTSD Treatment Guidelines Task Force of the International Society for Traumatic Stress Studies, this comprehensive volume brings together leading authorities on psychological trauma to offer best practice guidelines for the treatment of PTSD. Approaches covered include acute interventions, cognitive-behavior therapy, pharmacotherapy, EMDR, group therapy, psychodynamic therapy, impatient treatment, psychosocial rehabilitation, hypnosis, creative therapies, marital and family treatment. *$42.00*

388 pages Year Founded: 1973 ISBN 1-572305-84-3

2907 Even from a Broken Web: Brief, Respectful Solution Oriented Therapy for Sexual Abuse and Trauma
WW Norton & Company
500 5th Avenue
New York, NY 10110-54
212-354-5500
800-233-4830; *Fax:* 212-869-0856
npb@wwnorton.com
www.books.wwnorton.com

Drake McFeely, CEO

Recent years have shown more people than ever coming to therapy with the after affects of sexual abuse. The authors provide therapists solution oriented treatment that considers a person's inner healing abilities. This method is less traumatic and disruptive to the patient's life than traditional therapies. *$16.95*

208 pages Year Founded: 1923 ISBN 0-393703-94-0

2908 Eye Movement Desensitization and Reprocessing: Basic Principles, Protocols, and Procedures
Guilford Press
72 Spring Street
New York, NY 10012-4068
212-431-9800
800-365-7006; *Fax:* 212-966-6708
info@guilford.com
www.www.guilford.com

Bob Matloff, President
Seymour Weingarten, Editor-in-Chief

Reviews research and development, discusses theoretical constructs and possible underlying mechanisms, and presents protocols and procedures for treatment of adults and children with a range of presenting complaints. Material is applicable for victims of sexual abuse, crime, combat and phobias. *$45.00*

398 pages Year Founded: 1973 ISBN 0-898629-60-8

2909 Group Treatments for Post-Traumatic Stress Disorder
Brunner/Routledge
7625 Empire Drive
Florence, KY 41042-2919
800-634-7064; *Fax:* 215-269-0363
orders@taylorandfrancis.com
www.www.routledgementalhealth.com

Contains contributions from renowned PTSD experts who provide group treatment to trauma survivors. It reviews the state-of-the-art applications of group therapy for such survivors of trauma as rape victims, combat veterans, adult survivors of childhood abuse, motor vehicle accident survivors, survivors of disaster, homicide witnesses and disaster relief workers. *$34.95*

216 pages ISBN 0-876309-83-X

2910 Life After Trauma: Workbook for Healing
Guilford Press
72 Spring Street
New York, NY 10012-4068
212-431-9800
800-365-7006; *Fax:* 212-966-6708
info@guilford.com
www.www.guilford.com

Bob Matloff, President
Seymour Weingarten, Editor-in-Chief

Useful exercises for clinicians and trauma survivors, very empowering. *$17.95*

352 pages Year Founded: 1973 ISBN 1-572302-39-9

2911 Memory, Trauma and the Law
WW Norton & Company
500 5th Avenue
New York, NY 10110-54
212-354-5500
800-233-4830; *Fax:* 212-869-0856
admalmud@wwnorton.com
www.books.wwnorton.com

Drake McFeely, CEO

Professionals need to be informed of memory in the legal context to avoid malpractice liability suits. Recovered memory research, trauma treatment and the controversy of false memory in some cases are covered. *$100.00*

960 pages Year Founded: 1923 ISSN 70254-5

2912 Overcoming Post-Traumatic Stress Disorder
New Harbinger Publications
5674 Shattuck Avenue
Oakland, CA 94609-1662
510-652-0215
800-748-6273; *Fax:* 510-652-5472
customerservice@newharbinger.com
www.newharbinger.com

Matthew McKay, Owner
Patrick Fanning, Co-Founder

An eleven to twenty four session treatment. *$11.95*

95 pages Year Founded: 1973 ISBN 1-572241-47-0

2913 Post Traumatic Stress Disorder
New Harbinger Publications
5674 Shattuck Avenue
Oakland, CA 94609-1662

510-652-0215
800-748-6273; *Fax:* 510-652-5472
customerservice@newharbinger.com
www.newharbinger.com

Matthew McKay, Owner
Patrick Fanning, Co-Founder

Includes techniques for managing flashbacks, anxiety attacks, nightmares, insomnia, and dissociation; working through layers of pain; and handling survivor guilt, secondary wounding, low self esteem, victim thinking, anger, and depression. *$49.95*

384 pages Year Founded: 1973 ISBN 1-879237-68-7

2914 Post Traumatic Stress Disorder: Complete Treatment Guide

200 E Joppa Road
PO Box 436
Brooklandville, MD 21022-0436
410-825-8888
888-825-8249; *Fax:* 410-560-0134
sidran@sidran.org
www.sidran.org

Esther Giller, President and Director
Sheila Sidran Giller, Secretary/Treasurer
J. G. Goellner, Director Emeritus
Tracy Howard, Book Sales/Office Manager

For clinicians who want to work more effectively with trauma survivors, this textbook provides a step by step description of PTSD treatment strategies. Includes chapters on definitions, diagnostic criteria and the biochemistry of PTSD. Reflects a generalized 'ideal' structure of the healing process. Includes cognitive and behavioral techniques for managing flashbacks, anxiety attacks, sleep disturbances and dissociation; a comprehensive program for working through deeper layers of pain; plus PTSD related problems such as survivor guilt, secondary wounding, low self esteem, victim thinking, anger and depression. Presents trauma issues clearly for both general audiences and trauma professionals. *$49.95*

345 pages Year Founded: 1986

2915 Post Traumatic Stress Disorders in Children and Adolescents Handbook
WW Norton & Company

500 5th Avenue
New York, NY 10110-54
212-354-5500
800-233-4830; *Fax:* 212-869-0856
npb@wwnorton.com
www.books.wwnorton.com

Drake McFeely, CEO

The 15 chapters gathered here address different aspects of childhood and adolescent trauma-some consider a distinct therapeutic situation (abuse and neglect), others pertain to standard clinical procedure (assessment), and still others focus on complex research issues (neurobiology and genetics of PSTD).

Year Founded: 1923 ISBN 0-393704-12-2

2916 Rebuilding Shattered Lives: Responsible Treatment of Complex Post-Traumatic and Dissociative Disorders
John Wiley & Sons

111 River Street
Hoboken, NJ 07030-5774

201-748-6000; *Fax:* 201-748-6088
info@wiley.com
www.www.wiley.com

Stephen M. Smith, President and Chief Executive Of
Ellis E. Cousens, Executive Vice President, Chief
John Kritzmacher, Executive Vice President, Chief
MJ O'Leary, Senior Vice President, Human Res

The most up-to-date, integrative and emperically sound account of trauma theory and practice availible. Based on more than a decade of clinical research and treatment experience at the Harvard Medical School, this comprehensive and nontechnical text offers a stage oriented approach to understanding and treating complex and difficult traumatized patients, integrating modern trauma theory with traditional theraputic interventions. *$47.50*

364 pages Year Founded: 1807 ISBN 0-471247-32-4

2917 Remembering Trauma: Psychotherapist's Guide to Memory & Illusion
John Wiley & Sons

111 River Street
Hoboken, NJ 07030-5774
201-748-6000; *Fax:* 201-748-6088
info@wiley.com
www.www.wiley.com

Stephen M. Smith, President and Chief Executive Of
Ellis E. Cousens, Executive Vice President, Chief
John Kritzmacher, Executive Vice President, Chief
MJ O'Leary, Senior Vice President, Human Res

364 pages Year Founded: 1807

2918 Standing in the Spaces: Essays on Clinical Process, Trauma, and Dissociation
Analytic Press

7625 Empire Drive
Florence, KY 41042-2919
800-634-7064; *Fax:* 215-269-0363
orders@taylorandfrancis.com
www.www.routledgementalhealth.com

Paul E Stepansky PhD, Managing Director
John Kerr PhD, Sr Editor

Bromberg's essays are delightfully unpredictable, as they strive to keep the reader continually abreast of how words can and cannot capture the subtle shifts in relatedness that characterize the clinical process. Radiating clinical wisdom infused with compassion and wit, Standing in the Spaces, is a classic destined to be read and reread by anlysts and therapists for decades to come. *$55.00*

376 pages Year Founded: 1998 ISBN 0-881632-46-5

2919 The Body Remembers Casebook: Unifying Methods and Models in the Treatment of Trauma and PTSD
WW Norton & Company

500 5th Avenue
New York, NY 10110-54
212-354-5500
800-233-4830; *Fax:* 212-869-0856
npb@wwnorton.com
www.books.wwnorton.com

Drake McFeely, CEO

Emphasizes the importance of tailoring every trauma therapy to the particular needs of each individual client. Each varied and complex case is approached with a combination of methods ranging from traditional psychodynamic approaches and applications of attachment theory to innovative trauma methods including EMDR and Levine's SIBAM model.

Year Founded: 1923 ISBN 0-393704-00-9

2920 The Body Remembers: The Psychphysiology of Trauma and Trauma Treatment
WW Norton & Company
500 5th Avenue
New York, NY 10110-54
212-354-5500
800-233-4830; *Fax: 212-869-0856*
npb@wwnorton.com
www.books.wwnorton.com

Drake McFeely, CEO

There is tremendous value in understanding the psychophysiology of trauma and knowing what to do about its manifestations. This book illuminates psychophysiology, casting light on the impact of trauma on the body and the phenomenon of somatic memory. Presents principles and non-touch techniques for giving the body its due.

Year Founded: 1923 ISBN 0-393703-27-4

2921 The Trauma Spectrum: Hidden Wounds and Human Resiliency
WW Norton & Company
500 5th Avenue
New York, NY 10110-54
212-354-5500
800-233-4830; *Fax: 212-869-0856*
npb@wwnorton.com
www.books.wwnorton.com

Drake McFeely, CEO

Scaer, a neurologist with over 30 years experience working with car accident victims, extends the conceptual and practical horizons of trauma treatment, redefining trauma as a continuum of variably negative life events occuring over a lifespan-including 'little traumas' such as car accidents, risky medical interventions, childhood abuse and neglect, and social discrimination and poverty-that shape every aspect of our existence.

Year Founded: 1923 ISBN 0-393704-66-1

2922 Transforming Trauma: EMDR
WW Norton & Company
500 5th Avenue
New York, NY 10110-54
212-354-5500; *Fax: 212-869-0856*
admalmud@wwnorton.com
www.books.wwnorton.com

Drake McFeely, CEO

Has helped thousands of people dealing with abuse histories or recent traumatic events. The author has a unique perspective, as she is both a client of EMDR and a therapist. *$14.95*

288 pages Year Founded: 1923 ISSN 31757-9

2923 Trauma Response
WW Norton & Company
500 5th Avenue
New York, NY 10110-54
212-354-5500; *Fax: 212-869-0856*
admalmud@wwnorton.com
www.books.wwnorton.com

Drake McFeely, CEO

Different causes of psychological trauma and modes of recovery. *$22.36*

240 pages Year Founded: 1923

Conferences & Meetings

2924 AAIDD Annual Meeting
501 3rd Street NW
Suite 200
Washington, DC 20001
202-387-1968
800-424-3688; *Fax: 202-387-2193*
anam@aaidd.org
www.aaidd.org

Margaret A. Nygren, EdD, Executive Director & CEO
Danielle Webber, MSW, Manager
Kathleen McLane, Director
Paul D. Aitken,CPA, Director

AAIDD promotes progressive policies, sound research, effective practices and universal human rights for people with intellectual and developmental disabilities.

1 per year

2925 AAMA Annual Conference
American Academy of Medical Administrators
330 N Wabash Ave
Suite 2000
Chicago, IL 60611
312-321-6815; *Fax: 312-673-6705*
info@aameda.org
www.aameda.org

Mrs. Linda Larin, MBA, FACCA, FAC, Chairman
Dr. Robert McKenney, PhD,FAAMA, Vice Chairman
Kevin Baliozian, Executive Director
Jennifer Schap, Program Coordinator

Learn the newest trends in healthcare administration; focus on your area of specialty or broaden your knowledge; become energized with new information and contacts in your field; and return to your organization ready to implement new ideas anad face new challenges.

Year Founded: 1999

2926 AMA's Annual Medical Communications Conference
American Medical Association
330 North Wabash Ave
Suite 39300
Chicago, IL 60611-5885
312-464-5000
800-262-3211; *Fax: 312-464-4184*
www.ama-assn.org

James L. Madara, MD, Chief Executive Officer & Execut
Bernard L. Hengesbaugh, Chief Operating Officer
Denise M. Hagerty, Senior Vice President & Chief Fi
Robert W. Davis, Senior Vice President

Provides hands-on communications training and hear from top-level medical communicators, government leaders and national journalists

Year Founded: 1847

2927 ASHA Annual Convention
American Speech-Language-Hearing Association
2200 Research Blvd
Rockville, MD 20850-3289
301-269-5700
800-638-8255; *Fax:* 301-296-8580
TTY: 301-296-5650
convention@asha.org
www.asha.org

Perry F. Flynn, MEd, CCC-SLP, Co-Chair
Wayne A. Foster, PhD, CCC-SLP/A, Co-Chair
Elizabeth S. McCrea, PhD, CCC-SLP, President
Barbara K. Cone, PhD, CCC-A, Vice President for
Academic Affa

ASHA is the professional, scientific and credentialing association for 140,000 members and affiliates who are audiologists, speech-language pathologists and speech, language and hearing scientists.

1 per year Year Founded: 1925

2928 American Academy of Child and Adolescent
Psychiatry (AACAP): Annual Meeting
3615 Wisconsin Avenue NW
Washington, DC 20016-3007
202-966-7300; *Fax:* 202-966-2891
communications@aacap.org
www.www.aacap.org

Warren Y.K. Ng, M.D., Chairman
Paramjit T. Joshi, M.D., President
Aradhana Bela Sood, M.D., Secretary
David G. Fassler, M.D., Treasurer

Professional society of physicians who have completed an additional five years of stimulate and advance medical contributions to the knowledge and treatment of psychiatric illnesses of children and adolescents. Annual meeting.

2929 American Academy of Psychiatry & Law
Annual Conference
American Academy of Psychiatry & Law
1 Regency Drive
PO Box 30
Bloomfield, CT 06002-30
860-242-5450
800-331-1389; *Fax:* 860-286-0787
execoff@aapl.org
www.aapl.org

Charles Scott, MD, President
Jacquelyn T. Coleman, Executive Director
Year Founded: 1969

2930 American Academy of Psychoanalysis
Preliminary Meeting
American Academy of Psychoanalysis and
Dynamic Psychiatry
One Regency Drive
PO Box 30
Bloomfield, CT 06002-30
888-691-8281; *Fax:* 860-286-0787
info@aapdp.org
www.aapdp.org

Michael Blumenfield, M.D., President
Jacquelyn T Coleman CAE, Executive Director
Carol Filiaci, Secretary

Annual meeting, Toronto, Canada.

Year Founded: 1956

2931 American Association of Children's Residential
Center Annual Conference
American Association of Children's Residential
Centers
11700 W Lake Park Drive
Milwaukee, WI 53224-3021
877-332-2272; *Fax:* 877-362-2272
kbehling@alliance1.org

Christopher Bellonci, M.D., President
William Powers, MHA, MPA, Chief Executive Officer
Joseph Whalen, Executive Director
Laurah Currey, Treasurer

Funded by the Mental Health Community Support Program. The purpose of the association is to share information about services, providers and ways to cope with mental illnesses. Available services include referrals, professional seminars, support groups and a variety of publications.

2932 American Association of Geriatric Psychiatry
Annual Meetings
7910 Woodmont Avenue
Suite 1050
Bethesda, MD 20814-3004
301-654-7850; *Fax:* 301-654-4137
main@aagponline.org
www.aagponline.org

David C. Steffens, MD, MHS, President
Christine M. deVries, CEO/Executive Vice President
Denise Disque, Office Manager/Executive Assista
Kate McDuffie, Director, Communications & Marke

Annual Meeting: March, Puerto Rico

Year Founded: 1978

2933 American Association on Intellectual and
Developmental Disabilities Annual Meeting
501 3rd Street NW
Suite 200
Washington, DC 20001
202-387-1968
800-424-3688; *Fax:* 202-387-2193
anam@aaidd.org
www.aaidd.org

Margaret A. Nygren, EdD, Executive Director & CEO
Danielle Webber, MSW, Manager
Kathleen McLane, Director
Paul D. Aitken, CPA, Director

Provides the opportunity of networking with old friends and colleagues, and is a wonderful opportunity to welcome students and new disability professionals to our Association. *$445.00*

2934 American Board of Disability Analysts Annual
Conference
770 Broadway
New York, NY 10003
212-206-4400
americanbd@aol.com
www.www.aol.com

Tim Armstrong, Chairman and Chief Executive Off
Curtis Brown, Executive Vice President and Chi
Karen Dykstra, Executive Vice President and Chi
Year Founded: 1985

2935 American College of Health Care Administrators (ACHCA) Annual Convocation & Exposition
1321 Duke Street
Suite 400
Alexandria, VA 22314
202-536-5120; *Fax:* 888-874-1585
www.achca.org

Marianna Kern Grachek, MSN, CNH, President & CEO
Becky Reisinger, Director, Membership and Busines
Whitney O'Donnell, Coordinator, Member Services
Chelsea Whitman-Rush, Coordinator, Member and Chapter

A non-profit professional membership association which provides superior educataional programming, professional certification, and career development opportunities for its members.

Year Founded: 1966

2936 American College of Healthcare Executives Educational Events
American College of Healthcare Executives
One N Franklin Street
Suite 1700
Chicago, IL 60606-3529
312-424-2800; *Fax:* 312-424-0023
contact@ache.org
www.ache.org

Diana L. Smalley, FACHE, Chairman
Deborah J. Bowen, FACHE, President and CEO

2937 American College of Psychiatrists Annual Meeting
122 S. Michigan Ave
Suite 1360
Chicago, IL 60603-6185
312-662-1020; *Fax:* 312-662-1025
angel@acpsych.org
www.acpsych.org

James H. Scully Jr., President
Frank W. Brown, First Vice President
Gail E. Robinson, Second Vice President
Maureen D. Shick, Executive Director

Nonprofit honorary association of psychiatrists who, through excellence in their chosen fields, have been recognized for their significant contributions to the profession. The society's goal is to promote and support the highest standards in psychiatry through education, research and clinical practice. Annual Meeting in February.

Year Founded: 1963

2938 American Group Psychotherapy Association Annual Conference
American Group Psychotherapy Association
25 E 21st Street
6th Floor
New York, NY 10010-6207
212-477-2677
877-668-2472; *Fax:* 212-979-6627
info@agpa.org
www.agpa.org

Les R. Greene, Ph.D., CGP, LF, President
Jeffrey Kleinberg, PhD, CGP, President
Marsha S. Block, CAE, CFRE, CEO
Lise Motherwell, Ph.D., Psy, Treasurer

Educational conference with a changing annual focus. February.

Year Founded: 1942

2939 American Health Care Association Annual Convention
1201 L Street NW
Washington, DC 20005-4046
202-842-4444; *Fax:* 202-842-3860
teyet@ahca.org
www.www.ahcancal.org

Leonard Russ, Chairman
Bruse Yarwood, President

Exhibits and educational workshops from the nonprofit federation of affiliated state health organizations, together representing nearly 12,000 nonprofit and for profit assisted living, nursing facility, developmentally disabled and sub-acute care providers that care for more than 1.5 million elderly and disabled individuals nationally. AHCA represents the long term care community at large — to government, business leaders and the general public. It also serves as a force for change within the long term care field, providing information, education, and administrative tools that enhance quality at every level.

2940 American Health Information Management Association Annual Exhibition and Conference
233 N Michigan Avenue
21st Floor
Chicago, IL 60601-5809
312-233-1100
800-335-5535; *Fax:* 312-233-1090
info@ahima.org
www.ahima.org

Angela Kennedy, EdD, MBA, RHI, President, Chairman
Cassi Birnbaum, MS. RHIA, CP, President / Chair-Elect
Becky Garris-Perry, Executive Vice President/CFO
Linda Kloss, Executive Director

Exhibits, business and educational conferences of the dynamic professional association that represents more than 46,000 specially educated health information management professionals who work throughout the healthcare industry. Health information management professionals serve the health care industry and the public by manageing, analyzing and utilizing data vital for patient care and making it accessible to healthcare providers when it is needed most.

2941 American Society of Addiction Medicine
American Society of Addiction Medicine
4601 N Park Avenue
Upper Arcade #101
Chevy Chase, MD 20815-4520
301-656-3920; *Fax:* 301-656-3815
email@asam.org
www.asam.org

Penny S Mills, Executive VP, CEO
Arlene C. Deverman, CAE, VP, Professional Development
Carolyn C. Lanham, CAE, Chief Operating Officer
Kate Volpe, Director, Marketing, Communicati

Goal is to present the most up-to-date information in the addictions field. to attain this goal, program sessions will focus on the latest developments in research and treatment issues and will tanslate them into clinically useful knowledge. Through a mix of symposia, courses, workshops, didactic lectures, and paper and poster presentations based on submitted abstracts, participants will have an opportunity to interact with experts in their field.

2942 Association for Child Psychoanalysis (ACP) Annual Meeting

900 East Pecan Street
Suite 300, PMB 254
Pflugerville, TX 78660
512-551-8769; *Fax:* 866-534-7555
childanalysis65@gmail.com
www.childanalysis.org

Kerry Kelly Novick, President
Anita Schmukler, D.O., President
Barbara Streeter, Treasurer
Tricia Hall, CAE, CMP, Administrator

An international not-for-profit organization in which all members are highly trained child and adolescent psychoanalysts. Provides a forum for the interchange of ideas and clinical experience in order to advance the psychological treatment and understanding of children and adolescents and their families.

2943 Association of Black Psychologists Annual Convention

7119 Allentown Road
Suite 203
Ft Washington, MD 20744
301-449-3082; *Fax:* 301-449-3084
abpsi@abpsi.org
www.abpsi.org

Cheryl Tawede Grills, PhD, President
Tassogle Daryl Rowe, President-Elect
Kevin Washington, Ph.D., President-Elect
Carolyn Moore, Ph.D, Treasurer

Feature presentations, exhibits and workshops held over a four day period focusing on the unique concerns of Black professionals.

2944 California Psychological Association's Annual Convention

1231 I Street
Suite 204
Sacramento, CA 95814-2933
916-286-7979; *Fax:* 916-286-7971
membership@cpapsych.org
www.cpapsych.org

Robert deMayo, PhD, ABPP, President
Stephen Pfeiffer, PhD, President-Elect
Jo Linder-Crow, Ph.D., CEO
Betsy Levine-Proctor, PhD, Treasurer / Chair - Finance Comm

Poster sessions, roundtable discussions, CE sessions, ethics discussions and featured speakers. *$680.00*

2945 Georgia Psychological Society Annual Conference

2200 Century Parkway
Suite 660
Atlanta, GA 30345
404-634-6272; *Fax:* 404-634-8230

Jennifer Stapel-Wax, President
Steven Perlow, PhD, President Elect
Mary Gresham, Vice President
Dr. Chuck Talor, Conference, Newsletter's and Jou

Proposals for symposia, papers, posters and workshops on topics in all areas of psychology are invited. Proposals should not exceed 500 words, and each proposal must include a summary that is no longer than 50 words.

2946 NADD Annual Conference & Exhibit Show
National Association for the Dually Diagnosed

132 Fair Street
Kingston, NY 12401-4802
845-331-4336
800-331-5362; *Fax:* 845-331-4569
info@thenadd.org
www.thenadd.org

Daniel Baker, Ph.D., Conference Chairperson, Presiden
Donna McNelis, Ph.D., President
Robert J. Fletcher DSW, CEO
Brian Tallant, Conference Chairperson

2947 National Alliance on Mental Illness

3803 North Fairfax Drive
Suite 100
Arlington, VA 22203
703-524-7600
800-950-6264; *Fax:* 703-524-9094
TDD: 703-516-7227
info@nami.org
www.nami.org

Marilyn Ricci, MS, MD, President
Janet Edelman, MS, First Vice President
Mary Giliberti, JD, Chief Executive Officer
David Levy, Chief Financial Officer

Grassroots mental health organization dedicated to improving the lives of all Americans affected by mental illness.
Year Founded: 1979

2948 National Multicultural Conference and Summit

Brakins Consulting & Psychological Svs
13805 60th Avenue North
Phymouth, MN 55446-3583
www.multiculturalsummit.com

Debra Kawahara, Lead Coordinator
Michael Mobley, Programming Coordinator
Julii Green, Keynote Coordinator
Roberta Nutt, Awards Coordinator

The mission is to convene students, practitioners, and scholars in psychology and related fields to inform and inspire multicultural research and practice.

2949 New England Educational Institute
New England Educational Institute

449 Pittsfield Road
Suite 201
Lenox, MA 01240
413-499-1489; *Fax:* 413-499-6584
learn@neei.org
www.neei.org

Designed to meet the educational needs of physicians (psychiatrists, family practitioners, general practitioners), psychologists, nurse practitioners, physician assistants, nurses and other health care professionals. Each half-day will provide practical and clinically relevant information for day-to-day problems. Morning lectures will be followed by panel discussions.

2950 Traumatic Incident Reduction Workshop
E-Productivity-Services.Net
Division of 21st Century Enterprises
13 NW Barry Rd PMB 214
Kansas City, MO 64155-2728
816-468-4945; *Fax:* 816-468-6656
www.espn.net

Frank A Gerbode, Subject Developer
Marian Volkman, President
John Durkin, Vice President
Robert H Moore, Board Member

Defines the Conditioned Response Phenomena, establishes a safe environment, analyzes and applies the Unblocking technique to resolve issues relating to emotionally charged persons, places, things and situations, and analyzes and applies Traumatic Incident Reduction (TIR) to resolve known and unknown past traumatic experiences and the unwanted feelings, emotions, sensations, attitutdes and pain associated with them.

2951 YAI/National Institute for People with Disabilities
460 W 34th Street
New York, NY 10001-2382
212-273-6100
866-292-4546; *Fax:* 212-947-7524
TDD: 212-290-2787
www.yai.org

Bridget Waldron, L.C.S.W., Senior Vice President, Quality E
Marco Damiani, M.A., Executive Vice President, Innova
Paul Smoller, M.A., Executive Vice President, Talent
Kelly Burke-Quinn, Vice President, Business Analysi

Annual conference "Advancing Services Across the Life Span in Intellectual and Developmental Disabilities". A major forum for the exchange of ideas and the introduction of new models and strategies that have a positive impact in the field.

Periodicals & Pamphlets

2952 AAMI Newsletter
Arizona Alliance for the Mentally Ill (NAMI Arizona)
2210 N 7th Street
Phoenix, AZ 85006-1604
602-244-8166
800-626-5022; *Fax:* 602-244-9264
www.namiaz.org

Diane McVicker, President
Cheryl Weiner, Educutive Director

Provides support, education, research, and advocacy for individuals and families affected by mental illness. Reports on legislative updates, conventions, psychiatry/psychological practices, and activities of the alliance. Newsletter with membership. *$10.00*

8 pages 4 per year

2953 AAPL Newsletter
American Academy of Psychiatry and the Law
One Regency Drive
PO Box 30
Bloomfield, CT 06002-30
860-242-5450
800-331-1389; *Fax:* 860-286-0787

office@aapl.org
www.aapl.org

Jacquelyn T. Coleman, Executive Director
Charles Scott, MD, President
Ezra Griffith, MD, Editor

Scholarly articles on forensice psychiatry. *$130.00*

4 per year ISSN 1093-6793

2954 APA Monitor
American Psychological Association
750 1st Street NE
Washington, DC 20002-4242
202-336-5500
800-374-2721; *Fax:* 202-336-5518
TDD: 202-336-6123
TTY: 202-336-6123
letters.monitor@apa.org
www.apa.org

Nadine J. Kaslow, Ph.D., President
Barry S. Anton, Ph.D., President-Elect
Donald N. Bersoff, PhD, JD, Past President
Norman B Anderson, Ph.D., CEO, EVP

Magazine of the American Psychological Association.

12 per year ISSN 1529-4978

2955 ASAP Newsletter
American Society for Adolescent Psychiatry
PO Box 570218
Dallas, TX 75357-218
972-613-0985; *Fax:* 972-613-5532
info@adolpsych.org
www.adolpsych.org

Mohan Nair, President
Gregg Dwyer, President
Sheldon Glass, President-Elect
Gregory P. Barclay, VP

Contains articles about adolescent psychiatry and society news. Recurring features include news of research, a calendar of events, and book reviews. *$10.00*

16-20 pages 4 per year

2956 Advocate: Autism Society of America
Autism Society of America
4340 East-West Hwy
Suite 350
Bethesda, MD 20814-3067
301-657-0881
800-328-8476; *Fax:* 301-657-0869
sbadesch@autism-society.org
www.autism-society.org

Scott Badesch, President, CEO
Jennifer Repella, VP, Programs
John Dabrowski, CFO
Rose Jochum, Director, Programs

Reports news and information of national significance for individuals, families, and professionals dealing with autism. Recurring features include personal features and profiles, research summaries, government updates, book reviews, statistics, news of research, and a calendar of events.

32-36 pages 6 per year ISSN 0047-9101

2957 Alcohol & Drug Abuse Weekly
John Wiley & Sons
111 River Street
Hoboken, NJ 07030-5774
201-748-6000; *Fax:* 201-748-6088
info@wiley.com
www.wiley.com

Stephen M. Smith, President, CEO
MJ O'Leary, SVP, Human Resources
Edward J. Melando, SVP, Corporate Controller
Gary M. Rinck, SVP, General Counsel

48-issue subsrciption offers significant news and analysis of federal and state policy developments. A resource for directors of addiction treatment centers, managed care executives, federal and state policy makers and healthcare consultants. Topics include the latest findings in treatment and prevention; funding and survival issues for providers; the impact of state and federal policy on treatment and prevention; working under managed care; and co-occurring disorders.

8 pages 48 per year Year Founded: 1992 ISSN 1042-1394

2958 Alliance for Children and Families
Insider
1020 19th St. N.W.
Suite 500
Washington, DC 20036-1540
202-429-0400
800-220-1016; *Fax:* 202-429-0178
policy@alliance1.org
www.www.alliance1.org

Susan Dreyfus, CEO, President
Polina Makievsky, SVP, Knowledge, Leadership, and
Robert Cacase, Chief Information Officer
Tracy Wareing, Executive Director

Alliance for Children and Families' tool for providing members with accurate and up-to-date information on current legislation, issues the Alliance is advocating on Capitol Hill, summaries of how proposed bills will affect member organizations and the people they serve, and suggestions for local advocacy efforts.

12 per year

2959 American Academy of Child and Adolescent Psychiatry
AACAP
3615 Wisconsin Avenue Northwest
Washington, DC 20016-3007
202-966-7300; *Fax:* 202-464-0131
communications@aacap.org
www.aacap.org

Kristin Kroeger-Ptakowski, Director, Sr Deputy Director
Elizabeth DiLauro, Advocacy Manager
Emma Jellen, Policy Coordinator

The American Academy of Child and Adolescent Psychiatry, (AACAP) publishes a newsletter which focuses events within the Academy, child and adolescent psychiatrists, and AACAP members.

36-64 pages 6 per year

2960 American Association of Community Psychiatrists (AACP)
PO Box 570218
Dallas, TX 75357-0218

972-613-0985
972-613-3997; *Fax:* 972-613-5532
frda1@airmail.net
www.www.communitypsychiatry.org

Wesley Sowers MD, President
Anita Everett, M.D., President
Annelle Primm, Vice President
Stephanie Le Melle, M.D., Vice President

Psychiatrists and psychiatry residents practicing in community mental health centers or similar programs that provide care to the mentally ill regardless of their ability to pay. Addresses issues faced by psychiatrists who practice within CMHCs. Publications: AACP Membership Directory, annual. Community Psychiatrist, quarterly newsletter. Annual meeting, in conjunction with American Psychiatric Association in May. Annual meeting, in conjunction with Institute on Hospital and Community in fall.

4 per year

2961 American Institute for Preventive Medicine
American Institute for Preventive Medicine Press
30445 Northwestern Highway
Suite 350
Farmington Hills, MI 48334-3107
248-539-1800
800-345-2476; *Fax:* 248-539-1808
www.healthylife.com

Don R Powell, Ph.D., President, CEO
Sue Jackson, VP
Elaine Frank, M.Ed., R.D., VP
Jeanette Karwan, Director, Product Development

AIPM is an internationally renowned developer and provider of wellness programs and publications that address both mental and physical health issues. It works with over 11,500 corporations, hospitals, MCOs, universities, and goverment agencies to reduce health care costs, lower absenteeism, and improve productivity. The Institute has a number of publications that address mental health issues, including stress management, depression, self - esteem, and EAP issues.

Year Founded: 1999

2962 Behavioral Health Management
3800 Lakeside Avenue
Suite 201
Cleveland, OH 44114
216-391-9100; *Fax:* 216-391-9200
info@vendomegrp.com
www.behavioral.net

Richard Peck, Editorial Director
Douglas J Edwards, Managing Editor, Publisher
Kathi Homenick, Director
Judi Zeng, Traffic Manager

Informs decision makers in managed behavioral healthcare organizations, provider groups, and treatment centers of the ever-changing demands of their field. The magazine publishes analyses, editorials, and organizations case studies to give readers the information they need for best practices in a challenging marketplace.

2963 Biology of Sex Differences
Society for Women's Health Research (SWHR)
1025 Connecticut Avenue NW
Suite 601
Washington, DC 20036-5447

202-466-6069; *Fax:* 202-833-3472
www.bsd-journal.com

Phyllis Greenberger, MSW, President
Mary V. Hornig, VP Finance & Operations
Arthur Arnold, Univ. CA, Editor

Biology of Sex Differences considers manuscripts on all aspects of the effect of sex on biology and disease. It is an online, open access, peer-reviewed journal published in conjunction with BioMed Central.

Year Founded: 1990

2964 Brown University: Child & Adolescent Psychopharmacology Update
John Wiley & Sons
111 River Street
Hoboken, NJ 07030-5774
201-748-6000; *Fax:* 201-748-6088
info@wiley.com
www.wiley.com

Stephen M. Smith, President, CEO
MJ O'Leary, SVP, Human Resources
Edward J. Melando, SVP, Corporate Controller
Gary M. Rinck, SVP, General Counsel

Monthly newsletter that gives information on children and adolescent's unique psychotropic medication needs. Delivers updates on new drugs, their uses, typical doses, side effects and interactions, examines generic vs. name brand drugs, reports on new research and new indications for existing medications. Each issue also includes case studies, references for future reading, industry news notes, abstracts of current research and a patient psychotropic medication handout. *$ 190.00*

12 per year Year Founded: 1992 ISSN 1527-8395

2965 Brown University: Digest of Addiction Theory and Application (DATA)
John Wiley & Sons
111 River Street
Hoboken, NJ 07030-5774
201-748-6000; *Fax:* 201-748-6088
info@wiley.com
www.wiley.com

Stephen M. Smith, President, CEO
MJ O'Leary, SVP, Human Resources
Edward J. Melando, SVP, Corporate Controller
Gary M. Rinck, SVP, General Counsel

Monthly synopsis of critical research developments in the treatment and prevention of alcoholism and drug abuse, including dozens of research abstracts chosen from over 75 medical journals. *$129.00*

8 pages 12 per year Year Founded: 1992 ISSN 1040-6328

2966 Brown University: Geriatric Psychopharmacology Update
John Wiley & Sons
111 River Street
Hoboken, NJ 07030-5774
201-748-6000; *Fax:* 201-748-6088
info@wiley.com
www.wiley.com

Stephen M. Smith, President, CEO
MJ O'Leary, SVP, Human Resources
Edward J. Melando, SVP, Corporate Controller
Gary M. Rinck, SVP, General Counsel

This monthly report is an easy way to keep up to date on the newest breakthroughs in geriatric medicine that have an impact on psychiatric practice. *$190.00*

12 per year Year Founded: 1992 ISSN 1529-2584

2967 Brown University: Psychopharmacology Update
John Wiley & Sons
111 River Street
Hoboken, NJ 07030-5774
201-748-6000; *Fax:* 201-748-6088
info@wiley.com
www.wiley.com

Stephen M. Smith, President, CEO
MJ O'Leary, SVP, Human Resources
Edward J. Melando, SVP, Corporate Controller
Gary M. Rinck, SVP, General Counsel

Each issue examines the pros and cons of specific drugs, drug-drug interactions, side effects, street drugs, warning signs, case reports and more. *$199.00*

12 per year Year Founded: 1992 ISSN 1608-5308

2968 Bulletin of Menninger Clinic
Guilford Press
72 Spring Street
New York, NY 10012-4068
212-431-9800
800-288-3950; *Fax:* 212-966-6708

Bob Matloff, President

Valuable, practical information for clinicans. Recent topical issues have focused on rekindling the psychodynamic vision, treatment of different clinical populations with panic disorder, and treatment of complicated personality disorders in an era of managed care. All in an integrated, psychodynamic approach. *$75.00*

ISSN 0025-9284

2969 Bulletin of Psychological Type
Association for Psychological Type
2415 Westwood Ave.
Suite B
Richmond, VA 23230
804-523-2907
800-847-9943; *Fax:* 804-288-3551
www.aptinternational.org

Jane Kise, President
Susan Nash, President
Linda Berens, Past President
Maryanne DiMarzo, President-Elect

Provides information on regional, national, and international events to keep professionals up-to-date in the study and application of psychological type theory and the Myers-Briggs Type Indicator. Contains announcements of training workshops; international, national, and regional conferences; and awards, along with articles on issues directly related to type theory.

2970 Capitation Report
National Health Information
PO Box 15429
Atlanta, GA 30333-429
404-607-9500
800-597-6300; *Fax:* 404-607-0095
www.nhionline.net

NHI publishes specialized, targeted information for health care executives on a variety of topics from capitation to disease management.

2971 Child and Adolescent Psychiatry
American Academy of Child and Adolescent Psychiatry
3615 Wisconsin Avenue NW
Washington, DC 20016-3007
202-966-7300; *Fax:* 202-966-2891
communications@aacap.org
www.www.aacap.org

Robert Hendren, President
William Bernet, Treasurer
Michael Linsky, Assistant Director
David Herzog, Secretary

Journal focusing on today's psychiatric research and treatment of the child and adolescent. *$175.00*

36-64 pages 12 per year ISSN 0890-8567

2972 Clinical Psychiatry News
International Medical News Group
5635 Fishers Lane
Suite 6100
Rockville, MD 20852-1886
240-221-4500; *Fax:* 240-221-4400
aimhoff@frontlinemedcom.com

Stephen Stoneburn, Chairman
Alan J. Imhoff, President, CEO, Medical News Div
JoAnn Wahl, President, Custom Solutions
Marcy Holeton, President, CEO, Clinical Content

A leading independent newspaper for the Psychiatrist.

2973 Clinical Psychiatry Quarterly
AACP
PO Box 458
Glastonbury, CT 06033-458
860-633-6023; *Fax:* 866-668-9858
www.aacp.com

Donald W. Black, MD, President
Richard Balon, MD, VP
Sanjay Gupta, MD, Immediate Past President
James Wilcox, DO, PhD, Treasurer/Secretary

Informs members of of news and events. Recurring features include letters to the editor, news of research, a calendar of events, reports of meetings, and book reviews.

4 per year

2974 Couples Therapy in Managed Care
Haworth Press
10 Alice Street
Binghamton, NY 13904-1503
607-722-5857
800-429-6784; *Fax:* 607-722-1424
www.haworthpress.com

Provides social workers, psychologists and counselors with an overview of the negative effects of the managed care industry on the quality of marital health care.

ISBN 7-890078-86-6

2975 Current Directions in Psychological Science
Association for Psychological Science
1133 15th Street NW
Suite 1000
Washington, DC 20005

202-293-9300; *Fax:* 202-293-9350
www.psychologicalscience.org

Linda Bartoshuk, President
Elizabeth A. Phelps, President
Mahzarin R Banaji, President-Elect
Nancy Eisenberg, President-Elect

Current Directions publishes reviews by leading experts covering all of scientific psychology and its applications. Each issue features a diverse mix of reports on various topics such as language, memory and cognition, development, the neural basis of behavior and emotions, various aspects of psychopathology, and theory of mind. The articles keep readers apprised of important developments across subfields. The articles are also written to be accessible to non-experts, making them suited for classroom teaching supplements.

6 per year ISSN 0963-7214

2976 Development & Psychopathology
Cambridge University Press
40 W 20th Street
New York, NY 10011-4211
212-924-3900; *Fax:* 212-691-3239
marketing@cup.org
www.cup.org

This multidisciplinary journal is devoted to the publication of original, empirical, theoretical and review papers which address the interrelationship of normal and pathological development in adults and children. It is intended to serve and intergrate the emerging field of developmental psychopathology which strives to understand patterns of adaptation and maladaptation throughout the lifespan. This journal is of vital interest to psychologists, psychiatrists, social scientists, neuroscientists, pediatricians and researchers. *$66.00*

4 per year ISSN 0954-5794

2977 EAPA Exchange
Employee Assistance Professionals Association
4350 North Fairfax Drive
Suite 740
Arlington, VA 22203
703-387-1000; *Fax:* 703-522-4585
admanager@eapassn.org
www.www.eapassn.org

Steven Haught, President
Lucy Henry, President-Elect
Pam Ruster, Treasurer, Secretary
John Maynard, CEO

2978 ETR Associates
Health Education, Research, Training Curriculum
4 Carbonero Way
Scotts Valley, CA 95066-4200
831-438-4060
800-321-4407; *Fax:* 831-438-4284
www.etr.org

John Henry Ledwith, National Sales Director
Pamela Anderson, PhD, Senior Reasearch Associate
Eric Blanke, BS, Director, Solutions
Erin Cassidy-Eagle, PhD, Director, Research

Publishes a complete line of innovative materials covering the full spectrum of health education topics, including maternal/child health, HIV/STD prevention, risk and injury prevention, self esteem, fitness and nutrition, college health, and wellness education, engaging in both extensive training and research endeavors and a comprehensive K-12 health curriculum.

2979 Elsevier
Customer Support Department
1600 John F Kennedy Boulevard
Suite 1800
Philadelphia, PA 19103-2879
212-633-3730
888-437-4636; *Fax:* 212-633-3680
newsroom@elsevier.com
www.elsevier.com

Youngsuk (Y.S.) Chi, Chairman
Mark Seeley, SVP, General Counsel
David Ruth, SVP, Global Communications
Adriaan Roosen, EVP, Operations

 ISSN 0165-3806

2980 Employee Benefits Journal
International Foundation of Employee Benefit Plans
18700 W. Bluemound Rd.
PO Box 69
Brookfield, WI 53045
414-786-6700
888-334-3327; *Fax:* 414-786-8670
marybr@ifebp.org
www.ifebp.org

Kenneth R. Boyd, President, Chairman
Richard Lyall, Past President
Thomas T. Holsman, President-Elect
Regina C. Reardon, Treasurer

Contains articles on all aspects of employee benefits and related topics. *$70.00*

32-48 pages 4 per year   ISSN 0361-4050

2981 Exceptional Parent
416 Main Street
Johnstown, PA 15901
814-361-3860; *Fax:* 814-361-3861
www.eparent.com

Joseph M Valenzano, Jr., President,Publisher, CEO
James McGinnis, VP of Operations, CEO
Rick Rader, MD, Editor-in-Chief
Hamilton Maher, Director of Circulation & Busine

Magazine for parents and professionals involved in the care and development of children and young adults with special needs, including physical disabilities, developmental disabilities, autism, epilepsy, learning disabilities, hearing/vision impairments, emotional problems, and chronic illnesses. *$36.00*

12 per year

2982 Focal Point: Research, Policy and Practice in Children's Mental Health
Regional Research Institue-Portland State University
PO Box 751
Portland, OR 97207-0751
503-725-3000
800-547-8887; *Fax:* 503-725-4882
rtcpubs@pdx.edu

Janet Walker, Editor

Features information on research, interventions, organizations, strategies, and conferences to aid families that have children with emotional, mental, and/or behavioral disorders.

24 pages

2983 From the Couch
Behavioral Health Record Section-AMRA
919 N Michigan Avenue
Suite 1400
Chicago, IL 60611-1692
312-787-2672; *Fax:* 312-787-5926

From the couch, the newsletter for the Behavioral Health Record section of the American Medical Record Association, covers aspects of the medical records industry that pertain to mental health records.

 4 per year

2984 Frontiers of Health Services Management
American College of Healthcare Executives
1 N Franklin Street
Suite 1700
Chicago, IL 60606-3529
312-424-2800; *Fax:* 312-424-0023
contact@ache.org
www.ache.org

Christine M. Candio, RN, FACHE, Chairman
Richard D. Cordova, FACHE, Chairman-Elect
Diana L. Smalley, FACHE, Immediate Past Chairman
Deborah J. Bowen, FACHE, President, CEO

Enhanced by special access to today's healthcare leaders. Frontiers provides you with the cutting edge insight you want. Each quarterly issue engages you in a vigorous debate on a hot healthcare topic. One stimulating article leads the debate, followed by commentaries and perspectives from recognized experts. Unique combination of opinion, practice and research stimulate you to develop new management strategies. *$70.00*

4 per year   ISSN 0748-8157

2985 General Hospital Psychiatry: Psychiatry, Medicine and Primary Care
Elsevier
1600 John F Kennedy Boulevard
Suite 1800
Philadelphia, PA 19103-2879
314-447-8070
888-615-4500
newsroom@elsevier.com
www.elsevier.com

Youngsuk (Y.S.) Chi, Chairman
Mark Seeley, SVP, General Counsel
David Ruth, SVP, Global Communications
Adriaan Roosen, EVP, Operations

Journal that explores the linkages and interfaces between psychiatry, medicine and primary care. As a peer-reviewed journal, it provides a forum for communication among professionals with clinical, academic and research interests in psychiatry's essential function in the mainstream of medicine. *$195.00*

84 pages 6 per year   ISSN 01638343

2986 Geriatrics
Advanstar Communications
7500 Old Oak Boulevard
Cleveland, OH 44130-3343
440-243-8100; *Fax:* 440-891-2740

David Briemer, Sales Manager
Rich Ehrlich, Associate Publisher

Peer-reviewed clinical journal for primary care physicians
who care for patients age 50 and older.

100 pages 12 per year

2987 Group Practice Journal
Amerian Medical Group Association
One Prince Street
Alexandria, VA 22314-3318
703-838-0033; *Fax:* 703-548-1890
roconnor@amga.org
www.amga.org

Donald W. Fisher, Ph.D., CAE, President, CEO
Clyde L. Woody Morris, C.P.A., CFO
April L. Noland, Assistant to the President and C
Michael J. Pomeroy, C.P.A., Senior Assistant to the CFO

Penned by healthcare professionals, articles in the Group
Practice Journal give a view from the trenches of modern
medicine on a wide variety of topics, including innovative
disease management and clinical best practices. Readers
look to the publication to learn strategies and solutions
from peers in the profession, healthcare thought leaders,
and industry experts.

10 per year

2988 Harvard Mental Health Letter
Harvard Health Publications
10 Shattuck Street
2nf Floor
Boston, MA 02115-6030
617-432-4714
mental_health@hms.harvard.edu
www.www.health.harvard.edu

Anthony Komaroff, Owner

Delivers information on current thinking and debate on
mental health issues that concern professionals and layment
a like. In the ever-changing and complex field of mental
health care, the newsletter has become a trusted source for
psychiatrists, psychologists, social workers and therapists
of all kinds. *$59.00*

8 pages 12 per year Year Founded: 1983 ISSN 08843783

2989 Harvard Review of Psychiatry
Taylor and Francis
01650 Toebben Drive
Independence, KY 41051
800-634-7064; *Fax:* 800-248-4724

An authoritative source for scholarly reviews and perspectives on important topics in psychiatry. Founded by the
Harvard Medical School's Department of Psychiatry, the
Harvard Review of Psychiatry features review papares that
summarize and synthesize the key literature in a scholarly
and clinically relevant manner. *$185.00*

6 per year

2990 Health & Social Work
National Association of Social Workers
750 1st Street NE
Suite 700
Washington, DC 20002-4241
202-408-8600; *Fax:* 202-336-8312
press@naswdc.org
www.naswpress.org

Elvira Craig De Silva, President
Cheryl Y. Bradley, Publisher
Sharon Fletcher, Publications Marketing Manager
Kiera White, Marketing Coordinator

Articles cover research, policy, specialized servies, quality
assurance, inservice training and other topics that affect the
delivery of health care services. *$125.00*

2991 Health Data Management
Faulkner & Gray
11 Penn Plaza
New York, NY 10001-2006
212-967-7000; *Fax:* 212-239-4993
www.www.healthdatamanagement.com

Gary Baldwin, Editorial Director
Greg Gillespie, Editor-in-Chief
Joe Goedert, News Editor

2992 International Drug Therapy Newsletter
Lippincott Williams & Wilkins
351 W Camden Street
Baltimore, MD 21201-2436
410-528-4000
800-882-0483; *Fax:* 410-528-4414
korourke@lww.com
www.lww.com

J Arnold Anthony, Operations

Newsletter that focuses on psychotropic drugs, discussing
individual drugs, their effectiveness, and history. Examines
illnesses and the drugs used to treat them, studies done on
various drugs, their chemical make-up, and new developments and changes in drugs. *$149.00*

8 pages ISSN 0020-6571

2993 International Journal of
Neuropsychopharmacology
Cambridge University Press
40 W 20th Street
New York, NY 10011-4211
212-924-3900; *Fax:* 212-691-3239
marketing@cup.org
www.cup.org

2994 International Journal of Aging and Human
Developments
Baywood Publishing Company
26 Austin Avenue
Box 337
Amityville, NY 11701-3052
631-691-1270
800-638-7819; *Fax:* 631-691-1770
info@baywood.com
www.baywood.com

Stuart Cohen, Owner

$218.00

8 per year Year Founded: 1973 ISSN 0091-4150

2995 International Journal of Health Services
Baywood Publishing Company
26 Austin Avenue
Box 337
Amityville, NY 11701-3052
631-691-1270
800-638-7819; *Fax:* 631-691-1770
info@baywood.com
www.baywood.com

Stuart Cohen, Owner

$160.00

4 per year Year Founded: 1970

2996 International Journal of Psychiatry in Medicine
Baywood Publishing Company
26 Austin Avenue
Box 337
Amityville, NY 11701-3052
631-691-1270
800-638-7819; *Fax:* 631-691-1770
info@baywood.com
www.baywood.com

Stuart Cohen, Owner

$160.00

4 per year Year Founded: 1970 ISSN 0091274

2997 Journal of AHIMA
American Health Information Management
Association
233 N Michigan Avenue
21st Floor
Chicago, IL 60601-5809
312-233-1100; *Fax:* 312-233-1090
info@ahima.org
www.ahima.org

Angela Kennedy, EdD, MBA, RHI, President, Chairman
Cassi Birnbaum, MS. RHIA, CP, President / Chair-Elect
Jennifer McManis, RHIT, Speaker of the House
Lynne Thomas Gordon, CEO

Monthly magazine with articles, news and event
annoucements from the nonprofit federation of affiliated
state health organizations, together representing nearly
12,000 nonprofit and for profit assisted living, nursing facility, developmentally disabled and subacute care providers that care for more than 1.5 million elderly and disabled
individuals nationally.

2998 Journal of American Health Information
Management Association
American Health Information Management
Association
233 N Michigan Avenue
21st Floor
Chicago, IL 60601-5809
312-233-1100; *Fax:* 312-233-1090
info@ahima.org
www.ahima.org

Angela Kennedy, EdD, MBA, RHI, President, Chairman
Cassi Birnbaum, MS. RHIA, CP, President / Chair-Elect
Jennifer McManis, RHIT, Speaker of the House
Lynne Thomas Gordon, CEO

2999 Journal of American Medical Information
Association
Hanley & Befus
4720 Montgomery Lane
Suite 500
Bethesda, MD 20814
301-657-1291; *Fax:* 301-657-1296
mail@amia.org
www.www.amia.org

Karen Greenwood, EVP, COO
Ross D. Martin, MD, MHA, Vice President of Policy and
Dev
Jeffrey Williamson, M.Ed, Vice President, Education and
Ac
Pesha Rubinstein, MPH, CCMEP, Director of Education

3000 Journal of Drug Education
Baywood Publishing Company
26 Austin Avenue
Box 337
Amityville, NY 11701-3052
631-691-2048
800-638-7819; *Fax:* 631-691-1770
www.baywood.com

Stuart Cohen, Owner

$160.00

4 per year Year Founded: 1970

3001 Journal of Education Psychology
American Psychological Association
750 1st Street NE
Washington, DC 20002-4242
202-336-5500
800-374-2721; *Fax:* 202-336-5500
TDD: 202-336-6123
TTY: 202-336-6123
order@apa.org
www.apa.org

Nadine J. Kaslow, Ph.D., President
Barry S. Anton, Ph.D., President-Elect
Donald N. Bersoff, PhD, JD, Past President
Norman B Anderson, Ph.D., CEO, EVP

$102.00

4 per year ISSN 0022-0663

3002 Journal of Emotional and Behavioral Disorders
Pro-Ed Publications
8700 Shoal Creek Boulevard
Austin, TX 78757-6897
512-451-3246
800-897-3202; *Fax:* 512-451-8542
info@proedinc.com

Donald D Hammill, Owner

An international, multidisciplinary journal featuring articles on research, practice and theory related to individuals
with emotional and behavioral disorders and to the professionals who serve them. Presents topics of interest to individuals representing a wide range of disciplines including
corrections, psychiatry, mental health, counseling, rehabilitation, education, and psychology. *$39.00*

64 pages 4 per year ISSN 1063-4266

3003 Journal of Intellectual & Development Disability
Taylor & Francis Publishing
711 3rd Avenue
8th Floor
New York, NY 10017
212-216-7800
800-634-7064; *Fax:* 212-564-7854
orders@taylorandfrancis.com
www.taylorandfrancis.com

3004 Journal of Neuropsychiatry and Clinical Neurosciences
American Neuropsychiatric Association
700 Ackerman Road
Suite 625
Columbus, OH 43202-4505
614-447-2077
anpa@osu.edu

Sandy Bornstein, Executive Director
C. Edward Coffey, Treasurer

Official publication of the organization and a benefit of membership. Our mission is to apply neuroscience for the benefit of people. Three core values have been identified for the association: advancing knowledge of brain-behavior relationships, providing a forum for learning, and promoting excellent, scientific and compassionate health care.

3005 Journal of Personality Assessment
Society for Personality Assessment
6109H Arlington Boulevard
Falls Church, VA 22044-2708
703-534-4772; *Fax:* 703-534-6905
manager@spaonline.org
www.personality.org

Ronald J. Ganellen, Ph.D., President
Robert Bornstein, Ph.D., President-Elect
Radhika Krishnamurthy, Psy.D., Past President
John McNulty, Ph.D., Treasurer

Publishes articles dealing with the development, evaluation, refinement and application of personality assessment methods.

102 pages   ISSN 0022-3891

3006 Journal of Positive Behavior Interventions
Pro-Ed Publications
8700 Shoal Creek Boulevard
Austin, TX 78757-6897
512-451-3246
800-897-3202; *Fax:* 512-451-8542
info@proedinc.com

Donald D Hammill, Owner

Deals with principles of positive behavioral support in school, home, and community settings for people with challenges in behavioral adaptation. *$39.00*

64 pages 4 per year ISSN 1098-3007

3007 Journal of Practical Psychiatry
Williams & Wilkins
351 W Camden Street
Baltimore, MD 21201-2436
410-528-4000
800-882-0483; *Fax:* 410-528-4414
korourke@lww.com
www.lww.com

J Arnold Anthony, Operations
8 pages

3008 Journal of Professional Counseling: Practice, Theory & Research
Texas Counseling Association (TCA)
1204 San Antonio
Suite 201
Austin, TX 78701-1870
512-472-3403
800-580-8144; *Fax:* 512-472-3756
jan@txca.org
www.txca.org

Jan Friese, Executive Director

The Texas Counseling Association is dedicated to providing leadership, advocacy and education to promote the growth and development of the counseling profession and those that are served. *$150.00*

50 pages 2 per year

3009 Journal of the American Medical Informatics Association
American Medical Informatics Association
4720 Montgomery Lane
Suite 500
Bethesda, MD 20814-6052
301-657-1291; *Fax:* 301-657-1296
mail@amia.org
www.amia.org

Karen Greenwood, EVP, COO
Ross D. Martin, MD, MHA, Vice President of Policy and Dev
Jeffrey Williamson, M.Ed, Vice President, Education and Ac
Pesha Rubinstein, MPH, CCMEP, Director of Education

JAMIA is a bi-monthly journal that presents peer-reviewed articles on the spectrum of health care informatics in research, teaching, and application. *$212.00*

3010 Journal of the American Psychiatric Nurses Association
Sage Publications
2455 Teller Road
Thousand Oaks, CA 91320-2234
805-499-0721
800-818-7243; *Fax:* 800-583-2665
journals@sagepub.com
www.sagepub.com

Blaise R Simqu, CEO, President
Tracey A Ozmina, EVP, COO
Chris Hickok, SVP, CFO
Phil Denvir, Global Chief Information Officer

Official Journal of the American Psychiatric Nurses Association *$128.00*

ISSN 1078-3903

3011 Journal of the American Psychoanalytic Association
Analytic Press
101 W Street
Hillsdale, NJ 07642-1421
201-358-9477
800-926-6579; *Fax:* 201-358-4700
www.analyticpress.com

Paul E Stepansky PhD, Managing Director
John Kerr PhD, Sr Editor

JAPA is one of the preeminent psychoanalytic journals. Recognized for the quality of its clinical and theoretical contributions, JAPA is now a major publication source for scientists and humanists whose work elaborates, applies, critiques or impinges on psychoanalysis. Topics include child psychoanalysis and the effectiveness of the intensive treatment of children, boundary violations, problems of memory and false memory syndrome, the concept of working through, the scientific status of psychoanalysis and the relevance or irrevance of infant observation for adult analysis. *$115.00*

300 pages 4 per year Year Founded: 1952 ISSN 0003-0651

3012 Journal of the International Neuropsychological Society
Cambridge University Press
40 W 20th Street
New York, NY 10011-4211
212-924-3900; *Fax:* 212-691-3239
marketing@cup.org
www.cup.org

3013 Key
National Mental Health Consumers Self-Help
1211 Chestnut Street
Lobby 100
Philadelphia, PA 19107-4112
215-751-1810
800-553-4539; *Fax:* 215-636-6310
TTY: 215-751-9655
info@mhselfhelp.org
www.mhselfhelp.org

Violet Phillips, Editor

Provides information for consumers of mental health services/psychiatric survivors on mental health issues, including advocacy and alternative mental health services. *$15.00*

12 pages 4 per year

3014 Mayo Clinic Health Letter
Mayo Clinic
200 1st Street SW
Rochester, MN 55905-2
507-284-2511
healthletter@mayo.edu
www.mayoclinic.org

Marilyn Carlson Nelson, Chairman
John H Noseworthy, M.D., President, CEO
Shirley A. Weis, VP, CAO
William C. Rupp, M.D., VP

Helping our subscribers achieve healthier lives by providing useful, easy to understand health information that is timely and of broad interest.

ISSN 0741-6245

3015 Mental & Physical Disability Law Reporter
American Bar Association
1050 Connecticut Ave. N.W.
Suite 400
Washington, DC 20036
202-662-1000
800-285-2221; *Fax:* 202-662-1032

TTY: 202-662-1012
CMPDL@abanet.org
www.abanet.org

James R. Silkenat, President
Robert M. Carlson, Chair, House of Delegates
William C. Hubbard, President-Elect
Lucian T. Pera, Treasurer

Contains bylined articles and summaries of federal and state court opinions and legislative developments addressing persons with mental and physical disabilities.

6 per year Year Founded: 1976 ISSN 0883-7902

3016 Mental Health Law Reporter
Business Publishers Inc.
2222 Sedwick Drive
Suite 101
Durham, NC 27713
301-587-6300
800-223-8720; *Fax:* 800-508-2592
custserv@bpinews.com
www.bpinews.com

Nancy Biglin, Director Marketing

Summary of court cases pertaining to mental health professionals. *$273.00*

12 per year ISSN 0741-5141

3017 Mental Health Report
Business Publishers Inc.
2222 Sedwick Drive
Suite 101
Durham, NC 27713
301-587-6300
800-223-8720; *Fax:* 800-508-2592
custserv@bpinews.com
www.bpinews.com

Nancy Biglin, Director Marketing

Independent, inside Washington coverage of mental health administration, legislation and regulation, state policy plus research and trends. *$396.00*

26 per year ISSN 0191-6750

3018 Mentally Disabled and the Law
William S. Hein & Co.
2350 North Forest Rd.
Getzville, NY 14068
716-882-2600
800-828-7571; *Fax:* 716-883-8100
mail@wshein.com
www.wshein.com

William Hein, Chairman
Kevin Marmion, President
Daniel Rosati, SVP
Dick Spinelli, EVP

Offers information on treatment rights, the provider-patient relationship, and the rights of mentally disabled persons in the community. *$80.00*

3019 NAAP Newsletter
National Association for Advancement of Psychoanalysis
80 Eighth Avenue
Suite 1501
New York, NY 10011-5126

212-741-0515; *Fax:* 212-366-4347
NAAP@NAAP.org
www.naap.org

Douglas F. Maxwell, President
Margery Quackenbush, Executive Director
Kirsty Cardinale, NAAP News Editor
Elliott Hom, Art Director

Members: 1400 Institute Members: 40 *$24.00*

16 pages 4x per year

3020 NAMI Advocate
National Alliance for the Mentally Ill
3803 N. Fairfax Dr.
Suite 100
Arlington, VA 22203
703-524-7600
888-999-6264; *Fax:* 703-524-9094
TDD: 703-516-7227
frieda@nami.org
www.nami.org

David Levy, CFO
Lynn Borton, COO
Jean Michel Texier, Chief Information Officer
Katrina Gay, National Director, Communication

Newsletter that provides information on latest research, treatment, and medications for brain disorders. Reviews status major policy and legislation at federal, state, and local levels. Recurring features include interviews, news of research, news of educational opportunities, book reviews, politics, legal issues, and columns titled President's Column, Ask the Doctor, and News You Can Use. Included as NAMI membership benefit.

24-28 pages 24 per year

3021 NAMI Beginnings
National Alliance on Mental Illness
3803 N. Fairfax Dr.
Suite 100
Arlington, VA 22203
703-524-7600
888-999-6264; *Fax:* 703-524-9094
TDD: 703-516-7227
david@nami.org
www.nami.org

David Levy, CFO
Lynn Borton, COO
Jean Michel Texier, Chief Information Officer
Katrina Gay, National Director, Communication

A publication dedicated to the Young Minds of America from the Child and Adolescent Action Center, a free newsletter about children and adolescents living with mental illnesses.

4 per year

3022 NASW News
National Association of Social Works
750 1st Street NE
Suite 700
Washington, DC 20002-4241
202-408-8600; *Fax:* 202-336-8312
press@naswdc.org
www.naswpress.org

Elvira Craig De Silva, President
Cheryl Y. Bradley, Publisher

Sharon Fletcher, Publications Marketing Manager
Kiera White, Marketing Coordinator

3023 Newsletter of the American Psychoanalytic Association
Analytic Press
101 W Street
Hillsdale, NJ 07642-1421
201-358-9477
800-926-6579; *Fax:* 201-358-4700
www.analyticpress.com

Paul E Stepansky PhD, Managing Director
John Kerr PhD, Sr Editor

A scholarly and clinical resource for all analytic practitioners and students of the field. Articles and essays focused on contemporary social, political and cultural forces as they relate to the practice of psychoanalysis, regular interviews with leading proponents of analysis, essays and reminiscences that chart the evolution of anlaysis in America. The newsletter publishes articles that are rarely if ever found in the journal literature. Sample copies available. *$29.50*

4 per year

3024 North American Society of Adlerian Psychology Newsletter
NASAP
429 E. Dupont Road
#276
Fort Wayne, IN 46825
260-267-8807; *Fax:* 260-818-2098
nasap@msn.com
www.alfredadler.org

Richard Watts, President
Susan Belangee, VP
Steven J. Stein, Past-President
Susan Burak, Treasurer

Relates news and events of the North American Society of Alderian Psychology and regional news of affiliated associations. Recurring features include lists of courses and workshops offered by affiliated associations, reviews of new publications in the field, professional employment opportunities, a calendar of events, and a column titled President's Message. *$20.00*

8 pages 24 per year ISSN 0889-9428

3025 ORTHO Update
American Orthopsychiatric Association
PO Box 202798
Denver, CO 80220
720-708-0187; *Fax:* 303-366-3471
amerortho@aol.com
www.www.aoatoday.com

Mary I. Armstrong, MSW, PhD, President
Deborah Klein Walker, EdD, President-Elect
Donald Wertlieb, PhD, Past President
John Sargent, MD, Treasurer

Intended for members of the Association, who are concerned with the early signs of mental and behavioral disorder and preventive psychiatry. Provides news notes and feature articles on the trends, issues and events that concern mental health, as well as Association news.

6-16 pages 3 per year

3026 Open Minds
Behavioral Health Industry News
163 York Street
Gettysburg, PA 17325-1933
717-334-1329
877-350-6463; *Fax:* 717-334-0538
info@openminds.com
www.openminds.com

Monica Oss, Owner
Casey A. Miller, VP, Administration
Aida Porras, Senior Associate
Jim Jenkins, Senior Associate

Provides information on marketing, financial, and legal trends in the delivery of mental health and chemical dependency benefits and services. Recurring features include interviews, news of research, a calendar of events, job listings, book reviews, notices of publications available, and industry statistics. *$185.00*

12 pages 12 per year ISSN 1043-3880

3027 OpenMinds
Open Minds
163 York Street
Gettysburg, PA 17325-1933
717-334-1329
877-350-6463; *Fax:* 717-334-0538
info@openminds.com
www.openminds.com

Monica Oss, Owner
Casey A. Miller, VP, Administration
Aida Porras, Senior Associate
Jim Jenkins, Senior Associate

Provides information on marketing, financial, and legal trends in the delivery of mental health and chemical dependency benefits and services. Recurring features include interviews, news of research, a calendar of events, job listings, book reviews, notices of publications available, and industry statistics. *$185.00*

12 pages 12 per year ISSN 1043-3880

3028 Perspective on Psychological Science
Association for Psychological Science
1133 15th Street NW
Suite 1000
Washington, DC 20005
202-293-9300; *Fax:* 202-293-9350
akraut@psychologicalscience.org
www.psychologicalscience.org

Linda Bartoshuk, President
Elizabeth A. Phelps, President
Mahzarin R Banaji, President-Elect
Nancy Eisenberg, President-Elect

Perspectives publishes an eclectic mix of provocative reports and articles, including board integrative reviews, overviews of research programs, meta-analysis, theoretical statements, book reviews, and articles on topics such as the philosophy of science, opinion pieces about major issues in the field, autobiographical reflections of senior members in the field, and the occasional humorous essay and sketch.

6 per year Year Founded: 1988 ISSN 1745-6916

3029 Professional Counselor
3201 SW 15th Street
Deerfield Beach, FL 33442-8157

954-360-0909
800-851-9100; *Fax:* 954-570-8506
Gary.Seidler@usjt.com
www.professionalcounselor.com

Robert Ackerman, Editor
Gary Seidler, Executive Consulting Editor
Leah Honarbakhsh, Associate Editor
Lorrie Keip, Director of Continuing Education

The number one publication serving the addictions and mental health fields.

3030 Provider Magazine
American Health Care Association
1201 L Street NW
Washington, DC 20005-4046
202-842-4444
888-656-6669; *Fax:* 202-842-3860
sales@ahca.org
www.www.providermagazine.com

Bruse Yarwood, President
Bill Myers, Senior Editor
Meg LaPorte, Managing Editor
Joanne Erickson, Editor in Chief

Of interest to the professionals who work for the nearly 12,000 nonprofit and for profit assisted living, nursing facility, developmentally disabled and subacute care providers that care for more than 1.5 million elderly and disabled individuals nationally. Provides information, education, and administrative tools that enhance quality at every level.

3031 PsycINFO News
American Psychological Association
750 1st Street NE
Washington, DC 20002-4242
202-336-5500
800-374-2721; *Fax:* 202-336-5518
TDD: 202-336-6123
TTY: 202-336-6123
psycinfo@apa.org
www.apa.org

Nadine J. Kaslow, Ph.D., President
Barry S. Anton, Ph.D., President-Elect
Donald N. Bersoff, PhD, JD, Past President
Norman B Anderson, Ph.D., CEO, EVP

Free newsletter that keeps you up to date on enhancements to PsycINFO products.

4 per year

3032 PsycSCAN Series
American Psychological Association
750 1st Street NE
Washington, DC 20002-4242
202-336-5500
800-374-2721; *Fax:* 202-336-5518
TDD: 202-336-6123
TTY: 202-336-6123
psycinfo@apa.org
www.apa.org

Nadine J. Kaslow, Ph.D., President
Barry S. Anton, Ph.D., President-Elect
Donald N. Bersoff, PhD, JD, Past President
Norman B Anderson, Ph.D., CEO, EVP

Quarterly current awareness print publications in the fields of clinical, developmental, and applied psychology, as well as learning disorders and behavior analysis and therapy.

Contains relevant citations and abstracts from the PsycINFO database. PyscScan: Psychopharmacology is an electronic only publication.

4 per year

3033 Psych Discourse
The Association of Black Psychologists
7119 Allentown Road
Suite 203
Washington, MD 20744
301-449-3082; *Fax:* 301-449-3084
abpsi@abpsi.org
www.abpsi.org

Taasogle Daryl Rowe, Ph.D., President
Kevin Washington, Ph.D., President-Elect
Carolyn Moore, Ph.D., Treasurer
Anisha Lewis, Executive Director

Publishes news of the Association. Recurring features include editorials, news of research, letters to the editor, a calendar of events, and columns titled Social Actions, Chapter News, Publications, and Members in the News. *$110.00*

32-64 pages 12 per year Year Founded: 1969 ISSN 1091-4781

3034 Psychiatric News
American Psychiatric Publishing, Inc.
1000 Wilson Boulevard
Suite 1825
Arlington, VA 22209-3901
703-907-7322
800-368-5777; *Fax:* 703-907-1091
appi@psych.org
www.appi.org

Saul Levin, M.D., M.P.A., CEO, Medical Director
Ron McMillen, Chief Executive Officer
Robert E Hales, M.D., M.B.A., Editor-in-Chief
Rebecca D. Rinehart, Publisher

Psychiatric News is the official newspaper for the American Psychiatric Association. It is published twice a month and mailed to all APA members as a member benefit as well as to about 2,000 subscribers.

3035 Psychiatric Times
Continuing Medical Education
806 Plaza Three
Jersey City, NJ 07311-1112
949-250-1008
800-993-2632; *Fax:* 949-250-0445
www.psychiatrictimes.com

John L. Schwartz MD, Founder and Editor Emeritus
Ronald Pies, MD, Editor Emeritus
James L. Knoll, MD, Editor in Chief
George I. Papakostas, M.D., Director, Treatment-Resistant De

Allows you to earn CME credit every month with a clinical article, as well as keeping you up to date on the current news in the field. *$54.95*

12 per year

3036 Psychiatry Drug Alerts
MJ Powers & Company
65 Madison Avenue
Ssite 220
Morristown, NJ 07960-7354

973-889-5398
800-875-0058
psych@alertpubs.com

Evelyn Powers, Owner

Discusses drugs used in the psychiatric field, including side effects and risks. *$63.00*

8 pages 12 per year ISSN 0894-4873

3037 Psychiatry Research
Customer Support Department
PO Box 945
New York, NY 10159-945
212-633-3730
888-437-4636; *Fax:* 212-633-3680
www.elsevier.nl/locate/psychres

ISSN 0165-1781

3038 Psychological Abstracts
PsycINFO/American Psychological Association
750 1st Street NE
Washington, DC 20002-4242
202-336-5500
800-374-2721; *Fax:* 202-336-5518
TDD: 202-336-6123
TTY: 202-336-6123
psycinfo@apa.org
www.apa.org

Nadine J. Kaslow, Ph.D., President
Barry S. Anton, Ph.D., President-Elect
Donald N. Bersoff, PhD, JD, Past President
Norman B Anderson, Ph.D., CEO, EVP

Print index containing citations and abstracts for journal articles, books, and book chapters in psychology and related disciplines. Annual indexes.

12 per year

3039 Psychological Assessment Resources INC
16130 North Florida Avenue
Lutz, FL 33549
813-449-4065
800-331-8378; *Fax:* 800-725-9329
www.www4.parinc.com

R. Bob Smith III, PhD, Chairman, CEO
Cathy Smith, VP, Community Relations

3040 Psychological Science
Association for Psychological Science
1133 15th Street NW
Suite 1000
Washington, DC 20005
202-293-9300; *Fax:* 202-293-9350
akraut@psychologicalscience.org
www.psychologicalscience.org

Linda Bartoshuk, President
Elizabeth A. Phelps, President
Mahzarin R Banaji, President-Elect
Nancy Eisenberg, President-Elect

The flagship journal of the APS, it publishes cutting edge research articles, short reports, and research reports spanning the entire spectrum of the science of psychology. The Journal is the source for the latest findings in cognitive, social, developmental and health psychology, as well as behavioral neuroscience and biopsychology.

12 per year Year Founded: 1988 ISSN 0956-7976

3041 Psychological Science Agenda
American Psychological Association
750 1st Street NE
Washington, DC 20002-4242
202-336-5500
800-374-2721; *Fax:* 202-336-5518
TDD: 202-336-6123
TTY: 202-336-6123
psycinfo@apa.org

Nadine J. Kaslow, Ph.D., President
Barry S. Anton, Ph.D., President-Elect
Donald N. Bersoff, PhD, JD, Past President
Norman B Anderson, Ph.D., CEO, EVP

This newsletter disseminates information on scientific psychology, including news on activities of the Association and congressional and federal advocacy efforts of the Directorate. Recurring features include reports of meetings, news of research, notices of publications available, interviews, and the columns titled Science Directorate News, On Behalf of Science, Science Briefs, Announcements, and Funding Opportunities.

16-20 pages 6 per year ISSN 1040-404X

3042 Psychological Science in the Public Interest
Association for Psychological Science
1133 15th Street NW
Suite 1000
Washington, DC 20005
202-293-9300; *Fax:* 202-293-9350
akraut@psychologicalscience.org
www.psychologicalscience.org

Linda Bartoshuk, President
Elizabeth A. Phelps, President
Mahzarin R Banaji, President-Elect
Nancy Eisenberg, President-Elect

PSPI is a unique journal featuring comprehensive and compelling views of issues that are of direct relevance to the general public. Reviews are written by teams of award-winning specialists representing a range of viewpoints, and are intended to assess the current state-of-the-science with regard to the topic.

3 per year Year Founded: 1988 ISSN 1529-1006

3043 Psychology Teacher Network Education Directorate
American Psychological Association
750 1st Street NE
Washington, DC 20002-4242
202-336-5500
800-374-2721; *Fax:* 202-336-5518
TDD: 202-336-6123
TTY: 202-336-6123
psycinfo@apa.org
www.apa.org

Nadine J. Kaslow, Ph.D., President
Barry S. Anton, Ph.D., President-Elect
Donald N. Bersoff, PhD, JD, Past President
Norman B Anderson, Ph.D., CEO, EVP

Provides descriptions of experiments and demonstrations aimed at introducing topics as a basis for classroom lectures or discussion. Recurring features include news and announcements of courses, workshops, funding sources, and meetings; reviews of teaching aids; and reports of innovative programs or curricula occurring in schools, inter-

views and brief reports from prominent psychologists.
$15.00

16 pages 5 per year

3044 Psychophysiology
Cambridge University Press
40 W 20th Street
New York, NY 10011-4211
212-924-3900; *Fax:* 212-691-3239
marketing@cup.org
www.cup.org

3045 Psychosomatic Medicine
American Psychosomatic Society
6728 Old McLean Village Drive
McLean, VA 22101-3906
703-556-9222; *Fax:* 703-556-8729
info@psychosomatic.org
www.psychosomatic.org

William Lovallo, President
Karen L. Weihs, M.D., President
Mustafa al'Absi, Ph.D., President-Elect
George K. Degnon, CAE, Executive Director

News and event annoucements, examines the scientific understanding of the interrelationships among biological, psychological, social and behavioral factors in human health and disease, and the integration of the fields of science that separately examine each.

3046 Psychotherapy Bulletin
American Psychological Association
750 First Street NE
Washington, DC 20002-4242
202-336-5500
800-374-2721; *Fax:* 202-336-5518
TDD: 202-336-6123
TTY: 202-336-6123
psycinfo@apa.org
www.apa.org

Nadine J. Kaslow, Ph.D., President
Barry S. Anton, Ph.D., President-Elect
Donald N. Bersoff, PhD, JD, Past President
Norman B Anderson, Ph.D., CEO, EVP

Recurring features include letters to the editor, news of research, reports of meetings, news of educational opportunities, committee reports, legislative issues, and columns titled Washington Scene, Finance, Marketing, Professional Liability, Medical Psychology Update, and Substance Abuse. *$8.00*

50 pages 4 per year

3047 Psychotherapy Finances
Managed Care Strategies & Psychotherapy Finances
14255 U.S. Highway 1
Suite 286
Juno Beach, FL 33408-1612
561-624-1155
800-869-8450; *Fax:* 561-743-3504
www.www.psyfin.com

John Klein, Editor
John Nelander, Managing Editor
Anne Marie Church, Marketing Director
Herbert E. Klein, Publisher

3048 Research and Training for Children's Mental Health-Update
University of South Florida
13301 Bruce B Downs Boulevard
Florida Mental Health Institute
Tampa, FL 33612-3807
813-974-4565

Services and research on children with emotional disorders.

2 per year

3049 Rural Mental Health Journal
NARMH
25 Massachusetts Ave NW
Suite 500
Washington, DC 20001
202-942-4276
info@narmh.org
www.narmh.org

Jerry Parker, President
Paul Mackie, President-Elect
Linda Werlein, Past-President
David Weden, Treasurer

Provides a information for rural mental health professionals and advocates.

4 per year

3050 Smooth Sailing
Depression and Related Affective Disorders Association
600 N Wolfe Street
John Hopkins Hospital Meyer 3-181
Baltimore, MD 21287-5
Fax: 410-614-3241
www.med.jhu.edu/drada/

Outreach to students and parents through schools.

4 per year

3051 Social Work
NASW Press
750 1st Street NE
Suite 700
Washington, DC 20002-4241
202-408-8600; *Fax:* 202-336-8312
press@naswdc.org
www.naswpress.org

Elvira Craig De Silva, President
Cheryl Y. Bradley, Publisher
Sharon Fletcher, Publications Marketing Manager
Kiera White, Marketing Coordinator

3052 Social Work Abstracts
NASW Press
750 1st Street NE
Suite 700
Washington, DC 20002-4241
202-408-8600; *Fax:* 202-336-8312
press@naswdc.org
www.naswpress.org

Elvira Craig De Silva, President
Cheryl Y. Bradley, Publisher
Sharon Fletcher, Publications Marketing Manager
Kiera White, Marketing Coordinator

3053 Social Work Research
NASW Press
750 1st Street NE
Suite 700
Washington, DC 20002-4241
202-408-8600; *Fax:* 202-336-8312
press@naswdc.org
www.naswpress.org

Elvira Craig De Silva, President
Cheryl Y. Bradley, Publisher
Sharon Fletcher, Publications Marketing Manager
Kiera White, Marketing Coordinator

3054 Social Work in Education
NASW Press
750 1st Street NE
Suite 700
Washington, DC 20002-4241
202-408-8600; *Fax:* 202-336-8312
press@naswdc.org
www.naswpress.org

Elvira Craig De Silva, President
Cheryl Y. Bradley, Publisher
Sharon Fletcher, Publications Marketing Manager
Kiera White, Marketing Coordinator

3055 Society for Adolescent Psychiatry Newsletter
PO Box 570218
Dallas, TX 75357-218
972-613-0985; *Fax:* 972-613-5532
www.adolpsych.org

Mohan Nair, President
Gregg Dwyer, President
Sheldon Glass, President Elect
Gregory P. Barclay, VP

Puts psychiatrists in touch with an informed cross-section of the profession from all over North America. Dedicated to education development and advocacy of adolescents and the adolescent psychiatric field.

3056 The Bulletin
American Society of Psychoanalytic Physicians
13528 Wisteria Drive
Germantown, MD 20874-1049
301-540-3197

Christine Cotter, Executive Director

The Bulletin of the American Society of Psychoanalustic Physicians is a professional publication containing articles by members, meeting speakers and other professionals in addition to newes about the society. Papers are accepted based on a peer review process.

15 pages 1 per year

3057 World Federation for Mental Health Newsletter
World Federation for Mental Health
PO Box 807
Occoquania, VA 22125
703-838-7525; *Fax:* 703-490-6926
info@wfmh.com
www.wfmh.com

George Christodoulou, President, Greece
Deborah Wan, Hong Kong, Immediate Past President
Gabriel Ivbijaro, President Elect, U.K.
Gwen Dixon, Office Administrator

World-wide mental health reports. Education and advocacy on mental health issues. Working to protect the human rights of those defined as mentally ill.

8 pages 1 per year Year Founded: 1984

Testing & Evaluation

3058 Assessment of Neuropsychiatry and Mental Health Services
American Psychiatric Publishing, Inc.
1000 Wilson Boulevard
Suite 1825
Arlington, VA 22209-3901
703-907-7322
800-368-5777; *Fax:* 703-907-1091
appi@psych.org
www.appi.org

Ron McMillen, Chief Executive Officer
Robert E. Hales MD, M.B.A, Editor-in-Chief
John McDuffie, Editorial Director, Associate Pu
Rebecca D. Rinehart, Publisher

Examines the importance of an integrated approach to neuropsychiatric conditions and looks at ways to overcome the difficulties in assessing medical disorders in psychiatric populations. Addresses neuropsychiatric disorders and their costs and implications on policy. *$94.00*

448 pages Year Founded: 1999 ISBN 0-880487-30-5

3059 Attention-Deficit/Hyperactivity Disorder Test: a Method for Identifying Individuals with ADHD
Pro.Ed
8700 Shoal Creek Boulevard
Austin, TX 78757-6897
512-451-3246
800-897-3202; *Fax:* 512-451-8542
general@proedinc.com
www.www.proedinc.com

Donald D Hammill, Owner

An effective instrument for identifying and evaluating attention - deficit disorders in persons ages three to twenty-three. Designed for use in schools and clinics, the test is easily completed by teachers, parents and others who are knowledgeable about the referred individual. *$110.00*

Year Founded: 1995

3060 Behavioral and Emotional Rating Scale
Pro.Ed
8700 Shoal Creek Boulevard
Austin, TX 78757-6897
512-451-3246
800-897-3202; *Fax:* 512-451-8542
general@proedinc.com
www.www.proedinc.com

Donald D Hammill, Owner

Helps to measure the personal strengths of children ages five through eighteen. Contains 52 items that measure five aspects of a child's strength: interpersonal strength, involvement with family, intrapersonal strength, school functioning, and affective strength. Provides overall strength score and five subtest scores. Identifies individual behavioral and emotional strengths of children, the areas in which individual strengths need to be developed, and the goals for individual treatment plans. *$165.00*

Year Founded: 1998

3061 Childhood History Form for Attention Disorders
A.D.D. Warehouse
300 NW 70th Avenue
Suite 102
Plantation, FL 33317-2360
954-792-8100
800-233-9273; *Fax:* 954-792-8545
websales@addwarehouse.com
www.addwarehouse.com

Harvey C Parker, Owner

This form is completed by parents prior to a history taking session. It is designed to be used in conjunction with standardized assessment questionaires utilized in the evaluation of attention disorders. 25 per package. *$45.00*

10 pages

3062 Children's Depression Inventory
A.D.D. Warehouse
300 NW 70th Avenue
Suite 102
Plantation, FL 33317-2360
954-792-8100
800-233-9273; *Fax:* 954-792-8545
websales@addwarehouse.com
www.addwarehouse.com

Harvey C Parker, Owner

A self-report, symptom-oriented scale which requires at least a first grade reading level and was designed for school-aged children and adolescents. The CDI has 27 items, each of which consists of three choices. Quickscore form scoring make the inventories easy and economical to administer. The profile contains the following five factors plus a total score normed according to age and sex: negative mood, interpersonal problems, ineffectiveness, anhedonia and negative self-esteem. Contains ten items and provides a general indication of depressive symptoms. *$148.00*

3063 Clinical Evaluations of School Aged Children
Professional Resource Press
PO Box 3197
Sarasota, FL 34230-3197
941-343-9601
800-443-3364; *Fax:* 941-343-9201
cs.prpress@gmail.com
www.prpress.com

Laurie Girsch, Managing Editor

This book delineates the specific symptoms and behaviors associated with each DSM - IV diagnostic syndrome and provides an exceptionally well designed system for communicating diagnostic findings with great clarity when working with parents and professionals from different disciplines. *$34.95*

376 pages Year Founded: 1998 ISBN 1-568870-27-2

3064 Clinical Interview of the Adolescent: From Assessment and Formulation to Treatment Planning
Charles C Thomas Publisher Ltd.
2600 S 1st Street
Springfield, IL 62704-4730
217-789-8980
800-258-8980; *Fax:* 217-789-9130

books@ccthomas.com
www.ccthomas.com

Michael P Thomas, President

This book addresses the process of interviewing troubled and psychologically disturbed adolescents who are seen in hospital settings, schools, courts, clinics, and residential facilities. Interviews with adolescents, younger children or adults should follow a logical, sequential and integrated procedure, accomplishing diagnostic closure and the development of a treatment formulation. The nine chapters cover the theoretical and developmental concerns of adolescence; the initial referral; meeting with parents; the therapist; getting acquainted; getting to the heart of the matter; making order out of disorder; the reasons and rationale for the behavior problems. *$59.95*

234 pages Year Founded: 1997 ISBN 0-398067-79-1

3065 Concise Guide to Assessment and Management of Violent Patients
American Psychiatric Publishing, Inc.
1000 Wilson Boulevard
Suite 1825
Arlington, VA 22209-3901
703-907-7322
800-368-5777; *Fax:* 703-907-1091
appi@psych.org
www.appi.org

Ron McMillen, Chief Executive Officer
Robert E. Hales MD, M.B.A, Editor-in-Chief
John McDuffie, Editorial Director, Associate Pu
Rebecca D. Rinehart, Publisher

Written by an expert on violence, this edition provides current information on psychopharmacology, safety of clinicians and how to deal with threats of violence to the clinician. *$32.95*

180 pages Year Founded: 1996 ISBN 0-880483-44-X

3066 Conducting Insanity Evaluations
Guilford Press
72 Spring Street
New York, NY 10012-4068
212-431-9800
800-365-7006; *Fax:* 212-966-6708
info@guilford.com
www.www.guilford.com

Bob Matloff, President
Seymour Weingarten, Editor-in-Chief

Great resource for both psychologists and lawyers. Covers legal standards and their applications to clinical work. Mental health professionals who evaluate defendants or consult to courts on criminal matters will find this a useful resource. *$50.00*

342 pages Year Founded: 2000 ISBN 1-572305-21-5

3067 Conners' Rating Scales
Pro.Ed
8700 Shoal Creek Boulevard
Austin, TX 78757-6897
512-451-3246
800-897-3202; *Fax:* 512-451-8542
general@proedinc.com
www.www.proedinc.com

Donald D Hammill, Owner

Conner's Rating Scales are a result of 30 years of research on childhood and adolescent psychopathology and problem behavior. This revision adds a number of enhancements to a set of measures that has long been the standard instruments for the measurement of attention-deficit/hyperactivity disorder in children and adolescents. *$153.00*

Year Founded: 1997

3068 Depression and Anxiety in Youth Scale
Pro.Ed
8700 Shoal Creek Boulevard
Austin, TX 78757-6897
512-451-3246
800-897-3202; *Fax:* 512-451-8542
general@proedinc.com
www.www.proedinc.com

Donald D Hammill, Owner

A unique battery of three norm-referenced scales useful in identifying major depressive disorder and overanxious disorders in children and adolescents. *$150.00*

Year Founded: 1994

3069 Diagnosis and Treatment of Multiple Personality Disorder
Guilford Press
72 Spring Street
New York, NY 10012-4068
212-431-9800
800-365-7006; *Fax:* 212-966-6708
info@guilford.com
www.www.guilford.com

Bob Matloff, President
Seymour Weingarten, Editor-in-Chief

Comprehensive and integrated approach to a complex psychotherapeutic process. From first interview to crisis management to final post-integrative treatment each step is systematically reviewed, with detailed instructions on specific diagnostic and therapeutic techniques and examples of clinical applications. Specially geared to the needs of therapists, novice or expert alike, struggling with their first MPD case. *$48.00*

351 pages Year Founded: 1989 ISBN 0-898621-77-1

3070 Diagnosis and Treatment of Sociopaths and Clients with Sociopathic Traits
NewHarbinger Publications
5674 Shattuck Avenue
Oakland, CA 94609-1662
510-652-0215
800-748-6273; *Fax:* 800-652-1613
customerservice@newharbinger.com
www.newharbinger.com

Matthew McKay, Owner

This text presents a full course of treatment, with special attention to safety issues and other concerns for different client populations in a range of treatment settings. *$49.95*

208 pages Year Founded: 1996 ISBN 1-572240-47-4

3071 Draw a Person: Screening Procedure for Emotional Disturbance
Pro.Ed
8700 Shoal Creek Boulevard
Austin, TX 78757-6897

512-451-3246
800-897-3202; *Fax:* 512-451-8542
general@proedinc.com
www.www.proedinc.com

Donald D Hammill, Owner

Helps identify children and adolescents ages six through
seventeen who have emotional problems and require further evaluation. *$140.00*

Year Founded: 1991

3072 Handbook of Psychological Assessment
John Wiley & Sons
111 River Street
Hoboken, NJ 07030-5774
201-748-6000; *Fax:* 201-748-6088
info@wiley.com
www.wiley.com

Stephen M. Smith, President, CEO
MJ O'Leary, SVP, Human Resources
Edward J. Melando, SVP, Corporate Controller
Gary M. Rinck, SVP, General Counsel

Classic, revised and new psychological tests are all considered for validity and overall reliability in the light of current clinical thought and scientific development. The new
edition has expanded coverage of neuropsychological assessment and reports on assessment and treatment planning
in the age of managed care. *$95.00*

862 pages Year Founded: 1997 ISBN 0-471419-79-6

3073 Harvard Medical School Guide to Suicide Assessment and Intervention
Jossey-Bass Publishers
989 Market Street
San Francisco, CA 94103-1708
415-433-1740; *Fax:* 415-433-0499
www.leadertoleader.org

Debra Hunter, President

The definitive guide for helping mental health professionals
determine the risk for suicide and appropriate treatment
strategies for suicidal or at-risk patients. *$85.00*

736 pages ISBN 0-787943-03-7

3074 Health Watch
28 Maple Avenue
Medford, MA 02155-7118
781-395-5515
800-643-2757; *Fax:* 781-395-6547
www.healthwatch.cc

Bill Govostes, Owner

On site performer of preventative health screening services
and disease risk management programming. Specializing in
point of care testing, we perform fast and accurate health
screening tests and services to assist in indentifying partici-
pant's risk for developing future disease.

Year Founded: 1987

3075 Scale for Assessing Emotional Disturbance
Pro.Ed
8700 Shoal Creek Boulevard
Austin, TX 78757-6897
512-451-3246
800-897-3202; *Fax:* 512-451-8542
general@proedinc.com
www.www.proedinc.com

Donald D Hammill, Owner

Helps you identify children and adolescents who qualify
for the federal special education category Emotional Disturbance. *$100.00*

Year Founded: 1998

3076 Screening for Brain Dysfunction in Psychiatric Patients
Charles C Thomas Publisher Ltd.
2600 S 1st Street
Springfield, IL 62704-4730
217-789-8980
800-258-8980; *Fax:* 217-789-9130
books@ccthomas.com
www.ccthomas.com

Michael P Thomas, President

This book presents how medical diseases can be
misdiagnosed as psychiatric disorders and how clinicians
without extensive training in the neurosciences can do a
competent job of screening psychiatric clients for possible
brain disorders. The research cited in this book, dating back
to the 1890's, establishes beyond a doubt that such
misdiagnoses are more common than most clinicians would
guess. This book focuses on one type of medical condition
that is likely to be misdiagnosed: brain injuries and illnesses. *$36.95*

148 pages Year Founded: 1998 ISBN 0-398069-21-2

3077 Sexual Dysfunction: Guide for Assessment and Treatment
Guilford Press
72 Spring Street
New York, NY 10012-4068
212-431-9800
800-365-7006; *Fax:* 212-966-6708
info@guilford.com
www.www.guilford.com

Bob Matloff, President
Seymour Weingarten, Editor-in-Chief

Designed as a succinct guide to contemporary sex therapy,
this book provides an empirically based overview of the
most common sexual dysfunctions and a step-by-step manual for their assessment and treatment. Provides a
biopsychosocial model of sexual function and dysfunction
and describes the authors' general approach to management
of sexual difficulties. *$25.00*

212 pages Year Founded: 1991 ISBN 0-898622-07-7

3078 Social-Emotional Dimension Scale
Pro.Ed
8700 Shoal Creek Boulevard
Austin, TX 78757-6897
512-451-3246
800-897-3202; *Fax:* 512-451-8542
general@proedinc.com
www.www.proedinc.com

Donald D Hammill, Owner

A rating scale for teachers, counselors, and psychologists to
screen age 5 1/2 through 18 1/2 who are at risk for conduct
disorders, behavior problems, or emotional disturbance. It
assesses physical/fear reaction, depressive reaction, avoidance of peer interaction, avoidance of teacher interaction,
aggressive interaction, and inappropriate behaviors.
$149.00

Year Founded: 1986

3079 Test Collection at ETS
Educational Testing Service
660 Rosedale Road
Princeton, NJ 08541-1
609-921-9000; *Fax:* 609-734-5410
www.www.ets.org

Kurt M Landgraf, CEO

Provides 1,200 plus tests available in microfiche or downloadable for reaserch.

Training & Recruitment

3080 Ackerman Institute for the Family
936 Broadway
2nd Floor
New York, NY 10010
212-879-4900; *Fax:* 21- 74- 020
ackerman@ackerman.org
www.ackerman.org

Lois Braverman, LCSW, President, CEO
Marcia Sheinberg, LCSW, Director of Training and Clinica
Martha E. Edwards, PhD, Director of the Center for the D
Peter Fraenkel, PhD, Director of the Center for Work

A not-for-profit agency devoted to the treatment and study of families and to the training of family therapists. One of the first training institutions in the United States committed to promoting family functioning and family mental health, Acker is dedicated to helping all families at all stages of family life.

3081 Alfred Adler Institute (AAI)
372 Central Park West
New York, NY 10025
212-254-1048
director@alfredadler-ny.org
www.www.aai-ny.org

Ellen Mendel, M.Ed., M.S., M, President, Chair of the Board
Brock Hotaling, BSc, Executive Director
Fredrica Levinson, M.A., C.R.C., Dean of Students
Ellen Mendel, M.Ed., M.S., M, Director, Admissions

Offers training in psychotherapy and analysis to psychiatrists, psychologists, social workers, teachers, clergymen and other related professional persons. Conducts three-year program to provide an understanding of the dynamics of personality and interpersonal relationships and to teach therapeutic methods and techniques. Presents the theory of Individual Psychology as formulated by Alfred Adler. Publications: Journal of Individual Psychology, quarterly. Annual meeting. Semi-annual seminar.

3082 Alliance Behavioral Care: University of Cincinnati Psychiatric Services
222 Piedmont Avenue
Suite 8800
Cincinnati, OH 45219-4231
513-475-8622
800-926-8862
www.alliancebehavioral.com

A regional managed behavioral healthcare organization committed to continuously improving the resources and programs that serve their members and providers. Their goal is to provide resources that improve the well-being of those they serve and to integrate the behavioral healthcare within the overall healthcare systems.

3083 Alliant International University
Los Angeles Campus
1000 South Fremont Avenue, Unit 5
Alhambra, CA 91803-8835
626-270-3300
866-825-5426
TDD: 800-585-5087
admissions@alliant.edu
www.alliant.edu

Geoffrey Cox PhD, President

Offers industry-specific training to mid-management and supervisory personnel employed in behavioral healthcare organizations.

3084 Alton Ochsner Medical Foundation, Psychiatry Residency
1514 Jefferson Highway
New Orleans, LA 70121-2429
504-842-3000; *Fax:* 504-736-4978
gme@ochsner.org

Doris Ratcliff, Manager

3085 American Academy of Child and Adolescent Psychiatry
3615 Wisconsin Avenue Northwest
Washington, DC 20016-3007
202-966-7300; *Fax:* 202-464-0131
communications@aacap.org
www.aacap.org

Karen Wagner, MD, PhD, President
Andres Martin, MD, MPH, Secretary
Bennett L. Leventha, MD, Treasurer
Heidi B. Fordi, CAE, Executive Director

A nonprofit membership based organization composed of over 7,500 child and adolescent psychiatrists and other interested physicians. Promotes mentally healthy children, adolescents, and families through research, training, advocacy, prevention, comprehensive diagnosis and treatment, peer support, and collaboration.

Year Founded: 1953

3086 American College of Healthcare Executives
One N Franklin Street
Suite 1700
Chicago, IL 60606-3529
312-424-2800; *Fax:* 312-424-0023
contact@ache.org
www.ache.org

Christine M. Candio, RN, FACHE, Chairman
Richard D. Cordova, FACHE, Chairman-Elect
Diana L. Smalley, FACHE, Immediate Past Chairman
Deborah J. Bowen, FACHE, President, CEO

International professional society of nearly 30,000 healthcare executives. ACHE is known for its prestigious credentialing and educational programs. ACHE is also known for its journal, Journal of Healthcare Management, and magazine, Healthcare Executive, as well as ground-breaking research and career development programs. Through its efforts, ACHE works toward its goal of improving the health status of society by advancing healthcare management excellence.

3087 American College of Legal Medicine
1100 E Woodfield Road
Suite 350
Schaumburg, IL 60173-5125
847-969-0283; *Fax:* 847-517-7229
info@aclm.org
www.aclm.org

Thomas R. McLean, MD, MS, JD, FC, President-Elect
Victoria Green, MD, JD, MBA, MH, Past President
Daniel L. Orr, II, DDS PhD JD MD, Treasurer
Charles W. Hinnant, Jr., MD, JD,, Secretary

The mission of ACWHP is to advance women-centered healthcare.

3088 Andrus Children's Center
Julia Dyckman Andrus Memorial
1156 N Broadway
Yonkers, NY 10701-1108
914-965-3700

Tecla Critelli, President/CEO

Vision is to 'give opportunity to youth.' A private, non-profit community agency that provides assessment, treatment, education and preventive services for children and their families in residential, day and other restorative programs. Mission is to serve families, without regard to background or financial status, who have or are at risk for developing behavioral health problems. A highly qualified and caring staff uses established techniques and innovative programs to accomplish these purposes.

3089 Asian Pacific Development Center for Human Development
1537 Alton Street
Aurora, CO 80010
303-923-2920; *Fax:* 303-388-1172
info@apdc.org
www.apdc.org

Christine Wanifuchi, CEO
Eri Asano, Clinic Director
Jinny Kim, Director of Strategic Developmen
Edward McCarthy, Office Coordinator

A community-based non-profit organization that serves the needs of a growing population of Asian American and Pacific Islander residents throughout Colorado. APDC operates a licensed Community Mental Health Clinic and a multicultural Interpreters Bank.

Year Founded: 1980

3090 Behavioral Healthcare Center
464 Commonwealth Street
#147
Belmont, MA 02478
617-393-3935; *Fax:* 617-393-1808
cberney@mah.harvard.edu
www.academicpsychiatry.org

Carole Berney, Administrative Director
Joan Anzia, President

A behavioral health facility providing consultation in psychiatry, psychopharmacology and psychotherapy to primary care physicians and their patients.

3091 Behavioral Medicine and Biofeedback Consultants
150 SW 12th Avenue
Suite 207
Pompano Beach, FL 33069-3238
954-202-6200
info@behavioralmedicine.com
www.behavioralmedicine.com

Gary S Traub, Owner, Director

3092 Bowling Green University Psychology Department
Bowling Green State University
Bowling Green, OH 43403-0001
419-372-2531; *Fax:* 419-372-6013
www.www.bgsu.edu

Sherideen S. Stoll, VP, Finance and Administration,
Steve Krakoff, Associate VP, Capital Planning a
John Ellinger, Chief Information Officer
Bradley Leigh, Executive Director, Business Ope

3093 Brandeis University/Heller School
415 South Street
Waltham, MA 02453-2700
781-736-2000; *Fax:* 781-736-4416
www.brandeis.edu

Fred M. Lawrence, President
David A. Bunis, Senior Vice President, Chief of
Marianne Cwalina, Senior Vice President for Financ
Ellen de Graffenreid, Senior Vice President for Commun

3094 Brandeis University: Schneider Institute for Health Policy
Brandeis University
415 South Street, Mailstop 035
Waltham, MA 02454-9110
781-736-3900; *Fax:* 781-736-3905
colnon@brandeis.edu
www.sihp.brandeis.edu

Stanley S Wallack, Ph.D., Executive Director

Committed to developing an objective, university-based entity capable of providing research assistance to the Federal government on the major problems it faced in financing and delivering care to the elderly, disabled and poor. Our role has always been to solve complex health care problems, and to link research studies to policy change.

3095 Breining Institute College for the Advanced Study of Addictive Disorders
8894 Greenback Lane
Orangevale, CA 95662-4019
916-987-0662
college@breining.edu
www.breininginstitute.net

Kathy Breining, Administrator

The mission of Breining Institute faculty and staff is to ensure a consistent standard of higher education, training, testing and certification of professionals working in the field of addictions.

Year Founded: 1986

3096 California Institute of Behavioral Sciences
701 Welch Road
Suite #B 203
Palo Alto, CA 94304-1705

650-325-1501
info@ecibs.net
www.www.ecibs.net

Sanjay Jasuja, Medical Director

Provides the following services for children, adolescents, adults and families on national and international level: Objective testing and comprehensive treatment for ADHD/ADD, depression, manic depressive disorder or Bipolar disorder, anxiety disorders, including obsessive compulsive disorder, panic attacks, phobias, post-traumatic stress disorder, Tourette's syndrome, stuttering, psychopharmacology, stress and anger control, violence and workplace issues, learning and behavior problems, and parenting support groups.

3097 Cambridge Hospital: Department of Psychiatry

1493 Cambridge Street
Cambridge, MA 02139-1047
617-665-1000
webmaster@challiance.org
www.www.challiance.org

Jay Burke, MD, MPH, Chairman, Chief of Psychiatry
Joy Curtis, SVP, Human Resources
Elizabeth Cadigan, RN, MSN, Senior Vice President, Patient C
Judith Klickstein, SVP, Information Technology and

3098 Center for Health Policy Studies

10440 Little Patuxent Parkway
10th Floor
Columbia, MD 21044-3561
410-715-9400

3099 College of Health and Human Services: SE Missouri State

901 S National Ave
Springfield, MO 65897-27
417-836-5000
www.missouristate.edu

Dr.Frank Einhellig, Provost
Dr.Chris Craig, Associate Provost, Faculty & Aca
Dr.Rachelle Darabi, Associate Provost for Student De
Dr.Joye Norris, Associate Provost for Access and

3100 College of Southern Idaho

315 Falls Avenue
PO Box 1238
Twin Falls, ID 83303-1238
208-732-6221
800-680-0274; *Fax:* 208-736-4705
info@csi.edu
www.csi.edu

Jerry Beck, President
Dr.Jeff Fox, President
Jerry Gee, Executive VP/CAO
Dr.Todd Schwarz, EVP, CAO

Addiction Studies

3101 Colonial Services Board

1657 Merrimac Trail
Williamsburg, VA 23185-5624
757-220-3200; *Fax:* 757-229-7173
TDD: 757-253-4377
www.colonialcsb.org

David Coe, Executive Director
Keith German, Director, Administrative Service

Dan Longo, Director, Behavioural Services
Nancy Shackleford, Director, Human Resources

MR and substance abuse

3102 Daniel and Yeager Healthcare Staffing Solutions

6767 Old Madison Pike
Suite 690
Huntsville, AL 35806-2198
256-551-1070
800-955-1919; *Fax:* 256-551-5075
info@dystaffing.com
www.dystaffing.com

Mark Kingsley, VP
Susie Brown, COO
Mike Williams, CFO
Hans Edenfield, Director, Human Resources

Setting the standard for excellence in health care staffing.

3103 Dartmouth Univerisity: Department of Psychiatry

Dartmouth-Hitchcock Medical School
One Medical Center Drive
Lebanon, NH 03756
603-650-7075; *Fax:* 603-650-5842
www.geiselmed.dartmouth.edu/psych

3104 East Carolina University Department of Psychiatric Medicine

600 Moye Boulevard
Room 4E-98
Greenville, NC 27834-4300
252-744-4440

Joseph B Webster

3105 Emory University School of Medicine, Psychology and Behavior

1440 Clifton Road NE
Atlanta, GA 30322-1053
404-727-5630; *Fax:* 404-727-0473

3106 Emory University: Psychological Center

36 Eagle Row
Room 270
Atlanta, GA 30322-1122
404-727-7438; *Fax:* 404-727-0372
psych@emory.edu
www.psychology.emory.edu

Harold Gouzoules, Ph.D., Department Chair
Nancy Feng, Research Financial Analyst
Kelly Yates, Program Coordinator
Kate Coblin, Assistant Program Director

Nonprofit community clinic providing low cost counseling and psychological testing services for children and adults.

3107 Fletcher Allen Health Care

111 Colchester Avenue
Burlington, VT 05401-1416
802-847-0000
800-358-1144

Fletcher Allen Health Care is both a community hospital and, in partnership with the University of Vermont, the state's academic health center. Their mission is to improve the health of the people in the communities they serve by integrating patient care, education and research in a caring environment.

3108 Genesis Learning Center (Devereux)

430 Allied Drive
Nashville, TN 37211-3304
615-832-4222; *Fax:* 615-832-4577
admin@genesislearn.org
www.genesislearn.org

Terance Adams, Executive Director
Chuck Goon, PHR, Human Resource Director

3109 George Washington University

2121 Eye Street, NW
Washington, DC 20052-1
202-994-1000
www.www.gwu.edu

Steven Knapp, President
Steve R. Lerman, Provost, EVP, Academic Affairs
Beth Nolan, SVP, General Counsel
Louis H. Katz, EVP, Treasurer

3110 Haymarket Center, Professional Development

932 W Washington
Chicago, IL 60607-2217
312-226-7984; *Fax:* 312-226-0047
info@hcenter.org
www.hcenter.org

Raymond F. Soucek, President
Donald E. Musil, Executive VP
Dan Lustig, VP, Clinical Services
Leo C. Miller, VP, Support Services

Drug and alcohol treatment programs.

3111 Heartshare Human Services

12 Metro Tech Center
29th Floor
Brooklyn, NY 11201-3858
718-422-4200
info@heartshare.org
www.heartshare.org

Ralph A. Subbiondo, Chairman
William R. Guarinello, MS, President/ Ceo
Mia Higgins, Executive VP, Operations, Genera
Evelyn Alvarez, SVP, Developmental Disablilities

A nonprofit human services agency dedicated to improving the lives of people in need of special services and support.

3112 Hillcrest Utica Psychiatric Services

1120 S Utica Street
South Physician Bldg Suite 1000
Tulsa, OK 74104-4012
918-579-8000
www.helmerichwomenscenter.com

Steve Dobbs, CEO

3113 Institute for Behavioral Healthcare

PO Box 5710
Santa Rosa, CA 95402
650-851-8411
800-258-8411; *Fax:* 707-566-7474
staff@iahb.org
www.iahb.org

Gerry Piaget, Ph.D., President
Joan Piaget, Executive Director
Jen Dames, Director, Operations

Non-profit educational organization that is a fully accredited sponsor of continuing education and continuing medical education for mental health, chemical dependency, and substance abuse treatment providers in the United States and Canada. Mission is to provide high-quality training to healthcare professionals as well as to companies and individuals with healthcare-related interests.

3114 Jacobs Institute of Women's Health

950 New Hampshire Avenue
NW, 2nd Floor
Washington, DC 20052
202-994-4184; *Fax:* 202-296-0025
whieditor@gwu.edu
www.jiwh.org

Richard Mauery, MS, MPH, Managing Staff Director
Susan Wood, PhD, Executive Director
Chloe E. Bird, PhD, Editor In Chief
Carol Weisman, PhD, Associate Editor

Working to improve health care for women through research, dialogue and information dissemination. Mission is to identify and study women's health care issues involving the interaction of medical and social systems; facilitate informed dialogue and foster awareness among consumers and providers alike; and promote problem resolution, interdisciplinary coordination and information dissemination at the regional, national and international levels.

3115 John A Burns School of Medicine Department of Psychiatry

651 Ilalo Street
Medical Education Building
Honolulu, HI 96813-2409
808-692-0899; *Fax:* 808-586-2940
inip@hawaii.edu
www.jabsom.hawaii.edu

Naleen Andrade, Chair
Jerris Hedges, MD, MS, MMM, Dean and Professor of Medicine
Nancy Foster, CFO
A. Roy Magnusson, MD, Associate Dean, Clinical Affairs

Medical School Programs and Residency Programs, general, geriatric, addictive and, child and adolescent.

3116 Langley Porter Psych Institute at UCSF Parnassus Campus

401 Parnassus Avenue
San Francisco, CA 94143-2211
415-476-7500; *Fax:* 415-502-6361
www.psych.ucsf.edu/lpphc.aspx

Alissa M Peterson
Sam Hawgood, MBBS, Interim Chancellor

3117 Laurelwood Hospital and Counseling Centers

35900 Euclid Avenue
Willoughby, OH 44094-4648
440-953-3000
800-438-4673; *Fax:* 440-602-3938
www.www.windsorlaurelwood.com

Farshid Afsarifard, Administrator
Leonard Barley, M.D., MBA, Chief Medical Officer
Theodore Parran, M.D., Director, Addiction Medicine
Noah Miller, M.D., Director, Child and Adolescent S

Full-service behavioral healthcare system-(comprehensive outpatient and inpatient services).

3118 Life Science Associates
1 Fenimore Road
Bayport, NY 11705-2115
631-472-2111; *Fax:* 631-472-8146
www.lifesciassoc.home.pipeline.com

Joann Mandriota, President
Frank Mandriota, Vice President

Publishes over fifty computer programs for individuals impaired by head trauma and stroke. Also programs for personal memory care, GSSS (Get sharp stay sharp)

3119 Locumtenens.com
2655 Northwinds Parkway
Alpharetta, GA 30009
800-930-0748
customerservice@locumtenens.com
www.locumtenens.com

Shane Jackson, President, COO
Kevin Thill, SVP, Psychiatry
Chris Franklin, EVP
Katie Thill, EVP

Specializing in temporary and permanant placement of psychiatrists. Physicians tell us where and when they want to work and locumtenens.com will find a jop that fits those needs.

3120 MCG Telemedicine Center
1120 15th Street
Augusta, GA 30912-6
706-721-2231
mcgdean@gru.edu

Daniel W. Rahn, President
Ricardo Azziz, MD, MPH, MBA, President / Ceo
Susan L. Barcus, FAHP, SVP, Advancement, Chief Developm
David L. Brond, MBA, MHA, SVP, Communications and Marketin

3121 MCW Department of Psychiatry and Behavioral Medicine
8701 Watertown Plank Road
Milwaukee, WI 53226-3548
414-955-8296
webmaster@mcw.edu
www.www.mcw.edu

John R. Raymond, Sr., President, CEO
Joseph E. Kerschner, MD, Deean, EVP
G. Allen Bolton, Jr., SVP, COO

3122 Market Research Alliance
1109 Spring St
Suite 704
Silver Spring, MD 20910-4032
301-588-8732; *Fax:* 301-625-3001
www.mr-twg.com

Frank Black Jr., Partner,President
John Marty, Managing Director
Nick Campbell, Member
Tom Bergan, Member

3123 Marsh Foundation
1229 Lincoln Highway
PO Box 150
Van Wert, OH 45891-150

419-238-1695; *Fax:* 419-238-1747
marshfound@embarqmail.com
www.marshfoundation.org

Jeff Grothouse, Executive Secretary/Treasurer
Kim Mullins, P.C.C., Executive Director
Kathleen Davis, L.S.W., Director, Residential Services
Sherry Grone, Activities Coordinator

Nonprofit center serving children and families with special emphasis in juvenile sex offender population. Services include individual therapy, group therapy, case management and diagnostic assessment.

3124 Medical College of Georgia
1120 15th Street
Augusta, GA 30912-5563
706-721-0211; *Fax:* 706-721-6126
info@gru.edu

Daniel W. Rahn, President
Ricardo Azziz, MD, MPH, MBA, President / Ceo
Susan L. Barcus, FAHP, SVP, Advancement, Chief Developm
David L. Brond, MBA, MHA, SVP, Communications and Marketin

The mission of the Medical College of Georgia is to improve health and resuce the burden of illness in society by discovering, disseminating, and applying knowledge of human health and disease.

3125 Medical College of Ohio
3000 Arlington Avenue
Toledo, OH 43614-2595
419-383-4000
800-321-8383; *Fax:* 419-383-6140
utmc.webmaster@utoledo.edu
www.utmc.utoledo.edu

Mission is to improve the human condition through the creation, dissemination and application of knowledge using wisdom and compassion as our guides.

3126 Medical College of Pennsylvania
3300 Henry Avenue
Philadelphia, PA 19129-1191
215-842-6000

A tertiary care educational facility that reaches out to a regional referral base for select specialty services while continuing to offer primary and secondary service to the residents of its immediate community.

3127 Medical College of Wisconsin
8701 Watertown Plank Road
Milwaukee, WI 53226-3548
414-955-8296
webmaster@mcw.edu
www.mcw.edu

John R. Raymond, Sr., President, CEO
Joseph E. Kerschner, MD, Deean, EVP
G. Allen Bolton, Jr., SVP, COO
Douglas R. Campbell, Finance Executive

3128 Medical Doctor Associates
145 Technology Parkway NW
Norcross, GA 30092-2913
770-246-9191
800-780-3500; *Fax:* 770-246-0882
www.mdainc.com

Ken Shumard, President
Mike Pretiger, Cfo

Committed to providing the most complete staffing services available to the healthcare industry. The family of services offered by Medical Doctor Associates includes Locum Tenens, Contract, and Permanent Placement staffing for physicians, allied health and rehabilitation staffing, and credentials verification and licensing services.

3129 Medical University of South Carolina Institute of Psychiatry, Psychiatry Access Center

104 Colcock Hall
MSC - 003
Charleston, SC 29425-100
843-792-5050
800-296-0269; *Fax:* 843-792-4975
www.academicdepartments.musc.edu/musc/

Mark S. Sothmann, Ph.D., Interim President, VP, Academic
Lisa Montgomery, EVP, Finance and Operations
Patrick J. Wamsley, CPA, CFO
Stewart Mixon, COO

3130 Meharry Medical College

1005-David B Todd Boulevard
Nashville, TN 37208-3501
615-327-6000; *Fax:* 615-321-2932
admissions@mmc.edu
www.mmc.edu

A. Cherrie Epps, Ph.D., President, CEO
Saletta Holloway, MSP, SVP, Borad of Trustees Relations
Robert Poole, B.A., SVP, Institutional Advancement
Ivanetta Davis Samuels, J.D., SVP, General Counsel and Corpora

3131 Menninger Clinic

12301 Main Street
Houston, TX 77035
713-275-5000
800-351-9058; *Fax:* 713-275-5107
www.www.menningerclinic.com

Tony Gaglio, CPA, MBA, Acting President and CEO
Tony Gaglio, CPA, MBA, Senior VP and CFO
Bella Schanzer, MD, MPH, Chief of Staff
Avni Cirpili, RN, DNP, Sr. VP and Chief Nursing Officer

Menninger is a leading psychiatric hospital dedicated to treating individuals with mood, personality, anxiety, and addictive disorders; teaching mental health professionals; and advancing mental healthcare through research.

3132 Nathan S Kline Institute for Psychiatric Research

140 Old Orangeburg Road
Orangeburg, NY 10962-1157
845-398-5500; *Fax:* 845-398-5510
webmaster@nki.rfmh.org
www.www.rfmh.org/nki/

Bennet L Leventhal, MD, Deputy Director
Donald C. Goff, M.D., Director
Antonio Convit, M.D., Deputy Director
Thomas O. O'Hara, M.B.A., Deputy Director

Research programs in Alzheimers disease, analytical psychopharmacology, basic and clinical neuroimaging, cellular and molecular neurobiology, clinical trial data management, co-occuring disorders and many other mental health studies.

3133 National Association of Alcholism and Drug Abuse Counselors

1001 N. Fairfax Street
Suite 201
Alexandria, VA 22314-1535
703-741-7686
800-548-0497; *Fax:* 703-741-7698
naadac@naadac.org
www.naadac.org

Robert C. Richards, MA, NCAC II,, President
Kirk Bowden, PhD, MAC, LISA, President Elect
Cynthia Moreno Tuohy, NCAC II,, Executive Director
Autumn Kramer, Director, Operations

NAADAC is the only professional membership organization that serves counselors who specialize in addiction treatment. With 14,000 members and 47 state affiliates representing more than 80,000 addiction counselors, it is the nation's largest network of alcoholism and drug abuse treatment professionals. Among the organization's national certifacation programs are the National Certified Addiction Counselor and the Masters Addiction Counselor designations.

3134 National Association of School Psychologists

4340 E West Highway
Suite 402
Bethesda, MD 20814-4468
301-657-0270
866-331-6277; *Fax:* 301-657-0275
www.nasponline.org

Sally Baas, President
Stephen E. Brock, President Elect
Amy R. Smith, Past President
Susan Gorin, Executive Director

3135 New York University Behavioral Health Programs

530 1st Avenue
Suite 7D (at 30th Street)
New York, NY 10016-6402
212-263-7419; *Fax:* 212-263-7460
www.www.med.nyu.edu/nyubhp/

David Ginsberg, Director
Robert Cancro, MD, Professor of Psychiatry and Chai
Norman Sussman, MD, Clinical Professor of Psychiatry
Virginia Sadock, MD, Clinical Professor of Psychiatry

Outpatient psychiatry group for Tisch Hospital at NYU Medical Center. Our multidisciplinary team of licensed psychiatrists and social workers offers you the most up-to-date and scientifically validated treatments.

3136 Northeastern Ohio Universities College of Medicine

4209 State Route 44
PO Box 95
Rootstown, OH 44272-95
800-686-2511

Jay A. Gershen, D.D.S., Ph.D., President
John R. Wray, Vice President, Administration a
Daniel Blain, Vice President, Advancement, Pre
Michael A. Wolff, J.D., Senior Development Officer

Mission is to graduate qualified physicians who are passionate about serving their communities. All of our graduates, regardless of specialty, have a solid background in community and public health. NEOUCOM strives to improve the quality of health care throughout northeast Ohio by instilling in each graduate the desire to serve the public and the highest ideals of the medical profession.

3137 Northwestern University Medical School Feinberg School of Medicine
420 East Superior Street
Chicago, IL 60611-3128
312-503-8194; *Fax:* 312-503-8700
clinpsych@northwestern.edu
www.www.feinberg.northwestern.edu

Eric G. Neilson, MD, Dean, VP - Medical Affairs
Eva Erskine, Manager
Jim Baker, Ph.D., Science in Medicine Element Co-C
John X. Thomas, Ph.D., Teamwork & Leadership Thread Cha

The Mental Health Services and Policy Program is a multidisciplinary research/educational program on the development and implementation of outcomes management technology.

3138 Ochester Psychological Service
1924 Copper Oaks Circle
Blue Springs, MO 64015-8300
816-224-6500

Jeffery L Miller PhD, Psychologist/Owner

Offers a full range of outpatient mental health services including individuals, couples and family therapy. Offers psychological testing and evaluation. Adults, adolescents and children served.

3139 PRIMA ADD Corp.
12160 N. Abrams Rd
Suite 615
Dallas, TX 75243-4547
972-386-8599; *Fax:* 972-386-8597
robinbinnig@gmail.com
www.primaadd.com; drbinnig.wordpress.com

Robin Binnig, PhD, Owner

Prima ADD Corp specializes in the diagnosis and treatment of Attention-Deficit/Hyperactivity Disorder (ADHD). We treat children and adults. Services include: psychological assessment (including intellectual, achievement and pesonality testing), counseling, coaching and consultation. We also carry books and CD's concerning ADHD.

3140 Parent Child Center
2001 W Blue Heron Blvd
Riviera Beach, FL 33404-5003
561-841-3500
800-955-8770; *Fax:* 561-844-3577
TTY: 800-955-8771
information@parent-childcenter.org
www.www.gocpg.org

Patrick Mc Namara, President, CEO
Laura Barry, Vice Presidentof Community Serv
Pamela Figoras, Vice President of Child & Family
Laura Morse, Vice Presidentof Development

3141 Penn State Hershey Medical Center
500 University Drive
Hershey, PA 17033-2390
717-531-6955
800-731-3032; *Fax:* 717-531-4077
TTY: 717-531-4395

Harold L Paz, M.D., M.S., CEO, SVP, Dean
Jeff Miller, M.D., Associate Dean for Administratio
Lisa Abbott, M.B.A., S.P.H., Associate Vice President for Hum
Sean Young, Chief Marketing Officer

3142 Pepperdine University Graduate School of Education and Psychology
6100 Center Drive
Los Angeles, CA 90045-9200
310-506-4000
800-347-4849

Andrew Benton, President

Offers graduate degree programs designed to prepare psychologists, marriage and family therapists, and mental health practitioners. Many programs accommodate a full-time work schedule with evening and weekend classes available in a trimester schedule. The average class size is 15. There are five educational centers in southern California and three community counseling clinics available to the surrounding community.

3143 Portland University Regional Research Institute for Human Services
1600 Sw 4th Ave
Suite 900
Portland, OR 97201-5521
503-725-4040; *Fax:* 503-725-4180
www.rri.pdx.edu

Tom Keller, Interim Director
Diane Yatchmenoff, Ph.D., Associate Director
Jennifer Williams, Assistant to the Director

3144 Postgraduate Center for Mental Health
71 W 23rd St
New York, NY 10010-4102
212-576-4168
crichards@pgcmh.org
www.pgcmh.org

Jacob Barak, Ph.D., MBA, President, CEO
Marcia B. Holman, L.C.S.W., VP for Ambulatory Operations
Harold Moss, L.M.S.W., MA, VP for Residential Operations
John McMasters, Executive Assistant

Information on mental health.

3145 Pressley Ridge
5500 Corporate Drive
Suite 400
Pittsburgh, PA 15237
412-872-9400; *Fax:* 412-872-9478

Susanna L. Cole, MA, President, CEO
Laurah Currey, MA, LPC, LSW, Chief Operating Officer
Douglas A. Mullins, CPA, CFO
Edward J. Yongo, MBA, Chief Development and External R

Founded in 1832. Provides an array of social services, special education programs, and mental health services for troubled children and their families in Delaware, Maryland, Ohio, Pennsylvania, Virginia, Washngton, DC and West Virginia as well as worldwide.

3146 PsychTemps
2404 Auburn Avenue
Cincinnati, OH 45219-2735
513-651-9500
888-651-8367; *Fax:* 513-651-9558

info@psychpros.com
www.psychtemps.com

Holly Dorna MA LPCC, President/CEO
Timberline Knolls, HR Director
Lauren Kofod, M.D., Member
Paul J. Schwartz, M.D., Member

Specialized recruiting and staffing company that fills temporary, permanent, and temp-to-hire job placement for the behavioral healthcare field.

3147 Psychiatric Associates

2216 W Alto Road
Kokomo, IN 46902
765-453-9338

3148 Psychological Center

135 Oakland Street
Pasadena, CA 91101
626-584-5500

Winston Gooden, Manager

3149 QuadraMed Corporation

12110 Sunset Hills Road
Suite 600
Reston, VA 20190-5852
703-709-2300
800-393-0278; *Fax:* 703-709-2490
boardofdirectors@quadramed.com
www.quadramed.com

Daniel Desaulniers, CA, President, Harris Quebec Public
Jim Dowling, Executive Vice President, Enterp
Sandi Williams, Executive Vice President, Clinic
Duncan W James, CEO

3150 Skills Unlimited

2060 Ocean Ave
Suite 3
Ronkonkoma, NY 11779-6533
631-580-5319; *Fax:* 631-580-5394
success@skillsunlimited.org
www.skillsunlimited.org

Jeffrey Koppelson, Program Director
Richard Kassnove, Executive Director

SUCCESS provides rehabilitative services to indivduals who are recovering from mental illness. In addition to offering clinical treatment, SUCCESS has a schedule of classes and other services that help to identify and achieve personally meaningful goals in the areas of employment, housing, education, health and socialization. Transportation is generally available free of charge. The program is open Monday through Saturday and has ectended hours two evenings per week.

3151 Southern Illinois University School of Medicine: Department of Psychiatry

PO Box 19620
Springfield, IL 62794-9620
217-545-8000
www.siumed.edu

Stephen M Soltys MD, Pfr/Chair Dpt. of Psychiatry
Philip Pan MD, Division Chief
Connie Poole, Associate Dean for Information R
Klamen Debra, MD, MHPE, Associate Dean for Education and

3152 Southern Illinois University School of Medicine
SIU School of Medicine

PO Box 19620
Springfield, IL 62794-9620
217-545-8000
www.siumed.edu

Stephen M Soltys MD, Pfr/Chair Dpt. of Psychiatry
Philip Pan MD, Division Chief
Connie Poole, Associate Dean for Information R
Klamen Debra, MD, MHPE, Associate Dean for Education and

Provides high quality clinical treatment,outstanding teaching and solid efforts in research and community service.

3153 Specialzed Alternatives for Family and Youth (SAFY)

10100 Elida Road
Delphos, OH 45833-9056
419-695-8010
800-532-7239; *Fax:* 419-695-0004
webmaster@safy.org
www.safy.org

Scott Spangler, MSW, President, CEO
Jim Sherman, MA, LPC, SVP, Administrative Services
John Hollenkamp, CPA, VP, Contracts and Procurement
Marc Bloomingdale, M.S., VP, Operations

SAFY's mission is to foster an environment that possibly impacts the lives of youth and their families, whether they are with us an hour or a lifetime.

3154 St. Frnacis Medical Psych-Med Association

2616 Wilmington Road
New Castle, PA 16105-1504
724-652-2323

3155 St. Louis Behavioral Medicine Institute

1129 Macklind Avenue
Saint Louis, MO 63110-1440
314-289-9411
877-245-2688
www.slbmi.com

Ronald B. Margolis, Ph.D., President, CEO
Debbie Milfelt, Manager
Geeta Aatre-Prashar, Psy.D., Psychologist
Gelene Adkins, Ph.D., Psychologist

Offers exceptional quality, result-focused treatment. Have remained true to our commitment of providing excellence in clinical care and customer service. We offer comprehensive treatment plans to meet the individual needs of children, adolescents, adults, older adults, and their families suffering from emotional and behavioral problems.

3156 Stonington Institute

75 Swantown Hill Road
N Stonington, CT 06359-1022
860-535-1010
800-832-1022; *Fax:* 860-445-3030
andrea.keeney@uhsinc.com
www.stoningtoninstitute.com

William A. Aniskovich, M.A., J.D., CEO
Jerome M Schnitt, M.D., Medical Director
Georganna Georgie Koppermann, Director, Business Development a
Andrea Keeney, Director of Admissions

3157 Topeka Institute for Psychoanalysis
PO Box 829
Topeka, KS 66601-829
800-288-3950

A training facility for health care professionals, the Topeka Institute for Psychoanalysis has the tripartite mission of promoting research to expand the knowledge base in its field of expertise; providing didactic education and clinical supervision to trainees; and caring for patients in need of its services through a low-fee clinic.

3158 UCLA Neuropsychiatric Institute and Hospital
760 Westwood Plaza
Los Angeles, CA 90095
310-825-0291
www.www.semel.ucla.edu

Peter Whybrow, Director
Fawzy Fawzy, Associate Director
Mark Wheeler, Media Relations
Alan Han, Director of Development

Multidisciplinary institute of human neurosciences, and is unifying focus of scholarly activity at UCLA in this area. Scientific advances recent decades have shown the value in approaches that cut across traditional academic departments, and which emphasize interdisciplinary collaborations.

3159 UCLA School of Nursing
PO Box 951702
Los Angeles, CA 90095-1702
310-825-3109; *Fax:* 310-267-0330
sonsaff@sonnet.ucla.edu
www.nursing.ucla.edu

Courtney H. Lyder, ND, ScD(Hon), F, Professor, Dean
Rene Dennis, Director Development
Rhonda Flenoy-Younger, Director of Recruitment, Outreac
Mark Covin, Recruitment and Admissions Coord

3160 UCSF Department of Psychiatry, Cultural Competence
3 Regent Street
Livingston, NJ 07039
973-436-5000
973-436-5004
www.reprogenetics.com

Santiago Munne, Founder, Director
Jacques Cohen, Laboratory Director, Embryologis
Kelly Ketterson, Director of Operations
Pere Colls, Laboratory Director

3161 USC School of Medicine
Health Sciences Campuses
Name/Department USC
Los Angeles, CA 90089-1
323-442-1100
www.usc.edu/schools/medicine/

3162 Ulster County Department of Health and Mental Health
239 Golden Hill Lane
Kingston, NY 12401
845-340-4110; *Fax:* 845-340-4094
www.ulstercountyny.gov/health/health-mental-health

Dr. Carol Smith, Commissioner
Tara McDonald, Deputy Commissioner

Responsible for planning, funding and monitoring of community mental health, developmental disability and alcohol and substance abuse services in Ulster County.

3163 Union County Psychiatric Clinic
117 Roosevelt Avenue
Plainfield, NJ 07060-1331
908-756-6870
www.www.ucpcbhc.org

Rosalind Hunt Doctor, President
Gerard Kiely, VP
Richard L. Rodgers, MSW, LCSW, Executive Director
Joseph Daniel, MA, LPC, Associate Executive Director

3164 University Behavioral Healthcare
671 Hoes Lane
Piscataway, NJ 08855
732-235-5900
800-969-5300; *Fax:* 732-235-4594
www.ubhc.rutgers.edu

Christopher Kosseff, President

3165 University of California Davis Psychiatry and Behavioral Sciences Department
2315 Stockton Boulevard
Sacramento, CA 95817-2201
916-734-2011

Offers opportunities for students and faculty for clinical and research applications in all aspects of psychiatry and behavioral sciences.

3166 University of Cincinnati College of Medical Department of Psychiatry
260 Stelson Street
Suite 3200
Cincinnati, OH 45221
513-558-7700; *Fax:* 513-558-0187
uchealthnews@uc.edu
www.www.psychiatry.uc.edu

Stephen M. Strakowski, MD, Chair
Charles Collins, MD, Senior Vice Chair and Director o
Paul Keck, MD, Executive Vice Chair
Henry A. Nasrallah, MD, Vice Chair of Education and Trai

Researches eating disorders, bipolar disorder, and chemical dependency.

3167 University of Colorado Health Sciences Center
1250 14th Street
Denver, CO 80217
303-556-2400
877-472-2586
www.www.ucdenver.edu/pages/ucdwelcomepage.aspx

John C Slocumb

3168 University of Connecticut Health Center
263 Farmington Avenue
Farmington, CT 06030-1
860-679-2000
TDD: 860-679-2242
www.www.uchc.edu

Susan Herbst, President
Frank M. Torti, M.D., M.P.H., Executive VP for health affairs
Elizabeth Bolt, Vice President, Human Resources
Marianne Dess-Santoro, VP, Ambulatory Care

3169 University of Iowa Hospital
200 Hawkins Drive
Iowa City, IA 52242-1007
319-356-1616
800-777-8442
TDD: 319-356-4999
uihc-webcomments@uiowa.edu
www.www.uihealthcare.org

Kenneth P. Kates, CEO
Kenneth L. Fisher, CFO
Ann Williamson, PhD, RN, Chief Nursing Officer
Theresa Brennan, MD, Chief Medical Officer

3170 University of Kansas Medical Center
3901 Rainbow Boulevard
Kansas City, KS 66160-1
913-588-5000
TDD: 913-588-7963
kusmw@kumc.edu
www.www.kumc.edu

Douglas A. Girod, M.D., Executive Vice Chancellor
Barbara Atkinson, Executive Vice Chancellor
Tim Caboni, Vice Chancellor for Public Affai
David Vranicar, M.B.A., Vice Chancellor for Finance/CFO

An integral and unique component of the University of Kansas and the Kansas Board of Regents system, is composed of the School of Medicine, the School of Nursing, the School of Allied Health, the University of Kansas Hospital, and a Graduate School. KU Medical Center is a complex institution whose basic functions include research, education, patient care, and community service involving multiple constituencies at state and national levels.

3171 University of Kansas School of Medicine
3901 Rainbow Boulevard
Kansas City, KS 66160-1
913-588-5000
TDD: 913-588-7963
kusmw@kumc.edu
www.kumc.edu

Douglas A. Girod, M.D., Executive Vice Chancellor
Barbara Atkinson, Executive Vice Chancellor
Tim Caboni, Vice Chancellor for Public Affai
David Vranicar, M.B.A., Vice Chancellor for Finance/CFO

3172 University of Louisville School of Medicine
Abell Administration Center
323 E. Chestnut Street
Louisville, KY 40202
502-562-3000
meddean@louisville.edu
www.louisville.edu/medicine

Dean Ganzel, Dean
Wes Allison

Mission is to be a vital component in the University of Louisville's quest to become a premier, nationally recognized metropolitan research university, to excel in the education of physicians and scientists for careers in teching, research, patient care and community service, and to bring the fundamental discoveries of our basic and clinical scientists to the bedside.

3173 University of Maryland Medical Systems
22 S. Greene Street
Baltimore, MD 21201-1023
410-328-2132
800-492-5538
TDD: 800-735-2258
www.umm.edu

Robert A. Chrencik, MBA, CPA, President, CEO
Henry J. Franey, MBA, EVP, CFO
Megan M. Arthur, SVP, General Counsel
Janice J. Eisele, SVP, Development

3174 University of Maryland School of Medicine
655 West Baltimore Street
Baltimore, MD 21201-1509
410-706-3681
webmaster@som.umaryland.edu
www.medschool.umaryland.edu

Nancy Ryan Lowitt, Dean/Vp Medical Affairs
E. Albert Reece, MD, PhD, MBA, Dean, VP of Medical Affairs
Richard Pierson III, MD, Senior Associate Dean for Academ
Milford M. Foxwell, Jr., MD, Associate Dean for Admissions

Dedicated to providing excellence in biomedical education, basic and clinical research, quality patient care and service to improve the health of the citizens of Maryland and beyond.

3175 University of Massachusetts Medical Center
55 Lake Avenue N
Worcester, MA 01655-1
508-856-8989
www.www.umassmed.edu

Terence R. Flotte, MD, Dean of School of Medicine, Prov
Michael F. Collins, MD, FACP, Senior Vice President for the He
Mariann M. Manno, MD, Interim Associate Dean for Admis
Aaron Lazare, Administrator

Mission is to serve the people of the commonwealth through national distinction in health sciences, education, research, public service and clinical care.

3176 University of Michigan
500 S. State Street
Ann Arbor, MI 48109
734-764-1817
info@umich.edu
www.www.umich.edu

Mary Sue Coleman, President
Martha Pollack, Provost
Sally J. Churchill, VP, Secretary
Jerry A. May, VP, Development

3177 University of Minnesota Fairview Health Systems
2450 Riverside Ave
Minneapolis, MN 55454-1450
612-273-2229; *Fax:* 612-273-2211
TTY: 612-672-7300
www.fairview.org

Gordon Alexander, President
Rulon F. Stacey, PhD, FACHE, President, CEO
Daniel K. Anderson, President of Fairview Community
Daniel Fromm, SVP, CFO

Mission is to improve the health of the communities we serve. We commit our skills and resources to the benefit of the whole person by providing the finest in healthcare, while addressing the physical, emotional and spiritual needs of individuals and their families. Pledge to support the research and education efforts of our partner, the University of Minnesota, and its tradition of excellence.

3178 University of North Carolina School of Social Work

Behavioral Healthcare Resource Institute
301 Pittsboro Street
Cb # 3550
Chapel Hill, NC 27599-1
919-843-3018
bhrinstitute@listserv.unc.edu

3179 University of Pennsylvania Health System

399 S 34th Street
Suite 2002 Penn Tower
Philadelphia, PA 19104-4316
215-662-6995
800-789-PENN

3180 University of South Florida Research Center for Children's Mental Health

13301 Bruce B Downs Boulevard
Tampa, FL 33612-3807
813-974-4565

Robert M. Friedman, Ph.D., Center Director
Albert Duchnowski, Ph.D., Deputy Director
Krista Kutash, Ph.D., Deputy Director
Mary Armstrong, PhD, Center Staff

The center conducts research, synthesized and shared existingknowledge, provided training and consultation, and served as a resource for other researchers, policy makers, administrators in the public system, and organizations representing parents, consumers, advocates, professional societies and practitioners.

3181 University of Texas Medical Branch Managed Care

301 University Boulevard
Galveston, TX 77555-5302
409-772-1506
800-917-8906; *Fax:* 409-772-6216
public.affairs@utmb.edu
www.utmb.edu

David L. Callender, MD, MBA, FA, President
Danny O. Jacobs, MD, MPH, EVP, Provost, Dean
Carolee Carrie King, JD, SVP, General Counsel
David W. Niesel, PhD, VP, Dean

3182 University of Utah Neuropsychiatric

501 Chipeta Way
Salt Lake City, UT 84108-1222
801-583-2500
sarah.latta@hsc.utah.edu
www.healthcare.utah.edu/uni

Kristin Fontaine, Manager

Located in the University's Research Park, is a full service 90-bed psychiatric hospital providing mental health and substance abuse treatment. Services include inpatient, day treatment, intensive outpatient, and ooutpatient services for children, adolescents and adults. Confidential assessments, referrals, and intervention education are available.

3183 Wake Forest University

1834 Wake Forest Road
Winston Salem, NC 27106
336-758-5000; *Fax:* 336-759-6074
www.wfu.edu

Nathan O. Hatch, President
Rogan Kersh, Provost
Hof Milam, SVP of Finance and Administratio
James J. Dunn, VP, Chief Investment Officer

3184 West Jefferson Medical Center

1101 Medical Center Boulevard
Marrero, LA 70072-3191
504-347-5511
guestservicesweb@wjmc.org
www.wjmc.org

A Gary Muller, CEO

Not-for-profit community hospital on the West Bank of Jefferson Parish. Continues to strengthen its community base while maintaining its mission and values. Dedicated to considerate and respectful quality healthcare, the institution welcomes patient, family, and visitor feedback regarding programs, services, and community needs.

3185 Western Psychiatric Institute and Clinic

3811 Ohara Street
Pittsburgh, PA 15213-2597
412-624-2100
877-624-4100
www.www.upmc.com

Rizwan Parvez

A national leader in the diagnosis, management, and treatment of mental health and addictive disorders. Providing the most comprehensive range of behavioral health services available today, but also shaping tomorrow's behavioral health care through clinical innovation, research, and education.

3186 Wordsworth

3905 Ford Road
Philadelphia, PA 19131-2824
215-643-5400
800-769-0088
info@wordsworth.org
www.www.wordsworth.org

Debra Lacks, President, CEO
Amir Malek, CFO
Andrew Gross, Executive Director of Community
Jennifer Nickels, Executive Director of Residentia

The mission of Wordsworth, a not-for-profit institution, is to provide quality education, treatment and care to children and families with special needs.

Year Founded: 1952

Video & Audio

3187 Asperger's Diagnostic Assessment with Dr. Tony Attwood

Program Development Associates PO Box 2038 Syracuse, NY 13220-2038
315-452-0643; *Fax:* 315-452-0710
info@disabilitytraining.com
www.disabilitytraining.com

New from acclaimed autism expert Dr. Tony Attwood, this 4-hour DVD set with program guide offers diagnostic characteristics of Asperger's Syndrome in children and adults, patient interviews and impacts on girls. An essential guide for Child Psychologists, Special Ed teachers and Parents. *$129.95*

3188 Cognitive Behavioral Assessment
NewHarbinger Publications
5674 Shattuck Avenue
Oakland, CA 94609-1662
510-652-0215
800-748-6273; *Fax:* 800-652-1613
customerservice@newharbinger.com
www.newharbinger.com

Matthew McKay, Owner

A videotape that guides three clients through PAC (Problem, Antecedents, Consequences) method of cognitive behavioral assessment. *$49.95*

Year Founded: 1996 ISBN 1-572243-15-5

3189 Couples and Infertility - Moving Beyond Loss
Guilford Press
72 Spring Street
New York, NY 10012-4068
212-431-9800
800-365-7006; *Fax:* 212-966-6708
info@guilford.com
www.www.guilford.com

Bob Matloff, President
Seymour Weingarten, Editor-in-Chief

A VHS video explores the biological and resulting psychological and social issues of infertility. *$95.00*

Year Founded: 1995 ISBN 1-572302-86-0

3190 Educating Clients about the Cognitive Model
NewHarbinger Publications
5674 Shattuck Avenue
Oakland, CA 94609-1662
510-652-0215
800-748-6273; *Fax:* 800-652-1613
customerservice@newharbinger.com
www.newharbinger.com

Matthew McKay, Owner

Videotape that helps three clients understand their symptoms as they work toward developing a working contract to begin cognitive restructing. *$49.95*

Year Founded: 1996 ISBN 1-572243-19-8

3191 Gender Differences in Depression: Marital Therapy Approach
Guilford Press
72 Spring Street
New York, NY 10012-4068
212-431-9800
800-365-7006; *Fax:* 212-966-6708
info@guilford.com
www.www.guilford.com

Bob Matloff, President
Seymour Weingarten, Editor-in-Chief

Male-female treatment team is shown working with a markedly depressed couple to improve communication and sense of well being in their marriage. *$85.50*

Year Founded: 1996 ISBN 1-572302-87-9

3192 Group Work for Eating Disorders and Food Issues
American Counseling Association
5999 Stevenson Avenue
Alexandria, VA 22304-3304
703-823-9800
800-347-6647; *Fax:* 703-823-0252
webmaster@counseling.org
www.counseling.org

Cirecie A. West-Olatunji, President
Robert L. Smith, President Elect
Bradley T. Erford, Past President
Richard Yep, Executive Director

A plan for working with high school and college age females who are at risk for eating disorders. This video provides a method for identifying at-risk clients, a session-by-session desciption of the group, exercises and information on additional resources. *$89.95*

Year Founded: 1995 ISSN 79801

3193 Help This Kid's Driving Me Crazy - the Young Child with Attention Deficit Disorder
Pro-Ed Publications
8700 Shoal Creek Boulevard
Austin, TX 78757-6897
512-451-3246
800-897-3202; *Fax:* 512-451-8542
general@proedinc.com
www.www.proedinc.com

Donald D Hammill, Owner

This videotape provides information about the behavior and special needs of young children with ADD and offers suggestions on fostering appropriate behaviors. *$89.00*

3194 I Love You Like Crazy: Being a Parent with Mental Illness
Mental Illness Education Project
25 West Street
Westborough, MA Westb-roug
617-562-1111
800-343-5540; *Fax:* 617-779-0061
info@miepvideos.org
www.miepvideos.org

Christine Ledoux, Executive Director

In this videotape, eight mothers and fathers who have mental illness discuss the challenges they face as parents. Most of these parents have faced enormous obstacles from homelessness, addictions, legal difficulties and hospitalizations, yet have maintained a positive and loving relationship with their children. The tape introduces issues of work, fear, stigma, relationships with children and the rest of the family, with professionals, and with the community at large. Discounted price for families/consumers. *$79.95*

Year Founded: 1999

3195 Inner Health Incorporated
Christopher Alsten, PhD
1260 Lincoln Avenue
San Diego, CA 92103-2322
619-299-7273
800-283-4679; *Fax:* 619-291-7753
sleepenhancement@aol.com

Provides a series of prerecorded therapeutic audio programs for anxiety, insomnia and chemical dependency, both for adults and children. Developed over a 15 year period by a practicing psychiatrist and recording engineer they employ state-of-the-art 3-D sound technologies and the latest relaxation and psychological techniques (but no stimulants). Clients include: US Air Force, US Navy, National Institute of Health, National Institute of Aging and various psychiatric and chemical dependency facilities and companies with shiftworkers.

3196 Know Your Rights: Mental Health Private Practice & the Law
American Counseling Association
5999 Stevenson Avenue
Alexandria, VA 22304-3304
703-823-9800
800-347-6647; *Fax:* 703-823-0252
webmaster@counseling.org
www.counseling.org

Cirecie A. West-Olatunji, President
Robert L. Smith, President Elect
Bradley T. Erford, Past President
Richard Yep, Executive Director

Whether you are in private practice or are thinking about opening your own practice, this forum lead by national experts, offers answers to important questions and provides invaluable information for every practitioner. Helps to orientate practitioners on the legally permissible boundaries, legal liabilities that are seldom known and how to respond in the face of legal action. *$145.00*

ISSN 79062

3197 Life Is Hard: Audio Guide to Healing Emotional Pain
Impact Publishers
PO Box 6016
Atascadero, CA 93423-6016
805-466-5917
800-246-7228; *Fax:* 805-466-5919
info@impactpublishers.com
www.impactpublishers.com

In a very warm and highly personal style, psychologist Preston offers listeners powerful advice — realistic, practical, effective, on dealing with the emotional pain life often inflicts upon us. *$11.95*

Year Founded: 1996 ISBN 0-915166-99-2

3198 Life Passage in the Face of Death, Vol II: Psychological Engagement of the Physically Ill Patient
American Psychiatric Publishing, Inc.
1000 Wilson Boulevard
Suite 1825
Arlington, VA 22209-3901
703-907-7322
800-368-5777; *Fax:* 703-907-1091
appi@psych.org
www.appi.org

Ron McMillen, Chief Executive Officer
Robert E. Hales MD, M.B.A, Editor-in-Chief
John McDuffie, Editorial Director, Associate Pu
Rebecca D. Rinehart, Publisher

Ongoing explanation of therapy from a recognized expert. Valuable to clinicians and students alike.

3199 Life Passage in the Face of Death, Volume I: A Brief Psychotherapy
American Psychiatric Publishing, Inc.
1000 Wilson Boulevard
Suite 1825
Arlington, VA 22209-3901
703-907-7322
800-368-5777; *Fax:* 703-907-1091
appi@psych.org
www.appi.org

Ron McMillen, Chief Executive Officer
Robert E. Hales MD, M.B.A, Editor-in-Chief
John McDuffie, Editorial Director, Associate Pu
Rebecca D. Rinehart, Publisher

A senior psychoanalyst demonstrates the extraordinary impact of a very brief dynamic psychotherapy on a patient in a time of crisis — the terminal illness and death of a spouse. We not only meet the patient and observe the therapy, but our understanding is guided by the therapist's ongoing explanation of the process. He vividly illustrates concepts such as transference, clarification, interpretation, insight, denial, isolation and above all the relevance of understanding the past for changing the present. This unique opportunity to see a psychotherapy as it is conducted will be of immense value for all mental health clinicians and trainees.

3200 Medical Aspects of Chemical Dependency The Neurobiology of Addiction
Hazelden
15251 Pleasant Valley Road
PO Box 176
Center City, MN 55012-176
651-213-4200
800-257-7810; *Fax:* 651-213-4590
info@hazelden.org
www.hazelden.org

Mark Mishek, President, CEO of Hazelden Betty
Nick Motu, VP of Marketing and Communicatio
William C. Moyers, VP of Foundation Relations
James A. Blaha, VP of Finance and Administration

This interactive curriculum helps professionals educate clients in treatment and other settings about medical effects of chemical use and abuse. The program includes a video that explains body and brain changes that can occur when using alcohol or other drugs, a workbook that helps clients apply the information from the video to their own situations, a handbook that provides in-depth information on addiction, brain chemistry and the physiological effects of chemical dependency and a pamphlet that answers critical questions clients have about the medical effects of chemical dependency. Total price of $244.70, available to purchase separately. Program value packages available for $395.00, with 25 workbooks, two handbooks, two video and 25 pamphlets. *$225.00*

Year Founded: 2003 ISBN 1-568389-87-6

3201 Mental Health Media
25 West Street
Westborough, MA 01581
617-562-1111
www.www.mentalhealth-media.org/

Mental Health Media, formerly The Mental Illness Education Project, is engaged in the production of video-based educational and support materials for the following specific populations: people with psychiatric disabilities, families, mental health professionals, special audiences, and the general public. The videos are designed to be used in hospital, clinical, and educational settings, and at home by individuals and families.

Year Founded: 1995

3202 Physicians Living with Depression
American Psychiatric Publishing, Inc.
1000 Wilson Boulevard
Suite 1825
Arlington, VA 22209-3901
703-907-7322
800-368-5777; *Fax:* 703-907-1091
appi@psych.org
www.appi.org

Ron McMillen, Chief Executive Officer
Robert E. Hales MD, M.B.A, Editor-in-Chief
John McDuffie, Editorial Director, Associate Pu
Rebecca D. Rinehart, Publisher

Designed to help doctors see the signs of depression in their fellow physicians and to alert psychiatrists to the severity of the illness in their physician patients, the tape contains two fifteen-minute interviews, one with an emergency physician and one with a pediatrician. *$25.00*

ISBN 0-890422-78-8

3203 Rational Emotive Therapy
Research Press
PO Box 7886
Champaign, IL 61826-9177
217-352-3273
800-519-2707; *Fax:* 217-352-1221
rp@researchpress.com
www.researchpress.com

Robert W. Parkinson, Founder
Dennis Wiziecki, Marketing
Dr Albert Ellis, Author
Arnold Goldstein, Author

This video illustrates the basic concepts of Rational Emotive Therapy (RET). It includes demonstrations of RET procedures, informative discussions and unstaged counseling sessions. Viewers will see Albert Ellis and his colleagues help clients overcome such problems as guilt, social anxiety, and jealousy. Also, Dr. Ellis shares his perspectives on the evolution of RET. *$195.00*

3204 Solutions Step by Step - Substance Abuse
Treatment Videotape
WW Norton & Company
500 5th Avenue
New York, NY 10110-54
212-354-2907; *Fax:* 212-869-0856
admalmud@wwnorton.com

Drake McFeely, CEO

Quick tips, questions and examples focusing on successes that can be experienced helping substance abusers help themselves. *$ 100.00*

Year Founded: 1997 ISSN 70260-X

3205 Testing Automatic Thoughts with Thought
Records
NewHarbinger Publications
5674 Shattuck Avenue
Oakland, CA 94609-1662

510-652-0215
800-748-6273; *Fax:* 800-652-1613
customerservice@newharbinger.com
www.newharbinger.com

Matthew McKay, Owner

Videotape that helps a client explore the hot thoughts that contribute to depression. *$49.95*

ISBN 1-572243-17-1

Web Sites

3206 www.42online.org
Psychologists In Independent Practice - American
Psych Assn (APADIP)
E-mail: div42apa@cox.net
www.42online.org

Members of the American Psychological Association engaged in independent practice. Works to ensure that the needs and concerns of independent psychology practitioners are considered by the APA. Gathers and disseminates information on legislation affecting the practice of psychology, managed care, and other developments in the health care industries, office management, malpractice risk and insurance, hospital management. Offers continuing professional and educational programs. Semiannual convention, with board meeting.

3207 www.aacap.org Psychiatry
American Academy of Child and Adolescent
Psychiatry
3615 Wisconsin Avenue NW
Washington, DC 20016-3007
202-966-7300; *Fax:* 202-966-2891
communications@aacap.org
www.aacap.org

Kristin Kroeger-Ptakowski, Director, Sr Deputy Director
Elizabeth DiLauro, Advocacy Manager
Emma Jellen, Policy Coordinator

Represents over 6,000 child and adolescent psychiatrists, brochures availible online which provide concise and up-to-date material on issues ranging from children who suffer from depression and teen suicide to stepfamily problems and child sexual abuse.

3208 www.aan.com
American Academy of Neurology
201 Chicago Avenue
Minneapolis, MN 55415
612-928-6000
800-879-1960; *Fax:* 612-454-2746
memberservices@aan.com
www.www.aan.com

Timothy A. Pedley, MD, FAAN, President
Catherine M. Rydell, CAE, Executive Director, CEO

Provides information for both professionals and the public on neurology subjects, covering Alzheimer's and Parkinson's diseases to stroke and migraine, includes comprehensive fact sheets.

3209 www.aapb.org
Association for Applied Psychophysiology and
Biofeedback
10200 West 44th Avenue
Suite 304
Wheat Ridge, CO 80033

303-422-8436
800-477-8892
info@aapb.org
www.www.aapb.org

Richard Sherman, PhD, Board of Director, President
Stuart C. Donaldson, PhD, BCB, Board of Director,
President-Ele
Jeffrey Bolek, PhD, Board of Director, Past-Presiden
Richard Harvey, PhD, Board od Director, Treasurer

Represents clinicians interested in psychopsysiology or
biofeedback, offers links to their mission statement, membership information, research, FAQ about biofeedback,
conference listings, and links.

3210 www.abecsw.org
American Board of Examiners in Clinical Social
Work
241 Humphrey Street
Marblehead, MA 01945
781-639-5270
800-694-5285; *Fax:* 781-639-5278
abe@abecsw.org
www.www.abecsw.org

Bob Booth, CEO
Robert Booth, Executive Director
Michael Brooks, MSW, BCD, Director of Policy and
Business
Kathleen Bodoni, Credentials Manager

Information about the American Board of Examiners,
credentialing, and ethics.

3211 www.about.com
About.Com

Network of comprehensive Web sites for over 600 mental
health topics.

3212 www.abpsi.org
American Association of Black Psychologists
7119 Allentown Road
Suite 203
Fort Washington, MD 20744
301-449-3082; *Fax:* 301-449-3084
abpsi@abpsi.org
www.www.abpsi.org

Cheryl Tawede Grills, PhD, President
Tassogle Daryl Rowe, President-Elect
Kevin Washington, Ph.D., President-Elect
Carolyn Moore, Ph.D, Treasurer

Includes information about the Association's history and
objectives, contact and member information, upcoming
events, and publications of interest.

3213 www.ama-assn.org
American Medical Association
330 N. Wabash Ave.
Chicago, IL 60611-5885
800-621-8335
www.www.ama-assn.org

Denise M. Hagerty, SVP, CFO
James L. Madara, MD, EVP, CEO
Robert W. Davis, SVP, Human Resources and Corpora
Leslie M. Stokes, SVP, Physician Engagement

Offers a wide range of medical information and links,
full-text abstracts of each journal's current and past articles.

3214 www.apa.org
American Psychological Association
750 First St. NE
Washington, DC 20002-4242
202-336-5500
800-374-2721; *Fax:* 202-336-5518
TDD: 202-336-6123
TTY: 202-336-6123
psycinfo@apa.org
www.www.apa.org

Nadine J. Kaslow, Ph.D., President
Barry S. Anton, Ph.D., President-Elect
Donald N. Bersoff, PhD, JD, Past President
Norman B Anderson, Ph.D., CEO, EVP

Information about journals, press releases, professional and
consumer information related to the psychological profession; resources include ethical principles and guidelines,
science advocacy, awards and funding programs, testing
and assessment information, other on-line and real world
resources.

3215 www.apna.org
American Psychiatric Nurses Association
3141 Fairview Park Drive
Suite 625
Falls Church, Vi 22042
571-533-1919
855-863-APNA; *Fax:* 855-883-APNA
www.www.apna.org

Nicholas Croce Jr., MS, Executive Director
Patricia L. Black, PhD, RN, Associate Executive Director
Karla Lewis, Director, Finance and Administra
Lisa Deffenbaugh Nguyen, MS, Director, Operations

Includes membership information, contact information, organizational information, announcements and related links.

3216 www.appi.org
American Psychiatric Publishing Inc
1000 Wilson Boulevard
Suite 1825
Arlington, VA 22209-3901
703-907-7322
800-368-5777; *Fax:* 703-907-1091
appi@psych.org
www.www.appi.org

Ron McMillen, Chief Executive Officer
Robert E. Hales MD, M.B.A, Editor-in-Chief
John McDuffie, Editorial Director, Associate Pu
Rebecca D. Rinehart, Publisher

Informational site about mental disorders, 'Lets Talk Facts'
brochure series.

3217 www.apsa.org
American Psychoanalytic Asssociation
309 East 49th Street
New York, NY 10017-1601
212-752-0450; *Fax:* 212-593-0571
info@apsa.org
www.www.apsa.org

Robert L. Pyles, M.D., President
Mark Smaller, Ph.D., President-Elect
William A. Myerson, Ph.D., Treasurer
Ralph E. Fishkin, D.O., Secretary

Includes searchable bibliographic database containing books, reviews and articles of a psychoanalytical orientation, links and member information.

3218 www.askdrlloyd.wordpress.com
Ask Dr Lloyd
www.www.askdrlloyd.wordpress.com

Helps individuals understand mental illnesses and addictions, what treatments and services have been proven scientifically effective, how to manage yourself or help your loved one, and how to beat a mental health system.

3219 www.assc.caltech.edu
Association for the Scientific Study of Consciousness
The Associates of the California Institu
1200 East California Boulevard
Pasadena, CA 91125
626-395-3919; *Fax:* 626-395-5890
caltechassociates@caltech.edu
www.associates.caltech.edu

Catherine Reeves, Executive Director
Paula R. Elliott, Associate Director
Jerri Price-Gaines, Associate Director
Nicola Wilkins-Miller, Assistant Director

Electronic journal dedicated to interdisciplinary exploration on the nature of consciousness and its relationship to the brain, congnitive science, philosophy, psychology, physics, neuroscience, and artificial intelligence.

3220 www.blarg.net/~charlatn/voices
Compilation of Writings by People Suffering from Depression

3221 www.bpso.org
BPSO-Bipolar Significant Others
www.www.bpso.org

3222 www.bpso.org/nomania.htm
How to Avoid a Manic Episode

3223 www.cape.org
Cape Cod Institute
Professional Learning Network, LLC
270 Greenwich Avenue
Greenwich, CT 06830
203-422-0535
888-394-9293; *Fax:* 203-629-6048
institute@cape.org
www.www.cape.org

Offers symposia every summer for keeping mental health professionals up-to-date on the latest developments in psychology, treatment, psychiatry, and mental health, outlines available workshops, links and other relevant information.

3224 www.chadd.org
CHADD
4601 Presidents Drive
Suite 300
Lanham, MD 20706
301-306-7070
800-233-4050; *Fax:* 301-306-7090
www.www.chadd.org

Ruth Hughes, PhD, CEO
Susan Buningh, MRE, Executive Editor

Christine Hoch, Director of Development
Peg Nichols, Director Communications

National non-profit organization representing children and adults with attention deficit/hyperactivity disorder (AD/HD).

3225 www.cnn.com/Health
CNN Health Section
www.www.cnn.com/Health

Updated with health and mental health-related stories three to four times weekly.

3226 www.compuserve.com
IQuest/Knowledge Index
www.www.compuserve.com

On-line research and database information provider.

3227 www.counselingforloss.com
Counseling for Loss and Life Changes
420 West Main Street
Kent, OH 44240
E-mail: jbissler@counselingforwellness.com
www.www.counselingforloss.com

Jane Vair Bissler, Ph.D., L, Counselor, Teacher, Writer and S

Look under articles for reprints of writings and links.

3228 www.cyberpsych.org
CyberPsych
www.www.cyberpsych.org

Hosts the American Psychoanalyists Foundation, American Association of Suicideology, Society for the Exploration of Psychotherapy Intergration, and Anxiety Disorders Association of America. Also subcategories of the anxiety disorders, as well as general information, including panic disorder, phobias, obsessive compulsive disorder (OCD), social phobia, generalized anxiety disorder, post traumatic stress disorder, and phobias of childhood. Book reviews and links to web pages sharing the topics.

3229 www.goaskalice.columbia.edu
GoAskAlice/Healthwise Columbia University
www.www.goaskalice.columbia.edu

Oriented toward students, information on sexuality, sexual health, general health, alcohol and other drugs, fitness and nutrition, emotional wellbeing and relationships.

3230 www.grieftalk.com/help1.html
Grief Journey
800-TAL-

Short readings for clients.

3231 www.healthgate.com/
HealthGate
770-754-4513
www.www.healthgate.com

Max Shapiro, M.D., Doctor
Judith Dennis, M.D., Doctor
Richard Dukes, M.D., Doctor
Steven Richman, M.D., Doctor

On-line reference and database information service, $.75/record.

3232 www.healthtouch.com
Healthtouch Online
3500 Westgate Drive
Suite 504
Durham, NC 27707
919-490-4656
www.www.healthtouchnc.com

Anya Adams, Referral Practitioners
Petra Gustin, Referral Practitioners
Ruth Hamilton, Referral Practitioners
Mara Bishop, Referral Practitioners

Healthtouch Online is a resource that brings together valuable information from trusted health organizations.

3233 www.healthy.net
HealthWorld Online
www.www.healthy.net

Consumer-oriented articles on a wide range of health and mental health topics, including: Welcome Center, QuickN'Dex, Site Search, Free Medline, Health Conditions, Alternative Medicine, Referral Network, Health Columns, Global Calendar, Discussion, Cybrarian, Professional Center, Free Newsletter, Opportunities, Healthy Travel, Homepage, Library, University, Marketplace, Health Clinic, Wellness Center, Fitness Center, News Room, Association Network, Public Health, Self Care Central, and Nutrition Center.

3234 www.helix.com
GlaxoSmithKline
5 Crescent Drive
Philadelphia, PA 19112
888-825-5249
www.www.gsk.com

Roger Connor, President, Global Manufacturing
Deirdre Connelly, President, North America Pharmac
Abbas Hussain, President, Europe, Japan and EMA
Bill Louv, SVP, Core Business Services

Helix is an Education, Learning and Information exchange. Developed especially for healthcare practitioners by GlaxoSmithKline, HELIX is a premire source of on-line education and professional resources on a range of therapeutic and practice-management issues.

3235 www.human-nature.com/odmh
On-line Dictonary of Mental Health

Global information resource and research tool. It is compiled by Internet mental health resource users for Internet mental health resource users, and covers all the disciplines contributing to our understanding of mental health.

3236 www.infotrieve.com
Infotrieve Medline Services Provider
20 Westport Road
PO Box 7102
Wilton, CT 06897
203-423-2130; *Fax:* 203-423-2155
marketing@infotrieve.com
www.www.infotrieve.com

Kenneth J. Benvenuto, President, CEO
Richard H. Dick Weaver, SVP
Donna Pouliot, VP, Sales
Eileen Green, VP, Finance

Infotrieve is a library services company offering full-service document delivery, databases on the web and a variety of tools to simplify the process of identifying, retrieving and paying for published literature.

3237 www.intelihealth.com
InteliHealth

3238 www.krinfo.com
DataStar/Dialog

Information provider: reference and databases.

3239 www.lollie.com/blue/suicide.html
Comprehensive Approach to Suicide Prevention
E-mail: LollieDotCom@gmail.com

Readings for anyone contemplating suicide.

3240 www.mayohealth.org/mayo
Mayo Clinic Health Oasis Library
4500 San Pablo Road
Jacksonville, FL 32224
904-953-2000; *Fax:* 904-953-7329
www.www.mayoclinic.org

John H. Noseworthy, M.D., President
Andy Abril, M.D., Rheumatology, Medical Staff
Michael Albus, M.D., Emergency Medicine
Francisco Alvarez, M.D., Pulmonary Medicine

Healthcare library and resources.

3241 www.med.nyu.edu/Psych/index.html
NYU Department of Psychiatry

General mental health information, screening tests, reference desk, continuing educations in psychiatry program, interactive testing in psychiatry, augmentation of antidepressants, NYU Psychoanalytic Institute, Psychology Internship Program, Internet Mental Health Resources links.

3242 www.medscape.com
WebMD Health Professional Network
825 Eighth Avenue
11th Floor
New York, NY 10019
212-301-6700
FirstInitialLastName@webmd.net
www.www.medscape.com

Steven L. Zatz M.D., President
Michael B. Glick, EVP, Co-General Counsel
David J. Schlanger, CEO
Peter Anevski, CFO

Oriented toward physicians and medical topics, but also carries information relevant to the field of psychology and mental health.

3243 www.members.aol.com/dswgriff
Now Is Not Forever: A Survival Guide

Print out a no-suicide contract, do problem solving, and other exercises.

3244 www.mentalhealth.com/p20-grp.html
Manic-Depressive Illness

Click on Bipolar and then arrow down to Booklets.

3245 www.mentalhealth.com/story
How to Help a Person with Depression

Valuable family education.

3246 www.mentalhealthamerica.net
Mental Health America
2000 N. Beauregard Street
6th Floor
Alexandria, VA 22311
703-684-7722
800-969-6642; *Fax:* 703-684-5968
www.www.mentalhealthamerica.net

David L. Shern, Ph.D., Interim President, CEO
Mike Turner, VP, Development
Dianne Felton, Chief Operating Officer
Julio Abreu, Senior Director of Public Policy

Mental Health America is the nation's largest and oldest community-based network dedicated to helping all Americans live mentally healthier lives. With more than 300 affiliates across the country, Mental Health America touches the lives of millions - advocating for changes in policy; educating the public and providing critical information; & delivering urgently needed programs and services.

3247 www.metanoia.org/suicide/
If You Are Thinking about Suicide...Read This First
www.www.metanoia.org/suicide

Excellent suggestions, information and links for the suicidal.

3248 www.mhsource.com
CME Mental Health InfoSource

Mental health information and education, fully accredited for all medical specialties.

3249 www.mhsource.com/
CME Psychiatric Time

Select articles published online from the Psychiatric Times, topics relevant to all mental health professionals.

3250 www.mindfreedom.org
Support Coalition Human Rights & Psychiatry Home Page
454 Willamette, PO Box 11284
Suite 216
Eugene, OR 97440-3484
541-345-9106
877-MAD-PRID
www.www.mindfreedom.org

Celia Brown, Board President
Thomas E. Wittick, MFI Member
Mary Maddock, Founder, MindFreedom Ireland
Al Galves, PhD, Psychologist, Mental Health Cons

Support Coalition is an independent alliance of several dozen grassroots groups in the USA, Canada, Europe, New Zealand; has used protests, publications, letter-writing, e-mail, workshops, Dendron News, the arts and performances. Led by psychiatric survivors, and open to the public, membership is open to anyone who supports its mission and goals.

3251 www.mirror-mirror.org/eatdis.htm
Mirror, Mirror

Relapse prevention for eating disorders.

3252 www.naphs.org
National Association of Psychiatric Health Systems
900 17th Street NW
Suite 420
Washington, DC 20006-2507
202-393-6700; *Fax:* 202-783-6041
www.www.naphs.org

Mark J. Covall, President, CEO
Kathleen McCann, RN, PhD, Director, Quality and Regulatory
Nancy Trenti, JD, Director, Congressional Affairs
Carole Szpak, Director, Operations and Communi

The NAPHS advocates for behavioral health and represents provider systems that are committed to the delivery of responsive, accountable and clinically effective prevention, treatment and care for children, adolescents and adults with mental and substance use disorders.

3253 www.naswdc.org/
National Associaton of Social Workers
750 First Street, NE
Suite 700
Washington, DC 20002-4241
202-408-8600
800-742-4089
press@naswdc.org
www.www.naswdc.org/

Jeane W. Anastas, PhD, LMSW, President
Darrell P. Wheeler, PhD, ACSW, MP, President-Elect
E. Jane Middleton, DSW, MSW, VP
Mary L. McCarthy, PhD, LMSW, Treasurer

Central resource for clinical social workers, includes information about the federation, a conference and workshop calender, information on how to subscribe to social worker mailing lists, legislative and news updates, links to state agencies and social work societies, and publications.

3254 www.ndmda.org/justmood.htm
Just a Mood...or Something Else

A brochure for teens.

3255 www.nimh.nih.gov
National Institute of Mental Health (NIMH)
6001 Executive Boulevard
Rockville, MD 20852
301-443-4513
866-615-6464; *Fax:* 301-443-4279
TTY: 866-415-8051
NIMHinfo@mail.nih.gov
www.www.nimh.nih.gov

Dianne M. Rausch, Ph.D., Director, Office on AIDS
Gemma Weiblinger, Director, Office of Constituency
Suzanne M. Murrin, Associate Director for Managemen
Pamela Y. Collins, M.D., M.P.H., Director, Office of Rural Mental

The mission of NIMH is to diminish the burden of mental illness through research of the biological, behavioral, clinical, epidemiological, economic, and social science aspects of mental illnesses.

3256 www.nmha.org
National Mental Health Association
2000 N. Beauregard Street
6th Floor
Alexandria, VA 22311

703-684-7722
800-969-6642; *Fax:* 703-684-5968
www.www.mentalhealthamerica.net

David L. Shern, Ph.D., Interim President, CEO
Mike Turner, VP, Development
Dianne Felton, Chief Operating Officer
Julio Abreu, Senior Director of Public Policy

Dedicated to promoting mental health, preventing mental disorders and achieving victory over mental illness through advocacy, education, research and service. NMHA's collaboration with the National GAINS Center for People with Co-Occuring Disorders in the Justice System has produced the Justice for Juveniles Initiative. This program battles to reform the juvenile justice system so that the inmates mental needs are addressed. Envisions a just, humane and healthy society in which all people are accorded respect, dignity and the opportunity to achieve their full potential free from stigma and prejudice.

3257 www.oclc.org
EPIC
6565 Kilgour Place
Dublin, OH 43017-3395
614-764-6000
800-848-5878
oclc@oclc.org
www.www.oclc.org

Skip Prichard, President, CEO
Rick Schwieterman, EVP, CFO, Treasurer
Bruce Crocco, VP, Library Services for the Ame
Lorcan Dempsey, VP, OCLC Research and Chief Stra

On-line reference and database information provider, $40/hour (plus connection fees) and $.75/record.

3258 www.oznet.ksu.edu/library/famlf2/
Family Life Library
24 Umberger Hall
Kansas State University
Manhattan, KS 66506-3402
785-532-5830; *Fax:* 785-532-7938
orderpub@k-state.edu
www.www.oznet.ksu.edu/library/famlf2/

3259 www.pace-custody.org
Professional Academy of Custody Evaluators
Furlong, PA 18925
800-633-7223; *Fax:* 215-794-3386
www.pace411.com

Dr. Barry Bricklin, Ph.D., Chair, Founding Member
Dr. Gail Elliot, Ph.D., Vice Chair, Founding Member
John J. Hare, Jr., Treasurer, Secretary

Nonprofit corporation and membership organization to acknowledge and strengthen the professionally prepared comprehensive custody evaluation; psychologicals legal knowledge base, assessment procedures, courtroom testimony, provides continuing education courses, conferences, conventions and seminars.

3260 www.paperchase.com
PaperChase
PO Box 54
Hood, VA 22723
781-325-6086
800-722-2075; *Fax:* 540-948-4841
support@paperchase.com
www.www.paperchase.com

Searches may be conducted through a browsable list of topics, search engine recognizes queries made in natural language.

3261 www.parenthoodweb.com
Blended Families

Resolving conflicts.

3262 www.planetpsych.com
Planetpsych.com
E-mail: webmaster@planetpsych.com
www.www.planetpsych.com

Learn about disorders, their treatments and other topics in psychology. Articles are listed under the related topic areas. Ask a therapist a question for free, or view the directory of professionals in your area. If you are a therapist sign up for the directory. Current features, self-help, interactive, and newsletter archives.

3263 www.positive-way.com/step.htm
Stepfamily Information
www.www.positive-way.com/step.htm

Introduction and tips for stepfathers, stepmothers and re-married parents.

3264 www.psych.org
American Psychiatric Association
1000 Wilson Boulevard
Suite 1825
Arlington, VA 22209-3901
703-907-7322
800-368-5777; *Fax:* 703-907-1091
appi@psych.org
www.www.psych.org

Ron McMillen, Chief Executive Officer
Robert E. Hales MD, M.B.A, Editor-in-Chief
John McDuffie, Editorial Director, Associate Pu
Rebecca D. Rinehart, Publisher

A medical specialty society recognized world-wide. Its 40,500 US and international physicians specializing in the diagnosis and treatment of mental and emotional illness and substance use disorders.

384 pages Year Founded: 1993

3265 www.psychcentral.com
Psych Central
www.psychcentral.com

Personalized one-stop index for psychology, support, and mental health issues, resources, and people on the Internet.

3266 www.psychcrawler.com
American Psychological Association
750 1st Street NE
Washington, DC 20002-4242
202-336-5500
800-374-2721; *Fax:* 202-336-5518
TDD: 202-336-6123
TTY: 202-336-6123
psycinfo@apa.org
www.psycnet.apa.org

Nadine J. Kaslow, Ph.D., President
Barry S. Anton, Ph.D., President-Elect
Donald N. Bersoff, PhD, JD, Past President
Norman B Anderson, Ph.D., CEO, EVP

Indexing the web for the links in psychology.

16 pages

3267 www.psychology.com/therapy.htm
Therapist Directory
800-935-3277; *Fax:* 847-792-7500
www.therapist.psychology.com

Therapists listed geographically plus answers to frequently asked questions.

3268 www.psycom.net/depression.central.html
Dr. Ivan's Depression Central

Medication-oriented site.

3269 www.recovery-inc.com
Recovery

Describes the organizations approach.

3270 www.reutershealth.com
Reuters Health

Relevant and useful clinical information on mental disorders, news briefs updated daily.

3271 www.save.org
SA/VE - Suicide Awareness/Voices of Education
8120 Penn Ave. S.
Suite 470
Bloomington, MN 55431
952-946-7998
800-273-8255
dreidenberg@save.org
www.www.save.org

Daniel J. Reidenberg, PSY.D.,FA, Executive Director
Francene Young Rolstad, Business Manager
Linda Mars, Events Coordinator
Jennifer Owens, Program Coordinator

3272 www.schizophrenia.com
Schizophrenia.com
E-mail: szwebmaster@yahoo.com
www.www.schizophrenia.com

Brian Chiko, BSc, Executive Director
J. Megginson Hollister, PhD, Editor
Erin Hawkes, MSc, Writer/Contributor
Marvin Ross, Science Writer - Freelance

Offers basic and in-depth information, discussion and chat.

3273 www.schizophrenia.com/ami
Alliance for the Mentally Ill
E-mail: szwebmaster@yahoo.com
www.www.schizophrenia.com

Brian Chiko, BSc, Executive Director
J. Megginson Hollister, PhD, Editor
Erin Hawkes, MSc, Writer/Contributor
Marvin Ross, Science Writer - Freelance

Information on mental disorders, reducing the stigmatization of them in our society today, and how you can be more active in your local community. Includes articles, press information, media kits, mental disorder diagnostic and treatment information, coping issues, advocacy guides and announcements.

3274 www.schizophrenia.com/newsletter
Schizophrenia.com

Comprehensive psychoeducational site on schizophrenia.

3275 www.shpm.com
Self-Help and Psychology Magazine

General psychology and self-help magazine online, offers informative articles on general well being and psychology topics. Features Author of the Month, Breaking News Stories of the Month, Most Popular Pages, What's Hot, Departments, and Soundoff (articles and opinion page). This online compendium of hundreds of readers and professionals.

3276 www.shpm.com/articles/depress
Placebo Effect Accounts for Fifty Percent of Improvement

3277 www.siop.org
Society for Industrial and Organizational Psychology
440 E Poe Rd
Suite 101
Bowling Green, OH 43402
419-353-0032; *Fax:* 419-352-2645
SIOP@siop.org
www.www.siop.org

Tammy Allen, President
David Nershi, Executive Director
Linda Lentz, Administrative Services Director
Larry Nader, IT Manager

Home to the Industrial-Organizational Pyschologist newsletter, links and resources, member information, contact information for doctoral and master's level program in I/O psychology, and announcements of various events and conferences.

3278 www.stepfamily.org/tensteps.htm
Ten Steps for Steps
310 West 85th St.
Suite 1B
New York, NY 10024
212-877-3244
Stepfamily@aol.com
www.www.stepfamily.org

Jeannette Lofas, PhD, LCSW, President

Guidelines for stepfamilies.

3279 www.stepfamilyinfo.org/sitemap.htm
Stepfamily in Formation
310 West 85th St.
Suite 1B
New York, NY 10024
212-877-3244
Stepfamily@aol.com
www.www.stepfamily.org

Jeannette Lofas, PhD, LCSW, President

3280 www.usatoday.com
USA Today

'Mental Health' category includes news and in-depth reports.

3281 www.webmd.com
WebMD

Kristy Hammam, SVP, Programming and Content Str
Michael W. Smith, MD, Chief Medical Editor
Brunilda Nazario, MD, Lead Medical Editor
Hansa Bhargava, MD, Medical Editor

3282 www.wingofmadness.com
Wing of Madness: A Depression Guide

Accurate information, advice, support, and personal experiences.

Workbooks & Manuals

3283 Activities for Adolescents in Therapy
Charles C Thomas Publisher Ltd.
2600 S 1st Street
Springfield, IL 62704-4730
217-789-8980
800-258-8980; *Fax:* 217-789-9130
books@ccthomas.com
www.ccthomas.com

Michael P Thomas, President
Susan T. Dennison, Author
Connie M. Knight, Author
Richar J. Laban, Author

In this practical resource manual, professionals will find more than 100 therapeutic group activities for use in counseling troubled adolescents. This new edition provides specifics on establishing an effective group program while, at the same time, outlining therapeutic activities that can be used in each phase of a therapy group. Step-by-step instructions have been provided for setting up, planning and facilitating adolescent groups with social and emotional problems. The interventions provided have been designed specifically for initial, middle and termination phases of group. $39.95 $46.95

264 pages Year Founded: 1998 ISBN 0-398068-07-0

3284 Activities for Children in Therapy: Guide for
Planning and Facilitating Therapy with
Troubled Children
Charles C Thomas Publisher Ltd.
2600 S 1st Street
Springfield, IL 62704-4730
217-789-8980
800-258-8980; *Fax:* 217-789-9130
books@ccthomas.com
www.ccthomas.com

Michael P Thomas, President
Susan T. Dennison, Author
Connie M. Knight, Author
Richar J. Laban, Author

Provides the mental health professional with a wide variety of age-appropriate activities which are simultaneously fun and therapeutic for the five-to-twelve-year-old troubled child. Activities have been designed as enjoyable games in the context of therapy. Provides a comprehensive listing of books with other therapeutic intervention ideas, bibliotherapy materials, assessment scales for evaluating youngsters, and a sample child assessment for individual therapy. For professionals who provide counseling to children, such as social workers, psychologists, guidance counselors, speech/language pathologists, and art therapists. $52.95

302 pages Year Founded: 1999 ISBN 0-398069-71-9

3285 Chemical Dependency Treatment Planning
Handbook
Charles C Thomas Publisher Ltd.
2600 S 1st Street
Springfield, IL 62704-4730

217-789-8980
800-258-8980; *Fax:* 217-789-9130
books@ccthomas.com
www.ccthomas.com

Michael P Thomas, President
Richar J. Laban, Author
Connie M. Knight, Author
Susan T. Dennison, Author

Provides the entry-level clinician with a broad data base of treatment planning illustrations from which unpretentious treatment plans for the chemically dependent client can be generated. They are simple, largely measurable, and purposefully, with language that is cognizant of comprehension and learning needs of clients. It will be of interest to drug and alcohol counselors. $39.95

174 pages Year Founded: 1997 ISBN 0-398067-76-7

3286 Clinical Manual of Supportive Psychotherapy
American Psychiatric Publishing, Inc.
1000 Wilson Boulevard
Suite 1825
Arlington, VA 22209-3901
703-907-7322
800-368-5777; *Fax:* 703-907-1091
appi@psych.org
www.appi.org

Ron McMillen, Chief Executive Officer
Robert E. Hales MD, M.B.A, Editor-in-Chief
John McDuffie, Editorial Director, Associate Pu
Rebecca D. Rinehart, Publisher

New approaches and ideas for your practice. $101.00

384 pages Year Founded: 1993 ISBN 0-880484-03-9

3287 Concise Guide to Laboratory and Diagnostic
Testing in Psychiatry
American Psychiatric Publishing, Inc.
1000 Wilson Boulevard
Suite 1825
Arlington, VA 22209-3901
703-907-7322
800-368-5777; *Fax:* 703-907-1091
appi@psych.org
www.appi.org

Ron McMillen, Chief Executive Officer
Robert E. Hales MD, M.B.A, Editor-in-Chief
John McDuffie, Editorial Director, Associate Pu
Rebecca D. Rinehart, Publisher

Basic strategies for applying laboratory testing and evaluation. $19.50

176 pages Year Founded: 1989 ISBN 0-880483-33-4

3288 Creating and Implementing Your Strategic
Plan: Workbook for Public and Nonprofit
Organizations
John Wiley & Sons
111 River Street
Hoboken, NJ 07030-5774
201-748-6000; *Fax:* 201-748-6088
info@wiley.com
www.wiley.com

Stephen M. Smith, President, CEO
MJ O'Leary, SVP, Human Resources
Edward J. Melando, SVP, Corporate Controller
Gary M. Rinck, SVP, General Counsel

Step-by-step workbook to conducting strategic planning in public and nonprofit organizations. *$30.00*

Year Founded: 1992 ISBN 0-787967-54-8

3289 Handbook for the Study of Mental Health
Cambridge University Press
40 W 20th Street
New York, NY 10011-4211
212-924-3900; *Fax:* 212-691-3239

Offers the first comprehensive presentation of the sociology of mental health illness, including original, contemporary contributions by experts in the relevant aspects of the field. Divided into three sections, the chapters cover the general perspectives in the field, the social determinants of mental health and current policy areas affecting mental health services. Designed for classroom use in sociology, social work, human relations, human services and psychology. With its useful definitions, overview of the historical, social and institutional frameworks for understanding mental health and illness, and nontechnical style, the text is suitable for advanced undergraduate or lower level graduate students. *$90.00*

694 pages Year Founded: 1999 ISBN 0-521561-33-7

3290 Handbook of Clinical Psychopharmacology for Therapists
NewHarbinger Publications
5674 Shattuck Avenue
Oakland, CA 94609-1662
510-652-0215
800-748-6273; *Fax:* 800-652-1613
customerservice@newharbinger.com
www.newharbinger.com

Matthew McKay, Owner

This newly revised classic includes updates on new medications, and expanded quick reference section, and new material on bipolar illness, the treatment of psychosis, and the effect of severe trauma. *$55.95*

264 pages Year Founded: 2005 ISBN 1-572240-94-6

3291 Handbook of Constructive Therapies
John Wiley & Sons
111 River Street
Hoboken, NJ 07030-5774
201-748-6000; *Fax:* 201-748-6088
info@wiley.com
www.wiley.com

Stephen M. Smith, President, CEO
MJ O'Leary, SVP, Human Resources
Edward J. Melando, SVP, Corporate Controller
Gary M. Rinck, SVP, General Counsel

Learn techniques that focus on the strengths and resources of your clients and look to where they want to go rather than where they have been. *$64.00*

Year Founded: 1992 ISBN 0-787940-44-5

3292 Handbook of Counseling Psychology
John Wiley & Sons
111 River Street
Hoboken, NJ 07030-5774
201-748-6000; *Fax:* 201-748-6088
info@wiley.com
www.wiley.com

Stephen M. Smith, President, CEO
MJ O'Leary, SVP, Human Resources

Edward J. Melando, SVP, Corporate Controller
Gary M. Rinck, SVP, General Counsel

Provides a cross-disciplinary survey of the entire field and offers analysis of important areas of counseling psychology activity. the book elaborates on future directions for research, highlighting suggestions that may advance knowledge and stimulate further inquiry. Specific advice is presented from the literature in counseling psychology and related disciplines to help improve one's counseling practice. *$ 120.00*

Year Founded: 1992 ISBN 0-471254-58-4

3293 Handbook of Managed Behavioral Healthcare
John Wiley & Sons
111 River Street
Hoboken, NJ 07030-5774
201-748-6000; *Fax:* 201-748-6088
info@wiley.com
www.wiley.com

Stephen M. Smith, President, CEO
MJ O'Leary, SVP, Human Resources
Edward J. Melando, SVP, Corporate Controller
Gary M. Rinck, SVP, General Counsel

A comprehensive curriculum to understanding managed care. *$43.00*

Year Founded: 1992 ISBN 0-787941-53-0

3294 Handbook of Medical Psychiatry
Mosby
11830 Westline Industrial Drive
Saint Louis, MO 63146-3318
314-872-8370
800-325-4177; *Fax:* 314-432-1380

This large-format handbook covers almost every psychiatric, neurologic and general medical condition capable of causing disturbances in thought, feeling, or behavior and includes almost every psychopharmacologic agent available in America today. *$61.95*

544 pages Year Founded: 1996 ISBN 0-323029-11-6

3295 Handbook of Psychiatric Education and Faculty Development
American Psychiatric Publishing, Inc.
1000 Wilson Boulevard
Suite 1825
Arlington, VA 22209-3901
703-907-7322
800-368-5777; *Fax:* 703-907-1091
appi@psych.org
www.www.appi.org

Saul Levin, M.D., M.P.A., CEO and Medical Director
Jerald Kay, M.D., Co-Editor
Edward K. Silberman, M.D., Co-Editor
Linda Pessar, M.D., Co-Editor

Putting education to work in the real world. *$68.50*

680 pages Year Founded: 1999 ISBN 0-880487-80-1

3296 Handbook of Psychiatric Practice in the Juvenile Court
American Psychiatric Publishing, Inc.
1000 Wilson Boulevard
Suite 1825
Arlington, VA 22209-3901
703-907-7322
800-368-5777; *Fax:* 703-907-1091

appi@psych.org
www.www.appi.org

Robert E Hales M.D., M.B.A., Editor-in-Chief
Saul Levin, M.D., M.P.A., CEO and Medical Director
John McDuffie, Associate Publisher, Acquisition
Rebecca D. Rinehart, Publisher

How your practice can work with the court system, so your patients can get the help they need. *$27.95*

212 pages Year Founded: 1991 ISBN 0-890422-33-8

3297 Living Skills Recovery Workbook
Elsevier Science
PO Box 28430
Saint Louis, MO 63146-930
314-453-7010
800-545-2522; *Fax:* 314-453-7095
www.store.elsevier.com

Katie Hennessy, Medical Promotions Coordinator

Provides clinicians with the tools necessary to help patients with dual diagnoses acquire basic living skills. Focusing on stress management, time management, activities of daily living, and social skills training, each living skill is taught in relation to how it aids in recovery and relapse prevention for each patient's individual lifestyle and pattern of addiction.

224 pages ISBN 0-750671-18-1

3298 On the Client's Path: A Manual for the Practice of Brief Solution - Focused Therapy
NewHarbinger Publications
5674 Shattuck Avenue
Oakland, CA 94609-1662
510-652-0215
800-748-6273; *Fax:* 800-652-1613
customerservice@newharbinger.com
www.newharbinger.com

Matthew McKay, Owner

Provides everything you need to master the solution - focused model. *$49.95*

157 pages Year Founded: 1995 ISBN 1-572240-21-0

3299 Relaxation & Stress Reduction Workbook
NewHarbinger Publications
5674 Shattuck Avenue
Oakland, CA 94609-1662
510-652-0215
800-748-6273; *Fax:* 800-652-1613
customerservice@newharbinger.com
www.newharbinger.com

Matthew McKay, Owner

Details effective stress reduction methods such as breathing exercises, meditation, visualization, and time management. Widely reccomended by therapists, nurses, and physicians throughout the US, this fourth edition has been substantially revised and updated to reflect current research. Line drawings and charts. *$19.95*

276 pages Year Founded: 2005 ISBN 1-879237-82-2

3300 Skills Training Manual for Treating Borderline Personality Disorder, Companion Workbook
Guilford Press
72 Spring Street
New York, NY 10012-4068

212-431-9800
800-365-7006; *Fax:* 212-966-6708
info@guilford.com
www.www.guilford.com

Bob Matloff, President
Seymour Weingarten, Editor-in-Chief

A vital component in Dr. Linehan's comprehensive treatment program, this step-by-step manual details precisely how to implement the skills training procedures and includes practical pointers on when to use the other treatment strategies described. It includes useful, clear-cut handouts that may be readily photocopied. *$27.95*

180 pages Year Founded: 1993 ISBN 0-898620-34-1

3301 Step Workbook for Adolescent Chemical Dependency Recovery
American Psychiatric Publishing, Inc.
1000 Wilson Boulevard
Suite 1825
Arlington, VA 22209-3901
703-907-7322
800-368-5777; *Fax:* 703-907-1091
appi@psych.org
www.appi.org

Ron McMillen, Chief Executive Officer
Robert E. Hales MD, M.B.A, Editor-in-Chief
John McDuffie, Editorial Director, Associate Pu
Rebecca D. Rinehart, Publisher

Strategies for younger patients in your practice. *$ 62.00*

72 pages Year Founded: 1990 ISBN 0-882103-00-9

3302 Stress Management Training: Group Leader's Guide
Professional Resource Press
PO Box 3197
Sarasota, FL 34230-3197
941-343-9601
800-443-3364; *Fax:* 941-343-9201
cs.prpress@gmail.com
www.prpress.com

Laurie Girsch, Managing Editor

This practical guide will help you define the concept of stress for group members and teach them various intervention techniques ranging from relaxation training to communication skills. Includes specific exercises, visual aids, stress response index, stress analysis form and surveys for evaluating program effectiveness. *$13.95*

96 pages Year Founded: 1990 ISBN 0-943158-33-8

3303 Stress Owner's Manual: Meaning, Balance and Health in Your Life
Impact Publishers
PO Box 6016
Atascadero, CA 93423-6016
805-466-5917
800-246-7228; *Fax:* 805-466-5919
info@impactpublishers.com
www.impactpublishers.com

Offers specific solutions: maps, checklists and rating scales to help you assess your life; dozens of stress buffer activities to help you deal with stress on the spot; life-changing strategies to prepare you for a lifetime of effective stress management. *$15.95*

224 pages Year Founded: 2003 ISBN 1-886230-54-4

3304 The Comprehensive Directory
Resources For Children with Special Needs
116 E 16th Street
5th Floor
New York, NY 10003-2164
212-677-4650; *Fax:* 212-254-4070
info@resourcesnyc.org
www.resourcesnyc.org

Rachel Howard, Executive Director
Stephen Stern, Director , Finance and Administr
Todd Dorman, Director, Communications and Out
Helen Murphy, Director, Program and Fund Devel

The directory for everyone who needs to find services for children with disabilities and special needs. Designed for parents, caregivers and professionals, it includes more than 2,500 agencies providing more than 4,000 services and programs. *$30.00*

1200 pages ISBN 0-967836-51-4

3305 Therapist's Workbook
John Wiley & Sons
111 River Street
Hoboken, NJ 07030-5774
201-748-6000; *Fax:* 201-748-6088
info@wiley.com
www.wiley.com

Stephen M. Smith, President, CEO
MJ O'Leary, SVP, Human Resources
Edward J. Melando, SVP, Corporate Controller
Gary M. Rinck, SVP, General Counsel

This workbook nourishes and challenges counselors, guiding them on a journey of self-reflection and renewal. *$35.00*

Year Founded: 1992 ISBN 0-787945-23-4

3306 Treating Alcohol Dependence: a Coping Skills Training Guide
Guilford Press
72 Spring Street
New York, NY 10012-4068
212-431-9800
800-365-7006; *Fax:* 212-966-6708
info@guilford.com
www.www.guilford.com

Bob Matloff, President
Seymour Weingarten, Editor-in-Chief

Treatment program based on a cognitive-social learning theory of alcohol abuse. Presents a straight-forward treatment strategy that copes with how to stop drinking and provides the training skills to make it possible. *$21.95*

240 pages Year Founded: 1989 ISBN 0-898622-15-8

Directories & Databases

3307 AAHP/Dorland Directory of Health Plans
Dorland Health
1500 Walnut Street
Suite 1000
Philadelphia, PA 19102-3512
215-875-1212
855-CAL- DH1; *Fax:* 301-287-2535
info@dorlandhealth.com
www.dorlandhealth.com

Carol Brault, VP
Yolanda Matthews, Product Manager
Anne Llewellyn, Editor in Chief
Richard Scott, Managing Editor

Paperback, published yearly. *$215.00*

3308 American Academy of Child and Adolescent Psychiatry - Membership Directory
3615 Wisconsin Avenue NW
Washington, DC 20016-3007
202-966-7300
800-333-7636; *Fax:* 202-966-2891
communications@aacap.org
www.aacap.org

Robert Hendren, President
Kristin Kroeger-Ptakowski, Director, Sr Deputy Director
Elizabeth DiLauro, Advocacy Manager
Emma Jellen, Policy Coordinator

$30.00

179 pages 2 per year

3309 American Academy of Psychoanalysis and Dynamic Psychiatry
American Academy of Psychoanalysis and Dynamic Psychiatry
One Regency Drive
PO Box 30
Bloomfield, CT 06002-30
888-691-8281; *Fax:* 860-286-0787
info@aapdp.org
www.aapsa.org

Michael Blumenfield, MD, President
Sherry Katz-Bearnot, President
Jacquelyn T Coleman CAE, Executive Director
Carol Filiaci, Secretary

The journal of the American Academy of Psychoanalysis and Dynamic Psychiatry. Publishes articles by members and other authors who have a significant contribution to make to the community of scholars or practitioners interested in a psychodynamic understanding of human behavior. *$50.00*

70 pages

3310 American Network of Community Options and Resources-Directory of Members
ANCOR
1101 King Street
Suite 380
Alexandria, VA 22314-2962
703-535-7850; *Fax:* 703-535-7860
ancor@ancor.org
www.ancor.org

Barbara Merrill, VP, Public Policy
Renee L Pietrangelo, CEO
Katherine Berland, Director, Government Relations
Tony Yu, Director, Web and I.T.

Covers 650 agencies serving people with developmental disabilities. *$25.00*

179 pages 1 per year

3311 American Psychiatric Association-Membership Directory
Harris Publishing
2500 Westchester Avenue
Suite 400
Purchase, NY 10577-2515
800-326-6600; *Fax:* 914-641-3501

$59.95

816 pages

3312 American Psychoanalytic Association - Roster
American Psychological Association
750 1st Street NE
Washington, DC 20002-4242
202-336-5500
800-374-2721; *Fax:* 202-336-5518
TDD: 202-336-6123
TTY: 202-336-6123
webmaster@apa.org
www.apa.org

Nadine J. Kaslow, Ph.D., President
Barry S. Anton, Ph.D., President-Elect
Donald N. Bersoff, PhD, JD, Past President
Norman B Anderson, Ph.D., CEO, EVP

$40.00

194 pages

3313 Association for Advancement of Behavior Therapy: Membership Directory
305 Seventh Avenue
16th Floor
New York, NY 10001-6008
212-647-1890; *Fax:* 212-647-1865
www.www.abct.org

Mary Jane Eimer, Executive Director
Mary Ellen Brown, Administration/Convention
Rosemary Park, Membership Services

Covers over 4,500 psychologists, psychiatrists, social workers and other interested in behavior therapy. *$50.00*

240 pages 2 per year

3314 At Health
488 Woody Road
Rogersville, MO 65742
417-241-0553
888-284-3258
support@athealth.com
www.athealth.com

Andy Michaels, President
Jill Michaels, Vice President

Providing trustworthy online information, tools, and training that enhance the ability of practitioners to furnish high quality, personalized care to those they serve. For the meantl health consumer, find practitioners, treatment center, learn about disorders and conditions, and about medications being used, news and resources.

3315 CARF International
Rehabilitation Accreditation Commission
6951East Southpoint Road
Tucson, AZ 85756-9407
520-325-1044
888-281-6531; *Fax:* 520-318-1129
TTY: 888-281-6531
www.carf.org

Brian J. Boon, Ph.D., President/CEO
Amanda E. Birch, Administrator Of Operations
Cindy L. Johnson, CPA, Chief Resource and Strategic Dev
Leslie Ellis-Lang, Managing Director

Covers about three thousand organizations in seven thousand locations offering more than eighteen hundred medical rehabilitation, behavioral health, and employment and community support services that have been accredited by CARF. *$100.00*

200 pages 1 per year Year Founded: 1999

3316 Case Management Resource Guide
Dorland Health
1500 Walnut Street
Suite 1000
Philadelphia, PA 19102-3512
215-875-1212
855-CAL- DH1; *Fax:* 301-287-2535
info@dorlandhealth.com
www.dorlandhealth.com

Carol Brault, VP
Yolanda Matthews, Product Manager
Anne Llewellyn, Editor in Chief
Richard Scott, Managing Editor

In four volumes, over 110,000 health care facilities and support services are listed, including homecare, rehabilitation, psychiatric and addiction treatment programs, hospices, adult day care and burn and cancer centers.

5,200 pages 1 per year ISBN 1-880874-84-9

3317 Case Manager Database
Dorland Health
1500 Walnut Street
Suite 1000
Philadelphia, PA 19102-3512
215-875-1212
855-CAL- DH1; *Fax:* 301-287-2535
info@dorlandhealth.com
www.dorlandhealth.com

Carol Brault, VP
Yolanda Matthews, Product Manager
Anne Llewellyn, Editor in Chief
Richard Scott, Managing Editor

Largest database of information on case managers in US, especially of case managers who work for health plans and health insurers. Covers over 15,000 case managers and includes detailed data such as work setting and clinical specialty, which can be used to carefully target marketing communications. $2500 for full database, other prices available.

3318 Complete Directory for People with Disabilities
Grey House Publishing
4919 Route 22
PO Box 56
Amenia, NY 12501
518-789-8700
800-562-2139; *Fax:* 518-789-0556
books@greyhouse.com
www.greyhouse.com

Richard Gottlieb, President
Leslie Mackenzie, Publisher

This one-stop annual resource provides immediate access to the latest products and services available for people with disabilities, such as Periodicals & Books, Assistive Devices, Employment & Education Programs, Camps and Travel Groups. *$165.00*

1200 pages ISBN 1-592370-07-1

3319 Complete Learning Disabilities Directory
Grey House Publishing
4919 Route 22
PO Box 56
Amenia, NY 12501
518-789-8700
800-562-2139; *Fax:* 518-789-0556
books@greyhouse.com
www.greyhouse.com

Richard Gottlieb, President
Leslie Mackenzie, Publisher

This annual resource includes information about Associations & Organizations, Schools, Colleges & Testing Materials, Government Agencies, Legal Resources and much more. *$195.00*

745 pages ISBN 1-930956-79-7

3320 Complete Mental Health Directory
Grey House Publishing
4919 Route 22
PO Box 56
Amenia, NY 12501
518-789-8700
800-562-2139; *Fax:* 518-789-0556
books@greyhouse.com
www.greyhouse.com

Richard Gottlieb, President
Leslie Mackenzie, Publisher

This bi-annual directory offers understandable descriptions of 25 Mental Health Disorders as well as detailed information on Associations, Media, Support Groups and Mental Health Facilities. *$ 165.00*

800 pages ISBN 1-592370-46-2

3321 DSM-IV Psychotic Disorders: New Diagnostic Issue
American Psychiatric Publishing, Inc.
1000 Wilson Boulevard
Suite 1825
Arlington, VA 22209-3901
703-907-7322
800-368-5777; *Fax:* 703-907-1091
appi@psych.org
www.appi.org

Ron McMillen, Chief Executive Officer
Robert E. Hales MD, M.B.A, Editor-in-Chief
John McDuffie, Editorial Director, Associate Pu
Rebecca D. Rinehart, Publisher

Updates on clinical findings. *$39.95*

Year Founded: 1995

3322 Detwiler's Directory of Health and Medical Resources
Dorland Health
1500 Walnut Street
Suite 1000
Philadelphia, PA 19102-3512
215-875-1212
855-CAL- DH1; *Fax:* 301-287-2535
info@dorlandhealth.com
www.dorlandhealth.com

Carol Brault, VP
Yolanda Matthews, Product Manager
Anne Llewellyn, Editor in Chief
Richard Scott, Managing Editor

An invaluable guide to healthcare information sources. This directory lists information on over 2,000 sources of information on the medical and healthcare industry. *$195.00*

1 per year Year Founded: 1999 ISBN 1-880874-57-1

3323 Directory for People with Chronic Illness
Grey House Publishing
4919 Route 22
PO Box 56
Amenia, NY 12501
518-789-8700
800-562-2139; *Fax:* 845-373-5390
books@greyhouse.com
www.greyhouse.com

Richard Gottlieb, President
Leslie Mackenzie, Publisher

This bi-annual resource provides a comprehensive overview of the support services and information resources available for people diagnosed with a chronic illness. Includes 12,000 entries. *$165.00*

1200 pages ISBN 1-592370-81-0

3324 Directory of Developmental Disabilities Services
Nebraska Health and Human Services System
PO Box 94728
Department of Services
Lincoln, NE 68509-4728
402-471-2851
800-833-7352; *Fax:* 402-479-5094

Covers agencies and organizations that provide developmental disability services and programs in Nebraska.

28 pages

3325 Directory of Health Care Professionals
Dorland Health
1500 Walnut Street
Suite 1000
Philadelphia, PA 19102-3512
215-875-1212
855-CAL- DH1; *Fax:* 301-287-2535
customer@decisionhealth.com
www.dorlandhealth.com

Carol Brault, VP
Yolanda Matthews, Product Manager
Anne Llewellyn, Editor in Chief
Richard Scott, Managing Editor

Helps you easily locate the key personnel and facilities you want by hospital name, system head-quarters, or job title. Valuable for locating industry professionals, recruiting, networking, and prospecting for industry business. *$299.00*

1 per year Year Founded: 1998 ISBN 1-573721-40-9

3326 Directory of Hospital Personnel
Grey House Publishing
4919 Route 22
PO Box 56
Amenia, NY 12501
518-789-8700
800-562-2139; *Fax:* 518-789-0556

books@greyhouse.com
www.greyhouse.com

Richard Gottlieb, President
Leslie Mackenzie, Publisher

Best annual resource for researching or marketing a product or service to the hospital industry. Includes 6,000 hospitals and over 80,000 key contacts. *$275.00*

2400 pages ISBN 1-592370-26-8

3327 Directory of Physician Groups and Networks
Dorland Health
1500 Walnut Street
Suite 1000
Philadelphia, PA 19102-3512
215-875-1212
855-CAL- DH1; *Fax:* 301-287-2535
info@dorlandhealth.com
www.dorlandhealth.com

Carol Brault, VP
Yolanda Matthews, Product Manager
Anne Llewellyn, Editor in Chief
Richard Scott, Managing Editor

Reference tool with over 4,000 entries covering IPAs, PHOs, large medical group practices with 20 or more physicians, MSOs and PPMCs. Paperback, published yearly. *$345.00*

Year Founded: 1998 ISBN 1-880874-50-4

3328 Dorland's Medical Directory
Dorland Health
1500 Walnut Street
Suite 1000
Philadelphia, PA 19102-3512
215-875-1212
855-CAL- DH1; *Fax:* 301-287-2535
info@dorlandhealth.com
www.dorlandhealth.com

Carol Brault, VP
Yolanda Matthews, Product Manager
Anne Llewellyn, Editor in Chief
Richard Scott, Managing Editor

Contains expanded coverage of healthcare facilities with profiles of 616 group practices, 661 hospitals and 750 rehabilitation, subacute, hospice and long term care facilities. *$699.00*

1 per year ISBN 1-880874-82-2

3329 Drug Information Handbook for Psychiatry
Lexicomp Inc.
1100 Terex Road
Hudson, OH 44236-4438
330-650-6506
800-837-5394; *Fax:* 330-656-4307
www.lexi.com

Steven Kerscher, Owner
Arvind Subramanian, President, CEO, Wolters Kluwer H
Cheri Palmer, Vice President of Commercial Pro
John Pins, Vice President, Finance, Clinica

Written specifically for mental health professionals. Addresses the fact that mental health patients may be taking additional medication for the treatment of another medical condition in combination with their psychtropic agents. With that in mind, this book contains information on all drugs, not just the psychotropic agents. Specific fields of

information contained within the drug monograph include Effects on Mental Status and Effects on Psychiatric Treatment. *$38.75*

1 per year ISBN 1-591951-14-3

3330 HMO & PPO Database & Directory
Dorland Health
1500 Walnut Street
Suite 1000
Philadelphia, PA 19102-3512
215-875-1212
855-CAL- DH1; *Fax:* 301-287-2535
info@dorlandhealth.com
www.dorlandhealth.com

Carol Brault, VP
Yolanda Matthews, Product Manager
Anne Llewellyn, Editor in Chief
Richard Scott, Managing Editor

Delivers comprehensive and current information on senior-level individuals at virtually all US HMOs and PPOs at an affordable price. *$400.00*

3331 HMO/PPO Directory
Grey House Publishing
4919 Route 22
PO Box 56
Amenia, NY 12501
518-789-8700
800-562-2139; *Fax:* 518-789-0556
books@greyhouse.com
www.greyhouse.com

Richard Gottlieb, President
Leslie Mackenzie, Publisher

This annual resource provides detailed information about health maintenance organizations and preferred provider organizations nationwide. *$275.00*

500 pages ISBN 1-592370-22-5

3332 Innovations in Clinical Practice: Source Book - Volumes 4-20
Professional Resource Press
PO Box 3197
Sarasota, FL 34230-3197
941-343-9601
800-443-3364; *Fax:* 941-343-9201
cs.prpress@gmail.com
www.prpress.com

Laurie Girsch, Managing Editor

Provides a comprehensive source of practical information and applied techniques that can be put to immediate use in your practice. *$64.95*

524 pages Year Founded: 1999

3333 Medical & Healthcare Marketplace Guide Directory
Dorland Health
1500 Walnut Street
Suite 1000
Philadelphia, PA 19102-3512
215-875-1212
855-CAL- DH1; *Fax:* 301-287-2535
info@dorlandhealth.com
www.dorlandhealth.com

Carol Brault, VP
Yolanda Matthews, Product Manager

Anne Llewellyn, Editor in Chief
Richard Scott, Managing Editor

Contains valuable data on pharmaceutical, medical advice, and clinical and non-clinical healthcare service companies worldwide. *$499.00*

3334 Medical Psychoterapist and Disability Analysts
Americel Board of Medical Psychoterapists &
Psychodiagnosticians
4525 Harding Pike
Nashville, TN 37205
615-327-2984; *Fax:* 615-327-9235
americanbd@aol.com

Official newsletter of the American Board of Medical Psychoterapists and Psychodiagnosticians.

3335 Mental Health Directory
Office of Consumer, Family & Public Information
5600 Fishers Lane, Room 15-99
Center For Mental Health Services
Rockville, MD 20857-1
301-443-2792; *Fax:* 301-443-5163

Covers hospitals, treatment centers, outpatient clinics, day/night facilities, residential treatment centers for emotionally disturbed children, residential supportive programs such as halfway houses, and mental health centers offering mental health assistance. *$23.00*

468 pages

3336 National Association of Psychiatric Health
Systems: Membership Directory
900 17th Street, NW
Suite 420
Washington, DC 20006
202-393-6700; *Fax:* 202-783-6041
naphs@naphs.org
www.naphs.org

Mark J. Covall, President, CEO, Executive Direct
Carole Szpak, Director Communications and Oper
Nancy Trenti, JD, Director, Congressional Affairs
Kathleen McCann, RN, PhD, Director, Quality and
Regulatory

Contact information of professional groups working to co-ordinate a full spectrum of treatment services, including in-patient, residential, partial hospitalization and outpatient programs as well as prevention and management services. *$32.10*

48 pages 1 per year Year Founded: 1933

3337 National Register of Health Service Providers in
Psychology
1200 New York Avenue NW
Suite 800
Washington, DC 20005-3873
202-783-7663; *Fax:* 202-347-0550
andrew@nationalregister.org
www.nationalregister.org

Greg Hurley, Vice President/Vice-Chair
Judy E Hall, CEO
Andrew P. Boucher, Assistant Director
Julia Bernstein, Membership Coordinator

Psychologists who are licensed or certified by a state/pro-vincial board of examiners of psychology and who have met council criteria as health service providers in psychology.

Year Founded: 1974

3338 National Registry of Psychoanalysts
National Association for the Advancement of
Psychoanalysis
80 8th Avenue
Suite 1501
New York, NY 10011-5126
212-741-0515; *Fax:* 212-366-4347
dfmaxwell@mac.com
www.naap.org

Douglas Maxwell, President
Margery Quackenburh, Executive Director
Kirsty Cardinale, Editor
Elliott Hom, Art Director

NAAP provides information to the public on psychoanaly-sis. Publishes quarterly NAAP News, annual Registry of Psychoanalysts. *$ 15.00*

175 pages

3339 Patient Guide to Mental Health Issues: Desk
Chart
Lexicomp Inc.
1100 Terex Road
Hudson, OH 44236-4438
330-650-6506
800-837-5394; *Fax:* 330-656-4307
www.lexi.com

Steven Kerscher, Owner
Arvind Subramanian, President, CEO, Wolters Kluwer H
Cheri Palmer, Vice President of Commercial Pro
John Pins, Vice President, Finance, Clinica

Designed specifically for healthcare professionals dealing with mental health patients. Combines eight of our popular Patient Chart titles into one, convienient desktop presenta-tion. This will assist in explaining the most common mental health issue to your patients on a level that they will under-stand. *$38.75*

1 per year ISBN 1-591950-54-6

3340 PsycINFO Database
PsycINFO, American Psychological Association
750 1st Street NE
Washington, DC 20002-4242
202-336-5500
800-374-2721; *Fax:* 202-336-5518
TDD: 202-336-6123
TTY: 202-336-6123
psycinfo@apa.org
www.apa.org

Nadine J. Kaslow, Ph.D., President
Barry S. Anton, Ph.D., President-Elect
Donald N. Bersoff, PhD, JD, Past President
Norman B Anderson, Ph.D., CEO, EVP

PsycINFO is a database that contains citations and summa-ries of journal articles, book chapters, books, dissertations and technical reports in the field of psychology and the psychological aspects of related disciplines, such as medi-cine, psychiatry, nursing, sociology, education, pharmacol-ogy, physiology, linguistics, anthropology, business and law. Journal coverage, spanning 1887 to present, includes international material from 1,800 periodicals written in over 30 languages. Current chapter and book coverage in-cludes worldwide English language material published from 1987 to present. Over 75,000 references are added annually through weekly updates.

52 per year

3341 Rating Scales in Mental Health
Lexicomp Inc.
1100 Terex Road
Hudson, OH 44236-4438
330-650-6506
800-837-5394; *Fax:* 330-656-4307
www.lexi.com

Steven Kerscher, Owner
Arvind Subramanian, President, CEO, Wolters Kluwer H
Cheri Palmer, Vice President of Commercial Pro
John Pins, Vice President, Finance, Clinica

Ideal for clinicians as well as administrators, this title provides an overview of over 100 recommended rating scales for mental health assessment. This book is also a great tool to assist mental healthcare professionals determine the appropriate psychiatric rating scale when assessing their clients. *$38.75*

1 per year ISBN 1-591950-52-X

3342 Roster: Centers for the Developmentally Disabled
Nebraska Department of Health and Human Services
301 Centennial Mall S
Lincoln, NE 68508-2529
402-471-3121
800-254-4202; *Fax:* 402-471-0555
TDD: 070-119-99
www.dhhs.ne.gov

Joann Erickson RN, Program Manager

Covers approximately 160 licensed facilities in Nebraska for the developmentally disabled.

40 pages 1 per year

3343 Roster: Health Clinics
Nebraska Department of Health and Human Services
301 Centennial Mall S
Lincoln, NE 68508-2529
402-471-3121
800-254-4202; *Fax:* 402-471-0555
www.dhhs.ne.gov

Joann Erickson RN, Section Administrator

Covers approximately 90 licensed health clinic facilities in Nebraska.

11 pages 1 per year

3344 Roster: Substance Abuse Treatment Centers
Nebraska Department of Health and Human Services
301 Centennial Mall S
Lincoln, NE 68508-2529
402-471-3121
800-254-4202; *Fax:* 402-471-0555
www.dhhs.ne.gov

Joann Erickson RN, Program Manager

Covers approximately 56 licensed substance abuse treatment centers in Nebraska.

12 pages 1 per year

Publishers

Books

3345 ABC-CLIO
88 Post Road West
Westport, CT 06880-4208
203-226-3571; *Fax:* 203-222-1502
webmaster@greenwood.com
www.www.abc-clio.com/

Wayne Smith, President

Publisher of reference titles, academic and general interest books, texts, books for librarians and other profesionals, and electronic resources.

3346 Active Parenting Publishers
1220 Kennestone Circle
Suite 130
Marietta, GA 30066-6022
770-429-0565
800-825-0060; *Fax:* 770-429-0334
cservice@activeparenting.com
www.ActiveParenting.com

Michael H Popkin,PhD, Founder and President
Gabrielle Tingley, Art Director,Marketing Departmen
Melody Popkin, Manager of Christian Resources
Cathie Jordet, Accounting Manager,Finance Depar

Delivers quality education programs for parents, children and teachers to schools, hospitals, social service organizations, churches and corporate market. Innovator in the educational market.

Year Founded: 1980

3347 American Psychiatric Publishing (APPI)
1000 Wilson Boulevard
Suite 1825
Arlington, VA 22209-3924
703-907-7322
800-368-5777; *Fax:* 703-907-1091
appi@psych.org
www.appi.org

Saul Levin, M.D., M.P.A, CEO and Medical Director
Robert E Hales, M.D., M.B.A, Editor-in-Chief, Books
RebeccaD Rinehart, Publisher
John McDuffie, Editorial Director

Publisher of books, journals, and multi-media on psychiatry, mental healths and behavioral science. Offers authoratative, up-to-date and affordable information geared toward psychiatrists, other mental health professionals, psychiatric residents, medical students and the general public.

3348 Analytic Press
10 Industrial Avenue
Mahwah, NJ 07430-2253
201-258-2200; *Fax:* 201-760-3735

Publishes works of substance and originality that constitute genuine contributions to their respective disciplines and professions.

3349 Brookes Publishing
PO Box 10624
Baltimore, MD 21285-0624
410-337-9580
800-638-3775; *Fax:* 410-337-8539

custserv@brookespublishing.com
www.brookespublishing.com

Jeffrey D. Brookes, President
Melissa A. Behm, Vice President
George Stamathis, Vice President

Publishes highly respected resources in early childhood, early interventions, inclusive and special education, developmental disabilities, learning disabilities, communication and language, behavior, and mental health

Year Founded: 1978

3350 Brookline Books/Lumen Editions
34 University Road
Brookline, MA 02445-4533
617-734-6772; *Fax:* 617-734-3952

Publishes books on learning disabilities, study skills, self-advocacy for the disabled, early childhood intervention, and more, in readable language that reaches beyond the academic community.

3351 Brunner-Routledge Mental Health
270 Madison Avenue
New York, NY 10016-601
212-695-6599
800-634-7064

Maura May, Publisher

The Routledge imprint publishes books and journals on clinical psychology, psychiatry, psychoanalysis, analytical psychology, psychotherapy, counseling, mental health and other professional subjects.

3352 Bull Publishing Company
PO Box 1377
Boulder, CO 80306-1377
303-545-6350
800-676-2855; *Fax:* 303-545-6354
jim.bullpubco@comcast.net

Emily Sewell, Vice President of Operations
Claire Cameron, Director of Marketing

Publisher of books focused on addressing the growing need for sound health information and good advice.

3353 Cambridge University Press
32 Avenue of the Americas
New York, NY 10013-2473
212-337-5000
www.www.cambridge.org

Printing and publishing house that is an integral part of the University and has similar charitable objectives in advancing knowledge, education, learning and research.

3354 Castal Harlan
150 East 58th Street
New York, NY 10155
212-644-8600
800-775-1800; *Fax:* 212-207-8042
info@castleharlan.com
www.www.castleharlan.com

Leonard M Harlan, Chairman of the Executive Commun
John K Castle, Chairman,CEO
Howard D Morgan, Co-President
William M Pruellage, Co-President

Provides quality information and entertainment services. Worldwide distributor of books, videos, music and games in all disciplines.

Year Founded: 1987

3355 Charles C Thomas Publishers
2600 South First Street
Springfield, IL 62704
217-789-8980
800-258-8980; *Fax:* 217-789-9130
books@ccthomas.com
www.ccthomas.com

Producing a strong list of specialty titles and textbooks in the biomedical sciences. Also very active in producing books for the behavioral sciences, education and special education, speech language and hearing, as well as rehabilitation and long-term care. One of the largest producers of books in all areas of criminal justice and law enforcement.

Year Founded: 1927

3356 Crossroad Publishing
831 Chestnut Ridge Rd
Spring Valley, NY 10977-6356
212-868-1801; *Fax:* 212-868-2171
www.cpcbooks.com

Publishes words of thoughtfulness and hope. A leading independent publishing house.

3357 EBSCO Publishing
10 Estes Street
Ipswich, MA 01938-2106
978-356-6500
800-653-2726; *Fax:* 978-356-6565
www.www.ebsco.com/

Timothy S Collins, President
Daniel Boutchie, Inside Sales Representative
Jeffery Greaves, Inside Sales Representative

EBSCO Publishing offers electronic access to a variety of health data: full text databases containing aggregate journals, access to publishers' electronic journals, and the citational databases produced by the American Psychiatric Association to name just a few. Offers a free, nonobligation, on-line trial.

3358 Family Experiences Productions
PO Box 5879
Austin, TX 78763-5879
512-494-0338; *Fax:* 512-494-0340
todd@fepi.com
www.fepi.com

R Geyer, Executive Producer

Consumers Health videos; available individually, or in large volume (private branded) for health providers to give to patients, professionals, staff. Postpartum Emotions, Parenting Preschoolers, Facing Death (5-tape series) and teen grief English and Spanish.

ISSN 1-930772-00-9

3359 Franklin Electronic Publishers
3 Terri Lane
Suite 6
Burlington, NJ 08016-4907
609-386-2500
800-266-5626; *Fax:* 609-239-5950
www.franklin.com

Barry J Lipsky, CEO

Publishes materials for healthcare.

3360 Free Spirit Publishing
217 Fifth Avenue North
Suite 200
Minneapolis, MN 55401-1299
612-338-2068
866-703-7322; *Fax:* 866-419-5199
www.freespirit.com

Judy Galbraith, Founder

Publisher of learning tools that support young people's social and emotional health. Known for unique understanding of what young adults want and need to know to navigate life successfully.

Year Founded: 1983

3361 Grey House Publishing
4919 Route 22
PO Box 56
Amenia, NY 12501
518-789-8700
800-562-2139; *Fax:* 845-373-6360
books@greyhouse.com
www.greyhouse.com

Richard Gottlieb, President

Publishes over 100 titles including reference directories in the areas of business, education, health, statistics and demographics, as well as educational encyclopedias and business handbooks. All titles offer detailed information in well-organized formats. Many titles available online.

Year Founded: 1981

3362 Guilford Publications
72 Spring Street
New York, NY 10012-4068
212-431-9800
800-365-7006; *Fax:* 212-966-6708
info@guilford.com
www.www.guilford.com/

Bob Matloff, President

Publisher of books, periodicals, software and audiovisual programs in mental health, education, and the social sciences.

Year Founded: 1973

3363 Gurze Books
5145 B Avenida Encinas
Carisbad, CA 92008
760-434-7533
800-756-7533; *Fax:* 760-434-5476
www.www.gurzebooks.com

Lindsay Cohn, Co-Owner
Leigh Cohn, Co-Owner

Publishing company that specializes in resources and education on eating disorders. Offers high quality materials on understanding and overcoming eating disorders of all kinds.

Year Founded: 1980

3364 Harper Collins Publishers
10 East 53rd Street
New York, NY 10022-5299
212-207-7000; *Fax:* 212-207-6964
feedback2@harpercollins.com
www.harpercollins.com

Brian Murray, President and CEO
Susan Katz, President/publisher,Harper Colli
Chantal Restivo-Alessi, Chief Digital Officer
Larry Nevins, Executive Vice Preisdent,Operati

A subsidiary of News Corporation, Harper Collins produces literary and commercial fiction, business books, children's books, cookbooks, mystery, romance, reference, religious, healthcare and spiritual books.

Year Founded: 1817

3365 Harvard University Press

79 Garden Street
Cambridge, MA 02138-1400
617-495-2600
800-405-1619; *Fax:* 617-495-5898
contact_hup@harvard.edu
www.www.hup.harvard.edu

William Sisler, President

Publishes material on varied topics including healthcare.

Year Founded: 1913

3366 Hazelden

PO Box 11
Center City, MN 55012-0011
651-213-4200
800-257-7810; *Fax:* 651-213-4793
info@hazelden.org
www.hazelden.org

Mark Mishek, President and CEO,Hazeldon Betty
James A Blaha, VP Finance,Administration/CFO
Marvin D Seppala,MD, Chief Medical Officer
Mark Sheets, Execurive Director,Regional serv

A nonprofit organization that helps people transform their lives by providing the highest quality treatment and continuing care services, education, research, and publishing products available today.

Year Founded: 1949

3367 Health Communications

3201 SouthWest 15th Street
Deerfield Beach, FL 33442-8157
954-360-0909
800-441-5569; *Fax:* 954-360-0034

Peter Vegso, CEO

Original publisher of informational pamphlets for the recovery community; publishes inspiration, soul/spirituality, relationships, recovery/healing, women's issues and self-help material.

Year Founded: 1977

3368 High Tide Press

Ste 2N
2081 Calistoga Dr
New Lenox, IL 60451-4833
815-206-2054
800-469-9461
www.www.hightidepress.com/

Art Dykstra, Executive Director
Steve Baker, Director

Provides high quality books, training materials and seminars to people working in the field of human services. Seek to provide the best resources in developmental, mental and learning disabilities, as well as psychology, leadership and management.

3369 Hogrefe Publishing

38 Chauncy Street
Suite 485
Boston, MA 02111
866-823-4726; *Fax:* 617-354-6875
www.www.hogrefe.com

Publisher of journals and books of all different variety titles including healthcare.

3370 Hope Press

110 Mill Run
Monrovia, CA 91016-1658
626-303-0644
800-321-4039; *Fax:* 626-358-3520
www.hopepress.com

Specializes in the publication of books on Tourette Syndrome, Attention Deficit Hyperactivity Disorder (ADHD, ADD), Conduct Disorder, Oppositional Defiant Disorder and other psychological, psychiatric and behavioral problems.

3371 Hyperion Books

237 Park Avenue
New York, NY 10017
Fax: 212-456-1980
www.hyperionbooks.com

Publishes general-interest fiction and nonfiction books for adults including healthcare titles. Includes the Miramax, ESPN Books, ABC Daytime Press, Hyperion East and Hyperion Audiobooks.

3372 Icarus Films

32 Court Street
21st Floor
Brooklyn, NY 11201
718-488-8900
800-937-4113; *Fax:* 718-488-8642
info@fanlight.com
www.www.icarusfilms.com

Distributor of innovative film and video works on the social issues of our time, with a special focus on healthcare, mental health, profesional ethics, aging and gerontology, disabilites, the workplace, and gender and family issues.

Year Founded: 1978

3373 Impact Publishers

PO Box 6016
Atascadero, CA 93423-6016
805-466-5917
800-246-7228
info@impactpublishers.com
www.impactpublishers.com

Produces a select list of psychology and self improvement books and audio-tapes for adults, children, families, organizations, and communities. Written by highly respected psychologists and other human service professionals.

Year Founded: 1970

3374 Jerome M Sattler Publisher

PO Box 1060
La Mesa, CA 91944-1060
619-460-3667
888-815-2898; *Fax:* 619-460-2489
sattlerpublisher@sbcglobal.net
www.sattlerpublisher.com

Publishes books that represent the cutting edge of clinical assessment of children and families. Designed for students in training as well as for practitioners ans clinicians.

3375 John Wiley & Sons
111 River Street
Hoboken, NJ 07030-5774
201-748-6000; *Fax:* 201-748-6088
info@wiley.com
www.wiley.com

Peter B Wiley, Chairman of the Board
Stephen M Smith, President and Chief Executive Of
John Kritzmacher, Executive Vice President and CFO
Ellis E Cousens, Executive Vice President and COO

A global publisher of print and electronic products, specializing in scientific, technical, and medical books and journals professional and consumer books and subscription services; also textbooks and other educational materials for undergraduate and graduate students as well as lifelong learners.

3376 John Wiley & Sons, Inc.
111 River Street
Hoboken, NJ 07030-5774
201-748-6000; *Fax:* 201-748-6088
info@wiley.com
www.wiley.com

Peter B Wiley, Chairman of the Board
Stephen M Smith, President and Chief Executive Of
John Kritzmacher, Executive Vice President and CFO
Ellis E Cousens, Executive Vice President and COO

Jossey-Bass publishes books, periodicals, and other media to inform and inspire those interested in developing themselves, their organizations and their communities. The publications feature the work of some of the world's best-known authors in leadership, business, education, religion and spirituality, parenting, nonprofit, public health and health administration, conflict resolution and relationships.

3377 Johns Hopkins University Press
2715 North Charles Street
Baltimore, MD 21218-4363
410-516-6900; *Fax:* 410-516-6968
webmaster@jhupress.jhu.edu
www.www.press.jhu.edu/

William Brody, President

Publishes 58 scholarly periodicals and more than 200 new books each year. A leading online provider of scholarly journals, bringing more than 250 periodicals to the desktops of 9 million students, scholars, and others worldwide.

Year Founded: 1878

3378 Lexington Books
4501 Forbes Boulevard
Suite 200
Lanham, MD 20706-4346
301-459-3366
800-462-6420; *Fax:* 301-429-5748
pzline@rowman.com
www.lexingtonbooks.com

Julie E. Kirsch, Vice President/Publisher
Jonathan Raeder, Senior Marketing manager
Kelly Quarrington, Publicity and Advertising

Publisher of specialized new work by established and emerging scholars, including material for the healthcare community.

3379 Lippincott Williams & Wilkins
351 West Camden Street
Baltimore, MD 21201
410-528-4000; *Fax:* 215-521-8902

Gordon Macomber, CEO

Publishes specialized publications and software for physicians, nurses, students and specialized clinicians. Products include drug guides, medical journals, nursing journals, medical textbooks and medical pda software.

Year Founded: 1998

3380 Love Publishing
9101 East Kenyon Avenue
Suite 2200
Denver, CO 80237-1854
303-221-7333; *Fax:* 303-221-7444
www.lovepublishing.com

Stan Love, Owner

Publishes books that offer therapy options to children of all ages, adults, and adolescents.

Year Founded: 1968

3381 Mason Crest Publishers
450 Parkway Drive
Suite D
Broomall, PA 19008-4017
610-543-6200
866-627-2665; *Fax:* 610-543-3878
www.masoncrest.com

Dan Hilferty, President
Louis Cohen, Principal And Creative Director
Michelle Luke, International Rights and Marketi
Becki Stewart, Business Development

Publishes core-related materials for grades K-12. Current catalog includes many titles for health care and mental health curriculums.

3382 New Harbinger Publications
5674 Shattuck Avenue
Oakland, CA 94609-1662
510-652-0215
800-748-6273; *Fax:* 800-652-1613
customerservice@newharbinger.com
www.newharbinger.com

Matthew McKay, Owner
Patrick Fanning, Co-Founder

Publisher of self-help books that teach the reader skills they could use to significantly improve the quality of their lives.

Year Founded: 1973

3383 New World Library
14 Pamaron Way
Nopvato, CA 94949-6215
415-884-2100
800-972-6657; *Fax:* 415-884-2199
www.newworldlibrary.com

Marc Allen, CEO

Publishes books and audios that inspire and challenge us to improve the quality of our lives and our world.

3384 New York University Press
838 Broadway
3rd Floor
New York, NY 10003-4812
212-998-2575
800-996-6987; *Fax:* 212-995-3833
nyupressinfo@nyu.edu
www.www.nyupress.org

Ellen Chodosh, Director
Eric Zinner, Associate Director
Mary Beth Jarrad, Marketing and Sales Director
Laura Bisberg, Buisness/Finance Director

Publishes approximately 100 new books each year, and enjoys a backlist of over 1500 titles that includes health care and academic materials.

Year Founded: 1916

3385 Omnigraphics
155 West Congress
Suite 200
Detroit, MI 48226
313-961-1340
800-234-1340; *Fax:* 313-961-1383
contact@omnigraphics.com
www.omnigraphics.com

Fred Ruffner, Co-Founder
Peter Ruffner, Co-Founder

Quality reference resources for libraries and schools.

Year Founded: 1985

3386 Oxford University Press
2001 Evans Road
Cary, NC 27513-2010
919-677-0977
800-445-9714; *Fax:* 919-677-2673
custserv.us@oup.com
www.www.global.oup.com/

Publishes works that further Oxford University's objective of excellence in research, scholarship, and education, including titles in the health care and mental health field.

Year Founded: 1896

3387 Penguin Group
345 Hudson Street
New York, NY 10014-4592
212-366-2372; *Fax:* 212-366-2933
librariansden@us.penguingroup.com
www.www.penguin.com/

John Makinson, Chairman and Chief Executive
Coram Williams, Chief Financial Officer
David Shanks, Chief Executive Officer
Susan Petersen Kennedy, President

Publishes under a wide range of prominent imprints and trademarks, among them Berkeley Books, Dutton, Grosset & Dunlap, New American Library, Penguin, Philomel, G.P. Putnam's Sons, Riverhead Books, Viking and Frederick Warne. Includes a variety of titles in health care and mental health subjects.

3388 Perseus Books Group
210 American Drive
Jackson, TN 38301
731-423-1973
800-343-4499; *Fax:* 800-351-5073
www.www.perseusbooksgroup.com/

Chris Wagner, VP

Titles include science, public issues, military history, modern maternity, health care and mental health.

3389 Princeton University Press
41 William Street
Princeton, NJ 08540-5223
609-883-1759
800-777-4726; *Fax:* 609-258-6305
www.www.press.princeton.edu/

Peter Dougherty, Director
Martha Camp, Administrative Assistant to the
Patrick Carroll, Associate Director and Controlle
Brigitta van Rheinberg, Assistant Director, Editor in Ch

Independent publisher with close connection to Princeton Unviersity. Fundamental mission is to disseminate through books, journals, and electronic media, with both academia and society at large on a variety of social issues, including health care and mental health.

3390 Pro-Ed Publications
8700 Shoal Creek Blvd
Austin, TX 78757-6897
512-451-3246
800-897-3202; *Fax:* 512-451-8542
feedback@proedinc.com
www.www.proedinc.com/

Donald D Hammill, Owner

Leading publisher of nationally standardized tests, resource and reference texts, curricular and therapy materials, and professional journals covering: speech, language and hearing; psychology and counseling; special education including developmental disabilities, rehabilitation, and gifted education; early childhood intervention; and occupational and physical therapy.

3391 Professional Resource Press
PO Box 3197
Sarasota, FL 34230-3197
941-343-9601
800-443-3364; *Fax:* 941-343-9201
cs.prpress@gmail.com
www.prpress.com

Laurie Girsch, Managing Editor

Publisher of books, continuing education programs and other applied resources for mental health professionals, including psychologists, psychiatrists, clinical social workers, counselors, OTs, and recreational therapists.

Year Founded: 1980

3392 Rapid Psychler Press
2014 Holland Avenue
Suite 374
Port Huron, MI 48060-1994
888-779-2453; *Fax:* 888-779-2457
rapid@psychler.com
www.psychler.com

Produces textbooks and presentation graphics for use in mental health education (mainly psychiatry). Products are thoroughly researched and clinically oriented. Designed by students, instructors and clinicians.

3393 Research Press Publishers
PO Box-7886
Champaign, IL 61826

217-352-3273
800-519-2707; *Fax:* 217-352-1221
rp@researchpress.com
www.researchpress.com

Publishes books and videos in school counseling, special education, psychology, counseling and therapy, parenting, death and dying, and developmental disabilities.

Year Founded: 1968

3394 Riverside Publishing
3800 Golf Road
Suite 200
Rolling Meadows, IL 60008
630-467-7000
800-323-9540; *Fax:* 630-467-7192
RPC_Customer_Service@hmco.com
www.riverpub.com

Dedicated to providing society with the finest professional testing products and services available. Division of Houghton Mifflin Company.

Year Founded: 1979

3395 Rowman & Littlefield
4501 Forbes Boulevard
Suite 200
Lanham, MD 20706-4346
301-459-3366
800-462-6420; *Fax:* 301-429-5748
pzline@rowman.com
www.www.rowman.com

Oliver Gadsby, President and Publisher
Karen Allman, Vice President, Marketing/Sales
Jared Hughes, Senior Marketing Manager
Lindsey Reinstrom, Marketing Manager

Publisher of entertaining and informative books for general readers, as well as academic works by established and emerging scholars, in the areas of Health, Fitness, Sexuality, and Psychology.

3396 Sage Publications
2455 Teller Road
Thousand Oaks, CA 91320-2234
805-499-0721
800-818-7243; *Fax:* 800-583-2665
info@sagepub.com
www.sagepub.com

Sara Miller McCune, Founder,Chairman,Publisher
Blaise R Simqu, President and Chief Exeutive Off
Chris Hickok, Senior VP and Chief Financial Of
Tracey A Ozmina, Executive VP and Chief Operating

An independent international publisher of journals, books, and electronic media, known for commitment to quality and innovation in scholarly, educational and professional markets.

3397 Sidran Traumatic Stress Institute
PO Box 436
Brooklandville, MD 21022-0436
410-825-8888; *Fax:* 410-825-8888
www.sidran.org

Esther Giller, President and Director
Sheila Giller, Secretary and Treasurer
Ruta Mazelis, Editor, The Cutting Edge/Trainer
Stephanie Muszelik, Accountant

Sidran Institute is a leader in traumatic stress education and advocacy. Devoted to helping people who have experienced traumatic life events by publishing books and educational materials on traumatic stress and dissociative conditions.

Year Founded: 1986

3398 Simon & Schuster
1230 Avenue of the Americas
New York, NY 10020
212-698-7000; *Fax:* 856-824-2402
www.simonandschuster.com

Carolyn Reidy, President and Chief Executive Of
Dennis Ealau, Executive VP,Operations and Chie
Elinor Hirschhorn, Executive VP,Chief Digital Offic
Adam Rothberg, Sr VP,Director of Corporate Comm

Leader in the field of general interest publishing, providing consumers worldwide with a diverse range of quality books and multimedia products across a wide variety of genres and formats, including health care and mental health.

Year Founded: 1924

3399 Springer Science and Business Media
233 Spring Street
New York, NY 10013-1578
212-460-1500; *Fax:* 212-460-1575
service-ny@springer.com
www.www.springer.com/

William Curtis, President
Martin Mos, COO

Develops, manages and disseminates knowledge through books, journals and the internet in a variety of subjects, including health care and mental health.

3400 St. Martin's Press
175 Fifth Avenue
New York, NY 10010
212-674-5151; *Fax:* 212-677-7456
permissions@stmartins.com
www.us.macmillan.com

John Sargent, CEO

Publishes 700 titles a year, including those titles in a variety of health care and mental health subjects.

3401 Taylor & Francis Group
711 3rd Avenue
8th Floor
New York, NY 10017
212-216-7800
800-634-7064; *Fax:* 212-564-7854
beverley.acreman@tandf.co.uk
www.taylorandfrancis.com

Kevin Bradley, CEO

Publishes more than 1000 journals and 1800 new books each year with a books backlist in excess of 20,000 specialty titles. Providers of quality information and knowledge that enable our customers to perform their jobs efficiently, continue their education, and help contribute to the advancement of their chosen markets.

Year Founded: 1936

3402 Therapeutic Resources
PO Box 16814
Cleveland, OH 44116-814

888-331-7114; *Fax:* 440-331-7118
contactus@therapeuticresources.com
www.therapeuticresources.com

Publishers of a variety of titles including ADD/ADHD, Alzheimer/Dimentia, Anger Management, Autism/PDD, Bereavement/Adjustment Disorders, Substance Abuse and more.

3403 Underwood Books

PO Box 1919
Nevada City, CA 95959-1919
800-788-3123
contact@underwoodbooks.com
www.underwoodbooks.com

A publisher specializing in fantasy art, science fiction, and self-help/health related titles.

3404 University of California Press

155 Grand Avenue
Suite 400
Oakland, CA 94612-3758
510-883-8232; *Fax:* 510-836-8910
www.ucpress.edu

Alison Mudditt, Director

Distinguished university press that enriches lives around the world by advancing scholarships in the humanities, social sciences, and natural sciences.

3405 University of Chicago Press

1427 East 60th Street
Chicago, IL 60637-2902
773-702-7700
marketing@press.uchicago.edu
www.www.press.uchicago.edu/

Holds an obligation to disseminate scholarship of the highest standard and to publish serious works that promote education, foster public understanding, and enrich cultural life.

Year Founded: 1891

3406 University of Minnesota Press

111 Third Avenue South
Suite 290
Minneapolis, MN 55401-2520
612-627-1970; *Fax:* 612-627-1980
ump@umn.edu
www.upress.umn.edu

Douglas Armato, Director,Administrative
Susan Doerr, Operations Manager,Administrativ
Daniel Oschner, Production Manager
John Henderson, IT Manager

Publisher of groundbreaking work in social and cultural thought, critical theory, race and ethnic studies, urbanism, feminist criticism, and media studies.

Year Founded: 1925

3407 WW Norton

500 Fifth Avenue
New York, NY 10110
212-354-5500
800-233-4830; *Fax:* 212-869-0856
www.www.wwnorton.com

Drake McFeely, CEO

Publishing house owned by its employees, and publishes books in fiction, nonfiction, poetry, college, cookbooks, art,

and professional subjects, including health care and mental health.

3408 Woodbine House

6510 Bells Mill Road
Bethesda, MD 20817-1636
301-897-3570
800-843-7323; *Fax:* 301-897-5838
info@woodbinehouse.com
www.woodbinehouse.com

Irv Shapell, Owner

Publishes special needs books for parents, children, teachers and professionals.

Year Founded: 1985

Facilities

State

Alabama

3409 Taylor Hardin Secure Medical Facility
100 North Union Street
Montgomery, AL 36130-1410
334-242-3454
800-367-0955; *Fax:* 334-242-0725
webmaster@mh.alabama.gov
www.mh.alabama.gov

Michelle Vilamaa, Staff Development Coordinator
Ella White, Staff Development Administrative

Alaska

3410 Alaska Psychiatric Institute
3700 Piper Street
Anchorage, AK 99508-4677
907-269-7100; *Fax:* 907-269-7251
www.dhss.alaska.gov/dbh/Pages/api/default.aspx

Ronald Adler, CEO
R Duane Hopson MD, Medical Director

In partnership with individuals, their families and the community, natural network and providers, API's Alaska Recovery Center provides therapeutic services which assist individuals to achieve a personal level of satisfaction and success in their recovery.

Arizona

3411 Arizona State Hospital
2500 East Van Buren
Phoenix, AZ 85008-6079
602-244-1331; *Fax:* 602-220-6355
www.www.azdhs.gov/azsh

John C Cooper, CEO
M Megan Mitscher LMSW, Admissions & Tribal Liaison

The Arizona State Hospital provides specialized psychiatric services to support people in achieving mental health recovery in a safe and respectful environment.

Year Founded: 1887

Arkansas

3412 Arkansas State Hospital
305 South Palm Street
Little Rock, AR 72205
501-686-9000; *Fax:* 501-686-9464
barbra.brooks@arkansas.gov
www.humanservices.arkansas.gov/dbhs/Pages/ArStateHosp
i

Steven Henson, Interim Administrator
Steven Domon, MD, Medical Director
April Coe-Hout, MD, Clinical Director
Hillary Hunt, Internship Training Director

The Arkansas State Hospital is a psychiatric inpatient treatment facility for those with mental or emotional disorders which includes 90 beds for acute psychiatric admission; a 60-bed forensic treatment services program which offers assistance to circuit courts throughout the state; a 16-bed adolescent treatment program for youth 13-18; and a program for juvenile sex offenders.

3413 Center for Outcomes and Evidence
Agency for Healthcare Research and Quality
540 Gaither Road
Suite 2000
Rockville, MD 20850
301-427-1104; *Fax:* 301-427-1520
www.ahrq.gov

Richard Kronick, Ph.D., Director
Boyce Ginieczki, Ph.D., Acting Deputy Director

Formerly the Center for Outcomes and Effectiveness Research. Conducts and supports research and assessment of health care practices, technologies, processes, and systems.

3414 UAMS Psychiatric Research Institute
4301 West Markham
Suite 605
Little Rock, AR 72205
501-660-7559; *Fax:* 501-660-7542
kramerteresal@uams.edu
www.uams.edu

Combining research, education and clinical services into one facility, PRI offers inpatiend and outpatient services, with 40 psychiatric beds, therapy options, and specialized treatment for specific disorders, including: addictive eating, anxiety, deppressive and post-traumatic stress disorders. Research focuses on evidence-based care takes into consideration the education of future medical personnel while relying on research scientists to provide innovative forms of treatment. PRI includes the Center for Addiction Research as well as a methadone clinic.

California

3415 ANKA Behavioral Health
1875 Willow Pass Road
Suite 300
Concord, CA 94520-2527
925-825-4700; *Fax:* 925-825-2610
info@ankabhi.org
www.www.ankabhi.org

Naja W. Boyd, PsyD, Chief Operating Officer
Chris Withrow, Chief Executive Officer
Nzinga Harrison, Chief Medical Officer
Yolanda Braxton, PsyD, VP of Business Development

Offers comprehensive services and programs designed to promote a client's overall wellness and to attain an enhanced quality of life.

3416 Atascadero State Hospital
10333 El Camino Real
Atascadero, CA 93422-5808
805-468-2009; *Fax:* 805-466-6011
craig.dacus@ash.dsh.ca.gov
www.dsh.ca.gov

Craig Dacus, Public Information Officer
Joyce Ladwig, Human Resources Department

A maximum security forensic hosptial, providing inpatient forensic services for adult males who are court committed throughout the State of California. The staff members of Atascadero State Hospital (ASH) proudly serve the people of the State of California by providing protection for the community, expert evaluations for the courts, and state-of-the-science psychiatric recovery services for individuals referred to us from across the state.

Year Founded: 1954

3417 Campobello Chemical Dependency Treatment Services
3250 Guerneville Road
Santa Rosa, CA 95401-4030
707-579-4066
800-806-1833; *Fax:* 707-579-1603
www.campobello.org

Jim Cody, Executive Director
Kathy Leigh Willis, Executive Director

Innovative chemical dependency treatment center with the belief in the 12 step self-help programs of Alcoholics Anonymous, Narcotics Anonymous and Al-Anon for friends and family.

3418 Changing Echoes
7632 Pool Station Road
Angels Camp, CA 95222-9620
209-785-3666
800-633-7066; *Fax:* 209-785-5238
www.changingechoes.com

J R Maughan, Executive Director

Established as a social model chemical dependency facility with the intent to render high-quality treatment for affordable prices to men and women who suffer from the disease of addiction.

Year Founded: 1989

3419 Department of Mental Health Vacaville Psychiatric Program
1600 California Drive
PO Box 2297
Vacaville, CA 95696-2297
707-449-6504; *Fax:* 707-453-7047
www.dsh.ca.gov

Victor Brewer, Executive Director

The mission of Vacaville Psychiatric Program is to provide quality mental health evaluation and treatment to in-mate-patients. This is accomplished in a safe and therapeutic environment, and as part of a continuum of care.

3420 Exodus Recovery Center
9808 Venice Blvd.
Suite 700
Culver City, CA 90232
310-945-3350
800-829-3923; *Fax:* 310-840-7023
lezlie@exodusrecovery.com
www.exodusrecoveryinc.com

Luana Murphy, MBA, President /Chief Executive Offic
LeeAnn Skorohod, CHC - CCEP, Senior Vice President of Operati
Lezlie Murch, MA, LPCC, Senior Vice President of Program
Grace Lee, MBA, Vice President of Finance

Mission is that we believe that chemically dependent men and women can achieve freedom from the bondage of drugs and alcohol. Teaching patients and their families that the devastation of addiction can be overcome. Produce personal action plans that can produce a lifetime of recovery.

3421 Family Service Agency
123 W Gutierrez Street
Santa Barbara, CA 93101-3424

805-965-1001; *Fax:* 805-965-2178
hr@fsacares.org
www.fsacares.org

Stephanie Wilson, Co-President
Robert Manning, Co-President
Lisa Brabo, Ph.D., Executive Director
Denise Cicourel, MAOM, Director of Administration

A non-profit human service agency whose programs help people help themselves. FSA services prevent family breakdown, intervene effectively where problems are known to exist and help individuals and families build on existing strengt

Year Founded: 1899

3422 Fremont Hospital
Psychiatric Solutions
39001 Sundale Drive
Fremont, CA 94538-2005
510-796-1100
www.fremonthospital.com

Joey A Jacobs, President/CEO/Chairman

A private, modern 96-bed behavioral healthcare facility that provides services to adolescents (ages 12-17) and adults.

3423 Life Steps Pasos de Vida
1431 Pomeroy Road
Arroyo Grande, CA 93420-5943
805-481-2505
800-530-5433
www.lifestepsfoundation.org

Sue Horowitz, President
Virginia Franco, Founder/CEO
Allen C Haile, Secretary

Develops innovative programs that target underserved populations. Goal is to help participants develop healthy lifestyles free of alcohol and drugs.

3424 Lincoln Child Center
4368 Lincoln Avenue
Oakland, CA 94602-2529
510-531-3111; *Fax:* 510-530-8083
www.lincolncc.org

Diana Netherton, Chairman
Christine Stoner-Mertz, President/CEO
Peggy Padilla, Chief Administrative Officer
Allison Becwar, Chief Program Officer

Enables vulnerable and emotionally troubled children and their families to lead independent and fulfilling live

3425 Mental Health Association of Orange County
822 Town & Country Road
Orange, CA 92868
714-547-7559; *Fax:* 717-543-4431
www.mhaoc.org

Dedicated to improving the quality of life of Orange County residents impacted by mental illness through direct service, advocacy, education and information dissemination.

Year Founded: 1958

3426 Metropolitan State Hospital
11401 Bloomfield Avenue
Norwalk, CA 90650-2015

562-863-7011; *Fax:* 562-929-3131
TDD: 562-863-1743
www.dsh.ca.gov

Sharon Smith Nevins, Executive Director

The mission of Metropolitan State Hospital is to work in partnership with individuals to assist in their recovery by using rehabilitation services as their tool, thus preparing clients for community living.

Year Founded: 1915

3427 Napa State Hospital

2100 Napa-Vallejo Highway
Napa, CA 94558-6293
707-253-5000; *Fax:* 707-253-5379
TDD: 707-253-5768
nshcontact@dmhnsh.state.ca.us
www.dsh.ca.gov

Jennifer Marshall CTRS, RTC, Chief, Rehabilitation Therapy

Napa State Hospital provides treatment and support to adults with serious mental illness, and assists each individual in achieving his/her highest potential for independence and quality of life, leading to recovery and integrating safely and successfully into society.

3428 New Life Recovery Centers

782 Park Avenue
Suite 1
San Jose, CA 95126-4800
408-297-1182
866-894-6572; *Fax:* 408-297-7450
www.newliferecoverycenters.com

Kevin Richardson, President
Gary Ruble, Founder

Strives to provide our clients with the very best services available. We value our employees as our greatest asset, while collectively and continuously working to adopt and implement the latest and most effective medical, clinical, and social model treatment modalities.

Year Founded: 2004

3429 Northridge Hospital Medical Center

18300 Roscoe Boulevard
Northridge, CA 91328
818-885-8500; *Fax:* 818-885-5439
www.northridgehospital.org

Mike Wall, President, CEO

Northridge Hospital Medical Center offers a comprehensive Behavioral Health program for both adults and adolescents. Founded in 1955.

3430 PacifiCare Behavioral Health PO Box 31053 Laguna Hills, CA 92654-1053

800-999-9585

Richard J Kelliher PsyD, Clinical Director

Provides behavioral health services to children, adolescents, adults, and seniors.

3431 Patton State Hospital
California Department of Mental Health

3102 E Highland Avenue
Patton, CA 92369
909-425-7000; *Fax:* 909-425-6169
TDD: 909-862-5730

cbarrett@dmhpsh.state.ca.us
www.dsh.ca.gov

Harry Oreol, Executive Director
Nitin Kulkarni, Medical Director
Angela Fiore, Forensic Services Manager
Nancy Verela, Director, Human Resources

Patton State Hospital's mission is to empower forensic and civilly committed individuals to recover from mental illness utilizing Recovery principles and evidenced based practices within a safe, structured, and secure environment.

3432 Phoenix Programs Inc

90 E. Leslie Lane
Columbia, MO 65202-1535
573-442-3830; *Fax:* 925-778-7412
www.www.phoenixprogramsinc.org

Nelly Roach, President
Brock Bukowsky, Vice President/Treasurer
Deborah Beste, Executive Director
Rhiannon Pearson, Chief Financial Officer

Offers an array of services and programs designed to promote overall wellness while making it possible for all to obtain a higher quality of life.

3433 Presbyterian Intercommunity Hospital Mental Health Center

12401 Washington Boulevard
Whittier, CA 90602-1006
562-698-0811
TDD: 562-696-9267
TTY: 562-696-9267
www.www.pihhealth.org

Kenton Woods, Chair
Rich Atwood, Vice Chair
Efrain Aceves, Secretary
Jane Dicus, Treasurer

Offers an inpatient program for those with a variety of mental disorders.

Year Founded: 1959

3434 Twin Town Treatment Centers

4388 E Katella Avenue
Los Alamitos, CA 90720-3565
562-596-0050; *Fax:* 562-596-0058
www.twintowntreatmentcenters.com

David Lisonbee, President, CEO
Tiran Davidi-Durian, CFO
Ted Williams, MD, ASAM, Medical Director
Debbie Muehl, CATC II, Supervising Counselor

Mission is to introduce new solutions for people who find that chemically induced coping no longer works.

Colorado

3435 Centennial Mental Health Center

211 W Main Street
Sterling, CO 80751-3168
970-522-4392
webmaster@centennialmhc.org
www.centennialmhc.org

Daniel D Hammond, Manager

A non-profit organization dedicated to providing the highest quality comprehensive mental health services to the rural communities of northeastern Colorado.

3436 Colorado Mental Health Institute at Fort Logan
3520 West Oxford Avenue
Denver, CO 80236-3108
303-866-7066; *Fax:* 303-866-7048
www.colorado.gov

Keith Lagrenade, CEO

The mission of the Colorado Mental Health Institute at Fort Logan is to provide the highest quality mental health services to persons of all ages with complex, serious and persistent mental illness within the resources available.

3437 Colorado Mental Health Institute at Pueblo
1600 West 24th Street
Pueblo, CO 81003-1411
303-866-5700; *Fax:* 719-546-4484

John De Quardo, Administrator

Provides quality mental health services focused on sustaining hope and promoting recovery.

3438 Emily Griffith Center
1724 Gilpin Street
Denver, CO 80218
303-237-6865; *Fax:* 303-237-6873
www.www.griffithcenters.org

Howard Shiffman, CEO
Beth Miller, Deputy Director/COO
John Smrcka, Program Director

Provides troubled children the environment and opportunities to become healthy, participating and productive members of society.

Connecticut

3439 Daytop Residential Services Division
425 Grant Street
Bridgeport, CT 06610-3222
203-337-9943; *Fax:* 203-337-9986

David Parachini, Chairperson
Janet Ryan, Vice Chairperson
Peter Loomis, Treasurer
Jay Broderick, Secretary

Long-term substance abuse treatment facility based on the Therapeutic Community model. Combines current research and treatment methods with traditional therapeutic community concepts.

Year Founded: 1970

3440 Jewish Family Service
733 Summer Street
Suite 602
Stamford, CT 06901-1035
203-921-4161
www.www.ctjfs.org/

Michael Alexander, President
Matt Greenberg, CEO
Iris Morrison, Associate Executive Director
Saul Cohen, Vice President

Offers a wide range of innovative programs designed to address contemporary problems and issues through counseling and therapy, crisis intervention, Jewish Family Life Education, Depression, Aging and senior mental health, Obsessions and compulsions.

Year Founded: 1978

3441 Klingberg Family Centers
370 Linwood Street
New Britain, CT 06052-1998
860-832-5504; *Fax:* 860-832-8221
www.klingberg.org

Lynne V. Roe, Director of Intake

To uphold, preserve and restore families in a therapeutic environment, valuing the absolute worth of every child, while adhering to the highest ethical principles in accordance with our Judaeo-Christian heritage.

3442 McCall Foundation
58 High Street
PO Box 806
Torrington, CT 06790-806
860-496-2100; *Fax:* 860-496-2111
www.www.mccall-foundation.org

D'Arcy Lovetere, President
Roxanne Bachand, Vice President
Marie Wallace, Secretary/Treasurer

Provides outpatient, partial hospital, intensive outpatient, residential, parenting and prevention programs for substance abusers and/or their family members; and helps to reduce area substance abuse in the local community. Funding is provided by the United Way.

3443 Mountainside Treatment Center
187 South Canaan Road
Route 7
Canaan, CT 06018-717
860-824-1397
800-762-5433; *Fax:* 888-749-8752
admissions@mountainside.org
www.mountainside.org

Maureen O'Neill Biggs, LPC, LA, Clinical Director
Brittanie Decker, Continuing Care Case Manager
Bruce Dechert, LADC, ICADC, Director, Family Wellness
Susan Watso, CAC, Extended Care Counselor

Program is based on strategies and principles that promote healing and enhance the quality of life. Through the utilization of Motivational Interviewing, Directional Therapy, Gender-Specific Groups, the 12-Step Principles and Adventure Based Initiatives, individuals qwill encounter, confront and experience the challenges of recovery.

Year Founded: 1998

3444 Silver Hill Hospital
208 Valley Road
New Canaan, CT 06840-3899
203-966-1380
800-899-4455
www.silverhillhospital.org

Siguard Ackerman, President and Medical Director
Elizabeth Moore, Chief Operating Officer
Ruurd Leegstra, JD, CPA, Chief Financial Officer
Missy Fallon, Chief Development Officer

A nationally recognized, independent, not-for-profit psychiatric hospital that is focused exclusively on providing patients the best possible treatment of psychiatric illnesses and substance use disorders, in the best possible environment.

Year Founded: 1931

3445 Yale University School of Medicine: Child Study Center
230 S Frontage Road
New Haven, CT 06519-1124
203-785-2540
www.www.childstudycenter.yale.edu/index.aspx

Fred R Volkmar, MD, Director

Provides a comprehensive range of in-depth diagnostic and treatment services for children with psychiatric and developmental disorders. These services include specialized developmental evaluations for children ages zero-four, and psychological and psychiatric evaluations for children 5-18. Individualized treatment plans following evaluation make use for a range of theraputic interventions, including psychotherapy, group therapy, family therapy, psycho-pharmacological treatment, parent counseling, consultation and service planning. Immediate access for children needing to be seen within 24 hours and walk-in service is also available.

Florida

3446 Archways-A Bridge To A Brighter Future
919 NE 13th Street
Fort Lauderdale, FL 33304-2009
954-763-2030; *Fax:* 954-763-9847
intake@archways.org
www.archways.org

Andrea Katz, CEO

A not-for-profit, privately-governed organization whose mission is to provide quality comprehensive behavioral health care to individuals and families who are in need of improving their quality of life.

3447 Fairwinds Treatment Center
1569 South Fort Harrison
Clearwater, FL 33756-2004
727-449-0300
800-226-0300; *Fax:* 727-446-1022
fairwinds@fairwindstreatment.com
www.fairwindstreatment.com

Jess Loven, Clinical Director, CAP
Thomas H Lewis, Clinical Director

As a dually licensed psychiatric and substance abuse center, reaches far beyond standard treatment to offer medical services for substance abuse, eating disorders, and emotional/mental health issues.

3448 First Step of Sarasota
4579 Northgate Court
Sarasota, FL 34234
941-366-5333
800-266-6866; *Fax:* 941-351-5161
gethelp@fsos.org
www.www.fsos.org/

Richard Carlson, Chair
Peter Abbott, Vice Chair
Elizabeth LaBoone, Secretary

Provides high quality, affordable substance abuse treatment and recovery programs on Florida's Gulf Coast. Offers a variety of programs including a medical detox, residential and outpatient services for adolescents, adults and families.

Year Founded: 1967

3449 Florida State Hospital
1317 Winewood Blvd.
Building 1, Room 202
Tallahassee, FL 32399-0700
850-487-1111; *Fax:* 850-922-2993
www.www.myflfamilies.com

Diane James, Administrator

FSH provides person-centered treatment and rehabilitations in order to propel the client toward their personal recovery and to prepare for roles and environments that have personal and social value.

Year Founded: 1876

3450 Gateway Community Services
555 Stockton Street
Jacksonville, FL 32204-2597
904-387-4661; *Fax:* 904-384-5753
info@gatewaycommunity.com
www.gatewaycommunity.com

Candace Hodgkins, Ph.D., LMHC, President/Chief Executive Office
Laura Dale, CFO
Randy Jennings, Sr VP Operations
Dr. Yvonne Kennedy, Senior Vice President of Profess

Provides a full continuum of care that delivers effective treatment and rehabilitation services to individuals suffering from alcoholism, substance abuse and related mental health problems.

3451 Genesis House Recovery Residence
4865 40th Way South
Lake Worth, FL 33461-5301
561-439-4070
800-737-0933; *Fax:* 561-439-4864
info@genesishouse.net
www.genesishouse.net

James Dodge, Founder/CEO
Kathryn Shafer, Clinical Director

Works closely with both local and out of state courts. Provides the suffering person with a safe, secure, professional environment to glean the care, answers and support they so desperately need in their lives.

3452 Manatee Glens
391 6th Avenue W
Bradenton, FL 34205-8820
941-782-4299; *Fax:* 941-782-4301
Sondra.Guffey@manateeglens.org
www.www.manateeglens.org/

Paul M Duck, Chair
Mary Ruiz, CEO/President
Deborah Kostroun, COO
Thomas P Nolan, Vice Chair

Helps families in crisis with mental health and addictions services and supports the community through prevention and recovery.

3453 New Horizons of the Treasure Coast
4500 W Midway Road
Ft Pierce, FL 34981-4823
772-468-5600
888-468-5600; *Fax:* 772-468-5606
www.nhtcinc.org

John Wolsiefer, Chairman
Garry Wilson, Vice Chair

Robert Zomok, Treasurer
Patricia Austin-Novak, Secretary

To improve the quality of life in the community through the provision of accessible, person-centered behavioral health resources.

Year Founded: 1958

3454 North Florida Evaluation and Treatment Center
1200 NE 55th Boulevard
Gainesville, FL 32641-2759
352-375-8484; *Fax:* 352-264-8305
www.www.dcf.state.fl.us/facilities/nfetc/

William Baxter, Administrator

Dedicated to serving you while fulfilling our responsibilities for safety, security and a positive, caring environment.

Year Founded: 1976

3455 North Star Centre
9033 Glades Road
Boca Raton, FL 33434-3939
561-361-0500; *Fax:* 561-479-0384
inquiry@northstar-centre.com
www.northstar-centre.com

Ira Kaufman, Executive Director
Randi Katz, Administrative Assistant

A uniquely comprehensive facility dedicated to restoring your sense of emotional and physical well being.

3456 Northeast Florida State Hospital
7487 South State Road 121
MacClenny, FL 32063-5480
904-259-6211; *Fax:* 904-259-7101

Joe Infantino, Administrator
Rufus Johnson, Evening Administrator

To provide comprehensive mental health treatment services to ensure a timely transition to the community.

Year Founded: 1959

3457 Renaissance Manor
509 Berry Street
Punta Gorda, FL 33950
941-916-9621; *Fax:* 941-460-5119
www.www.renaissancemanor.org/

Heather Eller, Administrator

Community based assisted living facility with a limited mental health license, specializes in serving adults with neuro-biological disorders and mood disorders along with other special mental health needs. Our not-for-profit organization is a program designed to encourage positive mental health while meeting the various interest of our residents.

3458 Seminole Community Mental Health Center
237 Fernwood Blvd
Fern Park, FL 32730-2116
407-831-2411; *Fax:* 407-831-0195
scmhc@scmhc.com

Jim Berko, Manager

A private, nonprofit organization whose goal is to provide comprehensive, biopsychosocial rehabilitation programming in the areas of mental health and substance abuse.

3459 Starting Place
351 North State Road 7
Suite 200
Plantation, FL 33317
954-327-4060

Dr. Tammy Tucker, Chair
Marsha L. Currant, M.S.W,, CEO

Improves the lives through education, treatment and support services related to substance abuse, mental illness and co-occurring disorders

3460 The Transition House
3800 5th Street
St Cloud, FL 34769
407-892-5700
www.thetransitionhouse.org

Thomas Griffin, PhD, Chief Executive Officer
Jennifer R. Dellasanta, ICADC, CAP, Chief Operating Officer
Jeffrey Wainwright, Director of Work Release Program
Brett ms D'Aoust, MSW, CAP, Executive Director of Correction

The adress above is the men's house. The address for the women's house is: 505 N Clyde Street Kissimmee, FL 34741. All other information is the same. Mission is to provide a milieu of comprehensive educational, health, prevention and human services to Central Florida's most disenfranchised populations.

Year Founded: 1993

Georgia

3461 Central State Hospital
620 Broad Street
Milledgeville, GA 31062-7525
478-445-4128; *Fax:* 478-445-6034
info@centralstatehospital.org
www.dbhdd.georgia.gov

Dan Howell, Regional Hospital Administrator
Kay Brooks, Chief Nurse Executive
Lee Ann Molini, Director of Nursing

3462 Georgia Regional Hospital at Atlanta
Two Peachtree Street, N.W.
24th Floor
Atlanta, GA 30303
404-657-2252; *Fax:* 404-212-4621
www.dbhdd.georgia.gov

Susan Trueblood, CEO
Gwen Skinner, Director

Located on 174 Acres in DeKalb County, Georgia Regional Hospital/Atlanta operates 366 licensed, accredited inpatient beds in five major program areas: Adult Mental Health, Adolescent Mental Health, Child Mental Health, Forensic Services, and Developmental Disabilities. In addition, GRH/Atlanta also offers inpatient and outpatient Dental Services and an Outpatient Forensic Evaluation Program for juveniles and adults. Finally, GRH/Atlanta operates the Fulton County Collaborative Crisis Service System which provides mobile crisis and residential services to adults experiencing mental health problems in Fulton County.

3463 Georgia Regional Hospital at Augusta
3405 Mike Padgett Highway
Augusta, GA 30906-3897
706-792-7000; *Fax:* 706-792-7030

Ben Waker EdD, Contact

3464 Georgia Regional Hospital at Savannah
1915 Eisenhower Drive
Savannah, GA 31406
912-356-2011; *Fax:* 912-356-2691
www.www.garegionalsavannah.com/

Douglas Osborne, Contact

3465 Southwestern State Hospital
400 Pinetree Boulevard
PO Box 1378
Thomasville, GA 31792-1378
229-227-2850

Hillary Hooyou, Manager

Provides extensive behavioral healthcare services in community and hospital settings, including: residential MRDD services; inpatient, residential and case management psychiatric services; and residential care for dual-diagnosed persons.

3466 West Central Georgia Regional Hospital
3000 Schatulga Road
Columbus, GA 31907
706-568-5000
wcgrh@dhr.state.ga.us
www.dbhdd.georgia.gov/

Mission is to treat customers with respect and dignity while providing comprehensive, person-centered behavioral healthcare.

Year Founded: 1974

Idaho

3467 Children of Hope Family Hospital
PO Box 1829
Boise, ID 83701-1829
208-703-8688
drharper@afo.net
www.childofhope.org

Rev Anthony R Harper PhD, Founder
Craig Hardesty, M.B.A., Treasurer
Penny Nygaard, Secretary

Illinois

3468 Advocate Ravenswood Hospital Medical Center
3075 Highland Parkway Suite 600
Downers Grove, IL 60515
630-572-9393; *Fax:* 630-990-4752
www.advocatehealth.com

Kelly Jo Golson, CMO, Public Affairs & Marketing
Linda Williger, Manager, Public Affairs & Market
Vincent Pierri, Manager, Public Affairs & Market
Sarah Scroggins, Coordinator, Public Affairs & Ma

Provides a comprehensive array of services for inpatient (Adult, Adolescent, Substance Abuse), Partial Hospital, Intensive Outpatient, Psychological Rehabilitation, Emergency-Crisis, Assertive Community Outreach, Case Management, Program for Deaf and Hard of Hearing at multiple sites on the Northside of Chicago.

3469 Alexian Brothers Bonaventure House
825 W Wellington Avenue
Chicago, IL 60657-9249

773-327-9921; *Fax:* 773-327-9113
info@abam.org
www.www.alexianbrothershousing.org/

Bart Winters, CEO
Marty Hansen, Director Programs/Services

Offers adult men and women with HIV/AIDS-who are homeless or at-risk for homelessness- a chance to rebuild and reclaim their lives. Bonaventure House has a wide array of on-site supportive services-case management, occupational therapy, recovery, and spiritual care-most residents are able to return to independent life in the community within a 24-month period.

3470 Alton Mental Health Center
4500 College Avenue
Alton, IL 62002-5099
618-474-3273; *Fax:* 618-474-3967
www.illinois.gov

Susan Shobe, Administrator

3471 Andrew McFarland Mental Health Center
901 Southwind Road
Springfield, IL 62703-5125
217-786-6900; *Fax:* 217-786-7167

Karen Schweighart, Administrator

3472 Delta Center
1400 Commercial Avenue
Cairo, IL 62914-1978
618-734-3626; *Fax:* 618-734-1999
TTY: 618-734-1350
www.deltacenter.org

Lisa Tolbert, Executive Director

A non-profit mental health center, substance abuse counseling facility, and also provides various community services to Alexander and Pulaski County, Illinois

3473 FHN Family Counseling Center
421 W Exchange Street
Freeport, IL 61032-4008
815-599-6900; *Fax:* 815-599-6106
www.www.fhn.org/

Lisa Mahoney, VP

3474 Habilitative Systems
415 S Kilpatrick Avenue
Chicago, IL 60644-4958
773-854-1680; *Fax:* 773-854-8300
TDD: 773-854-8364
hsi@habilitative.org
www.www.habilitative.org

Donald Dew, President
Joyce Wade, VP Finance
Karen Barbee-Dixon, EdD, COO

To provide integrated human services to children, adults, families, and persons with disabling conditions that help them to achieve their highest level of self-sufficiency

Year Founded: 1978

3475 John R Day and Associates
3716 W Brighton Avenue
Peoria, IL 61615-2938
309-692-7755; *Fax:* 309-692-2262
www.christianpsychological.org

John R Day, Partner

Year Founded: 1974

3476 Keys To Recovery

100 North River Road
Des Plaines, IL 60016-1209
847-298-9355
www.www.reshealth.org

Philip Kolski, Director
Debra Ayanian, Nurse Manager

A leading Alcoholism and Drug Treatment Center in the Midwest, providing innovative and effective Alcoholism and Drug Treatment.

3477 MacNeal Hospital

3249 S. Oak Park Avenue
Berwyn, IL 60402
708-783-9100
888-622-6325
TTY: 708-783-3058
inf@macnealfp.com
www.www.macneal.com/

Randall K Mc Givney, Program Director
Davis Yang, Center Director
John Gong, Clinical Faculty
Edward C Foley MD, Director Of Research

The MacNeal Family Practice Residency Program was one of the first family practice programs in the country and the first in Illinois. We have continue a progressive tradition in all aspects of our curriculum. Our program is at the forefront of contemporary family medicine offering diverse academic and clinical opportunites and building on the innovative ideas of our residents.

3478 McHenry County Mental Health Board

620 Dakota Street
Crystal Lake, IL 60012-3732
815-455-2828; *Fax:* 815-455-2925
www.mc708.org

To Provide leadership and ensure the prevention and treatment of mental illness, developmental disabilities and chemical abuse by coordinating, developing and contracting for quality services for all citizens of McHenry County, Illinois. This is not a provider organization.

3479 Pfeiffer Treatment Center and Health Research Institute

3S 721 West Ave
Warrenville, IL 60555-4039
630-505-0300
866-504-6076; *Fax:* 630-836-0667
info@hriptc.org
www.hriptc.org

Scott Filer, MPH, Executive Director
Allen Lewis MD, Medical Director
William Walsh, PhD, Research/Found Dir/Co-Founder

A not-for-profit, outpatient medical facility for children, teens and adults seeking a biochemical assessment and treatment for their symptons caused by a biochemical imbalance, or to support health and promote wellness. PTC physician precribes individualized program of vitamins, minerals, and amino acids to address the patient's unique biochemical needs. Common conditions: anxiety, ADHA, autism spectrum disorder, post traumatic stress syndrome, depression, bipolar disorder, schozophrenia and Alzheimer's disease.

3480 Riveredge Hospital

8311 W Roosevelt
Forest Park, IL 60130-2500
708-771-7000; *Fax:* 708-209-2280
www.riveredgehospital.com

Carey Carlock, CEO
Lucyna Puszkarska, MD, Medical Director
Sheila Orr, JD, RN, Chief Nursing Officer and Chief
Ginny Trainor, LCSW, CADC, Director of Business Development

Striving to foster an environment that demonstrates compassion and caring with timely and effective communication through comprehensive behavioral health care services of clinical excellence.

3481 Sonia Shankman Orthogenic School

1365 E 60th Street
Chicago, IL 60637-2890
773-702-1203; *Fax:* 773-702-1304
www.orthogenicschool.uchicago.edu

Henry J Roth PhD, Executive Director

A coeducational residential treatment program for children and adolescents in need of support for emotional issues which cause the student to act in disruptive ways and experience unfulfilling social and educational experiences

Year Founded: 1915

3482 Stepping Stones Recovery Center

1621 Theodore Street
Joliet, IL 60435-1958
815-744-4555; *Fax:* 815-744-4670
info@steppingstonestreatment.com
www.steppingstonestreatment.com

Pat Fera, President
Pete McLenighan, Executive Director

Dedicated to providing effective treatment for persons suffering from the illness of addiction to alcohol and/or other drugs, even if these persons are unable to pay for the cost of such services.

3483 Way Back Inn-Grateful House

1915 W Roosevelt Road
Braodview, IL 60155-2925
708-344-3301; *Fax:* 708-344-2944
frankl@waybackinn.org
www.waybackinn.org

Frank Lieggi, Executive Director
Anita Pindiur, Clinical Director

Provides a high level clinical treatment program specializing in addressing the needs of men and women suffering from both chemical dependence (Alcohol and Drugs) and also Gambling Dependence.

3484 Wells Center

1300 Lincoln Avenue
Jacksonville, IL 62650-4007
217-243-1871; *Fax:* 217-243-2278
TDD: 217-243-0470
bcarter@wellscenter.org

Bruce Carter, Executive Director

Mission has been to improve the health and welfare of individuals and families affected by the ause of alcohol and other substances and by mental health issues. Dedicates its efforts to providing levels of care and support services in settings approval to the individual needs of the patient.

Year Founded: 1974

3485 White Oaks Companies of Illinois

130 Richard Pryor Place
Peoria, IL 61605-2484
309-671-8960
800-475-0257
www.whiteoaks.com

Non profit agency offering comprehensive, state-of-the-art chemical dependency services, individually designed for each client.

Indiana

3486 Community Hospital Anderson

1515 N Madison Avenue
Anderson, IN 46011-3457
765-298-4242
www.www.communityanderson.com

Beth Tharp, President/CEO

The mission of Community Hospital is to serve the medical, health and human service needs to the people in Anderson-Madison County and contiguous counties with compassion dignity, repect and excellence. Service, although focused on injury, illness and disease will also embrace prevention, education and alternative systems of health care delivery.

Year Founded: 1962

3487 Crossroad: Fort Wayne's Children's Home

2525 Lake Avenue
Fort Wayne, IN 46805-5457
260-484-4153
800-976-2306; *Fax:* 260-484-2337
www.crossroad-fwch.org

Patrick T Houlihan, Chair
Randall J. Rider, President/CEO
Kyle Zanker, Chief Development Officer
Beth McNeal, Director of Human Resources

A not-for-profit treatment center for emotionally troubled youth.

Year Founded: 1883

3488 Hamilton Center

620 Eighth Avenue
Terre Haute, IN 47804-2771
812-231-8200
800-742-0787
HumanResources@hamiltoncenter.org
www.www.hamiltoncenter.org/

Gaylan Good, CEO
Richard Pittelkow, Vice President
Cary Sparks, Treasurer
Virginia Gilman, Secretary

Provides the full continuum of psychological health and addiction services to children, adolescents, adults and families.

3489 Mental Health America of Indiana

1431 North Delaware Street
Indianapolis, IN 46202
317-638-3501
800-555-6424; *Fax:* 317-638-3540
www.mhai.net

Stephen C McCaffrey, JD, President and CEO
Lisa Hutcheson, MEd, VP, Policy and Programs

A statewide organization focused on mental illness and addictive disorder recovery and prevention through education, advocacy, and public health reform.

Year Founded: 1915

3490 Parkview Hospital Rehabilitation Center

2200 Randilla Drive
Ft. Wayne, IN 46805-4638
260-373-4000
888-480-5151
www.parkview.com

Sue Ehinger, CEO

31 bed inpatient rehabilitation unit serving a wide variety of diagnoses. CARF accredited for both comprehensive and B1 programs. Outpatient services are offered at several sites throughout the community.

Year Founded: 1995

3491 Richmond State Hospital

498 NW 18th Street
Richmond, IN 47374-2851
765-966-0511; *Fax:* 765-935-9504
www.richmondstatehospital.org

Jeff Butler, Superintendent
Terresa Bradburn, Human Resources Director
David Shelford, Assistant Superintendent
Josh Nolan, Clinical Director

A public behavioral health facility operated by the State of Indiana that provides psychiatric and chemical dependency treatment to citizens on a state wide basis.

Iowa

3492 Cherokee Mental Health Institute

1251 W Cedar Loop
Cherokee, IA 51012-1599
712-225-6927; *Fax:* 712-225-6925
rmoller@dhs.state.ia.us
www.www.dhs.state.ia.us/Consumers/Facilities/Cherokee.

Tony Morris, Manager

3493 Four Seasons Counseling Clinic

2015 West Bay Drive
Muscatine, IA 52761-2228
563-263-3869; *Fax:* 563-263-3869
www.www.fourseasonscounselingclinic.com/

Ruth Evans, Owner

3494 Independence Mental Health Institute

2277 Iowa Avenue
Independence, IA 50644-9215
319-334-2583
tmain@dhs.state.ia.us
www.www.dhs.state.ia.us/Consumers/Facilities/Independe

Bhasker Dave, Manager

3495 Mount Pleasant Mental Health Institute

1200 E Washington Street
Mount Pleasant, IA 52641-1898
319-385-7231; *Fax:* 319-385-8465
karla.sandoval@iowa.gov
www.www.dhs.state.ia.us/Consumers/Facilities/MtPleasan

Karla Sandoval, Contact

Kansas

3496 Prairie View
1901 E First Street
Newton, KS 67114-5010
316-284-6400
800-362-0180
info@pvi.org
www.www.prairieview.org/

Dee Donatelli-Reber, Chair
Jessie Kaye, President and CEO
Gary Fast, MD, Medical Director
Dorothy Nickel Friesen, Secretary

A behavioral and mental health facility which consists of the main campus in Newton that consists of outpatient services, a 38-bed inpatient hospital and various other divisions of our organization. Also maintain outpatient offices in Hutchinson, KS; Marion, KS; McPherson, KS; along with two outpatient offices in Wichita, KS.

Year Founded: 1954

3497 Via Christi Research
1100 N St. Francis Street
Suite 300
Wichita, KS 67214-2871
316-291-4774
800-362-0070; *Fax:* 316-291-7704

Joe Carrithers, Manager
Joe Carrithers, PhD, Research Operations Director

Provide people with mental health conditions such as depression, suicidal thoughts, schizophrenia or dementia have a unique set of needs. They receive highly skilled, compassionate treatment.

Kentucky

3498 Eastern State Hospital
1351 Newtown Pike
Building 1
Lexington, KY 40511-1277
859-253-1686
mjdaniluk@bluegrass.org
www.bluegrass.org

Carolyn Siegel, Chair
David E. Hanna, Interim President & CEO
Dee Werline, Vice President Administration &
Dana Royse, Chief Financial Officer

3499 Our Lady of Bellefonte Hospital
St. Christopher Drive
Ashland, KY 41101
606-833-3333
866-910-6524; *Fax:* 606-833-3946
www.careyoucantrust.com

Tim O'Toole, Manager

Louisiana

3500 Medical Center of LA: Mental Health Services
1532 Tulane Avenue
New Orleans, LA 70112-2860
504-903-3000

Genaro F Arriola Jr, Contact

3501 New Orleans Adolescent Hospital
210 State Street
New Orleans, LA 70118
504-897-3400; *Fax:* 504-896-4959
www.dhh.louisiana.gov

Provides a fully integrated hospital and community based continuum of mental health services for children and adolescents, with serious emotional and behavioral problems, residing in Louisiana.

3502 River Oaks Hospital
1525 River Oaks Road W
New Orleans, LA 70123-2199
504-734-1740
800-366-1740; *Fax:* 504-733-7020
www.www.riveroakshospital.com/

Evelyn Nolting, CEO

A private psychiatric facility for adults, adolescents and children.

3503 Southeast Louisiana Hospital
23515 Highway 190
PO Box 3850
Mandeville, LA 70470-3850
985-626-6300; *Fax:* 985-626-6658
www.dhh.louisiana.gov

Patricia Gonzalez, Facility Director

Maine

3504 Dorthea Dix Psychiatric Center
656 State Street
PO Box 926
Bangor, ME 04402-926
207-941-4000
TTY: 888-774-5290
www.www.maine.gov/dhhs

N Lawrence Ventura, Contact

DDPC is a 100 bed psychiatric hospital serving two-thirds of the State's geographic area that provides services for people with severe mental illness.

3505 Good Will-Hinckley Homes for Boys and Girls
PO Box 159
Hinckley, ME 04944
207-238-4000
info@gwh.org
www.gwh.org

Jack Moore, Chairman
Glenn Cummings, Ed.D, President and Executive Director
Robert Moody, Vice President of Operations
Valerie Cote, Human Resource Generalist

Provides a home for the reception and support of needy boys and girls who are in needs maintaining and operates a school for them; attends to the physical, industrial, moral and spiritual development of those who shall be placed in its care.

3506 Riverview Psychiatric Center
250 Arsenal Street
11 State House Station
Augusta, ME 04333-0011
207-624-3900
888-261-6684; *Fax:* 207-287-6123
www.maine.gov/dhhs/riverview/index.shtml

Mary Louise McEwen, Superintendent
William Nelson MD, Medical Director
Lauret Grommett RN, Director of Nursing

Acute care psychiatric hospital owned and operated by the state of Maine.

3507 Spring Harbor Hospital

123 Andover Road
Westbrook, ME 04092-3850
207-761-2200
866-857-6644
www.www.springharbor.org/

Tracy Hawkins, Chair
Dennis King, Chief Executive Officer
Nancy Hasenfus, M.D., Vice Chair
Anna H Wells, Secretary

Southern Maine's premier provider of inpatient services for individuals who experience acute mental illness or dual disorders issues.

Maryland

3508 Clifton T Perkins Hospital Center

One Renaissance Boulevard
8450 Dorsey Run Road
Oakbrook Terrace, IL 60181
410-724-3000
800-994-6610; *Fax:* 630-792-5636
complaint@jcaho.org
www.dhmh.maryland.gov

Sheilah Davenport, JD,MS,RN, CEO
Muhammed M Ajanah MD, Clinical Director
Steve Mason, COO

CTPHC is a maximum security facility. The mission of the facilty is to perform timely pretrial evaluations of defendants referred by the judicial circuit of Maryland, provide quality assessment of and treatment for all patients, and provide maximum security custody of patients to ensure public safety.

3509 Eastern Shore Hospital Center

PO Box 800
Cambridge, MD 21613
410-221-2300
888-216-8110; *Fax:* 410-221-2534
www.dhmh.maryland.gov/eshc/SitePages/Home.aspx

Mary K Noren, Contact

3510 John L. Gildner Regional Institute for Children and Adolescents

201 West Preston Street
Baltimore, MD 21201
410-767-6500
877-463-3464; *Fax:* 301-309-9004
www.dhmh.state.md.us/jlgrica/

Thomas E. Pukalski, CEO
Claudette Bernstein, Medical Director
Debra K. VanHorn, Director of Comm. Res. & Dev.

John L. Gildner Regional Institute for Children and Adolescents (JLG-RICA) is a community-based, public residential, clinical, and educational facility serving children and adolescents with severe emotional disabilities. The program is designed to provide residential and day treatment for students in grades 5-12. JLG-RICA's goal is to successfully return its students to an appropriate family, commu-

nity, and academic or vocational setting that will lead to happy and successful lives.

3511 Kennedy Krieger Institute

707 North Broadway
Baltimore, MD 21205-1888
443-923-9200
800-873-3377
TTY: 443-923-2645
info@kennedykrieger.org
www.www.kennedykrieger.org/

Gary W Goldstein, CEO

Dedicated to improving the lives of children and adolescents with pediatric developmental disabilities through patient care, special education, research, and professional training.

Year Founded: 1937

3512 RICA: Southern Maryland

9400 Surratts Road
Cheltenham, MD 20623
301-372-1840; *Fax:* 301-372-1906
www.pgcps.org/~rica/

Mary Sheperd, Contact

3513 Sheppard Pratt at Ellicott City

4100 College Avenue
PO Box 0836
Ellicott City, MD 21041-836
443-364-5500
800-883-3322; *Fax:* 443-364-5501
www.taylorhealth.com

To provide personal, high quality mental health services for your family, by our family of health care professionals.

Year Founded: 1939

3514 Spring Grove Hospital Center

55 Wade Avenue
Catonsville, MD 21228
410-402-6000
www.www.springgrove.com/

Patrick Sokas, Contact

3515 Springfield Hospital Center

6655 Sykesville Road
Sykesville, MD 21784-7966
410-795-2100
800-333-7564
www.dhmh.state.md.us

Paula Langmead, CEO
Janice Bowen, COO
Jonathan Book, Clinical Director

A regional psychiatric hospital operated by the State of Maryland, Department of Health and Mental Hygiene, Mental Hygiene Administration.

Year Founded: 1894

Massachusetts

3516 Arbour-Fuller Hospital

200 May Street
S Attleboro, MA 02703-5520
508-761-8500
800-828-3934; *Fax:* 508-761-4240

TTY: 800-974-6006
www.www.arbourhealth.com

Robert Mansfield, CEO
Frank Kahr MD, Medical Director
Judith Merel, Director Marketing

Psychiatric hospital providing services to adults, adolesents and adults with developmental disabilities.

3517 Baldpate Hospital
83 Baldpate Road
Georgetown, MA 01833-2303
978-352-2131; *Fax:* 978-352-6755
www.www.detoxma.com/

Lucille M Batal, President

3518 Concord Family and Adolescent Services
A Division of Justice Resource Institute, Inc
160 Gould Street
Suite 300
Needham, MA 02494-2300
781-559-4900; *Fax:* 978-263-3088
www.jri.org

Arden O'Connor, Chairperson
Andy Pond, MSW, MAT, President
Gregory Canfield, MSW, Executive Vice President
Deborah Reuman, MBA, Chief Financial Officer

Provides professional residential schools, group home, residence for homeless teens, alternative, therapeutic high school, education and parenting programs for children, adults and families throughout Massachusetts.

3519 First Connections and Healthy Families
A Division of Justice Resource Institute, Inc
160 Gould Street
Suite 300
Needham, MA 02494-2300
781-559-4900
www.jri.org

Arden O'Connor, Chairperson
Andy Pond, MSW, MAT, President
Gregory Canfield, MSW, Executive Vice President
Deborah Reuman, MBA, Chief Financial Officer

First Conneections provides resources, education and support to families with children birth through age three. First Connections is dedicated to providing quality, comprehensive parenting support services to a diverse communities seeking resources to compliment and enrich their parenting experience.

3520 Grip Project
A Division of Justice Resource Institute, Inc
319 Wilder St
Suite 433
Lowell, MA 01852-1926
978-452-4522
www.jri.org

Cindy Powers, Program Director

A by teens, for teens young people's program with residential services as a foundation. Grip serves young people, ages 16-20, who are homeless or aging out of foster-care/group homes and are committed to being independent. There is a separate residence for young women and men, both located in Lowell, MA.

3521 Littleton Group Home
A Division of Justice Resource Institute, Inc
22 King Street
Littleton, MA 01460-1519
978-952-6809; *Fax:* 978-952-8607
www.jri.org

Timothy Considine, Program Director

Prepares young men, ages 13-18 for independent living by helping them to live respectful, dignified and increasingly responsible lives. The young men participate in after school activities and have daily access to the community.

3522 Meadowridge Pelham Academy
A Division of Justice Resource Institute, Inc
160 Gould Street
Suite 300
Needham, MA 02494-2300
781-559-4900
www.jri.org

Arden O'Connor, Chairperson
Andy Pond, MSW, MAT, President
Gregory Canfield, MSW, Executive Vice President
Deborah Reuman, MBA, Chief Financial Officer

A residential treatment program that focuses on the special challenges of adolescent girls with emotional and behavioral difficulties. The students, between the ages of 12-22, have typically experienced trauma and poor functioning in their personal, educational and/or family life.

3523 Meadowridge Walden Street School
A Division of Justice Resource Institute, Inc
160 Gould Street
Suite 300
Needham, MA 02494-2300
781-559-4900
www.jri.org

Arden O'Connor, Chairperson
Andy Pond, MSW, MAT, President
Gregory Canfield, MSW, Executive Vice President
Deborah Reuman, MBA, Chief Financial Officer

A residential school program that focuses on the challenges and special needs of adolescent females age 12-22 whom are coping with educational, emotional and behavioral difficulties.

3524 Sleep Disorders Unit of Beth Israel Hospital
330 Brookline Avenue
Boston, MA 02215-5400
617-667-7000; *Fax:* 617-667-1134
www.bidmc.org/

Jean K Matheson MD, Contact

Provides testing and treatment for those with sleep disorders and offers educational workshops, plus support for their families.

3525 The Home for Little Wanderers
271 Huntington Avenue
Boston, MA 02115-4554
617-267-3700
888-466-3321; *Fax:* 617-267-8142
www.thehome.org

Joan Wallace-Benjamin, President/CEO
Michael L. Pearis, Executive Vice President and Chi
Meredith Bryan, Vice President for Development a
Thomas L. Durling, Vice President for Finance

To ensure the healthy, emotional, mental and social development of children at risk, their families and communities.

Year Founded: 1799

3526 Victor School
A Division of Justice Resource Institute, Inc
160 Gould Street
Suite 300
Needham, MA 02494-2300
781-559-4900
www.jri.org

Arden O'Connor, Chairperson
Andy Pond, MSW, MAT, President
Gregory Canfield, MSW, Executive Vice President
Deborah Reuman, MBA, Chief Financial Officer

A private, co-ed, therapeutic day school for students in grades 8-12 with a school philosophy that children learn when they can. Provides innovative and specialized educational and emotional support and treatment.

3527 Windhorse Integrative Mental Health
211 North Street
Suite 1
Northampton, MA 01060-2386
413-586-0207
877-844-8181; *Fax:* 413-585-1521
admissions@windhorseimh.org
www.windhorseimh.org

Eric Friedland-Kays, MA, Admissions Manager
Jeff Bliss MSW, Director, Admissions/Marketing
Sara Watters MA, LMHC, Director, Clinical Operations

Windhorse is a nonprofit treatment and education organization with a whole person approach to recovery from serious psychiatric distress. Services are tailored in close communication with each client and their family.

Year Founded: 1981

Michigan

3528 Hawthorn Center
234 West Baraga Avenue
Marquette, MI 49855
906-228-2850; *Fax:* 248-349-6893
www.michigan.gov

Shobhana Joshi, Executive Director

To provide high quality inpatient mental health services to emotionally disturbed children and adolescents.

3529 Samaritan Counseling Center
29887 W Eleventh Mile Road
Farmington Hills, MI 48336
248-474-4701; *Fax:* 248-474-1518
info@samaritancounselingmichigan.com
www.samaritancounselingmichigan.com

Robert A. Martin, Executive Director
Sara Kirsten, B.A., Administrative Manager

Provides professional therapeutic counseling and educational services to all God's people seeking wholeness through emotional and spiritual growth.

Minnesota

3530 River City Mental Health Clinic
1360 Energy Park Drive
Suite 340
Saint Paul, MN 55108
651-646-8985; *Fax:* 651-646-3959
www.rivercityclinic.com

Doug Jensen, Owner

Psychotherapy and assessment for all ages.

Mississippi

3531 East Mississippi State Hospital
PO Box 4128, W Station
Meridian, MS 39304-4128
601-482-6186; *Fax:* 601-483-5543
www.www.emsh.state.ms.us

Charles Carlisle, Director

To provide a continuum of behavioral health and long term care services for adults and adolescents in a caring, compassionate environment in which ethical principles guide decision making and resources are used responsibly and creatively.

Year Founded: 1882

3532 Mississippi State Hospital
PO Box 157-A
Whitfield, MS 39193-157
601-351-8018
info@msh.state.ms.us
www.msh.state.ms.us

Facilitates improvement in the quality of life for Mississippians who are in need of psychiatric, chemical dependency or nursing home survices by rehabilitating to the least restrictive environment utilizing a reange of psychiatric and medical services that reflect the accepted standard of care and are in compliance with statutory and regulatory guidlelines.

3533 North Mississippi State Hospital
1937 Briar Ridge Road
Tupelo, MS 38804-5963
662-690-4200; *Fax:* 662-690-4227
TDD: 662-690-4239
info@nmsh.state.ms.us

Paul Callens, Executive Director

3534 South Mississippi State Hospital
823 Highway 589
Purvis, MS 39475-4194
601-794-0100; *Fax:* 601-794-0210
www.www.smsh.state.ms.us

Wynona Winfield, Executive Director

Provides the highest quality acute psychiatric care for adults who live in southern Mississippi

Missouri

3535 Northwest Missouri Psychiatric Rehabilitation Center
3505 Frederick Avenue
Saint Joseph, MO 64506-2914
816-387-2300; *Fax:* 816-387-2329
www.mo.gov

Mary Attebury, Manager

Inpatient care for long-term psychiatric/adult.

3536 Southeast Missouri Mental Health Center
1010 W Columbia Street
Farmington, MO 63640-2902
573-218-6792; *Fax:* 573-218-6703
cynthia.forsythe@dmh.mo.gov
www.www.dmh.mo.gov/smmhc/

Karen Adams, CEO

People shall receive services focusing on strenghts and promoting opportunities beyond the limitations of mental illness.

Nebraska

3537 Norfolk Regional Center
1700 N Victory Road
PO Box 1209
Norfolk, NE 68702-1209
402-370-3400; *Fax:* 402-370-3194
www.dhhs.ne.gov

William Gibson, CEO
TyLynne Bauer, Facility Operating Officer

A progressive 120-bed state psychiatric hospital providing specialized psychiatric care to adults.

Nevada

3538 Behavioral Health Options: Sierra Health Services
2724 N Tenaya Way
Las Vegas, NV 89128-424
877-393-6094

Anthony M Marlon, Chairman/CEO

to manage behavioral health services in the private and public sectors on a national basis, creating value for our customers, including brokers, employers, members, providers and shareholders

3539 Northern Nevada Adult Mental Health Services
480 Galletti Way
Sparks, NV 89431-5564
775-688-2001; *Fax:* 775-688-2192

David Rosin MD, Contact

3540 Southern Nevada Adult Mental Health Services
6161 W Charleston Boulevard
Las Vegas, NV 89146-1148
702-486-6000
www.mhds.state.nv.us

Anuranjan Bist, Contact

New Hampshire

3541 Hampstead Hospital
218 E Road
Hamptead, NH 03841-5303
603-329-5311; *Fax:* 603-329-4746

Phillip Kubiak, Chief Executive Officer
Cynthia Gove, Chief Operating Officer
Scott Ranks, Director Support Services
Lisa Ryan, Human Resources Coordinator

Provides a full range of psychiatric and chemical dependency services for children, adolescents, adults and the elderly.

3542 New Hampshire State Hospital
29 Pleasant Street
Concord, NH 03301-3852
603-271-5300; *Fax:* 603-271-5395

Chester G Batchelder, CEO

A state operated, publicly funded hospital providing a range of specialized psychiatric services. NHH advocates for and provides services that support an individual's recovery.

New Jersey

3543 Ancora Psychiatric Hospital
301 Spring Garden Road
Hammonton, NJ 08037
609-561-1700; *Fax:* 609-567-7294
donna.ingram@dhs.state.nj.us
www.www.state.nj.us

John M. Lubitsky, CEO

Provides quality comprehensive psychiatric, medical and rehabilitative services that encourage maximun patient independence and movement towards community reintegration with an enviroment that is safe and caring.

3544 Ann Klein Forensic Center
Sullivan Way
PO Box 7717
W Trenton, NJ 08628-717
609-633-0900; *Fax:* 609-633-0971
mhs.affc-infoline@dhs.state.nj.us
www.www.state.nj.us/humanservices/dmhs/oshm/akfc/

Glenn Ferguson, Ph.D., CEO

A 200-bed psychiatric hospital serving a unique population that requires a secured environment. The facility provides care and treatment to individuals suffering from mental illness who are also within the legal system.

3545 Greystone Park Psychiatric Hospital
59 Koch Avenue
Morris Plains, NJ 07950
973-538-1800; *Fax:* 973-993-8782
william.lanni@dhs.state.nj.us
www.www.state.nj.us/humanservices/dmhs/oshm/gpph/

Janet Monroe, CEO

A 550 bed psychiattric hospital.

New Mexico

3546 Life Transition Therapy
110 Delgado Street
Santa Fe, NM 87501-2781
505-982-4183
800-547-2574
therapy@lifetransitiontherapy.com
www.www.lifetransitiontherapy.com

Ralph Steele, Founder
Ralph Steele, Founder

To eliminate the fear, ignorance and conditioning that fuel racism and social injustice within the individual as well as in relationships, families, communities, and the world at large.

3547 Sequoyah Adolescent Treatment Center
3405 W Pan American Freeway NE
Albuquerque, NM 87107-4786
505-222-0355
www.nmsatc.org

Henry Gardner, Manager

A 36 bed residential treatment center whose purpose is to provide care, treatment, and reintegration into society for adolescents who are violent or who have a history of violence and have a mental disorder and who are amenable to treatment.

New York

3548 Arms Acres
75 Seminary Hill Road
Carmel, NY 10512-1921
845-225-3400
888-227-4641; *Fax:* 845-698-4046
www.www.armsacres.com

Frederick R Hesse, CEO
Sultan Niazi, CFO
Michele Saari, Health Information Management

A private health care system providing high quality, cost-effective care to those suffering from alcoholism and chemical dependency and to the many whose lives are affected by the diseases of addiction.

3549 Berkshire Farm Center and Services for Youth
13640 State Route 22
Canaan, NY 12029-3506
518-781-4567; *Fax:* 518-781-0507
info@berkshirefarm.org
www.berkshirefarm.org

Mr. Robert A Kandel, Board Chairman
Timothy Giacchetta, President and CEO
Mr. Charles Mott, Chairman Emeritus

Mission is to strengthen children and their families so they can lives safely, independently and productively within their home communities.

3550 Bronx Psychiatric Center
1500 Waters Place
Bronx, NY 10461-2796
718-931-0600; *Fax:* 718-862-4879
www.www.omh.ny.gov

Pamela Turner, Executive Director
Joseph Battaglia, MD, Clinical Director
Roy Thomas, Deputy Director

A 360 bed facility that has three impatient services and a comprehensive outpatient program.

3551 Brooklyn Children's Center
1819 Bergen Street
Brooklyn, NY 11233-4513
718-221-4500; *Fax:* 718-221-4581
www.www.omh.ny.gov

Provides high quality comprehensive individualized mental health treatment services to serious emotionally disturbed children and adolescents in Brooklyn, and to continuously strive to improve the quality of those services.

3552 BryLin Behavioral Health System
1263 Delaware Avenue
Buffalo, NY 14209-2497

716-886-8200
800-727-9546; *Fax:* 716-886-1986
info@brylin.com
www.brylin.com

Eric D. Pleskow, President and CEO
E. Paul Hettich, Senior Vice President and CFO

Founded in 1955. Provides inpatient psychiatric services for children, adolescents, adults and geriatric patients. Outpatient substance abuse services for adolescents and adults. Outpatient mental health services for adults.

3553 Buffalo Psychiatric Center
400 Forest Avenue
Buffalo, NY 14213-1298
716-885-2261; *Fax:* 716-885-4852
www.omh.ny.gov

Kimberly Karalus, Chief of Outpatient Services
Nancy Johnson, Director of Residential Services

Provides psychiatric quality inpatient, outpatient, residential, vocational, and wellness services to adults with serious mental illnesses

3554 Capital District Psychiatric Center
75 New Scotland Avenue
Albany, NY 12208-3474
518-549-6000; *Fax:* 518-549-6804
www.www.omh.ny.gov

Lewis Campbell, CEO

Provides inpatient psychiatric treatment and rehabilitation to patients who have been diagnosed with serious and persistenet mental illnesses and for whom brief or short-term treatment in a community hospital mental health unit has been unable to provide sympton stability.

3555 Central New York Psychiatric Center
9005 Old River Road
PO Box 300
Marcy, NY 13403
315-765-3600; *Fax:* 315-765-3629
www.www.omh.ny.gov

A comprehensive mental health service delivery system providing a full range of care and treatment to persons incarcerated in the New York State and county correctional system.

3556 Cornerstone of Rhinebeck
500 Milan Hollow Road
Rhinebeck, NY 12572-2970
845-266-3481
800-266-4410; *Fax:* 845-266-8335
admin@cornerstoneny.com
www.cornerstoneny.com

Eileen Mc Curdy, Senior VP

Provides inpatient chemical dependency treatment and offers a comprehensive range of inpatient and outpatient treatment services for alcohol and substance abuse.

Year Founded: 1974

3557 Creedmoor Psychiatric Center
79-25 Winchester Boulevard
Queens Village, NY 11427-2128
718-464-7500; *Fax:* 718-264-3636
www.www.omh.ny.gov

William Fisher, MD, Clinical Director
Susan Chin, Deputy Director

John Holmes, Deputy Director
Renee Anderson, Chief Nursing Officer

Provides a continuum of inpatient, outpatient and related psychiatric services with inpatient hospitalization at the main campus and five outpatient sites in the boroughs of Queens.

3558 Elmira Psychiatric Center

100 Washington Street
Elmira, NY 14901-2898
607-737-4711; *Fax:* 607-737-4722
www.www.omh.ny.gov

Mark Stephany, Manager

Provides a wide array of comprehensive psychiatric services.

3559 Freedom Ranch

Freedom Village USA
5275 Rt. 14, PO Box 24
Lakemont, NY 14857-24
607-243-8126
800-842-8679; *Fax:* 607-243-5521
77pastor@fvusa.com
www.freedomvillageusa.com

Dr Fletcher Brothers, Founder

An extension of Freedom Village, Freedom Ranch offers a residential program for men 21 and older with substance abuse and emotional problems. Freedom Ranch is a faith-based program seeking to help men become productive members of society.

Year Founded: 1948

3560 Freedom Village USA

Freedom Village USA
5275 Rt. 14, PO Box 24
Lakemont, NY 14857-24
607-243-8126
800-842-8679; *Fax:* 607-243-5521
77pastor@fvusa.com
www.freedomvillageusa.com

Dr Fletcher Brothers, Founder

A not-for-profit residential campus for troubled teens. Offers a faith-based approach to teenagers in crisis or at risk. Students are required to make a voluntary one-year commitment to the program. Freedom Village has an 80% success rate with troubled teenagers.

3561 Gift of Life Home

Freedom Village USA
5275 Rt. 14, PO Box 24
Lakemont, NY 14857-24
607-243-8126
800-842-8679; *Fax:* 607-243-5521
77pastor@fvusa.com
www.freedomvillageusa.com

Dr Fletcher Brothers, Founder

An affiliate program of Freedom Village, USA, a residential program for troubled teenagers, the Gift of Life Home offers pregnant girls a safe haven, a place of refuge, where they can come and have their baby while transforming their life as well. Freedom Village is a faith-based alternative to other residential placements.

3562 Greater Binghamton Health Center

425 Robinson Street
Binghamton, NY 13904-1775
607-724-1391; *Fax:* 607-773-4387
www.www.omh.ny.gov

Pamela Vredenburgh, Manager

Provides comprehensive outpatient and inpatient services for adults and children who are seriously mentally ill.

3563 Hope House

573 Livingston Ave.
Albany, NY 12206
518-482-4673; *Fax:* 518-482-0873
www.hopehouseinc.org

Kevin M. Connally, Executive Director
Catherine Dowdell, Executive Assistant
Lynda Tymeson, Director of Program Services
Courtney Lerman, Quality Assurance Manager

Started helping the community in need of education, intervention and treatment for the persons affected by substance abuse.

3564 Hutchings Psychiatric Center

620 Madison Street
Syracuse, NY 13210-2338
315-426-3600; *Fax:* 315-426-3603
www.www.omh.ny.gov

Colleen Sawyer, Executive Director

A comprehensive, community-based mental health facility providing an integrated network of inpatient and outpatient services for children and adults residing in the Central New York Region.

3565 Kingsboro Psychiatric Center

681 Clarkson Avenue
Brooklyn, NY 11203-2199
718-221-7700; *Fax:* 718-221-7206
www.www.omh.ny.gov

Mark Lerman, Manager

Provides competent compassionate psychiatric care to people with serious mental illness with a purpose of reintegrating them to the community.

3566 Kirby Forensic Psychiatric Center

600 E 125th Street
New York, NY 10035-6000
646-672-5800; *Fax:* 646-672-6446
www.www.omh.ny.gov

Steve Rabinowitz, Manager

A maximum security hospital of the New York State Office of Mental Health that provides secure treatment and evaluation for the forensic patients and courts of New York City and Long Island.

Year Founded: 1985

3567 Manhattan Psychiatric Center

600 E 125th Street
New York, NY 10035-6000
646-672-6767; *Fax:* 646-672-6446
www.www.omh.ny.gov

Steve Rabinowitz, Manager

Offers inpatient and outpatient treatment for adults with mental illness.

3568 Mid-Hudson Forensic Psychiatric Center
2834 Route 17-M
New Hampton, NY 10958
845-374-8700; *Fax:* 845-374-8860
www.www.omh.ny.gov

Barbara Daria, Manager

A secure adult psychiatric center that provides a comprehensive program of evaluation, treatment, and rehabilitation for patients admitted by court order.

3569 Mohawk Valley Psychiatric Center
1400 Noyes at York
Utica, NY 13502
315-738-3800; *Fax:* 315-738-4414
www.www.omh.ny.gov

Sarah Rudes, CEO

Provides quality, individualized psychiatric treatment and rehabilitation services that promote recovery.

3570 Nathan S. Kline Institute for Psychiatric Research
140 Old Orangeburg Road
Orangeburg, NY 10962
845-398-5500; *Fax:* 845-398-5510
webmaster@nki.rfmh.org
www.www.rfmh.org/nki

Donald C. Goff, MD, Director
Antonio Convit, MD, Deputy Director
Thomas O. O'Hara, MBA, Deputy Director Administration

A facility of the New York State Office of Mental Health that has earned a national and international reputation for its pioneering contributions in psychiatric research, especially in the areas of psychopharmacological treatments for schizophrenia and major mood disorders, and in the application of computer technology to mental health services. A broad range of studies are conducted at NKI, including basic, clinical, and services research. All work is intended to improve care for people suffering from these complex, psychobiologically-based, severely disabling mental disorders.

Year Founded: 1952

3571 New York Psychiatric Institute
1051 Riverside Drive
New York, NY 10032-1098
212-543-6283
www.www.nyspi.org/

Jeffrey Lieberman, MD, Chairman
Anke Ehrhardt, PhD, Vice Chair for Academic Affairs
Avalon Lance, MHA, Vice Chair for Administration an
Harold A. Pincus, MD, Vice Chair for Strategic Initiat

3572 Odyssey House
120 Wall Street
New York, NY 10005
212-361-1600; *Fax:* 212-361-1666
info@odysseyhouseinc.org
www.odysseyhouseinc.org

Peter Provet, President & Chief Executive Offi
John Tavolacci, Executive Vice President & Chief
Durga Vallabhaneni, Senior Vice President & Chief Fi
Isobelle Surface, Senior Vice President & Director

Develops innovative treatment models to ensure that our systems take into account current research, utilizing what works most effectively to help these individuals overcome their difficulties and build a stable, produicitve, drug-free life.

Year Founded: 1967

3573 Pahl Transitional Apartments
559-565 Sixth Avenue
Troy, NY 12182-2620
518-237-9891; *Fax:* 518-237-9409
michael_kennedy@pahlinc.org
www.pahlinc.org

Michael Kennedy, Clinical Director

A 9-12 month residential, chemical dependency treatment facility for males ages 16-25. The goal for the residents is to learn the skills necessary for long-term recovery and independent living.

3574 Phoenix House
164 West 74th Street
New York, NY 10023-2301
646-505-2000; *Fax:* 646-721-2164
www.phoenixhouse.org

Alan Hargrove, Program Director
Brian Gillam, Managing Director
Christine Balzano, Program Director
Dan Boylan, Program Director

Reclaims disordered lives, encourages individual responsibility, positive behavior, and personal growth, also strengthens families and communities, and safeguards public health. Also, promotes a drug-free society through prevention, treatment, education and training, research, and advocacy.

3575 Pilgrim Psychiatric Center
998 Crooked Hill Road
West Brentwood, NY 11717-1019
631-761-3500; *Fax:* 631-761-2600
www.www.omh.ny.gov

Dean Wienstock, Manager

Provides excellent, integrated care in evaluation, treatment, crisis intervention, rehabilitation, support, and self help/empowerment service to individuals with serious psychiatric illness.

3576 Queens Children's Psychiatric Center
74-03 Commonwealth Boulevard
Bellerose, NY 11426-1839
718-264-4500
www.www.omh.ny.gov

Keith Little, Executive Director

Serves seriously emotionally disturbed children and adolescents from the ages of 5 through 18 in a range of programs including Inpatient hospitalization, outpatient clinic treatment, intensive case management, homemaker services and community education and consultation services.

3577 Rochester Psychiatric Center
1111 Elmwood Avenue
Rochester, NY 14620-3090
585-241-1200; *Fax:* 585-241-1424
TTY: 585-241-1982
www.www.omh.ny.gov

Elizabeth Suhre, R.N., B.S., MBA, Executive Director and Director
Philip Griffin, Director for Quality Improvement

Laurence Guttmacher, M.D., Clinical Director
Christopher Kirisits, R.N., M.S.N., Chief Nursing Officer

Provides quality comprehensive treatment and rehabilitation services to people with psychiatric disabilities working toward recovery.

3578 Rockland Children's Psychiatric Center
2 First Avenue
Orangeburg, NY 10962
845-359-7400
800-597-8481; *Fax:* 845-680-8900
www.www.omh.ny.gov

Josefina M Moneda

A psychiatric hospital exclusively for children and adolescents

3579 Rockland Psychiatric Center
140 Old Orangeburg Road
Orangeburg, NY 10962
845-359-1000; *Fax:* 845-680-5580
www.www.omh.ny.gov

Provides treatment, rehabilitation, and support to adults 18 and older with severe and complex mental illness.

3580 Sagamore Children's Psychiatric Center
197 Half Hollow Road
Dix Hills, NY 11746-5859
631-370-1700; *Fax:* 631-370-1714
www.www.omh.ny.gov

Dennis Dubey, Executive Director

Programs for youngsters and their families include inpatient hospitalization, day hospitalization, day treatment, outpatient clinic treatment, mobile mental health team crisis services, information and referral, and community consultation and training.

3581 Samaritan Village
138-02 Queens Blvd
Briarwood, NY 11435-2647
718-206-2000
800-532-4357
www.samaritanvillage.org

Tino Hernandez, President/CEO
Douglas Apple, Executive Vice President and Chi
John Iammatteo, Senior Vice President for Financ
Sheila Greene, Vice President of Communications

Mission is to eliminate the devastating impact of substance abuse on individuals, families and communities by helping addicted men and women take responsibility for their own recovery.

3582 South Beach Psychiatric Center
777 Seaview Avenue
Staten Island, NY 10305-3409
718-667-2300; *Fax:* 718-667-2344
www.www.omh.ny.gov

Rosanne Gaylor, MD, Executive Director
Rosanne Gaylor, MD, Director, Clinical Services
Doreen Piazza, R.N.C., MS, Director, Nursing
Titus Mathew, BE, Deputy Director, Administration

Provides intermediate level inpatient services to persons living in western Brooklyn, southern Staten Island, and Manhattan south of 42nd street.

3583 St. Lawrence Psychiatric Center
1 Chimney Point Drive
Ogdensburg, NY 13669-2291
315-541-2001; *Fax:* 315-541-2041
www.www.omh.ny.gov

Sam Bastien, Executive Director

3584 Veritas Villa
5 Ridgeview Road
Kerhonkson, NY 12446-1555
845-626-3555; *Fax:* 845-626-3840

Joseph Stoeckeler, CEO

Inpatient rehabilitation and wellness center
Year Founded: 1957

3585 Western New York Children's Psychiatric Center
1010 E & W Road
W Seneca, NY 14224-3698
716-677-7000; *Fax:* 716-675-6455
www.www.omh.ny.gov

Deborah Shiffner, Manager

Provides high quality, comprehensive behavioral health care services to seriously emotionally disturbed children and adolescents, and to partner with their families throughout the continuum of care.

North Carolina

3586 Broughton Hospital
1000 S Sterling Street
Morganton, NC 28655-3999
828-433-2111
BH.Information@NCMail.net
www.www.ncdhhs.gov/dsohf/broughton/

Dr Art Robarge, Interim Hospital Director/CEO

3587 Central Regional Hospital
803 Biggs Drive
Raleigh, NC 27699
919-575-7100
www.www.ncdhhs.gov/dsohf

Dale C. Armstrong, MBA, FACHE, Director
Laura White, Team Leader, Hospitals
Carol Donin, Team Leader, Developmental Cente
Wendi McDaniel, Team Leader, Facility Advocates

Formed by the merger of Dorothea Dix Hospital and John Umstead Hospital. Services include adult psychiatric services, clinical research services, child and adolescent services, medical services, and geropsychiatric services.

3588 Cherry Hospital
201 Stevens Mill Road
Goldsboro, NC 27530-1057
919-731-3411; *Fax:* 919-731-3788
www.www.ncdhhs.gov

J. Luckey Welsh, Jr., CEO
Nathaniel Carmichael, COO
Jim Mayo, MD, Clinical Director
Scott Mann, MD, Medical Director

North Dakota

3589 North Dakota State Hospital
2605 Circle Drive
Jamestown, ND 58401-6905
701-253-3650; *Fax:* 701-253-3999
TTY: 701-253-3880
www.nd.gov

Alex Schweitzer, CEO

Ohio

3590 Central Behavioral Healthcare
5965 Renaissance Place
Toledo, OH 43623-4728
419-882-5678; *Fax:* 419-882-7446
info@cbhpsych.com
www.cbhpsych.com

Dennis W. Kogut, PhD, Owner

Provides patients with a broad range of high-quality behavioral healthcare in a professional and personal matter.

Year Founded: 1986

3591 Heartland Behavioral Healthcare
3000 Erie Street S
Massillon, OH 44646-7976
330-833-3135
800-783-9301; *Fax:* 330-833-6564
TDD: 330-832-9991
www.mha.ohio.gov

Jeffrey L. Sims, CEO
Dr. Emmanuel Nwajei, Chief Clinical Officer
Michael Waggoner, Nurse Executive
John Stocker, Client Rights Specialist

3592 Northcoast Behavioral Healthcare System
PO Box 678003
1756 Sagamore Road
Northfield, OH 44067
330-467-7131; *Fax:* 330-467-2420
TDD: 330-467-5522
www.www.mha.ohio.gov

Doug Kern, Chief Executive Officer
Michael Emerick, Nurse Executive
Muhammad Momen, M.D., Lead Chief Clinical Officer (CCO
Joi Chapman, Client Rights Specialist

3593 Northcoast Behavioral Healthcare System
PO Box 678003
1756 Sagamore Road
Northfield, OH 44067
330-467-7131; *Fax:* 330-467-2420
TDD: 330-467-5522
www.www.mha.ohio.gov

Doug Kern, Chief Executive Officer
Michael Emerick, Nurse Executive
Muhammad Momen, M.D., Lead Chief Clinical Officer (CCO
Joi Chapman, Client Rights Specialist

3594 Twin Valley Behavioral Healthcare
Columbus Campus, 2200 W Broad Street
Columbus, OH 43223

614-752-0333
877-301-8824; *Fax:* 614-752-0087
TDD: 614-274-7137
www.www.mha.ohio.gov

Veronica Lofton, CEO
Dr. Alan Freeland, Chief Clinical Officer (CCO)
David Blahnik, Chief Operations Officer
Susan Cross, Client Rights Specialist

State operated BHD serving severley mentally ill adults in partnership with the community.

Oklahoma

3595 Griffin Memorial Hospital
900 E Main Street
PO Box 151
Norman, OK 73070-151
405-573-6623; *Fax:* 405-522-8320
www.www.ok.gov

Don Bowen, Contact

3596 Oklahoma Forensic Center
PO Box 69
Vinita, OK 74301-0069
918-256-7841; *Fax:* 918-256-4491
www.www.ok.gov/

William Burkett, Contact

3597 Willow Crest Hospital
130 A Street Southwest
Miami, OK 74354-6800
918-542-1836; *Fax:* 918-542-6060
aanthony@willowcresthospital.com
www.willowcresthospital.com

Anne Anthony, CEO

Oregon

3598 Blue Mountain Recovery Center
2600 Westgate
Pendleton, OR 97801-9604
541-276-0810; *Fax:* 541-278-2209
Kerry.Kelly@state.or.us
www.www.oregon.gov

Kerry Kelly, Contact

3599 Oregon State Hospital: Portland
1121 NE 2nd Avenue
Portland, OR 97232-2043
503-731-8620
www.www.oregon.gov

Nena Strickland, Executive Director
Year Founded: 1883

3600 Oregon State Hospital: Salem
2600 Center Street NE
Salem, OR 97301-2682
503-945-2800
www.www.oregon.gov

Pam Dickinson, Manager
Year Founded: 1883

3601 Riverside Center
671 Sw Main
PO Box 2259
Winston, OR 97496-2259
541-679-6129; *Fax:* 541-679-5285
www.riversidecenter.org

3602 St. Mary's Home for Boys
16535 SW Tualatin Valley Highway
Beaverton, OR 97006-5143
503-649-5651; *Fax:* 503-649-7405
reception@stmaryshomeforboys.org
www.www.stmaryshomeforboys.org

Francis Maher, Executive Director

Founded in 1889 as an orphanage for abandoned and wayward children, today St. Mary's is a private, non-profit organization that offers comprehensive residential, day treatment and mental health services to at-risk boys between the ages of 10 and 17 who are emotionally disturbed and/or disruptive behavior disordered.

Year Founded: 1889

Pennsylvania

3603 MHNet
9606 N. Mopac Expressway
Stonebridge Plaza 1, Suite 600
Austin, TX 78759
888-646-6889; *Fax:* 724-741-4552
edwynl@integra-ease.com
www.www.mhnet.com

Wesley J Brockhoeft, PhD, President/CEO
Peter Harris, MD, Corporate Medical Director
Robert Wilson, CFO
Richard T Wright, SVP Business Development

MHNet is an outgrowth of the Center for Individual and Family Counseling, a multi-disciplinary outpatient treatment clinic with a full spectrum behavioral health organization with national service delivery capability.

Year Founded: 1981

3604 National Mental Health Self-Help Clearinghouse
1211 Chestnut Street
Suite 1207
Philadephia, PA 19107-4103
215-751-1810
800-553-4539; *Fax:* 215-636-6312
www.mhselfhelp.org

Joseph Rogers, Executive Director
Susan Rogers, Director
Christa Burkett, Technical Assistance Coordinator
Britani Nestel, Program Specialist

A national consumer technical assistance center, has played a major role in the development of the mental health consumer movement.

Year Founded: 1986

3605 Renfrew Center Foundation
475 Spring Lane
Philadelphia, PA 19128-3918
215-482-5353; *Fax:* 215-482-7390
foundation@renfrew.org
www.renfrewcenter.com

Sam Menaged, President

A tax-exempt, nonprofit organization advancing the education, prevention, research, and treatment of eating disorders.

Year Founded: 1985

3606 Torrance State Hospital
PO Box 111
Torrance, PA 15779-111
724-459-4406
www.www.dpw.state.pa.us

Lyle Gardner, Director

3607 Warren State Hospital
33 Main Drive
N Warren, PA 16365-5099
814-726-4219; *Fax:* 814-726-4447
www.www.dpw.state.pa.us

Charlotte M. Uber, LSW, Chief Executive Officer
Nancy Saullo, HR Director
Susan Cramer, Admissions Coordinator

3608 Wernersville State Hospital
PO Box 300
Wernersville, PA 19565-300
610-678-3411; *Fax:* 610-670-4101

Andrea Kepler, Chief Executive Officer
Year Founded: 1891

Rhode Island

3609 Butler Hospital
345 Blackstone Boulevard
Providence, RI 02906-4829
401-455-6200
info@butler.org
www.butler.org

Patricia Recupero, President

Rhode Island's only private, nonprofit psychiatric and substance abuse hospital for adults, adolescents, children and seniors.

Year Founded: 1844

3610 Gateway Healthcare
249 Roosevelt Avenue
Suite 205
Pawtucket, RI 02860-2134
401-724-8400
www.gatewayhealth.org

Richard Leclerc, President
Scott W DiChristofero, VP Finance
Stephen Chabot MD, Medical Director
Carolyn Kyle, Senior Vice President of Strateg

To promote resiliency and to assist people in their recovery from mental health, substance abuse, and behavioral and emotional disorder

3611 Groden Center
86 Mount Hope Avenue
Providence, RI 02906-1648
401-274-6310; *Fax:* 401-421-3280
grodencenter@grodencenter.org
www.grodencenter.org

June Groden, President

Groden Center has been providing day and residential treatment and educational services to children and youth who have developmental and behavioral difficulties and their families. By providing a broad range of individualized services in the most normal and least restrictive settings possible, children and youth learn skills that will help them engage in typical experiences and interact more successfully with others. Education and treatment take place in Groden Center classrooms, in the student's homes, and in the community with every effort made to maintain typical family and peer relationships. Call or visit our web site for more information about the Center and the publications and materials we have available.

Year Founded: 1976

South Carolina

3612 CM Tucker Jr Nursing Care Center
2200 Harden Street
Columbia, SC 29203-7107
803-737-5300
www.www.state.sc.us

Laura W. Hughes, RN, BSN, MPH, Facility Director

Provides excellence in resident care in an environment of concern and compassion that is respectful to others, adaptive to change and accountable for outcome.

Year Founded: 1970

3613 Columbia Counseling Center
900 St. Andrews Road
Columbia, SC 29210-5816
803-731-4708; *Fax: 803-798-7607*
www.columbiacounselingcenter.com

Darrel G Shaver, President

3614 Earle E Morris Jr Alcohol & Drug Treatment Center
610 Faison Drive
Columbia, SC 29203-3218
803-935-7200; *Fax: 803-935-7329*
www.scdmh.org

George Mc Connell, Manager

Provides effective treatment of chemical dependence through comprehensive evaluation, safe detoxification, and state-of-the-art treatment servies.

3615 G Werber Bryan Psychiatric Hospital
220 Faison Drive
Columbia, SC 29203-3210
803-935-5761; *Fax: 803-935-7110*
www.www.state.sc.us

Versie Bellamy RN, MN, Deputy Director
Kimberly B. Rudd, MD, Medical Director
Algie Bryant, RN, MSN, Director of Performance Improvem
Mesa Foard, Director of Information Technolo

A 277 bed short term intensive care facility that serves adult and geriatric patients ages 16 years and older. Provides therapeutic services in a warm and nurturing environment for individuals in crisis.

3616 Patrick B Harris Psychiatric Hospital
130 Highway 252
PO Box 2907
Anderson, SC 29622-2907

864-231-2600; *Fax: 864-225-3297*

John Fletcher, CEO

Provides intensive, short-term, psychiatric diagnostic and treatment services on a 24 hour, emergency voluntary and involuntary basis.

3617 South Carolina State Hospital
2414 Bull Street
Columbia, SC 29202
803-898-8581
www.www.state.sc.us

John H. Magill, State Director

Psychiatric hospital

Year Founded: 1995

3618 William S Hall Psychiatric Institute
1800 Colonial Drive
PO Box 202
Columbia, SC 29203
803-898-1662
www.www.state.sc.us

Angela Forand, Ph.D.,, Program Director
Dr. Phyllis Bryant-Mobley, Medical Director
Natasha Davis, RN (Interim), Director of Nursing Services

South Dakota

3619 South Dakota Human Services Center
3515 Broadway Avenue
PO Box 7600
Yankton, SD 57078-7600
605-668-3100; *Fax: 605-668-3460*
infohsc@state.sd.us
www.dss.sd.gov/behavioralhealthservices/hsc/

Doug Dix, Deputy Financial Officer
Laura Schaeffer, Deputy Financial Officer
Amy Iversen-Pollreisz, Deputy Secretary

To provide persons who are mentally ill or chemically dependent with effective, individualized professional treatment that enables them to achieve their highest level of personal independence in the most therapeutic environment.

Tennessee

3620 Cherokee Health Systems
2018 Weestern Avenue
Knoxville, TN 37921-5718
865-934-6734
www.cherokeehealth.com

Tracey Trench, Manager

Uses an integrated model to provide behavioral health and primary care services in a community-based setting.

Year Founded: 1960

3621 Lakeshore Mental Health Institute
5908 Lyons View Drive
Knoxville, TN 37919-7598
865-584-1561; *Fax: 865-450-5203*
OCA.TDMHSAS@tn.gov.
www.www.tn.gov/

Richard L Thomas, CEO

3622 Memphis Mental Health Institute
951 Court Avenue
Memphis, TN 38103-2813
901-577-1800; *Fax:* 901-577-1434
www.www.tn.gov

Lisa A. Daniel, CEO
Tammy D. Ali-Carr, Psychiatric Hosp. Asst. Supt.
Lori Minor, Nurse Executive
Scott Baymiller, MD, Clinical Director

55 bed acute adult psychiatric facility operated by the State of Tennessee Department of Mental Health & Substance Abuse Services.

3623 Middle Tennessee Mental Health Institute
221 Stewarts Ferry Pike
Nashville, TN 37214-3325
615-902-7400; *Fax:* 615-902-7571
www.tennessee.gov

Candance Gilligan, Manager

3624 Moccasin Bend Mental Health Institute
100 Moccasin Bend Road
Chattanooga, TN 37405
423-265-2271; *Fax:* 423-785-3347
www.tennessee.gov

William Ventress, CEO

3625 Western Mental Health Institute
11100 U.S. Highway 64
Bolivar, TN 38008
731-228-2000
www.www.tn.gov/

Roger Pursley, Chief Officer

3626 Woodridge Hospital
403 State of Franklin Road
Johnson City, TN 37604-6034
423-928-7111
800-346-8899
www.msha.com

Kim Moore, Manager
Kim Cudebec, Clinical Director

Texas

3627 Austin State Hospital
4110 Guadalupe Street
Austin, TX 78751-4223
512-452-0381; *Fax:* 512-419-2812
www.www.dshs.state.tx.us

Carl Schock, CEO

Provides adult psychiatric services, specialty adult services and child and adolescent psychiatric services.

3628 Big Spring State Hospital
1901 N Highway 87
Big Spring, TX 79720-283
432-267-8216
www.www.dshs.state.tx.us

Ed Mougon, CEO

A 195-bed psychiatric hospital that provides hospitalization for people 18 years of age and older with psychiatric illnesses in a 57-county area in West Texas and the Texas Panhandle.

Year Founded: 1938

3629 Choices Adolescent Treatment Center
4521 Karnack Hwy
Marshall, TX 75670
903-938-4455
800-638-0880; *Fax:* 903-938-8906
choices@sydcom.net
www.choicestreatment.com

C G Bowman, CEO

Choices residential treatment program focuses on adolescents which abuse substances and addresses related psychiatric disorders.

3630 Dallas Metrocare Services
1380 Riverbend Drive
Dallas, TX 75247
214-743-1200
877-283-2121; *Fax:* 214-630-3469
metrocare@metrocareservices.org
www.metrocareservices.org

Julia P. Noble, Chair
Jill Martinez, Vice Chair
Judy N. Myers, Secretary

North Texas' leading nonprofit dedicated to helping people with mental illness, developmental disabilities, and severe emotional problems live healthier lives. Provides a comprehensive array of individually-tailored services to help the people we serve toward meaningful and satisfying lives.

Year Founded: 1967

3631 El Paso Psychiatric Center
4615 Alameda Avenue
El Paso, TX 79905-2702
915-532-2202
zulema.carrillo@dshs.state.tx.us
www.dshs.state.tx.us

Zulema C. Carrillo, Superintendent
Raul Luna, Chief Nurse Executive
Amber Bechtel, Quality Oversight Director
David Osterhout, Assistant Superintendent

A 74-bed psychiatric hospital that provides hospitalization to the citizens of far West Texas.

3632 Green Oaks Behavioral Healthcare Service
7808 Clodus Fields Drive
Dallas, TX 75251-2206
972-991-9504
800-866-6554; *Fax:* 972-789-1865
www.greenoakspsych.com

Committed to developing and emulating the latest, most effective clinical practices always, and, in all things, to promote dignity, holding compassion and respect for patients and their families as the absolute standard.

3633 Homeward Bound, Inc.
5300 University Hills Boulevard
Dallas, TX 75241
214-941-3500; *Fax:* 214-941-3517
ddenton@homewardboundinc.org
www.homewardboundinc.org

Jesse Oliver, Board Chair
Douglas W. Denton, MA, LCDC, LCCA, Executive Director
Nancy Pryor, Director of Grants Management
Sonny Gaither, Information Systems

Offers chemical dependence treatment for the indigent population anad those referred by the criminal justice system, local hospitals and private practitioners.

Year Founded: 1980

3634 Jewish Family and Children's Services

12500 NW Military Highway
Suite 250
San Antonio, TX 78231-1871
210-302-6920; *Fax:* 210-302-6952
www.jfs-sa.org

Ilene Kramer, President
Marion Bernstein, 1st Vice-President
Scott McLean, 2nd Vice-President
David Scotch, Treasurer

To strengthen community values, promote human dignity and enhance self-sufficiency of individuals and families through social, psychological, health educaitonal and financial support programs.

Year Founded: 1974

3635 Kerrville State Hospital

721 Thompson Drive
Kerrville, TX 78028-5199
830-896-2211; *Fax:* 830-792-4926
www.www.dshs.state.tx.us

Linda Highsmith, President

provides care for persons with major mental illnesses who need the safety, structure, and resources of an in-patient setting

3636 La Hacienda Treatment Center Hunt, TX 78024

800-749-6160
info@lahacienda.com
www.lahacienda.com

Provides treatment for alcoholism and other chemical dependencies

Year Founded: 1972

3637 Laurel Ridge Treatment Center

17720 Corporate Woods Drive
San Antonio, TX 78259-3500
210-491-9400
800-624-7975; *Fax:* 210-491-3550
www.laurelridgetc.com

Dan Thomas, CEO

A psychiatric hospital offering a comprehensive continuum of behavioral healthcare services including acute programs for children, adolescents and adults and residential treatment for children and adolescents.

3638 New Horizons Ranch and Center

PO Box 549
Goldthwaite, TX 76844-549
915-938-5518; *Fax:* 325-938-5665
www.newhorizonsinc.com

Gary Webb, President
Mark Horn, Vice President
JB Morgan, Secretary
Michael Redden, Executive Director

To provide an environment where children, families and staff are able to heal and grow through caring relationships and unconditional love and acceptance.

Year Founded: 1971

3639 North Texas State Hospital: Vernon Campus

4730 College Drive
Vernon, TX 76384-4009
940-552-9901; *Fax:* 940-553-2500
jamese.smith@dshs.state.tx.us
www.dshs.state.tx.us

James E Smith, Superintendent
Bill Lowery, Financial Officer
Kim Hays, Assistant to Financial Officer
Sheila Sidlauskas, Director, Quality Management

3640 North Texas State Hospital: Wichita Falls Campus

6515 Lake Road
Wichita Falls, TX 76308-5419
940-692-1220; *Fax:* 940-689-5538
jamese.smith@dshs.state.tx.us
www.www.dshs.state.tx.us

Jim Smith, Administrator

1917 pages

3641 Rio Grande State Center

1401 South Rangerville
Harlingen, TX 78552-7638
956-364-8000
www.www.dshs.texas.gov

The only public provider south of San Antonio, Texas that offers healthcare, inpatient mental health services and long-term services for individuals with intellectual and developmental disabilities.

1956 pages

3642 Rusk State Hospital

805 North Dickinson Drive
Rusk, TX 75785
903-683-3421
www.www.dshs.state.tx.us

Brenda Slaton, Superintendent
Michelle Foster, Assistant Superintendent
Frances L. Long, Financial Officer
Joe Bates, M.D., Clinical Director

An inpatient hospital providing psychiatric treatment and care for citizens primarily from the East Texas region.

3643 San Antonio State Hospital

6711 South New Braunfels
Suite 100
San Antonio, TX 78223-3006
210-532-8811; *Fax:* 210-531-7780
robert.arizpe@dshs.state.tx.us
www.dshs.state.tx.us

Bob Arizpe, Superintendent
Valerie Kroll, Assistant to Superintendent
Jessica Gutierrez-Rodriguez, Assistant Superintendent
Glenda Armstrong Huff, Assistant Superintendent

Provides intensive inpatient diagnostic, treatment, rehabilitative, and referral servious for seriously mentally ill persons from South Texas regardless of their financial status.

3644 Shades of Hope Treatment Center

402-A Mulberry Street
Buffalo Gap, TX 79508

800-588-4673
www.shadesofhope.com

Tennie McCarty, Founder/CEO
Carrie Willey, PhD, LPC, Clinical Director
Camela Balcomb, Executive Director
Becky Forrest, Admission Coordinator

A residential and outpatient all-addictions treatment center specializing in the intensive treatment of eating disorders.

3645 Starlite Recovery Center

230 Mesa Verde Drive East
PO Box 317
Center Point, TX 78010-317
866-220-1626; *Fax:* 830-634-2532
info@starliterecovery.com
www.starliterecovery.com

Amy J. Swetnam, LPC, LCDC, CE, Executive Director
Bryan M. Davis, D.O., MSPH, Medical Director
Shannon Malish, LMSW, Director of Counseling Services
Nancy Kneupper, L.V.N., Director of Nursing

Provides the highest quality of care in a cost-effective manner, insuring that our valued clients receive treatment that will allow them to return to a productive way of life.

3646 Terrell State Hospital

1200 East Brin
Terrell, TX 75160-2938
972-563-6452
www.www.dshs.state.tx.us

Dorothy Floyd, Ph.D., Superintendent
Nancy Drake, Assistant to Superintendent
Mike Verseckes, Financial Officer
Judy Tanner, Assistant to Financial Officer

A 316 bed, Joint Commission accredited and Medicare certified, psychiatric inpatient hospital, that is responsible for providing services for individuals with mental illnesses residing within a 19 county, 12,052 square mile service region, with a population of over 3 million.

3647 Waco Center for Youth

3501 N 19th Street
Waco, TX 76708-2097
254-756-2171; *Fax:* 254-745-5398
www.dshs.state.tx.us

Eddie Greenfield, Executive Director

A psychiatric residential treatment facility that serves teen-agers, ages 13 through 17, with emotional difficulties and/or behavioral problems.

Utah

3648 Copper Hills Youth Center

5899 Rivendell Drive
West Jordan, UT 84081-6500
801-561-3377
800-776-7116; *Fax:* 801-569-2959
www.www.copperhillsyouthcenter.com

Phil Sheridan, CEO
Daren Woolstenhulme, CFO
Rebekah Schuler, Director of Clinical Services
Dave Anderton, Director of Risk Management

Residential treatment center for boys and girls ages 12-17. Mental health and substance abuse treatment. Also specialized programs for Autism and sexual misconduct

3649 Utah State Hospital

1300 E Center Street
Provo, UT 84606-3554
801-344-4400; *Fax:* 801-344-4225
jgierisch@utah.gov

Mark I Payne, Manager

provides excellent care in a safe and respectful environment to promote hope and quality of life for individuals with mental illness

1885 pages

Vermont

3650 Brattleboro Retreat

Anna Marsh Lane
PO Box 803
Brattleboro, VT 05302-803
802-257-7785; *Fax:* 802-258-3770
www.www.brattlebororetreat.org

Robert E Simpson Jr, President/CEO
John E. Blaha, MBA, Senior Vice President & Chief Fi
Peter Albert, LICSW, Senior Vice President of Governm
Frederick Engstrom, MD, Chief Medical Officer

A not-for-profit health services organization which, above all else, is committed to assisting individuals to improve their health and functioning.

3651 Spring Lake Ranch Therapeutic Community

1169 Spring Lake Road
Cuttingville, VT 05738-4418
802-492-3322; *Fax:* 802-492-3331
info@springlakeranch.org
www.springlakeranch.org

Rachel Stark, Admissions
Ed Oechslie, Executive Director

Offers an alternative therapeutic treatment program for adults with mental illness and/or substance abuse. Our work program and community life help residents grow and recover in the beautiful Green Mountains of Vermont. Our goal is to help people move from hospitalization or period of crisis to an independent life.

Year Founded: 1932

Virginia

3652 Catawba Hospital

5525 Catawba Hospital Drive
Catawba, VA 24070-0200
540-375-4200
800-451-5544; *Fax:* 540-375-4394
www.www.catawba.dmhmrsas.virginia.gov/

Jack Wood, CEO

To support the continuous process of recovery by providing quality psychiatric services to those individuals entrusted to our care

1909 pages

3653 Central State Hospital

26317 West Washington Street
PO Box 4030
Petersburg, VA 23803-30
804-524-7000

to provide state of the art mental health care and treatment to forensic and civilly committed patients in need of a structured, secure environment. The major components of the hospital's mission include Evaluation, Treatment, Protection, and Disposition

3654 Commonwealth Center for Children & Adolescents
PO Box 4000
Staunton, VA 24402-4000
540-332-2100; *Fax:* 540-332-2201

William J Tuell, Contact

CCCA is an acute care mental health facility for minors under the age of 18 years, operated by the State of Virginia, Department of Behavioral Health and Developmental Services.

Year Founded: 1996

3655 Dominion Hospital
2960 Sleepy Hollow Road
Falls Church, VA 22044-2082
703-536-2000; *Fax:* 703-533-9650
Dominion.DLCares@HCAHealthcare.com
www.dominionhospital.com

Trula Minton, CEO

Offers individuals and families hope and help. Treats children, adolescents and adults who suffer from debilitating disorders such as anxiety, panic, depression, delusions, eating disorders, schizophrenia, school refusal, and self-injurious behavior.

3656 Eastern State Hospital
4601 Ironbound Road
Williamsburg, VA 23188-2652
757-253-5161; *Fax:* 757-253-5065
eshinfo@dshs.wa.gov
www.www.esh.dbhds.virginia.gov

David M. Lyon, Director

3657 Northern Virginia Mental Health Institute
3302 Gallows Road
Falls Church, VA 22042-3398
703-207-7100; *Fax:* 703-207-7160

Jim Newton, Facility Director

Actively promoting recovery of individuals with serious mental illness through the use of safe, efficient, and effective treatment

3658 Piedmont Geriatric Hospital
5001 East Patrick Henry Highway
PO Box 427
Burkeville, VA 23922-427
434-767-4401; *Fax:* 434-767-2346
TDD: 434-767-4454

Stephen Herrick, Director

A 135-bed psychiatric hospital that provides recovery based MH services to enable the elderly to thrive in the community.

3659 Southern Virginia Mental Health Institute
382 Taylor Drive
Danville, VA 24541-4096
434-799-6220; *Fax:* 434-773-4241
naomi.gibson@dbhds.virginia.gov

David Lyon, Manager

To be an inpatient mental health service provider within our Regional Service Area that responds to the patient's and area needs.

3660 Southwestern Virginia Mental Health Institute
340 Bagley Circle
Marion, VA 24354-3126
276-783-1200; *Fax:* 276-783-9712
TDD: 276-783-1365

Cynthia Mc Clure, CEO

3661 Western State Hospital
1301 Richmond Avenue
PO Box 2500
Staunton, VA 24402-2500
540-332-8000; *Fax:* 540-332-8144
TDD: 540-332-8000
www.www.wsh.dbhds.virginia.gov

Jack W Barber, Hospital Director
Year Founded: 1825

Washington

3662 Child Study & Treatment Center
2142 10th Ave West.
Seattle, WA 98119
206-298-9641
800-283-8639; *Fax:* 206-298-9655
ContactCLIP@CLIPadministration.org
www.clipadministration.org

Rick Mehlman, CEO

Treats children from age 5 to 17 who can not be served in less restrictive setting within the community.

3663 Eastern State Hospital
4601 Ironbound Road
PO Box 800 Mail Stop B 32-23
Williamsburg, VA 23188-2652
757-253-5161; *Fax:* 509-565-4705
eshinfo@dshs.wa.gov
www.www.esh.dbhds.virginia.gov

David M. Lyon, Director

Eastern State Hospital is a key partner in assisting adults with psychiatric illness in their recovery through expert inpatient treatment whenever needs exceed community resources.

3664 Ryther Child Center
2400 NE 95th Street
Seattle, WA 98115-2499
206-525-5050; *Fax:* 206-525-9795
TDD: 800-883-6388
www.ryther.org

Lee Grogg, Executive Director

Offers and develops safe places and opportunities for children, youth and families to heal and grow so that they can reach their highest potential.

West Virginia

3665 Highland Hospital
300 56th Street SE
Charleston, WV 25304-2361

304-926-1600
800-250-3806; *Fax:* 304-925-1524
www.highlandhosp.com

James H. Dissen, Chairman

Our mission is to identify and respond to mental health needs, and promote physical, social emotional and intellectual well-being.

3666 Mildred Mitchell-Bateman Hospital

1530 Norway Avenue
PO Box 448
Huntington, WV 25709-448
304-525-7801
800-644-9318
MMBHospital@wv.gov
www.www.batemanhospital.org

Roy Frasher, Volunteer Services Director

Provides inpatient psychiatric treatment for the adult citizens of southern West Virginia.

3667 Weirton Medical Center

601 Colliers Way
Weirton, WV 26062-5091
304-797-6000
www.weirtonmedical.com

Joseph Endrich, CEO

Weirton Medical Center is a 238 bed, non-profit, acute-care, general community hospital located in the city of Weirton in Brooke County, West Virginia. Weirton Medical Center offers health care services to the residents of West Virginia, Ohio and Pennsylvania.

3668 William R Sharpe, Jr Hospital

936 Sharpe Hospital Road
Weston, WV 26452-8550
304-269-1210; *Fax:* 304-269-6235
www.www.dhhr.wv.gov

D. Parker Haddix, CEO

1994 pages

Wisconsin

3669 Bellin Psychiatric Center

744 South Webster Avenue
PO Box 23400
Green Bay, WI 54305-3400
920-433-3500
www.bellin.org/psych

Year Founded: 1907

3670 Mendota Mental Health Institute

301 Troy Drive
Madison, WI 53704-1599
608-301-1000; *Fax:* 608-301-1358
TDD: 888-241-9442
TTY: 888-241-9442
www.www.dhs.wisconsin.gov

A psychiatric hospital operated by the Wisconsin Department of Health and Family Services, Division of Disability and Elder Services, specializes in serving patients with complex psychiatric conditions, often combined with certain problem behaviors.

1860 pages

3671 Wheaton Franciscan Healthcare: Elmbrook Memorial

19333 W North Avenue
Brookfield, WI 53045-4132
262-785-2000
www.www.mywheaton.org/elmbrook-memorial

3672 Winnebago Mental Health Institute

1300 South Drive
PO Box 9
Winnebago, WI 54985-9
920-235-4910; *Fax:* 920-237-2043
TDD: 888-241-9438

Winnebago Mental Health Institute (WMHI) serves as a specialized component in a community-based mental health delivery system.

Wyoming

3673 Wyoming State Hospital

831 Highway 150 South
Evanston, WY 82930-5340
307-789-3464; *Fax:* 307-789-7373

William L Matchinski, Manager

A center for treatment, rehabilitation and recovery.

Clinical Management

Management Companies

3674 ABE American Board of Examiners in Clinical Social Work

27 Congress Street Suite 501
Shetland Park
Salem, MA 01970-5577
978-825-9311
800-694-5285; *Fax: 978-740-5395*
abe@abecsw.org

Robert Booth, CEO
Robert Booth, Executive Director
Leonard Hill MSW BCD, Vice President

The American Board of Examiners in Clinical Social Work (ABE) sets national practice standards, issues an advanced-practice credential, and publishes reference information about its board-certified clinicians

3675 Academy of Managed Care Providers

1945 Palo Verde Avenue
Suite 202
Long Beach, CA 90815-3445
562-682-3559
800-297-2627; *Fax: 562-799-3355*
www.academymcp.org

Dr. John Russell, President
William Adams, Ph.D., Advisory Board Member
Brad Bangerter, Advisory Board Member
Ellen Betts, Ph.D., Advisory Board Member

National organization of clinicans and MCO professionals. Provides many services to members including continuing education, diplomate certification, notification of panel openings and practice opportunities, newsletter, group health insurance and many other benefits.

3676 Action Healthcare Management

6245 N. 24th Parkway
Suite 112
Phoenix, AZ 85016-2029
602-265-0681
800-433-6915; *Fax: 602-265-0202*
www.actionhealthcare.com

Jean Rice, President

Action Healthcare Management has been an independent healthcare management company offering a full range of services that can be tailored to meet your organization's needs-from pre-certification and utilization review, management of high risk pregnancy and workers' compensation cases, to cases involving serious illness, catastrophic injury and cases requiring transplants. AHM works within your budget to assure provision of quality, affordable healthcare, negotiation of provider agreements and cost containment in the structuring of quality utilization management plans. In today's complicated healthcare system, Action Healthcare Management is a partner to both your organization and your insured. We're by your side, every step of the way.

3677 Adanta Group-Behavioral Health Services

130 Southern School Road
Somerset, KY 42501-3152
606-679-4782; *Fax: 606-678-5296*
TDD: 800-633-5599
TTY: 800-633-5599

klworley@adanta.org
www.adanta.org

Jamie Burton, CEO

Adanta is composed of three major divisions which include Human Development Services, Clinical Services and the Regional Prevention Center. While each division is responsible for providing separate and distinct services, each relies on the expertise and resources available within the overall corporation. The three major divisions are made up of many smaller specialized areas, each of which include many professionals, staff and support personnel who take great pride in the quality of their work. Their professional skills, combined with time, energy and caring, have yielded and continue to yield positive results and many success stories across the region.

3678 Adult Learning Systems

1954 S Industrial Highway
Suite A
Ann Arbor, MI 48104-8601
734-668-7447

Sherri Turner, Contact

3679 Alcohol Justice

24 Belvedere Street
San Rafael, CA 94901
415-456-5692; *Fax: 415-456-0491*
www.alcoholjustice.org

Bruce Lee Livingston, Executive Director
Michael Scippa, Public Affairs Director
Sarah M. Mart, MS, MPH, Director of Research
Karen Kuhn, Administrative Director

3680 Aldrich and Cox

3075 Southwestern Boulevard
Suite 202
Orchard Park, NY 14127-1287
716-675-6300; *Fax: 716-675-2098*
cox@aldrichandcox.com
www.aldrichandcox.com

Herbert C. Cox, Chairman
Charles H. Cox, President
James B. Hood, Jr, Exec. VP/ Secretary
Daniel C. Buser, J.D., CPCU, EVP

Aldrich and Cox provides independent, fee-based Risk Management, Insurance and Employee Benefit Consulting services to a wide range of clientele.

3681 Alliance Behavioral Care

PO Box 19947
Cincinnati, OH 45219-947
513-475-8622
800-926-8862
www.alliancebehavioral.com

Allen Daniels, CEO

Alliance Behavioral Care is a regional managed behavioral healthcare organization located in Cincinnati, Ohio. They are committed to continuously improving the resources and programs that serve their members and providers. Their goal is to provide resources that improve the well-being of those they serve and to integrate the behavioral healthcare within the overall healthcare systems.

3682 Allina Hospitals & Clinics Behavioral Health Services
2925 Chicago Avenue
Minneapolis, MN 55407-1321
612-775-5000
800-877-7878
www.www.allinahealth.org

Penny Ann Wheeler, MD, President, Chief Clinical Office
Duncan P. Gallagher, EVP, Administration, CFO
Christine Bent, SVP, Clinical Service Lines
Kenneth Paulus, CEO

Provides clinically and geographically integrated care delivery. Innovative programs and services across comprehensive continuum of care. Practicing guideline development, outcomes data and quality managment programs to enhance care delivery.

3683 American Managed Behavioral Healthcare Association
1325 G Street, NW
Suite 500
Washington, DC 20005
202-449-7660; *Fax:* 202-449-7659
info@abhw.org
www.www.abhw.org

Pamela Greenberg, MPP, President/CEO
Rebecca Murow Klein, Associate Director, Government A
Tim Murphy, President, CEO, Beacon Health St
Larry Tallman, President, MHN

Year Founded: 1994

3684 Analysis Group
111 Huntington Avenue
Tenth Floor
Boston, MA 02199
617-425-8000; *Fax:* 617-425-8001
agweb@analysisgroup.com
www.analysisgroup.com

Martha Samuelson, President/CEO
Bruce F Deal, Managing Principal
Stephen Cacciola, VP
Brian Ellman, VP

Provides economic, financial, and business strategy consulting to law firms, corporations and government agencies

Year Founded: 1981

3685 Aon Consulting Group
200 East Randolph Street
14th Floor
Chicago, IL 60601-6408
312-381-2738; *Fax:* 312-701-3100
www.aon.com

Mike Bungert, Chariman, AON Benfield
Gregory C Case, President, CEO
Laurel Meissner, SVP, Global Controller
Christa Davies, EVP, CFO

Aon Corporation is a leading provider of risk management services, insurance and reinsurance brokerage, human capital and management consulting, and specialty insurance underwriting.

3686 Arthur S Shorr and Associates
98 Golden Eye Lane
Port Monmouth, NJ 07758

818-225-7055
800-530-5728; *Fax:* 732-201-0794
expert@hospitalexperts.com

Arthur S Shorr, MBA, FACHE, Owner
Nancy Daniels, Senior Consultant-Principal
Tom Bojko, MD, MS, JD, Managing Partner
Debra Petracca, MBA, Executive Director

Consultants to health care providers.

3687 Associated Counseling Services
8 Roberta Drive
Dartmouth, MA 02748-2020
508-992-9376

Douglas Riley, Owner

3688 Barbanell Associates
3629 Sacramento Street
San Francisco, CA 94118-1731
415-929-1155; *Fax:* 415-929-8485

Harriet Barbanell, Owner

3689 Barry Associates
6807 Knotty Pine Drive
PO Box 3069
Chapel Hill, NC 27515-3069
919-490-8474; *Fax:* 765-381-1100
www.barry-online.com

John S Barry MSW MBA, President

Provides technical assistance services to behavioral health and social service organizations in the areas of performance measurement, survey research, program evaluation, compensation system design and other selected human resource management areas.

3690 Behavioral Health Care
155 Inverness Drive West
Suite 201
Englewood, CO 80112-1411
720-490-4400
877-349-7379; *Fax:* 720-490-4395
TTY: 855-364-1799
www.www.bhicares.org

Julie Holtz, Chief Executive Officer
Joe Pastor M.D., Medical Director

BHI is committed to excellence in mental health service delivery. They strive to promote recovery by focusing on the unique needs, strengths and hopes of consumers and families.

3691 Behavioral Health Care Consultants
12 Windham Lane
Beverly, MA 01915-1568
978-921-5968
mkatzenstein@bhcconsult.com
www.bhcconsult.com

Michael L Katzenstein, President
Robert A. DeNoble, Staff
Lincoln Williams, Staff

3692 Behavioral Health Management Group
1025 Main Street
Suite 708
Wheeling, WV 26003-2726
304-232-7232; *Fax:* 304-232-7245
user655349@aol.com

William R Coburn, Practice Manager

They offer a wide range of services for men, women, adolescents, and children. The professional staff specializes in mental and emotional disorders, marital and family counseling, group therapy, vocational counseling, alcohol and substance abuse, academic adjustment counseling, psychological testing, biofeedback, and hypnotherapy.

3693 Behavioral Health Services

2925 Chicago Avenue
Minneapolis, MN 55407-1321
612-775-5000
800-877-7878
www.allina.com

Penny Ann Wheeler, MD, President, Chief Clinical Office
Duncan P. Gallagher, EVP, Administration, CFO
Christine Bent, SVP, Clinical Service Lines
Kenneth Paulus, CEO

Provides clinically and geographically integrated delivery system, innovative programs and services across comprehensive continuum of care, practice guidelines development, outcomes data and quality management programs to enhance care delivery systems.

3694 Behavioral Health Systems

2 Metroplex Drive
Suite 500
Birmingham, AL 35209-6827
205-879-1150
800-245-1150; *Fax:* 205-879-1178
www.behavioralhealthsystems.com

Deborah L. Stephens, Founder, Chairman, CEO
Danny Cooner, President, Safety First
Kyle Strange, Executive Vice President/MCO
Mark Gordon, EVP, Finance and CFO

Provides managed psychiatric and substance abuse and drug testing services to more than 20,000 employees nationally through a network of 7,600 providers.

3695 Broward County Health Care Services

115 S Andrews Avenue
Room 302
Fort Lauderdale, FL 33301
954-357-6551; *Fax:* 954-468-3592
TTY: 800-995-8711
civilcitation@broward.org
www.broward.org/healthcare

Bertha Henry, County Administrator
Joni Armstrong Coffey, County Attorney
Evan Lukic, CPA, County Auditor

The Health Care Section of the Community Partnership Division provide mental health, primary health care, and special health care services, as well as funding, Mahogany Project, and the Ryan White Part A Program offices.

3696 Brown Consulting

121 N Erie Street
Toledo, OH 43604-5915
419-241-8547
800-495-6786; *Fax:* 419-241-8689
info@danbrownconsulting.com
www.danbrownconsulting.com

Daniel C Brown, Owner, President
Rhonda Willhight, VP, Operations
Ross Calvin, VP, Consulting
David Galbraith, CFO

Provides a full range of consulting services to behavioral healthcare providers. Has relationships with national, regional and state behavioral healthcare organizations.
Year Founded: 1987

3697 CBCA

10900 Hampshire Avenue S
Bloomington, MN 55438-2384
952-829-3500
800-824-3882; *Fax:* 952-946-7694
www.cbca.com

Mary Dixon, Senior VP

Provides total health plan management including 24 hours a day, seven days a week patient access and demand management, care management, behavioral health care management, disease management and disability workers' compensation management, all supported by QualityFIRST clinical decision guidelines. These services are electronically integrated with HRM's national provider networks and electronic claims management. HRM's clients include HMOs, hospital systems, insurance and self-insured plans, workers' compensation and disability plans and Medicare/Medicaid plans throughout the US, Canada and New Zealand.

3698 CIGNA Behavioral Care

11095 Viking Drive
Suite 350
Eden Prairie, MN 55344-7234
952-996-2000
800-334-8925; *Fax:* 952-996-2579

Keith Dixon, CEO

Provides behavioral care benefit management, EAPs, and work/life programs to consumers through health plans offered by large U.S. employers, national and regional HMOs, Taft-Hartley trusts and disability insurers.
Year Founded: 1974

3699 Cameron and Associates

6100 Lake Forrest Drive
Suite 550
Atlanta, GA 30328-3889
404-843-3399
800-334-6014; *Fax:* 404-843-3572

William Cameron, Owner

Assists troubled employees and their dependents in resolving personal problems in order to provide their employer a level of acceptable job performance and efficiency, and to provide a safe working environment for all employees.

3700 Carewise

1501 4th Avenue
Suite 700
Seattle, WA 98101-3624
206-749-1100
800-755-2136; *Fax:* 206-749-1125

Rishabh Mehrotra, President/CEO
John McCarty, Executive Vice President/CFO

3701 Casey Family Services

127 Church Street
New Haven, CT 06510-2001
203-401-6900; *Fax:* 203-401-6901
info@caseyfamilyservices.org
www.caseyfamilyservices.org

Raymond L Torres, Executive Director
Michael Brennan, Co-Chairman
Year Founded: 1976

3702 Center for the Advancement of Health
2000 Florida Avenue NW
Suite 210
Washington, DC 20009-1231
202-387-2829; *Fax:* 202-387-2857
info@cfah.org
www.cfah.org

Jessie C. Gruman, PhD, President, Founder
David Torresen, VP, Finance and Operations
Dorothy Jeffres, MBA.MSW, MA, Executive Director
Goldie Pyka, Communications Manager

3703 Century Financial Services
23 Maiden Lane
PO Box 98
North Haven, CT 06473
203-239-6364
www.www.centuryfinancialservices.com

William Giovanni, Sr., Director, Operations
Kim Colapietro, Director
William J. Giovanni, Jr., Director, Marketing and Sales
Donella Fields, Collection Manager

3704 Children's Home of the Wyoming Conference, Quality Improvement
1182 Chenango Street
Binghamton, NY 13901-1696
607-772-6904
800-772-6904; *Fax:* 607-723-2617
www.chowc.org

Robert K. Chip Houser, President and CEO
Maria Cali, VP, Education
Patricia Giglio, CFO/Chief Admin. Officer
Ann M. MacLaren, CFO

Works with social services, court systems, school systems for children who are at risk, have trouble in the home, or have been abused or abandoned.

3705 ChoiceCare
655 Eden Park Drive, Suite 400
Grand Baldwin Building
Cincinnati, OH 45202-6039
513-241-1400
800-543-7158; *Fax:* 513-684-7461
www.choicecare.com

3706 College Health IPA
5665 Plaza Drive
Suite 400
Cypress, CA 90630
562-467-5555
800-779-3825; *Fax:* 562-402-2666
TTY: 800-735-2929
info@chipa.com
www.chipa.com

Randy Davis, President/CEO
Kevin Gardiner, VP Of Financial Operations
Brian Wheelan, Executive Vice President for Cor
Dale Seamans, Director, Corporate Communicatio

Culturally sensitive mental health referral service.

3707 College of Dupage
425 Fawell Boulevard
Glen Ellyn, IL 60137-6599
630-942-2800; *Fax:* 630-942-2947
www.cod.edu

Sunil Chand, President
Robert L. Breuder, President
Thomas J. Glaser, SVP, Administration, Treasurer
Joseph Collins, EVP

3708 College of Southern Idaho
315 Falls Avenue
PO Box 1238
Twin Falls, ID 83303-1238
208-732-6221
800-680-0274; *Fax:* 208-736-4705
info@csi.edu
www.csi.edu

Jerry Beck, President
Dr. Jeff Fox, President
Jerry Gee, Executive VP/CAO
Mike Mason, VP, Administration

3709 Columbia Hospital M/H Services
2201 45th Street
W Palm Beach, FL 33407-2095
561-842-6141; *Fax:* 561-844-8955
www.columbiahospital.com

Valerie Jackson, CEO
Dana C. Oaks, CEO
Brenda Logan, CNO
Oon Soo Ung, CFO

250-bed acute-care facility with dedicated psychiatry, emergency psychiatry, geriatric psychiatry, inpatient and outpatient psychiatry, and partial day psychiatry units and programs.

3710 ComPsych
455 N City Front Plaza Drive
NBC Tower
Chicago, IL 60611-5322
312-595-4000
800-755-3050; *Fax:* 312-660-1057
mpaskell@compsych.com
www.compsych.com

Richard A Chaifetz, Chairman, CEO

Worlwide leader in guidance resources, including employee assistance programs, managed behavioral health, work-life, legal, financial, and personal convenience services. ComPsych provides services worldwide covering millions of individuals. Clients range from Fortune 100 to smaller public and private concerns, government entities, health plans and Taft-Hartley groups. Guidance Resources transforms traditionally separate services into a seamless integration of information, resources and creative solutions that address personal life challenges and improve workplace productivity and performance.

3711 Comprehensive Care Corporation
3405 W. Martin Luther King Jr. Blvd
Suite 101
Tampa, FL 33607
813-288-4808; *Fax:* 813-288-4844

John M Hill, CEO
Robert Landis, Chairman/CFO/Treasurer

Offers a flexible system of services to provide comprehensive, compassionate and cost-effective mental health and substance abuse services to managed care organizations both public and private. CompCare is committed to providing state-of-the-art comprehensive care management services for all levels and phases of behavioral health care.

3712 Consecra Housing Network
1900 Spring Road
Suite 300
Oak Brook, IL 60523-1480
630-766-3570

Tim Rhodes, President/CEO
Susan Sinderson, Vice President
Dave Opitz, Director of Business Development

Provides therapy services in Spanish for children, families and couples. Offers substance abuse treatment and educational groups for men who batter in English and Spanish. Provides comprehensive services to Latina victims of domestic violence and their children in Spanish.

3713 Corphealth
1300 Summit Avenue
6th Floor
Fort Worth, TX 76102-4414
817-333-6400
800-240-8388

Patrick Gotcher II, President/CEO
Brae Jacobson, COO
Michael Baker, CFO

3714 Corporate Health Systems
15153 Technology Drive
Suite B
Eden Prairie, MN 55344-2221
952-939-0911; *Fax:* 952-939-0990
www.corphealthsys.com

Bob Hanalon, President

Benefits consulting firm to partner with clients to find the most flexible and comprehensive benefits packages for their investments.

3715 Counseling Associates
106 Milford Street
Suite 501B
Salisbury, MD 21804
410-546-1692
888-546-1692; *Fax:* 410-548-9056

Anne Bass Kinlaw, MSW, LCSW, President
Janet Brown, Manager
Joan Guzi, LCPC, Staff
Carol Ireland, LCSW-C, Staff

Provides therapeutic counseling to help individuals lead productive and fulfilled lives.

3716 Counseling Corner
2116 Merrick Avenue
Suite 3008A
Merrick, NY 11566
917-670-6262

Cari Sans, Founder And Director
Shari D. Siegel, Counsellor

3717 Covenant Home Healthcare
3615 19th Street
Lubbock, TX 79410-1209

806-725-2328
806-725-0000
www.covenanthealth.org

Melinda Clark, CEO

Provides quality home care to patients when hospitalization may be unneccessary, or when the length of stay may be shorter than expected.

3718 Coventry Health Care of Iowa
211 Lake Drive
Newark, DE 19702-3320
302-283-6500
800-752-7242

Al Redmen, CEO

3719 Creative Health Concepts
One Grand Central Place
Suite 2022
New York, NY 10165-2017
212-697-7207; *Fax:* 212-697-3509
www.creativegroupny.com

Harry F. Blair, Vice Chairman
Ira N. Gottlieb, President/CEO
Sharon S. Adair, SVP
Dan Pfeiffer, SVP

3720 Cypruss Communications
430 Myrtle Ave
Suite A
Fort Lee, NJ 07024-3913
201-735-7730
800-750-5231
peterm@cypruss.com
www.cypruss.com

Peter Miller, VP/CFO

3721 Deloitte and Touche LLP Management Consulting
1700 Market Street
Philadelphia, PA 19103-3984
215-246-2300; *Fax:* 215-569-2441
www.www.deloitte.com/view/en_US/us/index.htm

Sharon Allen, Chairman
Barry Salzberg, CEO
Punit Renjen, Chairman of the Board, Deloitte
Joe Echevarria, CEO, Deloitte LLP

3722 DeltaMetrics
600 Public Ledger Building
150 S Independence Mall West
Philadelphia, PA 19106-3475
215-399-0988
800-238-2433; *Fax:* 215-399-0989
www.deltametrics.com

Jack Durell, M.D., President/CEO
John Cacciola, Ph.D., Senior Vice President, Scientifi
Paul Keller, VP, Business Development
Kathleen Geary, Director, Operations

National research, evaluation, and consulting organization dedicated to the improvement of substance abuse and other behavioral health care treatment.

3723 Diversified Group Administrators
6345 Flank Drive
PO Box 6250
Harrisburg, PA 17112-250
717-652-8040
800-877-6490; *Fax: 717-652-8328*

James Hoellman, Contact

3724 Dorenfest Group
455 N Cityfront Plaza Drive
NBC Tower Suite 2725
Chicago, IL 60611-5555
312-464-3000; *Fax: 312-467-0541*
info@dorenfest.com
www.www.dorenfest.com

Sheldon Dorenfest, CEO
Xiao Liu, Manager, Consulting Services
Wei-Tih Cheng, Strategic Advisor
Michael Cohen, Strategic Advisor

3725 Dougherty Management Associates Health Strategies
9 Meriam Street
Suite 4
Lexington, MA 02420-5312
781-863-8003
800-817-7802; *Fax: 781-863-1519*
mail@dmahealth.com
www.dmahealth.com

Richard H. Dougherty, Ph.D., CEO, Owner
Wendy Holt, M.P.P., Principal
D. Russell Lyman, Ph.D., Senior Associate
Lisa Feldman Braude, Ph.D., Senior Associate

Providing the public and private sectors with superior management conusulting services to improve healthcare delivery systems and manage complex organizational change.

3726 Dupage County Health Department
111 North County Farm Road
Wheaton, IL 60187-3988
630-682-7400; *Fax: 630-462-9261*
TDD: 630-932-1447
www.dupagehealth.org

Linda A. Kurzawa, President
Dr. Lanny F. Wilson, VP
Maureen Mc Hugh, Executive Director
Scott J. Cross, Secretary

3727 Echo Management Group
15 Washington Street
PO Box 2150
Conway, NH 03818-2150
603-447-8600
800-635-8209; *Fax: 603-447-8680*
info@echoman.com
www.echoman.com

John Raden, CEO

Provides financial, clinical, and administrative software applications for behavioral health and social service agencies; comprehensive, fully-intergrated Human Service Information System is a powerful management tool that enables agencies to successfully operate their organizations within the stringent guidelines of managed care mandates. Provides implementation planning, training, support and systems consulting services.

3728 Elon Homes for Children
1717 Sharon Road West
Charlotte, NC 28210
704-369-2500; *Fax: 704-688-2960*
www.elonhomes.org

Dr Frederick Grosse, President/CEO
Andrea Rollins, VP, Administration
Rose Cooper, VP, Institutional Performance
Jane Grosse, VP, Institutional Advancement

Provides over 1,000 children and families a year in North Carolina an excellent opportunity for safe haven, life skills and education
Year Founded: 1907

3729 Employee Assistance Professionals
1234 Summer Street
Stamford, CT 06905-5558
203-977-2446

3730 Employee Benefit Specialists
PO Box 11657
Pleasanton, CA 94588
888-327-2770
800-229-7683
www.www.ebsbenefits.com

Alan Curtis, Chairman/CEO
Curtis Fankhouser, President

3731 Employee Network
1040 Vestal Parkway E
Vestal, NY 13850-2354
607-754-1043
800-364-4748; *Fax: 607-754-1629*
www.eniweb.com

Gene Raymondi, Owner, Founder, CEO
Towhee V. Shupka, President, COO

3732 Entropy Limited
345 South Great Road
Lincoln, MA 01773-4303
781-259-8901; *Fax: 781-259-1255*
clientservices@entropylimited.com
www.entropylimited.com

Ron Christensen, Owner

Uses pattern recognition, statistics, and computer simulation to track past behavior, see current behavior and predict future behavior. Used by insuranch companies and the healthcare industry.

3733 Essi Systems
70 Otis Street
San Francisco, CA 94103-1236
415-252-8224
800-252-3774; *Fax: 415-252-5732*
essi@essisystems.com
www.sesystems.com

Esther Orioli, CEO
Karen Trocki, Research Director

3734 Ethos Consulting
3219 E Camelback Road
Suite 515
Phoenix, AZ 85018-2307
480-296-3801
conrad@ethosconsulting.com
www.ethosconsulting.com

Conrad E Prusak, President, Co-Founder
Julie Prusak, CEO, Co-Founder

3735 FCS
1711 Ashley Circle
Suite 6
Bowling Green, KY 42104-5801
502-782-9152
800-783-9152; *Fax:* 270-782-1055
admin@fcspsy.com
www.fcspsy.com

Bob Toth, President, CEO
Brian Browning, VP Of Client Services
Dale Taylor, VP, Client Services
Jason Honshell, VP, Client Services

3736 Findley, Davies and Company
One SeaGate
Suite 2050
Toledo, OH 43604-1525
419-255-1360; *Fax:* 419-259-5685
www.findleydavies.com

Marc Stockwell, VP, Market Leader

3737 First Consulting Group
1160 West Swedesford Road
Building One, Suite 200
Berwyn, PA 19312
800-345-7672
www.csc.com

Larry Ferguson, CEO
Thomas Watford, COO/CFO

Around the world and across the healthcare spectrum, First Consulting Group is transforming healthcare with better information for better decisions.

3738 Fowler Healthcare Affiliates
2000 Riveredge Parkway
Suite 920
Atlanta, GA 30328-4600
770-635-8758
800-784-9829; *Fax:* 770-261-6361

Frances J Fowler, Owner, President
Denese Estep, Senior Consultant
Elizabeth Forro, Director
Joanne Judge, Legal Consultant

Developed innovative solutions for managing cost of high cost patients.

3739 GMR Group
755 Business Center Drive
Suite 250
Horsham, PA 19044-3491
215-653-7401; *Fax:* 215-653-7982
www.gmrgroup.com

Barron J Ginnetti, CEO
Thomas Bishop, Vice President/COO

Provides strategic and tactical solutions to the marketing and sales challenges their clients face in the managed healthcare environment.

3740 Garner Consulting
630 North Rosemead Blvd
Suite 300
Pasadena, CA 91107-2138

626-351-2300; *Fax:* 626-351-2331
info@garnerconsulting.com
www.garnerconsulting.com

Gerti Reagan Garner, GBA, FL, President
John C. Garner, CEBS, CLU, CFC, CEO
Carl Isaacs, Principal
Zaven K. Kazazian, JD, CBC, Principal

Provides innovative consultation, which produces immediate, bottom line results and long term value.

3741 Gaynor and Associates
100 Whitney Avenue
New Haven, CT 06510-1265
203-865-0865; *Fax:* 203-865-0093
mlg110@columbia.edu

Mark Gaynor LCSW, Principal

Clinical social work provider, EAP services, and clinical practice. Specialty weight management
Year Founded: 1980

3742 Geauga Board of Mental Health, Alcohol and Drug Addiction Services
13244 Ravenna Road
Chardon, OH 44024-9012
440-285-2282
800-750-0750; *Fax:* 440-285-9617
mhrs@geauga.org
www.geauga.org

Jim Adams, Executive Director, CEO
Beth Matthews, Associate Director
Jim Mausser, Finance Manager
Sandy Cohn, Information Coordinator

3743 Glazer Medical Solutions
PO Box 121
Beach Plum Lane
Menemsha, MA 02552
508-645-9635; *Fax:* 508-645-3212
glazermedicalsol@aol.com
www.glazmedsol.com

William M. Glazer, M.D., President/Founder

Glazer Medical Solutions is a national medical education consortium that has facilitated a comprehensive matrix of medical education services since 1994.

3744 HCA Healthcare
1 Park Plaza
Nashville, TN 37203-6527
615-344-9551
www.hcahealthcare.com

Richard M. Bracken, Chairman
Samuel N. Hazen, VP, Operations
R. Milton Johnson, President, CEO
David G. Anderson, SVP, Finance and Treasurer

3745 HPN Worldwide
119 W Vallette Street
Elmhurst, IL 60126-4419
630-941-9030; *Fax:* 630-941-9064
info@hpn.com
www.hpn.com

Bob Gorsky, PhD, Owner
Rick Suray, Staff
Ben Gorsky, Staff
Jennifer Toreja, Staff

Year Founded: 1983

3746 HSP Verified
National Register of Health Service Psychologists
1200 New York Avenue NW
Suite 800
Washington, DC 20005-3893
202-783-7663; *Fax:* 202-347-0550
www.nationalregister.org

Judy E Hall, CEO
Andrew P. Boucher, Assistant Director
Julia Bernstein, Membership Coordinator
Katie Huppi, Finance and Administration Coord

Offers comprehensive, innovative credential verification services designed to help you find that precious time. It relieves health care providers and management of tedious administrative activities-leaving time and resources to focus on quality health care. Provides valuable information and cultivates alliances between cutting edge health care organizations/plans and qualified health care providers.

3747 Hays Group
1133 20th Street NW
Suite 450
Washington, DC 20036-3452
202-263-4000
info@hayscompanies.com

3748 Health Alliance Plan
2850 W Grand Boulevard
Detroit, MI 48202-2692
313-872-8100
800-422-4641; *Fax:* 313-664-8479
TDD: 800-649-3777
msweb1@hap.org
www.www.hap.org

James Connelly, President, CEO
Ronald Berry, Senior Vice President/CFO
Christopher Pike, SVP, COO
Mary Ann Tournoux, SVP, Chief Marketing Officer

3749 Health Capital Consultants
1143 Olivette Executive Pkwy
Saint Louis, MO 63132-3205
314-994-7641
800-394-8258; *Fax:* 314-991-3435
solutions@healthcapital.com
www.healthcapital.com

Robert James Cimasi, MHA, ASA, President, CEO
Todd Zigrang, MBA, MHA, ASA, President
Matthew J. Wagner, MBA, VP
John R. Chwarzinski, MSF, MAE, VP

3750 Health Decisions
409 Plymouth Road
Suite 220
Plymouth, MI 48170-1834
734-451-2230; *Fax:* 734-451-2835
www.healthdecisions.com

Si Nahra, PhD, Owner, President
Judy L. Mardigian, CEO
Michael Falis, Senior Software Engineer
Tina Pelland, MA, Audit Practice Leader

3751 Health Management Associates
5811 Pelican Bay Boulevard
Suite 500
Naples, FL 34108-2711
239-598-3131; *Fax:* 239-597-5794

Gary D Newsome, President, CFO
Kelly E Curry, Chief Financial Officer
Kerry Gillespie, EVP, Operations Finance

3752 HealthPartners
2701 University Avenue SE
Minneapolis, MN 55414-3233
952-967-7992
TTY: 612-627-3584

Mary Brainerd, President/CEO

3753 Healthwise
2601 N Bogus Basin Road
Boise, ID 83702-909
208-345-1161
800-706-9646; *Fax:* 208-345-1897
www.healthwise.org

Donald W Kemper, MPH, Founder, CEO
Jim Giuffre, MPH, President/COO
Molly Mettler, MSW, SVP
Karen Baker, MHS, SVP

3754 Healthy Companies
2101 Wilson Boulevard
Suite 1002
Arlington, VA 22201-3048
703-351-9901
www.healthycompanies.com

Robert Rosen, Owner, Chairman, CEO
Jim Mathews, Vice Chairman
Tony Rutigliano, President
Eric Sass, COO

3755 HeartMath
14700 W Park Avenue
Boulder Creek, CA 95006-9318
831-338-8500
800-711-6221; *Fax:* 831-338-8504
info@heartmath.org
www.www.heartmath.org

Bruce Cryer, President
Sara Childre, President, CEO
Rollin McCraty, Ph.D., EVP, Director of Research
Brian Kabaker, CFO, Director of Sales and Marke

HeartMath's Freze-Framer Interactive Learning System is an innovative approach to stress relief based on learning to change the heart rhythm pattern and create physiological coherence in the body. The Freeze-Framer has been widely used with clients to help them develop internal awareness, self-recognition and emotional management skills. Clients can learn to prevent stress by becoming aware of when the stress response starts and stopping it in the moment and taking a more active role in preventing stress, managing the emotions associated with stress, creating better health and improving performance.

3756 Helms & Company
1 Pillsbury Street
Suite 200
Concord, NH 03301-3556

603-225-6633; *Fax:* 603-225-4739
info@helmsco.com
www.helmsco.com

J Michael Degnan, President, Co-Founder
Deborah J. White, Senior Consultant, Principal
Susan A. Cambria, Associate
Jeffrey G. White, Associate

They are a New Hampshire based behavioral health management company offering managed behavioral healthcare services, community service programs, and employee assistance programs for health care insurers, members, employers and their employees.

3757 Horizon Behavioral Services

2941 South Lake Vista Drive
Lewisville, TX 75067-3801
972-420-8300
800-931-4646; *Fax:* 972-420-8252

Mike Saul, President

Provider of national managed care, utilization management and employee assistance programs. Horizon will work in collaboration with HMOs, insurance companies, employers and hospitals to develop seamless, cost-effective managed care services including practitioner panel formation, information system development, utilization management services, EAPs, outcomes measurement systems and sales and marketing functions.

3758 Horizon Mental Health Management

2941 South Lake Vista Drive
Lewisville, TX 75067-3801
972-420-8300
800-931-4646; *Fax:* 972-420-8383

Johan Smith, VP

Inpatient, outpatient, partial hospitalization and home health psychiatric programs.

3759 Human Behavior Associates

1350 Hayes Street
Suite B-100
Benicia, CA 94510
707-747-0117
800-937-7770; *Fax:* 707-747-6646
corporate@callhba.com
www.callhba.com

James Wallace PhD, President
Yolanda Calderon, Operations Manager

National provider of emploee assistance programs, managed behavioral healthcare services, critical incident stress management services, conflict management, organizational consultation, and substance abuse professional services. Maintains a network of 6500 licensed mental health care providers and 650 hospitals and treatment centers nationwide.

3760 Human Services Research Institute

2336 Massachusetts Avenue
Cambridge, MA 02140
617-876-0426
www.hsri.org

David Hughes, President
John Agosta, Executive Vice President
Julie Bershadsky, Dir., Aging and Disabilities
Teresita Camacho-Gonsalves, Co-Dir., Behavioral Health

Assists state and federal government to enhance services and support people with mental illness and people with developmental disabilities.

3761 Insurance Management Institute

6 Stafford Court
Mount Holly, NJ 08060-3281
609-267-8998; *Fax:* 609-267-2472
TIMInstitute@aol.com

Michael C Hill, Management Consultant/Author

3762 Interface EAP

10370 Richmond Avenue
Suite 1100
Houston, TX 77042
713-781-3364
800-324-4327; *Fax:* 713-784-0425
info@ieap.com
www.ieap.com

Fred Newman, CEO
Tina Pace, CFO

3763 Interlink Health Services

4660 Belknap Court
Suite 209
Hillsboro, OR 97124
503-640-2000
800-599-9119; *Fax:* 503-640-2028
administration@interlinkhealth.com
www.interlinkhealth.com

John M. Van Dyke, CEO
Sherrie Simmons, Director of Operations
Jill Miller, Assistant Vice President-Facilit
Elizabeth Grafton, Claims Director

3764 Intermountain Healthcare

36 S State Street
Salt Lake City, UT 84111
801-442-2000
contactus@imail.org
www.intermountainhealthcare.org

Charles W. Sorenson, MD, President, CEO
Laura S. Kaiser, Executive Vice President & COO
Greg Poulsen, Senior Vice President & CSO
Bert Zimmerli, Executive Vice President & CFO

3765 Jeri Davis International

PO Box 770534
Memphis, TN 38177-534
901-763-0696
jeri@jeridavis.com
www.jeridavis.com

Jeri Davis, Founder/President

3766 KAI Research, Inc.

11300 Rockville Pike
Suite 500
Rockville, MD 20852
301-770-2730; *Fax:* 301-770-4183
kai@kai-research.com
www.kai-research.com

Selma C. Kunitz, Ph D., President
Rene Kozloff, Executive Vice President
Patti Shugarts, Chief Operating Officer

3767 Lake Regional Health System
54 Hospital Drive
Osage Beach, MO 65065
573-348-8000
www.lakeregional.com

Michael E. Henze, CEO
Kevin McRoberts, SVP Of Operations
David Halsell, SVP of Financial Services, CFO
Joe Butts, SVP of Facility Services

3768 Lifespan
600 Frederick Street
Santa Cruz, CA 95062
831-469-4900; *Fax:* 831-469-4950
information@lifespancare.com
www.lifespancare.com

Pamela Goodman, President
Becky Peters, CEO
Saundie Isaak, Executive Director
Ute Howland, Lifespan Care Manager

Comprehensive care management for adults who need care.

Year Founded: 1983

3769 MCW Department of Psychiatry and Behavioral Medicine
8701 Watertown Plank Road
Milwaukee, WI 53226
414-955-8990; *Fax:* 414-955-6299

John R. Raymond, Sr., MD, President/CEO
Joseph Kerschner, MD, Dean/Executive Vice President
G. Allen Bolton, Jr., MPH, MBA, Senior Vice President & COO

3770 MHN
2370 Kerner Blvd.
San Rafael, CA 94901
415-491-7200
800-327-2133
TDD: 800-735-2929
mhnfeedback@mhn.com
www.mhn.com

Steven Sell, President/CEO
Juanell Hefner, COO

Provides high-quality, cost-effective behavioral health care services to the public sector.

3771 MHNet Behavioral Health
9606 N MoPac Expressway
Stonebridge Plaza I, Suite 600
Austin, TX 78759
888-646-6889; *Fax:* 724-741-4552
www.mhnet.com

Wesley Brockhoeft, President/CEO
Robert Wilson, CFO

Health care management and solutions company providing employee assistance programs (EAP), work life programs, managed behavioral health care and consulting services.

3772 Magellan Health Service
6950 Columbia Gateway Drive
Columbia, MD 21046-3308
410-953-1000
800-458-2740
www.magellanhealth.com

Barry M. Smith, Chairman / Chief Executive Offic
Jonathan N. Rubin, Chief Financial Officer
Gary D. Anderson, Chief Information Officer

Provides members with high quality, clinically appropriate, affordable health care which is tailored to each individual's needs.

3773 Managed Care Concepts
PO Box 812032
Boca Raton, FL 33481-2032
561-750-2240
800-899-3926; *Fax:* 561-750-4621
info@theemployeeassistanceprogram.com
www.theemployeeassistanceprogram.com

Beth Harrell, Corporate Contacts Director

Provides comprehensive EAP services to large and small companies in the United States and parts of Canada. Also provides child/elder care referrals, drug free workplace program services, consultation and training services.

3774 Maniaci Insurance Services
500 Silver Spur Road
Suite 121
Palos Verdes, CA 90275
310-541-4824
866-541-4824; *Fax:* 310-377-2016
mail@maniaciinsurance.com
www.maniaciinsurance.com

Dan Maniaci, Owner
Dan Maniaci, President
Kristy Maniaci, Director Of Operations

3775 McGladery
801 Nicollet Avenue
Suite 1100
Minneapolis, MN 55402
952-835-9930
800-274-3978; *Fax:* 952-921-7702
www.mcgladrey.com

Joe Adams, Managing Partner and Chief Execu
Mike Kirley, Chief Operating Officer
Doug Opheim, Chief Finance Officer
Bruce Jorth, Chief Risk Officer

3776 McKesson Technology Solutions
5995 Windwrad Parkway
Alphretta, GA 30005
404-338-6000; *Fax:* 404-338-5112

Patrick J. Blake, Executive Vice President and Gro
Jim Pesce, President, Enterprise Informatio
Patrick Leonard, President, McKesson Business Per
Emad Rizk, MD, President, McKesson Health Solut

3777 Mercer Consulting
200 Clarendon Street
Boston, MA 02116-5026
617-424-3930; *Fax:* 617-424-3300

M. Michele Burns, Chairman/CEO
Tom Elliott, Chief Operating Officer

3778 Midwst Center for Personal/Family Development
2550 University Avenue W
Suite 435-South
Saint Paul, MN 55114

651-647-1900; *Fax:* 651-647-1861
www.mentalhealthinc.com

Tim Quesnell, Administrator
Kari Droubic, Manager

3779 Mihalik Group

1300 W Belmont
Suite 500
Chicago, IL 60657
773-929-4276
www.themihalikgroup.com

Gary J. Mihalik, President and CEO
Melinda Orlando, Senior VP Operations
Michael Alcenius, VP, Accreditation Services
Cathie Abrahamsen, Senior Consultant

3780 Milliman, Inc

1301 Fifth Avenue
Suite 3800
Seattle, WA 98101-2646
206-624-7940; *Fax:* 206-340-1380
more.info@milliman.com
www.milliman.com

Jeremy Engdahl-Johnson, Media inquiries

Assist plans and payors in measuring and analyzing their healthcare costs arising from behavioral health conditions, identifying specific value opportunities, and designing innovative ways to obtain increased quality and value from behavioral health care delivery.

Year Founded: 1947

3781 Murphy-Harpst Children's Centers

740 Fletcher Street
Cedartown, GA 30125
770-748-1500; *Fax:* 770-749-1094
www.murphyharpst.org

Charles Troutman, Chief Executive Officer
Emily Saltino, Vice President Development
Shirley Richardson, Chief Financial Officer
Tia McKnight, Director of Compliance

3782 NASW-NC

412 Morson Street
Raleigh, NC 27601
919-828-9650; *Fax:* 919-828-1341
membership@naswdc.org

Kathy Boyd, Executive Director
Valerie Arendt, Associate Executive Director
Kay Castillo, Director of Advocacy, Policy & L
Kristen Carter, Office Manager

3783 National Empowerment Center

599 Canal Street
Lawrence, MA 01840
978-685-1494
800-769-3728; *Fax:* 978-681-6426
info4@power2u.org
www.power2u.org/

Daniel B. Fisher, MD, PhD, Chief Executive Officer
Oryx Cohen, MPA, Chief Operating Officer
Maria Ostheimer, Coordinator, Emotional CPR

A consumer/survivor/expatient-run organization that is dedicated to helping people with mental health issues, trauma, and/or extreme states. Their central message revolves around recovery, empowerment, and healing.

3784 Oher and Associates

10 Tanglewild Plaza
Suite 100
Chappaqua, NY 10514
917-880-6969
joher@oher.net
www.oherandassociates.com

Jim Oher, Founder
Joel Mausner, PhD, Associate
Sheryl Spanier, Associate
Janet Taylor MD, MPH, Associate

3785 Optimum Care Corporation

30011 Ivy Glenn Drive
Suite 219
Laguna Niguel, CA 92677-5018
949-495-1100; *Fax:* 949-495-4316
www.optimumcare.net

Edward A Johnson, CEO

3786 Options Health Care

240 Corporate Boulevard
Norfolk, VA 23502-4900
757-393-0859
www.valueoptions.com

Barbara B Hill, CEO
Michele Alfano, Chief Operating Officer

Specializes in creating innovative services for a full range of at-risk and administrative services only benefits, including behavioral health programs, customized provider and facility networks, utilization and case management, EAPs and youth services.

3787 PMHCC

123 S Broad Street
23rd Floor
Philadelphia, PA 19109-1029
215-546-0300; *Fax:* 215-732-1606
www.pmhcc.org

Bernard Borislow, Executive Director
Jay Centifanti, Treasurer

3788 PRO Behavioral Health

7600 E Eastman Avenue
Ste. 500
Denver, CO 80231-4375
303-695-8007
888-687-6755; *Fax:* 303-695-0100

Martin Dubin, Senior Vice President
Theodore Wirecki, Chair

A managed behavioral health care company dedicated to containing psychiatric and substance abuse costs while providing high-quality health care. Owned and operated by mental health care professionals, PRO has exclusive, multi-year contracts with HMOs and insurers on both coasts and in the Rocky Mountain region.

3789 PSIMED Corporation

725 Town & Country
Suite 200
Orange, CA 92868-4723
714-689-1544

Suzanne Beals, Contact

3790 Paris International Corporation
185 Great Neck Rd
Ste. 305
Great Neck, NY 11021-3352
516-487-2630; *Fax:* 516-466-6255
www.parisint.com

Stuart A. Paris, CIMA, AIF, Founder and President
Robert Testa, Vice President
Michael Paris, AIF
Mark Zigman, Investment Adviser Representativ

3791 Pearson
5601 Green Valley Drive
Bloomington, MN 55437-1187
952-681-3000
800-627-7271; *Fax:* 952-681-3549
pearsonassessments@pearson.com

Robert Whelan, President and Chief Executive Of
Gary Gates, PhD, Senior Vice President, Global Bu
Corey Hoesley, Vice President, Global Operation
Doug Kennedy, Senior Vice President, Finance a

pearson is a publisher of assessment tools and instructional materials in the special needs behavior management, speech, language, and mental health markets. Among their numerous products are the MMPI-2, million inventories, BASC-2, BASC monitor for ADHD, vineland adaptive behavior scales(vineland II) and the Peabody picture vocabulary test (PPVT-4).

3792 Persoma Management
2540 Monroeville Blvd
Monroeville, PA 15146-2329
412-823-5155; *Fax:* 412-823-8262
www.persoma.com

James Long, President
Richard Heil Jr., Staff Member

3793 Perspectives
20 N Clark Street
Suite 2650
Chicago, IL 60602-5104
312-558-5318
800-866-7556; *Fax:* 312-558-1570
info@perspectivesltd.com
www.perspectivesltd.com

Bernard S. Dyme, President & CEO, Principal
Terry Cahill, Vice President of Sales and Mark
Christopher Kunze, Chief Operations Officer
Maureen Dorgan-Clemens, Vice President of
Organizational

3794 Philadelphia Health Management
260 South Broad Street
18th Floor
Philadelphia, PA 19102-5085
215-985-2500; *Fax:* 215-985-2550
www.www.phmc.org

Richard J Cohen, President and Chief Executive Of
Wayne Pendleton, Chief Operating Officer
Marino Puliti, Chief Financial Officer
Tine Hansen-Turton, Chief Strategy Officer

3795 Pinal Gila Behavioral Health Association
2066 W Apache Trail
Suite 116
Apache Junction, AZ 85120-3733

480-982-1317
800-982-1317; *Fax:* 480-982-7320
www.pgbha.org

Sandie Smith, President
Bryan Chambers, Vice President

3796 Porter Novelli
7 World Trade Center
250 Greenwich Street, 36th floor
New York, NY 10007
212-601-8000; *Fax:* 212-601-8101
Darlan.Monterisi@porternovelli.com
www.porternovelli.com

Karen van Bergen, Chief Executive Officer, Senior
Brad MacAfee, President, North America, Senior
John Orme, Senior Partner, President, Asia-
Karen Ovseyevitz, President, Latin America, Senior

3797 Practice Management Resource Group
1564-A Fitzgerald Dr.
#246
Pinole, CA 94564
708-623-8202; *Fax:* 708-507-2932
info@medicalpmrg.com
www.medicalpmrg.com

Ron Rosenberg, President/Founder
Curt Hill, Chief Executive Officer
Donna Connolly, Vice President of Operations

3798 Preferred Mental Health Management
401 E. Douglas
Suite 505
Wichita, KS 67202-3411
316-262-0444
800-819-9571; *Fax:* 316-262-0003
www.pmhm.com

Courtney Ruthven, Owner

Offers managed care services and EAP services.

Year Founded: 1987

3799 ProMetrics CAREeval
480 American Avenue
King of Prussia, PA 19406-4060
610-265-6344; *Fax:* 610-265-8377
admin@prometrics.com
www.prometrics.com

Marc Duey, Owner

A joint venture formed by Father Flanagan's Home (Boys Town), Susquehanna Pathfinders and ProMetrics Consulting. These organizations combine years of experience as service providers and technical resource developers. Provides innovative ways to collect, store and analyze service outcome data to improve the effectiveness of your services.

3800 ProMetrics Consulting & Susquehanna PathFinders
480 American Avenue
King of Prussia, PA 19406-4060
610-265-6344; *Fax:* 610-265-8377
admin@prometrics.com
www.prometrics.com

Marc Duey, Owner

3801 Professional Risk Management Services
1401 Wilson Boulevard
Suite 700
Arlington, VA 22209-2434
703-907-3800
800-245-3333; *Fax:* 703-276-9530
www.prmsva.com

Martin Tracy, CEO
Joseph Detorie, Executive Vice President/CFO

3802 PsycHealth
PO Box 5312
Evanston, IL 60204-5312
847-864-4961
800-753-5456; *Fax:* 847-864-9930
administration@psychealthltd.com
www.psychealthltd.com

Janet O'Brien, Manager

Specialists providing mental health services, managed care
and referrals.

Year Founded: 1989

3803 Public Consulting Group
148 State Street
10th Floor
Boston, MA 02109-2589
617-426-2026
800-210-6113; *Fax:* 617-426-4632
info@publicconsultinggroup.com
www.www.publicconsultinggroup.com

Dan Heaney, Chief Financial Officer
Dina Wolfman Baker, Director of Marketing and Commun
Debra V. Clark, Corporate Facilities Director
Grant Blair, Director PCG Education

Year Founded: 1986

3804 Pyrce Healthcare Group
7325 Greenfield Street
River Forest, IL 60305-1256
708-383-7700; *Fax:* 708-383-7746
phg@pyrcehealthcare.com
www.www.pyrcehealthcare.com

Janice M Pyrce, President/Founder

A national consulting firm, founded in 1990, with a focus
on behavioral health. The firm specializes in strategic planning, market research, integrated delivery systems, business development, retreat facilitation and
management/organizational development. PHG offers significant depth of resources, with direct involvement of experienced senior staff. Clients include hospitals, healthcare
systems, academic medical centers, human service agencies, physician/allied practices, professional/trade associations and investor groups. The firm has over 200
organizations with locations in over 40 states.

3805 Quinco Behavioral Health Systems
720 North Marr Road
Columbus, IN 47201-6660
812-314-3400
800-266-2341; *Fax:* 812-376-4875
webmaster@centerstone.org
www.centerstone.org

Robert Williams, CEO

Nonprofit mental health care provider serving south central
Indiana. 24 hour crisis line and full continuum of mental
health services.

3806 Schafer Consulting
602 Hemlock Road
Coraopolis, PA 15108-9140
724-695-0652
ask@schaferconsulting.com
www.schaferconsulting.com

Steve Schafer, Owner

**3807 Seelig and Company: Child Welfare and
Behavioral Healthcare**
140 E 45th Street
19th Floor
New York, NY 10017-7143
212-655-3500; *Fax:* 212-655-3535
rmm@msf-law.com
www.meisterseelig.com

Mark J Seelig, President
Mercedes Medina, Operations Manager
Elizabeth Roe, Billing Manager
Yvette Pe¤a, HR Manager

Year Founded: 1994

3808 Specialized Therapy Associates
83 Summit Avenue
Hackensack, NJ 07601-1262
201-488-6678; *Fax:* 201-488-6224
Information@SpecializedTherapy.com
www.specializedtherapy.com

Dr.Vanessa Gourdine, PsyD, MSN, P, Director
Dr. Cynthia Orosy, Clinical Director
Polina Levit, LPC, Assistant Director
Rick Rothman, MSW, LCSW, Assistant Director

3809 Suburban Research Associates
107 Chesley Drive
Unit 4
Media, PA 19063-1760
610-891-7200; *Fax:* 610-891-9699
www.suburbanresearch.com

Nikki Thomas, Marketing Director
Maureen O'Donnell, Sr. Clinical Research Coordnator
Brett Brashers, Clinical Research Coordnator
Ashley Tegler, Clinical Research Coordnator

3810 Supportive Systems
25 Beachway Drive
Suite C
Indianapolis, IN 46224-8506
317-788-4111
800-660-6645; *Fax:* 317-788-7783
staff@supportivesystems.com

Pam Ruster, Owner

3811 The Kennion Group Inc
800 Corporate Parkway
Suite 100
Birmingham, AL 35242-2942
205-972-0110
866-241-1682; *Fax:* 205-969-1199
www.kennion.com

W. Hal Shepherd, President/CEO

3812 The Lewin Group
3130 Fairview Park Drive
Suite 500
Falls Church, VA 22042-4517
703-269-5500
877-227-5042; *Fax:* 703-269-5501
lisa.chimento@lewin.com
www.lewin.com

Lisa Chimento, CEO
Ann Osborn, Vice President
Robert Page, Vice President
Linda Shields, Vice President

The Lewin Group is a national health care and human service policy, research, and consulting firm with more than 40 years' experience delivering objective analyses and strategic counsel to federal, state, and local governments foundations, associations, hospitals and health systems providers and health plans.

Year Founded: 1970

3813 Towers Perrin Integrated Heatlh Systems Consulting
335 Madison Avenue
New York, NY 10017-4605
212-309-3400; *Fax:* 212-309-0975
www.towersperrin.com

John Haley, Chief Executive Officer
Julie Gebauer, Managing Director, Talent and Re
Tricia Guinn, Managing Director, Risk and Fina
Gene Wickes, Managing Director, Benefits

Managed behavorial health care consultants specializing in strategy and operations, clinical effectiveness, actuarial and reimbursement and human resources for both the provider and the payer sides.

3814 Traumatic Incident Reduction Newsletter
Traumatic Incident Reduction Association
5145 Pontiac Trail
Ann Arbor, MI 48105-9279
734-761-6268
800-499-2751; *Fax:* 734-663-6861
info@tir.org

Victor Volkam, Author

Traumatic Incident Reduction is a brief, person-sentered treatment for the affects of trauma and loss. This newsletter offers part of the larger subject of Applied Metapsychology, which addresses relationship, self-esteem and well-being issues of all sorts, including traumatic stress. Additional web site for TIR: www.tir.org.

16 pages 2 per year

3815 United Behavioral Health
425 Market Street
27th Floor
San Francisco, CA 94105-2406
415-547-5000
800-888-2998
www.unitedbehavioralhealth.com

Larry Renfro, CEO
Paul Bleicher, MD, PhD, Chief Executive Officer, Optum L
Stan Dennis, Executive Vice President, Physic
Karen Erickson, Executive Vice President, Chief

3816 University of North Carolina School of Social Work, Behavioral Healthcare
Tate-Turner-Kuralt Building
325 Pittsboro Street Cb#3550
Chapel Hill, NC 27599-3155
919-962-1225; *Fax:* 919-962-0890
ssw@unc.edu
www.http://ssw.unc.edu

Year Founded: 1920

3817 ValueOptions Jacksonville
10199 Southside Blvd
Building 100 Suite 300
Jacksonville, FL 32256-757
800-700-8646
www.valueoptions.com

Heyward R. Donigan, President and Chief Executive Of
Douglas Thompson, M.S., M.B.A., Executive Vice President and Chi
Kyle A. Raffaniello, Executive Vice President and Chi
Dan Risku, J.D., Executive Vice President and Gen

3818 ValueOptions Norfolk
240 Corporate Blvd
Norfolk, VA 23502-4900
757-459-5100
www.valueoptions.com

Heyward R. Donigan, President and Chief Executive Of
Douglas Thompson, M.S., M.B.A., Executive Vice President and Chi
Kyle A. Raffaniello, Executive Vice President and Chi
Dan Risku, J.D., Executive Vice President and Gen

Designs and operates innovative administrative and full-risk services for a wide range of behavioral health and chemical dependency programs, Medicaid, child welfare and other human services, and Employee Assistance Programs. Develops collaborative relationships with government agencies, community providers, consumer groups, health plans, insurers, and others to foster a deeper understanding of the needs of the various populations they serve. Develops child welfare programs based upon the principles of managed care.

3819 Vedder Price
222 North LaSalle Street
Chicago, IL 60601-1003
312-609-7500; *Fax:* 312-609-5005
www.vedderprice.com

Michael A. Nemeroff, President and CEO
Robert J. Stucker, Chairman
Dean N. Gerber, Vice Chair
Douglas M. Hambleton, Operating Shareholder

3820 VeriCare
4715 Viewridge Avenue
Suite 110
San Diego, CA 92123
858-454-3610
800-257-8715; *Fax:* 800-819-1655
contactus@vericare.com
www.vericare.com

Cindy Watson, President/CEO
Bennett O. Voit, Chief Financial Officer
Cammile C. Bird, Vice President, Sales and Market
Karim S. Chalhoub, Executive VP of Revenue and Syst

3821 VeriTrak
179 Niblick Road
Suite 149
Paso Robles, CA 93446-4845
800-370-2440
support@veritrak.com
www.veritrak.com

3822 Webman Associates
4 Brattle Street
Cambridge, MA 02138-3714
617-864-6769
www.webmanassociates.com

Dorothy Webman, Owner

3823 WellPoint Behavioral Health
9655 Graniteridge Drive
Sixth Floor
San Diego, CA 92123-2674
858-571-8100
800-728-9498

Lori Wright, Manager

Software Companies

3824 ADL Data Systems
9 Skyline Drive
Hawthorne, NY 10532-2100
914-591-1800; *Fax:* 914-591-1818
www.adldata.com

David Pollack, President
Aaron S. Weg, Software Development
Ulysses Fleming, Accounting Solutions
Dorothy Dreiher, Clinical Solutions

The most comprehensive software solution for MH/MRDD and the continuum of care. 38 modules to choose from. Designed to meet all financial, clinical, and administrative needs. For organizations requiring greater flexiblity and processing power. Ask about new Windows-based products utilizing the latest in technology, including bar coding, scanning, etc.

Year Founded: 1977

3825 AHMAC
4600 Linden Ave.
Mechanicsburg, PA 17055
717-730-7189

CareManager is a microcomputer based system targeted at small to medium sized HMOs, PPOs and PHOs as well as vertical markets such as Medicaid and managed mental health. Easily customized to meet the needs and requirements of the client.

Year Founded: 1983

3826 Accumedic Computer Systems
11 Grace Avenue
Suite 401
Great Neck, NY 11021-2427
516-466-6800
800-765-9300; *Fax:* 516-466-6880
info@accumedic.com
www.accumedic.com

Mark Kollenscher, President
John Teubner, Vice President

AccudMed EHR, is fully ONC certified. We know the complexities you encounter in your financial and clinical program management. Now you can focus on your mission of improving quality treatment.

3827 Agilent Technologies
5301 Stevens Creek Blvd
Santa Clara, CA 95051-7201
408-345-8886
877-424-4536; *Fax:* 408-345-8474
contact_us@agilent.com
www.agilent.com

William P. (Sullivan, President and Chief Executive Of
Ron Nersesian, Executive Vice President
Henrik Ancher-Jensen, Senior Vice President
Rick Burdsall, Senior Vice President

Clinical measurement and diagnostic solutions for healthcare organizations.

3828 American Medical Software
1180 South State
Route 157
Edwardsville, IL 62025-236
618-692-1300
800-423-8836; *Fax:* 618-692-1809
sales@americanmedical.com
www.americanmedical.com

Practice management software for billing, electronic claims, appointments and electronic medical records.

3829 American Psychiatric Press Reference Library CD-ROM
American Psychiatric Publishing, Inc.
1000 Wilson Boulevard
Suite 1825
Arlington, VA 22209-3901
703-907-7322
800-368-5777; *Fax:* 703-907-1091
appi@psych.org
www.appi.org

Robert E Hales, M.D., M.B.A., Editor-in-Chief
Saul Levin, M.D., M.P.A., CEO and Medical Director
Laura W. Roberts, M.D., Deputy Editor
John W. Barnhill, M.D., Associate Editor

$395.00

Year Founded: 1998

3830 Aries Systems Corporation
200 Sutton Street
North Andover, MA 01845-1656
978-975-7570; *Fax:* 978-975-3811
marketing@edmgr.com
www.www.editorialmanager.com

Lyndon Holmes, President

Provides technical innovations that empower all of the participants in the knowledge retrieval chain: publishers, database developers, librarians.

3831 Askesis Development Group
One Chatham Center
112 Washington Place, Suite 300
Pittsburgh, PA 15219-3458
412-803-2400; *Fax:* 412-803-2099
info@askesis.com
www.askesis.com

Sharon Hicks, President and Chief Executive Of
Bob Teitt, Vice President of Technology and
Beth Rotto, Vice President, Finance and Oper
Nicholas Carosella, MD, Physician Advisor

Askesis Development Group's PsychConsult is a complete informatics solution for behavioral health organizations: inpatient or outpatient behavioral health facilities, managed care organizations, and provider networks. PsychConsult is Windows NT based, and Y2K compliant. ADG development is guided by the PsychConsult Consortium, a collaborative effort of leading institutions in behavioral health.

3832 BOSS Inc
2639 N Downer Avenue
Suite 9
Milwaukee, WI 53211
414-967-9689
800-964-4789
bmiller@healthcareboss.com
www.healthcareboss.com

Bob Miller, President

Practice management software that is easy to use and is in more than 29,000 practices nationally. Outcome management software products for social workers and hospitals. *$1499.00*

Year Founded: 1986

3833 Beaver Creek Software
525 SW 6th Street
Corvallis, OR 97333-4323
541-752-5039
800-895-3344; *Fax:* 541-752-5221
www.www.beaverlog.com

Peter Gysegem, Owner

'The THERAPIST' practice management and billing software for Windows operating systems comes in Pro and EZ versions. The EZ version is powerful yet simple to use and is tailored to needs of smaller offices. The Pro version is designed to handle the complex needs of busy practices. Use Pro to create HIPAA compliant electronic insurance claims. Both versions let you have an unlimited number of providers at no additional cost. *$249.00*

Year Founded: 1989

3834 Behavioral Health Advisor
McKesson Clinical Reference Systems
One Post Street
San Francisco, CA 94104
415-983-8300
800-782-1334
consumerproducts@mckesson.com
www.mckesson.com

The Behavioral Health Advisor software program provides consumer health information for more than 600 topics covering pediatric and adult mental illness, disorders and behavioral problems. Includes behavioral health topics from the American Academy of Child and Adolescent Psychiatry. Many Spanish translations available. *$4.75*

Year Founded: 1998

3835 Behaviordata
20863 Stevens Creek Boulevard
Suite 580
Cupertino, CA 95014-2154

408-342-0600
800-627-2673; *Fax:* 408-342-0617
www.behaviordat.com

Diana Everstine, President
Dr David Nichols, Contact

3836 Bottomline Technologies
325 Corporate Drive
Portsmouth, NH 03801
603-436-0700
800-243-2528; *Fax:* 603-436-0300
info@bottomline.com
www.www.bottomline.com

Robert A. Eberle, President and Chief Executive Of
Kevin M. Donovan, Chief Financial Officer
Karen Brieger, Vice President, Human Resources
Eric Campbell, Senior Vice President, Strategic

Provides software solutions that enable organizations to achieve unprecedented speed, accuracy, functionality and quality in their document processes such as procure-to-pay, order-to-case, manufacturing and healthcare.

Year Founded: 1981

3837 Bull HN Information Systems
285 Billerica Road
Chelmsford, MA 01824
978-294-6000; *Fax:* 978-244-0085
www.www.bull.us

David W Bradbury, President

Provides solutions and services to key markets, including the public sector, finance, manufacturing, and telecommunications.

3838 CSI Software
3333 Richmond
2nd Floor
Houston, TX 77098-3007
713-942-7779
800-247-3431; *Fax:* 713-942-7731
sales@csisoftwareusa.com
www.csisoftwareusa.com

Frank Mc Duff, VP

CSI Software designs software for the membership industry utilizing the most sophisticated software technologies, coupled with unsurpassed and experience and support.

3839 Center for Health Policy Studies
214 Massachusetts Ave NE
Washington, DC 20002-4999
202-546-4400
info@heritage.org
www.heritage.org

Thomas A. Saunders III, Chairman
Richard M. Scaife, Vice Chairman
J. Frederic Rench, Secretary
David S. Addington, Group Vice President, Research

3840 Ceridian Corporation
3311 E Old Shackopee Road
Minneapolis, MN 55425-1640
952-548-5000
800-729-7655; *Fax:* 952-548-5100
www.ceridian.com

Stuart C. Harvey, Jr., Chairman
David Ossip, Chief Executive Officer

Dave MacKay, President
Lois M. Martin, Executive Vice President and Chi

A computer services and manufacturing company.

Year Founded: 1957

3841 Cincom Systems

55 Merchant Street
Cincinnati, OH 45246-3761
513-612-2769
800-224-6266; *Fax:* 513-612-2000
info@cincom.com
www.www.cincom.com

Thomas M Nies, Founder and CEO

Cincom provides software and service solutions that help our clients create, manage and grow relationships with their customers through adaptive e-business information systems.

3842 Client Management Information System
WilData Systems Group

255 Bradenton Avenue
Dublin, OH 43017-2546
614-734-4719
800-860-4222; *Fax:* 614-734-1063
cmis@wildatainc.com

A total Electronic Health Records (EHR) solution for behavioral health care organization like mental health centers, substance abuse providers, human service organizations, and family service agencies. Become 100% paperless by using CMIS in-house or by accessing our web based version called e-CMIS to minimize the up front capital expenditure and ongoing maintenance costs.

3843 CliniSphere version 2.0
Facts and Comparisons

77 Westport Plaza
Suite 450
Saint Louis, MO 63146-3125
317-735-5300
800-223-0554
www.factsandcomparisons.com

Arvind Subramanian, President & CEO
John Pins, Vice President, Finance
Denise Basow, MD, Vice President, General Manager
David A. Del Toro, Vice President and General Manag

Access to all information in a clinical drug reference library, by drug, disease, side-effects; thousands of drugs (prescription, OTC, investigational) all included; contains information from Drug Facts and Comparisons, most definitive and comprehensive source for comparative drug information.

3844 Clinical Nutrition Center

7555 E Hampden Avenue
Suite 301
Denver, CO 80231-4834
303-750-9454
www.clinicalnutritioncenter.com

Ethan Lazarus, M.D., President
Heather Thomas, P.A. -C., Physician Assistant

Our programs are based on the latest development in the field of nutrition, weight loss and weight control, behavior modification.

3845 CoCENTRIX

540 North Tamiami Trail
Sarasota, FL 34236-4823
941-306-4951; *Fax:* 941-954-2033
www.unicaresys.com

May Ahdab, Ph.D., Chief Executive Officer/Co-Found
Leigh Orlov, President/Co-Founder
Neal Tilghman, Senior Vice President, Product M
Jason Ochipa, CPA, Chief Financial Officer

UNI/CARE's mission is to offer enterprise-based solutions designed to improve clinical recovery outcomes, standardize workflows and maximize revenue cycles within a technical environment, fostering collaboration and informed decision-making. Pro-Filer is a .NETcentric Human Service Enterprise (HSE) platform designed to support the requirements of data processing and use by healthcare organizations providing an array of clinical services. It's viable in a single organization or across a consortium, offering users customized workflows, best practice guides, revenue management tools, and the ability to concurrently meet clinical and financial compliance standards.

Year Founded: 1981

3846 Computer Transition Services

3223 S Loop
Suite 556
Lubbock, TX 79423
806-793-8961
800-687-2874; *Fax:* 806-793-8968
www.www.ctsinet.com

David Baucum, Owner

Improve the life and business success of clients by providing integrated solutions and professional services to meet their technological and organizational needs.

3847 Cornucopia Software

PO Box 6111
Albany, CA 94706-111
510-528-7000
supportstaff@practicemagic.com
www.practicemagic.com

Providers of Practice MAGIC, the billing and practice management software that counts for your psychotherapy practice.

3848 Creative Solutions Unlimited

203 Gilman Street
PO Box 550
Sheffield, IA 50475-550
641-892-4466
800-253-7697; *Fax:* 641-892-4333
mkoch@csumail.com
www.creativesolutionsunlimited.com

Martha Koch, Vp

Reliable, comprehensive, intuitive, fully-integrated clinical software able to manage MDS 2.0 electronic submission, RUGs/PPS, triggers, Quick RAP's, survey reports, QI's, assessments, care plans, Quick Plans, physician orders, CQI, census, and hundreds of reports. Creative Solutions Unlimited provides outstanding toll-free support, training, updates, user groups, newsletters, and continuing education.

Year Founded: 1988

3849 DB Consultants
1259 Cedar Crest Blvd.
Suite 328
Allentown, PA 18103
610-820-0440; *Fax:* 610-820-7651
sales@dbconsultants.com
www.dbconsultants.com

AS/PC includes electronic claims submission. Healtcare professionals rely on AS/PC every day to help them provide quality care.

Year Founded: 1980

3850 DST Output
2600 Sw Blvd
Kansas City, MO 64108-2349
816-221-1234
800-441-7587

Steven J Towle, CEO
Frank Delfer, CTO
Jim Reinert, EVP Business Development

Providing a customer communications solution offering myriad benefits to healthcare payor organizations, including the ability to manage both inbound and outbound communications; ensure document control and content compliance; integrate data from portal entry; distribute data, information, and material to the right place and audience with integrity.

3851 DeltaMetrics
600 Public Ledger Building
150 South Independence Mall West
Philadelphia, PA 19106-3475
215-399-0988; *Fax:* 215-399-0989
mail@deltametrics.com
www.deltametrics.com

Jack Durell, MD, President/CEO
John Cacciola, Ph.D., Senior Vice President & Scientif
Richard Weiss, Ph.D., Director of Research and Evaluat
Kathleen Geary, Director of Operations

DeltaMetrics is now assisting treatment agencies to design and implement programs of Continuous Quality Improvement (CQI) within their systems of care.

3852 Docu Trac
20140 Scholar Drive
Suite 218
Hagerstown, MD 21742-6575
301-766-4130
800-850-8510; *Fax:* 888-415-7939
sales@quicdoc.com
www.www.docutracinc.com

Arnie Schuster, Owner

Offering Quic Doc clinical documentation software, a comprehensive software system designed specifically for behavioral healthcare providers.

Year Founded: 1993

3853 DocuMed
3518 West Liberty Road
Ann Arbor, MI 48103-9013
734-930-9053
800-321-5595
info@documed.com
www.www.documed.com

DocuMed 2002 is a comprehensive system for automated documentation of physician/patient encounters in ambulatory settings for solo practitioners or multiple physician groups.

Year Founded: 1988

3854 E Services Group
5115 Pegasus Court
Suite N
Frederick, MD 21704
301-698-1901; *Fax:* 301-698-1909

Dave Walsh, Owner

Our primary focus is on finding that perfect marriage of savvy business logic and technologies so that our healthcare IT applications solve the real world business problems of our clients.

3855 EAP Technology Systems
PO Box 1650
Yreka, CA 96097-1650
800-755-6965; *Fax:* 530-842-4778
info@eaptechnology.com
www.eaptechnology.com

Tom Amaral, Ph.D., Founder/President & CEO/Board Me
Roland Alden, Technology Development Director
Bob Watson, Business Strategy Advisor/Board
Wayne Larocque, Business Development/Capital Rai

Provider of technologies that automate work flow and enhance the business value of Employee Assistance Programs.

3856 Echo Group
519 17th Street
Suite 400
Oakland, CA 94612-3461
603-447-8600
800-635-8209; *Fax:* 603-447-8680
info@echoman.com
www.echoman.com

David Allen, Manager

Echo Group has been helping behavioral healthcare organizations to succeed in their missions of healing.

3857 Electronic Healthcare Systems
Ehs One Metroplex Drive
Suite 500
Birmingham, AL 35209
205-871-1031
888-879-7302; *Fax:* 205-871-1185
marketing@ehsmed.com
www.ehsmed.com

EHS develops and markets system solutions to a select group of physicians who are leading the way to clinical excellence and practice efficiency trhough automation.

Year Founded: 1995

3858 Entre Technology Services
1501 14th St W
#201
Billings, MT 59102
406-256-5700; *Fax:* 406-256-0201
www.entremt.com

Mike Keene, Owner
Ben McClintock, Network Administrator

Veronica Smith, Partner Relations and Customer S
Mike Niles, Senior Systems Engineer

Software applications and website development; off site backup solutions and disaster recovery; managed services; product sales; seminar room and classroom rental; and computer training.

Year Founded: 1984

3859 Experior Corporation

5710 Coventry Lane
Fort Wayne, IN 46804-7141
260-432-2020
800-595-2020; *Fax:* 260-432-4753
sales@experior.com
www.experior.com

J. Richard Presser, President & CEO

Experior provides Innovative Information systems to practice management and ASC marketplace. Out products, SurgeOn and EMS provide scheduling, case costing and billing.

Year Founded: 1978

3860 Family Services of Delaware County

600 North Olive Street
Media, PA 19063-2418
610-566-7540; *Fax:* 610-566-7677
www.fcsdc.org

Tracy Segal, Director Development

The Where to Turn Database is the most comprehensive listing of Non-Profit Human Service programs in the Delaware County area, the Young Resources Database is a condensed version of the above.

3861 First Data Bank

701 Gateway Blvd.
Suite 600
South San Francisco, CA 94080
650-827-4564
800-633-3453; *Fax:* 650-588-4003
cs@fdbhealth.com
www.firstdatabank.com

Donald M Nielsen, CEO

Provides thousands of drug knowledge base implementations ranging from pharmacy dispensing and claims processing to emerging applications including computerized physician order entry (CPOE), electronic health records (EHR), e-Prescribing and electronic medication administration records (EMAR).

3862 Gelbart and Associates

423 S Pacific Coast Highway
Suite 102
Redondo Beach, CA 90277-3731
310-792-1823; *Fax:* 310-540-8904
www.www.gelbartandassociates.com

Robert Cutrow, Contact

Comprehensive Psychological and Psychiatric services for individuals, families, couples and groups, treating: anxiety, depression, relationship conflicts and medication management.

3863 Genelco Software Solutions

325 McDonnell Boulevard
Hazelwood, MO 63042-2513

800-548-2040; *Fax:* 314-593-3517
info@genelco.com

Offers its flagship software systems in an ASP financial model. An ASP arrangement allows an organization to maintain control over operations without maintaining the software onsite.

3864 HSA-Mental Health

1080 Emeline Avenue
Santa Cruz, CA 95060-1966
831-454-4000; *Fax:* 831-454-4770
TDD: 831-454-2123
info@santacruzhealth.org
www.santacruzhealth.org

Exists to protect and improve the health of the people in Santa Cruz County. Provides programs in environmental health, public health, medical care, substance abuse prevention and treatment, and mental health. Clients are entitled to information on the costs of care and their options for getting health insurance coverage through a variety of programs.

3865 Habilitation Software

204 N Sterling Street
Morganton, NC 28655-3345
828-438-9455; *Fax:* 828-438-9488
info@habsoft.com
www.habsoft.com

Randy Herson, President

Personal Planning System, Windows-based computer program which assists agencies serving people with developmental disabilities with the tasks of person-centered planning; tracks outcomes, services and supports, assists with assesments and quarterly reviews, and maintains a customizable library of training programs. Also includes a census system for agencies which must maintain an exact midnight census, as well as an Accident/Incident system.

3866 Hanover Insurance

440 Lincoln Street
Worcester, MA 01653-0002
508-855-1000
800-853-0456; *Fax:* 508-853-6332
www.www.hanover.com

Frederick H Eppinger Jr, President and Chief Executive Of
Bruce Bartell, Chief Underwriting Officer - Cha
Mark R. Desrochers, Senior Vice President, President
David Greenfield, Executive Vice President and Chi

Offers hospice programs, rehabilitation groups and mental health services.

3867 Health Probe

5693 Bear Wallow Road
Suite 100
Morgantown, IN 46160-9315
765-346-3332
support@healthprobe.com
www.healthprobe.com

EMR created to eliminate the need for paper with electronic medical records.

3868 HealthLine Systems

17085 Camino San Bernardo
San Diego, CA 92127-5709
858-673-1700
800-733-8737; *Fax:* 858-673-9866

cs@healthlinesystems.com
www.healthlinesystems.com

Dan Littrell, CEO

Provide peerless information management solutions and services that maximize the quality and delivery of healthcare.

3869 HealthSoft

PO Box 536489
Orlando, FL 32853-6489
407-648-4857
407-648-4857; *Fax:* 407-426-7440
admin@healthsoftonline.com

CD - ROM and web based software for professionals on mental health nursing and developmental disabilities nursing.

3870 Healthline Systems

17085 Camino San Bernardo
San Diego, CA 92127-5709
858-673-1700
800-254-7347; *Fax:* 858-673-9866
sales@healthlinesystems.com

Dan Littrell, CEO

Provider of Document Management and Physician Credentialing software solutions.

3871 Healthport

120 Bluegrass Valley Parkway
Alpharetta, GA 30005-2204
770-360-1700
800-367-1500
www.healthport.com

Michael J. Labedz, President and Chief Executive Of
Brian M. Grazzini, Chief Financial Officer
Matt Rohs, Vice President and General Manag
Bill Matits, Senior Vice President of Sales

Develops and sells Companion EMR, an electronic medical record system that eliminates paperwork, improves accuracy of information, provides instant access to patient and clinical information, and helps cuts costs while increasing revenue.

3872 Hogan Assessment Systems

2622 East 21st Street
Tulsa, OK 74114-1768
918-293-2300
800-756-0632; *Fax:* 918-749-0635
www.info.hoganassessments.com

Robert Hogan, President
Aaron Tracy, Chief Operating Officer
Rodney Warrentfeltz, Ph.D., Managing Partner
Ryan Ross, VP of Global Alliances

Focuses on five dimensions of personality including emotional stability, extroversion, likeability, conscientiousness and the degree to which a person needs stimulation.

3873 IBM Global Healthcare Industry

404 Wyman Street
Waltham, MA 02451-1212
781-895-2911; *Fax:* 617-361-2485
tgaffin@us.ibm.com
www.ibm.com/industries/healthcare

IBM has been strategically involved in assisting the healthcare industry in addressing numerous IT challenges.

IBM provides clients and partners with the industry's broadest portfolio of technology, services, skills, and insight.

3874 InfoMC

101 W Elm Street
Suite G10
Conshohocken, PA 19428-2075
484-530-0100; *Fax:* 484-530-0111
info@infomc.com
www.infomc.com

JJ Farook, Chairman & CEO
Donald Gravlin, EVP Product Startegy & COO
Rick Jackson, SVP Global Wellness Solutions
Susan Norris, Senior Vice Presodent of Clinica

Develops software solutions for Managed Care organizations, EAP/Work-Life organizations, and Health and Human Services agencies.

Year Founded: 1994

3875 Informix Software
IBM Corporation

1 New Orchard Road
Armonk, NY 10504-1722
914-499-1900
800-426-4968
TTY: 800-426-3383
ews@us.ibm.com
www.ibm.com/software

IBM Informix® software includes a comprehensive array of high-performance, stand-alone and integration tools that enable efficient application and Web development, information integration , and database administration.

3876 Inhealth Record Systems

5076 Winters Chapel Road
Atlanta, GA 30360-1832
770-396-4994
800-477-7374; *Fax:* 770-396-0475
sales@inhealth.us
www.inhealthrecords.com

Sue Kay, President

Provides variety of record keeping system products for health care practices and organizations.

Year Founded: 1979

3877 Innovative Data Solutions

386 Newberry Drive
Suite 100
Elk Grove Village, IL 60007-2778
847-923-1926
www.idsincp.com

Mark Parianos, President/CEO

Provide effective web based and software solutions for business, small offices and fortune 500 clients.

Year Founded: 1991

3878 Integrated Business Services

736 N Western Ave
125
Lake Forest, IL 60045-1820
847-735-1690
800-451-5478
info@medbase200.com
www.www.medbase200.com

Sam Tartamella, Manager

A medical research and information marketing firm providing access to highly selectable medical databases.

Year Founded: 1982

3879 Keane Care
8383 158th Avenue NE
Suite 100
Redmond, WA 98052-3846
425-869-9000
800-426-2675; *Fax:* 425-307-2220
kim_A_Allen@keane.com

Thomas Weitzel, Executive
Jim Ingalls, Director Sales

Develops, markets, and supports a range of clinical and financial software.

Year Founded: 1969

3880 MEDCOM Information Systems
2117 Stonington Avenue
Hoffman Estates, IL 60169-2016
847-885-1553
800-213-2161; *Fax:* 847-885-1591
medcom@emirj.com
www.emirj.com

John Holub, President

Provides a wide variety of products and services to the independent physician clinic as well as the hospital and private clinical laboratories.

Year Founded: 1991

3881 MEDecision
601 Lee Road
Chesterbrook Corporate Center
Wayne, PA 19087-5607
610-540-0202; *Fax:* 610-540-0270
salesinfo@medecision.com
www.medecision.com

Scott A Storrer, CEO

Providing managed care organizations with powerful and flexible care management solutions. MEDecision's tools help managed care organizations improve care management processes and align more closely with their members and providers to improve the quality and cost outcomes of healthcare.

Year Founded: 1988

3882 McKesson HBOC
2700 Snelling Ave N
Roseville, MN 55113-1719
651-697-5900; *Fax:* 651-697-5910

Chris Bauleke, VP

Our products and services are designed to meet the information needs of all participants in the integrated health system.

3883 MedPLus
4690 Parkway Drive
Mason, OH 45040-8172
513-229-5500
800-444-6235
info@medplus.com
www.www.questdiagnostics.com

Richard A Mahoney, President
Thomas R Wagner, CTO
Philip S Present, II, COO

Developer and integrator of clinical connectivity and data management solutions for health care organizations and clinicians.

Year Founded: 1991

3884 Medai
Millenia Park One
4901 Vineland Rd Suite 450
Orlando, FL 32811-7192
321-281-4480
866-422-5156; *Fax:* 321-281-4499
www.www.medai.com

Steve Epstein, Owner
Diane Lee, EVP/Co Founder
Swati Abbott, President

Provides solutions for the improvement of healthcare delivery. Utilizing cutting-edge technology, payers are able to predict patients at risk, identify cost drivers for their high-risk population, predict future health plan costs, evaluate patient patterns over time, and improve outcomes.

Year Founded: 1992

3885 Medcomp Software
PO Box 16687
Golden, CO 80402-6010
303-277-0772; *Fax:* 303-277-9801
www.medcompsoftware.com

Developing and designing case management systems for a wide variety of applications.

Year Founded: 1995

3886 Medi-Span
8425 Woodfield Crossing Boulevard
Suite 490
Indianapolis, IN 46240-7300
317-735-5300
855-539-7686; *Fax:* 317-735-5350
medispan-support@wolterskluwer.com
www.medi-span.com

Arvind Subramanian, President & CEO, Wolters Kluwer
John Pins, Vice President, Finance, Clinica
Denise Basow, MD, Vice President, General Manager
David A. Del Toro, Vice President and General Manag

Medi-Span offers a complete line of drug databases, including clinical decision support and disease suite modules, application programming interfaces, and stand-alone PC products.

3887 Medical Records Institute
425 Boylston Street
4th Floor
Boston, MA 02116-3315
617-964-3923; *Fax:* 617-964-3926
peter@medrecinst.com
www.medrecinst.com

Peter Waegemann, CEO

Promote and enhance the journey towards electronic health records, e-health, mobile health, mental health assessment, and related applications of information technologies (IT).

Year Founded: 1983

3888 Medix Systems Consultants
236 E 161st Place
Suite D
S Holland, IL 60473-3374
708-331-1271; *Fax:* 708-331-1272
sales@imsci.com
www.imsci.com

Systems integration and development company committed
to client/server multi vendor(open systems) solutions for a
diverse vertical market ranging from education and
healthcare.

Year Founded: 1987

3889 Mental Health Connections
21 Blossom Street
Lexington, MA 02421-8103
617-510-1318
www.mhc.com

Robert Patterson, MD, Founder/Principal

Developer of medical management software for physicians
and research scientists. Their primary product is desigend
to identify drug interactions based on the mainstream of
drug metabolism research.

Year Founded: 1983

3890 Mental Health Outcomes
2941 S Lake Vista Drive
Ste. 100
Lewisville, TX 75067-3801
800-266-4440; *Fax:* 972-420-8215
johan.smith@horizonhealth.com
www.mho-inc.net

Johan Smith, VP Operations/Development

Designs and implements custom outcome measurement
systems specifically for behavioral helath programs through
its CQI Outcomes Measurement System. This system provides information for a wide range of patient and treatment
focused variables for child, adolesent, adult, geriatric and
substance abuse programs in the inpatient, partial hospital,
residential treatment and outpatient settings.

Year Founded: 1994

3891 Micro Design International
40 Cain Dr.
Brentwood, NY 11717
631-273-4200
800-228-0891
sales@mdi.com
www.mdi.com

Martin Legat, President

Provides optical (CD/DVD/MO) storage solutions through
innovative achivements, easy-to-use data access, and exceptional service and support.

Year Founded: 1978

3892 Micro Office Systems
3825 Severn Road
Cleveland, OH 44118-1910
216-297-1240; *Fax:* 216-297-1241
info@micro-officesystems.com
www.www.micro-officesystems.com

Norman Efroymson, Chief Executive Officer
Yosef Gold, Manger, PCG Product Group

Michael Post, Integration Solutions/ Chief Sof
Daniel Ostroff, Manager, Data Conversions
Year Founded: 1985

3893 Micromedex
6200 S Syracuse Way
Suite 300
Greenwood Village, CO 80111-4705
303-486-6444
800-525-9083; *Fax:* 303-486-6450
www.micromedex.com

Roy Martin, Executive Vice President and Chi
Tina Moen, PharmD, Chief Clinical Officer
Jill Sutton, Senior Vice President of Solutio
Brandy O'Connor, Vice President, Sales

A comprehensive suite of alerts, answers, protocols, and interventions directly addresses clinicians need for evidence-based information. This vital information is used to
support patient care and improve outcomes.

Year Founded: 1974

3894 Misys Health Care Systems
8529 Six Forks Road
Forum IV
Raleigh, NC 27615-2963
800-877-5678
www.www.allscripts.com

Paul M. Black, Chief Executive Officer and Pres
Rick Poulton, Chief Financial Officer
Dennis Olis, Senior Vice President, Operation
Brian Farley, SVP and General Counsel

Develops and supports software and services for physicians
and caregivers.

3895 MphasiS(BPO)
5353 N 16th Street
Suite 400
Phoenix, AZ 85016-3228
602-604-3100
888-604-3100; *Fax:* 602-604-3115
selse@eldocomp.com
www.eldocomp.com

Sally Else, President
Len Miller, Chief Operating Officer
David J Hawkes, Executive Vice President
Hossein Abdollahi, Senior Vice President of Profess

Focused on financial services, logistics and technology
verticals and spans across architecture, application development and integration, application management and business process outsourcing, including the operation of large
scale customer contact centers.

3896 National Families in Action
PO Box 133136
Atlanta, GA 30333-3136
404-248-9676; *Fax:* 404-248-1312
nfia@nationalfamilies.org
www.nationalfamilies.org

William F. Carter, Chairman of the Board
Sue Rusche, President and Chief Executive Of
Carol S. Reeder, Treasurer
Paula C. Kemp, Secretary

An interactive database of ever-changing names of drugs
that people use and abuse for illnesses.

Year Founded: 1977

3897 NetMeeting
Microsoft Corporation
Customer Advocate Center
One Microsoft Way
Redmond, WA 98052-8300
425-882-8080
800-642-7676; *Fax:* 425-936-7329
www.microsoft.com

Steve Ballmer, CEO

NetMeeting delivers a complete Internet conferencing solution for all Window users with multi-point data conferencing, text chat, whiteboard, and file transfer, as well as point-to-point audio and video.

3898 Netsmart Technologies
570 Metro Place N
Dublin, OH 43017-5317
614-764-0143
800-434-2642; *Fax:* 614-764-0362
www.ntst.com

Kevin Scalia, Executive Vice President, Corpor
Michael Valentine, Chief Executive Officer
Frances Loshin-Turso, Senior Vice President, Child & F
Doug Abel, Executive Vice President, Soluti

Offers information systems for mental health, behavioral and public health organizations.

3899 Northwest Analytical
111 SW 5th Avenue
Suite 800
Portland, OR 97204-3606
503-224-7727
888-692-7638; *Fax:* 503-224-5236
nwa@nwasoft.com
www.nwasoft.com

Bob Ward, Chief Executive Officer
Jim Petrusich, Vice President of Sales
T. Olin Nichols, Chief Financial Officer
Louis K. Halvorsen, Chief Technology Officer

Provides comprehensive SPC software tools meeting technically stringent mental health industry requirements.

Year Founded: 1980

3900 OPTAIO-Optimizing Practice Through Assessment, Intervention and Outcome
Harcourt Assessment/PsychCorp
19500 Bulverde Road
San Antonio, TX 78259-3701
210-339-5000
800-622-3231; *Fax:* 210-339-5046

Mike Cook, Executive

Provides the clinical information necessary for proactive decision making.

3901 Oracle
4150 Network Circle
Santa Clara, CA 95054-1778
650-960-1300
800-633-0925; *Fax:* 650-786-4557
www.oracle.com

Gregory M Papadopoulos, Executive VP

Provider of healthcare software.

Year Founded: 1982

3902 Oracle Corporation
500 Oracle Parkway
Redwood Shores, CA 94065-1675
650-506-7000
800-392-2999; *Fax:* 650-506-7200
www.oracle.com

Lawrence J Ellison, Chief Executive Officer
Safra A. Catz, President and Chief Financial Of
Mark Hurd, President
Dorian Daley, Senior Vice President, General C

PeopleSoft provides a range of applications from traditional human resources, payroll and benefits to financials.

Year Founded: 1977

3903 Orion Healthcare Technology
18047 Oak Street
Omaha, NE 68130
402-341-8880
800-324-7966; *Fax:* 402-341-8911
info@orionhealthcare.com
www.myaccucare.com

Bill Allan, Owner

Orion provides technology solutions to meet the ever changing needs of the healthcare industry. To accomodate the behavioral health field, Orion developed the AccuCare software system, a highly integrated and adaptive approach to the clinical practice environment. AccuCare enables clinicians to quickly realize value, effiency and standardization without disrupting their primary focus to provide excellence in health care.

3904 Parrot Software
PO Box 250755
W Bloomfield, MI 48325-755
248-788-3223
800-727-7681; *Fax:* 248-788-3224
support@parrotsoftware.com
www.parrotsoftware.com

Provide 60 different software programs for the remediation of speech, cognitive, language, attention, and memory deficits seen in individuals who have suffered aphasia from stroke or head injury.

Year Founded: 1981

3905 Psychological Assessment Resources
16204 North Florida Avenue
Lutz, FL 33549-8119
813-449-4065
800-331-8378; *Fax:* 813-961-2196
www.www4.parinc.com

Robert Smith Iii, President

This program produces normative-based interpretive hypotheses based on your client's scores. It produces a profile of T scores, a listing of the associated raw and percentile scores, and interpretive hypotheses for each scale. Although this program is not designed to produce a finished clinical report, it allows you to integrate BRS and SRI data with other sources of information about your client. The report can be generated as a text file for editing.

Year Founded: 1978

3906 Psychological Software Services
3304 W 75th St
Indianapolis, IN 46268

317-257-9672; *Fax:* 317-257-9674
nsc@netdirect.net

Comprehensive and easy-to-use multimedia cognitive rehabilitation software. Packages include 64 computerized therapy tasks with modifiable parameters that will accommodate most requirements. Exercises extend from simple attention and executive skills, through multiple modalities of visuospatial and memory skills. For clinical and educational use with head injury, stroke, LD/ADD and other brain compromises. Price range: $260-$2,500.

Year Founded: 1984

3907 QuadraMed Corporation

12110 Sunset Hills Road
Suite 600
Reston, VA 20190-5852
703-709-2300
800-393-0278; *Fax:* 703-709-2490
www.quadramed.com

Daniel Desaulniers, CA, President, Harris Quebec Public
Jim Dowling, EVP, Enterprise Self-Service Sol
David L. Puckett, EVP, Revenue Cycle & Enterprise
Vicki Wheatley, EVP, Enterprise Master Person In

3908 RCF Information Systems

4200 Colonel Glenn Highway
Suite 100
Beavercreek, OH 45431-1670
937-427-5680; *Fax:* 937-427-5689
administrator@rcfinfo.com
www.rcfinfo.com

Roger Harris, President

Healthcare software.

3909 Raintree Systems

28765 Single Oak Drive
Suite 200
Temecula, CA 92590
951-252-9400
800-333-1033
www.raintreeinc.com

Richard Welty, President/CTO

Provides practice management software for commerical, not-for-profit, government healthcare providers, rehabilitation facilities, and social service agencies.

Year Founded: 1983

3910 SPSS

233 S Wacker Drive
11th Floor
Chicago, IL 60606-6306
312-651-3000
800-543-2185; *Fax:* 312-651-3668
www.spss.com

Jack Noonan, CEO

Worldwide provider of predictive analytics software and solutions.

Year Founded: 1968

3911 Saner Software

4198 13th ST NW
Garrison, ND 58540
630-762-9440; *Fax:* 630-562-9443
sales@sanersoftware.com
www.sanersoftware.com

John Parkinson, Owner

Develops health practice management software.

Year Founded: 1988

3912 Sanford Health

PO Box M.C
Fargo, ND 58122-1
701-234-2000
800-437-4010
www.www.sanfordhealth.org

Roger Gilbertson, CEO
Craig Hewitt, CIO

MeritCare is able to track your employees' health trends due to a new software program called Occusource.

3913 Stephens Systems Services

267 5th Avenue
Suite 812
New York, NY 10016-7506
212-545-7788; *Fax:* 212-545-9081
www.stephenssystems.com

Mike Stephens, Owner

Provides healthcare software.

3914 SumTime Software®

1152 Galvez Ct. SE
Los Lunas, NM 87031
505-990-8356
888-821-0771; *Fax:* 505-866-9041

Is the practice management solution for health care professionals. We offer the most comprehensive means for preparing billing statements and tracking payments and maintaining records.

3915 SunGard Pentamation

3 West Broad Street
Bethlehem, PA 18018-6799
610-691-3616
866-905-8989

Provides secure and reliable K-12 student information systems, special education management, financial and human resource management software to school districts.

Year Founded: 1992

3916 Synergistic Office Solutions (SOS Software)

17445 E Apshawa Road
Clermont, FL 34715-9049
352-242-9100; *Fax:* 888-609-5514
sales@sosoft.com
www.sosoft.com

Seth R Krieger, PhD, President

Produce patient management software for behavioral health service providers, including billing, scheduling and clinical records.

Year Founded: 1985

3917 Thomson ResearchSoft

1500 Spring Garden Street, Fourth Floor
Philadelphia, PA 19130
215-823-6600
800-722-1227; *Fax:* 215-386-6362
www.scientific.thomsonrueters.com

Software for wherever research is performed worldwide including all leading academic, corporate and government institutions, healthcare.

3918 TriZetto Group
9655 Maroon Circle
Englewood, CO 80112
949-718-4940
800-569-1222; *Fax:* 949-219-2197
salesinfo@trizetto.com
www.trizetto.com

R. Andrew Eckert, CEO
Jude Dieterman, President/COO
Douglas E. Barnett, Chief Financial Officer
John Schaefer, Senior Vice President, Chief Leg

Focuses on the business of healthcare and offers a broad portfolio of technology products and services.

Year Founded: 1997

3919 Turbo-Doc EMR
6480 Pentz Rd.
Suite A
Paradise, CA 95969
530-877-8650
800-977-4868; *Fax:* 530-877-8621
turbodoc@turbodoc.com
www.turbodoc.net

Lyle B Hunt, CEO

An electronic medical record system designed to assist physicians and other health care workers in completing medical record tasks.

3920 Vann Data Services
1801 Dunn Avenue
Daytona Beach, FL 32114-1250
386-310-1702; *Fax:* 386-238-1454
sales@vanndata.com
www.vanndata.com

Janice Huffstickler, President

Healthcare practice software.

Year Founded: 1978

3921 Velocity Healthcare Informatics
8441 Wayzata Boulevard
Suite 105
Minneapolis, MN 55426-1349
800-844-5648

Ellen B White, President/CEO

Provides outcomes management system.

3922 VersaForm Systems Corporation
2505 Carmel Ave
Suite 210
Brewster, NY 10509
800-448-6975; *Fax:* 845-207-3067
www.versaform.com

Electronic medical records and practice management.

3923 Virtual Software Systems
PO Box 815
Bethel Park, PA 15102-815
412-835-9417; *Fax:* 412-835-9419
sales@vss3.com
www.vss3.com

Thomas Palmquist, Contact

Easy to use practice management, billing, and scheduling software. *$3500.00*

Information Services

3924 3m Health Information Systems
575 West Murray Boulevard
Salt Lake City, UT 84123-4611
801-265-4400
800-367-2447; *Fax:* 801-263-3657
www.solutions.3m.com

George W Buckley, CEO

3925 Accumedic Computer Systems
11 Grace Avenue
Suite 401
Great Neck, NY 11021-2427
516-466-6800
800-765-9300; *Fax:* 516-466-6880
info@accumedic.com

Mark Kollenscher, President

Practice management solutions for mental health facilities: scheduling, billing, EMR, HIPAA.

Year Founded: 1977

3926 American Institute for Preventive Medicine
30445 Northwestern Highway
Suite 350
Farmington Hills, MI 48334-3107
248-539-1800
800-345-2476; *Fax:* 248-539-1808
aipm@healthylife.com
www.healthylife.com

Don R. Powell, Ph.D., President and CEO

Year Founded: 1983

3927 American Nurses Foundation: National Communications
8515 Georgia Avenue
Suite 400
Silver Spring, MD 20910-3492
301-628-5000
800-274-4262; *Fax:* 301-628-5001
anf@ana.org
www.nursingworld.org

Karen Daley, PhD, RN, FAAN, President
Marla J. Weston, PhD, RN, FAAN, Chief Executive Officer
Cindy R. Balkstra, MS, RN, CNS-, First Vice President
Jennifer S. Mensik, PhD, RN, NEA-B, Second Vice President

3928 Arbour Health System-Human Resource Institute Hospital
227 Babcock Street
Brookline, MA 02446-6773
617-731-3200
www.www.arbourhealth.com

Gary Gilberti, CEO

3929 Arservices, Limited
5904 Richmond Highway
Suite 550
Alexandria, VA 22303

703-820-9000; *Fax:* 703-824-6438
info@arslimited.com

Jerry (Jay) McCargo, President & CEO
Robert Mortis, Chief Operating Officer
Kevin Batchelor, Chief Financial Officer

3930 Association for Ambulatory Behavioral Healthcare

247 Douglas Ave
Portsmouth, VA 23707-1520
757-673-3741; *Fax:* 757-966-7734
www.www.aabh.org

Mickey Wright, Executive Director
Christopher McGowan, President

Powerful forum for people engaged in providing mental health services. Promoting the evolution of flexible models of responsive cost-effective ambulatory behavioral healthcare.

3931 Behavioral Intervention Planning: Completing a Functional Behavioral Assessment and Developing a Behavioral Intervention Plan
Pro-Ed Publications

8700 Shoal Creek Boulevard
Austin, TX 78757-6897
512-451-3246
800-897-3202; *Fax:* 512-451-8542
general@proedinc.com
www.www.proedinc.com

Donald D Hammill, Owner

Provides school personnel with all tools necessary to complete a functional behavioral assessment, determine whether a behavior is related to the disability of the student, and develop a behavioral intervention plan. *$22.00*

3932 Breining Institute College for the Advanced Study of Addictive Disorders

8894 Greenback Lane
Orangevale, CA 95662-4019
916-987-0662; *Fax:* 916-987-9384
Suggestions@Breining.edu
www.breininginstitute.net

Kathy Breining, Administrator

3933 Brief Therapy Institute of Denver

7800 S. Elati Street
Suite 230
Littleton, CO 80120
303-426-8757
tayers@btid.com
www.btid.com

Marne Wine, Therapist

Our form of psychotherapy emphasizes goals, active participation between therapist and client, client strengths, resources, resiliencies and accountability of the therapy process.

3934 Buckley Productions

238 E Blithedale Avenue
Mill Valley, CA 94941-2083
415-383-2009
877-508-3979; *Fax:* 415-383-5031
buckleypro@aol.com

Richard Buckley, Owner

Alcohol and drug education handbooks, videos, and web-based products for safety sensitive employers, supervisiors and employees who are covered by the Department of Transportaion rules. We provide training materials for Substance Abuse Professional (SAPs) and urine collectors.

3935 CareCounsel

101 Lucas Valley Road
Suite 360
San Rafael, CA 94903
415-472-2366
888-227-3334; *Fax:* 415-507-1906
staff@carecounsel.com
www.carecounsel.com

Lawrence N. Gelb, Founder, President & CEO

3936 Catholic Community Services of Western Washington

100 23rd Avenue S
Seattle, WA 98144-2302
206-328-5696; *Fax:* 206-324-4835
info@ccsww.org
www.ccsww.org

Michael Reichert, President

3937 Center for Creative Living

2635 Walnut St
Denver, CO 80205
303-893-0552; *Fax:* 303-892-0507
cclro@aol.com
www.centerforcreativeliving.com

Diane Braun, Owner

3938 Central Washington Comprehensive M/H

PO Box 959
402 S 4th Ave
Yakima, WA 98902-3546
509-575-4200
800-572-8122; *Fax:* 509-575-4811

Rick Weaver, CEO

3939 Child Welfare Information Gateway

1250 Maryland Avenue, SW
8th Floor
Washington, DC 20024-2141
703-385-7565
800-394-3366; *Fax:* 703-385-3206
info@childwelfare.gov
www.childwelfare.gov

The clearinghouse serves as a facilitator of information and knowledge exchange; the Children's Bureau and its training and technical assistant network; the child abuse and neglect, child welfare, and adoption communities; and allied agencies and professions.

3940 Cirrus Technology

403 Chris Drive
Building 4 Suite H
Huntsville, AL 35802
256-539-2241; *Fax:* 256-539-4266
info@cirrusti.com
www.cirrusti.com

Jerry T Harris, President/CEO
Larry Waller, Vice President Finance

Judy Dunivant, Accounting Manager
Machisa Gaither, Humnan Resources

3941 Community Solutions
9015 Murray Avenue
Suite 100
Gilroy, CA 90520
408-842-7138; *Fax:* 408-778-9672
cs@communitysolutions.org
www.communitysolutions.org

Greg Sellers, Chair
Janie Mardesich, Vice Chair
Nancy Miller, Secretary
Mike Thompson, Treasurer

3942 Consumer Health Information Corporation
8000 Wespark Drive
Suite 120
McLean, VA 22102-3661
703-734-0650; *Fax:* 703-734-1459
www.consumer-health.com

Dorothy L Smith, President

Specialists in development of evidence-based patient education programs that increase patient safety & patient adherence.

Year Founded: 1983

3943 Control-O-Fax Corporation
3070 W Airline Highway
Waterloo, IA 50703-9591
319-234-4651
800-553-0070; *Fax:* 319-236-7332
www.controlofax.com

Ken Weber, Manager

3944 DCC/The Dependent Care Connection
500 Nyla Farms
Westport, CT 06880-6270
203-226-2680

3945 Dean Foundation for Health, Research and Education
2711 Allen Boulevard
Suite 300
Middleton, WI 53562-2287
608-250-1393
800-576-8773
www.www.deancare.com

Todd Burchill, Vice President of Strategy, Comm
Carolyn J Ogland, Vice President of Medical Affair
Steve R Caldwell, Vice President of Finance
W Gehren Rall, Vice President of Finance

The Dean Foundation is the non-profit research and education entity of DHS. The Foundation currently encompasses Dean's Educational Services Department, supports community service and health education projects, funds research grants, and conducts its own ancillary research including several outcomes management studies and computer-assisted, voice-activated programs for behavioral medicine.

3946 Dorland Healthcare Information
PO Box 25128
Salt Lake City, UT 84125-128
800-784-2332; *Fax:* 801-365-2300
info@dorlandhealth.com
www.dorlandhealth.com

Carol Brault, Vice President
Yolanda Matthews, Product Manager
David J DeJulio, Account Executive
Anne Llewellyn, Editor in Chief

3947 FOCUS: Family Oriented Counseling Services
PO Box 921
1435 Hauck Drive
Rolla, MO 65401-2586
573-364-7551
800-356-5395; *Fax:* 573-364-4898
www.rollanet.org

3948 Federation of Families for Children's Mental Health
9605 Medical Center Drive
Suite 280
Rockville, MD 20850-6390
240-403-1901; *Fax:* 240-403-1909
ffcmh@ffcmh.org
www.ffcmh.org

Sandra Spencer, Executive Director
Lizette Albright, Finance Director
Lynda Gargan, Senior Managing Director
Barbara Huff, Social Marketing

National family-run organization dedicated exclusively to children and adolescents with mental health needs and their families. Our voice speaks through our work in policy, training and technical assistance programs. Publishes a quarterly newsletter and sponsors an annual conference and exhibits.

3949 HSA-Mental Health
1080 Emeline Avenue
Santa Cruz, CA 95060-1966
831-454-4000; *Fax:* 831-454-4770
TDD: 831-454-2123
www.santacruzhealth.org

Exists to protect and improve the health of the people in Santa Cruz County. Provides programs in environmental health, public health, medical care, substance abuse prevention and treatment, and mental health. Clients are entitled to information on the costs of care and their options for getting health insurance coverage through a variety of programs.

3950 Hagar and Associates
164 W Hospitality Lane
San Bernardino, CA 92408-3316
903-583-7202
www.hagarandassociates.com

Dennis Hagar, Owner
Matt Hager, Owner

Provides clients with data, from national databases, of outcomes, patient demographics, and benchmark data. Can provide technology and/or automated data connection. Provides support in objective outcomes measurement.

3951 Healthcheck
3954 Youngfield Street
Wheat Ridge, CO 80033-3865
916-556-1880
msalvatore@hsf.ca

3952 INMED/MotherNet America
20110 Ashbook Place
Suite 260
Ashburn, VA 20147
703-729-4951; *Fax:* 703-858-7253
www.inmed.org

Paul c Bosland, Chairman
James R Rutherford, Treasurer
Wendy balter, Secretary
Linda Pfieffer, President

3953 Information Access Technology
1100 E 6600 S
Suite 300
Salt Lake City, UT 84121-7411
801-265-8800
800-574-8801; *Fax:* 801-265-8880
www.iat-cti.com

David H Rudd, CEO

3954 Lad Lake
PO Box 158
W350 S1401 Waterville Rd
Dousman, WI 53118-9020
262-965-2131; *Fax:* 262-965-4107
www.ladlake.org

Phil Zweig, President
Hon. Derek Mosley, Vice President
Sara Walker, Treasurer
john Mikkelson, Secretary

3955 Lanstat Incorporated
4663 Mason Street
Port Townsend, WA 98368
425-377-2540
800-672-3166; *Fax:* 425-334-3124
info@lanstat.com
www.lanstat.com

Landon Kimbrough, President
Sherry Kimbrough, VP/Co-Founder

Provides quality technical assistance to behavioral health
treatment agencies nationwide, including tribal and government agencies.

3956 Liberty Healthcare Management Group
401 E City Avenue
Suite 820
Bala Cynwyd, PA 19004
610-688-800
800-331-7122
liberty@libertyhealth.com
www.www.libertyhealthcare.com

Liberty provides individualized programs and a continuum
of services for psychiatric and substance abuse treatment at
our centers located throughout the Northeast, Oklahoma
and Florida. Liberty's commitment to medical excellence
within an environment of results-oriented care is evident in
our outstanding record of clinical success.

3957 Managed Care Local Market Overviews
Dorland Health
PO Box 25128
Salt Lake City, UT 84125-128
800-784-2332; *Fax:* 801-365-2300

Carol Brault, Vice President
Yolanada Mathews, Product Manager

David DeJulio, Account Executive
Anne Llewellyn, Editor in Chief

Delivers valuable intelligence on local health and managed
care marekts. Each of these 71 reports describes key market participants and competitive environment in one US
market, including information on: local trends in events,
key players, alliances among MCOs and providers, legislative developments, regulatory development, statistics on
Managed Penetration. *$475.00*

3958 Manisses Communication Group
Manisses Communications Group
208 Governor Street
Providence, RI 02906-3246
401-831-6020; *Fax:* 401-861-6370
www.manisses.com

Fraser Lang, President/Publisher
Paul Newman, Director Of Sales

3959 Medical Data Research
5225 Wiley Post Way
Suite 500
Salt Lake City, UT 84116-2825
801-536-1110

Karen Beckstead, Contact

3960 Medipay
521 SW 11th Avenue
Suite 200
Portland, OR 97205-2620
503-227-6491

3961 Meridian Resource Corporation
1401 Enclave Parkway
Suite 300
Houston, TX 77077-2054
281-597-7000; *Fax:* 281-597-8880

Paul Ching, CEO

3962 Microsoft Corporation
1 Microsoft Way
Redmond, WA 98052-8300
425-882-8080
800-642-7676; *Fax:* 425-936-7329
www.microsoft.com

Steve Ballmer, CEO

3963 NASW West Virginia Chapter
750 First Street
Suite 700
Washinton, DC 20002-4241
304-345-6279
800-227-3590
naswwv@aol.com
www.naswpress.org

Sam Hickman, Executive Director

**3964 National Council on Alcoholism and Drug
Dependence**
217 Broadway
Suite 712
New York, NY 10007
212-269-7797
800-622-2255
national@ncadd.org
www.ncadd.org

Andrew N. Pucher, President and CEO
Leah Brock, Director of Affiliate Relations
Jill Price, Director of Administration
Paul Warren, Executive Assistant

3965 National Families in Action
PO Box 133136
Atlanta, GA 30333-3136
404-248-9676
nfia@nationalfamilies.org
www.nationalfamilies.org

William F Carter, Chairman
Sue Rusche, President/Chief Executive Office
Carol S Reeder, Treasurer
Paula C Kemp, Secretary

3966 National Mental Health Self-Help Clearinghouse
1211 Chestnut Street
Suite 1207
Philadelphia, PA 19107-4103
215-751-1810
800-553-4539; *Fax:* 215-636-6312
www.mhselfhelp.org

Joseph Rogers, Executive Director
Susan Rogers, Director
Christa Burkett, Technical Assistance Coordinator
Britani Nestel, Program Specialist

3967 North Bay Center for Behavioral Medicine
1100 Trancas Street
Suite 244
Napa, CA 94558-2960
707-255-7786
www.behavioralmed.org

Frank Lucchetti, Psychologist

Represents comprehensive assessment and a balanced schedule of medical and/or psychological treatments for individuals with disabilities needing relief from chronic pain, disabling conditions and stress related to depression, anxiety, and unhealthy work, community or family conditions.

3968 On-Line Information Services
PO Box 1489
Winterville, NC 28590-1489
252-758-4141
800-765-8268
TDD: 866-630-6400
www.onlineinfoservices.com

3969 Open Minds
Behavioral Health Industry News
163 York Street
Gettysburg, PA 17325-1933
717-334-0538
877-350-6463; *Fax:* 717-334-0538
openminds@openminds.com
www.openminds.com

Provides information on marketing, financial, and legal trends in the delivery of mental health and chemical dependency benefits and services. Recurring features include interviews, news of research, a calendar of events, job listings, book reviews, notices of publications available, and industry statistics. *$185.00*

12 pages 12 per year ISSN 1043-3880

3970 Optum
Mail Route MN010-S203
6300 Olson Memorial Highway
Golden Valley, MN 55427-4946
763-595-3200
800-788-4863; *Fax:* 763-595-3333

David Elton, Senior VP

A market leader in providing comprehensive information, education and support services that enhance quality of life through improved health and well-being. Through multiple access points-the telephone, audio tapes, print materials, in-person consultations and the Internet-Optum helps participants address daily living concerns, make appropriate health care decisions, and become more effective managers of their own health and well-being.

3971 Our Town Family Center
4131 E 5th Street
Tucson, AZ 85711
520-323-1706; *Fax:* 520-323-9077

Sue Eggleston, Executive Director

A general social services agency which focuses on serving children, youth, and their families. We offer low or no cost assistance with counseling, prevention, services for homeless youth and runaways (their families too) mediation, services for at risk youth, residential programs, parent mentoring, and much more. Our Town has made a conscious decision to keep its services focused in Pima County, in order to better serve our community. We are nonprofit, and funded by United Way, private donations, and grants with the state, county and city.

3972 Ovid Online
Ovid Technologies
333 7th Avenue
New York, NY 10001-5004
212-563-3006
800-950-2035; *Fax:* 212-674-6301
sales@ovid.com
www.ovid.com

Karen Abramson, CEO

Online reference and database information provider. $.50/record

3973 Patient Medical Records
901 Tahoka Road
Brownfield, TX 79316-3817
806-637-2556
800-285-7627

3974 Penelope Price
4281 MacDuff Pl
Dublin, OH 43016-9510
614-793-0165

3975 Physicians' ONLINE
560 White Plains Road
Tarrytown, NY 10591-5113
914-333-5800

3976 Quadramed
12110 Sunset Hills Road
Suite 600
Reston, VA 20190-5852

703-709-2300
800-393-0278; *Fax:* 703-709-2490
www.quadramed.com

Duncan W James, CEO

3977 SilverPlatter Information
100 River Ridge Drive
Suite 200
Norwood, MA 02062-5041
781-769-2599; *Fax:* 781-769-8763
www.www.silverplatter.info

3978 Stress Management Research Associates
10609-B Grant Road
Houston, TX 77070-4462
281-890-6395
relax@stresscontrol.com
www.stresscontrol.com

Edward Charlesworth, Contact

3979 Supervised Lifestyles
2505 Carmel Ave
Suite 210
Brewster, NY 10509-1122
845-279-5639
888-822-7348; *Fax:* 845-279-7678

3980 Technical Support Systems
775 E 3300 S
Suite 1
Salt Lake City, UT 84106-4078
801-484-1283; *Fax:* 801-486-8246
www.tssutah.com

Harry Heightman, Manager

Year Founded: 1984

3981 Traumatic Incident Reduction Association
5145 Pontiac Trail
Ann Arbor, MI 48105-9279
734-761-6268
800-499-2751; *Fax:* 734-663-6861
info@tir.org
www.tir.org

Marian Volkman, President
Margaret Nelson, Vice-President
Frank A Gerbode, Developer of the Subject

Traumatic Incident Reduction is a brief, person-sentered treatmetn for the affects of all sorts of trauma and loss. It is part of the larger subject of Applied Metapsychology, which addresses relationship, self-esteem and well-being issues of all sorts, including traumatic stress. Additional web site for TIR: www.tirbook.com

3982 UNISYS Corporation
8008 Westpark Drive
McLean, VA 22102-3109
703-847-2412
www.www.unisys.com

J Edward Coleman, Charman
Quincy Allen, Chuef Marketing And Strategy Off
Dominick Cavuoto, President
Janet B Haugen, Chief Financial Officer

3983 Virginia Beach Community Service Board
289 Independence Blvd
#138
Virginia Beach, VA 23462-5492
757-437-6150

3984 Well Mind Association
1201 Western Ave
Seattle, WA 98101-2936
206-728-9770
800-556-5829; *Fax:* 206-728-1500
www.speakeasy.net

Well Mind Association distributes information on current research and promotes alternative therapies for mental illness and related disorders. WMA believes that physical conditions and treatable biochemical imbalances are the causes of many mental, emotional and behavioral problems.

Pharmaceutical Companies

Manufacturers A-Z

3985 Abbott Laboratories
100 Abbott Park Road
Abbott Park, IL 60064-3500
847-937-6100
www.abbott.com

Miles D White, Chief Executive Officer
Wallace C Abbot, Founder

Founded in 1890. Manufactures the following psychological drugs: Cylert, Desoxyn, Depakote, Nembutal, Placidyl, Prosom, Tranxene.

3986 Actavis
400 Interpace Parkway
Parsippany, NJ 07054
862-261-7000
www.www.watson.com

Paul M Bisaro, CEO

Manufactures the following medications: Ferrlecit, Quasense, Androderm, Nicotine Polacrilex Gum USP, Trelstar, Oxycodone and Acetaminophen Tablets USP, Oxytrol.

3987 Astra Zeneca Pharmaceuticals
1800 Concord Pike
PO Box 15437
Wilmington, DE 19850-5437
302-886-3000; *Fax:* 302-886-3119
www.astrazeneca-us.com

David Brennan, Executive Director, CEO
Simon Lowth, Chief Financial Officer
Tony Zook, EVP, Global Commercial
Martin McKay, President

Full range of products in six therapeutic areas; gastrointestinal, oncology, anesthesia, cardiovascular, central nervous system and respiratory.

3988 Bristol-Myers Squibb
345 Park Avenue
New York, NY 10154-28
212-546-4000; *Fax:* 212-546-4020
www.bms.com

Lamberto Andreotti, Chief Executive Officer
Charles Bancroft, EVP, Chief Financial Officer
Brian Daniels MD, Senior Vice President
Sandra Leung, General Counsel, Corp Secretary

Manufactures the following psychological drugs: Avapro, Enfamil, Abilify, Provachol, and Serzone.

3989 Cephalon
41 Moores Road
Frazer, PA 19355-1113
610-344-0200; *Fax:* 610-738-6590
humanresources@cephalon.com
www.cephalon.com

Frank Baldino Jr, CEO
Frank Baldino, Chairman/CEO

Manufactures the following pharmaceuticals: Provigil, Amrix, Fentora, Vivitrol, Trisenox, Nuvigil.

3990 Edgemont Pharmaceuticals, LLC
1250 Capital of Texas
Site 400
Austin, TX 78746
512-550-8555
888-594-4332; *Fax:* 512-329-2094
www.edgemontpharma.com

Douglas A Saltel, President & CEO

Manufactures Fluoxetine 60 mg tablets

3991 Eli Lilly and Company
Lilly Corporate Center
Indianapolis, IN 46285
317-276-2000
www.lilly.com

John C Lechleiter, Chairman, President & CEO
Ralph Alvarez, Executive Chairman
Katherine Baicker, Professor of Health Economics
Sir Winfried Bischoff, Chairman

Manufactures the following psychological drugs: Prozac, Ceclor, Zyprexa, Cialis, Strattera, and Symbyax.

3992 Forest Laboratories
909 Third Avenue
New York, NY 10022-4748
212-421-7850
800-947-5227; *Fax:* 212-750-9152
www.frx.com

Howard Solomon, Chairman, CEO

Manufactures the following psychological drugs: Lexapro, Benicar, Campral, Celexa, Namenda, Tiazac, and Viibryd.

3993 GlaxoSmithKline
5 Moore Drive
PO Box 13398
Research Triangle Park, NC 27709-3398
888-825-5249; *Fax:* 919-483-5249
www.gsk.com

JP Garnier, CEO

Manufactures the following psychological drugs: Lamictal, Paxil, Parnate, Zyban.

3994 Janssen
1125 Trenton-Harbourton Road
PO Box 200
Titusville, NJ 08560-1002
609-730-2000
800-526-7736
www.janssen.com

Timothy Cost, Senior VP Corporate Affairs

Janssen markets prescription medications for the treatment of schizophrenia and bipolar disorder. Medications include: Invega and Risperdal.

3995 Jazz Pharmaceuticals plc
3180 Porter Drive
Palo Alto, CA 94304
650-496-3777; *Fax:* 650-496-3781
www.jazzpharma.com

Bruce C Cozadd, Chairman & CEO
Robert M Myers, President
Matthew Young, SVP & Chief Financial Officer
Russell J Cox, Executive Vice President & Chief

Manufactures the following medications: Xyrem, Prialt, FazaClo, LuvoxCR

3996 Johnson & Johnson
One Johnson & Johnson Plaza
New Brunswick, NJ 08933-1
732-524-0400
www.jnj.com

William C Weldon, CEO

Manufactures the following: Concerta, Haldol, Reminyl, Daktarin, Ertaczo, Levaquin.

3997 King Pharmaceuticals
132 Windsor Road
Tenafly, NJ 07670
423-989-8000
800-776-7637; *Fax:* 972-9 8-5 09
comments@king-pharma.com
www.king-pharma.com

Brian A Markison, CEO
David Robinson, Senior Dir. Corporate Affairs

Manufactures some of the following medications: Sonata, Corgard, Cytomel, Humatin, Levoxyl, Procanbid, and Septra.

3998 Mallinckrodt
675 McDonnell Boulevard
St. Louis, MO 63042-2379
314-654-2000
www.www.mallinckrodt.com

Mark Trudeau, President & CEO
Matthew Harbaugh, Senior Vice President & CFO
Peter Edwards, Senior Vice President & General
Dr. Frank Scholz, Senior Vice President, Global Op

Manufactures the following psychological drugs: Dexedrine, Methylin, Anafranil and Restoril for insomnia.

3999 Merck & Co.
One Merck Drive
PO Box 100
Whitehouse Station, NJ 08889-0100
908-423-1000
www.merck.com

Kenenth C Frazier, Chair, President & CEO
Willie A Deese, EVP & President
Leslie A Brun, Chairman & CEO

Manufactures the following drugs: Remeron™ and Saphris

4000 Mylan
1000 Mylan Blvd
Canonsburg, PA 15317
724-514-1800
www.mylan.com

Robert J Coury, Chairman & CEO
Heather Bresch, Chief Executive Officer
Rajiv Malik, President
John D Sheehan, Chief Financial Officer

Manufactures the following psychological drugs: Ativan, BuSpar, Clonopin, Tranxene, Valium, Xanax, Xanax XR

4001 Novartis
400 Technology Square
Cambridge, MA 02139-3545
617-871-8000; *Fax:* 617-871-8911
www.novartis.com

Joerg Reinhardt, Chairman
Ulrich Lehner, Vice Chairman
Enrico Vanni, Vice Chairman
Joseph Jimenez, Chief Executive Officer

Manufactures the following products: Diovan, Glivec, Lamisil, Zometa, Focalin and more.

4002 Noven Pharmaceuticals
Empire State Building
350 Fifth Avenue, 37th Floor
New York, NY 10118
212-682-4420
www.www.noven.com

Kazuhide Nakatomi, Chairman
Takehiko Noda, Vice Chairman
Jeffrey F Eisenberg, Director

Manufactures the following mood disorder drugs: Daytrana, Stravzor, Pexeva, Lithobid

4003 Ortho-McNeil Pharmaceutical
1125 Trenton Harbourton Road
PO Box 200
Titusville, NJ 08560-1002
800-526-7736
www.www.janssenpharmaceuticalsinc.com

Manufactures the following: Elmiron, Modicon, Ortho-Novum, and Terazol 3.

4004 Pfizer
235 E 42nd Street
New York, NY 10017-5703
212-573-2323
800-879-3477
www.pfizer.com

Ian C Read, Chairman & CEO
Frank D Amello, Executive VP & CFO
Rady Johnson, Executive VP & Chief Compliance
Doug Lankler, Executive VP, General Councel

Manufactures the following psychological drugs: Geodon, Halcion, Navane, Navane IM, Neurontin, Reboxetine, Relpax, Sinequan, Vistaril, Xanax, Zoloft.

4005 Purdue
1 Stamford Forum
201 Tresser Boulevard
Stamford, CT 06901-3431
203-588-8000
800-877-5666; *Fax:* 203-588-8850
www.purduepharma.com

Mark Timney, President & CEO
Stuart D Baker, EVP, Counsel to Board
Edward B Mahony, EVP & CFO
David Long, Senior Vice President

Manufactures the following drugs: Betadine, Betasept, Butrans, Colace, Dilaudid, Dilaudid-HP, Intermezzo, MS Contin Tablets, Oxycontin, OxyIR, Peri-Colace, Ryzolt, Senokot, SenokotXTRA, Slow-Mag

4006 Roxane Laboratories
1809 Wilson Road
PO Box 16532
Columbus, OH 43216-6532
614-276-4000
800-962-8364; *Fax:* 614-308-3540
www.www.roxane.com

Manufactures detoxification medication: Dolophine.

4007 Sanofi-Aventis

55 Corporate Drive
Bridgewater, NJ 08807-1265
908-981-5000
800-981-2491; *Fax:* 908-231-4744
www.www.sanofi.us

Thomas Zerzan, President
Gregory Irace, Senior Vice President
David Meeker, Chief Executive Officer

Manufacturer of medication for cardiovascular disease, thrombosis, oncology, diabetes, central nervous system, internal medicine, and vaccines. Medication includes Wellbutrin, Wellbutrin SR, and Wellbutrin XL.

4008 Sepracor Pharmaceuticals

84 Waterford Drive
Marlborough, MA 01752-7010
508-481-6700
800-586-3782; *Fax:* 508-357-7491
www.www.sunovion.com

Hiroshi Nomura, Vice Chair, EVP, CFO
Anthony Loebel, MD, EVP and Chief Medical Officer
Albert P Parker, EVP, General Councel & Corporate
Richard Russell, EVP and Chief Commercial Officer

Manufactures sleep disorder drug Lunesta,as well as other medications Xopenex, and Brovana.

4009 Shire Richwood

5 Riverwalk
City West Business Campus
Dublin, PA 19087-5649
484-595-8800; *Fax:* 484-595-8200
www.www.shire.com

Matthew Emmens, Chairman
Flemming Ornskov, Chief Executive Officer
James Bowling, Interim Financial Officer

Manufactures the following psychological drugs: Adderall, DextroStat.

4010 Solvay Pharmaceuticals

901 Sawyer Road
Marietta, GA 30062-2250
770-578-9000; *Fax:* 770-578-5597
www.www.solvay.com

Jean-Pierre Clamadieu, Chairman & CEO
Karim Hajjar, Chief Fianancial Officer
Michael Defourny, General Manager Communications

Manufactures the following psychological drugs: Klonopin, Lithobid, Lithonate.

4011 Sunovion Pharmaceuticals

84 Waterford Drive
Marlborough, MA 01752
508-481-6700
888-394-7377; *Fax:* 508-357-7491
info@sunovion.com
www.sunovion.com

Hiroshi Nomura, Vice Chair, EVP, CFO
Anthony Loebel, MD, EVP and Chief Medical Officer
Albert P Parker, EVP, General Councel & Corporate
Richard Russell, EVP and Chief Commercial Officer

Manufactures the following drugs: Lunesta, Latuda

4012 Synthon Pharmaceuticals

9000 Development Drive
PO Box 110487
Research Triangle, NC 27709-5487
919-493-6006; *Fax:* 919-493-6104
info@synthon.com
www.www.synthon.com

Develops, produces and sells high quality alternatives to innovative medicines. Our products are marketed at the earliest possible opportunity and we sell them at competitive prices.

4013 Takeda Pharmaceuticals North America

One Takeda Parkway
Deerfield, IL 60015-5713
224-554-6500
877-582-5332; *Fax:* 847-383-3080
openpayments@takeda.com
www.www.takeda.us

Shinji Honda, CEO

Manufacturer of Rozerem, Duetact, Amitiza, and Actos.

4014 Valeant Pharmaceuticals International

2150 St. Elzear Blvd.
West Laval
Quebec, CA H7l4A
514-744-6792
800-361-1448; *Fax:* 514-744-6272
www.valeant.com

J Michael Pearson, Chairman & CEO
G. Mason Morfit, Partner
Dr. Pavel Mirovsky, President & General Manager
Fred Hasan, Partnr & Managing Director

Develops, manufactures and markets pharmaceutical products primarily in the areas of neurology, dermatology and infectious disease.

4015 Validus Pharmaceuticals

119 Cherry Hill Road
Suite 310
Parsippany, NJ 07054
973-265-2777; *Fax:* 973-265-2770
jhunter@validuspharma.com
www.validuspharma.com

James R Hunter, President
Lee Rios, Chief Operating Officer
Richard Post, Vice President - Sales and Marke

Manufactures the following psychological drugs: Marplan, Equetro.

4016 Warner Chilcott

400 Interpace Parkway
Parsippany, NJ 07054
862-261-7488
800-521-8813; *Fax:* 973-442-3204
investor.relations@actavis.com

Manufactures Sarafem

ADHD

Adjustment Disorders

Anxiety Disorders

Associations & Organizations

Autism Spectrum Disorders

Bipolar and Related Disorders

Clinical Management

Depressive Disorders

Disruptive, Impulse-Control and Conduct Disorders

Neurodevelopmental Disorders

Obsessive Compulsive Disorder

Personality Disorders

Professional & Support Services

Schizophrenia Spectrum and Other Psychotic Disorde

Sexual Disorders

Sleep-Wake Disorders

Somatic Symptom and Related Disorders

Substance-Related and Addictive Disorders

Suicide

Tic Disorders

E

H

O

T

U

Y

Z

NAATP National Association of Addiction Treatment Providers, 1416

National Academy of Neuropsychology (NAN), 2409

PRO Behavioral Health, 3788

TriZetto Group, 3918

University of Colorado Health Sciences Center, 3167

Yellow Ribbon Suicide Prevention Program, 1593

Connecticut

American Academy of Clinical Psychiatrists, 2300

American Academy of Psychiatry & Law Annual Conference, 2929

American Academy of Psychiatry and the Law (AAPL), 2302

American Academy of Psychoanalysis Preliminary Meeting, 2930

American Academy of Psychoanalysis and Dynamic Psychiatry, 2303

Casey Family Services, 3701

Century Financial Services, 3703

Connecticut Department of Mental Health and Addiction Services, 2129

Connecticut Department of Children and Families, 2130

First Candle, 128

Gaynor and Associates, 3741

Infoline, 1521

Institute of Living-Anxiety Disorders Center; Center for Cognitive Behavioral Therapy, 1783

Joshua Center Programs, 1861

Purdue, 4005

Stonington Institute, 3156

University of Connecticut Health Center, 3168

Women's Support Services, 1863

Yale Mood Disorders Research Program, 521, 627

Delaware

Astra Zeneca Pharmaceuticals, 3987

Coventry Health Care of Iowa, 3718

Delaware Department of Health & Social Services, 2131

Delaware Division of Child Mental Health Services, 2132

Delaware Division of Family Services, 2133

Mental Health Association of Delaware, 1864

National P.O.L.I.C.E. Suicide Foundation, 1588

District of Columbia

AAIDD Annual Meeting, 2924

ASAA A.W.A.K.E. Network, 1335

Administration for Children and Families, 2063

Administration on Aging, 2064

Administration on Intellectual and Developmental Disabilities, 2065

American Academy of Child and Adolescent Psychiatry (AACAP): Annual Meeting, 2928

American Academy of Child & Adolescent Psychiatry, 2299

American Academy of Child and Adolescent Psychiatry, 968, 1746, 3085, 3085

American Association of Homes and Services for the Aging, 2311

American Association of Retired Persons, 2314

American Association of Suicidology, 1583

American Association on Intellectual and Developmental Disabilities Annual Meeting, 1749, 2315, 2933, 2933

American Health Care Association, 2329

American Health Care Association Annual Convention, 2939

American Humane Association, 2331

American Managed Behavioral Healthcare Association, 3683

American Pharmacists Association, 2339

American Psychiatric Association, 1753

American Psychiatric Association (APA), 2340

American Psychologial Association: Division of Family Psychology, 2344

American Psychological Association, 1754, 2345

American Psychological Association: Applied Experimental and Engineering Psychology, 2346

American Psychology- Law Society (AP-LS), 2347

American Public Human Services Association, 1407

Association for Behavioral Health and Wellness, 1756

Association for Psychological Science (APS), 2369

Association of Black Psychologists, 2373

Association of Maternal and Child Health Programs (AMCHP), 2067

Association of Reproductive Health Professionals, 1266

Bazelon Center for Mental Health Law, 1759, 2376

Caregiver Action Network, 918

Center for the Advancement of Health, 3702

Community Action Partnership, 2386

DC Commission on Mental Health Services, 2134

DC Department of Behavioral Health, 2072

DC Department of Human Services, 2135

Department of Health and Human Services/OAS, 1867

Equal Employment Opportunity Commission, 2073

Federation of Associations in Behavioral and Brain Sciences, 920

Genetic Alliance, 1779

George Washington University, 3109

Gerontoligical Society of America, 2394

HSP Verified, 3746

Hays Group, 3747

Health & Medicine Counsel of Washington DDNC Digestive Disease National Coalition, 2136

Health and Human Services Office of Assistant Secretary for Planning & Evaluation, 2075

Human Rights Campaign, 879

Jacobs Institute of Women's Health, 3114

National Association For Children's Behavioral Health, 2410

National Association for Rural Mental Health, 1796

National Association of Councils on Developmental Disabilities, 922

National Association of Psychiatric Health Systems, 2416

National Association of Social Workers, 1874, 1973, 2418, 2418

National Association of State Alcohol/Drug Abuse Directors, 1418

National Business Coalition Forum on Health (NBCH), 2420

National Center for the Prevention of Youth Suicide, 1586

National Coalition for LGBT Health, 881

National Coalition for the Homeless, 1419, 2421

National Committee for Quality Assurance, 2422

National Council for Behavioral Health, 207, 1080, 1420, 1420, 1801

National Council on Aging, 2424

National Disability Rights Network, Inc., 1802

National LGBTQ Task Force, 884

National Organization on Fetal Alcohol Syndrome, 1424

National Pharmaceutical Council, 2426

National Register of Health Service Providers in Psychology, 2293, 2428

National Technical Assistance Center for Children's Mental Health, 977

PFLAG, 886

Pharmaceutical Care Management Association, 2431

President's Committee for People with Intellectual Disabilities, 2092

Presidential Commission on Employment of the Disabled, 2093

Psychology of Religion, 2436

Public Health Foundation, 2095

Society for Women's Health Research (SWHR), 2445

Society for the Psychological Study of Social Issues (SPSSI), 2447

The Center for Workplace Mental Health, 1818

The World Bank Group, 1820

US Department of Health and Human Services: Office of Women's Health, 2099

ZERO TO THREE: National Center for Infants, Toddlers, and Families, 984, 1826

Florida

Alliance for Eating Disorders Awareness, 785

Association for Women in Psychology, 2371

Behavioral Medicine and Biofeedback Consultants, 3091

Best Buddies International (BBI), 1761

Broward County Health Care Services, 3695

Cenaps Corporation, 2283

Center for Applications of Psychological Type, 2380

CenterLink, 876

CoCENTRIX, 3845

Columbia Hospital M/H Services, 3709

Comprehensive Care Corporation, 3711

Developmental Disabilities Nurses Association, 2390

Family Network on Disabilities, 1868

Federation of Families of Central Florida, 1869

Florida Alcohol and Drug Abuse Association, 1870

Florida Department Health and Human Services: Substance Abuse Program, 2137

Florida Department of Children and Families, 2138

Florida Department of Health and Human Services, 2139

Florida Department of Mental Health and Rehabilitative Services, 2140

Florida Health Care Association, 1871

Florida Medicaid State Plan, 2141

Food Addicts Anonymous, 855

Goodwill's Community Employment Services, 201, 680, 1073, 1073, 1134, 1193, 1364, 1412, 1683

Gorski-Cenaps Corporation Training & Consultation, 2395

Health Management Associates, 3751

HealthSoft, 3869

KidsHealth, 1020, 1664

Managed Care Concepts, 3773

Med Advantage, 2290, 2404

Medai, 3884

Mental Health Association of West Florida, 1872

Mental Health Corporations of America, 2407

National Alliance on Mental Illness: Florida, 1873

National Association of Addiction Treatment Providers, 2413

Parent Child Center, 3140

Psychological Assessment Resources, 3905

Synergistic Office Solutions (SOS Software), 3916

The National Association for Males with Eating Disorders, Inc., 799

The Selective Mutism Foundation Inc., 217

University of South Florida Research Center for Children's Mental Health, 3180

ValueOptions Jacksonville, 3817

Vann Data Services, 3920

Georgia

Association of State and Provincial Psychology Boards, 2374

Cameron and Associates, 3699

Centers for Disease Control & Prevention, 1641, 2071

DailyStrength: Tourette Syndrome Support Forum, 1665

Emory University School of Medicine, Psychology and Behavior, 3105

Emory University: Psychological Center, 3106

Fowler Healthcare Affiliates, 3738

Georgia Department of Behavioral Health and Developmental Disabilities (DBHDD), 2142

Georgia Department of Human Resources, 2143

Holy Cross Children's Services, 1929
Kleptomaniacs Anonymous, 715
Macomb County Community Mental Health, 1930
Michigan Association for Children with Emotional
   Disorders: MACED, 1931
Michigan Association for Children's Mental
   Health, 1932
Michigan Department of Community Health, 2185
Michigan Department of Human Services, 2186
National Council on Alcoholism and Drug
   Dependence: Greater Detroit Area, 1421, 2187
Parrot Software, 3904
Rapid Psychler Press, 2438
Southwest Solutions, 1934
The Shulman Center for Compulsive Theft,
   Spending & Hoarding, 687
Thriving Minds, 218
TransYouth Family Allies, 899
Traumatic Incident Reduction Newsletter, 3814
University of Michigan, 3176
Woodlands Behavioral Healthcare Network, 1935

Minnesota

Allina Hospitals & Clinics Behavioral Health
   Services, 3682
Behavioral Health Services, 3693
CBCA, 3697
CIGNA Behavioral Care, 3698
Ceridian Corporation, 3840
Corporate Health Systems, 3714
Department of Human Services: Chemical Health
   Division, 2188
Emotions Anonymous International Service Center,
   283, 629, 1774, 1774
HealthPartners, 3752
Healtheast Behavioral Care, 2287
Impulse Control Disorders Clinic, 712
International Restless Legs Syndrome Study
   Group, 1305
International Society for the Study of Women's
   Sexual Health (ISSWSH), 748, 1270
Lake Area Youth Services Bureau, 2189
McGladery, 3775
McKesson HBOC, 3882
Midwest Center for Personal/Family Development,
   3778
Minnesota Department of Human Services, 2190
NASW Minnesota Chapter, 1936
National Multicultural Conference and Summit,
   2948
North American Training Institute, 1938
Pacer Center, 1939
Pearson, 3791
Sexual Medicine Society of North America, 1273
Suicide Awareness Voices of Education (SAVE),
   1590
University of Minnesota Fairview Health Systems,
   3177
Velocity Healthcare Informatics, 3921

Mississippi

Mississippi Alcohol Safety Education Program,
   2191
Mississippi Department of Human Services, 2192
Mississippi Department of Mental Health: Division
   of Alcohol and Drug Abuse, 2193
Mississippi Department of Mental Health, 2194
Mississippi Department of Mental Health: Division
   of Medicaid, 2195
Mississippi Department of Rehabilitation Services:
   Office of Vocational Rehabilitation (OVR), 2196

Missouri

Bereaved Parents of the USA, 151
CliniSphere version 2.0, 3843
College of Health and Human Services: SE
   Missouri State, 3099
DST Output, 3850

Genelco Software Solutions, 3863
Health Capital Consultants, 3749
Lake Regional Health System, 3767
Mallinckrodt, 3998
Missouri Coalition for Community Behavioral
   Healthcare, 1942
Missouri Department Health & Senior Services,
   2197
Missouri Department of Mental Health, 2198
Missouri Department of Public Safety, 2199
Missouri Department of Social Services, 2200
Missouri Department of Social Services: Medical
   Services Division, 2201
Missouri Division of Alcohol and Drug Abuse,
   2202
Missouri Division of Comprehensive Psychiatric
   Service, 2203
Missouri Division of Developmental Disabilities,
   2204
Missouri Institute of Mental Health, 1943
National Share Office, 154
Ochester Psychological Service, 3138
Pathways to Promise, 1527
St. Louis Behavioral Medicine Institute, 3155
Traumatic Incident Reduction Workshop, 2950

Montana

Entre Technology Services, 3858
Mental Health America of Montana, 1945
Montana Department of Health and Human
   Services: Child & Family Services Division,
   2205
Montana Department of Human & Community
   Services, 2206
Montana Department of Public Health & Human
   Services: Addictive and Mental Disorders, 2207
Montana Department of Public Health and Human
   Services: Montana Vocational Rehabilitation
   Programs, 2208
National Alliance on Mental Illness: Montana,
   1946

Nebraska

Department of Health and Human Services
   Division of Public Health, 1947
Mutual of Omaha's Health and Wellness Programs,
   1948
Nebraska Department of Health and Human
   Services (NHHS), 2209
Nebraska Family Support Network, 1951
Nebraska Health & Human Services: Medicaid and
   Managed Care Division, 2210
Nebraska Health and Human Services Division:
   Department of Mental Health, 2211
Nebraska Mental Health Centers, 2212
Orion Healthcare Technology, 3903
Parent to Parent of Omaha, 978, 1952
Wellness Councils of America, 2452

Nevada

National Alliance on Mental Illness: Western
   Nevada, 1953
National Council of Juvenile and Family Court
   Judges, 2423
Nevada Department of Health and Human Services,
   2213
Nevada Division of Mental Health &
   Developmental Services, 2214
Nevada Employment Training & Rehabilitation
   Department, 2215
Nevada Principals' Executive Program, 1954
Northern Nevada Adult Mental Health Services,
   2216
Southern Nevada Adult Mental Health Services,
   2217

New Hampshire

Bottomline Technologies, 3836
Dartmouth Univerisity: Department of Psychiatry,
   3103
Echo Management Group, 3727
Helms & Company, 3756
Monadnock Family Services, 1955
New Hampshire Department of Health & Human
   Services: Bureau of Community Health
   Services, 2218
New Hampshire Department of Health and Human
   Services: Bureau of Developmental Services,
   2219
New Hampshire Department of Health and Human
   Services: Bureau of Behavioral Health, 2220

New Jersey

Actavis, 3986
Advocates for Children of New Jersey, 1957
American Society of Group Psychotherapy &
   Psychodrama, 2353
Arthur S Shorr and Associates, 3686
Asperger Autism Spectrum Education Network,
   315
Community Resource Council, 1958
Cypruss Communications, 3720
Disability Rights New Jersey, 1959
Insurance Management Institute, 3761
Janssen, 3994
Jewish Family Service of Atlantic and Cape May
   Counties, 1960
Johnson & Johnson, 3996
Juvenile Justice Commission, 2221
King Pharmaceuticals, 3997
Mental Health Association in New Jersey, 1961
Merck & Co., 3999
New Hope Foundation, 1812
New Jersey Association of Mental Health and
   Addiction Agencies, 1963
New Jersey Department of Human Services, 2222
New Jersey Division of Mental Health Services,
   2223
New Jersey Psychiatric Association, 1964
Ortho-McNeil Pharmaceutical, 4003
Psychohistory Forum, 2435
Sanofi-Aventis, 4007
Specialized Therapy Associates, 3808
UCSF Department of Psychiatry, Cultural
   Competence, 3160
Union County Psychiatric Clinic, 3163
University Behavioral Healthcare, 3164
Validus Pharmaceuticals, 4015
Warner Chilcott, 4016

New Mexico

American College of Mental Health Administration
   (ACMHA), 2321
National Alliance on Mental Illness: New Mexico,
   1956, 1962, 1965, 1965
New Mexico Behavioral Health Collaborative,
   2224
New Mexico Department of Health, 2225
New Mexico Department of Human Services, 2226
New Mexico Health & Environment Department,
   2227
New Mexico Kids, Parents and Families Office of
   Child Development: Children, Youth and
   Families Department, 2228
Overeaters Anonymous General Service Office,
   858
SumTime Software®, 3914

New York

ADL Data Systems, 3824
AHRC New York City, 967
Accumedic Computer Systems, 3826
Achieve Beyond, 314

North Carolina

North Dakota

Ohio

Oklahoma

Oklahoma Mental Health Consumer Council, 1992, 2238
Oklahoma Office of Juvenile Affairs, 2239

Oregon

Association of the Advancement of Gestalt Therapy, 2375
Beaver Creek Software, 3833
Center for Women's Health, 1269
Interlink Health Services, 3763
Marion County Health Department, 2240
National Alliance on Mental Illness: Oregon, 1993
Northwest Analytical, 3899
Oregon Department of Human Resources: Division of Health Services, 2241
Oregon Family Support Network, 1994
Oregon Health Policy and Research: Policy and Analysis Unit, 2242
Oregon Psychiatric Physicians Association, 1995
Portland University Regional Research Institute for Human Services, 3143
Postpartum Support International, 554
Research and Training Center for Pathways to Positive Futures, 980

Pennsylvania

AHMAC, 3825
American Anorexia & Bulimia Association of Philadelphia, 1996
American Association of Chairs of Departments of Psychiatry (AACDP), 2306
American Association of Directors of Psychiatric Residency Training, 2308
Askesis Development Group, 3831
Association for Hospital Medical Education, 2365
Bipolar Research Program at University of Pennsylvania, 519
Cephalon, 3989
Consumer Satisfaction Team, 2285
DB Consultants, 3849
Deloitte and Touche LLP Management Consulting, 3721
DeltaMetrics, 3722, 3851
Diversified Group Administrators, 3723
Family Services of Delaware County, 3860
First Consulting Group, 3737
GMR Group, 3739
Health Federation of Philadelphia, 1997
InfoMC, 3874
Kidspeace National Centers, 1023
Learning Disabilities Association of America, 1787
MEDecision, 3881
Medical College of Pennsylvania, 3126
Mental Health Association of Southeastern Pennsylvania (MHASP), 1998
Mylan, 4000
National Mental Health Consumers' Self-Help Clearinghouse, 132, 208, 335, 335, 489, 553, 684, 750, 796, 885, 923, 1137, 1197, 1272, 1309, 1367, 1423
PMHCC, 3787
Penn State Hershey Medical Center, 3141
Pennsylvania Alliance for the Mentally Ill, 2000
Pennsylvania Department of Human Services: Office of Mental Health and Substance Abuse Services, 2243
Pennsylvania Psychiatric Society, 2001
Persoma Management, 3792
Philadelphia Health Management, 3794
Pressley Ridge, 3145
ProMetrics CAREeval, 3799
ProMetrics Consulting & Susquehanna PathFinders, 3800
Schafer Consulting, 3806
Selective Mutism Research Institute, 211
Shire Richwood, 4009
St. Frnacis Medical Psych-Med Association, 3154
Suburban Research Associates, 3809
SunGard Pentamation, 3915

The Children's and Adult Center for OCD and Anxiety, 215, 1083
The SMart Center: Selective Mutism, Anxiety, & Related Disorders Treatment Center, 216
Thomson ResearchSoft, 3917
UNITE, Inc., 137
University of Pennsylvania Health System, 3179
University of Pennsylvania Weight and Eating Disorders Program, 854
University of Pittsburgh Medical Center, 2002
Virtual Software Systems, 3923
Western Psychiatric Institute and Clinic, 3185
Wordsworth, 3186

Rhode Island

AMERSA The Association for Medical Education and Research in Substance Abuse, 1402
American Academy of Addiction Psychiatry (AAAP), 1405, 2298
Byron Peter Foundation for Hope, 1584
Parent Support Network of Rhode Island, 2004
Rhode Island Council on Alcoholism and Other Drug Dependence, 2244
Rhode Island Department of Behavioral Healthcare, Developmental Disabilities and Hospitals, 2245
Rhode Island Division of Substance Abuse, 2246

South Carolina

Association of Traumatic Stress Specialists, 1681
Federation of Families of South Carolina, 2005
Medical University of South Carolina Institute of Psychiatry, Psychiatry Access Center, 3129
Mental Health America of South Carolina, 2006
South Carolina Department of Alcohol and Other Drug Abuse Services, 2247
South Carolina Department of Mental Health, 2248
South Carolina Department of Social Services, 2249

South Dakota

National Alliance on Mental Illness: South Dakota, 2009
South Dakota Department of Social Services Office of Medical Services, 2250
South Dakota Human Services Center, 2251

Tennessee

Bureau of TennCare: State of Tennessee, 2252
Council for Alcohol & Drug Abuse Services (CADAS), 2253
Genesis Learning Center (Devereux), 3108
HCA Healthcare, 3744
Jeri Davis International, 3765
Meharry Medical College, 3130
Memphis Alcohol and Drug Council, 2254
Memphis Business Group on Health, 2010
Middle Tennessee Mental Health Institute, 2255
Tennessee Association of Mental Health Organization, 2012
Tennessee Commission on Children and Youth, 2256
Tennessee Department of Health, 2257
Tennessee Department of Human Services, 2258
Tennessee Mental Health Consumers' Association, 2013
Tennessee Voices for Children, 2014
The Jason Foundation, Inc., 1592
Vanderbilt University: John F Kennedy Center for Research on Human Development, 2015

Texas

American Association of Community Psychiatrists (AACP), 2305
American College of Psychoanalysts (ACPA), 2324

American Pediatric Society, 970, 1752
American Society for Adolescent Psychiatry (ASAP), 2349
Association for Child Psychoanalysis (ACP) Annual Meeting, 2364, 2942
CSI Software, 3838
Children's Mental Health Partnership, 2016
Computer Transition Services, 3846
Corphealth, 3713
Covenant Home Healthcare, 3717
Depression and Bipolar Support Alliance Greater Houston, 2017
Edgemont Pharmaceuticals, LLC, 3990
Eye Movement Desensitization and Reprocessing International Association (EMDRIA), 1775
Group for the Advancement of Psychiatry, 2396
Horizon Behavioral Services, 3757
Horizon Mental Health Management, 3758
Interface EAP, 3762
International Society for Developmental Psychobiology, 2400
Jewish Family Service of Dallas, 2018
Jewish Family Service of San Antonio, 2019
M.I.S.S. Foundation/Center for Loss & Trauma, 130
MADD-Mothers Against Drunk Drivers, 1523
MHNet Behavioral Health, 3771
Menninger Clinic, 1790, 3131
Mental Health America of Greater Dallas, 2020
Mental Health America of Southeast Texas, 2021
Mental Health America of Texas, 2022
Mental Health Outcomes, 3890
National Alliance on Mental Illness: Texas, 2023
OPTAIO-Optimizing Practice Through Assessment, Intervention and Outcome, 3900
PRIMA ADD Corp., 3139
Research Society on Alcoholism, 1425
Restless Legs Syndrome Foundation, Inc., 1311
Society for Pediatric Research, 981
Survivors of Loved Ones' Suicides (SOLOS), 135, 157, 1591, 1591
Texas Commission on Alcohol and Drug Abuse, 2259
Texas Counseling Association (TCA), 2024
Texas Department of Family and Protective Services, 2260
Texas Psychological Association, 2025
Texas Society of Psychiatric Physicians, 2026
The Harris Center for Mental Health and IDD, 2261
University of Texas Medical Branch Managed Care, 3181
University of Texas Southwestern Medical Center, 2027
University of Texas: Mental Health Clinical Research Center, 626

Utah

CompHealth Credentialing, 2284
Healthwise of Utah, 2028
Intermountain Healthcare, 3764
National Alliance on Mental Illness: Utah, 2029
University of Utah Neuropsychiatric, 3182
Utah Department of Health, 2262
Utah Department of Health: Health Care Financing, 2263
Utah Department of Human Services, 2264
Utah Department of Human Services: Division of Substance Abuse And Mental Health, 2265
Utah Division of Substance Abuse and Mental Health, 2266
Utah Parent Center, 2030
Utah Psychiatric Association, 2031

Vermont

Fletcher Allen Health Care, 2032, 3107
National Alliance on Mental Illness: Vermont, 2033
Retreat Healthcare, 2034

Vermont Federation of Families for Children's Mental Health, 2035

Virginia

Agoraphobics Building Independent Lives, 282
Al-Anon Family Group National Referral Hotline, 1516
Alateen and Al-Anon Family Groups, 1021, 1517
American Association for Geriatric Psychiatry, 1748
American Association for Marriage and Family Therapy, 2304
American Association of Pastoral Counselors, 2312
American Association of Pharmaceutical Scientists, 2313
American College of Health Care Administrators (ACHCA) Annual Convocation & Exposition, 2319, 2935
American Counseling Association, 2325
American Counseling Association (ACA), 2326
American Medical Group Association, 2334
American Mental Health Counselors Association (AMHCA), 2336
American Network of Community Options and Resources (ANCOR), 1751
American Psychiatric Nurses Association, 2341
American Psychiatric Press Reference Library CD-ROM, 3829
American Psychiatric Publishing, 2342
American Psychosomatic Society, 2348
American Society for Clinical Pharmacology & Therapeutics, 2350
American Society of Consultant Pharmacists, 2352
Association for Ambulatory Behavioral Healthcare, 2359
Association for Psychological Type, 2370
Beacon Health Options, 1901
Clinical Social Work Federation, 2383
Colonial Services Board, 3101
Community Anti-Drug Coalition of America, 1411
Community Anti-Drug Coalitions of America, 2387
Council on Social Work Education, 2286, 2389
Employee Assistance Professionals Association, 3729, 2392
Employee Assistance Society of North America, 2393
Family-to-Family: National Alliance on Mental Illness, 1240
Garnett Day Treatment Center, 2036
Healthy Companies, 3754
Institute on Psychiatric Services: American Psychiatric Association, 2398
Mental Health America, 202, 681, 1075, 1075, 1194, 1414, 1686, 1791, 2406
NAADAC, The Association for Addiction Professionals, 1415

National Alliance on Mental Illness, 204, 330, 486, 486, 550, 790, 1077, 1135, 1195, 1307, 1417, 1585, 1642, 1687, 1795, 2037, 2043
National Association of Alcholism and Drug Abuse Counselors, 3133
National Association of State Mental Health Program Directors (NASMHPD), 1798, 2419
National Nurses Association, 2425
National Rehabilitation Association, 1811
National Sleep Foundation, 1310
Options Health Care, 3786
Parent Resource Center, 2039
Professional Risk Management Services, 3801, 2433
QuadraMed Corporation, 3907, 3149
Society for Personality Assessment, 2443
Society of Multivariate Experimental Psychology (SMEP), 2449
The Lewin Group, 3812
United States Psychiatric Rehabilitation Organization (USPRA), 2451
ValueOptions Norfolk, 3818
Virginia Department of Behavioral Health and Developmental Services (DBHDS), 2267
Virginia Department of Medical Assistance Services, 2268
Virginia Department of Social Services, 2269
Virginia Office of the Secretary of Health and Human Resources, 2270
World Federation for Mental Health, 1824

Washington

A Common Voice, 2040
Carewise, 3700
Children's Alliance, 1902, 2041
Gender Diversity, 877
Keane Care, 3879
Lanstat Incorporated, 2289
Mental Health & Spirituality Support Group, 2042
Mental Health Matters, 682
Milliman, Inc, 3780
Narcolepsy Network, 1306
National Alliance on Mental Illness: Pierce County, 2045
NetMeeting, 3897
North Sound Regional Support Network, 2046
Nueva Esperanza Counseling Center, 2047
Sharing & Caring for Consumers, Families Alliance for the Mentally Ill, 2048
South King County Alliance for the Mentally Ill, 2049
Spanish Support Group Alliance for the Mentally Ill, 2050
Spokane Mental Health, 2051
Washington Advocates for the Mentally Ill, 2052
Washington Institute for Mental Illness Research and Training, 2053
Washington State Psychological Association, 2054

West Virginia

Behavioral Health Management Group, 3692
CAMC Family Medicine Center of Charleston, 2055
Mountain State Parent Child and Adolescent Contacts, 2056
West Virginia Bureau for Behavioral Health and Health Facilities, 2271
West Virginia Department of Health & Human Resources (DHHR), 2272
West Virginia Department of Welfare Bureau for Children and Families, 2273

Wisconsin

Alliance for Children and Families, 2297
American Association of Children's Residential Center Annual Conference, 677, 2307, 2931, 2931
BOSS Inc, 3832
Bethesda Lutheran Communities, 1762
International Society of Psychiatric-Mental Health Nurses, 1785
Journey Mental Health Center, 2274
MCW Department of Psychiatry and Behavioral Medicine, 3769, 3121
Medical College of Wisconsin, 3127
National Alliance on Mental Illness: Wisconsin, 1837, 1849, 1860, 1860, 1862, 1865, 1894, 1906, 1909, 1915, 1933, 1937, 1940, 1944, 1949, 1972, 1991
National Niemann-Pick Disease Foundation, 924
Society for Psychophysiological Research, 2444
Society of Behavioral Medicine, 2448
TOPS Take Off Pounds Sensibly, 797
University of Wisconsin Population Health Institute, 2275
Willowglen Academy-Wisconsin, Inc., 1823
Wisconsin Association of Family and Child Agency, 2058
Wisconsin Department of Health and Family Services, 2276
Wisconsin Family Ties, 2059

Wyoming

Central Wyoming Behavioral Health at Lander Valley, 2060
National Alliance on Mental Illness: Wyoming, 2061
Uplift, 2062
Wyoming Department of Family Services, 2277

Drugs A-Z, by Brand Name

Abilify
Generic: aripiprazole
Manufacturer: Bristol-Myers Squibb
Used in the treatment of psychotic disorders
and bipolar disorder

Adderall/Adderall XR
Generic: amphetamine/dextroamphetamine
Manufacturer: Shire US, Inc.
Used to manage anxiety disorders and some
cases of attention deficit hyperactivity
disorder

Ambien
Generic: zolpidem
Manufacturer: Sanofi-Aventis
Used to treat insomnia

Anafranil
Generic: clomipramine hydrochloride
Manufacturer: Mallinckrodt, Inc.
Used to treat obsessive-compulsive disorder
(OCD)

Antabuse
Generic: disulfiram
Manufacturer: Odyssey Pharmaceuticals,
Inc.
Used in the treatment of alcohol and
substance abuse

Aricept
Generic: donepezil
Manufacturer: Pfizer, Inc.
Used in the treatment of Alzheimer's disease

Ativan
Generic: lorazepam
Manufacturer: Wyeth-Ayerst Laboratories
Used in the treatment of anxiety and as a
preanesthetic medication in adults

BuSpar
Generic: buspirone
Manufacturer: Bristol-Myers Squibb
Used to treat anxiety

Butrans
Generic: buprenorphine
Manufacturer: Purdue
Used to treat pain as well as addiction to
narcotic pain relievers

Campral
Generic: acamprosate calcium
Manufacturer: Forest Laboratories, Inc.
Used to reduce the desire to drink alcohol
Celexa
Generic: citalopram
Manufacturer: Forest Laboratories, Inc.
Used in the treatment of depression

Clozaril
Generic: clozapine
Manufacturer: Novartis
Used in the treatment of severe
schizophrenia

Cylert
Generic: pemoline
Manufacturer: Abbott Laboratories
Used to treat attention-deficit hyperactivity
disorder (ADHD) and narcolepsy

Cymbalta
Generic: duloxetine
Manufacturer: Eli Lilly and Company
Used in the treatment of depression

Daytrana
Generic: methylphenidate transdermal
Manufacturer: Noven Pharmaceuticals
Used in the treatment of ADHD in children
6-17 years old

Depakote
Generic: valproic acid
Manufacturer: Abbott Laboratories
Used in the treatment of manic episodes
associated with bipolar disorder and mania

Desoxyn
Generic: methamphetamine hydrochloride
Manufacturer: Abbott Laboratories
Used in the treatment of attention deficit
hyperactivity disorder

Desyrel
Generic: trazodone hydrochloride
Manufacturer: Bristol-Myers Squibb
Used in the treatment of major depressive disorder

Dexedrine, DextroStat
Generic: dextroamphetamine
Manufacturer: Mallinckrodt, Inc.
Used in the treatment of attention deficit hyperactivity disorder and narcolepsy

Dolophine
Generic: methadone
Manufacturer: Eli Lilly and Company
May be used to treat or control withdrawal symptoms in patients being treated for narcotic drug addiction

Edronax
Generic: reboxetine
Manufacturer: Pfizer, Inc.
Used to treat depression

Effexor
Generic: venlafaxine
Manufacturer: Wyeth-Ayerst Laboratories
Used in the treatment of depression and generalized anxiety disorder

Elavil
Generic: amitriptyline
Manufacturer: Astra Zeneca Pharmaceuticals
Used in the treatment of depression

Emsam
Generic: selegiline
Manufacturer: Bristol-Myers Squibb
Used in the treatment of major depressive disorder

Equetro
Generic: carbamazepine
Manufacturer: Validus Pharmaceuticals LLC
Used to treat seizures, nerve pain, and bipolar disorder

Eskalith
Generic: lithium
Manufacturer: GlaxoSmithKline
Used in the treatment of bipolar disorder

Exelon
Generic: rivastigmine
Manufacturer: Novartis
Used in the treatment of Alzheimer's disease

Fanapt
Generic: iloperidone
Manufacturer: Novartis
Used to treat schizophrenia

FazaClo
Generic: clozapine
Manufacturer: Jazz Pharmaceuticals plc
Used in the treatment of Schizophrenia

Focalin/Focalin XR
Generic: dexmethylphenidate
Manufacturer: Novartis
Used in the treatment of attention deficit hyperactivity disorder

Geodone
Generic: ziprasidone
Manufacturer: Pfizer, Inc.
Antipsychotic drug to treat schizophrenia and bipolar disorder

Halcion
Generic: triazolam
Manufacturer: Pfizer, Inc.
Used to treat insomnia

Haldol
Generic: haloperidol
Manufacturer: Johnson & Johnson
Used in the treatment of Schizophrenia

Intermezzo
Generic: zolpidem
Manufacturer: Purdue
Used in the treatment of insomnia

Invega
Generic: paliperidone
Manufacturer: Janssen
Used in the treatment of Schizophrenia

Kapvay
Generic: clonidine hcl
Manufacturer: Concordia Pharmaceuticals Inc.
Used to treat attention deficit hyperactivity disorder (ADHD), and can also be used to help with withdrawal symptoms from

narcotic drugs, and to help people quit smoking

Klonopin
Generic: clonazepam
Manufacturer: Roche
Used to treat seizures, panic disorder, and anxiety

Lamictal
Generic: lamotrigine
Manufacturer: GlaxoSmithKline
Used in the treatment of bipolar disorder

Latuda
Generic: lurasidone hcl
Manufacturer: Sunovion Pharmaceuticals
Used in the treatment of schizophrenia

Lexapro
Generic: escitalopram
Manufacturer: Forest Laboratories, Inc.
Used in the treatment of depression

Librium
Generic: chlordiazepoxide hcl
Manufacturer: ICN Pharmaceuticals, Inc.
Used to treat anxiety and acute alcohol withdrawal

Lithobid, Lithonate
Generic: lithium carbonate
Manufacturer: Solvay Pharmaceuticals Inc.
Used in the treatment of bipolar disorder and depression

Lunesta
Generic: eszopiclone
Manufacturer: Sunovion Pharmaceuticals
Used in the treatment of insomnia

LuvoxCR
Generic: fluvoxamine maleate
Manufacturer: Jazz Pharmaceuticals plc
Used to treat obsessive-compulsive disorder (OCD)

Marplan
Generic: isocarboxazid
Manufacturer: Validus Pharmaceuticals LLC
Used to treat depression

Methylin
Generic: methylphenidate
Manufacturer: Mallinckrodt, Inc.
Used to treat ADHD and narcolepsy

Namenda
Generic: memantine
Manufacturer: Forest Laboratories, Inc.
Used in the treatment of dementia

Navane
Generic: thiothixene
Manufacturer: Pfizer, Inc.
Used to treat schizophrenia

Nembutal
Generic: pentobarbital
Manufacturer: Lundbeck
Used to treat tension, anxiety, nervousness, insomnia, epilepsy and other seizures

Neurontin
Generic: gabapentin
Manufacturer: Pfizer, Inc.
Used in the treatment of seizures and neuropathic pain

Niravam
Generic: alprazolam
Manufacturer: Jazz Pharmaceuticals plc
Used in the treatment of anxiety and panic disorder

Norpramin
Generic: desipramine hcl
Manufacturer: Sanofi-Aventis
Used to treat depression

Nuvigil
Generic: armodafinil
Manufacturer: Teva Pharmaceutical Industries Ltd.
Used to treat sleepiness from narcolepsy, sleep apnea, or night shift work

Orap
Generic: pimozide
Manufacturer: Teva Pharmaceutical Industries Ltd.
Used to reduce uncontrolled movements (motor tics) or outbursts of words/sounds (vocal tics) caused by Tourette syndrome

Parnate
Generic: tranylcypromine
Manufacturer: GlaxoSmithKline
Used to help manage depression

Paxil
Generic: paroxetine hcl
Manufacturer: GlaxoSmithKline
Used in the treatment of depression, and
anxiety disorders

Pexeva
Generic: paroxetine mesylate
Manufacturer: Noven Pharmaceuticals
Used in the treatment of depression, and
anxiety disorders

Pristiq
Generic: desvenlafaxine
Manufacturer: Pfizer, Inc.
Used in the treatment of depression

Prolixin
Generic: fluphenazine hcl
Manufacturer: Bristol-Myers Squibb
Used to treat schizophrenia

Prosom
Generic: estasolam
Manufacturer: Abbott Laboratories
Used to treat insomnia

Provigil
Generic: modafinil
Manufacturer: Teva Pharmaceutical
Industries Ltd.
Used to treat narcolepsy, sleep apnea, and
shift work sleep disorder

Prozac
Generic: fluoxetine
Manufacturer: Eli Lilly and Company
Used in the treatment of depression and
anxiety disorders

Remeron
Generic: mirtazapine
Manufacturer: Merck & Co
Used in the treatment of suicidality and
depression

Reminyl
Generic: galantamine
Manufacturer: Shire US, Inc.

Used to treat mild to moderate confusion
(dementia) related to Alzheimer's disease

Restoril
Generic: temazepam
Manufacturer: Mallinckrodt
Used in the treatment of insomnia

Risperdal
Generic: risperidone
Manufacturer: Janssen
Used in the treatment of schizophrenia and
other mental illnesses such as psychosis

Ritalin
Generic: methylphenidate
Manufacturer: Novartis
Used in the treatment of attention deficit
hyperactivity disorders and in some forms of
narcolepsy

Rozerem
Generic: ramelteon
Manufacturer: Takeda Pharmaceuticals
Used in the treatment of insomnia

Saphris
Generic: asenapine
Manufacturer: Merck & Co
Used in the treatment of Schizophrenia and
Bipolar Mania

Sarafem
Generic: fluoxetine
Manufacturer: Eli Lilly and Company
It can treat depression, obsessive-
compulsive disorder (OCD), bulimia
nervosa, and panic disorder

Serzone
Generic: nefazodone hydrochloride
Manufacturer: Bristol-Myers Squibb
Used to treat depression

Sinequan
Generic: doxepin
Manufacturer: Pfizer, Inc.
Used to treat depression, anxiety, and sleep
disorders

Stavzor
Generic: valproic acid
Manufacturer: Bristol-Myers Squibb

Used to treat seizures and bipolar disorder. It can also help prevent migraine headaches.

Strattera
Generic: atomoxetine
Manufacturer: Eli Lilly & Company
Used in the treatment of attention deficit disorder

Symbyax
Generic: fluoxetine/olanzapine
Manufacturer: Eli Lilly & Company
Used to treat depression

Tranxene
Generic: clorazepate dipotassium
Manufacturer: Recordati Rare Diseases, Inc.
Used to treat anxiety, acute alcohol withdrawal, and seizures

Valium
Generic: diazepam
Manufacturer: Roche
Used in the treatment of anxiety

Viibryd
Generic: vilazodone hydrochloride
Manufacturer: Forest Laboratories, Inc.
Used in the treatment of depression

Vistaril
Generic: hydroxyzine
Manufacturer: Pfizer, Inc.
Used as a sedative to treat anxiety and tension and to treat allergic skin reactions

Vivitrol
Generic: naltrexone
Manufacturer: Alkermes, plc
Used to help prevent relapses into alcohol or drug abuse

Vyvanse
Generic: lisdexamfetamine
Manufacturer: Shire US, Inc.
Used in the treatment of attention deficit hyperactivity disorder

Wellbutrin, Wellbutrin SR, Wellbutrin XL
Generic: bupropion
Manufacturer: Sanofi-Aventis
Used in the treatment of depression
Xanax, Xanax XR
Generic: alprazolam

Manufacturer: Pfizer, Inc.
Used in the treatment of anxiety

Xyrem
Generic: sodium oxybate
Manufacturer: Jazz Pharmaceuticals plc
Used in the treatment of narcolepsy

Zoloft
Generic: sertraline
Manufacturer: Pfizer, Inc.
Used in the treatment of depression and anxiety disorders

Zyban
Generic: bupropion
Manufacturer: GlaxoSmithKline
Used in the treatment of depression

Zyprexa
Generic: olanzapine
Manufacturer: Eli Lilly & Company
Used to treat mental disorders, including schizophrenia and bipolar disorder

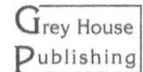
General Reference
America's College Museums
American Environmental Leaders: From Colonial Times to the Present
Encyclopedia of African-American Writing
Encyclopedia of Constitutional Amendments
Encyclopedia of Human Rights and the United States
Encyclopedia of Invasions & Conquests
Encyclopedia of Prisoners of War & Internment
Encyclopedia of Religion & Law in America
Encyclopedia of Rural America
Encyclopedia of the Continental Congress
Encyclopedia of the United States Cabinet, 1789-2010
Encyclopedia of War Journalism
Encyclopedia of Warrior Peoples & Fighting Groups
The Environmental Debate: A Documentary History
The Evolution Wars: A Guide to the Debates
From Suffrage to the Senate: America's Political Women
Gun Debate: An Encyclopedia of Gun Rights & Gun Control in the U.S.
Opinions throughout History: National Security vs. Civil and Privacy Rights
Opinions throughout History: Immigration
Opinions throughout History: Drug Abuse & Drug Epidemics
Political Corruption in America
Privacy Rights in the Digital Era
The Religious Right: A Reference Handbook
Speakers of the House of Representatives, 1789-2009
This is Who We Were: 1880-1900
This is Who We Were: A Companion to the 1940 Census
This is Who We Were: In the 1900s
This is Who We Were: In the 1910s
This is Who We Were: In the 1920s
This is Who We Were: In the 1940s
This is Who We Were: In the 1950s
This is Who We Were: In the 1960s
This is Who We Were: In the 1970s
This is Who We Were: In the 1980s
This is Who We Were: In the 1990s
This is Who We Were: In the 2000s
U.S. Land & Natural Resource Policy
The Value of a Dollar 1600-1865: Colonial Era to the Civil War
The Value of a Dollar: 1860-2014
Working Americans 1770-1869 Vol. IX: Revolutionary War to the Civil War
Working Americans 1880-1999 Vol. I: The Working Class
Working Americans 1880-1999 Vol. II: The Middle Class
Working Americans 1880-1999 Vol. III: The Upper Class
Working Americans 1880-1999 Vol. IV: Their Children
Working Americans 1880-2015 Vol. V: Americans At War
Working Americans 1880-2005 Vol. VI: Women at Work
Working Americans 1880-2006 Vol. VII: Social Movements
Working Americans 1880-2007 Vol. VIII: Immigrants
Working Americans 1880-2009 Vol. X: Sports & Recreation
Working Americans 1880-2010 Vol. XI: Inventors & Entrepreneurs
Working Americans 1880-2011 Vol. XII: Our History through Music
Working Americans 1880-2012 Vol. XIII: Education & Educators
Working Americans 1880-2016 Vol. XIV: Industry Through the Ages
Working Americans 1880-2017 Vol. XV: Politics & Politicians
World Cultural Leaders of the 20th & 21st Centuries

Education Information
Charter School Movement
Comparative Guide to American Elementary & Secondary Schools
Complete Learning Disabilities Directory
Educators Resource Handbook
Special Education: Policy and Curriculum Development

Health Information
Comparative Guide to American Hospitals
Complete Directory for Pediatric Disorders
Complete Directory for People with Chronic Illness
Complete Directory for People with Disabilities
Complete Mental Health Directory
Diabetes in America: Analysis of an Epidemic
Guide to Health Care Group Purchasing Organizations
Guide to U.S. HMO's & PPO's
Medical Device Market Place
Older Americans Information Directory

Business Information
Complete Television, Radio & Cable Industry Directory
Directory of Business Information Resources
Directory of Mail Order Catalogs
Directory of Venture Capital & Private Equity Firms
Environmental Resource Handbook
Financial Literacy Starter Kit
Food & Beverage Market Place
Grey House Homeland Security Directory
Grey House Performing Arts Directory
Grey House Safety & Security Directory
Hudson's Washington News Media Contacts Directory
New York State Directory
Sports Market Place Directory

Statistics & Demographics
American Tally
America's Top-Rated Cities
America's Top-Rated Smaller Cities
Ancestry & Ethnicity in America
The Asian Databook
Comparative Guide to American Suburbs
The Hispanic Databook
Profiles of America
"Profiles of" Series - State Handbooks
Weather America

Financial Ratings Series
Financial Literacy Basics
TheStreet Ratings' Guide to Bond & Money Market Mutual Funds
TheStreet Ratings' Guide to Common Stocks
TheStreet Ratings' Guide to Exchange-Traded Funds
TheStreet Ratings' Guide to Stock Mutual Funds
TheStreet Ratings' Ultimate Guided Tour of Stock Investing
Weiss Ratings' Consumer Guides
Weiss Ratings' Financial Literary Basic Guides
Weiss Ratings' Guide to Banks
Weiss Ratings' Guide to Credit Unions
Weiss Ratings' Guide to Health Insurers
Weiss Ratings' Guide to Life & Annuity Insurers
Weiss Ratings' Guide to Property & Casualty Insurers

Bowker's Books In Print® Titles
American Book Publishing Record® Annual
American Book Publishing Record® Monthly
Books In Print®
Books In Print® Supplement
Books Out Loud™
Bowker's Complete Video Directory™
Children's Books In Print®
El-Hi Textbooks & Serials In Print®
Forthcoming Books®
Law Books & Serials In Print™
Medical & Health Care Books In Print™
Publishers, Distributors & Wholesalers of the US™
Subject Guide to Books In Print®
Subject Guide to Children's Books In Print®

Canadian General Reference
Associations Canada
Canadian Almanac & Directory
Canadian Environmental Resource Guide
Canadian Parliamentary Guide
Canadian Venture Capital & Private Equity Firms
Canadian Who's Who
Financial Post Directory of Directors
Financial Services Canada
Governments Canada
Health Guide Canada
The History of Canada
Libraries Canada
Major Canadian Cities

Grey House Publishing | Salem Press | H.W. Wilson | 4919 Route, 22 PO Box 56, Amenia NY 12501-0056

2018 Title List

Visit www.SalemPress.com for Product Information, Table of Contents, and Sample Pages

Science, Careers & Mathematics

Ancient Creatures
Applied Science
Applied Science: Engineering & Mathematics
Applied Science: Science & Medicine
Applied Science: Technology
Biomes and Ecosystems
Careers in the Arts: Fine, Performing & Visual
Careers in Building Construction
Careers in Business
Careers in Chemistry
Careers in Communications & Media
Careers in Environment & Conservation
Careers in Financial Services
Careers in Green Energy
Careers in Healthcare
Careers in Hospitality & Tourism
Careers in Human Services
Careers in Law, Criminal Justice & Emergency Services
Careers in Manufacturing
Careers in Outdoor Jobs
Careers in Overseas Jobs
Careers in Physics
Careers in Sales, Insurance & Real Estate
Careers in Science & Engineering
Careers in Sports & Fitness
Careers in Social Media
Careers in Sports Medicine & Training
Careers in Technology Services & Repair
Computer Technology Innovators
Contemporary Biographies in Business
Contemporary Biographies in Chemistry
Contemporary Biographies in Communications & Media
Contemporary Biographies in Environment & Conservation
Contemporary Biographies in Healthcare
Contemporary Biographies in Hospitality & Tourism
Contemporary Biographies in Law & Criminal Justice
Contemporary Biographies in Physics
Earth Science
Earth Science: Earth Materials & Resources
Earth Science: Earth's Surface and History
Earth Science: Physics & Chemistry of the Earth
Earth Science: Weather, Water & Atmosphere
Encyclopedia of Energy
Encyclopedia of Environmental Issues
Encyclopedia of Environmental Issues: Atmosphere and Air Pollution
Encyclopedia of Environmental Issues: Ecology and Ecosystems
Encyclopedia of Environmental Issues: Energy and Energy Use
Encyclopedia of Environmental Issues: Policy and Activism
Encyclopedia of Environmental Issues: Preservation/Wilderness Issues
Encyclopedia of Environmental Issues: Water and Water Pollution
Encyclopedia of Global Resources
Encyclopedia of Global Warming
Encyclopedia of Mathematics & Society
Encyclopedia of Mathematics & Society: Engineering, Tech, Medicine
Encyclopedia of Mathematics & Society: Great Mathematicians
Encyclopedia of Mathematics & Society: Math & Social Sciences
Encyclopedia of Mathematics & Society: Math Development/Concepts
Encyclopedia of Mathematics & Society: Math in Culture & Society
Encyclopedia of Mathematics & Society: Space, Science, Environment
Encyclopedia of the Ancient World
Forensic Science
Geography Basics
Internet Innovators
Inventions and Inventors
Magill's Encyclopedia of Science: Animal Life
Magill's Encyclopedia of Science: Plant life
Notable Natural Disasters
Principles of Artificial Intelligence & Robotics
Principles of Astronomy
Principles of Biology
Principles of Biotechnology
Principles of Chemistry
Principles of Climatology
Principles of Physical Science
Principles of Physics
Principles of Programming & Coding
Principles of Research Methods
Principles of Sustainability
Science and Scientists
Solar System
Solar System: Great Astronomers

Solar System: Study of the Universe
Solar System: The Inner Planets
Solar System: The Moon and Other Small Bodies
Solar System: The Outer Planets
Solar System: The Sun and Other Stars
World Geography

Literature

American Ethnic Writers
Classics of Science Fiction & Fantasy Literature
Critical Approaches: Feminist
Critical Approaches: Multicultural
Critical Approaches: Moral
Critical Approaches: Psychological
Critical Insights: Authors
Critical Insights: Film
Critical Insights: Literary Collection Bundles
Critical Insights: Themes
Critical Insights: Works
Critical Survey of American Literature
Critical Survey of Drama
Critical Survey of Graphic Novels: Heroes & Super Heroes
Critical Survey of Graphic Novels: History, Theme & Technique
Critical Survey of Graphic Novels: Independents/Underground Classics
Critical Survey of Graphic Novels: Manga
Critical Survey of Long Fiction
Critical Survey of Mystery & Detective Fiction
Critical Survey of Mythology and Folklore: Heroes and Heroines
Critical Survey of Mythology and Folklore: Love, Sexuality & Desire
Critical Survey of Mythology and Folklore: World Mythology
Critical Survey of Novels into Film
Critical Survey of Poetry
Critical Survey of Poetry: American Poets
Critical Survey of Poetry: British, Irish & Commonwealth Poets
Critical Survey of Poetry: Cumulative Index
Critical Survey of Poetry: European Poets
Critical Survey of Poetry: Topical Essays
Critical Survey of Poetry: World Poets
Critical Survey of Science Fiction & Fantasy
Critical Survey of Shakespeare's Plays
Critical Survey of Shakespeare's Sonnets
Critical Survey of Short Fiction
Critical Survey of Short Fiction: American Writers
Critical Survey of Short Fiction: British, Irish, Commonwealth Writers
Critical Survey of Short Fiction: Cumulative Index
Critical Survey of Short Fiction: European Writers
Critical Survey of Short Fiction: Topical Essays
Critical Survey of Short Fiction: World Writers
Critical Survey of World Literature
Critical Survey of Young Adult Literature
Cyclopedia of Literary Characters
Cyclopedia of Literary Places
Holocaust Literature
Introduction to Literary Context: American Poetry of the 20th Century
Introduction to Literary Context: American Post-Modernist Novels
Introduction to Literary Context: American Short Fiction
Introduction to Literary Context: English Literature
Introduction to Literary Context: Plays
Introduction to Literary Context: World Literature
Magill's Literary Annual 2018
Masterplots
Masterplots II: African American Literature
Masterplots II: American Fiction Series
Masterplots II: British & Commonwealth Fiction Series
Masterplots II: Christian Literature
Masterplots II: Drama Series
Masterplots II: Juvenile & Young Adult Literature, Supplement
Masterplots II: Nonfiction Series
Masterplots II: Poetry Series
Masterplots II: Short Story Series
Masterplots II: Women's Literature Series
Notable African American Writers
Notable American Novelists
Notable Playwrights
Notable Poets
Recommended Reading: 600 Classics Reviewed
Short Story Writers

2018 Title List

Visit www.SalemPress.com for Product Information, Table of Contents, and Sample Pages

History and Social Science

The 2000s in America
50 States
African American History
Agriculture in History
American First Ladies
American Heroes
American Indian Culture
American Indian History
American Indian Tribes
American Presidents
American Villains
America's Historic Sites
Ancient Greece
The Bill of Rights
The Civil Rights Movement
The Cold War
Countries, Peoples & Cultures
Countries, Peoples & Cultures: Central & South America
Countries, Peoples & Cultures: Central, South & Southeast Asia
Countries, Peoples & Cultures: East & South Africa
Countries, Peoples & Cultures: East Asia & the Pacific
Countries, Peoples & Cultures: Eastern Europe
Countries, Peoples & Cultures: Middle East & North Africa
Countries, Peoples & Cultures: North America & the Caribbean
Countries, Peoples & Cultures: West & Central Africa
Countries, Peoples & Cultures: Western Europe
Defining Documents: American Revolution
Defining Documents: American West
Defining Documents: Ancient World
Defining Documents: Asia
Defining Documents: Civil Rights
Defining Documents: Civil War
Defining Documents: Court Cases
Defining Documents: Dissent & Protest
Defining Documents: Emergence of Modern America
Defining Documents: Exploration & Colonial America
Defining Documents: Immigration & Immigrant Communities
Defining Documents: LGBTQ
Defining Documents: Manifest Destiny
Defining Documents: Middle Ages
Defining Documents: Middle East
Defining Documents: Nationalism & Populism
Defining Documents: Native Americans
Defining Documents: Political Campaigns, Candidates & Discourse
Defining Documents: Postwar 1940s
Defining Documents: Reconstruction
Defining Documents: Renaissance & Early Modern Era
Defining Documents: Secrets, Leaks & Scandals
Defining Documents: 1920s
Defining Documents: 1930s
Defining Documents: 1950s
Defining Documents: 1960s
Defining Documents: 1970s
Defining Documents: The 17th Century
Defining Documents: The 18th Century
Defining Documents: The 19th Century
Defining Documents: The 20th Century: 1900-1950
Defining Documents: Vietnam War
Defining Documents: Women
Defining Documents: World War I
Defining Documents: World War II
Education Today
The Eighties in America
Encyclopedia of American Immigration
Encyclopedia of Flight
Encyclopedia of the Ancient World
Fashion Innovators
The Fifties in America
The Forties in America
Great Athletes
Great Athletes: Baseball
Great Athletes: Basketball
Great Athletes: Boxing & Soccer
Great Athletes: Cumulative Index
Great Athletes: Football
Great Athletes: Golf & Tennis
Great Athletes: Olympics

Great Athletes: Racing & Individual Sports
Great Contemporary Athletes
Great Events from History: 17th Century
Great Events from History: 18th Century
Great Events from History: 19th Century
Great Events from History: 20th Century (1901-1940)
Great Events from History: 20th Century (1941-1970)
Great Events from History: 20th Century (1971-2000)
Great Events from History: 21st Century (2000-2016)
Great Events from History: African American History
Great Events from History: Cumulative Indexes
Great Events from History: LGBTG
Great Events from History: Middle Ages
Great Events from History: Secrets, Leaks & Scandals
Great Events from History: Renaissance & Early Modern Era
Great Lives from History: 17th Century
Great Lives from History: 18th Century
Great Lives from History: 19th Century
Great Lives from History: 20th Century
Great Lives from History: 21st Century (2000-2017)
Great Lives from History: American Women
Great Lives from History: Ancient World
Great Lives from History: Asian & Pacific Islander Americans
Great Lives from History: Cumulative Indexes
Great Lives from History: Incredibly Wealthy
Great Lives from History: Inventors & Inventions
Great Lives from History: Jewish Americans
Great Lives from History: Latinos
Great Lives from History: Notorious Lives
Great Lives from History: Renaissance & Early Modern Era
Great Lives from History: Scientists & Science
Historical Encyclopedia of American Business
Issues in U.S. Immigration
Magill's Guide to Military History
Milestone Documents in African American History
Milestone Documents in American History
Milestone Documents in World History
Milestone Documents of American Leaders
Milestone Documents of World Religions
Music Innovators
Musicians & Composers 20th Century
The Nineties in America
The Seventies in America
The Sixties in America
Sociology Today
Survey of American Industry and Careers
The Thirties in America
The Twenties in America
United States at War
U.S. Court Cases
U.S. Government Leaders
U.S. Laws, Acts, and Treaties
U.S. Legal System
U.S. Supreme Court
Weapons and Warfare
World Conflicts: Asia and the Middle East

Health

Addictions & Substance Abuse
Adolescent Health & Wellness
Cancer
Complementary & Alternative Medicine
Community & Family Health
Genetics & Inherited Conditions
Health Issues
Infectious Diseases & Conditions
Magill's Medical Guide
Nutrition
Nursing
Psychology & Behavioral Health
Psychology Basics

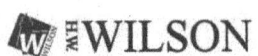 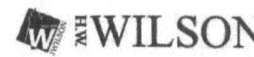
Current Biography
Current Biography Cumulative Index 1946-2013
Current Biography Monthly Magazine
Current Biography Yearbook: 2003
Current Biography Yearbook: 2004
Current Biography Yearbook: 2005
Current Biography Yearbook: 2006
Current Biography Yearbook: 2007
Current Biography Yearbook: 2008
Current Biography Yearbook: 2009
Current Biography Yearbook: 2010
Current Biography Yearbook: 2011
Current Biography Yearbook: 2012
Current Biography Yearbook: 2013
Current Biography Yearbook: 2014
Current Biography Yearbook: 2015
Current Biography Yearbook: 2016
Current Biography Yearbook: 2017

Core Collections
Children's Core Collection
Fiction Core Collection
Graphic Novels Core Collection
Middle & Junior High School Core
Public Library Core Collection: Nonfiction
Senior High Core Collection
Young Adult Fiction Core Collection

The Reference Shelf
Aging in America
Alternative Facts: Post Truth & the Information War
The American Dream
American Military Presence Overseas
The Arab Spring
Artificial Intelligence
The Brain
The Business of Food
Campaign Trends & Election Law
Conspiracy Theories
The Digital Age
Dinosaurs
Embracing New Paradigms in Education
Faith & Science
Families: Traditional and New Structures
The Future of U.S. Economic Relations: Mexico, Cuba, and Venezuela
Global Climate Change
Graphic Novels and Comic Books
Guns in America
Immigration
Immigration in the U.S.
Internet Abuses & Privacy Rights
Internet Safety
LGBTQ in the 21st Century
Marijuana Reform
The News and its Future
The Paranormal
Politics of the Ocean
Prescription Drug Abuse
Racial Tension in a "Postracial" Age
Reality Television
Representative American Speeches: 2008-2009
Representative American Speeches: 2009-2010
Representative American Speeches: 2010-2011
Representative American Speeches: 2011-2012
Representative American Speeches: 2012-2013
Representative American Speeches: 2013-2014
Representative American Speeches: 2014-2015
Representative American Speeches: 2015-2016
Representative American Speeches: 2016-2017
Representative American Speeches: 2017-2018
Rethinking Work
Revisiting Gender
Robotics
Russia
Social Networking
Social Services for the Poor
South China Seas Conflict
Space Exploration & Development
Sports in America

The Supreme Court
The Transformation of American Cities
U.S. Infrastructure
U.S. National Debate Topic: Educational Reform
U.S. National Debate Topic: Surveillance
U.S. National Debate Topic: The Ocean
U.S. National Debate Topic: Transportation Infrastructure
Whistleblowers

Readers' Guide
Abridged Readers' Guide to Periodical Literature
Readers' Guide to Periodical Literature

Indexes
Index to Legal Periodicals & Books
Short Story Index
Book Review Digest

Sears List
Sears List of Subject Headings
Sears: Lista de Encabezamientos de Materia

Facts About Series
Facts About American Immigration
Facts About China
Facts About the 20th Century
Facts About the Presidents
Facts About the World's Languages

Nobel Prize Winners
Nobel Prize Winners: 1901-1986
Nobel Prize Winners: 1987-1991
Nobel Prize Winners: 1992-1996
Nobel Prize Winners: 1997-2001

World Authors
World Authors: 1995-2000
World Authors: 2000-2005

Famous First Facts
Famous First Facts
Famous First Facts About American Politics
Famous First Facts About Sports
Famous First Facts About the Environment
Famous First Facts: International Edition

American Book of Days
The American Book of Days
The International Book of Days

Monographs
American Reformers
The Barnhart Dictionary of Etymology
Celebrate the World
Guide to the Ancient World
Indexing from A to Z
Nobel Prize Winners
The Poetry Break
Radical Change: Books for Youth in a Digital Age
Speeches of American Presidents

Wilson Chronology
Wilson Chronology of Asia and the Pacific
Wilson Chronology of Human Rights
Wilson Chronology of Ideas
Wilson Chronology of the Arts
Wilson Chronology of the World's Religions
Wilson Chronology of Women's Achievements

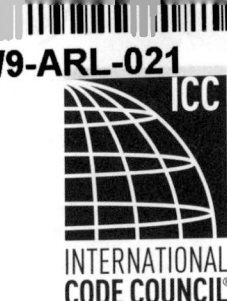

IRC®

INTERNATIONAL RESIDENTIAL CODE®
FOR ONE- AND TWO-FAMILY DWELLINGS

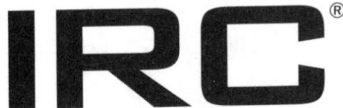

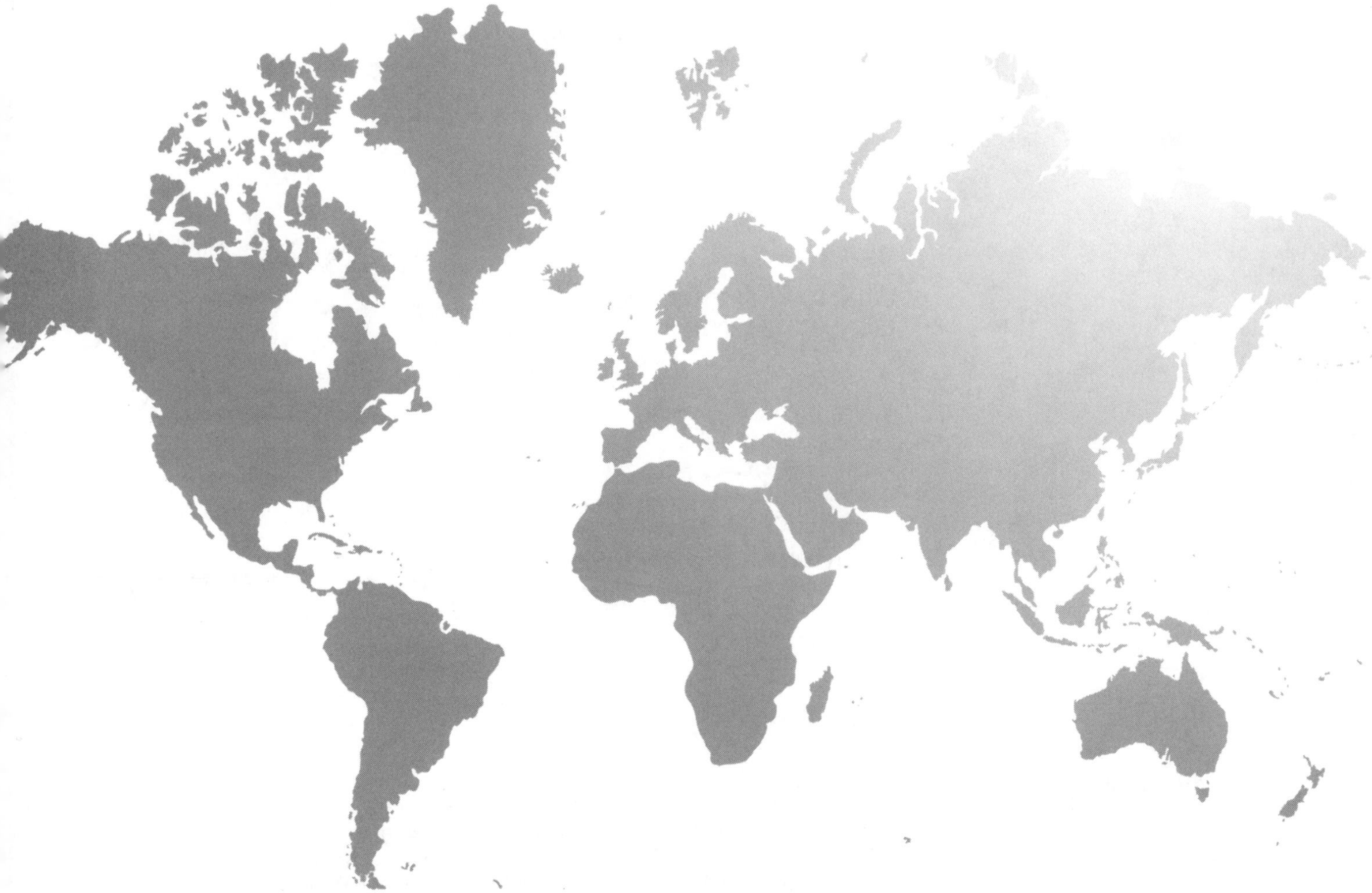

2009

Receive **FREE** updates, excerpts of code references, technical articles, and more when you register your code book. Go to
www.iccsafe.org/CodesPlus today!

2009 International Residential Code® for One- and Two-family Dwellings

First Printing: March 2009

ISBN: 978-1-58001-727-5 (soft-cover edition)
ISBN: 978-1-58001-726-8 (loose-leaf edition)

PRINTED IN THE U.S.A.

PREFACE

Introduction

Internationally, code officials recognize the need for a modern, up-to-date residential code addressing the design and construction of one- and two-family dwellings and townhouses. The *International Residential Code*®, in this 2009 edition, is designed to meet these needs through model code regulations that safeguard the public health and safety in all communities, large and small.

This comprehensive, stand-alone residential code establishes minimum regulations for one- and two-family dwellings and townhouses using prescriptive provisions. It is founded on broad-based principles that make possible the use of new materials and new building designs. This 2009 edition is fully compatible with all the *International Codes*® (I-Codes®) published by the International Code Council® (ICC)®, including the *International Building Code*®, *International Energy Conservation Code*®, *International Existing Building Code*®, *International Fire Code*®, *International Fuel Gas Code*®, *International Mechanical Code*®, ICC *Performance Code*®, *International Plumbing Code*®, *International Private Sewage Disposal Code*®, *International Property Maintenance Code*®, *International Wildland-Urban Interface Code*™ and *International Zoning Code*®.

The *International Residential Code* provisions provide many benefits, among which is the model code development process that offers an international forum for residential construction professionals to discuss prescriptive code requirements. This forum provides an excellent arena to debate proposed revisions. This model code also encourages international consistency in the application of provisions.

Development

The first edition of the *International Residential Code* (2000) was the culmination of an effort initiated in 1996 by ICC and consisting of representatives from the three statutory members of the International Code Council at the time, including: Building Officials and Code Administrators International, Inc. (BOCA), International Conference of Building Officials (ICBO) and Southern Building Code Congress International (SBCCI), and representatives from the National Association of Home Builders (NAHB). The intent was to draft a stand-alone residential code consistent with and inclusive of the scope of the existing model codes. Technical content of the 1998 *International One- and Two-Family Dwelling Code* and the latest model codes promulgated by BOCA, ICBO, SBCCI and ICC was used as the basis for the development, followed by public hearings in 1998 and 1999 to consider proposed changes. This 2009 edition represents the code as originally issued, with changes reflected in the 2006 edition, and further changes developed through the ICC Code Development Process through 2008. Residential electrical provisions are based on the 2008 *National Electrical Code*® (NFPA 70). A new edition such as this is promulgated every three years.

Fuel gas provisions have been included through an agreement with the American Gas Association (AGA). Electrical provisions have been included through an agreement with the National Fire Protection Association (NFPA).

This code is founded on principles intended to establish provisions consistent with the scope of a residential code that adequately protects public health, safety and welfare; provisions that do not unnecessarily increase construction costs; provisions that do not restrict the use of new materials, products or methods of construction; and provisions that do not give preferential treatment to particular types or classes of materials, products or methods of construction.

Adoption

The *International Residential Code* is available for adoption and use by jurisdictions internationally. Its use within a governmental jurisdiction is intended to be accomplished through adoption by reference in accordance with proceedings establishing the jurisdiction's laws. At the time of adoption, jurisdictions should insert the appropriate information in provisions requiring specific local information, such as the name of the adopting jurisdiction. These locations are shown in bracketed words in small capital letters in the code and in the sample ordinance. The sample adoption ordinance on page xiii addresses several key elements of a code adoption ordinance, including the information required for insertion into the code text.

Maintenance

The *International Residential Code* is kept up-to-date through the review of proposed changes submitted by code enforcing officials, industry representatives, design professionals and other interested parties. Proposed changes are carefully considered through an open code development process in which all interested and affected parties may participate.

The contents of this work are subject to change both through the Code Development Cycles and the governmental body that enacts the code into law. For more information regarding the code development process, contact the Code and Standard Development Department of the International Code Council.

The maintenance process for the fuel gas provisions is based upon the process used to maintain the *International Fuel Gas Code*, in conjunction with the American Gas Association. The maintenance process for the electrical provisions is undertaken by the National Fire Protection Association.

While the development procedure of the *International Residential Code* assures the highest degree of care, ICC, the founding members of ICC, its members and those participating in the development of this code do not accept any liability resulting from compliance or noncompliance with the provisions because ICC and its founding members do not have the power or authority to police or enforce compliance with the contents of this code. Only the governmental body that enacts the code into law has such authority.

Marginal Markings

Solid vertical lines in the margins within the body of the code indicate a technical change from the requirements of the 2006 edition. Deletion indicators in the form of an arrow (➡) are provided in the margin where an entire section, paragraph, exception or table has been deleted or an item in a list of items or a table has been deleted.

Italicized Terms

Selected terms set forth in Chapter 2, Definitions, are italicized where they appear in code text. Such terms are not italicized where the definition set forth in Chapter 2 does not impart the intended meaning in the use of the term. The terms selected have definitions which the user should read carefully to facilitate better understanding of the code.

Effective Use of the International Residential Code

The *International Residential Code*® (IRC®) was created to serve as a complete, comprehensive code regulating the construction of single-family houses, two-family houses (duplexes) and buildings consisting of three or more townhouse units. All buildings within the scope of the IRC are limited to three stories above grade plane. For example, a four-story single-family house would fall within the scope of the *International Building Code*® (IBC®), not the IRC. The benefits of devoting a separate code to residential construction include the fact that the user need not navigate through a multitude of code provisions that do not apply to residential construction in order to locate that which is applicable. A separate code also allows for residential and nonresidential code provisions to be distinct and tailored to the structures that fall within the appropriate code's scopes.

The IRC contains coverage for all components of a house or townhouse, including structural components, fireplaces and chimneys, thermal insulation, mechanical systems, fuel gas systems, plumbing systems and electrical systems.

The IRC is a prescriptive-oriented (specification) code with some examples of performance code language. It has been said that the IRC is the complete cookbook for residential construction. Section R301.1, for example, is written in performance language, but states that the prescriptive requirements of the code will achieve such performance.

It is important to understand that the IRC contains coverage for what is conventional and common in residential construction practice. While the IRC will provide all of the needed coverage for most residential construction, it might not address construction practices and systems that are atypical or rarely encountered in the industry. Sections such as R301.1.3, R301.2.2, R320.1, R322.1, N1101.2, M1301.1, G2401.1, P2601.1 and E3401.2 refer to other codes either as an alternative to the provisions of the IRC or where the IRC lacks coverage for a particular type of structure, design, system, appliance or method of construction. In other words, the IRC is meant to be all inclusive for typical residential construction and it relies on other codes only where alternatives are desired or where the code lacks coverage for the uncommon aspect of residential construction. Of course, the IRC constantly evolves to address new technologies and construction practices that were once uncommon, but now common.

The IRC is unique in that much of it, including Chapters 3 through 9 and Chapters 34 through 43, is presented in an ordered format that is consistent with the normal progression of construction, starting with the design phase and continuing through the final trim-out phase. This is consistent with the "cookbook" philosophy of the IRC.

The IRC is divided into eight main parts, specifically, Part I—Administration, Part II—Definitions, Part III—Building Planning and Construction, Part IV—Energy Conservation, Part V—Mechanical, Part VI—Fuel Gas, Part VII—Plumbing and Part VIII—Electrical.

The following provides a brief description of the content of each chapter and appendix of the IRC:

Chapter 1 Scope and Administration. This chapter contains provisions for the application, enforcement and administration of subsequent requirements of the code. In addition to establishing the scope of the code, Chapter 1 identifies which buildings and structures come under its purview. Chapter 1 is largely concerned with maintaining "due process of law" in enforcing the building criteria contained in the body of the code. Only through careful observation of the administrative provisions can the building official reasonably expect to demonstrate that "equal protection under the law" has been provided.

Chapter 2 Definitions. Terms defined in the code are listed alphabetically in Chapter 2. It is important to note that two chapters have their own definitions sections: Chapter 24 for the defined terms that are unique to fuel gas and Chapter 35 containing terms that are applicable to electrical Chapters 34 through 43. In the case where Chapter 2 and another chapter both define the same term differently, the definition found in Chapter 24 and/or 35 is intended to prevail where the term is used in Chapter 24 and/or 35 and the definition contained in Chapter 2 is intended to prevail where the term is used in all other locations in the code. Except where Chapter 24 or 35 has a definition that will prevail therein, the definitions in Chapter 2 are applicable throughout the code.

Additional definitions regarding skylights that are not listed in Chapter 2 are found in Section R308.6.1.

Where understanding a term's definition is key to or necessary for understanding a particular code provision, the term is shown in italics where it appears in the code. This is true only for those terms that have a meaning that is unique to the code. In other words, the generally understood meaning of a term or phrase might not be sufficient or consistent with the meaning prescribed by the code; therefore, it is essential that the code-defined meaning be known.

Guidance regarding not only tense, gender and plurality of defined terms, but also terms not defined in this code, is provided.

Chapter 3 Building Planning. Chapter 3 provides guidelines for a minimum level of structural integrity, life safety, fire safety and livability for inhabitants of dwelling units regulated by this code. Chapter 3 is a compilation of the code requirements specific to the building planning sector of the design and construction process. This chapter sets forth code requirements dealing with light, ventilation, sanitation, minimum room size, ceiling height and environmental comfort. Chapter 3 establishes life-safety provisions including limitations on glazing used in hazardous areas, specifications on stairways, use of guards at elevated surfaces and rules for means of egress. Snow, wind and seismic design and flood-resistant construction, as well as live and dead loads, are addressed in this chapter.

Chapter 4 Foundations. Chapter 4 provides the requirements for the design and construction of foundation systems for buildings regulated by this code. Provisions for seismic load, flood load and frost protection are contained in this chapter. A foundation system consists of two interdependent components: the foundation structure itself and the supporting soil.

The prescriptive provisions of this chapter provide requirements for constructing footings and walls for foundations of wood, masonry, concrete and precast concrete. In addition to a foundation's ability to support the required design loads, this chapter addresses several other factors that can affect foundation performance. These include controlling surface water and subsurface drainage, requiring soil tests where conditions warrant and evaluating proximity to slopes and minimum depth requirements. The chapter also provides requirements to minimize adverse effects of moisture, decay and pests in basements and crawl spaces.

Chapter 5 Floors. Chapter 5 provides the requirements for the design and construction of floor systems that will be capable of supporting minimum required design loads. This chapter covers four different types: wood floor framing, wood floors on the ground, cold-formed steel floor framing and concrete slabs on the ground. Allowable span tables are provided that greatly simplify the determination of joist, girder and sheathing sizes for raised floor systems of wood framing and cold-formed steel framing. This chapter also contains prescriptive requirements for attaching a deck to the main building.

Chapter 6 Wall Construction. Chapter 6 contains provisions that regulate the design and construction of walls. The wall construction covered in Chapter 6 consists of five different types: wood framed, cold-formed steel framed, masonry, concrete and structural insulated panel (SIP). The primary concern of this chapter is the structural integrity of wall construction and transfer of all imposed loads to the supporting structure. This chapter provides the requirements for the design and construction of wall systems that are capable of supporting the minimum design vertical loads (dead, live and snow loads) and lateral loads (wind or seismic loads). This chapter contains the prescriptive requirements for wall bracing and/or shear walls to resist the imposed lateral loads due to wind and seismic. Chapter 6 also contains requirements for the use of vapor retarders for moisture control in walls.

Chapter 6 also regulates exterior windows and doors installed in walls. The chapter contains criteria for the performance of exterior windows and doors and includes provisions for window sill height, testing and labeling, vehicular access doors, wind-borne debris protection and anchorage details.

Chapter 7 Wall Covering. Chapter 7 contains provisions for the design and construction of interior and exterior wall coverings. This chapter establishes the various types of materials, materials standards and methods of application permitted for use as interior coverings, including interior plaster, gypsum board, ceramic tile, wood veneer paneling, hardboard paneling, wood shakes and wood shingles.

Exterior wall coverings provide the weather-resistant exterior envelope that protects the building's interior from the elements. Chapter 7 provides the requirements for wind resistance and water-resistive barrier for exterior wall coverings. This chapter prescribes the exterior wall coverings as well as the water-resistive barrier required beneath the exterior materials. Exterior wall coverings regulated by this section include aluminum, stone and masonry veneer, wood, hardboard, particleboard, wood structural panel siding, wood shakes and shingles, exterior plaster, steel, vinyl, fiber cement and exterior insulation finish systems.

Chapter 8 Roof-ceiling Construction. Chapter 8 regulates the design and construction of roof-ceiling systems. This chapter contains two roof-ceiling framing systems: wood framing and cold-formed steel framing. Allowable span tables are provided to simplify the selection of rafter and ceiling joist size for wood roof framing and cold-formed steel framing. Chapter 8 also provides requirements for the application of ceiling finishes, the proper ventilation of concealed spaces in roofs (e.g., enclosed attics and rafter spaces), unvented attic assemblies, attic access and the proper clearance of combustible insulation from heat-producing devices.

Chapter 9 Roof Assemblies. Chapter 9 regulates the design and construction of roof assemblies. A roof assembly includes the roof deck, vapor retarder, substrate or thermal barrier, insulation, vapor retarder and roof covering. This chapter provides the requirement for wind resistance of roof coverings.

The types of roof covering materials and installation regulated by Chapter 9 are: asphalt shingles, clay and concrete tile, metal roof shingles, mineral-surfaced roll roofing, slate and slate-type shingles, wood shakes and shingles, built-up roofs, metal roof panels, modified bitumen roofing, thermoset and thermoplastic single-ply roofing, sprayed polyurethane foam roofing and liquid applied coatings. Chapter 9 also provides requirements for roof drainage, flashing, above deck thermal insulation and recovering or replacing an existing roof covering.

Chapter 10 Chimneys and Fireplaces. Chapter 10 contains requirements for the safe construction of masonry chimneys and fireplaces and establishes the standards for the use and installation of factory-built chimneys, fireplaces and masonry heaters. Chimneys and fireplaces constructed of masonry rely on prescriptive requirements for the details of their construction; the factory-built type relies on the listing and labeling method of approval. Chapter 10 provides the requirements for seismic reinforcing and anchorage of masonry fireplaces and chimneys.

Chapter 11 Energy Efficiency. Chapter 11 contains the energy-efficiency-related requirements for the design and construction of buildings regulated under this code. The applicable portions of the building must comply with the provisions within this chapter for energy efficiency. This chapter defines requirements for the portions of the building and building systems that impact energy use in new construction and promotes the effective use of energy. The provisions within the chapter promote energy efficiency in the building envelope, the heating and cooling system, the service water heating system and the lighting system of the building. This chapter also provides energy efficiency requirements for snow melt systems and pool heaters.

Chapter 12 Mechanical Administration. Chapter 12 establishes the limits of applicability of the code and describes how the code is to be applied and enforced. A mechanical code, like any other code, is intended to be adopted as a legally enforceable document and it cannot be effective without adequate provisions for its administration and enforcement. The provisions of Chapter 12 establish the authority and duties of the code official appointed by the jurisdiction having authority and also establish the rights and privileges of the design professional, contractor and property owner. It also relates this chapter to the administrative provisions in Chapter 1.

Chapter 13 General Mechanical System Requirements. Chapter 13 contains broadly applicable requirements related to appliance listing and labeling, appliance location and installation, appliance and systems access, protection of structural elements and clearances to combustibles, among others.

Chapter 14 Heating and Cooling Equipment. Chapter 14 is a collection of requirements for various heating and cooling appliances, dedicated to single topics by section. The common theme is that all of these types of appliances use energy in one form or another, and the improper installation of such appliances would present a hazard to the occupants of the dwellings, due to either the potential for fire or the accidental release of refrigerants. Both situations are undesirable in dwellings that are covered by this code.

Chapter 15 Exhaust Systems. Chapter 15 is a compilation of code requirements related to residential exhaust systems, including kitchens and bathrooms, clothes dryers and range hoods. The code regulates the materials used for constructing and installing such duct systems. Air brought into the building for ventilation, combustion or makeup purposes is protected from contamination by the provisions found in this chapter.

Chapter 16 Duct Systems. Chapter 16 provides requirements for the installation of ducts for supply, return and exhaust air systems. This chapter contains no information on the design of these systems from the standpoint of air movement, but is concerned with the structural integrity of the systems and the overall impact of the systems on the fire-safety performance of the building. This chapter regulates the materials and methods of construction which affect the performance of the entire air distribution system.

Chapter 17 Combustion Air. Complete combustion of solid and liquid fuel is essential for the proper operation of appliances, control of harmful emissions and achieving maximum fuel efficiency. If insufficient quantities of oxygen are supplied, the combustion process will be incomplete, creating dangerous byproducts and wasting energy in the form of unburned fuel (hydrocarbons). The byproducts of incomplete combustion are poisonous, corrosive and combustible, and can cause serious appliance or equipment malfunctions that pose fire or explosion hazards.

The combustion air provisions in this code from previous editions have been deleted from Chapter 17 in favor of a single section that directs the user to NFPA 31 for oil-fired appliance combustion air requirements and the manufacturer's installation instructions for solid fuel-burning appliances. If fuel gas appliances are used, the provisions of Chapter 24 must be followed.

Chapter 18 Chimneys and Vents. Chapter 18 regulates the design, construction, installation, maintenance, repair and approval of chimneys, vents and their connections to fuel-burning appliances. A properly designed chimney or vent system is needed to conduct the flue gases produced by a fuel-burning appliance to the outdoors. The provisions of this chapter are intended to minimize the hazards associated with high temperatures and potentially toxic and corrosive combustion gases. This chapter addresses factory-built and masonry chimneys, vents and venting systems used to vent oil-fired and solid fuel-burning appliances.

Chapter 19 Special Fuel-burning Equipment. Chapter 19 regulates the installation of fuel-burning appliances that are not covered in other chapters, such as ranges and ovens, sauna heaters, fuel cell power plants and hydrogen systems. Because the subjects in this chapter do not contain the volume of text necessary to warrant individual chapters, they have been combined into a single chapter. The only commonality is that the subjects use energy to perform some task or function. The intent is to provide a reasonable level of protection for the occupants of the dwelling.

Chapter 20 Boilers and Water Heaters. Chapter 20 regulates the installation of boilers and water heaters. Its purpose is to protect the occupants of the dwelling from the potential hazards associated with such appliances. A water heater is any appliance that heats potable water and supplies it to the plumbing hot water distribution system. A boiler either heats water or generates steam for space heating and is generally a closed system.

Chapter 21 Hydronic Piping. Hydronic piping includes piping, fittings and valves used in building space conditioning systems. Applications include hot water, chilled water, steam, steam condensate, brines and water/antifreeze mixtures. Chapter 21 regulates installation, alteration and repair of all hydronic piping systems to insure the reliability, serviceability, energy efficiency and safety of such systems.

Chapter 22 Special Piping and Storage Systems. Chapter 22 regulates the design and installation of fuel oil storage and piping systems. The regulations include reference to construction standards for above-ground and underground storage tanks, material standards for piping systems (both above-ground and underground) and extensive requirements for the proper assembly of system piping and components. The purpose of this chapter is to prevent fires, leaks and spills involving fuel oil storage and piping systems, whether inside or outside structures and above or underground.

Chapter 23 Solar Systems. Chapter 23 contains requirements for the construction, alteration and repair of all systems and components of solar energy systems used for space heating or cooling, and domestic hot water heating or processing. The provisions of this chapter are limited to those necessary to achieve installations that are relatively hazard free.

A solar energy system can be designed to handle 100 percent of the energy load of a building, although this is rarely accomplished. Because solar energy is a low-intensity energy source and dependent on the weather, it is usually necessary to supplement a solar energy system with traditional energy sources.

As our world strives to find alternate means of producing power for the future, the requirements of this chapter will become more and more important over time.

Chapter 24 Fuel Gas. Chapter 24 regulates the design and installation of fuel gas distribution piping and systems, appliances, appliance venting systems and combustion air provisions. The definition of "Fuel gas" includes natural, liquefied petroleum and manufactured gases and mixtures of these gases.

The purpose of this chapter is to establish the minimum acceptable level of safety and to protect life and property from the potential dangers associated with the storage, distribution and use of fuel gases and the byproducts of combustion of such fuels. This code also protects the personnel who install, maintain, service and replace the systems and appliances addressed herein.

Chapter 24 is composed entirely of text extracted from the IFGC; therefore, whether using the IFGC or the IRC, the fuel gas provisions will be identical. Note that to avoid the potential for confusion and conflicting definitions, Chapter 24 has its own definition section.

Chapter 25 Plumbing Administration. The requirements of Chapter 25 do not supersede the administrative provisions of Chapter 1. Rather, the administrative guidelines of Chapter 25 pertain to plumbing installations that are best referenced and located within the plumbing chapters. This chapter addresses how to apply the plumbing provisions of this code to specific types or phases of construction. This chapter also outlines the responsibilities of the applicant, installer and inspector with regard to testing plumbing installations.

Chapter 26 General Plumbing Requirements. The content of Chapter 26 is often referred to as "miscellaneous," rather than general plumbing requirements. This is the only chapter of the plumbing chapters of the code whose requirements do not interrelate. If a requirement cannot be located in another plumbing chapter, it should be located in this chapter. Chapter 26 contains safety requirements for the installation of plumbing systems and includes requirements for the identification of pipe, pipe fittings, traps, fixtures, materials and devices used in plumbing systems. If specific provisions do not demand that a requirement be located in another chapter, the requirement is located in this chapter.

Chapter 27 Plumbing Fixtures. Chapter 27 requires fixtures to be of the proper type, approved for the purpose intended and installed properly to promote usability and safe, sanitary conditions. This chapter regulates the quality of fixtures and faucets by requiring those items to comply with nationally recognized standards. Because fixtures must be properly installed so that they are usable by the occupants of the building, this chapter contains the requirements for the installation of fixtures.

Chapter 28 Water Heaters. Chapter 28 regulates the design, approval and installation of water heaters and related safety devices. The intent is to minimize the hazards associated with the installation and operation of water heaters. Although this chapter does not regulate the size of a water heater, it does regulate all other aspects of the water heater installation such as temperature and pressure relief valves, safety drip pans and connections. Where a water heater also supplies water for space heating, this chapter regulates the maximum water temperature supplied to the water distribution system.

Chapter 29 Water Supply and Distribution. This chapter regulates the supply of potable water from both public and individual sources to every fixture and outlet so that it remains potable and uncontaminated by cross connections. Chapter 29 also regulates the design of the water distribution system, which will allow fixtures to function properly. Because it is critical that the potable water supply system remain free of actual or potential sanitary hazards, this chapter has the requirements for providing backflow protection devices.

Chapter 30 Sanitary Drainage. The purpose of Chapter 30 is to regulate the materials, design and installation of sanitary drainage piping systems as well as the connections made to the system. The intent is to design and install sanitary drainage systems that will function reliably, are neither undersized nor oversized and are constructed from materials, fittings and connections whose quality is regulated by this section. This chapter addresses the proper use of fittings for directing the flow into and within the sanitary drain piping system. Materials and provisions necessary for servicing the drainage system are also included in this chapter.

Chapter 31 Vents. Venting protects the trap seal of each trap. The vents are designed to limit differential pressures at each trap to 1 inch of water column (249 Pa). Because waste flow in the drainage system creates pressure fluctuations that can negatively affect traps, the sanitary drainage system must have a properly designed venting system. Chapter 31 covers the requirements for vents and venting. All of the provisions set forth in this chapter are intended to limit the pressure differentials in the drainage system to a maximum of 1 inch of water column (249 Pa) above or below atmospheric pressure (i.e., positive or negative pressures).

Chapter 32 Traps. Traps prevent sewer gas from escaping from the drainage piping into the building. Water seal traps are the simplest and most reliable means of preventing sewer gas from entering the interior environment. This chapter lists prohibited trap types as well as specifies the minimum trap size for each type of fixture.

Chapter 33 Storm Drainage. Rainwater infiltration into the ground adjacent to a building can cause the interior of foundation walls to become wet. The installation of a subsoil drainage system prevents the build-up of rainwater on the exterior of the foundation walls. This chapter provides the specifications for subsoil drain piping. Where the discharge of the subsoil drain system is to a sump, this chapter also provides coverage for for sump construction, pumps and discharge piping.

Chapter 34 General Requirements. This chapter contains broadly applicable, general and miscellaneous requirements including scope, listing and labeling, equipment locations and clearances for conductor materials and connections and conductor identification.

Chapter 35 Electrical Definitions. Chapter 35 is the repository of the definitions of terms used in the body of Part VIII of the code. To avoid the potential for confusion and conflicting definitions, Part VIII, Electrical, has its own definition chapter.

Codes are technical documents and every word, term and punctuation mark can impact the meaning of the code text and the intended results. The code often uses terms that have a unique meaning in the code, which can differ substantially from the ordinarily understood meaning of the term as used outside of the code.

The terms defined in Chapter 35 are deemed to be of prime importance in establishing the meaning and intent of the electrical code text that uses the terms. The user of the code should be familiar with and consult this chapter because the definitions are essential to the correct interpretation of the code and because the user may not be aware that a term is defined.

Chapter 36 Services. This chapter covers the design, sizing and installation of the building's electrical service equipment and grounding electrode system. It includes an easy-to-use load calculation method and service conductor sizing table. The electrical service is generally the first part of the electrical system to be designed and installed.

Chapter 37 Branch Circuit and Feeder Requirements. Chapter 37 addresses the requirements for designing the power distribution system which consists of feeders and branch circuits emanating from the service equipment. This chapter dictates the ratings of circuits and the allowable loads, the number and types of branch circuits required, the wire sizing for such branch circuits and feeders and the requirements for protection from overcurrent for conductors. A load calculation method specific to feeders is also included. This chapter is used to design the electrical system on the load side of the service.

Chapter 38 Wiring Methods. Chapter 38 specifies the allowable wiring methods, such as cable, conduit and raceway systems, and provides the installation requirements for the wiring methods. This chapter is primarily applicable to the "rough-in" phase of construction.

Chapter 39 Power and Lighting Distribution. This chapter mostly contains installation requirements for the wiring that serves the lighting outlets, receptacle outlets, appliances and switches located throughout the building. The required distribution and spacing of receptacle outlets and lighting outlets is prescribed in this chapter, as well as the requirements for ground-fault and arc-fault circuit interrupter protection.

Chapter 40 Devices and Luminaires. This chapter focuses on the devices, including switches and receptacles, and lighting fixtures that are typically installed during the final phase of construction.

Chapter 41 Appliance Installation. Chapter 41 addresses the installation of appliances including HVAC appliances, water heaters, fixed space-heating equipment, dishwashers, garbage disposals, range hoods and suspended paddle fans.

Chapter 42 Swimming Pools. This chapter covers the electrical installation requirements for swimming pools, storable swimming pools, wading pools, decorative pools, fountains, hot tubs, spas and hydromassage bathtubs. The allowable wiring methods are specified along with the required clearances between electrical system components and pools, spas and tubs. This chapter includes the special grounding requirements related to pools, spas and tubs, and also prescribes the equipotential bonding requirements that are unique to pools, spas and tubs.

Chapter 43 Class 2 Remote-control, Signaling and Power-limited Circuits. This chapter covers the power supplies, wiring methods and installation requirements for the Class 2 circuits found in dwellings. Such circuits include thermostat wiring, alarm systems, security systems, automated control systems and doorbell systems.

Chapter 44 Referenced Standards. The code contains numerous references to standards that are used to regulate materials and methods of construction. Chapter 44 contains a comprehensive list of all standards that are referenced in the code. The standards are part of the code to the extent of the reference to the standard. Compliance with the referenced standard is necessary for compliance with this code. By providing specifically adopted standards, the construction and installation requirements necessary for compliance with the code can be readily determined. The basis for code compliance is, therefore, established and available on an equal basis to the code official, contractor, designer and owner.

Chapter 44 is organized in a manner that makes it easy to locate specific standards. It lists all of the referenced standards, alphabetically, by acronym of the promulgating agency of the standard. Each agency's standards are then listed in either alphabetical or numeric order based upon the standard identification. The list also contains the title of the standard; the edition (date) of the standard referenced; any addenda included as part of the ICC adoption; and the section or sections of this code that reference the standard.

Appendix A Sizing and Capacities of Gas Piping. This appendix is informative and not part of the code. It provides design guidance, useful facts and data and multiple examples of how to apply the sizing tables and sizing methodologies of Chapter 24.

Appendix B Sizing of Venting Systems Serving Appliances Equipped with Draft Hoods, Category I Appliances and Appliances Listed for Use with Type B Vents. This appendix is informative and not part of the code. It contains multiple examples of how to apply the vent and chimney tables and methodologies of Chapter 24.

Appendix C Exit Terminals of Mechanical Draft and Direct-venting Systems. This appendix is informative and not part of the code. It consists of a figure and notes that visually depict code requirements from Chapter 24 for vent terminals with respect to the openings found in building exterior walls.

Appendix D Recommended Procedure for Safety Inspection of an Existing Appliance Installation. This appendix is informative and not part of the code. It provides recommended procedures for testing and inspecting an appliance installation to determine if the installation is operating safely and if the appliance is in a safe condition.

Appendix E Manufactured Housing Used as Dwellings. The criteria for the construction of manufactured homes are governed by the National Manufactured Housing Construction and Safety Act. While this act may seem to cover the bulk of the construction of manufactured housing, it does not cover those areas related to the placement of the housing on the property. The provisions of Appendix E are not applicable to the design and construction of manufactured homes. Appendix E provides a complete set of regulations in conjunction with federal law for the installation of manufactured housing. This appendix also contains provisions for existing manufactured home installations.

Appendix F Radon Control Methods. Radon comes from the natural (radioactive) decay of the element radium in soil, rock and water and finds its way into the air. Appendix F contains requirements to mitigate the transfer of radon gases from the soil into the dwelling. The provisions of this appendix regulate the design and construction of radon-resistant measures intended to reduce the entry of radon gases into the living space of residential buildings.

Appendix G Swimming Pool, Spas and Hot Tubs. Appendix G provides the regulations for swimming pools, hot tubs and spas installed in or on the lot of a one- or two-family dwelling. This appendix contains provisions for an effective barrier surrounding the water area and entrapment protection for suction outlets to reduce the potential for drowning of young children.

Appendix H Patio Covers. Appendix H sets forth the regulations and limitations for patio covers. The provisions address those uses permitted in patio cover structures, the minimum design loads to be assigned for structural purposes, and the effect of the patio cover on egress and emergency escape or rescue from sleeping rooms. This appendix also contains the special provisions for aluminum screen enclosures in hurricane-prone regions.

Appendix I Private Sewage Disposal.

Appendix J Existing Buildings and Structures. Appendix J contains the provisions for the repair, renovation, alteration and reconstruction of existing buildings and structures that are within the scope of this code. To accomplish this objective and to make the rehabilitation process more available, this appendix allows for a controlled departure from full code compliance without compromising minimum life safety, fire safety, structural and environmental features of the rehabilitated existing building or structure.

Appendix K Sound Transmission. Appendix K regulates the sound transmission of wall and floor-ceiling assemblies separating dwelling units and townhouse units. Air-borne sound insulation is required for walls. Air-borne sound insulation and impact sound insulation are required for floor-ceiling assemblies. The provisions in Appendix K set forth a minimum Sound Transmission Class (STC) rating for common walls and floor-ceiling assemblies between dwelling units. In addition, a minimum Impact Insulation Class (IIC) rating is also established to limit structure-borne sound through common floor-ceiling assemblies separating dwelling units.

Appendix L Permit Fees. Appendix L provides guidance to jurisdictions for setting appropriate permit fees. This appendix will aid many jurisdictions to assess permit fees that will assist to fairly and properly administer the code. This appendix can be used for informational purposes only or may be adopted when specifically referenced in the adopting ordinance.

Appendix M Home Day Care—R3 Occupancy. Appendix M provides means of egress and smoke detection requirements for a Group R-3 Occupancy that is to be used as a home day care for more than five children who receive custodial care for less than 24 hours. This appendix is strictly for guidance and/or adoption by those jurisdictions that have Licensed Home Care Provider laws and statutes that allow more than five children to be cared for in a person's home. When a jurisdiction adopts this appendix, the provisions for day care and child care facilities in the IBC should be considered also.

Appendix N Venting Methods. Because venting of sanitary drainage systems is perhaps the most difficult concept to understand, and Chapter 31 uses only words to describe venting requirements, illustrations can offer greater insight into what the words mean. Appendix N has a number of illustrations for commonly installed sanitary drainage systems in order for the reader to gain a better understanding of this code's venting requirements.

Appendix O Gray Water Recycling Systems. Appendix O offers a method for utilizing gray water that is collected from certain fixtures such as lavatories, bathtubs, showers and clothes washing machines. Because many geographical areas of the world are in short supply of water resources, water that has already passed through these fixtures is an important resource that can lessen the demand for potable water. Where gray water is used for underground irrigation, no treatment other than basic filtering is required. In this application, gray water reuse offers savings in both potable water use and less wastewater to be treated. Gray water can also be reused for flushing water for water closets and urinals. In this application, the gray water requires disinfection and coloring in order to be safe for use in those fixtures. This appendix provides the user with basic information to choose the necessary components, size and construct a gray water system that suits the particular application.

Appendix P Sizing of Water Piping System. Appendix P provides two recognized methods for sizing the water service and water distribution piping for a building. The method under Section AP103 provides friction loss diagrams that require the user to "plot" points and read values from the diagrams in order to perform the required calculations and necessary checks. This method is the most accurate of the two presented in this appendix. The method under Section AP201 is known to be conservative; however, very few calculations are necessary in order to determine a pipe size that satisfies the flow requirements of any application.

Appendix Q ICC *International Residential Code Electrical Provisions/National Electrical Code* **Cross Reference.** This cross reference allows the code user to trace the code sections in Chapters 34 through 43 back to their source: the *National Electrical Code*. See the introduction to Chapter 34 for more information on the relationship between Part VIII of this code and the NEC, NFPA 70.

ORDINANCE

The *International Codes* are designed and promulgated to be adopted by reference by ordinance. Jurisdictions wishing to adopt the 2009 *International Residential Code* as an enforceable regulation governing one- and two-family dwellings and townhouses should ensure that certain factual information is included in the adopting ordinance at the time adoption is being considered by the appropriate governmental body. The following sample adoption ordinance addresses several key elements of a code adoption ordinance, including the information required for insertion into the code text.

SAMPLE ORDINANCE FOR ADOPTION OF THE
INTERNATIONAL RESIDENTIAL CODE

ORDINANCE NO._____

An ordinance of the **[JURISDICTION]** adopting the 2009 edition of the *International Residential Code*, regulating and governing the construction, alteration, movement, enlargement, replacement, repair, equipment, location, removal and demolition of detached one- and two-family dwellings and multiple single-family dwellings (townhouses) not more than threes stories in height with separate means of egress in the **[JURISDICTION]**; providing for the issuance of permits and collection of fees therefor; repealing Ordinance No. _____ of the **[JURISDICTION]** and all other ordinances and parts of the ordinances in conflict therewith.

The **[GOVERNING BODY]** of the **[JURISDICTION]** does ordain as follows:

Section 1. That a certain document, three (3) copies of which are on file in the office of the **[TITLE OF JURISDICTION'S KEEPER OF RECORDS]** of **[NAME OF JURISDICTION]**, being marked and designated as the *International Residential Code*, 2009 edition, including Appendix Chapters **[FILL IN THE APPENDIX CHAPTERS BEING ADOPTED]** (see *International Residential Code* Section R102.5, 2009 edition), as published by the International Code Council, be and is hereby adopted as the Residential Code of the **[JURISDICTION]**, in the State of **[STATE NAME]** for regulating and governing the construction, alteration, movement, enlargement, replacement, repair, equipment, location, removal and demolition of detached one- and two-family dwellings and multiple single-family dwellings (townhouses) not more than threes stories in height with separate means of egress as herein provided; providing for the issuance of permits and collection of fees therefor; and each and all of the regulations, provisions, penalties, conditions and terms of said Residential Code on file in the office of the **[JURISDICTION]** are hereby referred to, adopted, and made a part hereof, as if fully set out in this ordinance, with the additions, insertions, deletions and changes, if any, prescribed in Section 2 of this ordinance.

Section 2. The following sections are hereby revised:

Section R101.1. Insert: **[NAME OF JURISDICTION]**

Table R301.2 (1) Insert: **[APPROPRIATE DESIGN CRITERIA]**

Section P2603.6.1 Insert: **[NUMBER OF INCHES IN TWO LOCATIONS]**

Section 3. That Ordinance No. _____ of **[JURISDICTION]** entitled **[FILL IN HERE THE COMPLETE TITLE OF THE ORDINANCE OR ORDINANCES IN EFFECT AT THE PRESENT TIME SO THAT THEY WILL BE REPEALED BY DEFINITE MENTION]** and all other ordinances or parts of ordinances in conflict herewith are hereby repealed.

Section 4. That if any section, subsection, sentence, clause or phrase of this ordinance is, for any reason, held to be unconstitutional, such decision shall not affect the validity of the remaining portions of this ordinance. The **[GOVERNING BODY]** hereby declares that it would have passed this ordinance, and each section, subsection, clause or phrase thereof, irrespective of the fact that any one or more sections, subsections, sentences, clauses and phrases be declared unconstitutional.

Section 5. That nothing in this ordinance or in the Residential Code hereby adopted shall be construed to affect any suit or proceeding impending in any court, or any rights acquired, or liability incurred, or any cause or causes of action acquired or existing, under any act or ordinance hereby repealed as cited in Section 3 of this ordinance; nor shall any just or legal right or remedy of any character be lost, impaired or affected by this ordinance.

Section 6. That the **[JURISDICTION'S KEEPER OF RECORDS]** is hereby ordered and directed to cause this ordinance to be published. (An additional provision may be required to direct the number of times the ordinance is to be published and to specify that it is to be in a newspaper in general circulation. Posting may also be required.)

Section 7. That this ordinance and the rules, regulations, provisions, requirements, orders and matters established and adopted hereby shall take effect and be in full force and effect **[TIME PERIOD]** from and after the date of its final passage and adoption.

TABLE OF CONTENTS

Part I—Administrative

CHAPTER 1

SCOPE AND ADMINISTRATION

PART I—SCOPE AND APPLICATION

SECTION R101
GENERAL

R101.1 Title. These provisions shall be known as the *Residential Code for One- and Two-family Dwellings* of [NAME OF JURISDICTION], and shall be cited as such and will be referred to herein as "this code."

R101.2 Scope. The provisions of the *International Residential Code for One- and Two-family Dwellings* shall apply to the construction, *alteration*, movement, enlargement, replacement, repair, equipment, use and occupancy, location, removal and demolition of detached one- and two-family dwellings and townhouses not more than three stories above *grade plane* in height with a separate means of egress and their *accessory structures*.

> **Exception:** Live/work units complying with the requirements of Section 419 of the *International Building Code* shall be permitted to be built as one- and two-family *dwellings* or townhouses. Fire suppression required by Section 419.5 of the *International Building Code* when constructed under the *International Residential Code for One- and Two-family Dwellings* shall conform to Section 903.3.1.3 of the *International Building Code*.

R101.3 Intent. The purpose of this code is to establish minimum requirements to safeguard the public safety, health and general welfare through affordability, structural strength, means of egress facilities, stability, sanitation, light and ventilation, energy conservation and safety to life and property from fire and other hazards attributed to the built environment and to provide safety to fire fighters and emergency responders during emergency operations.

SECTION R102
APPLICABILITY

R102.1 General. Where there is a conflict between a general requirement and a specific requirement, the specific requirement shall be applicable. Where, in any specific case, different sections of this code specify different materials, methods of construction or other requirements, the most restrictive shall govern.

R102.2 Other laws. The provisions of this code shall not be deemed to nullify any provisions of local, state or federal law.

R102.3 Application of references. References to chapter or section numbers, or to provisions not specifically identified by number, shall be construed to refer to such chapter, section or provision of this code.

R102.4 Referenced codes and standards. The codes and standards referenced in this code shall be considered part of the requirements of this code to the prescribed extent of each such reference. Where differences occur between provisions of this code and referenced codes and standards, the provisions of this code shall apply.

> **Exception:** Where enforcement of a code provision would violate the conditions of the *listing* of the *equipment* or *appliance*, the conditions of the *listing* and manufacturer's instructions shall apply.

R102.5 Appendices. Provisions in the appendices shall not apply unless specifically referenced in the adopting ordinance.

R102.6 Partial invalidity. In the event any part or provision of this code is held to be illegal or void, this shall not have the effect of making void or illegal any of the other parts or provisions.

R102.7 Existing structures. The legal occupancy of any structure existing on the date of adoption of this code shall be permitted to continue without change, except as is specifically covered in this code, the *International Property Maintenance Code* or the *International Fire Code*, or as is deemed necessary by the *building official* for the general safety and welfare of the occupants and the public.

> **R102.7.1 Additions, alterations or repairs.** *Additions*, *alterations* or repairs to any structure shall conform to the requirements for a new structure without requiring the existing structure to comply with all of the requirements of this code, unless otherwise stated. *Additions*, *alterations* or repairs shall not cause an existing structure to become unsafe or adversely affect the performance of the building.

PART II—ADMINISTRATION AND ENFORCEMENT

SECTION R103
DEPARTMENT OF BUILDING SAFETY

R103.1 Creation of enforcement agency. The department of building safety is hereby created and the official in charge thereof shall be known as the *building official*.

R103.2 Appointment. The *building official* shall be appointed by the chief appointing authority of the *jurisdiction*.

R103.3 Deputies. In accordance with the prescribed procedures of this *jurisdiction* and with the concurrence of the appointing authority, the *building official* shall have the authority to appoint a deputy *building official*, the related technical officers, inspectors, plan examiners and other employees. Such employees shall have powers as delegated by the *building official*.

SECTION R104
DUTIES AND POWERS OF THE
BUILDING OFFICIAL

R104.1 General. The *building official* is hereby authorized and directed to enforce the provisions of this code. The *building official* shall have the authority to render interpretations of this code and to adopt policies and procedures in order to clarify the application of its provisions. Such interpretations, policies and procedures shall be in conformance with the intent and purpose of this code. Such policies and procedures shall not have the effect of waiving requirements specifically provided for in this code.

R104.2 Applications and permits. The *building official* shall receive applications, review *construction documents* and issue permits for the erection and alteration of buildings and structures, inspect the premises for which such permits have been issued and enforce compliance with the provisions of this code.

R104.3 Notices and orders. The *building official* shall issue all necessary notices or orders to ensure compliance with this code.

R104.4 Inspections. The *building official* is authorized to make all of the required inspections, or the *building official* shall have the authority to accept reports of inspection by *approved agencies* or individuals. Reports of such inspections shall be in writing and be certified by a responsible officer of such *approved* agency or by the responsible individual. The *building official* is authorized to engage such expert opinion as deemed necessary to report upon unusual technical issues that arise, subject to the approval of the appointing authority.

R104.5 Identification. The *building official* shall carry proper identification when inspecting structures or premises in the performance of duties under this code.

R104.6 Right of entry. Where it is necessary to make an inspection to enforce the provisions of this code, or where the *building official* has reasonable cause to believe that there exists in a structure or upon a premises a condition which is contrary to or in violation of this code which makes the structure or premises unsafe, dangerous or hazardous, the *building official* or designee is authorized to enter the structure or premises at reasonable times to inspect or to perform the duties imposed by this code, provided that if such structure or premises be occupied that credentials be presented to the occupant and entry requested. If such structure or premises be unoccupied, the *building official* shall first make a reasonable effort to locate the owner or other person having charge or control of the structure or premises and request entry. If entry is refused, the *building official* shall have recourse to the remedies provided by law to secure entry.

R104.7 Department records. The *building official* shall keep official records of applications received, permits and certificates issued, fees collected, reports of inspections, and notices and orders issued. Such records shall be retained in the official records for the period required for the retention of public records.

R104.8 Liability. The *building official*, member of the board of appeals or employee charged with the enforcement of this code, while acting for the *jurisdiction* in good faith and without malice in the discharge of the duties required by this code or other pertinent law or ordinance, shall not thereby be rendered liable personally and is hereby relieved from personal liability for any damage accruing to persons or property as a result of any act or by reason of an act or omission in the discharge of official duties. Any suit instituted against an officer or employee because of an act performed by that officer or employee in the lawful discharge of duties and under the provisions of this code shall be defended by legal representative of the *jurisdiction* until the final termination of the proceedings. The *building official* or any subordinate shall not be liable for cost in any action, suit or proceeding that is instituted in pursuance of the provisions of this code.

R104.9 Approved materials and equipment. Materials, *equipment* and devices *approved* by the *building official* shall be constructed and installed in accordance with such approval.

R104.9.1 Used materials and equipment. Used materials, *equipment* and devices shall not be reused unless *approved* by the *building official*.

R104.10 Modifications. Wherever there are practical difficulties involved in carrying out the provisions of this code, the *building official* shall have the authority to grant modifications for individual cases, provided the *building official* shall first find that special individual reason makes the strict letter of this code impractical and the modification is in compliance with the intent and purpose of this code and that such modification does not lessen health, life and fire safety requirements or structural. The details of action granting modifications shall be recorded and entered in the files of the department of building safety.

R104.10.1 Areas prone to flooding. The *building official* shall not grant modifications to any provision related to areas prone to flooding as established by Table R301.2(1) without the granting of a variance to such provisions by the board of appeals.

R104.11 Alternative materials, design and methods of construction and equipment. The provisions of this code are not intended to prevent the installation of any material or to prohibit any design or method of construction not specifically prescribed by this code, provided that any such alternative has been *approved*. An alternative material, design or method of construction shall be *approved* where the *building official* finds that the proposed design is satisfactory and complies with the intent of the provisions of this code, and that the material, method or work offered is, for the purpose intended, at least the equivalent of that prescribed in this code. Compliance with the specific performance-based provisions of the International Codes in lieu of specific requirements of this code shall also be permitted as an alternate.

R104.11.1 Tests. Whenever there is insufficient evidence of compliance with the provisions of this code, or evidence that a material or method does not conform to the requirements of this code, or in order to substantiate claims for alternative materials or methods, the *building official* shall have the authority to require tests as evidence of compliance to be made at no expense to the *jurisdiction*. Test methods shall be as specified in this code or by other recognized test standards. In the absence of recognized and accepted test methods, the *building official* shall approve the testing procedures. Tests shall be performed by an *approved* agency. Reports of such tests shall be retained by the *building official* for the period required for retention of public records.

SECTION R105
PERMITS

R105.1 Required. Any owner or authorized agent who intends to construct, enlarge, alter, repair, move, demolish or change the occupancy of a building or structure, or to erect, install, enlarge, alter, repair, remove, convert or replace any electrical, gas, mechanical or plumbing system, the installation of which is regulated by this code, or to cause any such work to be done, shall first make application to the *building official* and obtain the required *permit*.

R105.2 Work exempt from permit. *Permits* shall not be required for the following. Exemption from *permit* requirements of this code shall not be deemed to grant authorization for any work to be done in any manner in violation of the provisions of this code or any other laws or ordinances of this *jurisdiction*.

Building:

1. One-story detached *accessory structures* used as tool and storage sheds, playhouses and similar uses, provided the floor area does not exceed 200 square feet (18.58 m²).

2. Fences not over 6 feet (1829 mm) high.

3. Retaining walls that are not over 4 feet (1219 mm) in height measured from the bottom of the footing to the top of the wall, unless supporting a surcharge.

4. Water tanks supported directly upon *grade* if the capacity does not exceed 5,000 gallons (18 927 L) and the ratio of height to diameter or width does not exceed 2 to 1.

5. Sidewalks and driveways.

6. Painting, papering, tiling, carpeting, cabinets, counter tops and similar finish work.

7. Prefabricated swimming pools that are less than 24 inches (610 mm) deep.

8. Swings and other playground equipment.

9. Window awnings supported by an exterior wall which do not project more than 54 inches (1372 mm) from the exterior wall and do not require additional support.

10. Decks not exceeding 200 square feet (18.58 m²) in area, that are not more than 30 inches (762 mm) above *grade* at any point, are not attached to a *dwelling* and do not serve the exit door required by Section R311.4.

Electrical:

1. *Listed* cord-and-plug connected temporary decorative lighting.

2. Reinstallation of attachment plug receptacles but not the outlets therefor.

3. Replacement of branch circuit overcurrent devices of the required capacity in the same location.

4. Electrical wiring, devices, *appliances,* apparatus or *equipment* operating at less than 25 volts and not capable of supplying more than 50 watts of energy.

5. Minor repair work, including the replacement of lamps or the connection of *approved* portable electrical *equipment* to *approved* permanently installed receptacles.

Gas:

1. Portable heating, cooking or clothes drying *appliances*.

2. Replacement of any minor part that does not alter approval of *equipment* or make such *equipment* unsafe.

3. Portable-fuel-cell *appliances* that are not connected to a fixed piping system and are not interconnected to a power grid.

Mechanical:

1. Portable heating *appliances*.

2. Portable ventilation *appliances*.

3. Portable cooling units.

4. Steam, hot- or chilled-water piping within any heating or cooling *equipment* regulated by this code.

5. Replacement of any minor part that does not alter approval of *equipment* or make such *equipment* unsafe.

6. Portable evaporative coolers.

7. Self-contained refrigeration systems containing 10 pounds (4.54 kg) or less of refrigerant or that are actuated by motors of 1 horsepower (746 W) or less.

8. Portable-fuel-cell *appliances* that are not connected to a fixed piping system and are not interconnected to a power grid.

The stopping of leaks in drains, water, soil, waste or vent pipe; provided, however, that if any concealed trap, drainpipe, water, soil, waste or vent pipe becomes defective and it becomes necessary to remove and replace the same with new material, such work shall be considered as new work and a *permit* shall be obtained and inspection made as provided in this code.

The clearing of stoppages or the repairing of leaks in pipes, valves or fixtures, and the removal and reinstallation of water closets, provided such repairs do not involve or require the replacement or rearrangement of valves, pipes or fixtures.

R105.2.1 Emergency repairs. Where *equipment* replacements and repairs must be performed in an emergency situation, the *permit* application shall be submitted within the next working business day to the *building official*.

R105.2.2 Repairs. Application or notice to the *building official* is not required for ordinary repairs to structures, replacement of lamps or the connection of *approved* portable electrical *equipment* to *approved* permanently installed receptacles. Such repairs shall not include the cutting away of any wall, partition or portion thereof, the removal or cutting of any structural beam or load-bearing support, or the removal or change of any required means of egress, or rearrangement of parts of a structure affecting the egress requirements; nor shall ordinary repairs include *addition* to, *alteration* of, replacement or relocation of any water supply, sewer, drainage, drain leader, gas, soil, waste, vent or similar piping, electric wiring or mechanical or other work affecting public health or general safety.

R105.2.3 Public service agencies. A *permit* shall not be required for the installation, alteration or repair of generation, transmission, distribution, metering or other related *equipment* that is under the ownership and control of public service agencies by established right.

R105.3 Application for permit. To obtain a *permit*, the applicant shall first file an application therefor in writing on a form furnished by the department of building safety for that purpose. Such application shall:

1. Identify and describe the work to be covered by the *permit* for which application is made.

2. Describe the land on which the proposed work is to be done by legal description, street address or similar description that will readily identify and definitely locate the proposed building or work.

3. Indicate the use and occupancy for which the proposed work is intended.

4. Be accompanied by *construction documents* and other information as required in Section R106.1.

5. State the valuation of the proposed work.

6. Be signed by the applicant or the applicant's authorized agent.

7. Give such other data and information as required by the *building official*.

R105.3.1 Action on application. The *building official* shall examine or cause to be examined applications for permits and amendments thereto within a reasonable time after filing. If the application or the *construction documents* do not conform to the requirements of pertinent laws, the *building official* shall reject such application in writing stating the reasons therefor. If the *building official* is satisfied that the proposed work conforms to the requirements of this code and laws and ordinances applicable thereto, the *building official* shall issue a *permit* therefor as soon as practicable.

R105.3.1.1 Determination of substantially improved or substantially damaged existing buildings in flood hazard areas. For applications for reconstruction, rehabilitation, *addition* or other improvement of existing buildings or structures located in an area prone to flooding as established by Table R301.2(1), the *building official* shall examine or cause to be examined the *construction documents* and shall prepare a finding with regard to the value of the proposed work. For buildings that have sustained damage of any origin, the value of the proposed work shall include the cost to repair the building or structure to its predamaged condition. If the *building official* finds that the value of proposed work equals or exceeds 50 percent of the market value of the building or structure before the damage has occurred or the improvement is started, the finding shall be provided to the board of appeals for a determination of substantial improvement or substantial damage. Applications determined by the board of appeals to constitute substantial improvement or substantial damage shall require all existing portions of the entire building or structure to meet the requirements of Section R322.

R105.3.2 Time limitation of application. An application for a *permit* for any proposed work shall be deemed to have been abandoned 180 days after the date of filing unless such application has been pursued in good faith or a *permit* has been issued; except that the *building official* is authorized to grant one or more extensions of time for additional periods not exceeding 180 days each. The extension shall be requested in writing and justifiable cause demonstrated.

R105.4 Validity of permit. The issuance or granting of a *permit* shall not be construed to be a *permit* for, or an *approval* of, any violation of any of the provisions of this code or of any other ordinance of the *jurisdiction*. Permits presuming to give authority to violate or cancel the provisions of this code or other ordinances of the *jurisdiction* shall not be valid. The issuance of a *permit* based on *construction documents* and other data shall not prevent the *building official* from requiring the correction of errors in the *construction documents* and other data. The *building official* is also authorized to prevent occupancy or use of a structure where in violation of this code or of any other ordinances of this *jurisdiction*.

R105.5 Expiration. Every *permit* issued shall become invalid unless the work authorized by such *permit* is commenced within 180 days after its issuance, or if the work authorized by such *permit* is suspended or abandoned for a period of 180 days after the time the work is commenced. The *building official* is authorized to grant, in writing, one or more extensions of time, for periods not more than 180 days each. The extension shall be requested in writing and justifiable cause demonstrated.

R105.6 Suspension or revocation. The *building official* is authorized to suspend or revoke a *permit* issued under the provisions of this code wherever the *permit* is issued in error or on the basis of incorrect, inaccurate or incomplete information, or in violation of any ordinance or regulation or any of the provisions of this code.

R105.7 Placement of permit. The building *permit* or copy thereof shall be kept on the site of the work until the completion of the project.

R105.8 Responsibility. It shall be the duty of every person who performs work for the installation or repair of building, structure, electrical, gas, mechanical or plumbing systems, for which this code is applicable, to comply with this code.

R105.9 Preliminary inspection. Before issuing a *permit,* the *building official* is authorized to examine or cause to be examined buildings, structures and sites for which an application has been filed.

SECTION R106
CONSTRUCTION DOCUMENTS

R106.1 Submittal documents. Submittal documents consisting of *construction documents*, and other data shall be submitted in two or more sets with each application for a *permit*. The *construction documents* shall be prepared by a registered *design professional* where required by the statutes of the *jurisdiction* in which the project is to be constructed. Where special conditions exist, the *building official* is authorized to require additional *construction documents* to be prepared by a registered *design professional*.

> **Exception:** The *building official* is authorized to waive the submission of *construction documents* and other data not required to be prepared by a registered *design professional* if it is found that the nature of the work applied for is such that reviewing of *construction documents* is not necessary to obtain compliance with this code.

R106.1.1 Information on construction documents. *Construction documents* shall be drawn upon suitable material. Electronic media documents are permitted to be submitted when *approved* by the *building official*. *Construction documents* shall be of sufficient clarity to indicate the location, nature and extent of the work proposed and show in detail that it will conform to the provisions of this code and relevant laws, ordinances, rules and regulations, as determined by the *building official*. Where required by the *building official*, all braced wall lines, shall be identified on the *construction documents* and all pertinent information including, but not limited to, bracing methods, location and length of braced wall panels, foundation requirements of braced wall panels at top and bottom shall be provided.

R106.1.2 Manufacturer's installation instructions. Manufacturer's installation instructions, as required by this code, shall be available on the job site at the time of inspection.

R106.1.3 Information for construction in flood hazard areas. For buildings and structures located in whole or in part in flood hazard areas as established by Table R301.2(1), *construction documents* shall include:

1. Delineation of flood hazard areas, floodway boundaries and flood zones and the design flood elevation, as appropriate;

2. The elevation of the proposed lowest floor, including *basement*; in areas of shallow flooding (AO Zones), the height of the proposed lowest floor, including *basement*, above the highest adjacent *grade*;

3. The elevation of the bottom of the lowest horizontal structural member in coastal high hazard areas (V Zone); and

4. If design flood elevations are not included on the community's Flood Insurance Rate Map (FIRM), the *building official* and the applicant shall obtain and reasonably utilize any design flood elevation and floodway data available from other sources.

R106.2 Site plan or plot plan. The *construction documents* submitted with the application for *permit* shall be accompanied by a site plan showing the size and location of new construction and existing structures on the site and distances from *lot lines*. In the case of demolition, the site plan shall show construction to be demolished and the location and size of existing structures and construction that are to remain on the site or plot. The *building official* is authorized to waive or modify the requirement for a site plan when the application for permit is for alteration or repair or when otherwise warranted.

R106.3 Examination of documents. The *building official* shall examine or cause to be examined *construction documents* for code compliance.

R106.3.1 Approval of construction documents. When the *building official* issues a *permit*, the *construction documents* shall be *approved* in writing or by a stamp which states "REVIEWED FOR CODE COMPLIANCE." One set of *construction documents* so reviewed shall be retained by the *building official*. The other set shall be returned to the applicant, shall be kept at the site of work and shall be open to inspection by the *building official* or his or her authorized representative.

R106.3.2 Previous approvals. This code shall not require changes in the *construction documents*, construction or designated occupancy of a structure for which a lawful *permit* has been heretofore issued or otherwise lawfully authorized, and the construction of which has been pursued in good faith within 180 days after the effective date of this code and has not been abandoned.

R106.3.3 Phased approval. The *building official* is authorized to issue a *permit* for the construction of foundations or any other part of a building or structure before the *construction documents* for the whole building or structure have been submitted, provided that adequate information and detailed statements have been filed complying with pertinent requirements of this code. The holder of such *permit* for the foundation or other parts of a building or structure shall proceed at the holder's own risk with the building operation and without assurance that a *permit* for the entire structure will be granted.

R106.4 Amended construction documents. Work shall be installed in accordance with the *approved construction documents*, and any changes made during construction that are not in compliance with the *approved construction documents* shall be resubmitted for approval as an amended set of *construction documents*.

R106.5 Retention of construction documents. One set of *approved construction documents* shall be retained by the *building official* for a period of not less than 180 days from date of completion of the permitted work, or as required by state or local laws.

SECTION R107
TEMPORARY STRUCTURES AND USES

R107.1 General. The *building official* is authorized to issue a *permit* for temporary structures and temporary uses. Such permits shall be limited as to time of service, but shall not be permitted for more than 180 days. The *building official* is authorized to grant extensions for demonstrated cause.

R107.2 Conformance. Temporary structures and uses shall conform to the structural strength, fire safety, means of egress, light, ventilation and sanitary requirements of this code as necessary to ensure the public health, safety and general welfare.

R107.3 Temporary power. The *building official* is authorized to give permission to temporarily supply and use power in part of an electric installation before such installation has been fully completed and the final certificate of completion has been issued. The part covered by the temporary certificate shall comply with the requirements specified for temporary lighting, heat or power in NFPA 70.

R107.4 Termination of approval. The *building official* is authorized to terminate such *permit* for a temporary structure or use and to order the temporary structure or use to be discontinued.

SECTION R108
FEES

R108.1 Payment of fees. A *permit* shall not be valid until the fees prescribed by law have been paid. Nor shall an amendment to a *permit* be released until the additional fee, if any, has been paid.

R108.2 Schedule of permit fees. On buildings, structures, electrical, gas, mechanical and plumbing systems or *alterations* requiring a *permit*, a fee for each *permit* shall be paid as required, in accordance with the schedule as established by the applicable governing authority.

R108.3 Building permit valuations. Building *permit* valuation shall include total value of the work for which a *permit* is being issued, such as electrical, gas, mechanical, plumbing equipment and other permanent systems, including materials and labor.

R108.4 Related fees. The payment of the fee for the construction, alteration, removal or demolition for work done in connection with or concurrently with the work authorized by a building *permit* shall not relieve the applicant or holder of the *permit* from the payment of other fees that are prescribed by law.

R108.5 Refunds. The *building official* is authorized to establish a refund policy.

R108.6 Work commencing before permit issuance. Any person who commences work requiring a *permit* on a building, structure, electrical, gas, mechanical or plumbing system before obtaining the necessary permits shall be subject to a fee established by the applicable governing authority that shall be in addition to the required *permit* fees.

SECTION R109
INSPECTIONS

R109.1 Types of inspections. For onsite construction, from time to time the *building official*, upon notification from the *permit* holder or his agent, shall make or cause to be made any necessary inspections and shall either approve that portion of the construction as completed or shall notify the *permit* holder or his or her agent wherein the same fails to comply with this code.

R109.1.1 Foundation inspection. Inspection of the foundation shall be made after poles or piers are set or trenches or *basement* areas are excavated and any required forms erected and any required reinforcing steel is in place and supported prior to the placing of concrete. The foundation inspection shall include excavations for thickened slabs intended for the support of bearing walls, partitions, structural supports, or *equipment* and special requirements for wood foundations.

R109.1.2 Plumbing, mechanical, gas and electrical systems inspection. Rough inspection of plumbing, mechanical, gas and electrical systems shall be made prior to covering or concealment, before fixtures or *appliances* are set or installed, and prior to framing inspection.

> **Exception:** Back-filling of ground-source heat pump loop systems tested in accordance with Section M2105.1 prior to inspection shall be permitted.

R109.1.3 Floodplain inspections. For construction in areas prone to flooding as established by Table R301.2(1), upon placement of the lowest floor, including *basement*, and prior to further vertical construction, the *building official* shall require submission of documentation, prepared and sealed by a registered *design professional*, of the elevation of the lowest floor, including *basement*, required in Section R322.

R109.1.4 Frame and masonry inspection. Inspection of framing and masonry construction shall be made after the roof, masonry, all framing, firestopping, draftstopping and bracing are in place and after the plumbing, mechanical and electrical rough inspections are *approved*.

R109.1.5 Other inspections. In addition to the called inspections above, the *building official* may make or require any other inspections to ascertain compliance with this code and other laws enforced by the *building official*.

R109.1.5.1 Fire-resistance-rated construction inspection. Where fire-resistance-rated construction is required between *dwelling units* or due to location on property, the *building official* shall require an inspection of such construction after all lathing and/or wallboard is in place, but before any plaster is applied, or before wallboard joints and fasteners are taped and finished.

R109.1.6 Final inspection. Final inspection shall be made after the permitted work is complete and prior to occupancy.

R109.2 Inspection agencies. The *building official* is authorized to accept reports of *approved* agencies, provided such agencies satisfy the requirements as to qualifications and reliability.

R109.3 Inspection requests. It shall be the duty of the *permit* holder or their agent to notify the *building official* that such work is ready for inspection. It shall be the duty of the person requesting any inspections required by this code to provide access to and means for inspection of such work.

R109.4 Approval required. Work shall not be done beyond the point indicated in each successive inspection without first obtaining the approval of the *building official*. The *building official* upon notification, shall make the requested inspections and shall either indicate the portion of the construction that is satisfactory as completed, or shall notify the *permit* holder or an agent of the *permit* holder wherein the same fails to comply with this code. Any portions that do not comply shall be corrected and such portion shall not be covered or concealed until authorized by the *building official*.

SECTION R110
CERTIFICATE OF OCCUPANCY

R110.1 Use and occupancy. No building or structure shall be used or occupied, and no change in the existing occupancy classification of a building or structure or portion thereof shall be made until the *building official* has issued a certificate of occupancy therefor as provided herein. Issuance of a certificate of occupancy shall not be construed as an approval of a violation of the provisions of this code or of other ordinances of the *jurisdiction*. Certificates presuming to give authority to violate or cancel the provisions of this code or other ordinances of the *jurisdiction* shall not be valid.

Exceptions:

1. Certificates of occupancy are not required for work exempt from permits under Section R105.2.

2. Accessory buildings or structures.

R110.2 Change in use. Changes in the character or use of an existing structure shall not be made except as specified in Sections 3406 and 3407 of the *International Building Code*.

R110.3 Certificate issued. After the *building official* inspects the building or structure and finds no violations of the provisions of this code or other laws that are enforced by the department of building safety, the *building official* shall issue a certificate of occupancy which shall contain the following:

1. The building *permit* number.

2. The address of the structure.

3. The name and address of the owner.

4. A description of that portion of the structure for which the certificate is issued.

5. A statement that the described portion of the structure has been inspected for compliance with the requirements of this code.

6. The name of the *building official*.

7. The edition of the code under which the *permit* was issued.

8. If an automatic sprinkler system is provided and whether the sprinkler system is required.

9. Any special stipulations and conditions of the building *permit*.

R110.4 Temporary occupancy. The *building official* is authorized to issue a temporary certificate of occupancy before the completion of the entire work covered by the *permit*, provided that such portion or portions shall be occupied safely. The *building official* shall set a time period during which the temporary certificate of occupancy is valid.

R110.5 Revocation. The *building official* shall, in writing, suspend or revoke a certificate of occupancy issued under the provisions of this code wherever the certificate is issued in error, or on the basis of incorrect information supplied, or where it is determined that the building or structure or portion thereof is in violation of any ordinance or regulation or any of the provisions of this code.

SECTION R111
SERVICE UTILITIES

R111.1 Connection of service utilities. No person shall make connections from a utility, source of energy, fuel or power to any building or system that is regulated by this code for which a *permit* is required, until *approved* by the *building official*.

R111.2 Temporary connection. The *building official* shall have the authority to authorize and approve the temporary connection of the building or system to the utility, source of energy, fuel or power.

R111.3 Authority to disconnect service utilities. The *building official* shall have the authority to authorize disconnection of utility service to the building, structure or system regulated by this code and the referenced codes and standards set forth in Section R102.4 in case of emergency where necessary to eliminate an immediate hazard to life or property or when such utility connection has been made without the approval required by Section R111.1 or R111.2. The *building official* shall notify the serving utility and whenever possible the owner and occupant of the building, structure or service system of the decision to disconnect prior to taking such action if not notified prior to disconnection. The owner or occupant of the building, structure or service system shall be notified in writing as soon as practical thereafter.

SECTION R112
BOARD OF APPEALS

R112.1 General. In order to hear and decide appeals of orders, decisions or determinations made by the *building official* relative to the application and interpretation of this code, there shall be and is hereby created a board of appeals. The *building official* shall be an ex officio member of said board but shall have no vote on any matter before the board. The board of appeals shall be appointed by the governing body and shall hold office at its pleasure. The board shall adopt rules of procedure for conducting its business, and shall render all decisions and findings in writing to the appellant with a duplicate copy to the *building official*.

R112.2 Limitations on authority. An application for appeal shall be based on a claim that the true intent of this code or the rules legally adopted thereunder have been incorrectly interpreted, the provisions of this code do not fully apply, or an equally good or better form of construction is proposed. The board shall have no authority to waive requirements of this code.

R112.2.1 Determination of substantial improvement in areas prone to flooding. When the *building official* provides a finding required in Section R105.3.1.1, the board of appeals shall determine whether the value of the proposed work constitutes a substantial improvement. A substantial improvement means any repair, reconstruction, rehabilitation, *addition* or improvement of a building or structure, the cost of which equals or exceeds 50 percent of the market value of the building or structure before the improvement or repair is started. If the building or structure has sustained substantial damage, all repairs are considered substantial improvement regardless of the actual repair work performed. The term does not include:

1. Improvements of a building or structure required to correct existing health, sanitary or safety code violations identified by the *building official* and which are the minimum necessary to assure safe living conditions; or

2. Any alteration of an historic building or structure, provided that the alteration will not preclude the continued designation as an historic building or structure. For the purpose of this exclusion, an historic building is:

    2.1. *Listed* or preliminarily determined to be eligible for *listing* in the National Register of Historic Places; or

    2.2. Determined by the Secretary of the U.S. Department of Interior as contributing to the historical significance of a registered historic district or a district preliminarily determined to qualify as an historic district; or

    2.3. Designated as historic under a state or local historic preservation program that is *approved* by the Department of Interior.

R112.2.2 Criteria for issuance of a variance for areas prone to flooding. A variance shall be issued only upon:

1. A showing of good and sufficient cause that the unique characteristics of the size, configuration or topography of the site render the elevation standards in Section R322 inappropriate.

2. A determination that failure to grant the variance would result in exceptional hardship by rendering the *lot* undevelopable.

3. A determination that the granting of a variance will not result in increased flood heights, additional threats to public safety, extraordinary public expense, cause fraud on or victimization of the public, or conflict with existing local laws or ordinances.

4. A determination that the variance is the minimum necessary to afford relief, considering the flood hazard.

5. Submission to the applicant of written notice specifying the difference between the design flood elevation and the elevation to which the building is to be built, stating that the cost of flood insurance will be commensurate with the increased risk resulting from the reduced floor elevation, and stating that construction below the design flood elevation increases risks to life and property.

R112.3 Qualifications. The board of appeals shall consist of members who are qualified by experience and training to pass on matters pertaining to building construction and are not employees of the *jurisdiction*.

R112.4 Administration. The *building official* shall take immediate action in accordance with the decision of the board.

SECTION R113
VIOLATIONS

R113.1 Unlawful acts. It shall be unlawful for any person, firm or corporation to erect, construct, alter, extend, repair, move, remove, demolish or occupy any building, structure or *equipment* regulated by this code, or cause same to be done, in conflict with or in violation of any of the provisions of this code.

R113.2 Notice of violation. The *building official* is authorized to serve a notice of violation or order on the person responsible for the erection, construction, alteration, extension, repair, moving, removal, demolition or occupancy of a building or structure in violation of the provisions of this code, or in violation of a detail statement or a plan *approved* thereunder, or in violation of a *permit* or certificate issued under the provisions of this code. Such order shall direct the discontinuance of the illegal action or condition and the abatement of the violation.

R113.3 Prosecution of violation. If the notice of violation is not complied with in the time prescribed by such notice, the *building official* is authorized to request the legal counsel of the *jurisdiction* to institute the appropriate proceeding at law or in equity to restrain, correct or abate such violation, or to require the removal or termination of the unlawful occupancy of the building or structure in violation of the provisions of this code or of the order or direction made pursuant thereto.

R113.4 Violation penalties. Any person who violates a provision of this code or fails to comply with any of the requirements thereof or who erects, constructs, alters or repairs a building or structure in violation of the *approved construction documents* or directive of the *building official,* or of a *permit* or certificate issued under the provisions of this code, shall be subject to penalties as prescribed by law.

SECTION R114
STOP WORK ORDER

R114.1 Notice to owner. Upon notice from the *building official* that work on any building or structure is being prosecuted contrary to the provisions of this code or in an unsafe and dangerous manner, such work shall be immediately stopped. The stop work order shall be in writing and shall be given to the owner of the property involved, or to the owner's agent or to the person doing the work and shall state the conditions under which work will be permitted to resume.

R114.2 Unlawful continuance. Any person who shall continue any work in or about the structure after having been served with a stop work order, except such work as that person is directed to perform to remove a violation or unsafe condition, shall be subject to penalties as prescribed by law.

Part II—Definitions

CHAPTER 2
DEFINITIONS

SECTION R201
GENERAL

R201.1 Scope. Unless otherwise expressly stated, the following words and terms shall, for the purposes of this code, have the meanings indicated in this chapter.

R201.2 Interchangeability. Words used in the present tense include the future; words in the masculine gender include the feminine and neuter; the singular number includes the plural and the plural, the singular.

R201.3 Terms defined in other codes. Where terms are not defined in this code such terms shall have meanings ascribed to them as in other code publications of the International Code Council.

R201.4 Terms not defined. Where terms are not defined through the methods authorized by this section, such terms shall have ordinarily accepted meanings such as the context implies.

SECTION R202
DEFINITIONS

ACCESSIBLE. Signifies access that requires the removal of an access panel or similar removable obstruction.

ACCESSIBLE, READILY. Signifies access without the necessity for removing a panel or similar obstruction.

ACCESSORY STRUCTURE. A structure not greater than 3,000 square feet (279 m²) in floor area, and not over two stories in height, the use of which is customarily accessory to and incidental to that of the dwelling(s) and which is located on the same *lot*.

ADDITION. An extension or increase in floor area or height of a building or structure.

ADHERED STONE OR MASONRY VENEER. Stone or masonry veneer secured and supported through the adhesion of an *approved* bonding material applied to an *approved* backing.

AIR ADMITTANCE VALVE. A one-way valve designed to allow air into the plumbing drainage system when a negative pressure develops in the piping. This device shall close by gravity and seal the terminal under conditions of zero differential pressure (no flow conditions) and under positive internal pressure.

AIR BARRIER. Material(s) assembled and joined together to provide a barrier to air leakage through the building envelope. An air barrier may be a single material, or a combination of materials.

AIR BREAK (DRAINAGE SYSTEM). An arrangement in which a discharge pipe from a fixture, *appliance* or device drains indirectly into a receptor below the flood-level rim of the receptor, and above the trap seal.

AIR CIRCULATION, FORCED. A means of providing space conditioning utilizing movement of air through ducts or plenums by mechanical means.

AIR-CONDITIONING SYSTEM. A system that consists of heat exchangers, blowers, filters, supply, exhaust and return-air systems, and shall include any apparatus installed in connection therewith.

AIR GAP, DRAINAGE SYSTEM. The unobstructed vertical distance through free atmosphere between the outlet of a waste pipe and the flood-level rim of the fixture or receptor into which it is discharging.

AIR GAP, WATER-DISTRIBUTION SYSTEM. The unobstructed vertical distance through free atmosphere between the lowest opening from a water supply discharge to the flood-level rim of a plumbing fixture.

AIR-IMPERMEABLE INSULATION. An insulation having an air permanence equal to or less than 0.02 L/s-m² at 75 Pa pressure differential tested according to ASTM E 2178 or E 283.

ALTERATION. Any construction or renovation to an existing structure other than repair or addition that requires a *permit*. Also, a change in a mechanical system that involves an extension, addition or change to the arrangement, type or purpose of the original installation that requires a *permit*.

ANCHORED STONE OR MASONRY VENEER. Stone or masonry veneer secured with *approved* mechanical fasteners to an approved backing.

ANCHORS. See "Supports."

ANTISIPHON. A term applied to valves or mechanical devices that eliminate siphonage.

APPLIANCE. A device or apparatus that is manufactured and designed to utilize energy and for which this code provides specific requirements.

APPROVED. Acceptable to the *building official*.

APPROVED AGENCY. An established and recognized agency regularly engaged in conducting tests or furnishing inspection services, when such agency has been *approved* by the *building official*.

ASPECT RATIO. The ratio of longest to shortest perpendicular dimensions, or for wall sections, the ratio of height to length.

ATTIC. The unfinished space between the ceiling assembly of the top *story* and the roof assembly.

ATTIC, HABITABLE. A finished or unfinished area, not considered a *story*, complying with all of the following requirements:

1. The occupiable floor area is at least 70 square feet (17 m²), in accordance with Section R304,

2. The occupiable floor area has a ceiling height in accordance with Section R305, and

3. The occupiable space is enclosed by the roof assembly above, knee walls (if applicable) on the sides and the floor-ceiling assembly below.

BACKFLOW, DRAINAGE. A reversal of flow in the drainage system.

BACKFLOW PREVENTER. A device or means to prevent backflow.

BACKFLOW PREVENTER, REDUCED–PRESSURE-ZONE TYPE. A backflow-prevention device consisting of two independently acting check valves, internally force loaded to a normally closed position and separated by an intermediate chamber (or zone) in which there is an automatic relief means of venting to atmosphere internally loaded to a normally open position between two tightly closing shutoff valves and with means for testing for tightness of the checks and opening of relief means.

BACKFLOW, WATER DISTRIBUTION. The flow of water or other liquids into the potable water-supply piping from any sources other than its intended source. Backsiphonage is one type of backflow.

BACKPRESSURE. Pressure created by any means in the water distribution system, which by being in excess of the pressure in the water supply mains causes a potential backflow condition.

BACKPRESSURE, LOW HEAD. A pressure less than or equal to 4.33 psi (29.88 kPa) or the pressure exerted by a 10-foot (3048 mm) column of water.

BACKSIPHONAGE. The flowing back of used or contaminated water from piping into a potable water-supply pipe due to a negative pressure in such pipe.

BACKWATER VALVE. A device installed in a drain or pipe to prevent backflow of sewage.

BASEMENT. That portion of a building that is partly or completely below *grade* (see "*Story above grade*").

BASEMENT WALL. The opaque portion of a wall that encloses one side of a *basement* and has an average below *grade* wall area that is 50 percent or more of the total opaque and non-opaque area of that enclosing side.

BASIC WIND SPEED. Three-second gust speed at 33 feet (10 058 mm) above the ground in Exposure C (see Section R301.2.1) as given in Figure R301.2(4).

BATHROOM GROUP. A group of fixtures, including or excluding a bidet, consisting of a water closet, lavatory, and bathtub or shower. Such fixtures are located together on the same floor level.

BEND. A drainage fitting, designed to provide a change in direction of a drain pipe of less than the angle specified by the amount necessary to establish the desired slope of the line (see "Elbow" and "Sweep").

BOILER. A self-contained *appliance* from which hot water is circulated for heating purposes and then returned to the boiler, and which operates at water pressures not exceeding 160 pounds per square inch gage (psig) (1102 kPa gauge) and at water temperatures not exceeding 250°F (121°C).

BOND BEAM. A horizontal grouted element within masonry in which reinforcement is embedded.

BRACED WALL LINE. A straight line through the building plan that represents the location of the lateral resistance provided by the wall bracing.

BRACED WALL LINE, CONTINUOUSLY SHEATHED. A *braced wall line* with structural sheathing applied to all sheathable surfaces including the areas above and below openings.

BRACED WALL PANEL. A full-height section of wall constructed to resist in-plane shear loads through interaction of framing members, sheathing material and anchors. The panel's length meets the requirements of its particular bracing method, and contributes toward the total amount of bracing required along its *braced wall line* in accordance with Section R602.10.1.

BRANCH. Any part of the piping system other than a riser, main or stack.

BRANCH, FIXTURE. See "Fixture branch, drainage."

BRANCH, HORIZONTAL. See "Horizontal branch, drainage."

BRANCH INTERVAL. A vertical measurement of distance, 8 feet (2438 mm) or more in *developed length*, between the connections of horizontal branches to a drainage stack. Measurements are taken down the stack from the highest horizontal branch connection.

BRANCH, MAIN. A water-distribution pipe that extends horizontally off a main or riser to convey water to branches or fixture groups.

BRANCH, VENT. A vent connecting two or more individual vents with a vent stack or stack vent.

BTU/H. The *listed* maximum capacity of an *appliance*, absorption unit or burner expressed in British thermal units input per hour.

BUILDING. Building shall mean any one- and two-family dwelling or portion thereof, including *townhouses*, that is used, or designed or intended to be used for human habitation, for living, sleeping, cooking or eating purposes, or any combination thereof, and shall include accessory structures thereto.

BUILDING DRAIN. The lowest piping that collects the discharge from all other drainage piping inside the house and extends 30 inches (762 mm) in *developed length* of pipe, beyond the *exterior walls* and conveys the drainage to the *building sewer*.

BUILDING, EXISTING. Existing building is a building erected prior to the adoption of this code, or one for which a legal building *permit* has been issued.

BUILDING LINE. The line established by law, beyond which a building shall not extend, except as specifically provided by law.

BUILDING OFFICIAL. The officer or other designated authority charged with the administration and enforcement of this code.

BUILDING SEWER. That part of the drainage system that extends from the end of the *building drain* and conveys its discharge to a public sewer, private sewer, individual sewage-disposal system or other point of disposal.

BUILDING THERMAL ENVELOPE. The *basement walls*, *exterior walls*, floor, roof and any other building element that enclose *conditioned spaces*.

BUILT-UP ROOF COVERING. Two or more layers of felt cemented together and surfaced with a cap sheet, mineral aggregate, smooth coating or similar surfacing material.

CAP PLATE. The top plate of the double top plates used in structural insulated panel (SIP) construction. The cap plate is cut to match the panel thickness such that it overlaps the wood structural panel facing on both sides.

CEILING HEIGHT. The clear vertical distance from the finished floor to the finished ceiling.

CEMENT PLASTER. A mixture of portland or blended cement, portland cement or blended cement and hydrated lime, masonry cement or plastic cement and aggregate and other *approved* materials as specified in this code.

CHIMNEY. A primary vertical structure containing one or more flues, for the purpose of carrying gaseous products of combustion and air from a fuel-burning *appliance* to the outside atmosphere.

CHIMNEY CONNECTOR. A pipe that connects a fuel-burning *appliance* to a chimney.

CHIMNEY TYPES.

> **Residential-type appliance.** An *approved* chimney for removing the products of combustion from fuel-burning, residential-type *appliances* producing combustion gases not in excess of 1,000°F (538°C) under normal operating conditions, but capable of producing combustion gases of 1,400°F (760°C) during intermittent forces firing for periods up to 1 hour. All temperatures shall be measured at the *appliance* flue outlet. Residential-type *appliance* chimneys include masonry and factory-built types.

CIRCUIT VENT. A vent that connects to a horizontal drainage branch and vents two traps to a maximum of eight traps or trapped fixtures connected into a battery.

CLADDING. The exterior materials that cover the surface of the building envelope that is directly loaded by the wind.

CLEANOUT. An accessible opening in the drainage system used for the removal of possible obstruction.

CLOSET. A small room or chamber used for storage.

COMBINATION WASTE AND VENT SYSTEM. A specially designed system of waste piping embodying the horizontal wet venting of one or more sinks or floor drains by means of a common waste and vent pipe adequately sized to provide free movement of air above the flow line of the drain.

COMBUSTIBLE MATERIAL. Any material not defined as noncombustible.

COMBUSTION AIR. The air provided to fuel-burning *equipment* including air for fuel combustion, draft hood dilution and ventilation of the *equipment* enclosure.

COMMON VENT. A single pipe venting two trap arms within the same *branch interval*, either back-to-back or one above the other.

CONDENSATE. The liquid that separates from a gas due to a reduction in temperature, e.g., water that condenses from flue gases and water that condenses from air circulating through the cooling coil in air conditioning *equipment*.

CONDENSING APPLIANCE. An *appliance* that condenses water generated by the burning of fuels.

CONDITIONED AIR. Air treated to control its temperature, relative humidity or quality.

CONDITIONED AREA. That area within a building provided with heating and/or cooling systems or *appliances* capable of maintaining, through design or heat loss/gain, 68°F (20°C) during the heating season and/or 80°F (27°C) during the cooling season, or has a fixed opening directly adjacent to a conditioned area.

CONDITIONED FLOOR AREA. The horizontal projection of the floors associated with the *conditioned space*.

CONDITIONED SPACE. For energy purposes, space within a building that is provided with heating and/or cooling *equipment* or systems capable of maintaining, through design or heat loss/gain, 50°F (10°C) during the heating season and 85°F (29°C) during the cooling season, or communicates directly with a *conditioned space*. For mechanical purposes, an area, room or space being heated or cooled by any *equipment* or *appliance*.

CONSTRUCTION DOCUMENTS. Written, graphic and pictorial documents prepared or assembled for describing the design, location and physical characteristics of the elements of a project necessary for obtaining a building *permit*. Construction drawings shall be drawn to an appropriate scale.

CONTAMINATION. An impairment of the quality of the potable water that creates an actual hazard to the public health through poisoning or through the spread of disease by sewage, industrial fluids or waste.

CONTINUOUS WASTE. A drain from two or more similar adjacent fixtures connected to a single trap.

CONTROL, LIMIT. An automatic control responsive to changes in liquid flow or level, pressure, or temperature for limiting the operation of an *appliance*.

CONTROL, PRIMARY SAFETY. A safety control responsive directly to flame properties that senses the presence or absence of flame and, in event of ignition failure or unintentional flame extinguishment, automatically causes shutdown of mechanical equipment.

CONVECTOR. A system-incorporating heating element in an enclosure in which air enters an opening below the heating element, is heated and leaves the enclosure through an opening located above the heating element.

CORE. The light-weight middle section of the structural insulated panel composed of foam plastic insulation, which provides the link between the two facing shells.

CORROSION RESISTANCE. The ability of a material to withstand deterioration of its surface or its properties when exposed to its environment.

COURT. A space, open and unobstructed to the sky, located at or above *grade* level on a *lot* and bounded on three or more sides by walls or a building.

CRIPPLE WALL. A framed wall extending from the top of the foundation to the underside of the floor framing of the first *story above grade plane*.

CROSS CONNECTION. Any connection between two otherwise separate piping systems whereby there may be a flow from one system to the other.

DALLE GLASS. A decorative composite glazing material made of individual pieces of glass that are embedded in a cast matrix of concrete or epoxy.

DAMPER, VOLUME. A device that will restrict, retard or direct the flow of air in any duct, or the products of combustion of heat-producing *equipment*, vent connector, vent or chimney.

DEAD END. A branch leading from a DWV system terminating at a *developed length* of 2 feet (610 mm) or more. Dead ends shall be prohibited except as an *approved* part of a rough-in for future connection.

DEAD LOADS. The weight of all materials of construction incorporated into the building, including but not limited to walls, floors, roofs, ceilings, stairways, built-in partitions, finishes, cladding, and other similarly incorporated architectural and structural items, and fixed service *equipment*.

DECORATIVE GLASS. A carved, leaded or Dalle glass or glazing material whose purpose is decorative or artistic, not functional; whose coloring, texture or other design qualities or components cannot be removed without destroying the glazing material; and whose surface, or assembly into which it is incorporated, is divided into segments.

DESIGN PROFESSIONAL. See *"Registered design professional."*

DEVELOPED LENGTH. The length of a pipeline measured along the center line of the pipe and fittings.

DIAMETER. Unless specifically stated, the term "diameter" is the nominal diameter as designated by the *approved* material standard.

DIAPHRAGM. A horizontal or nearly horizontal system acting to transmit lateral forces to the vertical resisting elements. When the term *"diaphragm"* is used, it includes horizontal bracing systems.

DILUTION AIR. Air that enters a draft hood or draft regulator and mixes with flue gases.

DIRECT-VENT APPLIANCE. A fuel-burning *appliance* with a sealed combustion system that draws all air for combustion from the outside atmosphere and discharges all flue gases to the outside atmosphere.

DRAFT. The pressure difference existing between the *appliance* or any component part and the atmosphere, that causes a continuous flow of air and products of combustion through the gas passages of the *appliance* to the atmosphere.

> **Induced draft.** The pressure difference created by the action of a fan, blower or ejector, that is located between the *appliance* and the chimney or vent termination.

> **Natural draft.** The pressure difference created by a vent or chimney because of its height, and the temperature difference between the flue gases and the atmosphere.

DRAFT HOOD. A device built into an *appliance*, or a part of the vent connector from an *appliance*, which is designed to provide for the ready escape of the flue gases from the *appliance* in the event of no draft, backdraft or stoppage beyond the draft hood; prevent a backdraft from entering the *appliance*; and neutralize the effect of stack action of the chimney or gas vent on the operation of the *appliance*.

DRAFT REGULATOR. A device that functions to maintain a desired draft in the *appliance* by automatically reducing the draft to the desired value.

DRAFT STOP. A material, device or construction installed to restrict the movement of air within open spaces of concealed areas of building components such as crawl spaces, floor-ceiling assemblies, roof-ceiling assemblies and *attics*.

DRAIN. Any pipe that carries soil and water-borne wastes in a building drainage system.

DRAINAGE FITTING. A pipe fitting designed to provide connections in the drainage system that have provisions for establishing the desired slope in the system. These fittings are made from a variety of both metals and plastics. The methods of coupling provide for required slope in the system (see "Durham fitting").

DUCT SYSTEM. A continuous passageway for the transmission of air which, in addition to ducts, includes duct fittings, dampers, plenums, fans and accessory air-handling *equipment* and *appliances*.

DURHAM FITTING. A special type of drainage fitting for use in the durham systems installations in which the joints are made with recessed and tapered threaded fittings, as opposed to bell and spigot lead/oakum or solvent/cemented or soldered joints. The tapping is at an angle (not 90 degrees) to provide for proper slope in otherwise rigid connections.

DURHAM SYSTEM. A term used to describe soil or waste systems where all piping is of threaded pipe, tube or other such rigid construction using recessed drainage fittings to correspond to the types of piping.

DWELLING. Any building that contains one or two *dwelling units* used, intended, or designed to be built, used, rented, leased, let or hired out to be occupied, or that are occupied for living purposes.

DWELLING UNIT. A single unit providing complete independent living facilities for one or more persons, including permanent provisions for living, sleeping, eating, cooking and sanitation.

DWV. Abbreviated term for drain, waste and vent piping as used in common plumbing practice.

EFFECTIVE OPENING. The minimum cross-sectional area at the point of water-supply discharge, measured or expressed in terms of diameter of a circle and if the opening is not circular, the diameter of a circle of equivalent cross-sectional area. (This is applicable to air gap.)

ELBOW. A pressure pipe fitting designed to provide an exact change in direction of a pipe run. An elbow provides a sharp turn in the flow path (see "Bend" and "Sweep").

EMERGENCY ESCAPE AND RESCUE OPENING. An operable exterior window, door or similar device that provides for a means of escape and access for rescue in the event of an emergency.

EQUIPMENT. All piping, ducts, vents, control devices and other components of systems other than *appliances* that are permanently installed and integrated to provide control of environmental conditions for buildings. This definition shall also include other systems specifically regulated in this code.

EQUIVALENT LENGTH. For determining friction losses in a piping system, the effect of a particular fitting equal to the friction loss through a straight piping length of the same nominal diameter.

ESCARPMENT. With respect to topographic wind effects, a cliff or steep slope generally separating two levels or gently sloping areas.

ESSENTIALLY NONTOXIC TRANSFER FLUIDS. Fluids having a Gosselin rating of 1, including propylene glycol; mineral oil; polydimenthyoil oxane; hydrochlorofluorocarbon, chlorofluorocarbon and hydrofluorocarbon refrigerants; and FDA-*approved* boiler water additives for steam boilers.

ESSENTIALLY TOXIC TRANSFER FLUIDS. Soil, water or gray water and fluids having a Gosselin rating of 2 or more including ethylene glycol, hydrocarbon oils, ammonia refrigerants and hydrazine.

EVAPORATIVE COOLER. A device used for reducing air temperature by the process of evaporating water into an airstream.

EXCESS AIR. Air that passes through the combustion chamber and the *appliance* flue in excess of that which is theoretically required for complete combustion.

EXHAUST HOOD, FULL OPENING. An exhaust hood with an opening at least equal to the diameter of the connecting vent.

EXISTING INSTALLATIONS. Any plumbing system regulated by this code that was legally installed prior to the effective date of this code, or for which a *permit* to install has been issued.

EXTERIOR INSULATION AND FINISH SYSTEMS (EIFS). EIFS are nonstructural, nonload-bearing *exterior wall* cladding systems that consist of an insulation board attached either adhesively or mechanically, or both, to the substrate; an integrally reinforced base coat; and a textured protective finish coat.

EXTERIOR INSULATION AND FINISH SYSTEMS (EIFS) WITH DRAINAGE. An EIFS that incorporates a means of drainage applied over a water-resistive barrier.

EXTERIOR WALL. An above-*grade* wall that defines the exterior boundaries of a building. Includes between-floor spandrels, peripheral edges of floors, roof and *basement* knee walls, dormer walls, gable end walls, walls enclosing a mansard roof and *basement walls* with an average below-*grade* wall area that is less than 50 percent of the total opaque and nonopaque area of that enclosing side.

FACING. The wood structural panel facings that form the two outmost rigid layers of the structural insulated panel.

FACTORY-BUILT CHIMNEY. A *listed* and *labeled* chimney composed of factory-made components assembled in the field in accordance with the manufacturer's instructions and the conditions of the listing.

FENESTRATION. Skylights, roof windows, vertical windows (whether fixed or moveable); opaque doors; glazed doors; glass block; and combination opaque/glazed doors.

FIBER-CEMENT SIDING. A manufactured, fiber-reinforcing product made with an inorganic hydraulic or calcium silicate binder formed by chemical reaction and reinforced with discrete organic or inorganic nonasbestos fibers, or both. Additives which enhance manufacturing or product performance are permitted. Fiber-cement siding products have either smooth or textured faces and are intended for *exterior wall* and related applications.

FIREBLOCKING. Building materials or materials *approved* for use as fireblocking, installed to resist the free passage of flame to other areas of the building through concealed spaces.

FIREPLACE. An assembly consisting of a hearth and fire chamber of noncombustible material and provided with a chimney, for use with solid fuels.

> **Factory-built fireplace.** A *listed* and *labeled* fireplace and chimney system composed of factory-made components, and assembled in the field in accordance with manufacturer's instructions and the conditions of the listing.

> **Masonry chimney.** A field-constructed chimney composed of solid masonry units, bricks, stones or concrete.

> **Masonry fireplace.** A field-constructed fireplace composed of solid masonry units, bricks, stones or concrete.

FIREPLACE STOVE. A free-standing, chimney-connected solid-fuel-burning heater designed to be operated with the fire chamber doors in either the open or closed position.

FIREPLACE THROAT. The opening between the top of the firebox and the smoke chamber.

FIRE-RETARDANT-TREATED WOOD. Pressure-treated lumber and plywood that exhibit reduced surface burning characteristics and resist propagation of fire.

Other means during manufacture. A process where the wood raw material is treated with a fire-retardant formulation while undergoing creation as a finished product.

Pressure process. A process for treating wood using an initial vacuum followed by the introduction of pressure above atmospheric.

FIRE SEPARATION DISTANCE. The distance measured from the building face to one of the following:

1. To the closest interior *lot line*; or

2. To the centerline of a street, an alley or public way; or

3. To an imaginary line between two buildings on the *lot*.

FIXTURE. See "Plumbing fixture."

FIXTURE BRANCH, DRAINAGE. A drain serving two or more fixtures that discharges into another portion of the drainage system.

FIXTURE BRANCH, WATER-SUPPLY. A water-supply pipe between the fixture supply and a main water-distribution pipe or fixture group main.

FIXTURE DRAIN. The drain from the trap of a fixture to the junction of that drain with any other drain pipe.

FIXTURE FITTING.

Supply fitting. A fitting that controls the volume and/or directional flow of water and is either attached to or accessible from a fixture or is used with an open or atmospheric discharge.

Waste fitting. A combination of components that conveys the sanitary waste from the outlet of a fixture to the connection of the sanitary drainage system.

FIXTURE GROUP, MAIN. The main water-distribution pipe (or secondary branch) serving a plumbing fixture grouping such as a bath, kitchen or laundry area to which two or more individual fixture branch pipes are connected.

FIXTURE SUPPLY. The water-supply pipe connecting a fixture or fixture fitting to a fixture branch.

FIXTURE UNIT, DRAINAGE (d.f.u.). A measure of probable discharge into the drainage system by various types of plumbing fixtures, used to size DWV piping systems. The drainage fixture-unit value for a particular fixture depends on its volume rate of drainage discharge, on the time duration of a single drainage operation and on the average time between successive operations.

FIXTURE UNIT, WATER-SUPPLY (w.s.f.u.). A measure of the probable hydraulic demand on the water supply by various types of plumbing fixtures used to size water-piping systems. The water-supply fixture-unit value for a particular fixture depends on its volume rate of supply, on the time duration of a single supply operation and on the average time between successive operations.

FLAME SPREAD. The propagation of flame over a surface.

FLAME SPREAD INDEX. A comparative measure, expressed as a dimensionless number, derived from visual measurements of the spread of flame versus time for a material tested in accordance with ASTM E 84.

FLIGHT. A continuous run of rectangular treads or winders or combination thereof from one landing to another.

FLOOD-LEVEL RIM. The edge of the receptor or fixture from which water overflows.

FLOOR DRAIN. A plumbing fixture for recess in the floor having a floor-level strainer intended for the purpose of the collection and disposal of waste water used in cleaning the floor and for the collection and disposal of accidental spillage to the floor.

FLOOR FURNACE. A self-contained furnace suspended from the floor of the space being heated, taking air for combustion from outside such space, and with means for lighting the *appliance* from such space.

FLOW PRESSURE. The static pressure reading in the water-supply pipe near the faucet or water outlet while the faucet or water outlet is open and flowing at capacity.

FLUE. See "Vent."

FLUE, APPLIANCE. The passages within an *appliance* through which combustion products pass from the combustion chamber to the flue collar.

FLUE COLLAR. The portion of a fuel-burning *appliance* designed for the attachment of a draft hood, vent connector or venting system.

FLUE GASES. Products of combustion plus excess air in *appliance* flues or heat exchangers.

FLUSH VALVE. A device located at the bottom of a flush tank that is operated to flush water closets.

FLUSHOMETER TANK. A device integrated within an air accumulator vessel that is designed to discharge a predetermined quantity of water to fixtures for flushing purposes.

FLUSHOMETER VALVE. A flushometer valve is a device that discharges a predetermined quantity of water to fixtures for flushing purposes and is actuated by direct water pressure.

FOAM BACKER BOARD. Foam plastic used in siding applications where the foam plastic is a component of the siding.

FOAM PLASTIC INSULATION. A plastic that is intentionally expanded by the use of a foaming agent to produce a reduced-density plastic containing voids consisting of open or closed cells distributed throughout the plastic for thermal insulating or acoustic purposes and that has a density less than 20 pounds per cubic foot (320 kg/m^3) unless it is used as interior trim.

FOAM PLASTIC INTERIOR TRIM. Exposed foam plastic used as picture molds, chair rails, crown moldings, baseboards, handrails, ceiling beams, door trim and window trim and similar decorative or protective materials used in fixed applications.

FUEL-PIPING SYSTEM. All piping, tubing, valves and fittings used to connect fuel utilization *equipment* to the point of fuel delivery.

FULLWAY VALVE. A valve that in the full open position has an opening cross-sectional area equal to a minimum of 85 percent of the cross-sectional area of the connecting pipe.

FURNACE. A vented heating *appliance* designed or arranged to discharge heated air into a *conditioned space* or through a duct or ducts.

GLAZING AREA. The interior surface area of all glazed fenestration, including the area of sash, curbing or other framing elements, that enclose *conditioned space*. Includes the area of glazed fenestration assemblies in walls bounding conditioned *basements*.

GRADE. The finished ground level adjoining the building at all *exterior walls*.

GRADE FLOOR OPENING. A window or other opening located such that the sill height of the opening is not more than 44 inches (1118 mm) above or below the finished ground level adjacent to the opening.

GRADE, PIPING. See "Slope."

GRADE PLANE. A reference plane representing the average of the finished ground level adjoining the building at all *exterior walls*. Where the finished ground level slopes away from the *exterior walls*, the reference plane shall be established by the lowest points within the area between the building and the *lot line* or, where the *lot line* is more than 6 ft (1829 mm) from the building between the structure and a point 6 ft (1829 mm) from the building.

GRIDDED WATER DISTRIBUTION SYSTEM. A water distribution system where every water distribution pipe is interconnected so as to provide two or more paths to each fixture supply pipe.

GROSS AREA OF EXTERIOR WALLS. The normal projection of all *exterior walls*, including the area of all windows and doors installed therein.

GROUND-SOURCE HEAT PUMP LOOP SYSTEM. Piping buried in horizontal or vertical excavations or placed in a body of water for the purpose of transporting heat transfer liquid to and from a heat pump. Included in this definition are closed loop systems in which the liquid is recirculated and open loop systems in which the liquid is drawn from a well or other source.

GUARD. A building component or a system of building components located near the open sides of elevated walking surfaces that minimizes the possibility of a fall from the walking surface to the lower level.

HABITABLE SPACE. A space in a building for living, sleeping, eating or cooking. Bathrooms, toilet rooms, closets, halls, storage or utility spaces and similar areas are not considered *habitable spaces*.

HANDRAIL. A horizontal or sloping rail intended for grasping by the hand for guidance or support.

HANGERS. See "Supports."

HAZARDOUS LOCATION. Any location considered to be a fire hazard for flammable vapors, dust, combustible fibers or other highly combustible substances.

HEAT PUMP. An *appliance* having heating or heating/cooling capability and that uses refrigerants to extract heat from air, liquid or other sources.

HEATING DEGREE DAYS (HDD). The sum, on an annual basis, of the difference between 65°F (18°C) and the mean temperature for each day as determined from "NOAA Annual Degree Days to Selected Bases Derived from the 1960-1990 Normals" or other weather data sources acceptable to the code official.

HEIGHT, BUILDING. The vertical distance from *grade plane* to the average height of the highest roof surface.

HEIGHT, STORY. The vertical distance from top to top of two successive tiers of beams or finished floor surfaces; and, for the topmost *story*, from the top of the floor finish to the top of the ceiling joists or, where there is not a ceiling, to the top of the roof rafters.

HIGH-EFFICACY LAMPS. Compact fluorescent lamps, T-8 or smaller diameter linear fluorescent lamps or lamps with a minimum efficacy of:

1. 60 lumens per watt for lamps over 40 watts.
2. 50 lumens per watt for lamps over 15 watts to 40 watts.
3. 40 lumens per watt for lamps 15 watts or less.

HIGH-TEMPERATURE (H.T.) CHIMNEY. A high temperature chimney complying with the requirements of UL 103. A Type H.T. chimney is identifiable by the markings "Type H.T." on each chimney pipe section.

HILL. With respect to topographic wind effects, a land surface characterized by strong relief in any horizontal direction.

HORIZONTAL BRANCH, DRAINAGE. A drain pipe extending laterally from a soil or waste stack or *building drain*, that receives the discharge from one or more *fixture drains*.

HORIZONTAL PIPE. Any pipe or fitting that makes an angle of less than 45 degrees (0.79 rad) with the horizontal.

HOT WATER. Water at a temperature greater than or equal to 110°F (43°C).

HURRICANE-PRONE REGIONS. Areas vulnerable to hurricanes, defined as the U.S. Atlantic Ocean and Gulf of Mexico coasts where the basic wind speed is greater than 90 miles per hour (40 m/s), and Hawaii, Puerto Rico, Guam, Virgin Islands, and America Samoa.

HYDROGEN GENERATING APPLIANCE. A self-contained package or factory-matched packages of integrated systems for generating gaseous hydrogen. Hydrogen generating *appliances* utilize electrolysis, reformation, chemical, or other processes to generate hydrogen.

IGNITION SOURCE. A flame, spark or hot surface capable of igniting flammable vapors or fumes. Such sources include *appliance* burners, burner ignitions and electrical switching devices.

INDIRECT WASTE PIPE. A waste pipe that discharges into the drainage system through an air gap into a trap, fixture or receptor.

INDIVIDUAL SEWAGE DISPOSAL SYSTEM. A system for disposal of sewage by means of a septic tank or mechanical treatment, designed for use apart from a public sewer to serve a single establishment or building.

INDIVIDUAL VENT. A pipe installed to vent a single-*fixture drain* that connects with the vent system above or terminates independently outside the building.

INDIVIDUAL WATER SUPPLY. A supply other than an *approved* public water supply that serves one or more families.

INSULATING CONCRETE FORM (ICF). A concrete forming system using stay-in-place forms of rigid foam plastic insulation, a hybrid of cement and foam insulation, a hybrid of cement and wood chips, or other insulating material for constructing cast-in-place concrete walls.

INSULATING SHEATHING. An insulating board having a minimum thermal resistance of R-2 of the core material.

JURISDICTION. The governmental unit that has adopted this code under due legislative authority.

KITCHEN. Kitchen shall mean an area used, or designated to be used, for the preparation of food.

LABEL. An identification applied on a product by the manufacturer which contains the name of the manufacturer, the function and performance characteristics of the product or material, and the name and identification of an *approved agency* and that indicates that the representative sample of the product or material has been tested and evaluated by an *approved agency*. (See also "Manufacturer's designation" and "Mark.")

LABELED. *Equipment*, materials or products to which have been affixed a *label*, seal, symbol or other identifying *mark* of a nationally recognized testing laboratory, inspection agency or other organization concerned with product evaluation that maintains periodic inspection of the production of the above-*labeled* items and whose labeling indicates either that the *equipment*, material or product meets identified standards or has been tested and found suitable for a specified purpose.

LIGHT-FRAME CONSTRUCTION. A type of construction whose vertical and horizontal structural elements are primarily formed by a system of repetitive wood or cold-formed steel framing members.

LISTED. *Equipment*, materials, products or services included in a list published by an organization acceptable to the code official and concerned with evaluation of products or services that maintains periodic inspection of production of *listed equipment* or materials or periodic evaluation of services and whose listing states either that the *equipment*, material, product or service meets identified standards or has been tested and found suitable for a specified purpose.

LIVE LOADS. Those loads produced by the use and occupancy of the building or other structure and do not include construction or environmental loads such as wind load, snow load, rain load, earthquake load, flood load or dead load.

LIVING SPACE. Space within a *dwelling unit* utilized for living, sleeping, eating, cooking, bathing, washing and sanitation purposes.

LOT. A portion or parcel of land considered as a unit.

LOT LINE. A line dividing one *lot* from another, or from a street or any public place.

MACERATING TOILET SYSTEMS. A system comprised of a sump with macerating pump and with connections for a water closet and other plumbing fixtures, that is designed to accept, grind and pump wastes to an *approved* point of discharge.

MAIN. The principal pipe artery to which branches may be connected.

MAIN SEWER. See "Public sewer."

MANIFOLD WATER DISTRIBUTION SYSTEMS. A fabricated piping arrangement in which a large supply main is fitted with multiple branches in close proximity in which water is distributed separately to fixtures from each branch.

MANUFACTURED HOME. *Manufactured home* means a structure, transportable in one or more sections, which in the traveling mode is 8 body feet (2438 body mm) or more in width or 40 body feet (12 192 body mm) or more in length, or, when erected on site, is 320 square feet (30 m^2) or more, and which is built on a permanent chassis and designed to be used as a *dwelling* with or without a permanent foundation when connected to the required utilities, and includes the plumbing, heating, air-conditioning and electrical systems contained therein; except that such term shall include any structure that meets all the requirements of this paragraph except the size requirements and with respect to which the manufacturer voluntarily files a certification required by the secretary (HUD) and complies with the standards established under this title. For mobile homes built prior to June 15, 1976, a *label* certifying compliance to the Standard for Mobile Homes, NFPA 501, in effect at the time of manufacture is required. For the purpose of these provisions, a mobile home shall be considered a *manufactured home*.

MANUFACTURER'S DESIGNATION. An identification applied on a product by the manufacturer indicating that a product or material complies with a specified standard or set of rules. (See also "*Mark*" and "*Label*.")

MANUFACTURER'S INSTALLATION INSTRUCTIONS. Printed instructions included with *equipment* as part of the conditions of listing and labeling.

MARK. An identification applied on a product by the manufacturer indicating the name of the manufacturer and the function of a product or material. (See also "Manufacturer's designation" and "*Label*.")

MASONRY CHIMNEY. A field-constructed chimney composed of solid masonry units, bricks, stones or concrete.

MASONRY HEATER. A masonry heater is a solid fuel burning heating *appliance* constructed predominantly of concrete or solid masonry having a mass of at least 1,100 pounds (500 kg), excluding the chimney and foundation. It is designed to absorb and store a substantial portion of heat from a fire built in the firebox by routing exhaust gases through internal heat exchange channels in which the flow path downstream of the firebox includes at least one 180-degree (3.14-rad) change in flow direction before entering the chimney and which deliver heat by radiation through the masonry surface of the heater.

MASONRY, SOLID. Masonry consisting of solid masonry units laid contiguously with the joints between the units filled with mortar.

MASONRY UNIT. Brick, tile, stone, glass block or concrete block conforming to the requirements specified in Section 2103 of the *International Building Code*.

> **Clay.** A building unit larger in size than a brick, composed of burned clay, shale, fire clay or mixtures thereof.

> **Concrete.** A building unit or block larger in size than 12 inches by 4 inches by 4 inches (305 mm by 102 mm by 102 mm) made of cement and suitable aggregates.

> **Glass.** Nonload-bearing masonry composed of glass units bonded by mortar.

> **Hollow.** A masonry unit whose net cross-sectional area in any plane parallel to the loadbearing surface is less than 75 percent of its gross cross-sectional area measured in the same plane.

> **Solid.** A masonry unit whose net cross-sectional area in every plane parallel to the loadbearing surface is 75 percent or more of its cross-sectional area measured in the same plane.

MASS WALL. Masonry or concrete walls having a mass greater than or equal to 30 pounds per square foot (146 kg/m²), solid wood walls having a mass greater than or equal to 20 pounds per square foot (98 kg/m²), and any other walls having a heat capacity greater than or equal to 6 Btu/ft² · °F [266 J/(m² · K)].

MEAN ROOF HEIGHT. The average of the roof eave height and the height to the highest point on the roof surface, except that eave height shall be used for roof angle of less than or equal to 10 degrees (0.18 rad).

MECHANICAL DRAFT SYSTEM. A venting system designed to remove flue or vent gases by mechanical means, that consists of an induced draft portion under nonpositive static pressure or a forced draft portion under positive static pressure.

> **Forced-draft venting system.** A portion of a venting system using a fan or other mechanical means to cause the removal of flue or vent gases under positive static pressure.

> **Induced draft venting system.** A portion of a venting system using a fan or other mechanical means to cause the removal of flue or vent gases under nonpositive static vent pressure.

> **Power venting system.** A portion of a venting system using a fan or other mechanical means to cause the removal of flue or vent gases under positive static vent pressure.

MECHANICAL EXHAUST SYSTEM. A system for removing air from a room or space by mechanical means.

MECHANICAL SYSTEM. A system specifically addressed and regulated in this code and composed of components, devices, *appliances* and *equipment*.

METAL ROOF PANEL. An interlocking metal sheet having a minimum installed weather exposure of at least 3 square feet (0.28 m²) per sheet.

METAL ROOF SHINGLE. An interlocking metal sheet having an installed weather exposure less than 3 square feet (0.28 m²) per sheet.

MEZZANINE, LOFT. An intermediate level or levels between the floor and ceiling of any *story* with an aggregate floor area of not more than one-third of the area of the room or space in which the level or levels are located.

MODIFIED BITUMEN ROOF COVERING. One or more layers of polymer modified asphalt sheets. The sheet materials shall be fully adhered or mechanically attached to the substrate or held in place with an *approved* ballast layer.

MULTIPLE STATION SMOKE ALARM. Two or more single station alarm devices that are capable of interconnection such that actuation of one causes all integral or separate audible alarms to operate.

NATURAL DRAFT SYSTEM. A venting system designed to remove flue or vent gases under nonpositive static vent pressure entirely by natural draft.

NATURALLY DURABLE WOOD. The heartwood of the following species with the exception that an occasional piece with corner sapwood is permitted if 90 percent or more of the width of each side on which it occurs is heartwood.

> **Decay resistant.** Redwood, cedar, black locust and black walnut.

> **Termite resistant.** Alaska yellow cedar, redwood, Eastern red cedar and Western red cedar including all sapwood of Western red cedar.

NONCOMBUSTIBLE MATERIAL. Materials that pass the test procedure for defining noncombustibility of elementary materials set forth in ASTM E 136.

NONCONDITIONED SPACE. A space that is not a *conditioned space* by insulated walls, floors or ceilings.

NOSING. The leading edge of treads of stairs and of landings at the top of stairway flights.

OCCUPIED SPACE. The total area of all buildings or structures on any *lot* or parcel of ground projected on a horizontal plane, excluding permitted projections as allowed by this code.

OFFSET. A combination of fittings that makes two changes in direction bringing one section of the pipe out of line but into a line parallel with the other section.

OWNER. Any person, agent, firm or corporation having a legal or equitable interest in the property.

PANEL THICKNESS. Thickness of core plus two layers of structural wood panel facings.

PELLET FUEL-BURNING APPLIANCE. A closed combustion, vented *appliance* equipped with a fuel feed mechanism for burning processed pellets of solid fuel of a specified size and composition.

PELLET VENT. A vent *listed* and *labeled* for use with a *listed* pellet fuel-burning *appliance*.

PERMIT. An official document or certificate issued by the authority having *jurisdiction* that authorizes performance of a specified activity.

PERSON. An individual, heirs, executors, administrators or assigns, and also includes a firm, partnership or corporation, its or their successors or assigns, or the agent of any of the aforesaid.

PITCH. See "Slope."

PLATFORM CONSTRUCTION. A method of construction by which floor framing bears on load bearing walls that are not continuous through the *story* levels or floor framing.

PLENUM. A chamber that forms part of an air-circulation system other than the *occupied space* being conditioned.

PLUMBING. For the purpose of this code, plumbing refers to those installations, repairs, maintenance and *alterations* regulated by Chapters 25 through 33.

PLUMBING APPLIANCE. An energized household *appliance* with plumbing connections, such as a dishwasher, food-waste grinder, clothes washer or water heater.

PLUMBING APPURTENANCE. A device or assembly that is an adjunct to the basic plumbing system and demands no additional water supply nor adds any discharge load to the system. It is presumed that it performs some useful function in the operation, maintenance, servicing, economy or safety of the plumbing system. Examples include filters, relief valves and aerators.

PLUMBING FIXTURE. A receptor or device that requires both a water-supply connection and a discharge to the drainage system, such as water closets, lavatories, bathtubs and sinks. Plumbing *appliances* as a special class of fixture are further defined.

PLUMBING SYSTEM. Includes the water supply and distribution pipes, plumbing fixtures, supports and appurtenances; soil, waste and vent pipes; sanitary drains and *building sewers* to an *approved* point of disposal.

POLLUTION. An impairment of the quality of the potable water to a degree that does not create a hazard to the public health but that does adversely and unreasonably affect the aesthetic qualities of such potable water for domestic use.

PORTABLE-FUEL-CELL APPLIANCE. A fuel cell generator of electricity, which is not fixed in place. A portable-fuel-cell *appliance* utilizes a cord and plug connection to a grid-isolated load and has an integral fuel supply.

POSITIVE ROOF DRAINAGE. The drainage condition in which consideration has been made for all loading deflections of the roof deck, and additional slope has been provided to ensure drainage of the roof within 48 hours of precipitation.

POTABLE WATER. Water free from impurities present in amounts sufficient to cause disease or harmful physiological effects and conforming in bacteriological and chemical quality to the requirements of the public health authority having *jurisdiction*.

PRECAST CONCRETE. A structural concrete element cast elsewhere than its final position in the structure.

PRECAST CONCRETE FOUNDATION WALLS. Preengineered, precast concrete wall panels that are designed to withstand specified stresses and used to build below-*grade* foundations.

PRESSURE-RELIEF VALVE. A pressure-actuated valve held closed by a spring or other means and designed to automatically relieve pressure at the pressure at which it is set.

PUBLIC SEWER. A common sewer directly controlled by public authority.

PUBLIC WATER MAIN. A water-supply pipe for public use controlled by public authority.

PUBLIC WAY. Any street, alley or other parcel of land open to the outside air leading to a public street, which has been deeded, dedicated or otherwise permanently appropriated to the public for public use and that has a clear width and height of not less than 10 feet (3048 mm).

PURGE. To clear of air, gas or other foreign substances.

QUICK-CLOSING VALVE. A valve or faucet that closes automatically when released manually or controlled by mechanical means for fast-action closing.

R-VALUE, THERMAL RESISTANCE. The inverse of the time rate of heat flow through a *building thermal envelope* element from one of its bounding surfaces to the other for a unit temperature difference between the two surfaces, under steady state conditions, per unit area (h · ft^2 · °F/Btu).

RAMP. A walking surface that has a running slope steeper than 1 unit vertical in 20 units horizontal (5-percent slope).

RECEPTOR. A fixture or device that receives the discharge from indirect waste pipes.

REFRIGERANT. A substance used to produce refrigeration by its expansion or evaporation.

REFRIGERANT COMPRESSOR. A specific machine, with or without accessories, for compressing a given refrigerant vapor.

REFRIGERATING SYSTEM. A combination of interconnected parts forming a closed circuit in which refrigerant is circulated for the purpose of extracting, then rejecting, heat. A direct refrigerating system is one in which the evaporator or condenser of the refrigerating system is in direct contact with the air or other substances to be cooled or heated. An indirect refrigerating system is one in which a secondary coolant cooled or heated by the refrigerating system is circulated to the air or other substance to be cooled or heated.

REGISTERED DESIGN PROFESSIONAL. An individual who is registered or licensed to practice their respective design profession as defined by the statutory requirements of the professional registration laws of the state or *jurisdiction* in which the project is to be constructed.

RELIEF VALVE, VACUUM. A device to prevent excessive buildup of vacuum in a pressure vessel.

REPAIR. The reconstruction or renewal of any part of an existing building for the purpose of its maintenance.

REROOFING. The process of recovering or replacing an existing roof covering. See "Roof recover."

RETURN AIR. Air removed from an *approved conditioned space* or location and recirculated or exhausted.

RIDGE. With respect to topographic wind effects, an elongated crest of a hill characterized by strong relief in two directions.

RISER. A water pipe that extends vertically one full *story* or more to convey water to branches or to a group of fixtures.

ROOF ASSEMBLY. A system designed to provide weather protection and resistance to design loads. The system consists of a roof covering and roof deck or a single component serving as both the roof covering and the roof deck. A roof assembly includes the roof deck, vapor retarder, substrate or thermal barrier, insulation, vapor retarder, and roof covering.

ROOF COVERING. The covering applied to the roof deck for weather resistance, fire classification or appearance.

ROOF COVERING SYSTEM. See "Roof assembly."

ROOF DECK. The flat or sloped surface not including its supporting members or vertical supports.

ROOF RECOVER. The process of installing an additional roof covering over a prepared existing roof covering without removing the existing roof covering.

ROOF REPAIR. Reconstruction or renewal of any part of an existing roof for the purposes of its maintenance.

ROOFTOP STRUCTURE. An enclosed structure on or above the roof of any part of a building.

ROOM HEATER. A freestanding heating *appliance* installed in the space being heated and not connected to ducts.

ROUGH-IN. The installation of all parts of the plumbing system that must be completed prior to the installation of fixtures. This includes DWV, water supply and built-in fixture supports.

RUNNING BOND. The placement of masonry units such that head joints in successive courses are horizontally offset at least one-quarter the unit length.

SANITARY SEWER. A sewer that carries sewage and excludes storm, surface and groundwater.

SCUPPER. An opening in a wall or parapet that allows water to drain from a roof.

SEISMIC DESIGN CATEGORY (SDC). A classification assigned to a structure based on its occupancy category and the severity of the design earthquake ground motion at the site.

SEPTIC TANK. A water-tight receptor that receives the discharge of a building sanitary drainage system and is constructed so as to separate solids from the liquid, digest organic matter through a period of detention, and allow the liquids to discharge into the soil outside of the tank through a system of open joint or perforated piping or a seepage pit.

SEWAGE. Any liquid waste containing animal matter, vegetable matter or other impurity in suspension or solution.

SEWAGE PUMP. A permanently installed mechanical device for removing sewage or liquid waste from a sump.

SHALL. The term, when used in the code, is construed as mandatory.

SHEAR WALL. A general term for walls that are designed and constructed to resist racking from seismic and wind by use of masonry, concrete, cold-formed steel or wood framing in

accordance with Chapter 6 of this code and the associated limitations in Section R301.2 of this code.

SIDE VENT. A vent connecting to the drain pipe through a fitting at an angle less than 45 degrees (0.79 rad) to the horizontal.

SINGLE PLY MEMBRANE. A roofing membrane that is field applied using one layer of membrane material (either homogeneous or composite) rather than multiple layers.

SINGLE STATION SMOKE ALARM. An assembly incorporating the detector, control *equipment* and alarm sounding device in one unit that is operated from a power supply either in the unit or obtained at the point of installation.

SKYLIGHT AND SLOPED GLAZING. See Section R308.6.1.

SKYLIGHT, UNIT. See Section R308.6.1.

SLIP JOINT. A mechanical-type joint used primarily on fixture traps. The joint tightness is obtained by compressing a friction-type washer such as rubber, nylon, neoprene, lead or special packing material against the pipe by the tightening of a (slip) nut.

SLOPE. The fall (pitch) of a line of pipe in reference to a horizontal plane. In drainage, the slope is expressed as the fall in units vertical per units horizontal (percent) for a length of pipe.

SMOKE-DEVELOPED INDEX. A comparative measure, expressed as a dimensionless number, derived from measurements of smoke obscuration versus time for a material tested in accordance with ASTM E 84.

SOIL STACK OR PIPE. A pipe that conveys sewage containing fecal material.

SOLAR HEAT GAIN COEFFICIENT (SHGC). The solar heat gain through a fenestration or glazing assembly relative to the incident solar radiation (Btu/h · ft^2 · °F).

SOLID MASONRY. Load-bearing or nonload-bearing construction using masonry units where the net cross-sectional area of each unit in any plane parallel to the bearing surface is not less than 75 percent of its gross cross-sectional area. Solid masonry units shall conform to ASTM C 55, C 62, C 73, C 145 or C 216.

SPLINE. A strip of wood structural panel cut from the same material used for the panel facings, used to connect two structural insulated panels. The strip (spline) fits into a groove cut into the vertical edges of the two structural insulated panels to be joined. Splines are used behind each facing of the structural insulated panels being connected as shown in Figure R613.8.

STACK. Any main vertical DWV line, including offsets, that extends one or more stories as directly as possible to its vent terminal.

STACK BOND. The placement of masonry units in a bond pattern is such that head joints in successive courses are vertically aligned. For the purpose of this code, requirements for stack bond shall apply to all masonry laid in other than running bond.

STACK VENT. The extension of soil or waste stack above the highest horizontal drain connected.

STACK VENTING. A method of venting a fixture or fixtures through the soil or waste stack without individual fixture vents.

STAIR. A change in elevation, consisting of one or more risers.

STAIRWAY. One or more flights of stairs, either interior or exterior, with the necessary landings and platforms connecting them to form a continuous and uninterrupted passage from one level to another within or attached to a building, porch or deck.

STANDARD TRUSS. Any construction that does not permit the roof/ceiling insulation to achieve the required R-value over the *exterior walls*.

STATIONARY FUEL CELL POWER PLANT. A self-contained package or factory-matched packages which constitute an automatically-operated assembly of integrated systems for generating useful electrical energy and recoverable thermal energy that is permanently connected and fixed in place.

STORM SEWER, DRAIN. A pipe used for conveying rainwater, surface water, subsurface water and similar liquid waste.

STORY. That portion of a building included between the upper surface of a floor and the upper surface of the floor or roof next above.

STORY ABOVE GRADE PLANE. Any *story* having its finished floor surface entirely above *grade plane*, except that a *basement* shall be considered as a *story above grade plane* where the finished surface of the floor above the *basement* meets any one of the following:

1. Is more than 6 feet (1829 mm) *above grade plane*.

2. Is more than 6 feet (1829 mm) above the finished ground level for more than 50 percent of the total building perimeter.

3. Is more than 12 feet (3658 mm) above the finished ground level at any point.

STRUCTURAL INSULATED PANEL (SIP). A structural sandwich panel that consists of a light-weight foam plastic core securely laminated between two thin, rigid wood structural panel facings.

STRUCTURE. That which is built or constructed.

SUBSOIL DRAIN. A drain that collects subsurface water or seepage water and conveys such water to a place of disposal.

SUMP. A tank or pit that receives sewage or waste, located below the normal *grade* of the gravity system and that must be emptied by mechanical means.

SUMP PUMP. A pump installed to empty a sump. These pumps are used for removing storm water only. The pump is selected for the specific head and volume of the load and is usually operated by level controllers.

SUNROOM. A one-story structure attached to a *dwelling* with a *glazing area* in excess of 40 percent of the gross area of the structure's *exterior walls* and roof.

SUPPLY AIR. Air delivered to a *conditioned space* through ducts or plenums from the heat exchanger of a heating, cooling or ventilating system.

SUPPORTS. Devices for supporting, hanging and securing pipes, fixtures and *equipment*.

SWEEP. A drainage fitting designed to provide a change in direction of a drain pipe of less than the angle specified by the amount necessary to establish the desired slope of the line. Sweeps provide a longer turning radius than bends and a less turbulent flow pattern (see "Bend" and "Elbow").

TEMPERATURE- AND PRESSURE-RELIEF (T AND P) VALVE. A combination relief valve designed to function as both a temperature-relief and pressure-relief valve.

TEMPERATURE-RELIEF VALVE. A temperature-actuated valve designed to discharge automatically at the temperature at which it is set.

TERMITE-RESISTANT MATERIAL. Pressure-preservative treated wood in accordance with the AWPA standards in Section R318.1, naturally durable termite-resistant wood, steel, concrete, masonry or other *approved* material.

THERMAL ISOLATION. Physical and space conditioning separation from *conditioned space(s)* consisting of existing or new walls, doors and/or windows. The *conditioned space(s)* shall be controlled as separate zones for heating and cooling or conditioned by separate *equipment*.

THERMAL RESISTANCE, *R*-VALUE. The inverse of the time rate of heat flow through a body from one of its bounding surfaces to the other for a unit temperature difference between the two surfaces, under steady state conditions, per unit area (h · ft^2 · °F/Btu).

THERMAL TRANSMITTANCE, *U*-FACTOR. The coefficient of heat transmission (air to air) through a building envelope component or assembly, equal to the time rate of heat flow per unit area and unit temperature difference between the warm side and cold side air films (Btu/h · ft^2 · °F).

TOWNHOUSE. A single-family *dwelling unit* constructed in a group of three or more attached units in which each unit extends from foundation to roof and with a *yard* or public way on at least two sides.

TRAP. A fitting, either separate or built into a fixture, that provides a liquid seal to prevent the emission of sewer gases without materially affecting the flow of sewage or waste water through it.

TRAP ARM. That portion of a *fixture drain* between a trap weir and the vent fitting.

TRAP PRIMER. A device or system of piping to maintain a water seal in a trap, typically installed where infrequent use of the trap would result in evaporation of the trap seal, such as floor drains.

TRAP SEAL. The trap seal is the maximum vertical depth of liquid that a trap will retain, measured between the crown weir and the top of the dip of the trap.

TRIM. Picture molds, chair rails, baseboards, handrails, door and window frames, and similar decorative or protective materials used in fixed applications.

TRUSS DESIGN DRAWING. The graphic depiction of an individual truss, which describes the design and physical characteristics of the truss.

TYPE L VENT. A *listed* and *labeled* vent conforming to UL 641 for venting oil-burning *appliances listed* for use with Type L vents or with gas *appliances listed* for use with Type B vents.

***U*-FACTOR, THERMAL TRANSMITTANCE.** The coefficient of heat transmission (air to air) through a building envelope component or assembly, equal to the time rate of heat flow per unit area and unit temperature difference between the warm side and cold side air films (Btu/h · ft^2 · °F).

➤ **UNDERLAYMENT.** One or more layers of felt, sheathing paper, nonbituminous saturated felt, or other *approved* material over which a roof covering, with a slope of 2 to 12 (17-percent slope) or greater, is applied.

➤ **VACUUM BREAKERS.** A device which prevents back-siphonage of water by admitting atmospheric pressure through ports to the discharge side of the device.

VAPOR PERMEABLE MEMBRANE. A material or covering having a permeance rating of 5 perms (2.9 · 10^{-10} kg/Pa · s · m^2) or greater, when tested in accordance with the desiccant method using Procedure A of ASTM E 96. A vapor permeable material permits the passage of moisture vapor.

VAPOR RETARDER CLASS. A measure of the ability of a material or assembly to limit the amount of moisture that passes through that material or assembly. Vapor retarder class shall be defined using the desiccant method with Procedure A of ASTM E 96 as follows:

Class I: 0.1 perm or less

Class II: 0.1 < perm ≤ 1.0 perm

Class III: 1.0 < perm ≤ 10 perm

VEHICULAR ACCESS DOOR. A door that is used primarily for vehicular traffic at entrances of buildings such as garages and parking lots, and that is not generally used for pedestrian traffic.

VENT. A passageway for conveying flue gases from fuel-fired *appliances*, or their vent connectors, to the outside atmosphere.

VENT COLLAR. See "Flue collar."

VENT CONNECTOR. That portion of a venting system which connects the flue collar or draft hood of an *appliance* to a vent.

VENT DAMPER DEVICE, AUTOMATIC. A device intended for installation in the venting system, in the outlet of an individual, automatically operated fuel burning *appliance* and that is designed to open the venting system automatically when the *appliance* is in operation and to close off the venting system automatically when the *appliance* is in a standby or shutdown condition.

VENT GASES. Products of combustion from fuel-burning *appliances*, plus excess air and dilution air, in the venting system above the draft hood or draft regulator.

VENT STACK. A vertical vent pipe installed to provide circulation of air to and from the drainage system and which extends through one or more stories.

VENT SYSTEM. Piping installed to equalize pneumatic pressure in a drainage system to prevent trap seal loss or blow-back due to siphonage or back pressure.

VENTILATION. The natural or mechanical process of supplying conditioned or unconditioned air to, or removing such air from, any space.

VENTING. Removal of combustion products to the outdoors.

VENTING SYSTEM. A continuous open passageway from the flue collar of an *appliance* to the outside atmosphere for the purpose of removing flue or vent gases. A venting system is usually composed of a vent or a chimney and vent connector, if used, assembled to form the open passageway.

VERTICAL PIPE. Any pipe or fitting that makes an angle of 45 degrees (0.79 rad) or more with the horizontal.

VINYL SIDING. A shaped material, made principally from rigid polyvinyl chloride (PVC), that is used to cover exterior walls of buildings.

WALL, RETAINING. A wall not laterally supported at the top, that resists lateral soil load and other imposed loads.

WALLS. Walls shall be defined as follows:

Load-bearing wall is a wall supporting any vertical load in addition to its own weight.

Nonbearing wall is a wall which does not support vertical loads other than its own weight.

WASTE. Liquid-borne waste that is free of fecal matter.

WASTE PIPE OR STACK. Piping that conveys only liquid sewage not containing fecal material.

WATER-DISTRIBUTION SYSTEM. Piping which conveys water from the service to the plumbing fixtures, *appliances*, appurtenances, *equipment*, devices or other systems served, including fittings and control valves.

WATER HEATER. Any heating *appliance* or *equipment* that heats potable water and supplies such water to the potable hot water distribution system.

WATER MAIN. A water-supply pipe for public use.

WATER OUTLET. A valved discharge opening, including a hose bibb, through which water is removed from the potable water system supplying water to a plumbing fixture or plumbing *appliance* that requires either an air gap or backflow prevention device for protection of the supply system.

WATER-RESISTIVE BARRIER. A material behind an *exterior wall* covering that is intended to resist liquid water that has penetrated behind the exterior covering from further intruding into the *exterior wall* assembly.

WATER-SERVICE PIPE. The outside pipe from the water main or other source of potable water supply to the water-distribution system inside the building, terminating at the service valve.

WATER-SUPPLY SYSTEM. The water-service pipe, the water-distributing pipes and the necessary connecting pipes, fittings, control valves and all appurtenances in or adjacent to the building or premises.

WET VENT. A vent that also receives the discharge of wastes from other fixtures.

WIND-BORNE DEBRIS REGION. Areas within *hurricane-prone regions* within one mile of the coastal mean high water line where the basic wind speed is 110 miles per hour (49 m/s) or greater; or where the basic wind speed is equal to or greater than 120 miles per hour (54 m/s); or Hawaii.

WINDER. A tread with nonparallel edges.

WOOD/PLASTIC COMPOSITE. A composite material made primarily from wood or cellulose-based materials and plastic.

WOOD STRUCTURAL PANEL. A panel manufactured from veneers; or wood strands or wafers; bonded together with waterproof synthetic resins or other suitable bonding systems. Examples of wood structural panels are plywood, OSB or composite panels.

YARD. An open space, other than a court, unobstructed from the ground to the sky, except where specifically provided by this code, on the *lot* on which a building is situated.

Part III—Building Planning and Construction

CHAPTER 3

BUILDING PLANNING

SECTION R301
DESIGN CRITERIA

R301.1 Application. Buildings and structures, and all parts thereof, shall be constructed to safely support all loads, including dead loads, live loads, roof loads, flood loads, snow loads, wind loads and seismic loads as prescribed by this code. The construction of buildings and structures in accordance with the provisions of this code shall result in a system that provides a complete load path that meets all requirements for the transfer of all loads from their point of origin through the load-resisting elements to the foundation. Buildings and structures constructed as prescribed by this code are deemed to comply with the requirements of this section.

R301.1.1 Alternative provisions. As an alternative to the requirements in Section R301.1 the following standards are permitted subject to the limitations of this code and the limitations therein. Where engineered design is used in conjunction with these standards, the design shall comply with the *International Building Code.*

1. American Forest and Paper Association (AF&PA) *Wood Frame Construction Manual* (WFCM).

2. American Iron and Steel Institute (AISI) *Standard for Cold-Formed Steel Framing—Prescriptive Method for One- and Two-Family Dwellings* (AISI S230).

3. ICC-400 *Standard on the Design and Construction of Log Structures.*

R301.1.2 Construction systems. The requirements of this code are based on platform and balloon-frame construction for light-frame buildings. The requirements for concrete and masonry buildings are based on a balloon framing system. Other framing systems must have equivalent detailing to ensure force transfer, continuity and compatible deformations.

R301.1.3 Engineered design. When a building of otherwise conventional construction contains structural elements exceeding the limits of Section R301 or otherwise not conforming to this code, these elements shall be designed in accordance with accepted engineering practice. The extent of such design need only demonstrate compliance of nonconventional elements with other applicable provisions and shall be compatible with the performance of the conventional framed system. Engineered design in accordance with the *International Building Code* is permitted for all buildings and structures, and parts thereof, included in the scope of this code.

R301.2 Climatic and geographic design criteria. Buildings shall be constructed in accordance with the provisions of this code as limited by the provisions of this section. Additional criteria shall be established by the local *jurisdiction* and set forth in Table R301.2(1).

R301.2.1 Wind limitations. Buildings and portions thereof shall be limited by wind speed, as defined in Table R301.2(1) and construction methods in accordance with this code. Basic wind speeds shall be determined from Figure R301.2(4). Where different construction methods and structural materials are used for various portions of a building, the applicable requirements of this section for each portion shall apply. Where loads for wall coverings, curtain walls, roof coverings, exterior windows, skylights, garage doors and exterior doors are not otherwise specified, the loads listed in Table R301.2(2) adjusted for height and exposure using Table R301.2(3) shall be used to determine design load performance requirements for wall coverings, curtain walls, roof coverings, exterior windows, skylights, garage doors and exterior doors. Asphalt shingles shall be designed for wind speeds in accordance with Section R905.2.6.

R301.2.1.1 Design criteria. In regions where the basic wind speeds from Figure R301.2(4) equal or exceed 100 miles per hour (45 m/s) in *hurricane-prone regions*, or 110 miles per hour (49 m/s) elsewhere, the design of buildings shall be in accordance with one of the following methods. The elements of design not addressed by those documents in Items 1 through 4 shall be in accordance with this code.

1. American Forest and Paper Association (AF&PA) *Wood Frame Construction Manual for One- and Two-Family Dwellings* (WFCM); or

2. International Code Council (ICC) *Standard for Residential Construction in High Wind Regions* (ICC-600); or

3. *Minimum Design Loads for Buildings and Other Structures* (ASCE-7); or

4. American Iron and Steel Institute (AISI), *Standard for Cold-Formed Steel Framing—Prescriptive Method For One- and Two-Family Dwellings* (AISI S230).

5. Concrete construction shall be designed in accordance with the provisions of this code.

6. Structural insulated panel (SIP) walls shall be designed in accordance with the provisions of this code.

TABLE R301.2(1)
CLIMATIC AND GEOGRAPHIC DESIGN CRITERIA

GROUND SNOW LOAD	WIND DESIGN		SEISMIC DESIGN CATEGORY[f]	SUBJECT TO DAMAGE FROM			WINTER DESIGN TEMP[e]	ICE BARRIER UNDERLAYMENT REQUIRED[h]	FLOOD HAZARDS[g]	AIR FREEZING INDEX[i]	MEAN ANNUAL TEMP[j]
	Speed[d] (mph)	Topographic effects[k]		Weathering[a]	Frost line depth[b]	Termite[c]					

For SI: 1 pound per square foot = 0.0479 kPa, 1 mile per hour = 0.447 m/s.

a. Weathering may require a higher strength concrete or grade of masonry than necessary to satisfy the structural requirements of this code. The weathering column shall be filled in with the weathering index (i.e., "negligible," "moderate" or "severe") for concrete as determined from the Weathering Probability Map [Figure R301.2(3)]. The grade of masonry units shall be determined from ASTM C 34, C 55, C 62, C 73, C 90, C 129, C 145, C 216 or C 652.

b. The frost line depth may require deeper footings than indicated in Figure R403.1(1). The jurisdiction shall fill in the frost line depth column with the minimum depth of footing below finish grade.

c. The jurisdiction shall fill in this part of the table to indicate the need for protection depending on whether there has been a history of local subterranean termite damage.

d. The jurisdiction shall fill in this part of the table with the wind speed from the basic wind speed map [FigureR301.2(4)].Wind exposure category shall be determined on a site-specific basis in accordance with Section R301.2.1.4.

e. The outdoor design dry-bulb temperature shall be selected from the columns of 97$^1/_2$-percent values for winter from Appendix D of the *International Plumbing Code*. Deviations from the Appendix D temperatures shall be permitted to reflect local climates or local weather experience as determined by the building official.

f. The jurisdiction shall fill in this part of the table with the seismic design category determined from Section R301.2.2.1.

g. The jurisdiction shall fill in this part of the table with (a) the date of the jurisdiction's entry into the National Flood Insurance Program (date of adoption of the first code or ordinance for management of flood hazard areas), (b) the date(s) of the Flood Insurance Study and (c) the panel numbers and dates of all currently effective FIRMs and FBFMs or other flood hazard map adopted by the authority having jurisdiction, as amended.

h. In accordance with Sections R905.2.7.1, R905.4.3.1, R905.5.3.1, R905.6.3.1, R905.7.3.1 and R905.8.3.1, where there has been a history of local damage from the effects of ice damming, the jurisdiction shall fill in this part of the table with "YES." Otherwise, the jurisdiction shall fill in this part of the table with "NO."

i. The jurisdiction shall fill in this part of the table with the 100-year return period air freezing index (BF-days) from Figure R403.3(2) or from the 100-year (99%) value on the National Climatic Data Center data table "Air Freezing Index- USA Method (Base 32°)" at www.ncdc.noaa.gov/fpsf.html.

j. The jurisdiction shall fill in this part of the table with the mean annual temperature from the National Climatic Data Center data table "Air Freezing Index-USA Method (Base 32°F)" at www.ncdc.noaa.gov/fpsf.html.

k. In accordance with Section R301.2.1.5, where there is local historical data documenting structural damage to buildings due to topographic wind speed-up effects, the jurisdiction shall fill in this part of the table with "YES." Otherwise, the jurisdiction shall indicate "NO" in this part of the table.

TABLE R301.2(2)
COMPONENT AND CLADDING LOADS FOR A BUILDING WITH A MEAN ROOF HEIGHT OF 30 FEET LOCATED IN EXPOSURE B (psf)[a, b, c, d, e]

Each wind-speed cell lists the positive and negative pressure, separated by a comma.

	ZONE	EFFECTIVE WIND AREA (feet²)	85	90	100	105	110	120	125	130	140	145	150	170
Roof > 0 to 10 degrees	1	10	10.0, -13.0	10.0, -14.6	10.0, -18.0	10.0, -19.8	10.0, -21.8	10.5, -25.9	11.4, -28.1	12.4, -30.4	14.3, -35.3	15.4, -37.8	16.5, -40.5	21.1, -52.0
	1	20	10.0, -12.7	10.0, -14.2	10.0, -17.5	10.0, -19.3	10.0, -21.2	10.0, -25.2	10.7, -27.4	11.6, -29.6	13.4, -34.4	14.4, -36.9	15.4, -39.4	19.8, -50.7
	1	50	10.0, -12.2	10.0, -13.7	10.0, -16.9	10.0, -18.7	10.0, -20.5	10.0, -24.4	10.0, -26.4	10.6, -28.6	12.3, -33.2	13.1, -35.6	14.1, -38.1	18.1, -48.9
	1	100	10.0, -11.9	10.0, -13.3	10.0, -16.5	10.0, -18.2	10.0, -19.9	10.0, -23.7	10.0, -25.7	10.0, -27.8	11.4, -32.3	12.2, -34.6	13.0, -37.0	16.7, -47.6
	2	10	10.0, -21.8	10.0, -24.4	10.0, -30.2	10.0, -33.3	10.0, -36.5	10.5, -43.5	11.4, -47.2	12.4, -51.0	14.3, -59.2	15.4, -63.5	16.5, -67.9	21.1, -87.2
	2	20	10.0, -19.5	10.0, -21.8	10.0, -27.0	10.0, -29.7	10.0, -32.6	10.0, -38.8	10.7, -42.1	11.6, -45.6	13.4, -52.9	14.4, -56.7	15.4, -60.7	19.8, -78.0
	2	50	10.0, -16.4	10.0, -18.4	10.0, -22.7	10.0, -25.1	10.0, -27.5	10.0, -32.7	10.0, -35.5	10.6, -38.4	12.3, -44.5	13.1, -47.8	14.1, -51.1	18.1, -65.7
	2	100	10.0, -14.1	10.0, -15.8	10.0, -19.5	10.0, -21.5	10.0, -23.6	10.0, -28.1	10.0, -30.5	10.0, -33.0	11.4, -38.2	12.2, -41.0	13.0, -43.9	16.7, -56.4
	3	10	10.0, -32.8	10.0, -36.8	10.0, -45.4	10.0, -50.1	10.0, -55.0	10.5, -65.4	11.4, -71.0	12.4, -76.8	14.3, -89.0	15.4, -95.5	16.5, -102.2	21.1, -131.3
	3	20	10.0, -27.2	10.0, -30.5	10.0, -37.6	10.0, -41.5	10.0, -45.5	10.0, -54.2	10.7, -58.8	11.6, -63.6	13.4, -73.8	14.4, -79.1	15.4, -84.7	19.8, -108.7
	3	50	10.0, -19.7	10.0, -22.1	10.0, -27.3	10.0, -30.1	10.0, -33.1	10.0, -39.3	10.0, -42.7	10.6, -46.2	12.3, -53.5	13.1, -57.4	14.1, -61.5	18.1, -78.9
	3	100	10.0, -14.1	10.0, -15.8	10.0, -19.5	10.0, -21.5	10.0, -23.6	10.0, -28.1	10.0, -30.5	10.0, -33.0	11.4, -38.2	12.2, -41.0	13.0, -43.9	16.7, -56.4
Roof > 10 to 30 degrees	1	10	10.0, -11.9	10.0, -13.3	10.4, -16.5	11.4, -18.2	12.5, -19.9	14.9, -23.7	16.2, -25.7	17.5, -27.8	20.3, -32.3	21.8, -34.6	23.3, -37.0	30.0, -47.6
	1	20	10.0, -11.6	10.0, -13.0	10.0, -16.0	10.4, -17.6	11.4, -19.4	13.6, -23.0	14.8, -25.0	16.0, -27.0	18.5, -31.4	19.9, -33.7	21.3, -36.0	27.3, -46.3
	1	50	10.0, -11.1	10.0, -12.5	10.0, -15.4	10.0, -17.0	10.0, -18.6	11.9, -22.2	12.9, -24.1	13.9, -26.0	16.1, -30.2	17.3, -32.4	18.5, -34.6	23.8, -44.5
	1	100	10.0, -10.8	10.0, -12.1	10.0, -14.9	10.0, -16.5	10.0, -18.1	10.5, -21.5	11.4, -23.3	12.4, -25.2	14.3, -29.3	15.4, -31.4	16.5, -33.6	21.1, -43.2
	2	10	10.0, -25.1	10.0, -28.2	10.4, -34.8	11.4, -38.3	12.5, -42.1	14.9, -50.1	16.2, -54.3	17.5, -58.7	20.3, -68.1	21.8, -73.1	23.3, -78.2	30.0, -100.5
	2	20	10.0, -22.8	10.0, -25.6	10.0, -31.5	10.4, -34.8	11.4, -38.2	13.6, -45.4	14.8, -49.3	16.0, -53.3	18.5, -61.8	19.9, -66.3	21.3, -71.0	27.3, -91.2
	2	50	10.0, -19.7	10.0, -22.1	10.0, -27.3	10.0, -30.1	10.0, -33.0	11.9, -39.3	12.9, -42.7	13.9, -46.1	16.1, -53.5	17.3, -57.4	18.5, -61.4	23.8, -78.9
	2	100	10.0, -17.4	10.0, -19.5	10.0, -24.1	10.0, -26.6	10.0, -29.1	10.5, -34.7	11.4, -37.6	12.4, -40.7	14.3, -47.2	15.4, -50.6	16.5, -54.2	21.1, -69.6
	3	10	10.0, -25.1	10.0, -28.2	10.4, -34.8	11.4, -38.3	12.5, -42.1	14.9, -50.1	16.2, -54.3	17.5, -58.7	20.3, -68.1	21.8, -73.1	23.3, -78.2	30.0, -100.5
	3	20	10.0, -22.8	10.0, -25.6	10.0, -31.5	10.4, -34.8	11.4, -38.2	13.6, -45.4	14.8, -49.3	16.0, -53.3	18.5, -61.8	19.9, -66.3	21.3, -71.0	27.3, -91.2
	3	50	10.0, -19.7	10.0, -22.1	10.0, -27.3	10.0, -30.1	10.0, -33.0	11.9, -39.3	12.9, -42.7	13.9, -46.1	16.1, -53.5	17.3, -57.4	18.5, -61.4	23.8, -78.9
	3	100	10.0, -17.4	10.0, -19.5	10.0, -24.1	10.0, -26.6	10.0, -29.1	10.5, -34.7	11.4, -37.6	12.4, -40.7	14.3, -47.2	15.4, -50.6	16.5, -54.2	21.1, -69.6
Roof > 30 to 45 degrees	1	10	11.9, -13.0	13.3, -14.6	16.5, -18.0	18.2, -19.8	19.9, -21.8	23.7, -25.9	25.7, -28.1	27.8, -30.4	32.3, -35.3	34.6, -37.8	37.0, -40.5	47.6, -52.0
	1	20	11.6, -12.3	13.0, -13.8	16.0, -17.1	17.6, -18.8	19.4, -20.7	23.0, -24.6	25.0, -26.7	27.0, -28.9	31.4, -33.5	33.7, -35.9	36.0, -38.4	46.3, -49.3
	1	50	11.1, -11.5	12.5, -12.8	15.4, -15.9	17.0, -17.5	18.6, -19.2	22.2, -22.8	24.1, -24.8	26.0, -25.8	30.2, -31.1	32.4, -33.3	34.6, -35.7	44.5, -45.8
	1	100	10.8, -10.8	12.1, -12.1	14.9, -14.9	16.5, -16.5	18.1, -18.1	21.5, -21.5	23.3, -23.3	25.2, -25.2	29.3, -29.3	31.4, -31.4	33.6, -33.6	43.2, -43.2
	2	10	11.9, -15.2	13.3, -17.0	16.5, -21.0	18.2, -23.2	19.9, -25.5	23.7, -30.3	25.7, -32.9	27.8, -35.6	32.3, -41.2	34.6, -44.2	37.0, -47.3	47.6, -60.8
	2	20	11.6, -14.5	13.0, -16.3	16.0, -20.1	17.6, -22.2	19.4, -24.3	23.0, -29.0	25.0, -31.4	27.0, -34.0	31.4, -39.4	33.7, -42.3	36.0, -45.3	46.3, -58.1
	2	50	11.1, -13.7	12.5, -15.3	15.4, -18.9	17.0, -20.8	18.6, -22.9	22.2, -27.2	24.1, -29.5	26.0, -32.0	30.2, -37.1	32.4, -39.8	34.6, -42.5	44.5, -54.6
	2	100	10.8, -13.0	12.1, -14.6	14.9, -18.0	16.5, -19.8	18.1, -21.8	21.5, -25.9	23.3, -28.1	25.2, -30.4	29.3, -35.3	31.4, -37.8	33.6, -40.5	43.2, -52.0
	3	10	11.9, -15.2	13.3, -17.0	16.5, -21.0	18.2, -23.2	19.9, -25.5	23.7, -30.3	25.7, -32.9	27.8, -35.6	32.3, -41.2	34.6, -44.2	37.0, -47.3	47.6, -60.8
	3	20	11.6, -14.5	13.0, -16.3	16.0, -20.1	17.6, -22.2	19.4, -24.3	23.0, -29.0	25.0, -31.4	27.0, -34.0	31.4, -39.4	33.7, -42.3	36.0, -45.3	46.3, -58.1
	3	50	11.1, -13.7	12.5, -15.3	15.4, -18.9	17.0, -20.8	18.6, -22.9	22.2, -27.2	24.1, -29.5	26.0, -32.0	30.2, -37.1	32.4, -39.8	34.6, -42.5	44.5, -54.5
	3	100	10.8, -13.0	12.1, -14.6	14.9, -18.0	16.5, -19.8	18.1, -21.8	21.5, -25.9	23.3, -28.1	25.2, -30.4	29.3, -35.3	31.4, -37.8	33.6, -40.5	43.2, -52.0
Wall	4	10	13.0, -14.1	14.6, -15.8	18.0, -19.5	19.8, -21.5	21.8, -23.6	25.9, -28.1	28.1, -30.5	30.4, -33.0	35.3, -38.2	37.8, -41.0	40.5, -43.9	52.0, -56.4
	4	20	12.4, -13.5	13.9, -15.1	17.2, -18.7	18.9, -20.6	20.8, -22.6	24.7, -26.9	26.8, -29.2	29.0, -31.6	33.7, -36.7	36.1, -39.3	38.7, -42.1	49.6, -54.1
	4	50	11.6, -12.7	13.0, -14.3	16.1, -17.6	17.8, -19.4	19.5, -21.3	23.2, -25.4	25.2, -27.5	27.2, -29.8	31.6, -34.6	33.9, -37.1	36.2, -39.7	46.6, -51.0
	4	100	11.1, -12.2	12.4, -13.6	15.3, -16.8	16.9, -18.5	18.5, -20.4	22.0, -24.2	23.9, -26.3	25.9, -28.4	30.0, -33.0	32.2, -35.4	34.4, -37.8	44.2, -48.6
	5	10	13.0, -17.4	14.6, -19.5	18.0, -24.1	19.8, -26.6	21.8, -29.1	25.9, -34.7	28.1, -37.6	30.4, -40.7	35.3, -47.2	37.8, -50.6	40.5, -54.2	52.0, -69.6
	5	20	12.4, -16.2	13.9, -18.2	17.2, -22.5	18.9, -24.8	20.8, -27.2	24.7, -32.4	26.8, -35.1	29.0, -38.0	33.7, -44.0	36.1, -47.2	38.7, -50.5	49.6, -64.9
	5	50	11.6, -14.7	13.0, -16.5	16.1, -20.3	17.8, -22.4	19.5, -24.6	23.2, -29.3	25.2, -31.8	27.2, -34.3	31.6, -39.8	33.9, -42.7	36.2, -45.7	46.6, -58.7
	5	100	11.1, -13.5	12.4, -15.1	15.3, -18.7	16.9, -20.6	18.5, -22.6	22.0, -26.9	23.9, -29.2	25.9, -31.6	30.0, -36.7	32.2, -39.3	34.4, -42.1	44.2, -54.1

For SI: 1 foot = 304.8 mm, 1 square foot = 0.0929 m², 1 mile per hour = 0.447 m/s, 1 pound per square foot = 0.0479 kPa.

Notes:

a. The effective wind area shall be equal to the span length multiplied by an effective width. This width shall be permitted to be not less than one-third the span length. For cladding fasteners, the effective wind area shall not be greater than the area that is tributary to an individual fastener.

b. For effective areas between those given above, the load may be interpolated; otherwise, use the load associated with the lower effective area.

c. Table values shall be adjusted for height and exposure by multiplying by the adjustment coefficient in Table R301.2(3).

d. See Figure R301.2(7) for location of zones.

e. Plus and minus signs signify pressures acting toward and away from the building surfaces.

TABLE R301.2(3)
HEIGHT AND EXPOSURE ADJUSTMENT COEFFICIENTS FOR TABLE R301.2(2)

MEAN ROOF HEIGHT	EXPOSURE		
	B	C	D
15	1.00	1.21	1.47
20	1.00	1.29	1.55
25	1.00	1.35	1.61
30	1.00	1.40	1.66
35	1.05	1.45	1.70
40	1.09	1.49	1.74
45	1.12	1.53	1.78
50	1.16	1.56	1.81
55	1.19	1.59	1.84
60	1.22	1.62	1.87

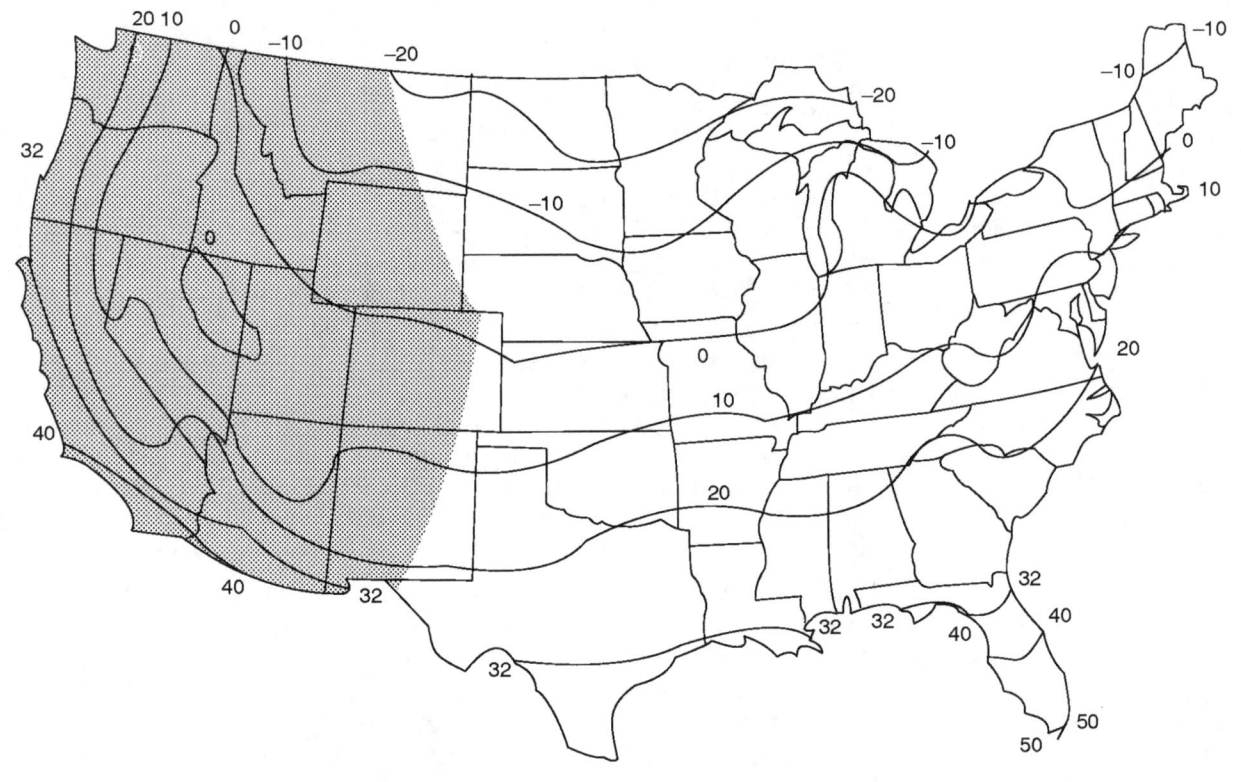

DESIGN TEMPERATURES IN THIS AREA MUST BE BASED ON ANALYSIS OF LOCAL CLIMATE AND TOPOGRAPHY

For SI: °C = [(°F)-32]/1.8.

FIGURE R301.2(1)
ISOLINES OF THE 97$^1/_2$ PERCENT WINTER (DECEMBER, JANUARY AND FEBRUARY) DESIGN TEMPERATURES (°F)

2009 INTERNATIONAL RESIDENTIAL CODE®

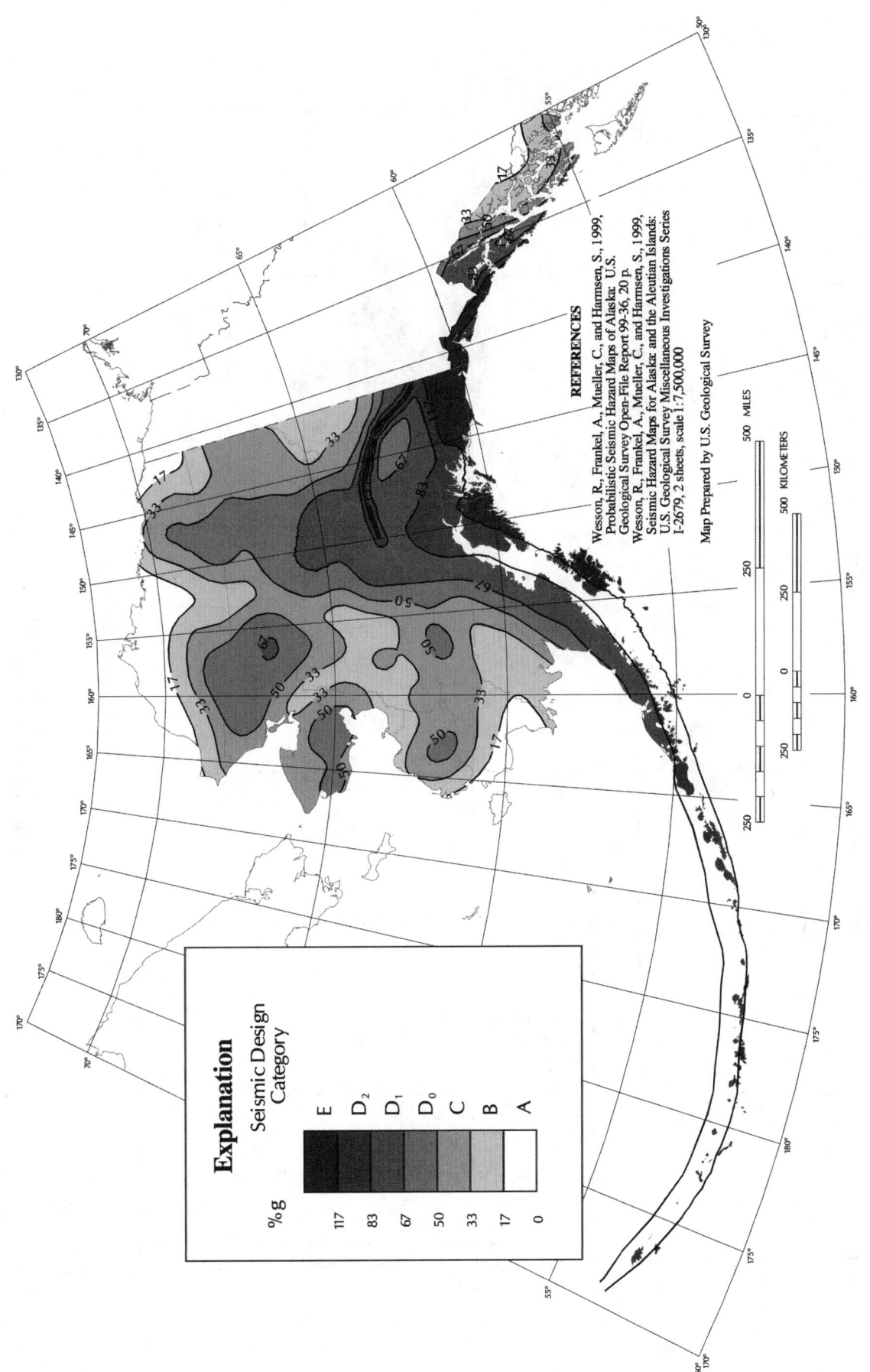

FIGURE R301.2(2)
SEISMIC DESIGN CATEGORIES—SITE CLASS D
(continued)

For SI: 1 mile = 1.61 km.

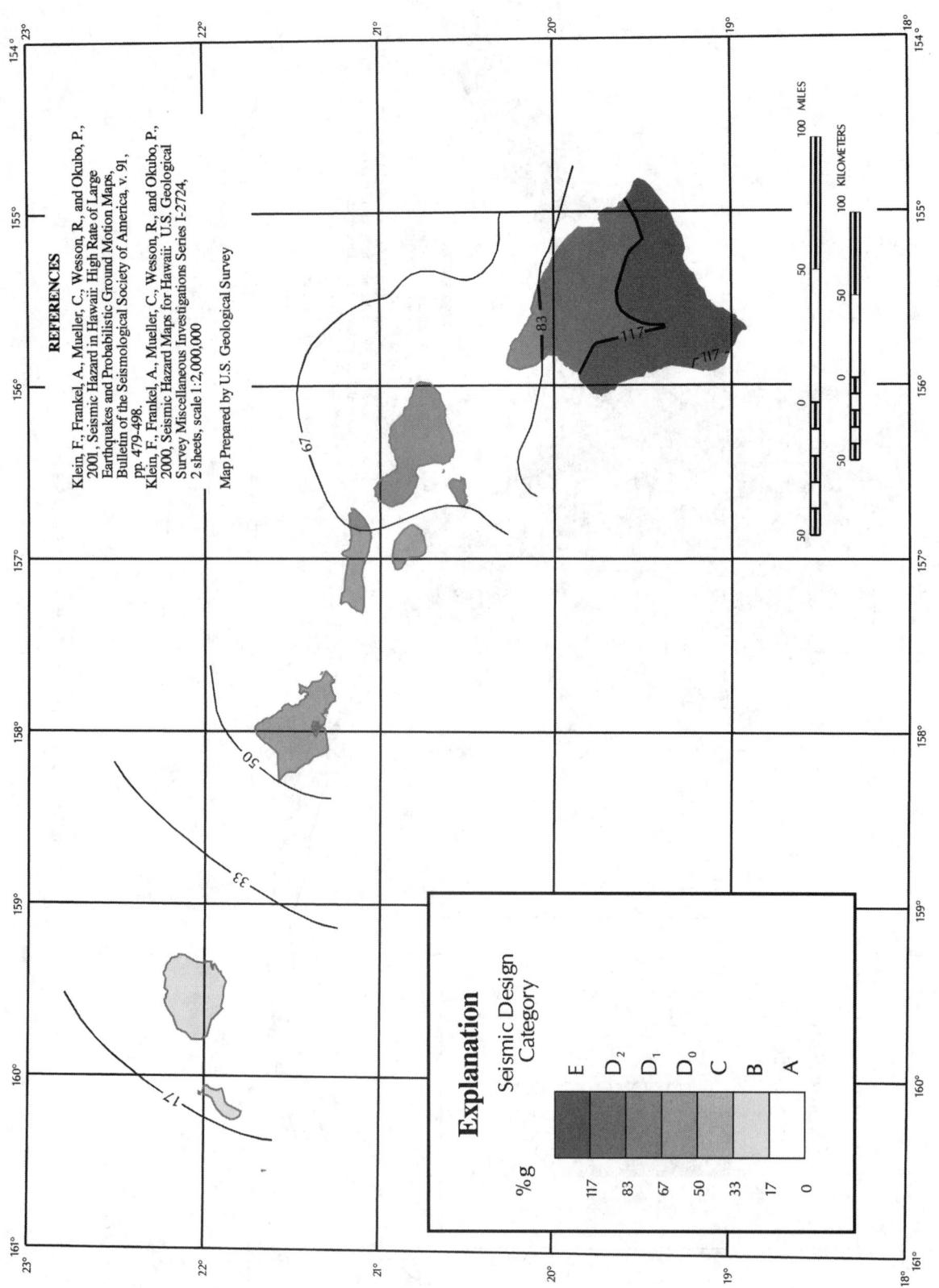

FIGURE R301.2(2)—continued
SEISMIC DESIGN CATEGORIES—SITE CLASS D
(continued)

For SI: 1 mile = 1.61 km.

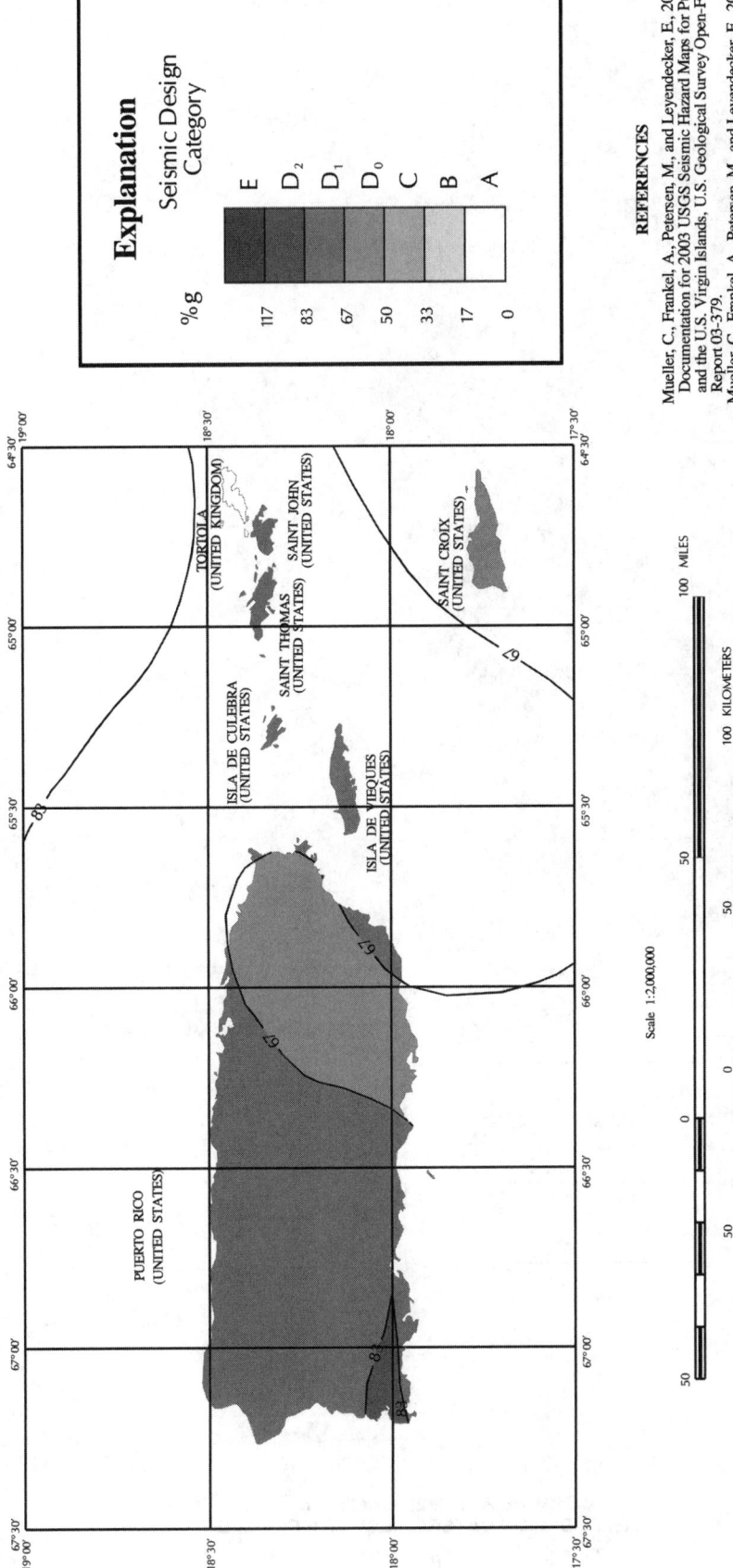

REFERENCES

Mueller, C., Frankel, A., Petersen, M., and Leyendecker, E., 2003, Documentation for 2003 USGS Seismic Hazard Maps for Puerto Rico and the U.S. Virgin Islands, U.S. Geological Survey Open-File Report 03-379.

Mueller, C., Frankel, A., Petersen, M., and Leyendecker, E., 2004, Seismic-Hazard Maps for Puerto Rico and the U.S. Virgin Island, Sheet 2 - 2% Probability of Exceedance in 50 Years for Peak Horizontal Acceleration and Horizontal Spectral Response Acceleration for 0.2, 0.3, and 1.0 Second Periods U.S. Geological Survey Geologic Investigation Series (in progress).

Map Prepared by U.S. Geological Survey

FIGURE R301.2(2)—continued
SEISMIC DESIGN CATEGORIES—SITE CLASS D

(continued)

For SI: 1 mile = 1.61 km.

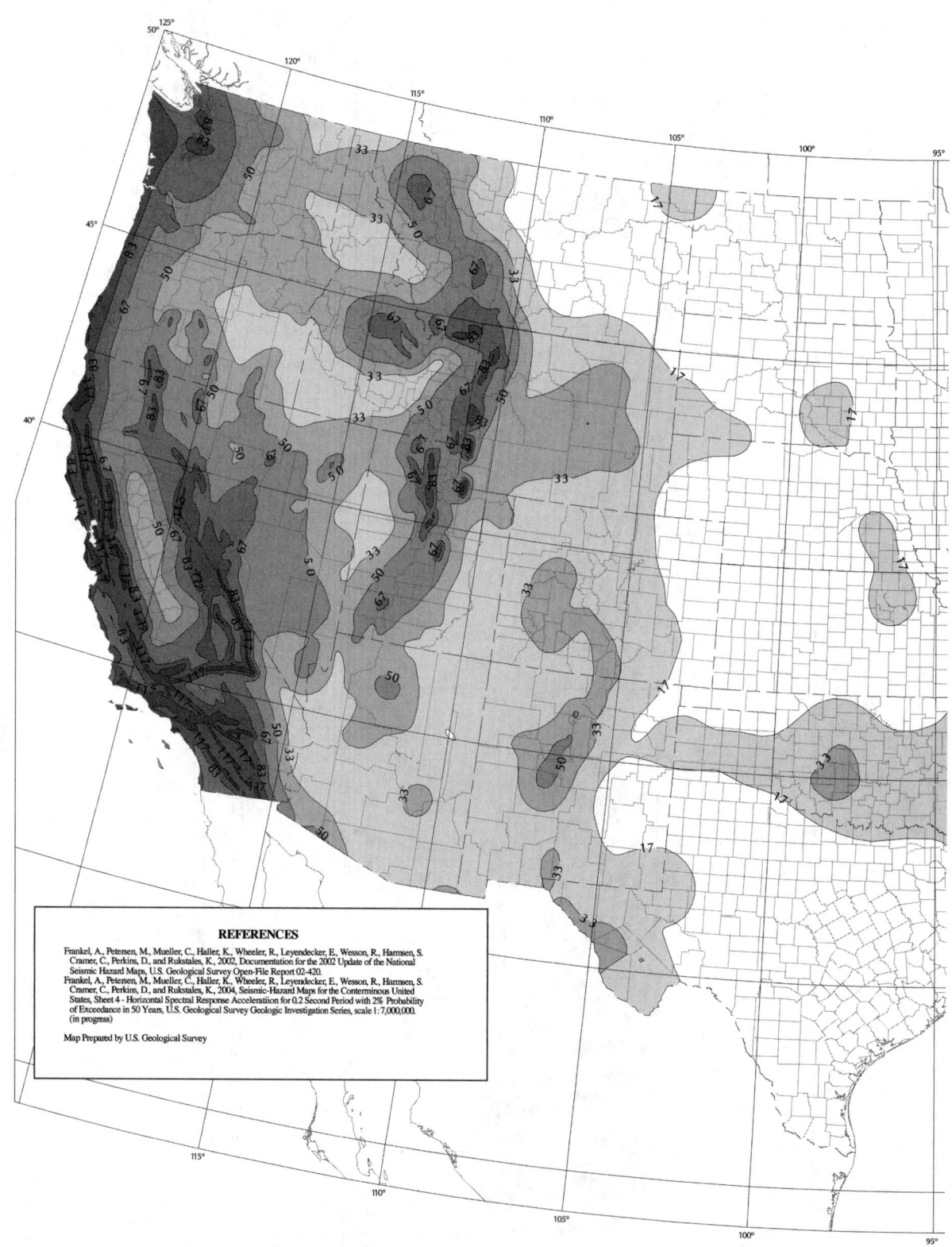

FIGURE R301.2(2)—continued
SEISMIC DESIGN CATEGORIES—SITE CLASS D

(continued)

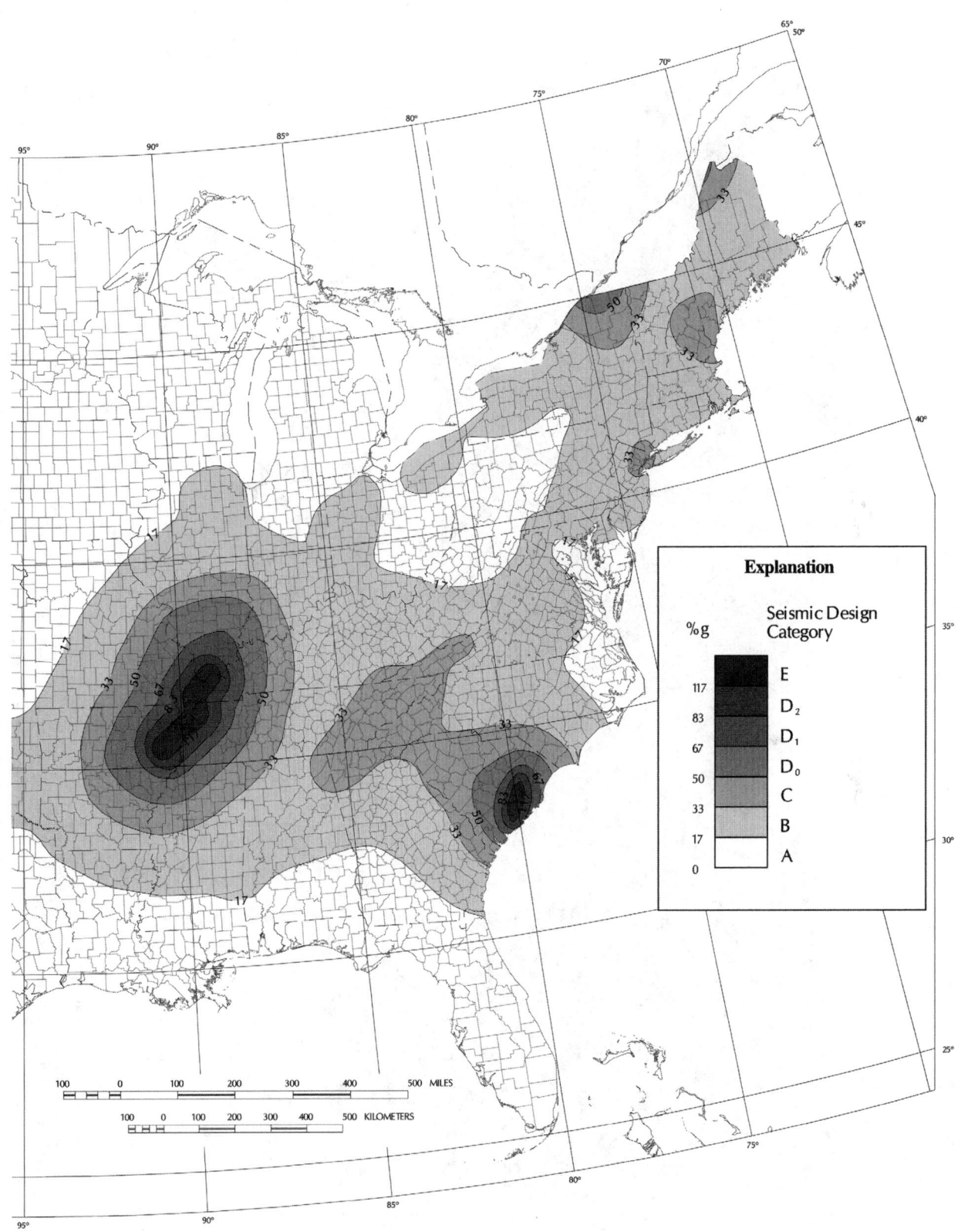

FIGURE R301.2(2)—continued
SEISMIC DESIGN CATEGORIES—SITE CLASS D

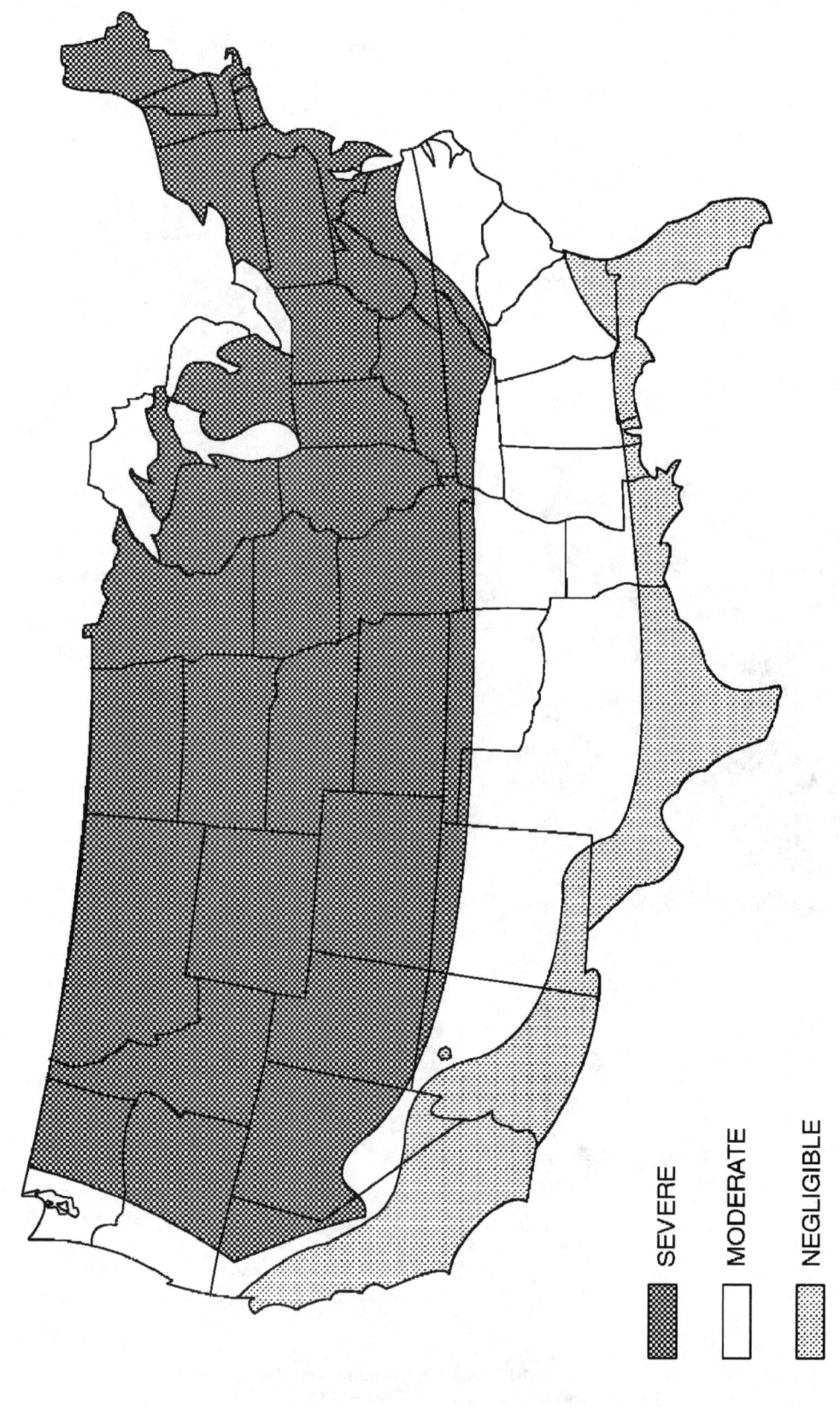

a. Alaska and Hawaii are classified as severe and negligible, respectively.

b. Lines defining areas are approximate only. Local conditions may be more or less severe than indicated by region classification. A severe classification is where weather conditions result in significant snowfall combined with extended periods during which there is little or no natural thawing causing deicing salts to be used extensively.

FIGURE R301.2(3)
WEATHERING PROBABILITY MAP FOR CONCRETE

SEVERE

MODERATE

NEGLIGIBLE

Location	V mph	(m/s)
Hawaii	105	(47)
Puerto Rico	145	(65)
Guam	170	(76)
Virgin Islands	145	(65)
American Samoa	125	(56)

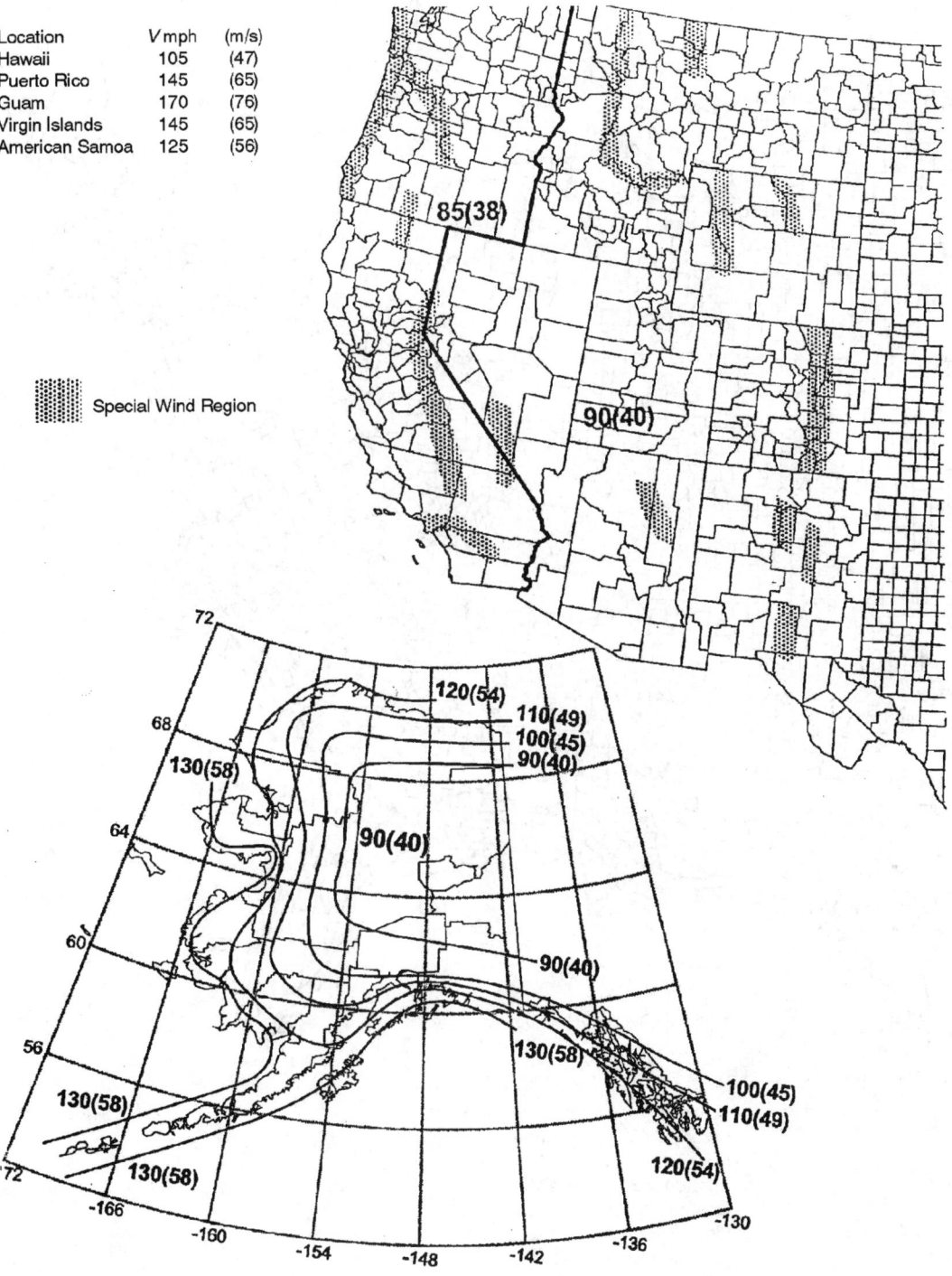

FIGURE R301.2(4)
BASIC WIND SPEEDS FOR 50-YEAR MEAN RECURRENCE INTERVAL

(continued)

For SI: 1 foot = 304.8 mm, 1 mile per hour = 0.447 m/s.

a. Values are nominal design 3-second gust wind speeds in miles per hour at 33 feet above ground for Exposure C category.

b. Linear interpolation between wind contours is permitted.

c. Islands and coastal areas outside the last contour shall use the last wind speed contour of the coastal area.

d. Mountainous terrain, gorges, ocean promontories and special wind regions shall be examined for unusual wind conditions.

e. Enlarged view of Eastern and Southern seaboards are on the following pages.

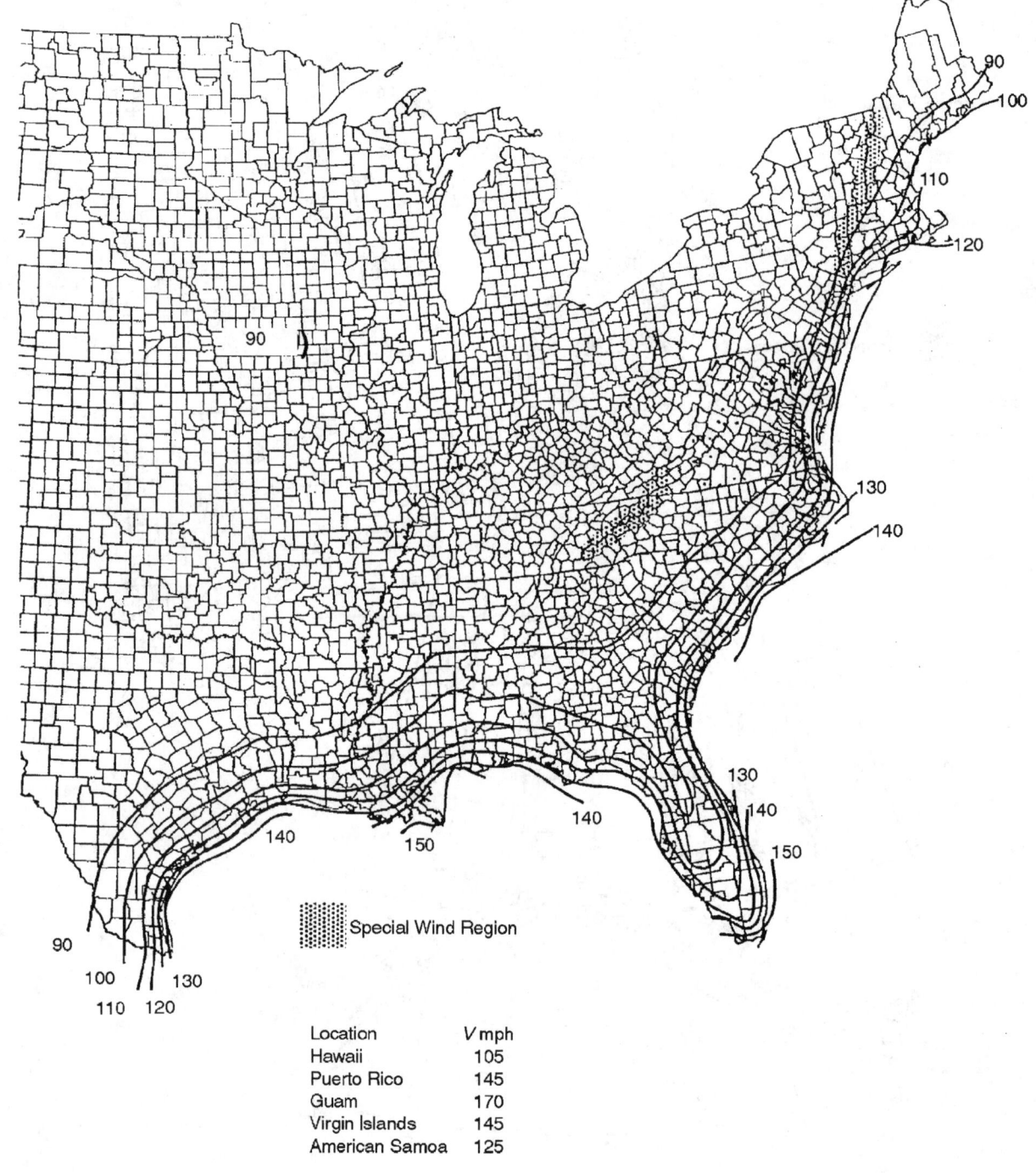

Location	V mph
Hawaii	105
Puerto Rico	145
Guam	170
Virgin Islands	145
American Samoa	125

FIGURE R301.2(4)—continued
BASIC WIND SPEEDS FOR 50-YEAR MEAN RECURRENCE INTERVAL

(continued)

For SI: 1 foot = 304.8 mm, 1 mile per hour = 0.447 m/s.

a. Values are nominal design 3-second gust wind speeds in miles per hour at 33 feet above ground for Exposure C category.

b. Linear interpolation between wind contours is permitted.

c. Islands and coastal areas outside the last contour shall use the last wind speed contour of the coastal area.

d. Mountainous terrain, gorges, ocean promontories and special wind regions shall be examined for unusual wind conditions.

e. Enlarged view of Eastern and Southern seaboards are on the following pages.

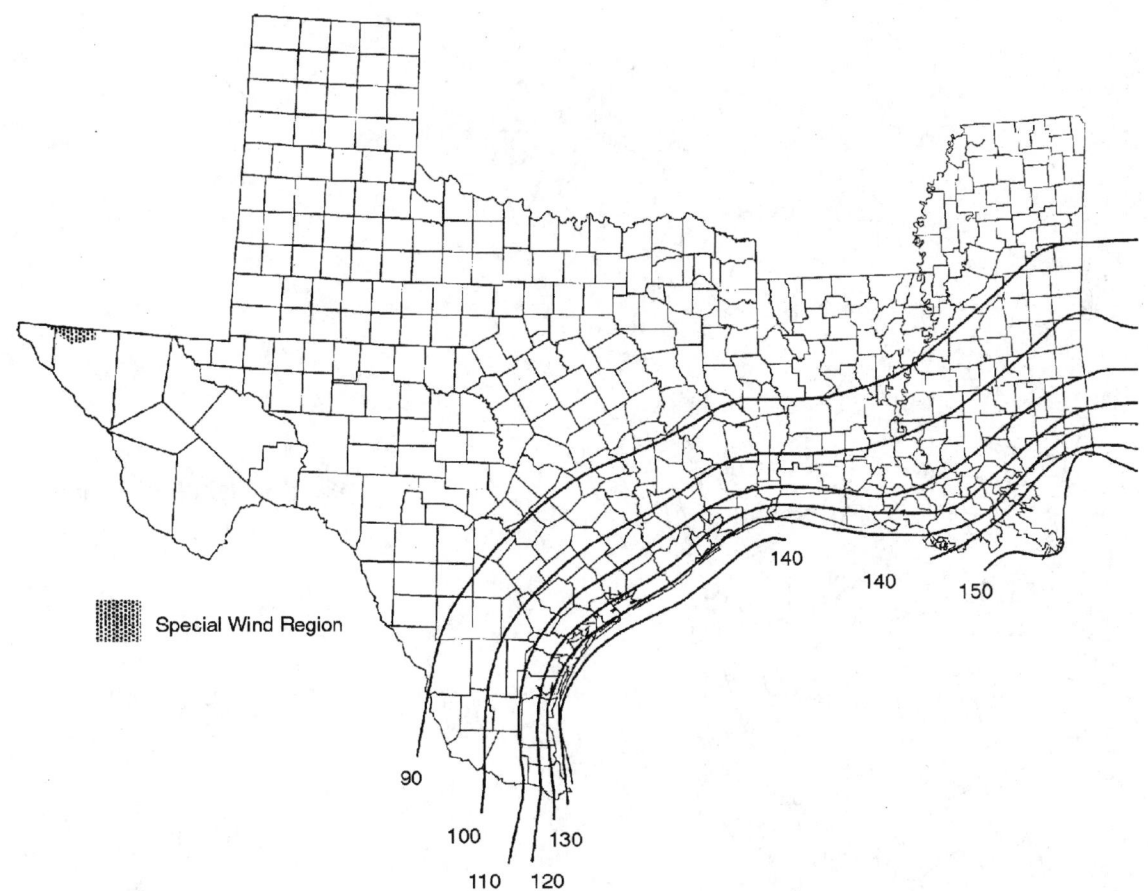

FIGURE R301.2(4)—continued
BASIC WIND SPEEDS FOR 50-YEAR MEAN RECURRENCE INTERVAL

(continued)

For SI: 1 foot = 304.8 mm, 1 mile per hour = 0.447 m/s.

a. Values are nominal design 3-second gust wind speeds in miles per hour at 33 feet above ground for Exposure C category.

b. Linear interpolation between wind contours is permitted.

c. Islands and coastal areas outside the last contour shall use the last wind speed contour of the coastal area.

d. Mountainous terrain, gorges, ocean promontories and special wind regions shall be examined for unusual wind conditions.

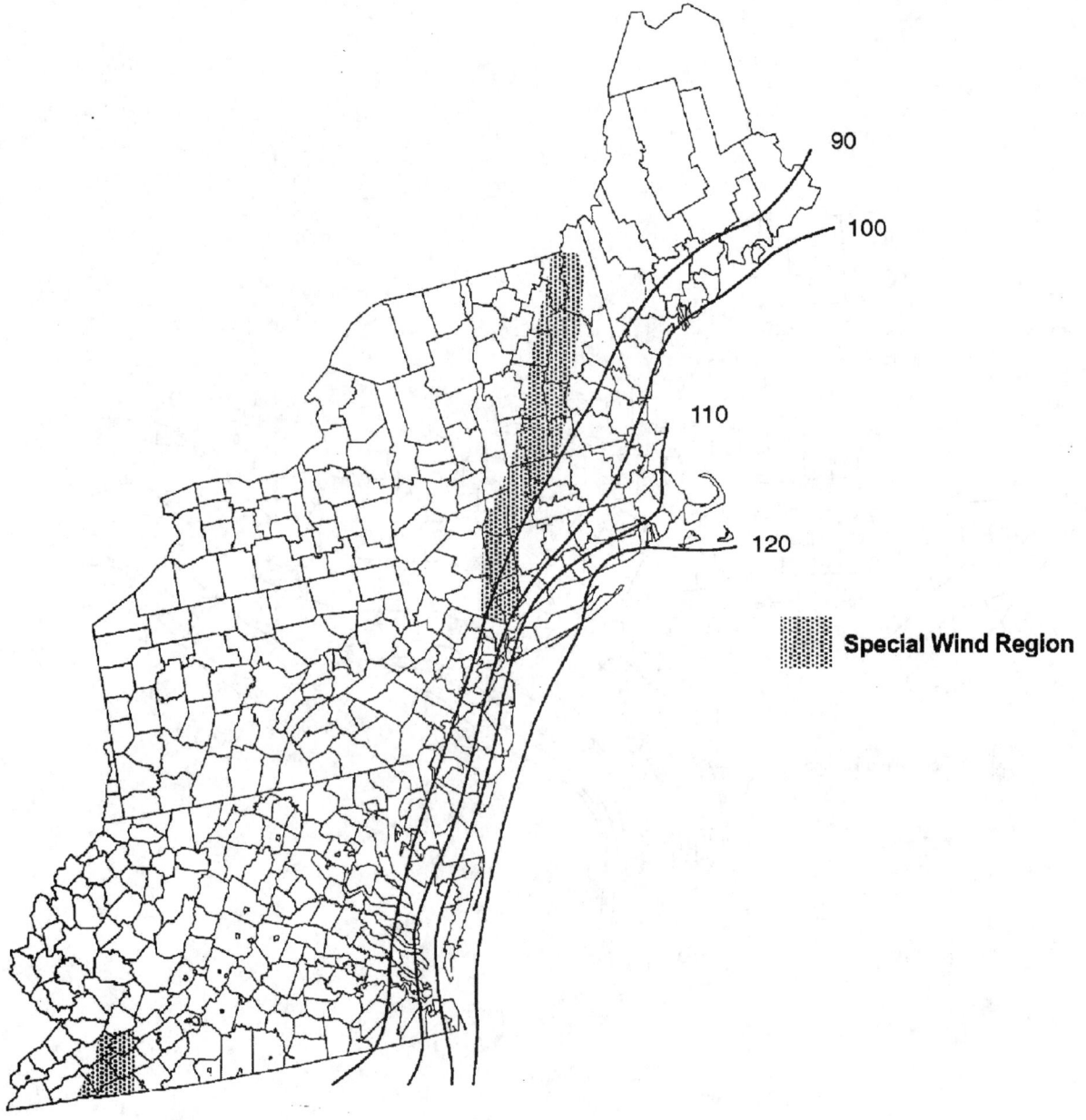

90

100

110

120

Special Wind Region

FIGURE R301.2(4)—continued
BASIC WIND SPEEDS FOR 50-YEAR MEAN RECURRENCE INTERVAL

(continued)

For SI: 1 foot = 304.8 mm, 1 mile per hour = 0.447 m/s.

a. Values are nominal design 3-second gust wind speeds in miles per hour at 33 feet above ground for Exposure C category.

b. Linear interpolation between wind contours is permitted.

c. Islands and coastal areas outside the last contour shall use the last wind speed contour of the coastal area.

d. Mountainous terrain, gorges, ocean promontories and special wind regions shall be examined for unusual wind conditions.

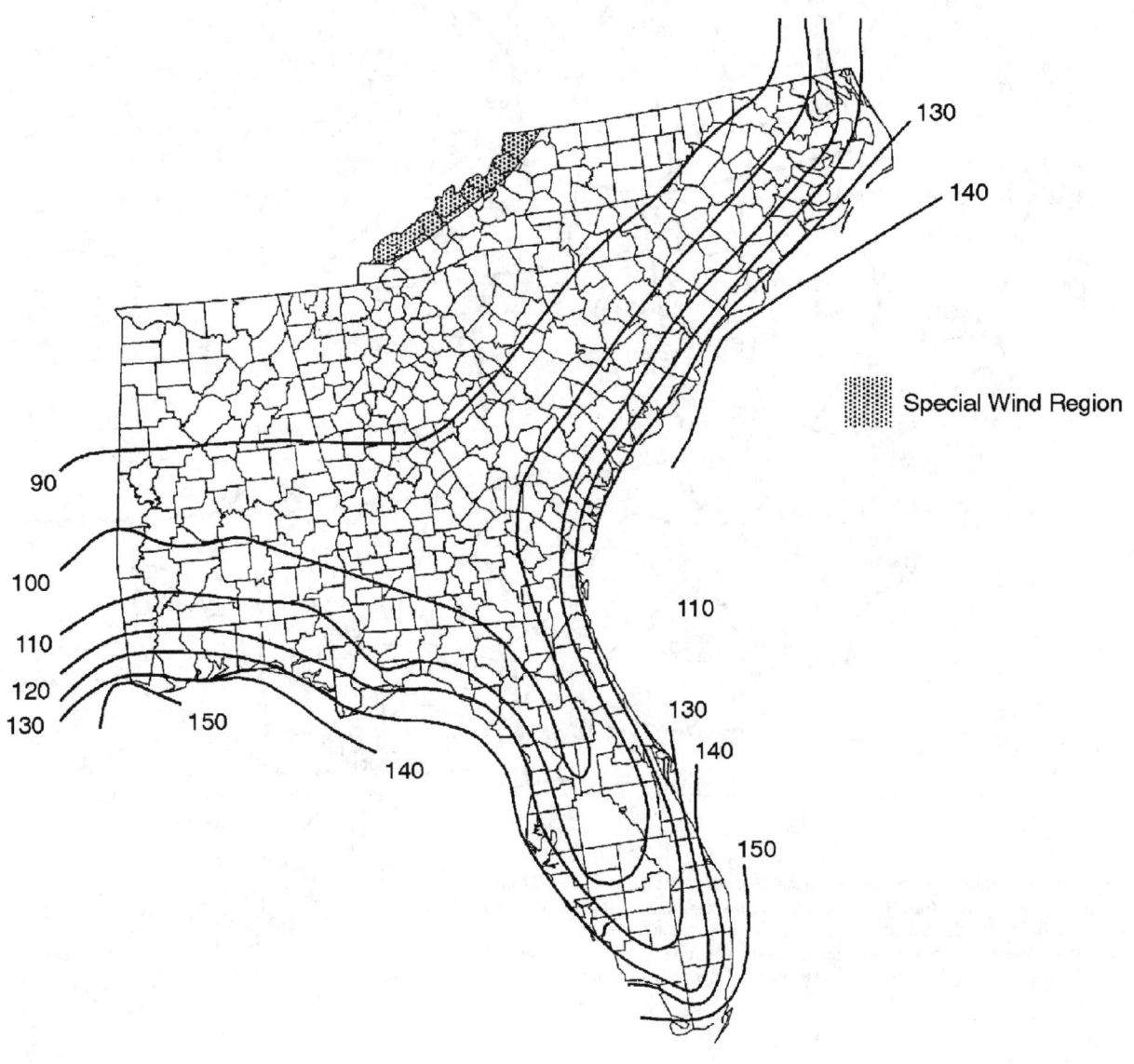

FIGURE R301.2(4)—continued
BASIC WIND SPEEDS FOR 50-YEAR MEAN RECURRENCE INTERVAL

For SI: 1 foot = 304.8 mm, 1 mile per hour = 0.447 m/s.

a. Values are nominal design 3-second gust wind speeds in miles per hour at 33 feet above ground for Exposure C category.

b. Linear interpolation between wind contours is permitted.

c. Islands and coastal areas outside the last contour shall use the last wind speed contour of the coastal area.

d. Mountainous terrain, gorges, ocean promontories and special wind regions shall be examined for unusual wind conditions.

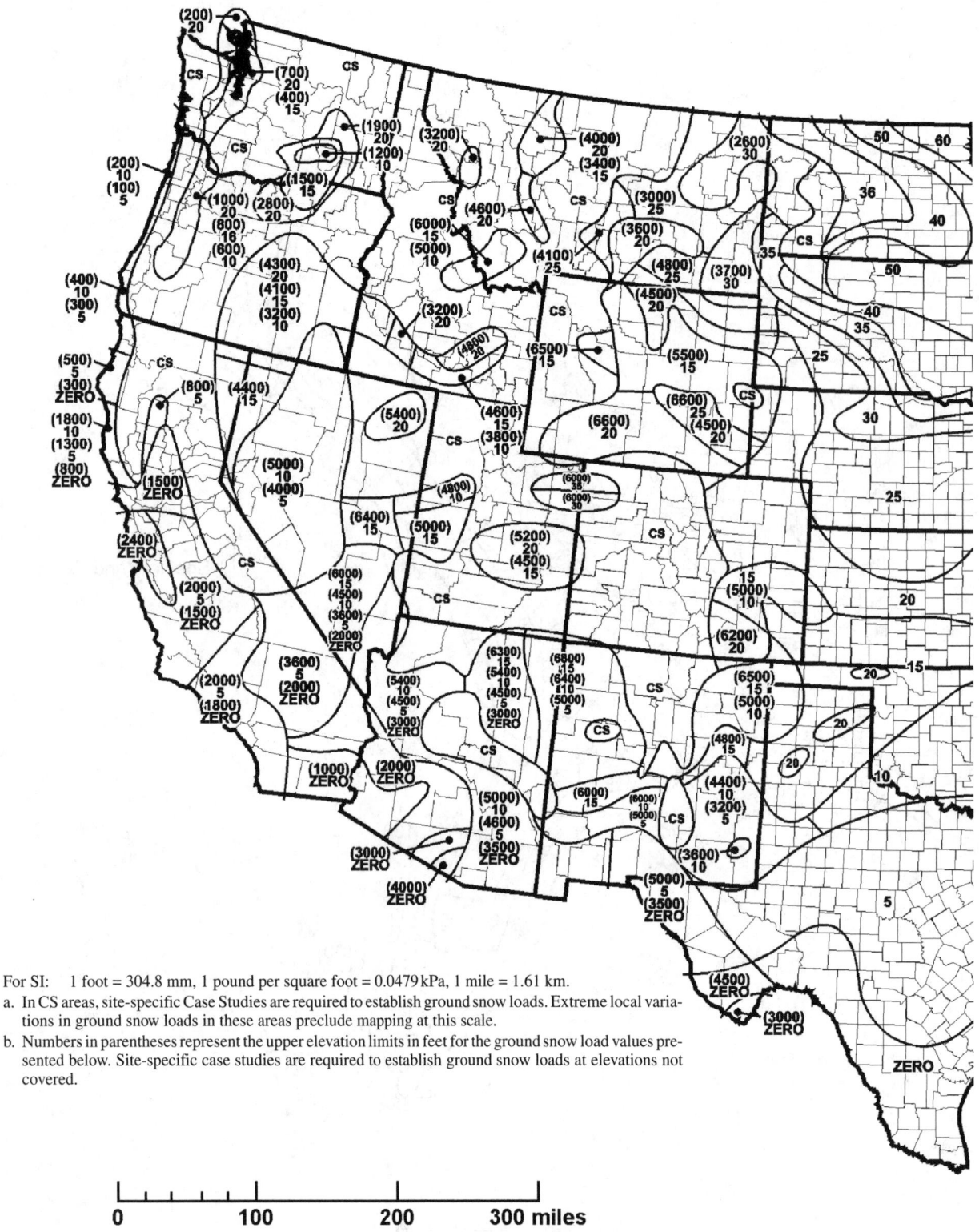

For SI: 1 foot = 304.8 mm, 1 pound per square foot = 0.0479 kPa, 1 mile = 1.61 km.

a. In CS areas, site-specific Case Studies are required to establish ground snow loads. Extreme local variations in ground snow loads in these areas preclude mapping at this scale.

b. Numbers in parentheses represent the upper elevation limits in feet for the ground snow load values presented below. Site-specific case studies are required to establish ground snow loads at elevations not covered.

FIGURE R301.2(5)
GROUND SNOW LOADS, P_g, FOR THE UNITED STATES (lb/ft^2)

(continued)

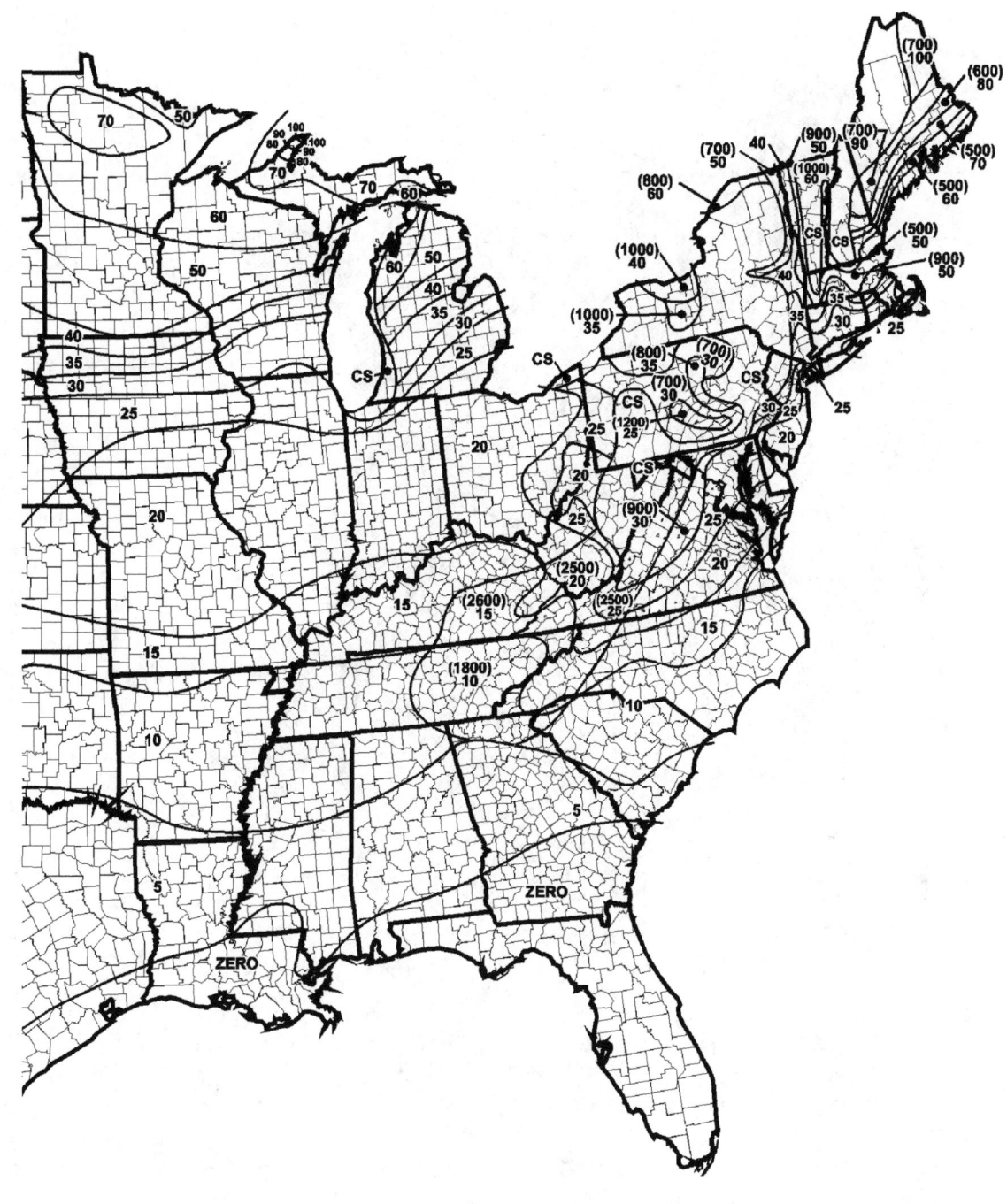

For SI: 1 foot = 304.8 mm, 1 pound per square foot = 0.0479 kPa.

FIGURE R301.2(5)—continued
GROUND SNOW LOADS, P_g, FOR THE UNITED STATES (lb/ft^2)

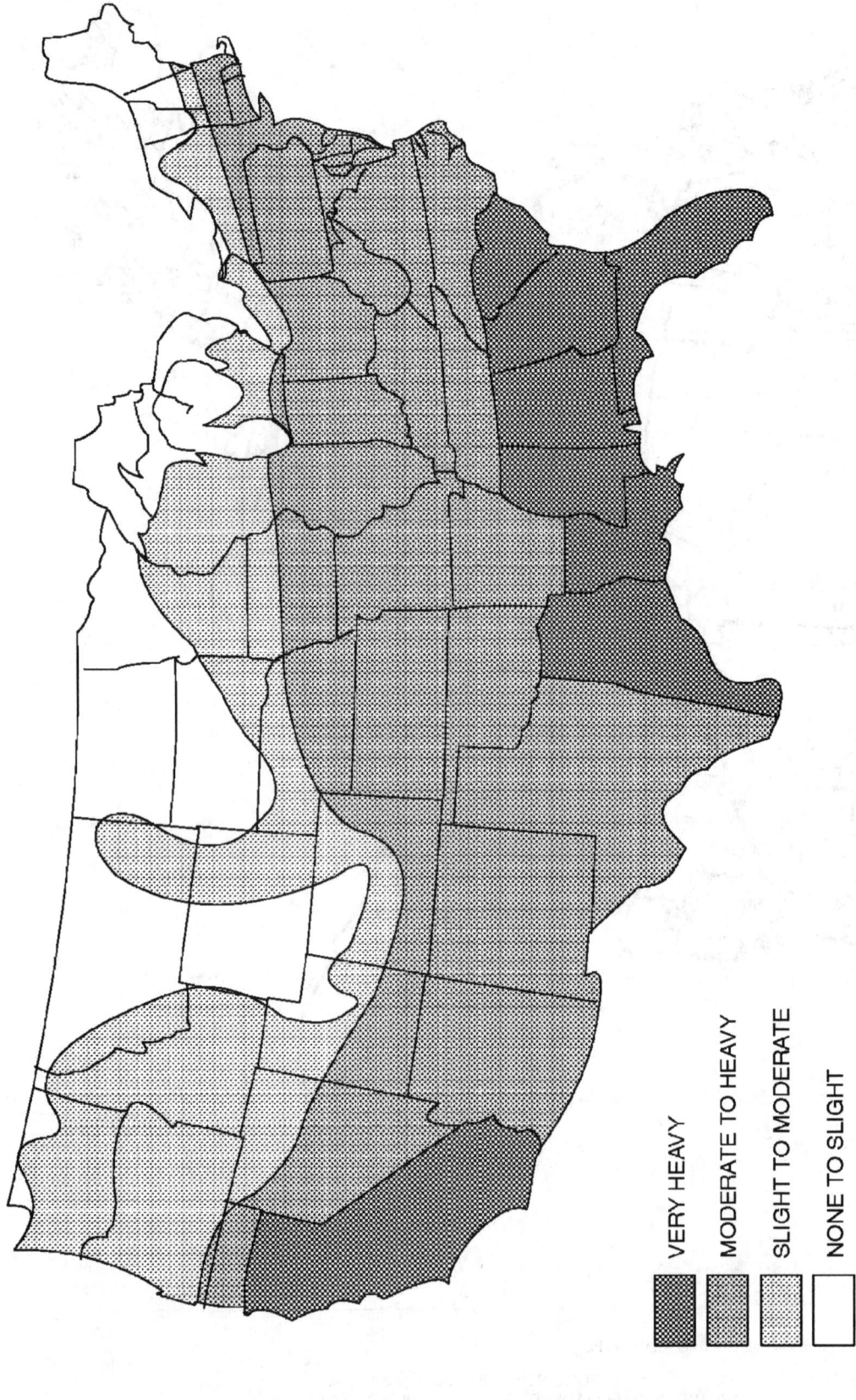

VERY HEAVY

MODERATE TO HEAVY

SLIGHT TO MODERATE

NONE TO SLIGHT

NOTE: Lines defining areas are approximate only. Local conditions may be more or less severe than indicated by the region classification.

FIGURE R301.2(6)
TERMITE INFESTATION PROBABILITY MAP

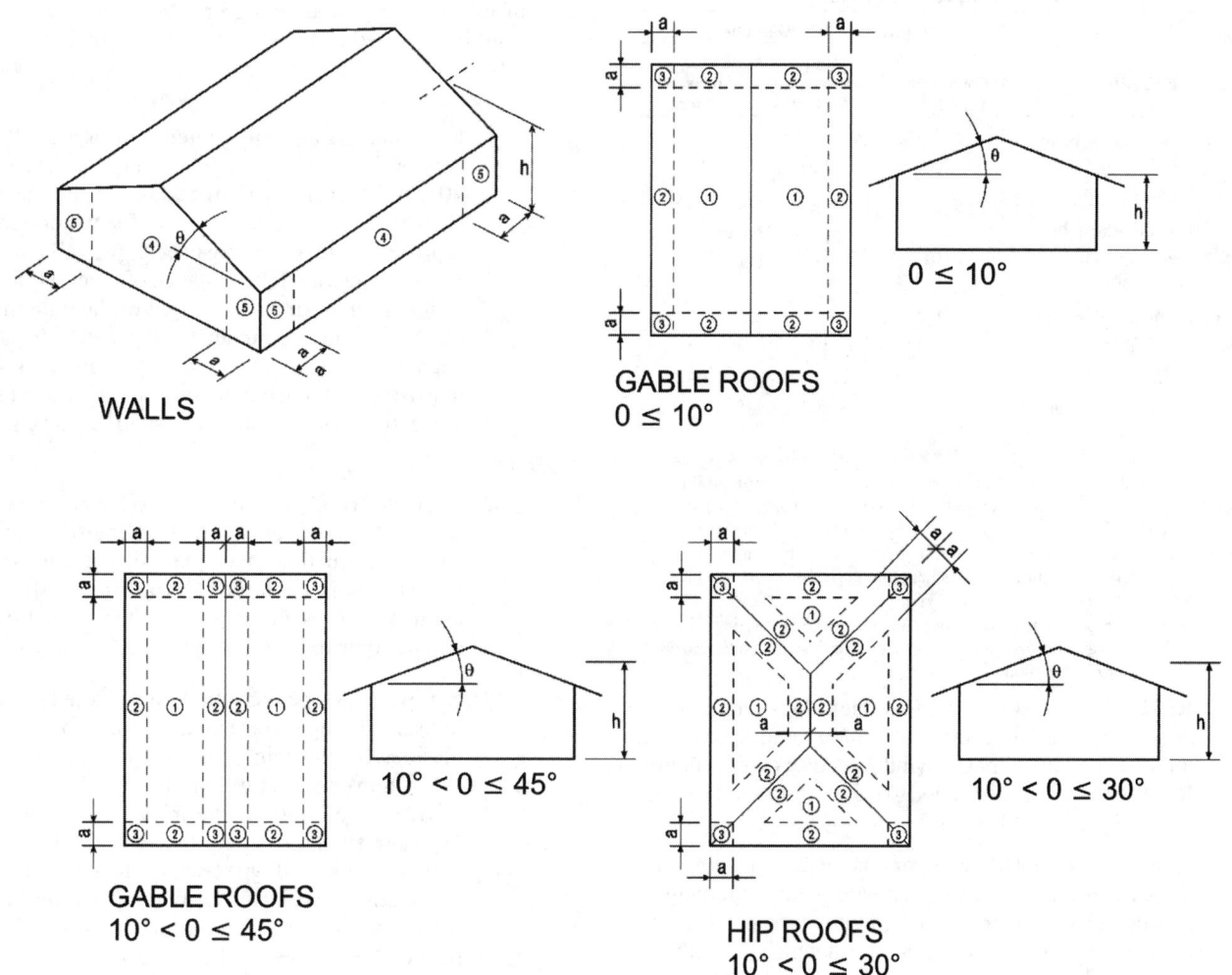

WALLS

GABLE ROOFS
0 ≤ 10°

0 ≤ 10°

GABLE ROOFS
10° < 0 ≤ 45°

10° < 0 ≤ 45°

HIP ROOFS
10° < 0 ≤ 30°

10° < 0 ≤ 30°

For SI: 1 foot = 304.8 mm, 1 degree = 0.0175 rad.
Note: a = 4 feet in all cases.

FIGURE R301.2(7)
COMPONENT AND CLADDING PRESSURE ZONES

R301.2.1.2 Protection of openings. Windows in buildings located in windborne debris regions shall have glazed openings protected from windborne debris. Glazed opening protection for windborne debris shall meet the requirements of the Large Missile Test of ASTM E 1996 and ASTM E 1886 referenced therein. Garage door glazed opening protection for windborne debris shall meet the requirements of an *approved* impact resisting standard or ANSI/DASMA 115.

Exception: Wood structural panels with a minimum thickness of $^7/_{16}$ inch (11 mm) and a maximum span of 8 feet (2438 mm) shall be permitted for opening protection in one- and two-story buildings. Panels shall be precut and attached to the framing surrounding the opening containing the product with the glazed opening. Panels shall be predrilled as required for the anchorage method and shall be secured with the attachment hardware provided. Attachments shall be designed to resist the component and cladding loads determined in accordance with either Table R301.2(2) or ASCE 7, with the permanent corrosion-resistant attachment hardware provided and anchors permanently installed on the building. Attachment in accordance with Table R301.2.1.2 is permitted for buildings with a mean roof height of 33 feet (10 058 mm) or less where windspeeds do not exceed 130 miles per hour (58 m/s).

TABLE R301.2.1.2
WINDBORNE DEBRIS PROTECTION FASTENING SCHEDULE
FOR WOOD STRUCTURAL PANELS[a, b, c, d]

FASTENER TYPE	FASTENER SPACING (inches)[a, b]		
	Panel span ≤ 4 feet	4 feet < panel span ≤ 6 feet	6 feet < panel span ≤ 8 feet
No. 8 wood screw based anchor with 2-inch embedment length	16	10	8
No. 10 wood screw based anchor with 2-inch embedment length	16	12	9
$^{1}/_{4}$-inch lag screw based anchor with 2-inch embedment length	16	16	16

For SI: 1 inch = 25.4 mm, 1 foot = 304.8 mm, 1 pound = 4.448 N, 1 mile per hour = 0.447 m/s.

a. This table is based on 130 mph wind speeds and a 33-foot mean roof height.

b. Fasteners shall be installed at opposing ends of the wood structural panel. Fasteners shall be located a minimum of 1 inch from the edge of the panel.

c. Anchors shall penetrate through the exterior wall covering with an embedment length of 2 inches minimum into the building frame. Fasteners shall be located a minimum of $2^{1}/_{2}$ inches from the edge of concrete block or concrete.

d. Where panels are attached to masonry or masonry/stucco, they shall be attached using vibration-resistant anchors having a minimum ultimate withdrawal capacity of 1500 pounds.

R301.2.1.3 Wind speed conversion. When referenced documents are based on fastest mile wind speeds, the three-second gust basic wind speeds, V_{3s}, of Figure R301.2(4) shall be converted to fastest mile wind speeds, V_{fm}, using Table R301.2.1.3.

R301.2.1.4 Exposure category. For each wind direction considered, an exposure category that adequately reflects the characteristics of ground surface irregularities shall be determined for the site at which the building or structure is to be constructed. For a site located in the transition zone between categories, the category resulting in the largest wind forces shall apply. Account shall be taken of variations in ground surface roughness that arise from natural topography and vegetation as well as from constructed features. For a site where multiple detached one- and two-family dwellings, *townhouses* or other structures are to be constructed as part of a subdivision, master-planned community, or otherwise designated as a developed area by the authority having jurisdiction, the exposure category for an individual structure shall be based upon the site conditions that will exist at the time when all adjacent structures on the site have been constructed, provided their construction is expected to begin within one year of the start of construction for the structure for which the exposure category is determined. For any given wind direction, the exposure in which a specific building or other structure is sited shall be assessed as being one of the following categories:

1. **Exposure A.** Large city centers with at least 50 percent of the buildings having a height in excess of 70 feet (21 336 mm). Use of this exposure category shall be limited to those areas for which terrain representative of Exposure A prevails in the upwind direction for a distance of at least 0.5 mile (0.8 km) or 10 times the height of the building or other structure, whichever is greater. Possible channeling effects or increased velocity pressures due to the building or structure being located in the wake of adjacent buildings shall be taken into account.

2. **Exposure B.** Urban and suburban areas, wooded areas, or other terrain with numerous closely spaced obstructions having the size of single-family dwellings or larger. Exposure B shall be assumed unless the site meets the definition of another type exposure.

3. **Exposure C.** Open terrain with scattered obstructions, including surface undulations or other irregularities, having heights generally less than 30 feet (9144 mm) extending more than 1,500 feet (457 m) from the building site in any quadrant. This exposure shall also apply to any building located within Exposure B type terrain where the building is directly adjacent to open areas of Exposure C type terrain in any quadrant for a distance of more than 600 feet (183 m). This category includes flat open country, grasslands and shorelines in hurricane prone regions.

4. **Exposure D.** Flat, unobstructed areas exposed to wind flowing over open water (excluding shorelines in hurricane prone regions) for a distance of at least 1 mile (1.61 km). Shorelines in Exposure D include inland waterways, the Great Lakes, and coastal areas of California, Oregon, Washington and Alaska. This exposure shall apply only to those buildings and other structures exposed to the wind coming from over the water. Exposure D extends inland from the shoreline a distance of 1500 feet (457 m) or 10 times the height of the building or structure, whichever is greater.

TABLE R301.2.1.3
EQUIVALENT BASIC WIND SPEEDS[a]

3-second gust, V_{3s}	85	90	100	105	110	120	125	130	140	145	150	160	170
Fastest mile, V_{fm}	71	76	85	90	95	104	109	114	123	128	133	142	152

For SI: 1 mile per hour = 0.447 m/s.

a. Linear interpolation is permitted.

R301.2.1.5 Topographic wind effects. In areas designated in Table R301.2(1) as having local historical data documenting structural damage to buildings caused by wind speed-up at isolated hills, ridges and escarpments that are abrupt changes from the general topography of the area, topographic wind effects shall be considered in the design of the building in accordance with Section R301.2.1.5.1 or in accordance with the provisions of ASCE 7. See Figure R301.2.1.5.1(1) for topographic features for wind speed-up effect.

In these designated areas, topographic wind effects shall apply only to buildings sited on the top half of an isolated hill, ridge or escarpment where all of the following conditions exist:

1. The average slope of the top half of the hill, ridge or escarpment is 10 percent or greater.

2. The hill, ridge or escarpment is 60 feet (18 288 mm) or greater in height for Exposure B, 30 feet (9144 mm) or greater in height for Exposure C, and 15 feet (4572 mm) or greater in height for Exposure D.

3. The hill, ridge or escarpment is isolated or unobstructed by other topographic features of similar height in the upwind direction for a distance measured from its high point of 100 times its height or 2 miles, whichever is less. See Figure R301.2.1.5.1(3) for upwind obstruction.

4. The hill, ridge or escarpment protrudes by a factor of two or more above the height of other upwind topographic features located in any quadrant within a radius of 2 miles measured from its high point.

R301.2.1.5.1 Simplified topographic wind speed-up method. As an alternative to the ASCE 7 topographic wind provisions, the provisions of Section R301.2.1.5.1 shall be permitted to be used to design for wind speed-up effects, where required by Section R301.2.1.5.

Structures located on the top half of isolated hills, ridges or escarpments meeting the conditions of Section R301.2.1.5 shall be designed for an increased basic wind speed as determined by Table R301.2.1.5.1. On the high side of an escarpment, the increased basic wind speed shall extend horizontally downwind from the edge of the escarpment 1.5 times the horizontal length of the upwind slope (1.5L) or 6 times the height of the escarpment (6H), whichever is greater. See Figure R301.2.1.5.1(2) for where wind speed increase is applied.

TABLE R301.2.1.5.1
BASIC WIND MODIFICATION FOR TOPOGRAPHIC WIND EFFECT

BASIC WIND SPEED FROM FIGURE R301.2(4) (mph)	AVERAGE SLOPE OF THE TOP HALF OF HILL, RIDGE OR ESCARPMENT (percent)						
	0.10	0.125	0.15	0.175	0.20	0.23	0.25 or greater
	Required basic wind speed-up, modified for topographic wind speed up (mph)						
85	100	100	100	110	110	110	120
90	100	100	110	110	120	120	120
100	110	120	120	130	130	130	140
110	120	130	130	140	140	150	150
120	140	140	150	150	N/A	N/A	N/A
130	150	N/A	N/A	N/A	N/A	N/A	N/A

For SI: 1 mile per hour = 0.447 m/s.

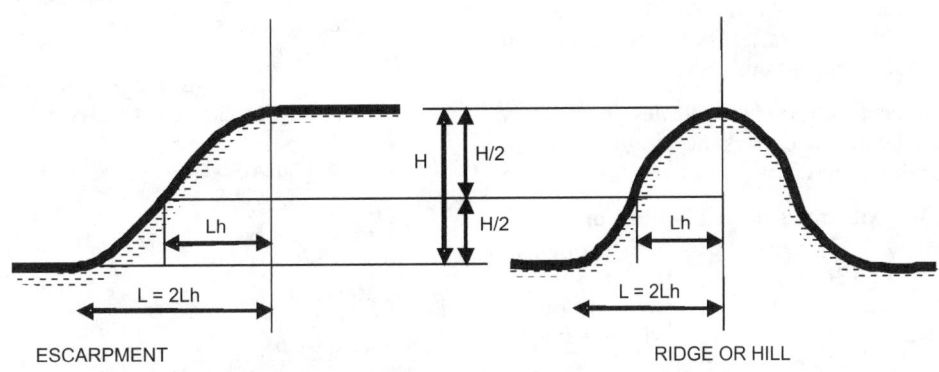

ESCARPMENT   RIDGE OR HILL

Note: H/2 determines the measurement point for Lh. L is twice Lh.

FIGURE R301.2.1.5.1(1)
TOPOGRAPHIC FEATURES FOR WIND SPEED-UP EFFECT

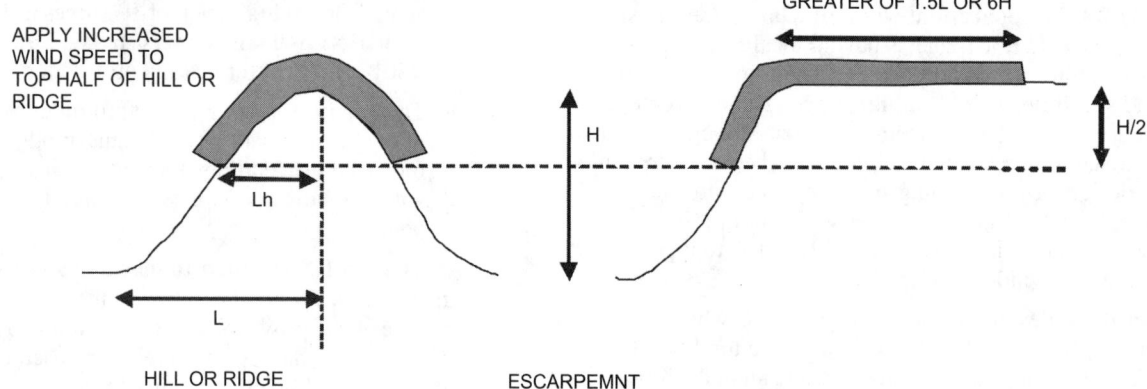

FIGURE R301.2.1.5.1(2)
ILLUSTRATION OF WHERE ON A TOPOGRAPHIC FEATURE, WIND SPEED INCREASE IS APPLIED

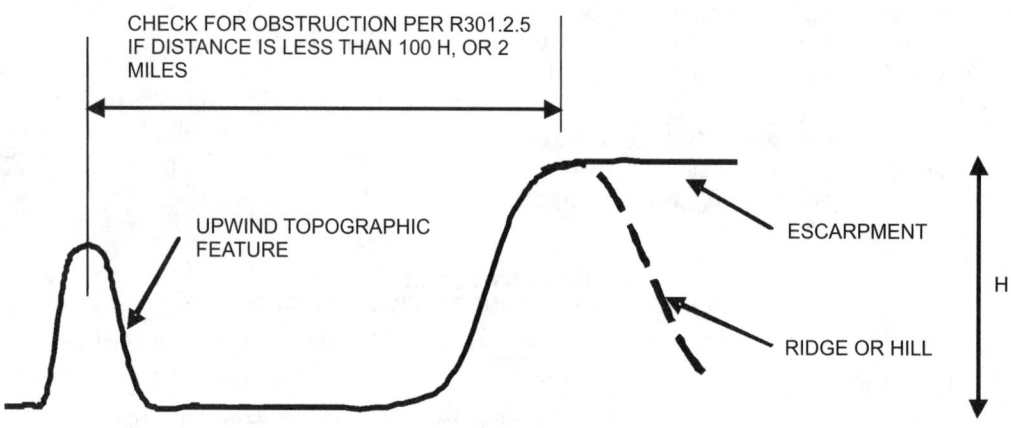

FIGURE R301.2.1.5.1(3)
ILLUSTRATION OF WHERE ON A TOPOGRAPHIC FEATURE, WIND SPEED INCREASE IS APPLIED

R301.2.2 Seismic provisions. The seismic provisions of this code shall apply to buildings constructed in Seismic Design Categories C, D_0, D_1 and D_2, as determined in accordance with this section.

Exception: Detached one- and two-family *dwellings* located in Seismic Design Category C are exempt from the seismic requirements of this code.

R301.2.2.1 Determination of seismic design category. Buildings shall be assigned a seismic design category in accordance with Figure R301.2(2).

R301.2.2.1.1 Alternate determination of seismic design category. The Seismic Design Categories and corresponding Short Period Design Spectral Response Accelerations, S_{DS} shown in Figure R301.2(2) are based on soil Site Class D, as defined in Section 1613.5.2 of the *International Building Code*. If soil conditions are other than Site Class D, the Short Period Design Spectral Response Accelerations, S_{DS}, for a site can be determined according to Section 1613.5 of the *International Building Code*. The value

of S_{DS} determined according to Section 1613.5 of the *International Building Code* is permitted to be used to set the seismic design category according to Table R301.2.2.1.1, and to interpolate between values in Tables R602.10.1, R603.7 and other seismic design requirements of this code.

TABLE R301.2.2.1.1
SEISMIC DESIGN CATEGORY DETERMINATION

CALCULATED S_{DS}	SEISMIC DESIGN CATEGORY
$S_{DS} \le 0.17g$	A
$0.17g < S_{DS} \le 0.33g$	B
$0.33g < S_{DS} \le 0.50g$	C
$0.50g < S_{DS} \le 0.67g$	D_0
$0.67g < S_{DS} \le 0.83g$	D_1
$0.83g < S_{DS} \le 1.17g$	D_2
$1.17g < S_{Ds}$	E

R301.2.2.1.2 Alternative determination of Seismic Design Category E. Buildings located in Seismic Design Category E in accordance with Figure R301.2(2) are permitted to be reclassified as being in Seismic Design Category D_2 provided one of the following is done:

1. A more detailed evaluation of the seismic design category is made in accordance with the provisions and maps of the *International Building Code*. Buildings located in Seismic Design Category E per Table R301.2.2.1.1, but located in Seismic Design Category D per the *International Building Code*, may be designed using the Seismic Design Category D_2 requirements of this code.

2. Buildings located in Seismic Design Category E that conform to the following additional restrictions are permitted to be constructed in accordance with the provisions for Seismic Design Category D_2 of this code:

    2.1. All exterior shear wall lines or *braced wall panels* are in one plane vertically from the foundation to the uppermost story.

    2.2. Floors shall not cantilever past the exterior walls.

    2.3. The building is within all of the requirements of Section R301.2.2.2.5 for being considered as regular.

R301.2.2.2 Seismic Design Category C. Structures assigned to Seismic Design Category C shall conform to the requirements of this section.

R301.2.2.2.1 Weights of materials. Average dead loads shall not exceed 15 pounds per square foot (720 Pa) for the combined roof and ceiling assemblies (on a horizontal projection) or 10 pounds per square foot (480 Pa) for floor assemblies, except as further limited by Section R301.2.2. Dead loads for walls above *grade* shall not exceed:

1. Fifteen pounds per square foot (720 Pa) for exterior light-frame wood walls.

2. Fourteen pounds per square foot (670 Pa) for exterior light-frame cold-formed steel walls.

3. Ten pounds per square foot (480 Pa) for interior light-frame wood walls.

4. Five pounds per square foot (240 Pa) for interior light-frame cold-formed steel walls.

5. Eighty pounds per square foot (3830 Pa) for 8-inch-thick (203 mm) masonry walls.

6. Eighty-five pounds per square foot (4070 Pa) for 6-inch-thick (152 mm) concrete walls.

7. Ten pounds per square foot (480 Pa) for SIP walls.

Exceptions:

1. Roof and ceiling dead loads not exceeding 25 pounds per square foot (1190 Pa) shall be permitted provided the wall bracing amounts in Chapter 6 are increased in accordance with Table R301.2.2.2.1.

2. Light-frame walls with stone or masonry veneer shall be permitted in accordance with the provisions of Sections R702.1 and R703.

3. Fireplaces and chimneys shall be permitted in accordance with Chapter 10.

TABLE R301.2.2.2.1
WALL BRACING ADJUSTMENT FACTORS BY ROOF COVERING DEAD LOAD[a]

WALL SUPPORTING	ROOF/CEILING DEAD LOAD	
	15 psf or less	25 psf
Roof only	1.0	1.2
Roof plus one or two stories	1.0	1.1

For SI: 1 pound per square foot = 0.0479 kPa.
a. Linear interpolation shall be permitted.

R301.2.2.2.2 Stone and masonry veneer. Anchored stone and masonry veneer shall comply with the requirements of Sections R702.1 and R703.

R301.2.2.2.3 Masonry construction. Masonry construction shall comply with the requirements of Section R606.11.2.

R301.2.2.2.4 Concrete construction. Detached one- and two-family *dwellings* with exterior above-*grade* concrete walls shall comply with the requirements of Section R611, PCA 100 or shall be designed in accordance with ACI 318. *Townhouses* with above-*grade* exterior concrete walls shall comply with the requirements of PCA 100 or shall be designed in accordance with ACI 318.

R301.2.2.2.5 Irregular buildings. Prescriptive construction as regulated by this code shall not be used for irregular structures located in Seismic Design Categories C, D_0, D_1 and D_2. Irregular portions of structures shall be designed in accordance with accepted engineering practice to the extent the irregular features affect the performance of the remaining structural system. When the forces associated with the irregularity are resisted by a structural system designed in accordance with accepted engineering practice, design of the remainder of the building shall be permitted using the provisions of this code. A building or portion of a building shall be considered to be irregular when one or more of the following conditions occur:

1. When exterior shear wall lines or *braced wall panels* are not in one plane vertically from the foundation to the uppermost *story* in which they are required.

    Exception: For wood light-frame construction, floors with cantilevers or setbacks not exceeding four times the nominal depth of the wood floor joists are permitted to support *braced wall panels* that are out of plane with *braced wall panels* below provided that:

1. Floor joists are nominal 2 inches by 10 inches (51 mm by 254 mm) or larger and spaced not more than 16 inches (406 mm) on center.

2. The ratio of the back span to the cantilever is at least 2 to 1.

3. Floor joists at ends of *braced wall panels* are doubled.

4. For wood-frame construction, a continuous rim joist is connected to ends of all cantilever joists. When spliced, the rim joists shall be spliced using a galvanized metal tie not less than 0.058 inch (1.5 mm) (16 gage) and $1^1/_2$ inches (38 mm) wide fastened with six 16d nails on each side of the splice or a block of the same size as the rim joist of sufficient length to fit securely between the joist space at which the splice occurs fastened with eight 16d nails on each side of the splice; and

5. Gravity loads carried at the end of cantilevered joists are limited to uniform wall and roof loads and the reactions from headers having a span of 8 feet (2438 mm) or less.

2. When a section of floor or roof is not laterally supported by shear walls or *braced wall lines* on all edges.

    Exception: Portions of floors that do not support shear walls or *braced wall panels* above, or roofs, shall be permitted to extend no more than 6 feet (1829 mm) beyond a shear wall or *braced wall line*.

3. When the end of a *braced wall panel* occurs over an opening in the wall below and ends at a horizontal distance greater than 1 foot (305 mm) from the edge of the opening. This provision is applicable to shear walls and *braced wall panels* offset in plane and to *braced wall panels* offset out of plane as permitted by the exception to Item 1 above.

    Exception: For wood light-frame wall construction, one end of a *braced wall panel* shall be permitted to extend more than 1 foot (305 mm) over an opening not more than 8 feet (2438 mm) wide in the wall below provided that the opening includes a header in accordance with the following:

    1. The building width, loading condition and framing member species limitations of Table R502.5(1) shall apply; and

    2. Not less than one 2 × 12 or two 2 × 10 for an opening not more than 4 feet (1219 mm) wide; or

    3. Not less than two 2 × 12 or three 2 × 10 for an opening not more than 6 feet (1829 mm) wide; or

    4. Not less than three 2 × 12 or four 2 × 10 for an opening not more than 8 feet (2438 mm) wide; and

    5. The entire length of the *braced wall panel* does not occur over an opening in the wall below.

4. When an opening in a floor or roof exceeds the lesser of 12 feet (3658 mm) or 50 percent of the least floor or roof dimension.

5. When portions of a floor level are vertically offset.

    Exceptions:

    1. Framing supported directly by continuous foundations at the perimeter of the building.

    2. For wood light-frame construction, floors shall be permitted to be vertically offset when the floor framing is lapped or tied together as required by Section R502.6.1.

6. When shear walls and *braced wall lines* do not occur in two perpendicular directions.

7. When stories above-*grade* partially or completely braced by wood wall framing in accordance with Section R602 or steel wall framing in accordance with Section R603 include masonry or concrete construction.

    Exception: Fireplaces, chimneys and masonry veneer as permitted by this code. When this irregularity applies, the entire *story* shall be designed in accordance with accepted engineering practice.

R301.2.2.3 Seismic Design Categories D_0, D_1 and D_2. Structures assigned to Seismic Design Categories D_0, D_1 and D_2 shall conform to the requirements for Seismic Design Category C and the additional requirements of this section.

R301.2.2.3.1 Height limitations. Wood framed buildings shall be limited to three stories above *grade* or the limits given in Table R602.10.1.2(2). Cold-formed steel framed buildings shall be limited to less than or equal to three stories above *grade* in accordance with AISI S230. Mezzanines as defined in Section R202 shall not be considered as stories. Structural insulated panel buildings shall be limited to two stories above *grade*.

R301.2.2.3.2 Stone and masonry veneer. Anchored stone and masonry veneer shall comply with the requirements of Sections R702.1 and R703.

R301.2.2.3.3 Masonry construction. Masonry construction in Seismic Design Categories D₀ and D₁ shall comply with the requirements of Section R606.11.3. Masonry construction in Seismic Design Category D₂ shall comply with the requirements of Section R606.11.4.

R301.2.2.3.4 Concrete construction. Buildings with exterior above-*grade* concrete walls shall comply with PCA 100 or shall be designed in accordance with ACI 318.

R301.2.2.3.5 Cold-formed steel framing in Seismic Design Categories D₀, D₁ and D₂. In Seismic Design Categories D₀, D₁ and D₂ in addition to the requirements of this code, cold-formed steel framing shall comply with the requirements of AISI S230.

R301.2.2.3.6 Masonry chimneys. Masonry chimneys shall be reinforced and anchored to the building in accordance with Sections R1003.3 and R1003.4.

R301.2.2.3.7 Anchorage of water heaters. Water heaters shall be anchored against movement and overturning in accordance with Section M1307.2.

R301.2.2.4 Seismic Design Category E. Buildings in Seismic Design Category E shall be designed in accordance with the *International Building Code*, except when the seismic design category is reclassified to a lower seismic design category in accordance with Section R301.2.2.1.

R301.2.3 Snow loads. Wood framed construction, cold-formed steel framed construction and masonry and concrete construction, and structural insulated panel construction in regions with ground snow loads 70 pounds per square foot (3.35 kPa) or less, shall be in accordance with Chapters 5, 6 and 8. Buildings in regions with ground snow loads greater than 70 pounds per square foot (3.35 kPa) shall be designed in accordance with accepted engineering practice.

R301.2.4 Floodplain construction. Buildings and structures constructed in whole or in part in flood hazard areas (including A or V Zones) as established in Table R301.2(1) shall be designed and constructed in accordance with Section R322.

> **Exception:** Buildings and structures located in whole or in part in identified floodways shall be designed and constructed in accordance with ASCE 24.

R301.2.4.1 Alternative provisions. As an alternative to the requirements in Section R322.3 for buildings and structures located in whole or in part in coastal high hazard areas (V Zones), ASCE 24 is permitted subject to the limitations of this code and the limitations therein.

R301.3 Story height. Buildings constructed in accordance with these provisions shall be limited to *story heights* of not more than the following:

1. For wood wall framing, the laterally unsupported bearing wall stud height permitted by Table R602.3(5) plus a height of floor framing not to exceed 16 inches (406 mm).

   > **Exception:** For wood framed wall buildings with bracing in accordance with Tables R602.10.1.2(1) and R602.10.1.2(2), the wall stud clear height used to determine the maximum permitted *story height* may be increased to 12 feet (3658 mm) without requiring an engineered design for the building wind and seismic force resisting systems provided that the length of bracing required by Table R602.10.1.2(1) is increased by multiplying by a factor of 1.10 and the length of bracing required by Table R602.10.1.2(2) is increased by multiplying by a factor of 1.20. Wall studs are still subject to the requirements of this section.

2. For steel wall framing, a stud height of 10 feet (3048 mm), plus a height of floor framing not to exceed 16 inches (406 mm).

3. For masonry walls, a maximum bearing wall clear height of 12 feet (3658 mm) plus a height of floor framing not to exceed 16 inches (406 mm).

   > **Exception:** An additional 8 feet (2438 mm) is permitted for gable end walls.

4. For insulating concrete form walls, the maximum bearing wall height per *story* as permitted by Section R611 tables plus a height of floor framing not to exceed 16 inches (406 mm).

5. For structural insulated panel (SIP) walls, the maximum bearing wall height per *story* as permitted by Section 614 tables shall not exceed 10 feet (3048 mm) plus a height of floor framing not to exceed 16 inches (406 mm).

Individual walls or walls studs shall be permitted to exceed these limits as permitted by Chapter 6 provisions, provided *story heights* are not exceeded. Floor framing height shall be permitted to exceed these limits provided the *story height* does not exceed 11 feet 7 inches (3531 mm). An engineered design shall be provided for the wall or wall framing members when they exceed the limits of Chapter 6. Where the *story height* limits are exceeded, an engineered design shall be provided in accordance with the *International Building Code* for the overall wind and seismic force resisting systems.

R301.4 Dead load. The actual weights of materials and construction shall be used for determining dead load with consideration for the dead load of fixed service *equipment*.

R301.5 Live load. The minimum uniformly distributed live load shall be as provided in Table R301.5.

TABLE R301.5
MINIMUM UNIFORMLY DISTRIBUTED LIVE LOADS
(in pounds per square foot)

USE	LIVE LOAD
Attics without storage[b]	10
Attics with limited storage[b, g]	20
Habitable attics and attics served with fixed stairs	30
Balconies (exterior) and decks[e]	40
Fire escapes	40
Guardrails and handrails[d]	200[h]
Guardrail in-fill components[f]	50[h]
Passenger vehicle garages[a]	50[a]
Rooms other than sleeping room	40
Sleeping rooms	30
Stairs	40[c]

For SI: 1 pound per square foot = 0.0479 kPa, 1 square inch = 645 mm², 1 pound = 4.45 N.

a. Elevated garage floors shall be capable of supporting a 2,000-pound load applied over a 20-square-inch area.

b. Attics without storage are those where the maximum clear height between joist and rafter is less than 42 inches, or where there are not two or more adjacent trusses with the same web configuration capable of containing a rectangle 42 inches high by 2 feet wide, or greater, located within the plane of the truss. For attics without storage, this live load need not be assumed to act concurrently with any other live load requirements.

c. Individual stair treads shall be designed for the uniformly distributed live load or a 300-pound concentrated load acting over an area of 4 square inches, whichever produces the greater stresses.

d. A single concentrated load applied in any direction at any point along the top.

e. See Section R502.2.2 for decks attached to exterior walls.

f. Guard in-fill components (all those except the handrail), balusters and panel fillers shall be designed to withstand a horizontally applied normal load of 50 pounds on an area equal to 1 square foot. This load need not be assumed to act concurrently with any other live load requirement.

g. For attics with limited storage and constructed with trusses, this live load need be applied only to those portions of the bottom chord where there are two or more adjacent trusses with the same web configuration capable of containing a rectangle 42 inches high or greater by 2 feet wide or greater, located within the plane of the truss. The rectangle shall fit between the top of the bottom chord and the bottom of any other truss member, provided that each of the following criteria is met.

  1. The attic area is accessible by a pull-down stairway or framed in accordance with Section R807.1.

  2. The truss has a bottom chord pitch less than 2:12.

  3. Required insulation depth is less than the bottom chord member depth.

  The bottom chords of trusses meeting the above criteria for limited storage shall be designed for the greater of the actual imposed dead load or 10 psf, uniformly distributed over the entire span.

h. Glazing used in handrail assemblies and guards shall be designed with a safety factor of 4. The safety factor shall be applied to each of the concentrated loads applied to the top of the rail, and to the load on the in-fill components. These loads shall be determined independent of one another, and loads are assumed not to occur with any other live load.

R301.6 Roof load. The roof shall be designed for the live load indicated in Table R301.6 or the snow load indicated in Table R301.2(1), whichever is greater.

TABLE R301.6
MINIMUM ROOF LIVE LOADS IN POUNDS-FORCE PER SQUARE FOOT OF HORIZONTAL PROJECTION

ROOF SLOPE	TRIBUTARY LOADED AREA IN SQUARE FEET FOR ANY STRUCTURAL MEMBER		
	0 to 200	201 to 600	Over 600
Flat or rise less than 4 inches per foot (1:3)	20	16	12
Rise 4 inches per foot (1:3) to less than 12 inches per foot (1:1)	16	14	12
Rise 12 inches per foot (1:1) and greater	12	12	12

For SI: 1 square foot = 0.0929 m², 1 pound per square foot = 0.0479 kPa, 1 inch per foot = 83.3 mm/m.

R301.7 Deflection. The allowable deflection of any structural member under the live load listed in Sections R301.5 and R301.6 shall not exceed the values in Table R301.7.

TABLE R301.7
ALLOWABLE DEFLECTION OF STRUCTURAL MEMBERS[a, b, c, d, e]

STRUCTURAL MEMBER	ALLOWABLE DEFLECTION
Rafters having slopes greater than 3:12 with no finished ceiling attached to rafters	L/180
Interior walls and partitions	H/180
Floors and plastered ceilings	L/360
All other structural members	L/240
Exterior walls with plaster or stucco finish	H/360
Exterior walls—wind loads[a] with brittle finishes	H/240
Exterior walls—wind loads[a] with flexible finishes	L/120[d]
Lintels supporting masonry veneer walls[e]	L/600

Note: L = span length, H = span height.

a. The wind load shall be permitted to be taken as 0.7 times the Component and Cladding loads for the purpose of the determining deflection limits herein.

b. For cantilever members, *L* shall be taken as twice the length of the cantilever.

c. For aluminum structural members or panels used in roofs or walls of sunroom additions or patio covers, not supporting edge of glass or sandwich panels, the total load deflection shall not exceed L/60. For continuous aluminum structural members supporting edge of glass, the total load deflection shall not exceed L/175 for each glass lite or L/60 for the entire length of the member, whichever is more stringent. For sandwich panels used in roofs or walls of sunroom additions or patio covers, the total load deflection shall not exceed L/120.

d. Deflection for exterior walls with interior gypsum board finish shall be limited to an allowable deflection of H/180.

e. Refer to Section R703.7.2.

R301.8 Nominal sizes. For the purposes of this code, where dimensions of lumber are specified, they shall be deemed to be nominal dimensions unless specifically designated as actual dimensions.

SECTION R302
FIRE-RESISTANT CONSTRUCTION

R302.1 Exterior walls. Construction, projections, openings and penetrations of *exterior walls* of *dwellings* and accessory buildings shall comply with Table R302.1.

Exceptions:

1. Walls, projections, openings or penetrations in walls perpendicular to the line used to determine the *fire separation distance*.

2. Walls of *dwellings* and *accessory structures* located on the same *lot*.

3. Detached tool sheds and storage sheds, playhouses and similar structures exempted from permits are not required to provide wall protection based on location on the *lot*. Projections beyond the *exterior wall* shall not extend over the *lot line*.

4. Detached garages accessory to a *dwelling* located within 2 feet (610 mm) of a *lot line* are permitted to have roof eave projections not exceeding 4 inches (102 mm).

5. Foundation vents installed in compliance with this code are permitted.

R302.2 Townhouses. Each *townhouse* shall be considered a separate building and shall be separated by fire-resistance-rated wall assemblies meeting the requirements of Section R302.1 for exterior walls.

Exception: A common 1-hour fire-resistance-rated wall assembly tested in accordance with ASTM E 119 or UL 263 is permitted for townhouses if such walls do not contain plumbing or mechanical equipment, ducts or vents in the cavity of the common wall. The wall shall be rated for fire exposure from both sides and shall extend to and be tight against exterior walls and the underside of the roof sheathing. Electrical installations shall be installed in accordance with Chapters 34 through 43. Penetrations of electrical outlet boxes shall be in accordance with Section R302.4.

R302.2.1 Continuity. The fire-resistance-rated wall or assembly separating *townhouses* shall be continuous from the foundation to the underside of the roof sheathing, deck or slab. The fire-resistance rating shall extend the full length of the wall or assembly, including wall extensions through and separating attached enclosed *accessory structures*.

R302.2.2 Parapets. Parapets constructed in accordance with Section R302.2.3 shall be constructed for *townhouses* as an extension of exterior walls or common walls in accordance with the following:

1. Where roof surfaces adjacent to the wall or walls are at the same elevation, the parapet shall extend not less than 30 inches (762 mm) above the roof surfaces.

2. Where roof surfaces adjacent to the wall or walls are at different elevations and the higher roof is not more than 30 inches (762 mm) above the lower roof, the parapet shall extend not less than 30 inches (762 mm) above the lower roof surface.

   Exception: A parapet is not required in the two cases above when the roof is covered with a minimum class C roof covering, and the roof decking or sheathing is of noncombustible materials or *approved* fire-retardant-treated wood for a distance of 4 feet (1219 mm) on each side of the wall or walls, or one layer of $^5/_8$-inch (15.9 mm) Type X gypsum board is installed directly beneath the roof decking or sheathing, supported by a minimum of nominal 2-inch (51 mm) ledgers attached to the sides of the roof framing members, for a minimum distance of 4 feet (1219 mm) on each side of the wall or walls.

3. A parapet is not required where roof surfaces adjacent to the wall or walls are at different elevations and the higher roof is more than 30 inches (762 mm) above the lower roof. The common wall construction from the lower roof to the underside of the higher roof deck shall have not less than a 1-hour fire-resistance rating. The wall shall be rated for exposure from both sides.

TABLE R302.1
EXTERIOR WALLS

EXTERIOR WALL ELEMENT		MINIMUM FIRE-RESISTANCE RATING	MINIMUM FIRE SEPARATION DISTANCE
Walls	(Fire-resistance rated)	1 hour-tested in accordance with ASTM E 119 or UL 263 with exposure form both sides	< 5 feet
	(Not fire-resistance rated)	0 hours	≥ 5 feet
Projections	(Fire-resistance rated)	1 hour on the underside	≥ 2 feet to 5 feet
	(Not fire-resistance rated)	0 hours	5 feet
Openings in walls	Not allowed	N/A	< 3 feet
	25% maximum of wall area	0 hours	3 feet
	Unlimited	0 hours	5 feet
Penetrations	All	Comply with Section R317.3	< 5 feet
		None required	5 feet

For SI: 1 foot = 304.8 mm.

N/A = Not Applicable.

R302.2.3 Parapet construction. Parapets shall have the same fire-resistance rating as that required for the supporting wall or walls. On any side adjacent to a roof surface, the parapet shall have noncombustible faces for the uppermost 18 inches (457 mm), to include counterflashing and coping materials. Where the roof slopes toward a parapet at slopes greater than 2 units vertical in 12 units horizontal (16.7-percent slope), the parapet shall extend to the same height as any portion of the roof within a distance of 3 feet (914 mm), but in no case shall the height be less than 30 inches (762 mm).

R302.2.4 Structural independence. Each individual *townhouse* shall be structurally independent.

Exceptions:

1. Foundations supporting *exterior walls* or common walls.

2. Structural roof and wall sheathing from each unit may fasten to the common wall framing.

3. Nonstructural wall and roof coverings.

4. Flashing at termination of roof covering over common wall.

5. *Townhouses* separated by a common 1-hour fire-resistance-rated wall as provided in Section R302.2.

R302.3 Two-family dwellings. *Dwelling units* in two-family dwellings shall be separated from each other by wall and/or floor assemblies having not less than a 1-hour fire-resistance rating when tested in accordance with ASTM E 119 or UL 263. Fire-resistance-rated floor-ceiling and wall assemblies shall extend to and be tight against the *exterior wall*, and wall assemblies shall extend from the foundation to the underside of the roof sheathing.

Exceptions:

1. A fire-resistance rating of $^1/_2$ hour shall be permitted in buildings equipped throughout with an automatic sprinkler system installed in accordance with NFPA 13.

2. Wall assemblies need not extend through *attic* spaces when the ceiling is protected by not less than $^5/_8$-inch (15.9 mm) Type X gypsum board and an *attic* draft stop constructed as specified in Section R302.12.1 is provided above and along the wall assembly separating the *dwellings*. The structural framing supporting the ceiling shall also be protected by not less than $^1/_2$-inch (12.7 mm) gypsum board or equivalent.

R302.3.1 Supporting construction. When floor assemblies are required to be fire-resistance rated by Section R302.3, the supporting construction of such assemblies shall have an equal or greater fire-resistance rating.

R302.4 Dwelling unit rated penetrations. Penetrations of wall or floor/ceiling assemblies required to be fire-resistance rated in accordance with Section R302.2 or R302.3 shall be protected in accordance with this section.

R302.4.1 Through penetrations. Through penetrations of fire-resistance-rated wall or floor assemblies shall comply with Section R302.4.1.1 or R302.4.1.2.

Exception: Where the penetrating items are steel, ferrous or copper pipes, tubes or conduits, the annular space shall be protected as follows:

1. In concrete or masonry wall or floor assemblies, concrete, grout or mortar shall be permitted where installed to the full thickness of the wall or floor assembly or the thickness required to maintain the fire-resistance rating, provided:

    1.1. The nominal diameter of the penetrating item is a maximum of 6 inches (152 mm); and

    1.2. The area of the opening through the wall does not exceed 144 square inches (92 900 mm²).

2. The material used to fill the annular space shall prevent the passage of flame and hot gases sufficient to ignite cotton waste where subjected to ASTM E 119 or UL 263 time temperature fire conditions under a minimum positive pressure differential of 0.01 inch of water (3 Pa) at the location of the penetration for the time period equivalent to the fire resistance rating of the construction penetrated.

R302.4.1.1 Fire-resistance-rated assembly. Penetrations shall be installed as tested in the *approved* fire-resistance-rated assembly.

R302.4.1.2 Penetration firestop system. Penetrations shall be protected by an *approved* penetration firestop system installed as tested in accordance with ASTM E 814 or UL 1479, with a minimum positive pressure differential of 0.01 inch of water (3 Pa) and shall have an F rating of not less than the required fire-resistance rating of the wall or floor/ceiling assembly penetrated.

R302.4.2 Membrane penetrations. Membrane penetrations shall comply with Section R302.4.1. Where walls are required to have a fire-resistance rating, recessed fixtures shall be installed so that the required fire-resistance rating will not be reduced.

Exceptions:

1. Membrane penetrations of maximum 2-hour fire-resistance-rated walls and partitions by steel electrical boxes that do not exceed 16 square inches (0.0103 m²) in area provided the aggregate area of the openings through the membrane does not exceed 100 square inches (0.0645 m²) in any 100 square feet (9.29 m)² of wall area. The annular space between the wall membrane and the box shall not exceed $^1/_8$ inch (3.1 mm). Such boxes on opposite sides of the wall shall be separated by one of the following:

    1.1. By a horizontal distance of not less than 24 inches (610 mm) where the wall or partition is constructed with individual noncommunicating stud cavities;

1.2. By a horizontal distance of not less than the depth of the wall cavity when the wall cavity is filled with cellulose loose-fill, rockwool or slag mineral wool insulation;

1.3. By solid fire blocking in accordance with Section R302.11;

1.4. By protecting both boxes with listed putty pads; or

1.5. By other listed materials and methods.

2. Membrane penetrations by listed electrical boxes of any materials provided the boxes have been tested for use in fire-resistance-rated assemblies and are installed in accordance with the instructions included in the listing. The annular space between the wall membrane and the box shall not exceed $^1/_8$ inch (3.1 mm) unless listed otherwise. Such boxes on opposite sides of the wall shall be separated by one of the following:

2.1. By the horizontal distance specified in the listing of the electrical boxes;

2.2. By solid fireblocking in accordance with Section R302.11;

2.3. By protecting both boxes with listed putty pads; or

2.4. By other listed materials and methods.

3. The annular space created by the penetration of a fire sprinkler provided it is covered by a metal escutcheon plate.

R302.5 Dwelling/garage opening/penetration protection. Openings and penetrations through the walls or ceilings separating the *dwelling* from the garage shall be in accordance with Sections R302.5.1 through R302.5.3.

R302.5.1 Opening protection. Openings from a private garage directly into a room used for sleeping purposes shall not be permitted. Other openings between the garage and residence shall be equipped with solid wood doors not less than $1^3/_8$ inches (35 mm) in thickness, solid or honeycomb core steel doors not less than $1^3/_8$ inches (35 mm) thick, or 20-minute fire-rated doors.

R302.5.2 Duct penetration. Ducts in the garage and ducts penetrating the walls or ceilings separating the *dwelling* from the garage shall be constructed of a minimum No. 26 gage (0.48 mm) sheet steel or other *approved* material and shall have no openings into the garage.

R302.5.3 Other penetrations. Penetrations through the separation required in Section R309.2 shall be protected as required by Section R302.11, Item 4.

R302.6 Dwelling/garage fire separation. The garage shall be separated as required by Table R302.6. Openings in garage walls shall comply with Section R302.5. This provision does not apply to garage walls that are perpendicular to the adjacent *dwelling unit* wall.

R302.7 Under-stair protection. Enclosed accessible space under stairs shall have walls, under-stair surface and any soffits protected on the enclosed side with $^1/_2$-inch (12.7 mm) gypsum board.

R302.8 Foam plastics. For requirements for foam plastics see Section R316.

R302.9 Flame spread index and smoke-developed index for wall and ceiling finishes. Flame spread and smoke index for wall and ceiling finishes shall be in accordance with Sections R302.9.1 through R302.9.4.

R302.9.1 Flame spread index. Wall and ceiling finishes shall have a flame spread index of not greater than 200.

Exception: Flame spread index requirements for finishes shall not apply to trim defined as picture molds, chair rails, baseboards and handrails; to doors and windows or their frames; or to materials that are less than $^1/_{28}$ inch (0.91 mm) in thickness cemented to the surface of walls or ceilings if these materials exhibit flame spread index values no greater than those of paper of this thickness cemented to a noncombustible backing.

R302.9.2 Smoke-developed index. Wall and ceiling finishes shall have a smoke-developed index of not greater than 450.

R302.9.3 Testing. Tests shall be made in accordance with ASTM E 84 or UL 723.

R302.9.4 Alternate test method. As an alternate to having a flame-spread index of not greater than 200 and a smoke developed index of not greater than 450 when tested in accordance with ASTM E 84 or UL 723, wall and ceiling finishes, other than textiles, shall be permitted to be tested in

TABLE R302.6
DWELLING/GARAGE SEPARATION

SEPARATION	MATERIAL
From the residence and attics	Not less than $^1/_2$-inch gypsum board or equivalent applied to the garage side
From all habitable rooms above the garage	Not less than $^5/_8$-inch Type X gypsum board or equivalent
Structure(s) supporting floor/ceiling assemblies used for separation required by this section	Not less than $^1/_2$-inch gypsum board or equivalent
Garages located less than 3 feet from a dwelling unit on the same lot	Not less than $^1/_2$-inch gypsum board or equivalent applied to the interior side of exterior walls that are within this area

For SI: 1 inch = 25.4 mm, 1 foot = 304.8 mm.

accordance with NFPA 286. Materials tested in accordance with NFPA 286 shall meet the following criteria:

During the 40 kW exposure, the interior finish shall comply with Item 1. During the 160 kW exposure, the interior finish shall comply with Item 2. During the entire test, the interior finish shall comply with Item 3.

1. During the 40 kW exposure, flames shall not spread to the ceiling.

2. During the 160 kW exposure, the interior finish shall comply with the following:

    2.1. Flame shall not spread to the outer extremity of the sample on any wall or ceiling.

    2.2. Flashover, as defined in NFPA 286, shall not occur.

3. The total smoke released throughout the NFPA 286 test shall not exceed 1,000 m².

R302.10 Flame spread index and smoke developed index for insulation. Flame spread and smoke developed index for insulation shall be in accordance with Sections R302.10.1 through R302.10.5.

R302.10.1 Insulation. Insulation materials, including facings, such as vapor retarders and vapor-permeable membranes installed within floor-ceiling assemblies, roof-ceiling assemblies, wall assemblies, crawl spaces and *attics* shall have a flame spread index not to exceed 25 with an accompanying smoke-developed index not to exceed 450 when tested in accordance with ASTM E 84 or UL 723.

Exceptions:

1. When such materials are installed in concealed spaces, the flame spread index and smoke-developed index limitations do not apply to the facings, provided that the facing is installed in substantial contact with the unexposed surface of the ceiling, floor or wall finish.

2. Cellulose loose-fill insulation, which is not spray applied, complying with the requirements of Section R302.10.3, shall only be required to meet the smoke-developed index of not more than 450.

R302.10.2 Loose-fill insulation. Loose-fill insulation materials that cannot be mounted in the ASTM E 84 or UL 723 apparatus without a screen or artificial supports shall comply with the flame spread and smoke-developed limits of Section R302.10.1 when tested in accordance with CAN/ULC S102.2.

Exception: Cellulose loose-fill insulation shall not be required to be tested in accordance with CAN/ULC S102.2, provided such insulation complies with the requirements of Section R302.10.1 and Section R302.10.3.

R302.10.3 Cellulose loose-fill insulation. Cellulose loose-fill insulation shall comply with CPSC 16 CFR, Parts 1209 and 1404. Each package of such insulating material shall be clearly *labeled* in accordance with CPSC 16 CFR, Parts 1209 and 1404.

R302.10.4 Exposed attic insulation. All exposed insulation materials installed on *attic* floors shall have a critical radiant flux not less than 0.12 watt per square centimeter.

R302.10.5 Testing. Tests for critical radiant flux shall be made in accordance with ASTM E 970.

R302.11 Fireblocking. In combustible construction, fireblocking shall be provided to cut off all concealed draft openings (both vertical and horizontal) and to form an effective fire barrier between stories, and between a top *story* and the roof space.

Fireblocking shall be provided in wood-frame construction in the following locations:

1. In concealed spaces of stud walls and partitions, including furred spaces and parallel rows of studs or staggered studs, as follows:

    1.1. Vertically at the ceiling and floor levels.

    1.2. Horizontally at intervals not exceeding 10 feet (3048 mm).

2. At all interconnections between concealed vertical and horizontal spaces such as occur at soffits, drop ceilings and cove ceilings.

3. In concealed spaces between stair stringers at the top and bottom of the run. Enclosed spaces under stairs shall comply with Section R302.7.

4. At openings around vents, pipes, ducts, cables and wires at ceiling and floor level, with an *approved* material to resist the free passage of flame and products of combustion. The material filling this annular space shall not be required to meet the ASTM E 136 requirements.

5. For the fireblocking of chimneys and fireplaces, see Section R1003.19.

6. Fireblocking of cornices of a two-family *dwelling* is required at the line of *dwelling unit* separation.

R302.11.1 Fireblocking materials. Except as provided in Section R302.11, Item 4, fireblocking shall consist of the following materials.

1. Two-inch (51 mm) nominal lumber.

2. Two thicknesses of 1-inch (25.4 mm) nominal lumber with broken lap joints.

3. One thickness of $^{23}/_{32}$-inch (18.3 mm) wood structural panels with joints backed by $^{23}/_{32}$-inch (18.3 mm) wood structural panels.

4. One thickness of $^{3}/_{4}$-inch (19.1 mm) particleboard with joints backed by $^{3}/_{4}$-inch (19.1 mm) particleboard.

5. One-half-inch (12.7 mm) gypsum board.

6. One-quarter-inch (6.4 mm) cement-based millboard.

7. Batts or blankets of mineral wool or glass fiber or other *approved* materials installed in such a manner as to be securely retained in place.

R302.11.1.1 Batts or blankets of mineral or glass fiber. Batts or blankets of mineral or glass fiber or other *approved* nonrigid materials shall be permitted for compliance with the 10-foot (3048 mm) horizontal fireblocking in walls constructed using parallel rows of studs or staggered studs.

R302.11.1.2 Unfaced fiberglass. Unfaced fiberglass batt insulation used as fireblocking shall fill the entire cross section of the wall cavity to a minimum height of 16 inches (406 mm) measured vertically. When piping, conduit or similar obstructions are encountered, the insulation shall be packed tightly around the obstruction.

R302.11.1.3 Loose-fill insulation material. Loose-fill insulation material shall not be used as a fireblock unless specifically tested in the form and manner intended for use to demonstrate its ability to remain in place and to retard the spread of fire and hot gases.

R302.11.2 Fireblocking integrity. The integrity of all fireblocks shall be maintained.

R302.12 Draftstopping. In combustible construction where there is usable space both above and below the concealed space of a floor/ceiling assembly, draftstops shall be installed so that the area of the concealed space does not exceed 1,000 square feet (92.9 m²). Draftstopping shall divide the concealed space into approximately equal areas. Where the assembly is enclosed by a floor membrane above and a ceiling membrane below, draftstopping shall be provided in floor/ceiling assemblies under the following circumstances:

1. Ceiling is suspended under the floor framing.

2. Floor framing is constructed of truss-type open-web or perforated members.

R302.12.1 Materials. Draftstopping materials shall not be less than ¹/₂-inch (12.7 mm) gypsum board, ³/₈-inch (9.5 mm) wood structural panels or other *approved* materials adequately supported. Draftopping shall be installed parallel to the floor framing members unless otherwise *approved* by the *building official*. The integrity of the draftstops shall be maintained.

R302.13 Combustible insulation clearance. Combustible insulation shall be separated a minimum of 3 inches (76 mm) from recessed luminaires, fan motors and other heat-producing devices.

Exception: Where heat-producing devices are listed for lesser clearances, combustible insulation complying with the listing requirements shall be separated in accordance with the conditions stipulated in the listing.

Recessed luminaires installed in the *building thermal envelope* shall meet the requirements of Section N1102.4.5.

SECTION R303
LIGHT, VENTILATION AND HEATING

R303.1 Habitable rooms. All habitable rooms shall have an aggregate glazing area of not less than 8 percent of the floor area of such rooms. Natural *ventilation* shall be through windows, doors, louvers or other *approved* openings to the outdoor air. Such openings shall be provided with ready access or shall otherwise be readily controllable by the building occupants.

The minimum openable area to the outdoors shall be 4 percent of the floor area being ventilated.

Exceptions:

1. The glazed areas need not be openable where the opening is not required by Section R310 and an *approved* mechanical *ventilation* system capable of producing 0.35 air change per hour in the room is installed or a whole-house mechanical *ventilation* system is installed capable of supplying outdoor *ventilation* air of 15 cubic feet per minute (cfm) (78 L/s) per occupant computed on the basis of two occupants for the first bedroom and one occupant for each additional bedroom.

2. The glazed areas need not be installed in rooms where Exception 1 above is satisfied and artificial light is provided capable of producing an average illumination of 6 footcandles (65 lux) over the area of the room at a height of 30 inches (762 mm) above the floor level.

3. Use of sunroom *additions* and patio covers, as defined in Section R202, shall be permitted for natural *ventilation* if in excess of 40 percent of the exterior sunroom walls are open, or are enclosed only by insect screening.

R303.2 Adjoining rooms. For the purpose of determining light and *ventilation* requirements, any room shall be considered as a portion of an adjoining room when at least one-half of the area of the common wall is open and unobstructed and provides an opening of not less than one-tenth of the floor area of the interior room but not less than 25 square feet (2.3 m²).

Exception: Openings required for light and/or *ventilation* shall be permitted to open into a thermally isolated sunroom *addition* or patio cover, provided that there is an openable area between the adjoining room and the sunroom *addition* or patio cover of not less than one-tenth of the floor area of the interior room but not less than 20 square feet (2 m²). The minimum openable area to the outdoors shall be based upon the total floor area being ventilated.

R303.3 Bathrooms. Bathrooms, water closet compartments and other similar rooms shall be provided with aggregate glazing area in windows of not less than 3 square feet (0.3 m²), one-half of which must be openable.

Exception: The glazed areas shall not be required where artificial light and a mechanical *ventilation* system are provided. The minimum *ventilation* rates shall be 50 cubic feet per minute (24 L/s) for intermittent *ventilation* or 20 cubic feet per minute (10 L/s) for continuous *ventilation*. *Ventilation* air from the space shall be exhausted directly to the outside.

R303.4 Opening location. Outdoor intake and exhaust openings shall be located in accordance with Sections R303.4.1 and R303.4.2.

R303.4.1 Intake openings. Mechanical and gravity outdoor air intake openings shall be located a minimum of 10 feet (3048 mm) from any hazardous or noxious contaminant, such as vents, chimneys, plumbing vents, streets, alleys, parking lots and loading docks, except as otherwise specified in this code. Where a source of contaminant is located within 10 feet (3048 mm) of an intake opening, such opening shall be located a minimum of 2 feet (610 mm) below the contaminant source.

For the purpose of this section, the exhaust from *dwelling* unit toilet rooms, bathrooms and kitchens shall not be considered as hazardous or noxious.

R303.4.2 Exhaust openings. Exhaust air shall not be directed onto walkways.

R303.5 Outside opening protection. Air exhaust and intake openings that terminate outdoors shall be protected with corrosion-resistant screens, louvers or grilles having a minimum opening size of $^1/_4$ inch (6 mm) and a maximum opening size of $^1/_2$ inch (13 mm), in any dimension. Openings shall be protected against local weather conditions. Outdoor air exhaust and intake openings shall meet the provisions for *exterior wall* opening protectives in accordance with this code.

R303.6 Stairway illumination. All interior and exterior stairways shall be provided with a means to illuminate the stairs, including the landings and treads. Interior stairways shall be provided with an artificial light source located in the immediate vicinity of each landing of the stairway. For interior stairs the artificial light sources shall be capable of illuminating treads and landings to levels not less than 1 foot-candle (11 lux) measured at the center of treads and landings. Exterior stairways shall be provided with an artificial light source located in the immediate vicinity of the top landing of the stairway. Exterior stairways providing access to a *basement* from the outside *grade* level shall be provided with an artificial light source located in the immediate vicinity of the bottom landing of the stairway.

Exception: An artificial light source is not required at the top and bottom landing, provided an artificial light source is located directly over each stairway section.

R303.6.1 Light activation. Where lighting outlets are installed in interior stairways, there shall be a wall switch at each floor level to control the lighting outlet where the stairway has six or more risers. The illumination of exterior stairways shall be controlled from inside the *dwelling* unit.

Exception: Lights that are continuously illuminated or automatically controlled.

R303.7 Required glazed openings. Required glazed openings shall open directly onto a street or public alley, or a *yard* or court located on the same *lot* as the building.

Exceptions:

1. Required glazed openings may face into a roofed porch where the porch abuts a street, *yard* or court and the longer side of the porch is at least 65 percent unobstructed and the ceiling height is not less than 7 feet (2134 mm).

2. Eave projections shall not be considered as obstructing the clear open space of a *yard* or court.

3. Required glazed openings may face into the area under a deck, balcony, bay or floor cantilever provided a clear vertical space at least 36 inches (914 mm) in height is provided.

R303.7.1 Sunroom additions. Required glazed openings shall be permitted to open into sunroom *additions* or patio covers that abut a street, *yard* or court if in excess of 40 percent of the exterior sunroom walls are open, or are enclosed only by insect screening, and the ceiling height of the sunroom is not less than 7 feet (2134 mm).

R303.8 Required heating. When the winter design temperature in Table R301.2(1) is below 60°F (16°C), every *dwelling unit* shall be provided with heating facilities capable of maintaining a minimum room temperature of 68°F (20°C) at a point 3 feet (914 mm) above the floor and 2 feet (610 mm) from exterior walls in all habitable rooms at the design temperature. The installation of one or more portable space heaters shall not be used to achieve compliance with this section.

SECTION R304
MINIMUM ROOM AREAS

R304.1 Minimum area. Every *dwelling* unit shall have at least one habitable room that shall have not less than 120 square feet (11 m²) of gross floor area.

R304.2 Other rooms. Other habitable rooms shall have a floor area of not less than 70 square feet (6.5 m²).

Exception: Kitchens.

R304.3 Minimum dimensions. Habitable rooms shall not be less than 7 feet (2134 mm) in any horizontal dimension.

Exception: Kitchens.

R304.4 Height effect on room area. Portions of a room with a sloping ceiling measuring less than 5 feet (1524 mm) or a furred ceiling measuring less than 7 feet (2134 mm) from the finished floor to the finished ceiling shall not be considered as contributing to the minimum required habitable area for that room.

SECTION R305
CEILING HEIGHT

R305.1 Minimum height. *Habitable space*, hallways, bathrooms, toilet rooms, laundry rooms and portions of *basements* containing these spaces shall have a ceiling height of not less than 7 feet (2134 mm).

Exceptions:

1. For rooms with sloped ceilings, at least 50 percent of the required floor area of the room must have a ceiling height of at least 7 feet (2134 mm) and no portion of the required floor area may have a ceiling height of less than 5 feet (1524 mm).

2. Bathrooms shall have a minimum ceiling height of 6 feet 8 inches (2032 mm) at the center of the front clearance area for fixtures as shown in Figure R307.1. The ceiling height above fixtures shall be such that the fixture is capable of being used for its intended purpose. A shower or tub equipped with a showerhead shall have a minimum ceiling height of 6 feet 8 inches (2032 mm) above a minimum area 30 inches (762 mm) by 30 inches (762 mm) at the showerhead.

R305.1.1 Basements. Portions of *basements* that do not contain *habitable space*, hallways, bathrooms, toilet rooms and laundry rooms shall have a ceiling height of not less than 6 feet 8 inches (2032 mm).

Exception: Beams, girders, ducts or other obstructions may project to within 6 feet 4 inches (1931 mm) of the finished floor.

SECTION R306
SANITATION

R306.1 Toilet facilities. Every *dwelling* unit shall be provided with a water closet, lavatory, and a bathtub or shower.

R306.2 Kitchen. Each *dwelling* unit shall be provided with a kitchen area and every kitchen area shall be provided with a sink.

R306.3 Sewage disposal. All plumbing fixtures shall be connected to a sanitary sewer or to an *approved* private sewage disposal system.

R306.4 Water supply to fixtures. All plumbing fixtures shall be connected to an *approved* water supply. Kitchen sinks, lavatories, bathtubs, showers, bidets, laundry tubs and washing machine outlets shall be provided with hot and cold water.

SECTION R307
TOILET, BATH AND SHOWER SPACES

R307.1 Space required. Fixtures shall be spaced in accordance with Figure R307.1, and in accordance with the requirements of Section P2705.1.

R307.2 Bathtub and shower spaces. Bathtub and shower floors and walls above bathtubs with installed shower heads and in shower compartments shall be finished with a nonabsorbent surface. Such wall surfaces shall extend to a height of not less than 6 feet (1829 mm) above the floor.

SECTION R308
GLAZING

R308.1 Identification. Except as indicated in Section R308.1.1 each pane of glazing installed in hazardous locations as defined in Section R308.4 shall be provided with a manufacturer's designation specifying who applied the designation, designating the type of glass and the safety glazing standard with which it complies, which is visible in the final installation. The designation shall be acid etched, sandblasted, ceramic-fired, laser etched, embossed, or be of a type which once applied cannot be removed without being destroyed. A *label* shall be permitted in lieu of the manufacturer's designation.

Exceptions:

1. For other than tempered glass, manufacturer's designations are not required provided the *building official*

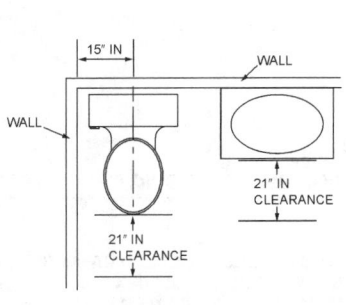
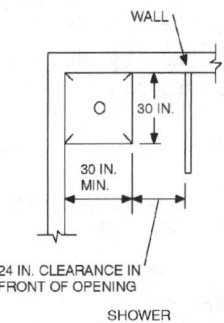
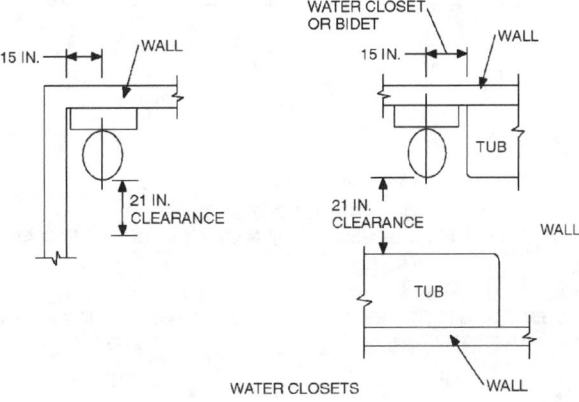

For SI: 1 inch = 25.4 mm.

**FIGURE R307.1
MINIMUM FIXTURE CLEARANCES**

approves the use of a certificate, affidavit or other evidence confirming compliance with this code.

2. Tempered spandrel glass is permitted to be identified by the manufacturer with a removable paper designation.

R308.1.1 Identification of multiple assemblies. Multipane assemblies having individual panes not exceeding 1 square foot (0.09 m²) in exposed area shall have at least one pane in the assembly identified in accordance with Section R308.1. All other panes in the assembly shall be *labeled* "CPSC 16 CFR 1201" or "ANSI Z97.1" as appropriate.

R308.2 Louvered windows or jalousies. Regular, float, wired or patterned glass in jalousies and louvered windows shall be no thinner than nominal $^{3}/_{16}$ inch (5 mm) and no longer than 48 inches (1219 mm). Exposed glass edges shall be smooth.

R308.2.1 Wired glass prohibited. Wired glass with wire exposed on longitudinal edges shall not be used in jalousies or louvered windows.

R308.3 Human impact loads. Individual glazed areas, including glass mirrors in hazardous locations such as those indicated as defined in Section R308.4, shall pass the test requirements of Section R308.3.1.

Exceptions:

1. Louvered windows and jalousies shall comply with Section R308.2.

2. Mirrors and other glass panels mounted or hung on a surface that provides a continuous backing support.

3. Glass unit masonry complying with Section R610.

R308.3.1 Impact test. Where required by other sections of the code, glazing shall be tested in accordance with CPSC 16 CFR 1201. Glazing shall comply with the test criteria for Category I or II as indicated in Table R308.3.1(1).

Exception: Glazing not in doors or enclosures for hot tubs, whirlpools, saunas, steam rooms, bathtubs and showers shall be permitted to be tested in accordance with ANSI Z97.1. Glazing shall comply with the test criteria for Class A or B as indicated in Table R308.3.1 (2).

R308.4 Hazardous locations. The following shall be considered specific hazardous locations for the purposes of glazing:

1. Glazing in all fixed and operable panels of swinging, sliding and bifold doors.

   Exceptions:

   1. Glazed openings of a size through which a 3-inch diameter (76 mm) sphere is unable to pass.

   2. Decorative glazing.

2. Glazing in an individual fixed or operable panel adjacent to a door where the nearest vertical edge is within a 24-inch (610 mm) arc of the door in a closed position and whose bottom edge is less than 60 inches (1524 mm) above the floor or walking surface.

   Exceptions:

   1. Decorative glazing.

   2. When there is an intervening wall or other permanent barrier between the door and the glazing.

   3. Glazing in walls on the latch side of and perpendicular to the plane of the door in a closed position.

TABLE R308.3.1(1)
MINIMUM CATEGORY CLASSIFICATION OF GLAZING USING CPSC 16 CFR 1201

EXPOSED SURFACE AREA OF ONE SIDE OF ONE LITE	GLAZING IN STORM OR COMBINATION DOORS (Category Class)	GLAZING IN DOORS (Category Class)	GLAZED PANELS REGULATED BY ITEM 7 OF SECTION R308.4 (Category Class)	GLAZED PANELS REGULATED BY ITEM 6 OF SECTION R308.4 (Category Class)	GLAZING IN DOORS AND ENCLOSURES REGULATED BY ITEM 5 OF SECTION R308.4 (Category Class)	SLIDING GLASS DOORS PATIO TYPE (Category Class)
9 square feet or less	I	I	NR	I	II	II
More than 9 square feet	II	II	II	II	II	II

For SI: 1 square foot = 0.0929 m².
NR means "No Requirement."

TABLE R308.3.1(2)
MINIMUM CATEGORY CLASSIFICATION OF GLAZING USING ANSI Z97.1

EXPOSED SURFACE AREA OF ONE SIDE OF ONE LITE	GLAZED PANELS REGULATED BY ITEM 7 OF SECTION R308.4 (Category Class)	GLAZED PANELS REGULATED BY ITEM 6 OF SECTION R308.4 (Category Class)	DOORS AND ENCLOSURES REGULATED BY ITEM 5 OF SECTION R308.4[a] (Category Class)
9 square feet or less	No requirement	B	A
More than 9 square feet	A	A	A

For SI: 1 square foot = 0.0929 m².
a. Use is permitted only by the exception to Section R308.3.1.

4. Glazing adjacent to a door where access through the door is to a closet or storage area 3 feet (914 mm) or less in depth.

5. Glazing that is adjacent to the fixed panel of patio doors.

3. Glazing in an individual fixed or operable panel that meets all of the following conditions:

3.1. The exposed area of an individual pane is larger than 9 square feet (0.836 m^2); and

3.2. The bottom edge of the glazing is less than 18 inches (457 mm) above the floor; and

3.3. The top edge of the glazing is more than 36 inches (914 mm) above the floor; and

3.4. One or more walking surfaces are within 36 inches (914 mm), measured horizontally and in a straight line, of the glazing.

Exceptions:

1. Decorative glazing.

2. When a horizontal rail is installed on the accessible side(s) of the glazing 34 to 38 inches (864 to 965) above the walking surface. The rail shall be capable of withstanding a horizontal load of 50 pounds per linear foot (730 N/m) without contacting the glass and be a minimum of $1^1/_2$ inches (38 mm) in cross sectional height.

3. Outboard panes in insulating glass units and other multiple glazed panels when the bottom edge of the glass is 25 feet (7620 mm) or more above *grade*, a roof, walking surfaces or other horizontal [within 45 degrees (0.79 rad) of horizontal] surface adjacent to the glass exterior.

4. All glazing in railings regardless of area or height above a walking surface. Included are structural baluster panels and nonstructural infill panels.

5. Glazing in enclosures for or walls facing hot tubs, whirlpools, saunas, steam rooms, bathtubs and showers where the bottom exposed edge of the glazing is less than 60 inches (1524 mm) measured vertically above any standing or walking surface.

Exception: Glazing that is more than 60 inches (1524 mm), measured horizontally and in a straight line, from the waters edge of a hot tub, whirlpool or bathtub.

6. Glazing in walls and fences adjacent to indoor and outdoor swimming pools, hot tubs and spas where the bottom edge of the glazing is less than 60 inches (1524 mm) above a walking surface and within 60 inches (1524 mm), measured horizontally and in a straight line, of the water's edge. This shall apply to single glazing and all panes in multiple glazing.

7. Glazing adjacent to stairways, landings and ramps within 36 inches (914 mm) horizontally of a walking sur-

face when the exposed surface of the glazing is less than 60 inches (1524 mm) above the plane of the adjacent walking surface.

Exceptions:

1. When a rail is installed on the accessible side(s) of the glazing 34 to 38 inches (864 to 965 mm) above the walking surface. The rail shall be capable of withstanding a horizontal load of 50 pounds per linear foot (730 N/m) without contacting the glass and be a minimum of $1^1/_2$ inches (38 mm) in cross sectional height.

2. The side of the stairway has a guardrail or handrail, including balusters or in-fill panels, complying with Sections R311.7.6 and R312 and the plane of the glazing is more than 18 inches (457 mm) from the railing; or

3. When a solid wall or panel extends from the plane of the adjacent walking surface to 34 inches (863 mm) to 36 inches (914 mm) above the walking surface and the construction at the top of that wall or panel is capable of withstanding the same horizontal load as a *guard*.

8. Glazing adjacent to stairways within 60 inches (1524 mm) horizontally of the bottom tread of a stairway in any direction when the exposed surface of the glazing is less than 60 inches (1524 mm) above the nose of the tread.

Exceptions:

1. The side of the stairway has a guardrail or handrail, including balusters or in-fill panels, complying with Sections R311.7.6 and R312 and the plane of the glass is more than 18 inches (457 mm) from the railing; or

2. When a solid wall or panel extends from the plane of the adjacent walking surface to 34 inches (864 mm) to 36 inches (914 mm) above the walking surface and the construction at the top of that wall or panel is capable of withstanding the same horizontal load as a *guard*.

R308.5 Site built windows. Site built windows shall comply with Section 2404 of the *International Building Code*.

R308.6 Skylights and sloped glazing. Skylights and sloped glazing shall comply with the following sections.

R308.6.1 Definitions.

SKYLIGHTS AND SLOPED GLAZING. Glass or other transparent or translucent glazing material installed at a slope of 15 degrees (0.26 rad) or more from vertical. Glazing materials in skylights, including unit skylights, solariums, sunrooms, roofs and sloped walls are included in this definition.

UNIT SKYLIGHT. A factory assembled, glazed fenestration unit, containing one panel of glazing material, that allows for natural daylighting through an opening in the roof assembly while preserving the weather-resistant barrier of the roof.

R308.6.2 Permitted materials. The following types of glazing may be used:

1. Laminated glass with a minimum 0.015-inch (0.38 mm) polyvinyl butyral interlayer for glass panes 16 square feet (1.5 m²) or less in area located such that the highest point of the glass is not more than 12 feet (3658 mm) above a walking surface or other accessible area; for higher or larger sizes, the minimum interlayer thickness shall be 0.030 inch (0.76 mm).

2. Fully tempered glass.

3. Heat-strengthened glass.

4. Wired glass.

5. *Approved* rigid plastics.

R308.6.3 Screens, general. For fully tempered or heat-strengthened glass, a retaining screen meeting the requirements of Section R308.6.7 shall be installed below the glass, except for fully tempered glass that meets either condition listed in Section R308.6.5.

R308.6.4 Screens with multiple glazing. When the inboard pane is fully tempered, heat-strengthened or wired glass, a retaining screen meeting the requirements of Section R308.6.7 shall be installed below the glass, except for either condition listed in Section R308.6.5. All other panes in the multiple glazing may be of any type listed in Section R308.6.2.

R308.6.5 Screens not required. Screens shall not be required when fully tempered glass is used as single glazing or the inboard pane in multiple glazing and either of the following conditions are met:

1. Glass area 16 square feet (1.49 m²) or less. Highest point of glass not more than 12 feet (3658 mm) above a walking surface or other accessible area, nominal glass thickness not more than $^3/_{16}$ inch (4.8 mm), and (for multiple glazing only) the other pane or panes fully tempered, laminated or wired glass.

2. Glass area greater than 16 square feet (1.49 m²). Glass sloped 30 degrees (0.52 rad) or less from vertical, and highest point of glass not more than 10 feet (3048 mm) above a walking surface or other accessible area.

R308.6.6 Glass in greenhouses. Any glazing material is permitted to be installed without screening in the sloped areas of greenhouses, provided the greenhouse height at the ridge does not exceed 20 feet (6096 mm) above *grade*.

R308.6.7 Screen characteristics. The screen and its fastenings shall be capable of supporting twice the weight of the glazing, be firmly and substantially fastened to the framing members, and have a mesh opening of no more than 1 inch by 1 inch (25 mm by 25 mm).

R308.6.8 Curbs for skylights. All unit skylights installed in a roof with a pitch flatter than three units vertical in 12 units horizontal (25-percent slope) shall be mounted on a curb extending at least 4 inches (102 mm) above the plane of the roof unless otherwise specified in the manufacturer's installation instructions.

R308.6.9 Testing and labeling. Unit skylights shall be tested by an *approved* independent laboratory, and bear a *label* identifying manufacturer, performance *grade* rating and *approved* inspection agency to indicate compliance with the requirements of AAMA/WDMA/CSA 101/I.S.2/A440.

SECTION R309
GARAGES AND CARPORTS

R309.1 Floor surface. Garage floor surfaces shall be of *approved* noncombustible material.

The area of floor used for parking of automobiles or other vehicles shall be sloped to facilitate the movement of liquids to a drain or toward the main vehicle entry doorway.

R309.2 Carports. Carports shall be open on at least two sides. Carport floor surfaces shall be of *approved* noncombustible material. Carports not open on at least two sides shall be considered a garage and shall comply with the provisions of this section for garages.

Exception: Asphalt surfaces shall be permitted at ground level in carports.

The area of floor used for parking of automobiles or other vehicles shall be sloped to facilitate the movement of liquids to a drain or toward the main vehicle entry doorway.

R309.3 Flood hazard areas. For buildings located in flood hazard areas as established by Table R301.2(1), garage floors shall be:

1. Elevated to or above the design flood elevation as determined in Section R322; or

2. Located below the design flood elevation provided they are at or above *grade* on at least one side, are used solely for parking, building access or storage, meet the requirements of Section R322 and are otherwise constructed in accordance with this code.

R309.4 Automatic garage door openers. Automatic garage door openers, if provided, shall be listed in accordance with UL 325.

SECTION R310
EMERGENCY ESCAPE AND RESCUE OPENINGS

R310.1 Emergency escape and rescue required. *Basements,* habitable attics and every sleeping room shall have at least one operable emergency escape and rescue opening. Where *basements* contain one or more sleeping rooms, emergency egress and rescue openings shall be required in each sleeping room. Where emergency escape and rescue openings are provided they shall have a sill height of not more than 44 inches (1118 mm) above the floor. Where a door opening having a threshold below the adjacent ground elevation serves as an emergency escape and rescue opening and is provided with a bulkhead enclosure, the bulkhead enclosure shall comply with Section R310.3. The net clear opening dimensions required by this section shall be obtained by the normal operation of the emergency escape and rescue opening from the inside. Emergency escape and rescue openings with a finished sill height below the adjacent ground elevation shall be provided with a window well in accordance with Section R310.2. Emergency escape and rescue openings shall open directly into a public way, or to a *yard* or court that opens to a public way.

Exception: *Basements* used only to house mechanical *equipment* and not exceeding total floor area of 200 square feet (18.58 m²).

R310.1.1 Minimum opening area. All emergency escape and rescue openings shall have a minimum net clear opening of 5.7 square feet (0.530 m²).

Exception: *Grade* floor openings shall have a minimum net clear opening of 5 square feet (0.465 m²).

R310.1.2 Minimum opening height. The minimum net clear opening height shall be 24 inches (610 mm).

R310.1.3 Minimum opening width. The minimum net clear opening width shall be 20 inches (508 mm).

R310.1.4 Operational constraints. Emergency escape and rescue openings shall be operational from the inside of the room without the use of keys, tools or special knowledge.

R310.2 Window wells. The minimum horizontal area of the window well shall be 9 square feet (0.9 m²), with a minimum horizontal projection and width of 36 inches (914 mm). The area of the window well shall allow the emergency escape and rescue opening to be fully opened.

Exception: The ladder or steps required by Section R310.2.1 shall be permitted to encroach a maximum of 6 inches (152 mm) into the required dimensions of the window well.

R310.2.1 Ladder and steps. Window wells with a vertical depth greater than 44 inches (1118 mm) shall be equipped with a permanently affixed ladder or steps usable with the window in the fully open position. Ladders or steps required by this section shall not be required to comply with Sections R311.7 and R311.8. Ladders or rungs shall have an inside width of at least 12 inches (305 mm), shall project at least 3 inches (76 mm) from the wall and shall be spaced not more than 18 inches (457 mm) on center vertically for the full height of the window well.

R310.3 Bulkhead enclosures. Bulkhead enclosures shall provide direct access to the *basement*. The bulkhead enclosure with the door panels in the fully open position shall provide the minimum net clear opening required by Section R310.1.1. Bulkhead enclosures shall also comply with Section R311.7.8.2.

R310.4 Bars, grilles, covers and screens. Bars, grilles, covers, screens or similar devices are permitted to be placed over emergency escape and rescue openings, bulkhead enclosures, or window wells that serve such openings, provided the minimum net clear opening size complies with Sections R310.1.1 to R310.1.3, and such devices shall be releasable or removable from the inside without the use of a key, tool, special knowledge or force greater than that which is required for normal operation of the escape and rescue opening.

R310.5 Emergency escape windows under decks and porches. Emergency escape windows are allowed to be installed under decks and porches provided the location of the deck allows the emergency escape window to be fully opened and provides a path not less than 36 inches (914 mm) in height to a *yard* or court.

SECTION R311
MEANS OF EGRESS

R311.1 Means of egress. All *dwellings* shall be provided with a means of egress as provided in this section. The means of egress shall provide a continuous and unobstructed path of vertical and horizontal egress travel from all portions of the *dwelling* to the exterior of the *dwelling* at the required egress door without requiring travel through a garage.

R311.2 Egress door. At least one egress door shall be provided for each *dwelling* unit. The egress door shall be side-hinged, and shall provide a minimum clear width of 32 inches (813 mm) when measured between the face of the door and the stop, with the door open 90 degrees (1.57 rad). The minimum clear height of the door opening shall not be less than 78 inches (1981 mm) in height measured from the top of the threshold to the bottom of the stop. Other doors shall not be required to comply with these minimum dimensions. Egress doors shall be readily openable from inside the *dwelling* without the use of a key or special knowledge or effort.

R311.3 Floors and landings at exterior doors. There shall be a landing or floor on each side of each exterior door. The width of each landing shall not be less than the door served. Every landing shall have a minimum dimension of 36 inches (914 mm) measured in the direction of travel. Exterior landings shall be permitted to have a slope not to exceed ¹/₄ unit vertical in 12 units horizontal (2-percent).

Exception: Exterior balconies less than 60 square feet (5.6 m²) and only accessible from a door are permitted to have a landing less than 36 inches (914 mm) measured in the direction of travel.

R311.3.1 Floor elevations at the required egress doors. Landings or floors at the required egress door shall not be more than 1¹/₂ inches (38 mm) lower than the top of the threshold.

Exception: The exterior landing or floor shall not be more than 7³/₄ inches (196 mm) below the top of the threshold provided the door does not swing over the landing or floor.

When exterior landings or floors serving the required egress door are not at *grade*, they shall be provided with access to *grade* by means of a ramp in accordance with Section R311.8 or a stairway in accordance with Section R311.7.

R311.3.2 Floor elevations for other exterior doors. Doors other than the required egress door shall be provided with landings or floors not more than 7³/₄ inches (196 mm) below the top of the threshold.

Exception: A landing is not required where a stairway of two or fewer risers is located on the exterior side of the door, provided the door does not swing over the stairway.

R311.3.3 Storm and screen doors. Storm and screen doors shall be permitted to swing over all exterior stairs and landings.

R311.4 Vertical egress. Egress from habitable levels including habitable attics and *basements* not provided with an egress door in accordance with Section R311.2 shall be by a ramp in accordance with Section R311.8 or a stairway in accordance with Section R311.7.

R311.5 Construction.

R311.5.1 Attachment. Exterior landings, decks, balconies, stairs and similar facilities shall be positively anchored to the primary structure to resist both vertical and lateral forces or shall be designed to be self-supporting. Attachment shall not be accomplished by use of toenails or nails subject to withdrawal.

R311.6 Hallways. The minimum width of a hallway shall be not less than 3 feet (914 mm).

R311.7 Stairways.

R311.7.1 Width. Stairways shall not be less than 36 inches (914 mm) in clear width at all points above the permitted handrail height and below the required headroom height. Handrails shall not project more than 4.5 inches (114 mm) on either side of the stairway and the minimum clear width of the stairway at and below the handrail height, including treads and landings, shall not be less than 31^1/$_2$ inches (787 mm) where a handrail is installed on one side and 27 inches (698 mm) where handrails are provided on both sides.

Exception: The width of spiral stairways shall be in accordance with Section R311.7.9.1.

R311.7.2 Headroom. The minimum headroom in all parts of the stairway shall not be less than 6 feet 8 inches (2032 mm) measured vertically from the sloped line adjoining the tread nosing or from the floor surface of the landing or platform on that portion of the stairway.

Exception: Where the nosings of treads at the side of a flight extend under the edge of a floor opening through which the stair passes, the floor opening shall be allowed to project horizontally into the required headroom a maximum of 4^3/$_4$ inches (121 mm).

R311.7.3 Walkline. The walkline across winder treads shall be concentric to the curved direction of travel through the turn and located 12 inches (305 mm) from the side where the winders are narrower. The 12-inch (305 mm) dimension shall be measured from the widest point of the clear stair width at the walking surface of the winder. If winders are adjacent within the flight, the point of the widest clear stair width of the adjacent winders shall be used.

R311.7.4 Stair treads and risers. Stair treads and risers shall meet the requirements of this section. For the purposes of this section all dimensions and dimensioned surfaces shall be exclusive of carpets, rugs or runners.

R311.7.4.1 Riser height. The maximum riser height shall be 7^3/$_4$ inches (196 mm). The riser shall be measured vertically between leading edges of the adjacent treads. The greatest riser height within any flight of stairs shall not exceed the smallest by more than ^{3}/$_8$ inch (9.5 mm).

R311.7.4.2 Tread depth. The minimum tread depth shall be 10 inches (254 mm). The tread depth shall be measured horizontally between the vertical planes of the foremost projection of adjacent treads and at a right angle to the tread's leading edge. The greatest tread depth within any flight of stairs shall not exceed the smallest by more than ^{3}/$_8$ inch (9.5 mm). Consistently shaped winders at the walkline shall be allowed within the same flight of stairs as rectangular treads and do not have to be within ^{3}/$_8$ inch (9.5 mm) of the rectangular tread depth.

Winder treads shall have a minimum tread depth of 10 inches (254 mm) measured between the vertical planes of the foremost projection of adjacent treads at the intersections with the walkline. Winder treads shall have a minimum tread depth of 6 inches (152 mm) at any point within the clear width of the stair. Within any flight of stairs, the largest winder tread depth at the walkline shall not exceed the smallest winder tread by more than ^{3}/$_8$ inch (9.5 mm).

R311.7.4.3 Profile. The radius of curvature at the nosing shall be no greater than ^{9}/$_{16}$ inch (14 mm). A nosing not less than ^{3}/$_4$ inch (19 mm) but not more than 1^1/$_4$ inches (32 mm) shall be provided on stairways with solid risers. The greatest nosing projection shall not exceed the smallest nosing projection by more than ^{3}/$_8$ inch (9.5 mm) between two stories, including the nosing at the level of floors and landings. Beveling of nosings shall not exceed ^{1}/$_2$ inch (12.7 mm). Risers shall be vertical or sloped under the tread above from the underside of the nosing above at an angle not more than 30 degrees (0.51 rad) from the vertical. Open risers are permitted, provided that the opening between treads does not permit the passage of a 4-inch diameter (102 mm) sphere.

Exceptions:

1. A nosing is not required where the tread depth is a minimum of 11 inches (279 mm).

2. The opening between adjacent treads is not limited on stairs with a total rise of 30 inches (762 mm) or less.

R311.7.4.4 Exterior wood/plastic composite stair treads. Wood/plastic composite stair treads shall comply with the provisions of Section R317.4.

R311.7.5 Landings for stairways. There shall be a floor or landing at the top and bottom of each stairway.

Exception: A floor or landing is not required at the top of an interior flight of stairs, including stairs in an enclosed garage, provided a door does not swing over the stairs. A flight of stairs shall not have a vertical rise larger than 12 feet (3658 mm) between floor levels or landings. The width of each landing shall not be less than the width of the stairway served. Every landing shall have a minimum dimension of 36 inches (914 mm) measured in the direction of travel.

R311.7.6 Stairway walking surface. The walking surface of treads and landings of stairways shall be sloped no steeper than one unit vertical in 48 inches horizontal (2-percent slope).

R311.7.7 Handrails. Handrails shall be provided on at least one side of each continuous run of treads or flight with four or more risers.

R311.7.7.1 Height. Handrail height, measured vertically from the sloped plane adjoining the tread nosing, or finish surface of ramp slope, shall be not less than 34 inches (864 mm) and not more than 38 inches (965 mm).

Exceptions:

1. The use of a volute, turnout or starting easing shall be allowed over the lowest tread.

2. When handrail fittings or bendings are used to provide continuous transition between flights, the transition from handrail to guardrail, or used at the start of a flight, the handrail height at the fittings or bendings shall be permitted to exceed the maximum height.

R311.7.7.2 Continuity. Handrails for stairways shall be continuous for the full length of the flight, from a point directly above the top riser of the flight to a point directly above the lowest riser of the flight. Handrail ends shall be returned or shall terminate in newel posts or safety terminals. Handrails adjacent to a wall shall have a space of not less than $1^1/_2$ inch (38 mm) between the wall and the handrails.

Exceptions:

1. Handrails shall be permitted to be interrupted by a newel post at the turn.

2. The use of a volute, turnout, starting easing or starting newel shall be allowed over the lowest tread.

R311.7.7.3 Grip-size. All required handrails shall be of one of the following types or provide equivalent graspability.

1. Type I. Handrails with a circular cross section shall have an outside diameter of at least $1^1/_4$ inches (32 mm) and not greater than 2 inches (51 mm). If the handrail is not circular, it shall have a perimeter dimension of at least 4 inches (102 mm) and not greater than $6^1/_4$ inches (160 mm) with a maximum cross section of dimension of $2^1/_4$ inches (57 mm). Edges shall have a minimum radius of 0.01 inch (0.25 mm).

2. Type II. Handrails with a perimeter greater than $6^1/_4$ inches (160 mm) shall have a graspable finger recess area on both sides of the profile. The finger recess shall begin within a distance of $3/_4$ inch (19 mm) measured vertically from the tallest portion of the profile and achieve a depth of at least $5/_{16}$ inch (8 mm) within $7/_8$ inch (22 mm) below the widest portion of the profile. This required depth shall continue for at least $3/_8$ inch (10 mm) to a level that is not less than $1^3/_4$ inches (45 mm) below the tallest portion of the profile. The minimum width of the handrail above the recess shall be $1^1/_4$ inches (32 mm) to a maximum of $2^3/_4$ inches (70 mm). Edges shall have a minimum radius of 0.01 inch (0.25 mm).

R311.7.7.4 Exterior wood/plastic composite handrails. Wood/plastic composite handrails shall comply with the provisions of Section R317.4.

R311.7.8 Illumination. All stairs shall be provided with illumination in accordance with Section R303.6.

R311.7.9 Special stairways. Spiral stairways and bulkhead enclosure stairways shall comply with all requirements of Section R311.7 except as specified below.

R311.7.9.1 Spiral stairways. Spiral stairways are permitted, provided the minimum clear width at and below the handrail shall be 26 inches (660 mm) with each tread having a $7^1/_2$-inch (190 mm) minimum tread depth at 12 inches (914 mm) from the narrower edge. All treads shall be identical, and the rise shall be no more than $9^1/_2$ inches (241 mm). A minimum headroom of 6 feet 6 inches (1982 mm) shall be provided.

R311.7.9.2 Bulkhead enclosure stairways. Stairways serving bulkhead enclosures, not part of the required building egress, providing access from the outside *grade* level to the *basement* shall be exempt from the requirements of Sections R311.3 and R311.7 where the maximum height from the *basement* finished floor level to *grade* adjacent to the stairway does not exceed 8 feet (2438 mm) and the *grade* level opening to the stairway is covered by a bulkhead enclosure with hinged doors or other *approved* means.

R311.8 Ramps.

R311.8.1 Maximum slope. Ramps shall have a maximum slope of 1 unit vertical in 12 units horizontal (8.3 percent slope).

Exception: Where it is technically infeasible to comply because of site constraints, ramps may have a maximum slope of one unit vertical in eight horizontal (12.5 percent slope).

R311.8.2 Landings required. A minimum 3-foot-by-3-foot (914 mm by 914 mm) landing shall be provided:

1. At the top and bottom of ramps.

2. Where doors open onto ramps.

3. Where ramps change direction.

R311.8.3 Handrails required. Handrails shall be provided on at least one side of all ramps exceeding a slope of one unit vertical in 12 units horizontal (8.33-percent slope).

R311.8.3.1 Height. Handrail height, measured above the finished surface of the ramp slope, shall be not less than 34 inches (864 mm) and not more than 38 inches (965 mm).

R311.8.3.2 Grip size. Handrails on ramps shall comply with Section R311.7.7.3.

R311.8.3.3 Continuity. Handrails where required on ramps shall be continuous for the full length of the ramp. Handrail ends shall be returned or shall terminate in newel posts or safety terminals. Handrails adjacent to a wall shall have a space of not less than $1^1/_2$ inches (38 mm) between the wall and the handrails.

SECTION R312
GUARDS

R312.1 Where required. *Guards* shall be located along open-sided walking surfaces, including stairs, ramps and landings, that are located more than 30 inches (762 mm) measured vertically to the floor or *grade* below at any point within 36 inches (914 mm) horizontally to the edge of the open side. Insect screening shall not be considered as a *guard*.

R312.2 Height. Required *guards* at open-sided walking surfaces, including stairs, porches, balconies or landings, shall be not less than 36 inches (914 mm) high measured vertically above the adjacent walking surface, adjacent fixed seating or the line connecting the leading edges of the treads.

Exceptions:

1. *Guards* on the open sides of stairs shall have a height not less than 34 inches (864 mm) measured vertically from a line connecting the leading edges of the treads.

2. Where the top of the *guard* also serves as a handrail on the open sides of stairs, the top of the *guard* shall not be not less than 34 inches (864 mm) and not more than 38 inches (965 mm) measured vertically from a line connecting the leading edges of the treads.

R312.3 Opening limitations. Required *guards* shall not have openings from the walking surface to the required *guard* height which allow passage of a sphere 4 inches (102 mm) in diameter.

Exceptions:

1. The triangular openings at the open side of a stair, formed by the riser, tread and bottom rail of a *guard*, shall not allow passage of a sphere 6 inches (153 mm) in diameter.

2. *Guards* on the open sides of stairs shall not have openings which allow passage of a sphere $4^3/_8$ inches (111 mm) in diameter.

R312.4 Exterior woodplastic composite guards. Woodplastic composite *guards* shall comply with the provisions of Section R317.4.

SECTION R313
AUTOMATIC FIRE SPRINKLER SYSTEMS

R313.1 Townhouse automatic fire sprinkler systems. An automatic residential fire sprinkler system shall be installed in *townhouses*.

Exception: An automatic residential fire sprinkler system shall not be required when *additions* or *alterations* are made to existing *townhouses* that do not have an automatic residential fire sprinkler system installed.

R313.1.1 Design and installation. Automatic residential fire sprinkler systems for *townhouses* shall be designed and installed in accordance with Section P2904.

R313.2 One- and two-family dwellings automatic fire systems. Effective January 1, 2011, an automatic residential fire sprinkler system shall be installed in one- and two- family *dwellings*.

Exception: An automatic residential fire sprinkler system shall not be required for *additions* or *alterations* to existing buildings that are not already provided with an automatic residential sprinkler system.

R313.2.1 Design and installation. Automatic residential fire sprinkler systems shall be designed and installed in accordance with Section P2904 or NFPA 13D.

SECTION R314
SMOKE ALARMS

R314.1 Smoke detection and notification. All smoke alarms shall be listed in accordance with UL 217 and installed in accordance with the provisions of this code and the household fire warning *equipment* provisions of NFPA 72.

R314.2 Smoke detection systems. Household fire alarm systems installed in accordance with NFPA 72 that include smoke alarms, or a combination of smoke detector and audible notification device installed as required by this section for smoke alarms, shall be permitted. The household fire alarm system shall provide the same level of smoke detection and alarm as required by this section for smoke alarms. Where a household fire warning system is installed using a combination of smoke detector and audible notification device(s), it shall become a permanent fixture of the occupancy and owned by the homeowner. The system shall be monitored by an *approved* supervising station and be maintained in accordance with NFPA 72.

Exception: Where smoke alarms are provided meeting the requirements of Section R314.4.

R314.3 Location. Smoke alarms shall be installed in the following locations:

1. In each sleeping room.

2. Outside each separate sleeping area in the immediate vicinity of the bedrooms.

3. On each additional *story* of the *dwelling*, including *basements* and habitable attics but not including crawl spaces and uninhabitable *attics*. In *dwellings* or *dwelling units* with split levels and without an intervening door between the adjacent levels, a smoke alarm installed on the upper level shall suffice for the adjacent lower level provided that the lower level is less than one full *story* below the upper level.

When more than one smoke alarm is required to be installed within an individual *dwelling* unit the alarm devices shall be interconnected in such a manner that the actuation of one alarm will activate all of the alarms in the individual unit.

R314.3.1 Alterations, repairs and additions. When *alterations*, repairs or *additions* requiring a *permit* occur, or when one or more sleeping rooms are added or created in existing *dwellings*, the individual *dwelling unit* shall be equipped with smoke alarms located as required for new *dwellings*.

Exceptions:

1. Work involving the exterior surfaces of *dwellings*, such as the replacement of roofing or siding, or the *addition* or replacement of windows or doors, or

the *addition* of a porch or deck, are exempt from the requirements of this section.

2. Installation, *alteration* or repairs of plumbing or mechanical systems are exempt from the requirements of this section.

R314.4 Power source. Smoke alarms shall receive their primary power from the building wiring when such wiring is served from a commercial source, and when primary power is interrupted, shall receive power from a battery. Wiring shall be permanent and without a disconnecting switch other than those required for overcurrent protection. Smoke alarms shall be interconnected.

Exceptions:

1. Smoke alarms shall be permitted to be battery operated when installed in buildings without commercial power.

2. Interconnection and hard-wiring of smoke alarms in existing areas shall not be required where the *alterations* or repairs do not result in the removal of interior wall or ceiling finishes exposing the structure, unless there is an *attic*, crawl space or *basement* available which could provide access for hard wiring and interconnection without the removal of interior finishes.

SECTION R315
CARBON MONOXIDE ALARMS

R315.1 Carbon monoxide alarms. For new construction, an approved carbon monoxide alarm shall be installed outside of each separate sleeping area in the immediate vicinity of the bedrooms in *dwelling units* within which fuel-fired *appliances* are installed and in dwelling units that have attached garages.

R315.2 Where required in existing dwellings. Where work requiring a *permit* occurs in existing *dwellings* that have attached garages or in existing dwellings within which fuel-fired *appliances* exist, carbon monoxide alarms shall be provided in accordance with Section R315.1.

R315.3 Alarm requirements. Single station carbon monoxide alarms shall be listed as complying with UL 2034 and shall be installed in accordance with this code and the manufacturer's installation instructions.

SECTION R316
FOAM PLASTIC

R316.1 General. The provisions of this section shall govern the materials, design, application, construction and installation of foam plastic materials.

R316.2 Labeling and identification. Packages and containers of foam plastic insulation and foam plastic insulation components delivered to the job site shall bear the *label* of an *approved agency* showing the manufacturer's name, the product listing, product identification and information sufficient to determine that the end use will comply with the requirements.

R316.3 Surface burning characteristics. Unless otherwise allowed in Section R316.5 or R316.6, all foam plastic or foam plastic cores used as a component in manufactured assemblies used in building construction shall have a flame spread index of not more than 75 and shall have a smoke-developed index of not more than 450 when tested in the maximum thickness intended for use in accordance with ASTM E 84 or UL 723. Loose-fill type foam plastic insulation shall be tested as board stock for the flame spread index and smoke-developed index.

Exception: Foam plastic insulation more than 4 inches (102 mm) thick shall have a maximum flame spread index of 75 and a smoke-developed index of 450 where tested at a minimum thickness of 4 inches (102 mm), provided the end use is *approved* in accordance with Section R316.6 using the thickness and density intended for use.

R316.4 Thermal barrier. Unless otherwise allowed in Section R316.5 or Section R316.6, foam plastic shall be separated from the interior of a building by an *approved* thermal barrier of minimum $^1/_2$ inch (12.7 mm) gypsum wallboard or an *approved* finish material equivalent to a thermal barrier material that will limit the average temperature rise of the unexposed surface to no more than 250°F (139°C) after 15 minutes of fire exposure complying with the ASTM E 119 or UL 263 standard time temperature curve. The thermal barrier shall be installed in such a manner that it will remain in place for 15 minutes based on NFPA 286 with the acceptance criteria of Section R302.9.4, FM 4880, UL 1040 or UL 1715.

R316.5 Specific requirements. The following requirements shall apply to these uses of foam plastic unless specifically *approved* in accordance with Section R316.6 or by other sections of the code or the requirements of Sections R316.2 through R316.4 have been met.

R316.5.1 Masonry or concrete construction. The thermal barrier specified in Section R316.4 is not required in a masonry or concrete wall, floor or roof when the foam plastic insulation is separated from the interior of the building by a minimum 1-inch (25 mm) thickness of masonry or concrete.

R316.5.2 Roofing. The thermal barrier specified in Section R316.4 is not required when the foam plastic in a roof assembly or under a roof covering is installed in accordance with the code and the manufacturer's installation instructions and is separated from the interior of the building by tongue-and-groove wood planks or wood structural panel sheathing in accordance with Section R803, not less than $^{15}/_{32}$ inch (11.9 mm) thick bonded with exterior glue and identified as Exposure 1, with edges supported by blocking or tongue-and-groove joints or an equivalent material. The smoke-developed index for roof applications shall not be limited.

R316.5.3 Attics. The thermal barrier specified in Section R316.4 is not required where all of the following apply:

1. *Attic* access is required by Section R807.1.

2. The space is entered only for purposes of repairs or maintenance.

3. The foam plastic insulation is protected against ignition using one of the following ignition barrier materials:

    3.1. $1^1/_2$-inch-thick (38 mm) mineral fiber insulation;

    3.2. $^1/_4$-inch-thick (6.4 mm) wood structural panels;

    3.3. $^3/_8$-inch (9.5 mm) particleboard;

    3.4. $^1/_4$-inch (6.4 mm) hardboard;

    3.5. $^3/_8$-inch (9.5 mm) gypsum board; or

    3.6. Corrosion-resistant steel having a base metal thickness of 0.016 inch (0.406 mm).

The above ignition barrier is not required where the foam plastic insulation has been tested in accordance with Section R316.6.

R316.5.4 Crawl spaces. The thermal barrier specified in Section R316.4 is not required where all of the following apply:

1. Crawlspace access is required by Section R408.4

2. Entry is made only for purposes of repairs or maintenance.

3. The foam plastic insulation is protected against ignition using one of the following ignition barrier materials:

    3.1. $1^1/_2$-inch-thick (38 mm) mineral fiber insulation;

    3.2. $^1/_4$-inch-thick (6.4 mm) wood structural panels;

    3.3. $^3/_8$-inch (9.5 mm) particleboard;

    3.4. $^1/_4$-inch (6.4 mm) hardboard;

    3.5. $^3/_8$-inch (9.5 mm) gypsum board; or

    3.6. Corrosion-resistant steel having a base metal thickness of 0.016 inch (0.406 mm).

The above ignition barrier is not required where the foam plastic insulation has been tested in accordance with Section R316.6.

R316.5.5 Foam-filled exterior doors. Foam-filled exterior doors are exempt from the requirements of Sections R316.3 and R316.4.

R316.5.6 Foam-filled garage doors. Foam-filled garage doors in attached or detached garages are exempt from the requirements of Sections R316.3 and R316.4.

R316.5.7 Foam backer board. The thermal barrier specified in Section R316.4 is not required where siding backer board foam plastic insulation has a maximum thickness of 0.5 inch (12.7 mm) and a potential heat of not more than 2000 Btu per square foot (22 720 kJ/m²) when tested in accordance with NFPA 259 provided that:

1. The foam plastic insulation is separated from the interior of the building by not less than 2 inches (51 mm) of mineral fiber insulation or

2. The foam plastic insulation is installed over existing *exterior wall* finish in conjunction with re-siding or

3. The foam plastic insulation has been tested in accordance with Section R316.6.

R316.5.8 Re-siding. The thermal barrier specified in Section R316.4 is not required where the foam plastic insulation is installed over existing *exterior wall* finish in conjunction with re-siding provided the foam plastic has a maximum thickness of 0.5 inch (12.7 mm) and a potential heat of not more than 2000 Btu per square foot (22 720 kJ/m²) when tested in accordance with NFPA 259.

R316.5.9 Interior trim. The thermal barrier specified in Section R316.4 is not required for exposed foam plastic interior trim, provided all of the following are met:

1. The minimum density is 20 pounds per cubic foot (320 kg/m³).

2. The maximum thickness of the trim is 0.5 inch (12.7 mm) and the maximum width is 8 inches (204 mm).

3. The interior trim shall not constitute more than 10 percent of the aggregate wall and ceiling area of any room or space.

4. The flame spread index does not exceed 75 when tested per ASTM E 84. The smoke-developed index is not limited.

R316.5.10 Interior finish. Foam plastics shall be permitted as interior finish where *approved* in accordance with Section R316.6 Foam plastics that are used as interior finish shall also meet the flame spread index and smoke-developed index requirements of Sections R302.9.1 and R302.9.2.

R316.5.11 Sill plates and headers. Foam plastic shall be permitted to be spray applied to a sill plate and header without the thermal barrier specified in Section R316.4 subject to all of the following:

1. The maximum thickness of the foam plastic shall be $3^1/_4$ inches (83 mm).

2. The density of the foam plastic shall be in the range of 0.5 to 2.0 pounds per cubic foot (8 to 32 kg/m³).

3. The foam plastic shall have a flame spread index of 25 or less and an accompanying smoke developed index of 450 or less when tested in accordance with ASTM E 84.

R316.5.12 Sheathing. Foam plastic insulation used as sheathing shall comply with Section R316.3 and Section R316.4. Where the foam plastic sheathing is exposed to the *attic* space at a gable or kneewall, the provisions of Section R316.5.3 shall apply.

R316.6 Specific approval. Foam plastic not meeting the requirements of Sections R316.3 through R316.5 shall be specifically *approved* on the basis of one of the following *approved* tests: NFPA 286 with the acceptance criteria of Section R302.9.4, FM4880, UL 723, UL 1040 or UL 1715, or fire tests related to actual end-use configurations. The specific approval shall be based on the actual end use configuration and shall be performed on the finished foam plastic assembly in the maximum thickness intended for use. Assemblies tested shall include seams, joints and other typical details used in the installation of the assembly and shall be tested in the manner intended for use.

R316.7 Termite damage. The use of foam plastics in areas of "very heavy" termite infestation probability shall be in accordance with Section R318.4.

SECTION R317
PROTECTION OF WOOD AND WOOD BASED PRODUCTS AGAINST DECAY

R317.1 Location required. Protection of wood and wood based products from decay shall be provided in the following locations by the use of naturally durable wood or wood that is preservative-treated in accordance with AWPA U1 for the species, product, preservative and end use. Preservatives shall be listed in Section 4 of AWPA U1.

1. Wood joists or the bottom of a wood structural floor when closer than 18 inches (457 mm) or wood girders when closer than 12 inches (305 mm) to the exposed ground in crawl spaces or unexcavated area located within the periphery of the building foundation.

2. All wood framing members that rest on concrete or masonry exterior foundation walls and are less than 8 inches (203 mm) from the exposed ground.

3. Sills and sleepers on a concrete or masonry slab that is in direct contact with the ground unless separated from such slab by an impervious moisture barrier.

4. The ends of wood girders entering exterior masonry or concrete walls having clearances of less than $^1/_2$ inch (12.7 mm) on tops, sides and ends.

5. Wood siding, sheathing and wall framing on the exterior of a building having a clearance of less than 6 inches (152 mm) from the ground or less than 2 inches (51 mm) measured vertically from concrete steps, porch slabs, patio slabs, and similar horizontal surfaces exposed to the weather.

6. Wood structural members supporting moisture-permeable floors or roofs that are exposed to the weather, such as concrete or masonry slabs, unless separated from such floors or roofs by an impervious moisture barrier.

7. Wood furring strips or other wood framing members attached directly to the interior of exterior masonry walls or concrete walls below *grade* except where an *approved* vapor retarder is applied between the wall and the furring strips or framing members.

R317.1.1 Field treatment. Field-cut ends, notches and drilled holes of preservative-treated wood shall be treated in the field in accordance with AWPA M4.

R317.1.2 Ground contact. All wood in contact with the ground, embedded in concrete in direct contact with the ground or embedded in concrete exposed to the weather that supports permanent structures intended for human occupancy shall be *approved* pressure-preservative-treated wood suitable for ground contact use, except untreated

wood may be used where entirely below groundwater level or continuously submerged in fresh water.

R317.1.3 Geographical areas. In geographical areas where experience has demonstrated a specific need, *approved* naturally durable or pressure-preservative-treated wood shall be used for those portions of wood members that form the structural supports of buildings, balconies, porches or similar permanent building appurtenances when those members are exposed to the weather without adequate protection from a roof, eave, overhang or other covering that would prevent moisture or water accumulation on the surface or at joints between members. Depending on local experience, such members may include:

1. Horizontal members such as girders, joists and decking.
2. Vertical members such as posts, poles and columns.
3. Both horizontal and vertical members.

R317.1.4 Wood columns. Wood columns shall be *approved* wood of natural decay resistance or *approved* pressure-preservative-treated wood.

Exceptions:

1. Columns exposed to the weather or in *basements* when supported by concrete piers or metal pedestals projecting 1 inch (25.4 mm) above a concrete floor or 6 inches (152 mm) above exposed earth and the earth is covered by an *approved* impervious moisture barrier.

2. Columns in enclosed crawl spaces or unexcavated areas located within the periphery of the building when supported by a concrete pier or metal pedestal at a height more than 8 inches (203mm) from exposed earth and the earth is covered by an impervious moisture barrier.

R317.1.5 Exposed glued-laminated timbers. The portions of glued-laminated timbers that form the structural supports of a building or other structure and are exposed to weather and not properly protected by a roof, eave or similar covering shall be pressure treated with preservative, or be manufactured from naturally durable or preservative-treated wood.

R317.2 Quality mark. Lumber and plywood required to be pressure-preservative-treated in accordance with Section R318.1 shall bear the quality *mark* of an *approved* inspection agency that maintains continuing supervision, testing and inspection over the quality of the product and that has been *approved* by an accreditation body that complies with the requirements of the American Lumber Standard Committee treated wood program.

R317.2.1 Required information. The required quality *mark* on each piece of pressure-preservative-treated lumber or plywood shall contain the following information:

1. Identification of the treating plant.
2. Type of preservative.
3. The minimum preservative retention.
4. End use for which the product was treated.
5. Standard to which the product was treated.

6. Identity of the *approved* inspection agency.

7. The designation "Dry," if applicable.

> **Exception:** Quality *mark*s on lumber less than 1 inch (25.4 mm) nominal thickness, or lumber less than nominal 1 inch by 5 inches (25.4 mm by 127 mm) or 2 inches by 4 inches (51 mm by 102 mm) or lumber 36 inches (914 mm) or less in length shall be applied by stamping the faces of exterior pieces or by end labeling not less than 25 percent of the pieces of a bundled unit.

R317.3 Fasteners and connectors in contact with preservative-treated and fire-retardant-treated wood. Fasteners and connectors in contact with preservative-treated wood and fire-retardant-treated wood shall be in accordance with this section. The coating weights for zinc-coated fasteners shall be in accordance with ASTM A 153.

R317.3.1 Fasteners for preservative-treated wood. Fasteners for preservative-treated wood shall be of hot dipped zinc-coated galvanized steel, stainless steel, silicon bronze or copper. Coating types and weights for connectors in contact with preservative-treated wood shall be in accordance with the connector manufacturer's recommendations. In the absence of manufacturer's recommendations, a minimum of ASTM A 653 type G185 zinc-coated galvanized steel, or equivalent, shall be used.

Exceptions:

1. One-half-inch (12.7 mm) diameter or greater steel bolts.

2. Fasteners other than nails and timber rivets shall be permitted to be of mechanically deposited zinc coated steel with coating weights in accordance with ASTM B 695, Class 55 minimum.

R317.3.2 Fastenings for wood foundations. Fastenings for wood foundations shall be as required in AF&PA Technical Report No. 7.

R317.3.3 Fasteners for fire-retardant-treated wood used in exterior applications or wet or damp locations. Fasteners for fire-retardant-treated wood used in exterior applications or wet or damp locations shall be of hot-dipped zinc-coated galvanized steel, stainless steel, silicon bronze or copper. Fasteners other than nails and timber rivets shall be permitted to be of mechanically deposited zinc-coated steel with coating weights in accordance with ASTM B 695, Class 55 minimum.

R317.3.4 Fasteners for fire-retardant-treated wood used in interior applications. Fasteners for fire-retardant-treated wood used in interior locations shall be in accordance with the manufacturer's recommendations. In the absence of manufacturer's recommendations, Section R317.3.3 shall apply.

R317.4 Wood/plastic composites. Wood/plastic composites used in exterior deck boards, stair treads, handrails and guardrail systems shall bear a *label* indicating the required performance levels and demonstrating compliance with the provisions of ASTM D 7032.

R317.4.1 Wood/plastic composites shall be installed in accordance with the manufacturer's instructions.

SECTION R318
PROTECTION AGAINST
SUBTERRANEAN TERMITES

R318.1 Subterranean termite control methods. In areas subject to damage from termites as indicated by Table R301.2(1), methods of protection shall be one of the following methods or a combination of these methods:

1. Chemical termiticide treatment, as provided in Section R318.2.

2. Termite baiting system installed and maintained according to the *label*.

3. Pressure-preservative-treated wood in accordance with the provisions of Section R317.1.

4. Naturally durable termite-resistant wood.

5. Physical barriers as provided in Section R318.3 and used in locations as specified in Section R318.1.

6. Cold-formed steel framing in accordance with Sections R505.2.1 and R603.2.1.

R318.1.1 Quality mark. Lumber and plywood required to be pressure-preservative-treated in accordance with Section R318.1 shall bear the quality *mark* of an *approved* inspection agency which maintains continuing supervision, testing and inspection over the quality of the product and which has been *approved* by an accreditation body which complies with the requirements of the American Lumber Standard Committee treated wood program.

R318.1.2 Field treatment. Field-cut ends, notches, and drilled holes of pressure-preservative-treated wood shall be retreated in the field in accordance with AWPA M4.

R318.2 Chemical termiticide treatment. Chemical termiticide treatment shall include soil treatment and/or field applied wood treatment. The concentration, rate of application and method of treatment of the chemical termiticide shall be in strict accordance with the termiticide *label*.

R318.3 Barriers. *Approved* physical barriers, such as metal or plastic sheeting or collars specifically designed for termite prevention, shall be installed in a manner to prevent termites from entering the structure. Shields placed on top of an exterior foundation wall are permitted to be used only if in combination with another method of protection.

R318.4 Foam plastic protection. In areas where the probability of termite infestation is "very heavy" as indicated in Figure R301.2(6), extruded and expanded polystyrene, polyisocyanurate and other foam plastics shall not be installed on the exterior face or under interior or exterior foundation walls or slab foundations located below *grade*. The clearance between foam plastics installed above *grade* and exposed earth shall be at least 6 inches (152 mm).

Exceptions:

1. Buildings where the structural members of walls, floors, ceilings and roofs are entirely of noncom-

bustible materials or pressure-preservative-treated wood.

2. When in *addition* to the requirements of Section R318.1, an *approved* method of protecting the foam plastic and structure from subterranean termite damage is used.

3. On the interior side of *basement walls*.

SECTION R319
SITE ADDRESS

R319.1 Address numbers. Buildings shall have *approved* address numbers, building numbers or *approved* building identification placed in a position that is plainly legible and visible from the street or road fronting the property. These numbers shall contrast with their background. Address numbers shall be Arabic numbers or alphabetical letters. Numbers shall be a minimum of 4 inches (102 mm) high with a minimum stroke width of $^1/_2$ inch (12.7 mm). Where access is by means of a private road and the building address cannot be viewed from the public way, a monument, pole or other sign or means shall be used to identify the structure.

SECTION R320
ACCESSIBILITY

R320.1 Scope. Where there are four or more *dwelling* units or sleeping units in a single structure, the provisions of Chapter 11 of the *International Building Code* for Group R-3 shall apply.

SECTION R321
ELEVATORS AND PLATFORM LIFTS

R321.1 Elevators. Where provided, passenger elevators, limited-use/limited-application elevators or private residence elevators shall comply with ASME A17.1.

R321.2 Platform lifts. Where provided, platform lifts shall comply with ASME A18.1.

R321.3 Accessibility. Elevators or platform lifts that are part of an accessible route required by Chapter 11 of the *International Building Code*, shall comply with ICC A117.1.

SECTION R322
FLOOD-RESISTANT CONSTRUCTION

R322.1 General. Buildings and structures constructed in whole or in part in flood hazard areas (including A or V Zones) as established in Table R301.2(1) shall be designed and constructed in accordance with the provisions contained in this section.

> **Exception:** Buildings and structures located in whole or in part in identified floodways shall be designed and constructed in accordance with ASCE 24.

R322.1.1 Alternative provisions. As an alternative to the requirements in Section R322.3 for buildings and structures located in whole or in part in coastal high-hazard areas (V

Zones), ASCE 24 is permitted subject to the limitations of this code and the limitations therein.

R322.1.2 Structural systems. All structural systems of all buildings and structures shall be designed, connected and anchored to resist flotation, collapse or permanent lateral movement due to structural loads and stresses from flooding equal to the design flood elevation.

R322.1.3 Flood-resistant construction. All buildings and structures erected in areas prone to flooding shall be constructed by methods and practices that minimize flood damage.

R322.1.4 Establishing the design flood elevation. The design flood elevation shall be used to define areas prone to flooding. At a minimum, the design flood elevation is the higher of:

1. The base flood elevation at the depth of peak elevation of flooding (including wave height) which has a 1 percent (100-year flood) or greater chance of being equaled or exceeded in any given year, or

2. The elevation of the design flood associated with the area designated on a flood hazard map adopted by the community, or otherwise legally designated.

R322.1.4.1 Determination of design flood elevations. If design flood elevations are not specified, the *building official* is authorized to require the applicant to:

1. Obtain and reasonably use data available from a federal, state or other source; or

2. Determine the design flood elevation in accordance with accepted hydrologic and hydraulic engineering practices used to define special flood hazard areas. Determinations shall be undertaken by a registered *design professional* who shall document that the technical methods used reflect currently accepted engineering practice. Studies, analyses and computations shall be submitted in sufficient detail to allow thorough review and approval.

R322.1.4.2 Determination of impacts. In riverine flood hazard areas where design flood elevations are specified but floodways have not been designated, the applicant shall demonstrate that the effect of the proposed buildings and structures on design flood elevations, including fill, when combined with all other existing and anticipated flood hazard area encroachments, will not increase the design flood elevation more than 1 foot (305 mm) at any point within the jurisdiction.

R322.1.5 Lowest floor. The lowest floor shall be the floor of the lowest enclosed area, including *basement*, but excluding any unfinished flood-resistant enclosure that is useable solely for vehicle parking, building access or limited storage provided that such enclosure is not built so as to render the building or structure in violation of this section.

R322.1.6 Protection of mechanical and electrical systems. Electrical systems, *equipment* and components; heating, ventilating, air conditioning; plumbing *appliances* and plumbing fixtures; *duct systems*; and other service *equipment* shall be located at or above the elevation required in Section R322.2 (flood hazard areas including A Zones) or R322.3 (coastal high-hazard areas including V Zones). If replaced as part of a substantial improvement, electrical systems, *equipment* and components; heating, ventilating, air conditioning and plumbing *appliances* and plumbing fixtures; *duct systems*; and other service *equipment* shall meet the requirements of this section. Systems, fixtures, and *equipment* and components shall not be mounted on or penetrate through walls intended to break away under flood loads.

> **Exception:** Locating electrical systems, *equipment* and components; heating, ventilating, air conditioning; plumbing *appliances* and plumbing fixtures; *duct systems*; and other service *equipment* is permitted below the elevation required in Section R322.2 (flood hazard areas including A Zones) or R322.3 (coastal high-hazard areas including V Zones) provided that they are designed and installed to prevent water from entering or accumulating within the components and to resist hydrostatic and hydrodynamic loads and stresses, including the effects of buoyancy, during the occurrence of flooding to the design flood elevation in accordance with ASCE 24. Electrical wiring systems are permitted to be located below the required elevation provided they conform to the provisions of the electrical part of this code for wet locations.

R322.1.7 Protection of water supply and sanitary sewage systems. New and replacement water supply systems shall be designed to minimize or eliminate infiltration of flood waters into the systems in accordance with the plumbing provisions of this code. New and replacement sanitary sewage systems shall be designed to minimize or eliminate infiltration of floodwaters into systems and discharges from systems into floodwaters in accordance with the plumbing provisions of this code and Chapter 3 of the *International Private Sewage Disposal Code*.

R322.1.8 Flood-resistant materials. Building materials used below the elevation required in Section R322.2 (flood hazard areas including A Zones) or R322.3 (coastal high-hazard areas including V Zones) shall comply with the following:

1. All wood, including floor sheathing, shall be pressure-preservative-treated in accordance with AWPA U1 for the species, product, preservative and end use or be the decay-resistant heartwood of redwood, black locust or cedars. Preservatives shall be listed in Section 4 of AWPA U1.

2. Materials and installation methods used for flooring and interior and *exterior walls* and wall coverings shall conform to the provisions of FEMA/FIA-TB-2.

R322.1.9 Manufactured homes. New or replacement *manufactured homes* shall be elevated in accordance with Section R322.2 or Section R322.3 in coastal high-hazard areas (V Zones). The anchor and tie-down requirements of Sections AE604 and AE605 of Appendix E shall apply. The foundation and anchorage of *manufactured homes* to be located in identified floodways shall be designed and constructed in accordance with ASCE 24.

R322.1.10 As-built elevation documentation. A registered *design professional* shall prepare and seal documentation of the elevations specified in Section R322.2 or R322.3.

R322.2 Flood hazard areas (including A Zones). All areas that have been determined to be prone to flooding but not subject to high velocity wave action shall be designated as flood hazard areas. Flood hazard areas that have been delineated as subject to wave heights between $1^1/_2$ feet (457 mm) and 3 feet (914 mm) shall be designated as Coastal A Zones. All building and structures constructed in whole or in part in flood hazard areas shall be designed and constructed in accordance with Sections R322.2.1 through R322.2.3.

R322.2.1 Elevation requirements.

1. Buildings and structures in flood hazard areas not designated as Coastal A Zones shall have the lowest floors elevated to or above the design flood elevation.

2. Buildings and structures in flood hazard areas designated as Coastal A Zones shall have the lowest floors elevated to or above the base flood elevation plus 1 foot (305 mm), or to the design flood elevation, whichever is higher.

3. In areas of shallow flooding (AO Zones), buildings and structures shall have the lowest floor (including *basement*) elevated at least as high above the highest adjacent *grade* as the depth number specified in feet on the FIRM, or at least 2 feet (610 mm) if a depth number is not specified.

4. Basement floors that are below *grade* on all sides shall be elevated to or above the design flood elevation.

Exception: Enclosed areas below the design flood elevation, including *basements* whose floors are not below *grade* on all sides, shall meet the requirements of Section R322.2.2.

R322.2.2 Enclosed area below design flood elevation. Enclosed areas, including crawl spaces, that are below the design flood elevation shall:

1. Be used solely for parking of vehicles, building access or storage.

2. Be provided with flood openings that meet the following criteria:

   2.1. There shall be a minimum of two openings on different sides of each enclosed area; if a building has more than one enclosed area below the design flood elevation, each area shall have openings on exterior walls.

   2.2. The total net area of all openings shall be at least 1 square inch (645 mm^2) for each square foot (0.093 m^2) of enclosed area, or the openings shall be designed and the *construction documents* shall include a statement by a registered *design professional* that the design of the openings will provide for equalization of hydrostatic flood forces on exterior walls by allowing for the automatic entry and exit of floodwaters as specified in Section 2.6.2.2 of ASCE 24.

2.3. The bottom of each opening shall be 1 foot (305 mm) or less above the adjacent ground level.

2.4. Openings shall be not less than 3 inches (76 mm) in any direction in the plane of the wall.

2.5. Any louvers, screens or other opening covers shall allow the automatic flow of floodwaters into and out of the enclosed area.

2.6. Openings installed in doors and windows, that meet requirements 2.1 through 2.5, are acceptable; however, doors and windows without installed openings do not meet the requirements of this section.

R322.2.3 Foundation design and construction. Foundation walls for all buildings and structures erected in flood hazard areas shall meet the requirements of Chapter 4.

Exception: Unless designed in accordance with Section R404:

1. The unsupported height of 6-inch (152 mm) plain masonry walls shall be no more than 3 feet (914 mm).

2. The unsupported height of 8-inch (203 mm) plain masonry walls shall be no more than 4 feet (1219 mm).

3. The unsupported height of 8-inch (203 mm) reinforced masonry walls shall be no more than 8 feet (2438 mm).

For the purpose of this exception, unsupported height is the distance from the finished *grade* of the under-floor space and the top of the wall.

R322.3 Coastal high-hazard areas (including V Zones). Areas that have been determined to be subject to wave heights in excess of 3 feet (914 mm) or subject to high-velocity wave action or wave-induced erosion shall be designated as coastal high-hazard areas. Buildings and structures constructed in whole or in part in coastal high-hazard areas shall be designed and constructed in accordance with Sections R322.3.1 through R322.3.6.

R322.3.1 Location and site preparation.

1. New buildings and buildings that are determined to be substantially improved pursuant to Section R105.3.1.1, shall be located landward of the reach of mean high tide.

2. For any alteration of sand dunes and mangrove stands the *building official* shall require submission of an engineering analysis which demonstrates that the proposed *alteration* will not increase the potential for flood damage.

R322.3.2 Elevation requirements.

1. All buildings and structures erected within coastal high hazard areas shall be elevated so that the lowest portion of all structural members supporting the low-

est floor, with the exception of mat or raft foundations, piling, pile caps, columns, grade beams and bracing, is:

1.1. Located at or above the design flood elevation, if the lowest horizontal structural member is oriented parallel to the direction of wave approach, where parallel shall mean less than or equal to 20 degrees (0.35 rad) from the direction of approach, or

1.2. Located at the base flood elevation plus 1 foot (305 mm), or the design flood elevation, whichever is higher, if the lowest horizontal structural member is oriented perpendicular to the direction of wave approach, where perpendicular shall mean greater than 20 degrees (0.35 rad) from the direction of approach.

2. Basement floors that are below *grade* on all sides are prohibited.

3. The use of fill for structural support is prohibited.

4. Minor grading, and the placement of minor quantities of fill, shall be permitted for landscaping and for drainage purposes under and around buildings and for support of parking slabs, pool decks, patios and walkways.

Exception: Walls and partitions enclosing areas below the design flood elevation shall meet the requirements of Sections R322.3.4 and R322.3.5.

R322.3.3 Foundations. Buildings and structures erected in coastal high-hazard areas shall be supported on pilings or columns and shall be adequately anchored to those pilings or columns. Pilings shall have adequate soil penetrations to resist the combined wave and wind loads (lateral and uplift). Water loading values used shall be those associated with the design flood. Wind loading values shall be those required by this code. Pile embedment shall include consideration of decreased resistance capacity caused by scour of soil strata surrounding the piling. Pile systems design and installation shall be certified in accordance with Section R322.3.6. Mat, raft or other foundations that support columns shall not be permitted where soil investigations that are required in accordance with Section R401.4 indicate that soil material under the mat, raft or other foundation is subject to scour or erosion from wave-velocity flow conditions. Slabs, pools, pool decks and walkways shall be located and constructed to be structurally independent of buildings and structures and their foundations to prevent transfer of flood loads to the buildings and structures during conditions of flooding, scour or erosion from wave-velocity flow conditions, unless the buildings and structures and their foundation are designed to resist the additional flood load.

R322.3.4 Walls below design flood elevation. Walls and partitions are permitted below the elevated floor, provided that such walls and partitions are not part of the structural support of the building or structure and:

1. Electrical, mechanical, and plumbing system components are not to be mounted on or penetrate through

walls that are designed to break away under flood loads; and

2. Are constructed with insect screening or open lattice; or

3. Are designed to break away or collapse without causing collapse, displacement or other structural damage to the elevated portion of the building or supporting foundation system. Such walls, framing and connections shall have a design safe loading resistance of not less than 10 (479 Pa) and no more than 20 pounds per square foot (958 Pa); or

4. Where wind loading values of this code exceed 20 pounds per square foot (958 Pa), the *construction documents* shall include documentation prepared and sealed by a registered *design professional* that:

    4.1. The walls and partitions below the design flood elevation have been designed to collapse from a water load less than that which would occur during the design flood.

    4.2. The elevated portion of the building and supporting foundation system have been designed to withstand the effects of wind and flood loads acting simultaneously on all building components (structural and nonstructural). Water loading values used shall be those associated with the design flood. Wind loading values shall be those required by this code.

R322.3.5 Enclosed areas below design flood elevation. Enclosed areas below the design flood elevation shall be used solely for parking of vehicles, building access or storage.

R322.3.6 Construction documents. The *construction documents* shall include documentation that is prepared and sealed by a registered *design professional* that the design and methods of construction to be used meet the applicable criteria of this section.

SECTION R323
STORM SHELTERS

R323.1 General. This section applies to the construction of storm shelters when constructed as separate detached buildings or when constructed as safe rooms within buildings for the purpose of providing safe refuge from storms that produce high winds, such as tornados and hurricanes. In addition to other applicable requirements in this code, storm shelters shall be constructed in accordance with ICC/NSSA-500.

CHAPTER 4

FOUNDATIONS

SECTION R401
GENERAL

R401.1 Application. The provisions of this chapter shall control the design and construction of the foundation and foundation spaces for all buildings. In addition to the provisions of this chapter, the design and construction of foundations in areas prone to flooding as established by Table R301.2(1) shall meet the provisions of Section R322. Wood foundations shall be designed and installed in accordance with AF&PA PWF.

> **Exception:** The provisions of this chapter shall be permitted to be used for wood foundations only in the following situations:
>
> 1. In buildings that have no more than two floors and a roof.
>
> 2. When interior *basement* and foundation walls are constructed at intervals not exceeding 50 feet (15 240 mm).

Wood foundations in Seismic Design Category D_0, D_1 or D_2 shall be designed in accordance with accepted engineering practice.

R401.2 Requirements. Foundation construction shall be capable of accommodating all loads according to Section R301 and of transmitting the resulting loads to the supporting soil. Fill soils that support footings and foundations shall be designed, installed and tested in accordance with accepted engineering practice. Gravel fill used as footings for wood and precast concrete foundations shall comply with Section R403.

R401.3 Drainage. Surface drainage shall be diverted to a storm sewer conveyance or other *approved* point of collection that does not create a hazard. *Lots* shall be graded to drain surface water away from foundation walls. The *grade* shall fall a minimum of 6 inches (152 mm) within the first 10 feet (3048 mm).

> **Exception:** Where *lot lines*, walls, slopes or other physical barriers prohibit 6 inches (152 mm) of fall within 10 feet (3048 mm), drains or swales shall be constructed to ensure drainage away from the structure. Impervious surfaces within 10 feet (3048 mm) of the building foundation shall be sloped a minimum of 2 percent away from the building.

R401.4 Soil tests. Where quantifiable data created by accepted soil science methodologies indicate expansive, compressible, shifting or other questionable soil characteristics are likely to be present, the *building official* shall determine whether to require a soil test to determine the soil's characteristics at a particular location. This test shall be done by an *approved agency* using an *approved* method.

R401.4.1 Geotechnical evaluation. In lieu of a complete geotechnical evaluation, the load-bearing values in Table R401.4.1 shall be assumed.

TABLE R401.4.1
PRESUMPTIVE LOAD-BEARING VALUES OF
FOUNDATION MATERIALS[a]

CLASS OF MATERIAL	LOAD-BEARING PRESSURE (pounds per square foot)
Crystalline bedrock	12,000
Sedimentary and foliated rock	4,000
Sandy gravel and/or gravel (GW and GP)	3,000
Sand, silty sand, clayey sand, silty gravel and clayey gravel (SW, SP, SM, SC, GM and GC)	2,000
Clay, sandy clay, silty clay, clayey silt, silt and sandy silt (CL, ML, MH and CH)	1,500[b]

For SI: 1 pound per square foot = 0.0479 kPa.

a. When soil tests are required by Section R401.4, the allowable bearing capacities of the soil shall be part of the recommendations.

b. Where the building official determines that in-place soils with an allowable bearing capacity of less than 1,500 psf are likely to be present at the site, the allowable bearing capacity shall be determined by a soils investigation.

R401.4.2 Compressible or shifting soil. Instead of a complete geotechnical evaluation, when top or subsoils are compressible or shifting, they shall be removed to a depth and width sufficient to assure stable moisture content in each active zone and shall not be used as fill or stabilized within each active zone by chemical, dewatering or presaturation.

SECTION R402
MATERIALS

R402.1 Wood foundations. Wood foundation systems shall be designed and installed in accordance with the provisions of this code.

R402.1.1 Fasteners. Fasteners used below *grade* to attach plywood to the exterior side of exterior *basement* or crawlspace wall studs, or fasteners used in knee wall construction, shall be of Type 304 or 316 stainless steel. Fasteners used above *grade* to attach plywood and all lumber-to-lumber fasteners except those used in knee wall construction shall be of Type 304 or 316 stainless steel, silicon bronze, copper, hot-dipped galvanized (zinc coated) steel nails, or hot-tumbled galvanized (zinc coated) steel nails. Electrogalvanized steel nails and galvanized (zinc coated) steel staples shall not be permitted.

R402.1.2 Wood treatment. All lumber and plywood shall be pressure-preservative treated and dried after treatment in accordance with AWPA U1 (Commodity Specification A, Use Category 4B and Section 5.2), and shall bear the *label* of an accredited agency. Where lumber and/or plywood is cut or drilled after treatment, the treated surface shall be field treated with copper naphthenate, the concentration of which shall contain a minimum of 2 percent copper metal, by repeated brushing, dipping or soaking until the wood absorbs no more preservative.

R402.2 Concrete. Concrete shall have a minimum specified compressive strength of f'_c, as shown in Table R402.2. Concrete subject to moderate or severe weathering as indicated in Table R301.2(1) shall be air entrained as specified in Table R402.2. The maximum weight of fly ash, other pozzolans, silica fume, slag or blended cements that is included in concrete mixtures for garage floor slabs and for exterior porches, carport slabs and steps that will be exposed to deicing chemicals shall not exceed the percentages of the total weight of cementitious materials specified in Section 4.2.3 of ACI 318. Materials used to produce concrete and testing thereof shall comply with the applicable standards listed in Chapter 3 of ACI 318 or ACI 332.

R402.3 Precast concrete. Precast concrete foundations shall be designed in accordance with Section R404.5 and shall be installed in accordance with the provisions of this code and the manufacturer's installation instructions.

R402.3.1 Precast concrete foundation materials. Materials used to produce precast concrete foundations shall meet the following requirements.

1. All concrete used in the manufacture of precast concrete foundations shall have a minimum compressive strength of 5,000 psi (34 470 kPa) at 28 days. Concrete exposed to a freezing and thawing environment shall be air entrained with a minimum total air content of 5 percent.

2. Structural reinforcing steel shall meet the requirements of ASTM A 615, A 706 or A 996. The minimum yield strength of reinforcing steel shall be 40,000 psi (Grade 40) (276 MPa). Steel reinforce-

ment for precast concrete foundation walls shall have a minimum concrete cover of $3/4$ inch (19.1 mm).

3. Panel-to-panel connections shall be made with Grade II steel fasteners.

4. The use of nonstructural fibers shall conform to ASTM C 1116.

5. Grout used for bedding precast foundations placed upon concrete footings shall meet ASTM C 1107.

SECTION R403
FOOTINGS

R403.1 General. All exterior walls shall be supported on continuous solid or fully grouted masonry or concrete footings, crushed stone footings, wood foundations, or other *approved* structural systems which shall be of sufficient design to accommodate all loads according to Section R301 and to transmit the resulting loads to the soil within the limitations as determined from the character of the soil. Footings shall be supported on undisturbed natural soils or engineered fill. Concrete footing shall be designed and constructed in accordance with the provisions of Section R403 or in accordance with ACI 332.

R403.1.1 Minimum size. Minimum sizes for concrete and masonry footings shall be as set forth in Table R403.1 and Figure R403.1(1). The footing width, W, shall be based on the load-bearing value of the soil in accordance with Table R401.4.1. Spread footings shall be at least 6 inches (152 mm) in thickness, T. Footing projections, P, shall be at least 2 inches (51 mm) and shall not exceed the thickness of the footing. The size of footings supporting piers and columns shall be based on the tributary load and allowable soil pressure in accordance with Table R401.4.1. Footings for wood foundations shall be in accordance with the details set forth in Section R403.2, and Figures R403.1(2) and R403.1(3).

TABLE R402.2
MINIMUM SPECIFIED COMPRESSIVE STRENGTH OF CONCRETE

TYPE OR LOCATION OF CONCRETE CONSTRUCTION	MINIMUM SPECIFIED COMPRESSIVE STRENGTH[a] (f'_c)		
	Weathering Potential[b]		
	Negligible	Moderate	Severe
Basement walls, foundations and other concrete not exposed to the weather	2,500	2,500	2,500[c]
Basement slabs and interior slabs on grade, except garage floor slabs	2,500	2,500	2,500[c]
Basement walls, foundation walls, exterior walls and other vertical concrete work exposed to the weather	2,500	3,000[d]	3,000[d]
Porches, carport slabs and steps exposed to the weather, and garage floor slabs	2,500	3,000[d, e, f]	3,500[d, e, f]

For SI: 1 pound per square inch = 6.895 kPa.

a. Strength at 28 days psi.

b. See Table R301.2(1) for weathering potential.

c. Concrete in these locations that may be subject to freezing and thawing during construction shall be air-entrained concrete in accordance with Footnote d.

d. Concrete shall be air-entrained. Total air content (percent by volume of concrete) shall be not less than 5 percent or more than 7 percent.

e. See Section R402.2 for maximum cementitious materials content.

f. For garage floors with a steel troweled finish, reduction of the total air content (percent by volume of concrete) to not less than 3 percent is permitted if the specified compressive strength of the concrete is increased to not less than 4,000 psi.

TABLE R403.1
MINIMUM WIDTH OF CONCRETE, PRECAST OR MASONRY FOOTINGS
(inches)[a]

	LOAD-BEARING VALUE OF SOIL (psf)			
	1,500	2,000	3,000	≥ 4,000
Conventional light-frame construction				
1-story	12	12	12	12
2-story	15	12	12	12
3-story	23	17	12	12
4-inch brick veneer over light frame or 8-inch hollow concrete masonry				
1-story	12	12	12	12
2-story	21	16	12	12
3-story	32	24	16	12
8-inch solid or fully grouted masonry				
1-story	16	12	12	12
2-story	29	21	14	12
3-story	42	32	21	16

For SI: 1 inch = 25.4 mm, 1 pound per square foot = 0.0479 kPa.

a. Where minimum footing width is 12 inches, use of a single wythe of solid or fully grouted 12-inch nominal concrete masonry units is permitted.

R403.1.2 Continuous footing in Seismic Design Categories D_0, D_1 and D_2. The *braced wall panels* at exterior walls of buildings located in Seismic Design Categories D_0, D_1 and D_2 shall be supported by continuous footings. All required interior *braced wall panels* in buildings with plan dimensions greater than 50 feet (15 240 mm) shall also be supported by continuous footings.

R403.1.3 Seismic reinforcing. Concrete footings located in Seismic Design Categories D_0, D_1 and D_2, as established in Table R301.2(1), shall have minimum reinforcement. Bottom reinforcement shall be located a minimum of 3 inches (76 mm) clear from the bottom of the footing.

In Seismic Design Categories D_0, D_1 and D_2 where a construction joint is created between a concrete footing and a stem wall, a minimum of one No. 4 bar shall be installed at not more than 4 feet (1219 mm) on center. The vertical bar shall extend to 3 inches (76 mm) clear of the bottom of the footing, have a standard hook and extend a minimum of 14 inches (357 mm) into the stem wall.

In Seismic Design Categories D_0, D_1 and D_2 where a grouted masonry stem wall is supported on a concrete footing and stem wall, a minimum of one No. 4 bar shall be installed at not more than 4 feet (1219 mm) on center. The vertical bar shall extend to 3 inches (76 mm) clear of the bottom of the footing and have a standard hook.

In Seismic Design Categories D_0, D_1 and D_2 masonry stem walls without solid grout and vertical reinforcing are not permitted.

Exception: In detached one- and two-family *dwellings* which are three stories or less in height and constructed with stud bearing walls, plain concrete footings without longitudinal reinforcement supporting walls and isolated plain concrete footings supporting columns or pedestals are permitted.

R403.1.3.1 Foundations with stemwalls. Foundations with stem walls shall have installed a minimum of one No. 4 bar within 12 inches (305 mm) of the top of the wall and one No. 4 bar located 3 inches (76 mm) to 4 inches (102 mm) from the bottom of the footing.

R403.1.3.2 Slabs-on-ground with turned-down footings. Slabs on ground with turned down footings shall have a minimum of one No. 4 bar at the top and the bottom of the footing.

Exception: For slabs-on-ground cast monolithically with the footing, locating one No. 5 bar or two No. 4 bars in the middle third of the footing depth shall be permitted as an alternative to placement at the footing top and bottom.

Where the slab is not cast monolithically with the footing, No. 3 or larger vertical dowels with standard hooks on each end shall be provided in accordance with Figure R403.1.3.2. Standard hooks shall comply with Section R611.5.4.5.

R403.1.4 Minimum depth. All exterior footings shall be placed at least 12 inches (305 mm) below the undisturbed ground surface. Where applicable, the depth of footings shall also conform to Sections R403.1.4.1 through R403.1.4.2.

R403.1.4.1 Frost protection. Except where otherwise protected from frost, foundation walls, piers and other permanent supports of buildings and structures shall be protected from frost by one or more of the following methods:

1. Extended below the frost line specified in Table R301.2.(1);

2. Constructing in accordance with Section R403.3;

3. Constructing in accordance with ASCE 32; or

4. Erected on solid rock.

Exceptions:

1. Protection of freestanding *accessory structures* with an area of 600 square feet (56 m²) or less, of light-frame construction, with an eave height of 10 feet (3048 mm) or less shall not be required.

2. Protection of freestanding *accessory structures* with an area of 400 square feet (37 m²) or less, of other than light-frame construction, with an eave height of 10 feet (3048 mm) or less shall not be required.

3. Decks not supported by a dwelling need not be provided with footings that extend below the frost line.

Footings shall not bear on frozen soil unless the frozen condition is permanent.

R403.1.4.2 Seismic conditions. In Seismic Design Categories D_0, D_1 and D_2, interior footings supporting bearing or bracing walls and cast monolithically with a slab on *grade* shall extend to a depth of not less than 12 inches (305 mm) below the top of the slab.

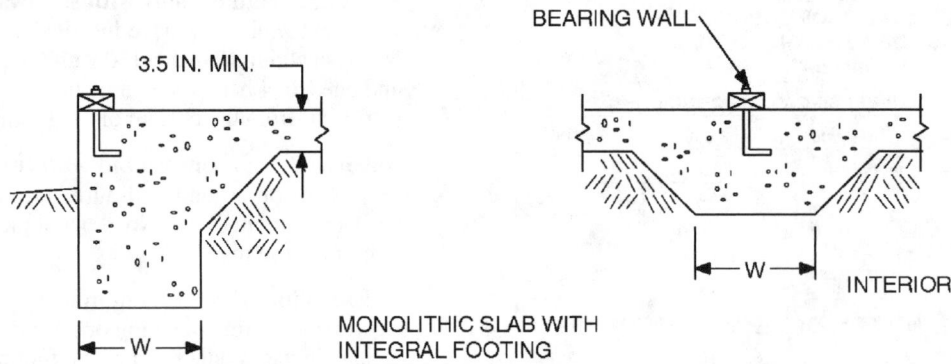

MONOLITHIC SLAB WITH
INTEGRAL FOOTING

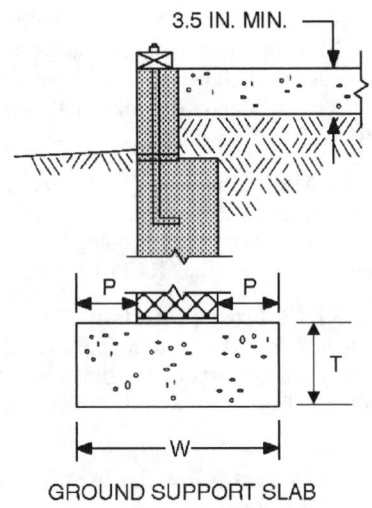

GROUND SUPPORT SLAB
WITH MASONRY WALL
AND SPREAD FOOTING

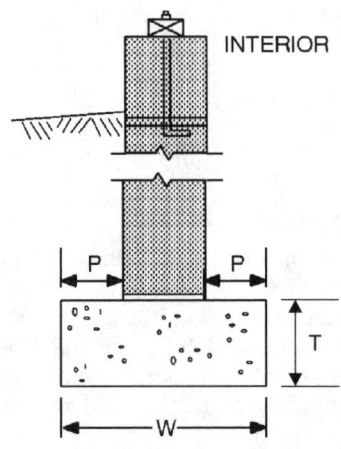

BASEMENT OR CRAWL SPACE
WITH MASONRY WALL AND
SPREAD FOOTING

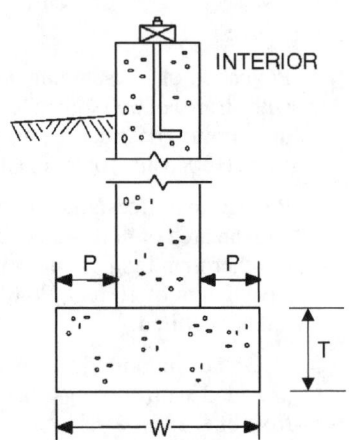

BASEMENT OR CRAWL SPACE
WITH CONCRETE WALL AND
SPREAD FOOTING

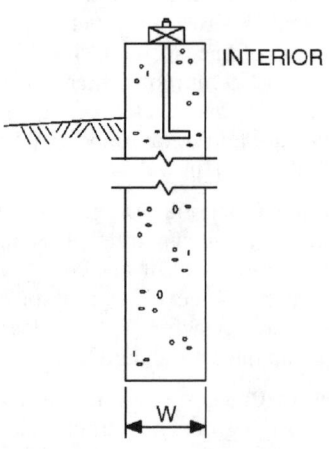

BASEMENT OR CRAWL SPACE
WITH FOUNDATION WALL
BEARING DIRECTLY ON SOIL

For SI: 1 inch = 25.4 mm.

FIGURE R403.1(1)
CONCRETE AND MASONRY FOUNDATION DETAILS

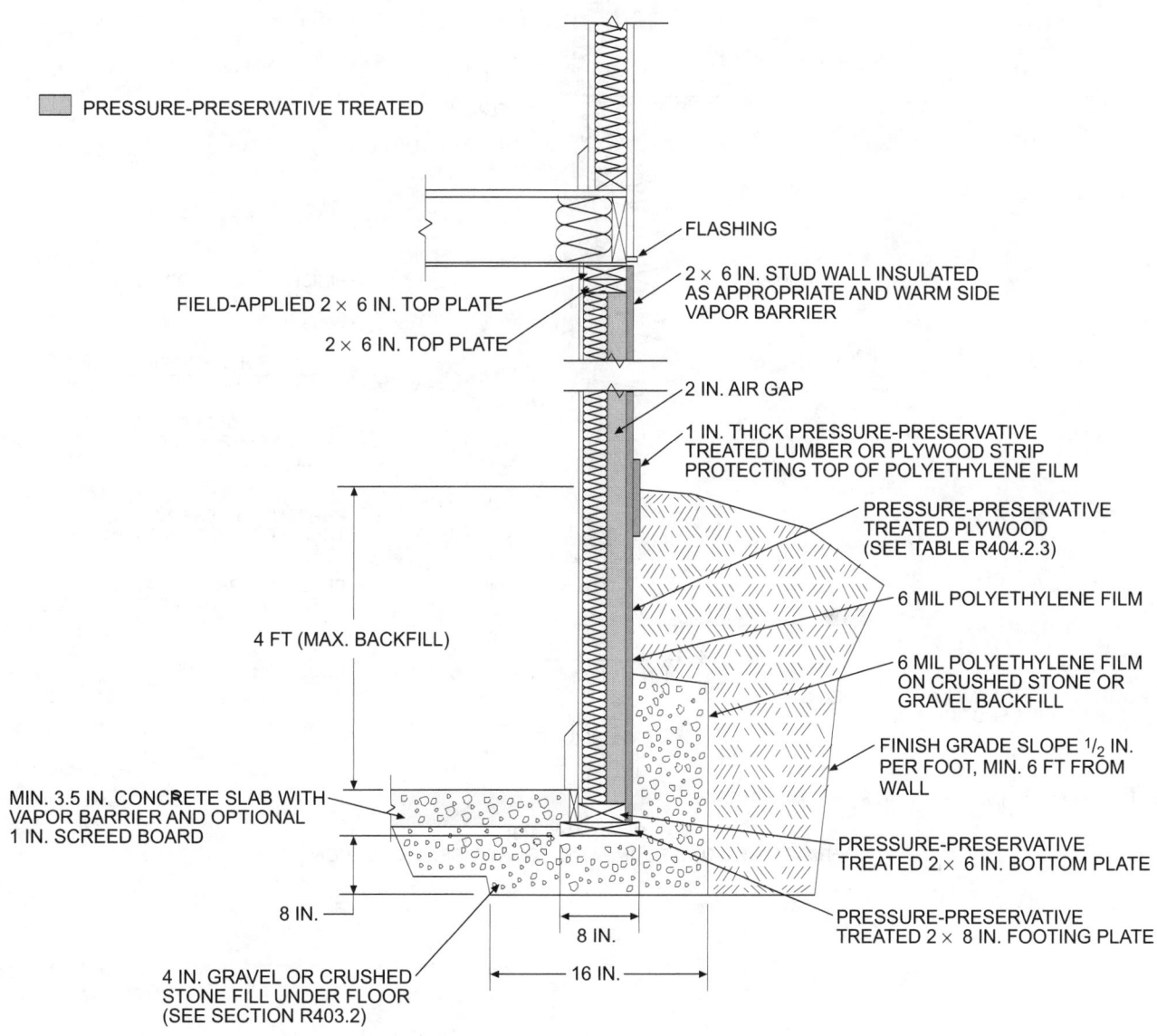

PRESSURE-PRESERVATIVE TREATED

FLASHING

2 × 6 IN. STUD WALL INSULATED AS APPROPRIATE AND WARM SIDE VAPOR BARRIER

FIELD-APPLIED 2 × 6 IN. TOP PLATE

2 × 6 IN. TOP PLATE

2 IN. AIR GAP

1 IN. THICK PRESSURE-PRESERVATIVE TREATED LUMBER OR PLYWOOD STRIP PROTECTING TOP OF POLYETHYLENE FILM

PRESSURE-PRESERVATIVE TREATED PLYWOOD (SEE TABLE R404.2.3)

6 MIL POLYETHYLENE FILM

6 MIL POLYETHYLENE FILM ON CRUSHED STONE OR GRAVEL BACKFILL

4 FT (MAX. BACKFILL)

FINISH GRADE SLOPE 1/2 IN. PER FOOT, MIN. 6 FT FROM WALL

MIN. 3.5 IN. CONCRETE SLAB WITH VAPOR BARRIER AND OPTIONAL 1 IN. SCREED BOARD

PRESSURE-PRESERVATIVE TREATED 2 × 6 IN. BOTTOM PLATE

PRESSURE-PRESERVATIVE TREATED 2 × 8 IN. FOOTING PLATE

8 IN.

8 IN.

4 IN. GRAVEL OR CRUSHED STONE FILL UNDER FLOOR (SEE SECTION R403.2)

16 IN.

For SI: 1 inch = 25.4 mm, 1 foot = 304.8 mm, 1 mil = 0.0254 mm.

FIGURE R403.1(2)
PERMANENT WOOD FOUNDATION BASEMENT WALL SECTION

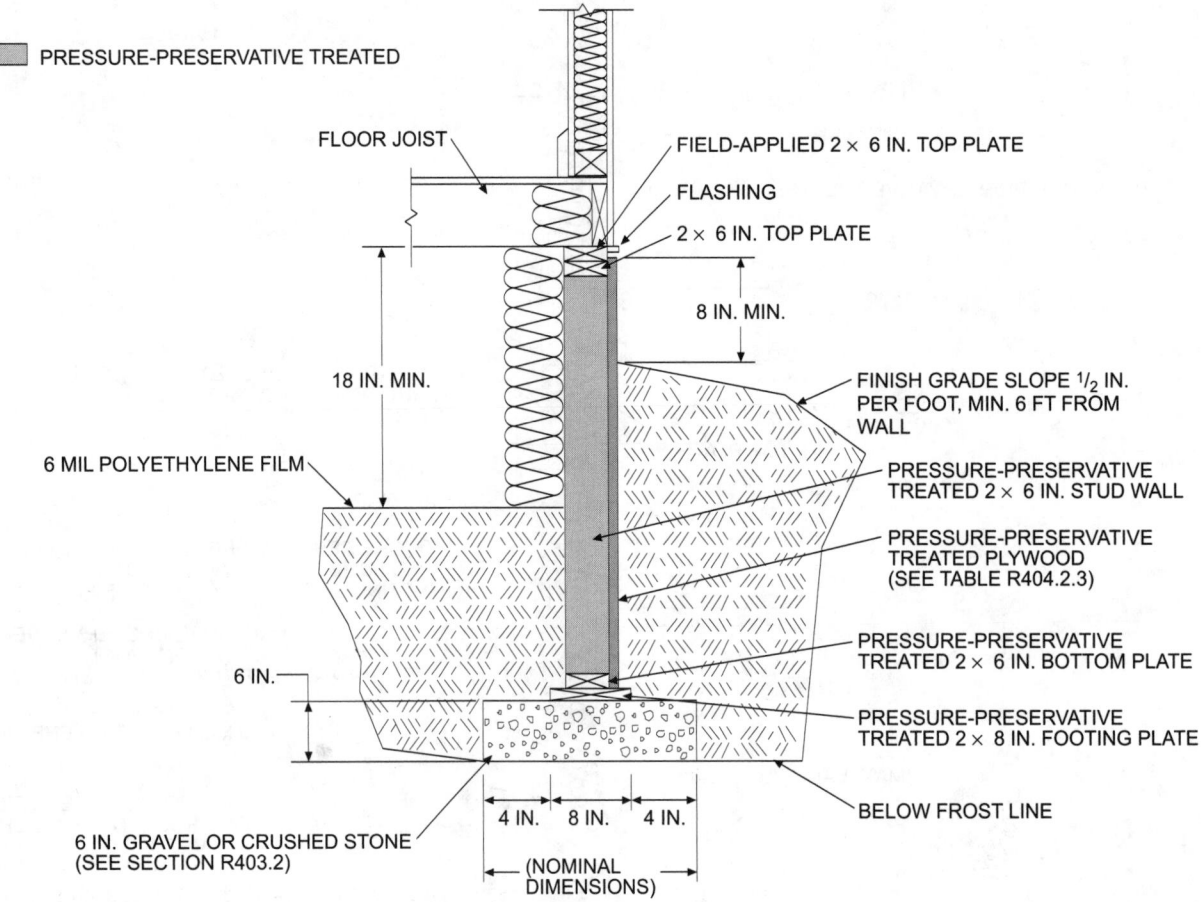

☐ PRESSURE-PRESERVATIVE TREATED

FLOOR JOIST

FIELD-APPLIED 2 × 6 IN. TOP PLATE

FLASHING

2 × 6 IN. TOP PLATE

8 IN. MIN.

18 IN. MIN.

FINISH GRADE SLOPE 1/2 IN. PER FOOT, MIN. 6 FT FROM WALL

6 MIL POLYETHYLENE FILM

PRESSURE-PRESERVATIVE TREATED 2 × 6 IN. STUD WALL

PRESSURE-PRESERVATIVE TREATED PLYWOOD (SEE TABLE R404.2.3)

PRESSURE-PRESERVATIVE TREATED 2 × 6 IN. BOTTOM PLATE

6 IN.

PRESSURE-PRESERVATIVE TREATED 2 × 8 IN. FOOTING PLATE

BELOW FROST LINE

6 IN. GRAVEL OR CRUSHED STONE (SEE SECTION R403.2)

4 IN.   8 IN.   4 IN.

(NOMINAL DIMENSIONS)

For SI: 1 inch = 25.4 mm, 1 foot = 304.8 mm, 1 mil = 0.0254 mm.

FIGURE R403.1(3)
PERMANENT WOOD FOUNDATION CRAWL SPACE SECTION

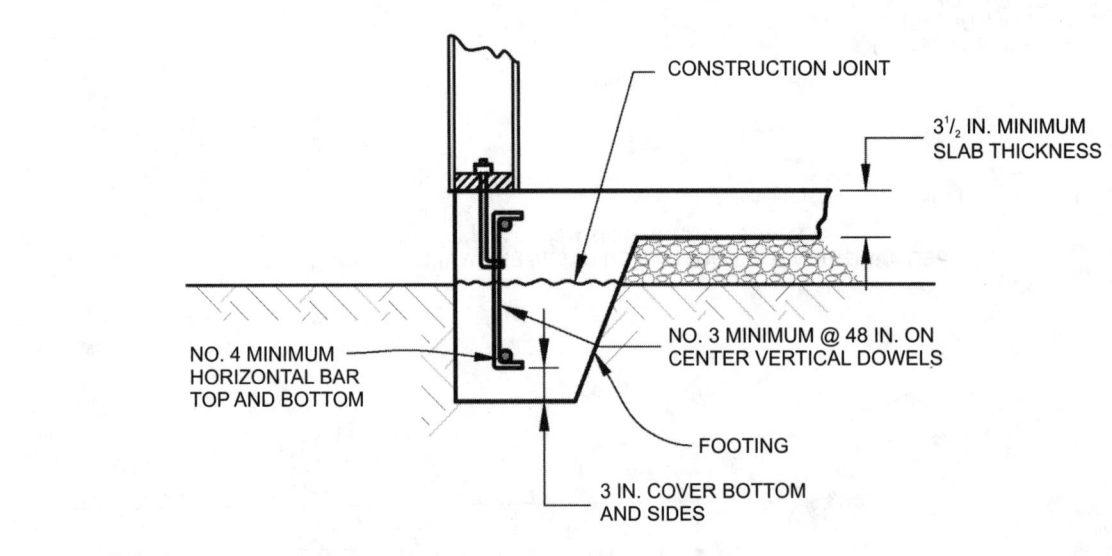

CONSTRUCTION JOINT

3 1/2 IN. MINIMUM SLAB THICKNESS

NO. 4 MINIMUM HORIZONTAL BAR TOP AND BOTTOM

NO. 3 MINIMUM @ 48 IN. ON CENTER VERTICAL DOWELS

FOOTING

3 IN. COVER BOTTOM AND SIDES

For SI: 1 inch = 25.4 mm.

FIGURE R403.1.3.2
DOWELS FOR SLABS-ON-GROUND WITH TURNED-DOWN FOOTINGS

R403.1.5 Slope. The top surface of footings shall be level. The bottom surface of footings shall not have a slope exceeding one unit vertical in 10 units horizontal (10-percent slope). Footings shall be stepped where it is necessary to change the elevation of the top surface of the footings or where the slope of the bottom surface of the footings will exceed one unit vertical in ten units horizontal (10-percent slope).

R403.1.6 Foundation anchorage. Sill plates and walls supported directly on continuous foundations shall be anchored to the foundation in accordance with this section.

Wood sole plates at all exterior walls on monolithic slabs, wood sole plates of *braced wall panels* at building interiors on monolithic slabs and all wood sill plates shall be anchored to the foundation with anchor bolts spaced a maximum of 6 feet (1829 mm) on center. Bolts shall be at least $^{1}/_{2}$ inch (12.7 mm) in diameter and shall extend a minimum of 7 inches (178 mm) into concrete or grouted cells of concrete masonry units. A nut and washer shall be tightened on each anchor bolt. There shall be a minimum of two bolts per plate section with one bolt located not more than 12 inches (305 mm) or less than seven bolt diameters from each end of the plate section. Interior bearing wall sole plates on monolithic slab foundation that are not part of a *braced wall panel* shall be positively anchored with *approved* fasteners. Sill plates and sole plates shall be protected against decay and termites where required by Sections R317 and R318. Cold-formed steel framing systems shall be fastened to wood sill plates or anchored directly to the foundation as required in Section R505.3.1 or R603.3.1.

Exceptions:

1. Foundation anchorage, spaced as required to provide equivalent anchorage to $^{1}/_{2}$-inch-diameter (12.7 mm) anchor bolts.

2. Walls 24 inches (610 mm) total length or shorter connecting offset *braced wall panels* shall be anchored to the foundation with a minimum of one anchor bolt located in the center third of the plate section and shall be attached to adjacent *braced wall panels* at corners as shown in Figure R602.10.4.4(1).

3. Connection of walls 12 inches (305 mm) total length or shorter connecting offset *braced wall panels* to the foundation without anchor bolts shall be permitted. The wall shall be attached to adjacent *braced wall panels* at corners as shown in Figure R602.10.4.4(1).

R403.1.6.1 Foundation anchorage in Seismic Design Categories C, D_0, D_1 and D_2. In addition to the requirements of Section R403.1.6, the following requirements shall apply to wood light-frame structures in Seismic Design Categories D_0, D_1 and D_2 and wood light-frame townhouses in Seismic Design Category C.

1. Plate washers conforming to Section R602.11.1 shall be provided for all anchor bolts over the full length of required *braced wall lines* except where *approved* anchor straps are used. Properly sized cut washers shall be permitted for anchor bolts in wall lines not containing *braced wall panels*.

2. Interior braced wall plates shall have anchor bolts spaced at not more than 6 feet (1829 mm) on center and located within 12 inches (305 mm) of the ends of each plate section when supported on a continuous foundation.

3. Interior bearing wall sole plates shall have anchor bolts spaced at not more than 6 feet (1829 mm) on center and located within 12 inches (305 mm) of the ends of each plate section when supported on a continuous foundation.

4. The maximum anchor bolt spacing shall be 4 feet (1219 mm) for buildings over two stories in height.

5. Stepped cripple walls shall conform to Section R602.11.2.

6. Where continuous wood foundations in accordance with Section R404.2 are used, the force transfer shall have a capacity equal to or greater than the connections required by Section R602.11.1 or the *braced wall panel* shall be connected to the wood foundations in accordance with the *braced wall panel*-to-floor fastening requirements of Table R602.3(1).

R403.1.7 Footings on or adjacent to slopes. The placement of buildings and structures on or adjacent to slopes steeper than one unit vertical in three units horizontal (33.3-percent slope) shall conform to Sections R403.1.7.1 through R403.1.7.4.

R403.1.7.1 Building clearances from ascending slopes. In general, buildings below slopes shall be set a sufficient distance from the slope to provide protection from slope drainage, erosion and shallow failures. Except as provided in Section R403.1.7.4 and Figure R403.1.7.1, the following criteria will be assumed to provide this protection. Where the existing slope is steeper than one unit vertical in one unit horizontal (100-percent slope), the toe of the slope shall be assumed to be at the intersection of a horizontal plane drawn from the top of the foundation and a plane drawn tangent to the slope at an angle of 45 degrees (0.79 rad) to the horizontal. Where a retaining wall is constructed at the toe of the slope, the height of the slope shall be measured from the top of the wall to the top of the slope.

R403.1.7.2 Footing setback from descending slope surfaces. Footings on or adjacent to slope surfaces shall be founded in material with an embedment and setback from the slope surface sufficient to provide vertical and lateral support for the footing without detrimental settlement. Except as provided for in Section R403.1.7.4 and Figure R403.1.7.1, the following setback is deemed adequate to meet the criteria. Where the slope is steeper than one unit vertical in one unit horizontal (100-percent slope), the required setback shall be measured from an imaginary plane 45 degrees (0.79 rad) to the horizontal, projected upward from the toe of the slope.

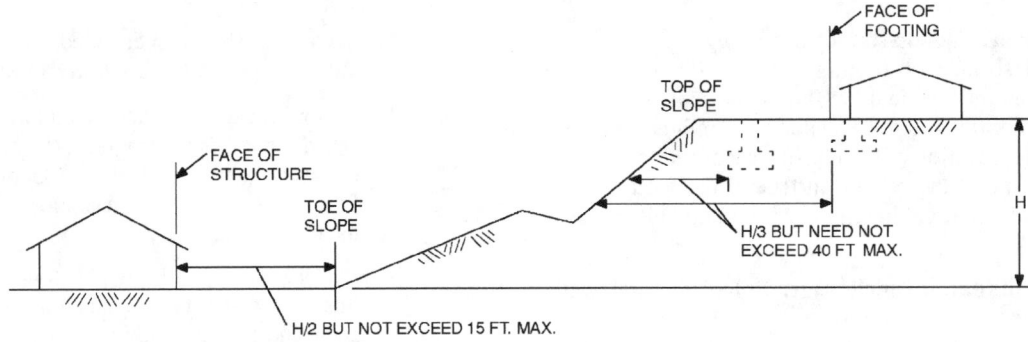

For SI: 1 foot = 304.8 mm.

FIGURE R403.1.7.1
FOUNDATION CLEARANCE FROM SLOPES

R403.1.7.3 Foundation elevation. On graded sites, the top of any exterior foundation shall extend above the elevation of the street gutter at point of discharge or the inlet of an *approved* drainage device a minimum of 12 inches (305 mm) plus 2 percent. Alternate elevations are permitted subject to the approval of the *building official*, provided it can be demonstrated that required drainage to the point of discharge and away from the structure is provided at all locations on the site.

R403.1.7.4 Alternate setback and clearances. Alternate setbacks and clearances are permitted, subject to the approval of the *building official*. The *building official* is permitted to require an investigation and recommendation of a qualified engineer to demonstrate that the intent of this section has been satisfied. Such an investigation shall include consideration of material, height of slope, slope gradient, load intensity and erosion characteristics of slope material.

R403.1.8 Foundations on expansive soils. Foundation and floor slabs for buildings located on expansive soils shall be designed in accordance with Section 1805.8 of the *International Building Code*.

Exception: Slab-on-ground and other foundation systems which have performed adequately in soil conditions similar to those encountered at the building site are permitted subject to the approval of the *building official*.

R403.1.8.1 Expansive soils classifications. Soils meeting all four of the following provisions shall be considered expansive, except that tests to show compliance with Items 1, 2 and 3 shall not be required if the test prescribed in Item 4 is conducted:

1. Plasticity Index (PI) of 15 or greater, determined in accordance with ASTM D 4318.

2. More than 10 percent of the soil particles pass a No. 200 sieve (75 µm), determined in accordance with ASTM D 422.

3. More than 10 percent of the soil particles are less than 5 micrometers in size, determined in accordance with ASTM D 422.

4. Expansion Index greater than 20, determined in accordance with ASTM D 4829.

R403.2 Footings for wood foundations. Footings for wood foundations shall be in accordance with Figures R403.1(2) and R403.1(3). Gravel shall be washed and well graded. The maximum size stone shall not exceed $^3/_4$ inch (19.1 mm). Gravel shall be free from organic, clayey or silty soils. Sand shall be coarse, not smaller than $^1/_{16}$-inch (1.6 mm) grains and shall be free from organic, clayey or silty soils. Crushed stone shall have a maximum size of $^1/_2$ inch (12.7 mm).

R403.3 Frost protected shallow foundations. For buildings where the monthly mean temperature of the building is maintained at a minimum of 64°F (18°C), footings are not required to extend below the frost line when protected from frost by insulation in accordance with Figure R403.3(1) and Table R403.3(1). Foundations protected from frost in accordance with Figure R403.3(1) and Table R403.3(1) shall not be used for unheated spaces such as porches, utility rooms, garages and carports, and shall not be attached to basements or crawl spaces that are not maintained at a minimum monthly mean temperature of 64°F (18°C).

Materials used below *grade* for the purpose of insulating footings against frost shall be *labeled* as complying with ASTM C 578.

R403.3.1 Foundations adjoining frost protected shallow foundations. Foundations that adjoin frost protected shallow foundations shall be protected from frost in accordance with Section R403.1.4.

R403.3.1.1 Attachment to unheated slab-on-ground structure. Vertical wall insulation and horizontal insulation of frost protected shallow foundations that adjoin a slab-on-ground foundation that does not have a monthly mean temperature maintained at a minimum of 64°F (18°C) shall be in accordance with Figure R403.3(3) and Table R403.3(1). Vertical wall insulation shall extend between the frost protected shallow foundation and the adjoining slab foundation. Required horizontal insulation shall be continuous under the adjoining slab foundation and through any foundation walls adjoining the frost protected shallow foundation. Where insulation passes through a foundation wall, it shall either be of a type complying with this section and having bearing capacity equal to or greater than the structural loads imposed by the building, or the building shall be designed and constructed using beams, lintels, cantilevers or other means of transferring building loads such that the structural loads of the building do not bear on the insulation.

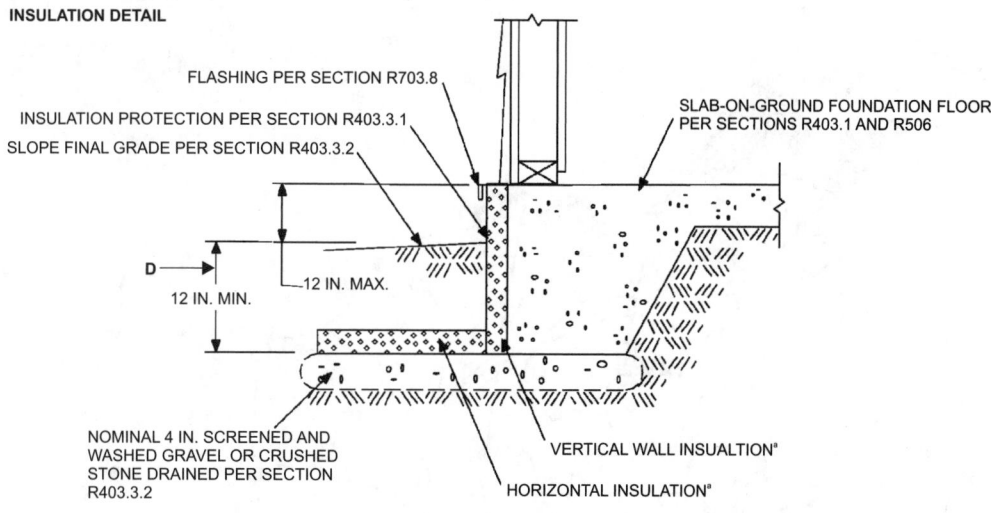

INSULATION DETAIL

FLASHING PER SECTION R703.8

INSULATION PROTECTION PER SECTION R403.3.1

SLOPE FINAL GRADE PER SECTION R403.3.2

SLAB-ON-GROUND FOUNDATION FLOOR PER SECTIONS R403.1 AND R506

D

12 IN. MIN.

12 IN. MAX.

NOMINAL 4 IN. SCREENED AND WASHED GRAVEL OR CRUSHED STONE DRAINED PER SECTION R403.3.2

VERTICAL WALL INSUALTION[a]

HORIZONTAL INSULATION[a]

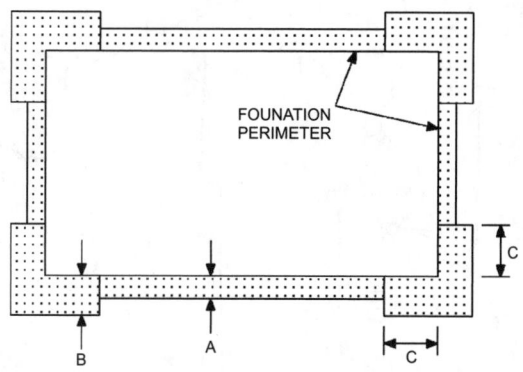

HORIZONTAL INSULATION PLAN

FOUNATION PERIMETER

C

B   A   C

For SI: 1 inch = 25.4 mm.

a. See Table R403.3(1) for required dimensions and *R*-values for vertical and horizontal insulation and minimum footing depth.

FIGURE R403.3(1)
INSULATION PLACEMENT FOR FROST PROTECTED FOOTINGS IN HEATED BUILDINGS

TABLE R403.3(1)
MINIMUM FOOTING DEPTH AND INSULATION REQUIREMENTS FOR FROST-PROTECTED FOOTINGS IN HEATED BUILDINGS[a]

AIR FREEZING INDEX (°F-days)[b]	MINIMUM FOOTING DEPTH, *D* (inches)	VERTICAL INSULATION *R*-VALUE[c, d]	HORIZONTAL INSULATION *R*-VALUE[c, e]		HORIZONTAL INSULATION DIMENSIONS PER FIGURE R403.3(1) (inches)		
			Along walls	At corners	A	B	C
1,500 or less	12	4.5	Not required	Not required	Not required	Not required	Not required
2,000	14	5.6	Not required	Not required	Not required	Not required	Not required
2,500	16	6.7	1.7	4.9	12	24	40
3,000	16	7.8	6.5	8.6	12	24	40
3,500	16	9.0	8.0	11.2	24	30	60
4,000	16	10.1	10.5	13.1	24	36	60

a. Insulation requirements are for protection against frost damage in heated buildings. Greater values may be required to meet energy conservation standards.

b. See Figure R403.3(2) or Table R403.3(2) for Air Freezing Index values.

c. Insulation materials shall provide the stated minimum *R*-values under long-term exposure to moist, below-ground conditions in freezing climates. The following *R*-values shall be used to determine insulation thicknesses required for this application: Type II expanded polystyrene—2.4*R* per inch; Type IV extruded polystyrene—4.5*R* per inch; Type VI extruded polystyrene—4.5*R* per inch; Type IX expanded polystyrene—3.2*R* per inch; Type X extruded polystyrene—4.5*R* per inch.

d. Vertical insulation shall be expanded polystyrene insulation or extruded polystyrene insulation.

e. Horizontal insulation shall be extruded polystyrene insulation.

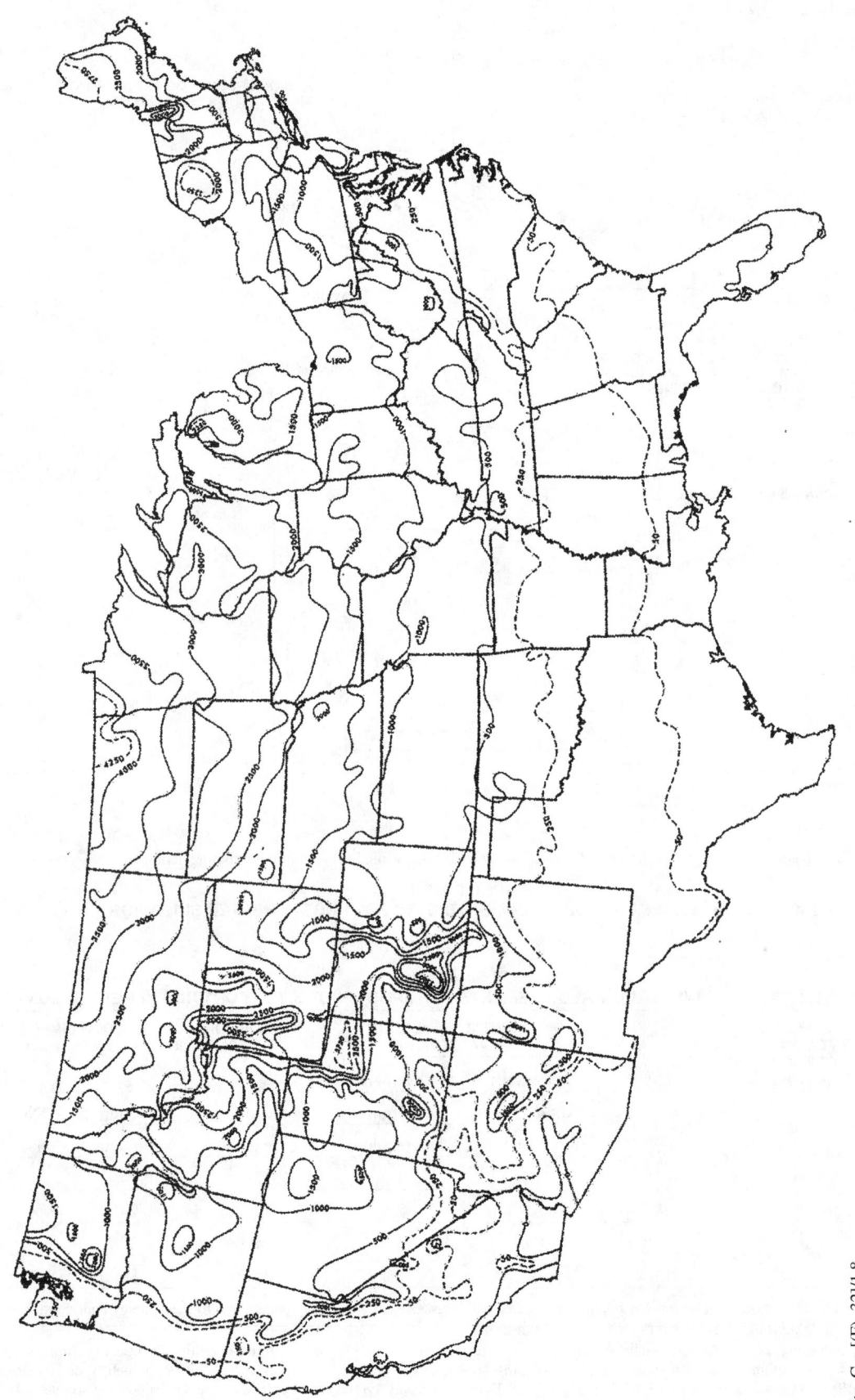

FIGURE R403.3(2)
AIR-FREEZING INDEX
AN ESTIMATE OF THE 100-YEAR RETURN PERIOD

For SI: C = [(F) -32]/1.8.

Note: The air-freezing index is defined as cumulative degree days below 32F. It is used as a measure of the combined magnitude and duration of air temperature below freezing. The index was computed over a 12-month period (July-June) for each of the 3,044 stations used in the above analysis. Date from the 1951-80 period were fitted to a Weibull probability distribution to produce an estimate of the 100-year return period.

TABLE R403.3(2)
AIR-FREEZING INDEX FOR U.S. LOCATIONS BY COUNTY

STATE	AIR-FREEZING INDEX					
	1500 or less	2000	2500	3000	3500	4000
Alabama	All counties	—	—	—	—	—
Alaska	Ketchikan Gateway, Prince of Wales-Outer Ketchikan (CA), Sitka, Wrangell-Petersburg (CA)	—	Aleutians West (CA), Haines, Juneau, Skagway-Hoonah-Angoon (CA), Yakutat	—	—	All counties not listed
Arizona	All counties	—	—	—	—	—
Arkansas	All counties	—	—	—	—	—
California	All counties not listed	Nevada, Sierra	—	—	—	—
Colorado	All counties not listed	Archuleta, Custer, Fremont, Huerfano, Las Animas, Ouray, Pitkin, San Miguel	Clear Creek, Conejos, Costilla, Dolores, Eagle, La Plata, Park, Routt, San Juan, Summit	Alamosa, Grand, Jackson, Larimer, Moffat, Rio Blanco, Rio Grande	Chaffee, Gunnison, Lake, Saguache	Hinsdale, Mineral
Connecticut	All counties not listed	Hartford, Litchfield	—	—	—	—
Delaware	All counties	—	—	—	—	—
District of Columbia	All counties	—	—	—	—	—
Florida	All counties	—	—	—	—	—
Georgia	All counties	—	—	—	—	—
Hawaii	All counties	—	—	—	—	—
Idaho	All counties not listed	Adams, Bannock, Blaine, Clearwater, Idaho, Lincoln, Oneida, Power, Valley, Washington	Bingham, Bonneville, Camas, Caribou, Elmore, Franklin, Jefferson, Madison, Teton	Bear Lake, Butte, Custer, Fremont, Lemhi	Clark	
Illinois	All counties not listed	Boone, Bureau, Cook, Dekalb, DuPage, Fulton, Grundy, Henderson, Henry, Iroquois, Jo Daviess, Kane, Kankakee, Kendall, Knox, La Salle, Lake, Lee, Livingston, Marshall, Mason, McHenry, McLean, Mercer, Peoria, Putnam, Rock Island, Stark Tazewell, Warren, Whiteside, Will, Woodford	Carroll, Ogle, Stephenson, Winnebago	—	—	—
Indiana	All counties not listed	Allen, Benton, Cass, Fountain, Fulton, Howard, Jasper, Kosciusko, La Porte, Lake, Marshall, Miami, Newton, Porter, Pulaski, Starke, Steuben, Tippecanoe, Tipton, Wabash, Warren, White	—	—	—	—

(continued)

TABLE R403.3(2)—continued
AIR-FREEZING INDEX FOR U.S. LOCATIONS BY COUNTY

STATE	AIR-FREEZING INDEX					
	1500 or less	2000	2500	3000	3500	4000
Iowa	Appanoose, Davis, Fremont, Lee, Van Buren	All counties not listed	Allamakee, Black Hawk, Boone, Bremer, Buchanan, Buena Vista, Butler, Calhoun, Cerro Gordo, Cherokee, Chickasaw, Clay, Clayton, Delaware, Dubuque, Fayette, Floyd, Franklin, Grundy, Hamilton, Hancock, Hardin, Humboldt, Ida, Jackson, Jasper, Jones, Linn, Marshall, Palo Alto, Plymouth, Pocahontas, Poweshiek, Sac, Sioux, Story, Tama, Webster, Winnebago, Woodbury, Worth, Wright	Dickinson, Emmet, Howard, Kossuth, Lyon, Mitchell, O'Brien, Osceola, Winneshiek	—	—
Kansas	All counties	—	—	—	—	—
Kentucky	All counties	—	—	—	—	—
Louisiana	All counties	—	—	—	—	—
Maine	York	Knox, Lincoln, Sagadahoc	Androscoggin, Cumberland, Hancock, Kennebec, Waldo, Washington	Aroostook, Franklin, Oxford, Penobscot, Piscataquis, Somerset	—	—
Maryland	All counties	—	—	—	—	—
Massachusetts	All counties not listed	Berkshire, Franklin, Hampden, Worcester	—	—	—	—
Michigan	Berrien, Branch, Cass, Kalamazoo, Macomb, Ottawa, St. Clair, St. Joseph	All counties not listed	Alger, Charlevoix, Cheboygan, Chippewa, Crawford, Delta, Emmet, Iosco, Kalkaska, Lake, Luce, Mackinac, Menominee, Missaukee, Montmorency, Ogemaw, Osceola, Otsego, Roscommon, Schoolcraft, Wexford	Baraga, Dickinson, Iron, Keweenaw, Marquette	Gogebic, Houghton, Ontonagon	—
Minnesota	—	—	Houston, Winona	All counties not listed	Aitkin, Big Stone, Carlton, Crow Wing, Douglas, Itasca, Kanabec, Lake, Morrison, Pine, Pope, Stearns, Stevens, Swift, Todd, Wadena	Becker, Beltrami, Cass, Clay, Clearwater, Grant, Hubbard, Kittson, Koochiching, Lake of the Woods, Mahnomen, Marshall, Norman, Otter Tail, Pennington, Polk, Red Lake, Roseau, St Louis, Traverse, Wilkin
Mississippi	All counties	—	—	—	—	—
Missouri	All counties not listed	Atchison, Mercer, Nodaway, Putnam	—	—	—	—

(continued)

TABLE R403.3(2)—continued
AIR-FREEZING INDEX FOR U.S. LOCATIONS BY COUNTY

STATE	AIR-FREEZING INDEX					
	1500 or less	2000	2500	3000	3500	4000
Montana	Mineral	Broadwater, Golden Valley, Granite, Lake, Lincoln, Missoula, Ravalli, Sanders, Sweet Grass	Big Horn, Carbon, Jefferson, Judith Basin, Lewis and Clark, Meagher, Musselshell, Powder River, Powell, Silver Bow, Stillwater, Westland	Carter, Cascade, Deer Lodge, Falcon, Fergus, Flathead, Gallanting, Glacier, Madison, Park, Petroleum, Ponder, Rosebud, Teton, Treasure, Yellowstone	Beaverhead, Blaine, Chouteau, Custer, Dawson, Garfield, Liberty, McCone, Prairie, Toole, Wibaux	Daniels, Hill, Phillips, Richland, Roosevelt, Sheridan, Valley
Nebraska	Adams, Banner, Chase, Cheyenne, Clay, Deuel, Dundy, Fillmore, Franklin, Frontier, Furnas, Gage, Garden, Gosper, Harlan, Hayes, Hitchcock, Jefferson, Kimball, Morrill, Nemaha, Nuckolls, Pawnee, Perkins, Phelps, Red Willow, Richardson, Saline, Scotts Bluff, Seward, Thayer, Webster	All counties not listed	Boyd, Burt, Cedar, Cuming, Dakota, Dixon, Dodge, Knox, Thurston	—	—	—
Nevada	All counties not listed	Elko, Eureka, Nye, Washoe, White Pine	—	—	—	—
New Hampshire	—	All counties not listed	—	—	—	Carroll, Coos, Grafton
New Jersey	All counties	—	—	—	—	—
New Mexico	All counties not listed	Rio Arriba	Colfax, Mora, Taos	—	—	—
New York	Albany, Bronx, Cayuga, Columbia, Cortland, Dutchess, Genessee, Kings, Livingston, Monroe, Nassau, New York, Niagara, Onondaga, Ontario, Orange, Orleans, Putnam, Queens, Richmond, Rockland, Seneca, Suffolk, Wayne, Westchester, Yates	All counties not listed	Clinton, Essex, Franklin, Hamilton, Herkimer, Jefferson, Lewis, St. Lawrence, Warren	—	—	—
North Carolina	All counties	—	—	—	—	—
North Dakota	—	—	—	Billings, Bowman	Adams, Dickey, Golden Valley, Hettinger, LaMoure, Oliver, Ransom, Sargent, Sioux, Slope, Stark	All counties not listed
Ohio	All counties not listed	Ashland, Crawford, Defiance, Holmes, Huron, Knox, Licking, Morrow, Paulding, Putnam, Richland, Seneca, Williams	—	—	—	—

(continued)

TABLE R403.3(2)—continued
AIR-FREEZING INDEX FOR U.S. LOCATIONS BY COUNTY

STATE	AIR-FREEZING INDEX					
	1500 or less	2000	2500	3000	3500	4000
Oklahoma	All counties	—	—	—	—	—
Oregon	All counties not listed	Baker, Crook, Grant, Harney	—	—	—	—
Pennsylvania	All counties not listed	Berks, Blair, Bradford, Cambria, Cameron, Centre, Clarion, Clearfield, Clinton, Crawford, Elk, Forest, Huntingdon, Indiana, Jefferson, Lackawanna, Lycoming, McKean, Pike, Potter, Susquehanna, Tioga, Venango, Warren, Wayne, Wyoming	—	—	—	—
Rhode Island	All counties	—	—	—	—	—
South Carolina	All counties	—	—	—	—	—
South Dakota	—	Bennett, Custer, Fall River, Lawrence, Mellette, Shannon, Todd, Tripp	Bon Homme, Charles Mix, Davison, Douglas, Gregory, Jackson, Jones, Lyman	All counties not listed	Beadle, Brookings, Brown, Campbell, Codington, Corson, Day, Deuel, Edmunds, Faulk, Grant, Hamlin, Kingsbury, Marshall, McPherson, Perkins, Roberts, Spink, Walworth	—
Tennessee	All counties	—	—	—	—	—
Texas	All counties	—	—	—	—	—
Utah	All counties not listed	Box Elder, Morgan, Weber	Garfield, Salt Lake, Summit	Carbon, Daggett, Duchesne, Rich, Sanpete, Uintah, Wasatch	—	—
Vermont	—	Bennington, Grand Isle, Rutland, Windham	Addison, Chittenden, Franklin, Orange, Washington, Windsor	Caledonia, Essex, Lamoille, Orleans	—	—
Virginia	All counties	—	—	—	—	—
Washington	All counties not listed	Chelan, Douglas, Ferry, Okanogan	—	—	—	—
West Virginia	All counties	—	—	—	—	—
Wisconsin	—	Kenosha, Kewaunee, Racine, Sheboygan, Walworth	All counties not listed	Ashland, Barron, Burnett, Chippewa, Clark, Dunn, Eau Claire, Florence, Forest, Iron, Jackson, La Crosse, Langlade, Marathon, Monroe, Pepin, Polk, Portage, Price, Rust, St. Croix, Taylor, Trempealeau, Vilas, Wood	Bayfield, Douglas, Lincoln, Oneida, Sawyer, Washburn	—
Wyoming	Goshen, Platte	Converse, Crook, Laramie, Niobrara	Campbell, Carbon, Hot Springs, Johnson, Natrona, Sheridan, Uinta, Weston	Albany, Big Horn, Park, Washakie	Fremont, Teton	Lincoln, Sublette, Sweetwater

INSULATION DETAIL

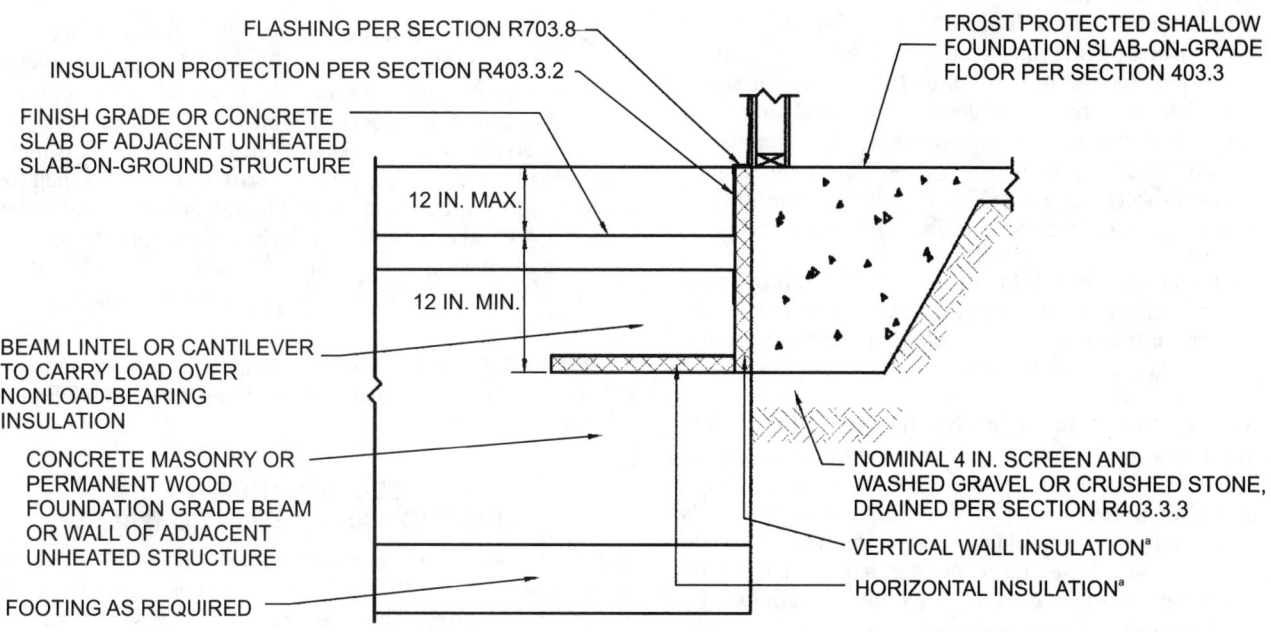

FLASHING PER SECTION R703.8

INSULATION PROTECTION PER SECTION R403.3.2

FINISH GRADE OR CONCRETE SLAB OF ADJACENT UNHEATED SLAB-ON-GROUND STRUCTURE

FROST PROTECTED SHALLOW FOUNDATION SLAB-ON-GRADE FLOOR PER SECTION 403.3

12 IN. MAX.

12 IN. MIN.

BEAM LINTEL OR CANTILEVER TO CARRY LOAD OVER NONLOAD-BEARING INSULATION

CONCRETE MASONRY OR PERMANENT WOOD FOUNDATION GRADE BEAM OR WALL OF ADJACENT UNHEATED STRUCTURE

FOOTING AS REQUIRED

NOMINAL 4 IN. SCREEN AND WASHED GRAVEL OR CRUSHED STONE, DRAINED PER SECTION R403.3.3

VERTICAL WALL INSULATION[a]

HORIZONTAL INSULATION[a]

HORIZONTAL INSULATION PLAN

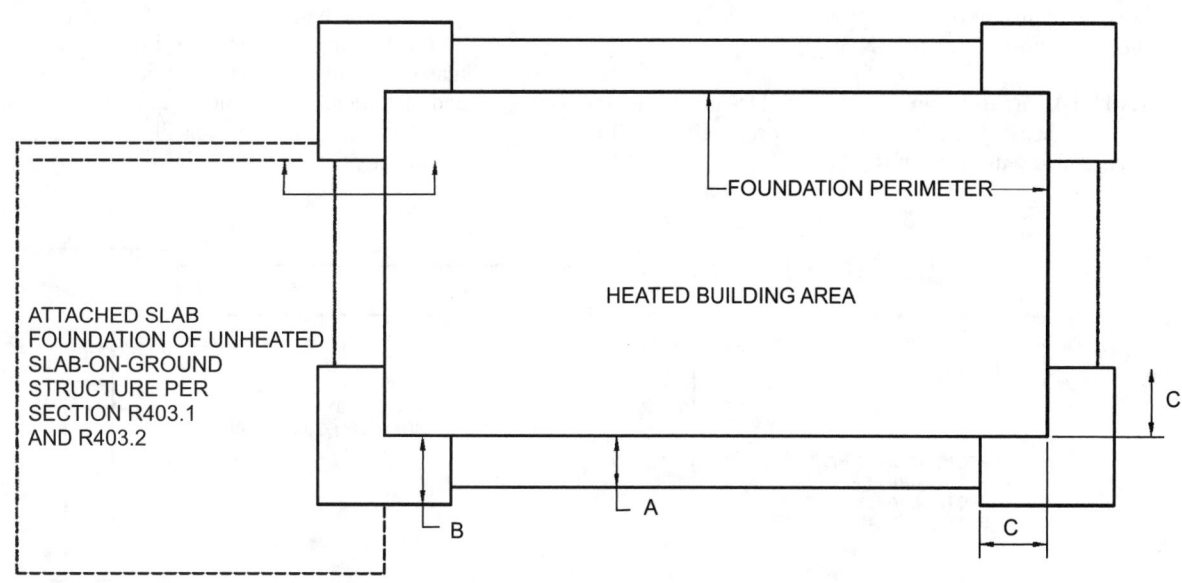

FOUNDATION PERIMETER

HEATED BUILDING AREA

ATTACHED SLAB FOUNDATION OF UNHEATED SLAB-ON-GROUND STRUCTURE PER SECTION R403.1 AND R403.2

B

A

C

C

For SI: 1 inch = 25.4 mm.

a. See Table R403.3(1) for required dimensions and *R*-values for vertical and horizontal insulation.

FIGURE R403.3(3)
INSULATION PLACEMENT FOR FROST-PROTECTED FOOTINGS ADJACENT TO UNHEATED SLAB-ON-GROUND STRUCTURE

R403.3.1.2 Attachment to heated structure. Where a frost protected shallow foundation abuts a structure that has a monthly mean temperature maintained at a minimum of 64°F (18°C), horizontal insulation and vertical wall insulation shall not be required between the frost protected shallow foundation and the adjoining structure. Where the frost protected shallow foundation abuts the heated structure, the horizontal insulation and vertical wall insulation shall extend along the adjoining foundation in accordance with Figure R403.3(4) a distance of not less than Dimension A in Table R403.3(1).

> **Exception:** Where the frost protected shallow foundation abuts the heated structure to form an inside corner, vertical insulation extending along the adjoining foundation is not required.

R403.3.2 Protection of horizontal insulation below ground. Horizontal insulation placed less than 12 inches (305 mm) below the ground surface or that portion of horizontal insulation extending outward more than 24 inches (610 mm) from the foundation edge shall be protected against damage by use of a concrete slab or asphalt paving on the ground surface directly above the insulation or by cementitious board, plywood rated for below-ground use, or other *approved* materials placed below ground, directly above the top surface of the insulation.

R403.3.3 Drainage. Final *grade* shall be sloped in accordance with Section R401.3. In other than Group I Soils, as detailed in Table R405.1, gravel or crushed stone beneath horizontal insulation below ground shall drain to daylight or into an *approved* sewer system.

R403.3.4 Termite damage. The use of foam plastic in areas of "very heavy" termite infestation probability shall be in accordance with Section R318.4.

R403.4 Footings for precast concrete foundations. Footings for precast concrete foundations shall comply with Section R403.4.

R403.4.1 Crushed stone footings. Clean crushed stone shall be free from organic, clayey or silty soils. Crushed stone shall be angular in nature and meet ASTM C 33, with the maximum size stone not to exceed $^1/_2$ inch (12.7 mm) and the minimum stone size not to be smaller than $^1/_{16}$-inch (1.6 mm). Crushed stone footings for precast foundations shall be installed in accordance with Figure R403.4(1) and Table R403.4. Crushed stone footings shall be consolidated using a vibratory plate in a maximum of 8-inch lifts. Crushed stone footings shall be limited to Seismic Design Categories A, B and C.

R403.4.2 Concrete footings. Concrete footings shall be installed in accordance with Section R403.1 and Figure R403.4(2).

SECTION R404
FOUNDATION AND RETAINING WALLS

R404.1 Concrete and masonry foundation walls. Concrete foundation walls shall be selected and constructed in accordance with the provisions of Section R404.1.2. Masonry foundation walls shall be selected and constructed in accordance with the provisions of Section R404.1.1.

R404.1.1 Design of masonry foundation walls. Masonry foundation walls shall be designed and constructed in accordance with the provisions of this section or in accordance with the provisions of ACI530/ASCE 5/TMS 402 or NCMA TR68-A. When ACI530/ASCE 5/TMS 402, NCMA TR68-A or the provisions of this section are used to design masonry foundation walls, project drawings, typical details and specifications are not required to bear the seal of the architect or engineer responsible for design, unless otherwise required by the state law of the *jurisdiction* having authority.

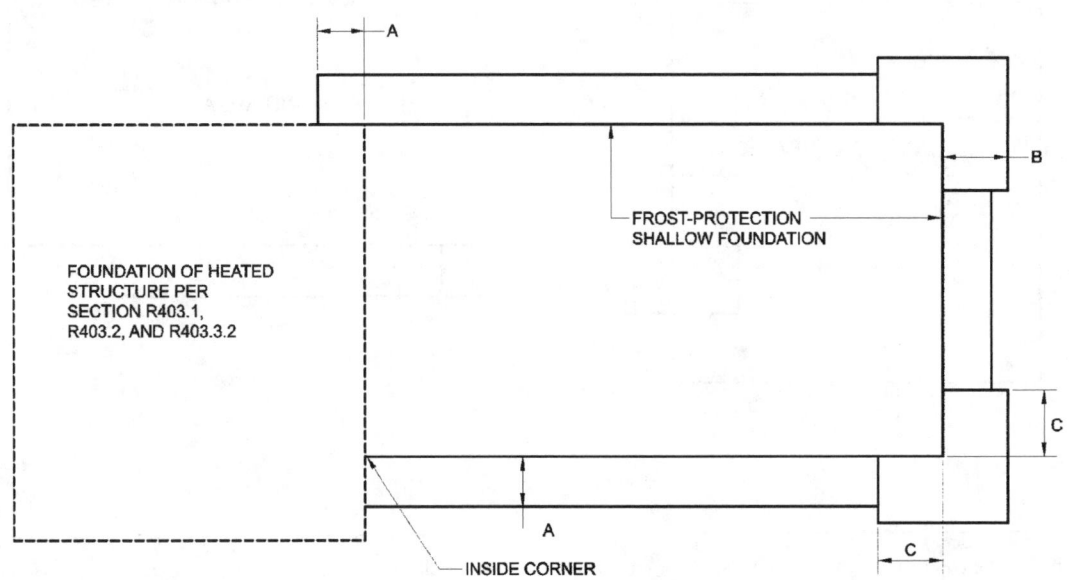

FIGURE R403.3(4)
INSULATION PLACEMENT FOR FROST-PROTECTED FOOTINGS ADJACENT TO HEATED STRUCTURE

TABLE R403.4
MINIMUM DEPTH OF CRUSHED STONE FOOTINGS (*D*), (inches)

		LOAD BEARING VALUE OF SOIL (psf)															
		1500				2000				3000				4000			
		MH, CH, CL, ML				SC, GC, SM, GM, SP, SW				GP, GW							
		Wall width (inches)				Wall width (inches)				Wall width (inches)				Wall width (inches)			
		6	8	10	12	6	8	10	12	6	8	10	12	6	8	10	12
Conventional light-frame construction																	
1-story	1100 plf	6	4	4	4	6	4	4	4	6	4	4	4	6	4	4	4
2-story	1800 plf	8	6	4	4	6	4	4	4	6	4	4	4	6	4	4	4
3-story	2000 plf	16	14	12	10	10	8	6	6	6	4	4	4	6	4	4	4
4-inch brick veneer over light-frame or 8-inch hollow concrete masonry																	
1-story	1500 plf	6	4	4	4	6	4	4	4	6	4	4	4	6	4	4	4
2-story	2700 plf	14	12	10	8	10	8	6	4	6	4	4	4	6	4	4	4
3-story	4000 plf	22	22	20	18	16	14	12	10	10	8	6	4	6	4	4	4
8-inch solid or fully grouted masonry																	
1-story	2000 plf	10	8	6	4	6	4	4	4	6	4	4	4	6	4	4	4
2-story	3600 plf	20	18	16	16	14	12	10	8	8	6	4	4	6	4	4	4
3-story	5300 plf	32	30	28	26	22	22	20	18	14	12	10	8	10	8	6	4

For SI: 1 inch = 25.4 mm, 1 pound per square inch = 6.89 kPa.

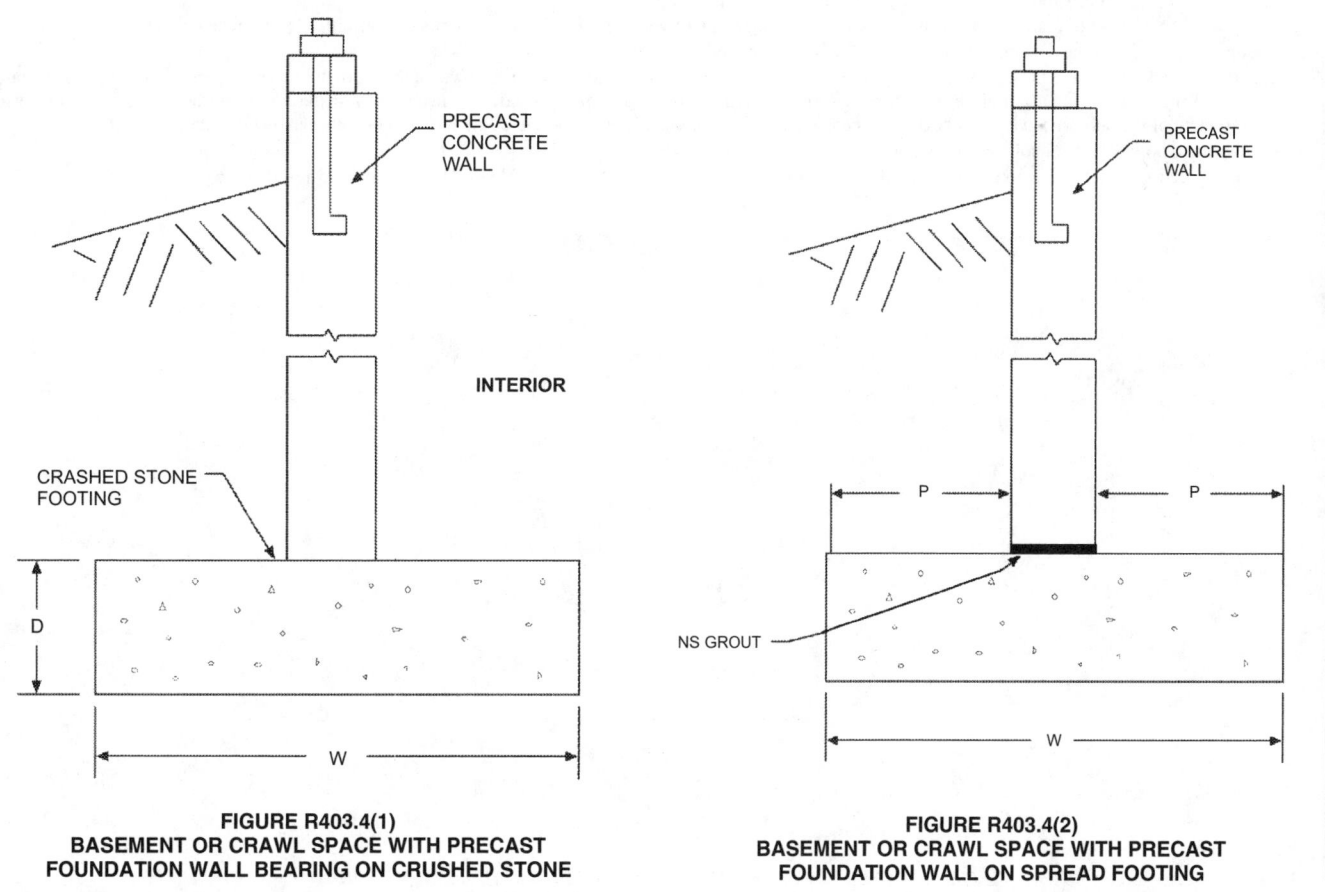

FIGURE R403.4(1)
BASEMENT OR CRAWL SPACE WITH PRECAST
FOUNDATION WALL BEARING ON CRUSHED STONE

FIGURE R403.4(2)
BASEMENT OR CRAWL SPACE WITH PRECAST
FOUNDATION WALL ON SPREAD FOOTING

TABLE R404.1.1(1)
PLAIN MASONRY FOUNDATION WALLS

MAXIMUM WALL HEIGHT (feet)	MAXIMUM UNBALANCED BACKFILL HEIGHT[c] (feet)	PLAIN MASONRY[a] MINIMUM NOMINAL WALL THICKNESS (inches)		
		Soil classes[b]		
		GW, GP, SW and SP	GM, GC, SM, SM-SC and ML	SC, MH, ML-CL and inorganic CL
5	4	6 solid[d] or 8	6 solid[d] or 8	6 solid[d] or 8
	5	6 solid[d] or 8	8	10
6	4	6 solid[d] or 8	6 solid[d] or 8	6 solid[d] or 8
	5	6 solid[d] or 8	8	10
	6	8	10	12
7	4	6 solid[d] or 8	8	8
	5	6 solid[d] or 8	10	10
	6	10	12	10 solid[d]
	7	12	10 solid[d]	12 solid[d]
8	4	6 solid[d] or 8	6 solid[d] or 8	8
	5	6 solid[d] or 8	10	12
	6	10	12	12 solid[d]
	7	12	12 solid[d]	Footnote e
	8	10 solid[d]	12 solid[d]	Footnote e
9	4	6 solid[d] or 8	6 solid[d] or 8	8
	5	8	10	12
	6	10	12	12 solid[d]
	7	12	12 solid[d]	Footnote e
	8	12 solid[d]	Footnote e	Footnote e
	9	Footnote e	Footnote e	Footnote e

For SI: 1 inch = 25.4 mm, 1 foot = 304.8 mm, 1 pound per square inch = 6.895 Pa.

a. Mortar shall be Type M or S and masonry shall be laid in running bond. Ungrouted hollow masonry units are permitted except where otherwise indicated.

b. Soil classes are in accordance with the Unified Soil Classification System. Refer to Table R405.1.

c. Unbalanced backfill height is the difference in height between the exterior finish ground level and the lower of the top of the concrete footing that supports the foundation wall or the interior finish ground level. Where an interior concrete slab-on-grade is provided and is in contact with the interior surface of the foundation wall, measurement of the unbalanced backfill height from the exterior finish ground level to the top of the interior concrete slab is permitted.

d. Solid grouted hollow units or solid masonry units.

e. Wall construction shall be in accordance with either Table R404.1.1(2), Table R404.1.1(3), Table R404.1.1(4), or a design shall be provided.

TABLE R404.1.1(2)
8-INCH MASONRY FOUNDATION WALLS WITH REINFORCING
WHERE d > 5 INCHES[a, c]

WALL HEIGHT	HEIGHT OF UNBALANCED BACKFILL[e]	MINIMUM VERTICAL REINFORCEMENT AND SPACING (INCHES)[b, c]		
		Soil classes and lateral soil load[d] (psf per foot below grade)		
		GW, GP, SW and SP soils 30	GM, GC, SM, SM-SC and ML soils 45	SC, ML-CL and inorganic CL soils 60
6 feet 8 inches	4 feet (or less)	#4 at 48	#4 at 48	#4 at 48
	5 feet	#4 at 48	#4 at 48	#4 at 48
	6 feet 8 inches	#4 at 48	#5 at 48	#6 at 48
7 feet 4 inches	4 feet (or less)	#4 at 48	#4 at 48	#4 at 48
	5 feet	#4 at 48	#4 at 48	#4 at 48
	6 feet	#4 at 48	#5 at 48	#5 at 48
	7 feet 4 inches	#5 at 48	#6 at 48	#6 at 40
8 feet	4 feet (or less)	#4 at 48	#4 at 48	#4 at 48
	5 feet	#4 at 48	#4 at 48	#4 at 48
	6 feet	#4 at 48	#5 at 48	#5 at 48
	7 feet	#5 at 48	#6 at 48	#6 at 40
	8 feet	#5 at 48	#6 at 48	#6 at 32
8 feet 8 inches	4 feet (or less)	#4 at 48	#4 at 48	#4 at 48
	5 feet	#4 at 48	#4 at 48	#5 at 48
	6 feet	#4 at 48	#5 at 48	#6 at 48
	7 feet	#5 at 48	#6 at 48	#6 at 40
	8 feet 8 inches	#6 at 48	#6 at 32	#6 at 24
9 feet 4 inches	4 feet (or less)	#4 at 48	#4 at 48	#4 at 48
	5 feet	#4 at 48	#4 at 48	#5 at 48
	6 feet	#4 at 48	#5 at 48	#6 at 48
	7 feet	#5 at 48	#6 at 48	#6 at 40
	8 feet	#6 at 48	#6 at 40	#6 at 24
	9 feet 4 inches	#6 at 40	#6 at 24	#6 at 16
10 feet	4 feet (or less)	#4 at 48	#4 at 48	#4 at 48
	5 feet	#4 at 48	#4 at 48	#5 at 48
	6 feet	#4 at 48	#5 at 48	#6 at 48
	7 feet	#5 at 48	#6 at 48	#6 at 32
	8 feet	#6 at 48	#6 at 32	#6 at 24
	9 feet	#6 at 40	#6 at 24	#6 at 16
	10 feet	#6 at 32	#6 at 16	#6 at 16

For SI: 1 inch = 25.4 mm, 1 foot = 304.8 mm, 1 pound per square foot per foot = 0.157 kPa/mm.

a. Mortar shall be Type M or S and masonry shall be laid in running bond.

b. Alternative reinforcing bar sizes and spacings having an equivalent cross-sectional area of reinforcement per lineal foot of wall shall be permitted provided the spacing of the reinforcement does not exceed 72 inches.

c. Vertical reinforcement shall be Grade 60 minimum. The distance, d, from the face of the soil side of the wall to the center of vertical reinforcement shall be at least 5 inches.

d. Soil classes are in accordance with the Unified Soil Classification System and design lateral soil loads are for moist conditions without hydrostatic pressure. Refer to Table R405.1.

e. Unbalanced backfill height is the difference in height between the exterior finish ground level and the lower of the top of the concrete footing that supports the foundation wall or the interior finish ground level. Where an interior concrete slab-on-grade is provided and is in contact with the interior surface of the foundation wall, measurement of the unbalanced backfill height from the exterior finish ground level to the top of the interior concrete slab is permitted.

TABLE R404.1.1(3)
10-INCH FOUNDATION WALLS WITH REINFORCING
WHERE d > 6.75 INCHES[a, c]

WALL HEIGHT	HEIGHT OF UNBALANCED BACKFILL[e]	MINIMUM VERTICAL REINFORCEMENT AND SPACING (INCHES)[b, c]		
		Soil classes and later soil load[d] (psf per foot below grade)		
		GW, GP, SW and SP soils 30	GM, GC, SM, SM-SC and ML soils 45	SC, ML-CL and inorganic CL soils 60
6 feet 8 inches	4 feet (or less)	#4 at 56	#4 at 56	#4 at 56
	5 feet	#4 at 56	#4 at 56	#4 at 56
	6 feet 8 inches	#4 at 56	#5 at 56	#5 at 56
7 feet 4 inches	4 feet (or less)	#4 at 56	#4 at 56	#4 at 56
	5 feet	#4 at 56	#4 at 56	#4 at 56
	6 feet	#4 at 56	#4 at 56	#5 at 56
	7 feet 4 inches	#4 at 56	#5 at 56	#6 at 56
8 feet	4 feet (or less)	#4 at 56	#4 at 56	#4 at 56
	5 feet	#4 at 56	#4 at 56	#4 at 56
	6 feet	#4 at 56	#4 at 56	#5 at 56
	7 feet	#4 at 56	#5 at 56	#6 at 56
	8 feet	#5 at 56	#6 at 56	#6 at 48
8 feet 8 inches	4 feet (or less)	#4 at 56	#4 at 56	#4 at 56
	5 feet	#4 at 56	#4 at 56	#4 at 56
	6 feet	#4 at 56	#4 at 56	#5 at 56
	7 feet	#4 at 56	#5 at 56	#6 at 56
	8 feet 8 inches	#5 at 56	#6 at 48	#6 at 32
9 feet 4 inches	4 feet (or less)	#4 at 56	#4 at 56	#4 at 56
	5 feet	#4 at 56	#4 at 56	#4 at 56
	6 feet	#4 at 56	#5 at 56	#5 at 56
	7 feet	#4 at 56	#5 at 56	#6 at 56
	8 feet	#5 at 56	#6 at 56	#6 at 40
	9 feet 4 inches	#6 at 56	#6 at 40	#6 at 24
10 feet	4 feet (or less)	#4 at 56	#4 at 56	#4 at 56
	5 feet	#4 at 56	#4 at 56	#4 at 56
	6 feet	#4 at 56	#5 at 56	#5 at 56
	7 feet	#5 at 56	#6 at 56	#6 at 48
	8 feet	#5 at 56	#6 at 48	#6 at 40
	9 feet	#6 at 56	#6 at 40	#6 at 24
	10 feet	#6 at 48	#6 at 32	#6 at 24

For SI: 1 inch = 25.4 mm, 1 foot = 304.8 mm, 1 pound per square foot per foot = 0.157 kPa/mm.

a. Mortar shall be Type M or S and masonry shall be laid in running bond.

b. Alternative reinforcing bar sizes and spacings having an equivalent cross-sectional area of reinforcement per lineal foot of wall shall be permitted provided the spacing of the reinforcement does not exceed 72 inches.

c. Vertical reinforcement shall be Grade 60 minimum. The distance, d, from the face of the soil side of the wall to the center of vertical reinforcement shall be at least 6.75 inches.

d. Soil classes are in accordance with the Unified Soil Classification System and design lateral soil loads are for moist conditions without hydrostatic pressure. Refer to Table R405.1.

e. Unbalanced backfill height is the difference in height between the exterior finish ground level and the lower of the top of the concrete footing that supports the foundation wall or the interior finish ground level. Where an interior concrete slab-on-grade is provided and is in contact with the interior surface of the foundation wall, measurement of the unbalanced backfill height from the exterior finish ground level to the top of the interior concrete slab is permitted.

TABLE R404.1.1(4)
12-INCH MASONRY FOUNDATION WALLS WITH REINFORCING
WHERE d > 8.75 INCHES[a, c]

WALL HEIGHT	HEIGHT OF UNBALANCED BACKFILL[e]	MINIMUM VERTICAL REINFORCEMENT AND SPACING (INCHES)[b, c]		
		Soil classes and lateral soil load[d] (psf per foot below *grade*)		
		GW, GP, SW and SP soils 30	GM, GC, SM, SM-SC and ML soils 45	SC, ML-CL and inorganic CL soils 60
6 feet 8 inches	4 feet (or less)	#4 at 72	#4 at 72	#4 at 72
	5 feet	#4 at 72	#4 at 72	#4 at 72
	6 feet 8 inches	#4 at 72	#4 at 72	#5 at 72
7 feet 4 inches	4 feet (or less)	#4 at 72	#4 at 72	#4 at 72
	5 feet	#4 at 72	#4 at 72	#4 at 72
	6 feet	#4 at 72	#4 at 72	#5 at 72
	7 feet 4 inches	#4 at 72	#5 at 72	#6 at 72
8 feet	4 feet (or less)	#4 at 72	#4 at 72	#4 at 72
	5 feet	#4 at 72	#4 at 72	#4 at 72
	6 feet	#4 at 72	#4 at 72	#5 at 72
	7 feet	#4 at 72	#5 at 72	#6 at 72
	8 feet	#5 at 72	#6 at 72	#6 at 64
8 feet 8 inches	4 feet (or less)	#4 at 72	#4 at 72	#4 at 72
	5 feet	#4 at 72	#4 at 72	#4 at 72
	6 feet	#4 at 72	#4 at 72	#5 at 72
	7 feet	#4 at 72	#5 at 72	#6 at 72
	8 feet 8 inches	#5 at 72	#7 at 72	#6 at 48
9 feet 4 inches	4 feet (or less)	#4 at 72	#4 at 72	#4 at 72
	5 feet	#4 at 72	#4 at 72	#4 at 72
	6 feet	#4 at 72	#5 at 72	#5 at 72
	7 feet	#4 at 72	#5 at 72	#6 at 72
	8 feet	#5 at 72	#6 at 72	#6 at 56
	9 feet 4 inches	#6 at 72	#6 at 48	#6 at 40
10 feet	4 feet (or less)	#4 at 72	#4 at 72	#4 at 72
	5 feet	#4 at 72	#4 at 72	#4 at 72
	6 feet	#4 at 72	#5 at 72	#5 at 72
	7 feet	#4 at 72	#6 at 72	#6 at 72
	8 feet	#5 at 72	#6 at 72	#6 at 48
	9 feet	#6 at 72	#6 at 56	#6 at 40
	10 feet	#6 at 64	#6 at 40	#6 at 32

For SI: 1 inch = 25.4 mm, 1 foot = 304.8 mm, 1 pound per square foot per foot = 0.157 kPa/mm.

a. Mortar shall be Type M or S and masonry shall be laid in running bond.

b. Alternative reinforcing bar sizes and spacings having an equivalent cross-sectional area of reinforcement per lineal foot of wall shall be permitted provided the spacing of the reinforcement does not exceed 72 inches.

c. Vertical reinforcement shall be Grade 60 minimum. The distance, d, from the face of the soil side of the wall to the center of vertical reinforcement shall be at least 8.75 inches.

d. Soil classes are in accordance with the Unified Soil Classification System and design lateral soil loads are for moist conditions without hydrostatic pressure. Refer to Table R405.1.

e. Unbalanced backfill height is the difference in height between the exterior finish ground level and the lower of the top of the concrete footing that supports the foundation wall or the interior finish ground levels. Where an interior concrete slab-on-grade is provided and in contact with the interior surface of the foundation wall, measurement of the unbalanced backfill height is permitted to be measured from the exterior finish ground level to the top of the interior concrete slab is permitted.

R404.1.1.1 Masonry foundation walls. Concrete masonry and clay masonry foundation walls shall be constructed as set forth in Table R404.1.1(1), R404.1.1(2), R404.1.1(3) or R404.1.1(4) and shall also comply with applicable provisions of Sections R606, R607 and R608. In buildings assigned to Seismic Design Categories D_0, D_1 and D_2, concrete masonry and clay masonry foundation walls shall also comply with Section R404.1.4.1. Rubble stone masonry foundation walls shall be constructed in accordance with Sections R404.1.8 and R607.2.2. Rubble stone masonry walls shall not be used in Seismic Design Categories D_0, D_1 and D_2.

R404.1.2 Concrete foundation walls. Concrete foundation walls that support light-frame walls shall be designed and constructed in accordance with the provisions of this section, ACI 318, ACI 332 or PCA 100. Concrete foundation walls that support above-grade concrete walls that are within the applicability limits of Section R611.2 shall be designed and constructed in accordance with the provisions of this section, ACI 318, ACI 332 or PCA 100. Concrete foundation walls that support above-grade concrete walls that are not within the applicability limits of Section R611.2 shall be designed and constructed in accordance with the provisions of ACI 318, ACI 332 or PCA 100. When ACI 318, ACI 332, PCA 100 or the provisions of this section are used to design concrete foundation walls, project drawings, typical details and specifications are not required to bear the seal of the architect or engineer responsible for design, unless otherwise required by the state law of the *jurisdiction* having authority.

R404.1.2.1 Concrete cross-section. Concrete walls constructed in accordance with this code shall comply with the shapes and minimum concrete cross-sectional dimensions required by Table R611.3. Other types of forming systems resulting in concrete walls not in compliance with this section and Table R611.3 shall be designed in accordance with ACI 318.

R404.1.2.2 Reinforcement for foundation walls. Concrete foundation walls shall be laterally supported at the top and bottom. Horizontal reinforcement shall be provided in accordance with Table R404.1.2(1). Vertical reinforcement shall be provided in accordance with Table R404.1.2(2), R404.1.2(3), R404.1.2(4), R404.1.2(5), R404.1.2(6), R404.1.2(7) or R404.1.2(8). Vertical reinforcement for flat *basement* walls retaining 4 feet (1219 mm) or more of unbalanced backfill is permitted to be determined in accordance with Table R404.1.2(9). For *basement* walls supporting above-grade concrete walls, vertical reinforcement shall be the greater of that required by Tables R404.1.2(2) through R404.1.2(8) or by Section R611.6 for the above-grade wall. In buildings assigned to Seismic Design Category D_0, D_1 or D_2, concrete foundation walls shall also comply with Section R404.1.4.2.

R404.1.2.2.1 Concrete foundation stem walls supporting above-grade concrete walls. Foundation stem walls that support above-grade concrete walls shall be designed and constructed in accordance with this section.

1. Stem walls not laterally supported at top. Concrete stem walls that are not monolithic with slabs-on-ground or are not otherwise laterally supported by slabs-on-ground shall comply with this section. Where unbalanced backfill retained by the stem wall is less than or equal to 18 inches (457 mm), the stem wall and above-grade wall it supports shall be provided with vertical reinforcement in accordance with Section R611.6 and Table R611.6(1), R611.6(2) or R611.6(3) for above-grade walls. Where unbalanced backfill retained by the stem wall is greater than 18 inches (457 mm), the stem wall and above-grade wall it supports shall be provided with vertical reinforcement in accordance with Section R611.6 and Table R611.6(4).

2. Stem walls laterally supported at top. Concrete stem walls that are monolithic with slabs-on-ground or are otherwise laterally supported by slabs-on-ground shall be vertically reinforced in accordance with Section R611.6 and Table R611.6(1), R611.6(2) or R611.6(3) for above-grade walls. Where the unbalanced backfill retained by the stem wall is greater than 18 inches (457 mm), the connection between the stem wall and the slab-on-ground, and the portion of the slab-on-ground providing lateral support for the wall shall be designed in accordance with PCA 100 or in accordance with accepted engineering practice. Where the unbalanced backfill retained by the stem wall is greater than 18 inches (457 mm), the minimum nominal thickness of the wall shall be 6 inches (152 mm).

R404.1.2.2.2 Concrete foundation stem walls supporting light-frame above-grade walls. Concrete foundation stem walls that support light-frame above-grade walls shall be designed and constructed in accordance with this section.

1. Stem walls not laterally supported at top. Concrete stem walls that are not monolithic with slabs-on-ground or are not otherwise laterally supported by slabs-on-ground and retain 48 inches (1219 mm) or less of unbalanced fill, measured from the top of the wall, shall be constructed in accordance with Section R404.1.2. Foundation stem walls that retain more than 48 inches (1219 mm) of unbalanced fill, measured from the top of the wall, shall be designed in accordance with Sections R404.1.3 and R404.4.

2. Stem walls laterally supported at top. Concrete stem walls that are monolithic with slabs-on-ground or are otherwise laterally supported by slabs-on-ground shall be constructed in accordance with Section R404.1.2. Where the unbalanced backfill retained by the stem wall is greater than 48 inches (1219 mm), the connection between the stem wall and the slab-on- ground, and the portion of the slab-on-ground providing lateral support for the wall shall be designed in accordance with PCA 100 or in accordance with accepted engineering practice.

TABLE R404.1.2(1)
MINIMUM HORIZONTAL REINFORCEMENT FOR CONCRETE BASEMENT WALLS[a, b]

MAXIMUM UNSUPPORTED HEIGHT OF BASEMENT WALL (feet)	LOCATION OF HORIZONTAL REINFORCEMENT
≤ 8	One No. 4 bar within 12 inches of the top of the wall story and one No. 4 bar near mid-height of the wall story
> 8	One No. 4 bar within 12 inches of the top of the wall story and one No. 4 bar near third points in the wall story

For SI: 1 inch = 25.4 mm, 1 foot = 304.8 mm, 1 pound per square inch = 6.895 kPa.

a. Horizontal reinforcement requirements are for reinforcing bars with a minimum yield strength of 40,000 psi and concrete with a minimum concrete compressive strength 2,500 psi.

b. See Section R404.1.2.2 for minimum reinforcement required for foundation walls supporting above-grade concrete walls.

TABLE R404.1.2(2)
MINIMUM VERTICAL REINFORCEMENT FOR 6-INCH NOMINAL FLAT CONCRETE BASEMENT WALLS[b, c, d, e, g, h, i, j]

MAXIMUM UNSUPPORTED WALL HEIGHT (feet)	MAXIMUM UNBALANCED BACKFILL HEIGHT[f] (feet)	MINIMUM VERTICAL REINFORCEMENT—BAR SIZE AND SPACING (inches)		
		Soil classes[a] and design lateral soil (psf per foot of depth)		
		GW, GP, SW, SP 30	GM, GC, SM, SM-SC and ML 45	SC, ML-CL and inorganic CL 60
8	4	NR	NR	NR
	5	NR	6 @ 39	6 @ 48
	6	5 @ 39	6 @ 48	6 @ 35
	7	6 @ 48	6 @ 34	6 @ 25
	8	6 @ 39	6 @ 25	6 @ 18
9	4	NR	NR	NR
	5	NR	5 @ 37	6 @ 48
	6	5 @ 36	6 @ 44	6 @ 32
	7	6 @ 47	6 @ 30	6 @ 22
	8	6 @ 34	6 @ 22	6 @ 16
	9	6 @ 27	6 @ 17	DR
10	4	NR	NR	NR
	5	NR	5 @ 35	6 @ 48
	6	6 @ 48	6 @ 41	6 @ 30
	7	6 @ 43	6 @ 28	6 @ 20
	8	6 @ 31	6 @ 20	DR
	9	6 @ 24	6 @ 15	DR
	10	6 @ 19	DR	DR

For SI:1 foot = 304.8 mm; 1 inch = 25.4 mm; 1 pound per square foot per foot = 0.1571 kPa²/m, 1 pound per square inch = 6.895 kPa.

a. Soil classes are in accordance with the Unified Soil Classification System. Refer to Table R405.1.

b. Table values are based on reinforcing bars with a minimum yield strength of 60,000 psi concrete with a minimum specified compressive strength of 2,500 psi and vertical reinforcement being located at the centerline of the wall. See Section R404.1.2.3.7.2.

c. Vertical reinforcement with a yield strength of less than 60,000 psi and/or bars of a different size than specified in the table are permitted in accordance with Section R404.1.2.3.7.6 and Table R404.1.2(9).

d. Deflection criterion is $L/240$, where L is the height of the basement wall in inches.

e. Interpolation is not permitted.

f. Where walls will retain 4 feet or more of unbalanced backfill, they shall be laterally supported at the top and bottom before backfilling.

g. NR indicates no vertical wall reinforcement is required, except for 6-inch nominal walls formed with stay-in-place forming systems in which case vertical reinforcement shall be No. 4@48 inches on center.

h. See Section R404.1.2.2 for minimum reinforcement required for basement walls supporting above-grade concrete walls.

i. See Table R611.3 for tolerance from nominal thickness permitted for flat walls.

j. DR means design is required in accordance with the applicable building code, or where there is no code, in accordance with ACI 318.

R404.1.2.3 Concrete, materials for concrete, and forms. Materials used in concrete, the concrete itself and forms shall conform to requirements of this section or ACI 318.

R404.1.2.3.1 Compressive strength. The minimum specified compressive strength of concrete, f'$_c$, shall comply with Section R402.2 and shall be not less than 2,500 psi (17.2 MPa) at 28 days in buildings assigned to Seismic Design Category A, B or C and 3000 psi (20.5 MPa) in buildings assigned to Seismic Design Category D$_0$, D$_1$ or D$_2$.

R404.1.2.3.2 Concrete mixing and delivery. Mixing and delivery of concrete shall comply with ASTM C 94 or ASTM C 685.

R404.1.2.3.3 Maximum aggregate size. The nominal maximum size of coarse aggregate shall not exceed one-fifth the narrowest distance between sides of forms, or three-fourths the clear spacing between reinforcing bars or between a bar and the side of the form.

Exception: When *approved*, these limitations shall not apply where removable forms are used and workability and methods of consolidation permit concrete to be placed without honeycombs or voids.

TABLE R404.1.2(3)
MINIMUM VERTICAL REINFORCEMENT FOR 8-INCH (203 mm) NOMINAL FLAT CONCRETE BASEMENT WALLS[b, c, d, e, f, h, i]

| MAXIMUM UNSUPPORTED WALL HEIGHT (feet) | MAXIMUM UNBALANCED BACKFILL HEIGHT[g] (feet) | MINIMUM VERTICAL REINFORCEMENT—BAR SIZE AND SPACING (inches) | | |
| | | Soil classes[a] and design lateral soil (psf per foot of depth) | | |
		GW, GP, SW, SP 30	GM, GC, SM, SM-SC and ML 45	SC, ML-CL and inorganic CL 60
8	4	NR	NR	NR
	5	NR	NR	NR
	6	NR	NR	6 @ 37
	7	NR	6 @ 36	6 @ 35
	8	6 @ 41	6 @ 35	6 @ 26
9	4	NR	NR	NR
	5	NR	NR	NR
	6	NR	NR	6 @ 35
	7	NR	6 @ 35	6 @ 32
	8	6 @ 36	6 @ 32	6 @ 23
	9	6 @ 35	6 @ 25	6 @ 18
10	4	NR	NR	NR
	5	NR	NR	NR
	6	NR	NR	6 @ 35
	7	NR	6 @ 35	6 @ 29
	8	6 @ 35	6 @ 29	6 @ 21
	9	6 @ 34	6 @ 22	6 @ 16
	10	6 @ 27	6 @ 17	6 @ 13

For SI: 1 foot = 304.8 mm; 1 inch = 25.4 mm; 1 pound per square foot per foot = 0.1571 kPa^2/m, 1 pound per square inch = 6.895 kPa.

a. Soil classes are in accordance with the Unified Soil Classification System. Refer to Table R405.1.

b. Table values are based on reinforcing bars with a minimum yield strength of 60,000 psi (420 MPa), concrete with a minimum specified compressive strength of 2,500 psi and vertical reinforcement being located at the centerline of the wall. See Section R404.1.2.3.7.2.

c. Vertical reinforcement with a yield strength of less than 60,000 psi and/or bars of a different size than specified in the table are permitted in accordance with Section R404.1.2.3.7.6 and Table R404.1.2(9).

d. NR indicates no vertical reinforcement is required.

e. Deflection criterion is L/240, where L is the height of the basement wall in inches.

f. Interpolation is not permitted.

g. Where walls will retain 4 feet or more of unbalanced backfill, they shall be laterally supported at the top and bottom before backfilling.

h. See Section R404.1.2.2 for minimum reinforcement required for basement walls supporting above-grade concrete walls.

i. See Table R611.3 for tolerance from nominal thickness permitted for flat walls.

R404.1.2.3.4 Proportioning and slump of concrete. Proportions of materials for concrete shall be established to provide workability and consistency to permit concrete to be worked readily into forms and around reinforcement under conditions of placement to be employed, without segregation or excessive bleeding. Slump of concrete placed in removable forms shall not exceed 6 inches (152 mm).

Exception: When *approved*, the slump is permitted to exceed 6 inches (152 mm) for concrete mixtures that are resistant to segregation, and are in accordance with the form manufacturer's recommendations.

Slump of concrete placed in stay-in-place forms shall exceed 6 inches (152 mm). Slump of concrete shall be determined in accordance with ASTM C 143.

R404.1.2.3.5 Consolidation of concrete. Concrete shall be consolidated by suitable means during placement and shall be worked around embedded items and reinforcement and into corners of forms. Where stay-in-place forms are used, concrete shall be consolidated by internal vibration.

Exception: When *approved* for concrete to be placed in stay-in-place forms, self-consolidating concrete mixtures with slumps equal to or greater than 8 inches (203 mm) that are specifically designed for placement without internal vibration need not be internally vibrated.

TABLE R404.1.2(4)
MINIMUM VERTICAL REINFORCEMENT FOR 10-INCH NOMINAL FLAT CONCRETE BASEMENT WALLS[b, c, d, e, f, h, i]

MAXIMUM UNSUPPORTED WALL HEIGHT (feet)	MAXIMUM UNBALANCED BACKFILL HEIGHT[g] (feet)	MINIMUM VERTICAL REINFORCEMENT—BAR SIZE AND SPACING (inches)		
		Soil classes[a] and design lateral soil (psf per foot of depth)		
		GW, GP, SW, SP 30	GM, GC, SM, SM-SC and ML 45	SC, ML-CL and inorganic CL 60
8	4	NR	NR	NR
	5	NR	NR	NR
	6	NR	NR	NR
	7	NR	NR	NR
	8	6 @ 48	6 @ 35	6 @ 28
9	4	NR	NR	NR
	5	NR	NR	NR
	6	NR	NR	NR
	7	NR	NR	6 @ 31
	8	NR	6 @ 31	6 @ 28
	9	6 @ 37	6 @ 28	6 @ 24
10	4	NR	NR	NR
	5	NR	NR	NR
	6	NR	NR	NR
	7	NR	NR	6 @ 28
	8	NR	6 @ 28	6 @ 28
	9	6 @ 33	6 @ 28	6 @ 21
	10	6 @ 28	6 @ 23	6 @ 17

For SI: 1 foot = 304.8 mm; 1 inch = 25.4 mm; 1 pound per square foot per foot = 0.1571 kPa^2/m, 1 pound per square inch = 6.895 kPa.

a. Soil classes are in accordance with the Unified Soil Classification System. Refer to Table R405.1.

b. Table values are based on reinforcing bars with a minimum yield strength of 60,000 psi concrete with a minimum specified compressive strength of 2,500 psi and vertical reinforcement being located at the centerline of the wall. See Section R404.1.2.3.7.2.

c. Vertical reinforcement with a yield strength of less than 60,000 psi and/or bars of a different size than specified in the table are permitted in accordance with Section R404.1.2.3.7.6 and Table R404.1.2(9).

d. NR indicates no vertical reinforcement is required.

e. Deflection criterion is $L/240$, where L is the height of the basement wall in inches.

f. Interpolation is not permitted.

g. Where walls will retain 4 feet or more of unbalanced backfill, they shall be laterally supported at the top and bottom before backfilling.

h. See Section R404.1.2.2 for minimum reinforcement required for basement walls supporting above-grade concrete walls.

i. See Table R611.3 for tolerance from nominal thickness permitted for flat walls.

R404.1.2.3.6 Form materials and form ties. Forms shall be made of wood, steel, aluminum, plastic, a composite of cement and foam insulation, a composite of cement and wood chips, or other *approved* material suitable for supporting and containing concrete. Forms shall provide sufficient strength to contain concrete during the concrete placement operation.

Form ties shall be steel, solid plastic, foam plastic, a composite of cement and wood chips, a composite of cement and foam plastic, or other suitable material capable of resisting the forces created by fluid pressure of fresh concrete.

R404.1.2.3.6.1 Stay-in-place forms. Stay-in-place concrete forms shall comply with this section.

1. Surface burning characteristics. The flame-spread index and smoke-developed index of forming material, other than foam plastic, left exposed on the interior shall comply with Section R302. The surface burning characteristics of foam plastic used in insulating concrete forms shall comply with Section R316.3.

2. Interior covering. Stay-in-place forms constructed of rigid foam plastic shall be protected on the interior of the building as required by Section R316. Where gypsum board is used to protect the foam plastic, it shall be installed with a mechanical fastening system. Use of adhesives in addition to mechanical fasteners is permitted.

3. Exterior wall covering. Stay-in-place forms constructed of rigid foam plastics shall be

TABLE R404.1.2(5)
MINIMUM VERTICAL WALL REINFORCEMENT FOR 6-INCH WAFFLE-GRID BASEMENT WALLS[b, c, d, e, g, h, i]

MAXIMUM UNSUPPORTED WALL HEIGHT (feet)	MAXIMUM UNBALANCED BACKFILL HEIGHT[f] (feet)	MINIMUM VERTICAL REINFORCEMENT—BAR SIZE AND SPACING (inches)		
		Soil classes[a] and design lateral soil (psf per foot of depth)		
		GW, GP, SW, SP 30	GM, GC, SM, SM-SC and ML 45	SC, ML-CL and inorganic CL 60
8	4	4 @ 48	4 @ 46	6 @ 39
	5	4 @ 45	5 @ 46	6 @ 47
	6	5 @ 45	6 @ 40	DR
	7	6 @ 44	DR	DR
	8	6 @ 32	DR	DR
9	4	4 @ 48	4 @ 46	4 @ 37
	5	4 @ 42	5 @ 43	6 @ 44
	6	5 @ 41	6 @ 37	DR
	7	6 @ 39	DR	DR
	> 8	DR[i]	DR	DR
10	4	4 @ 48	4 @ 46	4 @ 35
	5	4 @ 40	5 @ 40	6 @ 41
	6	5 @ 38	6 @ 34	DR
	7	6 @ 36	DR	DR
	> 8	DR	DR	DR

For SI: 1 foot = 304.8 mm; 1 inch = 25.4 mm; 1 pound per square foot per foot = 0.1571 kPa^2/m, 1 pound per square inch = 6.895 kPa.

a. Soil classes are in accordance with the Unified Soil Classification System. Refer to Table R405.1.

b. Table values are based on reinforcing bars with a minimum yield strength of 60,000 psi concrete with a minimum specified compressive strength of 2,500 psi and vertical reinforcement being located at the centerline of the wall. See Section R404.1.2.3.7.2.

c. Maximum spacings shown are the values calculated for the specified bar size. Where the bar used is Grade 60 and the size specified in the table, the actual spacing in the wall shall not exceed a whole-number multiple of 12 inches (i.e., 12, 24, 36 and 48) that is less than or equal to the tabulated spacing. Vertical reinforcement with a yield strength of less than 60,000 psi and/or bars of a different size than specified in the table are permitted in accordance with Section R404.1.2.3.7.6 and Table R404.1.2(9).

d. Deflection criterion is L/240, where L is the height of the basement wall in inches.

e. Interpolation is not permitted.

f. Where walls will retain 4 feet or more of unbalanced backfill, they shall be laterally supported at the top and bottom before backfilling.

g. See Section R404.1.2.2 for minimum reinforcement required for basement walls supporting above-grade concrete walls.

h. See Table R611.3 for thicknesses and dimensions of waffle-grid walls.

i. DR means design is required in accordance with the applicable building code, or where there is no code, in accordance with ACI 318.

protected from sunlight and physical damage by the application of an *approved* exterior wall covering complying with this code. Exterior surfaces of other stay-in-place forming systems shall be protected in accordance with this code.

4. Termite hazards. In areas where hazard of termite damage is very heavy in accordance with Figure R301.2(6), foam plastic insulation shall be permitted below *grade* on foundation walls in accordance with one of the following conditions:

4.1. Where in addition to the requirements in Section R318.1, an *approved* method of protecting the foam plastic and structure from subterranean termite damage is provided.

4.2. The structural members of walls, floors, ceilings and roofs are entirely of noncombustible materials or pressure-preservative-treated wood.

4.3. On the interior side of *basement* walls.

TABLE R404.1.2(6)
MINIMUM VERTICAL REINFORCEMENT FOR 8-INCH WAFFLE-GRID BASEMENT WALLS[b, c, d, e, f, h, i, j]

MAXIMUM UNSUPPORTED WALL HEIGHT (feet)	MAXIMUM UNBALANCED BACKFILL HEIGHT[g] (feet)	MINIMUM VERTICAL REINFORCEMENT—BAR SIZE AND SPACING (inches)		
		Soil classes[a] and design lateral soil (psf per foot of depth)		
		GW, GP, SW, SP 30	GM, GC, SM, SM-SC and ML 45	SC, ML-CL and inorganic CL 60
8	4	NR	NR	NR
	5	NR	5 @ 48	5 @ 46
	6	5 @ 48	5 @ 43	6 @ 45
	7	5 @ 46	6 @ 43	6 @ 31
	8	6 @ 48	6 @ 32	6 @ 23
9	4	NR	NR	NR
	5	NR	5 @ 47	5 @ 46
	6	5 @ 46	5 @ 39	6 @ 41
	7	5 @ 42	6 @ 38	6 @ 28
	8	6 @ 44	6 @ 28	6 @ 20
	9	6 @ 34	6 @ 21	DR
10	4	NR	NR	NR
	5	NR	5 @ 46	5 @ 44
	6	5 @ 46	5 @ 37	6 @ 38
	7	5 @ 38	6 @ 35	6 @ 25
	8	6 @ 39	6 @ 25	DR
	9	6 @ 30	DR	DR
	10	6 @ 24	DR	DR

For SI: 1 foot = 304.8 mm; 1 inch = 25.4 mm; 1 pound per square foot per foot = 0.1571 kPa²/m, 1 pound per square inch = 6.895 kPa.

a. Soil classes are in accordance with the Unified Soil Classification System. Refer to Table R405.1.

b. Table values are based on reinforcing bars with a minimum yield strength of 60,000 psi concrete with a minimum specified compressive strength of 2,500 psi and vertical reinforcement being located at the centerline of the wall. See Section R404.1.2.3.7.2.

c. Maximum spacings shown are the values calculated for the specified bar size. Where the bar used is Grade 60 (420 MPa) and the size specified in the table, the actual spacing in the wall shall not exceed a whole-number multiple of 12 inches (i.e., 12, 24, 36 and 48) that is less than or equal to the tabulated spacing. Vertical reinforcement with a yield strength of less than 60,000 psi and/or bars of a different size than specified in the table are permitted in accordance with Section R404.1.2.3.7.6 and Table R404.1.2(9).

d. NR indicates no vertical reinforcement is required.

e. Deflection criterion is $L/240$, where L is the height of the basement wall in inches.

f. Interpolation shall not be permitted.

g. Where walls will retain 4 feet or more of unbalanced backfill, they shall be laterally supported at the top and bottom before backfilling.

h. See Section R404.1.2.2 for minimum reinforcement required for basement walls supporting above-grade concrete walls.

i. See Table R611.3 for thicknesses and dimensions of waffle-grid walls.

j. DR means design is required in accordance with the applicable building code, or where there is no code, in accordance with ACI 318.

TABLE R404.1.2(7)
MINIMUM VERTICAL REINFORCEMENT FOR 6-INCH (152 mm) SCREEN-GRID BASEMENT WALLS[b, c, d, e, g, h, i,]

MAXIMUM UNSUPPORTED WALL HEIGHT (feet)	MAXIMUM UNBALANCED BACKFILL HEIGHT[f] (feet)	MINIMUM VERTICAL REINFORCEMENT—BAR SIZE AND SPACING (inches)		
		Soil classes[a] and design lateral soil (psf per foot of depth)		
		GW, GP, SW, SP 30	GM, GC, SM, SM-SC and ML 45	SC, ML-CL and inorganic CL 60
8	4	4 @ 48	4 @ 48	5 @ 43
	5	4 @ 48	5 @ 48	5 @ 37
	6	5 @ 48	6 @ 45	6 @ 32
	7	6 @ 48	DR	DR
	8	6 @ 36	DR	DR
9	4	4 @ 48	4 @ 48	4 @ 41
	5	4 @ 48	5 @ 48	6 @ 48
	6	5 @ 45	6 @ 41	DR
	7	6 @ 43	DR	DR
	> 8	DR	DR	DR
10	4	4 @ 48	4 @ 48	4 @ 39
	5	4 @ 44	5 @ 44	6 @ 46
	6	5 @ 42	6 @ 38	DR
	7	6 @ 40	DR	DR
	> 8	DR	DR	DR

For SI: 1 foot = 304.8 mm; 1 inch = 25.4 mm; 1 pound per square foot per foot = 0.1571 kPa²/m, 1 pound per square inch = 6.895 kPa.

a. Soil classes are in accordance with the Unified Soil Classification System. Refer to Table R405.1.

b. Table values are based on reinforcing bars with a minimum yield strength of 60,000 psi (420 MPa), concrete with a minimum specified compressive strength of 2,500 psi and vertical reinforcement being located at the centerline of the wall. See Section R404.1.2.3.7.2.

c. Maximum spacings shown are the values calculated for the specified bar size. Where the bar used is Grade 60 and the size specified in the table, the actual spacing in the wall shall not exceed a whole-number multiple of 12 inches (i.e., 12, 24, 36 and 48) that is less than or equal to the tabulated spacing. Vertical reinforcement with a yield strength of less than 60,000 psi and/or bars of a different size than specified in the table are permitted in accordance with Section R404.1.2.3.7.6 and Table R404.1.2(9).

d. Deflection criterion is $L/240$, where L is the height of the basement wall in inches.

e. Interpolation is not permitted.

f. Where walls will retain 4 feet or more of unbalanced backfill, they shall be laterally supported at the top and bottom before backfilling.

g. See Sections R404.1.2.2 for minimum reinforcement required for basement walls supporting above-grade concrete walls.

h. See Table R611.3 for thicknesses and dimensions of screen-grid walls.

i. DR means design is required in accordance with the applicable building code, or where there is no code, in accordance with ACI 318.

R404.1.2.3.7 Reinforcement.

R404.1.2.3.7.1 Steel reinforcement. Steel reinforcement shall comply with the requirements of ASTM A 615, A 706, or A 996. ASTM A 996 bars produced from rail steel shall be Type R. In buildings assigned to Seismic Design Category A, B or C, the minimum yield strength of reinforcing steel shall be 40,000 psi (Grade 40) (276 MPa). In buildings assigned to Seismic Design Category D_0, D_1 or D_2, reinforcing steel shall comply with the requirements of ASTM A 706 for low-alloy steel with a minimum yield strength of 60,000 psi (Grade 60) (414 MPa).

R404.1.2.3.7.2 Location of reinforcement in wall. The center of vertical reinforcement in *basement* walls determined from Tables R404.1.2(3) through R404.1.2(7) shall be located at the center-line of the wall. Vertical reinforcement in *basement* walls determined from Tables R404.1.2(2) or R404.1.2(8) shall be located to provide a maximum cover of 1.25 inches (32 mm) measured from the inside face of the wall. Regardless of the table used to determine vertical wall reinforcement, the center of the steel shall not vary from the specified location by more than the greater of 10 percent of the wall thickness and $^3/_8$-inch (10 mm). Horizontal and vertical reinforcement shall be located in foundation walls to provide the minimum cover required by Section R404.1.2.3.7.4.

R404.1.2.3.7.3 Wall openings. Vertical wall reinforcement required by Section R404.1.2.2 that is interrupted by wall openings shall have additional vertical reinforcement of the same size placed within 12 inches (305 mm) of each side of the opening.

TABLE R404.1.2(8)
MINIMUM VERTICAL REINFORCEMENT FOR 6-, 8-, 10-INCH AND 12-INCH NOMINAL FLAT BASEMENT WALLS[b, c, d, e, f, h, i, k, n]

MAXIMUM WALL HEIGHT (feet)	MAXIMUM UNBALANCED BACKFILL HEIGHT[g] (feet)	MINIMUM VERTICAL REINFORCEMENT—BAR SIZE AND SPACING (inches)											
		Soil classes[a] and design lateral soil (psf per foot of depth)											
		GW, GP, SW, SP 30				GM, GC, SM, SM-SC and ML 45				SC, ML-CL and inorganic CL 60			
		Minimum nominal wall thickness (inches)											
		6	8	10	12	6	8	10	12	6	8	10	12
5	4	NR	NR	NR	NR	NR	NR	NR	NR	NR	NR	NR	NR
	5	NR	NR	NR	NR	NR	NR	NR	NR	NR	NR	NR	NR
6	4	NR	NR	NR	NR	NR	NR	NR	NR	NR	NR	NR	NR
	5	NR	NR	NR	NR	NR	NR[l]	NR	NR	4 @ 35	NR[l]	NR	NR
	6	NR	NR	NR	NR	5 @ 48	NR	NR	NR	5 @ 36	NR	NR	NR
7	4	NR	NR	NR	NR	NR	NR	NR	NR	NR	NR	NR	NR
	5	NR	NR	NR	NR	NR	NR	NR	NR	5 @ 47	NR	NR	NR
	6	NR	NR	NR	NR	5 @ 42	NR	NR	NR	6 @ 43	5 @ 48	NR[l]	NR
	7	5 @ 46	NR	NR	NR	6 @ 42	5 @ 46	NR[l]	NR	6 @ 34	6 @ 48	NR	NR
8	4	NR	NR	NR	NR	NR	NR	NR	NR	NR	NR	NR	NR
	5	NR	NR	NR	NR	4 @ 38	NR[l]	NR	NR	5 @ 43	NR	NR	NR
	6	4 @ 37	NR[l]	NR	NR	5 @ 37	NR	NR	NR	6 @ 37	5 @ 43	NR[l]	NR
	7	5 @ 40	NR	NR	NR	6 @ 37	5 @ 41	NR[l]	NR	6 @ 34	6 @ 43	NR	NR
	8	6 @ 43	5 @ 47	NR[l]	NR	6 @ 34	6 @ 43	NR	NR	6 @ 27	6 @ 32	6 @ 44	NR
9	4	NR	NR	NR	NR	NR	NR	NR	NR	NR	NR	NR	NR
	5	NR	NR	NR	NR	4 @ 35	NR[l]	NR	NR	5 @ 40	NR	NR	NR
	6	4 @ 34	NR[l]	NR	NR	6 @ 48	NR	NR	NR	6 @ 36	6 @ 39	NR[l]	NR
	7	5 @ 36	NR	NR	NR	6 @ 34	5 @ 37	NR	NR	6 @ 33	6 @ 38	5 @ 37	NR[l]
	8	6 @ 38	5 @ 41	NR[l]	NR	6 @ 33	6 @ 38	5 @ 37	NR[l]	6 @ 24	6 @ 29	6 @ 39	4 @ 48[m]
	9	6 @ 34	6 @ 46	NR	NR	6 @ 26	6 @ 30	6 @ 41	NR	6 @ 19	6 @ 23	6 @ 30	6 @ 39
10	4	NR	NR	NR	NR	NR	NR	NR	NR	NR	NR	NR	NR
	5	NR	NR	NR	NR	4 @ 33	NR[l]	NR	NR	5 @ 38	NR	NR	NR
	6	5 @ 48	NR[l]	NR	NR	6 @ 45	NR	NR	NR	6 @ 34	5 @ 37	NR	NR
	7	6 @ 47	NR	NR	NR	6 @ 34	6 @ 48	NR	NR	6 @ 30	6 @ 35	6 @ 48	NR[l]
	8	6 @ 34	5 @ 38	NR	NR	6 @ 30	6 @ 34	6 @ 47	NR[l]	6 @ 22	6 @ 26	6 @ 35	6 @ 45[m]
	9	6 @ 34	6 @ 41	4 @ 48	NR[l]	6 @ 23	6 @ 27	6 @ 35	4 @ 48[m]	DR	6 @ 22	6 @ 27	6 @ 34
	10	6 @ 28	6 @ 33	6 @ 45	NR	DR[j]	6 @ 23	6 @ 29	6 @ 38	DR	6 @ 22	6 @ 22	6 @ 28

For SI: 1 foot = 304.8 mm; 1 inch = 25.4 mm; 1 pound per square foot per foot = 0.1571 kPa^2/m, 1 pound per square inch = 6.895 kPa.

a. Soil classes are in accordance with the Unified Soil Classification System. Refer to Table R405.1.

b. Table values are based on reinforcing bars with a minimum yield strength of 60,000 psi.

c. Vertical reinforcement with a yield strength of less than 60,000 psi and/or bars of a different size than specified in the table are permitted in accordance with Section R404.1.2.3.7.6 and Table R404.1.2(9).

d. NR indicates no vertical wall reinforcement is required, except for 6-inch nominal walls formed with stay-in-place forming systems in which case vertical reinforcement shall be #4@48 inches on center.

e. Allowable deflection criterion is L/240, where L is the unsupported height of the basement wall in inches.

f. Interpolation is not permitted.

g. Where walls will retain 4 feet or more of unbalanced backfill, they shall be laterally supported at the top and bottom before backfilling.

h. Vertical reinforcement shall be located to provide a cover of 1.25 inches measured from the inside face of the wall. The center of the steel shall not vary from the specified location by more than the greater of 10 percent of the wall thickness or $^3/_8$-inch.

i. Concrete cover for reinforcement measured from the inside face of the wall shall not be less than $^3/_4$-inch. Concrete cover for reinforcement measured from the outside face of the wall shall not be less than $1^1/_2$ inches for No. 5 bars and smaller, and not less than 2 inches for larger bars.

j. DR means design is required in accordance with the applicable building code, or where there is no code in accordance with ACI 318.

k. Concrete shall have a specified compressive strength, f'_c, of not less than 2,500 psi at 28 days, unless a higher strength is required by footnote l or m.

l. The minimum thickness is permitted to be reduced 2 inches, provided the minimum specified compressive strength of concrete, f'_c, is 4,000 psi.

m. A plain concrete wall with a minimum nominal thickness of 12 inches is permitted, provided minimum specified compressive strength of concrete, f'_c, is 3,500 psi.

n. See Table R611.3 for tolerance from nominal thickness permitted for flat walls.

TABLE R404.1.2(9)
MINIMUM SPACING FOR ALTERNATE BAR SIZE AND/OR ALTERNATE GRADE OF STEEL[a, b, c]

BAR SPACING FROM APPLICABLE TABLE IN SECTION R404.1.2.2 (inches)	BAR SIZE FROM APPLICABLE TABLE IN SECTION R404.1.2.2														
	#4					#5					#6				
	Alternate bar size and/or alternate grade of steel desired														
	Grade 60		Grade 40			Grade 60		Grade 40			Grade 60		Grade 40		
	#5	#6	#4	#5	#6	#4	#6	#4	#5	#6	#4	#5	#4	#5	#6
	Maximum spacing for alternate bar size and/or alternate grade of steel (inches)														
8	12	18	5	8	12	5	11	3	5	8	4	6	2	4	5
9	14	20	6	9	13	6	13	4	6	9	4	6	3	4	6
10	16	22	7	10	15	6	14	4	7	9	5	7	3	5	7
11	17	24	7	11	16	7	16	5	7	10	5	8	3	5	7
12	19	26	8	12	18	8	17	5	8	11	5	8	4	6	8
13	20	29	9	13	19	8	18	6	9	12	6	9	4	6	9
14	22	31	9	14	21	9	20	6	9	13	6	10	4	7	9
15	23	33	10	16	22	10	21	6	10	14	7	11	5	7	10
16	25	35	11	17	23	10	23	7	11	15	7	11	5	8	11
17	26	37	11	18	25	11	24	7	11	16	8	12	5	8	11
18	28	40	12	19	26	12	26	8	12	17	8	13	5	8	12
19	29	42	13	20	28	12	27	8	13	18	9	13	6	9	13
20	31	44	13	21	29	13	28	9	13	19	9	14	6	9	13
21	33	46	14	22	31	14	30	9	14	20	10	15	6	10	14
22	34	48	15	23	32	14	31	9	15	21	10	16	7	10	15
23	36	48	15	24	34	15	33	10	15	22	10	16	7	11	15
24	37	48	16	25	35	15	34	10	16	23	11	17	7	11	16
25	39	48	17	26	37	16	35	11	17	24	11	18	8	12	17
26	40	48	17	27	38	17	37	11	17	25	12	18	8	12	17
27	42	48	18	28	40	17	38	12	18	26	12	19	8	13	18
28	43	48	19	29	41	18	40	12	19	26	13	20	8	13	19
29	45	48	19	30	43	19	41	12	19	27	13	20	9	14	19
30	47	48	20	31	44	19	43	13	20	28	14	21	9	14	20
31	48	48	21	32	45	20	44	13	21	29	14	22	9	15	21
32	48	48	21	33	47	21	45	14	21	30	15	23	10	15	21
33	48	48	22	34	48	21	47	14	22	31	15	23	10	16	22
34	48	48	23	35	48	22	48	15	23	32	15	24	10	16	23
35	48	48	23	36	48	23	48	15	23	33	16	25	11	16	23
36	48	48	24	37	48	23	48	15	24	34	16	25	11	17	24
37	48	48	25	38	48	24	48	16	25	35	17	26	11	17	25
38	48	48	25	39	48	25	48	16	25	36	17	27	12	18	25
39	48	48	26	40	48	25	48	17	26	37	18	27	12	18	26
40	48	48	27	41	48	26	48	17	27	38	18	28	12	19	27
41	48	48	27	42	48	26	48	18	27	39	19	29	12	19	27
42	48	48	28	43	48	27	48	18	28	40	19	30	13	20	28
43	48	48	29	44	48	28	48	18	29	41	20	30	13	20	29
44	48	48	29	45	48	28	48	19	29	42	20	31	13	21	29
45	48	48	30	47	48	29	48	19	30	43	20	32	14	21	30

(continued)

TABLE R404.1.2(9)—continued
MINIMUM SPACING FOR ALTERNATE BAR SIZE AND/OR ALTERNATE GRADE OF STEEL[a, b, c]

BAR SPACING FROM APPLICABLE TABLE IN SECTION R404.1.2.2 (inches)	BAR SIZE FROM APPLICABLE TABLE IN SECTION R404.1.2.2														
	#4					#5					#6				
	Alternate bar size and/or alternate grade of steel desired to be used														
	Grade 60		Grade 40			Grade 60		Grade 40			Grade 60		Grade 40		
	#5	#6	#4	#5	#6	#4	#6	#4	#5	#6	#4	#5	#4	#5	#6
	Maximum spacing for alternate bar size and/or alternate grade of steel (inches)														
46	48	48	31	48	48	30	48	20	31	44	21	32	14	22	31
47	48	48	31	48	48	30	48	20	31	44	21	33	14	22	31
48	48	48	32	48	48	31	48	21	32	45	22	34	15	23	32

For SI: 1 inch = 25.4 mm, 1 pound per square inch = 6.895 kPa.

a. This table is for use with tables in Section R404.1.2.2 that specify the minimum bar size and maximum spacing of vertical wall reinforcement for foundation walls and above-grade walls. Reinforcement specified in tables in Sections R404.1.2.2 is based on Grade 60 steel reinforcement.

b. Bar spacing shall not exceed 48 inches on center and shall not be less than one-half the nominal wall thickness.

c. For Grade 50 steel bars (ASTM A 996, Type R), use spacing for Grade 40 bars or interpolate between Grades 40 and 60.

R404.1.2.3.7.4 Support and cover. Reinforcement shall be secured in the proper location in the forms with tie wire or other bar support system to prevent displacement during the concrete placement operation. Steel reinforcement in concrete cast against the earth shall have a minimum cover of 3 inches (75 mm). Minimum cover for reinforcement in concrete cast in removable forms that will be exposed to the earth or weather shall be $1^{1}/_{2}$ inches (38 mm) for No. 5 bars and smaller, and 2 inches (50 mm) for No. 6 bars and larger. For concrete cast in removable forms that will not be exposed to the earth or weather, and for concrete cast in stay-in-place forms, minimum cover shall be $^{3}/_{4}$ inch (19 mm). The minus tolerance for cover shall not exceed the smaller of one-third the required cover or $^{3}/_{8}$ inch (10 mm).

R404.1.2.3.7.5 Lap splices. Vertical and horizontal wall reinforcement shall be the longest lengths practical. Where splices are necessary in reinforcement, the length of lap splice shall be in accordance with Table R611.5.4.(1) and Figure R611.5.4(1). The maximum gap between noncontact parallel bars at a lap splice shall not exceed the smaller of one-fifth the required lap length and 6 inches (152 mm). See Figure R611.5.4(1).

R404.1.2.3.7.6 Alternate grade of reinforcement and spacing. Where tables in Section R404.1.2.2 specify vertical wall reinforcement based on minimum bar size and maximum spacing, which are based on Grade 60 (414 MPa) steel reinforcement, different size bars and/or bars made from a different grade of steel are permitted provided an equivalent area of steel per linear foot of wall is provided. Use of Table R404.1.2(9) is permitted to determine the maximum bar spacing for different bar sizes than specified in the tables and/or bars made from a different grade of steel. Bars shall not be spaced less than one-half the wall thickness, or more than 48 inches (1219 mm) on center.

R404.1.2.3.7.7 Standard hooks. Where reinforcement is required by this code to terminate with a standard hook, the hook shall comply with Section R611.5.4.5 and Figure R611.5.4(3).

R404.1.2.3.7.8 Construction joint reinforcement. Construction joints in foundation walls shall be made and located to not impair the strength of the wall. Construction joints in plain concrete walls, including walls required to have not less than No. 4 bars at 48 inches (1219 mm) on center by Sections R404.1.2.2 and R404.1.4.2, shall be located at points of lateral support, and a minimum of one No. 4 bar shall extend across the construction joint at a spacing not to exceed 24 inches (610 mm) on center. Construction joint reinforcement shall have a minimum of 12 inches (305 mm) embedment on both sides of the joint. Construction joints in reinforced concrete walls shall be located in the middle third of the span between lateral supports, or located and constructed as required for joints in plain concrete walls.

Exception: Use of vertical wall reinforcement required by this code is permitted in lieu of construction joint reinforcement provided the spacing does not exceed 24 inches (610 mm), or the combination of wall reinforcement and No.4 bars described above does not exceed 24 inches (610 mm).

R404.1.2.3.8 Exterior wall coverings. Requirements for installation of masonry veneer, stucco and other wall coverings on the exterior of concrete walls and other construction details not covered in this section shall comply with the requirements of this code.

R404.1.2.4 Requirements for Seismic Design Category C. Concrete foundation walls supporting above-grade concrete walls in townhouses assigned to Seismic Design Category C shall comply with ACI 318, ACI 332 or PCA 100 (see Section R404.1.2).

R404.1.3 Design required. Concrete or masonry foundation walls shall be designed in accordance with accepted engineering practice when either of the following conditions exists:

1. Walls are subject to hydrostatic pressure from groundwater.

2. Walls supporting more than 48 inches (1219 mm) of unbalanced backfill that do not have permanent lateral support at the top or bottom.

R404.1.4 Seismic Design Category D_0, D_1 or D_2.

R404.1.4.1 Masonry foundation walls. In addition to the requirements of Table R404.1.1(1) plain masonry foundation walls in buildings assigned to Seismic Design Category D_0, D_1 or D_2, as established in Table R301.2(1), shall comply with the following.

1. Wall height shall not exceed 8 feet (2438 mm).

2. Unbalanced backfill height shall not exceed 4 feet (1219 mm).

3. Minimum nominal thickness for plain masonry foundation walls shall be 8 inches (203 mm).

4. Masonry stem walls shall have a minimum vertical reinforcement of one No. 3 (No. 10) bar located a maximum of 4 feet (1219 mm) on center in grouted cells. Vertical reinforcement shall be tied to the horizontal reinforcement in the footings.

Foundation walls in buildings assigned to Seismic Design Category D_0, D_1 or D_2, as established in Table R301.2(1), supporting more than 4 feet (1219 mm) of unbalanced backfill or exceeding 8 feet (2438 mm) in height shall be constructed in accordance with Table R404.1.1(2), R404.1.1(3) or R404.1.1(4). Masonry foundation walls shall have two No. 4 (No. 13) horizontal bars located in the upper 12 inches (305 mm) of the wall.

R404.1.4.2 Concrete foundation walls. In buildings assigned to Seismic Design Category D_0, D_1 or D_2, as established in Table R301.2(1), concrete foundation walls that support light-frame walls shall comply with this section, and concrete foundation walls that support above-grade concrete walls shall comply with ACI 318, ACI 332 or PCA 100 (see Section R404.1.2). In addition to the horizontal reinforcement required by Table R404.1.2(1), plain concrete walls supporting light-frame walls shall comply with the following.

1. Wall height shall not exceed 8 feet (2438 mm).

2. Unbalanced backfill height shall not exceed 4 feet (1219 mm).

3. Minimum thickness for plain concrete foundation walls shall be 7.5 inches (191 mm) except that 6 inches (152 mm) is permitted where the maximum wall height is 4 feet, 6 inches (1372 mm).

Foundation walls less than 7.5 inches (191 mm) in thickness, supporting more than 4 feet (1219 mm) of unbalanced backfill or exceeding 8 feet (2438 mm) in height shall be provided with horizontal reinforcement in

accordance with Table R404.1.2(1), and vertical reinforcement in accordance with Table R404.1.2(2), R404.1.2(3), R404.1.2(4), R404.1.2(5), R404.1.2(6), R404.1.2(7) or R404.1.2(8). Where Tables R404.1.2(2) through R404.1.2(8) permit plain concrete walls, not less than No. 4 (No. 13) vertical bars at a spacing not exceeding 48 inches (1219 mm) shall be provided.

R404.1.5 Foundation wall thickness based on walls supported. The thickness of masonry or concrete foundation walls shall not be less than that required by Section R404.1.5.1 or R404.1.5.2, respectively.

R404.1.5.1 Masonry wall thickness. Masonry foundation walls shall not be less than the thickness of the wall supported, except that masonry foundation walls of at least 8-inch (203 mm) nominal thickness shall be permitted under brick veneered frame walls and under 10-inch-wide (254 mm) cavity walls where the total height of the wall supported, including gables, is not more than 20 feet (6096 mm), provided the requirements of Section R404.1.1 are met.

R404.1.5.2 Concrete wall thickness. The thickness of concrete foundation walls shall be equal to or greater than the thickness of the wall in the *story* above. Concrete foundation walls with corbels, brackets or other projections built into the wall for support of masonry veneer or other purposes are not within the scope of the tables in this section.

Where a concrete foundation wall is reduced in thickness to provide a shelf for the support of masonry veneer, the reduced thickness shall be equal to or greater than the thickness of the wall in the *story* above. Vertical reinforcement for the foundation wall shall be based on Table R404.1.2(8) and located in the wall as required by Section R404.1.2.3.7.2 where that table is used. Vertical reinforcement shall be based on the thickness of the thinner portion of the wall.

Exception: Where the height of the reduced thickness portion measured to the underside of the floor assembly or sill plate above is less than or equal to 24 inches (610 mm) and the reduction in thickness does not exceed 4 inches (102 mm), the vertical reinforcement is permitted to be based on the thicker portion of the wall.

R404.1.5.3 Pier and curtain wall foundations. Use of pier and curtain wall foundations shall be permitted to support light-frame construction not more than two stories in height, provided the following requirements are met:

1. All load-bearing walls shall be placed on continuous concrete footings placed integrally with the exterior wall footings.

2. The minimum actual thickness of a load-bearing masonry wall shall be not less than 4 inches (102 mm) nominal or $3^3/_8$ inches (92 mm) actual thickness, and shall be bonded integrally with piers spaced in accordance with Section R606.9.

3. Piers shall be constructed in accordance with Section R606.6 and Section R606.6.1, and shall be

bonded into the load-bearing masonry wall in accordance with Section R608.1.1 or Section R608.1.1.2.

4. The maximum height of a 4-inch (102 mm) load-bearing masonry foundation wall supporting wood-frame walls and floors shall not be more than 4 feet (1219 mm).

5. Anchorage shall be in accordance with Section R403.1.6, Figure R404.1.5(1), or as specified by engineered design accepted by the *building official*.

6. The unbalanced fill for 4-inch (102 mm) foundation walls shall not exceed 24 inches (610 mm) for solid masonry or 12 inches (305 mm) for hollow masonry.

7. In Seismic Design Categories D_0, D_1 and D_2, prescriptive reinforcement shall be provided in the horizontal and vertical direction. Provide minimum horizontal joint reinforcement of two No.9 gage wires spaced not less than 6 inches (152 mm) or one $^1/_4$ inch (6.4 mm) diameter wire at 10 inches (254 mm) on center vertically. Provide minimum vertical reinforcement of one No. 4 bar at 48 inches (1220 mm) on center horizontally grouted in place.

R404.1.6 Height above finished grade. Concrete and masonry foundation walls shall extend above the finished *grade* adjacent to the foundation at all points a minimum of 4 inches (102 mm) where masonry veneer is used and a minimum of 6 inches (152 mm) elsewhere.

R404.1.7 Backfill placement. Backfill shall not be placed against the wall until the wall has sufficient strength and has been anchored to the floor above, or has been sufficiently braced to prevent damage by the backfill.

> **Exception:** Bracing is not required for walls supporting less than 4 feet (1219 mm) of unbalanced backfill.

R404.1.8 Rubble stone masonry. Rubble stone masonry foundation walls shall have a minimum thickness of 16 inches (406 mm), shall not support an unbalanced backfill exceeding 8 feet (2438 mm) in height, shall not support a soil pressure greater than 30 pounds per square foot per foot (4.71 kPa/m), and shall not be constructed in Seismic Design Categories D_0, D_1, D_2 or townhouses in Seismic Design Category C, as established in Figure R301.2(2).

R404.2 Wood foundation walls. Wood foundation walls shall be constructed in accordance with the provisions of Sections R404.2.1 through R404.2.6 and with the details shown in Figures R403.1(2) and R403.1(3).

R404.2.1 Identification. All load-bearing lumber shall be identified by the grade *mark* of a lumber grading or inspection agency which has been *approved* by an accreditation body that complies with DOC PS 20. In lieu of a grade *mark*,

a certificate of inspection issued by a lumber grading or inspection agency meeting the requirements of this section shall be accepted. Wood structural panels shall conform to DOC PS 1 or DOC PS 2 and shall be identified by a grade *mark* or certificate of inspection issued by an *approved agency*.

R404.2.2 Stud size. The studs used in foundation walls shall be 2-inch by 6-inch (51 mm by 152 mm) members. When spaced 16 inches (406 mm) on center, a wood species with an F_b value of not less than 1,250 pounds per square inch (8619 kPa) as listed in AF&PA/NDS shall be used. When spaced 12 inches (305 mm) on center, an F_b of not less than 875 psi (6033 kPa) shall be required.

R404.2.3 Height of backfill. For wood foundations that are not designed and installed in accordance with AF&PA PWF, the height of backfill against a foundation wall shall not exceed 4 feet (1219 mm). When the height of fill is more than 12 inches (305 mm) above the interior *grade* of a crawl space or floor of a *basement*, the thickness of the plywood sheathing shall meet the requirements of Table R404.2.3.

R404.2.4 Backfilling. Wood foundation walls shall not be backfilled until the *basement* floor and first floor have been constructed or the walls have been braced. For crawl space construction, backfill or bracing shall be installed on the interior of the walls prior to placing backfill on the exterior.

R404.2.5 Drainage and dampproofing. Wood foundation basements shall be drained and dampproofed in accordance with Sections R405 and R406, respectively.

R404.2.6 Fastening. Wood structural panel foundation wall sheathing shall be attached to framing in accordance with Table R602.3(1) and Section R402.1.1.

R404.3 Wood sill plates. Wood sill plates shall be a minimum of 2-inch by 4-inch (51 mm by 102 mm) nominal lumber. Sill plate anchorage shall be in accordance with Sections R403.1.6 and R602.11.

R404.4 Retaining walls. Retaining walls that are not laterally supported at the top and that retain in excess of 24 inches (610 mm) of unbalanced fill shall be designed to ensure stability against overturning, sliding, excessive foundation pressure and water uplift. Retaining walls shall be designed for a safety factor of 1.5 against lateral sliding and overturning.

404.5 Precast concrete foundation walls.

R404.5.1 Design. Precast concrete foundation walls shall be designed in accordance with accepted engineering practice. The design and manufacture of precast concrete foundation wall panels shall comply with the materials requirements of Section R402.3 or ACI 318. The panel design drawings shall be prepared by a registered design professional where required by the statutes of the *jurisdiction* in which the project is to be constructed in accordance with Section R106.1.

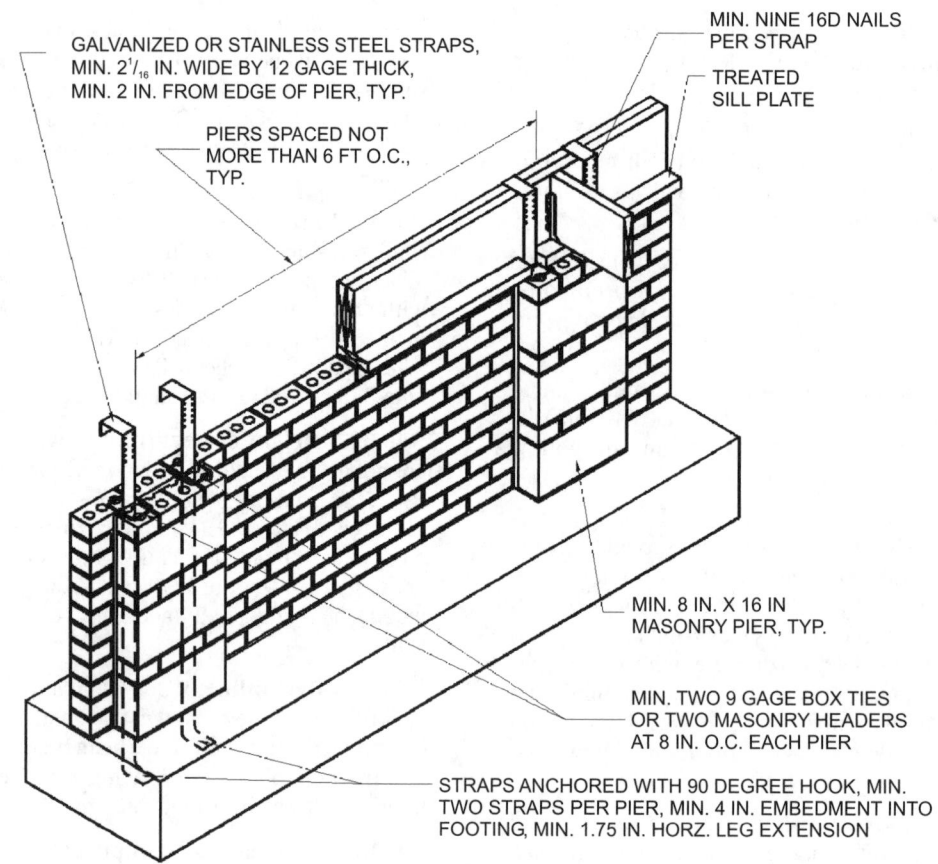

GALVANIZED OR STAINLESS STEEL STRAPS,
MIN. 2$^1/_{16}$ IN. WIDE BY 12 GAGE THICK,
MIN. 2 IN. FROM EDGE OF PIER, TYP.

PIERS SPACED NOT
MORE THAN 6 FT O.C.,
TYP.

MIN. NINE 16D NAILS
PER STRAP

TREATED
SILL PLATE

MIN. 8 IN. X 16 IN
MASONRY PIER, TYP.

MIN. TWO 9 GAGE BOX TIES
OR TWO MASONRY HEADERS
AT 8 IN. O.C. EACH PIER

STRAPS ANCHORED WITH 90 DEGREE HOOK, MIN.
TWO STRAPS PER PIER, MIN. 4 IN. EMBEDMENT INTO
FOOTING, MIN. 1.75 IN. HORZ. LEG EXTENSION

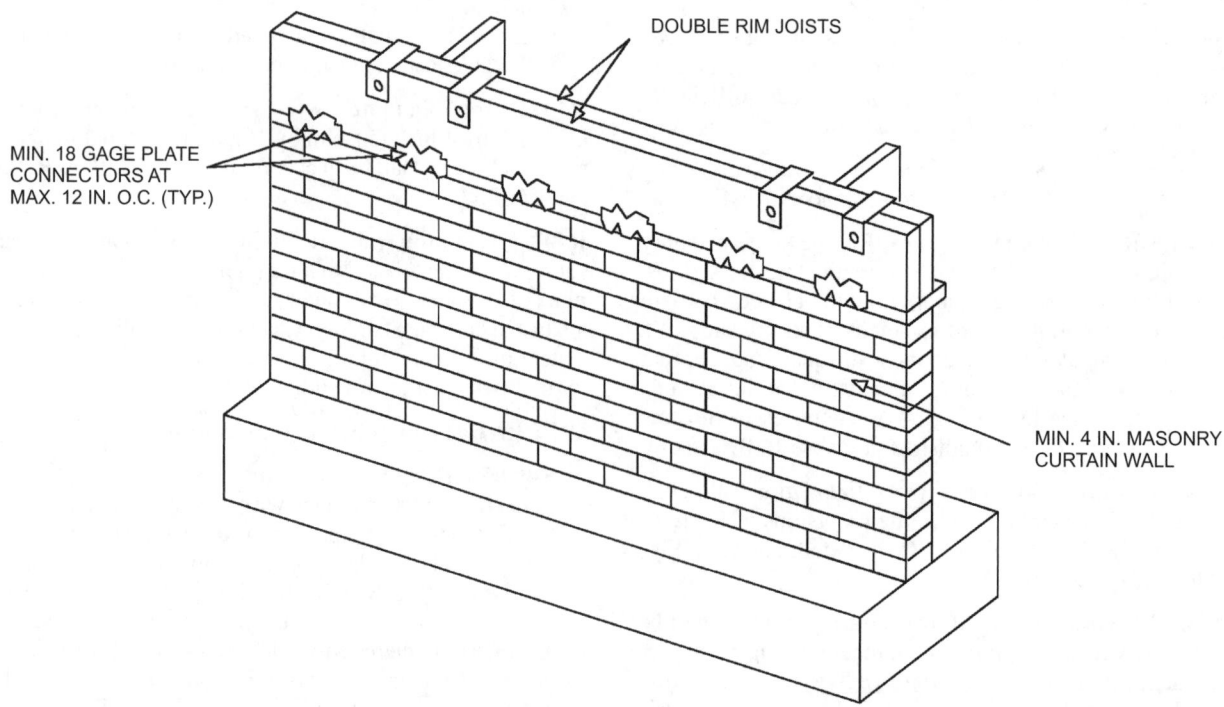

DOUBLE RIM JOISTS

MIN. 18 GAGE PLATE
CONNECTORS AT
MAX. 12 IN. O.C. (TYP.)

MIN. 4 IN. MASONRY
CURTAIN WALL

For SI: 1 inch = 25.4 mm, 1 foot = 304.8 mm, 1 degree = 0.0175 rad.

FIGURE R404.1.5(1)
FOUNDATION WALL CLAY MASONRY CURTAIN WALL WITH CONCRETE MASONRY PIERS

TABLE R404.2.3
PLYWOOD GRADE AND THICKNESS FOR WOOD FOUNDATION CONSTRUCTION
(30 pcf equivalent-fluid weight soil pressure)

HEIGHT OF FILL (inches)	STUD SPACING (inches)	FACE GRAIN ACROSS STUDS			FACE GRAIN PARALLEL TO STUDS		
		Grade[a]	Minimum thickness (inches)	Span rating	Grade[a]	Minimum thickness (inches)[b, c]	Span rating
24	12	B	$^{15}/_{32}$	32/16	A	$^{15}/_{32}$	32/16
					B	$^{15}/_{32}{}^c$	32/16
	16	B	$^{15}/_{32}$	32/16	A	$^{15}/_{32}{}^c$	32/16
					B	$^{19}/_{32}{}^c$ (4, 5 ply)	40/20
36	12	B	$^{15}/_{32}$	32/16	A	$^{15}/_{32}$	32/16
					B	$^{15}/_{32}{}^c$ (4, 5 ply)	32/16
					B	$^{19}/_{32}$ (4, 5 ply)	40/20
	16	B	$^{15}/_{32}{}^c$	32/16	A	$^{19}/_{32}$	40/20
					B	$^{23}/_{32}$	48/24
48	12	B	$^{15}/_{32}$	32/16	A	$^{15}/_{32}{}^c$	32/16
					B	$^{19}/_{32}{}^c$ (4, 5 ply)	40/20
	16	B	$^{19}/_{32}$	40/20	A	$^{19}/_{32}{}^c$	40/20
					A	$^{23}/_{32}$	48/24

For SI: 1 inch = 25.4 mm, 1 foot = 304.8 mm, 1 pound per cubic foot = 0.1572 kN/m³.

a. Plywood shall be of the following minimum grades in accordance with DOC PS 1 or DOC PS 2:

  1. DOC PS 1 Plywood grades marked:

    1.1. Structural I C-D (Exposure 1)

    1.2. C-D (Exposure 1)

  2. DOC PS 2 Plywood grades marked:

    2.1. Structural I Sheathing (Exposure 1)

    2.2. Sheathing (Exposure 1)

  3. Where a major portion of the wall is exposed above ground and a better appearance is desired, the following plywood grades marked exterior are suitable:

    3.1. Structural I A-C, Structural I B-C or Structural I C-C (Plugged) in accordance with DOC PS 1

    3.2. A-C Group 1, B-C Group 1, C-C (Plugged) Group 1 or MDO Group 1 in accordance with DOC PS 1

    3.3. Single Floor in accordance with DOC PS 1 or DOC PS 2

b. Minimum thickness $^{15}/_{32}$ inch, except crawl space sheathing may be $^3/_8$ inch for face grain across studs 16 inches on center and maximum 2-foot depth of unequal fill.

c. For this fill height, thickness and grade combination, panels that are continuous over less than three spans (across less than three stud spacings) require blocking 16 inches above the bottom plate. Offset adjacent blocks and fasten through studs with two 16d corrosion-resistant nails at each end.

R404.5.2 Precast concrete foundation design drawings. Precast concrete foundation wall design drawings shall be submitted to the *building official* and *approved* prior to installation. Drawings shall include, at a minimum, the information specified below:

  1. Design loading as applicable;

  2. Footing design and material;

  3. Concentrated loads and their points of application;

  4. Soil bearing capacity;

  5. Maximum allowable total uniform load;

  6. Seismic design category; and

  7. Basic wind speed.

R404.5.3 Identification. Precast concrete foundation wall panels shall be identified by a certificate of inspection *label* issued by an *approved* third party inspection agency.

SECTION R405
FOUNDATION DRAINAGE

R405.1 Concrete or masonry foundations. Drains shall be provided around all concrete or masonry foundations that retain earth and enclose habitable or usable spaces located below *grade*. Drainage tiles, gravel or crushed stone drains, perforated pipe or other *approved* systems or materials shall be installed at or below the area to be protected and shall discharge by gravity or mechanical means into an *approved* drainage system. Gravel or crushed stone drains shall extend at least 1 foot (305 mm) beyond the outside edge of the footing and 6 inches (152 mm) above the top of the footing and be covered with an *approved* filter membrane material. The top of open joints of drain tiles shall be protected with strips of building paper, and the drainage tiles or perforated pipe shall be placed on a minimum of 2 inches (51 mm) of washed gravel or crushed rock at least one sieve size larger than the tile joint opening or perforation and covered with not less than 6 inches (152 mm) of the same material.

Exception: A drainage system is not required when the foundation is installed on well-drained ground or sand-gravel mixture soils according to the Unified Soil Classification System, Group I Soils, as detailed in Table R405.1.

R405.1.1 Precast concrete foundation. Precast concrete walls that retain earth and enclose habitable or useable space located below-grade that rest on crushed stone footings shall have a perforated drainage pipe installed below the base of the wall on either the interior or exte-

rior side of the wall, at least one foot (305 mm) beyond the edge of the wall. If the exterior drainage pipe is used, an *approved* filter membrane material shall cover the pipe. The drainage system shall discharge into an *approved* sewer system or to daylight.

R405.2 Wood foundations. Wood foundations enclosing habitable or usable spaces located below *grade* shall be adequately drained in accordance with Sections R405.2.1 through R405.2.3.

R405.2.1 Base. A porous layer of gravel, crushed stone or coarse sand shall be placed to a minimum thickness of 4 inches (102 mm) under the *basement* floor. Provision shall be made for automatic draining of this layer and the gravel or crushed stone wall footings.

R405.2.2 Vapor retarder. A 6-mil-thick (0.15 mm) polyethylene vapor retarder shall be applied over the porous layer with the *basement* floor constructed over the polyethylene.

TABLE R405.1
PROPERTIES OF SOILS CLASSIFIED ACCORDING TO THE UNIFIED SOIL CLASSIFICATION SYSTEM

SOIL GROUP	UNIFIED SOIL CLASSIFICATION SYSTEM SYMBOL	SOIL DESCRIPTION	DRAINAGE CHARACTERISTICS[a]	FROST HEAVE POTENTIAL	VOLUME CHANGE POTENTIAL EXPANSION[b]
Group I	GW	Well-graded gravels, gravel sand mixtures, little or no fines	Good	Low	Low
	GP	Poorly graded gravels or gravel sand mixtures, little or no fines	Good	Low	Low
	SW	Well-graded sands, gravelly sands, little or no fines	Good	Low	Low
	SP	Poorly graded sands or gravelly sands, little or no fines	Good	Low	Low
	GM	Silty gravels, gravel-sand-silt mixtures	Good	Medium	Low
	SM	Silty sand, sand-silt mixtures	Good	Medium	Low
Group II	GC	Clayey gravels, gravel-sand-clay mixtures	Medium	Medium	Low
	SC	Clayey sands, sand-clay mixture	Medium	Medium	Low
	ML	Inorganic silts and very fine sands, rock flour, silty or clayey fine sands or clayey silts with slight plasticity	Medium	High	Low
	CL	Inorganic clays of low to medium plasticity, gravelly clays, sandy clays, silty clays, lean clays	Medium	Medium	Medium to Low
Group III	CH	Inorganic clays of high plasticity, fat clays	Poor	Medium	High
	MH	Inorganic silts, micaceous or diatomaceous fine sandy or silty soils, elastic silts	Poor	High	High
Group IV	OL	Organic silts and organic silty clays of low plasticity	Poor	Medium	Medium
	OH	Organic clays of medium to high plasticity, organic silts	Unsatisfactory	Medium	High
	Pt	Peat and other highly organic soils	Unsatisfactory	Medium	High

For SI: 1 inch = 25.4 mm.

a. The percolation rate for good drainage is over 4 inches per hour, medium drainage is 2 inches to 4 inches per hour, and poor is less than 2 inches per hour.

b. Soils with a low potential expansion typically have a plasticity index (PI) of 0 to 15, soils with a medium potential expansion have a PI of 10 to 35 and soils with a high potential expansion have a PI greater than 20.

R405.2.3 Drainage system. In other than Group I soils, a sump shall be provided to drain the porous layer and footings. The sump shall be at least 24 inches (610 mm) in diameter or 20 inches square (0.0129 m²), shall extend at least 24 inches (610 mm) below the bottom of the *basement* floor and shall be capable of positive gravity or mechanical drainage to remove any accumulated water. The drainage system shall discharge into an *approved* sewer system or to daylight.

SECTION R406
FOUNDATION WATERPROOFING AND DAMPPROOFING

R406.1 Concrete and masonry foundation dampproofing. Except where required by Section R406.2 to be waterproofed, foundation walls that retain earth and enclose interior spaces and floors below *grade* shall be dampproofed from the top of the footing to the finished *grade*. Masonry walls shall have not less than ³/₈ inch (9.5 mm) portland cement parging applied to the exterior of the wall. The parging shall be dampproofed in accordance with one of the following:

1. Bituminous coating.

2. Three pounds per square yard (1.63 kg/m²) of acrylic modified cement.

3. One-eighth inch (3.2 mm) coat of surface-bonding cement complying with ASTM C 887.

4. Any material permitted for waterproofing in Section R406.2.

5. Other *approved* methods or materials.

> **Exception:** Parging of unit masonry walls is not required where a material is *approved* for direct application to the masonry.

Concrete walls shall be dampproofed by applying any one of the above listed dampproofing materials or any one of the waterproofing materials listed in Section R406.2 to the exterior of the wall.

R406.2 Concrete and masonry foundation waterproofing. In areas where a high water table or other severe soil-water conditions are known to exist, exterior foundation walls that retain earth and enclose interior spaces and floors below *grade* shall be waterproofed from the top of the footing to the finished *grade*. Walls shall be waterproofed in accordance with one of the following:

1. Two-ply hot-mopped felts.

2. Fifty five pound (25 kg) roll roofing.

3. Six-mil (0.15 mm) polyvinyl chloride.

4. Six-mil (0.15 mm) polyethylene.

5. Forty-mil (1 mm) polymer-modified asphalt.

6. Sixty-mil (1.5 mm) flexible polymer cement.

7. One-eighth inch (3 mm) cement-based, fiber-reinforced, waterproof coating.

8. Sixty-mil (0.22 mm) solvent-free liquid-applied synthetic rubber.

> **Exception:** Organic-solvent-based products such as hydrocarbons, chlorinated hydrocarbons, ketones and esters shall not be used for ICF walls with expanded polystyrene form material. Use of plastic roofing cements, acrylic coatings, latex coatings, mortars and pargings to seal ICF walls is permitted. Cold-setting asphalt or hot asphalt shall conform to type C of ASTM D 449. Hot asphalt shall be applied at a temperature of less than 200°F (93°C).

All joints in membrane waterproofing shall be lapped and sealed with an adhesive compatible with the membrane.

R406.3 Dampproofing for wood foundations. Wood foundations enclosing habitable or usable spaces located below *grade* shall be dampproofed in accordance with Sections R406.3.1 through R406.3.4.

R406.3.1 Panel joint sealed. Plywood panel joints in the foundation walls shall be sealed full length with a caulking compound capable of producing a moisture-proof seal under the conditions of temperature and moisture content at which it will be applied and used.

R406.3.2 Below-grade moisture barrier. A 6-mil-thick (0.15 mm) polyethylene film shall be applied over the below-grade portion of exterior foundation walls prior to backfilling. Joints in the polyethylene film shall be lapped 6 inches (152 mm) and sealed with adhesive. The top edge of the polyethylene film shall be bonded to the sheathing to form a seal. Film areas at *grade* level shall be protected from mechanical damage and exposure by a pressure preservatively treated lumber or plywood strip attached to the wall several inches above finish *grade* level and extending approximately 9 inches (229 mm) below *grade*. The joint between the strip and the wall shall be caulked full length prior to fastening the strip to the wall. Other coverings appropriate to the architectural treatment may also be used. The polyethylene film shall extend down to the bottom of the wood footing plate but shall not overlap or extend into the gravel or crushed stone footing.

R406.3.3 Porous fill. The space between the excavation and the foundation wall shall be backfilled with the same material used for footings, up to a height of 1 foot (305 mm) above the footing for well-drained sites, or one-half the total back-fill height for poorly drained sites. The porous fill shall be covered with strips of 30-pound (13.6 kg) asphalt paper or 6-mil (0.15 mm) polyethylene to permit water seepage while avoiding infiltration of fine soils.

R406.3.4 Backfill. The remainder of the excavated area shall be backfilled with the same type of soil as was removed during the excavation.

R406.4 Precast concrete foundation system dampproofing. Except where required by Section R406.2 to be waterproofed, precast concrete foundation walls enclosing habitable or useable spaces located below *grade* shall be dampproofed in accordance with Section R406.1.

R406.4.1 Panel joints sealed. Precast concrete foundation panel joints shall be sealed full height with a sealant meeting ASTM C 920, Type S or M, *Grade* NS, Class 25, Use NT, M or A. Joint sealant shall be installed in accordance with the manufacturer's installation instructions.

SECTION R407
COLUMNS

R407.1 Wood column protection. Wood columns shall be protected against decay as set forth in Section R317.

R407.2 Steel column protection. All surfaces (inside and outside) of steel columns shall be given a shop coat of rust-inhibitive paint, except for corrosion-resistant steel and steel treated with coatings to provide corrosion resistance.

R407.3 Structural requirements. The columns shall be restrained to prevent lateral displacement at the bottom end. Wood columns shall not be less in nominal size than 4 inches by 4 inches (102 mm by 102 mm). Steel columns shall not be less than 3-inch-diameter (76 mm) Schedule 40 pipe manufactured in accordance with ASTM A 53 Grade B or *approved* equivalent.

Exception: In Seismic Design Categories A, B and C, columns no more than 48 inches (1219 mm) in height on a pier or footing are exempt from the bottom end lateral displacement requirement within under-floor areas enclosed by a continuous foundation.

SECTION R408
UNDER-FLOOR SPACE

R408.1 Ventilation. The under-floor space between the bottom of the floor joists and the earth under any building (except space occupied by a *basement*) shall have ventilation openings through foundation walls or exterior walls. The minimum net area of ventilation openings shall not be less than 1 square foot (0.0929 m²) for each 150 square feet (14 m²) of under-floor space area, unless the ground surface is covered by a Class 1 vapor retarder material. When a Class 1 vapor retarder material is used, the minimum net area of ventilation openings shall not be less than 1 square foot (0.0929 m²) for each 1,500 square feet (140 m²) of under-floor space area. One such ventilating opening shall be within 3 feet (914 mm) of each corner of the building.

R408.2 Openings for under-floor ventilation. The minimum net area of ventilation openings shall not be less than 1 square foot (0.0929 m²) for each 150 square feet (14 m²) of under-floor area. One ventilation opening shall be within 3 feet (915 mm) of each corner of the building. Ventilation openings shall be covered for their height and width with any of the following materials provided that the least dimension of the covering shall not exceed ¹/₄ inch (6.4 mm):

1. Perforated sheet metal plates not less than 0.070 inch (1.8 mm) thick.

2. Expanded sheet metal plates not less than 0.047 inch (1.2 mm) thick.

3. Cast-iron grill or grating.

4. Extruded load-bearing brick vents.

5. Hardware cloth of 0.035 inch (0.89 mm) wire or heavier.

6. Corrosion-resistant wire mesh, with the least dimension being ¹/₈ inch (3.2 mm) thick.

Exception: The total area of ventilation openings shall be permitted to be reduced to ¹/₁,₅₀₀ of the under-floor area where the ground surface is covered with an *approved* Class I vapor retarder material and the required openings are placed to provide cross ventilation of the space. The installation of operable louvers shall not be prohibited.

R408.3 Unvented crawl space. Ventilation openings in under-floor spaces specified in Sections R408.1 and R408.2 shall not be required where:

1. Exposed earth is covered with a continuous Class I vapor retarder. Joints of the vapor retarder shall overlap by 6 inches (152 mm) and shall be sealed or taped. The edges of the vapor retarder shall extend at least 6 inches (152 mm) up the stem wall and shall be attached and sealed to the stem wall; and

2. One of the following is provided for the under-floor space:

   2.1. Continuously operated mechanical exhaust ventilation at a rate equal to 1 cubic foot per minute (0.47 L/s) for each 50 square feet (4.7m²) of crawlspace floor area, including an air pathway to the common area (such as a duct or transfer grille), and perimeter walls insulated in accordance with Section N1102.2.9;

   2.2. *Conditioned air* supply sized to deliver at a rate equal to 1 cubic foot per minute (0.47 L/s) for each 50 square feet (4.7 m²) of under-floor area, including a return air pathway to the common area (such as a duct or transfer grille), and perimeter walls insulated in accordance with Section N1102.2.9;

   2.3. Plenum in existing structures complying with Section M1601.5, if under-floor space is used as a plenum.

R408.4 Access. Access shall be provided to all under-floor spaces. Access openings through the floor shall be a minimum of 18 inches by 24 inches (457 mm by 610 mm). Openings through a perimeter wall shall be not less than 16 inches by 24 inches (407 mm by 610 mm). When any portion of the through-wall access is below *grade*, an areaway not less than 16 inches by 24 inches (407 mm by 610 mm) shall be provided. The bottom of the areaway shall be below the threshold of the access opening. Through wall access openings shall not be located under a door to the residence. See Section M1305.1.4 for access requirements where mechanical *equipment* is located under floors.

R408.5 Removal of debris. The under-floor *grade* shall be cleaned of all vegetation and organic material. All wood forms used for placing concrete shall be removed before a building is occupied or used for any purpose. All construction materials shall be removed before a building is occupied or used for any purpose.

R408.6 Finished grade. The finished *grade* of under-floor surface may be located at the bottom of the footings; however, where there is evidence that the groundwater table can rise to within 6 inches (152 mm) of the finished floor at the building perimeter or where there is evidence that the surface water does not readily drain from the building site, the *grade* in the under-floor space shall be as high as the outside finished *grade*, unless an *approved* drainage system is provided.

R408.7 Flood resistance. For buildings located in areas prone to flooding as established in Table R301.2(1):

1. Walls enclosing the under-floor space shall be provided with flood openings in accordance with Section R322.2.2.

2. The finished ground level of the under-floor space shall be equal to or higher than the outside finished ground level on at least one side.

Exception: Under-floor spaces that meet the requirements of FEMA/FIA TB 11-1.

CHAPTER 5

FLOORS

SECTION R501
GENERAL

R501.1 Application. The provisions of this chapter shall control the design and construction of the floors for all buildings including the floors of *attic* spaces used to house mechanical or plumbing fixtures and *equipment*.

R501.2 Requirements. Floor construction shall be capable of accommodating all loads according to Section R301 and of transmitting the resulting loads to the supporting structural elements.

SECTION R502
WOOD FLOOR FRAMING

R502.1 Identification. Load-bearing dimension lumber for joists, beams and girders shall be identified by a grade *mark* of a lumber grading or inspection agency that has been *approved* by an accreditation body that complies with DOC PS 20. In lieu of a grade *mark*, a certificate of inspection issued by a lumber grading or inspection agency meeting the requirements of this section shall be accepted.

R502.1.1 Preservative-treated lumber. Preservative treated dimension lumber shall also be identified as required by Section R319.1.

R502.1.2 Blocking and subflooring. Blocking shall be a minimum of utility grade lumber. Subflooring may be a minimum of utility grade lumber or No. 4 common grade boards.

R502.1.3 End-jointed lumber. *Approved* end-jointed lumber identified by a grade *mark* conforming to Section R502.1 may be used interchangeably with solid-sawn members of the same species and grade.

R502.1.4 Prefabricated wood I-joists. Structural capacities and design provisions for prefabricated wood I-joists shall be established and monitored in accordance with ASTM D 5055.

R502.1.5 Structural glued laminated timbers. Glued laminated timbers shall be manufactured and identified as required in ANSI/AITC A190.1 and ASTM D 3737.

R502.1.6 Structural log members. Stress grading of structural log members of nonrectangular shape, as typically used in log buildings, shall be in accordance with ASTM D 3957. Such structural log members shall be identified by the grade *mark* of an *approved* lumber grading or inspection agency. In lieu of a grade *mark* on the material, a certificate of inspection as to species and grade issued by a lumber-grading or inspection agency meeting the requirements of this section shall be permitted to be accepted.

R502.1.7 Exterior wood/plastic composite deck boards. Wood/plastic composites used in exterior deck boards shall comply with the provisions of Section R317.4.

R502.2 Design and construction. Floors shall be designed and constructed in accordance with the provisions of this chapter, Figure R502.2 and Sections R317 and R318 or in accordance with AF&PA/NDS.

R502.2.1 Framing at braced wall lines. A load path for lateral forces shall be provided between floor framing and *braced wall panels* located above or below a floor, as specified in Section R602.10.6.

R502.2.2 Decks. Where supported by attachment to an exterior wall, decks shall be positively anchored to the primary structure and designed for both vertical and lateral loads as applicable. Such attachment shall not be accomplished by the use of toenails or nails subject to withdrawal. Where positive connection to the primary building structure cannot be verified during inspection, decks shall be self- supporting. For decks with cantilevered framing members, connections to exterior walls or other framing members, shall be designed and constructed to resist uplift resulting from the full live load specified in Table R301.5 acting on the cantilevered portion of the deck.

R502.2.2.1 Deck ledger connection to band joist. For decks supporting a total design load of 50 pounds per square foot (2394 Pa) [40 pounds per square foot (1915 Pa) live load plus 10 pounds per square foot (479 Pa) dead load], the connection between a deck ledger of pressure-preservative-treated Southern Pine, incised pressure-pre-servative-treated Hem-Fir or *approved* decay- resistant species, and a 2-inch (51 mm) nominal lumber band joist bearing on a sill plate or wall plate shall be constructed with $^1/_2$-inch (12.7 m) lag screws or bolts with washers in accordance with Table R502.2.2.1. Lag screws, bolts and washers shall be hot-dipped galvanized or stainless steel.

R502.2.2.1.1 Placement of lag screws or bolts in deck ledgers. The lag screws or bolts shall be placed 2 inches (51 mm) in from the bottom or top of the deck ledgers and between 2 and 5 inches (51 and 127 mm) in from the ends. The lag screws or bolts shall be staggered from the top to the bottom along the horizontal run of the deck ledger.

R502.2.2.2 Alternate deck ledger connections. Deck ledger connections not conforming to Table R502.2.2.1 shall be designed in accordance with accepted engineering practice. Girders supporting deck joists shall not be supported on deck ledgers or band joists. Deck ledgers shall not be supported on stone or masonry veneer.

R502.2.2.3 Deck lateral load connection. The lateral load connection required by Section R502.2.2 shall be permitted to be in accordance with Figure R502.2.2.3. Hold-down tension devices shall be installed in not less than two locations per deck, and each device shall have an allowable stress design capacity of not less than 1500 pounds (6672 N).

R502.2.2.4 Exterior wood/plastic composite deck boards. Wood/plastic composite deck boards shall be installed in accordance with the manufacturer's instructions.

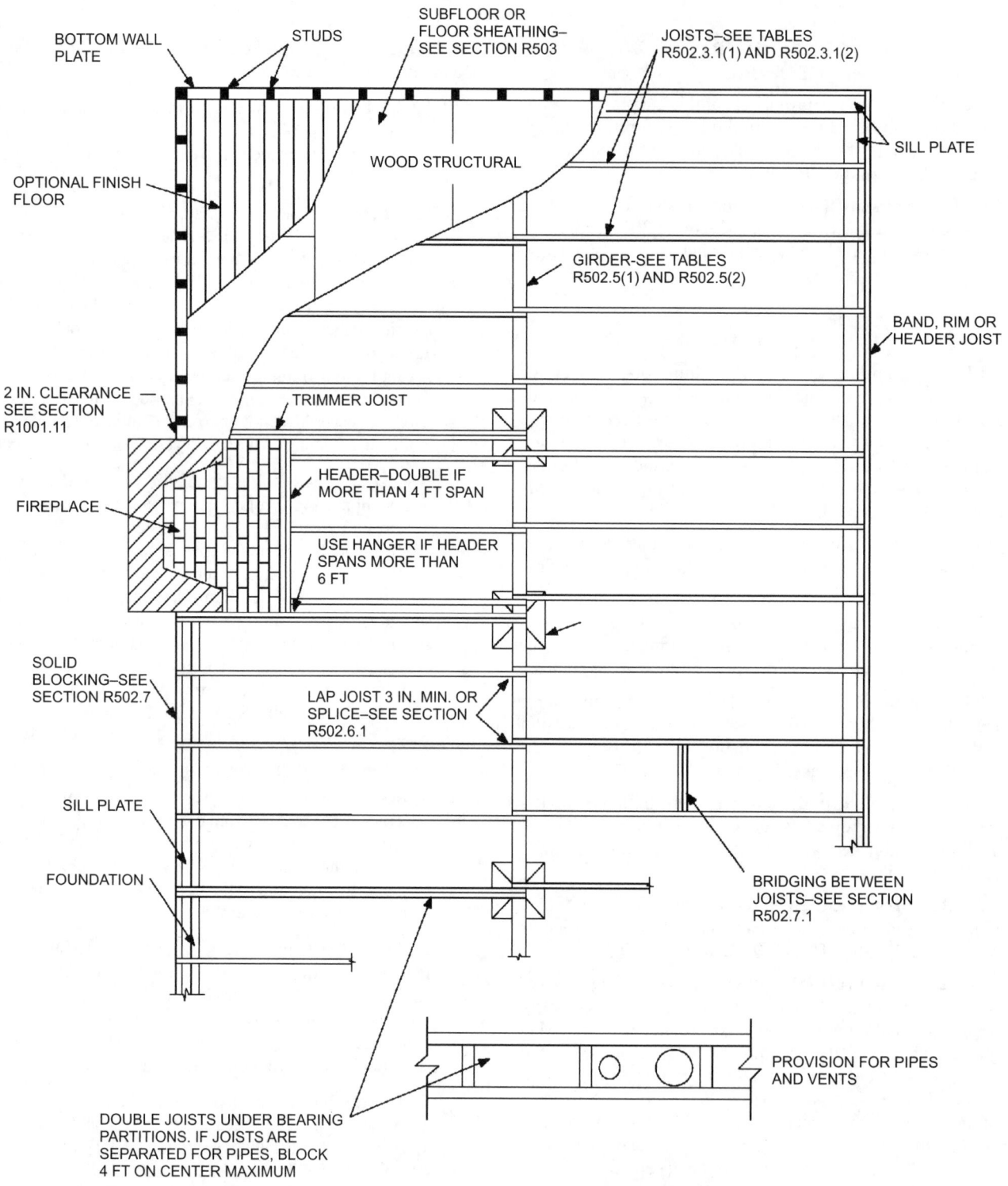

BOTTOM WALL PLATE

STUDS

SUBFLOOR OR FLOOR SHEATHING– SEE SECTION R503

JOISTS–SEE TABLES R502.3.1(1) AND R502.3.1(2)

SILL PLATE

WOOD STRUCTURAL

OPTIONAL FINISH FLOOR

GIRDER-SEE TABLES R502.5(1) AND R502.5(2)

BAND, RIM OR HEADER JOIST

2 IN. CLEARANCE — SEE SECTION R1001.11

TRIMMER JOIST

FIREPLACE

HEADER–DOUBLE IF MORE THAN 4 FT SPAN

USE HANGER IF HEADER SPANS MORE THAN 6 FT

SOLID BLOCKING–SEE SECTION R502.7

LAP JOIST 3 IN. MIN. OR SPLICE–SEE SECTION R502.6.1

SILL PLATE

FOUNDATION

BRIDGING BETWEEN JOISTS–SEE SECTION R502.7.1

PROVISION FOR PIPES AND VENTS

DOUBLE JOISTS UNDER BEARING PARTITIONS. IF JOISTS ARE SEPARATED FOR PIPES, BLOCK 4 FT ON CENTER MAXIMUM

For SI: 1 inch = 25.4 mm, 1 foot = 304.8 mm.

FIGURE R502.2
FLOOR CONSTRUCTION

TABLE R502.2.2.1
FASTENER SPACING FOR A SOUTHERN PINE OR HEM-FIR DECK LEDGER
AND A 2-INCH NOMINAL SOLID-SAWN SPRUCE-PINE-FIR BAND JOIST[c, f, g]
(Deck live load = 40 psf, deck dead load = 10 psf)

JOIST SPAN	6' and less	6'1" to 8'	8'1" to 10'	10'1" to 12'	12'1" to 14'	14'1" to 16'	16'1" to 18'
Connection details	On-center spacing of fasteners[d, e]						
$^{1}/_{2}$ inch diameter lag screw with $^{15}/_{32}$ inch maximum sheathing[a]	30	23	18	15	13	11	10
$^{1}/_{2}$ inch diameter bolt with $^{15}/_{32}$ inch maximum sheathing	36	36	34	29	24	21	19
$^{1}/_{2}$ inch diameter bolt with $^{15}/_{32}$ inch maximum sheathing and $^{1}/_{2}$ inch stacked washers[b, h]	36	36	29	24	21	18	16

For SI: 1 inch = 25.4 mm, 1 foot = 304.8 mm. 1 pound per square foot = 0.0479kPa.

a. The tip of the lag screw shall fully extend beyond the inside face of the band joist.

b. The maximum gap between the face of the ledger board and face of the wall sheathing shall be $^{1}/_{2}$".

c. Ledgers shall be flashed to prevent water from contacting the house band joist.

d. Lag screws and bolts shall be staggered in accordance with Section R502.2.2.1.1.

e. Deck ledger shall be minimum 2 × 8 pressure-preservative-treated No.2 grade lumber, or other approved materials as established by standard engineering practice.

f. When solid-sawn pressure-preservative-treated deck ledgers are attached to a minimum 1 inch thick engineered wood product (structural composite lumber, laminated veneer lumber or wood structural panel band joist), the ledger attachment shall be designed in accordance with accepted engineering practice.

g. A minimum 1 × 9$^{1}/_{2}$ Douglas Fir laminated veneer lumber rimboard shall be permitted in lieu of the 2-inch nominal band joist.

h. Wood structural panel sheathing, gypsum board sheathing or foam sheathing not exceeding 1 inch in thickness shall be permitted. The maximum distance between the face of the ledger board and the face of the band joist shall be 1 inch.

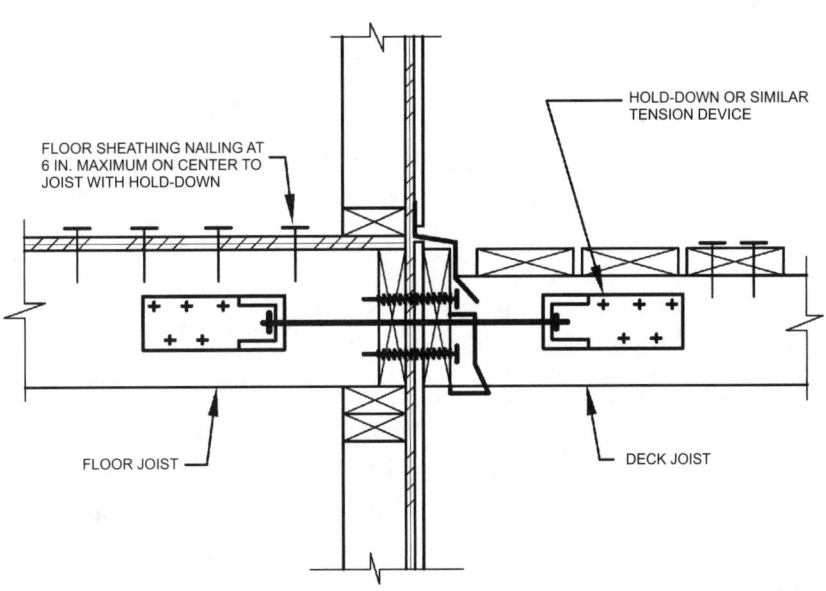

For SI: 1 inch = 25.4 mm.

FIGURE 502.2.2.3
DECK ATTACHMENT FOR LATERAL LOADS

R502.3 Allowable joist spans. Spans for floor joists shall be in accordance with Tables R502.3.1(1) and R502.3.1(2). For other grades and species and for other loading conditions, refer to the AF&PA Span Tables for Joists and Rafters.

R502.3.1 Sleeping areas and attic joists. Table R502.3.1(1) shall be used to determine the maximum allowable span of floor joists that support sleeping areas and *attics* that are accessed by means of a fixed stairway in accordance with Section R311.7 provided that the design live load does not exceed 30 pounds per square foot (1.44 kPa) and the design dead load does not exceed 20 pounds per square foot (0.96 kPa). The allowable span of ceiling joists that support *attics* used for limited storage or no storage shall be determined in accordance with Section R802.4.

R502.3.2 Other floor joists. Table R502.3.1(2) shall be used to determine the maximum allowable span of floor joists that support all other areas of the building, other than sleeping rooms and *attics*, provided that the design live load does not exceed 40 pounds per square foot (1.92 kPa) and the design dead load does not exceed 20 pounds per square foot (0.96 kPa).

R502.3.3 Floor cantilevers. Floor cantilever spans shall not exceed the nominal depth of the wood floor joist. Floor cantilevers constructed in accordance with Table R502.3.3(1) shall be permitted when supporting a light-frame bearing wall and roof only. Floor cantilevers supporting an exterior balcony are permitted to be constructed in accordance with Table R502.3.3(2).

R502.4 Joists under bearing partitions. Joists under parallel bearing partitions shall be of adequate size to support the load. Double joists, sized to adequately support the load, that are separated to permit the installation of piping or vents shall be full depth solid blocked with lumber not less than 2 inches (51 mm) in nominal thickness spaced not more than 4 feet (1219 mm) on center. Bearing partitions perpendicular to joists shall not be offset from supporting girders, walls or partitions more than the joist depth unless such joists are of sufficient size to carry the additional load.

R502.5 Allowable girder spans. The allowable spans of girders fabricated of dimension lumber shall not exceed the values set forth in Tables R502.5(1) and R502.5(2).

R502.6 Bearing. The ends of each joist, beam or girder shall have not less than 1.5 inches (38 mm) of bearing on wood or metal and not less than 3 inches (76 mm) on masonry or concrete except where supported on a 1-inch-by-4-inch (25.4 mm by 102 mm) ribbon strip and nailed to the adjacent stud or by the use of *approved* joist hangers.

R502.6.1 Floor systems. Joists framing from opposite sides over a bearing support shall lap a minimum of 3 inches (76 mm) and shall be nailed together with a minimum three 10d face nails. A wood or metal splice with strength equal to or greater than that provided by the nailed lap is permitted.

R502.6.2 Joist framing. Joists framing into the side of a wood girder shall be supported by *approved* framing anchors or on ledger strips not less than nominal 2 inches by 2 inches (51 mm by 51 mm).

R502.7 Lateral restraint at supports. Joists shall be supported laterally at the ends by full-depth solid blocking not less than 2 inches (51 mm) nominal in thickness; or by attachment to a full-depth header, band or rim joist, or to an adjoining stud or shall be otherwise provided with lateral support to prevent rotation.

Exceptions:

1. Trusses, structural composite lumber, structural glued-laminated members and I-joists shall be supported laterally as required by the manufacturer's recommendation.

2. In Seismic Design Categories D_0, D_1 and D_2, lateral restraint shall also be provided at each intermediate support.

R502.7.1 Bridging. Joists exceeding a nominal 2 inches by 12 inches (51 mm by 305 mm) shall be supported laterally by solid blocking, diagonal bridging (wood or metal), or a continuous 1-inch-by-3-inch (25.4 mm by 76 mm) strip nailed across the bottom of joists perpendicular to joists at intervals not exceeding 8 feet (2438 mm).

Exception: Trusses, structural composite lumber, structural glued-laminated members and I-joists shall be supported laterally as required by the manufacturer's recommendations.

R502.8 Drilling and notching. Structural floor members shall not be cut, bored or notched in excess of the limitations specified in this section. See Figure R502.8.

R502.8.1 Sawn lumber. Notches in solid lumber joists, rafters and beams shall not exceed one-sixth of the depth of the member, shall not be longer than one-third of the depth of the member and shall not be located in the middle one-third of the span. Notches at the ends of the member shall not exceed one-fourth the depth of the member. The tension side of members 4 inches (102 mm) or greater in nominal thickness shall not be notched except at the ends of the members. The diameter of holes bored or cut into members shall not exceed one-third the depth of the member. Holes shall not be closer than 2 inches (51 mm) to the top or bottom of the member, or to any other hole located in the member. Where the member is also notched, the hole shall not be closer than 2 inches (51 mm) to the notch.

R502.8.2 Engineered wood products. Cuts, notches and holes bored in trusses, structural composite lumber, structural glue-laminated members or I-joists are prohibited except where permitted by the manufacturer's recommendations or where the effects of such alterations are specifically considered in the design of the member by a *registered design professional*.

R502.9 Fastening. Floor framing shall be nailed in accordance with Table R602.3(1). Where posts and beam or girder construction is used to support floor framing, positive connections shall be provided to ensure against uplift and lateral displacement.

R502.10 Framing of openings. Openings in floor framing shall be framed with a header and trimmer joists. When the header joist span does not exceed 4 feet (1219 mm), the header joist may be a single member the same size as the floor joist. Single trimmer joists may be used to carry a single header joist that is located within 3 feet (914 mm) of the trimmer joist bearing. When the header joist span exceeds 4 feet (1219 mm), the trimmer joists and the header joist shall be doubled and of sufficient cross section to support the floor joists framing into the header. *Approved* hangers shall be used for the header joist to trimmer joist connections when the header joist span exceeds 6 feet (1829 mm). Tail joists over 12 feet (3658 mm) long shall be supported at the header by framing anchors or on ledger strips not less than 2 inches by 2 inches (51 mm by 51 mm).

TABLE R502.3.1(1)
FLOOR JOIST SPANS FOR COMMON LUMBER SPECIES
(Residential sleeping areas, live load = 30 psf, L/Δ = 360)[a]

JOIST SPACING (inches)	SPECIES AND *GRADE*		DEAD LOAD = 10 psf				DEAD LOAD = 20 psf			
			2×6	2×8	2×10	2×12	2×6	2×8	2×10	2×12
			Maximum floor joist spans							
			(ft - in.)	(ft - in.)	(ft - in.)	(ft - in.)	(ft - in.)	(ft - in.)	(ft - in.)	(ft - in.)
12	Douglas fir-larch	SS	12-6	16-6	21-0	25-7	12-6	16-6	21-0	25-7
	Douglas fir-larch	#1	12-0	15-10	20-3	24-8	12-0	15-7	19-0	22-0
	Douglas fir-larch	#2	11-10	15-7	19-10	23-0	11-6	14-7	17-9	20-7
	Douglas fir-larch	#3	9-8	12-4	15-0	17-5	8-8	11-0	13-5	15-7
	Hem-fir	SS	11-10	15-7	19-10	24-2	11-10	15-7	19-10	24-2
	Hem-fir	#1	11-7	15-3	19-5	23-7	11-7	15-2	18-6	21-6
	Hem-fir	#2	11-0	14-6	18-6	22-6	11-0	14-4	17-6	20-4
	Hem-fir	#3	9-8	12-4	15-0	17-5	8-8	11-0	13-5	15-7
	Southern pine	SS	12-3	16-2	20-8	25-1	12-3	16-2	20-8	25-1
	Southern pine	#1	12-0	15-10	20-3	24-8	12-0	15-10	20-3	24-8
	Southern pine	#2	11-10	15-7	19-10	24-2	11-10	15-7	18-7	21-9
	Southern pine	#3	10-5	13-3	15-8	18-8	9-4	11-11	14-0	16-8
	Spruce-pine-fir	SS	11-7	15-3	19-5	23-7	11-7	15-3	19-5	23-7
	Spruce-pine-fir	#1	11-3	14-11	19-0	23-0	11-3	14-7	17-9	20-7
	Spruce-pine-fir	#2	11-3	14-11	19-0	23-0	11-3	14-7	17-9	20-7
	Spruce-pine-fir	#3	9-8	12-4	15-0	17-5	8-8	11-0	13-5	15-7
16	Douglas fir-larch	SS	11-4	15-0	19-1	23-3	11-4	15-0	19-1	23-0
	Douglas fir-larch	#1	10-11	14-5	18-5	21-4	10-8	13-6	16-5	19-1
	Douglas fir-larch	#2	10-9	14-1	17-2	19-11	9-11	12-7	15-5	17-10
	Douglas fir-larch	#3	8-5	10-8	13-0	15-1	7-6	9-6	11-8	13-6
	Hem-fir	SS	10-9	14-2	18-0	21-11	10-9	14-2	18-0	21-11
	Hem-fir	#1	10-6	13-10	17-8	20-9	10-4	13-1	16-0	18-7
	Hem-fir	#2	10-0	13-2	16-10	19-8	9-10	12-5	15-2	17-7
	Hem-fir	#3	8-5	10-8	13-0	15-1	7-6	9-6	11-8	13-6
	Southern pine	SS	11-2	14-8	18-9	22-10	11-2	14-8	18-9	22-10
	Southern pine	#1	10-11	14-5	18-5	22-5	10-11	14-5	17-11	21-4
	Southern pine	#2	10-9	14-2	18-0	21-1	10-5	13-6	16-1	18-10
	Southern pine	#3	9-0	11-6	13-7	16-2	8-1	10-3	12-2	14-6
	Spruce-pine-fir	SS	10-6	13-10	17-8	21-6	10-6	13-10	17-8	21-4
	Spruce-pine-fir	#1	10-3	13-6	17-2	19-11	9-11	12-7	15-5	17-10
	Spruce-pine-fir	#2	10-3	13-6	17-2	19-11	9-11	12-7	15-5	17-10
	Spruce-pine-fir	#3	8-5	10-8	13-0	15-1	7-6	9-6	11-8	13-6
19.2	Douglas fir-larch	SS	10-8	14-1	18-0	21-10	10-8	14-1	18-0	21-0
	Douglas fir-larch	#1	10-4	13-7	16-9	19-6	9-8	12-4	15-0	17-5
	Douglas fir-larch	#2	10-1	12-10	15-8	18-3	9-1	11-6	14-1	16-3
	Douglas fir-larch	#3	7-8	9-9	11-10	13-9	6-10	8-8	10-7	12-4
	Hem-fir	SS	10-1	13-4	17-0	20-8	10-1	13-4	17-0	20-7
	Hem-fir	#1	9-10	13-0	16-4	19-0	9-6	12-0	14-8	17-0
	Hem-fir	#2	9-5	12-5	15-6	17-1	8-11	11-4	13-10	16-1
	Hem-fir	#3	7-8	9-9	11-10	13-9	6-10	8-8	10-7	12-4
	Southern pine	SS	10-6	13-10	17-8	21-6	10-6	13-10	17-8	21-6
	Southern pine	#1	10-4	13-7	17-4	21-1	10-4	13-7	16-4	19-6
	Southern pine	#2	10-1	13-4	16-5	19-3	9-6	12-4	14-8	17-2
	Southern pine	#3	8-3	10-6	12-5	14-9	7-4	9-5	11-1	13-2
	Spruce-pine-fir	SS	9-10	13-0	16-7	20-2	9-10	13-0	16-7	19-6
	Spruce-pine-fir	#1	9-8	12-9	15-8	18-3	9-1	11-6	14-1	16-3
	Spruce-pine-fir	#2	9-8	12-9	15-8	18-3	9-1	11-6	14-1	16-3
	Spruce-pine-fir	#3	7-8	9-9	11-10	13-9	6-10	8-8	10-7	12-4
24	Douglas fir-larch	SS	9-11	13-1	16-8	20-3	9-11	13-1	16-2	18-9
	Douglas fir-larch	#1	9-7	12-4	15-0	17-5	8-8	11-0	13-5	15-7
	Douglas fir-larch	#2	9-1	11-6	14-1	16-3	8-1	10-3	12-7	14-7
	Douglas fir-larch	#3	6-10	8-8	10-7	12-4	6-2	7-9	9-6	11-0
	Hem-fir	SS	9-4	12-4	15-9	19-2	9-4	12-4	15-9	18-5
	Hem-fir	#1	9-2	12-0	14-8	17-0	8-6	10-9	13-1	15-2
	Hem-fir	#2	8-9	11-4	13-10	16-1	8-0	10-2	12-5	14-4
	Hem-fir	#3	6-10	8-8	10-7	12-4	6-2	7-9	9-6	11-0
	Southern pine	SS	9-9	12-10	16-5	19-11	9-9	12-10	16-5	19-11
	Southern pine	#1	9-7	12-7	16-1	19-6	9-7	12-4	14-7	17-5
	Southern pine	#2	9-4	12-4	14-8	17-2	8-6	11-0	13-1	15-5
	Southern pine	#3	7-4	9-5	11-1	13-2	6-7	8-5	9-11	11-10
	Spruce-pine-fir	SS	9-2	12-1	15-5	18-9	9-2	12-1	15-0	17-5
	Spruce-pine-fir	#1	8-11	11-6	14-1	16-3	8-1	10-3	12-7	14-7
	Spruce-pine-fir	#2	8-11	11-6	14-1	16-3	8-1	10-3	12-7	14-7
	Spruce-pine-fir	#3	6-10	8-8	10-7	12-4	6-2	7-9	9-6	11-0

For SI: 1 inch = 25.4 mm, 1 foot = 304.8 mm, 1 pound per square foot = 0.0479 kPa.

Note: Check sources for availability of lumber in lengths greater than 20 feet.

a. Dead load limits for townhouses in Seismic Design Category C and all structures in Seismic Design Categories D_0, D_1 and D_2 shall be determined in accordance with Section R301.2.2.2.1.

TABLE R502.3.1(2)
FLOOR JOIST SPANS FOR COMMON LUMBER SPECIES
(Residential living areas, live load = 40 psf, L/Δ = 360)[b]

JOIST SPACING (inches)	SPECIES AND *GRADE*		DEAD LOAD = 10 psf				DEAD LOAD = 20 psf			
			2×6	2×8	2×10	2×12	2×6	2×8	2×10	2×12
						Maximum floor joist spans				
			(ft - in.)	(ft - in.)	(ft - in.)	(ft - in.)	(ft - in.)	(ft - in.)	(ft - in.)	(ft - in.)
12	Douglas fir-larch	SS	11-4	15-0	19-1	23-3	11-4	15-0	19-1	23-3
	Douglas fir-larch	#1	10-11	14-5	18-5	22-0	10-11	14-2	17-4	20-1
	Douglas fir-larch	#2	10-9	14-2	17-9	20-7	10-6	13-3	16-3	18-10
	Douglas fir-larch	#3	8-8	11-0	13-5	15-7	7-11	10-0	12-3	14-3
	Hem-fir	SS	10-9	14-2	18-0	21-11	10-9	14-2	18-0	21-11
	Hem-fir	#1	10-6	13-10	17-8	21-6	10-6	13-10	16-11	19-7
	Hem-fir	#2	10-0	13-2	16-10	20-4	10-0	13-1	16-0	18-6
	Hem-fir	#3	8-8	11-0	13-5	15-7	7-11	10-0	12-3	14-3
	Southern pine	SS	11-2	14-8	18-9	22-10	11-2	14-8	18-9	22-10
	Southern pine	#1	10-11	14-5	18-5	22-5	10-11	14-5	18-5	22-5
	Southern pine	#2	10-9	14-2	18-0	21-9	10-9	14-2	16-11	19-10
	Southern pine	#3	9-4	11-11	14-0	16-8	8-6	10-10	12-10	15-3
	Spruce-pine-fir	SS	10-6	13-10	17-8	21-6	10-6	13-10	17-8	21-6
	Spruce-pine-fir	#1	10-3	13-6	17-3	20-7	10-3	13-3	16-3	18-10
	Spruce-pine-fir	#2	10-3	13-6	17-3	20-7	10-3	13-3	16-3	18-10
	Spruce-pine-fir	#3	8-8	11-0	13-5	15-7	7-11	10-0	12-3	14-3
16	Douglas fir-larch	SS	10-4	13-7	17-4	21-1	10-4	13-7	17-4	21-0
	Douglas fir-larch	#1	9-11	13-1	16-5	19-1	9-8	12-4	15-0	17-5
	Douglas fir-larch	#2	9-9	12-7	15-5	17-10	9-1	11-6	14-1	16-3
	Douglas fir-larch	#3	7-6	9-6	11-8	13-6	6-10	8-8	10-7	12-4
	Hem-fir	SS	9-9	12-10	16-5	19-11	9-9	12-10	16-5	19-11
	Hem-fir	#1	9-6	12-7	16-0	18-7	9-6	12-0	14-8	17-0
	Hem-fir	#2	9-1	12-0	15-2	17-7	8-11	11-4	13-10	16-1
	Hem-fir	#3	7-6	9-6	11-8	13-6	6-10	8-8	10-7	12-4
	Southern pine	SS	10-2	13-4	17-0	20-9	10-2	13-4	17-0	20-9
	Southern pine	#1	9-11	13-1	16-9	20-4	9-11	13-1	16-4	19-6
	Southern pine	#2	9-9	12-10	16-1	18-10	9-6	12-4	14-8	17-2
	Southern pine	#3	8-1	10-3	12-2	14-6	7-4	9-5	11-1	13-2
	Spruce-pine-fir	SS	9-6	12-7	16-0	19-6	9-6	12-7	16-0	19-6
	Spruce-pine-fir	#1	9-4	12-3	15-5	17-10	9-1	11-6	14-1	16-3
	Spruce-pine-fir	#2	9-4	12-3	15-5	17-10	9-1	11-6	14-1	16-3
	Spruce-pine-fir	#3	7-6	9-6	11-8	13-6	6-10	8-8	10-7	12-4
19.2	Douglas fir-larch	SS	9-8	12-10	16-4	19-10	9-8	12-10	16-4	19-2
	Douglas fir-larch	#1	9-4	12-4	15-0	17-5	8-10	11-3	13-8	15-11
	Douglas fir-larch	#2	9-1	11-6	14-1	16-3	8-3	10-6	12-10	14-10
	Douglas fir-larch	#3	6-10	8-8	10-7	12-4	6-3	7-11	9-8	11-3
	Hem-fir	SS	9-2	12-1	15-5	18-9	9-2	12-1	15-5	18-9
	Hem-fir	#1	9-0	11-10	14-8	17-0	8-8	10-11	13-4	15-6
	Hem-fir	#2	8-7	11-3	13-10	16-1	8-2	10-4	12-8	14-8
	Hem-fir	#3	6-10	8-8	10-7	12-4	6-3	7-11	9-8	11-3
	Southern pine	SS	9-6	12-7	16-0	19-6	9-6	12-7	16-0	19-6
	Southern pine	#1	9-4	12-4	15-9	19-2	9-4	12-4	14-11	17-9
	Southern pine	#2	9-2	12-1	14-8	17-2	8-8	11-3	13-5	15-8
	Southern pine	#3	7-4	9-5	11-1	13-2	6-9	8-7	10-1	12-1
	Spruce-pine-fir	SS	9-0	11-10	15-1	18-4	9-0	11-10	15-1	17-9
	Spruce-pine-fir	#	8-9	11-6	14-1	16-3	8-3	10-6	12-10	14-10
	Spruce-pine-fir	#2	8-9	11-6	14-1	16-3	8-3	10-6	12-10	14-10
	Spruce-pine-fir	#3	6-10	8-8	10-7	12-4	6-3	7-11	9-8	11-3
24	Douglas fir-larch	SS	9-0	11-11	15-2	18-5	9-0	11-11	14-9	17-1
	Douglas fir-larch	#1	8-8	11-0	13-5	15-7	7-11	10-0	12-3	14-3
	Douglas fir-larch	#2	8-1	10-3	12-7	14-7	7-5	9-5	11-6	13-4
	Douglas fir-larch	#3	6-2	7-9	9-6	11-0	5-7	7-1	8-8	10-1
	Hem-fir	SS	8-6	11-3	14-4	17-5	8-6	11-3	14-4	16-10[a]
	Hem-fir	#1	8-4	10-9	13-1	15-2	7-9	9-9	11-11	13-10
	Hem-fir	#2	7-11	10-2	12-5	14-4	7-4	9-3	11-4	13-1
	Hem-fir	#3	6-2	7-9	9-6	11-0	5-7	7-1	8-8	10-1
	Southern pine	SS	8-10	11-8	14-11	18-1	8-10	11-8	14-11	18-1
	Southern pine	#1	8-8	11-5	14-7	17-5	8-8	11-3	13-4	15-11
	Southern pine	#2	8-6	11-0	13-1	15-5	7-9	10-0	12-0	14-0
	Southern pine	#3	6-7	8-5	9-11	11-10	6-0	7-8	9-1	10-9
	Spruce-pine-fir	SS	8-4	11-0	14-0	17-0	8-4	11-0	13-8	15-11
	Spruce-pine-fir	#1	8-1	10-3	12-7	14-7	7-5	9-5	11-6	13-4
	Spruce-pine-fir	#2	8-1	10-3	12-7	14-7	7-5	9-5	11-6	13-4
	Spruce-pine-fir	#3	6-2	7-9	9-6	11-0	5-7	7-1	8-8	10-1

For SI: 1 inch = 25.4 mm, 1 foot = 304.8 mm, 1 pound per square foot = 0.0479 kPa.

Note: Check sources for availability of lumber in lengths greater than 20 feet.

a. End bearing length shall be increased to 2 inches.

b. Dead load limits for townhouses in Seismic Design Category C and all structures in Seismic Design Categories D_0, D_1, and D_2 shall be determined in accordance with Section R301.2.2.2.1.

TABLE R502.3.3(1)
CANTILEVER SPANS FOR FLOOR JOISTS SUPPORTING LIGHT-FRAME EXTERIOR BEARING WALL AND ROOF ONLY[a, b, c, f, g, h]
(Floor Live Load ≤ 40 psf, Roof Live Load ≤ 20 psf)

Member & Spacing	Maximum Cantilever Span (Uplift Force at Backspan Support in Lbs.)[d, e]											
	Ground Snow Load											
	≤ 20 psf			30 psf			50 psf			70 psf		
	Roof Width			Roof Width			Roof Width			Roof Width		
	24 ft	32 ft	40 ft	24 ft	32 ft	40 ft	24 ft	32 ft	40 ft	24 ft	32 ft	40 ft
2 × 8 @ 12″	20″ (177)	15″ (227)	—	18″ (209)	—	—	—	—	—	—	—	—
2 × 10 @ 16″	29″ (228)	21″ (297)	16″ (364)	26″ (271)	18″ (354)	—	20″ (375)	—	—	—	—	—
2 × 10 @ 12″	36″ (166)	26″ (219)	20″ (270)	34″ (198)	22″ (263)	16″ (324)	26″ (277)	—	—	19″ (356)	—	—
2 × 12 @ 16″	—	32″ (287)	25″ (356)	36″ (263)	29″ (345)	21″ (428)	29″ (367)	20″ (484)	—	23″ (471)	—	—
2 × 12 @ 12″	—	42″ (209)	31″ (263)	—	37″ (253)	27″ (317)	36″ (271)	27″ (358)	17″ (447)	31″ (348)	19″ (462)	—
2 × 12 @ 8″	—	48″ (136)	45″ (169)	—	48″ (164)	38″ (206)	—	40″ (233)	26″ (294)	36″ (230)	29″ (304)	18″ (379)

For SI: 1 inch = 25.4 mm, 1 foot = 304.8 mm, 1 pound per square foot = 0.0479 kPa.

a. Tabulated values are for clear-span roof supported solely by exterior bearing walls.
b. Spans are based on No. 2 Grade lumber of Douglas fir-larch, hem-fir, southern pine, and spruce-pine-fir for repetitive (3 or more) members.
c. Ratio of backspan to cantilever span shall be at least 3:1.
d. Connections capable of resisting the indicated uplift force shall be provided at the backspan support.
e. Uplift force is for a backspan to cantilever span ratio of 3:1. Tabulated uplift values are permitted to be reduced by multiplying by a factor equal to 3 divided by the actual backspan ratio provided (3/backspan ratio).
f. See Section R301.2.2.2.5, Item 1, for additional limitations on cantilevered floor joists for detached one- and two-family dwellings in Seismic Design Category D_0, D_1, or D_2 and townhouses in Seismic Design Category C, D_0, D_1, or D_2.
g. A full-depth rim joist shall be provided at the unsupported end of the cantilever joists. Solid blocking shall be provided at the supported end.
h. Linear interpolation shall be permitted for building widths and ground snow loads other than shown.

TABLE R502.3.3(2)
CANTILEVER SPANS FOR FLOOR JOISTS SUPPORTING EXTERIOR BALCONY[a, b, e, f]

Member Size	Spacing	Maximum Cantilever Span (Uplift Force at Backspan Support in lb)[c, d]		
		Ground Snow Load		
		≤ 30 psf	50 psf	70 psf
2 × 8	12″	42″ (139)	39″ (156)	34″ (165)
2 × 8	16″	36″ (151)	34″ (171)	29″ (180)
2 × 10	12″	61″ (164)	57″ (189)	49″ (201)
2 × 10	16″	53″ (180)	49″ (208)	42″ (220)
2 × 10	24″	43″ (212)	40″ (241)	34″ (255)
2 × 12	16″	72″ (228)	67″ (260)	57″ (268)
2 × 12	24″	58″ (279)	54″ (319)	47″ (330)

For SI: 1 inch = 25.4 mm, 1 pound per square foot = 0.0479 kPa.

a. Spans are based on No. 2 Grade lumber of Douglas fir-larch, hem-fir, southern pine, and spruce-pine-fir for repetitive (3 or more) members.
b. Ratio of backspan to cantilever span shall be at least 2:1.
c. Connections capable of resisting the indicated uplift force shall be provided at the backspan support.
d. Uplift force is for a backspan to cantilever span ratio of 2:1. Tabulated uplift values are permitted to be reduced by multiplying by a factor equal to 2 divided by the actual backspan ratio provided (2/backspan ratio).
e. A full-depth rim joist shall be provided at the unsupported end of the cantilever joists. Solid blocking shall be provided at the supported end.
f. Linear interpolation shall be permitted for ground snow loads other than shown.

TABLE R502.5(1)
GIRDER SPANS[a] AND HEADER SPANS[a] FOR EXTERIOR BEARING WALLS
(Maximum spans for Douglas fir-larch, hem-fir, southern pine and spruce-pine-fir[b] and required number of jack studs)

GIRDERS AND HEADERS SUPPORTING	SIZE	GROUND SNOW LOAD (psf)[e]																	
		30						50						70					
		Building width[c] (feet)																	
		20		28		36		20		28		36		20		28		36	
		Span	NJ[d]	Span	NJ[d]	Span	NJ[d]	Span	NJ[d]	Span	NJ[d]	Span	NJ[d]	Span	NJ[d]	Span	NJ[d]	Span	NJ[d]
Roof and ceiling	2-2×4	3-6	1	3-2	1	2-10	1	3-2	1	2-9	1	2-6	1	2-10	1	2-6	1	2-3	1
	2-2×6	5-5	1	4-8	1	4-2	1	4-8	1	4-1	1	3-8	2	4-2	1	3-8	2	3-3	2
	2-2×8	6-10	1	5-11	2	5-4	2	5-11	2	5-2	2	4-7	2	5-4	2	4-7	2	4-1	2
	2-2×10	8-5	2	7-3	2	6-6	2	7-3	2	6-3	2	5-7	2	6-6	2	5-7	2	5-0	2
	2-2×12	9-9	2	8-5	2	7-6	2	8-5	2	7-3	2	6-6	2	7-6	2	6-6	2	5-10	3
	3-2×8	8-4	1	7-5	1	6-8	1	7-5	1	6-5	2	5-9	2	6-8	1	5-9	2	5-2	2
	3-2×10	10-6	1	9-1	2	8-2	2	9-1	2	7-10	2	7-0	2	8-2	2	7-0	2	6-4	2
	3-2×12	12-2	2	10-7	2	9-5	2	10-7	2	9-2	2	8-2	2	9-5	2	8-2	2	7-4	2
	4-2×8	9-2	1	8-4	1	7-8	1	8-4	1	7-5	1	6-8	1	7-8	1	6-8	1	5-11	2
	4-2×10	11-8	1	10-6	1	9-5	2	10-6	1	9-1	2	8-2	2	9-5	2	8-2	2	7-3	2
	4-2×12	14-1	1	12-2	2	10-11	2	12-2	2	10-7	2	9-5	2	10-11	2	9-5	2	8-5	2
Roof, ceiling and one center-bearing floor	2-2×4	3-1	1	2-9	1	2-5	1	2-9	1	2-5	1	2-2	1	2-7	1	2-3	1	2-0	1
	2-2×6	4-6	1	4-0	1	3-7	2	4-1	1	3-7	2	3-3	2	3-9	2	3-3	2	2-11	2
	2-2×8	5-9	2	5-0	2	4-6	2	5-2	2	4-6	2	4-1	2	4-9	2	4-2	2	3-9	2
	2-2×10	7-0	2	6-2	2	5-6	2	6-4	2	5-6	2	5-0	2	5-9	2	5-1	2	4-7	3
	2-2×12	8-1	2	7-1	2	6-5	2	7-4	2	6-5	2	5-9	3	6-8	2	5-10	3	5-3	3
	3-2×8	7-2	1	6-3	2	5-8	2	6-5	2	5-8	2	5-1	2	5-11	2	5-2	2	4-8	2
	3-2×10	8-9	2	7-8	2	6-11	2	7-11	2	6-11	2	6-3	2	7-3	2	6-4	2	5-8	2
	3-2×12	10-2	2	8-11	2	8-0	2	9-2	2	8-0	2	7-3	2	8-5	2	7-4	2	6-7	2
	4-2×8	8-1	1	7-3	1	6-7	1	7-5	1	6-6	1	5-11	2	6-10	1	6-0	2	5-5	2
	4-2×10	10-1	1	8-10	2	8-0	2	9-1	2	8-0	2	7-2	2	8-4	2	7-4	2	6-7	2
	4-2×12	11-9	2	10-3	2	9-3	2	10-7	2	9-3	2	8-4	2	9-8	2	8-6	2	7-7	2
Roof, ceiling and one clear span floor	2-2×4	2-8	1	2-4	1	2-1	1	2-7	1	2-3	1	2-0	1	2-5	1	2-1	1	1-10	1
	2-2×6	3-11	1	3-5	2	3-0	2	3-10	2	3-4	2	3-0	2	3-6	2	3-1	2	2-9	2
	2-2×8	5-0	2	4-4	2	3-10	2	4-10	2	4-2	2	3-9	2	4-6	2	3-11	2	3-6	2
	2-2×10	6-1	2	5-3	2	4-8	2	5-11	2	5-1	2	4-7	3	5-6	2	4-9	2	4-3	3
	2-2×12	7-1	2	6-1	3	5-5	3	6-10	2	5-11	3	5-4	3	6-4	2	5-6	3	5-0	3
	3-2×8	6-3	2	5-5	2	4-10	2	6-1	2	5-3	2	4-8	2	5-7	2	4-11	2	4-5	2
	3-2×10	7-7	2	6-7	2	5-11	2	7-5	2	6-5	2	5-9	2	6-10	2	6-0	2	5-4	2
	3-2×12	8-10	2	7-8	2	6-10	2	8-7	2	7-5	2	6-8	2	7-11	2	6-11	2	6-3	2
	4-2×8	7-2	1	6-3	2	5-7	2	7-0	1	6-1	2	5-5	2	6-6	1	5-8	2	5-1	2
	4-2×10	8-9	2	7-7	2	6-10	2	8-7	2	7-5	2	6-7	2	7-11	2	6-11	2	6-2	2
	4-2×12	10-2	2	8-10	2	7-11	2	9-11	2	8-7	2	7-8	2	9-2	2	8-0	2	7-2	2
Roof, ceiling and two center-bearing floors	2-2×4	2-7	1	2-3	1	2-0	1	2-6	1	2-2	1	1-11	1	2-4	1	2-0	1	1-9	1
	2-2×6	3-9	2	3-3	2	2-11	2	3-8	2	3-2	2	2-10	2	3-5	2	3-0	2	2-8	2
	2-2×8	4-9	2	4-2	2	3-9	2	4-7	2	4-0	2	3-8	2	4-4	2	3-9	2	3-5	2
	2-2×10	5-9	2	5-1	2	4-7	3	5-8	2	4-11	2	4-5	3	5-3	2	4-7	3	4-2	3
	2-2×12	6-8	2	5-10	3	5-3	3	6-6	2	5-9	3	5-2	3	6-1	3	5-4	3	4-10	3
	3-2×8	5-11	2	5-2	2	4-8	2	5-9	2	5-1	2	4-7	2	5-5	2	4-9	2	4-3	2
	3-2×10	7-3	2	6-4	2	5-8	2	7-1	2	6-2	2	5-7	2	6-7	2	5-9	2	5-3	2
	3-2×12	8-5	2	7-4	2	6-7	2	8-2	2	7-2	2	6-5	3	7-8	2	6-9	2	6-1	3
	4-2×8	6-10	1	6-0	2	5-5	2	6-8	1	5-10	2	5-3	2	6-3	2	5-6	2	4-11	2
	4-2×10	8-4	2	7-4	2	6-7	2	8-2	2	7-2	2	6-5	2	7-7	2	6-8	2	6-0	2
	4-2×12	9-8	2	8-6	2	7-8	2	9-5	2	8-3	2	7-5	2	8-10	2	7-9	2	7-0	2

(continued)

TABLE R502.5(1)—continued
GIRDER SPANS[a] AND HEADER SPANS[a] FOR EXTERIOR BEARING WALLS
(Maximum spans for Douglas fir-larch, hem-fir, southern pine and spruce-pine-fir[b] and required number of jack studs)

GIRDERS AND HEADERS SUPPORTING	SIZE	GROUND SNOW LOAD (psf)[e]																
		30						50						70				
		Building width[c] (feet)																
		20		28		36		20		28		36		20		28		36
		Span	NJ[d]	Span	NJ[d]	Span	NJ[d]	Span	NJ[d]	Span	NJ[d]	Span	NJ[d]	Span	NJ[d]	Span	NJ[d]	Span	NJ[d]
Roof, ceiling, and two clear span floors	2-2×4	2-1	1	1-8	1	1-6	2	2-0	1	1-8	1	1-5	2	2-0	1	1-8	1	1-5	2
	2-2×6	3-1	2	2-8	2	2-4	2	3-0	2	2-7	2	2-3	2	2-11	2	2-7	2	2-3	2
	2-2×8	3-10	2	3-4	2	3-0	3	3-10	2	3-4	2	2-11	3	3-9	2	3-3	2	2-11	3
	2-2×10	4-9	2	4-1	3	3-8	3	4-8	2	4-0	3	3-7	3	4-7	3	4-0	3	3-6	3
	2-2×12	5-6	3	4-9	3	4-3	3	5-5	3	4-8	3	4-2	3	5-4	3	4-7	3	4-1	4
	3-2×8	4-10	2	4-2	2	3-9	2	4-9	2	4-1	2	3-8	2	4-8	2	4-1	2	3-8	2
	3-2×10	5-11	2	5-1	2	4-7	3	5-10	2	5-0	2	4-6	3	5-9	2	4-11	2	4-5	3
	3-2×12	6-10	2	5-11	3	5-4	3	6-9	2	5-10	3	5-3	3	6-8	2	5-9	3	5-2	3
	4-2×8	5-7	2	4-10	2	4-4	2	5-6	2	4-9	2	4-3	2	5-5	2	4-8	2	4-2	2
	4-2×10	6-10	2	5-11	2	5-3	2	6-9	2	5-10	2	5-2	2	6-7	2	5-9	2	5-1	2
	4-2×12	7-11	2	6-10	2	6-2	3	7-9	2	6-9	2	6-0	3	7-8	2	6-8	2	5-11	3

For SI: 1 inch = 25.4 mm, 1 pound per square foot = 0.0479 kPa.

a. Spans are given in feet and inches.

b. Tabulated values assume #2 grade lumber.

c. Building width is measured perpendicular to the ridge. For widths between those shown, spans are permitted to be interpolated.

d. NJ - Number of jack studs required to support each end. Where the number of required jack studs equals one, the header is permitted to be supported by an approved framing anchor attached to the full-height wall stud and to the header.

e. Use 30 psf ground snow load for cases in which ground snow load is less than 30 psf and the roof live load is equal to or less than 20 psf.

TABLE R502.5(2)
GIRDER SPANS[a] AND HEADER SPANS[a] FOR INTERIOR BEARING WALLS
(Maximum spans for Douglas fir-larch, hem-fir, southern pine and spruce-pine-fir[b] and required number of jack studs)

HEADERS AND GIRDERS SUPPORTING	SIZE	BUILDING WIDTH[c] (feet)					
		20		28		36	
		Span	NJ[d]	Span	NJ[d]	Span	NJ[d]
One floor only	2-2×4	3-1	1	2-8	1	2-5	1
	2-2×6	4-6	1	3-11	1	3-6	1
	2-2×8	5-9	1	5-0	2	4-5	2
	2-2×10	7-0	2	6-1	2	5-5	2
	2-2×12	8-1	2	7-0	2	6-3	2
	3-2×8	7-2	1	6-3	1	5-7	2
	3-2×10	8-9	1	7-7	2	6-9	2
	3-2×12	10-2	2	8-10	2	7-10	2
	4-2×8	9-0	1	7-8	1	6-9	1
	4-2×10	10-1	1	8-9	1	7-10	2
	4-2×12	11-9	1	10-2	2	9-1	2
Two floors	2-2×4	2-2	1	1-10	1	1-7	1
	2-2×6	3-2	2	2-9	2	2-5	2
	2-2×8	4-1	2	3-6	2	3-2	2
	2-2×10	4-11	2	4-3	2	3-10	3
	2-2×12	5-9	2	5-0	3	4-5	3
	3-2×8	5-1	2	4-5	2	3-11	2
	3-2×10	6-2	2	5-4	2	4-10	2
	3-2×12	7-2	2	6-3	2	5-7	3
	4-2×8	6-1	1	5-3	2	4-8	2
	4-2×10	7-2	2	6-2	2	5-6	2
	4-2×12	8-4	2	7-2	2	6-5	2

For SI: 1 inch = 25.4 mm, 1 foot = 304.8 mm.

a. Spans are given in feet and inches.

b. Tabulated values assume #2 grade lumber.

c. Building width is measured perpendicular to the ridge. For widths between those shown, spans are permitted to be interpolated.

d. NJ - Number of jack studs required to support each end. Where the number of required jack studs equals one, the header is permitted to be supported by an approved framing anchor attached to the full-height wall stud and to the header.

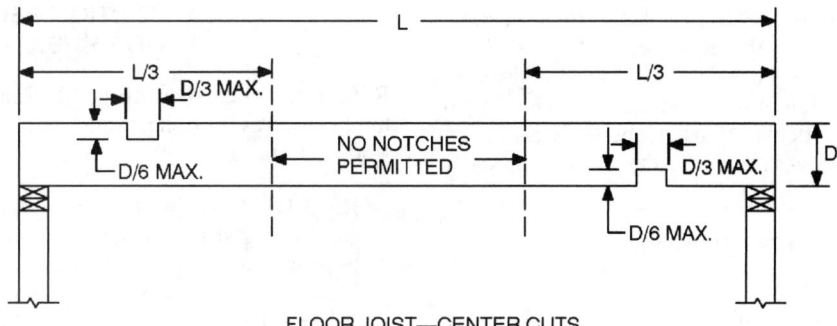

FLOOR JOIST—CENTER CUTS

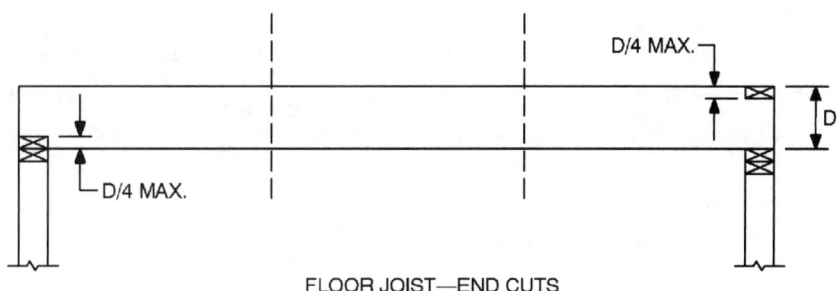

FLOOR JOIST—END CUTS

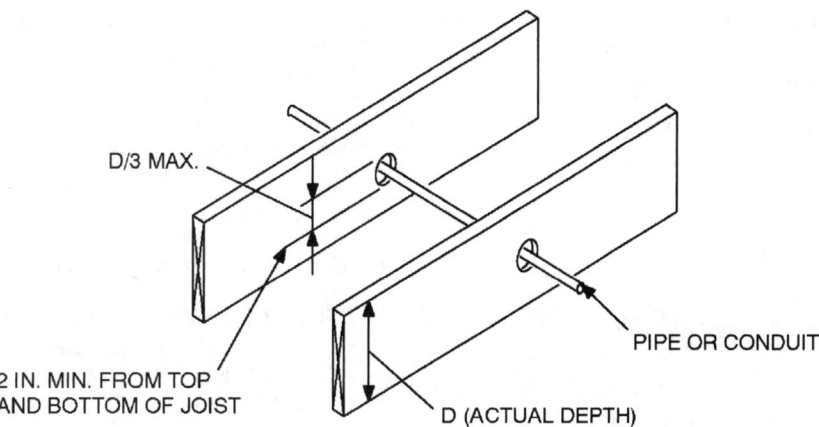

For SI: 1 inch = 25.4 mm.

FIGURE R502.8
CUTTING, NOTCHING AND DRILLING

R502.11 Wood trusses.

R502.11.1 Design. Wood trusses shall be designed in accordance with *approved* engineering practice. The design and manufacture of metal plate connected wood trusses shall comply with ANSI/TPI 1. The truss design drawings shall be prepared by a registered professional where required by the statutes of the *jurisdiction* in which the project is to be constructed in accordance with Section R106.1.

R502.11.2 Bracing. Trusses shall be braced to prevent rotation and provide lateral stability in accordance with the requirements specified in the *construction documents* for the building and on the individual truss design drawings. In the absence of specific bracing requirements, trusses shall be braced in accordance with the Building Component Safety Information (BCSI 1-03) Guide to Good Practice for Handling, Installing & Bracing of Metal Plate Connected Wood Trusses.

R502.11.3 Alterations to trusses. Truss members and components shall not be cut, notched, spliced or otherwise altered in any way without the approval of a registered *design professional. Alterations* resulting in the addition of load (e.g., HVAC *equipment*, water heater, etc.), that exceed the design load for the truss, shall not be permitted without verification that the truss is capable of supporting the additional loading.

R502.11.4 Truss design drawings. Truss design drawings, prepared in compliance with Section R502.11.1, shall be submitted to the *building official* and *approved* prior to installation. Truss design drawings shall be provided with the shipment of trusses delivered to the job site. Truss design drawings shall include, at a minimum, the information specified below:

1. Slope or depth, span and spacing.

2. Location of all joints.

3. Required bearing widths.

4. Design loads as applicable:

    4.1. Top chord live load;

    4.2. Top chord dead load;

    4.3. Bottom chord live load;

    4.4. Bottom chord dead load;

    4.5. Concentrated loads and their points of application; and

    4.6. Controlling wind and earthquake loads.

5. Adjustments to lumber and joint connector design values for conditions of use.

6. Each reaction force and direction.

7. Joint connector type and description, e.g., size, thickness or gauge, and the dimensioned location of each joint connector except where symmetrically located relative to the joint interface.

8. Lumber size, species and grade for each member.

9. Connection requirements for:

    9.1. Truss-to-girder-truss;

    9.2. Truss ply-to-ply; and

    9.3. Field splices.

10. Calculated deflection ratio and/or maximum description for live and total load.

11. Maximum axial compression forces in the truss members to enable the building designer to design the size, connections and anchorage of the permanent continuous lateral bracing. Forces shall be shown on the truss drawing or on supplemental documents.

12. Required permanent truss member bracing location.

R502.12 Draftstopping required. Draftstopping shall be provided in accordance with Section R302.12.

R502.13 Fireblocking required. Fireblocking shall be provided in accordance with Section R302.11.

SECTION R503
FLOOR SHEATHING

R503.1 Lumber sheathing. Maximum allowable spans for lumber used as floor sheathing shall conform to Tables R503.1, R503.2.1.1(1) and R503.2.1.1(2).

R503.1.1 End joints. End joints in lumber used as subflooring shall occur over supports unless end-matched lumber is used, in which case each piece shall bear on at least two joists. Subflooring may be omitted when joist spacing does not exceed 16 inches (406 mm) and a 1-inch (25.4 mm) nominal tongue-and-groove wood strip flooring is applied perpendicular to the joists.

TABLE R503.1
MINIMUM THICKNESS OF LUMBER FLOOR SHEATHING

JOIST OR BEAM SPACING (inches)	MINIMUM NET THICKNESS	
	Perpendicular to joist	Diagonal to joist
24	$^{11}/_{16}$	$^{3}/_{4}$
16	$^{5}/_{8}$	$^{5}/_{8}$
48[a]		
54[b]	$1^{1}/_{2}$ T & G	N/A
60[c]		

For SI: 1 inch = 25.4 mm, 1 pound per square inch = 6.895 kPa.

a. For this support spacing, lumber sheathing shall have a minimum F_b of 675 and minimum E of 1,100,000 (see AF&PA/NDS).

b. For this support spacing, lumber sheathing shall have a minimum F_b of 765 and minimum E of 1,400,000 (see AF&PA/NDS).

c. For this support spacing, lumber sheathing shall have a minimum F_b of 855 and minimum E of 1,700,000 (see AF&PA/NDS).

R503.2 Wood structural panel sheathing.

R503.2.1 Identification and grade. Wood structural panel sheathing used for structural purposes shall conform to DOC PS 1, DOC PS 2 or, when manufactured in Canada, CSA O437 or CSA O325. All panels shall be identified by a grade *mark* of certificate or inspection issued by an *approved agency.*

R503.2.1.1 Subfloor and combined subfloor underlayment. Where used as subflooring or combination subfloor underlayment, wood structural panels shall be of one of the grades specified in Table R503.2.1.1(1). When sanded plywood is used as combination subfloor underlayment, the grade shall be as specified in Table R503.2.1.1(2).

TABLE R503.2.1.1(1)
ALLOWABLE SPANS AND LOADS FOR WOOD STRUCTURAL PANELS FOR ROOF
AND SUBFLOOR SHEATHING AND COMBINATION SUBFLOOR UNDERLAYMENT[a, b, c]

SPAN RATING	MINIMUM NOMINAL PANEL THICKNESS (inch)	ALLOWABLE LIVE LOAD (psf)[h, l] SPAN @ 16″ o.c.	SPAN @ 24″ o.c.	MAXIMUM SPAN (inches) With edge support[d]	Without edge support	LOAD (pounds per square foot, at maximum span) Total load	Live load	MAXIMUM SPAN (inches)
Sheathing[e]					Roof[f]			Subfloor[j]
16/0	$^3/_8$	30	—	16	16	40	30	0
20/0	$^3/_8$	50	—	20	20	40	30	0
24/0	$^3/_8$	100	30	24	20[g]	40	30	0
24/16	$^7/_{16}$	100	40	24	24	50	40	16
32/16	$^{15}/_{32}, ^1/_2$	180	70	32	28	40	30	16[h]
40/20	$^{19}/_{32}, ^5/_8$	305	130	40	32	40	30	20[h, i]
48/24	$^{23}/_{32}, ^3/_{48}$	—	175	48	36	45	35	24
60/32	$^7/_8$	—	305	60	48	45	35	32
Underlayment, C-C plugged, single floor[e]					Roof[f]			**Combination subfloor underlayment[k]**
16 o.c.	$^{19}/_{32}, ^5/_8$	100	40	24	24	50	40	16[i]
20 o.c.	$^{19}/_{32}, ^5/_8$	150	60	32	32	40	30	20[i, j]
24 o.c.	$^{23}/_{32}, ^3/_4$	240	100	48	36	35	25	24
32 o.c.	$^7/_8$	—	185	48	40	50	40	32
48 o.c.	$1^3/_{32}, 1^1/_8$	—	290	60	48	50	40	48

For SI: 1 inch = 25.4 mm, 1 pound per square foot = 0.0479 kPa.

a. The allowable total loads were determined using a dead load of 10 psf. If the dead load exceeds 10 psf, then the live load shall be reduced accordingly.

b. Panels continuous over two or more spans with long dimension (strength axis) perpendicular to supports. Spans shall be limited to values shown because of possible effect of concentrated loads.

c. Applies to panels 24 inches or wider.

d. Lumber blocking, panel edge clips (one midway between each support, except two equally spaced between supports when span is 48 inches), tongue-and-groove panel edges, or other approved type of edge support.

e. Includes Structural 1 panels in these grades.

f. Uniform load deflection limitation: $^1/_{180}$ of span under live load plus dead load, $^1/_{240}$ of span under live load only.

g. Maximum span 24 inches for $^{15}/_{32}$-and $^1/_2$-inch panels.

h. Maximum span 24 inches where $^3/_4$-inch wood finish flooring is installed at right angles to joists.

i. Maximum span 24 inches where 1.5 inches of lightweight concrete or approved cellular concrete is placed over the subfloor.

j. Unsupported edges shall have tongue-and-groove joints or shall be supported with blocking unless minimum nominal $^1/_4$-inch thick underlayment with end and edge joints offset at least 2 inches or 1.5 inches of lightweight concrete or approved cellular concrete is placed over the subfloor, or $^3/_4$-inch wood finish flooring is installed at right angles to the supports. Allowable uniform live load at maximum span, based on deflection of $^1/_{360}$ of span, is 100 psf.

k. Unsupported edges shall have tongue-and-groove joints or shall be supported by blocking unless nominal $^1/_4$-inch-thick underlayment with end and edge joints offset at least 2 inches or $^3/_4$-inch wood finish flooring is installed at right angles to the supports. Allowable uniform live load at maximum span, based on deflection of $^1/_{360}$ of span, is 100 psf, except panels with a span rating of 48 on center are limited to 65 psf total uniform load at maximum span.

l. Allowable live load values at spans of 16″ o.c. and 24″ o.c taken from reference standard APA E30, APA Engineered Wood Construction Guide. Refer to reference standard for allowable spans not listed in the table.

TABLE R503.2.1.1(2)
ALLOWABLE SPANS FOR SANDED PLYWOOD
COMBINATION SUBFLOOR UNDERLAYMENT[a]

IDENTIFICATION	SPACING OF JOISTS (inches)		
	16	20	24
Species group[b]	—	—	—
1	$^1/_2$	$^5/_8$	$^3/_4$
2, 3	$^5/_8$	$^3/_4$	$^7/_8$
4	$^3/_4$	$^7/_8$	1

For SI: 1 inch = 25.4 mm, 1 pound per square foot = 0.0479 kPa.

a. Plywood continuous over two or more spans and face grain perpendicular to supports. Unsupported edges shall be tongue-and-groove or blocked except where nominal $^1/_4$-inch-thick underlayment or $^3/_4$-inch wood finish floor is used. Allowable uniform live load at maximum span based on deflection of $^1/_{360}$ of span is 100 psf.

b. Applicable to all grades of sanded exterior-type plywood.

R503.2.2 Allowable spans. The maximum allowable span for wood structural panels used as subfloor or combination subfloor underlayment shall be as set forth in Table R503.2.1.1(1), or APA E30. The maximum span for sanded plywood combination subfloor underlayment shall be as set forth in Table R503.2.1.1(2).

R503.2.3 Installation. Wood structural panels used as subfloor or combination subfloor underlayment shall be attached to wood framing in accordance with Table R602.3(1) and shall be attached to cold-formed steel framing in accordance with Table R505.3.1(2).

R503.3 Particleboard.

R503.3.1 Identification and grade. Particleboard shall conform to ANSI A208.1 and shall be so identified by a grade *mark* or certificate of inspection issued by an *approved agency*.

R503.3.2 Floor underlayment. Particleboard floor underlayment shall conform to Type PBU and shall not be less than $^1/_4$ inch (6.4 mm) in thickness.

R503.3.3 Installation. Particleboard underlayment shall be installed in accordance with the recommendations of the manufacturer and attached to framing in accordance with Table R602.3(1).

SECTION R504
PRESSURE PRESERVATIVELY TREATED-WOOD FLOORS (ON GROUND)

R504.1 General. Pressure preservatively treated-wood *basement* floors and floors on ground shall be designed to withstand axial forces and bending moments resulting from lateral soil pressures at the base of the exterior walls and floor live and dead loads. Floor framing shall be designed to meet joist deflection requirements in accordance with Section R301.

R504.1.1 Unbalanced soil loads. Unless special provision is made to resist sliding caused by unbalanced lateral soil loads, wood *basement* floors shall be limited to applications where the differential depth of fill on opposite exterior foundation walls is 2 feet (610 mm) or less.

R504.1.2 Construction. Joists in wood *basement* floors shall bear tightly against the narrow face of studs in the foundation wall or directly against a band joist that bears on the studs. Plywood subfloor shall be continuous over lapped joists or over butt joints between in-line joists. Sufficient blocking shall be provided between joists to transfer lateral forces at the base of the end walls into the floor system.

R504.1.3 Uplift and buckling. Where required, resistance to uplift or restraint against buckling shall be provided by interior bearing walls or properly designed stub walls anchored in the supporting soil below.

R504.2 Site preparation. The area within the foundation walls shall have all vegetation, topsoil and foreign material removed, and any fill material that is added shall be free of vegetation and foreign material. The fill shall be compacted to assure uniform support of the pressure preservatively treated-wood floor sleepers.

R504.2.1 Base. A minimum 4-inch-thick (102 mm) granular base of gravel having a maximum size of $^3/_4$ inch (19.1 mm) or crushed stone having a maximum size of $^1/_2$ inch (12.7 mm) shall be placed over the compacted earth.

R504.2.2 Moisture barrier. Polyethylene sheeting of minimum 6-mil (0.15 mm) thickness shall be placed over the granular base. Joints shall be lapped 6 inches (152 mm) and left unsealed. The polyethylene membrane shall be placed over the pressure preservatively treated-wood sleepers and shall not extend beneath the footing plates of the exterior walls.

R504.3 Materials. All framing materials, including sleepers, joists, blocking and plywood subflooring, shall be pressure-preservative treated and dried after treatment in accordance with AWPA U1 (Commodity Specification A, Use Category 4B and section 5.2), and shall bear the *label* of an accredited agency.

SECTION R505
STEEL FLOOR FRAMING

R505.1 Cold-formed steel floor framing. Elements shall be straight and free of any defects that would significantly affect structural performance. Cold-formed steel floor framing members shall comply with the requirements of this section.

R505.1.1 Applicability limits. The provisions of this section shall control the construction of cold-formed steel floor framing for buildings not greater than 60 feet (18 288 mm) in length perpendicular to the joist span, not greater than 40 feet (12 192 mm) in width parallel to the joist span, and less than or equal to three stories above *grade* plane. Cold-formed steel floor framing constructed in accordance with the provisions of this section shall be limited to sites subjected to a maximum design wind speed of 110 miles per hour (49 m/s), Exposure B or C, and a maximum ground snow load of 70 pounds per square foot (3.35 kPa).

R505.1.2 In-line framing. When supported by cold-formed steel framed walls in accordance with Section R603, cold-formed steel floor framing shall be constructed with floor joists located in-line with load-bearing studs located below the joists in accordance with Figure R505.1.2 and the tolerances specified as follows:

1. The maximum tolerance shall be $^3/_4$ inch (19.1 mm) between the centerline of the horizontal framing member and the centerline of the vertical framing member.

2. Where the centerline of the horizontal framing member and bearing stiffener are located to one side of the centerline of the vertical framing member, the maximum tolerance shall be $^1/_8$ inch (3 mm) between the web of the horizontal framing member and the edge of the vertical framing member.

R505.1.3 Floor trusses. Cold-formed steel trusses shall be designed, braced and installed in accordance with AISI S100, Section D4. Truss members shall not be notched, cut or altered in any manner without an *approved* design.

R505.2 Structural framing. Load-bearing cold-formed steel floor framing members shall comply with Figure R505.2(1) and with the dimensional and minimum thickness requirements specified in Tables R505.2(1) and R505.2(2). Tracks shall comply with Figure R505.2(2) and shall have a minimum flange width of $1^1/_4$ inches (32 mm). The maximum inside bend radius for members shall be the greater of $^3/_{32}$ inch (2.4 mm) minus half the base steel thickness or 1.5 times the base steel thickness.

R505.2.1 Material. Load-bearing cold-formed steel framing members shall be cold-formed to shape from structural quality sheet steel complying with the requirements of one of the following:

1. ASTM A 653: Grades 33 and 50 (Class 1 and 3).

2. ASTM A 792: Grades 33 and 50A.

3. ASTM A 1003: Structural Grades 33 Type H and 50 Type H.

R505.2.2 Identification. Load-bearing cold-formed steel framing members shall have a legible *label*, stencil, stamp or embossment with the following information as a minimum:

1. Manufacturer's identification.

2. Minimum base steel thickness in inches (mm).

3. Minimum coating designation.

4. Minimum yield strength, in kips per square inch (ksi) (MPa).

R505.2.3 Corrosion protection. Load-bearing cold-formed steel framing shall have a metallic coating complying with ASTM A 1003 and one of the following:

1. A minimum of G 60 in accordance with ASTM A 653.

2. A minimum of AZ 50 in accordance with ASTM A 792.

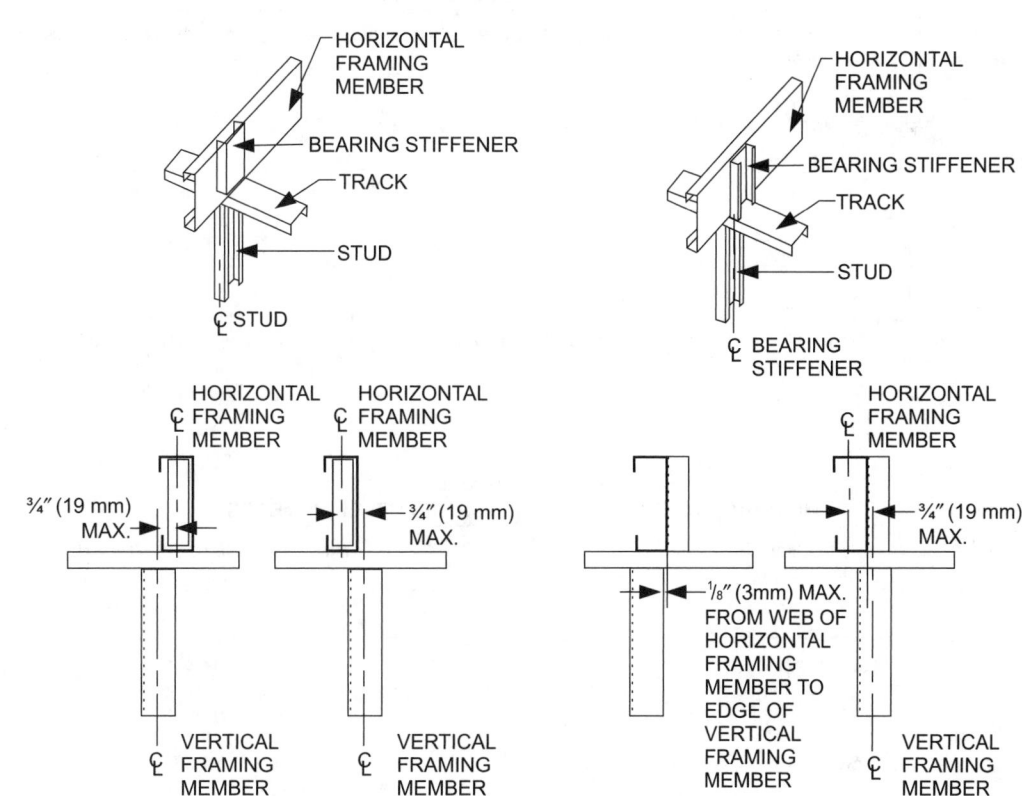

For SI: 1 inch = 25.4 mm.

FIGURE R505.1.2
IN-LINE FRAMING

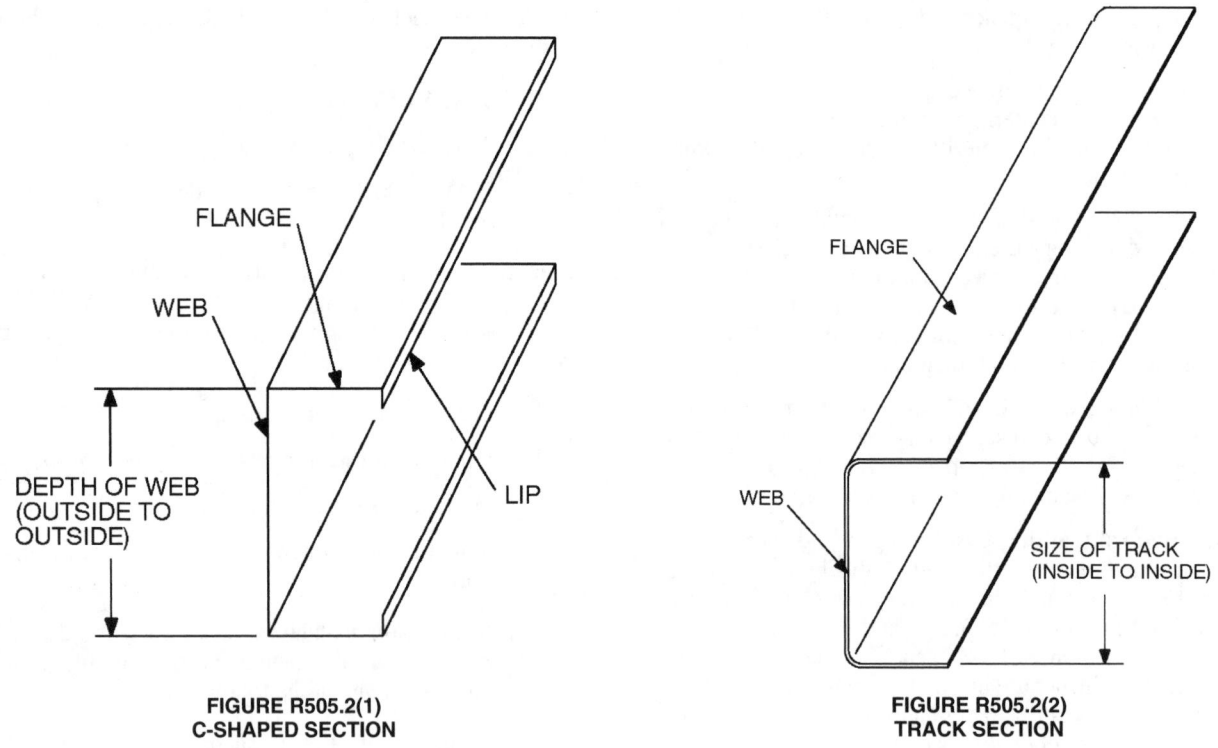

FIGURE R505.2(1)
C-SHAPED SECTION

FIGURE R505.2(2)
TRACK SECTION

TABLE R505.2(1)
COLD-FORMED STEEL JOIST SIZES

MEMBER DESIGNATION[a]	WEB DEPTH (inches)	MINIMUM FLANGE WIDTH (inches)	MAXIMUM FLANGE WIDTH (inches)	MINIMUM LIP SIZE (inches)
550S162-t	5.5	1.625	2	0.5
800S162-t	8	1.625	2	0.5
1000S162-t	10	1.625	2	0.5
1200S162-t	12	1.625	2	0.5

For SI: 1 inch = 25.4 mm, 1 mil = 0.0254 mm.

a. The member designation is defined by the first number representing the member depth in 0.01 inch, the letter "S" representing a stud or joist member, the second number representing the flange width in 0.01 inch, and the letter "t" shall be a number representing the minimum base metal thickness in mils [See Table R505.2(2)].

TABLE R505.2(2)
MINIMUM THICKNESS OF COLD-FORMED STEEL MEMBERS

DESIGNATION THICKNESS (mils)	MINIMUM BASE STEEL THICKNESS (inches)
33	0.0329
43	0.0428
54	0.0538
68	0.0677
97	0.0966

For SI: 1 inch = 25.4 mm, 1 mil = 0.0254 mm.

R505.2.4 Fastening requirements. Screws for steel-to-steel connections shall be installed with a minimum edge distance and center-to-center spacing of $^1/_2$ inch (12.7 mm), shall be self-drilling tapping, and shall conform to ASTM C 1513. Floor sheathing shall be attached to cold-formed steel joists with minimum No. 8 self-drilling tapping screws that conform to ASTM C 1513. Screws attaching floor-sheathing to cold-formed steel joists shall have a minimum head diameter of 0.292 inch (7.4 mm) with countersunk heads and shall be installed with a minimum edge distance of $^3/_8$ inch (9.5 mm). Gypsum board ceilings shall be attached to cold-formed steel joists with minimum No. 6 screws conforming to ASTM C 954 or ASTM C 1513 with a bugle head style and shall be installed in accordance with Section R702. For all connections, screws shall extend through the steel a minimum of three exposed threads. All fasteners shall have rust inhibitive coating suitable for the installation in which they are being used, or be manufactured from material not susceptible to corrosion.

Where No. 8 screws are specified in a steel-to-steel connection, the required number of screws in the connection is permitted to be reduced in accordance with the reduction factors in Table R505.2.4 when larger screws are used or when one of the sheets of steel being connected is thicker than 33 mils (0.84 mm). When applying the reduction factor, the resulting number of screws shall be rounded up.

TABLE R505.2.4
SCREW SUBSTITUTION FACTOR

SCREW SIZE	THINNEST CONNECTED STEEL SHEET (mils)	
	33	43
#8	1.0	0.67
#10	0.93	0.62
#12	0.86	0.56

For SI: 1 mil = 0.0254 mm.

R505.2.5 Web holes, web hole reinforcing and web hole patching. Web holes, web hole reinforcing, and web hole patching shall be in accordance with this section.

R505.2.5.1 Web holes. Web holes in floor joists shall comply with all of the following conditions:

1. Holes shall conform to Figure R505.2.5.1;

2. Holes shall be permitted only along the centerline of the web of the framing member;

3. Holes shall have a center-to-center spacing of not less than 24 inches (610 mm);

4. Holes shall have a web hole width not greater than 0.5 times the member depth, or $2^1/_2$ inches (64.5 mm);

5. Holes shall have a web hole length not exceeding $4^1/_2$ inches (114 mm); and

6. Holes shall have a minimum distance between the edge of the bearing surface and the edge of the web hole of not less than 10 inches (254 mm).

Framing members with web holes not conforming to the above requirements shall be reinforced in accordance with Section R505.2.5.2, patched in accordance with Section R505.2.5.3 or designed in accordance with accepted engineering practices.

R505.2.5.2 Web hole reinforcing. Reinforcement of web holes in floor joists not conforming to the requirements of Section R505.2.5.1 shall be permitted if the hole is located fully within the center 40 percent of the span and the depth and length of the hole does not exceed 65 percent of the flat width of the web. The reinforcing shall be a steel plate or C-shape section with a hole that does not exceed the web hole size limitations of Section R505.2.5.1 for the member being reinforced. The steel reinforcing shall be the same thickness as the receiving member and shall extend at least 1 inch (25.4 mm) beyond all edges of the hole. The steel reinforcing shall be fastened to the web of the receiving member with No.8 screws spaced no more than 1 inch (25.4 mm) center-to-center along the edges of the patch with minimum edge distance of $^1/_2$ inch (12.7 mm).

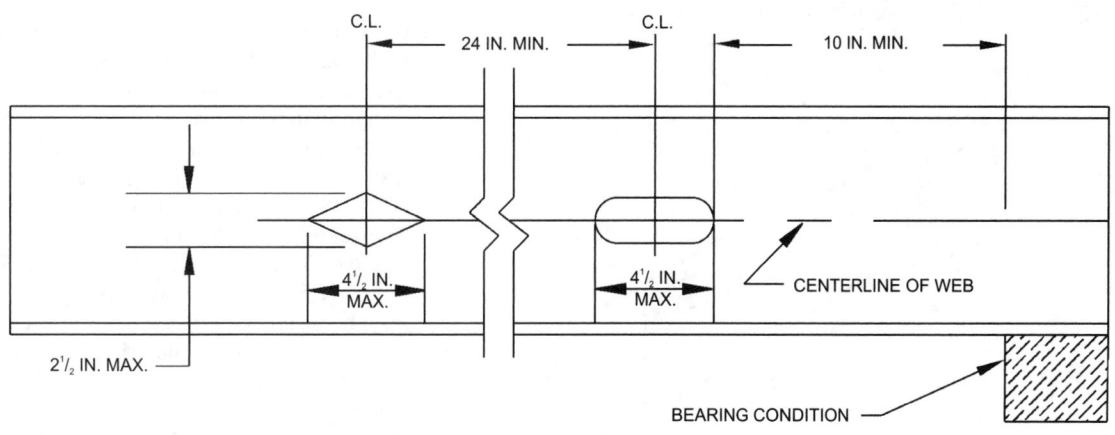

For SI: 1 inch = 25.4 mm.

FIGURE R505.2.5.1
FLOOR JOIST WEB HOLES

R505.2.5.3 Hole patching. Patching of web holes in floor joists not conforming to the requirements in Section R505.2.5.1 shall be permitted in accordance with either of the following methods:

1. Framing members shall be replaced or designed in accordance with accepted engineering practices where web holes exceed the following size limits:

    1.1. The depth of the hole, measured across the web, exceeds 70 percent of the flat width of the web; or

    1.2. The length of the hole measured along the web, exceeds 10 inches (254 mm) or the depth of the web, whichever is greater.

2. Web holes not exceeding the dimensional requirements in Section R505.2.5.3, Item 1, shall be patched with a solid steel plate, stud section, or track section in accordance with Figure R505.2.5.3. The steel patch shall, as a minimum, be of the same thickness as the receiving member and shall extend at least 1 inch (25 mm) beyond all edges of the hole. The steel patch shall be fastened to the web of the receiving member with No.8 screws spaced no more than 1 inch (25 mm) center-to-center along the edges of the patch with minimum edge distance of $^1/_2$ inch (13 mm).

R505.3 Floor construction. Cold-formed steel floors shall be constructed in accordance with this section.

R505.3.1 Floor to foundation or load-bearing wall connections. Cold-formed steel framed floors shall be anchored to foundations, wood sills or load-bearing walls in accordance with Table R505.3.1(1) and Figure R505.3.1(1), R505.3.1(2), R505.3.1(3), R505.3.1(4), R505.3.1(5) or R505.3.1(6). Anchor bolts shall be located not more than 12 inches (305 mm) from corners or the termination of bottom tracks. Continuous cold-formed steel joists supported by interior load-bearing walls shall be constructed in accordance with Figure R505.3.1(7). Lapped cold-formed steel joists shall be constructed in accordance with Figure R505.3.1(8). End floor joists constructed on foundation walls parallel to the joist span shall be doubled unless a C-shaped bearing stiffener, sized in accordance with Section R505.3.4, is installed web-to-web with the floor joist beneath each supported wall stud, as shown in Figure R505.3.1(9). Fastening of cold-formed steel joists to other framing members shall be in accordance with Section R505.2.4 and Table R505.3.1(2).

R505.3.2 Minimum floor joist sizes. Floor joist size and thickness shall be determined in accordance with the limits set forth in Table R505.3.2(1) for single spans, and Tables R505.3.2(2) and R505.3.2(3) for multiple spans. When continuous joist members are used, the interior bearing supports shall be located within 2 feet (610 mm) of mid-span of the cold-formed steel joists, and the individual spans shall not exceed the spans in Table R505.3.2(2) or R505.3.2(3), as applicable. Floor joists shall have a bearing support length of not less than $1^1/_2$ inches (38 mm) for exterior wall supports and $3^1/_2$ inches (89 mm) for interior wall supports. Tracks shall be a minimum of 33 mils (0.84 mm) thick except when used as part of a floor header or trimmer in accordance with Section R505.3.8. Bearing stiffeners shall be installed in accordance with Section R505.3.4.

R505.3.3 Joist bracing and blocking. Joist bracing and blocking shall be in accordance with this section.

R505.3.3.1 Joist top flange bracing. The top flanges of cold-formed steel joists shall be laterally braced by the application of floor sheathing fastened to the joists in accordance with Section R505.2.4 and Table R505.3.1(2).

R505.3.3.2 Joist bottom flange bracing/blocking. Floor joists with spans that exceed 12 feet (3658 mm) shall have the bottom flanges laterally braced in accordance with one of the following:

1. Gypsum board installed with minimum No. 6 screws in accordance with Section R702.

2. Continuous steel straps installed in accordance with Figure R505.3.3.2(1). Steel straps shall be spaced at a maximum of 12 feet (3658 mm) on center and shall be at least $1^1/_2$ inches (38 mm) in width and 33 mils (0.84 mm) in thickness. Straps shall be fastened to the bottom flange of each joist with one No. 8 screw, fastened to blocking with two No. 8 screws, and fastened at each end (of strap) with two No. 8 screws. Blocking in accordance with Figure R505.3.3.2(1) or Figure R505.3.3.2(2) shall be installed between joists at each end of the continuous strapping and at a maximum spacing of 12 feet (3658 mm) measured along the continuous strapping (perpendicular to the joist run). Blocking shall also be located at the termination of all straps. As an alternative to blocking at the ends, anchoring the strap to a stable building component with two No. 8 screws shall be permitted.

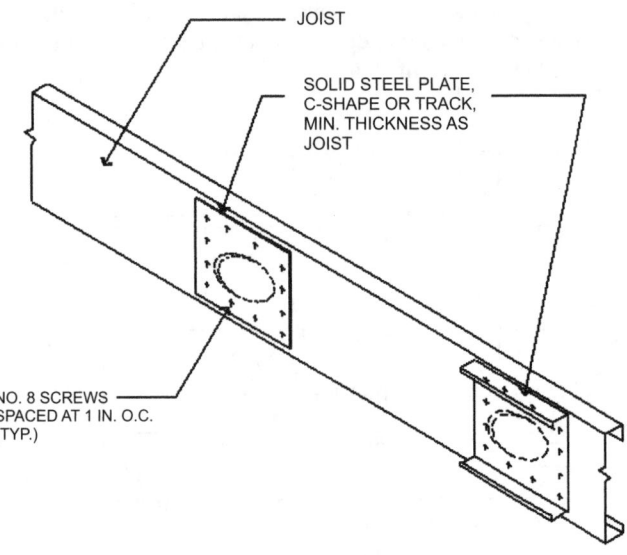

JOIST

SOLID STEEL PLATE, C-SHAPE OR TRACK, MIN. THICKNESS AS JOIST

NO. 8 SCREWS SPACED AT 1 IN. O.C. (TYP.)

FIGURE R505.2.5.3
WEB HOLE PATCH

TABLE R505.3.1(1)
FLOOR TO FOUNDATION OR BEARING WALL CONNECTION REQUIREMENTS[a, b]

FRAMING CONDITION	BASIC WIND SPEED (mph) AND EXPOSURE	
	85 mph Exposure C or less than 110 mph Exposure B	Less than 110 mph Exposure C
Floor joist to wall track of exterior wall per Figure R505.3.1(1)	2-No. 8 screws	3-No. 8 screws
Rim track or end joist to load-bearing wall top track per Figure R505.3.1(1)	1-No. 8 screw at 24 inches o.c.	1-No. 8 screw at 24 inches o.c.
Rim track or end joist to wood sill per Figure R505.3.1(2)	Steel plate spaced at 4 feet o.c. with 4-No. 8 screws and 4-10d or 6-8d common nails	Steel plate spaced at 2 feet o.c. with 4-No. 8 screws and 4-10d or 6-8d common nails
Rim track or end joist to foundation per Figure R505.3.1(3)	$^1/_2$ inch minimum diameter anchor bolt and clip angle spaced at 6 feet o.c. with 8-No. 8 screws	$^1/_2$ inch minimum diameter anchor bolt and clip angle spaced at 4 feet o.c. with 8-No. 8 screws
Cantilevered joist to foundation per Figure R505.3.1(4)	$^1/_2$ inch minimum diameter anchor bolt and clip angle spaced at 6 feet o.c. with 8-No. 8 screws	$^1/_2$ inch minimum diameter anchor bolt and clip angle spaced at 4 feet o.c. with 8-No. 8 screws
Cantilevered joist to wood sill per Figure R505.3.1(5)	Steel plate spaced at 4 feet o.c. with 4-No. 8 screws and 4-10d or 6-8d common nails	Steel plate spaced at 2 feet o.c. with 4-No. 8 screws and 4-10d or 6-8d common nails
Cantilevered joist to exterior load-bearing wall track per Figure R505.3.1(6)	2-No. 8 screws	3-No. 8 screws

For SI: 1 inch = 25.4 mm, 1 pound per square foot = 0.0479 kPa, 1 mile per hour = 0.447 m/s, 1 foot = 304.8 mm.

a. Anchor bolts are to be located not more than 12 inches from corners or the termination of bottom tracks (e.g., at door openings or corners). Bolts extend a minimum of 15 inches into masonry or 7 inches into concrete. Anchor bolts connecting cold-formed steel framing to the foundation structure are to be installed so that the distance from the center of the bolt hole to the edge of the connected member is not less than one and one-half bolt diameters.

b. All screw sizes shown are minimum.

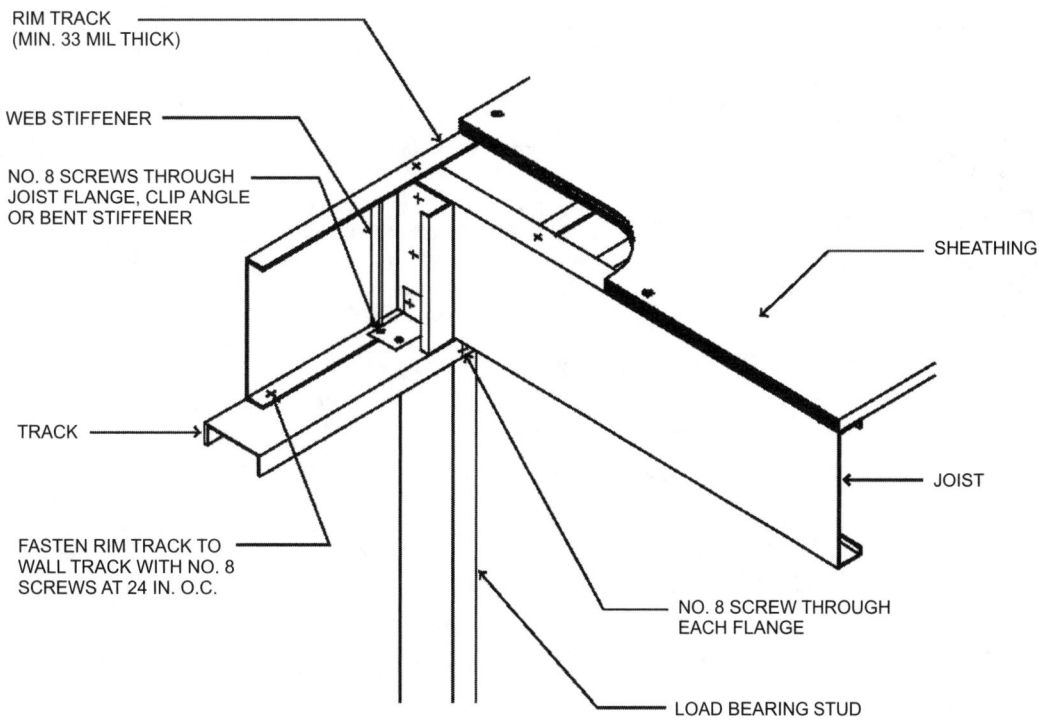

RIM TRACK (MIN. 33 MIL THICK)

WEB STIFFENER

NO. 8 SCREWS THROUGH JOIST FLANGE, CLIP ANGLE OR BENT STIFFENER

SHEATHING

TRACK

JOIST

FASTEN RIM TRACK TO WALL TRACK WITH NO. 8 SCREWS AT 24 IN. O.C.

NO. 8 SCREW THROUGH EACH FLANGE

LOAD BEARING STUD

For SI: 1 mil = 0.0254 mm, 1 inch = 25.4 mm.

FIGURE 505.3.1(1)
FLOOR TO EXTERIOR LOAD-BEARING WALL STUD CONNECTION

TABLE R505.3.1(2)
FLOOR FASTENING SCHEDULE[a]

DESCRIPTION OF BUILDING ELEMENTS	NUMBER AND SIZE OF FASTENERS	SPACING OF FASTENERS
Floor joist to track of an interior load-bearing wall per Figures R505.3.1(7) and R505.3.1(8)	2 No. 8 screws	Each joist
Floor joist to track at end of joist	2 No. 8 screws	One per flange or two per bearing stiffener
Subfloor to floor joists	No. 8 screws	6 in. o.c. on edges and 12 in. o.c. at intermediate supports

For SI: 1 inch = 25.4 mm.

a. All screw sizes shown are minimum.

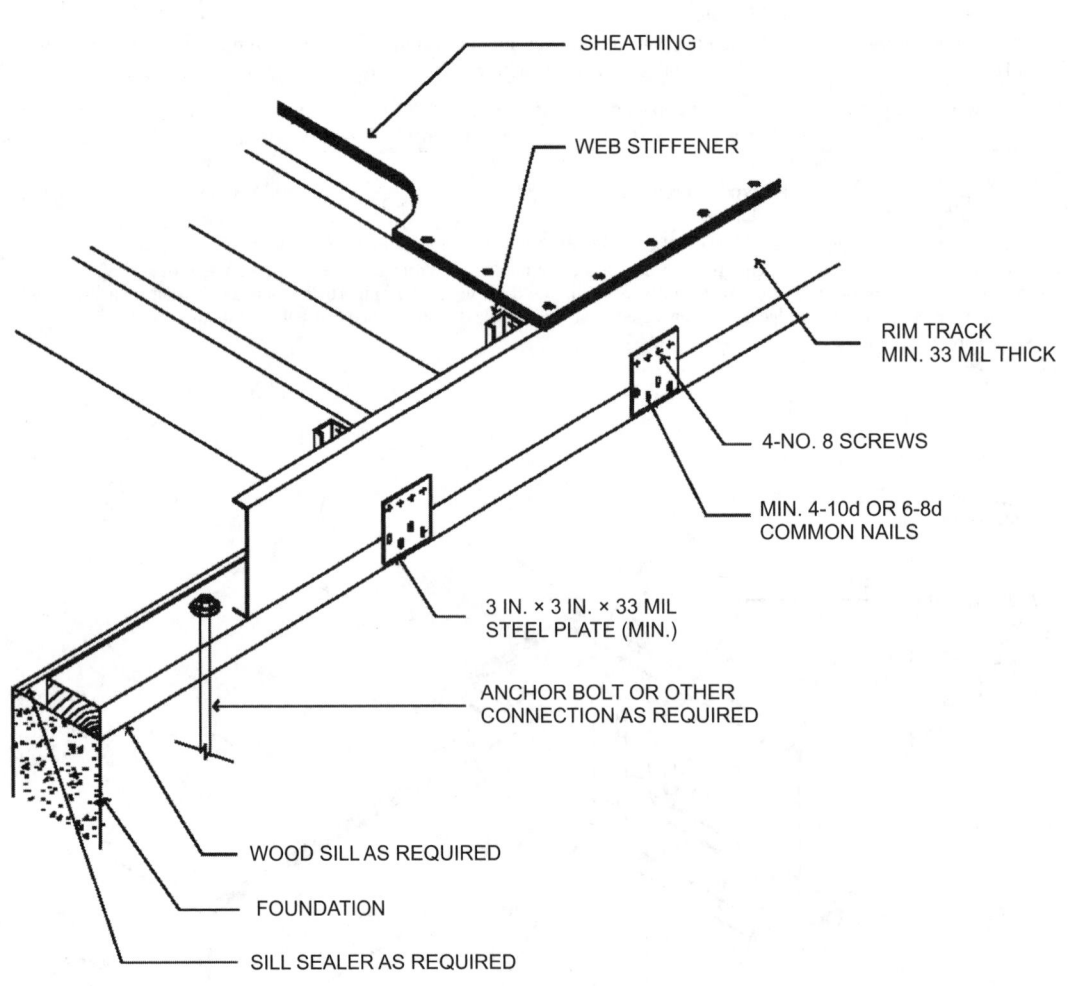

For SI: 1 mil = 0.0254 mm, 1 inch = 25.4 mm.

FIGURE R505.3.1(2)
FLOOR TO WOOD SILL CONNECTION

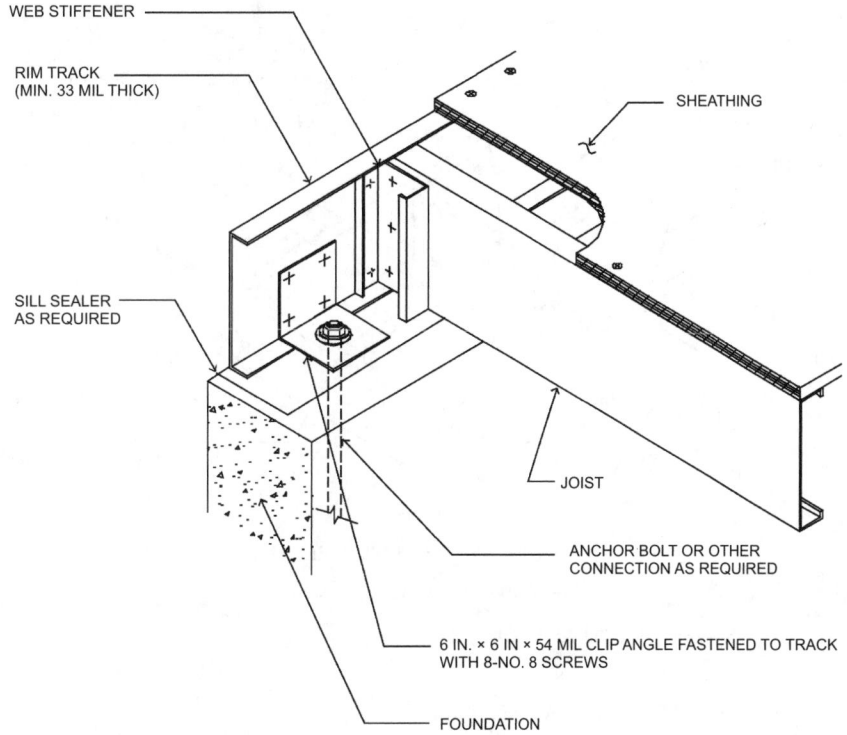

WEB STIFFENER

RIM TRACK
(MIN. 33 MIL THICK)

SHEATHING

SILL SEALER
AS REQUIRED

JOIST

ANCHOR BOLT OR OTHER
CONNECTION AS REQUIRED

6 IN. × 6 IN × 54 MIL CLIP ANGLE FASTENED TO TRACK
WITH 8-NO. 8 SCREWS

FOUNDATION

For SI: 1 mil = 0.0254 mm, 1 inch = 25.4 mm.

FIGURE R505.3.1(3)
FLOOR TO FOUNDATION CONNECTION

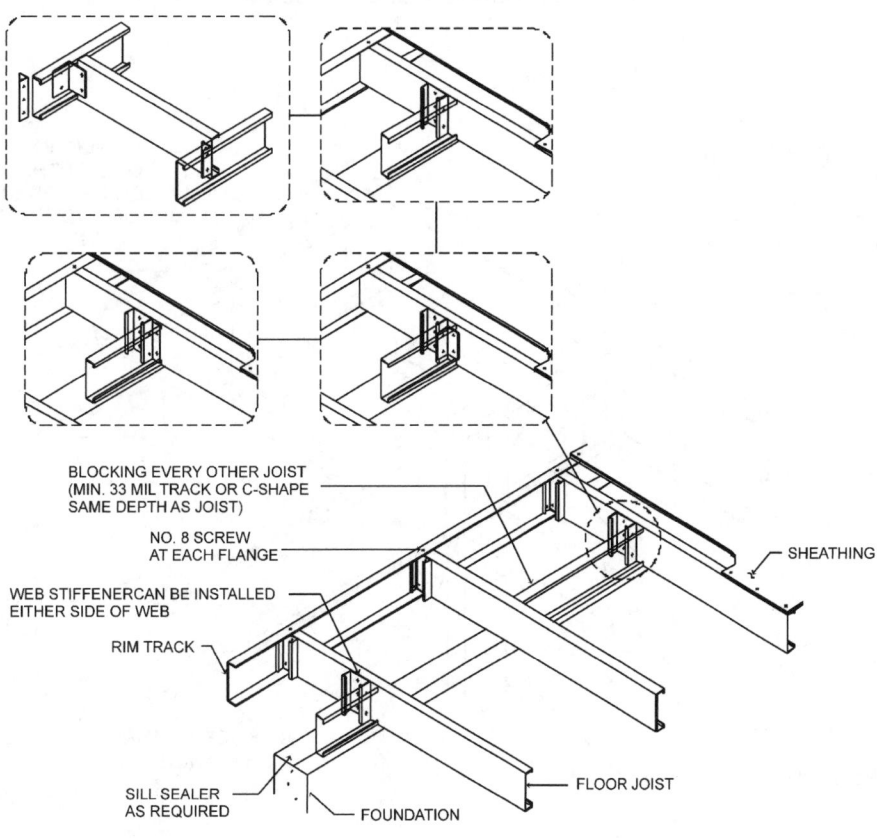

BLOCKING EVERY OTHER JOIST
(MIN. 33 MIL TRACK OR C-SHAPE
SAME DEPTH AS JOIST)

NO. 8 SCREW
AT EACH FLANGE

SHEATHING

WEB STIFFENERCAN BE INSTALLED
EITHER SIDE OF WEB

RIM TRACK

FLOOR JOIST

SILL SEALER
AS REQUIRED

FOUNDATION

For SI: 1 mil = 0.0254 mm.

FIGURE R505.3.1(4)
CANTILEVERED FLOOR TO FOUNDATION CONNECTION

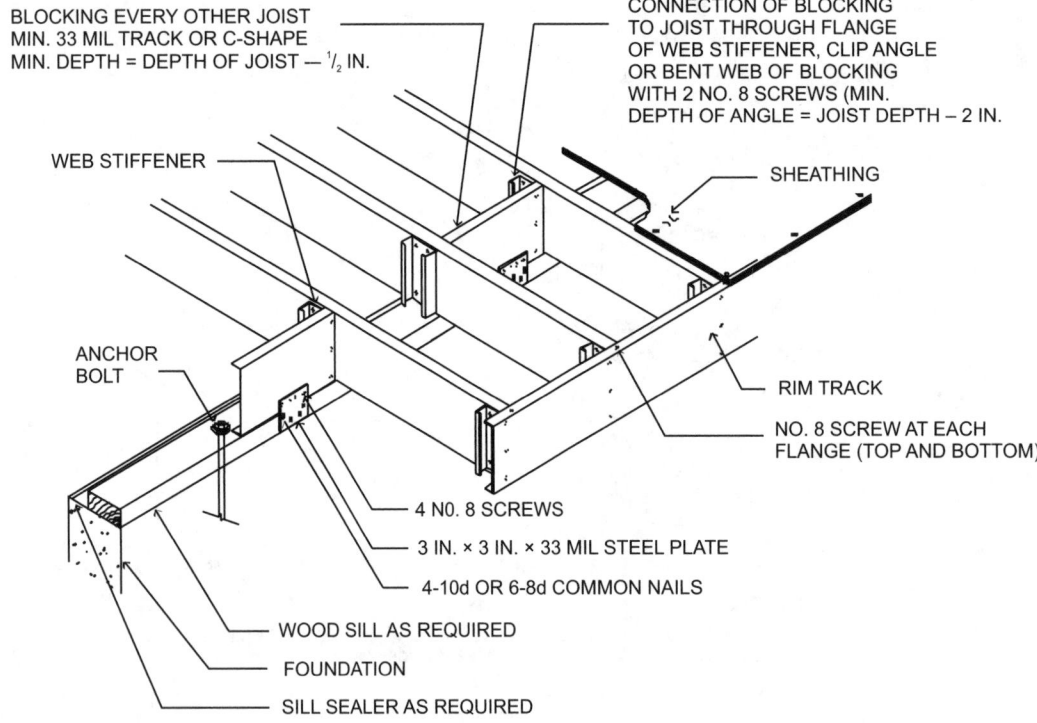

BLOCKING EVERY OTHER JOIST
MIN. 33 MIL TRACK OR C-SHAPE
MIN. DEPTH = DEPTH OF JOIST — $^1/_2$ IN.

CONNECTION OF BLOCKING
TO JOIST THROUGH FLANGE
OF WEB STIFFENER, CLIP ANGLE
OR BENT WEB OF BLOCKING
WITH 2 NO. 8 SCREWS (MIN.
DEPTH OF ANGLE = JOIST DEPTH – 2 IN.

WEB STIFFENER

SHEATHING

ANCHOR
BOLT

RIM TRACK

NO. 8 SCREW AT EACH
FLANGE (TOP AND BOTTOM)

4 NO. 8 SCREWS

3 IN. × 3 IN. × 33 MIL STEEL PLATE

4-10d OR 6-8d COMMON NAILS

WOOD SILL AS REQUIRED

FOUNDATION

SILL SEALER AS REQUIRED

For SI: 1 mil = 0.0254 mm, 1 inch = 25.4 mm.

FIGURE R505.3.1(5)
CANTILEVERED FLOOR TO WOOD SILL CONNECTION

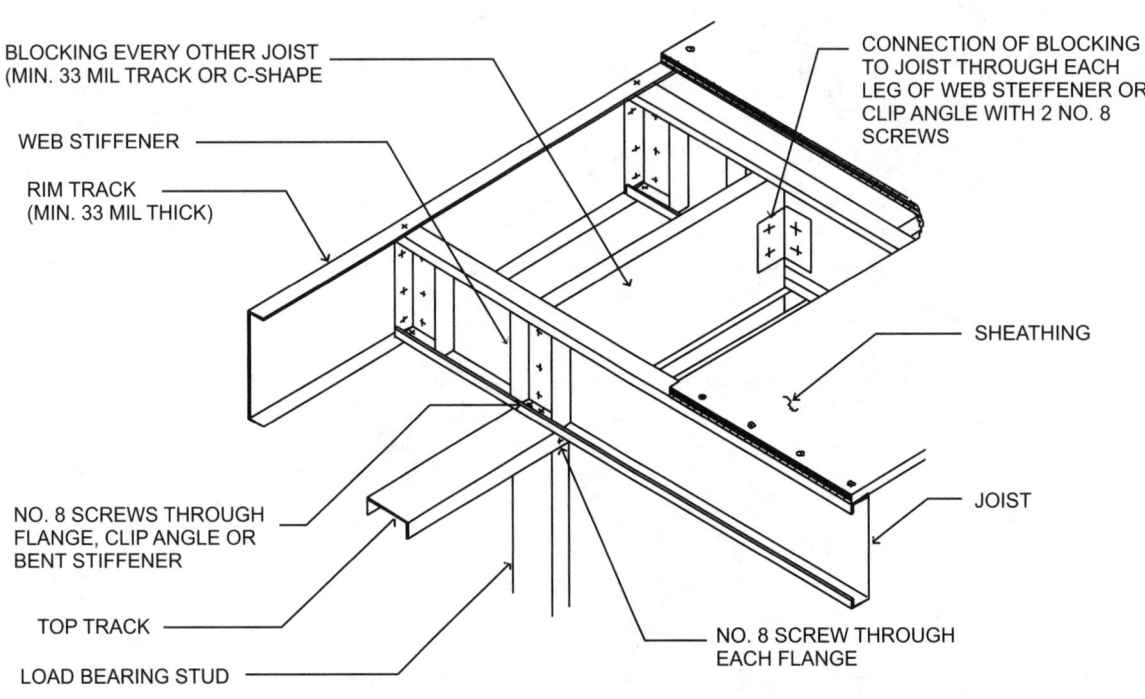

BLOCKING EVERY OTHER JOIST
(MIN. 33 MIL TRACK OR C-SHAPE)

WEB STIFFENER

RIM TRACK
(MIN. 33 MIL THICK)

CONNECTION OF BLOCKING
TO JOIST THROUGH EACH
LEG OF WEB STEFFENER OR
CLIP ANGLE WITH 2 NO. 8
SCREWS

SHEATHING

JOIST

NO. 8 SCREWS THROUGH
FLANGE, CLIP ANGLE OR
BENT STIFFENER

TOP TRACK

LOAD BEARING STUD

NO. 8 SCREW THROUGH
EACH FLANGE

For SI: 1 mil = 0.0254 mm.

FIGURE R505.3.1(6)
CANTILEVERED FLOOR TO EXTERIOR LOAD-BEARING WALL CONNECTION

2009 INTERNATIONAL RESIDENTIAL CODE®

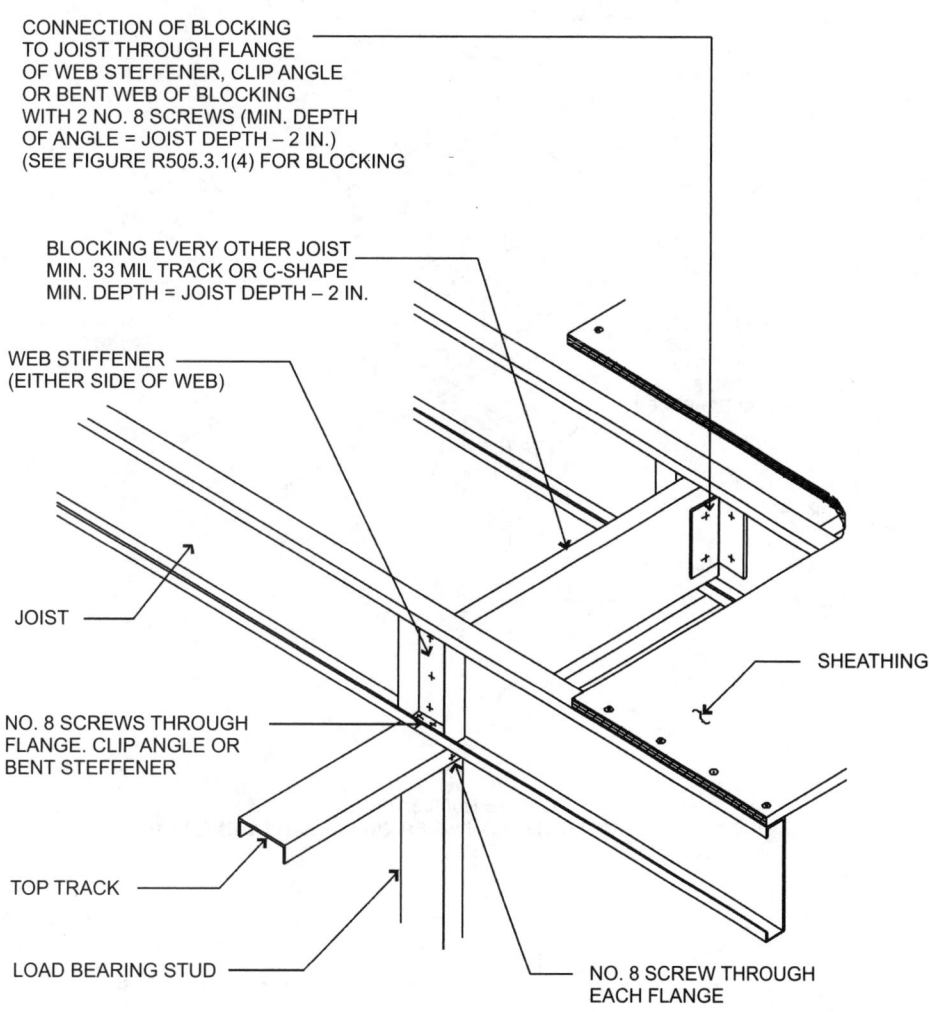

CONNECTION OF BLOCKING
TO JOIST THROUGH FLANGE
OF WEB STEFFENER, CLIP ANGLE
OR BENT WEB OF BLOCKING
WITH 2 NO. 8 SCREWS (MIN. DEPTH
OF ANGLE = JOIST DEPTH – 2 IN.)
(SEE FIGURE R505.3.1(4) FOR BLOCKING

BLOCKING EVERY OTHER JOIST
MIN. 33 MIL TRACK OR C-SHAPE
MIN. DEPTH = JOIST DEPTH – 2 IN.

WEB STIFFENER
(EITHER SIDE OF WEB)

JOIST

SHEATHING

NO. 8 SCREWS THROUGH
FLANGE. CLIP ANGLE OR
BENT STEFFENER

TOP TRACK

LOAD BEARING STUD

NO. 8 SCREW THROUGH
EACH FLANGE

For SI: 1 mil = 0.0254 mm, 1 inch = 25.4 mm.

FIGURE R505.3.1(7)
CONTINUOUS SPAN JOIST SUPPORTED ON INTERIOR LOAD-BEARING WALL

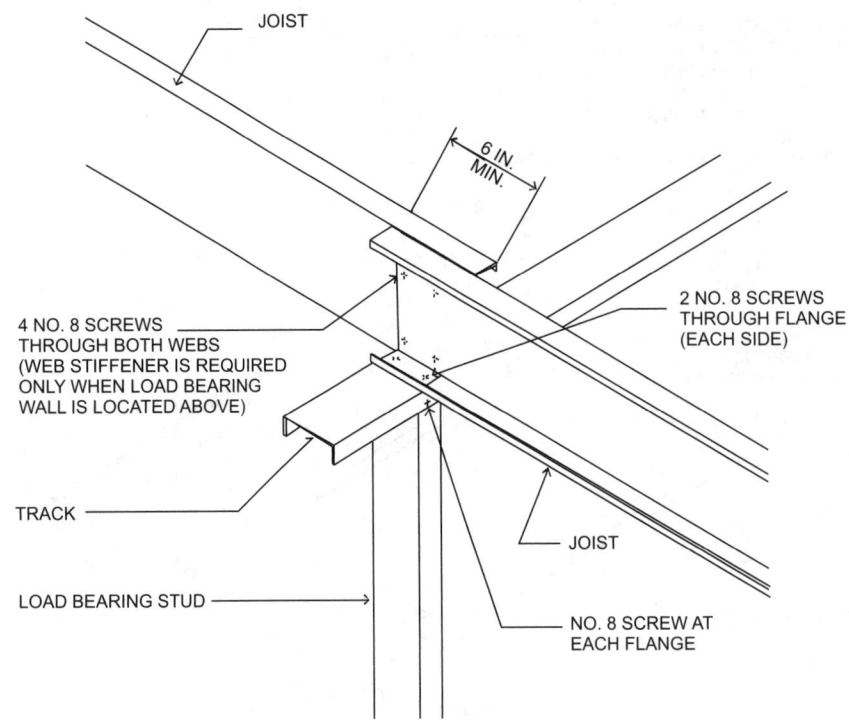

JOIST

6 IN.
MIN.

4 NO. 8 SCREWS
THROUGH BOTH WEBS
(WEB STIFFENER IS REQUIRED
ONLY WHEN LOAD BEARING
WALL IS LOCATED ABOVE)

2 NO. 8 SCREWS
THROUGH FLANGE
(EACH SIDE)

TRACK

JOIST

LOAD BEARING STUD

NO. 8 SCREW AT
EACH FLANGE

For SI: 1 inch = 25.4 mm.

FIGURE R505.3.1(8)
LAPPED JOISTS SUPPORTED ON INTERIOR LOAD-BEARING WALL

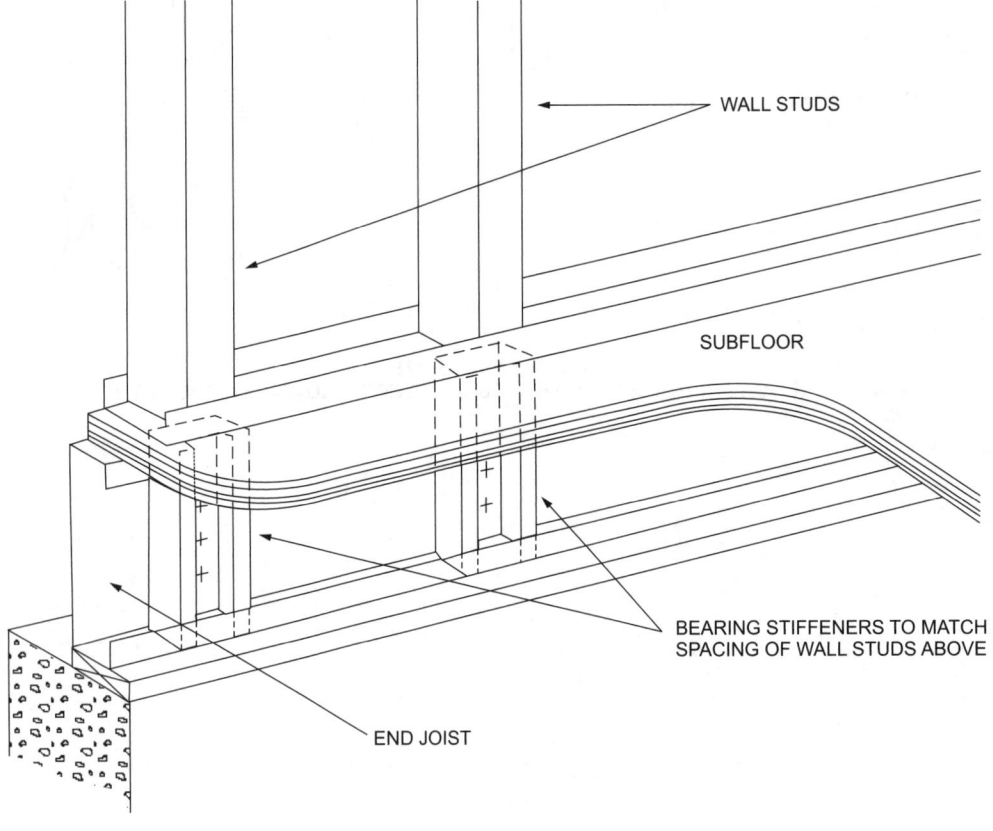

WALL STUDS

SUBFLOOR

BEARING STIFFENERS TO MATCH
SPACING OF WALL STUDS ABOVE

END JOIST

FIGURE R505.3.1(9)
BEARING STIFFENERS FOR END JOISTS

TABLE R505.3.2(1)
ALLOWABLE SPANS FOR COLD-FORMED STEEL JOISTS—SINGLE SPANS[a, b, c, d] 33 ksi STEEL

JOIST DESIGNATION	30 PSF LIVE LOAD				40 PSF LIVE LOAD			
	Spacing (inches)				Spacing (inches)			
	12	16	19.2	24	12	16	19.2	24
550S162-33	11'-7"	10'-7"	9'-6"	8'-6"	10'-7"	9'-3"	8'-6"	7'-6"
550S162-43	12'-8"	11'-6"	10'-10"	10'-2"	11'-6"	10'-5"	9'-10"	9'-1"
550S162-54	13'-7"	12'-4"	11'-7"	10'-9"	12'-4"	11'-2"	10'-6"	9'-9"
550S162-68	14'-7"	13'-3"	12'-6"	11'-7"	13'-3"	12'-0"	11'-4"	10'-6"
550S162-97	16'-2"	14'-9"	13'-10"	12'-10"	14'-9"	13'-4"	12'-7"	11'-8"
800S162-33	15'-8"	13'-11"	12'-9"	11'-5"	14'-3"	12'-5"	11'-3"	9'-0"
800S162-43	17'-1"	15'-6"	14'-7"	13'-7"	15'-6"	14'-1"	13'-3"	12'-4"
800S162-54	18'-4"	16'-8"	15'-8"	14'-7"	16'-8"	15'-2"	14'-3"	13'-3"
800S162-68	19'-9"	17'-11"	16'-10"	15'-8"	17'-11"	16'-3"	15'-4"	14'-2"
800S162-97	22'-0"	20'-0"	16'-10"	17'-5"	20'-0"	18'-2"	17'-1"	15'-10"
1000S162-43	20'-6"	18'-8"	17'-6"	15'-8"	18'-8"	16'-11"	15'-6"	13'-11"
1000S162-54	22'-1"	20'-0"	18'-10"	17'-6"	20'-0"	18'-2"	17'-2"	15'-11"
1000S162-68	23'- 9"	21'-7"	20'-3"	18'-10"	21'-7"	19'-7"	18'-5"	17'-1"
1000S162-97	26'-6"	24'-1"	22'-8"	21'-0"	24'-1"	21'-10"	20'-7"	19'-1"
1200S162-43	23'-9"	20'-10"	19'-0"	16'-8"	21'-5"	18'-6"	16'-6"	13'-2"
1200S162-54	25'-9"	23'-4"	22'-0"	20'-1"	23'-4"	21'-3"	20'-0"	17'-10"
1200S162-68	27'-8"	25'-1"	23'-8"	21'-11"	25'-1"	22'-10"	21'-6"	21'-1"
1200S162-97	30'-11"	28'-1"	26'-5"	24'-6"	28'-1"	25'-6"	24'-0"	22'-3"

For SI: 1 inch = 25.4 mm, 1 foot = 304.8 mm, 1 pound per square foot = 0.0479 kPa.

a. Deflection criteria: $L/480$ for live loads, $L/240$ for total loads.

b. Floor dead load = 10 psf.

c. Table provides the maximum clear span in feet and inches.

d. Bearing stiffeners are to be installed at all support points and concentrated loads.

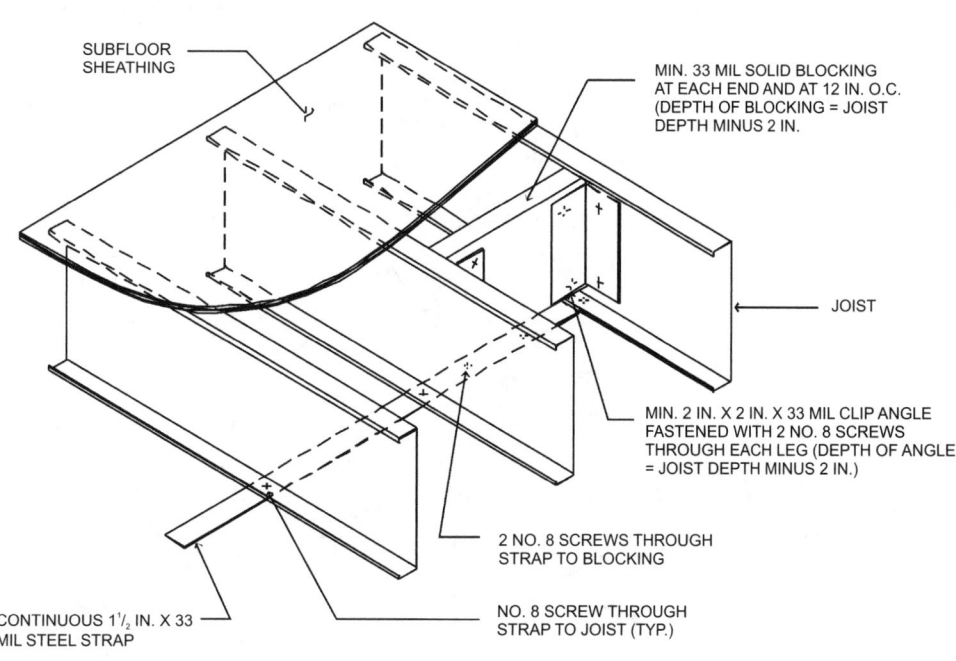

For SI: 1 mil = 0.0254 mm, 1 inch = 25.4 mm.

FIGURE R505.3.3.2(1)
JOIST BLOCKING (SOLID)

TABLE R505.3.2(2)
ALLOWABLE SPANS FOR COLD-FORMED STEEL JOISTS—MULTIPLE SPANS[a, b, c, d, e, f] 33 ksi STEEL

JOIST DESIGNATION	30 PSF LIVE LOAD				40 PSF LIVE LOAD			
	Spacing (inches)				Spacing (inches)			
	12	16	19.2	24	12	16	19.2	24
550S162-33	12'-1"	10'-5"	9'-6"	8'-6"	10'-9"	9'-3"	8'-6"	7'-6"
550S162-43	14'-5"	12'-5"	11'-4"	10'-2"	12'-9"	11'-11"	10'-1"	9'-0"
550S162-54	16'-3"	14'-1"	12'-10"	11'-6"	14'-5"	12'-6"	11'-5"	10'-2"
550S162-68	19'-7"	17'-9"	16'-9"	15'-6"	17'-9"	16'-2"	15'-2"	14'-1"
550S162-97	21'-9"	19'-9"	18'-7"	17'-3"	19'-9"	17'-11"	16'-10"	15'-4"
800S162-33	14'-8"	11'-10"	10'-4"	8'-8"	12'-4"	9'-11"	8'-7"	7'-2"
800S162-43	20'-0"	17'-4"	15'-9"	14'-1"	17'-9"	15'-4"	14'-0"	12'-0"
800S162-54	23'-7"	20'-5"	18'-8"	16'-8"	21'-0"	18'-2"	16'-7"	14'-10"
800S162-68	26'-5"	23'-1"	21'-0"	18'-10"	23'-8"	20'-6"	18'-8"	16'-9"
800S162-97	29'-6"	26'-10"	25'-3"	22'-8"	26'-10"	24'-4"	22'-6"	20'-2"
1000S162-43	22'-2"	18'-3"	16'-0"	13'-7"	18'-11"	15'-5"	13'-6"	11'-5"
1000S162-54	26'-2"	22'-8"	20'-8"	18'-6"	23'-3"	20'-2"	18'-5"	16'-5"
1000S162-68	31'- 5"	27'-2"	24'-10"	22'-2"	27'-11"	24'-2"	22'-1"	19'-9"
1000S162-97	35'-6"	32'-3"	29'-11"	26'-9"	32'-3"	29'-2"	26'-7"	23'-9"
1200S162-43	21'-8"	17'-6"	15'-3"	12'-10"	18'-3"	14'-8"	12'-8"	10'-6²
1200S162-54	28'-5"	24'-8"	22'-6"	19'-6"	25'-3"	21'-11"	19'-4"	16'-6"
1200S162-68	33'-7"	29'-1"	26'-6"	23'-9"	29'-10"	25'-10"	23'-7"	21'-1"
1200S162-97	41'-5"	37'-8"	34'-6"	30'-10"	37'-8"	33'-6"	30'-7"	27'-5"

For SI: 1 inch = 25.4 mm, 1 foot = 304.8 mm, 1 pound per square foot = 0.0479kPa.

a. Deflection criteria: $L/480$ for live loads, $L/240$ for total loads.
b. Floor dead load = 10 psf.
c. Table provides the maximum clear span in feet and inches to either side of the interior support.
d. Interior bearing supports for multiple span joists consist of structural (bearing) walls or beams.
e. Bearing stiffeners are to be installed at all support points and concentrated loads.
f. Interior supports shall be located within 2 feet of mid-span provided that each of the resulting spans does not exceed the appropriate maximum span shown in the table above.

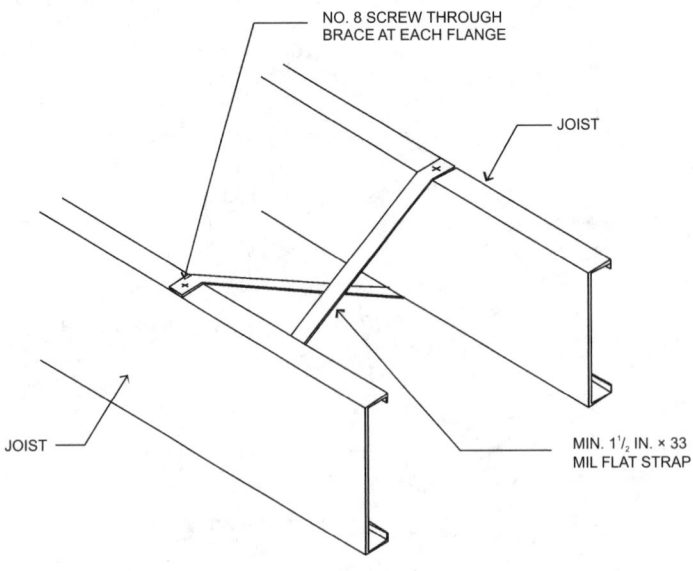

For SI: 1 mil = 0.0254 = 25.4 mm.

FIGURE R505.3.3.2(2)
JOIST BLOCKING (STRAP)

2009 INTERNATIONAL RESIDENTIAL CODE®

TABLE R505.3.2(3)
ALLOWABLE SPANS FOR COLD-FORMED STEEL JOISTS—MULTIPLE SPANS[a, b, c, d, e, f] 50 ksi STEEL

JOIST DESIGNATION	30 PSF LIVE LOAD				40 PSF LIVE LOAD			
	Spacing (inches)				Spacing (inches)			
	12	16	19.2	24	12	16	19.2	24
550S162-33	13'-11"	12'-0"	11'-0"	9'-3"	12'-3"	10'-8"	9'-7"	8'-4"
550S162-43	16'-3"	14'-1"	12'-10"	11'-6"	14'-6"	12'-6"	11'-5"	10'-3"
550S162-54	18'-2"	16'-6"	15'-4"	13'-8"	16'-6"	14'-11"	13'-7"	12'-2"
550S162-68	19'-6"	17'-9"	16'-8"	15'-6"	17'-9"	16'-1"	15'-2"	14'-0"
550S162-97	21'-9"	19'-9"	18'-6"	17'-2"	19'-8"	17'-10"	16'-8"	15'-8"
800S162-33	15'-6"	12'-6"	10'-10"	9'-1"	13'-0"	10'-5"	8'-11"	6'-9"
800S162-43	22'-0"	19'-1"	17'-5"	15'-0"	19'-7"	16'-11"	14'-10"	12'-8"
800S162-54	24'-6"	22'-4"	20'-6"	17'-11"	22'-5"	19'-9"	17'-11"	15'-10"
800S162-68	26'-6"	24'-1"	22'-8"	21'-0"	24'-1"	21'-10"	20'-7"	19'-2"
800S162-97	29'-9"	26'-8"	25'-2"	23'-5"	26'-8"	24'-3"	22'-11"	21'-4"
1000S162-43	23'-6"	19'-2"	16'-9"	14'-2"	19'-11"	16'-2"	14'-0"	11'-9"
1000S162-54	28'-2"	23'-10"	21'-7"	18'-11"	24'-8"	20'-11"	18'-9"	18'-4"
1000S162-68	31'-10"	28'-11"	27'-2"	25'-3"	28'-11"	26'-3"	24'-9"	22'-9"
1000S162-97	35'-4"	32'-1"	30'-3"	28'-1"	32'-1"	29'-2"	27'-6"	25'-6"
1200S162-43	22'-11"	18'-5"	16'-0"	13'-4"	19'-2"	15'-4"	13'-2"	10'-6"
1200S162-54	32'-8"	28'-1"	24'-9"	21'-2"	29'-0"	23'-10"	20'-11"	17'-9"
1200S162-68	37'-1"	32'-5"	29'-4"	25'-10"	33'-4"	28'-6"	25'-9"	22'-7"
1200S162-97	41'-2"	37'-6"	35'-3"	32'-9"	37'-6"	34'-1"	32'-1"	29'-9"

For SI: 1 inch = 25.4 mm, 1 foot = 304.8 mm, 1 pound per square foot = 0.0479kPa.

a. Deflection criteria: $L/480$ for live loads, $L/240$ for total loads.

b. Floor dead load = 10 psf.

c. Table provides the maximum clear span in feet and inches to either side of the interior support.

d. Interior bearing supports for multiple span joists consist of structural (bearing) walls or beams.

e. Bearing stiffeners are to be installed at all support points and concentrated loads.

f. Interior supports shall be located within 2 feet of mid-span provided that each of the resulting spans does not exceed the appropriate maximum span shown in the table above.

R505.3.3.3 Blocking at interior bearing supports. Blocking is not required for continuous back-to-back floor joists at bearing supports. Blocking shall be installed between every other joist for single continuous floor joists across bearing supports in accordance with Figure R505.3.1(7). Blocking shall consist of C-shape or track section with a minimum thickness of 33 mils (0.84 mm). Blocking shall be fastened to each adjacent joist through a 33-mil (0.84 mm) clip angle, bent web of blocking or flanges of web stiffeners with two No. 8 screws on each side. The minimum depth of the blocking shall be equal to the depth of the joist minus 2 inches (51 mm). The minimum length of the angle shall be equal to the depth of the joist minus 2 inches (51 mm).

R505.3.3.4 Blocking at cantilevers. Blocking shall be installed between every other joist over cantilever bearing supports in accordance with Figure R505.3.1(4), R505.3.1(5) or R505.3.1(6). Blocking shall consist of C-shape or track section with minimum thickness of 33 mils (0.84 mm). Blocking shall be fastened to each adjacent joist through bent web of blocking, 33 mil clip angle or flange of web stiffener with two No.8 screws at each end. The depth of the blocking shall be equal to the depth of the joist. The minimum length of the angle shall be equal to the depth of the joist minus 2 inches (51 mm). Blocking shall be fastened through the floor sheathing and to the support with three No.8 screws (top and bottom).

R505.3.4 Bearing stiffeners. Bearing stiffeners shall be installed at each joist bearing location in accordance with this section, except for joists lapped over an interior support not carrying a load-bearing wall above. Floor joists supporting jamb studs with multiple members shall have two bearing stiffeners in accordance with Figure R505.3.4(1). Bearing stiffeners shall be fabricated from a C-shaped, track or clip angle member in accordance with the one of following:

1. C-shaped bearing stiffeners:

    1.1. Where the joist is not carrying a load-bearing wall above, the bearing stiffener shall be a minimum 33 mil (0.84 mm) thickness.

1.2. Where the joist is carrying a load-bearing wall above, the bearing stiffener shall be at least the same designation thickness as the wall stud above.

2. Track bearing stiffeners:

2.1. Where the joist is not carrying a load-bearing wall above, the bearing stiffener shall be a minimum 43 mil (1.09 mm) thickness.

2.2. Where the joist is carrying a load-bearing wall above, the bearing stiffener shall be at least one designation thickness greater than the wall stud above.

3. Clip angle bearing stiffeners: Where the clip angle bearing stiffener is fastened to both the web of the member it is stiffening and an adjacent rim track using the fastener pattern shown in Figure R505.3.4(2), the bearing stiffener shall be a minimum 2-inch by 2-inch (51 mm by 51 mm) angle sized in accordance with Tables R505.3.4(1),R505.3.4(2),R505.3.4(3), and R505.3.4(4).

The minimum length of a bearing stiffener shall be the depth of member being stiffened minus $^{3}/_{8}$ inch (9.5 mm). Each bearing stiffener shall be fastened to the web of the member it is stiffening as shown in Figure R505.3.4(2). Each clip angle bearing stiffener shall also be fastened to the web of the adjacent rim track using the fastener pattern shown in Figure R505.3.4(2). No. 8 screws shall be used for C-shaped and track members of any thickness and for clip angle members with a designation thickness less than or equal to 54. No. 10 screws shall be used for clip angle members with a designation thickness greater than 54.

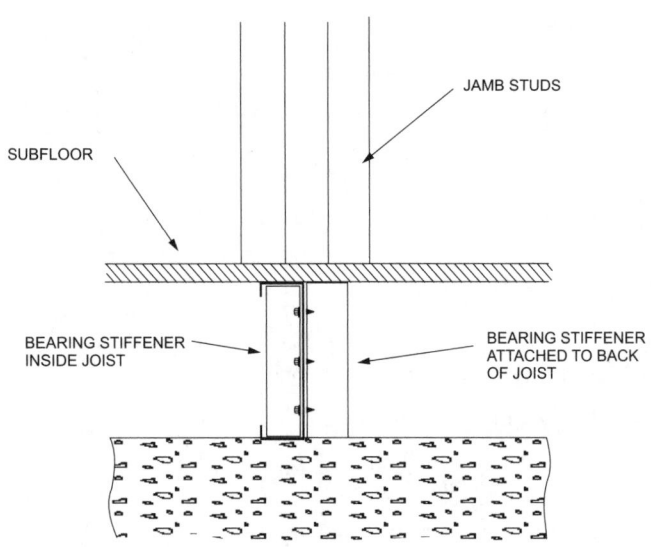

FIGURE R505.3.4(1)
BEARING STIFFENERS UNDER JAMB STUDS

TABLE R505.3.4(1)
CLIP ANGLE BEARING STIFFENERS
(20 psf equivalent snow load)

JOIST DESIGNATION	MINIMUM THICKNESS (mils) OF 2-INCH × 2-INCH (51 mm × 51 mm) CLIP ANGLE											
	Top floor				Bottom floor in 2 story Middle floor in 3 story				Bottom floor in 3 story			
	Joist spacing (inches)				Joist spacing (inches)				Joist spacing (inches)			
	12	16	19.2	24	12	16	19.2	24	12	16	19.2	24
800S162-33	43	43	43	43	43	54	68	68	68	97	97	—
800S162-43	43	43	43	43	54	54	68	68	97	97	97	97
800S162-54	43	43	43	43	43	54	68	68	68	97	97	—
800S162-68	43	43	43	43	43	43	54	68	54	97	97	—
800S162-97	43	43	43	43	43	43	43	43	43	43	54	97
1000S162-43	43	43	43	43	54	68	97	97	97	—	—	—
1000S162-54	43	43	43	43	54	68	68	97	97	97	—	—
1000S162-68	43	43	43	43	54	68	97	97	97	—	—	—
1000S162-97	43	43	43	43	43	43	43	54	43	68	97	—
1200S162-43	43	54	54	54	97	97	97	97	—	—	—	—
1200S162-54	54	54	54	54	97	97	97	97	—	—	—	—
1200S162-68	43	43	54	54	68	97	97	97	—	—	—	—
1200S162-97	43	43	43	43	43	54	68	97	97	—	—	—

For SI: 1 mil = 0.254 mm, 1 inch = 25.4 mm, 1 pound per square foot = 0.0479 kPa..

2009 INTERNATIONAL RESIDENTIAL CODE®

TABLE R505.3.4(2)
CLIP ANGLE BEARING STIFFENERS
(30 psf equivalent snow load)

JOIST DESIGNATION	MINIMUM THICKNESS (mils) OF 2-INCH × 2 INCH (51 mm × 51 mm) CLIP ANGLE											
	Top floor				Bottom floor in 2 story Middle floor in 3 story				Bottom floor in 3 story			
	Joist spacing (inches)				Joist spacing (inches)				Joist spacing (inches)			
	12	16	19.2	24	12	16	19.2	24	12	16	19.2	24
800S162-33	43	43	43	43	54	68	68	97	97	97	97	—
800S162-43	43	43	43	54	68	68	68	97	97	97	97	—
800S162-54	43	43	43	43	54	68	68	97	97	97	—	—
800S162-68	43	43	43	43	43	54	68	97	68	97	97	—
800S162-97	43	43	43	43	43	43	43	43	43	43	68	97
1000S162-43	54	54	54	54	68	97	97	97	97	—	—	—
1000S162-54	54	54	54	54	68	97	97	97	97	—	—	—
1000S162-68	43	43	54	68	68	97	97	—	97	—	—	—
1000S162-97	43	43	43	43	43	43	54	68	54	97	—	—
1200S162-43	54	68	68	68	97	97	97	—	—	—	—	—
1200S162-54	68	68	68	68	97	97	—	—	—	—	—	—
1200S162-68	68	68	68	68	97	97	97	—	—	—	—	—
1200S162-97	43	43	43	43	54	68	97	—	97	—	—	—

For SI: 1 mil = 0.0254 mm, 1 inch = 25.4 mm, 1 pound per square foot = 0.0479 kPa.

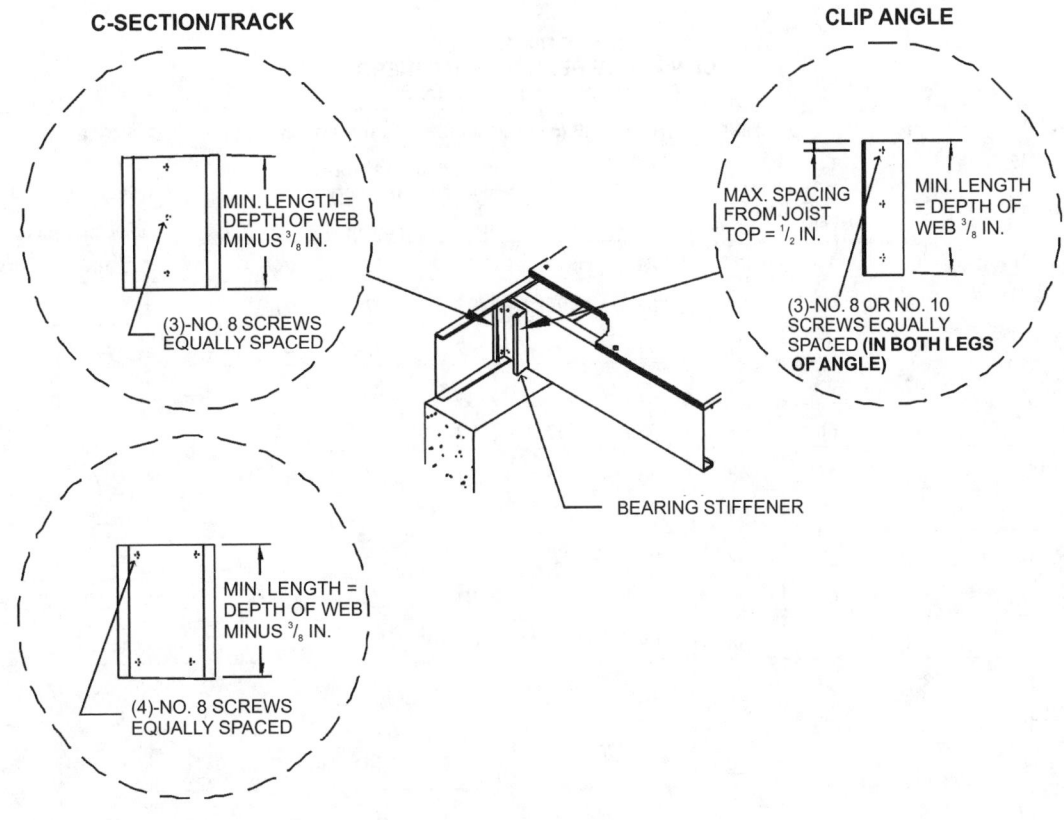

For SI: 1 inch = 25.4 mm.

FIGURE R505.3.4(2)
BEARING STIFFENER

TABLE R505.3.4(3)
CLIP ANGLE BEARING STIFFENERS
(50 psf equivalent snow load)

JOIST DESIGNATION	MINIMUM THICKNESS (mils) OF 2-INCH × 2-INCH (51 mm × 51 mm) CLIP ANGLE											
	Top floor				Bottom floor in 2 story Middle floor in 3 story				Bottom floor in 3 story			
	Joist spacing (inches)				Joist spacing (inches)				Joist spacing (inches)			
	12	16	19.2	24	12	16	19.2	24	12	16	19.2	24
800S162-33	54	54	54	54	68	97	97	97	97	—	—	—
800S162-43	68	68	68	68	97	97	97	97	—	—	—	—
800S162-54	54	68	68	68	97	97	97	97	—	—	—	—
800S162-68	43	43	54	54	68	97	97	97	97	—	—	—
800S162-97	43	43	43	43	43	43	43	54	54	68	97	—
1000S162-43	97	68	68	68	97	97	97	97	—	—	—	—
1000S162-54	97	97	68	68	97	97	97	—	—	—	—	—
1000S162-68	68	97	97	97	97	—	—	—	—	—	—	—
1000S162-97	43	43	43	43	54	68	97	97	—	—	—	—
1200S162-43	97	97	97	97	—	—	—	—	—	—	—	—
1200S162-54	—	97	97	97	—	—	—	—	—	—	—	—
1200S162-68	97	97	97	97	—	—	—	—	—	—	—	—
1200S162-97	54	68	68	97	97	—	—	—	—	—	—	—

For SI: 1 mil = 0.0254 mm, 1 inch = 25.4 mm, 1 pound per square foot = 0.0479 kPa.

TABLE R505.3.4(4)
CLIP ANGLE BEARING STIFFENERS
(70 psf equivalent snow load)

JOIST DESIGNATION	MINIMUM THICKNESS (mils) OF 2-INCH × 2-INCH (51 mm × 51 mm) CLIP ANGLE											
	Top floor				Bottom floor in 2 story Middle floor in 3 story				Bottom floor in 3 story			
	Joist spacing (inches)				Joist spacing (inches)				Joist spacing (inches)			
	12	16	19.2	24	12	16	19.2	24	12	16	19.2	24
800S162-33	68	68	68	68	97	97	97	97	—	—	—	—
800S162-43	97	97	97	97	97	97	97	—	—	—	—	—
800S162-54	97	97	97	97	97	—	—	—	—	—	—	—
800S162-68	68	68	68	97	97	97	97	—	—	—	—	—
800S162-97	43	43	43	43	43	54	68	97	97	97	—	—
1000S162-43	97	97	97	97	—	—	—	—	—	—	—	—
1000S162-54	—	97	97	97	—	—	—	—	—	—	—	—
1000S162-68	97	97	—	—	—	—	—	—	—	—	—	—
1000S162-97	68	68	68	68	97	97	—	—	—	—	—	—
1200S162-43	97	97	97	97	—	—	—	—	—	—	—	—
1200S162-54	—	—	—	—	—	—	—	—	—	—	—	—
1200S162-68	—	—	—	—	—	—	—	—	—	—	—	—
1200S162-97	97	97	97	—	—	—	—	—	—	—	—	—

For SI: 1 mil 0.0254 mm, 1 inch = 25.4 mm, 1 pound per square foot = 0.0479 kPa.

R505.3.5 Cutting and notching. Flanges and lips of load-bearing cold-formed steel floor framing members shall not be cut or notched.

R505.3.6 Floor cantilevers. Floor cantilevers for the top floor of a two- or three-story building or the first floor of a one-story building shall not exceed 24 inches (610 mm). Cantilevers, not exceeding 24 inches (610 mm) and supporting two stories and roof (i.e., first floor of a two-story building), shall also be permitted provided that all cantilevered joists are doubled (nested or back-to-back). The doubled cantilevered joists shall extend a minimum of 6 feet (1829 mm) toward the inside and shall be fastened with a minimum of two No.8 screws spaced at 24 inches (610 mm) on center through the webs (for back-to-back) or flanges (for nested joists).

R505.3.7 Splicing. Joists and other structural members shall not be spliced. Splicing of tracks shall conform to Figure R505.3.7.

R505.3.8 Framing of floor openings. Openings in floors shall be framed with header and trimmer joists. Header joist spans shall not exceed 6 feet (1829 mm) or 8 feet (2438 mm) in length in accordance with Figure R505.3.8(1) or R505.3.8(2), respectively. Header and trimmer joists shall be fabricated from joist and track members, having a minimum size and thickness at least equivalent to the adjacent floor joists and shall be installed in accordance with Figures R505.3.8(1), R505.3.8(2), R505.3.8(3), and R505.3.8(4). Each header joist shall be connected to trimmer joists with four 2-inch-by-2-inch (51mm by 51 mm) clip angles. Each clip angle shall be fastened to both the header and trimmer joists with four No. 8 screws, evenly spaced, through each leg of the clip angle. The clip angles shall have a thickness not less than that of the floor joist. Each track section for a built-up header or trimmer joist shall extend the full length of the joist (continuous).

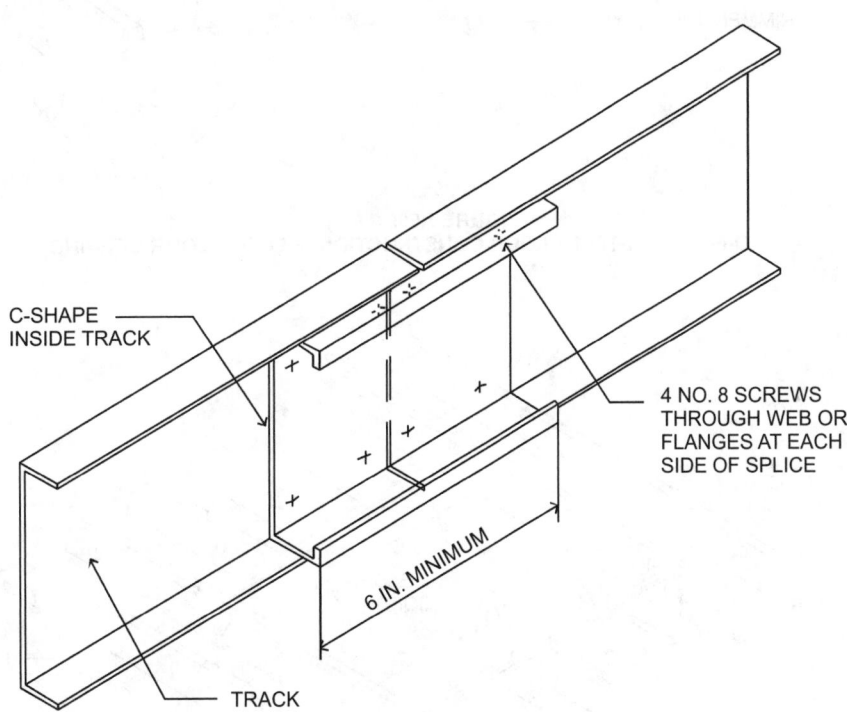

For SI: 1 inch = 25.4 mm.

FIGURE R505.3.7
TRACK SPLICE

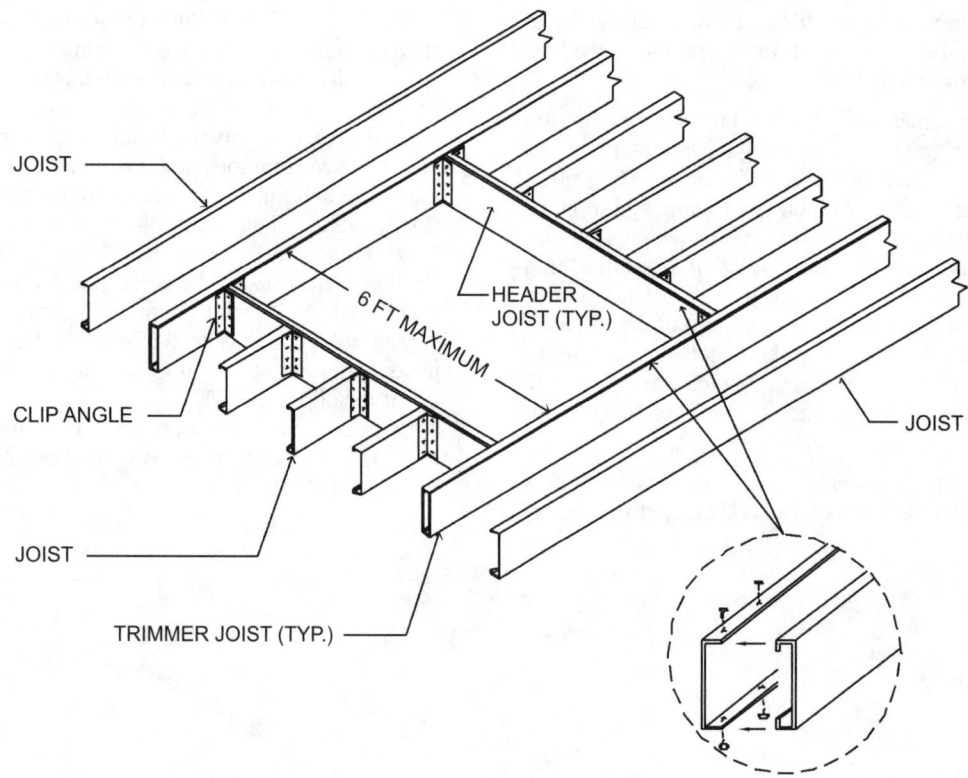

For SI: 1 foot = 304.8 mm.

FIGURE R505.3.8(1)
COLD-FORMED STEEL FLOOR CONSTRUCTION: 6-FOOT FLOOR OPENING

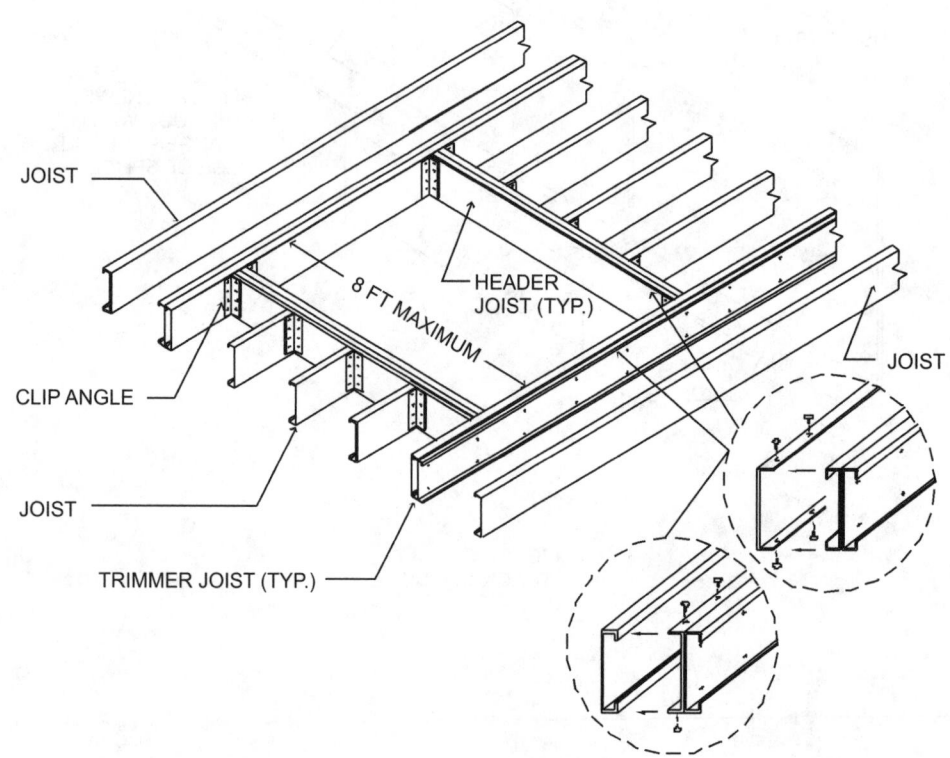

For SI: 1 foot = 304.8 mm.

FIGURE R505.3.8(2)
COLD-FORMED STEEL FLOOR CONSTRUCTION: 8-FOOT FLOOR OPENING

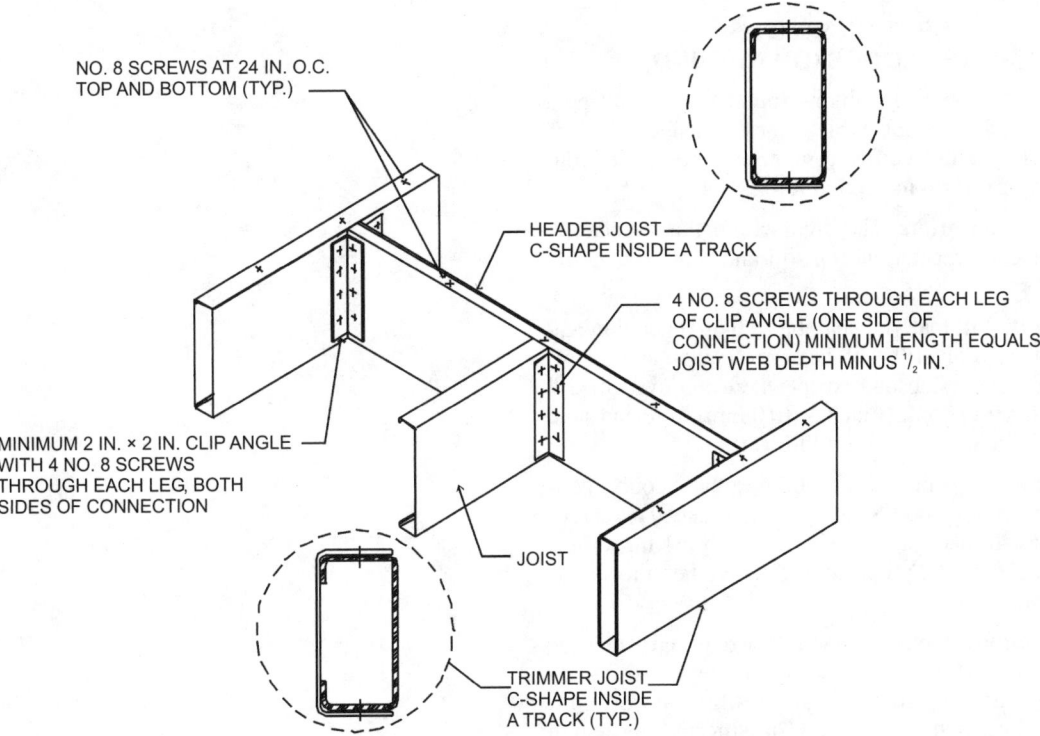

For SI: 1 inch = 25.4 mm.

FIGURE R505.3.8(3)
COLD-FORMED STEEL FLOOR CONSTRUCTION:
FLOOR HEADER TO TRIMMER CONNECTION—6-FOOT OPENING

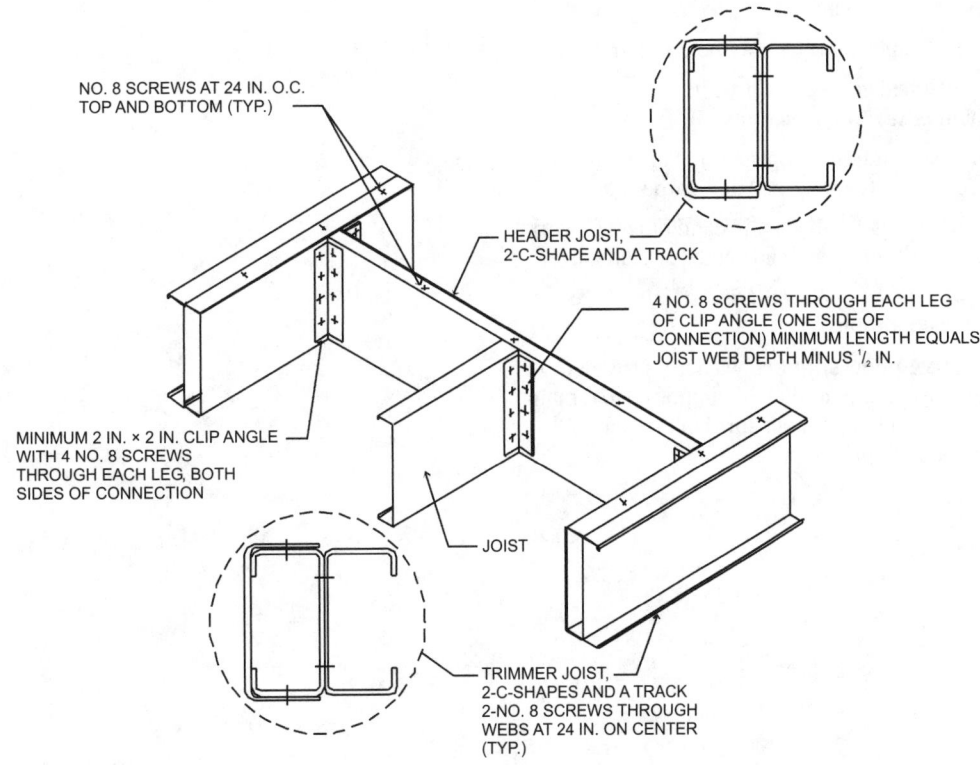

For SI: 1 inch = 25.4 mm.

FIGURE R505.3.8(4)
COLD-FORMED STEEL FLOOR CONSTRUCTION:
FLOOR HEADER TO TRIMMER CONNECTION—8-FOOT OPENING

SECTION R506
CONCRETE FLOORS (ON GROUND)

R506.1 General. Concrete slab-on-ground floors shall be a minimum 3.5 inches (89 mm) thick (for expansive soils, see Section R403.1.8). The specified compressive strength of concrete shall be as set forth in Section R402.2.

R506.2 Site preparation. The area within the foundation walls shall have all vegetation, top soil and foreign material removed.

R506.2.1 Fill. Fill material shall be free of vegetation and foreign material. The fill shall be compacted to assure uniform support of the slab, and except where *approved*, the fill depths shall not exceed 24 inches (610 mm) for clean sand or gravel and 8 inches (203 mm) for earth.

R506.2.2 Base. A 4-inch-thick (102 mm) base course consisting of clean graded sand, gravel, crushed stone or crushed blast-furnace slag passing a 2-inch (51 mm) sieve shall be placed on the prepared subgrade when the slab is below *grade*.

> **Exception:** A base course is not required when the concrete slab is installed on well-drained or sand-gravel mixture soils classified as Group I according to the United Soil Classification System in accordance with Table R405.1.

R506.2.3 Vapor retarder. A 6 mil (0.006 inch; 152 μm) polyethylene or *approved* vapor retarder with joints lapped not less than 6 inches (152 mm) shall be placed between the concrete floor slab and the base course or the prepared subgrade where no base course exists.

> **Exception:** The vapor retarder may be omitted:
>
> 1. From detached garages, utility buildings and other unheated *accessory structures*.
>
> 2. For unheated storage rooms having an area of less than 70 square feet (6.5 m²) and carports.
>
> 3. From driveways, walks, patios and other flatwork not likely to be enclosed and heated at a later date.
>
> 4. Where *approved* by the *building official*, based on local site conditions.

R506.2.4 Reinforcement support. Where provided in slabs on ground, reinforcement shall be supported to remain in place from the center to upper one third of the slab for the duration of the concrete placement.

CHAPTER 6

WALL CONSTRUCTION

SECTION R601
GENERAL

R601.1 Application. The provisions of this chapter shall control the design and construction of all walls and partitions for all buildings.

R601.2 Requirements. Wall construction shall be capable of accommodating all loads imposed according to Section R301 and of transmitting the resulting loads to the supporting structural elements.

R601.2.1 Compressible floor-covering materials. Compressible floor-covering materials that compress more than $^1/_{32}$ inch (0.8 mm) when subjected to 50 pounds (23 kg) applied over 1 inch square (645 mm) of material and are greater than $^1/_8$ inch (3 mm) in thickness in the uncompressed state shall not extend beneath walls, partitions or columns, which are fastened to the floor.

R601.3 Vapor retarders. Class I or II vapor retarders are required on the interior side of frame walls in Zones 5, 6, 7, 8 and Marine 4.

Exceptions:

1. *Basement walls.*
2. Below *grade* portion of any wall.
3. Construction where moisture or its freezing will not damage the materials.

R601.3.1 Class III vapor retarders. Class III vapor retarders shall be permitted where any one of the conditions in Table R601.3.1 is met.

R601.3.2 Material vapor retarder class. The vapor retarder class shall be based on the manufacturer's certified testing or a tested assembly.

The following shall be deemed to meet the class specified:

Class I: Sheet polyethylene, unperforated aluminum foil.

Class II: Kraft-faced fiberglass batts.

Class III: Latex or enamel paint.

R601.3.3 Minimum clear air spaces and vented openings for vented cladding. For the purposes of this section, vented cladding shall include the following minimum clear air spaces. Other openings with the equivalent vent area shall be permitted.

1. Vinyl lap or horizontal aluminum siding applied over a weather resistive barrier as specified in Table R703.4.
2. Brick veneer with a clear airspace as specified in Section R703.7.4.2.
3. Other *approved* vented claddings.

TABLE R601.3.1
CLASS III VAPOR RETARDERS

ZONE	CLASS III VAPOR RETARDERS PERMITTED FOR:[a]
Marine 4	Vented cladding over OSB Vented cladding over plywood Vented cladding over fiberboard Vented cladding over gypsum Insulated sheathing with R-value ≥ 2.5 over 2 × 4 wall Insulated sheathing with R-value ≥ 3.75 over 2 × 6 wall
5	Vented cladding over OSB Vented cladding over plywood Vented cladding over fiberboard Vented cladding over gypsum Insulated sheathing with R-value ≥ 5 over 2 × 4 wall Insulated sheathing with R-value ≥ 7.5 over 2 × 6 wall
6	Vented cladding over fiberboard Vented cladding over gypsum Insulated sheathing with R-value ≥ 7.5 over 2 × 4 wall Insulated sheathing with R-value ≥ 11.25 over 2 × 6 wall
7 and 8	Insulated sheathing with R-value ≥ 10 over 2 × 4 wall Insulated sheathing with R-value ≥ 15 over 2 × 6 wall

For SI: 1 pound per cubic foot = 16.02 kg/m^3.

a. Spray foam with a minimum density of 2 lb/ft^3 applied to the interior cavity side of OSB, plywood, fiberboard, insulating sheathing or gypsum is deemed to meet the insulating sheathing requirement where the spray foam R-value meets or exceeds the specified insulating sheathing R-value.

SECTION R602
WOOD WALL FRAMING

R602.1 Identification. Load-bearing dimension lumber for studs, plates and headers shall be identified by a grade mark of a lumber grading or inspection agency that has been *approved* by an accreditation body that complies with DOC PS 20. In lieu of a grade mark, a certification of inspection issued by a lumber grading or inspection agency meeting the requirements of this section shall be accepted.

R602.1.1 End-jointed lumber. *Approved* end-jointed lumber identified by a grade mark conforming to Section R602.1 may be used interchangeably with solid-sawn members of the same species and grade.

R602.1.2 Structural glued laminated timbers. Glued laminated timbers shall be manufactured and identified as required in ANSI/AITC A190.1 and ASTM D 3737.

R602.1.3 Structural log members. Stress grading of structural log members of nonrectangular shape, as typically used in log buildings, shall be in accordance with ASTM D 3957. Such structural log members shall be identified by the grade mark of an *approved* lumber grading or inspection agency. In lieu of a grade mark on the material, a certificate of inspection as to species and grade, issued by a lumber-grading or inspection agency meeting the requirements of this section, shall be permitted to be accepted.

R602.2 Grade. Studs shall be a minimum No. 3, standard or stud grade lumber.

Exception: Bearing studs not supporting floors and nonbearing studs may be utility grade lumber, provided the studs are spaced in accordance with Table R602.3(5).

R602.3 Design and construction. Exterior walls of wood-frame construction shall be designed and constructed in accordance with the provisions of this chapter and Figures R602.3(1) and R602.3.(2) or in accordance with AF&PA's NDS. Components of exterior walls shall be fastened in accordance with Tables R602.3(1) through R602.3(4). Structural wall sheathing shall be fastened directly to structural framing members. Exterior wall coverings shall be capable of resisting the wind pressures listed in Table R301.2(2) adjusted for height and exposure using Table R301.2(3). Wood structural panel sheathing used for exterior walls shall conform to the requirements of Table R602.3(3).

Studs shall be continuous from support at the sole plate to a support at the top plate to resist loads perpendicular to the wall. The support shall be a foundation or floor, ceiling or roof diaphragm or shall be designed in accordance with accepted engineering practice.

Exception: Jack studs, trimmer studs and cripple studs at openings in walls that comply with Tables R502.5(1) and R502.5(2).

R602.3.1 Stud size, height and spacing. The size, height and spacing of studs shall be in accordance with Table R602.3.(5).

Exceptions:

1. Utility grade studs shall not be spaced more than 16 inches (406 mm) on center, shall not support more than a roof and ceiling, and shall not exceed 8 feet (2438 mm) in height for exterior walls and load-bearing walls or 10 feet (3048 mm) for interior nonload-bearing walls.

2. Studs more than 10 feet (3048 mm) in height which are in accordance with Table R602.3.1.

R602.3.2 Top plate. Wood stud walls shall be capped with a double top plate installed to provide overlapping at corners and intersections with bearing partitions. End joints in top plates shall be offset at least 24 inches (610 mm). Joints in plates need not occur over studs. Plates shall be not less than 2-inches (51 mm) nominal thickness and have a width at least equal to the width of the studs.

Exception: A single top plate may be installed in stud walls, provided the plate is adequately tied at joints, corners and intersecting walls by a minimum 3-inch-by-6-inch by a 0.036-inch-thick (76 mm by 152 mm by 0.914 mm) galvanized steel plate that is nailed to each wall or segment of wall by six 8d nails on each side, provided the rafters or joists are centered over the studs with a tolerance of no more than 1 inch (25 mm). The top plate may be omitted over lintels that are adequately tied to adjacent wall sections with steel plates or equivalent as previously described.

R602.3.3 Bearing studs. Where joists, trusses or rafters are spaced more than 16 inches (406 mm) on center and the bearing studs below are spaced 24 inches (610 mm) on center, such members shall bear within 5 inches (127 mm) of the studs beneath.

Exceptions:

1. The top plates are two 2-inch by 6-inch (38 mm by 140 mm) or two 3-inch by 4-inch (64 mm by 89 mm) members.

2. A third top plate is installed.

3. Solid blocking equal in size to the studs is installed to reinforce the double top plate.

R602.3.4 Bottom (sole) plate. Studs shall have full bearing on a nominal 2-by (51 mm) or larger plate or sill having a width at least equal to the width of the studs.

R602.4 Interior load-bearing walls. Interior load-bearing walls shall be constructed, framed and fireblocked as specified for exterior walls.

R602.5 Interior nonbearing walls. Interior nonbearing walls shall be permitted to be constructed with 2-inch-by-3-inch (51 mm by 76 mm) studs spaced 24 inches (610 mm) on center or, when not part of a *braced wall line*, 2-inch-by-4-inch (51 mm by 102 mm) flat studs spaced at 16 inches (406 mm) on center. Interior nonbearing walls shall be capped with at least a single top plate. Interior nonbearing walls shall be fireblocked in accordance with Section R602.8.

TABLE R602.3(1)
FASTENER SCHEDULE FOR STRUCTURAL MEMBERS

ITEM	DESCRIPTION OF BUILDING ELEMENTS	NUMBER AND TYPE OF FASTENER[a, b, c]	SPACING OF FASTENERS
	Roof		
1	Blocking between joists or rafters to top plate, toe nail	3-8d $(2^1/_2'' \times 0.113'')$	—
2	Ceiling joists to plate, toe nail	3-8d $(2^1/_2'' \times 0.113'')$	—
3	Ceiling joists not attached to parallel rafter, laps over partitions, face nail	3-10d	—
4	Collar tie rafter, face nail or $1^1/_4'' \times 20$ gage ridge strap	3-10d $(3'' \times 0.128'')$	—
5	Rafter to plate, toe nail	2-16d $(3^1/_2'' \times 0.135'')$	—
6	Roof rafters to ridge, valley or hip rafters: toe nail, face nail	4-16d $(3^1/_2'' \times 0.135'')$, 3-16d $(3^1/_2'' \times 0.135'')$	—, —
	Wall		
7	Built-up corner studs	10d $(3'' \times 0.128'')$	24″ o.c.
8	Built-up header, two pieces with $^1/_2''$ spacer	16d $(3^1/_2'' \times 0.135'')$	16″ o.c. along each edge
9	Continued header, two pieces	16d $(3^1/_2'' \times 0.135'')$	16″ o.c. along each edge
10	Continuous header to stud, toe nail	4-8d $(2^1/_2'' \times 0.113'')$	—
11	Double studs, face nail	10d $(3'' \times 0.128'')$	24″ o.c.
12	Double top plates, face nail	10d $(3'' \times 0.128'')$	24″ o.c.
13	Double top plates, minimum 48-inch offset of end joints, face nail in lapped area	8-16d $(3^1/_2'' \times 0.135'')$	—
14	Sole plate to joist or blocking, face nail	16d $(3^1/_2'' \times 0.135'')$	16″ o.c.
15	Sole plate to joist or blocking at braced wall panels	3-16d $(3^1/_2'' \times 0.135'')$	16″ o.c.
16	Stud to sole plate, toe nail	3-8d $(2^1/_2'' \times 0.113'')$ or 2-16d $3^1/_2'' \times 0.135''$	—, —
17	Top or sole plate to stud, end nail	2-16d $(3^1/_2'' \times 0.135'')$	—
18	Top plates, laps at corners and intersections, face nail	2-10d $(3'' \times 0.128'')$	—
19	1″ brace to each stud and plate, face nail	2-8d $(2^1/_2'' \times 0.113'')$, 2 staples $1^3/_4''$	—, —
20	1″ × 6″ sheathing to each bearing, face nail	2-8d $(2^1/_2'' \times 0.113'')$, 2 staples $1^3/_4''$	—, —
21	1″ × 8″ sheathing to each bearing, face nail	2-8d $(2^1/_2'' \times 0.113'')$, 3 staples $1^3/_4''$	—, —
22	Wider than 1″ × 8″ sheathing to each bearing, face nail	3-8d $(2^1/_2'' \times 0.113'')$, 4 staples $1^3/_4''$	—, —
	Floor		
23	Joist to sill or girder, toe nail	3-8d $(2^1/_2'' \times 0.113'')$	—
24	1″ × 6″ subfloor or less to each joist, face nail	2-8d $(2^1/_2'' \times 0.113'')$, 2 staples $1^3/_4''$	—, —
25	2″ subfloor to joist or girder, blind and face nail	2-16d $(3^1/_2'' \times 0.135'')$	—
26	Rim joist to top plate, toe nail (roof applications also)	8d $(2^1/_2'' \times 0.113'')$	6″ o.c.
27	2″ planks (plank & beam – floor & roof)	2-16d $(3^1/_2'' \times 0.135'')$	at each bearing
28	Built-up girders and beams, 2-inch lumber layers	10d $(3'' \times 0.128'')$	Nail each layer as follows: 32″ o.c. at top and bottom and staggered. Two nails at ends and at each splice.
29	Ledger strip supporting joists or rafters	3-16d $(3^1/_2'' \times 0.135'')$	At each joist or rafter

(continued)

TABLE R602.3(1)—continued
FASTENER SCHEDULE FOR STRUCTURAL MEMBERS

ITEM	DESCRIPTION OF BUILDING MATERIALS	DESCRIPTION OF FASTENER[b, c, e]	SPACING OF FASTENERS	
			Edges (inches)[i]	Intermediate supports[c, e] (inches)
Wood structural panels, subfloor, roof and interior wall sheathing to framing and particleboard wall sheathing to framing				
30	$3/8''$ - $1/2''$	6d common (2″ × 0.113″) nail (subfloor wall)[j] 8d common (2$1/2$″ × 0.131″) nail (roof)	6	12[g]
31	$5/16''$ - $1/2''$	6d common (2″ × 0.113″) nail (subfloor, wall) 8d common (2$1/2$″ × 0.131″) nail (roof)[f]	6	12[g]
32	$19/32''$ - 1″	8d common nail (2$1/2$″ × 0.131″)	6	12[g]
33	1$1/8$″ - 1$1/4$″	10d common (3″ × 0.148″) nail or 8d (2$1/2$″ × 0.131″) deformed nail	6	12
Other wall sheathing[h]				
34	$1/2''$ structural cellulosic fiberboard sheathing	$1/2''$ galvanized roofing nail, $7/16''$ crown or 1″ crown staple 16 ga., 1$1/4$″ long	3	6
35	$25/32''$ structural cellulosic fiberboard sheathing	1$3/4$″ galvanized roofing nail, $7/16''$ crown or 1″ crown staple 16 ga., 1$1/2$″ long	3	6
36	$1/2''$ gypsum sheathing[d]	1$1/2$″ galvanized roofing nail; staple galvanized, 1$1/2$″ long; 1$1/4$ screws, Type W or S	7	7
37	$5/8''$ gypsum sheathing[d]	1$3/4$″ glavanized roofing nail; staple galvanized, 1$5/8$″ long; 1$5/8$″ screws, Type W or S	7	7
Wood structural panels, combination subfloor underlayment to framing				
38	$3/4''$ and less	6d deformed (2″ × 0.120″) nail or 8d common (2$1/2$″ × 0.131″) nail	6	12
39	$7/8''$ - 1″	8d common (2$1/2$″ × 0.131″) nail or 8d deformed (2$1/2$″ × 0.120″) nail	6	12
40	1$1/8$″ - 1$1/4$″	10d common (3″ × 0.148″) nail or 8d deformed (2$1/2$″ × 0.120″) nail	6	12

For SI: 1 inch = 25.4 mm, 1 foot = 304.8 mm, 1 mile per hour = 0.447 m/s; 1ksi = 6.895 MPa.

a. All nails are smooth-common, box or deformed shanks except where otherwise stated. Nails used for framing and sheathing connections shall have minimum average bending yield strengths as shown: 80 ksi for shank diameter of 0.192 inch (20d common nail), 90 ksi for shank diameters larger than 0.142 inch but not larger than 0.177 inch, and 100 ksi for shank diameters of 0.142 inch or less.

b. Staples are 16 gage wire and have a minimum $7/16$-inch on diameter crown width.

c. Nails shall be spaced at not more than 6 inches on center at all supports where spans are 48 inches or greater.

d. Four-foot-by-8-foot or 4-foot-by-9-foot panels shall be applied vertically.

e. Spacing of fasteners not included in this table shall be based on Table R602.3(2).

f. For regions having basic wind speed of 110 mph or greater, 8d deformed (2$1/2$″ × 0.120) nails shall be used for attaching plywood and wood structural panel roof sheathing to framing within minimum 48-inch distance from gable end walls, if mean roof height is more than 25 feet, up to 35 feet maximum.

g. For regions having basic wind speed of 100 mph or less, nails for attaching wood structural panel roof sheathing to gable end wall framing shall be spaced 6 inches on center. When basic wind speed is greater than 100 mph, nails for attaching panel roof sheathing to intermediate supports shall be spaced 6 inches on center for minimum 48-inch distance from ridges, eaves and gable end walls; and 4 inches on center to gable end wall framing.

h. Gypsum sheathing shall conform to ASTM C 1396 and shall be installed in accordance with GA 253. Fiberboard sheathing shall conform to ASTM C 208.

i. Spacing of fasteners on floor sheathing panel edges applies to panel edges supported by framing members and required blocking and at all floor perimeters only. Spacing of fasteners on roof sheathing panel edges applies to panel edges supported by framing members and required blocking. Blocking of roof or floor sheathing panel edges perpendicular to the framing members need not be provided except as required by other provisions of this code. Floor perimeter shall be supported by framing members or solid blocking.

TABLE R602.3(2)
ALTERNATE ATTACHMENTS

NOMINAL MATERIAL THICKNESS (inches)	DESCRIPTION[a, b] OF FASTENER AND LENGTH (inches)	SPACING[c] OF FASTENERS	
		Edges (inches)	Intermediate supports (inches)
Wood structural panels subfloor, roof and wall sheathing to framing and particleboard wall sheathing to framing[f]			
up to $^1/_2$	Staple 15 ga. $1^3/_4$	4	8
	0.097 - 0.099 Nail $2^1/_4$	3	6
	Staple 16 ga. $1^3/_4$	3	6
$^{19}/_{32}$ and $^5/_8$	0.113 Nail 2	3	6
	Staple 15 and 16 ga. 2	4	8
	0.097 - 0.099 Nail $2^1/_4$	4	8
$^{23}/_{32}$ and $^3/_4$	Staple 14 ga. 2	4	8
	Staple 15 ga. $1^3/_4$	3	6
	0.097 - 0.099 Nail $2^1/_4$	4	8
	Staple 16 ga. 2	4	8
1	Staple 14 ga. $2^1/_4$	4	8
	0.113 Nail $2^1/_4$	3	6
	Staple 15 ga. $2^1/_4$	4	8
	0.097 - 0.099 Nail $2^1/_2$	4	8

NOMINAL MATERIAL THICKNESS (inches)	DESCRIPTION[a,b] OF FASTENER AND LENGTH (inches)	SPACING[c] OF FASTENERS	
		Edges (inches)	Body of panel[d] (inches)
Floor underlayment; plywood-hardboard-particleboard[f]			
Plywood			
$^1/_4$ and $^5/_{16}$	$1^1/_4$ ring or screw shank nail—minimum $12^1/_2$ ga. (0.099″) shank diameter	3	6
	Staple 18 ga., $^7/_8$, $^3/_{16}$ crown width	2	5
$^{11}/_{32}$, $^3/_8$, $^{15}/_{32}$, and $^1/_2$	$1^1/_4$ ring or screw shank nail—minimum $12^1/_2$ ga. (0.099″) shank diameter	6	8[e]
$^{19}/_{32}$, $^5/_8$, $^{23}/_{32}$ and $^3/_4$	$1^1/_2$ ring or screw shank nail—minimum $12^1/_2$ ga. (0.099″) shank diameter	6	8
	Staple 16 ga. $1^1/_2$	6	8
Hardboard[f]			
0.200	$1^1/_2$ long ring-grooved underlayment nail	6	6
	4d cement-coated sinker nail	6	6
	Staple 18 ga., $^7/_8$ long (plastic coated)	3	6
Particleboard			
$^1/_4$	4d ring-grooved underlayment nail	3	6
	Staple 18 ga., $^7/_8$ long, $^3/_{16}$ crown	3	6
$^3/_8$	6d ring-grooved underlayment nail	6	10
	Staple 16 ga., $1^1/_8$ long, $^3/_8$ crown	3	6
$^1/_2$, $^5/_8$	6d ring-grooved underlayment nail	6	10
	Staple 16 ga., $1^5/_8$ long, $^3/_8$ crown	3	6

For SI: 1 inch = 25.4 mm.

a. Nail is a general description and may be T-head, modified round head or round head.

b. Staples shall have a minimum crown width of $^7/_{16}$-inch on diameter except as noted.

c. Nails or staples shall be spaced at not more than 6 inches on center at all supports where spans are 48 inches or greater. Nails or staples shall be spaced at not more than 12 inches on center at intermediate supports for floors.

d. Fasteners shall be placed in a grid pattern throughout the body of the panel.

e. For 5-ply panels, intermediate nails shall be spaced not more than 12 inches on center each way.

f. Hardboard underlayment shall conform to ANSI/AHA A135.4.

TABLE R602.3(3)
REQUIREMENTS FOR WOOD STRUCTURAL PANEL
WALL SHEATHING USED TO RESIST WIND PRESSURES[a,b,c]

MINIMUM NAIL		MINIMUM WOOD STRUCTURAL PANEL SPAN RATING	MINIMUM NOMINAL PANEL THICKNESS (inches)	MAXIMUM WALL STUD SPACING (inches)	PANEL NAIL SPACING		MAXIMUM WIND SPEED (mph)		
Size	Penetration (inches)				Edges (inches o.c.)	Field (inches o.c.)	Wind exposure category		
							B	C	D
6d Common (2.0″ × 0.113″)	1.5	24/0	3/8	16	6	12	110	90	85
8d Common (2.5″ × 0.131″)	1.75	24/16	7/16	16	6	12	130	110	105
				24	6	12	110	90	85

For SI: 1 inch = 25.4 mm, 1 mile per hour = 0.447 m/s.

a. Panel strength axis parallel or perpendicular to supports. Three-ply plywood sheathing with studs spaced more than 16 inches on center shall be applied with panel strength axis perpendicular to supports.

b. Table is based on wind pressures acting toward and away from building surfaces per Section R301.2. Lateral bracing requirements shall be in accordance with Section R602.10.

c. Wood Structural Panels with span ratings of Wall-16 or Wall-24 shall be permitted as an alternate to panels with a 24/0 span rating. Plywood siding rated 16 oc or 24 oc shall be permitted as an alternate to panels with a 24/16 span rating. Wall-16 and Plywood siding 16 oc shall be used with studs spaced a maximum of 16 inches on center.

TABLE R602.3(4)
ALLOWABLE SPANS FOR PARTICLEBOARD WALL SHEATHING[a]

THICKNESS (inch)	GRADE	STUD SPACING (inches)	
		When siding is nailed to studs	When siding is nailed to sheathing
3/8	M—1 Exterior glue	16	—
1/2	M—2 Exterior glue	16	16

For SI: 1 inch = 25.4 mm.

a. Wall sheathing not exposed to the weather. If the panels are applied horizontally, the end joints of the panel shall be offset so that four panels corners will not meet. All panel edges must be supported. Leave a 1/16-inch gap between panels and nail no closer than 3/8 inch from panel edges.

TABLE R602.3(5)
SIZE, HEIGHT AND SPACING OF WOOD STUDS[a]

STUD SIZE (inches)	BEARING WALLS					NONBEARING WALLS	
	Laterally unsupported stud height[a] (feet)	Maximum spacing when supporting a roof-ceiling assembly or a habitable attic assembly, only (inches)	Maximum spacing when supporting one floor, plus a roof-ceiling assembly or a habitable attic assembly (inches)	Maximum spacing when supporting two floors, plus a roof-ceiling assembly or a habitable attic assembly (inches)	Maximum spacing when supporting one floor height[a] (feet)	Laterally unsupported stud height[a] (feet)	Maximum spacing (inches)
2 × 3[b]	—	—	—	—	—	10	16
2 × 4	10	24[c]	16[c]	—	24	14	24
3 × 4	10	24	24	16	24	14	24
2 × 5	10	24	24	—	24	16	24
2 × 6	10	24	24	16	24	20	24

For SI: 1 inch = 25.4 mm, 1 foot = 304.8 mm, 1 square foot = 0.093 m².

a. Listed heights are distances between points of lateral support placed perpendicular to the plane of the wall. Increases in unsupported height are permitted where justified by analysis.

b. Shall not be used in exterior walls.

c. A habitable attic assembly supported by 2 × 4 studs is limited to a roof span of 32 feet. Where the roof span exceeds 32 feet, the wall studs shall be increased to 2 × 6 or the studs shall be designed in accordance with accepted engineering practice.

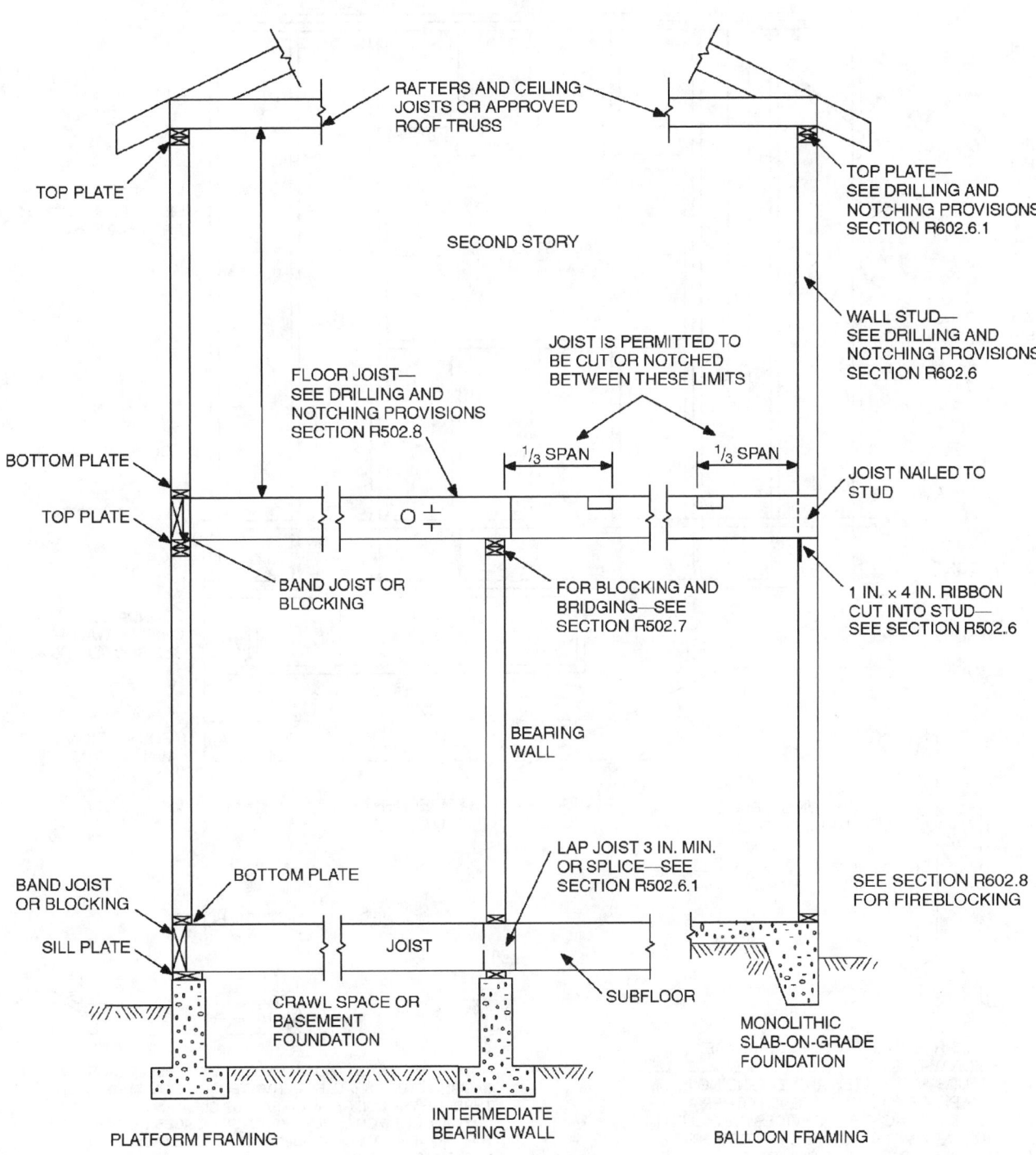

RAFTERS AND CEILING
JOISTS OR APPROVED
ROOF TRUSS

TOP PLATE

TOP PLATE—
SEE DRILLING AND
NOTCHING PROVISIONS
SECTION R602.6.1

SECOND STORY

WALL STUD—
SEE DRILLING AND
NOTCHING PROVISIONS
SECTION R602.6

JOIST IS PERMITTED TO
BE CUT OR NOTCHED
BETWEEN THESE LIMITS

FLOOR JOIST—
SEE DRILLING AND
NOTCHING PROVISIONS
SECTION R502.8

¹/₃ SPAN   ¹/₃ SPAN

BOTTOM PLATE

TOP PLATE

JOIST NAILED TO
STUD

BAND JOIST OR
BLOCKING

FOR BLOCKING AND
BRIDGING—SEE
SECTION R502.7

1 IN. × 4 IN. RIBBON
CUT INTO STUD—
SEE SECTION R502.6

BEARING
WALL

LAP JOIST 3 IN. MIN.
OR SPLICE—SEE
SECTION R502.6.1

SEE SECTION R602.8
FOR FIREBLOCKING

BAND JOIST
OR BLOCKING

BOTTOM PLATE

SILL PLATE

JOIST

SUBFLOOR

CRAWL SPACE OR
BASEMENT
FOUNDATION

MONOLITHIC
SLAB-ON-GRADE
FOUNDATION

PLATFORM FRAMING

INTERMEDIATE
BEARING WALL

BALLOON FRAMING

For SI: 1 inch = 25.4 mm.

FIGURE R602.3(1)
TYPICAL WALL, FLOOR AND ROOF FRAMING

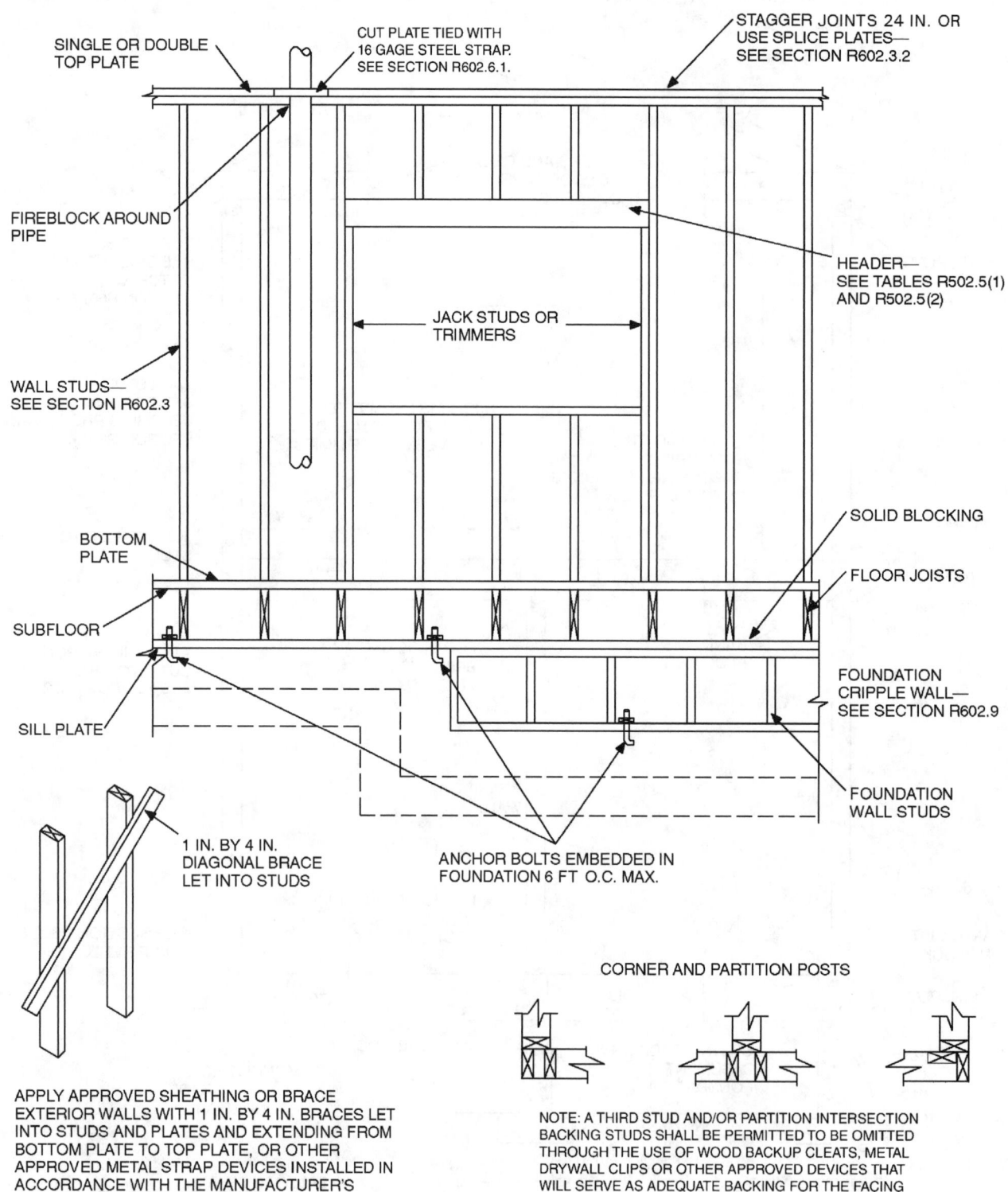

SINGLE OR DOUBLE TOP PLATE

CUT PLATE TIED WITH 16 GAGE STEEL STRAP. SEE SECTION R602.6.1.

STAGGER JOINTS 24 IN. OR USE SPLICE PLATES— SEE SECTION R602.3.2

FIREBLOCK AROUND PIPE

HEADER— SEE TABLES R502.5(1) AND R502.5(2)

JACK STUDS OR TRIMMERS

WALL STUDS— SEE SECTION R602.3

BOTTOM PLATE

SOLID BLOCKING

FLOOR JOISTS

SUBFLOOR

SILL PLATE

FOUNDATION CRIPPLE WALL— SEE SECTION R602.9

FOUNDATION WALL STUDS

1 IN. BY 4 IN. DIAGONAL BRACE LET INTO STUDS

ANCHOR BOLTS EMBEDDED IN FOUNDATION 6 FT O.C. MAX.

CORNER AND PARTITION POSTS

APPLY APPROVED SHEATHING OR BRACE EXTERIOR WALLS WITH 1 IN. BY 4 IN. BRACES LET INTO STUDS AND PLATES AND EXTENDING FROM BOTTOM PLATE TO TOP PLATE, OR OTHER APPROVED METAL STRAP DEVICES INSTALLED IN ACCORDANCE WITH THE MANUFACTURER'S SPECIFICATIONS. SEE SECTION R602.10.

NOTE: A THIRD STUD AND/OR PARTITION INTERSECTION BACKING STUDS SHALL BE PERMITTED TO BE OMITTED THROUGH THE USE OF WOOD BACKUP CLEATS, METAL DRYWALL CLIPS OR OTHER APPROVED DEVICES THAT WILL SERVE AS ADEQUATE BACKING FOR THE FACING MATERIALS.

For SI: 1 inch = 25.4 mm, 1 foot = 304.8 mm.

FIGURE R602.3(2)
FRAMING DETAILS

TABLE R602.3.1
MAXIMUM ALLOWABLE LENGTH OF WOOD WALL STUDS EXPOSED TO WIND SPEEDS OF 100 mph OR LESS
IN SEISMIC DESIGN CATEGORIES A, B, C, D_0, D_1 and D_2[b, c]

HEIGHT (feet)	ON-CENTER SPACING (inches)			
	24	16	12	8
Supporting a roof only				
>10	2 × 4	2 × 4	2 × 4	2 × 4
12	2 × 6	2 × 4	2 × 4	2 × 4
14	2 × 6	2 × 6	2 × 6	2 × 4
16	2 × 6	2 × 6	2 × 6	2 × 4
18	NA[a]	2 × 6	2 × 6	2 × 6
20	NA[a]	NA[a]	2 × 6	2 × 6
24	NA[a]	NA[a]	NA[a]	2 × 6
Supporting one floor and a roof				
>10	2 × 6	2 × 4	2 × 4	2 × 4
12	2 × 6	2 × 6	2 × 6	2 × 4
14	2 × 6	2 × 6	2 × 6	2 × 6
16	NA[a]	2 × 6	2 × 6	2 × 6
18	NA[a]	2 × 6	2 × 6	2 × 6
20	NA[a]	NA[a]	2 × 6	2 × 6
24	NA[a]	NA[a]	NA[a]	2 × 6
Supporting two floors and a roof				
>10	2 × 6	2 × 6	2 × 4	2 × 4
12	2 × 6	2 × 6	2 × 6	2 × 6
14	2 × 6	2 × 6	2 × 6	2 × 6
16	NA[a]	NA[a]	2 × 6	2 × 6
18	NA[a]	NA[a]	2 × 6	2 × 6
20	NA[a]	NA[a]	NA[a]	2 × 6
22	NA[a]	NA[a]	NA[a]	NA[a]
24	NA[a]	NA[a]	NA[a]	NA[a]

For SI: 1 inch = 25.4 mm, 1 foot = 304.8 mm, 1 pound per square foot = 0.0479 kPa,
1 pound per square inch = 6.895 kPa, 1 mile per hour = 0.447 m/s.

a. Design required.

b. Applicability of this table assumes the following: Snow load not exceeding 25 psf, f_b not less than 1310 psi determined by multiplying the AF&PA NDS tabular base design value by the repetitive use factor, and by the size factor for all species except southern pine, E not less than 1.6×10^6 psi, tributary dimensions for floors and roofs not exceeding 6 feet, maximum span for floors and roof not exceeding 12 feet, eaves not over 2 feet in dimension and exterior sheathing. Where the conditions are not within these parameters, design is required.

c. Utility, standard, stud and No. 3 grade lumber of any species are not permitted.

(continued)

TABLE R602.3.1—continued
MAXIMUM ALLOWABLE LENGTH OF WOOD WALL STUDS EXPOSED TO WIND SPEEDS OF 100 mph OR LESS
IN SEISMIC DESIGN CATEGORIES A, B, C, D$_0$, D$_1$ and D$_2$

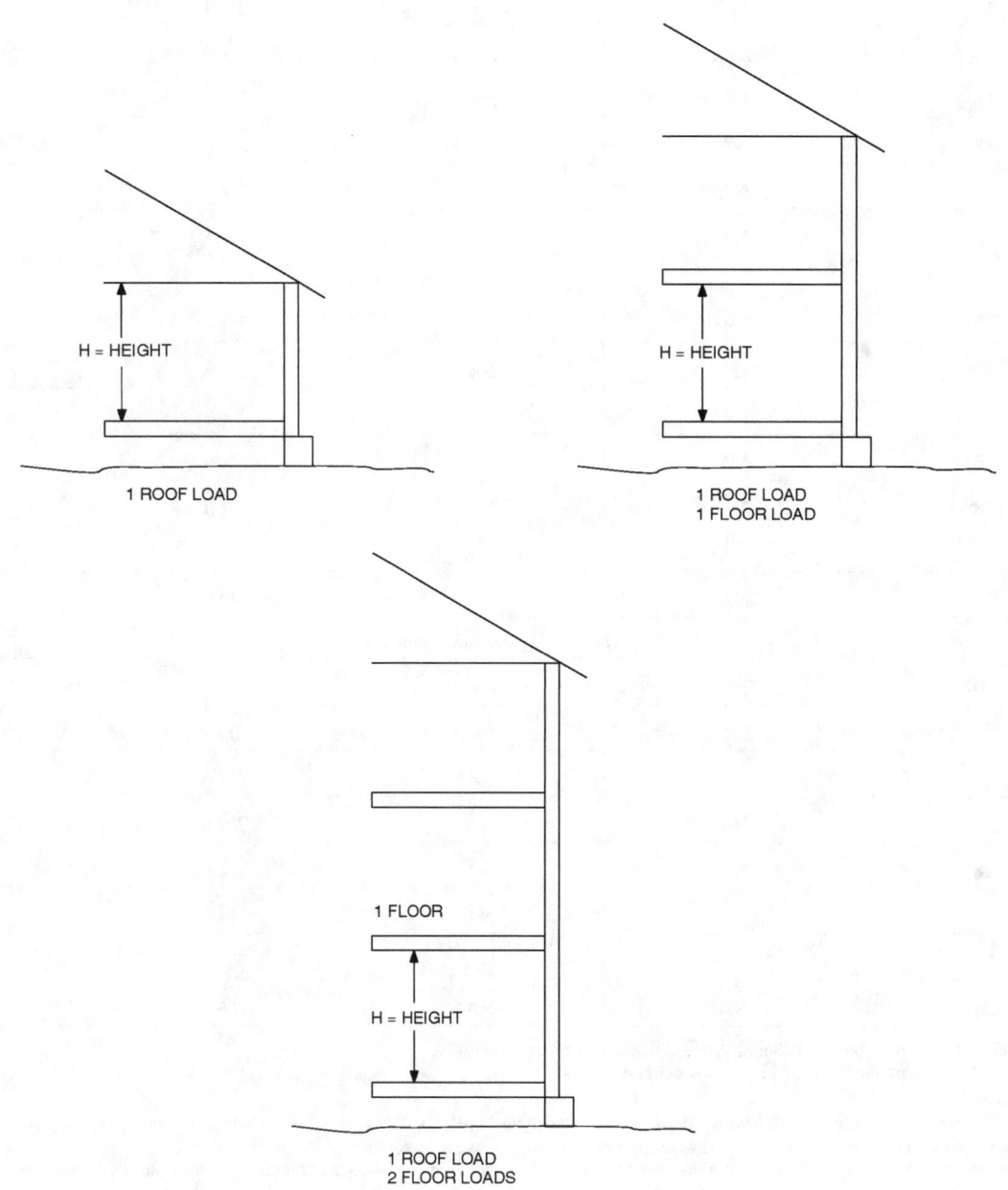

R602.6 Drilling and notching–studs. Drilling and notching of studs shall be in accordance with the following:

1. Notching. Any stud in an exterior wall or bearing partition may be cut or notched to a depth not exceeding 25 percent of its width. Studs in nonbearing partitions may be notched to a depth not to exceed 40 percent of a single stud width.

2. Drilling. Any stud may be bored or drilled, provided that the diameter of the resulting hole is no more than 60 percent of the stud width, the edge of the hole is no more than ⁵/₈ inch (16 mm) to the edge of the stud, and the hole is not located in the same section as a cut or notch. Studs located in exterior walls or bearing partitions drilled over 40 percent and up to 60 percent shall also be doubled with no more than two successive doubled studs bored. See Figures R602.6(1) and R602.6(2).

Exception: Use of *approved* stud shoes is permitted when they are installed in accordance with the manufacturer's recommendations.

R602.6.1 Drilling and notching of top plate. When piping or ductwork is placed in or partly in an exterior wall or interior load-bearing wall, necessitating cutting, drilling or notching of the top plate by more than 50 percent of its width, a galvanized metal tie not less than 0.054 inch thick (1.37 mm) (16 ga) and 1¹/₂ inches (38 mm) wide shall be fastened across and to the plate at each side of the opening with not less than eight 10d (0.148 inch diameter) having a minimum length of 1¹/₂ inches (38 mm) at each side or equivalent. The metal tie must extend a minimum of 6 inches past the opening. See Figure R602.6.1.

Exception: When the entire side of the wall with the notch or cut is covered by wood structural panel sheathing.

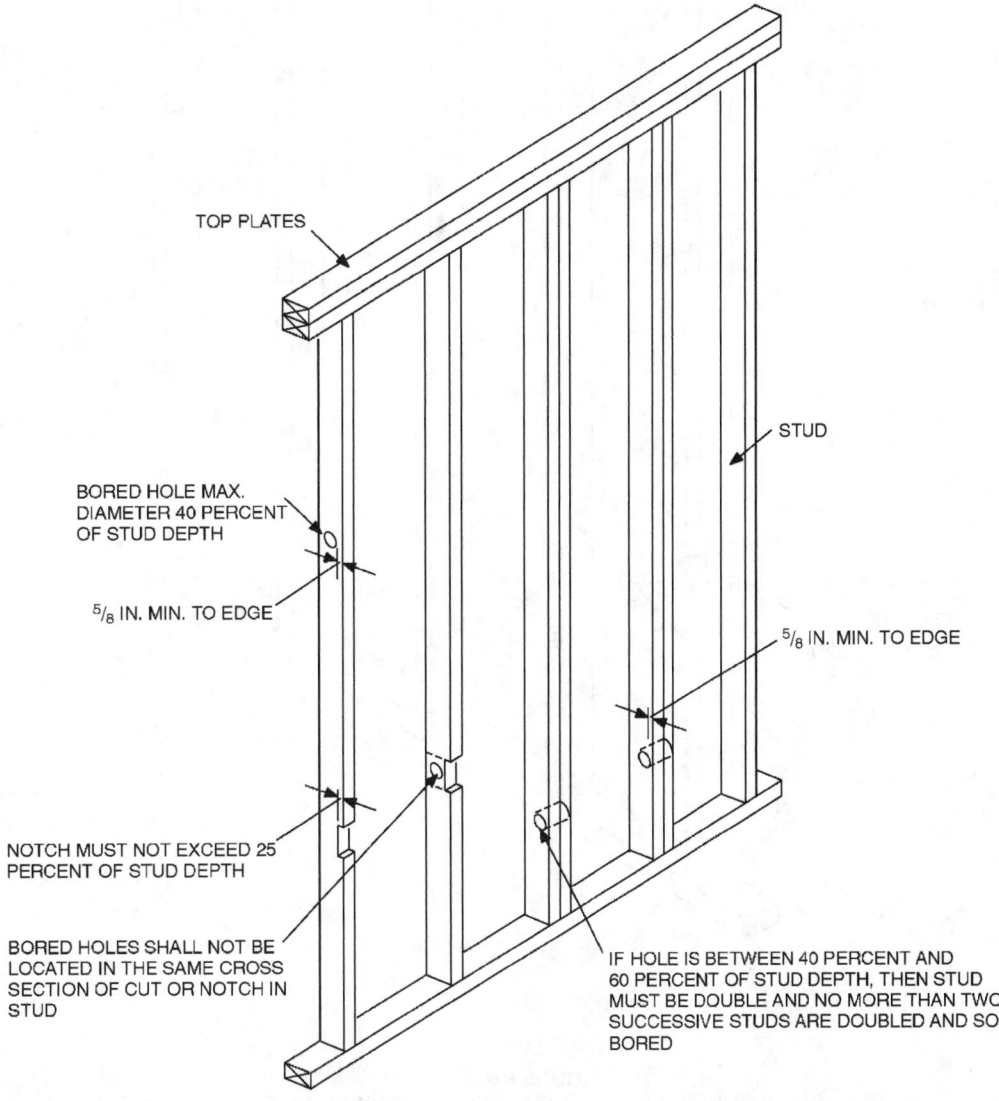

TOP PLATES

STUD

BORED HOLE MAX. DIAMETER 40 PERCENT OF STUD DEPTH

⁵/₈ IN. MIN. TO EDGE

⁵/₈ IN. MIN. TO EDGE

NOTCH MUST NOT EXCEED 25 PERCENT OF STUD DEPTH

BORED HOLES SHALL NOT BE LOCATED IN THE SAME CROSS SECTION OF CUT OR NOTCH IN STUD

IF HOLE IS BETWEEN 40 PERCENT AND 60 PERCENT OF STUD DEPTH, THEN STUD MUST BE DOUBLE AND NO MORE THAN TWO SUCCESSIVE STUDS ARE DOUBLED AND SO BORED

For SI: 1 inch = 25.4 mm.
NOTE: Condition for exterior and bearing walls.

FIGURE R602.6(1)
NOTCHING AND BORED HOLE LIMITATIONS FOR EXTERIOR WALLS AND BEARING WALLS

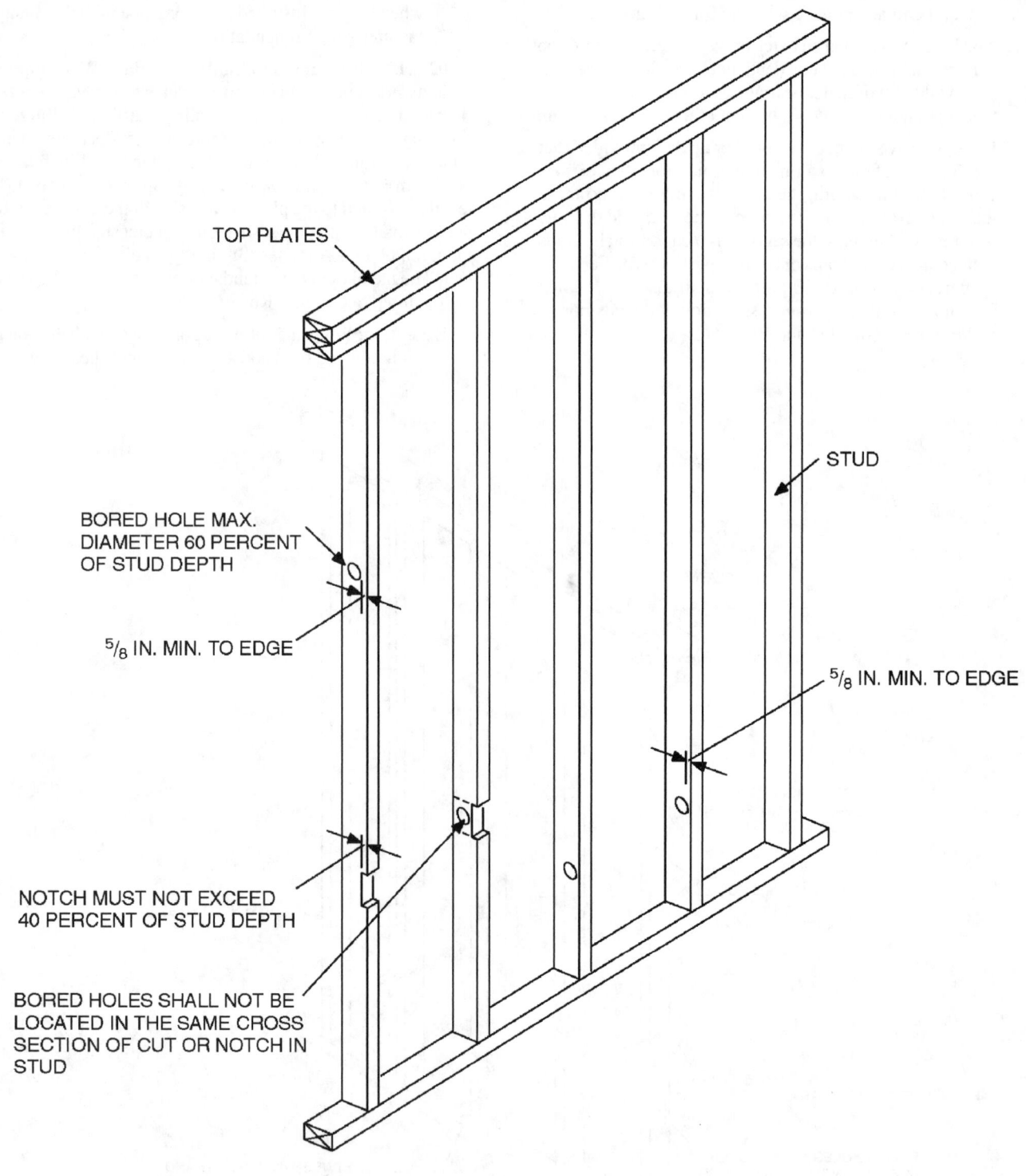

TOP PLATES

STUD

BORED HOLE MAX.
DIAMETER 60 PERCENT
OF STUD DEPTH

⁵/₈ IN. MIN. TO EDGE

⁵/₈ IN. MIN. TO EDGE

NOTCH MUST NOT EXCEED
40 PERCENT OF STUD DEPTH

BORED HOLES SHALL NOT BE
LOCATED IN THE SAME CROSS
SECTION OF CUT OR NOTCH IN
STUD

For SI: 1 inch = 25.4 mm.

FIGURE R602.6(2)
NOTCHING AND BORED HOLE LIMITATIONS FOR INTERIOR NONBEARING WALLS

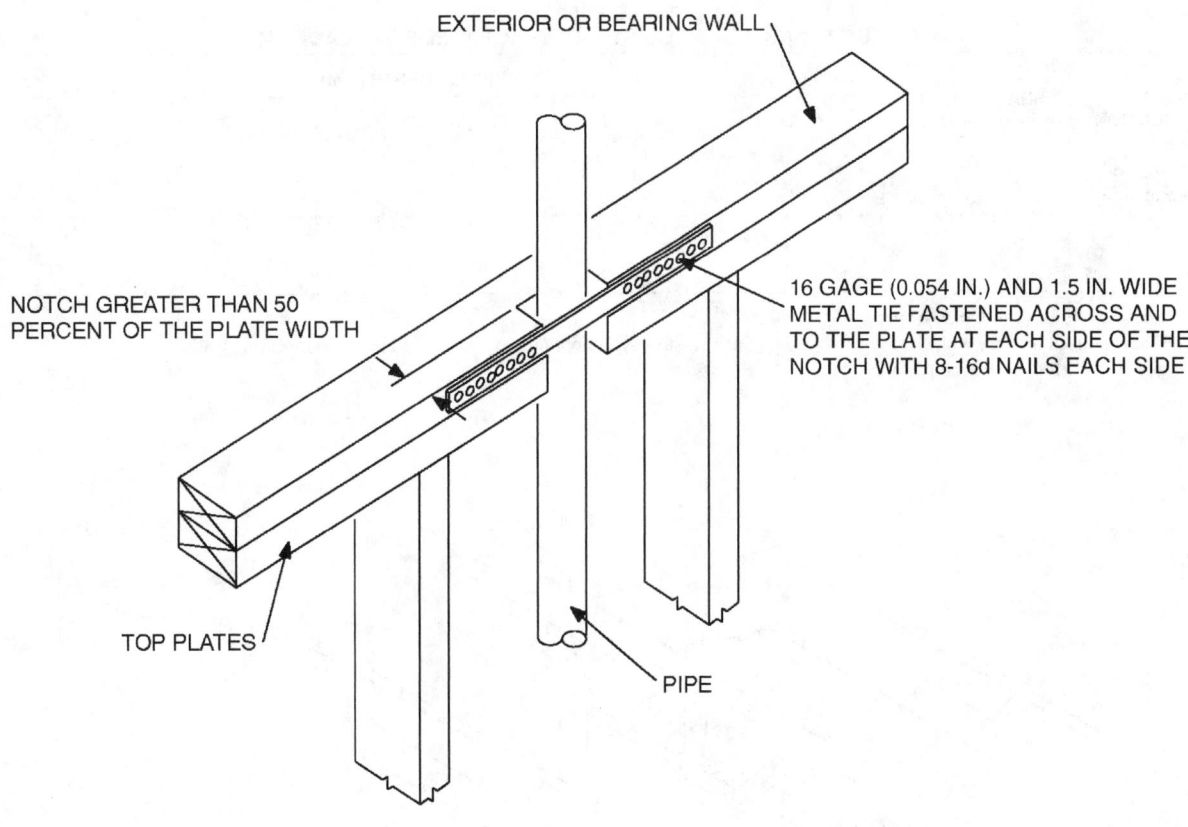

EXTERIOR OR BEARING WALL

NOTCH GREATER THAN 50 PERCENT OF THE PLATE WIDTH

16 GAGE (0.054 IN.) AND 1.5 IN. WIDE METAL TIE FASTENED ACROSS AND TO THE PLATE AT EACH SIDE OF THE NOTCH WITH 8-16d NAILS EACH SIDE

TOP PLATES

PIPE

For SI: 1 inch = 25.4 mm.

FIGURE R602.6.1
TOP PLATE FRAMING TO ACCOMMODATE PIPING

R602.7 Headers. For header spans see Tables R502.5(1) and R502.5(2).

R602.7.1 Wood structural panel box headers. Wood structural panel box headers shall be constructed in accordance with Figure R602.7.2 and Table R602.7.2.

R602.7.2 Nonbearing walls. Load-bearing headers are not required in interior or exterior nonbearing walls. A single flat 2-inch-by-4-inch (51 mm by 102 mm) member may be used as a header in interior or exterior nonbearing walls for openings up to 8 feet (2438 mm) in width if the vertical distance to the parallel nailing surface above is not more than 24 inches (610 mm). For such nonbearing headers, no cripples or blocking are required above the header.

R602.8 Fireblocking required. Fireblocking shall be provided in accordance with Section R302.11.

R602.9 Cripple walls. Foundation cripple walls shall be framed of studs not smaller than the studding above. When exceeding 4 feet (1219 mm) in height, such walls shall be framed of studs having the size required for an additional *story*.

Cripple walls with a stud height less than 14 inches (356 mm) shall be sheathed on at least one side with a wood structural panel that is fastened to both the top and bottom plates in accordance with Table R602.3(1), or the cripple walls shall be constructed of solid blocking. Cripple walls shall be supported on continuous foundations.

TABLE R602.7.2
MAXIMUM SPANS FOR WOOD STRUCTURAL PANEL BOX HEADERS[a]

HEADER CONSTRUCTION[b]	HEADER DEPTH (inches)	HOUSE DEPTH (feet)				
		24	26	28	30	32
Wood structural panel—one side	9	4	4	3	3	—
	15	5	5	4	3	3
Wood structural panel—both sides	9	7	5	5	4	3
	15	8	8	7	7	6

For SI: 1 inch = 25.4 mm, 1 foot = 304.8 mm.

a. Spans are based on single story with clear-span trussed roof or two-story with floor and roof supported by interior-bearing walls.

b. See Figure R602.7.2 for construction details.

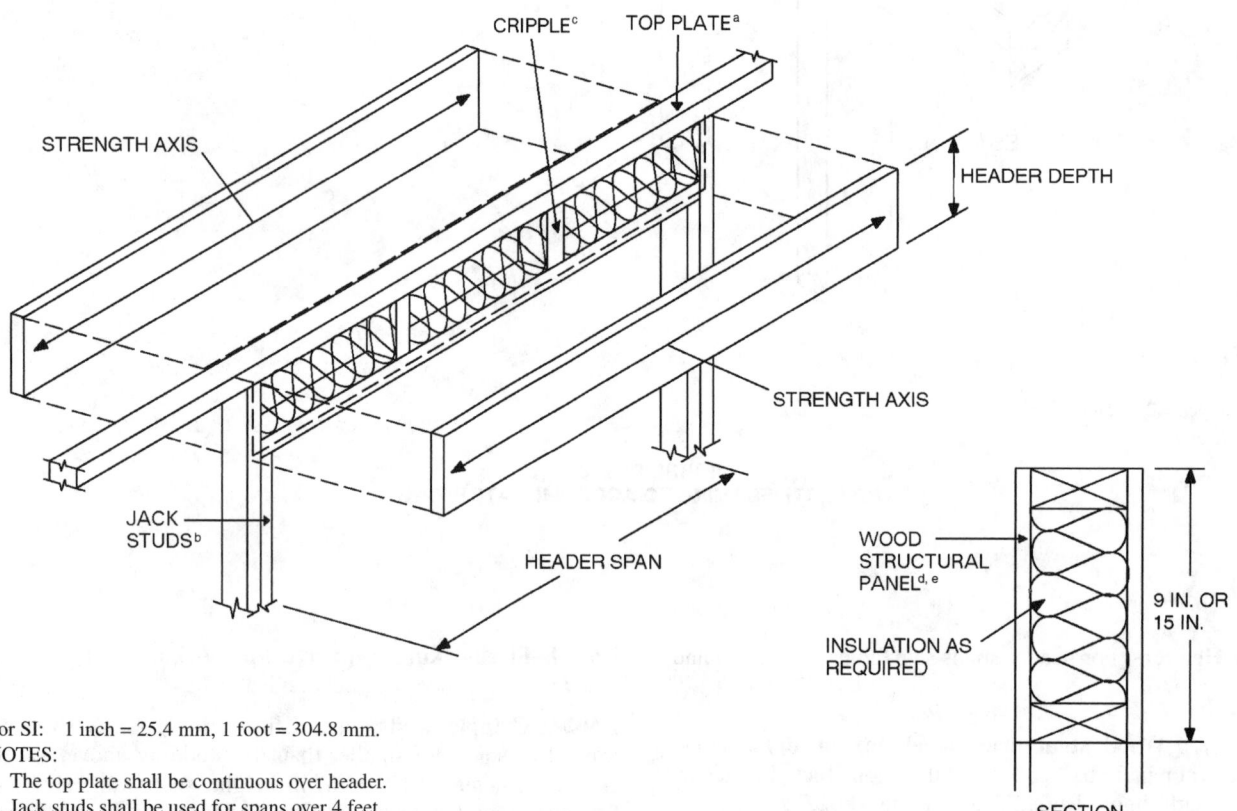

For SI: 1 inch = 25.4 mm, 1 foot = 304.8 mm.

NOTES:

a. The top plate shall be continuous over header.

b. Jack studs shall be used for spans over 4 feet.

c. Cripple spacing shall be the same as for studs.

d. Wood structural panel faces shall be single pieces of $^{15}/_{32}$-inch-thick Exposure 1 (exterior glue) or thicker, installed on the interior or exterior or both sides of the header.

e. Wood structural panel faces shall be nailed to framing and cripples with 8d common or galvanized box nails spaced 3 inches on center, staggering alternate nails $^{1}/_{2}$ inch. Galvanized nails shall be hot-dipped or tumbled.

FIGURE R602.7.2
TYPICAL WOOD STRUCTURAL PANEL BOX HEADER CONSTRUCTION

R602.10 Wall bracing. Buildings shall be braced in accordance with this section. Where a building, or portion thereof, does not comply with one or more of the bracing requirements in this section, those portions shall be designed and constructed in accordance with Section R301.1.

Exception: Detached one- and two-family *dwellings* located in Seismic Design Category C are exempt from the seismic bracing requirements of this section. Wind speed provisions for bracing shall be applicable to detached one- and two-family *dwellings*.

R602.10.1 Braced wall lines. *Braced wall lines* shall be provided in accordance with this section. The length of a *braced wall line* shall be measured as the distance between the ends of the wall line. The end of a *braced wall line* shall be considered to be either:

1. The intersection with perpendicular exterior walls or projection thereof,

2. The intersection with perpendicular *braced wall lines*.

The end of the *braced wall line* shall be chosen such that the maximum length results.

R602.10.1.1 Braced wall panels. *Braced wall panels* shall be constructed in accordance with the intermittent bracing methods specified in Section R602.10.2, or the continuous sheathing methods specified in Sections R602.10.4 and R602.10.5. Mixing of bracing method shall be permitted as follows:

1. Mixing bracing methods from *story* to *story* is permitted.

2. Mixing bracing methods from *braced wall line* to *braced wall line* within a *story* is permitted, except that continuous sheathing methods shall conform to the additional requirements of Sections R602.10.4 and R602.10.5.

3. Mixing bracing methods within a *braced wall line* is permitted only in Seismic Design Categories A and B, and detached *dwellings* in Seismic Design Category C. The length of required bracing for the *braced wall line* with mixed sheathing types shall have the higher bracing length requirement, in accordance with Tables R602.10.1.2(1) and R602.10.1.2(2), of all types of bracing used.

R602.10.1.2 Length of bracing. The length of bracing along each *braced wall line* shall be the greater of that required by the design wind speed and *braced wall line* spacing in accordance with Table R602.10.1.2(1) as adjusted by the factors in the footnotes or the Seismic Design Category and *braced wall line* length in accordance with Table R602.10.1.2(2) as adjusted by the factors in Table R602.10.1.2(3) or *braced wall panel* location requirements of Section R602.10.1.4. Only

walls that are parallel to the *braced wall line* shall be counted toward the bracing requirement of that line, except angled walls shall be counted in accordance with Section R602.10.1.3. In no case shall the minimum total length of bracing in a *braced wall line*, after all adjustments have been taken, be less than 48 inches (1219 mm) total.

R602.10.1.2.1 Braced wall panel uplift load path. *Braced wall panels* located at exterior walls that support roof rafters or trusses (including stories below top *story*) shall have the framing members connected in accordance with one of the following:

1. Fastening in accordance with Table R602.3(1) where:

   1.1. The basic wind speed does not exceed 90 mph (40 m/s), the wind exposure category is B, the roof pitch is 5:12 or greater, and the roof span is 32 feet (9754 mm) or less, or

   1.2. The net uplift value at the top of a wall does not exceed 100 plf. The net uplift value shall be determined in accordance with Section R802.11 and shall be permitted to be reduced by 60 plf (86 N/mm) for each full wall above.

2. Where the net uplift value at the top of a wall exceeds 100 plf (146 N/mm), installing *approved* uplift framing connectors to provide a continuous load path from the top of the wall to the foundation. The net uplift value shall be as determined in Item 1.2 above.

3. Bracing and fasteners designed in accordance with accepted engineering practice to resist combined uplift and shear forces.

R602.10.1.3 Angled corners. At corners, *braced wall lines* shall be permitted to angle out of plane up to 45 degrees with a maximum diagonal length of 8 feet (2438 mm). When determining the length of bracing required, the length of each *braced wall line* shall be determined as shown in Figure R602.10.1.3. The placement of bracing for the *braced wall lines* shall begin at the point where the *braced wall line*, which contains the angled wall adjoins the adjacent *braced wall line* (Point A as shown in Figure R602.10.1.3). Where an angled corner is constructed at an angle equal to 45 degrees (0.79 rad) and the diagonal length is no more than 8 feet (2438 mm), the angled wall may be considered as part of either of the adjoining *braced wall lines*, but not both. Where the diagonal length is greater than 8 feet (2438 mm), it shall be considered its own *braced wall line* and be braced in accordance with Section R602.10.1 and methods in Section R602.10.2.

TABLE R602.10.1.2(1)[a, b, c, d, e]
BRACING REQUIREMENTS BASED ON WIND SPEED
(as a function of braced wall line spacing)

EXPOSURE CATEGORY B, 30 FT MEAN ROOF HEIGHT, 10 FT EAVE TO RIDGE HEIGHT, 10 FT WALL HEIGHT, 2 BRACED WALL LINES			MINIMUM TOTAL LENGTH (feet) OF BRACED WALL PANELS REQUIRED ALONG EACH BRACED WALL LINE			
Basic Wind Speed (mph)	Story Location	Braced Wall Line Spacing (feet)	Method LIB[f, h]	Method GB (double sided)[g]	Methods DWB, WSP, SFB, PCP, HPS[f, i]	Continuous Sheathing
≤ 85 (mph)		10	3.5	3.5	2.0	1.5
		20	6.0	6.0	3.5	3.0
		30	8.5	8.5	5.0	4.5
		40	11.5	11.5	6.5	5.5
		50	14.0	14.0	8.0	7.0
		60	16.5	16.5	9.5	8.0
		10	6.5	6.5	3.5	3.0
		20	11.5	11.5	6.5	5.5
		30	16.5	16.5	9.5	8.0
		40	21.5	21.5	12.5	10.5
		50	26.5	26.5	15.0	13.0
		60	31.5	31.5	18.0	15.5
		10	NP	9.0	5.5	4.5
		20	NP	17.0	10.0	8.5
		30	NP	24.5	14.0	12.0
		40	NP	32.0	18.0	15.5
		50	NP	39.0	22.5	19.0
		60	NP	46.5	26.5	22.5
≤ 90 (mph)		10	3.5	3.5	2.0	2.0
		20	7.0	7.0	4.0	3.5
		30	9.5	9.5	5.5	5.0
		40	12.5	12.5	7.5	6.0
		50	15.5	15.5	9.0	7.5
		60	18.5	18.5	10.5	9.0
		10	7.0	7.0	4.0	3.5
		20	13.0	13.0	7.5	6.5
		30	18.5	18.5	10.5	9.0
		40	24.0	24.0	14.0	12.0
		50	29.5	29.5	17.0	14.5
		60	35.0	35.0	20.0	17.0
		10	NP	10.5	6.0	5.0
		20	NP	19.0	11.0	9.5
		30	NP	27.5	15.5	13.5
		40	NP	35.5	20.5	17.5
		50	NP	44.0	25.0	21.5
		60	NP	52.0	30.0	25.5

(continued)

TABLE R602.10.1.2(1)[a, b, c, d, e]—continued
BRACING REQUIREMENTS BASED ON WIND SPEED
(as a function of braced wall line spacing)

EXPOSURE CATEGORY B, 30 FT MEAN ROOF HEIGHT, 10 FT EAVE TO RIDGE HEIGHT, 10 FT WALL HEIGHT, 2 BRACED WALL LINES			MINIMUM TOTAL LENGTH (feet) OF BRACED WALL PANELS REQUIRED ALONG EACH BRACED WALL LINE			
Basic Wind Speed (mph)	Story Location	Braced wall Line Spacing (feet)	Method LIB[f, h]	Method GB (doubled sided)[g]	Method DWB, WSP, SFB, PCP, HPS[f, i]	Continuous Sheathing
≤ 100 (mph)		10	4.5	4.5	2.5	2.5
		20	8.5	8.5	5.0	4.0
		30	12.0	12.0	7.0	6.0
		40	15.5	15.5	9.0	7.5
		50	19.0	19.0	11.0	9.5
		60	22.5	22.5	13.0	11.0
		10	8.5	8.5	5.0	4.5
		20	16.0	16.0	9.0	8.0
		30	23.0	23.0	13.0	11.0
		40	29.5	29.5	17.0	14.5
		50	36.5	36.5	21.0	18.0
		60	43.5	43.5	25.0	21.0
		10	NP	12.5	7.5	6.0
		20	NP	23.5	13.5	11.5
		30	NP	34.0	19.5	16.5
		40	NP	44.0	25.0	21.5
		50	NP	54.0	31.0	26.5
		60	NP	64.0	36.5	31.0
≤ 110 (mph)		10	5.5	5.5	3.0	3.0
		20	10.0	10.0	6.0	5.0
		30	14.5	14.5	8.5	7.0
		40	18.5	18.5	11.0	9.0
		50	23.0	23.0	13.0	11.5
		60	27.5	27.5	15.5	13.5
		10	10.5	10.5	6.0	5.0
		20	19.0	19.0	11.0	9.5
		30	27.5	27.5	16.0	13.5
		40	36.0	36.0	20.5	17.5
		50	44.0	44.0	25.5	21.5
		60	52.5	52.5	30.0	25.5
		10	NP	15.5	9.0	7.5
		20	NP	28.5	16.5	14.0
		30	NP	41.0	23.5	20.0
		40	NP	53.0	30.5	26.0
		50	NP	65.5	37.5	32.0
		60	NP	77.5	44.5	37.5

(continued)

TABLE R602.10.1.2(1)[a, b, c, d, e]—continued
BRACING REQUIREMENTS BASED ON WIND SPEED
(as a function of braced wall line spacing)

For SI: 1 foot = 304.8 mm, 1 inch = 25.4 mm, 1 mile per hour = 0.447 m/s, 1 pound force = 4.448 N.

a. Tabulated bracing lengths are based on Wind Exposure Category B, a 30-ft mean roof height, a 10-ft eave to ridge height, a 10-ft wall height, and two braced wall lines sharing load in a given plan direction on a given story level. Methods of bracing shall be as described in Sections R602.10.2, R602.10.4 and R602.10.5. Interpolation shall be permitted.

NUMBER OF STORIES	EXPOSURE/HEIGHT FACTORS		
	Exposure B	Exposure C	Exposure D
1	1.0	1.2	1.5
2	1.0	1.3	1.6
3	1.0	1.4	1.7

b. For other mean roof heights and exposure categories, the required bracing length shall be multiplied by the appropriate factor from the following table:

c. For other roof-to-eave ridge heights, the required bracing length shall be multiplied by the appropriate factor from the following table: interpolation shall be permitted.

SUPPORT CONDITION	ROOF EAVE-TO-RIDGE HEIGHT			
	5 ft or less	10 ft	15 ft	20 ft
Roof only	0.7	1.0	1.3	1.6
Roof + floor	0.85	1.0	1.15	1.3
Roof + 2 floors	0.9	1.0	1.1	NP

d. For a maximum 9-foot wall height, multiplying the table values by 0.95 shall be permitted . For a maximum 8-foot wall height, multiplying, the table values by 0.90 shall be permitted. For a maximum 12-foot wall height, the table values shall be multiplied by 1.1.

e. For three or more braced wall lines in a given plan direction, the required bracing length on each braced wall line shall be multiplied by the appropriate factor from the following table:

NUMBER OF BRACED WALL LINES	ADJUSTMENT FACTOR
3	1.30
4	1.45
≥ 5	1.60

f. Bracing lengths are based on the application of gypsum board finish (or equivalent) applied to the inside face of a braced wall panel. When gypsum board finish (or equivalent) is not applied to the inside face of braced wall panels, the tabulated lengths shall be multiplied by the appropriate factor from the following table:

BRACING METHOD	ADJUSTMENT FACTOR
Method LIB	1.8
Methods DWB, WSP, SFB, PBS, PCP, HPS	1.4

g. Bracing lengths for Method GB are based on the application of gypsum board on both faces of a braced wall panel. When Method GB is provided on only one side of the wall, the required bracing amounts shall be doubled. When Method GB braced wall panels installed in accordance with Section R602.10.2 are fastened at 4 inches on center at panel edges, including top and bottom plates, and are blocked at all horizontal joints, multiplying the required bracing percentage for wind loading by 0.7 shall be permitted.

h. Method LIB bracing shall have gypsum board attached to at least one side according to the Section R602.10.2 Method GB requirements.

i. Required bracing length for Methods DWB, WSP, SFB, PBS, PCP and HPS in braced wall lines located in one-story buildings and in the top story of two or three story buildings shall be permitted to be multiplied by 0.80 when an approved hold-down device with a minimum uplift design value of 800 pounds is fastened to the end studs of each braced wall panel in the braced wall line and to the foundation or framing below.

TABLE R602.10.1.2(2)[a, b, c]
BRACING REQUIREMENTS BASED ON SEISMIC DESIGN CATEGORY
(AS A FUNCTION OF BRACED WALL LINE LENGTH)

SOIL CLASS D[a] WALL HEIGHT = 10 FT 10 PSF FLOOR DEAD LOAD 15 PSF ROOF/CEILING DEAD LOAD BRACED WALL LINE SPACING ≤ 25 FT			MINIMUM TOTAL LENGTH (feet) OF BRACED WALL PANELS REQUIRED ALONG EACH BRACED WALL LINE			
Seismic Design Category (SDC)	Story Location	Braced Wall Line Length	Method LIB	Methods DWB, SFB, GB, PBS, PCP, HPS	Method WSP	Continuous Sheathing
SDC A and B and Detached Dwellings in C			Exempt from Seismic Requirements Use Table R602.10.1.2(1) for Bracing Requirements			
SDC C		10	2.5	2.5	1.6	1.4
		20	5.0	5.0	3.2	2.7
		30	7.5	7.5	4.8	4.1
		40	10.0	10.0	6.4	5.4
		50	12.5	12.5	8.0	6.8
		10	NP	4.5	3.0	2.6
		20	NP	9.0	6.0	5.1
		30	NP	13.5	9.0	7.7
		40	NP	18.0	12.0	10.2
		50	NP	22.5	15.0	12.8
		10	NP	6.0	4.5	3.8
		20	NP	12.0	9.0	7.7
		30	NP	18.0	13.5	11.5
		40	NP	24.0	18.0	15.3
		50	NP	30.0	22.5	19.1
SDC D₀ or D₁		10	NP	3.0	2.0	1.7
		20	NP	6.0	4.0	3.4
		30	NP	9.0	6.0	5.1
		40	NP	12.0	8.0	6.8
		50	NP	15.0	10.0	8.5
		10	NP	6.0	4.5	3.8
		20	NP	12.0	9.0	7.7
		30	NP	18.0	13.5	11.5
		40	NP	24.0	18.0	15.3
		50	NP	30.0	22.5	19.1
		10	NP	8.5	6.0	5.1
		20	NP	17.0	12.0	10.2
		30	NP	25.5	18.0	15.3
		40	NP	34.0	24.0	20.4
		50	NP	42.5	30.0	25.5

(continued)

TABLE R602.10.1.2(2)[a, b, c]—continued
BRACING REQUIREMENTS BASED ON SEISMIC DESIGN CATEGORY
(AS A FUNCTION OF BRACED WALL LINE LENGTH)

SOIL CLASS D[a] WALL HEIGHT = 10 FT 10 PSF FLOOR DEAD LOAD 15 PSF ROOF/CEILING DEAD LOAD BRACED WALL LINE SPACING ≤ 25 FT			MINIMUM TOTAL LENGTH (feet) OF BRACED WALL PANELS REQUIRED ALONG EACH BRACED WALL LINE			
Seismic Design Category (SDC)	Story Location	Braced Wall Line Length	Method LIB	METHODS DWB, SFB, GB, PBS, PCP, HPS	Method WSP	Continuous Sheathing
SDC D₂		10	NP	4.0	2.5	2.1
		20	NP	8.0	5.0	4.3
		30	NP	12.0	7.5	6.4
		40	NP	16.0	10.0	8.5
		50	NP	20.0	12.5	10.6
		10	NP	7.5	5.5	4.7
		20	NP	15.0	11.0	9.4
		30	NP	22.5	16.5	14.0
		40	NP	30.0	22.0	18.7
		50	NP	37.5	27.5	23.4
		10	NP	NP	NP	NP
		20	NP	NP	NP	NP
		30	NP	NP	NP	NP
		40	NP	NP	NP	NP
		50	NP	NP	NP	NP

For SI: 1 foot = 304.8 mm, 1 pound per square foot = 47.89 Pa.

a. Wall bracing lengths are based on a soil site class "D." Interpolation of bracing length between the S_{ds} values associated with the seismic design categories shall be permitted when a site-specific S_{ds} value is determined in accordance with Section 1613.5 of the *International Building Code*.

b. Foundation cripple wall panels shall be braced in accordance with Section R602.10.9.

c. Methods of bracing shall be as described in Sections R602.10.2, R602.10.4 and R602.10.5.

TABLE R602.10.1.2(3)
ADJUSTMENT FACTORS TO THE LENGTH OF REQUIRED SEISMIC WALL BRACING[a]

ADJUSTMENT BASED ON:		MULTIPLY LENGTH OF BRACING PER WALL LINE BY:	APPLIES TO:
Story height[b] (Section R301.3)	≤10 ft	1.0	All bracing methods - Sections R602.10.2, R602.10.4 and R602.10.5
	> 10 ≤ 12 ft	1.2	
Braced wall line spacing townhouses in SDC A-C[b,c]	≤ 35 ft	1.0	
	> 35 ≤ 50 ft	1.43	
Wall dead load	> 8 ≤ 15 psf	1.0	
	≤ 8 psf	0.85	
Roof/ceiling dead load for wall supporting[b]	roof only or roof plus one story ≤ 15 psf	1.0	
	roof only < 15 psf ≤ 25 psf	1.1	
	roof plus one story < 15 psf ≤ 25 psf	1.2	
Walls with stone or masonry veneer in SDC C-D₂		See Section R703.7	
Cripple walls		See Section R602.10.9	

For SI: 1 foot = 304.8 mm, 1 pound per square foot = 47.89 Pa.

a. The total length of bracing required for a given wall line is the product of all applicable adjustment factors.

b. Linear interpolation shall be permitted.

c. Braced wall line spacing and adjustment to bracing length in SDC D₀, D₁, and D₂ shall comply with Section R602.10.1.5.

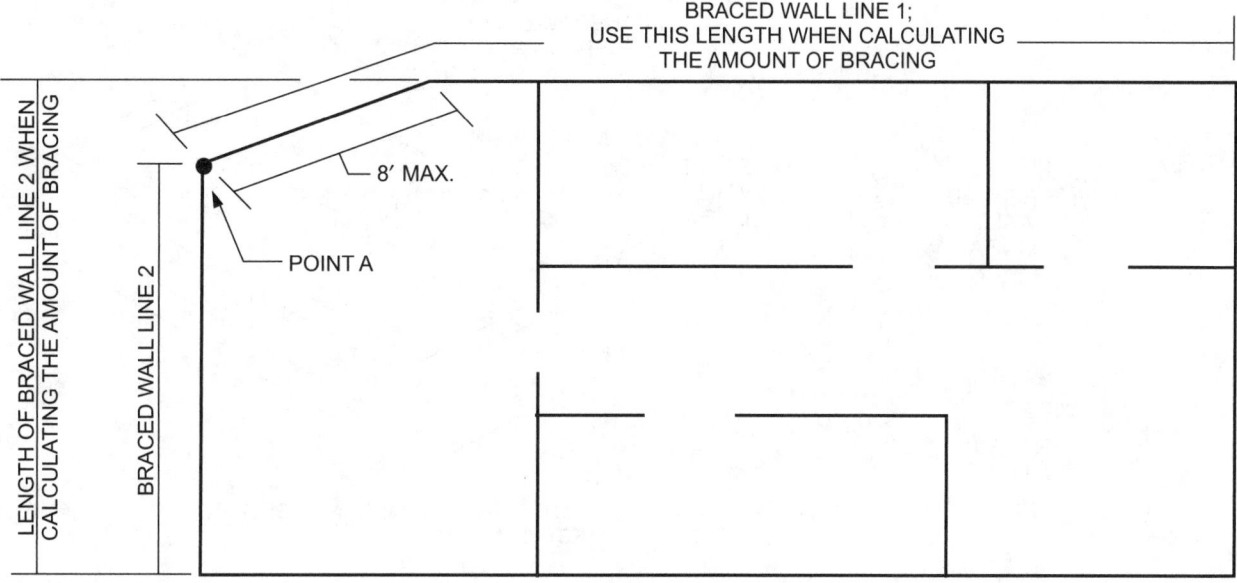

For SI: 1 foot = 304.8 mm.

**FIGURE R602.10.1.3
ANGLED CORNERS**

R602.10.1.4 Braced wall panel location. *Braced wall panels* shall be located in accordance with Figure R602.10.1.4(1). *Braced wall panels* shall be located not more than 25 feet (7620 mm) on center and shall be permitted to begin no more than 12.5 feet (3810 mm) from the end of a *braced wall line* in accordance with Section R602.10.1 and Figure R602.10.1.4(2). The total combined distance from each end of a *braced wall line* to the outermost *braced wall panel* or panels in the line shall not exceed 12.5 feet (3810 mm). *Braced wall panels* may be offset out-of-plane up to 4 feet (1219 mm) from the designated *braced wall line* provided that the total out-to-out offset of *braced wall panels* in a *braced wall line* is not more than 8 feet (2438 mm) in accordance with Figures R602.10.1.4(3) and R602.10.1.4(4). All *braced wall panels* within a *braced wall line* shall be permitted to be offset from the designated *braced wall line*.

R602.10.1.4.1 Braced wall panel location in Seismic Design Categories D_0, D_1 and D_2. *Braced wall lines* at exterior walls shall have a *braced wall panel* located at each end of the *braced wall line*.

Exception: For *braced wall panel* construction Method WSP of Section R602.10.2, the *braced wall panel* shall be permitted to begin no more than 8 feet (2438 mm) from each end of the *braced wall line* provided one of the following is satisfied in accordance with Figure R602.10.1.4.1:

1. A minimum 24-inch-wide (610 mm) panel is applied to each side of the building corner and the two 24-inch-wide (610 mm) panels

at the corner are attached to framing in accordance with Figure R602.10.4.4(1), or

2. The end of each *braced wall panel* closest to the corner shall have a hold-down device fastened to the stud at the edge of the *braced wall panel* closest to the corner and to the foundation or framing below. The hold-down device shall be capable of providing an uplift allowable design value of at least 1,800 pounds (8 kN). The hold-down device shall be installed in accordance with the manufacturer's recommendations.

R602.10.1.5 Braced wall line spacing for Seismic Design Categories D_0, D_1 and D_2. Spacing between *braced wall lines* in each *story* shall not exceed 25 feet (7620 mm) on center in both the longitudinal and transverse directions.

Exception: In one- and two-story buildings, spacing between two adjacent *braced wall lines* shall not exceed 35 feet (10 668 mm) on center in order to accommodate one single room not exceeding 900 square feet (84 m²) in each *dwelling unit*. Spacing between all other *braced wall lines* shall not exceed 25 feet (7620 mm). A spacing of 35 feet (10 668 mm) or less shall be permitted between *braced wall lines* where the length of wall bracing required by Table R602.10.1.2(2) is multiplied by the appropriate adjustment factor from Table R602.10.1.5, the length-to-width ratio for the floor/roof *diaphragm* does not exceed 3:1, and the top plate lap splice face nailing is twelve 16d nails on each side of the splice.

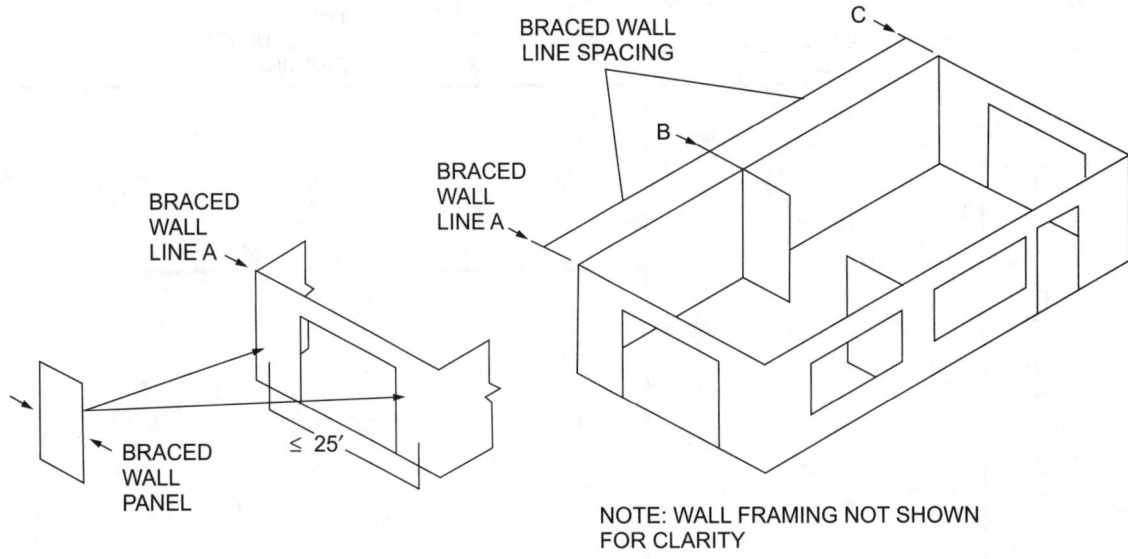

For SI: 1 foot = 304.8 mm.

FIGURE R602.10.1.4(1)
BRACED WALL PANELS AND BRACED WALL LINES

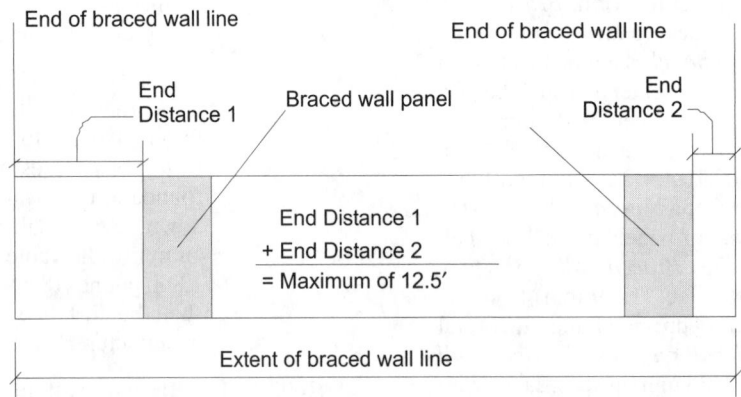

Braced wall panel shall be permitted to be located away from the end of a braced wall line, provided the total end distance from each end to the nearest braced wall panel does not exceed 12.5′. If braced wall panel is located at the end of the braced wall line, then end distance is 0′.

For SI: 1 foot = 304.8 mm.

FIGURE R602.10.1.4(2)
BRACED WALL PANEL END DISTANCE REQUIREMENTS (SDC A, B AND C)

R602.10.2 Intermittent braced wall panel construction methods. The construction of intermittent *braced wall panels* shall be in accordance with one of the methods listed in Table R602.10.2.

R602.10.2.1 Intermittent braced wall panel interior finish material. Intermittent *braced wall panels* shall have gypsum wall board installed on the side of the wall opposite the bracing material. Gypsum wall board shall be not less than $1/2$ inch (12.7 mm) in thickness and be fastened in accordance with Table R702.3.5 for interior gypsum wall board.

Exceptions:

1. Wall panels that are braced in accordance with Methods GB, ABW, PFG and PFH.

2. When an *approved* interior finish material with an in-plane shear resistance equivalent to gypsum board is installed.

3. For Methods DWB, WSP, SFB, PBS, PCP and HPS, omitting gypsum wall board is permitted provided the length of bracing in Tables R602.10.1.2(1) and R602.10.1.2(2) is multiplied by a factor of 1.5.

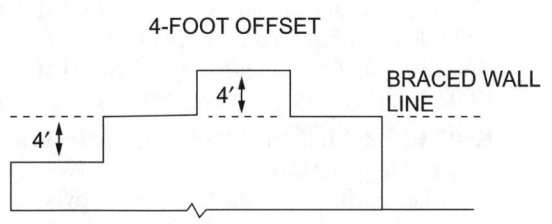

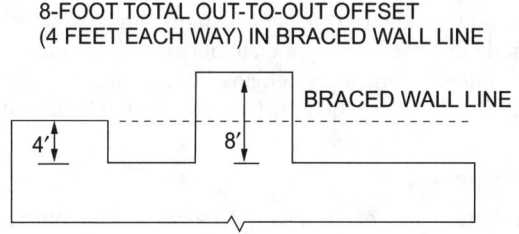

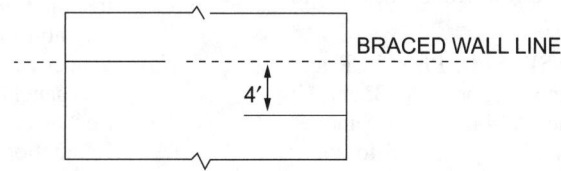

For SI: 1 foot = 304.8 mm.

FIGURE R602.10.1.4(3)
OFFSETS PERMITTED FOR BRACED WALL LINES

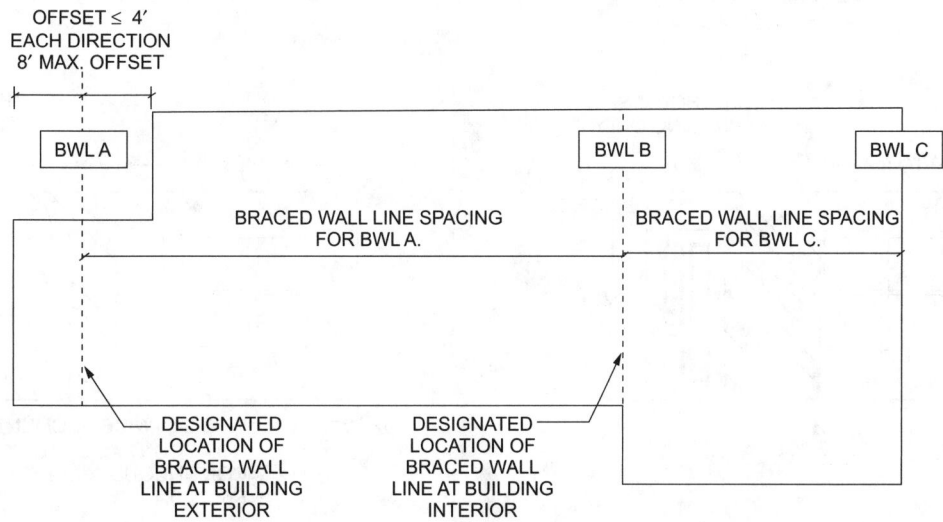

NOTE: BRACED WALL SPACING FOR BWL B IS THE GREATER OF THE DISTANCE FROM BWL A TO BWL B OR FROM BWL B TO BWL C.

For SI: 1 foot = 304.8 mm.

FIGURE R602.10.1.4(4)
BRACED WALL LINE SPACING

R602.10.2.2 Adhesive attachment of sheathing in Seismic Design Categories C, D_0, D_1 and D_2. Adhesive attachment of wall sheathing shall not be permitted in Seismic Design Categories C, D_0, D_1 and D_2.

R602.10.3 Minimum length of braced panels. For Methods DWB, WSP, SFB, PBS, PCP and HPS, each *braced wall panel* shall be at least 48 inches (1219 mm) in length, covering a minimum of three stud spaces where studs are spaced 16 inches (406 mm) on center and covering a minimum of two stud spaces where studs are spaced 24 inches (610 mm) on center. For Method GB, each *braced wall panel* and shall be at least 96 inches (2438 mm) in length where applied to one face of a *braced wall panel* and at least 48 inches (1219 mm) where applied to both faces. For Methods DWB, WSP, SFB, PBS, PCP and HPS, for purposes of computing the length of panel bracing required in Tables R602.10.1.2(1) and R602.10.1.2(2), the effective length of the *braced wall* panel shall be equal to the actual length of the panel. When Method GB panels are applied to only one face of a *braced wall panel*, bracing lengths required in Tables R602.10.1.2(1) and R602.10.1.2(2) for Method GB shall be doubled.

Exceptions:

1. Lengths of *braced wall panels* for continuous sheathing methods shall be in accordance with Table R602.10.4.2.

2. Lengths of Method ABW panels shall be in accordance with Sections R602.10.3.2.

3. Length of Methods PFH and PFG panels shall be in accordance with Section R602.10.3.3 and R602.10.3.4 respectively.

4. For Methods DWB, WSP, SFB, PBS, PCP and HPS in Seismic Design Categories A, B, and C: Panels between 36 inches (914 mm) and 48 inches (1219 mm) in length shall be permitted to count towards the required length of bracing in Tables R602.10.1.2(1) and R602.10.1.2(2), and the effective contribution shall comply with Table R602.10.3.

R602.10.3.1 Adjustment of length of braced panels. When *story height* (H), measured in feet, exceeds 10 feet (3048 mm), in accordance with Section R301.3, the minimum length of *braced wall panels* specified in Section R602.10.3 shall be increased by a factor H/10. See Table R602.10.3.1. Interpolation is permitted.

R602.10.3.2 Method ABW: Alternate braced wall panels. Method ABW *braced wall panels* constructed in accordance with one of the following provisions shall be permitted to replace each 4 feet (1219 mm) of *braced wall panel* as required by Section R602.10.3. The maximum height and minimum length and hold-down force of each panel shall be in accordance with Table R602.10.3.2:

1. In one-story buildings, each panel shall be installed in accordance with Figure R602.10.3.2. The hold-down device shall be installed in accordance with the manufacturer's recommendations. The panels shall be supported directly on a foundation or on floor framing supported directly on a foundation which is continuous across the entire length of the *braced wall line*.

2. In the first *story* of two-story buildings, each *braced wall panel* shall be in accordance with Item 1 above, except that the wood structural panel sheathing edge nailing spacing shall not exceed 4 inches (102 mm) on center.

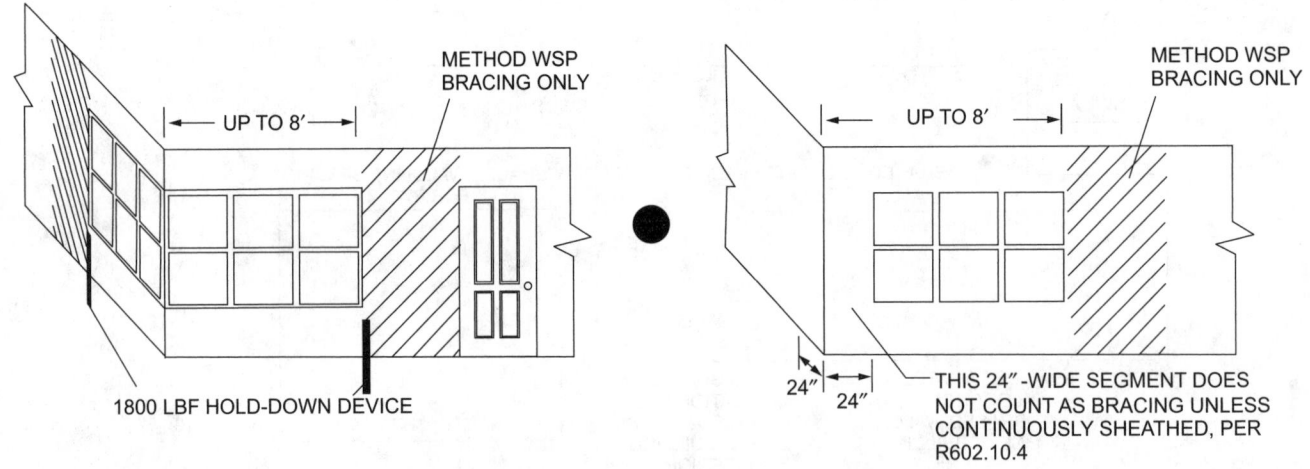

For SI: 1 inch = 25.4 mm, 1 foot = 304.8 mm, 1 pound force = 4,448 N.

FIGURE R602.10.1.4.1
BRACED WALL PANELS AT ENDS OF BRACED WALL LINES IN SEISMIC DESIGN CATEGORIES D_0, D_1 AND D_2

TABLE R602.10.1.5
ADJUSTMENTS OF BRACING LENGTH FOR BRACED WALL LINES GREATER THAN 25 FEET[a,b]

BRACED WALL LINE SPACING (feet)	MULTIPLY BRACING LENGTH IN TABLE R602.10.1.2(2) BY:
25	1.0
30	1.2
35	1.4

For SI: 1 foot = 304.8 mm.

a. Linear interpolation is permitted.

b. When a braced wall line has a parallel braced wall line on both sides, the larger adjustment factor shall be used.

TABLE R602.10.2
INTERMITTENT BRACING METHODS

METHOD	MATERIAL	MINIMUM THICKNESS	FIGURE	CONNECTION CRITERIA
LIB	Let-in-bracing	1 × 4 wood or approved metal straps at 45° to 60° angles for maximum 16″ stud spacing		Wood: 2-8d nails per stud including top and bottom plate metal: per manufacturer
DWB	Diagonal wood boards	$^3/_4$″ (1″ nominal) for maximum 24″ stud spacing		2-8d ($2^1/_2$″ × 0.113″) nails or 2 staples, $1^3/_4$″ per stud
WSP	Wood structural panel (see Section R604)	$^3/_8$″		For exterior sheathing see Table R602.3(3) For interior sheathing see Table R602.3(1)
SFB	Structural fiberboard sheathing	$^1/_2$″ or $^{25}/_{32}$″ for maximum 16″ stud spacing		$1^1/_2$″ galvanized roofing nails or 8d common ($2^1/_2$″ × 0.131) nails at 3″ spacing (panel edges) at 6″ spacing (intermediate supports)
GB	Gypsum board	$^1/_2$″		Nails or screws at 7″ spacing at panel edges including top and bottom plates; for all braced wall panel locations for exterior sheathing nail or screw size, see Table R602.3(1); for interior gypsum board nail or screw size, see Table R702.3.5
PBS	Particleboard sheathing (see Section R605)	$^3/_8$″ or $^1/_2$″ for maximum 16″ stud spacing		$1^1/_2$″ galvanized roofing nails or 8d common ($2^1/_2$″ × 0.131) nails at 3″ spacing (panel edges) at 6 spacing (intermediate supports)
PCP	Portland cement plaster	See Section R703.6 For maximum 16″ stud spacing		$1^1/_2$″, 11 gage, $^7/_{16}$″ head nails at 6″ spacing or $^7/_8$″, 16 gage staples at 6″ spacing
HPS	Hardboard panel siding	$^7/_{16}$″ For maximum 16″ stud spacing		0.092″ dia., 0.225″ head nails with length to accommodate $1^1/_2$″ penetration into studs at 4″ spacing (panel edges), at 8″ spacing (intermediate supports)
ABW	Alternate braced wall	See Section R602.10.3.2		See Section R602.10.3.2
PFH	Intermittent portal frame	See Section R602.10.3.3		See Section R602.10.3.3
PFG	Intermittent portal frame at garage	See Section R602.10.3.4		See Section R602.10.3.4

R602.10.3.3 Method PFH: Portal frame with hold-downs. Method PFH *braced wall panels* constructed in accordance with one of the following provisions are also permitted to replace each 4 feet (1219 mm) of *braced wall panel* as required by Section R602.10.3 for use adjacent to a window or door opening with a full-length header:

1. Each panel shall be fabricated in accordance with Figure R602.10.3.3. The wood structural panel sheathing shall extend up over the solid sawn or glued-laminated header and shall be nailed in accordance with Figure R602.10.3.3. A spacer, if used with a built-up header, shall be placed on the side of the built-up beam opposite the wood structural panel sheathing. The header

shall extend between the inside faces of the first full-length outer studs of each panel. One anchor bolt not less than $^5/_8$-inch-diameter (16 mm) and installed in accordance with Section R403.1.6 shall be provided in the center of each sill plate. The hold-down devices shall be an embedded-strap type, installed in accordance with the manufacturer's recommendations. The panels shall be supported directly on a foundation which is continuous across the entire length of the braced wall line. The foundation shall be reinforced as shown on Figure R602.10.3.2. This reinforcement shall be lapped not less than 15 inches (381 mm) with the reinforcement required in the continuous foundation located directly under the braced wall line.

TABLE R602.10.3
EFFECTIVE LENGTHS FOR BRACED WALL PANELS LESS THAN 48 INCHES IN ACTUAL LENGTH
(BRACE METHODS DWB, WSP, SFB, PBS, PCP AND HPS[a])

ACTUAL LENGTH OF BRACED WALL PANEL (inches)	EFFECTIVE LENGTH OF BRACED WALL PANEL (inches)		
	8-foot Wall Height	9-foot Wall Height	10-foot Wall Height
48	48	48	48
42	36	36	N/A
36	27	N/A	N/A

For SI: 1 inch = 25.4 mm, 1 foot = 304.8 mm.
a. Interpolation shall be permitted.

TABLE R602.10.3.1
MINIMUM LENGTH REQUIREMENTS FOR BRACED WALL PANELS

SEISMIC DESIGN CATEGORY AND WIND SPEED	BRACING METHOD	HEIGHT OF BRACED WALL PANEL				
		8 ft	9 ft	10 ft	11 ft	12 ft
SDC A, B, C, D$_0$, D$_1$ and D$_2$ Wind speed < 110 mph	DWB, WSP, SFB, PBS, PCP, HPS and Method GB when double sided	4' - 0"	4' - 0"	4' - 0"	4' - 5"	4' - 10"
	Method GB, single sided	8' - 0"	8' - 0"	8' - 0"	8' - 10"	9' - 8"

For SI: 1 inch = 25.4 mm, 1 foot = 304.8 mm.

TABLE R602.10.3.2
MINIMUM LENGTH REQUIREMENTS AND HOLD-DOWN FORCES FOR METHOD ABW BRACED WALL PANELS

SEISMIC DESIGN CATEGORY AND WIND SPEED		HEIGHT OF BRACED WALL PANEL				
		8 ft	9 ft	10 ft	11 ft	12 ft
SDC A, B and C Wind speed < 110 mph	Minimum sheathed length	2' - 4"	2' - 8"	2' - 10"	3' - 2"	3' - 6"
	R602.10.3.2, item 1 hold-down force (lb)	1800	1800	1800	2000	2200
	R602.10.3.2, item 2 hold-down force (lb)	3000	3000	3000	3300	3600
SDC D$_0$, D$_1$ and D$_2$ Wind speed < 110 mph	Minimum sheathed length	2' - 8"	2' - 8"	2' - 10"	NP[a]	NP[a]
	R602.10.3.2, item 1 hold-down force (lb)	1800	1800	1800	NP[a]	NP[a]
	R602.10.3.2, item 2 hold-down force (lb)	3000	3000	3000	NP[a]	NP[a]

For SI: 1 inch = 25.4 mm, 1 foot = 305 mm, 1 pound = 4.448 N.
a. NP = Not Permitted. Maximum height of 10 feet.

2. In the first *story* of two-story buildings, each wall panel shall be braced in accordance with item 1 above, except that each panel shall have a length of not less than 24 inches (610 mm).

R602.10.3.4 Method PFG: at garage door openings in Seismic Design Categories A, B and C. Where supporting a roof or one *story* and a roof, alternate *braced wall panels* constructed in accordance with the following provisions are permitted on either side of garage door openings. For the purpose of calculating wall bracing amounts to satisfy the minimum requirements of Table R602.10.1.2(1), the length of the alternate *braced wall panel* shall be multiplied by a factor of 1.5.

1. *Braced wall panel* length shall be a minimum of 24 inches (610 mm) and *braced wall panel* height shall be a maximum of 10 feet (3048 mm).

2. *Braced wall panel* shall be sheathed on one face with a single layer of $^7/_{16}$-inch-minimum (11 mm) thickness wood structural panel sheathing attached to framing with 8d common nails at 3 inches (76 mm) on center in accordance with Figure R602.10.3.4.

3. The wood structural panel sheathing shall extend up over the solid sawn or glued-laminated header and shall be nailed to the header at 3 inches (76 mm) on center grid in accordance with Figure R602.10.3.4.

4. The header shall consist of a minimum of two solid sawn 2×12s (51 by 305 mm) or a 3 inches × 11.25 inch (76 by 286 mm) glued-laminated header. The header shall extend between the inside faces of the first full-length outer studs of each panel in accordance with Figure R602.10.3.4. The clear span of the header between the inner studs of each panel shall be not less than 6 feet (1829 mm) and not more than 18 feet (5486 mm) in length.

5. A strap with an uplift capacity of not less than 1,000 pounds (4448 N) shall fasten the header to the side of the inner studs opposite the sheathing face. Where building is located in Wind Exposure Categories C or D, the strap uplift capacity shall be in accordance with Table R602.10.4.1.1.

6. A minimum of two bolts not less than $^1/_2$-inch (12.7 mm) diameter shall be installed in accordance with Section R403.1.6. A $^3/_{16}$-inch by $2^1/_2$-inch (4.8 by 63 by 63 mm) by $2^1/_2$-inch steel plate washer is installed between the bottom plate and the nut of each bolt.

7. *Braced wall panel* shall be installed directly on a foundation.

8. Where an alternate *braced wall panel* is located only on one side of the garage opening, the header shall be connected to a supporting jack stud on the opposite side of the garage opening with a metal strap with an uplift capacity of not less than 1,000 pounds. Where that supporting jack stud is not part of a *braced wall panel* assembly, another 1,000 pounds (4448 N) strap shall be installed to attach the supporting jack stud to the foundation.

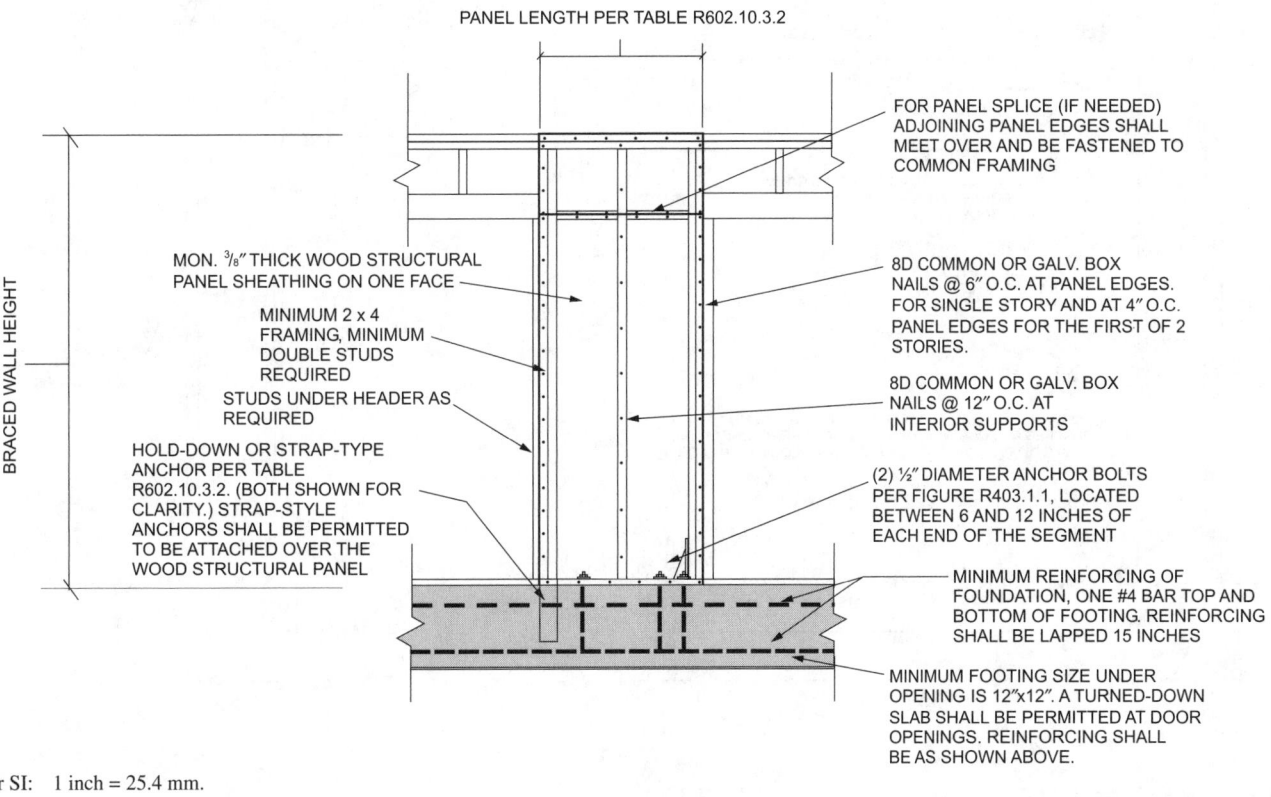

PANEL LENGTH PER TABLE R602.10.3.2

FOR PANEL SPLICE (IF NEEDED) ADJOINING PANEL EDGES SHALL MEET OVER AND BE FASTENED TO COMMON FRAMING

MON. $^3/_8$" THICK WOOD STRUCTURAL PANEL SHEATHING ON ONE FACE

MINIMUM 2 x 4 FRAMING, MINIMUM DOUBLE STUDS REQUIRED

STUDS UNDER HEADER AS REQUIRED

HOLD-DOWN OR STRAP-TYPE ANCHOR PER TABLE R602.10.3.2. (BOTH SHOWN FOR CLARITY.) STRAP-STYLE ANCHORS SHALL BE PERMITTED TO BE ATTACHED OVER THE WOOD STRUCTURAL PANEL

BRACED WALL HEIGHT

8D COMMON OR GALV. BOX NAILS @ 6" O.C. AT PANEL EDGES. FOR SINGLE STORY AND AT 4" O.C. PANEL EDGES FOR THE FIRST OF 2 STORIES.

8D COMMON OR GALV. BOX NAILS @ 12" O.C. AT INTERIOR SUPPORTS

(2) ½" DIAMETER ANCHOR BOLTS PER FIGURE R403.1.1, LOCATED BETWEEN 6 AND 12 INCHES OF EACH END OF THE SEGMENT

MINIMUM REINFORCING OF FOUNDATION, ONE #4 BAR TOP AND BOTTOM OF FOOTING. REINFORCING SHALL BE LAPPED 15 INCHES

MINIMUM FOOTING SIZE UNDER OPENING IS 12"x12". A TURNED-DOWN SLAB SHALL BE PERMITTED AT DOOR OPENINGS. REINFORCING SHALL BE AS SHOWN ABOVE.

For SI: 1 inch = 25.4 mm.

FIGURE R602.10.3.2
ALTERNATE BRACED WALL PANEL

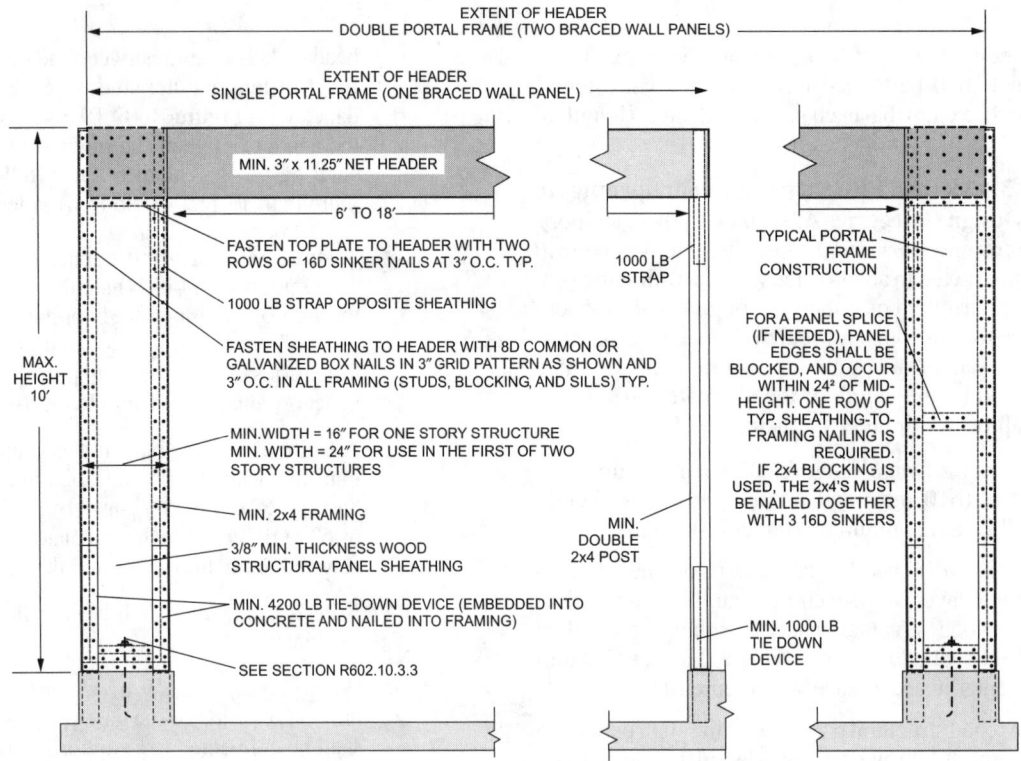

For SI: 1 inch = 25.4 mm, 1 foot = 304.8 mm, 1 pound force = 4.448 N.

FIGURE R602.10.3.3
METHOD PFH: PORTAL FRAME WITH HOLD-DOWNS

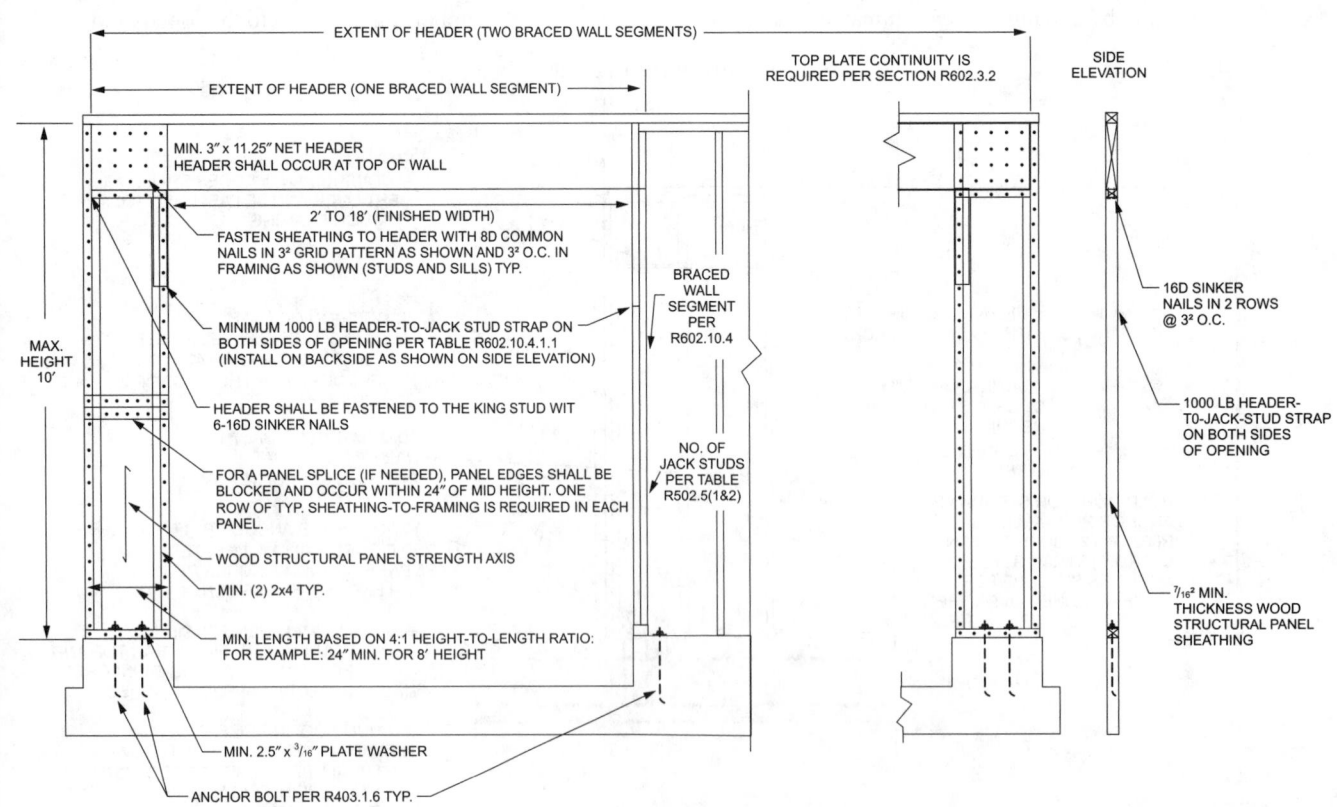

For SI: 1 inch = 25.4 mm, 1 foot = 304.8 mm, 1 pound force = 4.448 N.

FIGURE R602.10.3.4
METHOD PFG PORTAL FRAME AT GARAGE DOOR OPENINGS IN SEISMIC DESIGN CATEGORIES A, B AND C

2009 INTERNATIONAL RESIDENTIAL CODE®

R602.10.4 Continuous sheathing. *Braced wall lines* with continuous sheathing shall be constructed in accordance with this section. All *braced wall lines* along exterior walls on the same *story* shall be continuously sheathed.

Exception: Within Seismic Design Categories A, B and C or in regions where the basic wind speed is less than or equal to 100 mph (45 m/s), other bracing methods prescribed by this code shall be permitted on other *braced wall lines* on the same *story* level or on any *braced wall line* on different *story* levels of the building.

R602.10.4.1 Continuous sheathing braced wall panels. Continuous sheathing methods require structural panel sheathing to be used on all sheathable surfaces on one side of a *braced wall line* including areas above and below openings and gable end walls. *Braced wall panels* shall be constructed in accordance with one of the methods listed in Table R602.10.4.1. Different bracing methods, other than those listed in Table R602.10.4.1, shall not be permitted along a *braced wall line* with continuous sheathing.

R602.10.4.1.1 Continuous portal frame. Continuous portal frame *braced wall panels* shall be constructed in accordance with Figure R602.10.4.1.1. The number of continuous portal frame panels in a single *braced wall line* shall not exceed four. For purposes of resisting wind pressures acting perpendicular to the wall, the requirements of Figure R602.10.4.1.1 and Table R602.10.4.1.1 shall be met. There shall be a maximum of two braced wall segments per header and header length shall not exceed 22 feet (6706 mm). Tension straps shall be installed in accordance with the manufacturer's recommendations.

R602.10.4.2 Length of braced wall panels with continuous sheathing. *Braced wall panels* along a *braced wall line* with continuous sheathing shall be full-height with a length based on the adjacent clear opening height in accordance with Table R602.10.4.2 and Figure R602.10.4.2. Within a *braced wall line* when a panel has an opening on either side of differing heights, the taller opening height shall be used to determine the panel length from Table R602.10.4.2. For Method CS-PF, wall height shall be measured from the top of the header to the bottom of the bottom plate as shown in Figure R602.10.4.1.1.

R602.10.4.3 Length of bracing for continuous sheathing. *Braced wall lines* with continuous sheathing shall be provided with *braced wall panels* in the length required in Tables R602.10.1.2(1) and R602.10.1.2(2). Only those full-height *braced wall panels* complying with the length requirements of Table R602.10.4.2 shall be permitted to contribute to the minimum required length of bracing.

R602.10.4.4 Continuously sheathed braced wall panel location and corner construction. For all continuous sheathing methods, full-height *braced wall panels* complying with the length requirements of Table R602.10.4.2 shall be located at each end of a *braced wall line* with continuous sheathing and at least every 25 feet (7620 mm) on center. A minimum 24 inch (610 mm) wood structural panel corner return shall be provided at both ends of a *braced wall line* with continuous sheathing in accordance with Figures R602.10.4.4(1) and R602.10.4.4(2). In lieu of the corner return, a hold-down device with a minimum uplift design value of 800 pounds

TABLE R602.10.4.1
CONTINUOUS SHEATHING METHODS

METHOD	MATERIAL	MINIMUM THICKNESS	FIGURE	CONNECTION CRITERIA
CS-WSP	Wood structural panel	$^3/_8''$		6d common ($2'' \times 0.113''$) nails at 6″ spacing (panel edges) and at 12″ spacing (intermediate supports) or 16 ga. × 1³/₄ staples at 3″ spacing (panel edges) and 6″ spacing (intermediate supports)
CS-G	Wood structural panel adjacent to garage openings and supporting roof load only[a,b]	$^3/_8''$		See Method CS-WSP
CS-PF	Continuous portal frame	See Section R602.10.4.1.1		See Section R602.10.4.1.1

For SI: 1 inch = 25.4 mm, 1 pound per square foot = 47.89 Pa.

a. Applies to one wall of a garage only.
b. Roof covering dead loads shall be 3 psf or less.

(3560 N) shall be fastened to the corner stud and to the foundation or framing below in accordance with Figure R602.10.4.4(3).

Exception: The first *braced wall panel* shall be permitted to begin 12.5 feet (3810 mm) from each end of the *braced wall line* in Seismic Design Categories A, B and C and 8 feet (2438 mm) in Seismic Design Categories D_0, D_1 and D_2 provided one of the following is satisfied:

1. A minimum 24 inch (610 mm) long, full-height wood structural panel is provided at both sides

of a corner constructed in accordance with Figure R602.10.4.4(1) at the *braced wall line* ends in accordance with Figure R602.10.4.4(4), or

2. The *braced wall panel* closest to the corner shall have a hold-down device with a minimum uplift design value of 800 pounds (3560 N) fastened to the stud at the edge of the *braced wall panel* closest to the corner and to the foundation or framing below in accordance with Figure R602.10.4.4(5).

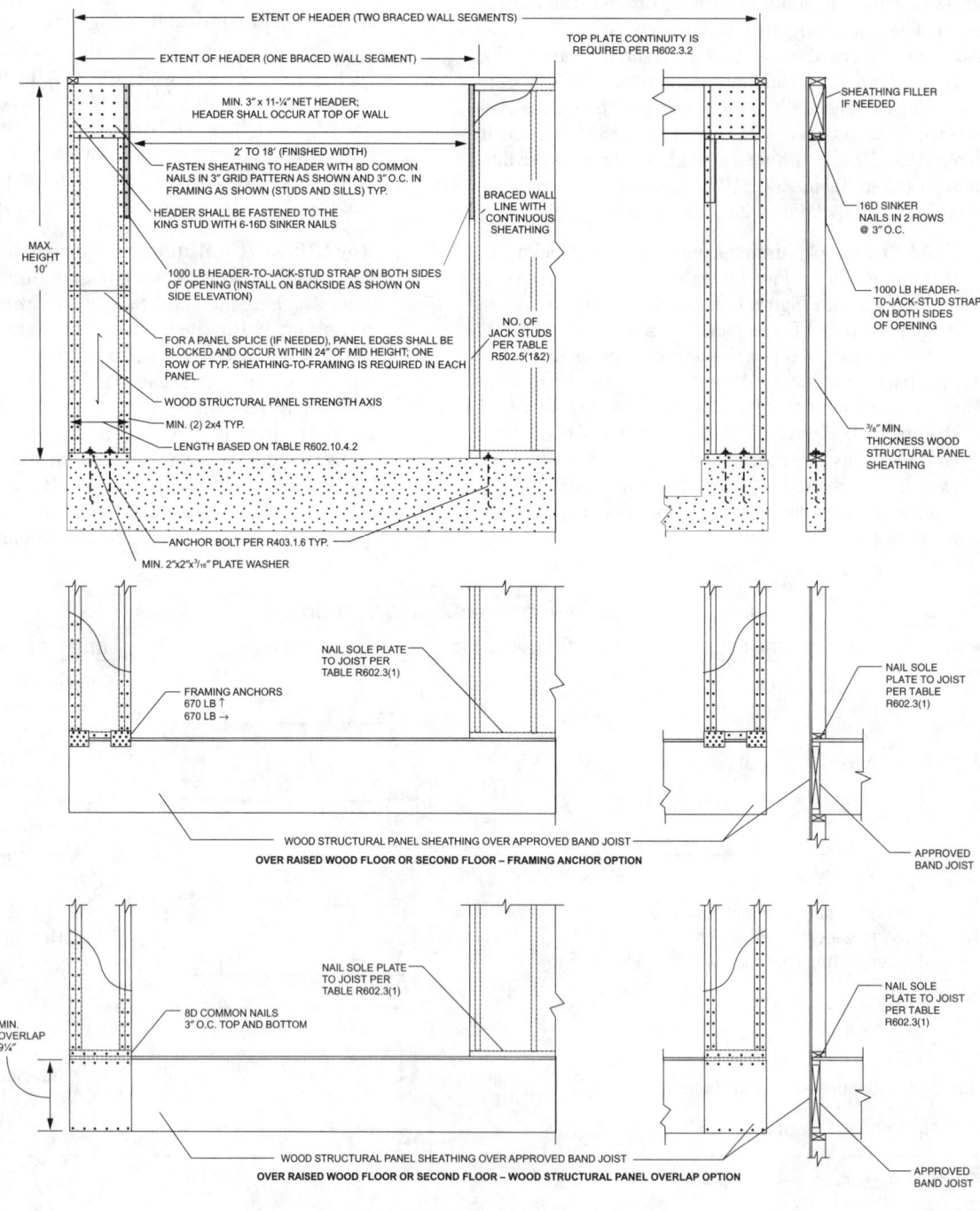

For SI: 1 inch = 25.4 mm, 1 foot = 304.8 mm, 1 pound force = 4.448 N.

FIGURE R602.10.4.1.1
METHOD CS-PF: CONTINUOUS PORTAL FRAME PANEL CONSTRUCTION

TABLE R602.10.4.1.1
TENSION STRAP CAPACITY REQUIRED FOR RESISTING WIND PRESSURES
PERPENDICULAR TO 6:1 ASPECT RATIO WALLS[a,b]

MINIMUM WALL STUD FRAMING NOMINAL SIZE AND GRADE	MAXIMUM PONY WALL HEIGHT (feet)	MAXIMUM TOTAL WALL HEIGHT (feet)	MAXIMUM OPENING WIDTH (feet)	BASIC WIND SPEED (mph)					
				85	90	100	85	90	100
				Exposure B			Exposure C		
				Tension strap capacity required (lbf)[a,b]					
2 × 4 No. 2 Grade	0	10	18	1000	1000	1000	1000	1000	1000
	1	10	9	1000	1000	1000	1000	1000	1275
			16	1000	1000	1750	1800	2325	3500
			18	1000	1200	2100	2175	2725	DR
	2	10	9	1000	1000	1025	1075	1550	2500
			16	1525	2025	3125	3200	3900	DR
			18	1875	2400	3575	3700	DR	DR
	2	12	9	1000	1200	2075	2125	2750	4000
			16	2600	3200	DR	DR	DR	DR
			18	3175	3850	DR	DR	DR	DR
	4	12	9	1775	2350	500	3550	DR	DR
			16	4175	DR	DR	DR	DR	DR
2 × 6 Stud Grade	2	12	9	1000	1000	1325	1375	1750	2550
			16	1650	2050	2925	3000	3550	DR
			18	2025	2450	3425	3500	4100	DR
	4	12	9	1125	1500	2225	2275	2775	3800
			16	2650	3150	DR	DR	DR	DR
			18	3125	3675	DR	DR	DR	DR

For SI: 1 inch = 25.4 mm, 1 foot = 304.8 mm, 1 pound force = 4.448 N.

a. DR = design required.

b. Strap shall be installed in accordance with manufacturer's recommendations.

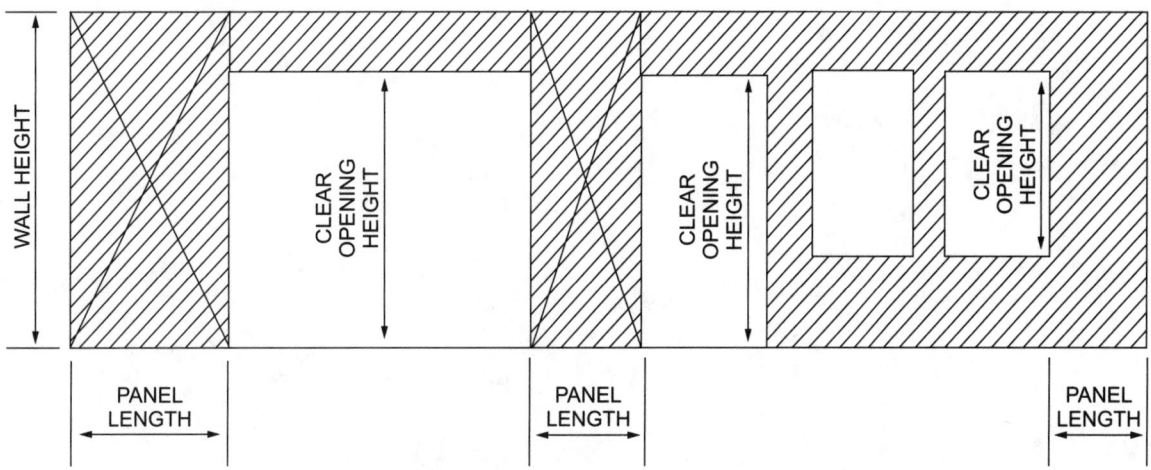

FIGURE R602.10.4.2
BRACED WALL PANELS WITH CONTINUOUS SHEATHING

TABLE R602.10.4.2
LENGTH REQUIREMENTS FOR BRACED WALL PANELS WITH CONTINUOUS SHEATHING[a] (inches)

METHOD	ADJACENT CLEAR OPENING HEIGHT (inches)	WALL HEIGHT (feet)				
		8	9	10	11	12
CS-WSP	64	24	27	30	33	36
	68	26	27	30	—	—
	72	28	27	30	—	—
	76	29	30	30	—	—
	80	31	33	30	—	—
	84	35	36	33	—	—
	88	39	39	36	—	—
	92	44	42	39	—	—
	96	48	45	42	—	—
	100	—	48	45	—	—
	104	—	51	48	—	—
	108	—	54	51	—	—
	112	—	—	54	44	—
	116	—	—	57	—	—
	120	—	—	60	—	—
	122	—	—	—	—	48
	132	—	—	—	66	—
	144	—	—	—	—	75
CS-G	≤ 120	24	27	30	—	—
CS-PF	≤ 120	16	18	20	—	—

For SI: 1 inch = 25.4 mm, 1 foot = 304.8 mm.
a. Interpolation shall be permitted.

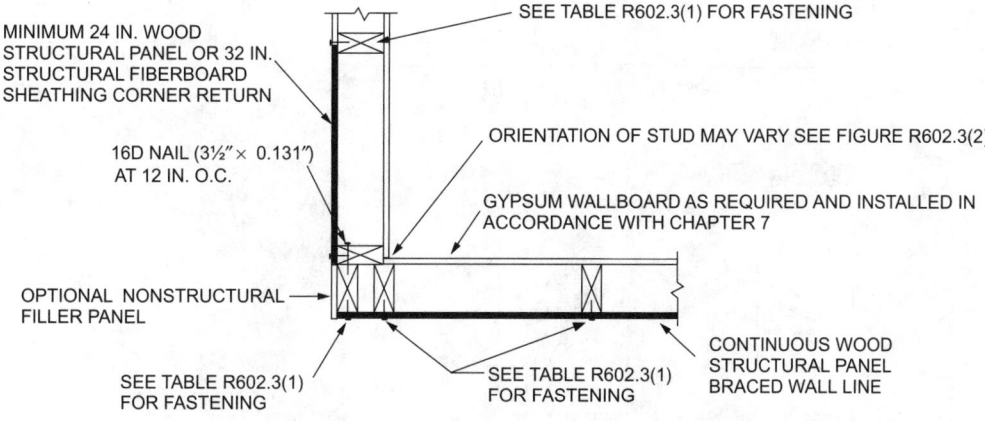

(a) OUTSIDE CORNER DETAIL

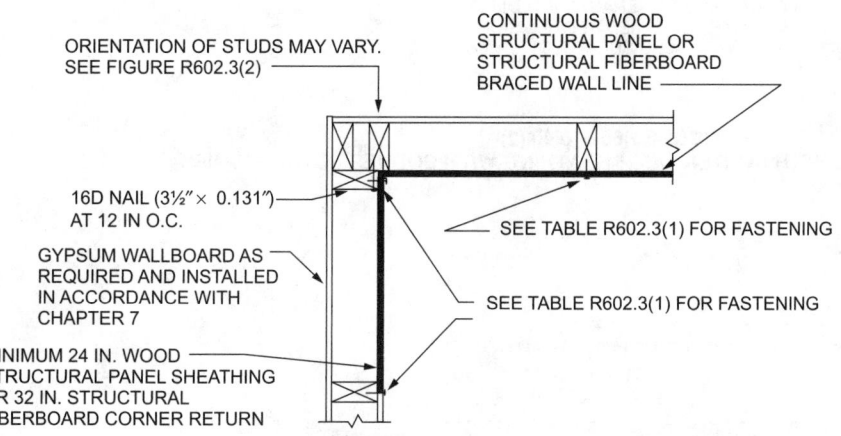

(b) INSIDE CORNER DETAIL

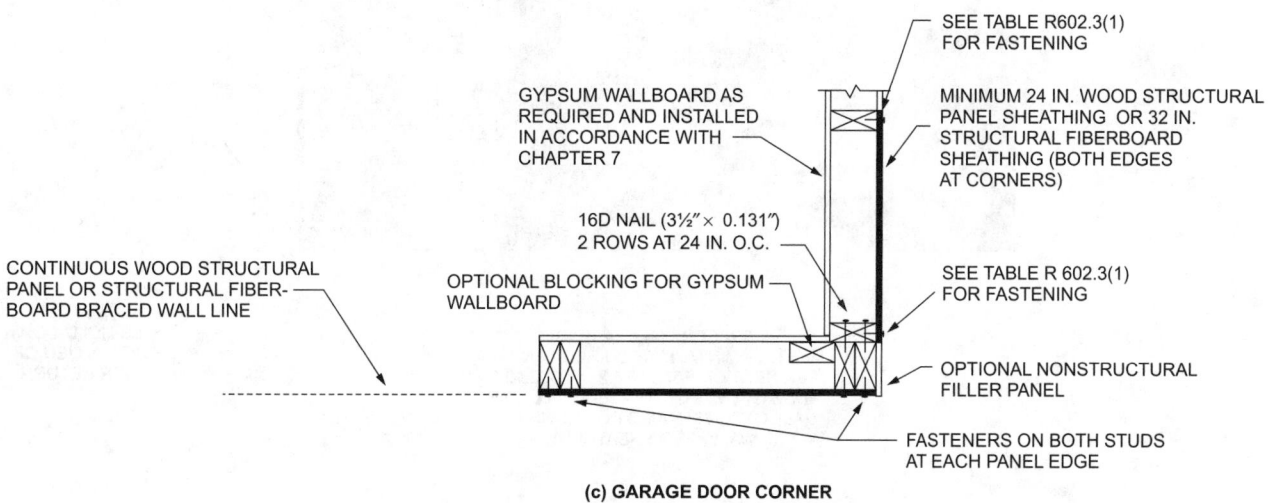

(c) GARAGE DOOR CORNER

For SI: 1 inch = 25.4 mm, 1 foot = 305 mm.

FIGURE R602.10.4.4(1)
TYPICAL EXTERIOR CORNER FRAMING FOR CONTINUOUS SHEATHING

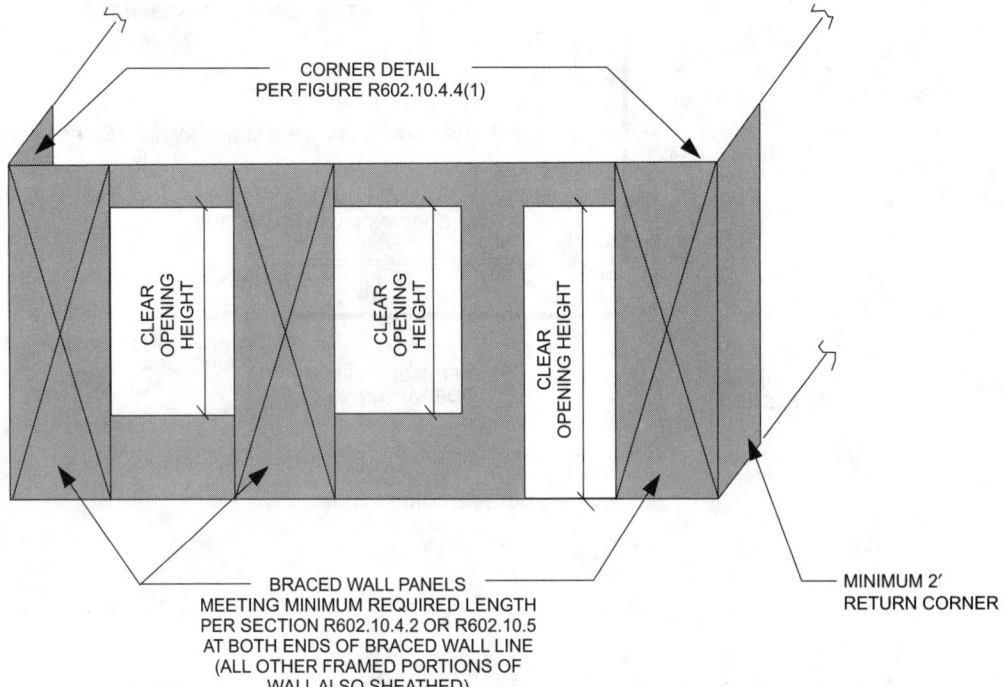

For SI: 1 foot = 304.8 mm.

FIGURE R602.10.4.4(2)
BRACED WALL LINE WITH CONTINUOUS SHEATHING WITH CORNER RETURN PANEL

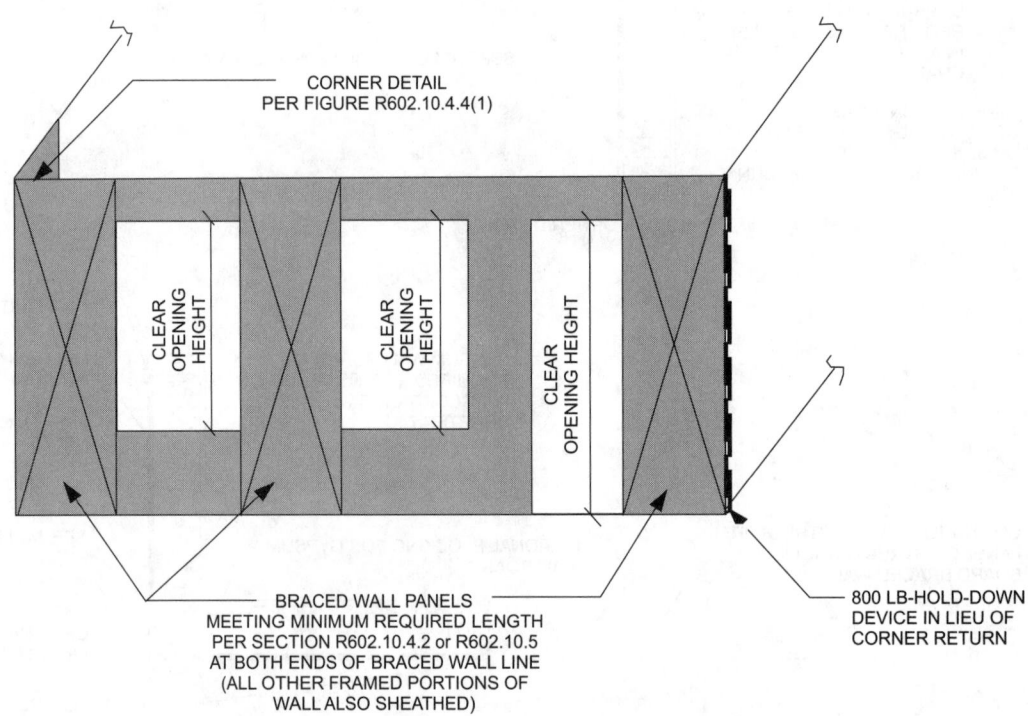

For SI: 1 inch = 25.4 mm, 1 pound = 4.448 N.

FIGURE R602.10.4.4(3)
BRACED WALL LINE WITH CONTINUOUS SHEATHING WITHOUT CORNER RETURN PANEL

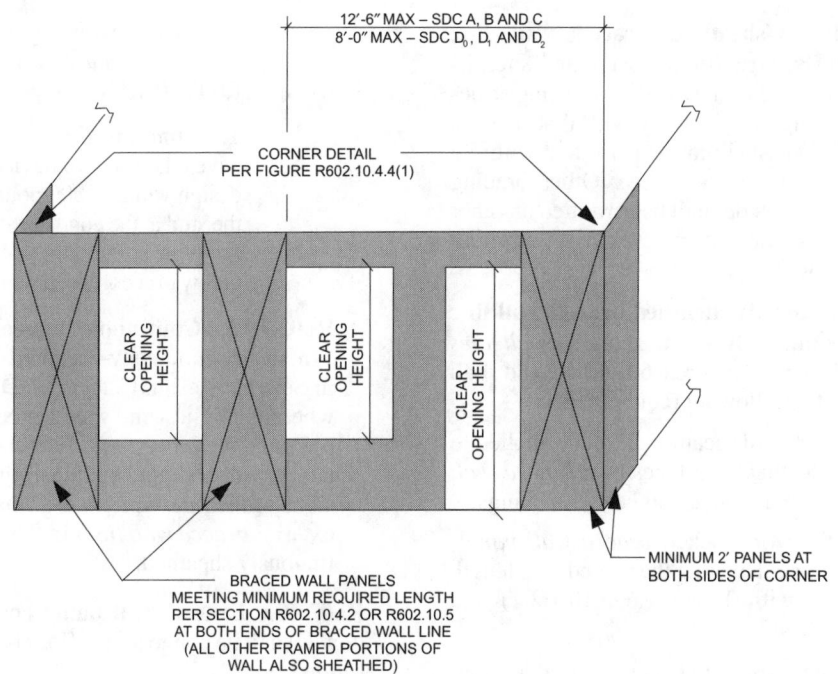

For SI: 1 inch = 25.4 mm.

FIGURE R602.10.4.4(4)
BRACED WALL LINE WITH CONTINUOUS SHEATHING FIRST BRACED WALL PANEL
AWAY FROM END OF WALL LINE WITHOUT TIE DOWN

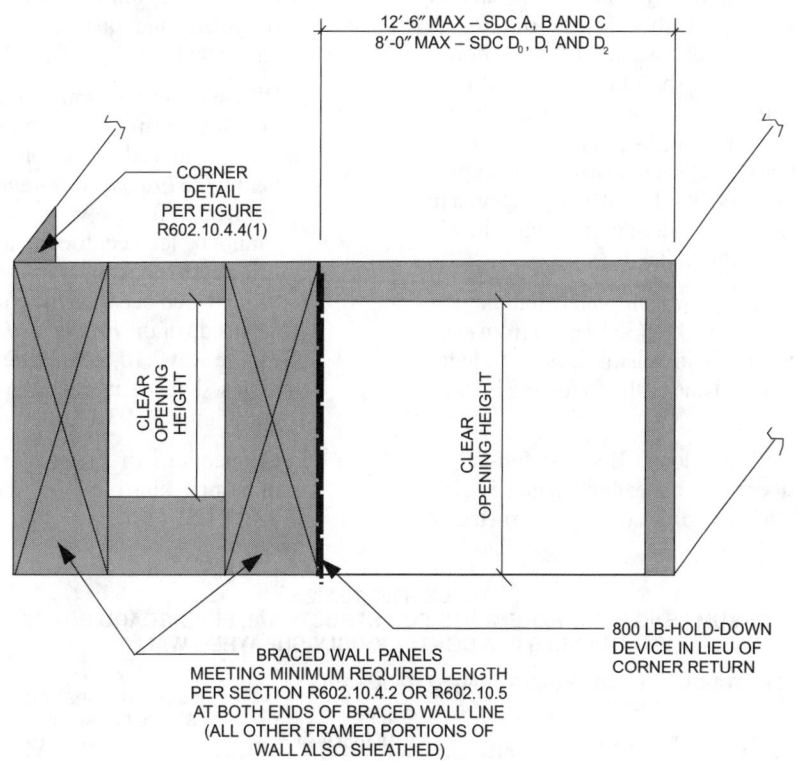

For SI: 1 foot = 305 mm. 1 pound = 4.448 N.

FIGURE R602.10.4.4(5)
BRACED WALL LINE WITH CONTINUOUS SHEATHING—FIRST BRACED WALL
PANEL AWAY FROM END OF WALL LINE WITH HOLD-DOWN

R602.10.5 Continuously-sheathed braced wall line using Method CS-SFB (structural fiberboard sheathing). Continuously sheathed *braced wall lines* using structural fiberboard sheathing shall comply with this section. Different bracing methods shall not be permitted within a continuously sheathed *braced wall line*. Other bracing methods prescribed by this code shall be permitted on other *braced wall lines* on the same *story* level or on different *story* levels of the building.

R602.10.5.1 Continuously sheathed braced wall line requirements. Continuously-sheathed *braced wall lines* shall be in accordance with Figure R602.10.4.2 and shall comply with all of the following requirements:

1. Structural fiberboard sheathing shall be applied to all exterior sheathable surfaces of a *braced wall line* including areas above and below openings.

2. Only full-height or blocked *braced wall panels* shall be used for calculating the braced wall length in accordance with Tables R602.10.1.2(1) and R602.10.1.2(2).

R602.10.5.2 Braced wall panel length. In a continuously-sheathed structural fiberboard *braced wall line*, the minimum *braced wall panel* length shall be in accordance with Table R602.10.5.2.

R602.10.5.3 Braced wall panel location and corner construction. A *braced wall panel* shall be located at each end of a continuously-sheathed *braced wall line*. A minimum 32-inch (813 mm) structural fiberboard sheathing panel corner return shall be provided at both ends of a continuously-sheathed *braced wall line* in accordance with Figure R602.10.4.4(1) In lieu of the corner return, a hold-down device with a minimum uplift design value of 800 pounds (3560 N) shall be fastened to the corner stud and to the foundation or framing below in accordance with Figure R602.10.4.4(3).

Exception: The first *braced wall panel* shall be permitted to begin 12 feet 6 inches (3810 mm) from each end of the *braced wall line* in Seismic Design Categories A, B and C provided one of the following is satisfied:

1. A minimum 32-inch-long (813 mm), full-height structural fiberboard sheathing panel is provided at both sides of a corner constructed in

accordance with Figure R602.10.4.4(1) at the *braced wall line* ends in accordance with Figure R602.10.4.4(4), or

2. The *braced wall panel* closest to the corner shall have a hold-down device with a minimum uplift design value of 800 pounds (3560 N) fastened to the stud at the edge of the *braced wall panel* closest to the corner and to the foundation or framing below in accordance with Figure R602.10.4.4(5).

R602.10.5.4 Continuously sheathed braced wall lines. Where a continuously-sheathed *braced wall line* is used in Seismic Design Categories D_0, D_1 and D_2 or regions where the basic wind speed exceeds 100 miles per hour (45 m/s), the *braced wall line* shall be designed in accordance with accepted engineering practice and the provisions of the *International Building Code*. Also, all other exterior *braced wall lines* in the same *story* shall be continuously sheathed.

R602.10.6 Braced wall panel connections. *Braced wall panels* shall be connected to floor framing or foundations as follows:

1. Where joists are perpendicular to a *braced wall panel* above or below, a rim joist, band joist or blocking shall be provided along the entire length of the *braced wall panel* in accordance with Figure R602.10.6(1). Fastening of top and bottom wall plates to framing, rim joist, band joist and/or blocking shall be in accordance with Table R602.3(1).

2. Where joists are parallel to a *braced wall panel* above or below, a rim joist, end joist or other parallel framing member shall be provided directly above and below the *braced wall panel* in accordance with Figure R602.10.6(2). Where a parallel framing member cannot be located directly above and below the panel, full-depth blocking at 16 inch (406 mm) spacing shall be provided between the parallel framing members to each side of the *braced wall panel* in accordance with Figure R602.10.6(2). Fastening of blocking and wall plates shall be in accordance with Table R602.3(1) and Figure R602.10.6(2).

3. Connections of *braced wall panels* to concrete or masonry shall be in accordance with Section R403.1.6.

TABLE R602.10.5.2
MINIMUM LENGTH REQUIREMENTS FOR STRUCTURAL FIBERBOARD BRACED WALL PANELS IN A CONTINUOUSLY-SHEATHED WALL[a]

MINIMUM LENGTH OF STRUCTURAL FIBERBOARD BRACED WALL PANEL (inches)			MINIMUM OPENING CLEAR HEIGHT NEXT TO THE STRUCTURAL FIBERBOARD BRACED WALL PANEL (% of wall height)
8-foot wall	9-foot wall	10-foot wall	
48	54	60	100
32	36	40	85
24	27	30	67

For SI: 1 inch = 25.4 mm, 1 foot = 304.8 mm.
a. Interpolation is permitted.

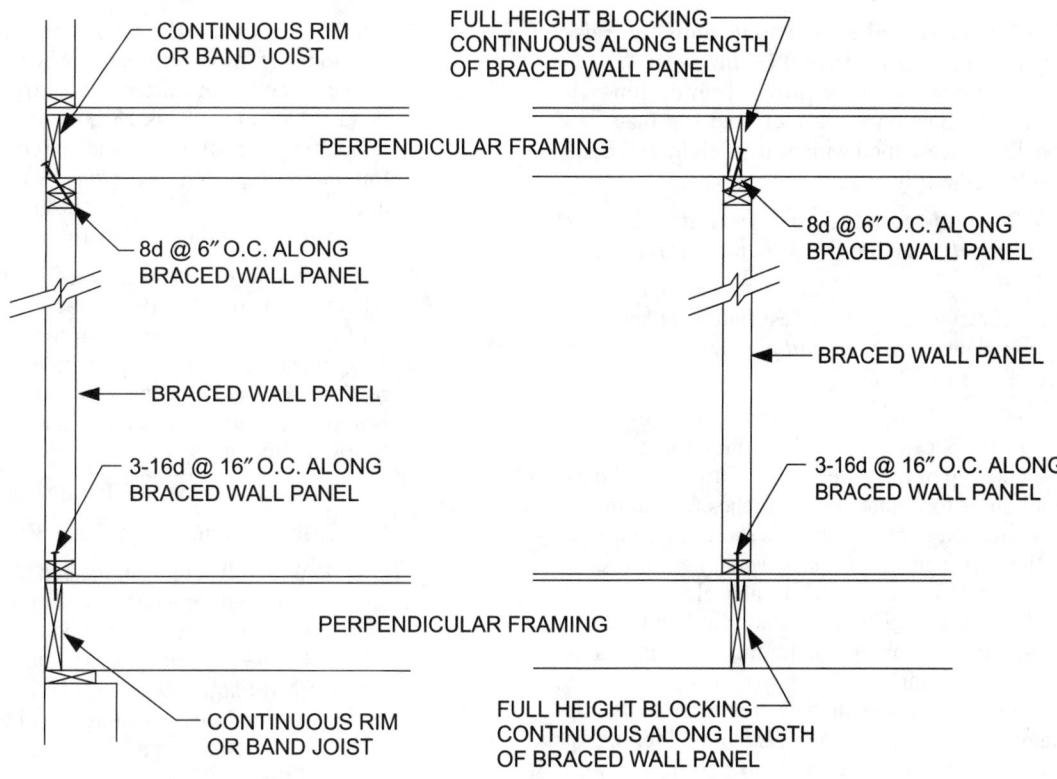

For SI: 1 inch = 25.4 mm.

FIGURE R602.10.6(1)
BRACED WALL PANEL CONNECTION WHEN PERPENDICULAR TO FLOOR/CEILING FRAMING

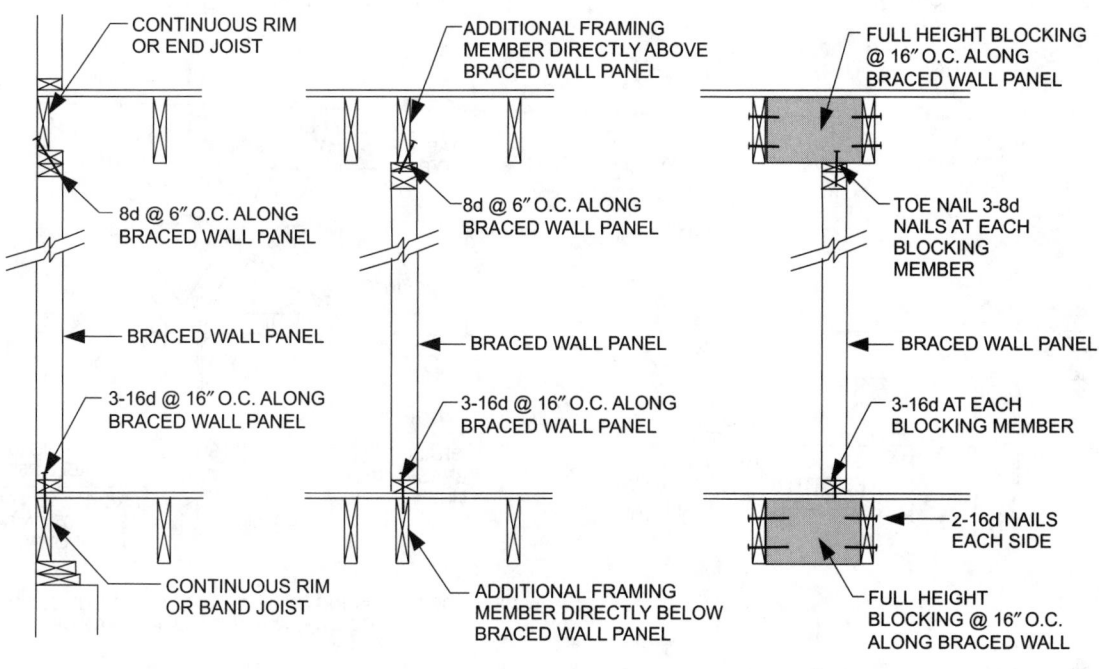

For SI: 1 inch = 25.4 mm.

FIGURE R602.10.6(2)
BRACED WALL PANEL CONNECTION WHEN PARALLEL TO FLOOR/CEILING FRAMING

R602.10.6.1 Braced wall panel connections for Seismic Design Categories D₀, D₁ and D₂. *Braced wall panels* shall be fastened to required foundations in accordance with Section R602.11.1, and top plate lap splices shall be face-nailed with at least eight 16d nails on each side of the splice.

R602.10.6.2 Connections to roof framing. Exterior *braced wall panels* shall be connected to roof framing as follows.

1. Parallel rafters or roof trusses shall be attached to the top plates of *braced wall panels* in accordance with Table R602.3(1).

2. For SDC A, B and C and wind speeds less than 100 miles per hour (45 m/s), where the distance from the top of the rafters or roof trusses and perpendicular top plates is 9¹/₄ inches (235 mm) or less, the rafters or roof trusses shall be connected to the top plates of *braced wall lines* in accordance with Table R602.3(1) and blocking need not be installed. Where the distance from the top of the rafters and perpendicular top plates is between 9¹/₄ inches (235 mm) and 15¹/₄ inches (387 mm) the rafters shall be connected to the top plates of *braced wall panels* with blocking in accordance with Figure R602.10.6.2(1) and attached in accordance with Table R602.3(1). Where the distance from the top of the roof trusses and perpendicular top plates is between 9¹/₄ inches (235 mm) and 15¹/₄ inches (387 mm) the roof trusses shall be connected to the top plates of *braced wall panels* with blocking in accordance with Table R602.3(1).

3. For SDC D₀, D₁ and D₂ or wind speeds of 100 miles per hour (45 m/s) or greater, where the distance between the top of rafters or roof trusses and perpendicular top plates is 15¹/₄ inches (387 mm) or less, rafters or roof trusses shall be connected to the top plates of *braced wall panels* with blocking in accordance with Figure R602.10.6.2(1) and attached in accordance with Table R602.3(1).

4. For all seismic design categories and wind speeds, where the distance between the top of rafters or roof trusses and perpendicular top plates exceeds 15¹/₄ inches (387 mm), perpendicular rafters or roof trusses shall be connected to the top plates of *braced wall panels* in accordance with one of the following methods:

   4.1. In accordance with Figure R602.10.6.2(2),

   4.2. In accordance with Figure R602.10.6.2(3),

   4.3. With full height engineered blocking panels designed for values listed in American Forest and Paper Association (AF&PA) Wood Frame Construction Manual for One- and Two-Family *Dwellings* (WFCM). Both the roof and floor sheathing shall be attached to the blocking panels in accordance with Table R602.3(1).

   4.4. Designed in accordance with accepted engineering methods.

Lateral support for the rafters and ceiling joists shall be provided in accordance with Section R802.8. Lateral support for trusses shall be provided in accordance with Section R802.10.3. Ventilation shall be provided in accordance with Section R806.1.

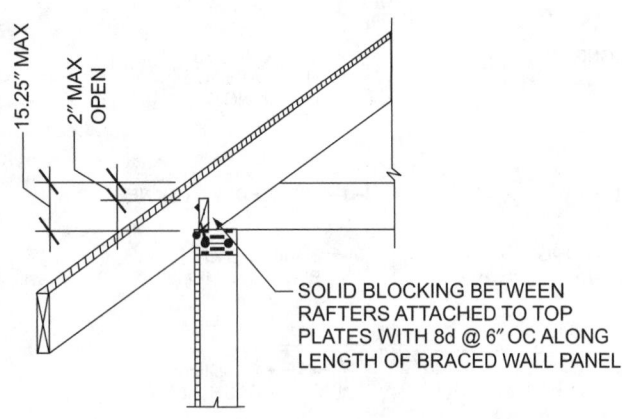

15.25" MAX

2" MAX OPEN

SOLID BLOCKING BETWEEN RAFTERS ATTACHED TO TOP PLATES WITH 8d @ 6" OC ALONG LENGTH OF BRACED WALL PANEL

For SI: 1 inch = 25.4 mm.

FIGURE R602.10.6.2(1)
BRACED WALL PANEL CONNECTION
TO PERPENDICULAR RAFTERS

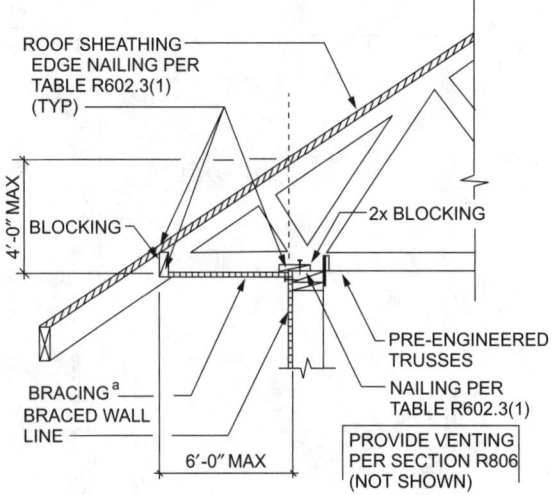

ROOF SHEATHING EDGE NAILING PER TABLE R602.3(1) (TYP)

4'-0" MAX

BLOCKING

2x BLOCKING

PRE-ENGINEERED TRUSSES

BRACING ᵃ BRACED WALL LINE

NAILING PER TABLE R602.3(1)

PROVIDE VENTING PER SECTION R806 (NOT SHOWN)

6'-0" MAX

a. METHODS OF BRACING SHALL BE AS DESCRIBED IN SECTION R602.10.2 METHOD DWB, WSP, SFB, GB, PBS, PCP OR HPS

For SI: 1 inch = 25.4 mm.

FIGURE R602.10.6.2(2)
BRACED WALL PANEL CONNECTION OPTION TO
PERPENDICULAR RAFTERS OR ROOF TRUSSES

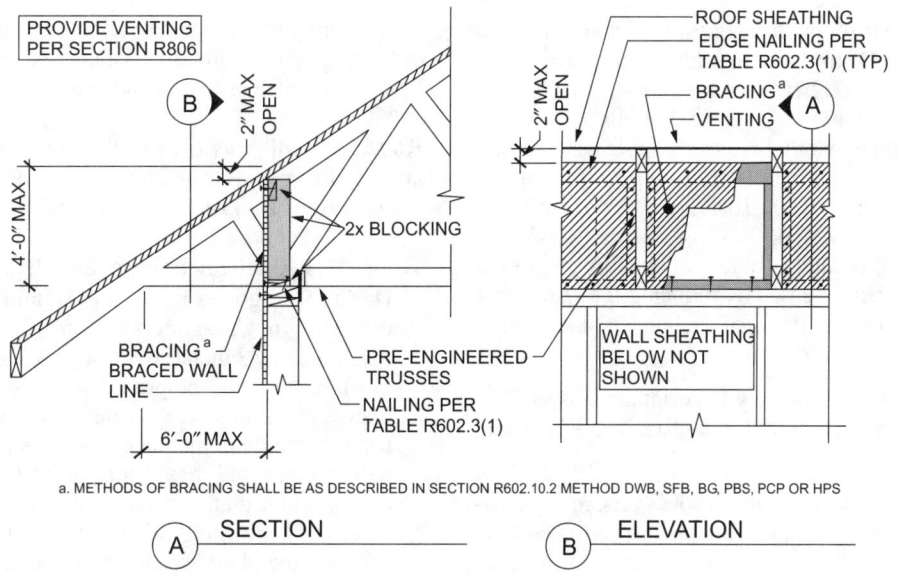

FIGURE R602.10.6.2(3)
BRACED WALL PANEL CONNECTION OPTION TO PERPENDICULAR RAFTERS OR ROOF TRUSSES

R602.10.7 Braced wall panel support. *Braced wall panel* support shall be provided as follows:

1. Cantilevered floor joists, supporting *braced wall lines*, shall comply with Section R502.3.3. Solid blocking shall be provided at the nearest bearing wall location. In Seismic Design Categories A, B and C, where the cantilever is not more than 24 inches (610 mm), a full height rim joist instead of solid blocking shall be provided.

2. Elevated post or pier foundations supporting *braced wall panels* shall be designed in accordance with accepted engineering practice.

3. Masonry stem walls with a length of 48 inches (1220 mm) or less supporting *braced wall panels* shall be reinforced in accordance with Figure R602.10.7. Masonry stem walls with a length greater than 48 inches (1220 mm) supporting *braced wall panels* shall be constructed in accordance with Section R403.1 *Braced wall panels* constructed in accordance with Sections R602.10.3.2 and R602.10.3.3 shall not be attached to masonry stem walls.

R602.10.7.1 Braced wall panel support for Seismic Design Category D$_2$. In one-story buildings located in Seismic Design Category D$_2$, *braced wall panels* shall be supported on continuous foundations at intervals not exceeding 50 feet (15 240 mm). In two-story buildings located in Seismic Design Category D$_2$, all *braced wall panels* shall be supported on continuous foundations.

Exception: Two-story buildings shall be permitted to have interior *braced wall panels* supported on continuous foundations at intervals not exceeding 50 feet (15 240 mm) provided that:

1. The height of cripple walls does not exceed 4 feet (1219 mm).

2. First-floor *braced wall panels* are supported on doubled floor joists, continuous blocking or floor beams.

3. The distance between bracing lines does not exceed twice the building width measured parallel to the *braced wall line*.

R602.10.8 Panel joints. All vertical joints of panel sheathing shall occur over, and be fastened to common studs. Horizontal joints in *braced wall panels* shall occur over, and be fastened to common blocking of a minimum 1^1/$_2$ inch (38 mm) thickness.

Exceptions:

1. Blocking at horizontal joints shall not be required in wall segments that are not counted as *braced wall panels*.

2. Where the bracing length provided is at least twice the minimum length required by Tables R602.10.1.2(1) and R602.10.1.2(2) blocking at horizontal joints shall not be required in *braced wall panels* constructed using Methods WSP, SFB, GB, PBS or HPS.

3. When Method GB panels are installed horizontally, blocking of horizontal joints is not required.

R602.10.9 Cripple wall bracing. In Seismic Design Categories other than D$_2$, cripple walls shall be braced with a length and type of bracing as required for the wall above in accordance with Tables R602.10.1.2(1) and R602.10.1.2(2) with the following modifications for cripple wall bracing:

1. The length of bracing as determined from Tables R602.10.1.2(1) and R602.10.1.2(2) shall be multiplied by a factor of 1.15, and

2. The wall panel spacing shall be decreased to 18 feet (5486 mm) instead of 25 feet (7620 mm).

R602.10.9.1 Cripple wall bracing in Seismic Design Categories D₀, D₁ and D₂. In addition to the requirements of Section R602.10.9, where *braced wall lines* at interior walls occur without a continuous foundation below, the length of parallel exterior cripple wall bracing shall be $1^1/_2$ times the length required by Tables R602.10.1.2(1) and R602.10.1.2(2). Where cripple walls braced using Method WSP of Section R602.10.2 cannot provide this additional length, the capacity of the sheathing shall be increased by reducing the spacing of fasteners along the perimeter of each piece of sheathing to 4 inches (102 mm) on center.

In Seismic Design Category D₂, cripple walls shall be braced in accordance with Tables R602.10.1.2(1) and R602.10.1.2(2).

R602.10.9.2 Redesignation of cripple walls. In any Seismic Design Category, cripple walls shall be permitted to be redesignated as the first *story* walls for purposes of deter-

mining wall bracing requirements. If the cripple walls are redesignated, the stories above the redesignated *story* shall be counted as the second and third stories, respectively.

R602.11 Wall anchorage. *Braced wall line* sills shall be anchored to concrete or masonry foundations in accordance with Sections R403.1.6 and R602.11.1.

602.11.1 Wall anchorage for all buildings in Seismic Design Categories D₀, D₁ and D₂ and townhouses in Seismic Design Category C. Plate washers, a minimum of 0.229 inch by 3 inches by 3 inches (5.8 mm by 76 mm by 76 mm) in size, shall be provided between the foundation sill plate and the nut except where *approved* anchor straps are used. The hole in the plate washer is permitted to be diagonally slotted with a width of up to $^3/_{16}$ inch (5 mm) larger than the bolt diameter and a slot length not to exceed $1^3/_4$ inches (44 mm), provided a standard cut washer is placed between the plate washer and the nut.

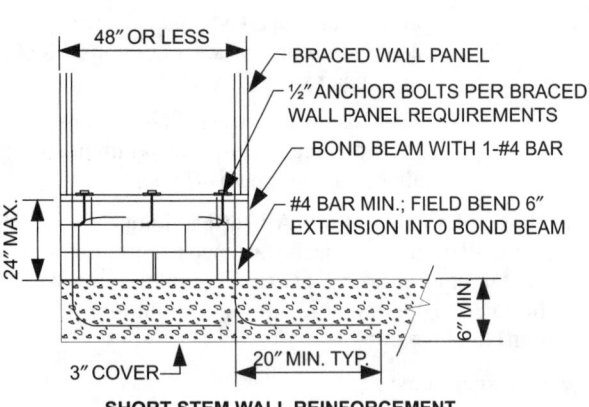

SHORT STEM WALL REINFORCEMENT

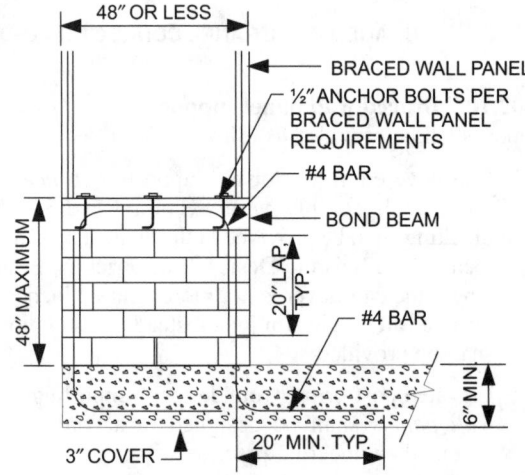

TALL STEM WALL REINFORCEMENT

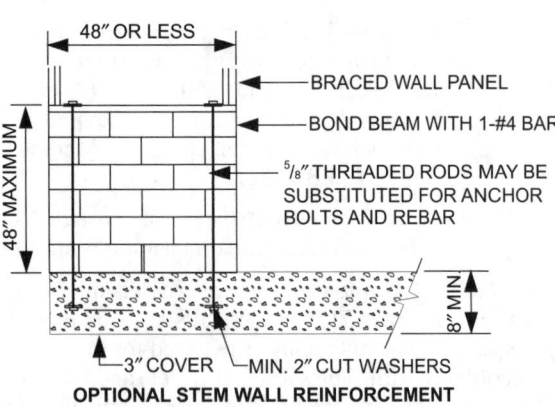

OPTIONAL STEM WALL REINFORCEMENT

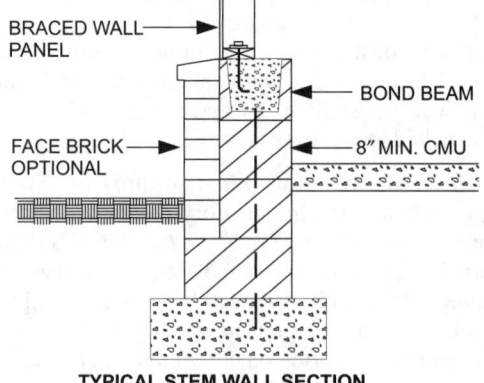

TYPICAL STEM WALL SECTION

NOTE: GROUT BOND BEAMS AND ALL CELLS WHICH CONTAIN REBAR, THREADED RODS AND ANCHOR BOLTS.

For SI: 1 inch = 25.4 mm.

FIGURE R602.10.7
MASONRY STEM WALLS SUPPORTING BRACED WALL PANELS

R602.11.2 Stepped foundations in Seismic Design Categories D₀, D₁ and D₂. In all buildings located in Seismic Design Categories D_0, D_1 or D_2, where the height of a required *braced wall line* that extends from foundation to floor above varies more than 4 feet (1219 mm), the *braced wall line* shall be constructed in accordance with the following:

1. Where the lowest floor framing rests directly on a sill bolted to a foundation not less than 8 feet (2440 mm) in length along a line of bracing, the line shall be considered as braced. The double plate of the cripple stud wall beyond the segment of footing that extends to the lowest framed floor shall be spliced by extending the upper top plate a minimum of 4 feet (1219 mm) along the foundation. Anchor bolts shall be located a maximum of 1 foot and 3 feet (305 and 914 mm) from the step in the foundation. See Figure R602.11.2.

2. Where cripple walls occur between the top of the foundation and the lowest floor framing, the bracing requirements of Sections R602.10.9 and R602.10.9.1 shall apply.

3. Where only the bottom of the foundation is stepped and the lowest floor framing rests directly on a sill bolted to the foundations, the requirements of Sections R403.1.6 and R602.11.1 shall apply.

R602.12 Wall bracing and stone and masonry veneer. Where stone and masonry veneer is installed in accordance with Section R703.7, wall bracing shall comply with this section.

For all buildings in Seismic Design Categories A, B and C, wall bracing at exterior and interior *braced wall lines* shall be in accordance with Section R602.10 and the additional requirements of Table R602.12(1).

For detached one- or two-family *dwellings* in Seismic Design Categories D_0, D_1 and D_2, wall bracing and hold downs at exterior and interior *braced wall lines* shall be in accordance with Sections R602.10 and R602.11 and the additional requirements of Section R602.12.1 and Table R602.12(2). In Seismic Design Categories D_0, D_1 and D_2, cripple walls are not permitted, and required interior *braced wall lines* shall be supported on continuous foundations.

R602.12.1 Seismic Design Categories D₀, D₁ and D₂. Wall bracing where stone and masonry veneer exceeds the first *story height* in Seismic Design Categories D_0, D_1 and D_2 shall conform to the requirements of Sections R602.10 and R602.11 and the following requirements.

R602.12.1.1 Length of bracing. The length of bracing along each *braced wall line* shall be in accordance with Table R602.12(2).

R602.12.1.2 Braced wall panel location. *Braced wall panels* shall begin no more than 8 feet (2440 mm) from each end of a *braced wall line* and shall be spaced a maximum of 25 feet (7620 mm) on center.

R602.12.1.3 Braced wall panel construction. *Braced wall panels* shall be constructed of sheathing with a thickness of not less than $^7/_{16}$ inch (11 mm) nailed with 8d common nails spaced 4 inches (102 mm) on center at all panel edges and 12 inches (305 mm) on center at intermediate supports. The end of each *braced wall panel* shall have a hold down device in accordance with Table R602.12(2) installed at each end. Size, height and spacing of wood studs shall be in accordance with Table R602.3(5).

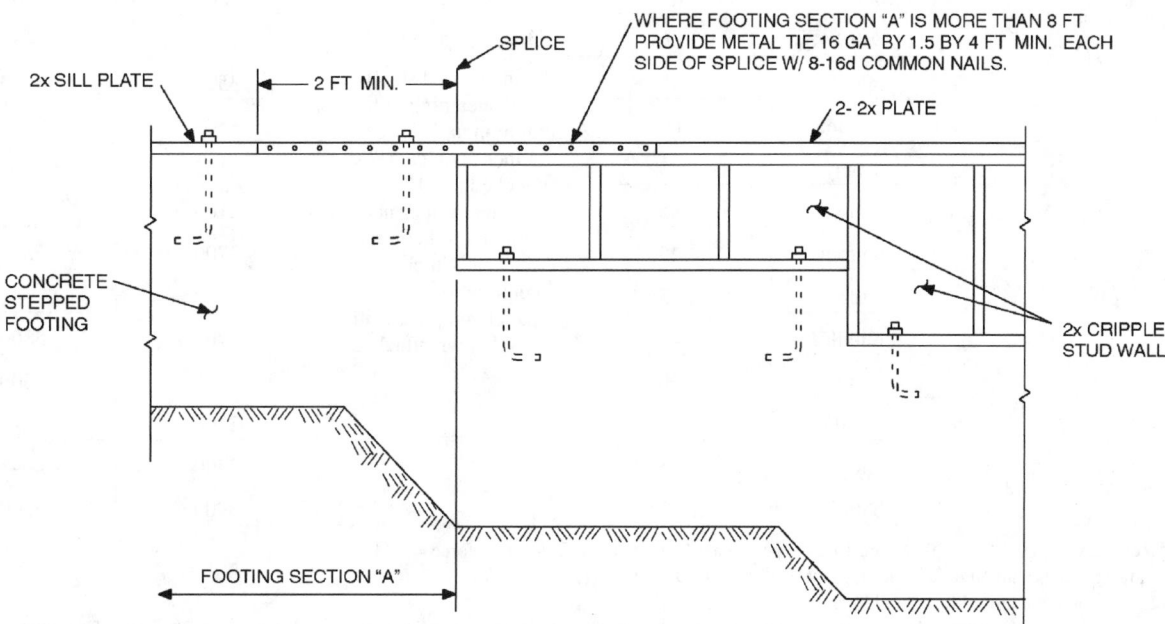

WHERE FOOTING SECTION "A" IS MORE THAN 8 FT PROVIDE METAL TIE 16 GA BY 1.5 BY 4 FT MIN. EACH SIDE OF SPLICE W/ 8-16d COMMON NAILS.

For SI: 1 inch = 25.4 mm, 1 foot = 304.8 mm.

Note: Where footing Section "A" is less than 8 feet long in a 25-foot-long wall, install bracing at cripple stud wall.

FIGURE R602.11.2
STEPPED FOUNDATION CONSTRUCTION

TABLE R602.12(1)
STONE OR MASONRY VENEER WALL BRACING REQUIREMENTS, WOOD
OR STEEL FRAMING, SEISMIC DESIGN CATEGORIES A, B and C

SEISMIC DESIGN CATEGORY	NUMBER OF WOOD FRAMED STORIES	WOOD FRAMED STORY	MINIMUM SHEATHING AMOUNT (length of braced wall line length)[a]
A or B	1, 2 or 3	all	Table R602.10.1.2(2)
C	1	1 only	Table R602.10.1.2(2)
	2	top	Table R602.10.1.2(2)
		bottom	1.5 times length required by Table R602.10.1.2(2)
	3	top	Table R602.10.1.2(2)
		middle	1.5 times length required by Table R602.10.1.2(2)
		bottom	1.5 times length required by Table R602.10.1.2(2)

a. Applies to exterior and interior braced wall lines.

TABLE R602.12(2)
STONE OR MASONRY VENEER WALL BRACING REQUIREMENTS,
ONE- AND TWO-FAMILY DETACHED DWELLINGS, SEISMIC DESIGN CATEGORIES D_0, D_1 and D_2

SEISMIC DESIGN CATEGORY	NUMBER OF STORIES[a]	STORY	MINIMUM SHEATHING AMOUNT (length of braced wall line length in feet)[b]	MINIMUM SHEATHING THICKNESS AND FASTENING	SINGLE STORY HOLD DOWN FORCE (lb)[c]	CUMULATIVE HOLD DOWN FORCE (lb)[d]
D_0	1	1 only	35		N/A	—
	2	top	35		1900	—
		bottom	45		3200	5100
	3	top	40		1900	—
		middle	45	$^7/_{16}$-inch wood structural panel sheathing with 8d common nails spaced at 4 inches on center at panel edges, 12 inches on center at intermediate supports; 8d common nails at 4 inches on center at braced wall panel end posts with hold down attached	3500	5400
		bottom	60		3500	8900
D_1	1	1 only	45		2100	—
	2	top	45		2100	—
		bottom	45		3700	5800
	3	top	45		2100	—
		middle	45		3700	5800
		bottom	60		3700	9500
D_2	1	1 only	55		2300	—
	2	top	55		2300	—
		bottom	55		3900	6200

For SI: 1 inch = 25.4 mm, 1 foot = 304.8 mm, 1 pound per square foot = 0.479 kPa, 1 pound-force = 4.448 N.

a. Cripple walls are not permitted in Seismic Design Categories D_0, D_1 and D_2.

b. Applies to exterior and interior braced wall lines.

c. Hold down force is minimum allowable stress design load for connector providing uplift tie from wall framing at end of braced wall panel at the noted story to wall framing at end of braced wall panel at the story below, or to foundation or foundation wall. Use single story hold down force where edges of braced wall panels do not align; a continuous load path to the foundation shall be maintained. [See Figure R602.12].

d. Where hold down connectors from stories above align with stories below, use cumulative hold down force to size middle and bottom story hold down connectors. (See Figure R602.12).

2009 INTERNATIONAL RESIDENTIAL CODE®

R602.12.1.4 Minimum length of braced panel. Each *braced wall panel* shall be at least 48 inches (1219 mm) in length, covering a minimum of 3 stud spaces where studs are spaced 16 inches (406 mm) on center and covering a minimum of 2 stud spaced where studs are spaced 24 inches on center.

R602.12.1.5 Alternate braced wall panel. Alternate *braced wall panels* described in Section R602.10.3.2 shall not replace the *braced wall panel* specification of this section.

R602.12.1.6 Continuously sheathed wall bracing. Continuously sheathed provisions of Section R602.10.4 shall not be used in conjunction with the wall bracing provisions of this section.

SECTION R603
STEEL WALL FRAMING

R603.1 General. Elements shall be straight and free of any defects that would significantly affect structural performance. Cold-formed steel wall framing members shall comply with the requirements of this section.

R603.1.1 Applicability limits. The provisions of this section shall control the construction of exterior cold-formed steel wall framing and interior load-bearing cold-formed steel wall framing for buildings not more than 60 feet (18 288 mm) long perpendicular to the joist or truss span, not more than 40 feet (12 192 mm) wide parallel to the joist or truss span, and less than or equal to three stories above *grade plane*. All exterior walls installed in accordance with the provisions of this section shall be considered as load-bearing walls. Cold-formed steel walls constructed in accordance with the provisions of this section shall be limited to sites subjected to a maximum design wind speed of 110 miles per hour (49 m/s) Exposure B or C and a maximum ground snow load of 70 pounds per square foot (3.35 kPa).

R603.1.2 In-line framing. Load-bearing cold-formed steel studs constructed in accordance with Section R603 shall be located in-line with joists, trusses and rafters in accordance with Figure R603.1.2 and the tolerances specified as follows:

1. The maximum tolerance shall be $^3/_4$ inch (19 mm) between the centerline of the horizontal framing member and the centerline of the vertical framing member.

2. Where the centerline of the horizontal framing member and bearing stiffener are located to one side of the centerline of the vertical framing member, the maximum tolerance shall be $^1/_8$ inch (3 mm) between the web of the horizontal framing member and the edge of the vertical framing member.

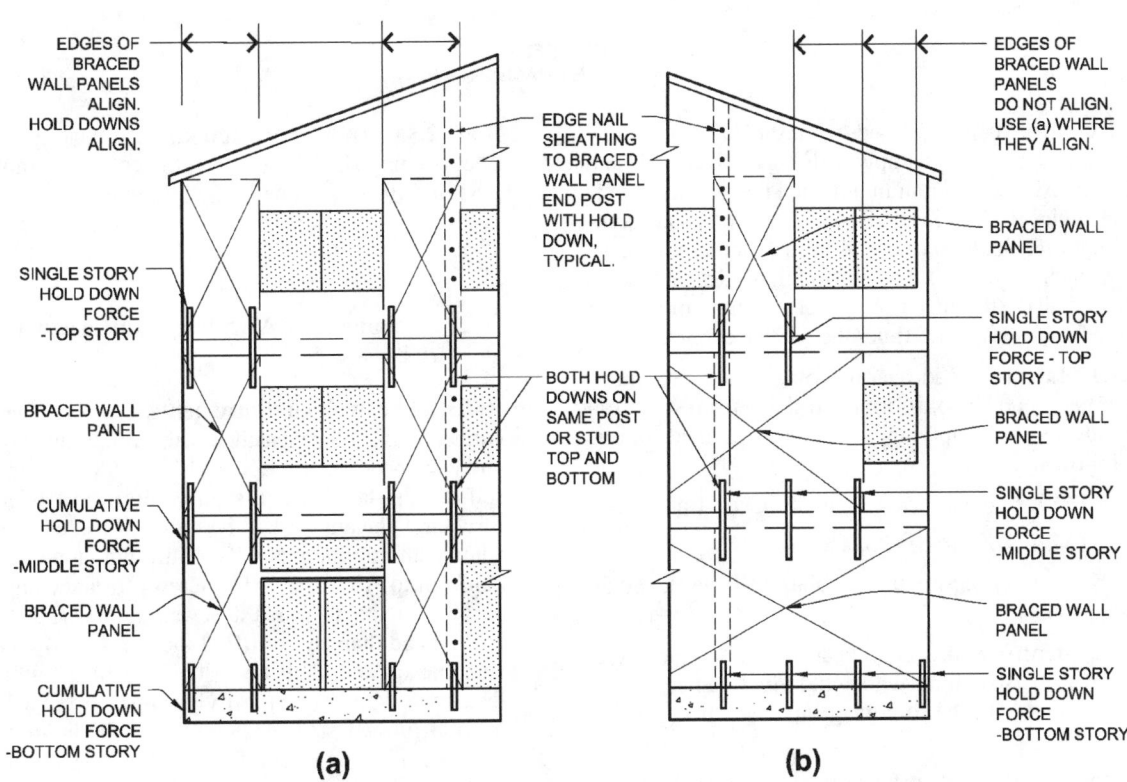

(a) Braced wall panels stacked (aligned story to story). Use cumulative hold down force.
(b) Braced wall panels not stacked. Use single story hold down force.

FIGURE R602.12
HOLD DOWNS AT EXTERIOR AND INTERIOR BRACED WALL PANELS

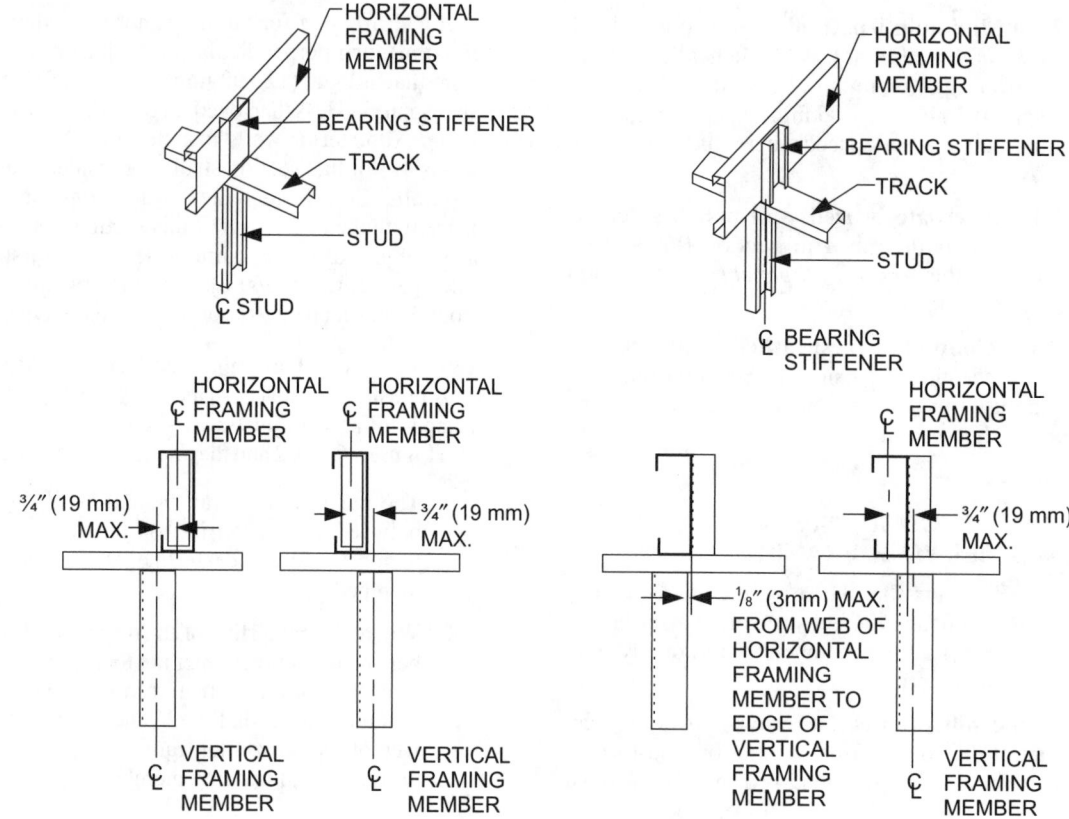

For SI: 1 inch = 25.4 mm,

FIGURE R603.1.2
IN-LINE FRAMING

R603.2 Structural framing. Load-bearing cold-formed steel wall framing members shall comply with Figure R603.2(1) and with the dimensional and minimum thickness requirements specified in Tables R603.2(1) and R603.2(2). Tracks shall comply with Figure R603.2(2) and shall have a minimum flange width of $1^1/_4$ inches (32 mm). The maximum inside bend radius for members shall be the greater of $^3/_{32}$ inch (2.4 mm) minus half the base steel thickness or 1.5 times the base steel thickness.

R603.2.1 Material. Load-bearing cold-formed steel framing members shall be cold-formed to shape from structural quality sheet steel complying with the requirements of one of the following:

1. ASTM A 653: Grades 33, and 50 (Class 1 and 3).

2. ASTM A 792: Grades 33, and 50A.

3. ASTM A 1003: Structural Grades 33 Type H, and 50 Type H.

R603.2.2 Identification. Load-bearing cold-formed steel framing members shall have a legible *label*, stencil, stamp or embossment with the following information as a minimum:

1. Manufacturer's identification.

2. Minimum base steel thickness in inches (mm).

3. Minimum coating designation.

4. Minimum yield strength, in kips per square inch (ksi) (MPa).

R603.2.3 Corrosion protection. Load-bearing cold-formed steel framing shall have a metallic coating complying with ASTM A 1003 and one of the following:

1. A minimum of G 60 in accordance with ASTM A 653.

2. A minimum of AZ 50 in accordance with ASTM A 792.

R603.2.4 Fastening requirements. Screws for steel-to-steel connections shall be installed with a minimum edge distance and center-to-center spacing of $^1/_2$ inch (12.7 mm), shall be self-drilling tapping and shall conform to ASTM C 1513. Structural sheathing shall be attached to cold-formed steel studs with minimum No. 8 self-drilling tapping screws that conform to ASTM C 1513. Screws for attaching structural sheathing to cold-formed steel wall framing shall have a minimum head diameter of 0.292 inch (7.4 mm) with countersunk heads and shall be installed with a minimum edge distance of $^3/_8$ inch (9.5 mm). Gypsum board shall be attached to cold-formed steel wall framing with minimum No. 6 screws conforming to ASTM C 954 or ASTM C 1513 with a bugle head style and shall be installed in accordance with Section R702. For all connections, screws shall extend through the steel a minimum of three exposed threads. All fasteners shall have rust inhibitive coating suitable for the installation in which they are being used, or be manufactured from material not susceptible to corrosion.

TABLE R603.2(1)
LOAD-BEARING COLD-FORMED STEEL STUD SIZES

MEMBER DESIGNATION[a]	WEB DEPTH (inches)	MINIMUM FLANGE WIDTH (inches)	MAXIMUM FLANGE WIDTH (inches)	MINIMUM LIP SIZE (inches)
350S162-t	3.5	1.625	2	0.5
550S162-t	5.5	1.625	2	0.5

For SI: 1 inch = 25.4 mm; 1 mil = 0.0254 mm.

a. The member designation is defined by the first number representing the member depth in hundredths of an inch "S" representing a stud or joist member, the second number representing the flange width in hundredths of an inch, and the letter "t" shall be a number representing the minimum base metal thickness in mils [See Table R603.2(2)].

TABLE R603.2(2)
MINIMUM THICKNESS OF COLD-FORMED STEEL MEMBERS

DESIGNATION THICKNESS (mils)	MINIMUM BASE STEEL THICKNESS (inches)
33	0.0329
43	0.0428
54	0.0538
68	0.0677
97	0.0966

For SI: 1 mil = 0.0254 mm, 1 inch = 25.4 mm.

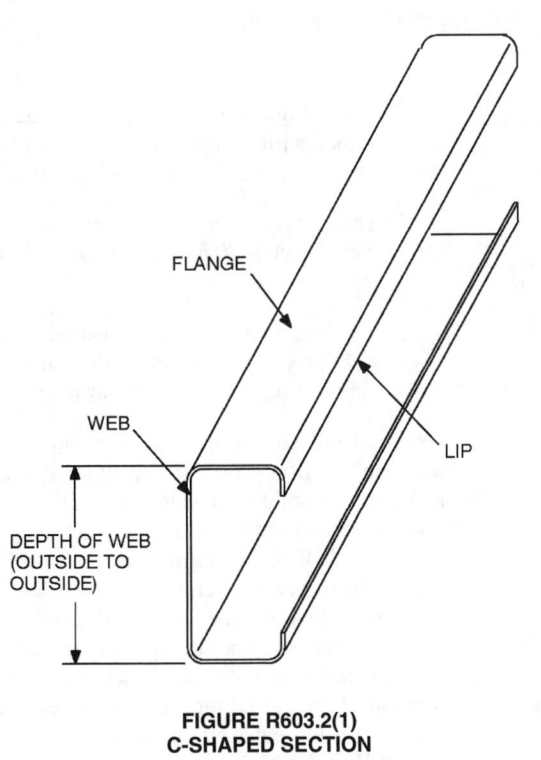

FIGURE R603.2(1)
C-SHAPED SECTION

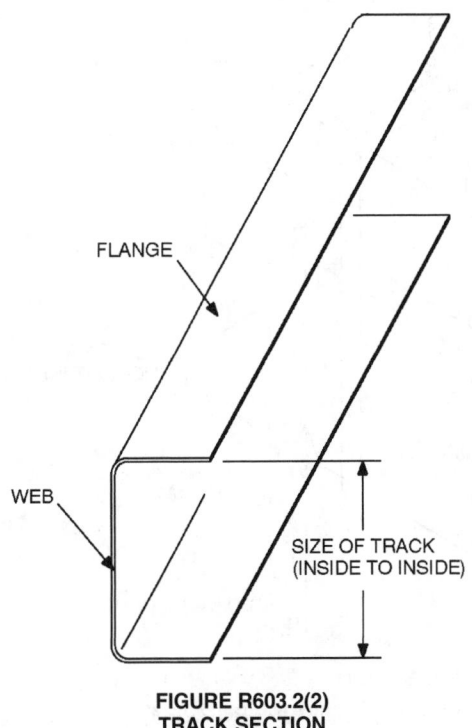

FIGURE R603.2(2)
TRACK SECTION

Where No. 8 screws are specified in a steel-to-steel connection, the required number of screws in the connection is permitted to be reduced in accordance with the reduction factors in Table R603.2.4, when larger screws are used or when one of the sheets of steel being connected is thicker than 33 mils (0.84 mm). When applying the reduction factor, the resulting number of screws shall be rounded up.

TABLE R603.2.4
SCREW SUBSTITUTION FACTOR

SCREW SIZE	THINNEST CONNECTED STEEL SHEET (mils)	
	33	43
#8	1.0	0.67
#10	0.93	0.62
#12	0.86	0.56

For SI: 1 mil = 0.0254 mm.

R603.2.5 Web holes, web hole reinforcing and web hole patching. Web holes, web hole reinforcing and web hole patching shall be in accordance with this section.

R603.2.5.1 Web holes. Web holes in wall studs and other structural members shall comply with all of the following conditions:

1. Holes shall conform to Figure R603.2.5.1;

2. Holes shall be permitted only along the centerline of the web of the framing member;

3. Holes shall have a center-to-center spacing of not less than 24 inches (610 mm);

4. Holes shall have a web hole width not greater than 0.5 times the member depth, or $1^1/_2$ inches (38 mm);

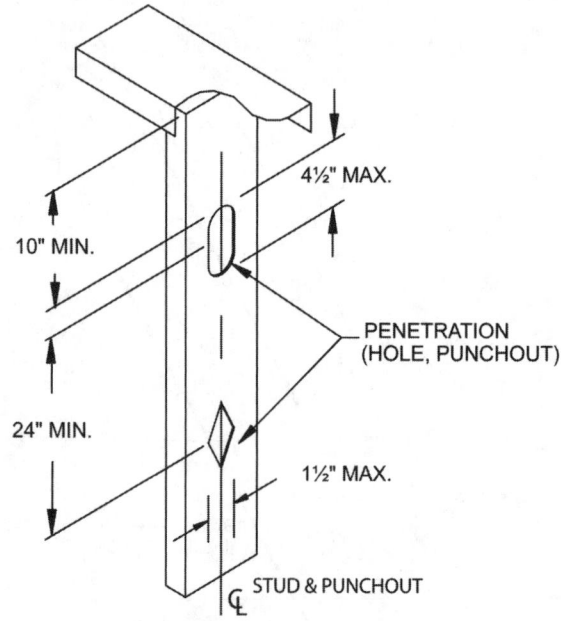

For SI: 1 inch = 25.4 mm.

FIGURE R603.2.5.1
WEB HOLES

5. Holes shall have a web hole length not exceeding $4^1/_2$ inches (114 mm); and

6. Holes shall have a minimum distance between the edge of the bearing surface and the edge of the web hole of not less than 10 inches (254 mm).

Framing members with web holes not conforming to the above requirements shall be reinforced in accordance with Section R603.2.5.2, patched in accordance with Section R603.2.5.3 or designed in accordance with accepted engineering practice.

R603.2.5.2 Web hole reinforcing. Web holes in gable endwall studs not conforming to the requirements of Section R603.2.5.1 shall be permitted to be reinforced if the hole is located fully within the center 40 percent of the span and the depth and length of the hole does not exceed 65 percent of the flat width of the web. The reinforcing shall be a steel plate or C-shape section with a hole that does not exceed the web hole size limitations of Section R603.2.5.1 for the member being reinforced. The steel reinforcing shall be the same thickness as the receiving member and shall extend at least 1 inch (25.4 mm) beyond all edges of the hole. The steel reinforcing shall be fastened to the web of the receiving member with No.8 screws spaced no more than 1 inch (25.4 mm) center-to-center along the edges of the patch with minimum edge distance of $^1/_2$ inch (12.7 mm).

R603.2.5.3 Hole patching. Web holes in wall studs and other structural members not conforming to the requirements in Section R603.2.5.1 shall be permitted to be patched in accordance with either of the following methods:

1. Framing members shall be replaced or designed in accordance with accepted engineering practice when web holes exceed the following size limits:

   1.1. The depth of the hole, measured across the web, exceeds 70 percent of the flat width of the web; or

   1.2. The length of the hole measured along the web exceeds 10 inches (254 mm) or the depth of the web, whichever is greater.

2. Web holes not exceeding the dimensional requirements in Section R603.2.5.3, Item 1 shall be patched with a solid steel plate, stud section or track section in accordance with Figure R603.2.5.3. The steel patch shall, as a minimum, be the same thickness as the receiving member and shall extend at least 1 inch (25.4 mm) beyond all edges of the hole. The steel patch shall be fastened to the web of the receiving member with No. 8 screws spaced no more than 1 inch (25.4 mm) center-to-center along the edges of the patch with a minimum edge distance of $^1/_2$ inch (12.7 mm).

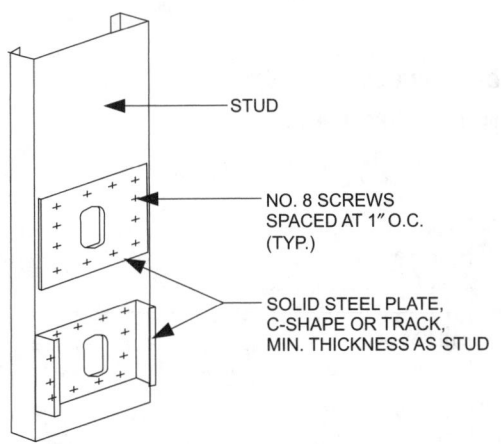

STUD

NO. 8 SCREWS
SPACED AT 1″ O.C.
(TYP.)

SOLID STEEL PLATE,
C-SHAPE OR TRACK,
MIN. THICKNESS AS STUD

For SI: 1 inch = 25.4 mm.

FIGURE R603.2.5.3
STUD WEB HOLE PATCH

R603.3 Wall construction. All exterior cold-formed steel framed walls and interior load-bearing cold-formed steel framed walls shall be constructed in accordance with the provisions of this section.

R603.3.1 Wall to foundation or floor connection. Cold-formed steel framed walls shall be anchored to foundations or floors in accordance with Table R603.3.1 and Figure R603.3.1(1), R603.3.1(2) or R603.3.1(3). Anchor bolts shall be located not more than 12 inches (305 mm) from corners or the termination of bottom tracks. Anchor bolts shall extend a minimum of 15 inches (381 mm) into masonry or 7 inches (178 mm) into concrete. Foundation anchor straps shall be permitted, in lieu of anchor bolts, if spaced as required to provide equivalent anchorage to the required anchor bolts and installed in accordance with manufacturer's requirements.

R603.3.1.1 Gable endwalls. Gable endwalls with heights greater than 10 feet (3048 mm) shall be anchored to foundations or floors in accordance with Tables R603.3.1.1(1) or R603.3.1.1(2).

R603.3.2 Minimum stud sizes. Cold-formed steel walls shall be constructed in accordance with Figures R603.3.1(1), R603.3.1(2), or R603.3.1(3), as applicable. Exterior wall stud size and thickness shall be determined in accordance with the limits set forth in Tables R603.3.2(2) through R603.3.2(31). Interior load-bearing wall stud size and thickness shall be determined in accordance with the limits set forth in Tables R603.3.2(2) through R603.3.2(31) based upon an 85 miles per hour (38 m/s) Exposure A/B wind value and the building width, stud spacing and snow load, as appropriate. Fastening requirements shall be in accordance with Section R603.2.4 and Table R603.3.2(1). Top and bottom tracks shall have the same minimum thickness as the wall studs.

Exterior wall studs shall be permitted to be reduced to the next thinner size, as shown in Tables R603.3.2(2) through R603.3.2(31), but not less than 33 mils (0.84 mm) ,where both of the following conditions exist:

1. Minimum of $^1/_2$ inch (12.7 mm) gypsum board is installed and fastened in accordance with Section R702 on the interior surface.

2. Wood structural sheathing panels of minimum $^7/_{16}$ inch (11 mm) thick oriented strand board or $^{15}/_{32}$ inch (12 mm) thick plywood is installed and fastened in accordance with Section R603.9.1 and Table R603.3.2(1) on the outside surface.

Interior load-bearing walls shall be permitted to be reduced to the next thinner size, as shown in Tables R603.3.2(2) through R603.3.2(31), but not less than 33 mils (0.84 mm), where a minimum of $^1/_2$ inch (12.7 mm) gypsum board is installed and fastened in accordance with Section R702 on both sides of the wall. The tabulated stud thickness for load-bearing walls shall be used when the *attic* load is 10 pounds per square feet (480 Pa) or less. A limited *attic* storage load of 20 pounds per square feet (960 Pa) shall be permitted provided that the next higher snow load column is used to select the stud size from Tables R603.3.2(2) through R603.3.2(31).

For two-story buildings, the tabulated stud thickness for walls supporting one floor, roof and ceiling shall be used when second floor live load is 30 pounds per square feet (1440 Pa). Second floor live loads of 40 psf (1920 pounds per square feet) shall be permitted provided that the next higher snow load column is used to select the stud size from Tables R603.3.2(2) through R603.3.2(21).

For three-story buildings, the tabulated stud thickness for walls supporting one or two floors, roof and ceiling shall be used when the third floor live load is 30 pounds per square feet (1440 Pa). Third floor live loads of 40 pounds per square feet (1920 Pa) shall be permitted provided that the next higher snow load column is used to select the stud size from Tables R603.3.2(22) through R603.3.2(31).

R603.3.2.1 Gable endwalls. The size and thickness of gable endwall studs with heights less than or equal to 10 feet (3048 mm) shall be permitted in accordance with the limits set forth in Tables R603.3.2.1(1) or R603.3.2.1(2). The size and thickness of gable endwall studs with heights greater than 10 feet (3048 mm) shall be determined in accordance with the limits set forth in Tables R603.3.2.1(3) or R603.3.2.1(4).

R603.3.3 Stud bracing. The flanges of cold-formed steel studs shall be laterally braced in accordance with one of the following:

1. Gypsum board on both sides, structural sheathing on both sides, or gypsum board on one side and structural sheathing on the other side of load-bearing walls with gypsum board installed with minimum No. 6 screws in accordance with Section R702 and structural sheathing installed in accordance with Section R603.9.1 and Table R603.3.2(1).

2. Horizontal steel straps fastened in accordance with Figure R603.3.3(1) on both sides at mid-height for 8-foot (2438 mm) walls, and at one-third points for 9-foot and 10-foot (2743 mm and 3048 mm) walls. Horizontal steel straps shall be at least 1.5 inches in width and 33 mils in thickness (38 mm by 0.84 mm). Straps shall be attached to the flanges of studs with one No. 8 screw. In-line blocking shall be installed between studs at the termination of all straps and at 12 foot (3658 mm) intervals along the strap. Straps shall be fastened to the blocking with two No. 8 screws.

TABLE R603.3.1
WALL TO FOUNDATION OR FLOOR CONNECTION REQUIREMENTS[a,b]

FRAMING CONDITION	WIND SPEED (mph) AND EXPOSURE					
	85 B	90 B	100 B / 85 C	110 B / 90 C	100 C	< 110 C
Wall bottom track to floor per Figure R603.3.1(1)	1-No. 8 screw at 12″ o.c.	1-No. 8 screw at 12″ o.c.	1-No. 8 screw at 12″ o.c.	1-No. 8 screw at 12″ o.c.	2-No. 8 screws at 12″ o.c.	2 No. 8 screws at 12″ o.c.
Wall bottom track to foundation per Figure R603.3.1(2)[d]	$^1/_2$″ minimum diameter anchor bolt at 6′ o.c.	$^1/_2$″ minimum diameter anchor bolt at 6′ o.c.	$^1/_2$″ minimum diameter anchor bolt at 4′ o.c.	$^1/_2$″ minimum diameter anchor bolt at 4′ o.c.	$^1/_2$″ minimum diameter anchor bolt at 4′ o.c.	$^1/_2$″ minimum diameter anchor bolt at 4′ o.c.
Wall bottom track to wood sill per Figure R603.3.1(3)	Steel plate spaced at 4′ o.c., with 4-No. 8 screws and 4-10d or 6-8d common nails	Steel plate spaced at 4′ o.c., with 4-No. 8 screws and 4-10d or 6-8d common nails	Steel plate spaced at 3′ o.c., with 4-No. 8 screws and 4-10d or 6-8d common nails	Steel plate spaced at 3′ o.c., with 4-No. 8 screws and 4-10d or 6-8d common nails	Steel plate spaced at 2′ o.c., with 4-No. 8 screws and 4-10d or 6-8d common nails	Steel plate spaced at 2′ o.c., with 4-No. 8 screws and 4-10d or 6-8d common nails
Wind uplift connector strength to 16″ stud spacing[c]	NR	NR	NR	NR	NR	65 lb per foot of wall length
Wind uplift connector strength for 24″ stud spacing[c]	NR	NR	NR	NR	NR	100 lb per foot of wall length

For SI: 1 inch = 25.4 mm, 1 mile per hour = 0.447 m/s, 1 foot = 304.8 mm, 1 lb = 4.45 N.

a. Anchor bolts are to be located not more than 12 inches from corners or the termination of bottom tracks (e.g., at door openings or corners). Bolts are to extend a minimum of 15 inches into masonry or 7 inches into concrete.

b. All screw sizes shown are minimum.

c. NR = uplift connector not required.

d. Foundation anchor straps are permitted in place of anchor bolts, if spaced as required to provide equivalent anchorage to the required anchor bolts and installed in accordance with manufacturer's requirements.

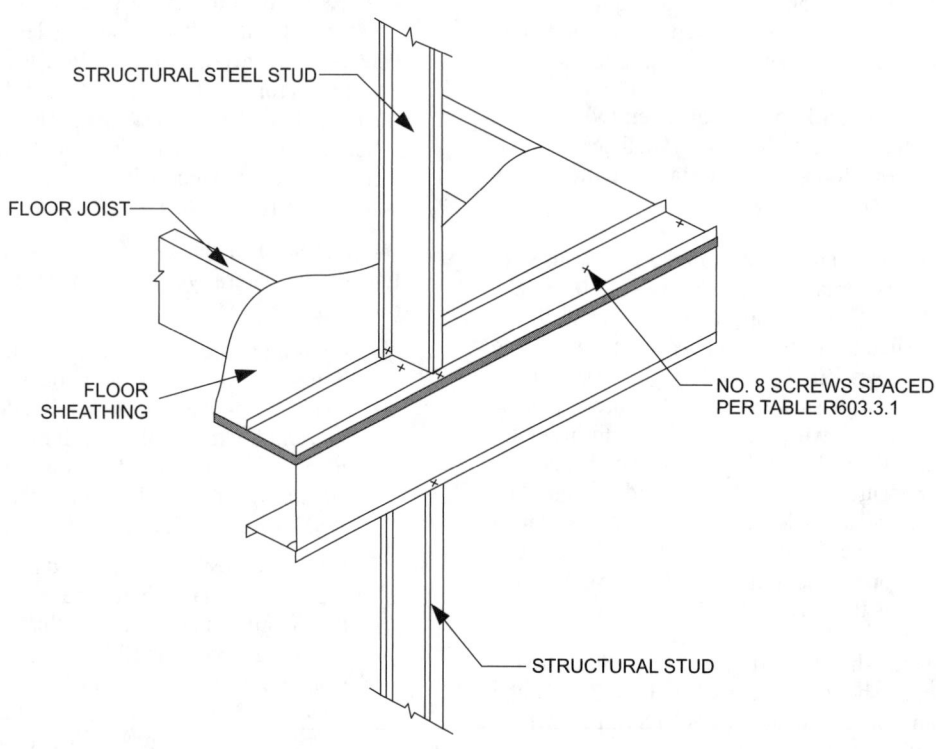

FIGURE R603.3.1(1)
WALL TO FLOOR CONNECTION

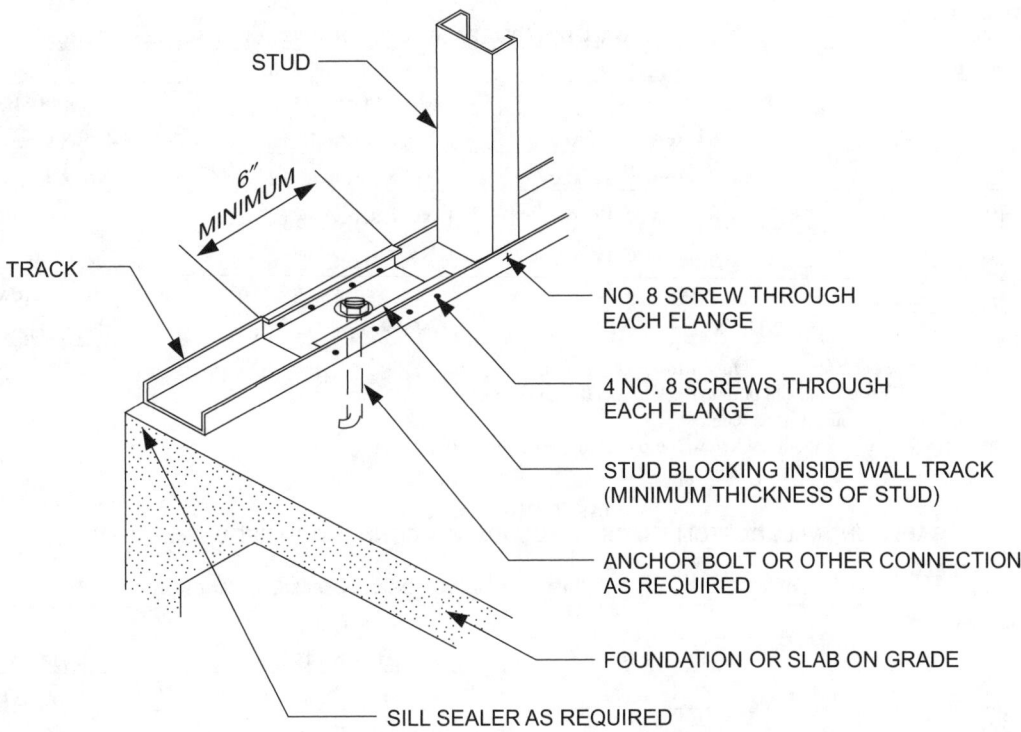

STUD

6" MINIMUM

TRACK

NO. 8 SCREW THROUGH EACH FLANGE

4 NO. 8 SCREWS THROUGH EACH FLANGE

STUD BLOCKING INSIDE WALL TRACK (MINIMUM THICKNESS OF STUD)

ANCHOR BOLT OR OTHER CONNECTION AS REQUIRED

FOUNDATION OR SLAB ON GRADE

SILL SEALER AS REQUIRED

For SI: 1 inch = 25.4 mm.

FIGURE R603.3.1(2)
WALL TO FOUNDATION CONNECTION

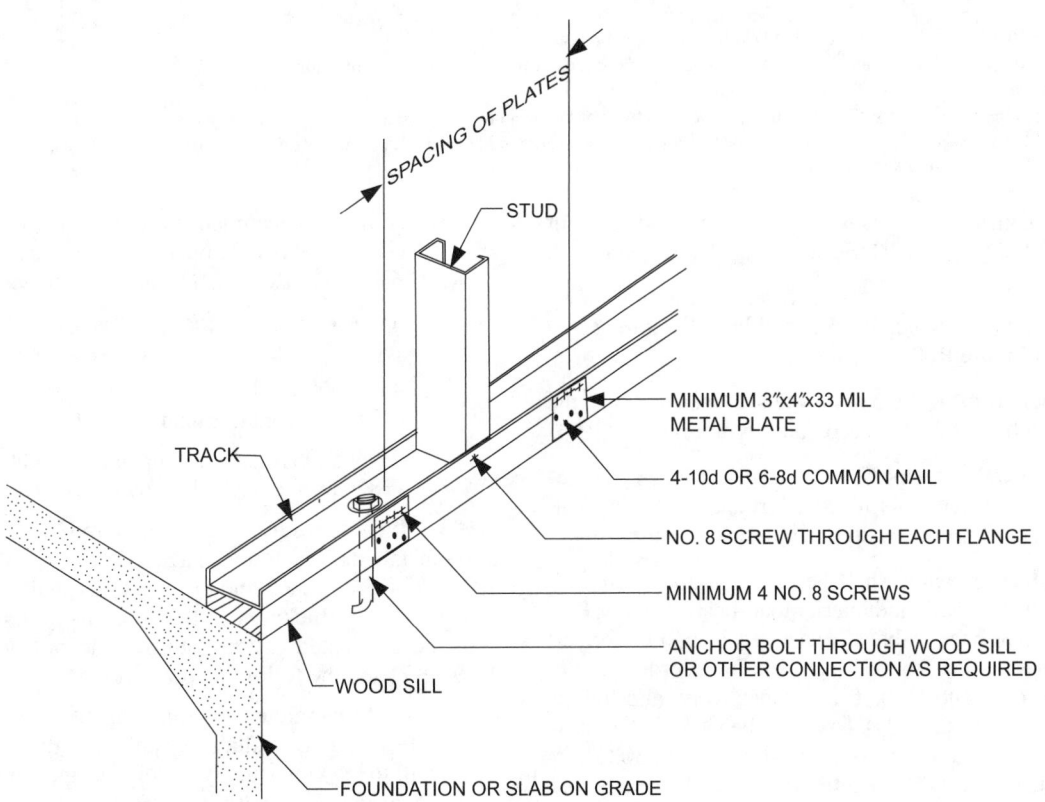

SPACING OF PLATES

STUD

TRACK

MINIMUM 3"x4"x33 MIL METAL PLATE

4-10d OR 6-8d COMMON NAIL

NO. 8 SCREW THROUGH EACH FLANGE

MINIMUM 4 NO. 8 SCREWS

ANCHOR BOLT THROUGH WOOD SILL OR OTHER CONNECTION AS REQUIRED

WOOD SILL

FOUNDATION OR SLAB ON GRADE

For SI: 1 mil = 0.0254 mm, 1 inch = 25.4 mm.

FIGURE R603.3.1(3)
WALL TO WOOD SILL CONNECTION

TABLE R603.3.1.1(1)
GABLE ENDWALL TO FLOOR CONNECTION REQUIREMENTS[a,b,c]

BASIC WIND SPEED (mph)		WALL BOTTOM TRACK TO FLOOR JOIST OR TRACK CONNECTION		
Exposure		Stud height, h (ft)		
B	C	10 < h ≤ 14	14 < h ≤ 18	18 < h ≤ 22
85	—	1-No. 8 screw @ 12″ o.c.	1-No. 8 screw @ 12″ o.c.	1-No. 8 screw @ 12″ o.c.
90	—	1-No. 8 screw @ 12″ o.c.	1-No. 8 screw @ 12″ o.c.	1-No. 8 screw @ 12″ o.c.
100	85	1-No. 8 screw @ 12″ o.c.	1-No. 8 screw @ 12″ o.c.	1-No. 8 screw @ 12″ o.c.
110	90	1-No. 8 screw @ 12″ o.c.	1-No. 8 screw @ 12″ o.c.	2-No. 8 screws @ 12″ o.c.
—	100	1-No. 8 screw @ 12″ o.c.	2-No. 8 screws @ 12″ o.c.	1-No. 8 screw @ 8″ o.c.
—	110	2-No. 8 screws @ 12″ o.c.	1-No. 8 screw @ 8″ o.c.	2-No. 8 screws @ 8″ o.c.

For SI: 1 inch = 25.4 mm, 1 mile per hour = 0.447 m/s, 1 foot = 304.8 mm.
a. Refer to Table R603.3.1.1(2) for gable endwall bottom track to foundation connections.
b. Where attachment is not given, special design is required.
c. Stud height, h, is measured from wall bottom track to wall top track or brace connection height.

TABLE R603.3.1.1(2)
GABLE ENDWALL BOTTOM TRACK TO FOUNDATION CONNECTION REQUIREMENTS[a,b,c]

BASIC WIND SPEED (mph)		MINIMUM SPACING FOR 1/2 IN. DIAMETER ANCHOR BOLTS[d]		
Exposure		Stud height, h (ft)		
B	C	10 < h ≤ 14	14 < h ≤ 18	18 < h ≤ 22
85	—	6′ - 0″ o.c.	6′ - 0″ o.c.	6′ - 0″ o.c.
90	—	6′ - 0″ o.c.	5′ - 7″ o.c.	6′ - 0″ o.c.
100	85	5′ - 10″ o.c.	6′ - 0″ o.c.	6′ - 0″ o.c.
110	90	4′ - 10″ o.c.	5′ - 6″ o.c.	6′ - 0″ o.c.
—	100	4′ - 1″ o.c.	6′ - 0″ o.c.	6′ - 0″ o.c.
—	110	5′ - 1″ o.c.	6′ - 0″ o.c.	5′ - 2″ o.c.

For SI: 1 inch = 25.4 mm, 1 mile per hour = 0.447 m/s, 1 foot = 304.8 mm.
a. Refer to Table R603.3.1.1(1) for gable endwall bottom track to floor joist or track connection connections.
b. Where attachment is not given, special design is required.
c. Stud height, h, is measured from wall bottom track to wall top track or brace connection height.
d. Foundation anchor straps are permitted in place of anchor bolts if spaced as required to provide equivalent anchorage to the required anchor bolts and installed in accordance with manufacturer's requirements.

R603.3.4 Cutting and notching. Flanges and lips of cold-formed steel studs and headers shall not be cut or notched.

R603.3.5 Splicing. Steel studs and other structural members shall not be spliced. Tracks shall be spliced in accordance with Figure R603.3.5.

R603.4 Corner framing. In exterior walls, corner studs and the top tracks shall be installed in accordance with Figure R603.4.

R603.5 Exterior wall covering. The method of attachment of exterior wall covering materials to cold-formed steel stud wall framing shall conform to the manufacturer's installation instructions.

R603.6 Headers. Headers shall be installed above all wall openings in exterior walls and interior load-bearing walls. Box beam headers and back-to-back headers each shall be formed from two equal sized C-shaped members in accordance with Figures R603.6(1) and R603.6(2), respectively, and Tables R603.6(1) through R603.6(24). L-shaped headers shall be permitted to be constructed in accordance with AISI S230. Alternately, headers shall be permitted to be designed and constructed in accordance with AISI S100, Section D4.

R603.6.1 Headers in gable endwalls. Box beam and back-to-back headers in gable endwalls shall be permitted to be constructed in accordance with Section R603.6 or with the header directly above the opening in accordance with Figures R603.6.1(1) and R603.6.1(2) and the following provisions:

1. Two 362S162-33 for openings less than or equal to 4 feet (1219 mm).

2. Two 600S162-43 for openings greater than 4 feet (1219 mm) but less than or equal to 6 feet (1830 mm).

3. Two 800S162-54 for openings greater than 6 feet (1829 mm) but less than or equal to 9 feet (2743 mm).

R603.7 Jack and king studs. The number of jack and king studs installed on each side of a header shall comply with Table R603.7(1). King, jack and cripple studs shall be of the same dimension and thickness as the adjacent wall studs. Headers shall be connected to king studs in accordance with Table R603.7(2) and the following provisions:

1. For box beam headers, one-half of the total number of required screws shall be applied to the header and one half to the king stud by use of C-shaped or track member in accordance with Figure R603.6(1). The track or C-shape sections shall extend the depth of the header minus 1/2 inch (12.7 mm) and shall have a minimum thickness not less than that of the wall studs.

2. For back-to-back headers, one-half the total number of screws shall be applied to the header and one-half to the king stud by use of a minimum 2-inch-by-2-inch (51 mm × 51 mm) clip angle in accordance with Figure R603.6(2). The clip angle shall extend the depth of the header minus $^1/_2$ inch (12.7 mm) and shall have a minimum thickness not less than that of the wall studs. Jack and king studs shall be interconnected with structural sheathing in accordance with Figures R603.6(1) and R603.6(2).

R603.8 Head and sill track. Head track spans above door and window openings and sill track spans beneath window openings shall comply with Table R603.8. For openings less than 4 feet (1219 mm) in height that have both a head track and a sill track, multiplying the spans by 1.75 shall be permitted in Table R603.8. For openings less than or equal to 6 feet (1829 mm) in height that have both a head track and a sill track, multiplying the spans in Table R603.8 by 1.50 shall be permitted.

R603.9 Structural sheathing. Structural sheathing shall be installed in accordance with Figure R603.9 and this section on all sheathable exterior wall surfaces, including areas above and below openings.

R603.9.1 Sheathing materials. Structural sheathing panels shall consist of minimum $^7/_{16}$-inch (11 mm) thick oriented strand board or $^{15}/_{32}$-inch (12 mm) thick plywood.

R603.9.2 Determination of minimum length of full height sheathing. The minimum length of full height sheathing on each *braced wall line* shall be determined by multiplying the length of the *braced wall line* by the percentage obtained from Table R603.9.2(1) and by the plan aspect-ratio adjustment factors obtained from Table R603.9.2(2). The minimum length of full height sheathing shall not be less than 20 percent of the *braced wall line* length.

To be considered full height sheathing, structural sheathing shall extend from the bottom to the top of the wall without interruption by openings. Only sheathed, full height wall sections, uninterrupted by openings, which are a minimum of 48 inches (1219 mm) wide, shall be counted toward meeting the minimum percentages in Table R603.9.2(1). In addition, structural sheathing shall comply with all of the following requirements:

1. Be installed with the long dimension parallel to the stud framing (i.e. vertical orientation) and shall cover the full vertical height of wall from the bottom of the bottom track to the top of the top track of each *story*. Installing the long dimension perpendicular to the stud framing or using shorter segments shall be permitted provided that the horizontal joint is blocked as described in Item 2 below.

2. Be blocked when the long dimension is installed perpendicular to the stud framing (i.e. horizontal orientation). Blocking shall be a minimum of 33 mil (0.84 mm) thickness. Each horizontal structural sheathing panel shall be fastened with No. 8 screws spaced at 6 inches (152 mm) on center to the blocking at the joint.

3. Be applied to each end (corners) of each of the exterior walls with a minimum 48 inch (1219 mm) wide panel.

R603.9.2.1 The minimum percentage of full-height structural sheathing shall be multiplied by 1.10 for 9 foot (2743 mm) high walls and multiplied by 1.20 for 10 foot (3048 mm) high walls.

R603.9.2.2 For hip roofed homes, the minimum percentages of full height sheathing in Table R603.9.2(1), based upon wind, shall be permitted to be multiplied by a factor of 0.95 for roof slopes not exceeding 7:12 and a factor of 0.9 for roof slopes greater than 7:12.

R603.9.2.3 In the lowest *story* of a *dwelling*, multiplying the percentage of full height sheathing required in Table R603.9.2(1) by 0.6, shall be permitted provided hold down anchors are provided in accordance with Section R603.9.4.2.

R603.9.3 Structural sheathing fastening. All edges and interior areas of structural sheathing panels shall be fastened to framing members and tracks in accordance with Figure R603.9 and Table R603.3.2(1). Screws for attachment of structural sheathing panels shall be bugle-head, flat-head, or similar head style with a minimum head diameter of 0.29 inch (8 mm).

For continuously-sheathed *braced wall lines* using wood structural panels installed with No. 8 screws spaced 4-inches (102 mm) on center at all panel edges and 12 inches (304.8 mm) on center on intermediate framing members, the following shall apply:

1. Multiplying the percentages of full height sheathing in Table R603.9.2(1) by 0.72 shall be permitted.

2. For bottom track attached to foundations or framing below, the bottom track anchor or screw connection spacing in Table R505.3.1(1) and Table R603.3.1 shall be multiplied by 2/3.

R603.9.4 Uplift connection requirements. Uplift connections shall be provided in accordance with this section.

R603.9.4.1 Where wind speeds are in excess of 100 miles per hour (45 m/s), Exposure C, walls shall be provided wind direct uplift connections in accordance with AISI S230, Section E13.3, and AISI S230, Section F7.2, as required for 110 miles per hour (49 m/s), Exposure C.

R603.9.4.2 Where the percentage of full height sheathing is adjusted in accordance with Section R603.9.2.3, a hold-down anchor, with a strength of 4,300 pounds (19 kN), shall be provided at each end of each full-height sheathed wall section used to meet the minimum percent sheathing requirements of Section R603.9.2. Hold down anchors shall be attached to back-to-back studs; structural sheathing panels shall have edge fastening to the studs, in accordance with Section R603.9.3 and AISI S230, Table E11-1.

A single hold down anchor, installed in accordance with Figure R603.9.2, shall be permitted at the corners of buildings.

R603.9.5 Structural sheathing for stone and masonry veneer. In Seismic Design Category C, where stone and masonry veneer is installed in accordance with Section R703.7, the length of structural sheathing for walls supporting one *story*, roof and ceiling shall be the greater of the amount required by Section R603.9.2 or 36 percent, modified by Section R603.9.2 except Section R603.9.2.2 shall not be permitted.

TABLE R603.3.2(1)
WALL FASTENING SCHEDULE[a]

DESCRIPTION OF BUILDING ELEMENT	NUMBER AND SIZE OF FASTENERS[a]	SPACING OF FASTENERS
Floor joist to track of load-bearing wall	2-No. 8 screws	Each joist
Wall stud to top or bottom track	2-No. 8 screws	Each end of stud, one per flange
Structural sheathing to wall studs	No. 8 screws[b]	6″ o.c. on edges and 12″ o.c. at intermediate supports
Roof framing to wall	Approved design or tie down in accordance with Section R802.11	

For SI: 1 inch = 25.4 mm.

a. All screw sizes shown are minimum.

b. Screws for attachment of structural sheathing panels are to be bugle-head, flat-head, or similar head styles with a minimum head diameter of 0.29 inch.

TABLE R603.3.2(2)
24-FOOT-WIDE BUILDING SUPPORTING ROOF AND CEILING ONLY[a, b, c]
33 ksi STEEL

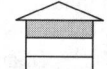

WIND SPEED		MEMBER SIZE	STUD SPACING (inches)	MINIMUM STUD THICKNESS (mils)											
				8-Foot Studs				9-Foot Studs				10-Foot Studs			
				Ground Snow Load (psf)											
Exp. B	Exp. C			20	30	50	70	20	30	50	70	20	30	50	70
85 mph	—	350S162	16	33	33	33	33	33	33	33	33	33	33	33	33
			24	33	33	33	43	33	33	33	43	33	33	43	43
		550S162	16	33	33	33	33	33	33	33	33	33	33	33	33
			24	33	33	33	33	33	33	33	33	33	33	33	33
90 mph	—	350S162	16	33	33	33	33	33	33	33	33	33	33	33	33
			24	33	33	33	43	33	33	33	43	33	33	43	43
		550S162	16	33	33	33	33	33	33	33	33	33	33	33	33
			24	33	33	33	33	33	33	33	33	33	33	33	33
100 mph	85 mph	350S162	16	33	33	33	33	33	33	33	33	33	33	33	33
			24	33	33	33	43	33	33	33	43	43	43	43	43
		550S162	16	33	33	33	33	33	33	33	33	33	33	33	33
			24	33	33	33	43	33	33	33	33	33	33	33	43
110 mph	90 mph	350S162	16	33	33	33	33	33	33	33	33	33	33	33	33
			24	33	33	33	43	43	43	43	43	43	43	43	54
		550S162	16	33	33	33	33	33	33	33	33	33	33	33	33
			24	33	33	33	43	33	33	33	33	43	43	43	43
—	100 mph	350S162	16	33	33	33	33	33	33	33	33	43	43	43	43
			24	43	43	43	43	43	43	43	43	54	54	54	54
		550S162	16	33	33	33	33	33	33	33	33	33	33	33	33
			24	33	33	33	43	43	43	43	43	43	43	43	43
—	110 mph	350S162	16	33	33	33	33	43	43	43	43	43	43	43	43
			24	43	43	43	43	54	54	54	54	68	68	68	68
		550S162	16	33	33	33	33	33	33	33	33	33	33	33	33
			24	33	43	43	43	43	43	43	43	43	43	43	43

For SI: 1 inch = 25.4 mm, 1 foot = 304.8 mm, 1 mil = 0.0254 mm, 1 mile per hour = 0.447 m/s, 1 pound per square foot = 0.0479 kPa,
1 ksi = 1000 psi = 6.895 MPa.

a. Deflection criterion: $L/240$.

b. Design load assumptions:
    Second floor dead load is 10 psf.
    Second floor live load is 30 psf.
    Roof/ceiling dead load is 12 psf.
    Attic live load is 10 psf.

c. Building width is in the direction of horizontal framing members supported by the wall studs.

TABLE R603.3.2(3)
24-FOOT-WIDE BUILDING SUPPORTING ROOF AND CEILING ONLY[a,b,c]
50 ksi STEEL

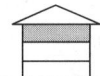

WIND SPEED		MEMBER SIZE	STUD SPACING (inches)	MINIMUM STUD THICKNESS (mils)											
				8-Foot Studs				9-Foot Studs				10-Foot Studs			
				Ground Snow Load (psf)											
Exp. B	Exp. C			20	30	50	70	20	30	50	70	20	30	50	70
85 mph	—	350S162	16	33	33	33	33	33	33	33	33	33	33	33	33
			24	33	33	33	43	33	33	33	33	33	33	33	43
		550S162	16	33	33	33	33	33	33	33	33	33	33	33	33
			24	33	33	33	33	33	33	33	33	33	33	33	33
90 mph	—	350S162	16	33	33	33	33	33	33	33	33	33	33	33	33
			24	33	33	33	43	33	33	33	33	33	33	33	43
		550S162	16	33	33	33	33	33	33	33	33	33	33	33	33
			24	33	33	33	33	33	33	33	33	33	33	33	33
100 mph	85 mph	350S162	16	33	33	33	33	33	33	33	33	33	33	33	33
			24	33	33	33	43	33	33	33	33	33	33	33	43
		550S162	16	33	33	33	33	33	33	33	33	33	33	33	33
			24	33	33	33	33	33	33	33	33	33	33	33	33
110 mph	90 mph	350S162	16	33	33	33	33	33	33	33	33	33	33	33	33
			24	33	33	33	43	33	33	33	43	43	43	43	43
		550S162	16	33	33	33	33	33	33	33	33	33	33	33	33
			24	33	33	33	33	33	33	33	33	33	33	33	33
—	100 mph	350S162	16	33	33	33	33	33	33	33	33	33	33	33	33
			24	33	33	33	43	43	43	43	43	43	43	43	43
		550S162	16	33	33	33	33	33	33	33	33	33	33	33	33
			24	33	33	33	33	33	33	33	33	33	33	33	33
—	110 mph	350S162	16	33	33	33	33	33	33	33	33	33	33	33	33
			24	33	33	33	43	43	43	43	43	54	54	54	54
		550S162	16	33	33	33	33	33	33	33	33	33	33	33	33
			24	33	33	33	33	33	33	33	33	33	33	33	33

For SI: 1 inch = 25.4 mm, 1 foot = 304.8 mm, 1 mil = 0.0254 mm, 1 mile per hour = 0.447 m/s, 1 pound per square foot = 0.0479kPa,
1 ksi = 1000 psi = 6.895 MPa.

a. Deflection criterion: L/240.

b. Design load assumptions:
   Second floor dead load is 10 psf.
   Second floor live load is 30 psf.
   Roof/ceiling dead load is 12 psf.
   Attic live load is 10 psf.

c. Building width is in the direction of horizontal framing members supported by the wall studs.

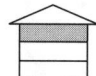

TABLE R603.3.2(4)
28-FOOT-WIDE BUILDING SUPPORTING ROOF AND CEILING ONLY[a,b,c]
33 ksi STEEL

WIND SPEED		MEMBER SIZE	STUD SPACING (inches)	MINIMUM STUD THICKNESS (mils)											
				8-Foot Studs				9-Foot Studs				10-Foot Studs			
				Ground Snow Load (psf)											
Exp. B	Exp. C			20	30	50	70	20	30	50	70	20	30	50	70
85 mph	—	350S162	16	33	33	33	33	33	33	33	33	33	33	33	33
			24	33	33	43	43	33	33	43	43	33	33	43	54
		550S162	16	33	33	33	33	33	33	33	33	33	33	33	33
			24	33	33	33	43	33	33	33	43	33	33	33	43
90 mph	—	350S162	16	33	33	33	33	33	33	33	33	33	33	33	33
			24	33	33	43	43	33	33	43	43	33	33	43	54
		550S162	16	33	33	33	33	33	33	33	33	33	33	33	33
			24	33	33	33	43	33	33	33	43	33	33	33	43
100 mph	85 mph	350S162	16	33	33	33	33	33	33	33	33	33	33	33	33
			24	33	33	43	43	33	33	43	43	43	43	43	54
		550S162	16	33	33	33	33	33	33	33	33	33	33	33	33
			24	33	33	33	43	33	33	33	43	33	33	33	43
110 mph	90 mph	350S162	16	33	33	33	33	33	33	33	33	33	33	33	43
			24	33	33	43	43	43	43	43	43	43	43	43	54
		550S162	16	33	33	33	33	33	33	33	33	33	33	33	33
			24	33	33	33	43	33	33	33	43	33	33	33	43
—	100 mph	350S162	16	33	33	33	33	33	33	33	33	43	43	43	43
			24	43	43	43	54	43	43	43	54	54	54	54	54
		550S162	16	33	33	33	33	33	33	33	33	33	33	33	33
			24	33	33	33	43	33	33	33	43	33	33	33	43
—	110 mph	350S162	16	33	33	33	33	43	43	43	43	43	43	43	43
			24	43	43	43	54	54	54	54	54	68	68	68	68
		550S162	16	33	33	33	33	33	33	33	33	33	33	33	33
			24	33	33	33	43	33	33	33	43	43	43	43	43

For SI: 1 inch = 25.4 mm, 1 foot = 304.8 mm, 1 mil = 0.0254 mm, 1 mile per hour = 0.447 m/s, 1 pound per square foot = 0.0479kPa,
1 ksi = 1000 psi = 6.895 MPa.

a. Deflection criterion: $L/240$.
b. Design load assumptions:
Second floor dead load is 10 psf.
Second floor live load is 30 psf.
Roof/ceiling dead load is 12 psf.
Attic live load is 10 psf.
c. Building width is in the direction of horizontal framing members supported by the wall studs.

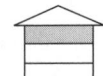

TABLE R603.3.2(5)
28-FOOT-WIDE BUILDING SUPPORTING ROOF AND CEILING ONLY[a,b,c]
50 ksi STEEL

WIND SPEED		MEMBER SIZE	STUD SPACING (inches)	MINIMUM STUD THICKNESS (mils)											
				8-Foot Studs				9-Foot Studs				10-Foot Studs			
				Ground Snow Load (psf)											
Exp. B	Exp. C			20	30	50	70	20	30	50	70	20	30	50	70
85 mph	—	350S162	16	33	33	33	33	33	33	33	33	33	33	33	33
			24	33	33	33	43	33	33	33	43	33	33	33	43
		550S162	16	33	33	33	33	33	33	33	33	33	33	33	33
			24	33	33	33	33	33	33	33	33	33	33	33	33
90 mph	—	350S162	16	33	33	33	33	33	33	33	33	33	33	33	33
			24	33	33	33	43	33	33	33	43	33	33	33	43
		550S162	16	33	33	33	33	33	33	33	33	33	33	33	33
			24	33	33	33	33	33	33	33	33	33	33	33	33
100 mph	85 mph	350S162	16	33	33	33	33	33	33	33	33	33	33	33	33
			24	33	33	33	43	33	33	33	43	33	33	43	43
		550S162	16	33	33	33	33	33	33	33	33	33	33	33	33
			24	33	33	33	33	33	33	33	33	33	33	33	33
110 mph	90 mph	350S162	16	33	33	33	33	33	33	33	33	33	33	33	33
			24	33	33	33	43	33	33	33	43	43	43	43	43
		550S162	16	33	33	33	33	33	33	33	33	33	33	33	33
			24	33	33	33	33	33	33	33	33	33	33	33	33
—	100 mph	350S162	16	33	33	33	33	33	33	33	33	33	33	33	33
			24	33	33	33	43	43	43	43	43	43	43	43	43
		550S162	16	33	33	33	33	33	33	33	33	33	33	33	33
			24	33	33	33	43	33	33	33	33	33	33	33	33
—	110 mph	350S162	16	33	33	33	33	33	33	33	33	33	33	33	33
			24	33	33	43	43	43	43	43	43	54	54	54	54
		550S162	16	33	33	33	33	33	33	33	33	33	33	33	33
			24	33	33	33	33	33	33	33	33	33	33	33	43

For SI: 1 inch = 25.4 mm, 1 foot = 304.8 mm, 1 mil = 0.0254 mm, 1 mile per hour = 0.447 m/s, 1 pound per square foot = 0.0479kPa,
        1 ksi = 1000 psi = 6.895 MPa.
a. Deflection criterion: *L*/240.
b. Design load assumptions:
    Second floor dead load is 10 psf.
    Second floor live load is 30 psf.
    Roof/ceiling dead load is 12 psf.
    Attic live load is 10 psf.
c. Building width is in the direction of horizontal framing members supported by the wall studs.

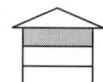

TABLE R603.3.2(6)
32-FOOT-WIDE BUILDING SUPPORTING ROOF AND CEILING ONLY[a,b,c]
33 ksi STEEL

WIND SPEED		MEMBER SIZE	STUD SPACING (inches)	MINIMUM STUD THICKNESS (mils)											
				8-Foot Studs				9-Foot Studs				10-Foot Studs			
				Ground Snow Load (psf)											
Exp. B	Exp. C			20	30	50	70	20	30	50	70	20	30	50	70
85 mph	—	350S162	16	33	33	33	33	33	33	33	33	33	33	33	43
			24	33	33	43	54	33	33	43	43	33	33	43	54
		550S162	16	33	33	33	33	33	33	33	33	33	33	33	33
			24	33	33	33	43	33	33	33	43	33	33	33	43
90 mph	—	350S162	16	33	33	33	33	33	33	33	33	33	33	33	43
			24	33	33	43	54	33	33	43	43	33	33	43	54
		550S162	16	33	33	33	33	33	33	33	33	33	33	33	33
			24	33	33	33	43	33	33	33	43	33	33	33	43
100 mph	85 mph	350S162	16	33	33	33	33	33	33	33	33	33	33	33	43
			24	33	33	43	54	33	33	43	54	43	43	43	54
		550S162	16	33	33	33	33	33	33	33	33	33	33	33	33
			24	33	33	33	43	33	33	33	43	33	33	33	43
110 mph	90 mph	350S162	16	33	33	33	43	33	33	33	33	33	33	33	43
			24	33	33	43	54	43	43	43	54	43	43	43	54
		550S162	16	33	33	33	33	33	33	33	33	33	33	33	33
			24	33	33	33	43	33	33	33	43	33	33	43	43
—	100 mph	350S162	16	33	33	33	43	33	33	33	43	43	43	43	43
			24	43	43	43	54	43	43	43	54	54	54	54	54
		550S162	16	33	33	33	33	33	33	33	33	33	33	33	33
			24	33	33	43	43	33	33	33	43	33	33	43	43
—	110 mph	350S162	16	33	33	33	43	43	43	43	43	43	43	43	43
			24	43	43	43	54	54	54	54	54	68	68	68	68
		550S162	16	33	33	33	33	33	33	33	33	33	33	33	33
			24	33	33	43	43	33	33	43	43	43	43	43	43

For SI: 1 inch = 25.4 mm, 1 foot = 304.8 mm, 1 mil = 0.0254 mm, 1 mile per hour = 0.447 m/s, 1 pound per square foot = 0.0479kPa, 1 ksi = 1000 psi = 6.895 MPa.

a. Deflection criterion: $L/240$.
b. Design load assumptions:
   Second floor dead load is 10 psf.
   Second floor live load is 30 psf.
   Roof/ceiling dead load is 12 psf.
   Attic live load is 10 psf.
c. Building width is in the direction of horizontal framing members supported by the wall studs.

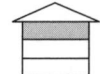

TABLE R603.3.2(7)
32-FOOT-WIDE BUILDING SUPPORTING ROOF AND CEILING ONLY[a,b,c]
50 ksi STEEL

WIND SPEED		MEMBER SIZE	STUD SPACING (inches)	MINIMUM STUD THICKNESS (mils)											
				8-Foot Studs				9-Foot Studs				10-Foot Studs			
				Ground Snow Load (psf)											
Exp. B	Exp. C			20	30	50	70	20	30	50	70	20	30	50	70
85 mph	—	350S162	16	33	33	33	33	33	33	33	33	33	33	33	33
			24	33	33	33	43	33	33	33	43	33	33	43	43
		550S162	16	33	33	33	33	33	33	33	33	33	33	33	33
			24	33	33	33	43	33	33	33	33	33	33	33	43
90 mph	—	350S162	16	33	33	33	33	33	33	33	33	33	33	33	33
			24	33	33	33	43	33	33	33	43	33	33	43	43
		550S162	16	33	33	33	33	33	33	33	33	33	33	33	33
			24	33	33	33	43	33	33	33	33	33	33	33	43
100 mph	85 mph	350S162	16	33	33	33	33	33	33	33	33	33	33	33	33
			24	33	33	43	43	33	33	33	43	33	33	43	43
		550S162	16	33	33	33	33	33	33	33	33	33	33	33	33
			24	33	33	33	43	33	33	33	33	33	33	33	43
110 mph	90 mph	350S162	16	33	33	33	33	33	33	33	33	33	33	33	33
			24	33	33	43	43	33	33	33	43	43	43	43	54
		550S162	16	33	33	33	33	33	33	33	33	33	33	33	33
			24	33	33	33	43	33	33	33	33	33	33	33	43
—	100 mph	350S162	16	33	33	33	33	33	33	33	33	33	33	33	33
			24	33	33	43	43	43	43	43	43	43	43	43	54
		550S162	16	33	33	33	33	33	33	33	33	33	33	33	33
			24	33	33	33	43	33	33	33	43	33	33	33	43
—	110 mph	350S162	16	33	33	33	33	33	33	33	33	33	33	33	43
			24	33	33	43	43	43	43	43	43	54	54	54	54
		550S162	16	33	33	33	33	33	33	33	33	33	33	33	33
			24	33	33	33	43	33	33	33	43	33	33	33	43

For SI: 1 inch = 25.4 mm, 1 foot = 304.8 mm, 1 mil = 0.0254 mm, 1 mile per hour = 0.447 m/s, 1 pound per square foot = 0.0479kPa,
1 ksi = 1000 psi = 6.895 MPa.

a. Deflection criterion: $L/240$.
b. Design load assumptions:
   Second floor dead load is 10 psf.
   Second floor live load is 30 psf.
   Roof/ceiling dead load is 12 psf.
   Attic live load is 10 psf.
c. Building width is in the direction of horizontal framing members supported by the wall studs.

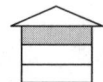

TABLE R603.3.2(8)
36-FOOT-WIDE BUILDING SUPPORTING ROOF AND CEILING ONLY[a,b,c]
33 ksi STEEL

WIND SPEED		MEMBER SIZE	STUD SPACING (inches)	MINIMUM STUD THICKNESS (mils)											
				8-Foot Studs				9-Foot Studs				10-Foot Studs			
				Ground Snow Load (psf)											
Exp. B	Exp. C			20	30	50	70	20	30	50	70	20	30	50	70
85 mph	—	350S162	16	33	33	33	43	33	33	33	43	33	33	33	43
			24	33	33	43	54	33	33	43	54	33	43	43	54
		550S162	16	33	33	33	33	33	33	33	33	33	33	33	33
			24	33	33	43	43	33	33	43	43	33	33	43	43
90 mph	—	350S162	16	33	33	33	43	33	33	33	43	33	33	33	43
			24	33	33	43	54	33	33	43	54	33	43	43	54
		550S162	16	33	33	33	33	33	33	33	33	33	33	33	33
			24	33	33	43	43	33	33	43	43	33	33	43	43
100 mph	85 mph	350S162	16	33	33	33	43	33	33	33	43	33	33	33	43
			24	33	33	43	54	33	33	43	54	43	43	54	54
		550S162	16	33	33	33	33	33	33	33	33	33	33	33	33
			24	33	33	43	43	33	33	43	43	33	33	43	43
110 mph	90 mph	350S162	16	33	33	33	43	33	33	33	33	33	33	33	43
			24	33	33	43	54	43	43	43	43	43	43	54	68
		550S162	16	33	33	33	33	33	33	33	33	33	33	33	33
			24	33	33	43	43	33	33	43	43	33	33	43	43
—	100 mph	350S162	16	33	33	33	43	33	33	33	43	43	43	43	43
			24	43	43	43	54	43	43	43	54	54	54	54	68
		550S162	16	33	33	33	33	33	33	33	33	33	33	33	33
			24	33	33	43	43	33	33	43	43	33	33	43	43
—	110 mph	350S162	16	33	33	33	43	43	43	43	43	43	43	43	43
			24	43	43	54	54	54	54	54	54	68	68	68	68
		550S162	16	33	33	33	33	33	33	33	33	33	33	33	33
			24	33	33	43	54	33	33	43	43	43	43	43	54

For SI: 1 inch = 25.4 mm, 1 foot = 304.8 mm, 1 mil = 0.0254 mm, 1 mile per hour = 0.447 m/s, 1 pound per square foot = 0.0479 kPa,
1 ksi = 1000 psi = 6.895 MPa.

a. Deflection criterion: $L/240$.
b. Design load assumptions:
  Second floor dead load is 10 psf.
  Second floor live load is 30 psf.
  Roof/ceiling dead load is 12 psf.
  Attic live load is 10 psf.
c. Building width is in the direction of horizontal framing members supported by the wall studs.

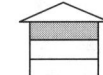

TABLE R603.3.2(9)
36-FOOT-WIDE BUILDING SUPPORTING ROOF AND CEILING ONLY[a,b,c]
50 ksi STEEL

WIND SPEED		MEMBER SIZE	STUD SPACING (inches)	MINIMUM STUD THICKNESS (mils)											
				8-Foot Studs				9-Foot Studs				10-Foot Studs			
				Ground Snow Load (psf)											
Exp. B	Exp. C			20	30	50	70	20	30	50	70	20	30	50	70
85 mph	—	350S162	16	33	33	33	33	33	33	33	33	33	33	33	33
			24	33	33	43	43	33	33	43	43	33	33	43	54
		550S162	16	33	33	33	33	33	33	33	33	33	33	33	33
			24	33	33	33	43	33	33	33	43	33	33	33	43
90 mph	—	350S162	16	33	33	33	33	33	33	33	33	33	33	33	33
			24	33	33	43	43	33	33	43	43	33	33	43	54
		550S162	16	33	33	33	33	33	33	33	33	33	33	33	33
			24	33	33	33	43	33	33	33	43	33	33	33	43
100 mph	85 mph	350S162	16	33	33	33	33	33	33	33	33	33	33	33	33
			24	33	33	43	43	33	33	43	43	33	33	43	54
		550S162	16	33	33	33	33	33	33	33	33	33	33	33	33
			24	33	33	33	43	33	33	33	43	33	33	33	43
110 mph	90 mph	350S162	16	33	33	33	33	33	33	33	33	33	33	33	43
			24	33	33	43	54	33	33	33	43	43	43	43	54
		550S162	16	33	33	33	33	33	33	33	33	33	33	33	33
			24	33	33	33	43	33	33	33	43	33	33	33	43
—	100 mph	350S162	16	33	33	33	33	33	33	33	33	33	33	33	43
			24	33	33	33	54	43	43	43	43	43	43	43	54
		550S162	16	33	33	33	33	33	33	33	33	33	33	33	33
			24	33	33	33	43	33	33	33	43	33	33	33	43
—	110 mph	350S162	16	33	33	33	43	33	33	33	33	33	33	33	43
			24	33	33	43	54	43	43	43	54	54	54	54	54
		550S162	16	33	33	33	33	33	33	33	33	33	33	33	33
			24	33	33	33	43	33	33	33	43	33	33	33	43

For SI: 1 inch = 25.4 mm, 1 foot = 304.8 mm, 1 mil = 0.0254 mm, 1 mile per hour = 0.447 m/s, 1 pound per square foot = 0.0479kPa, 1 ksi = 1000 psi = 6.895 MPa.

a. Deflection criterion: $L/240$.
b. Design load assumptions:
    Second floor dead load is 10 psf.
    Second floor live load is 30 psf.
    Roof/ceiling dead load is 12 psf.
    Attic live load is 10 psf.
c. Building width is in the direction of horizontal framing members supported by the wall studs.

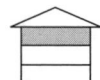

TABLE R603.3.2(10)
40-FOOT-WIDE BUILDING SUPPORTING ROOF AND CEILING ONLY[a,b,c]
33 ksi STEEL

WIND SPEED Exp. B	Exp. C	MEMBER SIZE	STUD SPACING (inches)	8-Foot Studs 20	30	50	70	9-Foot Studs 20	30	50	70	10-Foot Studs 20	30	50	70
85 mph	—	350S162	16	33	33	33	43	33	33	33	43	33	33	33	43
			24	33	33	43	54	33	33	43	54	43	43	54	68
		550S162	16	33	33	33	33	33	33	33	33	33	33	33	33
			24	33	33	43	54	33	33	43	43	33	33	43	54
90 mph	—	350S162	16	33	33	33	43	33	33	33	43	33	33	33	43
			24	33	33	43	54	33	33	43	54	43	43	54	68
		550S162	16	33	33	33	33	33	33	33	33	33	33	33	33
			24	33	33	43	54	33	33	43	43	33	33	43	54
100 mph	85 mph	350S162	16	33	33	33	43	33	33	33	43	33	33	33	43
			24	33	43	43	54	33	43	43	54	43	43	54	68
		550S162	16	33	33	33	43	33	33	33	33	33	33	33	33
			24	33	33	43	54	33	33	43	43	33	33	43	54
110 mph	90 mph	350S162	16	33	33	33	43	33	33	33	43	33	33	43	43
			24	33	43	43	54	43	43	43	54	43	43	54	68
		550S162	16	33	33	33	43	33	33	33	33	33	33	33	43
			24	33	33	43	54	33	33	43	43	33	33	43	54
—	100 mph	350S162	16	33	33	33	43	33	33	33	43	43	43	43	43
			24	43	43	54	68	43	43	54	54	54	54	54	68
		550S162	16	33	33	33	43	33	33	33	33	33	33	33	43
			24	33	33	43	54	33	33	43	54	33	33	43	54
—	110 mph	350S162	16	33	33	43	43	43	43	43	43	43	43	43	54
			24	43	43	54	68	54	54	54	68	68	68	68	68
		550S162	16	33	33	33	43	33	33	33	43	33	33	33	43
			24	33	33	43	54	33	33	43	54	43	43	43	54

For SI: 1 inch = 25.4 mm, 1 foot = 304.8 mm, 1 mil = 0.0254 mm, 1 mile per hour = 0.447 m/s, 1 pound per square foot = 0.0479 kPa, 1 ksi = 1000 psi = 6.895 MPa.

a. Deflection criterion: $L/240$.
b. Design load assumptions:
    Second floor dead load is 10 psf.
    Second floor live load is 30 psf.
    Roof/ceiling dead load is 12 psf.
    Attic live load is 10 psf.
c. Building width is in the direction of horizontal framing members supported by the wall studs.

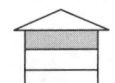

TABLE R603.3.2(11)
40-FOOT-WIDE BUILDING SUPPORTING ROOF AND CEILING ONLY[a,b,c]
50 ksi STEEL

WIND SPEED		MEMBER SIZE	STUD SPACING (inches)	MINIMUM STUD THICKNESS (mils)											
				8-Foot Studs				9-Foot Studs				10-Foot Studs			
				Ground Snow Load (psf)											
Exp. B	Exp. C			20	30	50	70	20	30	50	70	20	30	50	70
85 mph	—	350S162	16	33	33	33	33	33	33	33	33	33	33	33	43
			24	33	33	43	54	33	33	43	43	33	33	43	54
		550S162	16	33	33	33	33	33	33	33	33	33	33	33	33
			24	33	33	33	43	33	33	33	43	33	33	33	43
90 mph	—	350S162	16	33	33	33	33	33	33	33	33	33	33	33	43
			24	33	33	43	54	33	33	43	43	33	33	43	54
		550S162	16	33	33	33	33	33	33	33	33	33	33	33	33
			24	33	33	33	43	33	33	33	43	33	33	33	43
100 mph	85 mph	350S162	16	33	33	33	43	33	33	33	33	33	33	33	43
			24	33	33	43	54	33	33	43	54	33	33	43	54
		550S162	16	33	33	33	33	33	33	33	33	33	33	33	33
			24	33	33	33	43	33	33	33	43	33	33	33	43
110 mph	90 mph	350S162	16	33	33	33	43	33	33	33	33	33	33	33	43
			24	33	33	43	54	33	33	43	54	43	43	43	54
		550S162	16	33	33	33	33	33	33	33	33	33	33	33	33
			24	33	33	33	43	33	33	33	43	33	33	33	43
—	100 mph	350S162	16	33	33	33	43	33	33	33	43	33	33	33	43
			24	33	33	43	54	43	43	43	54	43	43	54	54
		550S162	16	33	33	33	33	33	33	33	33	33	33	33	33
			24	33	33	43	43	33	33	33	43	33	33	43	43
—	110 mph	350S162	16	33	33	33	43	33	33	33	43	33	33	33	43
			24	33	33	43	54	43	43	43	54	54	54	54	68
		550S162	16	33	33	33	33	33	33	33	33	33	33	33	33
			24	33	33	43	43	33	33	33	43	33	33	43	43

For SI: 1 inch = 25.4 mm, 1 foot = 304.8 mm, 1 mil = 0.0254 mm, 1 mile per hour = 0.447 m/s, 1 pound per square foot = 0.0479kPa,
   1 ksi = 1000 psi = 6.895 MPa.

a. Deflection criterion: $L/240$.

b. Design load assumptions:
   Second floor dead load is 10 psf.
   Second floor live load is 30 psf.
   Roof/ceiling dead load is 12 psf.
   Attic live load is 10 psf.

c. Building width is in the direction of horizontal framing members supported by the wall studs.

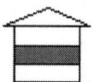

TABLE R603.3.2(12)
24-FOOT-WIDE BUILDING SUPPORTING ONE FLOOR, ROOF AND CEILING[a,b,c]
33 ksi STEEL

WIND SPEED		MEMBER SIZE	STUD SPACING (inches)	MINIMUM STUD THICKNESS (mils)											
				8-Foot Studs				9-Foot Studs				10-Foot Studs			
				Ground Snow Load (psf)											
Exp. B	Exp. C			20	30	50	70	20	30	50	70	20	30	50	70
85 mph	—	350S162	16	33	33	33	33	33	33	33	33	33	33	33	43
			24	33	33	43	43	33	43	43	43	43	43	43	54
		550S162	16	33	33	33	33	33	33	33	33	33	33	33	33
			24	33	33	33	43	33	33	33	43	33	33	33	43
90 mph	—	350S162	16	33	33	33	33	33	33	33	33	33	33	33	43
			24	33	33	43	43	33	43	43	43	43	43	43	54
		550S162	16	33	33	33	33	33	33	33	33	33	33	33	33
			24	33	33	33	43	33	33	33	43	33	33	33	43
100 mph	85 mph	350S162	16	33	33	33	33	33	33	33	33	33	33	33	43
			24	33	43	43	43	43	43	43	43	43	43	43	54
		550S162	16	33	33	33	33	33	33	33	33	33	33	33	33
			24	33	33	33	33	33	33	33	43	33	33	33	43
110 mph	90 mph	350S162	16	33	33	33	43	33	33	33	33	33	33	43	43
			24	43	43	43	43	43	43	43	43	54	54	54	54
		550S162	16	33	33	33	33	33	33	33	33	33	33	33	33
			24	33	33	33	43	33	33	33	43	43	43	43	43
—	100 mph	350S162	16	33	33	33	43	33	33	33	43	43	43	43	43
			24	43	43	43	54	43	43	54	54	54	54	54	54
		550S162	16	33	33	33	33	33	33	33	33	33	33	33	33
			24	33	33	33	43	43	43	43	43	43	43	43	43
—	110 mph	350S162	16	33	33	33	43	43	43	43	43	43	43	43	43
			24	43	43	43	54	54	54	54	54	68	68	68	68
		550S162	16	33	33	33	33	33	33	33	33	33	33	33	33
			24	43	43	43	43	43	43	43	43	43	43	43	43

For SI: 1 inch = 25.4 mm, 1 foot = 304.8 mm, 1 mil = 0.0254 mm, 1 mile per hour = 0.447 m/s, 1 pound per square foot = 0.0479kPa,
1 ksi = 1000 psi = 6.895 MPa.

a. Deflection criterion: $L/240$.
b. Design load assumptions:
    Second floor dead load is 10 psf.
    Second floor live load is 30 psf.
    Roof/ceiling dead load is 12 psf.
    Attic live load is 10 psf.
c. Building width is in the direction of horizontal framing members supported by the wall studs.

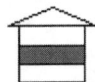

TABLE R603.3.2(13)
24-FOOT-WIDE BUILDING SUPPORTING ONE FLOOR, ROOF AND CEILING[a,b,c]
50 ksi STEEL

WIND SPEED		MEMBER SIZE	STUD SPACING (inches)	MINIMUM STUD THICKNESS (mils)											
				8-Foot Studs				9-Foot Studs				10-Foot Studs			
				Ground Snow Load (psf)											
Exp. B	Exp. C			20	30	50	70	20	30	50	70	20	30	50	70
85 mph	—	350S162	16	33	33	33	33	33	33	33	33	33	33	33	33
			24	33	33	33	43	33	33	33	43	33	33	43	43
		550S162	16	33	33	33	33	33	33	33	33	33	33	33	33
			24	33	33	33	33	33	33	33	33	33	33	33	33
90 mph	—	350S162	16	33	33	33	33	33	33	33	33	33	33	33	33
			24	33	33	33	43	33	33	33	43	33	33	43	43
		550S162	16	33	33	33	33	33	33	33	33	33	33	33	33
			24	33	33	33	33	33	33	33	33	33	33	33	33
100 mph	85 mph	350S162	16	33	33	33	33	33	33	33	33	33	33	33	33
			24	33	33	33	43	33	33	33	43	43	43	43	43
		550S162	16	33	33	33	33	33	33	33	33	33	33	33	33
			24	33	33	33	33	33	33	33	33	33	33	33	33
110 mph	90 mph	350S162	16	33	33	33	33	33	33	33	33	33	33	33	33
			24	33	33	43	43	33	33	43	43	43	43	43	43
		550S162	16	33	33	33	33	33	33	33	33	33	33	33	33
			24	33	33	33	33	33	33	33	33	33	33	33	33
—	100 mph	350S162	16	33	33	33	33	33	33	33	33	33	33	33	33
			24	33	33	43	43	43	43	43	43	43	43	43	54
		550S162	16	33	33	33	33	33	33	33	33	33	33	33	33
			24	33	33	33	43	33	33	33	33	33	33	33	43
—	110 mph	350S162	16	33	33	33	33	33	33	33	33	33	33	43	43
			24	43	43	43	43	43	43	43	43	54	54	54	54
		550S162	16	33	33	33	33	33	33	33	33	33	33	33	33
			24	33	33	33	43	33	33	33	33	33	33	33	43

For SI: 1 inch = 25.4 mm, 1 foot = 304.8 mm, 1 mil = 0.0254 mm, 1 mile per hour = 0.447 m/s, 1 pound per square foot = 0.0479 kPa,
 1 ksi = 1000 psi = 6.895 MPa.

a. Deflection criterion: $L/240$.

b. Design load assumptions:
  Second floor dead load is 10 psf.
  Second floor live load is 30 psf.
  Roof/ceiling dead load is 12 psf.
  Attic live load is 10 psf.

c. Building width is in the direction of horizontal framing members supported by the wall studs.

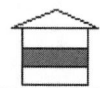

TABLE R603.3.2(14)
28-FOOT-WIDE BUILDING SUPPORTING ONE FLOOR, ROOF AND CEILING[a,b,c]
33 ksi STEEL

WIND SPEED		MEMBER SIZE	STUD SPACING (inches)	MINIMUM STUD THICKNESS (mils)											
				8-Foot Studs				9-Foot Studs				10-Foot Studs			
				Ground Snow Load (psf)											
Exp. B	Exp. C			20	30	50	70	20	30	50	70	20	30	50	70
85 mph	—	350S162	16	33	33	33	43	33	33	33	43	33	33	33	43
			24	43	43	43	54	43	43	43	54	43	43	43	54
		550S162	16	33	33	33	33	33	33	33	33	33	33	33	33
			24	33	33	43	43	33	33	43	43	33	33	43	43
90 mph	—	350S162	16	33	33	33	43	33	33	33	43	33	33	33	43
			24	43	43	43	54	43	43	43	54	43	43	43	54
		550S162	16	33	33	33	33	33	33	33	33	33	33	33	33
			24	33	33	43	43	33	33	43	43	33	33	43	43
100 mph	85 mph	350S162	16	33	33	33	43	33	33	33	43	33	33	43	43
			24	43	43	43	54	43	43	43	54	43	43	54	54
		550S162	16	33	33	33	33	33	33	33	33	33	33	33	33
			24	33	33	43	43	33	33	43	43	33	33	43	43
110 mph	90 mph	350S162	16	33	33	33	43	33	33	33	43	43	43	43	43
			24	43	43	43	54	43	43	43	54	54	54	54	54
		550S162	16	33	33	33	33	33	33	33	33	33	33	33	33
			24	33	33	43	43	33	33	43	43	43	43	43	43
—	100 mph	350S162	16	33	33	33	43	33	33	43	43	43	43	43	43
			24	43	43	43	54	54	54	54	54	54	54	54	68
		550S162	16	33	33	33	33	33	33	33	33	33	33	33	33
			24	33	33	43	43	43	43	43	43	43	43	43	43
—	110 mph	350S162	16	33	33	43	43	43	43	43	43	43	43	43	54
			24	43	43	54	54	54	54	54	54	68	68	68	68
		550S162	16	33	33	33	33	33	33	33	33	33	33	33	33
			24	43	43	43	43	43	43	43	43	43	43	43	43

For SI: 1 inch = 25.4 mm, 1 foot = 304.8 mm, 1 mil = 0.0254 mm, 1 mile per hour = 0.447 m/s, 1 pound per square foot = 0.0479 kPa,
1 ksi = 1000 psi = 6.895 MPa.

a. Deflection criterion: $L/240$.
b. Design load assumptions:
   Second floor dead load is 10 psf.
   Second floor live load is 30 psf.
   Roof/ceiling dead load is 12 psf.
   Attic live load is 10 psf.
c. Building width is in the direction of horizontal framing members supported by the wall studs.

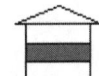

TABLE R603.3.2(15)
28-FOOT-WIDE BUILDING SUPPORTING ONE FLOOR, ROOF AND CEILING[a,b,c]
50 ksi STEEL

WIND SPEED		MEMBER SIZE	STUD SPACING (inches)	MINIMUM STUD THICKNESS (mils)											
				8-Foot Studs				9-Foot Studs				10-Foot Studs			
				Ground Snow Load (psf)											
Exp. B	Exp. C			20	30	50	70	20	30	50	70	20	30	50	70
85 mph	—	350S162	16	33	33	33	33	33	33	33	33	33	33	33	33
			24	33	33	43	43	33	33	43	43	43	43	43	54
		550S162	16	33	33	33	33	33	33	33	33	33	33	33	33
			24	33	33	33	43	33	33	33	43	33	33	33	43
90 mph	—	350S162	16	33	33	33	33	33	33	33	33	33	33	33	33
			24	33	33	43	43	33	33	43	43	43	43	43	54
		550S162	16	33	33	33	33	33	33	33	33	33	33	33	33
			24	33	33	33	43	33	33	33	43	33	33	33	43
100 mph	85 mph	350S162	16	33	33	33	33	33	33	33	33	33	33	33	43
			24	33	33	43	43	33	33	43	43	43	43	43	54
		550S162	16	33	33	33	33	33	33	33	33	33	33	33	33
			24	33	33	33	43	33	33	33	43	33	33	33	43
110 mph	90 mph	350S162	16	33	33	33	33	33	33	33	33	33	33	33	43
			24	33	33	43	43	43	43	43	43	43	43	43	54
		550S162	16	33	33	33	33	33	33	33	33	33	33	33	33
			24	33	33	33	43	33	33	33	43	33	33	33	43
—	100 mph	350S162	16	33	33	33	33	33	33	33	33	33	33	33	43
			24	43	43	43	54	43	43	43	43	43	43	54	54
		550S162	16	33	33	33	33	33	33	33	33	33	33	33	33
			24	33	33	33	43	33	33	33	43	33	33	33	43
—	110 mph	350S162	16	33	33	33	43	33	33	33	33	43	43	43	43
			24	43	43	43	54	43	43	43	43	54	54	54	54
		550S162	16	33	33	33	33	33	33	33	33	33	33	33	33
			24	33	33	33	43	33	33	33	43	33	33	33	43

For SI: 1 inch = 25.4 mm, 1 foot = 304.8 mm, 1 mil = 0.0254 mm, 1 mile per hour = 0.447 m/s, 1 pound per square foot = 0.0479kPa, 1 ksi = 1000 psi = 6.895 MPa.

a. Deflection criterion: $L/240$.
b. Design load assumptions:
  Second floor dead load is 10 psf.
  Second floor live load is 30 psf.
  Roof/ceiling dead load is 12 psf.
  Attic live load is 10 psf.
c. Building width is in the direction of horizontal framing members supported by the wall studs.

TABLE R603.3.2(16)
32-FOOT-WIDE BUILDING SUPPORTING ONE FLOOR, ROOF AND CEILING[a,b,c]
33 ksi STEEL

WIND SPEED		MEMBER SIZE	STUD SPACING (inches)	MINIMUM STUD THICKNESS (mils)											
				8-Foot Studs				9-Foot Studs				10-Foot Studs			
				Ground Snow Load (psf)											
Exp. B	Exp. C			20	30	50	70	20	30	50	70	20	30	50	70
85 mph	—	350S162	16	33	33	33	43	33	33	33	43	33	33	43	43
			24	43	43	43	54	43	43	43	54	43	43	54	54
		550S162	16	33	33	33	43	33	33	33	33	33	33	33	43
			24	33	43	43	54	33	33	43	43	33	33	43	43
90 mph	—	350S162	16	33	33	33	43	33	33	33	43	33	33	43	43
			24	43	43	43	54	43	43	43	54	43	43	54	54
		550S162	16	33	33	33	43	33	33	33	33	33	33	33	43
			24	33	43	43	54	33	33	43	43	33	33	43	43
100 mph	85 mph	350S162	16	33	33	33	43	33	33	33	43	33	43	43	43
			24	43	43	43	54	43	43	43	54	54	54	54	68
		550S162	16	33	33	33	43	33	33	33	33	33	33	33	43
			24	33	43	43	54	33	33	43	43	33	33	43	43
110 mph	90 mph	350S162	16	33	33	43	43	33	33	33	43	43	43	43	43
			24	43	43	54	54	43	43	54	54	54	54	54	68
		550S162	16	33	33	33	43	33	33	33	33	33	33	33	43
			24	33	43	43	54	33	33	43	43	43	43	43	54
—	100 mph	350S162	16	33	33	43	43	43	43	43	43	43	43	43	43
			24	43	43	54	54	54	54	54	54	54	54	54	54
		550S162	16	33	33	33	43	33	33	33	33	33	33	33	43
			24	33	43	43	54	43	43	43	43	43	43	43	54
—	110 mph	350S162	16	43	43	43	43	43	43	43	43	43	43	54	54
			24	54	54	54	68	54	54	54	68	68	68	68	68
		550S162	16	33	33	33	43	33	33	33	43	33	33	33	43
			24	43	43	43	54	43	43	43	43	43	43	43	54

For SI: 1 inch = 25.4 mm, 1 foot = 304.8 mm, 1 mil = 0.0254 mm, 1 mile per hour = 0.447 m/s, 1 pound per square foot = 0.0479kPa,
  1 ksi = 1000 psi = 6.895 MPa.

a. Deflection criterion: $L/240$.
b. Design load assumptions:
   Second floor dead load is 10 psf.
   Second floor live load is 30 psf.
   Roof/ceiling dead load is 12 psf.
   Attic live load is 10 psf.
c. Building width is in the direction of horizontal framing members supported by the wall studs.

TABLE R603.3.2(17)
32-FOOT-WIDE BUILDING SUPPORTING ONE FLOOR, ROOF AND CEILING[a,b,c]
50 ksi STEEL

WIND SPEED Exp. B	Exp. C	MEMBER SIZE	STUD SPACING (inches)	8-Foot Studs 20	30	50	70	9-Foot Studs 20	30	50	70	10-Foot Studs 20	30	50	70
85 mph	—	350S162	16	33	33	33	43	33	33	33	33	33	33	33	43
			24	33	33	43	54	33	33	43	43	43	43	43	54
		550S162	16	33	33	33	33	33	33	33	33	33	33	33	33
			24	33	33	43	43	33	33	33	43	33	33	33	43
90 mph	—	350S162	16	33	33	33	43	33	33	33	33	33	33	33	43
			24	33	33	43	54	33	33	43	43	43	43	43	54
		550S162	16	33	33	33	33	33	33	33	33	33	33	33	33
			24	33	33	43	43	33	33	33	43	33	33	33	43
100 mph	85 mph	350S162	16	33	33	33	43	33	33	33	33	33	33	33	43
			24	33	33	43	54	33	33	43	43	43	43	43	54
		550S162	16	33	33	33	33	33	33	33	33	33	33	33	33
			24	33	33	43	43	33	33	33	43	33	33	33	43
110 mph	90 mph	350S162	16	33	33	33	43	33	33	33	33	33	33	33	43
			24	43	43	43	54	43	43	43	54	43	43	54	54
		550S162	16	33	33	33	33	33	33	33	33	33	33	33	33
			24	33	33	43	43	33	33	33	43	33	33	33	43
—	100 mph	350S162	16	33	33	33	43	33	33	33	43	33	33	43	43
			24	43	43	43	54	43	43	43	54	54	54	54	54
		550S162	16	33	33	33	33	33	33	33	33	33	33	33	33
			24	33	33	43	43	33	33	33	43	33	33	43	43
—	110 mph	350S162	16	33	33	33	43	33	33	33	43	43	43	43	43
			24	43	43	43	54	43	43	43	54	54	54	54	54
		550S162	16	33	33	33	33	33	33	33	33	33	33	33	33
			24	33	33	43	43	33	33	33	43	33	33	43	43

For SI: 1 inch = 25.4 mm, 1 foot = 304.8 mm, 1 mil = 0.0254 mm, 1 mile per hour = 0.447 m/s, 1 pound per square foot = 0.0479 kPa, 1 ksi = 1000 psi = 6.895 MPa.

a. Deflection criterion: $L/240$.
b. Design load assumptions:
   Second floor dead load is 10 psf.
   Second floor live load is 30 psf.
   Roof/ceiling dead load is 12 psf.
   Attic live load is 10 psf.
c. Building width is in the direction of horizontal framing members supported by the wall studs.

TABLE R603.3.2(18)
36-FOOT-WIDE BUILDING SUPPORTING ONE FLOOR, ROOF AND CEILING[a,b,c]
33 ksi STEEL

WIND SPEED		MEMBER SIZE	STUD SPACING (inches)	MINIMUM STUD THICKNESS (mils)											
				8-Foot Studs				9-Foot Studs				10-Foot Studs			
				Ground Snow Load (psf)											
Exp. B	Exp. C			20	30	50	70	20	30	50	70	20	30	50	70
85 mph	—	350S162	16	33	33	43	43	33	33	43	43	33	33	43	43
			24	43	43	54	54	43	43	54	54	54	54	54	68
		550S162	16	33	33	33	43	33	33	33	43	33	33	33	43
			24	43	43	43	54	43	43	43	54	43	43	43	54
90 mph	—	350S162	16	33	33	43	43	33	33	43	43	33	33	43	43
			24	43	43	54	54	43	43	54	54	54	54	54	68
		550S162	16	33	33	33	43	33	33	33	43	33	33	33	43
			24	43	43	43	54	43	43	43	54	43	43	43	54
100 mph	85 mph	350S162	16	33	33	43	43	33	33	43	43	43	43	43	43
			24	43	43	54	68	43	43	54	54	54	54	54	68
		550S162	16	33	33	33	43	33	33	33	43	33	33	33	43
			24	43	43	43	54	43	43	43	54	43	43	43	54
110 mph	90 mph	350S162	16	33	33	43	43	33	33	43	43	43	43	43	54
			24	43	43	54	68	54	54	54	54	54	54	54	68
		550S162	16	33	33	33	43	33	33	33	43	33	33	33	43
			24	43	43	43	54	43	43	43	54	43	43	43	54
—	100 mph	350S162	16	33	33	43	43	43	43	43	43	43	43	43	54
			24	54	54	54	68	54	54	54	68	54	68	68	68
		550S162	16	33	33	33	43	33	33	33	43	33	33	33	43
			24	43	43	43	54	43	43	43	54	43	43	43	54
—	110 mph	350S162	16	43	43	43	43	43	43	43	43	43	54	54	54
			24	54	54	54	68	54	54	54	68	68	68	68	68
		550S162	16	33	33	33	43	33	33	33	43	33	33	33	43
			24	43	43	43	54	43	43	43	54	43	43	43	54

For SI: 1 inch = 25.4 mm, 1 foot = 304.8 mm, 1 mil = 0.0254 mm, 1 mile per hour = 0.447 m/s, 1 pound per square foot = 0.0479kPa,
1 ksi = 1000 psi = 6.895 MPa.

a. Deflection criterion: *L*/240.
b. Design load assumptions:
   Second floor dead load is 10 psf.
   Second floor live load is 30 psf.
   Roof/ceiling dead load is 12 psf.
   Attic live load is 10 psf.
c. Building width is in the direction of horizontal framing members supported by the wall studs.

TABLE R603.3.2(19)
36-FOOT-WIDE BUILDING SUPPORTING ONE FLOOR, ROOF AND CEILING[a,b,c]
50 ksi STEEL

WIND SPEED		MEMBER SIZE	STUD SPACING (inches)	MINIMUM STUD THICKNESS (mils)											
				8-Foot Studs				9-Foot Studs				10-Foot Studs			
				Ground Snow Load (psf)											
Exp. B	Exp. C			20	30	50	70	20	30	50	70	20	30	50	70
85 mph	—	350S162	16	33	33	33	43	33	33	33	43	33	33	33	43
			24	43	43	43	54	33	33	43	54	43	43	43	54
		550S162	16	33	33	33	33	33	33	33	33	33	33	33	33
			24	33	33	43	43	33	33	43	43	33	33	43	43
90 mph	—	350S162	16	33	33	33	43	33	33	33	43	33	33	33	43
			24	43	43	43	54	33	33	43	54	43	43	43	54
		550S162	16	33	33	33	33	33	33	33	33	33	33	33	33
			24	33	33	43	43	33	33	43	43	33	33	43	43
100 mph	85 mph	350S162	16	33	33	33	43	33	33	33	43	33	33	33	43
			24	43	43	43	54	43	43	43	54	43	43	54	54
		550S162	16	33	33	33	33	33	33	33	33	33	33	33	33
			24	33	33	43	43	33	33	43	43	33	33	43	43
110 mph	90 mph	350S162	16	33	33	33	43	33	33	33	43	33	33	43	43
			24	43	43	43	54	43	43	43	54	43	43	54	54
		550S162	16	33	33	33	33	33	33	33	33	33	33	33	33
			24	33	33	43	43	33	33	43	43	33	33	43	43
—	100 mph	350S162	16	33	33	33	43	33	33	33	43	43	43	43	43
			24	43	43	43	54	43	43	43	54	54	54	54	68
		550S162	16	33	33	33	33	33	33	33	33	33	33	33	33
			24	33	33	43	43	33	33	43	43	33	33	43	43
—	110 mph	350S162	16	33	33	43	43	33	33	33	43	43	43	43	43
			24	43	43	54	54	43	43	54	54	54	54	54	68
		550S162	16	33	33	33	33	33	33	33	33	33	33	33	33
			24	33	33	43	43	33	33	43	43	43	43	43	43

For SI: 1 inch = 25.4 mm, 1 foot = 304.8 mm, 1 mil = 0.0254 mm, 1 mile per hour = 0.447 m/s, 1 pound per square foot = 0.0479kPa,
1 ksi = 1000 psi = 6.895 MPa.

a. Deflection criterion: $L/240$.

b. Design load assumptions:
Second floor dead load is 10 psf.
Second floor live load is 30 psf.
Roof/ceiling dead load is 12 psf.
Attic live load is 10 psf.

c. Building width is in the direction of horizontal framing members supported by the wall studs.

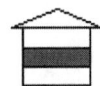

TABLE R603.3.2(20)
40-FOOT-WIDE BUILDING SUPPORTING ONE FLOOR, ROOF AND CEILING[a,b,c]
33 ksi STEEL

WIND SPEED		MEMBER SIZE	STUD SPACING (inches)	MINIMUM STUD THICKNESS (mils)											
				8-Foot Studs				9-Foot Studs				10-Foot Studs			
				Ground Snow Load (psf)											
Exp. B	Exp. C			20	30	50	70	20	30	50	70	20	30	50	70
85 mph	—	350S162	16	33	33	43	43	33	33	43	43	43	43	43	54
			24	43	43	54	68	43	43	54	68	54	54	54	68
		550S162	16	33	33	33	43	33	33	33	43	33	33	33	43
			24	43	43	54	54	43	43	43	54	43	43	43	54
90 mph	—	350S162	16	33	33	43	43	33	33	43	43	43	43	43	54
			24	43	43	54	68	43	43	54	68	54	54	54	68
		550S162	16	33	33	33	43	33	33	33	43	33	33	33	43
			24	43	43	54	54	43	43	43	54	43	43	43	54
100 mph	85 mph	350S162	16	33	33	43	43	33	33	43	43	43	43	43	54
			24	43	43	54	68	43	43	54	68	54	54	54	68
		550S162	16	33	33	33	43	33	33	33	43	33	33	33	43
			24	43	43	54	54	43	43	43	54	43	43	43	54
110 mph	90 mph	350S162	16	33	33	43	43	43	43	43	43	43	43	43	54
			24	43	43	54	68	54	54	54	68	54	54	68	68
		550S162	16	33	33	43	43	33	33	33	43	33	33	33	43
			24	43	43	54	54	43	43	43	54	43	43	43	54
—	100 mph	350S162	16	43	43	43	54	43	43	43	54	43	43	54	54
			24	54	54	54	68	54	54	54	68	68	68	68	97
		550S162	16	33	33	43	43	33	33	33	43	33	33	43	43
			24	43	43	54	54	43	43	43	54	43	43	54	54
—	110 mph	350S162	16	43	43	43	54	43	43	43	54	54	54	54	54
			24	54	54	54	68	54	54	68	68	68	68	68	97
		550S162	16	33	33	43	43	33	33	33	43	33	33	43	43
			24	43	43	54	54	43	43	43	54	43	43	54	54

For SI: 1 inch = 25.4 mm, 1 foot = 304.8 mm, 1 mil = 0.0254 mm, 1 mile per hour = 0.447 m/s, 1 pound per square foot = 0.0479kPa, 1 ksi = 1000 psi = 6.895 MPa.

a. Deflection criterion: L/240.
b. Design load assumptions:
   Second floor dead load is 10 psf.
   Second floor live load is 30 psf.
   Roof/ceiling dead load is 12 psf.
   Attic live load is 10 psf.
c. Building width is in the direction of horizontal framing members supported by the wall studs.

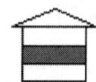

TABLE R603.3.2(21)
40-FOOT-WIDE BUILDING SUPPORTING ONE FLOOR, ROOF AND CEILING[a,b,c]
50 ksi STEEL

WIND SPEED		MEMBER SIZE	STUD SPACING (inches)	MINIMUM STUD THICKNESS (mils)											
				8-Foot Studs				9-Foot Studs				10-Foot Studs			
				Ground Snow Load (psf)											
Exp. B	Exp. C			20	30	50	70	20	30	50	70	20	30	50	70
85 mph	—	350S162	16	33	33	33	43	33	33	33	43	33	33	43	43
			24	43	43	43	54	43	43	43	54	43	43	54	54
		550S162	16	33	33	33	43	33	33	33	33	33	33	33	33
			24	33	43	43	54	33	33	43	43	33	33	43	43
90 mph	—	350S162	16	33	33	33	43	33	33	33	43	33	33	43	43
			24	43	43	43	54	43	43	43	54	43	43	54	54
		550S162	16	33	33	33	43	33	33	33	33	33	33	33	33
			24	33	43	43	54	33	33	43	43	33	33	43	43
100 mph	85 mph	350S162	16	33	33	33	43	33	33	33	43	33	33	43	43
			24	43	43	54	54	43	43	43	54	43	43	54	68
		550S162	16	33	33	33	43	33	33	33	33	33	33	33	33
			24	33	43	43	54	33	33	43	43	33	33	43	43
110 mph	90 mph	350S162	16	33	33	43	43	33	33	33	43	33	33	43	43
			24	43	43	54	54	43	43	43	54	54	54	54	68
		550S162	16	33	33	33	43	33	33	33	33	33	33	33	43
			24	33	43	43	54	33	33	43	43	33	33	43	43
—	100 mph	350S162	16	33	33	43	43	33	33	33	43	43	43	43	43
			24	43	43	54	54	43	43	54	54	54	54	54	68
		550S162	16	33	33	33	43	33	33	33	33	33	33	33	43
			24	33	43	43	54	33	33	43	43	33	43	43	43
—	110 mph	350S162	16	33	33	43	43	33	33	43	43	43	43	43	54
			24	43	43	54	68	54	54	54	54	54	54	54	68
		550S162	16	33	33	33	43	33	33	33	33	33	33	33	43
			24	33	43	43	54	33	33	43	43	43	43	43	54

For SI: 1 inch = 25.4 mm, 1 foot = 304.8 mm, 1 mil = 0.0254 mm, 1 mile per hour = 0.447 m/s, 1 pound per square foot = 0.0479 kPa, 1 ksi = 1000 psi = 6.895 MPa.

a. Deflection criterion: $L/240$.
b. Design load assumptions:
   Second floor dead load is 10 psf.
   Second floor live load is 30 psf.
   Roof/ceiling dead load is 12 psf.
   Attic live load is 10 psf.
c. Building width is in the direction of horizontal framing members supported by the wall studs.

TABLE R603.3.2(22)
24-FOOT-WIDE BUILDING SUPPORTING TWO FLOORS, ROOF AND CEILING[a,b,c]
33 ksi STEEL

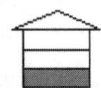

WIND SPEED		MEMBER SIZE	STUD SPACING (inches)	MINIMUM STUD THICKNESS (mils)											
				8-Foot Studs				9-Foot Studs				10-Foot Studs			
				Ground Snow Load (psf)											
Exp. B	Exp. C			20	30	50	70	20	30	50	70	20	30	50	70
85 mph	—	350S162	16	43	43	43	43	33	33	33	43	43	43	43	43
			24	54	54	54	54	43	43	54	54	54	54	54	54
		550S162	16	33	33	43	43	33	33	33	33	33	33	33	43
			24	43	43	54	54	43	43	43	43	43	43	43	54
90 mph	—	350S162	16	43	43	43	43	33	33	33	43	43	43	43	43
			24	54	54	54	54	43	43	54	54	54	54	54	54
		550S162	16	33	33	43	43	33	33	33	33	33	33	33	43
			24	43	43	54	54	43	43	43	43	43	43	43	54
100 mph	85 mph	350S162	16	43	43	43	43	33	33	33	43	43	43	43	43
			24	54	54	54	54	54	54	54	54	54	54	54	68
		550S162	16	33	33	43	43	33	33	33	33	33	33	33	43
			24	43	43	54	54	43	43	43	43	43	43	43	54
110 mph	90 mph	350S162	16	43	43	43	43	43	43	43	43	43	43	43	43
			24	54	54	54	54	54	54	54	54	54	54	68	68
		550S162	16	33	33	43	43	33	33	33	33	33	33	33	43
			24	43	43	54	54	43	43	43	43	43	43	43	54
—	100 mph	350S162	16	43	43	43	43	43	43	43	43	43	43	43	54
			24	54	54	54	54	54	54	54	54	68	68	68	68
		550S162	16	33	33	43	43	33	33	33	33	33	33	33	43
			24	43	43	54	54	43	43	43	43	43	43	43	54
—	110 mph	350S162	16	43	43	43	43	43	43	43	43	54	54	54	54
			24	54	54	54	68	54	54	68	68	68	68	68	97
		550S162	16	33	33	43	43	33	33	33	33	33	33	33	43
			24	43	43	54	54	43	43	43	43	43	43	43	54

For SI: 1 inch = 25.4 mm, 1 foot = 304.8 mm, 1 mil = 0.0254 mm, 1 mile per hour = 0.447 m/s, 1 pound per square foot = 0.0479kPa,
1 ksi = 1000 psi = 6.895 MPa.

a. Deflection criterion: $L/240$.

b. Design load assumptions:
   Top and middle floor dead load is 10 psf.
   Top floor live load is 30 psf.
   Middle floor live load is 40 psf.
   Roof/ceiling dead load is 12 psf.
   Attic live load is 10 psf.

c. Building width is in the direction of horizontal framing members supported by the wall studs.

2009 INTERNATIONAL RESIDENTIAL CODE®

TABLE R603.3.2(23)
24-FOOT-WIDE BUILDING SUPPORTING TWO FLOORS, ROOF AND CEILING[a,b,c]
50 ksi STEEL

WIND SPEED		MEMBER SIZE	STUD SPACING (inches)	MINIMUM STUD THICKNESS (mils)											
				8-Foot Studs				9-Foot Studs				10-Foot Studs			
				Ground Snow Load (psf)											
Exp. B	Exp. C			20	30	50	70	20	30	50	70	20	30	50	70
85 mph	—	350S162	16	33	33	33	43	33	33	33	33	33	33	33	33
			24	43	43	54	54	43	43	43	43	43	43	43	54
		550S162	16	33	33	33	33	33	33	33	33	33	33	33	33
			24	43	43	43	43	43	43	43	43	43	43	43	43
90 mph	—	350S162	16	33	33	33	43	33	33	33	33	33	33	33	33
			24	43	43	54	54	43	43	43	43	43	43	43	54
		550S162	16	33	33	33	33	33	33	33	33	33	33	33	33
			24	43	43	43	43	43	43	43	43	43	43	43	43
100 mph	85 mph	350S162	16	33	33	33	43	33	33	33	33	33	33	33	33
			24	43	43	54	54	43	43	43	43	43	43	54	54
		550S162	16	33	33	33	33	33	33	33	33	33	33	33	33
			24	43	43	43	43	43	43	43	43	43	43	43	43
110 mph	90 mph	350S162	16	33	33	33	43	33	33	33	33	33	33	43	43
			24	43	43	54	54	43	43	43	43	54	54	54	54
		550S162	16	33	33	33	33	33	33	33	33	33	33	33	33
			24	43	43	43	43	43	43	43	43	43	43	43	43
—	100 mph	350S162	16	33	33	33	43	33	33	33	33	43	43	43	43
			24	43	43	54	54	43	43	54	54	54	54	54	54
		550S162	16	33	33	33	33	33	33	33	33	33	33	33	33
			24	43	43	43	43	43	43	43	43	43	43	43	43
—	110 mph	350S162	16	33	33	33	43	33	33	33	43	43	43	43	43
			24	54	54	54	54	54	54	54	54	54	54	54	68
		550S162	16	33	33	33	33	33	33	33	33	33	33	33	33
			24	43	43	43	43	43	43	43	43	43	43	43	43

For SI: 1 inch = 25.4 mm, 1 foot = 304.8 mm, 1 mil = 0.0254 mm, 1 mile per hour = 0.447 m/s, 1 pound per square foot = 0.0479kPa, 1 ksi = 1000 psi = 6.895 MPa.

a. Deflection criterion: $L/240$.

b. Design load assumptions:
    Top and middle floor dead load is 10 psf.
    Top floor live load is 30 psf.
    Middle floor live load is 40 psf.
    Attic live load is 10 psf.

c. Building width is in the direction of horizontal framing members supported by the wall studs.

TABLE R603.3.2(24)
28-FOOT-WIDE BUILDING SUPPORTING TWO FLOORS, ROOF AND CEILING[a,b,c]
33 ksi STEEL

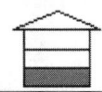

WIND SPEED		MEMBER SIZE	STUD SPACING (inches)	MINIMUM STUD THICKNESS (mils)											
				8-Foot Studs				9-Foot Studs				10-Foot Studs			
				Ground Snow Load (psf)											
Exp. B	Exp. C			20	30	50	70	20	30	50	70	20	30	50	70
85 mph	—	350S162	16	43	43	43	43	43	43	43	43	43	43	43	43
			24	54	54	54	68	54	54	54	54	54	54	54	68
		550S162	16	43	43	43	43	43	43	43	43	43	43	43	43
			24	54	54	54	54	54	54	54	54	54	54	54	54
90 mph	—	350S162	16	43	43	43	43	43	43	43	43	43	43	43	43
			24	54	54	54	68	54	54	54	54	54	54	54	68
		550S162	16	43	43	43	43	43	43	43	43	43	43	43	43
			24	54	54	54	54	54	54	54	54	54	54	54	54
100 mph	85 mph	350S162	16	43	43	43	43	43	43	43	43	43	43	43	43
			24	54	54	54	68	54	54	54	54	54	54	68	68
		550S162	16	43	43	43	43	43	43	43	43	43	43	43	43
			24	54	54	54	54	54	54	54	54	54	54	54	54
110 mph	90 mph	350S162	16	43	43	43	43	43	43	43	43	43	43	43	43
			24	54	54	54	68	54	54	54	54	68	68	68	68
		550S162	16	43	43	43	43	43	43	43	43	43	43	43	43
			24	54	54	54	54	54	54	54	54	54	54	54	54
—	100 mph	350S162	16	43	43	43	43	43	43	43	43	43	43	54	54
			24	54	54	54	68	54	54	68	68	68	68	68	97
		550S162	16	43	43	43	43	43	43	43	43	43	43	43	43
			24	54	54	54	54	54	54	54	54	54	54	54	54
—	110 mph	350S162	16	43	43	43	43	43	43	43	43	54	54	54	54
			24	54	68	68	68	68	68	68	68	68	68	97	97
		550S162	16	43	43	43	43	43	43	43	43	43	43	43	43
			24	54	54	54	54	54	54	54	54	54	54	54	54

For SI: 1 inch = 25.4 mm, 1 foot = 304.8 mm, 1 mil = 0.0254 mm, 1 mile per hour = 0.447 m/s, 1 pound per square foot = 0.0479kPa,
1 ksi = 1000 psi = 6.895 MPa.

a. Deflection criterion: $L/240$.
b. Design load assumptions:
Top and middle floor dead load is 10 psf.
Top floor live load is 30 psf.
Middle floor live load is 40 psf.
Roof/ceiling dead load is 12 psf.
Attic live load is 10 psf.
c. Building width is in the direction of horizontal framing members supported by the wall studs.

TABLE R603.3.2(25)
28-FOOT-WIDE BUILDING SUPPORTING TWO FLOORS, ROOF AND CEILING[a,b,c]
50 ksi STEEL

WIND SPEED		MEMBER SIZE	STUD SPACING (inches)	MINIMUM STUD THICKNESS (mils)											
				8-Foot Studs				9-Foot Studs				10-Foot Studs			
				Ground Snow Load (psf)											
Exp. B	Exp. C			20	30	50	70	20	30	50	70	20	30	50	70
85 mph	—	350S162	16	43	43	43	43	33	33	33	43	43	43	43	43
			24	54	54	54	54	43	43	54	54	54	54	54	54
		550S162	16	33	33	33	43	33	33	33	33	33	33	33	33
			24	43	43	43	54	43	43	43	43	43	43	43	43
90 mph	—	350S162	16	43	43	43	43	33	33	33	43	43	43	43	43
			24	54	54	54	54	43	43	54	54	54	54	54	54
		550S162	16	33	33	33	43	33	33	33	33	33	33	33	33
			24	43	43	43	54	43	43	43	43	43	43	43	43
100 mph	85 mph	350S162	16	43	43	43	43	33	33	33	43	43	43	43	43
			24	54	54	54	54	43	43	54	54	54	54	54	54
		550S162	16	33	33	33	43	33	33	33	33	33	33	33	33
			24	43	43	43	54	43	43	43	43	43	43	43	43
110 mph	90 mph	350S162	16	43	43	43	43	33	33	33	43	43	43	43	43
			24	54	54	54	54	43	43	54	54	54	54	54	54
		550S162	16	33	33	33	43	33	33	33	33	33	33	33	33
			24	43	43	43	54	43	43	43	43	43	43	43	43
—	100 mph	350S162	16	43	43	43	43	33	33	33	43	43	43	43	43
			24	54	54	54	54	54	54	54	54	54	54	54	68
		550S162	16	33	33	33	43	33	33	33	33	33	33	33	33
			24	43	43	43	54	43	43	43	43	43	43	43	43
—	110 mph	350S162	16	43	43	43	43	43	43	43	43	43	43	43	43
			24	54	54	54	54	54	54	54	54	68	68	68	68
		550S162	16	33	33	33	43	33	33	33	33	33	33	33	33
			24	43	43	43	54	43	43	43	43	43	43	43	43

For SI: 1 inch = 25.4 mm, 1 foot = 304.8 mm, 1 mil = 0.0254 mm, 1 mile per hour = 0.447 m/s, 1 pound per square foot = 0.0479kPa, 1 ksi = 1000 psi = 6.895 MPa.

a. Deflection criterion: $L/240$.
b. Design load assumptions:
   Top and middle floor dead load is 10 psf.
   Top floor live load is 30 psf.
   Middle floor live load is 40 psf.
   Roof/ceiling dead load is 12 psf.
   Attic live load is 10 psf.
c. Building width is in the direction of horizontal framing members supported by the wall studs.

TABLE R603.3.2(26)
32-FOOT-WIDE BUILDING SUPPORTING TWO FLOORS, ROOF AND CEILING[a,b,c]
33 ksi STEEL

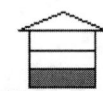

WIND SPEED		MEMBER SIZE	STUD SPACING (inches)	MINIMUM STUD THICKNESS (mils)											
				8-Foot Studs				9-Foot Studs				10-Foot Studs			
				Ground Snow Load (psf)											
Exp. B	Exp. C			20	30	50	70	20	30	50	70	20	30	50	70
85 mph	—	350S162	16	43	43	43	54	43	43	43	43	43	43	43	54
			24	68	68	68	68	54	54	68	68	68	68	68	68
		550S162	16	43	43	43	43	43	43	43	43	43	43	43	43
			24	54	54	54	68	54	54	54	54	54	54	54	54
90 mph	—	350S162	16	43	43	43	54	43	43	43	43	43	43	43	54
			24	68	68	68	68	54	54	68	68	68	68	68	68
		550S162	16	43	43	43	43	43	43	43	43	43	43	43	43
			24	54	54	54	68	54	54	54	54	54	54	54	54
100 mph	85 mph	350S162	16	43	43	43	54	43	43	43	43	43	43	43	54
			24	68	68	68	68	54	54	68	68	68	68	68	68
		550S162	16	43	43	43	43	43	43	43	43	43	43	43	43
			24	54	54	54	68	54	54	54	54	54	54	54	54
110 mph	90 mph	350S162	16	43	43	43	54	43	43	43	43	43	43	54	54
			24	68	68	68	68	54	54	68	68	68	68	68	68
		550S162	16	43	43	43	43	43	43	43	43	43	43	43	43
			24	54	54	54	68	54	54	54	54	54	54	54	54
—	100 mph	350S162	16	43	43	43	54	43	43	43	43	54	54	54	54
			24	68	68	68	68	68	68	68	68	68	68	97	97
		550S162	16	43	43	43	43	43	43	43	43	43	43	43	43
			24	54	54	54	68	54	54	54	54	54	54	54	54
—	110 mph	350S162	16	43	43	43	54	43	43	54	54	54	54	54	54
			24	68	68	68	68	68	68	68	68	97	97	97	97
		550S162	16	43	43	43	43	43	43	43	43	43	43	43	43
			24	54	54	54	68	54	54	54	54	54	54	54	54

For SI: 1 inch = 25.4 mm, 1 foot = 304.8 mm, 1 mil = 0.0254 mm, 1 mile per hour = 0.447 m/s, 1 pound per square foot = 0.0479kPa, 1 ksi = 1000 psi = 6.895 MPa.

a. Deflection criterion: $L/240$.

b. Design load assumptions:
    Top and middle floor dead load is 10 psf.
    Top floor live load is 30 psf.
    Middle floor live load is 40 psf.
    Roof/ceiling dead load is 12 psf.
    Attic live load is 10 psf.

c. Building width is in the direction of horizontal framing members supported by the wall studs.

TABLE R603.3.2(27)
32-FOOT-WIDE BUILDING SUPPORTING TWO FLOORS, ROOF AND CEILING[a,b,c]
50 ksi STEEL

WIND SPEED Exp. B	WIND SPEED Exp. C	MEMBER SIZE	STUD SPACING (inches)	8-Foot Studs 20	30	50	70	9-Foot Studs 20	30	50	70	10-Foot Studs 20	30	50	70
85 mph	—	350S162	16	43	43	43	43	43	43	43	43	43	43	43	43
			24	54	54	54	68	54	54	54	54	54	54	54	68
		550S162	16	43	43	43	43	33	33	33	43	33	33	43	43
			24	54	54	54	54	43	43	43	54	43	43	54	54
90 mph	—	350S162	16	43	43	43	43	43	43	43	43	43	43	43	43
			24	54	54	54	68	54	54	54	54	54	54	54	68
		550S162	16	43	43	43	43	33	33	33	43	33	33	43	43
			24	54	54	54	54	43	43	43	54	43	43	54	54
100 mph	85 mph	350S162	16	43	43	43	43	43	43	43	43	43	43	43	43
			24	54	54	54	68	54	54	54	54	54	54	54	68
		550S162	16	43	43	43	43	33	33	33	43	33	33	43	43
			24	54	54	54	54	43	43	43	54	43	43	54	54
110 mph	90 mph	350S162	16	43	43	43	43	43	43	43	43	43	43	43	43
			24	54	54	54	68	54	54	54	54	54	54	54	68
		550S162	16	43	43	43	43	33	33	33	43	33	33	43	43
			24	54	54	54	54	43	43	43	54	43	43	54	54
—	100 mph	350S162	16	43	43	43	43	43	43	43	43	43	43	43	43
			24	54	54	54	68	54	54	54	54	68	68	68	68
		550S162	16	43	43	43	43	33	33	33	43	33	33	43	43
			24	54	54	54	54	43	43	43	54	43	43	54	54
—	110 mph	350S162	16	43	43	43	43	43	43	43	43	43	43	43	54
			24	54	54	54	68	54	54	54	54	68	68	68	68
		550S162	16	43	43	43	43	33	33	33	43	33	33	43	43
			24	54	54	54	54	43	43	43	54	43	43	54	54

For SI: 1 inch = 25.4 mm, 1 foot = 304.8 mm, 1 mil = 0.0254 mm, 1 mile per hour = 0.447 m/s, 1 pound per square foot = 0.0479 kPa, 1 ksi = 1000 psi = 6.895 MPa.

a. Deflection criterion: L/240.
b. Design load assumptions:
   Top and middle floor dead load is 10 psf.
   Top floor live load is 30 psf.
   Middle floor live load is 40 psf.
   Roof/ceiling dead load is 12 psf.
   Attic live load is 10 psf.
c. Building width is in the direction of horizontal framing members supported by the wall studs.

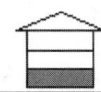

TABLE R603.3.2(28)
36-FOOT-WIDE BUILDING SUPPORTING TWO FLOORS, ROOF AND CEILING[a,b,c]
33 ksi STEEL

WIND SPEED		MEMBER SIZE	STUD SPACING (inches)	MINIMUM STUD THICKNESS (mils)											
				8-Foot Studs				9-Foot Studs				10-Foot Studs			
				Ground Snow Load (psf)											
Exp. B	Exp. C			20	30	50	70	20	30	50	70	20	30	50	70
85 mph	—	350S162	16	54	54	54	54	43	43	43	54	54	54	54	54
			24	68	68	68	97	68	68	68	68	68	68	68	97
		550S162	16	43	43	43	54	43	43	43	43	43	43	43	43
			24	68	68	68	68	54	54	54	68	54	54	68	68
90 mph	—	350S162	16	54	54	54	54	43	43	43	54	54	54	54	54
			24	68	68	68	97	68	68	68	68	68	68	68	97
		550S162	16	43	43	43	54	43	43	43	43	43	43	43	43
			24	68	68	68	68	54	54	54	68	54	54	68	68
100 mph	85 mph	350S162	16	54	54	54	54	43	43	43	54	54	54	54	54
			24	68	68	68	97	68	68	68	68	68	68	68	97
		550S162	16	43	43	43	54	43	43	43	43	43	43	43	43
			24	68	68	68	68	54	54	54	68	54	54	68	68
110 mph	90 mph	350S162	16	54	54	54	54	43	43	43	54	54	54	54	54
			24	68	68	68	97	68	68	68	68	68	68	97	97
		550S162	16	43	43	43	54	43	43	43	43	43	43	43	43
			24	68	68	68	68	54	54	54	68	54	54	68	68
—	100 mph	350S162	16	54	54	54	54	43	43	54	54	54	54	54	54
			24	68	68	68	97	68	68	68	68	97	97	97	97
		550S162	16	43	43	43	54	43	43	43	43	43	43	43	43
			24	68	68	68	68	54	54	54	68	54	54	68	68
—	110 mph	350S162	16	54	54	54	54	54	54	54	54	54	54	54	68
			24	68	68	68	97	68	68	68	97	97	97	97	97
		550S162	16	43	43	43	54	43	43	43	43	43	43	43	43
			24	68	68	68	68	54	54	54	68	54	54	68	68

For SI: 1 inch = 25.4 mm, 1 foot = 304.8 mm, 1 mil = 0.0254 mm, 1 mile per hour = 0.447 m/s, 1 pound per square foot = 0.0479 kPa, 1 ksi = 1000 psi = 6.895 MPa.

a. Deflection criterion: $L/240$.
b. Design load assumptions:
   Top and middle floor dead load is 10 psf.
   Top floor live load is 30 psf.
   Middle floor live load is 40 psf.
   Roof/ceiling dead load is 12 psf.
   Attic live load is 10 psf.
c. Building width is in the direction of horizontal framing members supported by the wall studs.

TABLE R603.3.2(29)
36-FOOT-WIDE BUILDING SUPPORTING TWO FLOORS, ROOF AND CEILING[a,b,c]
50 ksi STEEL

WIND SPEED		MEMBER SIZE	STUD SPACING (inches)	MINIMUM STUD THICKNESS (mils)											
				8-Foot Studs				9-Foot Studs				10-Foot Studs			
				Ground Snow Load (psf)											
Exp. B	Exp. C			20	30	50	70	20	30	50	70	20	30	50	70
85 mph	—	350S162	16	43	43	43	54	43	43	43	43	43	43	43	43
			24	68	68	68	68	54	54	54	68	68	68	68	68
		550S162	16	43	43	43	43	43	43	43	43	43	43	43	43
			24	54	54	54	54	54	54	54	54	54	54	54	54
90 mph	—	350S162	16	43	43	43	54	43	43	43	43	43	43	43	43
			24	68	68	68	68	54	54	54	68	68	68	68	68
		550S162	16	43	43	43	43	43	43	43	43	43	43	43	43
			24	54	54	54	54	54	54	54	54	54	54	54	54
100 mph	85 mph	350S162	16	43	43	43	54	43	43	43	43	43	43	43	43
			24	68	68	68	68	54	54	54	68	68	68	68	68
		550S162	16	43	43	43	43	43	43	43	43	43	43	43	43
			24	54	54	54	54	54	54	54	54	54	54	54	54
110 mph	90 mph	350S162	16	43	43	43	54	43	43	43	43	43	43	43	43
			24	68	68	68	68	54	54	54	68	68	68	68	68
		550S162	16	43	43	43	43	43	43	43	43	43	43	43	43
			24	54	54	54	54	54	54	54	54	54	54	54	54
—	100 mph	350S162	16	43	43	43	54	43	43	43	43	43	43	43	54
			24	68	68	68	68	54	54	54	68	68	68	68	68
		550S162	16	43	43	43	43	43	43	43	43	43	43	43	43
			24	54	54	54	54	54	54	54	54	54	54	54	54
—	110 mph	350S162	16	43	43	43	54	43	43	43	43	43	54	54	54
			24	68	68	68	68	54	54	68	68	68	68	68	68
		550S162	16	43	43	43	43	43	43	43	43	43	43	43	43
			24	54	54	54	54	54	54	54	54	54	54	54	54

For SI: 1 inch = 25.4 mm, 1 foot = 304.8 mm, 1 mil = 0.0254 mm, 1 mile per hour = 0.447 m/s, 1 pound per square foot = 0.0479kPa,
1 ksi = 1000 psi = 6.895 MPa.

a. Deflection criterion: *L*/240.

b. Design load assumptions:
   Top and middle floor dead load is 10 psf.
   Top floor live load is 30 psf.
   Middle floor live load is 40 psf.
   Roof/ceiling dead load is 12 psf.
   Attic live load is 10 psf.

c. Building width is in the direction of horizontal framing members supported by the wall studs.

TABLE R603.3.2(30)
40-FOOT-WIDE BUILDING SUPPORTING TWO FLOORS, ROOF AND CEILING[a,b,c]
3 ksi STEEL

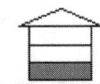

WIND SPEED		MEMBER SIZE	STUD SPACING (inches)	MINIMUM STUD THICKNESS (mils)											
				8-Foot Studs				9-Foot Studs				10-Foot Studs			
				Ground Snow Load (psf)											
Exp. B	Exp. C			20	30	50	70	20	30	50	70	20	30	50	70
85 mph	—	350S162	16	54	54	54	54	54	54	54	54	54	54	54	54
			24	97	97	97	97	68	68	68	97	97	97	97	97
		550S162	16	54	54	54	54	43	43	54	54	43	43	54	54
			24	68	68	68	68	68	68	68	68	68	68	68	68
90 mph	—	350S162	16	54	54	54	54	54	54	54	54	54	54	54	54
			24	97	97	97	97	68	68	68	97	97	97	97	97
		550S162	16	54	54	54	54	43	43	54	54	43	43	54	54
			24	68	68	68	68	68	68	68	68	68	68	68	68
100 mph	85 mph	350S162	16	54	54	54	54	54	54	54	54	54	54	54	54
			24	97	97	97	97	68	68	68	97	97	97	97	97
		550S162	16	54	54	54	54	43	43	54	54	43	43	54	54
			24	68	68	68	68	68	68	68	68	68	68	68	68
110 mph	90 mph	350S162	16	54	54	54	54	54	54	54	54	54	54	54	54
			24	97	97	97	97	68	68	68	97	97	97	97	97
		550S162	16	54	54	54	54	43	43	54	54	43	43	54	54
			24	68	68	68	68	68	68	68	68	68	68	68	68
—	100 mph	350S162	16	54	54	54	54	54	54	54	54	54	54	54	54
			24	97	97	97	97	68	68	68	97	97	97	97	97
		550S162	16	54	54	54	54	43	43	54	54	43	43	54	54
			24	68	68	68	68	68	68	68	68	68	68	68	68
—	110 mph	350S162	16	54	54	54	54	54	54	54	54	54	54	68	68
			24	97	97	97	97	68	68	97	97	97	97	97	97
		550S162	16	54	54	54	54	43	43	54	54	43	43	54	54
			24	68	68	68	68	68	68	68	68	68	68	68	68

For SI: 1 inch = 25.4 mm, 1 foot = 304.8 mm, 1 mil = 0.0254 mm, 1 mile per hour = 0.447 m/s, 1 pound per square foot = 0.0479kPa,
1 ksi = 1000 psi = 6.895 MPa.

a. Deflection criterion: $L/240$.
b. Design load assumptions:
   Top and middle floor dead load is 10 psf.
   Top floor live load is 30 psf.
   Middle floor live load is 40 psf.
   Roof/ceiling dead load is 12 psf.
   Attic live load is 10 psf.
c. Building width is in the direction of horizontal framing members supported by the wall studs.

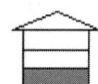

TABLE R603.3.2(31)
40-FOOT-WIDE BUILDING SUPPORTING TWO FLOORS, ROOF AND CEILING[a,b,c]
50 ksi STEEL

WIND SPEED		MEMBER SIZE	STUD SPACING (inches)	MINIMUM STUD THICKNESS (mils)											
				8-Foot Studs				9-Foot Studs				10-Foot Studs			
				Ground Snow Load (psf)											
Exp. B	Exp. C			20	30	50	70	20	30	50	70	20	30	50	70
85 mph	—	350S162	16	54	54	54	54	43	43	43	43	43	54	54	54
			24	68	68	68	68	68	68	68	68	68	68	68	68
		550S162	16	43	43	43	43	43	43	43	43	43	43	43	43
			24	54	54	54	68	54	54	54	54	54	54	54	54
90 mph	—	350S162	16	54	54	54	54	43	43	43	43	43	54	54	54
			24	68	68	68	68	68	68	68	68	68	68	68	68
		550S162	16	43	43	43	43	43	43	43	43	43	43	43	43
			24	54	54	54	68	54	54	54	54	54	54	54	54
100 mph	85 mph	350S162	16	54	54	54	54	43	43	43	43	43	54	54	54
			24	68	68	68	68	68	68	68	68	68	68	68	68
		550S162	16	43	43	43	43	43	43	43	43	43	43	43	43
			24	54	54	54	68	54	54	54	54	54	54	54	54
110 mph	90 mph	350S162	16	54	54	54	54	43	43	43	43	43	54	54	54
			24	68	68	68	68	68	68	68	68	68	68	68	68
		550S162	16	43	43	43	43	43	43	43	43	43	43	43	43
			24	54	54	54	68	54	54	54	54	54	54	54	54
—	100 mph	350S162	16	54	54	54	54	43	43	43	43	43	54	54	54
			24	68	68	68	68	68	68	68	68	68	68	68	68
		550S162	16	43	43	43	43	43	43	43	43	43	43	43	43
			24	54	54	54	68	54	54	54	54	54	54	54	54
—	110 mph	350S162	16	54	54	54	54	43	43	43	43	54	54	54	54
			24	68	68	68	68	68	68	68	68	68	68	68	97
		550S162	16	43	43	43	43	43	43	43	43	43	43	43	43
			24	54	54	54	68	54	54	54	54	54	54	54	54

For SI: 1 inch = 25.4 mm, 1 foot = 304.8 mm, 1 mil = 0.0254 mm, 1 mile per hour = 0.447 m/s, 1 pound per square foot = 0.0479kPa, 1 ksi = 1000 psi = 6.895 MPa.

a. Deflection criterion: $L/240$.

b. Design load assumptions:
    Top and middle floor dead load is 10 psf.
    Top floor live load is 30 psf.
    Middle floor live load is 40 psf.
    Roof/ceiling dead load is 12 psf.
    Attic live load is 10 psf.

c. Building width is in the direction of horizontal framing members supported by the wall studs.

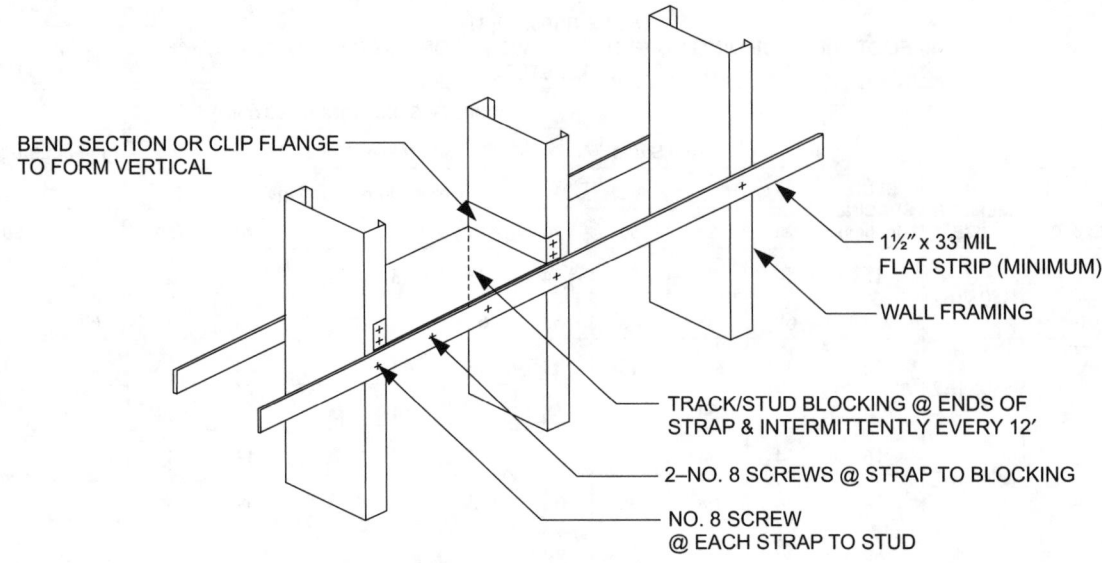

BEND SECTION OR CLIP FLANGE
TO FORM VERTICAL

1½" x 33 MIL
FLAT STRIP (MINIMUM)

WALL FRAMING

TRACK/STUD BLOCKING @ ENDS OF
STRAP & INTERMITTENTLY EVERY 12'

2–NO. 8 SCREWS @ STRAP TO BLOCKING

NO. 8 SCREW
@ EACH STRAP TO STUD

For SI: 1 mil = 0.0254 mm, 1 inch = 25.4 mm.

FIGURE R603.3.3(1)
STUD BRACING WITH STRAPPING ONLY

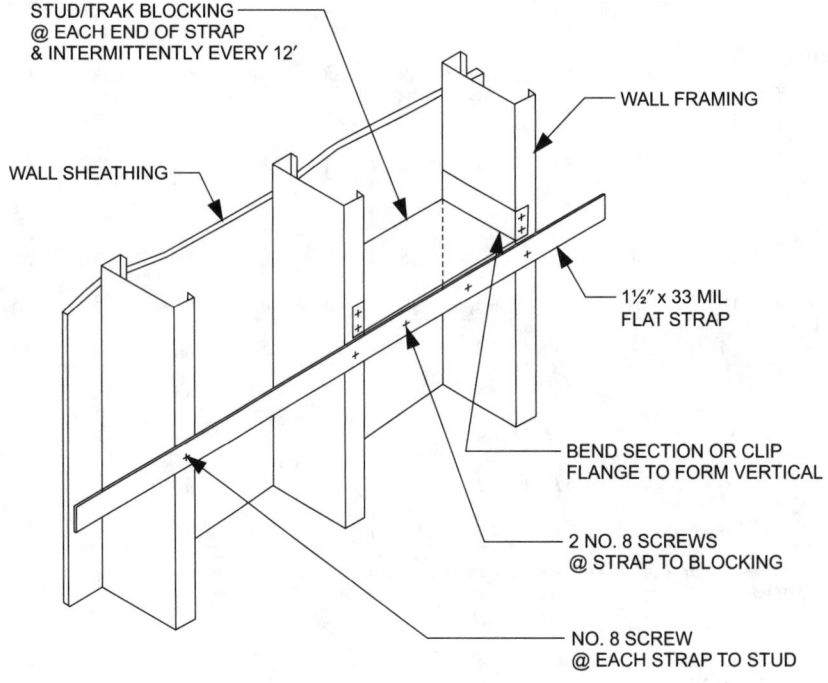

STUD/TRAK BLOCKING
@ EACH END OF STRAP
& INTERMITTENTLY EVERY 12'

WALL FRAMING

WALL SHEATHING

1½" x 33 MIL
FLAT STRAP

BEND SECTION OR CLIP
FLANGE TO FORM VERTICAL

2 NO. 8 SCREWS
@ STRAP TO BLOCKING

NO. 8 SCREW
@ EACH STRAP TO STUD

For SI: 1 mil = 0.0254 mm, 1 inch = 25.4 mm.

FIGURE R603.3.3(2)
STUD BRACING WITH STRAPPING AND SHEATHING MATERIAL

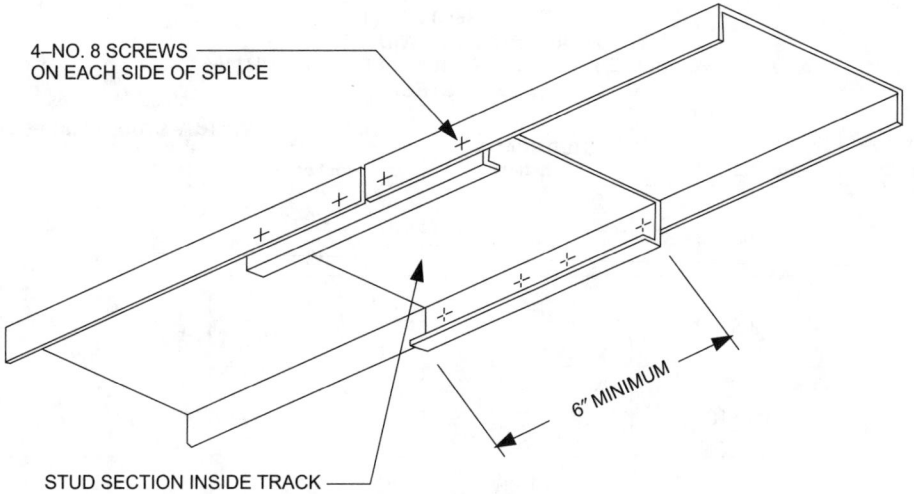

4–NO. 8 SCREWS
ON EACH SIDE OF SPLICE

6" MINIMUM

STUD SECTION INSIDE TRACK

For SI: 1 inch = 25.4 mm.

**FIGURE R603.3.5
TRACK SPLICE**

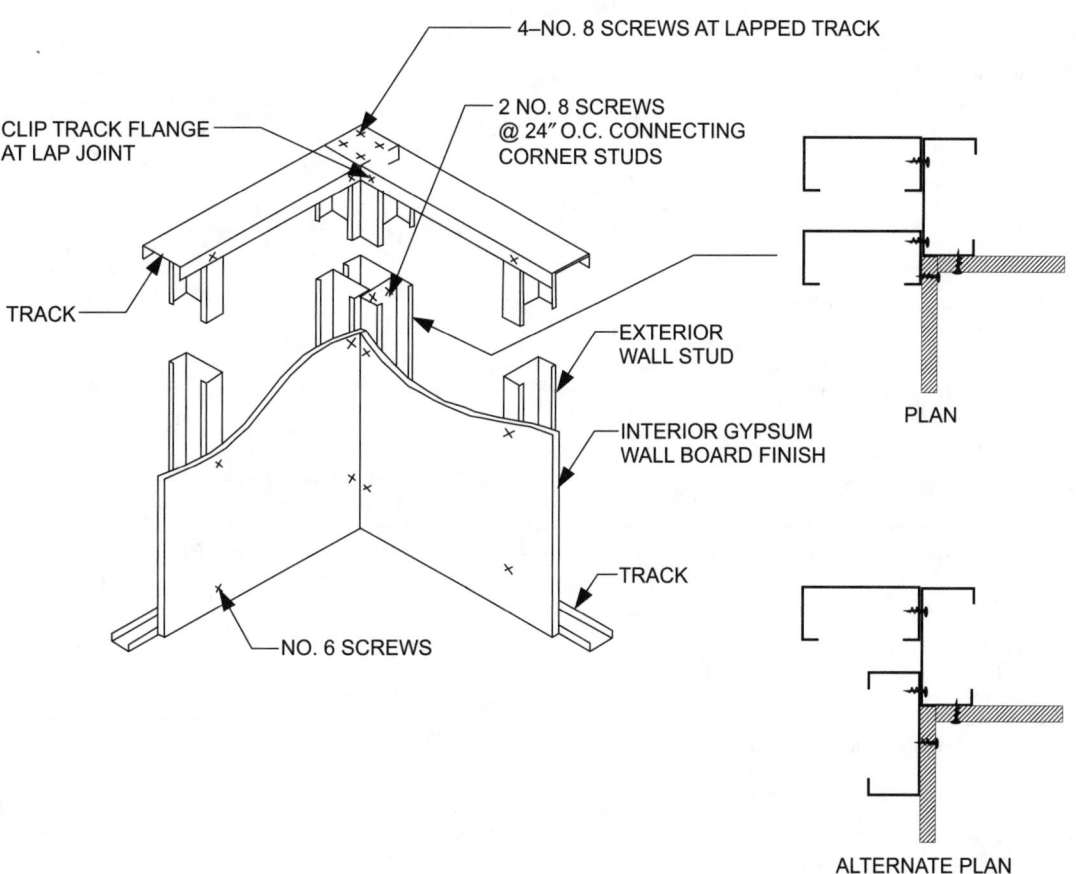

4–NO. 8 SCREWS AT LAPPED TRACK

CLIP TRACK FLANGE
AT LAP JOINT

2 NO. 8 SCREWS
@ 24" O.C. CONNECTING
CORNER STUDS

TRACK

EXTERIOR
WALL STUD

INTERIOR GYPSUM
WALL BOARD FINISH

TRACK

NO. 6 SCREWS

PLAN

ALTERNATE PLAN

For SI: 1 inch = 25.4 mm.

**FIGURE R603.4
CORNER FRAMING**

TABLE R603.3.2.1(1)
ALL BUILDING WIDTHS
GABLE ENDWALLS 8, 9 OR 10 FEET IN HEIGHT[a,b,c]
33 ksi STEEL

WIND SPEED		MEMBER SIZE	STUD SPACING (inches)	MINIMUM STUD THICKNESS (Mils)		
Exp. B	Exp. C			8-foot studs	9-foot studs	10-foot studs
85 mph	—	350S162	16	33	33	33
			24	33	33	33
		550S162	16	33	33	33
			24	33	33	33
90 mph	—	350S162	16	33	33	33
			24	33	33	33
		550S162	16	33	33	33
			24	33	33	33
100 mph	85 mph	350S162	16	33	33	33
			24	33	33	43
		550S162	16	33	33	33
			24	33	33	33
110 mph	90 mph	350S162	16	33	33	33
			24	33	33	43
		550S162	16	33	33	33
			24	33	33	33
—	100 mph	350S162	16	33	33	43
			24	43	43	54
		550S162	16	33	33	33
			24	33	33	33
—	110 mph	350S162	16	33	43	43
			24	43	54	54
		550S162	16	33	33	33
			24	33	33	43

For SI: 1 inch = 25.4, 1 foot = 304.8 mm, 1 mil = 0.0254 mm, 1 mile per hour = 0.447 m/s, 1 pound per square foot = 0.0479kPa, 1 ksi = 6.895 MPa.

a. Deflection criterion $L/240$.
b. Design load assumptions:
   Ground snow load is 70 psf.
   Roof and ceiling dead load is 12 psf.
   Floor dead load is 10 psf.
   Floor live load is 40 psf.
   Attic dead load is 10 psf.
c. Building width is in the direction of horizontal framing members supported by the wall studs.

TABLE R603.3.2.1(2)
ALL BUILDING WIDTHS
GABLE ENDWALLS 8, 9 OR 10 FEET IN HEIGHT[a,b,c]
50 ksi STEEL

WIND SPEED		MEMBER SIZE	STUD SPACING (inches)	MINIMUM STUD THICKNESS (Mils)		
Exp. B	Exp. C			8-foot studs	9-foot studs	10-foot studs
85 mph	—	350S162	16	33	33	33
			24	33	33	33
		550S162	16	33	33	33
			24	33	33	33
90 mph	—	350S162	16	33	33	33
			24	33	33	33
		550S162	16	33	33	33
			24	33	33	33
100 mph	85 mph	350S162	16	33	33	33
			24	33	33	33
		550S162	16	33	33	33
			24	33	33	33
110 mph	90 mph	350S162	16	33	33	33
			24	33	33	43
		550S162	16	33	33	33
			24	33	33	33
—	100 mph	350S162	16	33	33	33
			24	33	33	43
		550S162	16	33	33	33
			24	33	33	33
—	110 mph	350S162	16	33	33	33
			24	33	43	54
		550S162	16	33	33	33
			24	33	33	33

For SI: 1 inch = 25.4, 1 foot = 304.8 mm, 1 mil = 0.0254 mm, 1 mile per hour = 0.447 m/s, 1 pound per square foot = 0.0479kPa, 1 ksi = 6.895 MPa.

a. Deflection criterion L/240.

b. Design load assumptions:
    Ground snow load is 70 psf.
    Roof and ceiling dead load is 12 psf.
    Floor dead load is 10 psf.
    Floor live load is 40 psf.
    Attic dead load is 10 psf.

c. Building width is in the direction of horizontal framing members supported by the wall studs.

TABLE R603.3.2.1(3)
ALL BUILDING WIDTHS
GABLE ENDWALLS OVER 10 FEET IN HEIGHT[a,b,c]
33 ksi STEEL

WIND SPEED		MEMBER SIZE	STUD SPACING (inches)	MINIMUM STUD THICKNESS (Mils)					
				Stud Height, h (feet)					
Exp. B	Exp. C			10 < h ≤ 12	12 < h ≤ 14	14 < h ≤ 16	16 < h ≤ 18	18 < h ≤ 20	20 < h ≤ 22
85 mph	—	350S162	16	33	43	54	97	—	—
			24	43	54	97	—	—	—
		550S162	16	33	33	33	43	43	54
			24	33	33	43	54	68	97
90 mph	—	350S162	16	33	43	68	97	—	—
			24	43	68	97	—	—	—
		550S162	16	33	33	33	43	54	54
			24	33	33	43	54	68	97
100 mph	85 mph	350S162	16	43	54	97	—	—	—
			24	54	97	—	—	—	—
		550S162	16	33	33	43	54	54	68
			24	33	43	54	68	97	97
110 mph	90 mph	350S162	16	43	68	—	—	—	—
			24	68	—	—	—	—	—
		550S162	16	33	43	43	54	68	97
			24	43	54	68	97	97	—
—	100 mph	350S162	16	54	97	—	—	—	—
			24	97	—	—	—	—	—
		550S162	16	33	43	54	68	97	—
			24	43	68	97	97	—	—
—	110 mph	350S162	16	68	97	—	—	—	—
			24	97	—	—	—	—	—
		550S162	16	43	54	68	97	97	—
			24	54	68	97	—	—	—

For SI: 1 inch = 25.4, 1 foot = 304.8 mm, 1 mil = 0.0254 mm, 1 mile per hour = 0.447 m/s, 1 pound per square foot = 0.0479kPa, 1 ksi = 6.895 MPa.

a. Deflection criterion L/240.

b. Design load assumptions:
    Ground snow load is 70 psf.
    Roof and ceiling dead load is 12 psf.
    Floor dead load is 10 psf.
    Floor live load is 40 psf.
    Attic dead load is 10 psf.

c. Building width is in the direction of horizontal framing members supported by the wall studs.

TABLE R603.3.2.1(4)
ALL BUILDING WIDTHS
GABLE ENDWALLS OVER 10 FEET IN HEIGHT[a,b,c]
50 ksi STEEL

WIND SPEED		MEMBER SIZE	STUD SPACING (inches)	MINIMUM STUD THICKNESS (Mils)					
				Stud Height, h (feet)					
Exp. B	Exp. C			10 < h ≤ 12	12 < h ≤ 14	14 < h ≤ 16	16 < h ≤ 18	18 < h ≤ 20	20 < h ≤ 22
85 mph	—	350S162	16	33	43	54	97	—	—
			24	33	54	97	—	—	—
		550S162	16	33	33	33	33	43	54
			24	33	33	33	43	54	97
90 mph	—	350S162	16	33	43	68	97	—	—
			24	43	68	97	—	—	—
		550S162	16	33	33	33	33	43	54
			24	33	33	43	43	68	97
100 mph	85 mph	350S162	16	33	54	97	—	—	—
			24	54	97	—	—	—	—
		550S162	16	33	33	33	43	54	68
			24	33	33	43	54	97	97
110 mph	90 mph	350S162	16	43	68	—	—	—	—
			24	68	—	—	—	—	—
		550S162	16	33	33	43	43	68	97
			24	33	43	54	68	97	—
—	100 mph	350S162	16	54	97	—	—	—	—
			24	97	—	—	—	—	—
		550S162	16	33	33	43	54	97	—
			24	43	54	54	97	—	—
—	110 mph	350S162	16	54	97	—	—	—	—
			24	97	—	—	—	—	—
		550S162	16	33	43	54	68	97	—
			24	43	54	68	97	—	—

For SI: 1 inch = 25.4, 1 foot = 304.8 mm, 1 mil = 0.0254 mm, 1 mile per hour = 0.447 m/s, 1 pound per square foot = 0.0479kPa, 1 ksi = 6.895 MPa.

a. Deflection criterion $L/240$.
b. Design load assumptions:
    Ground snow load is 70 psf.
    Roof and ceiling dead load is 12 psf.
    Floor dead load is 10 psf.
    Floor live load is 40 psf.
    Attic dead load is 10 psf.
c. Building width is in the direction of horizontal framing members supported by the wall studs.

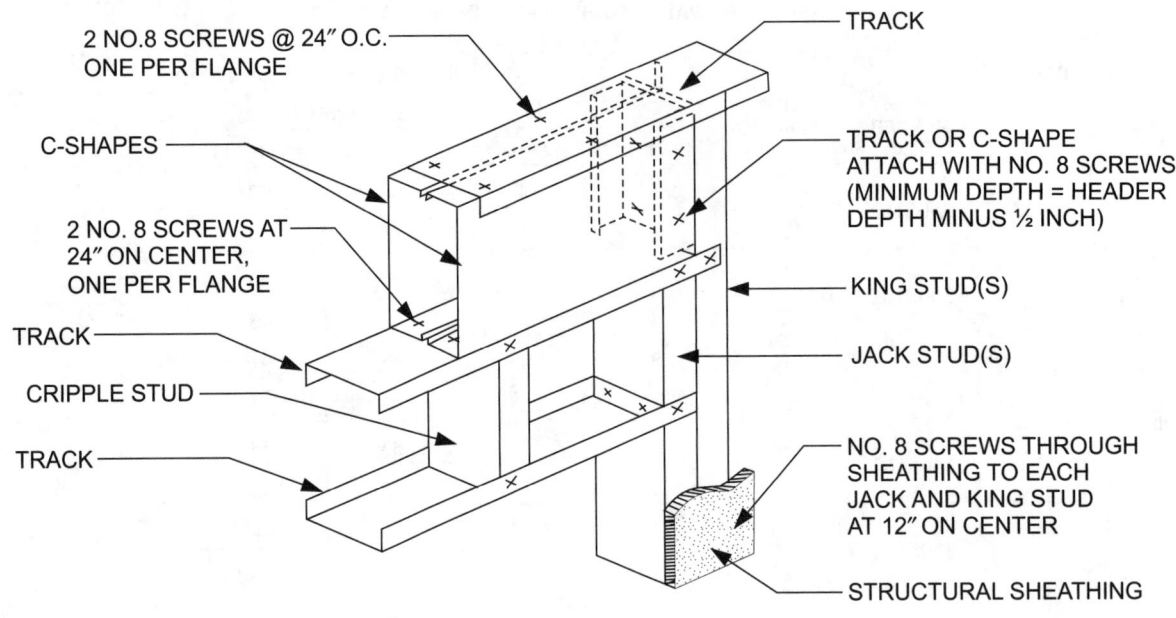

2 NO.8 SCREWS @ 24″ O.C.
ONE PER FLANGE

C-SHAPES

2 NO. 8 SCREWS AT
24″ ON CENTER,
ONE PER FLANGE

TRACK

CRIPPLE STUD

TRACK

TRACK

TRACK OR C-SHAPE
ATTACH WITH NO. 8 SCREWS
(MINIMUM DEPTH = HEADER
DEPTH MINUS ½ INCH)

KING STUD(S)

JACK STUD(S)

NO. 8 SCREWS THROUGH
SHEATHING TO EACH
JACK AND KING STUD
AT 12″ ON CENTER

STRUCTURAL SHEATHING

For SI: 1 inch = 25.4 mm.

FIGURE R603.6(1)
BOX BEAM HEADER

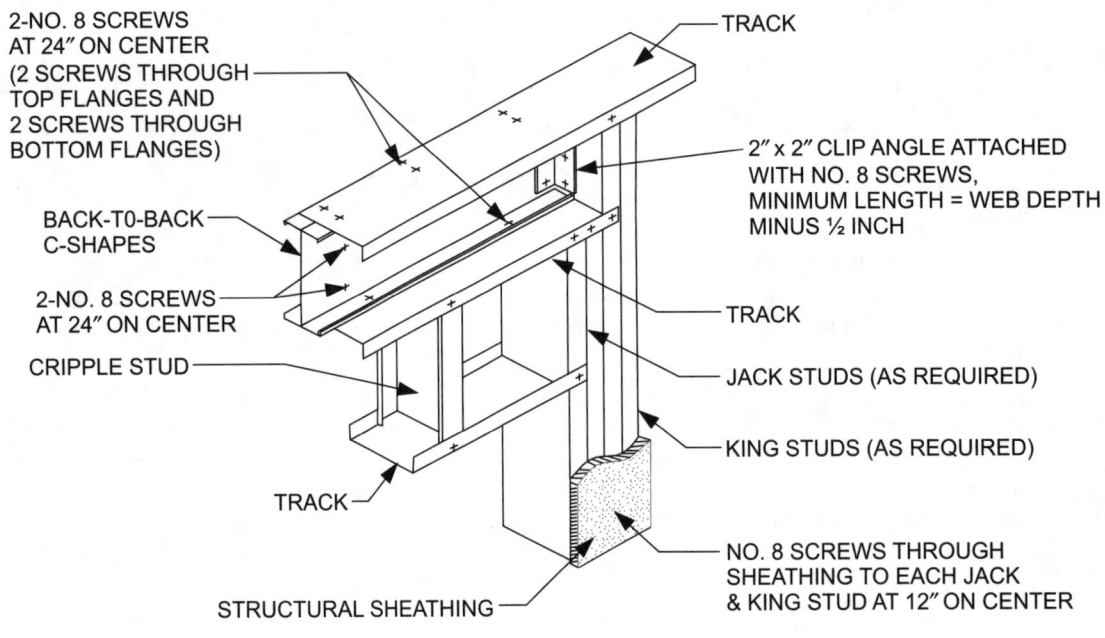

2-NO. 8 SCREWS
AT 24″ ON CENTER
(2 SCREWS THROUGH
TOP FLANGES AND
2 SCREWS THROUGH
BOTTOM FLANGES)

BACK-T0-BACK
C-SHAPES

2-NO. 8 SCREWS
AT 24″ ON CENTER

CRIPPLE STUD

TRACK

STRUCTURAL SHEATHING

TRACK

2″ x 2″ CLIP ANGLE ATTACHED
WITH NO. 8 SCREWS,
MINIMUM LENGTH = WEB DEPTH
MINUS ½ INCH

TRACK

JACK STUDS (AS REQUIRED)

KING STUDS (AS REQUIRED)

NO. 8 SCREWS THROUGH
SHEATHING TO EACH JACK
& KING STUD AT 12″ ON CENTER

For SI: 1 inch = 25.4 mm.

FIGURE 601.6(2)
BACK-TO-BACK HEADER

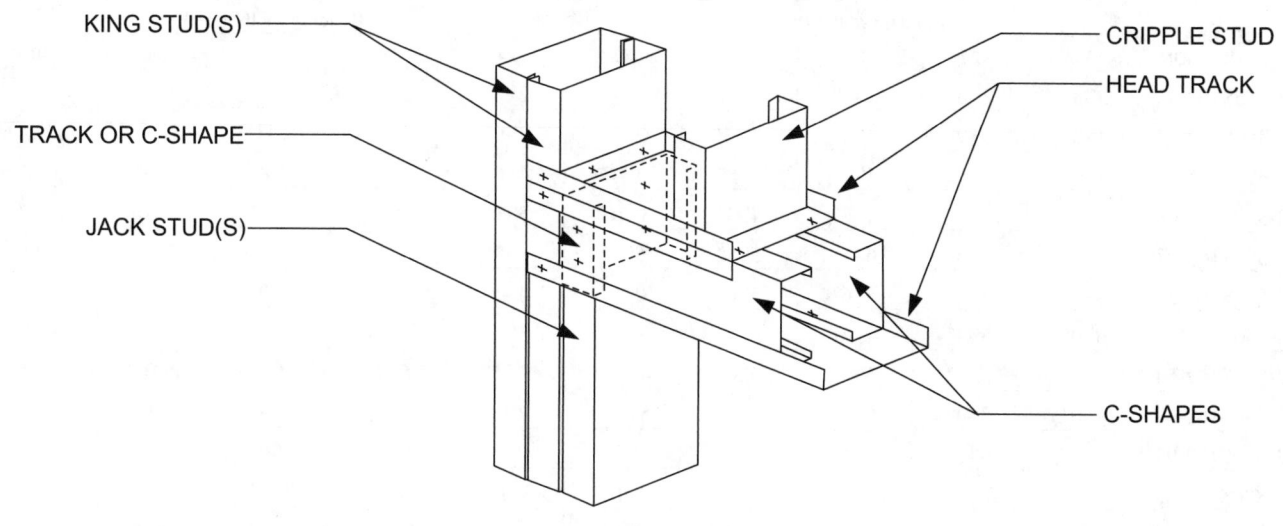

FIGURE R603.6.1(1)
BOX BEAM HEADER IN GABLE ENDWALL

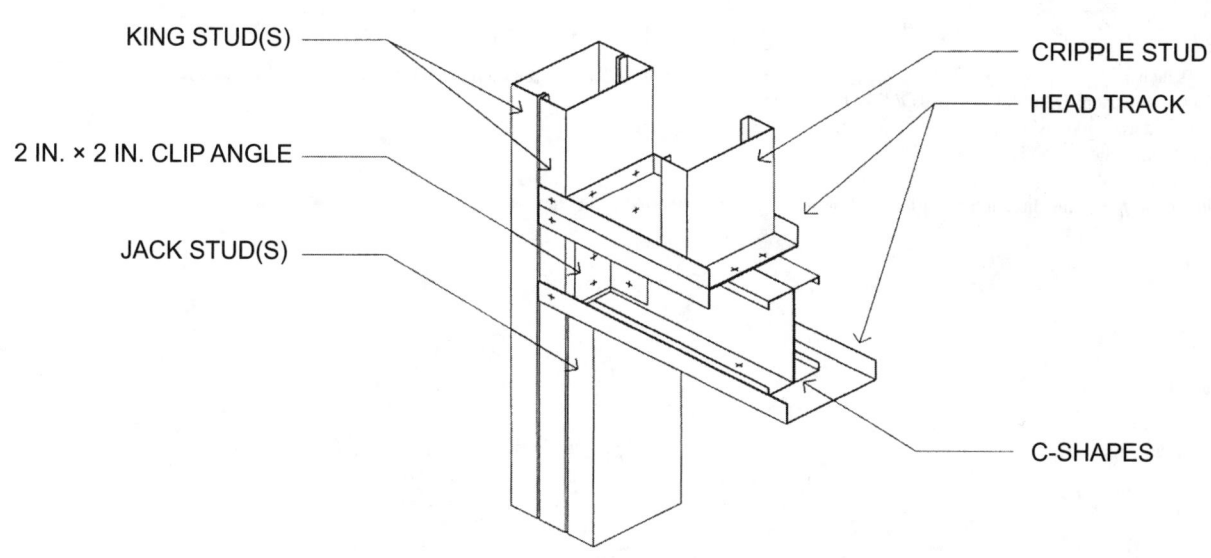

For SI: 1 inch = 25.4 mm.

FIGURE R603.6.1(2)
BACK-TO-BACK HEADER IN GABLE ENDWALL

TABLE R603.6(1)
BOX-BEAM HEADER SPANS
Headers Supporting Roof and Ceiling Only (33 ksi steel)[a, b]

MEMBER DESIGNATION	GROUND SNOW LOAD (20 psf) Building width[c] (feet)					GROUND SNOW LOAD (30 psf) Building width[c] (feet)				
	24	28	32	36	40	24	28	32	36	40
2-350S162-33	3'-3"	2'-8"	2'-2"	—	—	2'-8"	2'-2"	—	—	—
2-350S162-43	4'-2"	3'-9"	3'-4"	2'-11"	2'-7"	3'-9"	3'-4"	2'-11"	2'-7"	2'-2"
2-350S162-54	5'-0"	4'-6"	4'-1"	3'-8"	3'-4"	4'-6"	4'-1"	3'-8"	3'-3"	3'-0"
2-350S162-68	5'-7"	5'-1"	4'-7"	4'-3"	3'-10"	5'-1"	4'-7"	4'-2"	3'-10"	3'-5"
2-350S162-97	7'-1"	6'-6"	6'-1"	5'-8"	5'-3"	6'-7"	6'-1"	5'-7"	5'-3"	4'-11"
2-550S162-33	4'-8"	4'-0"	3'-6"	3'-0"	2'-6"	4'-1"	3'-6"	3'-0"	2'-6"	—
2-550S162-43	6'-0"	5'-4"	4'-10"	4'-4"	3'-11"	5'-5"	4'-10"	4'-4"	3'-10"	3'-5"
2-550S162-54	7'-0"	6'-4"	5'-9"	5'-4"	4'-10"	6'-5"	5'-9"	5'-3"	4'-10"	4'-5"
2-550S162-68	8'-0"	7'-4"	6'-9"	6'-3"	5'-10"	7'-5"	6'-9"	6'-3"	5'-9"	5'-4"
2-550S162-97	9'-11"	9'-2"	8'-6"	8'-0"	7'-6"	9'-3"	8'-6"	8'-0"	7'-5"	7'-0"
2-800S162-33	4'-5"	3'-11"	3'-5"	3'-1"	2'-10"	3'-11"	3'-6"	3'-1"	2'-9"	2'-3"
2-800S162-43	7'-3"	6'-7"	5'-11"	5'-4"	4'-10"	6'-7"	5'-11"	5'-4"	4'-9"	4'-3"
2-800S162-54	8'-10"	8'-0"	7'-4"	6'-9"	6'-2"	8'-1"	7'-4"	6'-8"	6'-1"	5'-7"
2-800S162-68	10'-5"	9'-7"	8'-10"	8'-2"	7'-7"	9'-8"	8'-10"	8'-1"	7'-6"	7'-0"
2-800S162-97	13'-1"	12'-1"	11'-3"	10'-7"	10'-0"	12'-2"	11'-4"	10'-6"	10'-0"	9'-4"
2-1000S162-43	7'-10"	6'-10"	6'-1"	5'-6"	5'-0"	6'-11"	6'-1"	5'-5"	4'-11"	4'-6"
2-1000S162-54	10'-0"	9'-1"	8'-3"	7'-7"	7'-0"	9'-2"	8'-4"	7'-7"	6'-11"	6'-4"
2-1000S162-68	11'-11"	10'-11"	10'-1"	9'-4"	8'-8"	11'-0"	10'-1"	9'-3"	8'-7"	8'-0"
2-1000S162-97	15'-3"	14'-3"	13'-5"	12'-6"	11'-10"	14'-4"	13'-5"	12'-6"	11'-9"	11'-0"
2-1200S162-54	11'-1"	10'-0"	9'-2"	8'-5"	7'-9"	10'-1"	9'-2"	8'-4"	7'-7"	7'-0"
2-1200S162-68	13'-3"	12'-1"	11'-2"	10'-4"	9'-7"	12'-3"	11'-2"	10'-3"	9'-6"	8'-10"
2-1200S162-97	16'-8"	15'-7"	14'-8"	13'-11"	13'-3"	15'-8"	14'-8"	13'-11"	13'-2"	12'-6"

For SI: 1 inch = 25.4 mm, 1 foot = 304.8 mm, 1 pound per square foot = 0.0479 kPa, 1 pound per square inch = 6.895 kPa.

a. Deflection criterion: $L/360$ for live loads, $L/240$ for total loads.

b. Design load assumptions:
   Roof/Ceiling dead load is 12 psf.
   Attic dead load is 10 psf.

c. Building width is in the direction of horizontal framing members supported by the header.

TABLE R603.6(2)
BOX-BEAM HEADER SPANS
Headers Supporting Roof and Ceiling Only (50 ksi steel)[a, b]

MEMBER DESIGNATION	GROUND SNOW LOAD (20 psf) Building width[c] (feet)					GROUND SNOW LOAD (30 psf) Building width[c] (feet)				
	24	28	32	36	40	24	28	32	36	40
2-350S162-33	4'-4"	3'-11"	3'-6"	3'-2"	2'-10"	3'-11"	3'-6"	3'-1"	2'-9"	2'-5"
2-350S162-43	5'-6"	5'-0"	4'-7"	4'-2"	3'-10"	5'-0"	4'-7"	4'-2"	3'-10"	3'-6"
2-350S162-54	6'-2"	5'-10"	5'-8"	5'-3"	4'-10"	5'-11"	5'-8"	5'-2"	4'-10"	4'-6"
2-350S162-68	6'-7"	6'-3"	6'-0"	5'-10"	5'-8"	6'-4"	6'-1"	5'-10"	5'-8"	5'-6"
2-350S162-97	7'-3"	6'-11"	6'-8"	6'-5"	6'-3"	7'-0"	6'-8"	6'-5"	6'-3"	6'-0"
2-550S162-33	6'-2"	5'-6"	5'-0"	4'-7"	4'-2"	5'-7"	5'-0"	4'-6"	4'-1"	3'-8"
2-550S162-43	7'-9"	7'-2"	6'-7"	6'-1"	5'-8"	7'-3"	6'-7"	6'-1"	5'-7"	5'-2"
2-550S162-54	8'-9"	8'-5"	8'-1"	7'-9"	7'-3"	8'-6"	8'-1"	7'-8"	7'-2"	6'-8"
2-550S162-68	9'-5"	9'-0"	8'-8"	8'-4"	8'-1"	9'-1"	8'-8"	8'-4"	8'-1"	7'-10"
2-550S162-97	10'-5"	10'-0"	9'-7"	9'-3"	9'-0"	10'-0"	9'-7"	9'-3"	8'-11"	8'-8"
2-800S162-33	4'-5"	3'-11"	3'-5"	3'-1"	2'-10"	3'-11"	3'-6"	3'-1"	2'-9"	2'-6"
2-800S162-43	9'-1"	8'-5"	7'-8"	6'-11"	6'-3"	8'-6"	7'-8"	6'-10"	6'-2"	5'-8"
2-800S162-54	10'-10"	10'-2"	9'-7"	9'-0"	8'-5"	10'-2"	9'-7"	8'-11"	8'-4"	7'-9"
2-800S162-68	12'-8"	11'-10"	11'-2"	10'-7"	10'-1"	11'-11"	11'-2"	10'-7"	10'-0"	9'-6"
2-800S162-97	14'-2"	13'-6"	13'-0"	12'-7"	12'-2"	13'-8"	13'-1"	12'-7"	12'-2"	11'-9"
2-1000S162-43	7'-10"	6'-10"	6'-1"	5'-6"	5'-0"	6'-11"	6'-1"	5'-5"	4'-11"	4'-6"
2-1000S162-54	12'-3"	11'-5"	10'-9"	10'-2"	9'-6"	11'-6"	10'-9"	10'-1"	9'-5"	8'-9"
2-1000S162-68	14'-5"	13'-5"	12'-8"	12'-0"	11'-6"	13'-6"	12'-8"	12'-0"	11'-5"	10'-10"
2-1000S162-97	17'-1"	16'-4"	15'-8"	14'-11"	14'-3"	16'-5"	15'-9"	14'-10"	14'-1"	13'-6"
2-1200S162-54	12'-11"	11'-3"	10'-0"	9'-0"	8'-2"	11'-5"	10'-0"	9'-0"	8'-1"	7'-4"
2-1200S162-68	15'-11"	14'-10"	14'-0"	13'-4"	12'-8"	15'-0"	14'-0"	13'-3"	12'-7"	11'-11"
2-1200S162-97	19'-11"	18'-7"	17'-6"	16'-8"	15'-10"	18'-9"	17'-7"	16'-7"	15'-9"	15'-0"

For SI: 1 inch = 25.4 mm, 1 foot = 304.8 mm, 1 pound per square foot = 0.0479 kPa, 1 pound per square inch = 6.895 kPa.

a. Deflection criterion: $L/360$ for live loads, $L/240$ for total loads.

b. Design load assumptions:
   Roof/Ceiling dead load is 12 psf.
   Attic dead load is 10 psf.

c. Building width is in the direction of horizontal framing members supported by the header.

TABLE R603.6(3)
BOX-BEAM HEADER SPANS
Headers Supporting Roof and Ceiling Only (33 ksi steel)[a, b]

MEMBER DESIGNATION	GROUND SNOW LOAD (50 psf)					GROUND SNOW LOAD (70 psf)				
	Building width[c] (feet)					Building width[c] (feet)				
	24	28	32	36	40	24	28	32	36	40
2-350S162-33	—	—	—	—	—	—	—	—	—	—
2-350S162-43	2'-4"	—	—	—	—	—	—	—	—	—
2-350S162-54	3'-1"	2'-8"	2'-3"	—	—	2'-1"	—	—	—	—
2-350S162-68	3'-7"	3'-2"	2'-8"	2'-3"	—	2'-6"	—	—	—	—
2-350S162-97	5'-1"	4'-7"	4'-3"	3'-11"	3'-7"	4'-1"	3'-8"	3'-4"	3'-0"	2'-8"
2-550S162-33	2'-2"	—	—	—	—	—	—	—	—	—
2-550S162-43	3'-8"	3'-1"	2'-6"	—	—	2'-3"	—	—	—	—
2-550S162-54	4'-7"	4'-0"	3'-6"	3'-0"	2'-6"	3'-3"	2'-8"	2'-1"	—	—
2-550S162-68	5'-6"	4'-11"	4'-5"	3'-11"	3'-6"	4'-3"	3'-8"	3'-1"	2'-7"	2'-1"
2-550S162-97	7'-3"	6'-7"	6'-1"	5'-8"	5'-3"	5'-11"	5'-4"	4'-11"	4'-6"	4'-1"
2-800S162-33	2'-7"	—	—	—	—	—	—	—	—	—
2-800S162-43	4'-6"	3'-9"	3'-1"	2'-5"	—	2'-10"	—	—	—	—
2-800S162-54	5'-10"	5'-1"	4'-6"	3'-11"	3'-4"	4'-3"	3'-6"	2'-9"	—	—
2-800S162-68	7'-2"	6'-6"	5'-10"	5'-3"	4'-8"	5'-7"	4'-10"	4'-2"	3'-7"	2'-11"
2-800S162-97	9'-7"	8'-9"	8'-2"	7'-7"	7'-0"	7'-11"	7'-2"	6'-7"	6'-0"	5'-7"
2-1000S162-43	4'-8"	4'-1"	3'-6"	2'-9"	—	3'-3"	2'-2"	—	—	—
2-1000S162-54	6'-7"	5'-10"	5'-1"	4'-5"	3'-9"	4'-10"	4'-0"	3'-2"	2'-3"	—
2-1000S162-68	8'-3"	7'-5"	6'-8"	6'-0"	5'-5"	6'-5"	5'-7"	4'-9"	4'-1"	3'-5"
2-1000S162-97	11'-4"	10'-5"	9'-8"	9'-0"	8'-5"	9'-5"	8'-6"	7'-10"	7'-2"	6'-7"
2-1200S162-54	7'-3"	6'-5"	5'-7"	4'-10"	4'-2"	5'-4"	4'-4"	3'-5"	2'-5"	—
2-1200S162-68	9'-2"	8'-2"	7'-5"	6'-8"	6'-0"	7'-1"	6'-2"	5'-4"	4'-6"	3'-9"
2-1200S162-97	12'-10"	11'-9"	10'-11"	10'-2"	9'-6"	10'-7"	9'-8"	8'-10"	8'-2"	7'-6"

For SI: 1 inch = 25.4 mm, 1 foot = 304.8 mm, 1 pound per square foot = 0.0479kPa, 1 pound per square inch = 6.895 kPa.

a. Deflection criterion: $L/360$ for live loads, $L/240$ for total loads.

b. Design load assumptions:
    Roof/Ceiling dead load is 12 psf.
    Attic dead load is 10 psf.

c. Building width is in the direction of horizontal framing members supported by the header.

TABLE R603.6(4)
BOX-BEAM HEADER SPANS
Headers Supporting Roof and Ceiling Only (50 ksi steel)[a, b]

MEMBER DESIGNATION	GROUND SNOW LOAD (50 psf)					GROUND SNOW LOAD (70 psf)				
	Building width[c] (feet)					Building width[c] (feet)				
	24	28	32	36	40	24	28	32	36	40
2-350S162-33	2'-7"	2'-2"	—	—	—	—	—	—	—	—
2-350S162-43	3'-8"	3'-3"	2'-10"	2'-6"	2'-1"	2'-8"	2'-3"	—	—	—
2-350S162-54	4'-8"	4'-2"	3'-9"	3'-5"	3'-1"	3'-7"	3'-2"	2'-9"	2'-5"	2'-0"
2-350S162-68	5'-7"	5'-2"	4'-9"	4'-4"	3'-11"	4'-7"	4'-1"	3'-7"	3'-2"	2'-10"
2-350S162-97	6'-2"	5'-11"	5'-8"	5'-6"	5'-4"	5'-8"	5'-5"	5'-3"	4'-11"	4'-7"
2-550S162-33	3'-11"	3'-4"	2'-10"	2'-4"	—	2'-7"	—	—	—	—
2-550S162-43	5'-4"	4'-10"	4'-4"	3'-10"	3'-5"	4'-2"	3'-7"	3'-1"	2'-7"	2'-1"
2-550S162-54	6'-11"	6'-3"	5'-9"	5'-3"	4'-9"	5'-6"	4'-11"	4'-5"	3'-11"	3'-5"
2-550S162-68	8'-0"	7'-6"	6'-11"	6'-5"	5'-11"	6'-9"	6'-1"	5'-6"	5'-0"	4'-7"
2-550S162-97	8'-11"	8'-6"	8'-2"	7'-11"	7'-8"	8'-1"	7'-9"	7'-6"	7'-1"	6'-7"
2-800S162-33	2'-8"	2'-4"	2'-1"	1'-11"	1'-9"	2'-0"	1'-9"	—	—	—
2-800S162-43	5'-10"	5'-2"	4'-7"	4'-2"	3'-10"	4'-5"	3'-11"	3'-6"	3'-0"	2'-6"
2-800S162-54	8'-0"	7'-3"	6'-8"	6'-1"	5'-7"	6'-5"	5'-9"	5'-1"	4'-7"	4'-0"
2-800S162-68	9'-9"	9'-0"	8'-3"	7'-8"	7'-1"	8'-0"	7'-3"	6'-7"	6'-0"	5'-6"
2-800S162-97	12'-1"	11'-7"	11'-2"	10'-8"	10'-2"	11'-0"	10'-4"	9'-9"	9'-2"	8'-7"
2-1000S162-43	4'-8"	4'-1"	3'-8"	3'-4"	3'-0"	3'-6"	3'-1"	2'-9"	2'-6"	2'-3"
2-1000S162-54	9'-1"	8'-2"	7'-3"	6'-7"	6'-0"	7'-0"	6'-2"	5'-6"	5'-0"	4'-6"
2-1000S162-68	11'-1"	10'-2"	9'-5"	8'-8"	8'-1"	9'-1"	8'-3"	7'-6"	6'-10"	6'-3"
2-1000S162-97	13'-9"	12'-11"	12'-2"	11'-7"	11'-1"	11'-11"	11'-3"	10'-7"	9'-11"	9'-4"
2-1200S162-54	7'-8"	6'-9"	6'-1"	5'-6"	5'-0"	5'-10"	5'-1"	4'-7"	4'-1"	3'-9"
2-1200S162-68	12'-3"	11'-3"	10'-4"	9'-7"	8'-11"	10'-1"	9'-1"	8'-3"	7'-6"	6'-10"
2-1200S162-97	15'-4"	14'-5"	13'-7"	12'-11"	12'-4"	13'-4"	12'-6"	11'-10"	11'-1"	10'-5"

For SI: 1 inch = 25.4 mm, 1 foot = 304.8 mm, 1 pound per square foot = 0.0479 kPa, 1 pound per square inch = 6.895 kPa.

a. Deflection criterion: $L/360$ for live loads, $L/240$ for total loads.

b. Design load assumptions:
Roof/Ceiling dead load is 12 psf.
Attic dead load is 10 psf.

c. Building width is in the direction of horizontal framing members supported by the header.

TABLE R603.6(5)
BOX-BEAM HEADER SPANS
Headers Supporting One Floor, Roof and Ceiling (33 ksi steel)[a, b]

MEMBER DESIGNATION	GROUND SNOW LOAD (20 psf)					GROUND SNOW LOAD (30 psf)				
	Building width[c] (feet)					Building width[c] (feet)				
	24	28	32	36	40	24	28	32	36	40
2-350S162-33	—	—	—	—	—	—	—	—	—	—
2-350S162-43	2′-2″	—	—	—	—	2′-1″	—	—	—	—
2-350S162-54	2′-11″	2′-5″	—	—	—	2′-10″	2′-4″	—	—	—
2-350S162-68	3′-8″	3′-2″	2′-9″	2′-4″	—	3′-7″	3′-1″	2′-8″	2′-3″	—
2-350S162-97	4′-11″	4′-5″	4′-2″	3′-8″	3′-5″	4′-10″	4′-5″	4′-0″	3′-8″	3′-4″
2-550S162-33	—	—	—	—	—	—	—	—	—	—
2-550S162-43	3′-5″	2′-9″	2′-1″	—	—	3′-3″	2′-7″	—	—	—
2-550S162-54	4′-4″	3′-9″	3′-2″	2′-7″	2′-1″	4′-3″	3′-7″	3′-1″	2′-6″	—
2-550S162-68	5′-3″	4′-8″	4′-1″	3′-7″	3′-2″	5′-2″	4′-7″	4′-0″	3′-6″	3′-1″
2-550S162-97	7′-0″	6′-5″	5′-10″	5′-5″	5′-0″	6′-11″	6′-4″	5′-9″	5′-4″	4′-11″
2-800S162-33	2′-1″	—	—	—	—	—	—	—	—	—
2-800S162-43	4′-2″	3′-4″	2′-7″	—	—	4′-0″	3′-3″	2′-5″	—	—
2-800S162-54	5′-6″	4′-9″	4′-1″	3′-5″	2′-9″	5′-5″	4′-8″	3′-11″	3′-3″	2′-8″
2-800S162-68	6′-11″	6′-2″	5′-5″	4′-10″	4′-3″	6′-9″	6′-0″	5′-4″	4′-8″	4′-1″
2-800S162-97	9′-4″	8′-6″	7′-10″	7′-3″	6′-8″	9′-2″	8′-4″	7′-8″	7′-1″	6′-7″
2-1000S162-43	4′-4″	3′-9″	2′-11″	—	—	4′-3″	3′-8″	2′-9″	—	—
2-1000S162-54	6′-3″	5′-5″	4′-7″	3′-11″	3′-2″	6′-1″	5′-3″	4′-6″	3′-9″	3′-0″
2-1000S162-68	7′-11″	7′-0″	6′-3″	5′-6″	4′-10″	7′-9″	6′-10″	6′-1″	5′-4″	4′-9″
2-1000S162-97	11′-0″	10′-1″	9′-3″	8′-7″	8′-0″	10′-11″	9′-11″	9′-2″	8′-5″	7′-10″
2-1200S162-54	6′-11″	5′-11″	5′-1″	4′-3″	3′-5″	6′-9″	5′-9″	4′-11″	4′-1″	3′-3″
2-1200S162-68	8′-9″	7′-9″	6′-11″	6′-1″	5′-4″	8′-7″	7′-7″	6′-9″	5′-11″	5′-3″
2-1200S162-97	12′-4″	11′-5″	10′-6″	9′-8″	9′-0″	12′-3″	11′-3″	10′-4″	9′-6″	8′-10″

For SI: 1 inch = 25.4 mm, 1 foot = 304.8 mm, 1 pound per square foot = 0.0479kPa, 1 pound per square inch = 6.895 kPa.

a. Deflection criterion: L/360 for live loads, L/240 for total loads.

b. Design load assumptions:
    Second floor dead load is 10 psf.
    Roof/Ceiling dead load is 12 psf.
    Second floor live load is 30 psf.
    Attic dead load is 10 psf.

c. Building width is in the direction of horizontal framing members supported by the header

TABLE R603.6(6)
BOX-BEAM HEADER SPANS
Headers Supporting One Floor, Roof and Ceiling (50 ksi steel)[a, b]

MEMBER DESIGNATION	GROUND SNOW LOAD (20 psf)					GROUND SNOW LOAD (30 psf)				
	Building width[c] (feet)					Building width[c] (feet)				
	24	28	32	36	40	24	28	32	36	40
2-350S162-33	2′-4″	—	—	—	—	2′-3″	—	—	—	—
2-350S162-43	3′-4″	2′-11″	2′-6″	2′-1″	—	3′-3″	2′-10″	2′-5″	2′-0″	—
2-350S162-54	4′-4″	3′-10″	3′-5″	3′-1″	2′-9″	4′-3″	2′-9″	3′-4″	3′-0″	2′-8″
2-350S162-68	5′-0″	4′-9″	4′-7″	4′-2″	3′-9″	4′-11″	4′-8″	4′-6″	4′-1″	3′-9″
2-350S162-97	5′-6″	5′-3″	5′-1″	4′-11″	2′-9″	5′-5″	5′-2″	5′-0″	4′-10″	4′-8″
2-550S162-33	3′-6″	2′-11″	2′-4″	—	—	3′-5″	2′-10″	2′-3″	—	—
2-550S162-43	5′-0″	4′-5″	3′-11″	3′-5″	3′-0″	4′-11″	4′-4″	3′-10″	3′-4″	2′-11″
2-550S162-54	6′-6″	5′-10″	5′-3″	4′-9″	4′-4″	6′-4″	5′-9″	5′-2″	4′-8″	4′-3″
2-550S162-68	7′-2″	6′-10″	6′-5″	5′-11″	5′-6″	7′-0″	6′-9″	6′-4″	5′-10″	5′-4″
2-550S162-97	7′-11″	7′-7″	7′-3″	7′-0″	6′-10″	7′-9″	7′-5″	7′-2″	6′-11″	6′-9″
2-800S162-33	2′-5″	2′-2″	1′-11″	1′-9″	—	2′-5″	2′-1″	1′-10″	1′-8″	—
2-800S162-43	5′-5″	4′-9″	4′-3″	3′-9″	3′-5″	5′-3″	4′-8″	4′-1″	3′-9″	3′-5″
2-800S162-54	7′-6″	6′-9″	6′-2″	5′-7″	5′-0″	7′-5″	6′-8″	6′-0″	5′-5″	4′-11″
2-800S162-68	9′-3″	8′-5″	7′-8″	7′-1″	6′-6″	9′-1″	8′-3″	7′-7″	7′-0″	6′-5″
2-800S162-97	10′-9″	10′-3″	9′-11″	9′-7″	9′-3″	10′-7″	10′-1″	9′-9″	9′-5″	9′-1″
2-1000S162-43	4′-4″	3′-9″	3′-4″	3′-0″	2′-9″	4′-3″	3′-8″	3′-3″	2′-11″	2′-8″
2-1000S162-54	8′-6″	7′-6″	6′-8″	6′-0″	5′-5″	8′-4″	7′-4″	6′-6″	5′-10″	5′-4″
2-1000S162-68	10′-6″	9′-7″	8′-9″	8′-0″	7′-5″	10′-4″	9′-5″	8′-7″	7′-11″	7′-3″
2-1000S162-97	12′-11″	12′-4″	11′-8″	11′-1″	10′-6″	12′-9″	12′-2″	11′-6″	10′-11″	10′-5″
2-1200S162-54	7′-1″	6′-2″	5′-6″	5′-0″	4′-6″	6′-11″	6′-1″	5′-5″	4′-10″	4′-5″
2-1200S162-68	11′-7″	10′-7″	9′-8″	8′-11″	8′-2″	11′-5″	10′-5″	9′-6″	8′-9″	8′-0″
2-1200S162-97	14′-9″	13′-9″	13′-0″	12′-4″	11′-9″	14′-7″	13′-8″	12′-10″	12′-3″	11′-8″

For SI: 1 inch = 25.4 mm, 1 foot = 304.8 mm, 1 pound per square foot = 0.0479kPa, 1 pound per square inch = 6.895 kPa.

a. Deflection criterion: $L/360$ for live loads, $L/240$ for total loads.

b. Design load assumptions:
    Second floor dead load is 10 psf.
    Roof/ceiling dead load is 12 psf.
    Second floor live load is 30 psf.
    Attic live load is 10 psf.

c. Building width is in the direction of horizontal framing members supported by the header.

TABLE R603.6(7)
BOX-BEAM HEADER SPANS
Headers Supporting One Floor, Roof and Ceiling (33 ksi steel)[a, b]

MEMBER DESIGNATION	GROUND SNOW LOAD (50 psf) Building width[c] (feet)					GROUND SNOW LOAD (70 psf) Building width[c] (feet)				
	24	28	32	36	40	24	28	32	36	40
2-350S162-33	—	—	—	—	—	—	—	—	—	—
2-350S162-43	—	—	—	—	—	—	—	—	—	—
2-350S162-54	—	—	—	—	—	—	—	—	—	—
2-350S162-68	2'-8"	2'-3"	—	—	—	—	—	—	—	—
2-350S162-97	4'-0"	3'-7"	3'-3"	2'-11"	2'-7"	3'-4"	2'-11"	2'-6"	2'-2"	—
2-550S162-33	—	—	—	—	—	—	—	—	—	—
2-550S162-43	2'-0"	—	—	—	—	—	—	—	—	—
2-550S162-54	3'-1"	2'-6"	—	—	—	—	—	—	—	—
2-550S162-68	4'-1"	3'-6"	2'-11"	2'-5"	—	3'-1"	2'-5"	—	—	—
2-550S162-97	5'-10"	5'-3"	4'-10"	4'-5"	4'-0"	4'-11"	4'-5"	3'-11"	3'-6"	3'-2"
2-800S162-33	—	—	—	—	—	—	—	—	—	—
2-800S162-43	2'-6"	—	—	—	—	—	—	—	—	—
2-800S162-54	4'-0"	3'-3"	2'-6"	—	—	2'-8"	—	—	—	—
2-800S162-68	5'-5"	4'-8"	4'-0"	3'-4"	2'-8"	4'-2"	3'-4"	2'-6"	—	—
2-800S162-97	7'-9"	7'-1"	6'-6"	5'-11"	5'-5"	6'-7"	5'-11"	5'-4"	4'-10"	4'-4"
2-1000S162-43	2'-10"	—	—	—	—	—	—	—	—	—
2-1000S162-54	4'-7"	3'-8"	2'-9"[c]	—	—	3'-0"	—	—	—	—
2-1000S162-68	6'-2"	5'-4"	4'-7"	3'-10"	3'-1"	4'-9"	3'-10"	2'-11"	—	—
2-1000S162-97	9'-3"	8'-5"	7'-8"	7'-1"	6'-6"	7'-10"	7'-1"	6'-5"	5'-9"	5'-2"
2-1200S162-54	5'-0"	4'-0"	3'-1"	—	—	3'-4"	—	—	—	—
2-1200S162-68	6'-10"	5'-11"	5'-0"	4'-3"	3'-5"	5'-3"	4'-3"	3'-2"	—	—
2-1200S162-97	10'-5"	9'-6"	8'-8"	8'-0"	7'-4"	8'-10"	8'-0"	7'-3"	6'-6"	5'-10"

For SI: 1 inch = 25.4 mm, 1 foot = 304.8 mm, 1 pound per square foot = 0.0479 kPa, 1 pound per square inch = 6.895 kPa.

a. Deflection criterion: $L/360$ for live loads, $L/240$ for total loads.

b. Design load assumptions:
   Second floor dead load is 10 psf.
   Roof/ceiling dead load is 12 psf.
   Second floor live load is 30 psf.
   Attic live load is 10 psf.

c. Building width is in the direction of horizontal framing members supported by the header.

TABLE R603.6(8)
BOX-BEAM HEADER SPANS
Headers Supporting One Floor, Roof and Ceiling (50 ksi steel)[a, b]

MEMBER DESIGNATION	GROUND SNOW LOAD (50 psf)					GROUND SNOW LOAD (70 psf)				
	Building width[c] (feet)					Building width[c] (feet)				
	24	28	32	36	40	24	28	32	36	40
2-350S162-33	—	—	—	—	—	—	—	—	—	—
2-350S162-43	2'-8"	—	—	—	—	—	—	—	—	—
2-350S162-54	3'-5"	3'-0"	2'-7"	2'-2"	—	2'-8"	2'-2"	—	—	—
2-350S162-68	4'-6"	4'-1"	3'-8"	3'-3"	2'-11"	3'-9"	3'-3"	2'-10"	2'-5"	2'-1"
2-350S162-97	5'-1"	4'-10"	4'-8"	4'-6"	4'-5"	4'-10"	4'-7"	4'-4"	4'-0"	3'-8"
2-550S162-33	2'-4"	—	—	—	—	—	—	—	—	—
2-550S162-43	3'-10"	3'-4"	2'-9"	2'-3"	—	2'-11"	2'-3"	—	—	—
2-550S162-54	5'-3"	3'-8"	4'-1"	3'-8"	3'-2"	4'-3"	3'-8"	3'-1"	2'-7"	2'-0"
2-550S162-68	6'-5"	5'-10"	5'-3"	4'-9"	4'-4"	5'-5"	4'-9"	4'-3"	3'-9"	3'-4"
2-550S162-97	7'-4"	7'-0"	6'-9"	6'-6"	6'-4"	6'-11"	6'-8"	6'-3"	5'-10"	5'-5"
2-800S162-33	1'-11"	1'-8"	—	—	—	—	—	—	—	—
2-800S162-43	4'-2"	3'-8"	3'-4"	2'-9"	2'-2"	3'-5"	2'-9"	—	—	—
2-800S162-54	6'-1"	5'-5"	4'-10"	4'-3"	3'-9"	4'-11"	4'-3"	3'-8"	3'-0"	2'-5"
2-800S162-68	7'-8"	6'-11"	6'-3"	5'-9"	5'-2"	6'-5"	5'-9"	5'-1"	4'-6"	4'-0"
2-800S162-97	9'-11"	9'-6"	9'-2"	8'-10"	8'-3"	9'-5"	8'-10"	8'-2"	7'-7"	7'-0"
2-1000S162-43	3'-4"	2'-11"	2'-7"	2'-5"	2'-2"	2'-8"	2'-5"	2'-2"	—	—
2-1000S162-54	6'-7"	5'-10"	5'-3"	4'-9"	4'-3"	5'-4"	4'-9"	4'-1"	3'-5"	2'-9"
2-1000S162-68	8'-8"	7'-10"	7'-2"	6'-6"	5'-11"	7'-4"	6'-6"	5'-9"	5'-1"	4'-6"
2-1000S162-97	11'-7"	10'-11"	10'-3"	9'-7"	9'-0"	10'-5"	9'-7"	8'-10"	8'-2"	7'-8"
2-1200S162-54	5'-6"	4'-10"	4'-4"	3'-11²"	3'-7"	4'-5"	3'-11"	3'-6"	3'-2"	2'-11"
2-1200S162-68	9'-7"	8'-8"	7'-11"	7'-2"	6'-6"	8'-1"	7'-2"	6'-4"	5'-8"	5'-0"
2-1200S162-97	12'-11"	12'-2"	11'-6"	10'-8"	10'-0"	11'-8"	10'-9"	9'-11"	9'-2"	8'-6"

For SI: 1 inch = 25.4 mm, 1 foot = 304.8 mm, 1 pound per square foot = 0.0479 kPa, 1 pound per square inch = 6.895 kPa.

a. Deflection criterion: $L/360$ for live loads, $L/240$ for total loads.

b. Design load assumptions:
    Second floor dead load is 10 psf.
    Roof/ceiling dead load is 12 psf.
    Second floor live load is 30 psf.
    Attic live load is 10 psf.

c. Building width is in the direction of horizontal framing members supported by the header.

TABLE R603.6(9)
BOX-BEAM HEADER SPANS
Headers Supporting Two Floors, Roof and Ceiling (33 ksi steel)[a]

| MEMBER DESIGNATION | GROUND SNOW LOAD (20 psf) | | | | | GROUND SNOW LOAD (30 psf) | | | | |
| | Building width[c] (feet) | | | | | Building width[c] (feet) | | | | |
	24	28	32	36	40	24	28	32	36	40
2-350S162-33	—	—	—	—	—	—	—	—	—	—
2-350S162-43	—	—	—	—	—	—	—	—	—	—
2-350S162-54	—	—	—	—	—	—	—	—	—	—
2-350S162-68	—	—	—	—	—	—	—	—	—	—
2-350S162-97	3'-1"	2'-8"	2'-3"	—	—	3'-1"	2'-7"	2'-2"	—	—
2-550S162-33	—	—	—	—	—	—	—	—	—	—
2-550S162-43	—	—	—	—	—	—	—	—	—	—
2-550S162-54	—	—	—	—	—	—	—	—	—	—
2-550S162-68	2'-9"	—	—	—	—	2'-8"	—	—	—	—
2-550S162-97	4'-8"	4'-1"	3'-7"	3'-2"	2'-9"	4'-7"	4'-0"	3'-6"	3'-1"	2'-8"
2-800S162-33	—	—	—	—	—	—	—	—	—	—
2-800S162-43	—	—	—	—	—	—	—	—	—	—
2-800S162-54	2'-1"	—	—	—	—	—	—	—	—	—
2-800S162-68	3'-8"	2'-9"	—	—	—	3'-7"	2'-8"	—	—	—
2-800S162-97	6'-3"	5'-6"	4'-11"	4'-4"	3'-9"	6'-2"	5'-5"	4'-10"	4'-3"	3'-9"
2-1000S162-43	—	—	—	—	—	—	—	—	—	—
2-1000S162-54	2'-5"	—	—	—	—	2'-3"	—	—	—	—
2-1000S162-68	4'-3"	3'-2"	2'-0"	—	—	4'-2"	3'-1"	—	—	—
2-1000S162-97	7'-5"	6'-7"	5'-10"	5'-2"	4'-7"	7'-4"	6'-6"	5'-9"	5'-1"	4'-6"
2-1200S162-54	2'-7"	—	—	—	—	2'-6"	—	—	—	—
2-1200S162-68	4'-8"	3'-6"	2'-2"	—	—	4'-7"	3'-5"	2'-0"	—	—
2-1200S162-97	8'-5"	7'-5"	6'-7"	5'-10"	5'-2"	8'-3"	7'-4"	6'-6"	5'-9"	5'-1"

For SI: 1 inch = 25.4 mm, 1 foot = 304.8 mm, 1 pound per square foot = 0.0479 kPa, 1 pound per square inch = 6.895 kPa.

a. Deflection criterion: $L/360$ for live loads, $L/240$ for total loads.

b. Design load assumptions:
   Second floor dead load is 10 psf.
   Roof/ceiling dead load is 12 psf.
   Second floor live load is 40 psf.
   Third floor live load is 30 psf.
   Attic live load is 10 psf.

c. Building width is in the direction of horizontal framing members supported by the header.

TABLE R603.6(10)
BOX-BEAM HEADER SPANS
Headers Supporting Two Floors, Roof and Ceiling (50 ksi steel)[a, b]

MEMBER DESIGNATION	GROUND SNOW LOAD (20 psf)					GROUND SNOW LOAD (30 psf)				
	Building width[c] (feet)					Building width[c] (feet)				
	24	28	32	36	40	24	28	32	36	40
2-350S162-33	—	—	—	—	—	—	—	—	—	—
2-350S162-43	—	—	—	—	—	—	—	—	—	—
2-350S162-54	2'-5"	—	—	—	—	2'-4"	—	—	—	—
2-350S162-68	3'-6"	3'-0"	2'-6"	2'-1"	—	3'-5"	2'-11"	2'-6"	2'-0"	—
2-350S162-97	4'-9"	4'-6"	4'-1"	3'-8"	3'-4"	4'-8"	4'-5"	4'-0"	3'-8"	3'-4"
2-550S162-33	—	—	—	—	—	—	—	—	—	—
2-550S162-43	2'-7"	—	—	—	—	2'-6"	—	—	—	—
2-550S162-54	3'-11"	3'-3"	2'-8"	2'-0"	—	3'-10"	3'-3"	2'-7"	—	—
2-550S162-68	5'-1"	4'-5"	3'-10"	3'-3"	2'-9"	5'-0"	4'-4"	3'-9"	3'-3"	2'-9"
2-550S162-97	6'-10"	6'-5"	5'-10"	5'-5"	4'-11"	6'-9"	6'-4"	5'-10"	5'-4"	4'-11"
2-800S162-33	—	—	—	—	—	—	—	—	—	—
2-800S162-43	3'-1"	2'-3"	—	—	—	3'-0"	2'-2"	—	—	—
2-800S162-54	4'-7"	3'-10"	3'-1"	2'-5"	—	4'-6"	3'-9"	3'-0"	2'-4"	—
2-800S162-68	6'-0"	5'-3"	4'-7"	3'-11"	3'-4"	6'-0"	5'-2"	4'-6"	3'-11"	3'-3"
2-800S162-97	9'-2"	8'-4"	7'-8"	7'-0"	6'-6"	9'-1"	8'-3"	7'-7"	7'-0"	6'-5"
2-1000S162-43	2'-6"	2'-2"	—	—	—	2'-6"	2'-2"	—	—	—
2-1000S162-54	5'-0"	4'-4"	3'-6"	2'-9"	—	4'-11"	4'-3"	3'-5"	2'-7"	—
2-1000S162-68	6'-10"	6'-0"	5'-3"	4'-6"	3'-10"	6'-9"	5'-11"	5'-2"	4'-5"	3'-9"
2-1000S162-97	10'-0"	9'-1"	8'-3"	7'-8"	7'-0"	9'-10"	9'-0"	8'-3"	7'-7"	7'-0"
2-1200S162-54	4'-2"	3'-7"	3'-3"	2'-11"	—	4'-1"	3'-7"	3'-2"	2'-10"	—
2-1200S162-68	7'-7"	6'-7"	5'-9"	5'-0"	4'-2"	7'-6"	6'-6"	5'-8"	4'-10"	4'-1"
2-1200S162-97	11'-2"	10'-1"	9'-3"	8'-6"	7'-10"	11'-0"	10'-0"	9'-2"	9'-2"	7'-9"

For SI: 1 inch = 25.4 mm, 1 foot = 304.8 mm, 1 pound per square foot = 0.0479 kPa, 1 pound per square inch = 6.895 kPa.

a. Deflection criterion: $L/360$ for live loads, $L/240$ for total loads.

b. Design load assumptions:
   Second floor dead load is 10 psf.
   Roof/ceiling dead load is 12 psf.
   Second floor live load is 40 psf.
   Third floor live load is 30 psf.
   Attic live load is 10 psf.

c. Building width is in the direction of horizontal framing members supported by the header.

TABLE R603.6(11)
BOX-BEAM HEADER SPANS
Headers Supporting Two Floors, Roof and Ceiling (33 ksi steel)[a, b]

MEMBER DESIGNATION	GROUND SNOW LOAD (50 psf) Building width[c] (feet)					GROUND SNOW LOAD (70 psf) Building width[c] (feet)				
	24	28	32	36	40	24	28	32	36	40
2-350S162-33	—	—	—	—	—	—	—	—	—	—
2-350S162-43	—	—	—	—	—	—	—	—	—	—
2-350S162-54	—	—	—	—	—	—	—	—	—	—
2-350S162-68	—	—	—	—	—	—	—	—	—	—
2-350S162-97	2'-11"	2'-5"	2'-0"	—	—	2'-7"	2'-2"	—	—	—
2-550S162-33	—	—	—	—	—	—	—	—	—	—
2-550S162-43	—	—	—	—	—	—	—	—	—	—
2-550S162-54	—	—	—	—	—	—	—	—	—	—
2-550S162-68	2'-5"	—	—	—	—	—	—	—	—	—
2-550S162-97	4'-4"	3'-10"	3'-4"	2'-10"	2'-5"	4'-0"	3'-6"	3'-1"	2'-7"	2'-2"
2-800S162-33	—	—	—	—	—	—	—	—	—	—
2-800S162-43	—	—	—	—	—	—	—	—	—	—
2-800S162-54	—	—	—	—	—	—	—	—	—	—
2-800S162-68	3'-3"	2'-3"	—	—	—	2'-8"	—	—	—	—
2-800S162-97	5'-11"	5'-2"	4'-6"	4'-0"	3'-5"	5'-6"	4'-10"	4'-3"	3'-8"	3'-2"
2-1000S162-43	—	—	—	—	—	—	—	—	—	—
2-1000S162-54	—	—	—	—	—	—	—	—	—	—
2-1000S162-68	3'-9"	2'-7"	—	—	—	3'-1"	—	—	—	—
2-1000S162-97	7'-0"	6'-2"	5'-5"	4'-9"	4'-2"	6'-6"	5'-9"	5'-1"	4'-5"	3'-10"
2-1200S162-54	—	—	—	—	—	—	—	—	—	—
2-1200S162-68	4'-2"	2'-10"	—	—	—	3'-5"	2'-0"	—	—	—
2-1200S162-97	7'-11"	7'-0"	6'-2"	5'-5"	4'-8"	7'-4"	6'-6"	5'-9"	5'-0"	4'-4"

For SI: 1 inch = 25.4 mm, 1 foot = 304.8 mm, 1 pound per square foot = 0.0479 kPa, 1 pound per square inch = 6.895 kPa.

a. Deflection criterion: $L/360$ for live loads, $L/240$ for total loads.

b. Design load assumptions:
    Second floor dead load is 10 psf.
    Roof/ceiling dead load is 12 psf.
    Second floor live load is 40 psf.
    Third floor live load is 30 psf.
    Attic live load is 10 psf.

c. Building width is in the direction of horizontal framing members supported by the header.

TABLE R603.6(12)
BOX-BEAM HEADER SPANS[a,b,c]
Headers Supporting Two Floors, Roof and Ceiling (50 ksi steel)[a,b]

MEMBER DESIGNATION	GROUND SNOW LOAD (50 psf) Building width[c] (feet)					GROUND SNOW LOAD (70 psf) Building width[c] (feet)				
	24	28	32	36	40	24	28	32	36	40
2-350S162-33	—	—	—	—	—	—	—	—	—	—
2-350S162-43	—	—	—	—	—	—	—	—	—	—
2-350S162-54	2'-2"	—	—	—	—	—	—	—	—	—
2-350S162-68	3'-3"	2'-9"	2'-3"	—	—	2'-11"	2'-5"	—	—	—
2-350S162-97	4'-6"	4'-3"	3'-10"	3'-6"	3'-2"	4'-3"	4'-0"	3'-7"	3'-3"	3'-0"
2-550S162-33	—	—	—	—	—	—	—	—	—	—
2-550S162-43	2'-3"	—	—	—	—	—	—	—	—	—
2-550S162-54	3'-7"	2'-11"	2'-3"	—	—	3'-3"	2'-7"	—	—	—
2-550S162-68	4'-9"	2'-1"	3'-6"	3'-0"	2'-5"	4'-4"	3'-9"	3'-2"	2'-8"	2'-1"
2-550S162-97	6'-5"	6'-1"	5'-7"	5'-1"	4'-8"	6'-3"	5'-10"	5'-4"	4'-10"	4'-5"
2-800S162-33	—	—	—	—	—	—	—	—	—	—
2-800S162-43	2'-8"	—	—	—	—	2'-2"	—	—	—	—
2-800S162-54	4'-3"	3'-5"	2'-8"	—	—	3'-9"	3'-0"	2'-3"	—	—
2-800S162-68	5'-8"	4'-11"	4'-2"	3'-7"	2'-11"	5'-3"	4'-6"	3'-10"	3'-3"	2'-7"
2-800S162-97	8'-9"	8'-0"	7'-3"	6'-8"	6'-2"	8'-4"	7'-7"	6'-11"	6'-4"	5'-10"
2-1000S162-43	2'-4"	2'-0"	—	—	—	2'-2"	—	—	—	—
2-1000S162-54	4'-8"	3'-11"	3'-1"	2'-2"	—	4'-3"	3'-5"	2'-7"	—	—
2-1000S162-68	6'-5"	5'-7"	4'-9"	4'-1"	3'-4"	5'-11"	5'-1"	4'-5"	3'-8"	2'-11"
2-1000S162-97	9'-6"	8'-8"	7'-11"	7'-3"	6'-8"	9'-0"	8'-3"	7'-6"	6'-11"	6'-4"
2-1200S162-54	3'-11"	3'-5"	3'-0"	2'-4"	—	3'-7"	3'-2"	2'-10"	—	—
2-1200S162-68	7'-1"	6'-2"	5'-3"	4'-6"	3'-8"	6'-6"	5'-8"	4'-10"	4'-0"	3'-3"
2-1200S162-97	10'-8"	9'-8"	8'-10"	8'-1"	7'-5"	10'-1"	9'-2"	8'-5"	7'-9"	7'-1"

For SI: 1 inch = 25.4 mm, 1 foot = 304.8 mm, 1 pound per square foot = 0.0479kPa, 1 pound per square inch = 6.895 kPa.

a. Deflection criterion: $L/360$ for live loads, $L/240$ for total loads.

b. Design load assumptions:
   Second floor dead load is 10 psf.
   Roof/ceiling dead load is 12 psf.
   Second floor live load is 40 psf.
   Third floor live load is 30 psf.
   Attic live load is 10 psf.

c. Building width is in the direction of horizontal framing members supported by the header.

TABLE R603.6(13)
BACK-TO-BACK HEADER SPANS
Headers Supporting Roof and Ceiling Only (33 ksi steel)[a,b]

MEMBER DESIGNATION	GROUND SNOW LOAD (20 psf)					GROUND SNOW LOAD (30 psf)				
	Building width[c] (feet)					Building width[c] (feet)				
	24	28	32	36	40	24	28	32	36	40
2-350S162-33	2'-11"	2'-4"	—	—	—	2'-5"	—	—	—	—
2-350S162-43	4'-8"	3'-10"	3'-5"	3'-1"	2'-9"	3'-11"	3'-5"	3'-0"	2'-8"	2'-4"
2-350S162-54	5'-3"	4'-9"	4'-4"	4'-1"	3'-8"	4'-10"	4'-4"	4'-0"	3'-8"	3'-4"
2-350S162-68	6'-1"	5'-7"	5'-2"	4'-10"	4'-6"	5'-8"	5'-3"	4'-10"	4'-6"	4'-2"
2-350S162-97	7'-3"	6'-10"	6'-5"	6'-0"	5'-8"	6'-11"	6'-5"	6'-0"	5'-8"	5'-4"
2-550S162-33	4'-5"	3'-9"	3'-1"	2'-6"	—	3'-9"	3'-2"	2'-6"	—	—
2-550S162-43	6'-2"	5'-7"	5'-0"	4'-7"	4'-2"	5'-7"	5'-0"	4'-6"	4'-1"	3'-8"
2-550S162-54	7'-5"	6'-9"	6'-3"	5'-9"	5'-4"	6'-10"	6'-3"	5'-9"	5'-4"	4'-11"
2-550S162-68	6'-7"	7'-11"	7'-4"	6'-10"	6'-5"	8'-0"	7'-4"	6'-10"	6'-5"	6'-0"
2-550S162-97	10'-5"	9'-8"	9'-0"	8'-6"	8'-0"	9'-9"	9'-0"	8'-6"	8'-0"	7'-7"
2-800S162-33	4'-5"	3'-11"	3'-5"	3'-1"	2'-4"	3'-11"	3'-6"	3'-0"	2'-3"	—
2-800S162-43	7'-7"	6'-10"	6'-2"	5'-8"	5'-2"	6'-11"	6'-2"	5'-7"	5'-1"	4'-7"
2-800S162-54	9'-3"	8'-7"	7'-11"	7'-4"	6'-10"	8'-8"	7'-11"	7'-4"	6'-9"	6'-3"
2-800S162-68	10'-7"	9'-10"	9'-4"	8'-10"	8'-5"	9'-11"	9'-4"	8'-10"	8'-4"	7'-11"
2-800S162-97	13'-9"	12'-9"	12'-0"	11'-3"	10'-8"	12'-10"	12'-0"	11'-3"	10'-7"	10'-0"
2-1000S162-43	7'-10"	6'-10"	6'-1"	5'-6"	5'-0"	6'-11"	6'-1"	5'-5"	4'-11"	4'-6"
2-1000S162-54	10'-5"	9'-9"	9'-0"	8'-4"	7'-9"	9'-10"	9'-0"	8'-4"	7'-9"	7'-2"
2-1000S162-68	12'-1"	11'-3"	10'-8"	10'-1"	9'-7"	11'-4"	10'-8"	10'-1"	9'-7"	9'-1"
2-1000S162-97	15'-3"	14'-3"	13'-5"	12'-9"	12'-2"	14'-4"	13'-5"	12'-8"	12'-1"	11'-6"
2-1200S162-54	11'-6"	10'-9"	10'-0"	9'-0"	8'-2"	10'-10"	10'-0"	9'-0"	8'-1"	7'-4"
2-1200S162-68	13'-4"	12'-6"	11'-9"	11'-2"	10'-8"	12'-7"	11'-10"	11'-2"	10'-7"	10'-1"
2-1200S162-97	16'-8"	15'-7"	14'-8"	13'-11"	13'-3"	15'-8"	14'-8"	13'-11"	13'-2"	12'-7"

For SI: 1 inch = 25.4 mm, 1 foot = 304.8 mm, 1 pound per square foot = 0.0479 kPa, 1 pound per square inch = 6.895 kPa.

a. Deflection criterion: $L/360$ for live loads, $L/240$ for total loads.

b. Design load assumptions:
   Second floor dead load is 12 psf.
   Attic live load is 10 psf.

c. Building width is in the direction of horizontal framing members supported by header.

TABLE R603.6(14)
BACK-TO-BACK HEADER SPANS
Headers Supporting Roof and Ceiling Only (50 ksi steel)[a,b]

MEMBER DESIGNATION	GROUND SNOW LOAD (20 psf)					GROUND SNOW LOAD (30 psf)				
	Building width[c] (feet)					Building width[c] (feet)				
	24	28	32	36	40	24	28	32	36	40
2-350S162-33	4'-2"	3'-8"	3'-3"	2'-10"	2'-6"	3'-8"	3'-3"	2'-10"	2'-5"	2'-1"
2-350S162-43	5'-5"	5'-0"	4'-6"	4'-2"	3'-10"	5'-0"	4'-7"	4'-2"	3'-10"	3'-6"
2-350S162-54	6'-2"	5'-10"	5'-8"	5'-4"	5'-0"	5'-11"	5'-8"	5'-4"	5'-0"	4'-8"
2-350S162-68	6'-7"	6'-3"	6'-0"	5'-10"	5'-8"	6'-4"	6'-1"	5'-10"	5'-8"	5'-6"
2-350S162-97	7'-3"	6'-11"	6'-8"	6'-5"	6'-3"	7'-0"	6'-8"	6'-5"	6'-3"	6'-0"
2-550S162-33	5'-10"	5'-3"	4'-8"	4'-3"	3'-9"	5'-3"	4'-9"	4'-2"	3'-9"	3'-3"
2-550S162-43	7'-9"	7'-2"	6'-7"	6'-1"	5'-8"	7'-3"	6'-7"	6'-1"	5'-8"	5'-3"
2-550S162-54	8'-9"	8'-5"	8'-1"	7'-9"	7'-5"	8'-6"	8'-1"	7'-9"	7'-5"	6'-11"
2-550S162-68	9'-5"	9'-0"	8'-8"	8'-4"	8'-1"	9'-1"	8'-8"	8'-4"	8'-1"	7'-10"
2-550S162-97	10'-5"	10'-0"	9'-7"	9'-3"	9'-0"	10'-0"	9'-7"	9'-3"	8'-11"	8'-8"
2-800S162-33	4'-5"	3'-11"	3'-5"	3'-1"	2'-10"	3'-11"	3'-6"	3'-1"	2'-9"	2'-6"
2-800S162-43	9'-1"	8'-5"	7'-8"	6'-11"	6'-3"	8'-6"	7'-8"	6'-10"	6'-2"	5'-8"
2-800S162-54	10'-10"	10'-2"	9'-7"	9'-1"	8'-8"	10'-2"	9'-7"	9'-0"	8'-7"	8'-1"
2-800S162-68	12'-8"	11'-10"	11'-2"	10'-7"	10'-1"	11'-11"	11'-2"	10'-7"	10'-0"	9'-7"
2-800S162-97	14'-2"	13'-6"	13'-0"	12'-7"	12'-2"	13'-8"	13'-1"	12'-7"	12'-2"	11'-9"
2-1000S162-43	7'-10"	6'-10"	6'-1"	5'-6"	5'-0"	6'-11"	6'-1"	5'-5"	4'-11"	4'-6"
2-1000S162-54	12'-3"	11'-5"	10'-9"	10'-3"	9'-9"	11'-6"	10'-9"	10'-2"	9'-8"	8'-11"
2-1000S162-68	14'-5"	13'-5"	12'-8"	12'-0"	11'-6"	13'-6"	12'-8"	12'-0"	11'-5"	10'-11"
2-1000S162-97	17'-1"	16'-4"	15'-8"	14'-11"	14'-3"	16'-5"	15'-9"	14'-10"	14'-1"	13'-6"
2-1200S162-54	12'-11"	11'-3"	10'-0"	9'-0"	8'-2"	11'-5"	10'-0"	9'-0"	8'-1"	7'-4"
2-1200S162-68	15'-11"	14'-10"	14'-0"	13'-4"	12'-8"	15'-0"	14'-0"	13'-3"	12'-7"	12'-0"
2-1200S162-97	19'-11"	18'-7"	17'-6"	16'-8"	15'-10"	18'-9"	17'-7"	16'-7"	15'-9"	15'-0"

For SI: 1 inch = 25.4 mm, 1 foot = 304.8 mm, 1 pound per square foot = 0.0479 kPa, 1 pound per square inch = 6.895 kPa.

a. Deflection criterion: $L/360$ for live loads, $L/240$ for total loads.

b. Design load assumptions:
Roof/ceiling dead load is 12 psf.
Attic live load is 10 psf.

c. Building width is in the direction of horizontal framing members supported by the header.

TABLE R603.6(15)
BACK-TO-BACK HEADER SPANS
Headers Supporting Roof and Ceiling Only (33 ksi steel)[a, b]

MEMBER DESIGNATION	GROUND SNOW LOAD (50 psf)					GROUND SNOW LOAD (70 psf)				
	Building width[c] (feet)					Building width[c] (feet)				
	24	28	32	36	40	24	28	32	36	40
2-350S162-33	—	—	—	—	—	—	—	—	—	—
2-350S162-43	2'-6"	—	—	—	—	—	—	—	—	—
2-350S162-54	3'-6"	3'-1"	2'-8"	2'-4"	2'-0"	2'-7"	2'-1"	—	—	—
2-350S162-68	4'-4"	3'-11"	3'-7"	3'-3"	2'-11"	3'-5"	3'-0"	2'-8"	2'-4"	2'-1"
2-350S162-97	5'-5"	5'-0"	4'-8"	4'-6"	4'-1"	4'-6"	4'-2"	3'-10"	3'-6"	3'-3"
2-550S162-33	—	—	—	—	—	—	—	—	—	—
2-550S162-43	3'-10"	3'-3"	2'-9"	2'-2"	—	2'-6"	—	—	—	—
2-550S162-54	5'-1"	4'-7"	4'-1"	3'-8"	3'-4"	3'-11"	3'-5"	2'-11"	2'-6"	2'-0"
2-550S162-68	6'-2"	5'-8"	5'-2"	4'-9"	4'-5"	5'-0"	4'-6"	4'-1"	3'-9"	3'-4"
2-550S162-97	7'-9"	7'-2"	6'-8"	6'-3"	5'-11"	6'-6"	6'-0"	5'-7"	5'-2"	4'-10"
2-800S162-33	—	—	—	—	—	—	—	—	—	—
2-800S162-43	4'-10"	4'-1"	3'-6"	2'-11"	2'-3"	3'-3"	2'-5"	—	—	—
2-800S162-54	6'-6"	5'-10"	5'-3"	4'-9"	4'-4"	5'-1"	4'-6"	3'-11"	3'-4"	2'-10"
2-800S162-68	8'-1"	7'-5"	6'-10"	6'-4"	5'-11"	6'-8"	6'-1"	5'-6"	5'-0"	4'-7"
2-800S162-97	10'-3"	9'-7"	8'-11"	8'-5"	7'-11"	8'-8"	8'-0"	7'-6"	7'-0"	6'-7"
2-1000S162-43	4'-8"	4'-1"	3'-8"	3'-4"	2'-8"	3'-6"	2'-10"	—	—	—
2-1000S162-54	7'-5"	6'-8"	6'-1"	5'-6"	5'-0"	5'-10"	5'-1"	4'-6"	3'-11"	3'-4"
2-1000S162-68	9'-4"	8'-7"	7'-11"	7'-4"	6'-10"	7'-8"	7'-0"	6'-4"	5'-10"	5'-4"
2-1000S162-97	11'-9"	11'-0"	10'-5"	9'-11"	9'-5"	10'-3"	9'-7"	8'-11"	8'-4"	7'-10"
2-1200S162-54	7'-8"	6'-9"	6'-1"	5'-6"	5'-0"	5'-10"	5'-1"	4'-7"	4'-1"	3'-9"
2-1200S162-68	10'-4"	9'-6"	8'-10"	8'-2"	7'-7"	8'-7"	7'-9"	7'-1"	6'-6"	6'-0"
2-1200S162-97	12'-10"	12'-1"	11'-5"	10'-10"	10'-4"	11'-2"	10'-6"	9'-11"	9'-5"	9'-0"

For SI: 1 inch = 25.4 mm, 1 foot = 304.8 mm, 1 pound per square foot = 0.0479 kPa, 1 pound per square inch = 6.895 kPa.

a. Deflection criterion: $L/360$ for live loads, $L/240$ for total loads.

b. Design load assumptions:
   Roof/ceiling dead load is 12 psf.
   Attic live load is 10 psf.

c. Building width is in the direction of horizontal framing members supported by the header.

TABLE R603.6(16)
BACK-TO-BACK HEADER SPANS
Headers Supporting Roof and Ceiling Only (50 ksi steel)[a, b]

MEMBER DESIGNATION	GROUND SNOW LOAD (50 psf)					GROUND SNOW LOAD (70 psf)				
	Building width[c] (feet)					Building width[c] (feet)				
	24	28	32	36	40	24	28	32	36	40
2-350S162-33	2'-3"	—	—	—	—	—	—	—	—	—
2-350S162-43	3'-8"	3'-3"	2'-10"	2'-6"	2'-2"	2'-8"	2'-3"	—	—	—
2-350S162-54	4'-9"	4'-4"	4'-0"	3'-8"	3'-8"	3'-10"	3'-5"	3'-1"	2'-9"	2'-5"
2-350S162-68	5'-7"	5'-4"	5'-2"	4'-11"	4'-7"	5'-1"	4'-8"	4'-3"	3'-11"	3'-8"
2-350S162-97	6'-2"	5'-11"	5'-8"	5'-6"	5'-4"	5'-8"	5'-5"	5'-3"	5'-0"	4'-11"
2-550S162-33	3'-6"	2'-10"	2'-3"	—	—	2'-0"	—	—	—	—
2-550S162-43	5'-5"	4'-10"	4'-4"	3'-11"	3'-6"	4'-2"	3'-8"	3'-2"	2'-8"	2'-3"
2-550S162-54	7'-2"	6'-6"	6'-0"	5'-7"	5'-2"	5'-10"	5'-3"	4'-10"	4'-5"	4'-0"
2-550S162-68	8'-0"	7'-8"	7'-3"	6'-11"	6'-6"	7'-2"	6'-7"	6'-1"	5'-8"	5'-4"
2-550S162-97	8'-11"	8'-6"	8'-2"	7'-11"	7'-8"	8'-1"	7'-9"	7'-6"	7'-2"	6'-11"
2-800S162-33	2'-8"	2'-4"	2'-1"	1'-11"	—	2'-0"	—	—	—	—
2-800S162-43	5'-10"	5'-2"	4'-7"	4'-2"	3'-10"	4'-5"	3'-11"	3'-6"	3'-2"	2'-9"
2-800S162-54	8'-4"	7'-8"	7'-1"	6'-7"	6'-1"	6'-10"	6'-3"	5'-8"	5'-2"	4'-9"
2-800S162-68	9'-9"	9'-2"	8'-8"	8'-3"	7'-10"	8'-6"	7'-11"	7'-4"	6'-10"	6'-5"
2-800S162-97	12'-1"	11'-7"	11'-2"	10'-8"	10'-2"	11'-0"	10'-4"	9'-9"	9'-3"	8'-10"
2-1000S162-43	4'-8"	4'-1"	2'-8"	3'-4"	3'-0"	3'-6"	10'-1"	2'-9"	2'-6"	2'-3"
2-1000S162-54	9'-3"	8'-2"	7'-3"	6'-7"	6'-0"	7'-0"	6'-2"	5'-6"	5'-0"	4'-6"
2-1000S162-68	11'-1"	10'-5"	9'-10"	9'-4"	8'-11"	9'-8"	9'-1"	8'-5"	7'-10"	7'-4"
2-1000S162-97	13'-9"	12'-11"	12'-2"	11'-7"	11'-1"	11'-11"	11'-3"	10'-7"	10'-1"	9'-7"
2-1200S162-54	7'-8"	6'-9"	6'-1"	5'-6"	5'-0"	5'-10"	5'-1"	4'-7"	4'-1"	3'-9"
2-1200S162-68	12'-3"	11'-6"	10'-11"	10'-4"	9'-11"	10'-8"	10'-0"	9'-2"	8'-4"	7'-7"
2-1200S162-97	15'-4"	14'-5"	13'-7"	12'-11"	12'-4"	13'-4"	12'-6"	11'-10"	11'-3"	10'-9"

For SI: 1 inch = 25.4 mm, 1 foot = 304.8 mm, 1 pound per square foot = 0.0479 kPa, 1 pound per square inch = 6.895 kPa.

a. Deflection criterion: $L/360$ for live loads, $L/240$ for total loads.

b. Design load assumptions:
    Roof/ceiling dead load is 12 psf.
    Attic live load is 10 psf.

c. Building width is in the direction of horizontal framing members supported by the header.

TABLE R603.6(17)
BACK-TO-BACK HEADER SPANS
Headers Supporting One Floor, Roof and Ceiling (33 ksi steel)[a, b]

MEMBER DESIGNATION	GROUND SNOW LOAD (20 psf)					GROUND SNOW LOAD (30 psf)				
	Building width[c] (feet)					Building width[c] (feet)				
	24	28	32	36	40	24	28	32	36	40
2-350S162-33	—	—	—	—	—	—	—	—	—	—
2-350S162-43	2'-2"	—	—	—	—	2'-1"	—	—	—	—
2-350S162-54	3'-3"	2'-9"	2'-5"	2'-0"	—	3'-2"	2'-9"	2'-4"	—	—
2-350S162-68	4'-4"	3'-8"	3'-3"	2'-11"	2'-8"	4'-0"	3'-7"	3'-2"	2'-11"	2'-7"
2-350S162-97	5'-2"	4'-9"	4'-4"	4'-1"	3'-9"	5'-1"	4'-8"	4'-4"	4'-0"	3'-9"
2-550S162-33	—	—	—	—	—	—	—	—	—	—
2-550S162-43	3'-6"	2'-10"	2'-3"	—	—	3'-5"	2'-9"	2'-2"	—	—
2-550S162-54	4'-9"	4'-2"	3'-9"	3'-3"	2'-10"	4'-8"	4'-1"	3'-8"	3'-2"	2'-9"
2-550S162-68	5'-10"	5'-3"	4'-10"	4'-5"	4'-1"	5'-9"	5'-3"	4'-9"	4'-4"	4'-0"
2-550S162-97	7'-4"	6'-9"	6'-4"	5'-11"	5'-6"	7'-3"	6'-9"	6'-3"	5'-10"	5'-5"
2-800S162-33	—	—	—	—	—	—	—	—	—	—
2-800S162-43	4'-4"	3'-8"	2'-11"	2'-3"	—	4'-3"	3'-6"	2'-10"	2'-1"	—
2-800S162-54	6'-1"	5'-5"	4'-10"	4'-4"	3'-10"	6'-0"	5'-4"	4'-9"	4'-3"	3'-9"
2-800S162-68	7'-8"	7'-0"	6'-5"	5'-11"	5'-5"	7'-7"	6'-11"	6'-4"	5'-10"	5'-4"
2-800S162-97	9'-10"	9'-1"	8'-5"	7'-11"	7'-5"	9'-8"	8'-11"	8'-4"	7'-10"	7'-4"
2-1000S162-43	4'-4"	3'-9"	3'-4"	2'-8"	—	4'-3"	3'-8"	3'-3"	2'-6"	—
2-1000S162-54	6'-11"	6'-2"	5'-6"	5'-0"	4'-5"	6'-10"	6'-1"	5'-5"	4'-10"	4'-4"
2-1000S162-68	8'-10"	8'-1"	7'-5"	6'-10"	6'-4"	8'-8"	7'-11"	7'-3"	6'-8"	6'-2"
2-1000S162-97	11'-3"	10'-7"	9'-11"	9'-5"	8'-10"	11'-2"	10'-5"	9'-10"	9'-3"	8'-9"
2-1200S162-54	7'-1"	6'-2"	5'-6"	5'-0"	4'-6"	6'-11"	6'-1"	5'-5"	4'-10"	4'-5"
2-1200S162-68	9'-10"	9'-0"	8'-3"	7'-7"	7'-0"	9'-8"	8'-10"	8'-1"[11]	7'-6"	6'-11"
2-1200S162-97	12'-4"	11'-7"	10'-11"	10'-4"	9'-10"	12'-3"	11'-5"	10'-9"	10'-3"	9'-9"

For SI: 1 inch = 25.4 mm, 1 foot = 304.8 mm, 1 pound per square foot = 0.0479 kPa, 1 pound per square inch = 6.895 kPa.

a. Deflection criterion: $L/360$ for live loads, $L/240$ for total loads.
b. Design load assumptions:
   Second floor dead load is 10 psf.
   Roof/ceiling dead load is 12 psf.
   Second floor live load is 30 psf.
   Attic live load is 10 psf.
c. Building width is in the direction of horizontal framing members supported by the header.

TABLE R603.6(18)
BACK-TO-BACK HEADER SPANS
Headers Supporting One Floor, Roof and Ceiling (50 ksi steel)[a, b]

MEMBER DESIGNATION	GROUND SNOW LOAD (20 psf) Building width[c] (feet)					GROUND SNOW LOAD (30 psf) Building width[c] (feet)				
	24	28	32	36	40	24	28	32	36	40
2-350S162-33	—	—	—	—	—	—	—	—	—	—
2-350S162-43	3'-4"	2'-11"	2'-6"	2'-2"	—	3'-3"	2'-10"	2'-5"	2'-1"	—
2-350S162-54	4'-6"	4'-1"	3'-8"	3'-4"	3'-0"	4'-5"	4'-0"	3'-7"	3'-3"	2'-11"
2-350S162-68	5'-0"	4'-9"	4'-7"	4'-5"	4'-3"	4'-11"	4'-8"	4'-6"	4'-4"	4'-2"
2-350S162-97	5'-6"	5'-3"	5'-1"	4'-11"	4'-9"	5'-5"	5'-2"	5'-0"	4'-10"	4'-8"
2-550S162-33	3'-1"	2'-5"	—	—	—	3'-0"	2'-3"	—	—	—
2-550S162-43	5'-1"	4'-6"	4'-0"	3'-6"	3'-1"	4'-11"	4'-5"	3'-11"	3'-5"	3'-0"
2-550S162-54	6'-8"	6'-2"	5'-7"	5'-2"	4'-9"	6'-6"	6'-0"	5'-6"	5'-1"	4'-8"
2-550S162-68	7'-2"	6'-10"	6'-7"	6'-4"	6'-1"	7'-0"	6'-9"	6'-6"	6'-3"	6'-0"
2-550S162-97	7'-11"	7'-7"	7'-3"	7'-0"	6'-10"	7'-9"	7'-5"	7'-2"	6'-11"	6'-9"
2-800S162-33	2'-5"	2'-2"	1'-11"	—	—	2'-5"	2'-1"	1'-10"	—	—
2-800S162-43	5'-5"	4'-9"	4'-3"	3'-9"	3'-5"	5'-3"	4'-8"	4'-1"	3'-9"	3'-5"
2-800S162-54	7'-11"	7'-2"	6'-7"	6'-1"	5'-7"	7'-9"	7'-1"	6'-6"	6'-0"	5'-6"
2-800S162-68	9'-5"	8'-9"	8'-3"	7'-9"	7'-4"	9'-3"	8'-8"	8'-2"	7'-8"	7'-3"
2-800S162-97	10'-9"	10'-3"	9'-11"	9'-7"	9'-3"	10'-7"	10'-1"	9'-9"	9'-5"	9'-1"
2-1000S162-43	4'-4"	3'-9"	3'-4"	3'-0"	2'-9"	4'-3"	3'-8"	3'-3"	2'-11"	2'-8"
2-1000S162-54	8'-6"	7'-5"	6'-8"	6'-0"	5'-5"	8'-4"	7'-4"	6'-6"	5'-10"	5'-4"
2-1000S162-68	10'-8"	10'-0"	9'-5"	8'-11"	8'-4"	10'-7"	9'-10"	9'-4"	8'-9"	8'-3"
2-1000S162-97	12'-11"	12'-4"	11'-8"	11'-1"	10'-6"	12'-9"	12'-2"	11'-6"	10'-11"	10'-5"
2-1200S162-54	7'-1"	6'-2"	5'-6"	5'-0"	4'-6"	6'-11"	6'-1"	5'-5"	4'-10"	4'-5"
2-1200S162-68	11'-9"	11'-0"	10'-5"	9'-10"	9'-1"	11'-8"	10'-11"	10'-3"	9'-9"	8'-11"
2-1200S162-97	14'-9"	13'-9"	13'-0"	12'-4"	11'-9"	14'-7"	13'-8"	12'-10"	12'-3"	11'-8"

For SI: 1 inch = 25.4 mm, 1 foot = 304.8 mm, 1 pound per square foot = 0.0479 kPa, 1 pound per square inch = 6.895 kPa.

a. Deflection criterion: $L/360$ for live loads, $L/240$ for total loads.

b. Design load assumptions:
  Second floor dead load is 10 psf.
  Roof/ceiling dead load is 12 psf.
  Second floor live load is 30 psf.
  Attic live load is 10 psf.

c. Building width is in the direction of horizontal framing members supported by the header.

TABLE R603.6(19)
BACK-TO-BACK HEADER SPANS
Headers Supporting One Floor, Roof and Ceiling (33 ksi steel)[a, b]

MEMBER DESIGNATION	GROUND SNOW LOAD (50 psf)					GROUND SNOW LOAD (70 psf)				
	Building width[c] (feet)					Building width[c] (feet)				
	24	28	32	36	40	24	28	32	36	40
2-350S162-33	—	—	—	—	—	—	—	—	—	—
2-350S162-43	—	—	—	—	—	—	—	—	—	—
2-350S162-54	2'-4"	—	—	—	—	—	—	—	—	—
2-350S162-68	3'-3"	2'-10"	2'-6"	2'-2"	—	2'-7"	2'-2"	—	—	—
2-350S162-97	4'-4"	4'-0"	3'-8"	3'-4"	3'-1"	3'-9"	3'-4"	3'-1"	2'-9"	2'-6"
2-550S162-33	—	—	—	—	—	—	—	—	—	—
2-550S162-43	2'-2"	—	—	—	—	—	—	—	—	—
2-550S162-54	3'-8"	3'-2"	2'-8"	2'-3"	—	2'-10"	2'-3"	—	—	—
2-550S162-68	4'-9"	4'-4"	3'-11"	3'-6"	3'-2"	4'-0"	3'-6"	3'-1"	2'-9"	2'-4"
2-550S162-97	6'-3"	5'-9"	5'-4"	5'-0"	4'-8"	5'-6"	5'-0"	4'-7"	4'-3"	3'-11"
2-800S162-33	—	—	—	—	—	—	—	—	—	—
2-800S162-43	2'-11"	2'-0"	—	—	—	—	—	—	—	—
2-800S162-54	4'-9"	4'-2"	3'-7"	3'-1"	2'-7"	3'-9"	3'-1"	2'-5"	—	—
2-800S162-68	6'-4"	5'-9"	5'-3"	4'-9"	4'-4"	5'-4"	4'-9"	4'-3"	3'-10"	3'-4"
2-800S162-97	8'-5"	7'-9"	7'-3"	6'-9"	6'-4"	7'-4"	6'-9"	6'-3"	5'-10"	5'-5"
2-1000S162-43	3'-4"	2'-5"	—	—	—	—	—	—	—	—
2-1000S162-54	5'-6"	4'-10"	4'-2"	3'-7"	3'-0"	4'-4"	3'-7"	2'-11"	2'-2"	—
2-1000S162-68	7'-4"	6'-8"	6'-1"	5'-7"	5'-1"	6'-3"	5'-7"	5'-0"	4'-5"	4'-0"
2-1000S162-97	9'-11"	8'-3"	8'-7"	8'-1"	7'-7"	8'-9"	8'-1"	7'-6"	7'-0"	6'-6"
2-1200S162-54	5'-6"	4'-10"	4'-4"	3'-11"	3'-5"	4'-5"	3'-11"	3'-3"	2'-6"	—
2-1200S162-68	8'-2"	7'-5"	6'-9"	6'-3"	5'-8"	6'-11"	6'-3"	5'-7"	5'-0"	4'-6"
2-1200S162-97	10'-10"	10'-2"	9'-8"	9'-2"	8'-7"	9'-9"	9'-2"	8'-6"	7'-11"	7'-5"

For SI: 1 inch = 25.4 mm, 1 foot = 304.8 mm, 1 pound per square foot = 0.0479kPa, 1 pound per square inch = 6.895 kPa.

a. Deflection criterion: $L/360$ for live loads, $L/240$ for total loads.

b. Design load assumptions:
   Second floor dead load is 10 psf.
   Roof/ceiling dead load is 12 psf.
   Second floor live load is 30 psf.
   Attic live load is 10 psf.

c. Building width is in the direction of horizontal framing members supported by the header.

TABLE R603.6(20)
BACK-TO-BACK HEADER SPANS
Headers Supporting One Floor, Roof and Ceiling (50 ksi steel)[a, b]

MEMBER DESIGNATION	GROUND SNOW LOAD (50 psf)					GROUND SNOW LOAD (70 psf)				
	Building width[c] (feet)					Building width[c] (feet)				
	24	28	32	36	40	24	28	32	36	40
2-350S162-33	—	—	—	—	—	—	—	—	—	—
2-350S162-43	2'-6"	2'-0"	—	—	—	—	—	—	—	—
2-350S162-54	3'-8"	3'-3"	2'-11"	2'-7"	2'-3"	3'-0"	2'-7"	2'-2"	—	—
2-350S162-68	4'-7"	4'-5"	4'-1"	3'-9"	3'-6"	4'-2"	3'-9"	3'-5"	3'-1"	2'-10"
2-350S162-97	5'-1"	4'-10"	4'-8"	4'-6"	4'-5"	4'-10"	4'-7"	4'-5"	4'-3"	4'-1"
2-550S162-33	—	—	—	—	—	—	—	—	—	—
2-550S162-43	3'-11"	3'-5"	2'-11"	2'-5"	—	3'-0"	2'-5"	—	—	—
2-550S162-54	5'-7"	5'-0"	4'-7"	4'-2"	3'-9"	4'-8"	4'-2"	3'-8"	3'-3"	2'-11"
2-550S162-68	6'-7"	6'-4"	5'-11"	5'-6"	5'-1"	6'-0"	5'-6"	5'-0"	4'-7"	4'-3"
2-550S162-97	7'-4"	7'-0"	6'-9"	6'-6"	6'-4"	6'-11"	6'-8"	6'-5"	6'-2"	6'-0"
2-800S162-33	1'-11"	—	—	—	—	—	—	—	—	—
2-800S162-43	4'-2"	3'-8"	3'-4"	3'-0"	2'-6"	3'-5"	3'-0"	2'-4"	—	—
2-800S162-54	6'-7"	5'-11"	5'-5"	4'-11"	4'-6"	5'-6"	4'-11"	4'-5"	3'-11"	3'-6"
2-800S162-68	8'-3"	7'-8"	7'-1"	6'-8"	6'-2"	7'-3"	6'-7"	6'-1"	5'-7"	5'-2"
2-800S162-97	9'-11"	9'-6"	9'-2"	8'-10"	8'-7"	9'-5"	9'-0"	8'-7"	8'-2"	7'-9"
2-1000S162-43	3'-4"	2'-11"	2'-7"	2'-5"	2'-2"	2'-8"	2'-5"	2'-2"	1'-11"	—
2-1000S162-54	6'-7"	5'-10"	5'-3"	4'-9"	4'-4"	5'-4"	4'-9"	4'-3"	3'-10"	3'-6"
2-1000S162-68	9'-4"	8'-9"	8'-1"	7'-7"	7'-1"	8'-3"	7'-7"	6'-11"	6'-5"	5'-11"
2-1000S162-97	11'-7"	10'-11"	10'-4"	9'-10"	9'-5"	10'-5"	9'-10"	9'-3"	8'-10"	8'-5"
2-1200S162-54	5'-6"	4'-10"	4'-4"	3'-11"	3'-7"	4'-5"	3'-11"	3'-6"	3'-2"	2'-11"
2-1200S162-68	10'-4"	9'-8"	8'-8"	7'-11"	7'-2"	8'-11"	7'-11"	7'-1"	6'-5"	5'-10"
2-1200S162-97	12'-11"	12'-2"	11'-6"	11'-0"	10'-6"	11'-8"	11'-0"	10'-5"	9'-10"	9'-5"

For SI: 1 inch = 25.4 mm, 1 foot = 304.8 mm, 1 pound per square foot = 0.0479 kPa, 1 pound per square inch = 6.895 kPa.

a. Deflection criterion: $L/360$ for live loads, $L/240$ for total loads.

b. Design load assumptions:
    Second floor dead load is 10 psf.
    Roof/ceiling dead load is 12 psf.
    Second floor live load is 30 psf.
    Attic live load is 10 psf.

c. Building width is in the direction of horizontal framing members supported by the header.

TABLE R603.6(21)
BACK-TO-BACK HEADER SPANS
Headers Supporting Two Floors, Roof and Ceiling (33 ksi steel)[a, b]

MEMBER DESIGNATION	GROUND SNOW LOAD (20 psf) Building width[c] (feet)					GROUND SNOW LOAD (30 psf) Building width[c] (feet)				
	24	28	32	36	40	24	28	32	36	40
2-350S162-33	—	—	—	—	—	—	—	—	—	—
2-350S162-43	—	—	—	—	—	—	—	—	—	—
2-350S162-54	—	—	—	—	—	—	—	—	—	—
2-350S162-68	2'-5"	—	—	—	—	2'-4"	—	—	—	—
2-350S162-97	3'-6"	3'-2"	2'-10"	2'-6"	2'-3"	3'-6"	3'-1"	2'-9"	2'-6"	2'-3"
2-550S162-33	—	—	—	—	—	—	—	—	—	—
2-550S162-43	—	—	—	—	—	—	—	—	—	—
2-550S162-54	2'-6"	—	—	—	—	2'-5"	—	—	—	—
2-550S162-68	3'-9"	3'-3"	2'-9"	2'-4"	—	3'-8"	3'-2"	2'-9"	2'-4"	—
2-550S162-97	5'-3"	4'-9"	4'-4"	3'-11"	3'-8"	5'-2"	4'-8"	4'-3"	3'-11"	3'-7"
2-800S162-33	—	—	—	—	—	—	—	—	—	—
2-800S162-43	—	—	—	—	—	—	—	—	—	—
2-800S162-54	3'-5"	2'-8"	—	—	—	3'-4"	2'-7"	—	—	—
2-800S162-68	5'-1"	4'-5"	3'-11"	3'-4"	2'-11"	5'-0"	4'-4"	3'-10"	3'-4"	2'-10"
2-800S162-97	7'-0"	6'-5"	5'-11"	5'-5"	5'-0"	7'-0"	6'-4"	5'-10"	5'-5"	5'-0"
2-1000S162-43	—	—	—	—	—	—	—	—	—	—
2-1000S162-54	3'-11"	3'-1"	2'-3"	—	—	3'-10"	3'-0"	2'-2"	—	—
2-1000S162-68	5'-10"	5'-2"	4'-6"	4'-0"	3'-5"	5'-9"	5'-1"	4'-6"	3'-11"	3'-4"
2-1000S162-97	8'-5"	7'-8"	7'-1"	6'-6"	6'-1"	8'-4"	7'-7"	7'-0"	6'-6"	6'-0"
2-1200S162-54	4'-2"	3'-6"	2'-7"	—	—	4'-1"	3'-5"	2'-6"	—	—
2-1200S162-68	6'-6"	5'-9"	5'-1"	4'-6"	3'-11"	6'-6"	5'-8"	5'-0"	4'-5"	3'-10"
2-1200S162-97	9'-5"	8'-8"	8'-0"	7'-5"	6'-11"	9'-5"	8'-7"	7'-11"	7'-4"	6'-10"

For SI: 1 inch = 25.4 mm, 1 foot = 304.8 mm, 1 pound per square foot = 0.0479 kPa, 1 pound per square inch = 6.895 kPa.

a. Deflection criterion: $L/360$ for live loads, $L/240$ for total loads.

b. Design load assumptions:
   Second floor dead load is 10 psf.
   Roof/ceiling dead load is 12 psf.
   Second floor live load is 40 psf.
   Third floor live load is 30 psf.
   Attic live load is 10 psf.

c. Building width is in the direction of horizontal framing members supported by the header.

TABLE R603.6(22)
BACK-TO-BACK HEADER SPANS
Headers Supporting Two Floors, Roof and Ceiling (50 ksi steel)[a, b]

MEMBER DESIGNATION	GROUND SNOW LOAD (20 psf) Building width[c] (feet)					GROUND SNOW LOAD (30 psf) Building width[c] (feet)				
	24	28	32	36	40	24	28	32	36	40
2-350S162-33	—	—	—	—	—	—	—	—	—	—
2-350S162-43	—	—	—	—	—	—	—	—	—	—
2-350S162-54	2'-9"	2'-3"	—	—	—	2'-8"	2'-3"	—	—	—
2-350S162-68	3'-11"	3'-6"	3'-2"	2'-10"	2'-6"	3'-11"	3'-6"	3'-1"	2'-9"	2'-6"
2-350S162-97	4'-9"	4'-6"	4'-4"	4'-1"	3'-10"	4'-8"	4'-6"	4'-4"	4'-1"	3'-9"
2-550S162-33	—	—	—	—	—	—	—	—	—	—
2-550S162-43	2'-9"	2'-0"	—	—	—	2'-8"	—	—	—	—
2-550S162-54	4'-5"	3'-10"	3'-4"	2'-11"	2'-5"	4'-4"	3'-9"	3'-3"	2'-10"	2'-5"
2-550S162-68	5'-8"	5'-2"	4'-8"	4'-3"	3'-11"	5'-8"	5'-1"	4'-8"	4'-3"	3'-10"
2-550S162-97	6'-10"	6'-6"	6'-3"	6'-0"	5'-7"	6'-9"	6'-5"	6'-3"	5'-11"	5'-6"
2-800S162-33	—	—	—	—	—	—	—	—	—	—
2-800S162-43	3'-2"	2'-7"	—	—	—	3'-1"	2'-6"	—	—	—
2-800S162-54	5'-2"	4'-7"	4'-0"	3'-6"	3'-0"	5'-2"	4'-6"	3'-11"	3'-5"	2'-11"
2-800S162-68	6'-11"	6'-3"	5'-8"	5'-2"	4'-9"	6'-10"	6'-2"	5'-7"	5'-2"	4'-8"
2-800S162-97	9'-3"	8'-8"	8'-3"	7'-9"	7'-4"	9'-2"	8'-8"	8'-2"	7'-9"	7'-4"
2-1000S162-43	2'-6"	2'-2"	2'-0"	—	—	2'-6"	2'-2"	1'-11"	—	—
2-1000S162-54	5'-0"	4'-4"	3'-11"	3'-6"	3'-2"	4'-11"	4'-4"	3'-10"	3'-6"	3'-2"
2-1000S162-68	7'-10"	7'-2"	6'-6"	5'-11"	5'-6"	7'-9"	7'-1"	6'-5"	5'-11"	5'-5"
2-1000S162-97	10'-1"	9'-5"	8'-11"	8'-6"	8'-0"	10'-0"	9'-5"	8'-10"	8'-5"	7'-11"
2-1200S162-54	—	—	—	—	—	—	—	—	—	—
2-1200S162-68	7'-4"	6'-8"	6'-1"	5'-6"	5'-1"	7'-3"	6'-7"	6'-0"	5'-6"	5'-0"
2-1200S162-97	9'-5"	8'-8"	8'-1"	7'-6"	7'-1"	9'-4"	8'-8"	8'-0"	7'-6"	7'-0"

For SI: 1 inch = 25.4 mm, 1 foot = 304.8 mm, 1 pound per square foot = 0.0479 kPa, 1 pound per square inch = 6.895 kPa.

a. Deflection criterion: $L/360$ for live loads, $L/240$ for total loads.

b. Design load assumptions:

   Second floor dead load is 10 psf.
   Roof/ceiling dead load is 12 psf.
   Second floor live load is 40 psf.
   Third floor live load is 30 psf.
   Attic live load is 10 psf.

c. Building width is in the direction of horizontal framing members supported by the header.

TABLE R603.6(23)
BACK-TO-BACK HEADER SPANS
Headers Supporting Two Floors, Roof and ceiling (50 ksi steel)[a, b]

MEMBER DESIGNATION	GROUND SNOW LOAD (50 psf) Building width[c] (feet)					GROUND SNOW LOAD (70 psf) Building width[c] (feet)				
	24	28	32	36	40	24	28	32	36	40
2-350S162-33	—	—	—	—	—	—	—	—	—	—
2-350S162-43	—	—	—	—	—	—	—	—	—	—
2-350S162-54	—	—	—	—	—	—	—	—	—	—
2-350S162-68	2'-2"	—	—	—	—	—	—	—	—	—
2-350S162-97	3'-3"	3'-0"	2'-8"	2'-4"	2'-1"	3'-1"	2'-9"	2'-6"	2'-2"	—
2-550S162-33	—	—	—	—	—	—	—	—	—	—
2-550S162-43	—	—	—	—	—	—	—	—	—	—
2-550S162-54	2'-2"	—	—	—	—	—	—	—	—	—
2-550S162-68	3'-6"	3'-0"	2'-6"	2'-1"	—	3'-2"	2'-9"	2'-3"	—	—
2-550S162-97	5'-0"	4'-6"	4'-1"	3'-9"	3'-5"	4'-8"	4'-3"	3'-11"	3'-7"	3'-3"
2-800S162-33	—	—	—	—	—	—	—	—	—	—
2-800S162-43	—	—	—	—	—	—	—	—	—	—
2-800S162-54	3'-0"	2'-3"	—	—	—	2'-7"	—	—	—	—
2-800S162-68	4'-9"	4'-2"	3'-7"	3'-1"	2'-7"	4'-5"	3'-10"	3'-3"	2'-9"	2'-3"
2-800S162-97	6'-9"	6'-1"	5'-7"	5'-2"	4'-9"	6'-4"	5'-10"	5'-4"	4'-11"	4'-7"
2-1000S162-43	—	—	—	—	—	—	—	—	—	—
2-1000S162-54	3'-6"	2'-8"	—	—	—	3'-1"	2'-2"	—	—	—
2-1000S162-68	5'-6"	4'-10"	4'-2"	3'-7"	3'-1"	5'-1"	4'-6"	3'-10"	3'-4"	2'-9"
2-1000S162-97	8'-0"	7'-4"	6'-9"	6'-3"	5'-9"	7'-7"	7'-0"	6'-5"	5'-11"	5'-6"
2-1200S162-54	3'-11"	3'-0"	2'-0"	—	—	3'-5"	2'-6"	—	—	—
2-1200S162-68	6'-2"	5'-5"	4'-9"	4'-1"	3'-6"	5'-9"	5'-0"	4'-4"	3'-9"	3'-2"
2-1200S162-97	9'-1"	8'-4"	7'-8"	7'-1"	6'-7"	8'-8"	7'-11"	7'-4"	6'-9"	6'-3"

For SI: 1 inch = 25.4 mm, 1 foot = 304.8 mm, 1 pound per square foot = 0.0479kPa, 1 pound per square inch = 6.895 kPa.

a. Deflection criterion: $L/360$ for live loads, $L/240$ for total loads.

b. Design load assumptions:
  Second floor dead load is 10 psf.
  Roof/ceiling dead load is 12 psf.
  Second floor live load is 40 psf.
  Third floor live load is 30 psf.
  Attic live load is 10 psf.

c. Building width is in the direction of horizontal framing members supported by the header.

TABLE R603.6(24)
BACK-TO-BACK HEADER SPANS
Headers Supporting Two Floors, Roof and Ceiling (50 ksi steel)[a, b]

MEMBER DESIGNATION	GROUND SNOW LOAD (50 psf)					GROUND SNOW LOAD (70 psf)				
	Building width[c] (feet)					Building width[c] (feet)				
	24	28	32	36	40	24	28	32	36	40
2-350S162-33	—	—	—	—	—	—	—	—	—	—
2-350S162-43	—	—	—	—	—	—	—	—	—	—
2-350S162-54	2′-6″	2′-1″	—	—	—	2′-3″	—	—	—	—
2-350S162-68	3′-9″	3′-4″	2′-11″	2′-7″	2′-4″	3′-6″	3′-1″	2′-9″	2′-5″	2′-2″
2-350S162-97	4′-6″	4′-4″	4′-2″	3′-11″	3′-8″	4′-4″	4′-2″	4′-0″	3′-9″	3′-6″
2-550S162-33	—	—	—	—	—	—	—	—	—	—
2-550S162-43	2′-5″	—	—	—	—	—	—	—	—	—
2-550S162-54	4′-1″	3′-7″	3′-1″	2′-7″	2′-2″	3′-10″	3′-3″	2′-10″	2′-4″	—
2-550S162-68	5′-5″	4′-11″	4′-5″	4′-0″	3′-8″	5′-1″	4′-7″	4′-2″	3′-10″	3′-5″
2-550S162-97	6′-5″	6′-2″	5′-11″	5′-9″	5′-4″	6′-3″	6′-0″	5′-9″	5′-6″	5′-2″
2-800S162-33	—	—	—	—	—	—	—	—	—	—
2-800S162-43	2′-11″	2′-2″	—	—	—	2′-6″	—	—	—	—
2-800S162-54	4′-11″	4′-3″	3′-8″	3′-2″	2′-8″	4′-6″	3′-11″	3′-5″	2′-11″	2′-4″
2-800S162-68	6′-7″	5′-11″	5′-4″	4′-11″	4′-6″	6′-2″	5′-7″	5′-1″	4′-8″	4′-3″
2-800S162-97	8′-9″	8′-5″	7′-11″	7′-6″	7′-0″	8′-5″	8′-1″	7′-9″	7′-3″	6′-10″
2-1000S162-43	2′-4″	2′-1″	—	—	—	2′-2″	1′-11″	—	—	—
2-1000S162-54	4′-8″	4′-1″	3′-8″	3′-3″	3′-0″	4′-4″	3′-10″	3′-5″	3′-1″	2′-9″
2-1000S162-68	7′-6″	6′-9″	6′-2″	5′-8″	5′-2″	7′-1″	6′-5″	5′-10″	5′-4″	4′-11″
2-1000S162-97	9′-9″	9′-2″	8′-7″	8′-2″	7′-8″	9′-5″	8′-10″	8′-5″	7′-11″	7′-5″
2-1200S162-54	—	—	—	—	—	—	—	—	—	—
2-1200S162-68	7′-0″	6′-4″	5′-9″	5′-3″	4′-9″	6′-7″	6′-0″	5′-5″	5′-0″	4′-6″
2-1200S162-97	9′-1″	8′-4″	7′-9″	7′-3″	6′-9″	8′-8″	8′-0″	7′-6″	7′-0″	6′-7″

For SI: 1 inch = 25.4 mm, 1 foot = 304.8 mm, 1 pound per square foot = 0.0479 kPa, 1 pound per square inch = 6.895 kPa.

a. Deflection criterion: $L/360$ for live loads, $L/240$ for total loads.

b. Design load assumptions:
   Second floor dead load is 10 psf.
   Roof/ceiling dead load is 12 psf.
   Second floor live load is 40 psf.
   Third floor live load is 30 psf.
   Attic live load is 10 psf.

c. Building width is in the direction of horizontal framing members supported by the header.

TABLE R603.7(1)
TOTAL NUMBER OF JACK AND KING STUDS REQUIRED AT EACH END OF AN OPENING

SIZE OF OPENING (feet-inches)	24″ O.C. STUD SPACING		16″ O.C. STUD SPACING	
	No. of jack studs	No. of king studs	No. of jack studs	No. of king studs
Up to 3'-6″	1	1	1	1
> 3'-6″ to 5'-0″	1	2	1	2
> 5'-0″ to 5'-6″	1	2	2	2
> 5'-6″ to 8'-0″	1	2	2	2
> 8'-0″ to 10'-6″	2	2	2	3
> 10'-6″ to 12'-0″	2	2	3	3
> 12'-0″ to 13'-0″	2	3	3	3
> 13'-0″ to 14'-0″	2	3	3	4
> 14'-0″ to 16'-0″	2	3	3	4
> 16'-0″ to 18'-0″	3	3	4	4

For SI: 1 inch = 25.4 mm, 1 foot = 304.8 mm.

TABLE R603.7(2)
HEADER TO KING STUD CONNECTION REQUIREMENTS[a, b, c, d]

HEADER SPAN (feet)	BASIC WIND SPEED (mph), EXPOSURE		
	85 B or Seismic Design Categories A, B, C, D_0, D_1 and D_2	85 C or less than 110 B	Less than 110 C
≤ 4'	4-No. 8 screws	4-No. 8 screws	6-No. 8 screws
> 4' to 8'	4-No. 8 screws	4-No. 8 screws	8-No. 8 screws
> 8' to 12'	4-No. 8 screws	6-No. 8 screws	10-No. 8 screws
> 12' to 16'	4-No. 8 screws	8-No. 8 screws	12-No. 8 screws

For SI: 1 inch = 25.4 mm, 1 foot = 304.8 mm, 1 mile per hour = 0.447 m/s, 1 pound = 4.448 N.

a. All screw sizes shown are minimum.

b. For headers located on the first floor of a two-story building or the first or second floor of a three-story building, the total number of screws is permitted to be reduced by 2 screws, but the total number of screws shall be no less than 4.

c. For roof slopes of 6:12 or greater, the required number of screws may be reduced by half, but the total number of screws shall be no less than four.

d. Screws can be replaced by an uplift connector which has a capacity of the number of screws multiplied by 164 pounds (e.g., 12-No. 8 screws can be replaced by an uplift connector whose capacity exceeds 12 × 164 pounds = 1,968 pounds).

TABLE R603.8
HEAD AND SILL TRACK SPAN
F_y = 33 ksi

BASIC WIND SPEED (mph)		ALLOWABLE HEAD AND SILL TRACK SPAN[a,b,c] (ft-in.)					
EXPOSURE		TRACK DESIGNATION					
B	C	350T125-33	350T125-43	350T125-54	550T125-33	550T125-43	550T125-54
85	—	5'-0"	5'-7"	6'-2"	5'-10"	6'-8"	7'-0"
90	—	4'-10"	5'-5"	6'-0"	5'-8"	6'-3"	6'-10"
100	85	4'-6"	5'-1"	5'-8"	5'-4"	5'-11"	6'-5"
110	90	4'-2"	4'-9"	5'-4"	5'-1"	5'-7"	6'-1"
120	100	3'-11"	4'-6"	5'-0"	4'-10"	5'-4"	5'-10"
130	110	3'-8"	4'-2"	4'-9"	4'-1"	5'-1"	5'-7"
140	120	3'-7"	4'-1"	4'-7"	3'-6"	4'-11"	5'-5"
150	130	3'-5"	3'-10"	4'-4"	2'-11"	4'-7"	5'-2"
—	140	3'-1"	3'-6"	4'-1"	2'-3"	4'-0"	4'-10"
—	150	2'-9"	3'-4"	3'-10"	2'-0"	3'-7"	4'-7"

For SI: 1 inch = 25.4 mm, 1 foot = 304.8 mm, 1 mile per hour = 0.447 m/s.

a. Deflection limit: $L/240$.

b. Head and sill track spans are based on components and cladding wind speeds and 48 inch tributary span.

c. For openings less than 4 feet in height that have both a head track and sill track, the above spans are permitted to be multiplied by 1.75. For openings less than or equal to 6 feet in height that have both a head track and a sill track, the above spans are permitted to be multiplied by a factor of 1.5.

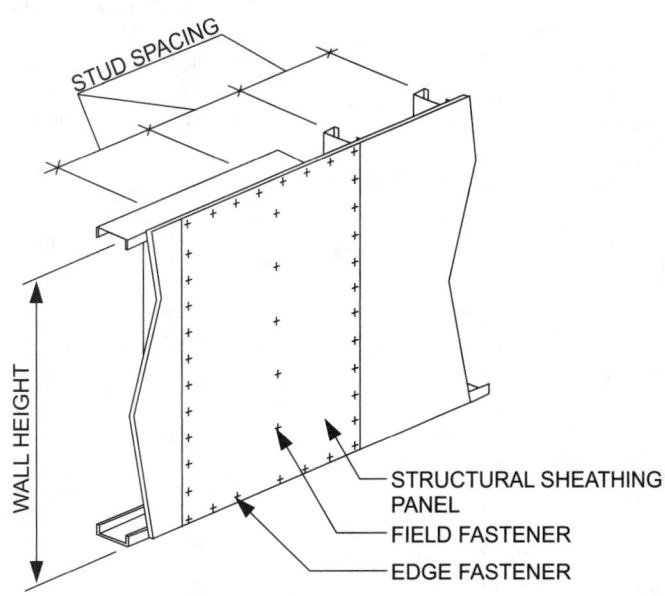

FIGURE R603.9
STRUCTURAL SHEATHING FASTENING PATTERN

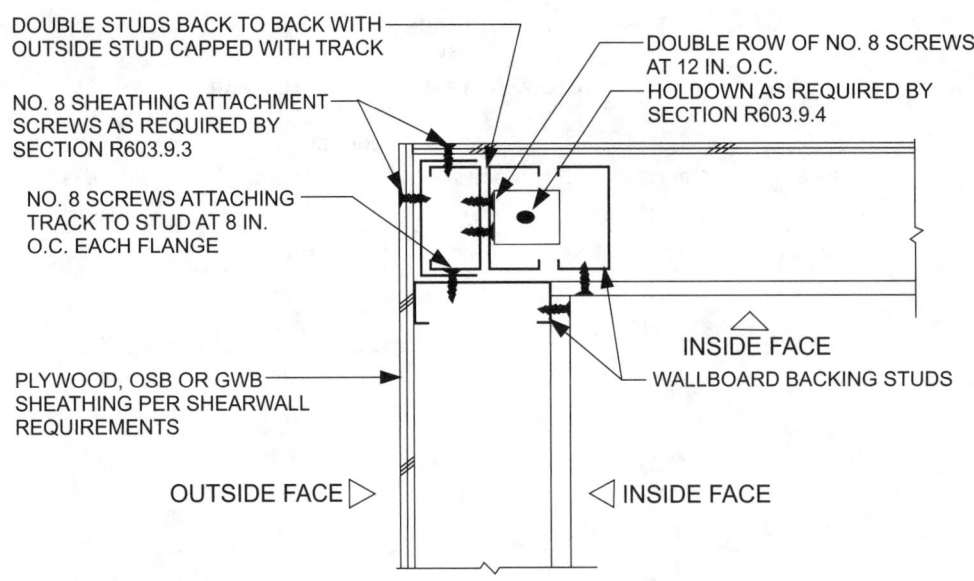

DOUBLE STUDS BACK TO BACK WITH OUTSIDE STUD CAPPED WITH TRACK

NO. 8 SHEATHING ATTACHMENT SCREWS AS REQUIRED BY SECTION R603.9.3

NO. 8 SCREWS ATTACHING TRACK TO STUD AT 8 IN. O.C. EACH FLANGE

DOUBLE ROW OF NO. 8 SCREWS AT 12 IN. O.C.

HOLDOWN AS REQUIRED BY SECTION R603.9.4

INSIDE FACE

WALLBOARD BACKING STUDS

PLYWOOD, OSB OR GWB SHEATHING PER SHEARWALL REQUIREMENTS

OUTSIDE FACE ▷

◁ INSIDE FACE

For SI: 1 inch = 25.4 mm.

FIGURE R603.9.2
CORNER STUD HOLD DOWN DETAIL

TABLE R603.9.2(1)
MINIMUM PERCENTAGE OF FULL HEIGHT
STRUCTURAL SHEATHING ON EXTERIOR WALLS[a,b]

WALL SUPPORTING	ROOF SLOPE	BASIC WIND SPEED AND EXPOSURE (mph)					
		85 B	90 B	100 B / 85 C	< 110 B / 90 C	100 C	< 110 C
Roof and ceiling only (One story or top floor of two or three story building)	3:12	8	9	9	12	16	20
	6:12	12	13	15	20	26	35
	9:12	21	23	25	30	50	58
	12:12	30	33	35	40	66	75
One story, roof and ceiling (First floor of a two-story building or second floor of a three story building)	3:12	24	27	30	35	50	66
	6:12	25	28	30	40	58	74
	9:12	35	38	40	55	74	91
	12:12	40	45	50	65	100	115
Two story, roof and ceiling (First floor of a three story building)	3:12	40	45	51	58	84	112
	6:12	38	43	45	60	90	113
	9:12	49	53	55	80	98	124
	12:12	50	57	65	90	134	155

For SI: 1 mile per hour = 0.447 m/s.

a. Linear interpolation is permitted.

b. For hip-roofed homes the minimum percentage of full height sheathing, based upon wind, is permitted to be multiplied by a factor of 0.95 for roof slopes not exceeding 7:12 and a factor of 0.9 for roof slopes greater than 7:12.

TABLE R603.9.2(2)
FULL HEIGHT SHEATHING LENGTH ADJUSTMENT FACTORS

PLAN ASPECT RATIO	LENGTH ADJUSTMENT FACTORS	
	Short wall	Long wall
1:1	1.0	1.0
1.5:1	1.5	0.67
2:1	2.0	0.50
3:1	3.0	0.33
4:1	4.0	0.25

SECTION R604
WOOD STRUCTURAL PANELS

R604.1 Identification and grade. Wood structural panels shall conform to DOC PS 1 or DOC PS 2 or, when manufactured in Canada, CSA O437 or CSA O325. All panels shall be identified by a grade mark or certificate of inspection issued by an *approved* agency.

R604.2 Allowable spans. The maximum allowable spans for wood structural panel wall sheathing shall not exceed the values set forth in Table R602.3(3).

R604.3 Installation. Wood structural panel wall sheathing shall be attached to framing in accordance with Table R602.3(1). Wood structural panels marked Exposure 1 or Exterior are considered water-repellent sheathing under the code.

SECTION R605
PARTICLEBOARD

R605.1 Identification and grade. Particleboard shall conform to ANSI A208.1 and shall be so identified by a grade mark or certificate of inspection issued by an *approved* agency. Particleboard shall comply with the grades specified in Table R602.3(4).

SECTION R606
GENERAL MASONRY CONSTRUCTION

R606.1 General. Masonry construction shall be designed and constructed in accordance with the provisions of this section or in accordance with the provisions of ACI 530/ASCE 5/TMS 402.

R606.1.1 Professional registration not required. When the empirical design provisions of ACI 530/ASCE 5/TMS 402 Chapter 5 or the provisions of this section are used to design masonry, project drawings, typical details and specifications are not required to bear the seal of the architect or engineer responsible for design, unless otherwise required by the state law of the *jurisdiction* having authority.

R606.2 Thickness of masonry. The nominal thickness of masonry walls shall conform to the requirements of Sections R606.2.1 through R606.2.4.

R606.2.1 Minimum thickness. The minimum thickness of masonry bearing walls more than one *story* high shall be 8 inches (203 mm). *Solid masonry* walls of one-story *dwellings* and garages shall not be less than 6 inches (152 mm) in thickness when not greater than 9 feet (2743 mm) in height, provided that when gable construction is used, an additional 6 feet (1829 mm) is permitted to the peak of the gable. Masonry walls shall be laterally supported in either the horizontal or vertical direction at intervals as required by Section R606.9.

R606.2.2 Rubble stone masonry wall. The minimum thickness of rough, random or coursed rubble stone masonry walls shall be 16 inches (406 mm).

R606.2.3 Change in thickness. Where walls of masonry of hollow units or masonry-bonded hollow walls are decreased in thickness, a course of *solid masonry* shall be constructed between the wall below and the thinner wall above, or special units or construction shall be used to transmit the loads from face shells or wythes above to those below.

R606.2.4 Parapet walls. Unreinforced *solid masonry* parapet walls shall not be less than 8 inches (203 mm) thick and their height shall not exceed four times their thickness. Unreinforced hollow unit masonry parapet walls shall be not less than 8 inches (203 mm) thick, and their height shall not exceed three times their thickness. Masonry parapet walls in areas subject to wind loads of 30 pounds per square foot (1.44 kPa) located in Seismic Design Category D_0, D_1 or D_2, or on townhouses in Seismic Design Category C shall be reinforced in accordance with Section R606.12.

R606.3 Corbeled masonry. Corbeled masonry shall be in accordance with Sections R606.3.1 through R606.3.3.

R606.3.1 Units. *Solid masonry* units or masonry units filled with mortar or grout shall be used for corbeling.

R606.3.2 Corbel projection. The maximum projection of one unit shall not exceed one-half the height of the unit or one-third the thickness at right angles to the wall. The maximum corbeled projection beyond the face of the wall shall not exceed:

1. One-half of the wall thickness for multiwythe walls bonded by mortar or grout and wall ties or masonry headers, or

2. One-half the wythe thickness for single wythe walls, masonry-bonded hollow walls, multiwythe walls with open collar joints and veneer walls.

R606.3.3 Corbeled masonry supporting floor or roof-framing members. When corbeled masonry is used to support floor or roof-framing members, the top course of the corbel shall be a header course or the top course bed joint shall have ties to the vertical wall.

R606.4 Support conditions. Bearing and support conditions shall be in accordance with Sections R606.4.1 and R606.4.2.

R606.4.1 Bearing on support. Each masonry wythe shall be supported by at least two-thirds of the wythe thickness.

R606.4.2 Support at foundation. Cavity wall or masonry veneer construction may be supported on an 8-inch (203 mm) foundation wall, provided the 8-inch (203 mm) wall is corbeled to the width of the wall system above with masonry constructed of *solid masonry* units or masonry units filled with mortar or grout. The total horizontal projection of the corbel shall not exceed 2 inches (51 mm) with individual corbels projecting not more than one-third the thickness of the unit or one-half the height of the unit. The hollow space behind the corbeled masonry shall be filled with mortar or grout.

R606.5 Allowable stresses. Allowable compressive stresses in masonry shall not exceed the values prescribed in Table R606.5. In determining the stresses in masonry, the effects of all loads and conditions of loading and the influence of all forces affecting the design and strength of the several parts shall be taken into account.

R606.5.1 Combined units. In walls or other structural members composed of different kinds or grades of units, materials or mortars, the maximum stress shall not exceed the allowable stress for the weakest of the combination of units, materials and mortars of which the member is composed. The net thickness of any facing unit that is used to resist stress shall be not less than 1.5 inches (38 mm).

R606.6 Piers. The unsupported height of masonry piers shall not exceed ten times their least dimension. When structural clay tile or hollow concrete masonry units are used for isolated piers to support beams and girders, the cellular spaces shall be filled solidly with concrete or Type M or S mortar, except that unfilled hollow piers may be used if their unsupported height is not more than four times their least dimension. Where hollow masonry units are solidly filled with concrete or Type M, S or N mortar, the allowable compressive stress shall be permitted to be increased as provided in Table R606.5.

R606.6.1 Pier cap. Hollow piers shall be capped with 4 inches (102 mm) of *solid masonry* or concrete or shall have cavities of the top course filled with concrete or grout or other *approved* methods.

R606.7 Chases. Chases and recesses in masonry walls shall not be deeper than one-third the wall thickness, and the maximum length of a horizontal chase or horizontal projection shall not exceed 4 feet (1219 mm), and shall have at least 8 inches (203 mm) of masonry in back of the chases and recesses and between adjacent chases or recesses and the jambs of openings. Chases and recesses in masonry walls shall be designed and constructed so as not to reduce the required strength or required fire resistance of the wall and in no case shall a chase or recess be permitted within the required area of a pier. Masonry directly above chases or recesses wider than 12 inches (305 mm) shall be supported on noncombustible lintels.

TABLE R606.5
ALLOWABLE COMPRESSIVE STRESSES FOR EMPIRICAL DESIGN OF MASONRY

CONSTRUCTION; COMPRESSIVE STRENGTH OF UNIT, GROSS AREA	ALLOWABLE COMPRESSIVE STRESSES[a] GROSS CROSS-SECTIONAL AREA[b]	
	Type M or S mortar	Type N mortar
Solid masonry of brick and other solid units of clay or shale; sand-lime or concrete brick:		
8,000+ psi	350	300
4,500 psi	225	200
2,500 psi	160	140
1,500 psi	115	100
Grouted[c] masonry, of clay or shale; sand-lime or concrete:		
4,500+ psi	225	200
2,500 psi	160	140
1,500 psi	115	100
Solid masonry of solid concrete masonry units:		
3,000+ psi	225	200
2,000 psi	160	140
1,200 psi	115	100
Masonry of hollow load-bearing units:		
2,000+ psi	140	120
1,500 psi	115	100
1,000 psi	75	70
700 psi	60	55
Hollow walls (cavity or masonry bonded[d]) solid units:		
2,500+ psi	160	140
1,500 psi	115	100
Hollow units	75	70
Stone ashlar masonry:		
Granite	720	640
Limestone or marble	450	400
Sandstone or cast stone	360	320
Rubble stone masonry:		
Coarse, rough or random	120	100

For SI: 1 pound per square inch = 6.895 kPa.

a. Linear interpolation shall be used for determining allowable stresses for masonry units having compressive strengths that are intermediate between those given in the table.

b. Gross cross-sectional area shall be calculated on the actual rather than nominal dimensions.

c. See Section R608.

d. Where floor and roof loads are carried upon one wythe, the gross cross-sectional area is that of the wythe under load; if both wythes are loaded, the gross cross-sectional area is that of the wall minus the area of the cavity between the wythes. Walls bonded with metal ties shall be considered as cavity walls unless the collar joints are filled with mortar or grout.

R606.8 Stack bond. In unreinforced masonry where masonry units are laid in stack bond, longitudinal reinforcement consisting of not less than two continuous wires each with a minimum aggregate cross-sectional area of 0.017 square inch (11 mm²) shall be provided in horizontal bed joints spaced not more than 16 inches (406 mm) on center vertically.

R606.9 Lateral support. Masonry walls shall be laterally supported in either the horizontal or the vertical direction. The maximum spacing between lateral supports shall not exceed the distances in Table R606.9. Lateral support shall be provided by cross walls, pilasters, buttresses or structural frame members when the limiting distance is taken horizontally, or by floors or roofs when the limiting distance is taken vertically.

TABLE R606.9
SPACING OF LATERAL SUPPORT FOR MASONRY WALLS

CONSTRUCTION	MAXIMUM WALL LENGTH TO THICKNESS OR WALL HEIGHT TO THICKNESS[a,b]
Bearing walls:	
Solid or solid grouted	20
All other	18
Nonbearing walls:	
Exterior	18
Interior	36

For SI: 1 foot = 304.8 mm.

a. Except for cavity walls and cantilevered walls, the thickness of a wall shall be its nominal thickness measured perpendicular to the face of the wall. For cavity walls, the thickness shall be determined as the sum of the nominal thicknesses of the individual wythes. For cantilever walls, except for parapets, the ratio of height to nominal thickness shall not exceed 6 for solid masonry, or 4 for hollow masonry. For parapets, see Section R606.2.4.

b. An additional unsupported height of 6 feet is permitted for gable end walls.

R606.9.1 Horizontal lateral support. Lateral support in the horizontal direction provided by intersecting masonry walls shall be provided by one of the methods in Section R606.9.1.1 or Section R606.9.1.2.

R606.9.1.1 Bonding pattern. Fifty percent of the units at the intersection shall be laid in an overlapping masonry bonding pattern, with alternate units having a bearing of not less than 3 inches (76 mm) on the unit below.

R606.9.1.2 Metal reinforcement. Interior nonload-bearing walls shall be anchored at their intersections, at vertical intervals of not more than 16 inches (406 mm) with joint reinforcement of at least 9 gage [0.148 in. (4mm)], or $^1/_4$ inch (6 mm) galvanized mesh hardware cloth. Intersecting masonry walls, other than interior nonloadbearing walls, shall be anchored at vertical intervals of not more than 8 inches (203 mm) with joint reinforcement of at least 9 gage and shall extend at least 30 inches (762 mm) in each direction at the intersection. Other metal ties, joint reinforcement or anchors, if used, shall be spaced to provide equivalent area of anchorage to that required by this section.

R606.9.2 Vertical lateral support. Vertical lateral support of masonry walls in Seismic Design Category A, B or C shall be provided in accordance with one of the methods in Section R606.9.2.1 or Section R606.9.2.2.

R606.9.2.1 Roof structures. Masonry walls shall be anchored to roof structures with metal strap anchors spaced in accordance with the manufacturer's instructions, $^1/_2$-inch (13 mm) bolts spaced not more than 6 feet (1829 mm) on center, or other *approved* anchors. Anchors shall be embedded at least 16 inches (406 mm) into the masonry, or be hooked or welded to bond beam reinforcement placed not less than 6 inches (152 mm) from the top of the wall.

R606.9.2.2 Floor diaphragms. Masonry walls shall be anchored to floor *diaphragm* framing by metal strap anchors spaced in accordance with the manufacturer's instructions, $^1/_2$-inch-diameter (13 mm) bolts spaced at intervals not to exceed 6 feet (1829 mm) and installed as shown in Figure R606.11(1), or by other *approved* methods.

R606.10 Lintels. Masonry over openings shall be supported by steel lintels, reinforced concrete or masonry lintels or masonry arches, designed to support load imposed.

R606.11 Anchorage. Masonry walls shall be anchored to floor and roof systems in accordance with the details shown in Figure R606.11(1), R606.11(2) or R606.11(3). Footings may be considered as points of lateral support.

R606.12 Seismic requirements. The seismic requirements of this section shall apply to the design of masonry and the construction of masonry building elements located in Seismic Design Category D_0, D_1 or D_2. Townhouses in Seismic Design Category C shall comply with the requirements of Section R606.12.2. These requirements shall not apply to glass unit masonry conforming to Section R610 or masonry veneer conforming to Section R703.7.

R606.12.1 General. Masonry structures and masonry elements shall comply with the requirements of Sections R606.12.2 through R606.12.4 based on the seismic design category established in Table R301.2(1). Masonry structures and masonry elements shall comply with the requirements of Section R606.12 and Figures R606.11(1), R606.11(2) and R606.11(3) or shall be designed in accordance with ACI 530/ASCE 5/TMS 402.

R606.12.1.1 Floor and roof diaphragm construction. Floor and roof *diaphragms* shall be constructed of wood structural panels attached to wood framing in accordance with Table R602.3(1) or to cold-formed steel floor framing in accordance with Table R505.3.1(2) or to cold-formed steel roof framing in accordance with Table R804.3. Additionally, sheathing panel edges perpendicular to framing members shall be backed by blocking, and sheathing shall be connected to the blocking with fasteners at the edge spacing. For Seismic Design Categories C, D_0, D_1 and D_2, where the width-to-thickness dimension of the *diaphragm* exceeds 2-to-1, edge spacing of fasteners shall be 4 inches (102 mm) on center.

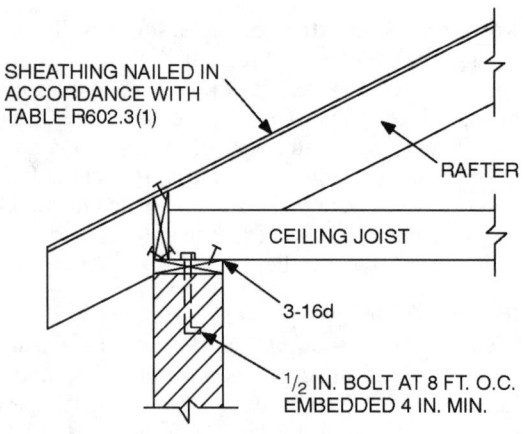

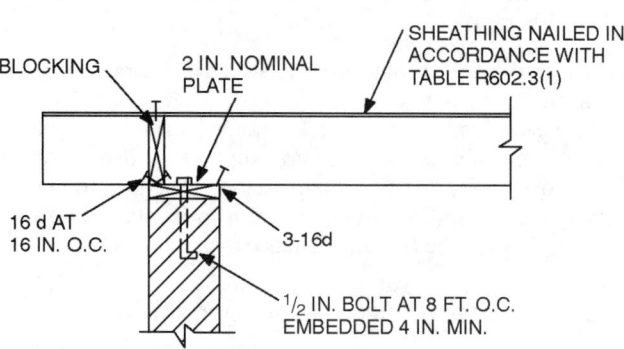

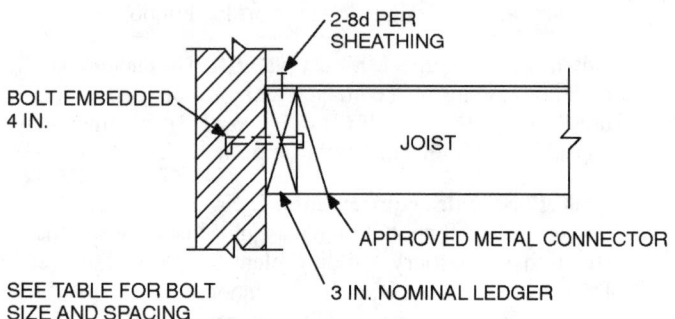

LEDGER BOLT SIZE AND SPACING

JOIST SPAN	BOLT SIZE AND SPACING	
	ROOF	FLOOR
10 FT.	$\frac{1}{2}$ AT 2 FT. 6 IN. $\frac{7}{8}$ AT 3 FT. 6 IN.	$\frac{1}{2}$ AT 2 FT. 0 IN. $\frac{7}{8}$ AT 2 FT. 9 IN.
10–15 FT.	$\frac{1}{2}$ AT 1 FT. 9 IN. $\frac{7}{8}$ AT 2 FT. 6 IN.	$\frac{1}{2}$ AT 1 FT. 4 IN. $\frac{7}{8}$ AT 2 FT. 0 IN.
15-20 FT.	$\frac{1}{2}$ AT 1 FT. 3 IN. $\frac{7}{8}$ AT 2 FT. 0 IN.	$\frac{1}{2}$ AT 1 FT. 0 IN. $\frac{7}{8}$ AT 1 FT. 6 IN.

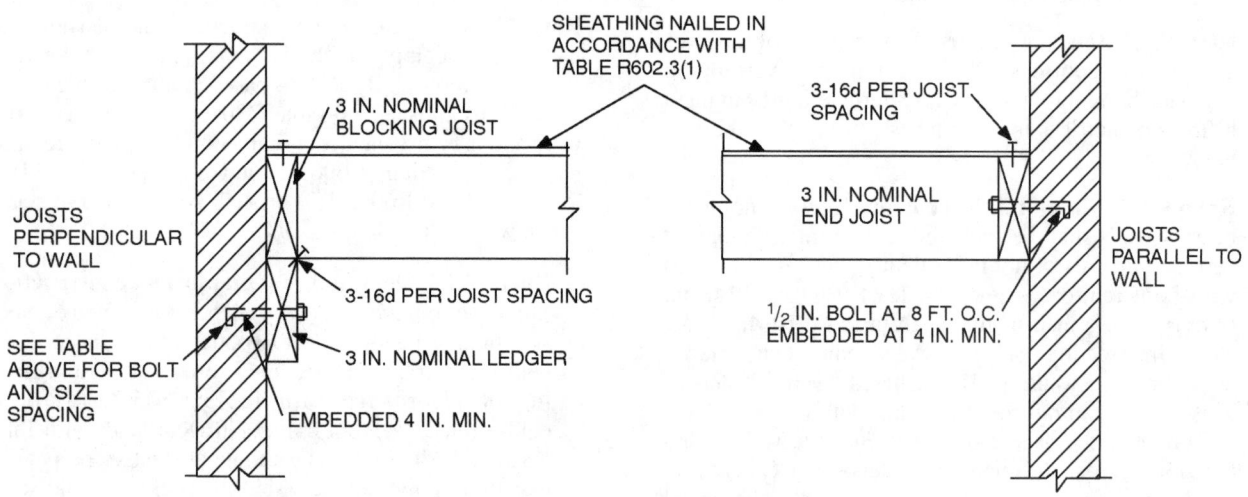

NOTE: Where bolts are located in hollow masonry, the cells in the courses receiving the bolt shall be grouted solid.

For SI: 1 inch = 25.4 mm, 1 foot = 304.8 mm, 1 pound per square foot = 0.0.479 kPa.

FIGURE R606.11(1)
ANCHORAGE REQUIREMENTS FOR MASONRY WALLS LOCATED IN SEISMIC
DESIGN CATEGORY A, B OR C AND WHERE WIND LOADS ARE LESS THAN 30 PSF

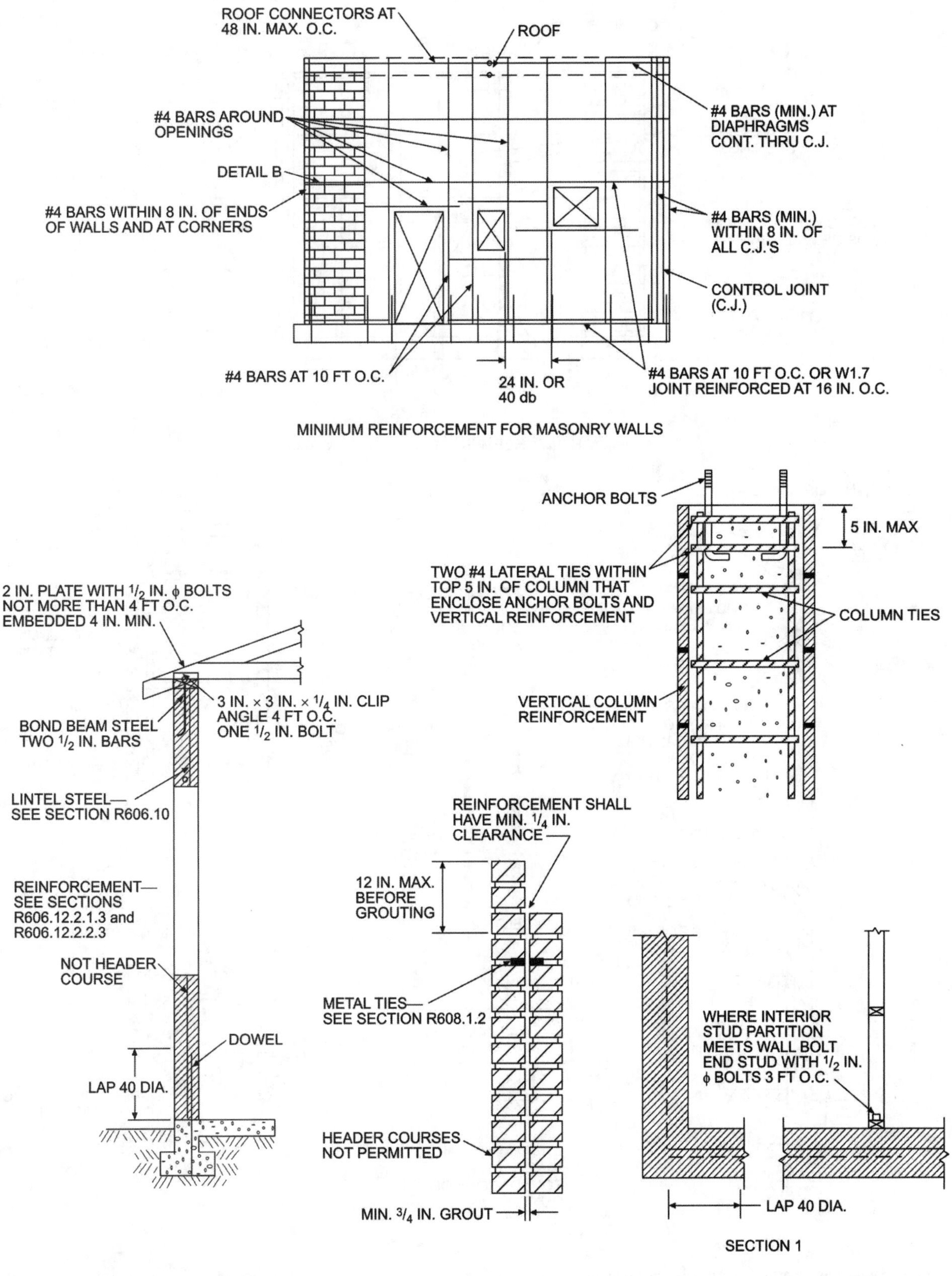

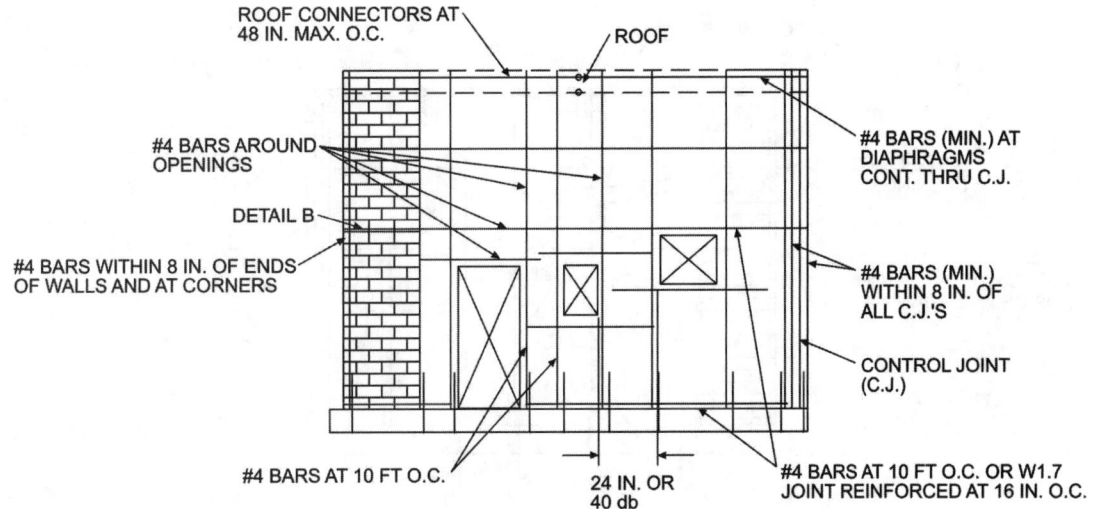

ROOF CONNECTORS AT 48 IN. MAX. O.C.

ROOF

#4 BARS AROUND OPENINGS

DETAIL B

#4 BARS WITHIN 8 IN. OF ENDS OF WALLS AND AT CORNERS

#4 BARS (MIN.) AT DIAPHRAGMS CONT. THRU C.J.

#4 BARS (MIN.) WITHIN 8 IN. OF ALL C.J.'S

CONTROL JOINT (C.J.)

#4 BARS AT 10 FT O.C.

24 IN. OR 40 db

#4 BARS AT 10 FT O.C. OR W1.7 JOINT REINFORCED AT 16 IN. O.C.

MINIMUM REINFORCEMENT FOR MASONRY WALLS

ANCHOR BOLTS

5 IN. MAX

TWO #4 LATERAL TIES WITHIN TOP 5 IN. OF COLUMN THAT ENCLOSE ANCHOR BOLTS AND VERTICAL REINFORCEMENT

COLUMN TIES

2 IN. PLATE WITH 1/2 IN. φ BOLTS NOT MORE THAN 4 FT O.C. EMBEDDED 4 IN. MIN.

3 IN. × 3 IN. × 1/4 IN. CLIP ANGLE 4 FT O.C. ONE 1/2 IN. BOLT

BOND BEAM STEEL TWO 1/2 IN. BARS

LINTEL STEEL— SEE SECTION R606.10

REINFORCEMENT— SEE SECTIONS R606.12.2.1.3 and R606.12.2.2.3

NOT HEADER COURSE

DOWEL

LAP 40 DIA.

VERTICAL COLUMN REINFORCEMENT

REINFORCEMENT SHALL HAVE MIN. 1/4 IN. CLEARANCE

12 IN. MAX. BEFORE GROUTING

METAL TIES— SEE SECTION R608.1.2

HEADER COURSES NOT PERMITTED

MIN. 3/4 IN. GROUT

WHERE INTERIOR STUD PARTITION MEETS WALL BOLT END STUD WITH 1/2 IN. φ BOLTS 3 FT O.C.

LAP 40 DIA.

SECTION 1

For SI: 1 inch = 25.4 mm, 1 foot = 304.8 mm.

FIGURE R606.11(2)
REQUIREMENTS FOR REINFORCED GROUTED MASONRY CONSTRUCTION IN SEISMIC DESIGN CATEGORY C

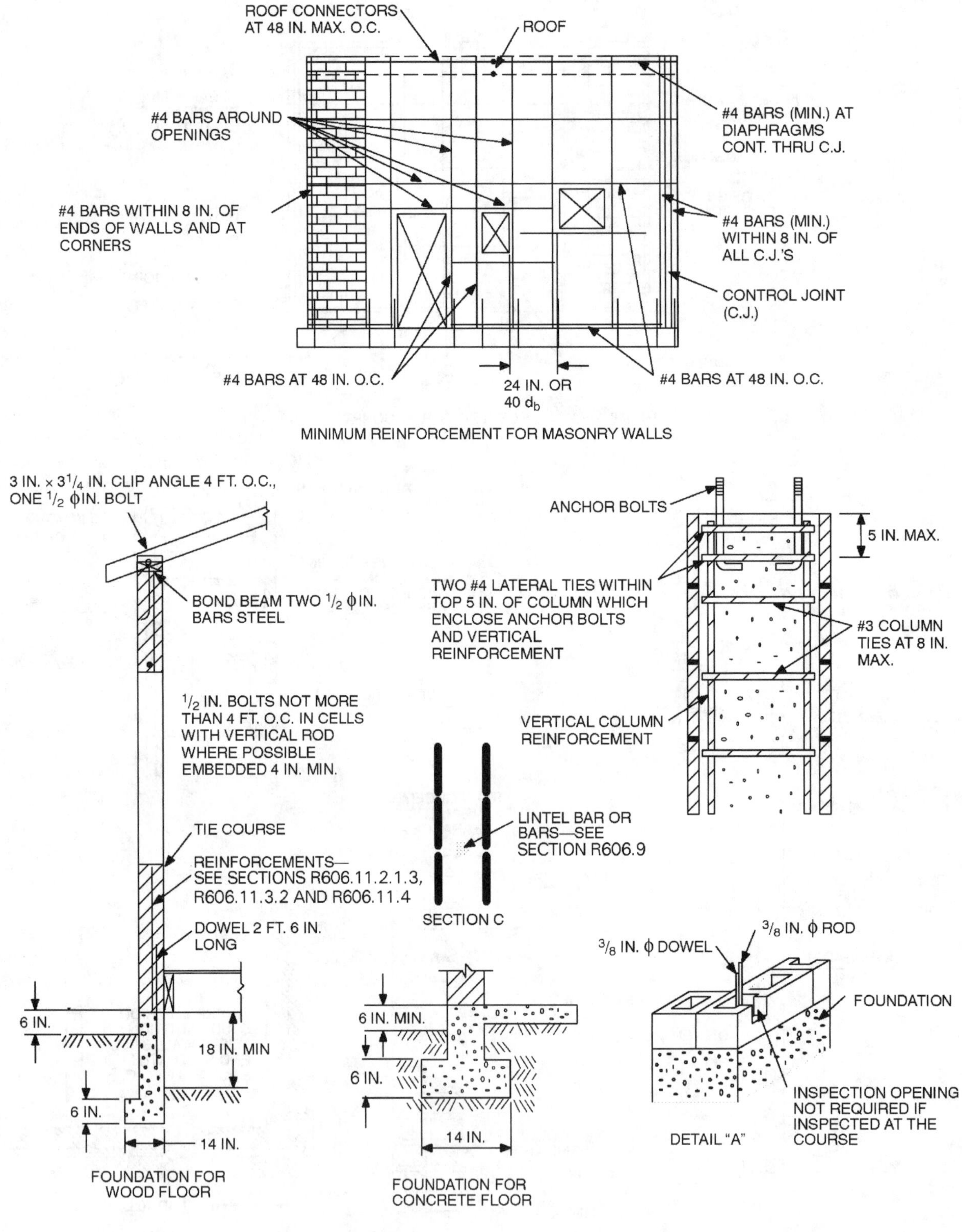

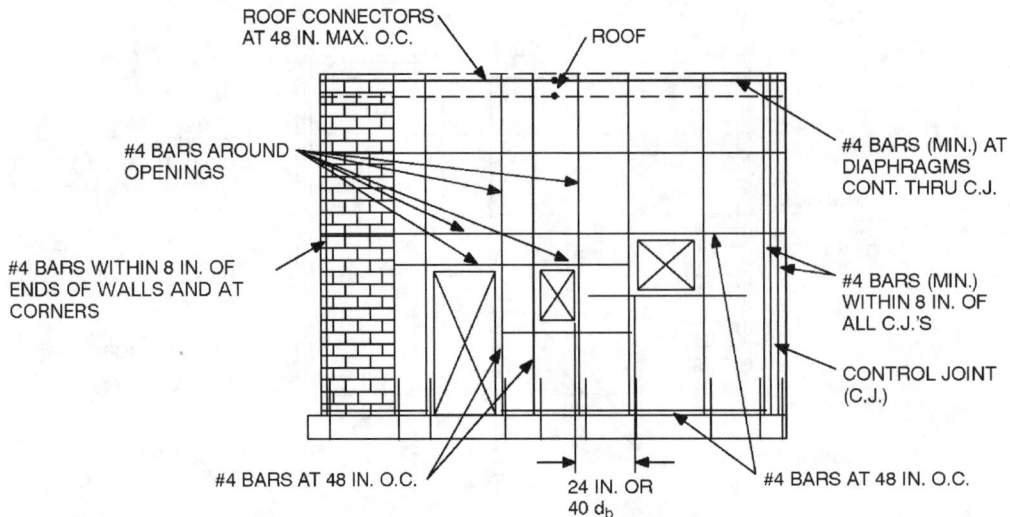

ROOF CONNECTORS AT 48 IN. MAX. O.C.

ROOF

#4 BARS (MIN.) AT DIAPHRAGMS CONT. THRU C.J.

#4 BARS AROUND OPENINGS

#4 BARS WITHIN 8 IN. OF ENDS OF WALLS AND AT CORNERS

#4 BARS (MIN.) WITHIN 8 IN. OF ALL C.J.'S

CONTROL JOINT (C.J.)

#4 BARS AT 48 IN. O.C.

24 IN. OR 40 d_b

#4 BARS AT 48 IN. O.C.

MINIMUM REINFORCEMENT FOR MASONRY WALLS

3 IN. × 3 1/4 IN. CLIP ANGLE 4 FT. O.C., ONE 1/2 ϕ IN. BOLT

BOND BEAM TWO 1/2 ϕ IN. BARS STEEL

1/2 IN. BOLTS NOT MORE THAN 4 FT. O.C. IN CELLS WITH VERTICAL ROD WHERE POSSIBLE EMBEDDED 4 IN. MIN.

TIE COURSE

REINFORCEMENTS— SEE SECTIONS R606.11.2.1.3, R606.11.3.2 AND R606.11.4

DOWEL 2 FT. 6 IN. LONG

6 IN.

18 IN. MIN

6 IN.

14 IN.

FOUNDATION FOR WOOD FLOOR

6 IN. MIN.

6 IN.

14 IN.

FOUNDATION FOR CONCRETE FLOOR

ANCHOR BOLTS

5 IN. MAX.

TWO #4 LATERAL TIES WITHIN TOP 5 IN. OF COLUMN WHICH ENCLOSE ANCHOR BOLTS AND VERTICAL REINFORCEMENT

#3 COLUMN TIES AT 8 IN. MAX.

VERTICAL COLUMN REINFORCEMENT

LINTEL BAR OR BARS—SEE SECTION R606.9

SECTION C

3/8 IN. ϕ DOWEL

3/8 IN. ϕ ROD

FOUNDATION

INSPECTION OPENING NOT REQUIRED IF INSPECTED AT THE COURSE

DETAIL "A"

NOTE: A full bed joint must be provided. All cells containing vertical bars are to be filled to the top of wall and provide inspection opening as shown on detail "A." Horizontal bars are to be laid as shown on detail "B." Lintel bars are to be laid as shown on Section C.

For SI: 1 inch = 25.4 mm, 1 foot = 304.8 mm.

FIGURE R606.11(3)
REQUIREMENTS FOR REINFORCED MASONRY CONSTRUCTION IN SEISMIC DESIGN CATEGORY D₀, D₁, OR D₂

R606.12.2 Seismic Design Category C. Townhouses located in Seismic Design Category C shall comply with the requirements of this section.

R606.12.2.1 Minimum length of wall without openings. Table R606.12.2.1 shall be used to determine the minimum required solid wall length without openings at each masonry exterior wall. The provided percentage of solid wall length shall include only those wall segments that are 3 feet (914 mm) or longer. The maximum clear distance between wall segments included in determining the solid wall length shall not exceed 18 feet (5486 mm). Shear wall segments required to meet the minimum wall length shall be in accordance with Section R606.12.2.2.3.

R606.12.2.2 Design of elements not part of the lateral force-resisting system.

R606.12.2.2.1 Load-bearing frames or columns. Elements not part of the lateral-force-resisting system shall be analyzed to determine their effect on the response of the system. The frames or columns shall be adequate for vertical load carrying capacity and induced moment caused by the design *story* drift.

R606.12.2.2.2 Masonry partition walls. Masonry partition walls, masonry screen walls and other masonry elements that are not designed to resist vertical or lateral loads, other than those induced by their own weight, shall be isolated from the structure so that vertical and lateral forces are not imparted to these elements. Isolation joints and connectors between these elements and the structure shall be designed to accommodate the design *story* drift.

R606.12.2.2.3 Reinforcement requirements for masonry elements. Masonry elements listed in Section R606.12.2.2.2 shall be reinforced in either the horizontal or vertical direction as shown in Figure R606.11(2) and in accordance with the following:

1. Horizontal reinforcement. Horizontal joint reinforcement shall consist of at least two longitudinal W1.7 wires spaced not more than 16 inches (406 mm) for walls greater than 4 inches (102 mm) in width and at least one longitudinal W1.7 wire spaced not more than 16 inches (406 mm) for walls not exceeding 4 inches (102 mm)

in width; or at least one No. 4 bar spaced not more than 48 inches (1219 mm). Where two longitudinal wires of joint reinforcement are used, the space between these wires shall be the widest that the mortar joint will accommodate. Horizontal reinforcement shall be provided within 16 inches (406 mm) of the top and bottom of these masonry elements.

2. Vertical reinforcement. Vertical reinforcement shall consist of at least one No. 4 bar spaced not more than 48 inches (1219 mm). Vertical reinforcement shall be located within 16 inches (406 mm) of the ends of masonry walls.

R606.12.2.3 Design of elements part of the lateral-force-resisting system.

R606.12.2.3.1 Connections to masonry shear walls. Connectors shall be provided to transfer forces between masonry walls and horizontal elements in accordance with the requirements of Section 2.1.8 of ACI 530/ASCE 5/TMS 402. Connectors shall be designed to transfer horizontal design forces acting either perpendicular or parallel to the wall, but not less than 200 pounds per linear foot (2919 N/m) of wall. The maximum spacing between connectors shall be 4 feet (1219 mm). Such anchorage mechanisms shall not induce tension stresses perpendicular to grain in ledgers or nailers.

R606.12.2.3.2 Connections to masonry columns. Connectors shall be provided to transfer forces between masonry columns and horizontal elements in accordance with the requirements of Section 2.1.8 of ACI 530/ASCE 5/TMS 402. Where anchor bolts are used to connect horizontal elements to the tops of columns, the bolts shall be placed within lateral ties. Lateral ties shall enclose both the vertical bars in the column and the anchor bolts. There shall be a minimum of two No. 4 lateral ties provided in the top 5 inches (127 mm) of the column.

R606.12.2.3.3 Minimum reinforcement requirements for masonry shear walls. Vertical reinforcement of at least one No. 4 bar shall be provided at corners, within 16 inches (406 mm) of each side of

TABLE R606.12.2.1
MINIMUM SOLID WALL LENGTH ALONG EXTERIOR WALL LINES

SESIMIC DESIGN CATEGORY	MINIMUM SOLID WALL LENGTH (percent)[a]		
	One Story or Top Story of Two Story	Wall Supporting Light-framed Second Story and Roof	Wall Supporting Masonry Second Story and Roof
Townhouses in C	20	25	35
D$_0$ or D$_1$	25	NP	NP
D$_2$	30	NP	NP

NP = Not permitted , except with design in accordance with the *International Building Code*.

a. For all walls, the minimum required length of solid walls shall be based on the table percent multiplied by the dimension, parallel to the wall direction under consideration, of a rectangle inscribing the overall building plan.

openings, within 8 inches (203 mm) of each side of movement joints, within 8 inches (203 mm) of the ends of walls, and at a maximum spacing of 10 feet (3048 mm).

Horizontal joint reinforcement shall consist of at least two wires of W1.7 spaced not more than 16 inches (406 mm); or bond beam reinforcement of at least one No. 4 bar spaced not more than 10 feet (3048 mm) shall be provided. Horizontal reinforcement shall also be provided at the bottom and top of wall openings and shall extend not less than 24 inches (610 mm) nor less than 40 bar diameters past the opening; continuously at structurally connected roof and floor levels; and within 16 inches (406 mm) of the top of walls.

R606.12.3 Seismic Design Category D_0 or D_1. Structures in Seismic Design Category D_0 or D_1 shall comply with the requirements of Seismic Design Category C and the additional requirements of this section.

R606.12.3.1 Design requirements. Masonry elements other than those covered by Section R606.12.2.2.2 shall be designed in accordance with the requirements of Chapter 1 and Sections 2.1 and 2.3 of ACI 530/ASCE 5/TMS 402 and shall meet the minimum reinforcement requirements contained in Sections R606.12.3.2 and R606.12.3.2.1.

Exception: Masonry walls limited to one *story* in height and 9 feet (2743 mm) between lateral supports need not be designed provided they comply with the minimum reinforcement requirements of Sections R606.12.3.2 and R606.12.3.2.1.

R606.12.3.2 Minimum reinforcement requirements for masonry walls. Masonry walls other than those covered by Section R606.12.2.2.3 shall be reinforced in both the vertical and horizontal direction. The sum of the cross-sectional area of horizontal and vertical reinforcement shall be at least 0.002 times the gross cross-sectional area of the wall, and the minimum cross-sectional area in each direction shall be not less than 0.0007 times the gross cross-sectional area of the wall. Reinforcement shall be uniformly distributed. Table R606.12.3.2 shows the minimum reinforcing

bar sizes required for varying thicknesses of masonry walls. The maximum spacing of reinforcement shall be 48 inches (1219 mm) provided that the walls are solid grouted and constructed of hollow open-end units, hollow units laid with full head joints or two wythes of solid units. The maximum spacing of reinforcement shall be 24 inches (610 mm) for all other masonry.

R606.12.3.2.1 Shear wall reinforcement requirements. The maximum spacing of vertical and horizontal reinforcement shall be the smaller of one-third the length of the shear wall, one-third the height of the shear wall, or 48 inches (1219 mm). The minimum cross-sectional area of vertical reinforcement shall be one-third of the required shear reinforcement. Shear reinforcement shall be anchored around vertical reinforcing bars with a standard hook.

R606.12.3.3 Minimum reinforcement for masonry columns. Lateral ties in masonry columns shall be spaced not more than 8 inches (203 mm) on center and shall be at least $3/8$ inch (9.5 mm) diameter. Lateral ties shall be embedded in grout.

R606.12.3.4 Material restrictions. Type N mortar or masonry cement shall not be used as part of the lateral-force-resisting system.

R606.12.3.5 Lateral tie anchorage. Standard hooks for lateral tie anchorage shall be either a 135-degree (2.4 rad) standard hook or a 180-degree (3.2 rad) standard hook.

R606.12.4 Seismic Design Category D_2. All structures in Seismic Design Category D_2 shall comply with the requirements of Seismic Design Category D_1 and to the additional requirements of this section.

R606.12.4.1 Design of elements not part of the lateral-force-resisting system. Stack bond masonry that is not part of the lateral-force-resisting system shall have a horizontal cross-sectional area of reinforcement of at least 0.0015 times the gross cross-sectional area of masonry. Table R606.12.4.1 shows minimum reinforcing bar sizes for masonry walls. The maximum spacing of horizontal reinforcement shall be 24 inches (610 mm). These elements shall be solidly grouted and shall be constructed of hollow open-end units or two wythes of solid units.

TABLE R606.12.3.2
MINIMUM DISTRIBUTED WALL REINFORCEMENT FOR BUILDING ASSIGNED TO SEISMIC DESIGN CATEGORY D_0 or D_1

NOMINAL WALL THICKNESS (inches)	MINIMUM SUM OF THE VERTICAL AND HORIZONTAL REINFORCEMENT AREAS[a] (square inches per foot)	MINIMUM REINFORCEMENT AS DISTRIBUTED IN BOTH HORIZONTAL AND VERTICAL DIRECTIONS[b] (square inches per foot)	MINIMUM BAR SIZE FOR REINFORCEMENT SPACED AT 48 INCHES
6	0.135	0.047	#4
8	0.183	0.064	#5
10	0.231	0.081	#6
12	0.279	0.098	#6

For SI: 1 inch = 25.4 mm, 1 foot = 304.8 mm, 1 square inch per foot = 2064 mm²/m.

a. Based on the minimum reinforcing ratio of 0.002 times the gross cross-sectional area of the wall.

b. Based on the minimum reinforcing ratio each direction of 0.0007 times the gross cross-sectional area of the wall.

TABLE R606.12.4.1
MINIMUM REINFORCING FOR STACKED BONDED
MASONRY WALLS IN SEISMIC DESIGN CATEGORY D$_2$

NOMINAL WALL THICKNESS (inches)	MINIMUM BAR SIZE SPACED AT 24 INCHES
6	#4
8	#5
10	#5
12	#6

For SI: 1 inch = 25.4 mm.

R606.12.4.2 Design of elements part of the lateral-force-resisting system. Stack bond masonry that is part of the lateral-force-resisting system shall have a horizontal cross-sectional area of reinforcement of at least 0.0025 times the gross cross-sectional area of masonry. Table R606.12.4.2 shows minimum reinforcing bar sizes for masonry walls. The maximum spacing of horizontal reinforcement shall be 16 inches (406 mm). These elements shall be solidly grouted and shall be constructed of hollow open-end units or two wythes of solid units.

TABLE R606.12.4.2
MINIMUM REINFORCING FOR STACKED BONDED MASONRY
WALLS IN SEISMIC DESIGN CATEGORY D$_2$

NOMINAL WALL THICKNESS (inches)	MINIMUM BAR SIZE SPACED AT 16 INCHES
6	#4
8	#5
10	#5
12	#6

For SI: 1 inch = 25.4 mm.

R606.13 Protection for reinforcement. Bars shall be completely embedded in mortar or grout. Joint reinforcement embedded in horizontal mortar joints shall not have less than $^5/_8$-inch (15.9 mm) mortar coverage from the exposed face. All other reinforcement shall have a minimum coverage of one bar diameter over all bars, but not less than $^3/_4$ inch (19 mm), except where exposed to weather or soil, in which case the minimum coverage shall be 2 inches (51 mm).

R606.14 Beam supports. Beams, girders or other concentrated loads supported by a wall or column shall have a bearing of at least 3 inches (76 mm) in length measured parallel to the beam upon *solid masonry* not less than 4 inches (102 mm) in thickness, or upon a metal bearing plate of adequate design and dimensions to distribute the load safely, or upon a continuous reinforced masonry member projecting not less than 4 inches (102 mm) from the face of the wall.

R606.14.1 Joist bearing. Joists shall have a bearing of not less than $1^1/_2$ inches (38 mm), except as provided in Section R606.14, and shall be supported in accordance with Figure R606.11(1).

R606.15 Metal accessories. Joint reinforcement, anchors, ties and wire fabric shall conform to the following: ASTM A 82 for wire anchors and ties; ASTM A 36 for plate, headed and bent-bar anchors; ASTM A 510 for corrugated sheet metal anchors and ties; ASTM A 951 for joint reinforcement; ASTM

B 227 for copper-clad steel wire ties; or ASTM A 167 for stainless steel hardware.

R606.15.1 Corrosion protection. Minimum corrosion protection of joint reinforcement, anchor ties and wire fabric for use in masonry wall construction shall conform to Table R606.15.1.

TABLE R606.15.1
MINIMUM CORROSION PROTECTION

MASONRY METAL ACCESSORY	STANDARD
Joint reinforcement, interior walls	ASTM A 641, Class 1
Wire ties or anchors in exterior walls completely embedded in mortar or grout	ASTM A 641, Class 3
Wire ties or anchors in exterior walls not completely embedded in mortar or grout	ASTM A 153, Class B-2
Joint reinforcement in exterior walls or interior walls exposed to moist environment	ASTM A 153, Class B-2
Sheet metal ties or anchors exposed to weather	ASTM A 153, Class B-2
Sheet metal ties or anchors completely embedded in mortar or grout	ASTM A 653, Coating Designation G60
Stainless steel hardware for any exposure	ASTM A 167, Type 304

SECTION R607
UNIT MASONRY

R607.1 Mortar. Mortar for use in masonry construction shall comply with ASTM C 270. The type of mortar shall be in accordance with Sections R607.1.1, R607.1.2 and R607.1.3 and shall meet the proportion specifications of Table R607.1 or the property specifications of ASTM C 270.

R607.1.1 Foundation walls. Masonry foundation walls constructed as set forth in Tables R404.1.1(1) through R404.1.1(4) and mortar shall be Type M or S.

R607.1.2 Masonry in Seismic Design Categories A, B and C. Mortar for masonry serving as the lateral-force-resisting system in Seismic Design Categories A, B and C shall be Type M, S or N mortar.

R607.1.3 Masonry in Seismic Design Categories D$_0$, D$_1$ and D$_2$. Mortar for masonry serving as the lateral-force- resisting system in Seismic Design Categories D$_0$, D$_1$ and D$_2$ shall be Type M or S portland cement-lime or mortar cement mortar.

R607.2 Placing mortar and masonry units.

R607.2.1 Bed and head joints. Unless otherwise required or indicated on the project drawings, head and bed joints shall be $^3/_8$ inch (10 mm) thick, except that the thickness of the bed joint of the starting course placed over foundations shall not be less than $^1/_4$ inch (7 mm) and not more than $^3/_4$ inch (19 mm).

TABLE R607.1
MORTAR PROPORTIONS[a, b]

MORTAR	TYPE	Portland cement or blended cement	Mortar cement M	Mortar cement S	Mortar cement N	Masonry cement M	Masonry cement S	Masonry cement N	Hydrated lime[c] or lime putty	Aggregate ratio (measured in damp, loose conditions)
Cement-lime	M	1	—	—	—	—	—	—	$1/4$	
	S	1	—	—	—	—	—	—	over $1/4$ to $1/2$	
	N	1	—	—	—	—	—	—	over $1/2$ to $1 1/4$	
	O	1	—	—	—	—	—	—	over $1 1/4$ to $2 1/2$	
Mortar cement	M	1	—	—	1	—	—	—	—	Not less than $2 1/4$ and not more than 3 times the sum of separate volumes of lime, if used, and cement
	M	—	1	—	—	—	—	—		
	S	$1/2$	—	—	1	—	—	—		
	S	—	—	1	—	—	—	—		
	N	—	—	—	1	—	—	—		
	O	—	—	—	1	—	—	—		
Masonry cement	M	1				—	—	1	—	
	M	—				1	—	—		
	S	$1/2$				—	—	1		
	S	—				—	1	—		
	N	—				—	—	1		
	O	—				—	—	1		

For SI: 1 cubic foot = 0.0283 m³, 1 pound = 0.454 kg.

a. For the purpose of these specifications, the weight of 1 cubic foot of the respective materials shall be considered to be as follows:

Portland Cement	94 pounds	Masonry Cement	Weight printed on bag
Mortar Cement	Weight printed on bag	Hydrated Lime	40 pounds
Lime Putty (Quicklime)	80 pounds	Sand, damp and loose	80 pounds of dry sand

b. Two air-entraining materials shall not be combined in mortar.

R607.2.1.1 Mortar joint thickness tolerance. Mortar joint thickness for load-bearing masonry shall be within the following tolerances from the specified dimensions:

1. Bed joint: + $1/8$ inch (3 mm).

2. Head joint: - $1/4$ inch (7 mm), + $3/8$ inch (10 mm).

3. Collar joints: - $1/4$ inch (7 mm), + $3/8$ inch (10 mm).

R607.2.2 Masonry unit placement. The mortar shall be sufficiently plastic and units shall be placed with sufficient pressure to extrude mortar from the joint and produce a tight joint. Deep furrowing of bed joints that produces voids shall not be permitted. Any units disturbed to the extent that initial bond is broken after initial placement shall be removed and relaid in fresh mortar. Surfaces to be in contact with mortar shall be clean and free of deleterious materials.

R607.2.2.1 Solid masonry. *Solid masonry* units shall be laid with full head and bed joints and all interior vertical joints that are designed to receive mortar shall be filled.

R607.2.2.2 Hollow masonry. For hollow masonry units, head and bed joints shall be filled solidly with mortar for a distance in from the face of the unit not less than the thickness of the face shell.

R607.3 Installation of wall ties. The installation of wall ties shall be as follows:

1. The ends of wall ties shall be embedded in mortar joints. Wall tie ends shall engage outer face shells of hollow units by at least $1/2$ inch (13 mm). Wire wall ties shall be embedded at least $1 1/2$ inches (38 mm) into the mortar bed of *solid masonry* units or solid grouted hollow units.

2. Wall ties shall not be bent after being embedded in grout or mortar.

SECTION R608
MULTIPLE WYTHE MASONRY

R608.1 General. The facing and backing of multiple wythe masonry walls shall be bonded in accordance with Section R608.1.1, R608.1.2 or R608.1.3. In cavity walls, neither the facing nor the backing shall be less than 3 inches (76 mm) nominal in thickness and the cavity shall not be more than 4 inches (102 mm) nominal in width. The backing shall be at least as thick as the facing.

Exception: Cavities shall be permitted to exceed the 4-inch (102 mm) nominal dimension provided tie size and tie spacing have been established by calculation.

R608.1.1 Bonding with masonry headers. Bonding with solid or hollow masonry headers shall comply with Sections R608.1.1.1 and R608.1.1.2.

R608.1.1.1 Solid units. Where the facing and backing (adjacent wythes) of *solid masonry* construction are bonded by means of masonry headers, no less than 4 percent of the wall surface of each face shall be composed of headers extending not less than 3 inches (76 mm) into the backing. The distance between adjacent full-length headers shall not exceed 24 inches (610 mm) either vertically or horizontally. In walls in which a single header does not extend through the wall, headers from the opposite sides shall overlap at least 3 inches (76 mm), or headers from opposite sides shall be covered with another header course overlapping the header below at least 3 inches (76 mm).

R608.1.1.2 Hollow units. Where two or more hollow units are used to make up the thickness of a wall, the stretcher courses shall be bonded at vertical intervals not exceeding 34 inches (864 mm) by lapping at least 3 inches (76 mm) over the unit below, or by lapping at vertical intervals not exceeding 17 inches (432 mm) with units that are at least 50 percent thicker than the units below.

R608.1.2 Bonding with wall ties or joint reinforcement. Bonding with wall ties or joint reinforcement shall comply with Sections R608.1.2.1 through R608.1.2.3.

R608.1.2.1 Bonding with wall ties. Bonding with wall ties, except as required by Section R610, where the facing and backing (adjacent wythes) of masonry walls are bonded with $^3/_{16}$-inch-diameter (5 mm) wall ties embedded in the horizontal mortar joints, there shall be at least one metal tie for each 4.5 square feet (0.418 m²) of wall area. Ties in alternate courses shall be staggered. The maximum vertical distance between ties shall not exceed 24 inches (610 mm), and the maximum horizontal distance shall not exceed 36 inches (914 mm). Rods or ties bent to rectangular shape shall be used with hollow masonry units laid with the cells vertical. In other walls, the ends of ties shall be bent to 90-degree (0.79 rad) angles to provide hooks no less than 2 inches (51 mm) long. Additional bonding ties shall be provided at all openings, spaced not more than 3 feet (914 mm) apart around the perimeter and within 12 inches (305 mm) of the opening.

R608.1.2.2 Bonding with adjustable wall ties. Where the facing and backing (adjacent wythes) of masonry are bonded with adjustable wall ties, there shall be at least one tie for each 2.67 square feet (0.248 m²) of wall area. Neither the vertical nor the horizontal spacing of the adjustable wall ties shall exceed 24 inches (610 mm). The maximum vertical offset of bed joints from one wythe to the other shall be 1.25 inches (32 mm). The maximum clearance between connecting parts of the ties shall be $^1/_{16}$ inch (2 mm). When pintle legs are used, ties shall have at least two $^3/_{16}$-inch-diameter (5 mm) legs.

R608.1.2.3 Bonding with prefabricated joint reinforcement. Where the facing and backing (adjacent wythes) of masonry are bonded with prefabricated joint reinforcement, there shall be at least one cross wire serving as a tie for each 2.67 square feet (0.248 m²) of wall area. The vertical spacing of the joint reinforcement shall not exceed 16 inches (406 mm). Cross wires on prefabricated joint reinforcement shall not be smaller than No. 9 gage. The longitudinal wires shall be embedded in the mortar.

R608.1.3 Bonding with natural or cast stone. Bonding with natural and cast stone shall conform to Sections R608.1.3.1 and R608.1.3.2.

R608.1.3.1 Ashlar masonry. In ashlar masonry, bonder units, uniformly distributed, shall be provided to the extent of not less than 10 percent of the wall area. Such bonder units shall extend not less than 4 inches (102 mm) into the backing wall.

R608.1.3.2 Rubble stone masonry. Rubble stone masonry 24 inches (610 mm) or less in thickness shall have bonder units with a maximum spacing of 3 feet (914 mm) vertically and 3 feet (914 mm) horizontally, and if the masonry is of greater thickness than 24 inches (610 mm), shall have one bonder unit for each 6 square feet (0.557 m²) of wall surface on both sides.

R608.2 Masonry bonding pattern. Masonry laid in running and stack bond shall conform to Sections R608.2.1 and R608.2.2.

R608.2.1 Masonry laid in running bond. In each wythe of masonry laid in running bond, head joints in successive courses shall be offset by not less than one-fourth the unit length, or the masonry walls shall be reinforced longitudinally as required in Section R608.2.2.

R608.2.2 Masonry laid in stack bond. Where unit masonry is laid with less head joint offset than in Section R607.2.1, the minimum area of horizontal reinforcement placed in mortar bed joints or in bond beams spaced not more than 48 inches (1219 mm) apart, shall be 0.0007 times the vertical cross-sectional area of the wall.

SECTION R609
GROUTED MASONRY

R609.1 General. Grouted multiple-wythe masonry is a form of construction in which the space between the wythes is solidly filled with grout. It is not necessary for the cores of masonry units to be filled with grout. Grouted hollow unit masonry is a form of construction in which certain cells of hollow units are continuously filled with grout.

R609.1.1 Grout. Grout shall consist of cementitious material and aggregate in accordance with ASTM C 476 and the proportion specifications of Table R609.1.1. Type M or Type S mortar to which sufficient water has been added to produce pouring consistency can be used as grout.

R609.1.2 Grouting requirements. Maximum pour heights and the minimum dimensions of spaces provided for grout placement shall conform to Table R609.1.2. If the work is stopped for one hour or longer, the horizontal construction joints shall be formed by stopping all tiers at the same elevation and with the grout 1 inch (25 mm) below the top.

R609.1.3 Grout space (cleaning). Provision shall be made for cleaning grout space. Mortar projections that project more than 0.5 inch (13 mm) into grout space and any other foreign matter shall be removed from grout space prior to inspection and grouting.

R609.1.4 Grout placement. Grout shall be a plastic mix suitable for pumping without segregation of the constituents and shall be mixed thoroughly. Grout shall be placed by pumping or by an *approved* alternate method and shall be placed before any initial set occurs and in no case more than $1^1/_2$ hours after water has been added. Grouting shall be done in a continuous pour, in lifts not exceeding 5 feet (1524 mm). It shall be consolidated by puddling or mechanical vibrating during placing and reconsolidated after excess moisture has been absorbed but before plasticity is lost.

R609.1.4.1 Grout pumped through aluminum pipes. Grout shall not be pumped through aluminum pipes.

R609.1.5 Cleanouts. Where required by the *building official*, cleanouts shall be provided as specified in this section. The cleanouts shall be sealed before grouting and after inspection.

R609.1.5.1 Grouted multiple-wythe masonry. Cleanouts shall be provided at the bottom course of the exterior wythe at each pour of grout where such pour exceeds 5 feet (1524 mm) in height.

R609.1.5.2 Grouted hollow unit masonry. Cleanouts shall be provided at the bottom course of each cell to be grouted at each pour of grout, where such pour exceeds 4 feet (1219 mm) in height.

R609.2 Grouted multiple-wythe masonry. Grouted multiple-wythe masonry shall conform to all the requirements specified in Section R609.1 and the requirements of this section.

R609.2.1 Bonding of backup wythe. Where all interior vertical spaces are filled with grout in multiple-wythe construction, masonry headers shall not be permitted. Metal wall ties shall be used in accordance with Section R608.1.2 to prevent spreading of the wythes and to maintain the vertical alignment of the wall. Wall ties shall be installed in accordance with Section R608.1.2 when the backup wythe in multiple-wythe construction is fully grouted.

R609.2.2 Grout spaces. Fine grout shall be used when interior vertical space to receive grout does not exceed 2 inches (51 mm) in thickness. Interior vertical spaces exceeding 2 inches (51 mm) in thickness shall use coarse or fine grout.

R609.2.3 Grout barriers. Vertical grout barriers or dams shall be built of *solid masonry* across the grout space the entire height of the wall to control the flow of the grout horizontally. Grout barriers shall not be more than 25 feet (7620 mm) apart. The grouting of any section of a wall between control barriers shall be completed in one day with no interruptions greater than one hour.

R609.3 Reinforced grouted multiple-wythe masonry. Reinforced grouted multiple-wythe masonry shall conform to all the requirements specified in Sections R609.1 and R609.2 and the requirements of this section.

R609.3.1 Construction. The thickness of grout or mortar between masonry units and reinforcement shall not be less than $1/4$ inch (7 mm), except that $1/4$-inch (7 mm) bars may be laid in horizontal mortar joints at least $1/2$ inch (13 mm) thick, and steel wire reinforcement may be laid in horizontal mortar joints at least twice the thickness of the wire diameter.

TABLE R609.1.1
GROUT PROPORTIONS BY VOLUME FOR MASONRY CONSTRUCTION

TYPE	PORTLAND CEMENT OR BLENDED CEMENT SLAG CEMENT	HYDRATED LIME OR LIME PUTTY	AGGREGATE MEASURED IN A DAMP, LOOSE CONDITION	
			Fine	Coarse
Fine	1	0 to 1/10	$2^1/_4$ to 3 times the sum of the volume of the cementitious materials	—
Coarse	1	0 to 1/10	$2^1/_4$ to 3 times the sum of the volume of the cementitious materials	1 to 2 times the sum of the volumes of the cementitious materials

TABLE R609.1.2
GROUT SPACE DIMENSIONS AND POUR HEIGHTS

GROUT TYPE	GROUT POUR MAXIMUM HEIGHT (feet)	MINIMUM WIDTH OF GROUT SPACES[a,b] (inches)	MINIMUM GROUT[b,c] SPACE DIMENSIONS FOR GROUTING CELLS OF HOLLOW UNITS (inches x inches)
Fine	1	0.75	1.5 × 2
	5	2	2 × 3
	12	2.5	2.5 × 3
	24	3	3 × 3
Coarse	1	1.5	1.5 × 3
	5	2	2.5 × 3
	12	2.5	3 × 3
	24	3	3 × 4

For SI: 1 inch = 25.4 mm, 1 foot = 304.8 mm.

a. For grouting between masonry wythes.

b. Grout space dimension is the clear dimension between any masonry protrusion and shall be increased by the horizontal projection of the diameters of the horizontal bars within the cross section of the grout space.

c. Area of vertical reinforcement shall not exceed 6 percent of the area of the grout space.

R609.4 Reinforced hollow unit masonry. Reinforced hollow unit masonry shall conform to all the requirements of Section R609.1 and the requirements of this section.

R609.4.1 Construction. Requirements for construction shall be as follows:

1. Reinforced hollow-unit masonry shall be built to preserve the unobstructed vertical continuity of the cells to be filled. Walls and cross webs forming cells to be filled shall be full-bedded in mortar to prevent leakage of grout. Head and end joints shall be solidly filled with mortar for a distance in from the face of the wall or unit not less than the thickness of the longitudinal face shells. Bond shall be provided by lapping units in successive vertical courses.

2. Cells to be filled shall have vertical alignment sufficient to maintain a clear, unobstructed continuous vertical cell of dimensions prescribed in Table R609.1.2.

3. Vertical reinforcement shall be held in position at top and bottom and at intervals not exceeding 200 diameters of the reinforcement.

4. Cells containing reinforcement shall be filled solidly with grout. Grout shall be poured in lifts of 8-foot (2438 mm) maximum height. When a total grout pour exceeds 8 feet (2438 mm) in height, the grout shall be placed in lifts not exceeding 5 feet (1524 mm) and special inspection during grouting shall be required.

5. Horizontal steel shall be fully embedded by grout in an uninterrupted pour.

SECTION R610
GLASS UNIT MASONRY

R610.1 General. Panels of glass unit masonry located in load-bearing and nonload-bearing exterior and interior walls shall be constructed in accordance with this section.

R610.2 Materials. Hollow glass units shall be partially evacuated and have a minimum average glass face thickness of $3/_{16}$ inch (5 mm). The surface of units in contact with mortar shall be treated with a polyvinyl butyral coating or latex-based paint. The use of reclaimed units is prohibited.

R610.3 Units. Hollow or solid glass block units shall be standard or thin units.

R610.3.1 Standard units. The specified thickness of standard units shall be at least $3^7/_8$ inches (98 mm).

R610.3.2 Thin units. The specified thickness of thin units shall be at least $3^1/_8$ inches (79 mm) for hollow units and at least 3 inches (76 mm) for solid units.

R610.4 Isolated panels. Isolated panels of glass unit masonry shall conform to the requirements of this section.

R610.4.1 Exterior standard-unit panels. The maximum area of each individual standard-unit panel shall be 144 square feet (13.4 m²) when the design wind pressure is 20 psf (958 Pa). The maximum area of such panels subjected to design wind pressures other than 20 psf (958 Pa) shall be in accordance with Figure R610.4.1. The maximum panel dimension between structural supports shall be 25 feet (7620 mm) in width or 20 feet (6096 mm) in height.

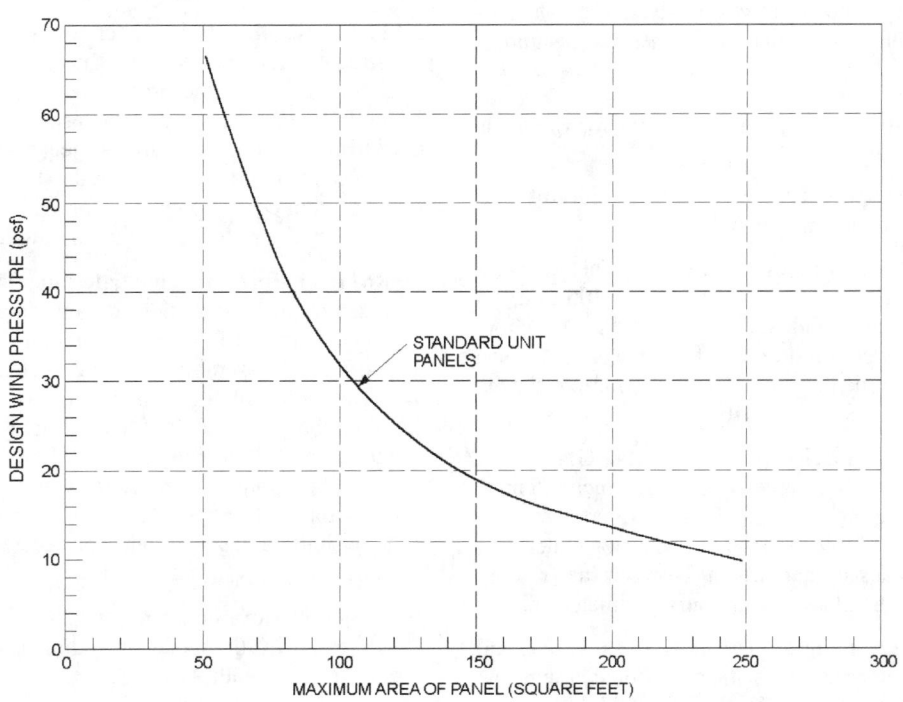

For SI: 1 square foot = 0.0929 m², 1 pound per square foot = 0.0479 kPa.

FIGURE R610.4.1
GLASS UNIT MASONRY DESIGN WIND LOAD RESISTANCE

R610.4.2 Exterior thin-unit panels. The maximum area of each individual thin-unit panel shall be 85 square feet (7.9 m²). The maximum dimension between structural supports shall be 15 feet (4572 mm) in width or 10 feet (3048 mm) in height. Thin units shall not be used in applications where the design wind pressure as stated in Table R301.2(1) exceeds 20 psf (958 Pa).

R610.4.3 Interior panels. The maximum area of each individual standard-unit panel shall be 250 square feet (23.2 m²). The maximum area of each thin-unit panel shall be 150 square feet (13.9 m²). The maximum dimension between structural supports shall be 25 feet (7620 mm) in width or 20 feet (6096 mm) in height.

R610.4.4 Curved panels. The width of curved panels shall conform to the requirements of Sections R610.4.1, R610.4.2 and R610.4.3, except additional structural supports shall be provided at locations where a curved section joins a straight section, and at inflection points in multicurved walls.

R610.5 Panel support. Glass unit masonry panels shall conform to the support requirements of this section.

R610.5.1 Deflection. The maximum total deflection of structural members that support glass unit masonry shall not exceed $^1/_{600}$.

R610.5.2 Lateral support. Glass unit masonry panels shall be laterally supported along the top and sides of the panel. Lateral supports for glass unit masonry panels shall be designed to resist a minimum of 200 pounds per lineal feet (2918 N/m) of panel, or the actual applied loads, whichever is greater. Except for single unit panels, lateral support shall be provided by panel anchors along the top and sides spaced a maximum of 16 inches (406 mm) on center or by channel-type restraints. Single unit panels shall be supported by channel-type restraints.

Exceptions:

1. Lateral support is not required at the top of panels that are one unit wide.

2. Lateral support is not required at the sides of panels that are one unit high.

R610.5.2.1 Panel anchor restraints. Panel anchors shall be spaced a maximum of 16 inches (406 mm) on center in both jambs and across the head. Panel anchors shall be embedded a minimum of 12 inches (305 mm) and shall be provided with two fasteners so as to resist the loads specified in Section R610.5.2.

R610.5.2.2 Channel-type restraints. Glass unit masonry panels shall be recessed at least 1 inch (25 mm) within channels and chases. Channel-type restraints shall be oversized to accommodate expansion material in the opening, packing and sealant between the framing restraints, and the glass unit masonry perimeter units.

R610.6 Sills. Before bedding of glass units, the sill area shall be covered with a water base asphaltic emulsion coating. The coating shall be a minimum of $^1/_8$ inch (3 mm) thick.

R610.7 Expansion joints. Glass unit masonry panels shall be provided with expansion joints along the top and sides at all structural supports. Expansion joints shall be a minimum of $^3/_8$ inch (10 mm) in thickness and shall have sufficient thickness to accommodate displacements of the supporting structure. Expansion joints shall be entirely free of mortar and other debris and shall be filled with resilient material.

R610.8 Mortar. Glass unit masonry shall be laid with Type S or N mortar. Mortar shall not be retempered after initial set. Mortar unused within $1^1/_2$ hours after initial mixing shall be discarded.

R610.9 Reinforcement. Glass unit masonry panels shall have horizontal joint reinforcement spaced a maximum of 16 inches (406 mm) on center located in the mortar bed joint. Horizontal joint reinforcement shall extend the entire length of the panel but shall not extend across expansion joints. Longitudinal wires shall be lapped a minimum of 6 inches (152 mm) at splices. Joint reinforcement shall be placed in the bed joint immediately below and above openings in the panel. The reinforcement shall have not less than two parallel longitudinal wires of size W1.7 or greater, and have welded cross wires of size W1.7 or greater.

R610.10 Placement. Glass units shall be placed so head and bed joints are filled solidly. Mortar shall not be furrowed. Head and bed joints of glass unit masonry shall be $^1/_4$ inch (6.4 mm) thick, except that vertical joint thickness of radial panels shall not be less than $^1/_8$ inch (3 mm) or greater than $^5/_8$ inch (16 mm). The bed joint thickness tolerance shall be minus $^1/_{16}$ inch (1.6 mm) and plus $^1/_8$ inch (3 mm). The head joint thickness tolerance shall be plus or minus $^1/_8$ inch (3 mm).

SECTION R611
EXTERIOR CONCRETE
WALL CONSTRUCTION

R611.1 General. Exterior concrete walls shall be designed and constructed in accordance with the provisions of this section or in accordance with the provisions of PCA 100 or ACI 318. When PCA 100, ACI 318 or the provisions of this section are used to design concrete walls, project drawings, typical details and specifications are not required to bear the seal of the architect or engineer responsible for design, unless otherwise required by the state law of the jurisdiction having authority.

R611.1.1 Interior construction. These provisions are based on the assumption that interior walls and partitions, both load-bearing and nonload-bearing, floors and roof/ceiling assemblies are constructed of *light-framed construction* complying with the limitations of this code and the additional limitations of Section R611.2. Design and construction of light-framed assemblies shall be in accordance with the applicable provisions of this code. Where second-story exterior walls are of *light-framed construction*, they shall be designed and constructed as required by this code.

Aspects of concrete construction not specifically addressed by this code, including interior concrete walls, shall comply with ACI 318.

R611.1.2 Other concrete walls. Exterior concrete walls constructed in accordance with this code shall comply with the shapes and minimum concrete cross-sectional dimensions of Table R611.3. Other types of forming systems resulting in concrete walls not in compliance with this section shall be designed in accordance with ACI 318.

R611.2 Applicability limits. The provisions of this section shall apply to the construction of exterior concrete walls for buildings not greater than 60 feet (18 288 mm) in plan dimensions, floors with clear spans not greater than 32 feet (9754 mm) and roofs with clear spans not greater than 40 feet (12 192 mm). Buildings shall not exceed 35 feet (10 668 mm) in mean roof height or two stories in height above-grade. Floor/ceiling dead loads shall not exceed 10 pounds per square foot (479 Pa), roof/ceiling dead loads shall not exceed 15 pounds per square foot (718 Pa) and *attic* live loads shall not exceed 20 pounds per square foot (958 Pa). Roof overhangs shall not exceed 2 feet (610 mm) of horizontal projection beyond the exterior wall and the dead load of the overhangs shall not exceed 8 pounds per square foot (383 Pa).

Walls constructed in accordance with the provisions of this section shall be limited to buildings subjected to a maximum design wind speed of 130 miles per hour (58 m/s) Exposure B, 110 miles per hour (49 m/s) Exposure C and 100 miles per hour (45 m/s) Exposure D. Walls constructed in accordance with the provisions of this section shall be limited to detached one- and two-family *dwellings* and townhouses assigned to Seismic Design Category A or B, and detached one- and two-family *dwellings* assigned to Seismic Design Category C.

Buildings that are not within the scope of this section shall be designed in accordance with PCA 100 or ACI 318.

R611.3 Concrete wall systems. Concrete walls constructed in accordance with these provisions shall comply with the shapes and minimum concrete cross-sectional dimensions of Table R611.3.

R611.3.1 Flat wall systems. Flat concrete wall systems shall comply with Table R611.3 and Figure R611.3(1) and have a minimum nominal thickness of 4 inches (102 mm).

R611.3.2 Waffle-grid wall systems. Waffle-grid wall systems shall comply with Table R611.3 and Figure R611.3(2). and shall have a minimum nominal thickness of 6 inches (152 mm) for the horizontal and vertical concrete members (cores). The core and web dimensions shall comply with Table R611.3. The maximum weight of waffle-grid walls shall comply with Table R611.3.

R611.3.3 Screen-grid wall systems. Screen-grid wall systems shall comply with Table R611.3 and Figure R611.3(3) and shall have a minimum nominal thickness of 6 inches (152 mm) for the horizontal and vertical concrete members (cores). The core dimensions shall comply with Table R611.3. The maximum weight of screen-grid walls shall comply with Table R611.3.

R611.4 Stay-in-place forms. Stay-in-place concrete forms shall comply with this section.

R611.4.1 Surface burning characteristics. The flame spread index and smoke-developed index of forming material, other than foam plastic, left exposed on the interior shall comply with Section R302.9. The surface burning

TABLE R611.3
DIMENSIONAL REQUIREMENTS FOR WALLS[a,b]

WALL TYPE AND NOMINAL THICKNESS	MAXIMUM WALL WEIGHT[c] (psf)	MINIMUM WIDTH, W, OF VERTICAL CORES (inches)	MINIMUM THICKNESS, T, OF VERTICAL CORES (inches)	MAXIMUM SPACING OF VERTICAL CORES (inches)	MAXIMUM SPACING OF HORIZONTAL CORES (inches)	MINIMUM WEB THICKNESS (inches)
4″ Flat[d]	50	N/A	N/A	N/A	N/A	N/A
6″ Flat[d]	75	N/A	N/A	N/A	N/A	N/A
8″ Flat[d]	100	N/A	N/A	N/A	N/A	N/A
10″ Flat[d]	125	N/A	N/A	N/A	N/A	N/A
6″ Waffle-grid	56	8[e]	5.5[e]	12	16	2
8″ Waffle-grid	76	8[f]	8[f]	12	16	2
6″ Screen-grid	53	6.25[g]	6.25[g]	12	12	N/A

For SI: 1 inch = 25.4 mm; 1 pound per square foot = 0.0479 kPa, 1 pound per cubic foot = 2402.77 kg/m³, 1 square inch = 645.16 mm².

a. Width "W," thickness "T," spacing and web thickness, refer to Figures R611.3(2) and R611.3(3).

b. N/A indicates not applicable.

c. Wall weight is based on a unit weight of concrete of 150 pcf. For flat walls the weight is based on the nominal thickness. The tabulated values do not include any allowance for interior and exterior finishes.

d. Nominal wall thickness. The actual as-built thickness of a flat wall shall not be more than $^1/_2$-inch less or more than $^1/_4$-inch more than the nominal dimension indicated.

e. Vertical core is assumed to be elliptical-shaped. Another shape core is permitted provided the minimum thickness is 5 inches, the moment of inertia, I, about the centerline of the wall (ignoring the web) is not less than 65 in⁴, and the area, A, is not less than 31.25 in². The width used to calculate A and I shall not exceed 8 inches.

f. Vertical core is assumed to be circular. Another shape core is permitted provided the minimum thickness is 7 inches, the moment of inertia, I, about the centerline of the wall (ignoring the web) is not less than 200 in⁴, and the area, A, is not less than 49 in². The width used to calculate A and I shall not exceed 8 inches.

g. Vertical core is assumed to be circular. Another shape core is permitted provided the minimum thickness is 5.5 inches, the moment of inertia, I, about the centerline of the wall is not less than 76 in⁴, and the area, A, is not less than 30.25 in². The width used to calculate A and I shall not exceed 6.25 inches.

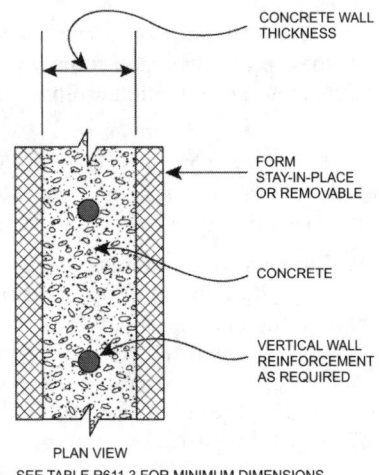

CONCRETE WALL THICKNESS

FORM STAY-IN-PLACE OR REMOVABLE

CONCRETE

VERTICAL WALL REINFORCEMENT AS REQUIRED

PLAN VIEW
SEE TABLE R611.3 FOR MINIMUM DIMENSIONS

FIGURE R611.3(1)
FLAT WALL SYSTEM

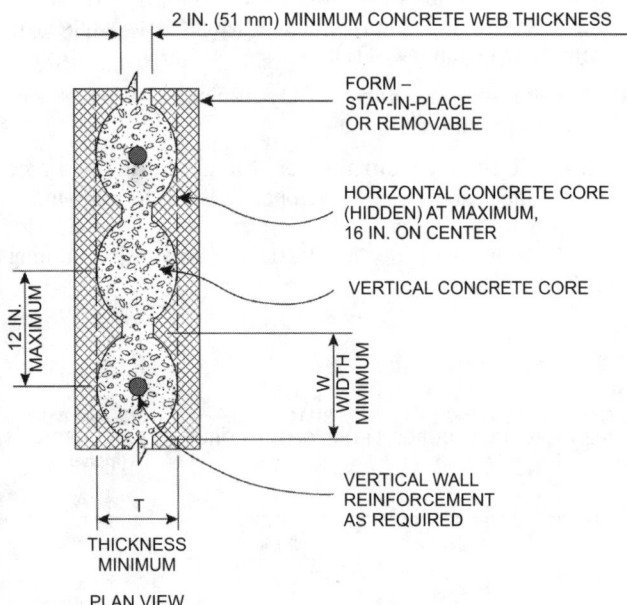

2 IN. (51 mm) MINIMUM CONCRETE WEB THICKNESS

FORM – STAY-IN-PLACE OR REMOVABLE

HORIZONTAL CONCRETE CORE (HIDDEN) AT MAXIMUM, 16 IN. ON CENTER

VERTICAL CONCRETE CORE

12 IN. MAXIMUM

W WIDTH MINIMUM

VERTICAL WALL REINFORCEMENT AS REQUIRED

T
THICKNESS MINIMUM

PLAN VIEW

SEE TABLE R611.3 FOR MINIMUM DIMENSIONS

For SI: 1 inch = 25.4 mm.

FIGURE R611.3(2)
WAFFLE-GRID WALL SYSTEM

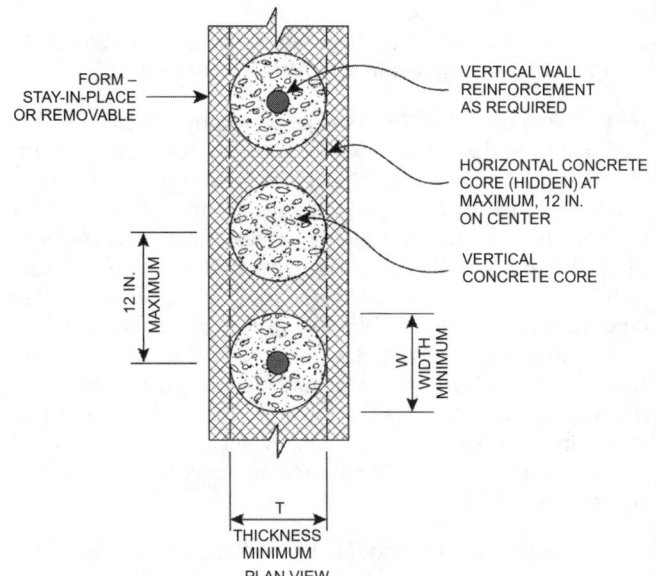

FORM – STAY-IN-PLACE OR REMOVABLE

VERTICAL WALL REINFORCEMENT AS REQUIRED

HORIZONTAL CONCRETE CORE (HIDDEN) AT MAXIMUM, 12 IN. ON CENTER

VERTICAL CONCRETE CORE

12 IN. MAXIMUM

W WIDTH MINIMUM

T
THICKNESS MINIMUM
PLAN VIEW

SEE TABLE R611.3 FOR MINIMUM DIMENSIONS.

For SI: 1 inch = 25.4 mm.

FIGURE R611.3(3)
SCREEN-GRID WALL SYSTEM

characteristics of foam plastic used in insulating concrete forms shall comply with Section R316.3.

R611.4.2 Interior covering. Stay-in-place forms constructed of rigid foam plastic shall be protected on the interior of the building as required by Sections R316.4 and R702.3.4. Where gypsum board is used to protect the foam plastic, it shall be installed with a mechanical fastening system. Use of adhesives is permitted in addition to mechanical fasteners.

R611.4.3 Exterior wall covering. Stay-in-place forms constructed of rigid foam plastics shall be protected from sunlight and physical damage by the application of an *approved* exterior wall covering complying with this code. Exterior surfaces of other stay-in-place forming systems shall be protected in accordance with this code.

Requirements for installation of masonry veneer, stucco and other finishes on the exterior of concrete walls and other construction details not covered in this section shall comply with the requirements of this code.

R611.5 Materials. Materials used in the construction of concrete walls shall comply with this section.

R611.5.1 Concrete and materials for concrete. Materials used in concrete, and the concrete itself, shall conform to requirements of this section, or ACI 318.

R611.5.1.1 Concrete mixing and delivery. Mixing and delivery of concrete shall comply with ASTM C 94 or ASTM C 685.

R611.5.1.2 Maximum aggregate size. The nominal maximum size of coarse aggregate shall not exceed one-fifth the narrowest distance between sides of forms, or three-fourths the clear spacing between reinforcing bars or between a bar and the side of the form.

Exception: When *approved*, these limitations shall not apply where removable forms are used and workability and methods of consolidation permit concrete to be placed without honeycombs or voids.

R611.5.1.3 Proportioning and slump of concrete. Proportions of materials for concrete shall be established to provide workability and consistency to permit concrete to be worked readily into forms and around reinforcement under conditions of placement to be employed, without segregation or excessive bleeding. Slump of concrete placed in removable forms shall not exceed 6 inches (152 mm).

Exception: When *approved*, the slump is permitted to exceed 6 inches (152 mm) for concrete mixtures that are resistant to segregation, and are in accordance with the form manufacturer's recommendations.

Slump of concrete placed in stay-in-place forms shall exceed 6 inches (152 mm). Slump of concrete shall be determined in accordance with ASTM C 143.

R611.5.1.4 Compressive strength. The minimum specified compressive strength of concrete, f'_c, shall comply with Section R402.2 and shall be not less than 2,500 pounds per square inch (17.2 MPa) at 28 days.

R611.5.1.5 Consolidation of concrete. Concrete shall be consolidated by suitable means during placement and shall be worked around embedded items and reinforcement and into corners of forms. Where stay-in-place forms are used, concrete shall be consolidated by internal vibration.

> **Exception:** When *approved*, self-consolidating concrete mixtures with slumps equal to or greater than 8 inches (203 mm) that are specifically designed for placement without internal vibration need not be internally vibrated.

R611.5.2 Steel reinforcement and anchor bolts.

R611.5.2.1 Steel reinforcement. Steel reinforcement shall comply with ASTM A 615, A 706, or A 996. ASTM A 996 bars produced from rail steel shall be Type R.

R611.5.2.2 Anchor bolts. Anchor bolts for use with connection details in accordance with Figures R611.9(1) through R611.9(12) shall be bolts with heads complying with ASTM A 307 or ASTM F 1554. ASTM A 307 bolts shall be Grade A (i.e., with heads). ASTM F 1554 bolts shall be Grade 36 minimum. Instead of bolts with heads, it is permissible to use rods with threads on both ends fabricated from steel complying with ASTM A 36. The threaded end of the rod to be embedded in the concrete shall be provided with a hex or square nut.

R611.5.2.3 Sheet steel angles and tension tie straps. Angles and tension tie straps for use with connection details in accordance with Figures R611.9(1) through R611.9(12) shall be fabricated from sheet steel complying with ASTM A 653 SS, ASTM A 792 SS, or ASTM A 875 SS. The steel shall be minimum Grade 33 unless a higher grade is required by the applicable figure.

R611.5.3 Form materials and form ties. Forms shall be made of wood, steel, aluminum, plastic, a composite of cement and foam insulation, a composite of cement and wood chips, or other *approved* material suitable for supporting and containing concrete. Forms shall provide sufficient strength to contain concrete during the concrete placement operation.

Form ties shall be steel, solid plastic, foam plastic, a composite of cement and wood chips, a composite of cement and foam plastic, or other suitable material capable of resisting the forces created by fluid pressure of fresh concrete.

R611.5.4 Reinforcement installation details.

R611.5.4.1 Support and cover. Reinforcement shall be secured in the proper location in the forms with tie wire or other bar support system such that displacement will not occur during the concrete placement operation. Steel reinforcement in concrete cast against the earth shall have a minimum cover of 3 inches (76 mm). Minimum cover for reinforcement in concrete cast in removable forms that will be exposed to the earth or weather shall be $1^1/_2$ inches (38 mm) for No. 5 bars and smaller, and 2 inches (50 mm) for No. 6 bars and larger. For concrete cast in removable forms that will not be exposed to the earth or weather, and for concrete cast in stay-in-place forms, minimum cover shall be $^3/_4$ inch (19 mm). The minus tolerance for cover shall not exceed the smaller of one-third the required cover and $^3/_8$ inch (10 mm). See Section R611.5.4.4 for cover requirements for hooks of bars developed in tension.

R611.5.4.2 Location of reinforcement in walls. For location of reinforcement in foundation walls and above-grade walls, see Sections R404.1.2.3.7.2 and R611.6.5, respectively.

R611.5.4.3 Lap splices. Vertical and horizontal wall reinforcement required by Sections R611.6 and R611.7 shall be the longest lengths practical. Where splices are necessary in reinforcement, the length of lap splices shall be in accordance with Table R611.5.4(1) and Figure R611.5.4 (1). The maximum gap between noncontact parallel bars at a lap splice shall not exceed the smaller of one-fifth the required lap length and 6 inches (152 mm). See Figure R611.5.4(1).

R611.5.4.4 Development of bars in tension. Where bars are required to be developed in tension by other provisions of this code, development lengths and cover for hooks and bar extensions shall comply with Table R611.5.4(1) and Figure R611.5.4 (2). The development lengths shown in Table R611.5.4(1) also apply to bundled bars in lintels installed in accordance with Section R611.8.2.2.

R611.5.4.5 Standard hooks. Where reinforcement is required by this code to terminate with a standard hook, the hook shall comply with Figure R611.5.4(3).

R611.5.4.6 Webs of waffle-grid walls. Reinforcement, including stirrups, shall not be placed in webs of waffle-grid walls, including lintels. Webs are permitted to have form ties.

R611.5.4.7 Alternate grade of reinforcement and spacing. Where tables in Sections R404.1.2 and R611.6 specify vertical wall reinforcement based on minimum bar size and maximum spacing, which are based on Grade 60 (420 MPa) steel reinforcement, different size bars and/or bars made from a different grade of steel are permitted provided an equivalent area of steel per linear foot of wall is provided. Use of Table R611.5.4(2) is permitted to determine the maximum bar spacing for different bar sizes than specified in the tables and/or bars made from a different grade of steel. Bars shall not be spaced less than one-half the wall thickness, or more than 48 inches (1219 mm) on center.

R611.5.5 Construction joints in walls. Construction joints shall be made and located to not impair the strength of the wall. Construction joints in plain concrete walls, including walls required to have not less than No. 4 bars at 48 inches (1219 mm) on center by Section R611.6, shall be located at points of lateral support, and a minimum of one No. 4 bar shall extend across the construction joint at a spacing not to exceed 24 inches (610 mm) on center. Construction joint reinforcement shall have a minimum of 12 inches (305 mm) embedment on both sides of the joint. Construction joints in reinforced concrete walls shall be located in the middle third of the span between lateral supports, or located and constructed as required for joints in plain concrete walls.

Exception: Vertical wall reinforcement required by this code is permitted to be used in lieu of construction joint reinforcement, provided the spacing does not exceed 24 inches (610 mm), or the combination of wall reinforcement and No. 4 bars described above does not exceed 24 inches (610 mm).

R611.6 Above-grade wall requirements.

R611.6.1 General. The minimum thickness of load-bearing and nonload-bearing above-grade walls and reinforcement shall be as set forth in the appropriate table in this section based on the type of wall form to be used. Where the wall or building is not within the limitations of Section

TABLE R611.5.4(1)
LAP SPLICE AND TENSION DEVELOPMENT LENGTHS

	BAR SIZE NO.	YIELD STRENGTH OF STEEL, f_y - psi (MPa)	
		40,000 (280)	60,000 (420)
		Splice length or tension development length (inches)	
Lap splice length–tension	4	20	30
	5	25	38
	6	30	45
Tension development length for straight bar	4	15	23
	5	19	28
	6	23	34
Tension development length for: a. 90-degree and 180-degree standard hooks with not less than $2^1/_2$ inches of side cover perpendicular to plane of hook, and b. 90-degree standard hooks with not less than 2 inches of cover on the bar extension beyond the hook.	4	6	9
	5	7	11
	6	8	13
Tension development length for bar with 90-degree or 180-degree standard hook having less cover than required above.	4	8	12
	5	10	15
	6	12	18

For SI: 1 inch = 25.4 mm, 1 degree = 0.0175 rad.

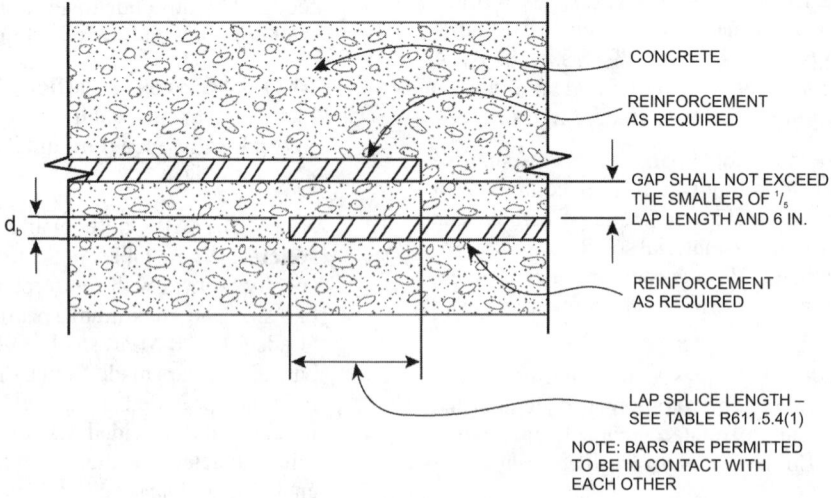

For SI: 1 inch = 25.4 mm.

FIGURE R611.5.4(1)
LAP SPLICES

R611.2, design is required by the tables in this section, or the wall is not within the scope of the tables in this section, the wall shall be designed in accordance with ACI 318.

Above-grade concrete walls shall be constructed in accordance with this section and Figure R611.6(1), R611.6(2), R611.6(3), or R611.6(4). Above-grade concrete walls that are continuous with stem walls and not laterally supported by the slab-on-ground shall be designed and constructed in accordance with this section. Concrete walls shall be supported on continuous foundation walls or slabs-on-ground that are monolithic with the footing in accordance with Section R403. The minimum length of solid wall without openings shall be in accordance with Section R611.7. Reinforcement around openings, including lintels, shall be in accordance with Section R611.8. Lateral support for above-grade walls in the out-of-plane direction shall be provided by connections to the floor framing system, if applicable, and to ceiling and roof framing systems

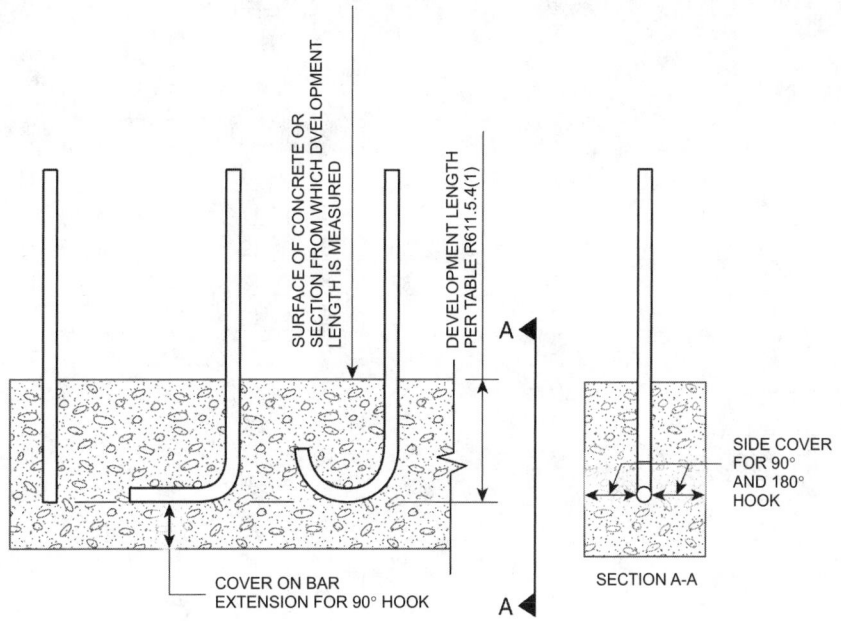

For SI: 1 degree = 0.0175 rad.

FIGURE R611.5.4(2)
DEVELOPMENT LENGTH AND COVER FOR HOOKS AND BAR EXTENSION

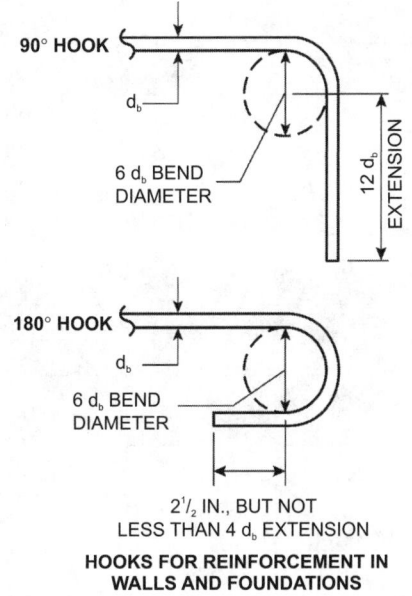

HOOKS FOR REINFORCEMENT IN WALLS AND FOUNDATIONS

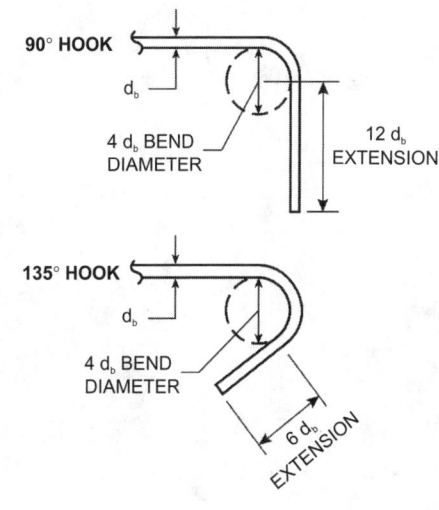

HOOKS FOR STIRRUPS IN LINTELS

For SI: 1 inch = 25.4 mm, 1 degree = 0.0175 rad.

FIGURE R611.5.4(3)
STANDARD HOOKS

TABLE R611.5.4(2)
MAXIMUM SPACING FOR ALTERNATE BAR SIZE AND/OR ALTERNATE GRADE OF STEEL[a, b, c]

BAR SPACING FROM APPLICABLE TABLE IN SECTION R611.6 (inches)	#4 Grade 60 #5	#4 Grade 60 #6	#4 Grade 40 #4	#4 Grade 40 #5	#4 Grade 40 #6	#5 Grade 60 #4	#5 Grade 60 #6	#5 Grade 40 #4	#5 Grade 40 #5	#5 Grade 40 #6	#6 Grade 60 #4	#6 Grade 60 #5	#6 Grade 40 #4	#6 Grade 40 #5	#6 Grade 40 #6
8	12	18	5	8	12	5	11	3	5	8	4	6	2	4	5
9	14	20	6	9	13	6	13	4	6	9	4	6	3	4	6
10	16	22	7	10	15	6	14	4	7	9	5	7	3	5	7
11	17	24	7	11	16	7	16	5	7	10	5	8	3	5	7
12	19	26	8	12	18	8	17	5	8	11	5	8	4	6	8
13	20	29	9	13	19	8	18	6	9	12	6	9	4	6	9
14	22	31	9	14	21	9	20	6	9	13	6	10	4	7	9
15	23	33	10	16	22	10	21	6	10	14	7	11	5	7	10
16	25	35	11	17	23	10	23	7	11	15	7	11	5	8	11
17	26	37	11	18	25	11	24	7	11	16	8	12	5	8	11
18	28	40	12	19	26	12	26	8	12	17	8	13	5	8	12
19	29	42	13	20	28	12	27	8	13	18	9	13	6	9	13
20	31	44	13	21	29	13	28	9	13	19	9	14	6	9	13
21	33	46	14	22	31	14	30	9	14	20	10	15	6	10	14
22	34	48	15	23	32	14	31	9	15	21	10	16	7	10	15
23	36	48	15	24	34	15	33	10	15	22	10	16	7	11	15
24	37	48	16	25	35	15	34	10	16	23	11	17	7	11	16
25	39	48	17	26	37	16	35	11	17	24	11	18	8	12	17
26	40	48	17	27	38	17	37	11	17	25	12	18	8	12	17
27	42	48	18	28	40	17	38	12	18	26	12	19	8	13	18
28	43	48	19	29	41	18	40	12	19	26	13	20	8	13	19
29	45	48	19	30	43	19	41	12	19	27	13	20	9	14	19
30	47	48	20	31	44	19	43	13	20	28	14	21	9	14	20
31	48	48	21	32	45	20	44	13	21	29	14	22	9	15	21
32	48	48	21	33	47	21	45	14	21	30	15	23	10	15	21
33	48	48	22	34	48	21	47	14	22	31	15	23	10	16	22
34	48	48	23	35	48	22	48	15	23	32	15	24	10	16	23
35	48	48	23	36	48	23	48	15	23	33	16	25	11	16	23
36	48	48	24	37	48	23	48	15	24	34	16	25	11	17	24
37	48	48	25	38	48	24	48	16	25	35	17	26	11	17	25
38	48	48	25	39	48	25	48	16	25	36	17	27	12	18	25
39	48	48	26	40	48	25	48	17	26	37	18	27	12	18	26
40	48	48	27	41	48	26	48	17	27	38	18	28	12	19	27
41	48	48	27	42	48	26	48	18	27	39	19	29	12	19	27
42	48	48	28	43	48	27	48	18	28	40	19	30	13	20	28
43	48	48	29	44	48	28	48	18	29	41	20	30	13	20	29
44	48	48	29	45	48	28	48	19	29	42	20	31	13	21	29
45	48	48	30	47	48	29	48	19	30	43	20	32	14	21	30
46	48	48	31	48	48	30	48	20	31	44	21	32	14	22	31
47	48	48	31	48	48	30	48	20	31	44	21	33	14	22	31
48	48	48	32	48	48	31	48	21	32	45	22	34	15	23	32

For SI: 1 inch = 25.4 mm.

a. This table is for use with tables in Section R611.6 that specify the minimum bar size and maximum spacing of vertical wall reinforcement for foundation walls and above-grade walls. Reinforcement specified in tables in Section R611.6 is based on Grade 60 (420 MPa) steel reinforcement.

b. Bar spacing shall not exceed 48 inches on center and shall not be less than one-half the nominal wall thickness.

c. For Grade 50 (350 MPa) steel bars (ASTM A 996, Type R), use spacing for Grade 40 (280 MPa) bars or interpolate between Grade 40 (280 MPa) and Grade 60 (420 MPa).

in accordance with Section R611.9. The wall thickness shall be equal to or greater than the thickness of the wall in the *story* above.

R611.6.2 Wall reinforcement for wind. Vertical wall reinforcement for resistance to out-of-plane wind forces shall be determined from Table R611.6(1), R611.6(2), R611.6(3) or R611.6(4). Also, see Sections R611.7.2.2.2 and R611.7.2.2.3. There shall be a vertical bar at all corners of exterior walls. Unless more horizontal reinforcement is required by Section R611.7.2.2.1, the minimum horizontal reinforcement shall be four No. 4 bars [Grade 40 (280 MPa)] placed as follows: top bar within 12 inches (305 mm) of the top of the wall, bottom bar within 12 inches (305 mm) of the finish floor, and one bar each at approximately one-third and two-thirds of the wall height.

R611.6.3 Continuity of wall reinforcement between stories. Vertical reinforcement required by this section shall be continuous between elements providing lateral support for the wall. Reinforcement in the wall of the *story* above shall be continuous with the reinforcement in the wall of the *story* below, or the foundation wall, if applicable. Lap splices, where required, shall comply with Section R611.5.4.3 and Figure R611.5.4(1). Where the above-grade wall is supported by a monolithic slab-on-ground and footing, dowel bars with a size and spacing to match the vertical above-grade concrete wall reinforcement shall be embedded in the monolithic slab-on-ground and footing the distance required to develop the dowel bar in tension in accordance with Section R611.5.4.4 and Figure R611.5.4(2) and lap-spliced with the above-grade wall reinforcement in accordance with Section R611.5.4.3 and Figure R611.5.4(1).

Exception: Where reinforcement in the wall above cannot be made continuous with the reinforcement in the wall below, the bottom of the reinforcement in the wall above shall be terminated in accordance with one of the following:

1. Extend below the top of the floor the distance required to develop the bar in tension in accordance with Section R611.5.4.4 and Figure R611.5.4(2).

2. Lap-spliced in accordance with Section R611.5.4.3 and Figure R611.5.4(1) with a dowel bar that extends into the wall below the distance required to develop the bar in tension in accordance with Section R611.5.4.4 and Figure R611.5.4(2).

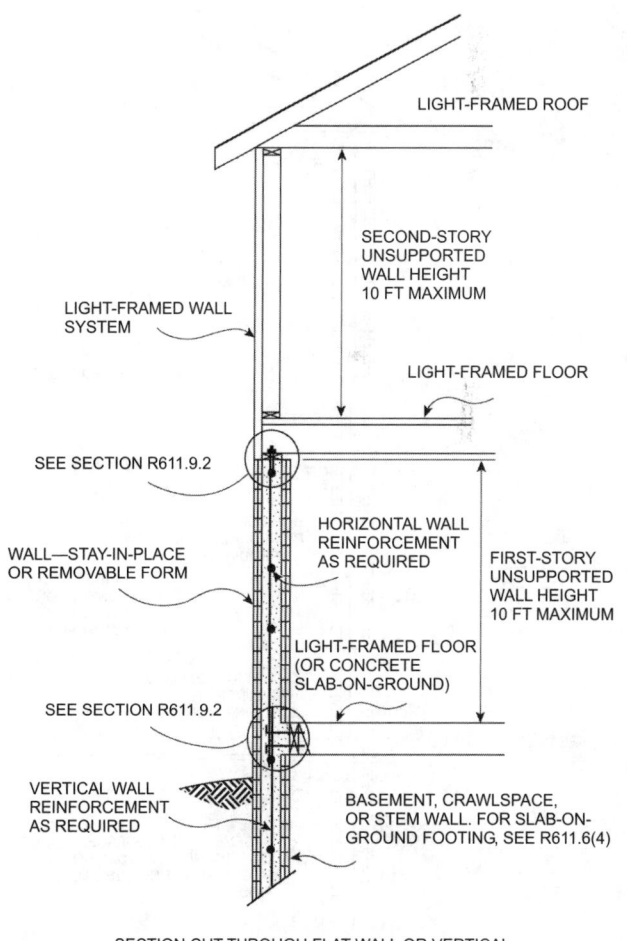

SECTION CUT THROUGH FLAT WALL OR VERTICAL CORE OF A WAFFLE—OR SCREEN-GRID WALL

For SI: 1 foot = 304.8 mm.

FIGURE R611.6(1)
ABOVE-GRADE CONCRETE WALL CONSTRUCTION ONE

SECTION CUT THROUGH FLAT WALL OR VERTICAL CORE OF A WAFFLE—OR SCREEN-GRID WALL

For SI: 1 foot = 304.8 mm.

FIGURE R611.6(2)
ABOVE-GRADE CONCRETE WALL CONSTRUCTION
CONCRETE FIRST-STORY AND
LIGHT-FRAMED SECOND-STORY

Where a construction joint in the wall is located below the level of the floor and less than the distance required to develop the bar in tension, the distance required to develop the bar in tension shall be measured from the top of the concrete below the joint. See Section R611.5.5.

R611.6.4 Termination of reinforcement. Where indicated in items 1 through 3 below, vertical wall reinforcement in the top-most *story* with concrete walls shall be terminated with a 90-degree (1.57 rad) standard hook complying with Section R611.5.4.5 and Figure R611.5.4(3).

1. Vertical bars adjacent to door and window openings required by Section R611.8.1.2.

2. Vertical bars at the ends of required solid wall segments. See Section R611.7.2.2.2.

3. Vertical bars (other than end bars – see item 2) used as shear reinforcement in required solid wall segments where the reduction factor for design strength, R_3, used is based on the wall having horizontal and vertical shear reinforcement. See Section R611.7.2.2.3.

The bar extension of the hook shall be oriented parallel to the horizontal wall reinforcement and be within 4 inches (102 mm) of the top of the wall.

Horizontal reinforcement shall be continuous around the building corners by bending one of the bars and lap-splicing it with the bar in the other wall in accordance with Section R611.5.4.3 and Figure R611.5.4(1).

Exception: In lieu of bending horizontal reinforcement at corners, separate bent reinforcing bars shall be permitted provided that the bent bar is lap-spliced with the horizontal reinforcement in both walls in accordance with Section R611.5.4.3 and Figure R611.5.4(1).

In required solid wall segments where the reduction factor for design strength, R_3, is based on the wall having horizontal and vertical shear reinforcement in accordance with Section R611.7.2.2.1, horizontal wall reinforcement shall be terminated with a standard hook complying with Section R611.5.4.5 and Figure R611.5.4(3) or in a lap-splice, except at corners where the reinforcement shall be continuous as required above.

R611.6.5 Location of reinforcement in wall. Except for vertical reinforcement at the ends of required solid wall segments, which shall be located as required by Section R611.7.2.2.2, the location of the vertical reinforcement shall not vary from the center of the wall by more than the greater of 10 percent of the wall thickness and $^3/_8$-inch (10 mm). Horizontal and vertical reinforcement shall be located to provide not less than the minimum cover required by Section R611.5.4.1.

LIGHT-FRAMED ROOF

SEE SECTION R611.9.3

SECOND-STORY UNSUPPORTED WALL HEIGHT 10 FT MAXIMUM

LIGHT-FRAMED FLOOR

SEE SECTION R611.9.2

WALL—STAY-IN-PLACE OR REMOVABLE FORM

HORIZONTAL WALL REINFORCEMENT AS REQUIRED

FIRST-STORY UNSUPPORTED WALL HEIGHT 10 FT MAXIMUM

LIGHT-FRAMED FLOOR (OR CONCRETE SLAB-ON-GROUND)

SEE SECTION R611.9.2

VERTICAL WALL REINFORCEMENT AS REQUIRED

BASEMENT, CRAWLSPACE, OR STEM WALL. fOR SLAB-ON-GROUND FOOTING SEE FIGURE R611.6(4)

SECTION CUT THROUGH FLAT WALL OR VERTICAL CORE OF A WAFFLE- OR SCREEN-GRID WALL

For SI: 1 foot = 304.8 mm.

FIGURE R611.6(3)
ABOVE-GRADE CONCRETE WALL CONSTRUCTION
TWO-STORY

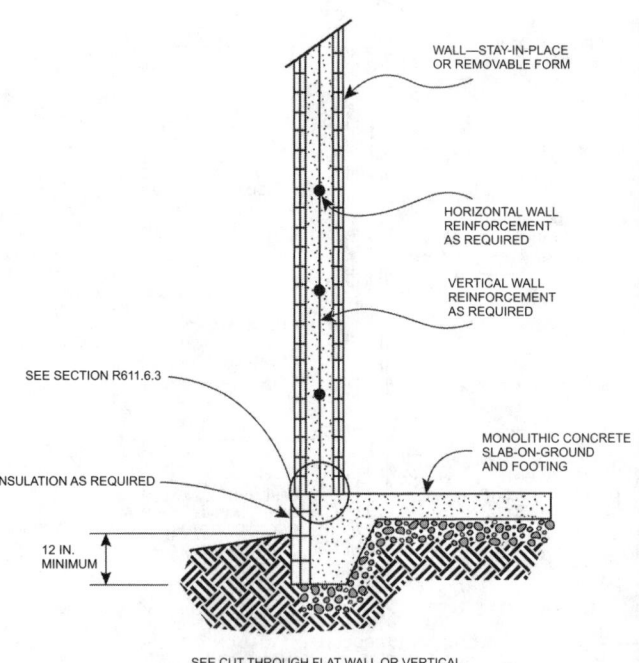

WALL—STAY-IN-PLACE OR REMOVABLE FORM

HORIZONTAL WALL REINFORCEMENT AS REQUIRED

VERTICAL WALL REINFORCEMENT AS REQUIRED

SEE SECTION R611.6.3

INSULATION AS REQUIRED

MONOLITHIC CONCRETE SLAB-ON-GROUND AND FOOTING

12 IN. MINIMUM

SEE CUT THROUGH FLAT WALL OR VERTICAL CORE OF A WAFFLE- OR SCREEN-GRID WALL

For SI: 1 inch = 25.4 mm.

FIGURE R611.6(4)
ABOVE-GRADE CONCRETE WALL SUPPORTED ON
MONOLITHIC SLAB-ON GROUND FOOTING

TABLE R611.6(1)
MINIMUM VERTICAL REINFORCEMENT FOR FLAT ABOVE-GRADE WALLS[a, b, c, d, e]

MAXIMUM WIND SPEED (mph) Exposure Category			MAXIMUM UNSUPPORTED WALL HEIGHT PER STORY (feet)	MINIMUM VERTICAL REINFORCEMENT—BAR SIZE AND SPACING (inches)[f, g] Nominal[h] wall thickness (inches)							
				4		6		8		10	
B	C	D		Top[i]	Side[i]	Top[i]	Side[i]	Top[i]	Side[i]	Top[i]	Side[i]
85	—	—	8	4@48	4@48	4@48	4@48	4@48	4@48	4@48	4@48
			9	4@48	4@43	4@48	4@48	4@48	4@48	4@48	4@48
			10	4@47	4@36	4@48	4@48	4@48	4@48	4@48	4@48
90	—	—	8	4@48	4@47	4@48	4@48	4@48	4@48	4@48	4@48
			9	4@48	4@39	4@48	4@48	4@48	4@48	4@48	4@48
			10	4@42	4@34	4@48	4@48	4@48	4@48	4@48	4@48
100	85	—	8	4@48	4@40	4@48	4@48	4@48	4@48	4@48	4@48
			9	4@42	4@34	4@48	4@48	4@48	4@48	4@48	4@48
			10	4@34	4@34	4@48	4@48	4@48	4@48	4@48	4@48
110	90	85	8	4@44	4@34	4@48	4@48	4@48	4@48	4@48	4@48
			9	4@34	4@34	4@48	4@48	4@48	4@48	4@48	4@48
			10	4@34	4@31	4@48	4@37	4@48	4@48	4@48	4@48
120	100	90	8	4@36	4@34	4@48	4@48	4@48	4@48	4@48	4@48
			9	4@34	4@32	4@48	4@38	4@48	4@48	4@48	4@48
			10	4@30	4@27	4@48	5@48	4@48	4@48	4@48	4@48
130	110	100	8	4@34	4@34	4@48	4@48	4@48	4@48	4@48	4@48
			9	4@32	4@28	4@48	4@33	4@48	4@48	4@48	4@48
			10	4@26	4@23	4@48	5@43	4@48	4@48	4@48	4@48

For SI:1 inch = 25.4 mm; 1 foot = 304.8 mm; 1 mile per hour = 0.447 m/s, 1 pound per square inch = 1.895kPa.

a. Table is based on ASCE 7 components and cladding wind pressures for an enclosed building using a mean roof height of 35 ft, interior wall area 4, an effective wind area of 10 ft², and topographic factor, K_{zt}, and importance factor, I, equal to 1.0.

b. Table is based on concrete with a minimum specified compressive strength of 2,500 psi.

c. See Section R611.6.5 for location of reinforcement in wall.

d. Deflection criterion is $L/240$, where L is the unsupported height of the wall in inches.

e. Interpolation is not permitted.

f. Where No. 4 reinforcing bars at a spacing of 48 inches are specified in the table, use of bars with a minimum yield strength of 40,000 psi or 60,000 psi is permitted.

g. Other than for No. 4 bars spaced at 48 inches on center, table values are based on reinforcing bars with a minimum yield strength of 60,000 psi. Vertical reinforcement with a yield strength of less than 60,000 psi and/or bars of a different size than specified in the table are permitted in accordance with Section R611.5.4.7 and Table R611.5.4(2).

h. See Table R611.3 for tolerances on nominal thicknesses.

i. Top means gravity load from roof and/or floor construction bears on top of wall. Side means gravity load from floor construction is transferred to wall from a wood ledger or cold-formed steel track bolted to side of wall. Where floor framing members span parallel to the wall, use of the top bearing condition is permitted.

TABLE R611.6(2)
MINIMUM VERTICAL REINFORCEMENT FOR WAFFLE-GRID ABOVE-GRADE WALLS[a, b, c, d, e]

MAXIMUM WIND SPEED (mph) Exposure Category			MAXIMUM UNSUPPORTED WALL HEIGHT PER STORY (feet)	MINIMUM VERTICAL REINFORCEMENT—BAR SIZE AND SPACING (inches)[f, g] Nominal[h] wall thickness (inches)			
				6		8	
B	C	D		Top[i]	Side[i]	Top[i]	Side[i]
85	—	—	8	4@48	4@36, 5@48	4@48	4@48
			9	4@48	4@30, 5@47	4@48	4@45
			10	4@48	4@26, 5@40	4@48	4@39
90	—	—	8	4@48	4@33, 5@48	4@48	4@48
			9	4@48	4@28, 5@43	4@48	4@42
			10	4@31, 5@48	4@24, 5@37	4@48	4@36
100	85	—	8	4@48	4@28, 5@44	4@48	4@43
			9	4@31, 5@48	4@24, 5@37	4@48	4@36
			10	4@25, 5@39	4@24, 5@37	4@48	4@31, 5@48
110	90	85	8	4@33, 5@48	4@25, 5@38	4@48	4@38
			9	4@26, 5@40	4@24, 5@37	4@48	4@31, 5@48
			10	4@24, 5@37	4@23, 5@35	4@48	4@27, 5@41
120	100	90	8	4@27, 5@42	4@24, 5@37	4@48	4@33, 5@48
			9	4@24, 5@37	4@23, 5@36	4@48	4@27, 5@43
			10	4@23, 5@35	4@19, 5@30	4@48	4@23, 5@36
130	110	100	8	4@24, 5@37	4@24, 5@37	4@48	4@29, 5@45
			9	4@24, 5@37	4@20, 5@32	4@48	4@24, 5@37
			10	4@19, 5@30	4@17, 5@26	4@23, 5@36	4@20, 5@31

For SI: 1 inch = 25.4 mm; 1 foot = 304.8 mm; 1 mile per hour = 0.447 m/s, 1 pound per square inch = 6.895 kPa.

a. Table is based on ASCE 7 components and cladding wind pressures for an enclosed building using a mean roof height of 35 ft (10 668 mm), interior wall area 4, an effective wind area of 10 ft^2 (0.9 m^2), and topographic factor, K_{zt}, and importance factor, I, equal to 1.0.

b. Table is based on concrete with a minimum specified compressive strength of 2,500 psi (17.2 MPa).

c. See Section R611.6.5 for location of reinforcement in wall.

d. Deflection criterion is $L/240$, where L is the unsupported height of the wall in inches.

e. Interpolation is not permitted.

f. Where No. 4 reinforcing bars at a spacing of 48 inches are specified in the table, use of bars with a minimum yield strength of 40,000 psi or 60,000 psi is permitted.

g. Other than for No. 4 bars spaced at 48 inches on center, table values are based on reinforcing bars with a minimum yield strength of 60,000 psi. Maximum spacings shown are the values calculated for the specified bar size. Where the bar used is Grade 60 (420 MPa) and the size specified in the table, the actual spacing in the wall shall not exceed a whole-number multiple of 12 inches (i.e., 12, 24, 36 and 48) that is less than or equal to the tabulated spacing. Vertical reinforcement with a yield strength of less than 60,000 psi and/or bars of a different size than specified in the table are permitted in accordance with Section R611.5.4.7 and Table R611.5.4(2).

h. See Table R611.3 for minimum core dimensions and maximum spacing of horizontal and vertical cores.

i. Top means gravity load from roof and/or floor construction bears on top of wall. Side means gravity load from floor construction is transferred to wall from a wood ledger or cold-formed steel track bolted to side of wall. Where floor framing members span parallel to the wall, the top bearing condition is permitted to be used.

TABLE R611.6(3)
MINIMUM VERTICAL REINFORCEMENT FOR 6-INCH SCREEN-GRID ABOVE-GRADE WALLS[a, b, c, d, e]

MAXIMUM WIND SPEED (mph)			MAXIMUM UNSUPPORTED WALL HEIGHT PER STORY (feet)	MINIMUM VERTICAL REINFORCEMENT—BAR SIZE AND SPACING (inches)[f, g]	
Exposure Category				Nominal[h] wall thickness (inches)	
				6	
B	C	D		Top[i]	Side[i]
85	—	—	8	4@48	4@34, 5@48
			9	4@48	4@29, 5@45
			10	4@48	4@25, 5@39
90	—	—	8	4@48	4@31, 5@48
			9	4@48	4@27, 5@41
			10	4@30, 5@47	4@23, 5@35
100	85	—	8	4@48	4@27, 5@42
			9	4@30, 5@47	4@23, 5@35
			10	4@24, 5@38	4@22, 5@34
110	90	85	8	4@48	4@24, 5@37
			9	4@25, 5@38	4@22, 5@34
			10	4@22, 5@34	4@22, 5@34
120	100	90	8	4@26, 5@41	4@22, 5@34
			9	4@22, 5@34	4@22, 5@34
			10	4@22, 6@34	4@19, 5@26
130	110	100	8	4@22, 5@35	4@22, 5@34
			9	4@22, 5@34	4@20, 5@30
			10	4@19, 5@29	4@16, 5@25

For SI: 1 inch = 25.4 mm; 1 foot = 304.8 mm; 1 mph = 0.447 m/s, pound per square inch = 6.895 kPa.

a. Table is based on ASCE 7 components and cladding wind pressures for an enclosed building using a mean roof height of 35 ft, interior wall area 4, an effective wind area of 10 ft², and topographic factor, K_{zt}, and importance factor, I, equal to 1.0.

b. Table is based on concrete with a minimum specified compressive strength of 2,500 psi.

c. See Section R611.6.5 for location of reinforcement in wall.

d. Deflection criterion is $L/240$, where L is the unsupported height of the wall in inches.

e. Interpolation is not permitted.

f. Where No. 4 reinforcing bars at a spacing of 48 inches are specified in the table, use of bars with a minimum yield strength of 40,000 psi or 60,000 psi is permitted.

g. Other than for No. 4 bars spaced at 48 inches on center, table values are based on reinforcing bars with a minimum yield strength of 60,000 psi (420 MPa). Maximum spacings shown are the values calculated for the specified bar size. Where the bar used is Grade 60 and the size specified in the table, the actual spacing in the wall shall not exceed a whole-number multiple of 12 inches (i.e., 12, 24, 36 and 48) that is less than or equal to the tabulated spacing. Vertical reinforcement with a yield strength of less than 60,000 psi and/or bars of a different size than specified in the table are permitted in accordance with Section R611.5.4.7 and Table R611.5.4(2).

h. See Table R611.3 for minimum core dimensions and maximum spacing of horizontal and vertical cores.

i. Top means gravity load from roof and/or floor construction bears on top of wall. Side means gravity load from floor construction is transferred to wall from a wood ledger or cold-formed steel track bolted to side of wall. Where floor framing members span parallel to the wall, use of the top bearing condition is permitted.

TABLE R611.6(4)
MINIMUM VERTICAL REINFORCEMENT FOR FLAT, WAFFLE- AND SCREEN-GRID ABOVE-GRADE WALLS DESIGNED CONTINUOUS WITH FOUNDATION STEM WALLS[a, b, c, d, e, k, l]

MAXIMUM WIND SPEED (mph) Exposure Category B	C	D	HEIGHT OF STEM WALL[h, i] (feet)	MAXIMUM DESIGN LATERAL SOIL LOAD (psf/ft)	MAXIMUM UNSUPPORTED HEIGHT OF ABOVE-GRADE WALL (feet)	MINIMUM VERTICAL REINFORCEMENT—BAR SIZE AND SPACING (inches)[f, g] Flat 4	6	8	10	Waffle 6	8	Screen 6
85	—	—	3	30	8	4@33	4@39	4@48	4@48	4@24	4@28	4@22
				30	10	4@26	5@48	4@41	4@48	4@19	4@22	4@18
				60	10	4@21	5@40	5@48	4@44	4@16	4@19	4@15
			6	30	10	DR	5@22	6@35	6@43	DR	4@11	DR
				60	10	DR	DR	6@26	6@28	DR	DR	DR
90	—	—	3	30	8	4@30	4@36	4@48	4@48	4@22	4@26	4@21
				30	10	4@24	5@44	4@38	4@48	4@17	4@21	4@17
				60	10	4@20	5@37	4@48	4@41	4@15	4@18	4@14
			6	30	10	DR	5@21	6@35	6@41	DR	4@10	DR
				60	10	DR	DR	6@26	6@28	DR	DR	DR
100	85	—	3	30	8	4@26	5@48	4@42	4@48	4@19	4@23	4@18
				30	10	4@20	5@37	4@33	4@41	4@15	4@18	4@14
				60	10	4@17	5@34	5@44	4@36	4@13	4@17	4@12
			6	30	10	DR	5@20	6@35	6@38	DR	4@9	DR
				60	10	DR	DR	6@24	6@28	DR	DR	DR
110	90	85	3	30	8	4@22	5@42	4@37	4@46	4@16	4@20	4@16
				30	10	4@17	5@34	5@44	4@35	4@12	4@17	4@12
				60	10	4@15	5@34	5@39	5@48	4@11	4@17	4@11
			6	30	10	DR	5@18	6@35	6@35	DR	4@9	DR
				60	10	DR	DR	6@23	6@28	DR	DR	DR
120	100	90	3	30	8	4@19	5@37	5@48	4@40	4@14	4@17	4@14
				30	10	4@14	5@34	5@38	5@48	4@11	4@17	4@10
				60	10	4@13	5@33	6@48	5@43	4@10	4@16	4@9
			6	30	10	DR	5@16	6@33	6@32	DR	4@8	DR
				60	10	DR	DR	6@22	6@28	DR	DR	DR
130	110	100	3	30	8	4@17	5@34	5@44	4@36	4@12	4@17	4@10
				30	10	DR	5@32	6@47	5@42	4@9	4@15	DR
				60	10	DR	5@29	6@43	5@39	DR	4@14	DR
			6	30	10	DR	5@15	6@30	6@29	DR	4@7	DR
				60	10	DR	DR	6@21	6@27	DR	DR	DR

For SI: 1 inch = 25.4 mm; 1 foot = 304.8 mm; 1 mile per hour = 0.447 m/s; 1 pound per square foot per foot = 0.1571kPa/m.

a. Table is based on ASCE 7 components and cladding wind pressures for an enclosed building using a mean roof height of 35 ft (10 668 mm), interior wall area 4, an effective wind area of 10 ft², and topographic factor, K_{zt}, and importance factor, I, equal to 1.0.

b. Table is based on concrete with a minimum specified compressive strength of 2,500 psi.

c. See Section R611.6.5 for location of reinforcement in wall.

d. Deflection criterion is $L/240$, where L is the height of the wall in inches from the exterior finish ground level to the top of the above-grade wall.

e. Interpolation is not permitted. For intermediate values of basic wind speed, heights of stem wall and above-grade wall, and design lateral soil load, use next higher value.

f. Where No. 4 reinforcing bars at a spacing of 48 inches are specified in the table, use of bars with a minimum yield strength of 40,000 psi or 60,000 psi is permitted.

g. Other than for No. 4 bars spaced at 48 inches on center, table values are based on reinforcing bars with a minimum yield strength of 60,000 psi. Maximum spacings shown are the values calculated for the specified bar size. In waffle and screen-grid walls where the bar used is Grade 60 and the size specified in the table, the actual spacing in the wall shall not exceed a whole-number multiple of 12 inches (i.e., 12, 24, 36 and 48) that is less than or equal to the tabulated spacing. Vertical reinforcement with a yield strength of less than 60,000 psi and/or bars of a different size than specified in the table are permitted in accordance with Section R611.5.4.7 and Table R611.5.4(2).

h. Height of stem wall is the distance from the exterior finish ground level to the top of the slab-on-ground.

i. Where the distance from the exterior finish ground level to the top of the slab-on-ground is equal to or greater than 4 feet, the stem wall shall be laterally supported at the top and bottom before backfilling. Where the wall is designed and constructed to be continuous with the above-grade wall, temporary supports bracing the top of the stem wall shall remain in place until the above-grade wall is laterally supported at the top by floor or roof construction.

j. See Table R611.3 for tolerances on nominal thicknesses, and minimum core dimensions and maximum spacing of horizontal and vertical cores for waffle- and screen-grid walls.

k. Tabulated values are applicable to construction where gravity loads bear on top of wall, and conditions where gravity loads from floor construction are transferred to wall from a wood ledger or cold-formed steel track bolted to side of wall. See Tables R611.6(1), R611.6(2) and R611.6(3).

l. DR indicates design required.

R611.7 Solid walls for resistance to lateral forces.

R611.7.1 Length of solid wall. Each exterior wall line in each *story* shall have a total length of solid wall required by Section R611.7.1.1. A solid wall is a section of flat, waffle-grid or screen-grid wall, extending the full *story height* without openings or penetrations, except those permitted by Section R611.7.2. Solid wall segments that contribute to the total length of solid wall shall comply with Section R611.7.2.

R611.7.1.1 Length of solid wall for wind. All buildings shall have solid walls in each exterior endwall line (the side of a building that is parallel to the span of the roof or floor framing) and sidewall line (the side of a building that is perpendicular to the span of the roof or floor framing) to resist lateral in-plane wind forces. The site-appropriate basic wind speed and exposure category shall be used in Tables R611.7(1A) through (1C) to determine the unreduced total length, UR, of solid wall required in each exterior endwall line and sidewall line. For buildings with a mean roof height of less than 35 feet (10 668 mm), the unreduced values determined from Tables R611.7(1A) though (1C) is permitted by multiplying by the applicable factor, R1, from Table R611.7(2); however, reduced values shall not be less than the minimum values in Tables R611.7(1A) through (1C). Where the floor-to-ceiling height of a *story* is less than 10 feet (3048 mm), the unreduced values determined from Tables R611.7(1A) through (C), including minimum values, is permitted to be reduced by multiplying by the applicable factor, R_2, from Table R611.7(3). To account for different design strengths than assumed in determining the values in Tables R611.7(1A) through (1C), the unreduced lengths determined from Tables R611.7(1A) through (1C), including minimum values, are permitted to be reduced by multiplying by the applicable factor, R_3, from Table R611.7(4). The reductions permitted by Tables R611.7(2), R611.7(3) and R611.7(4) are cumulative.

The total length of solid wall segments, TL, in a wall line that comply with the minimum length requirements of Section R611.7.2.1 [see Figure R611.7(1)] shall be equal to or greater than the product of the unreduced length of solid wall from Tables R611.7(1A) through (1C), UR and the applicable reduction factors, if any, from Tables R611.7(2), R611.7(3) and R611.7(4) as indicated by Equation R611-1.

$$TL \geq R_1 \cdot R_2 \cdot R_3 \cdot UR \qquad \textbf{(Equation R611-1)}$$

Where

TL = total length of solid wall segments in a wall line that comply with Section R611.7.2.1 [see Figure R611.7(1)], and

R_1 = 1.0 or reduction factor for mean roof height from Table R611.7(2),

R_2 = 1.0 or reduction factor for floor-to-ceiling wall height from Table R611.7(3),

R_3 = 1.0 or reduction factor for design strength from Table R611.7(4), and

UR = unreduced length of solid wall from Tables R611.7(1A) through (1C).

The total length of solid wall in a wall line, TL, shall not be less than that provided by two solid wall segments complying with the minimum length requirements of Section R611.7.2.1.

To facilitate determining the required wall thickness, wall type, number and *grade* of vertical bars at the each end of each solid wall segment, and whether shear reinforcement is required, use of Equation R611-2 is permitted.

$$R_3 \leq \frac{TL}{R_1 \cdot R_2 \cdot UR} \qquad \textbf{(Equation R611-2)}$$

After determining the maximum permitted value of the reduction factor for design strength, R_3, in accordance with Equation R611-2, select a wall type from Table R611.7(4) with R_3 less than or equal to the value calculated.

R611.7.2 Solid wall segments. Solid wall segments that contribute to the required length of solid wall shall comply with this section. Reinforcement shall be provided in accordance with Section R611.7.2.2 and Table R611.7(4). Solid wall segments shall extend the full story-height without openings, other than openings for the utilities and other building services passing through the wall. In flat walls and waffle-grid walls, such openings shall have an area of less than 30 square inches (19 355 mm²) with no dimension exceeding $6^1/_4$ inches (159 mm), and shall not be located within 6 inches (152 mm) of the side edges of the solid wall segment. In screen-grid walls, such openings shall be located in the portion of the solid wall segment between horizontal and vertical cores of concrete and opening size and location are not restricted provided no concrete is removed.

R611.7.2.1 Minimum length of solid wall segment and maximum spacing. Only solid wall segments equal to or greater than 24 inches (610 mm) in length shall be included in the total length of solid wall required by Section R611.7.1. In addition, no more than two solid wall segments equal to or greater than 24 inches (610 mm) in length and less than 48 inches (1219 mm) in length shall be included in the required total length of solid wall. The maximum clear opening width shall be 18 feet (5486 mm). See Figure R611.7(1).

R611.7.2.2 Reinforcement in solid wall segments.

R611.7.2.2.1 Horizontal shear reinforcement. Where reduction factors for design strength, R_3, from Table R611.7(4) based on horizontal and vertical shear reinforcement being provided are used, solid wall segments shall have horizontal reinforcement consisting of minimum No. 4 bars. Horizontal shear reinforcement shall be the same grade of steel required for the vertical reinforcement at the ends of solid wall segments by Section R611.7.2.2.2.

The spacing of horizontal reinforcement shall not exceed the smaller of one-half the length of the solid wall segment, minus 2 inches (51 mm), and 18 inches (457 mm). Horizontal shear reinforcement shall terminate in accordance with Section R611.6.4.

R611.7.2.2.2 Vertical reinforcement. Vertical reinforcement applicable to the reduction factor(s) for design strength, R_3, from Table R611.7(4) that is used, shall be located at each end of each solid wall segment in accordance with the applicable detail in Figure R611.7(2). The No. 4 vertical bar required on each side of an opening by Section R611.8.1.2 is permitted to be used as reinforcement at the ends of solid wall segments where installed in accordance with the applicable detail in Figure R611.7(2). There shall be not less than two No. 4 bars at each end of solid wall segments located as required by the applicable detail in Figure R611.7(2). One of the bars at each end of solid wall segments shall be deemed to meet the requirements for vertical wall reinforcement required by Section R611.6.

The vertical wall reinforcement at each end of each solid wall segment shall be developed below the bottom of the adjacent wall opening [see Figure R611.7(3)] by one of the following methods:

1. Where the wall height below the bottom of the adjacent opening is equal to or greater than 22 inches (559 mm) for No. 4 or 28 inches (711 mm) for No. 5 vertical wall reinforcement, reinforcement around openings in accordance with Section R611.8.1 shall be sufficient, or

2. Where the wall height below the bottom of the adjacent opening is less than required by Item 1 above, the vertical wall reinforcement adjacent to the opening shall extend into the footing far enough to develop the bar in tension in accordance with Section R611.5.4.4 and Figure R611.5.4(2), or shall be lap-spliced with a dowel that is embedded in the footing far enough to develop the dowel-bar in tension.

R611.7.2.2.3 Vertical shear reinforcement. Where reduction factors for design strength, R_3, from Table R611.7(4) based on horizontal and vertical shear reinforcement being provided are used, solid wall segments shall have vertical reinforcement consisting of minimum No. 4 bars. Vertical shear reinforcement shall be the same grade of steel required by Section R611.7.2.2.2 for the vertical reinforcement at the ends of solid wall segments. The spacing of vertical reinforcement throughout the length of the segment shall not exceed the smaller of one third the length of the segment, and 18 inches (457 mm). Vertical shear reinforcement shall be continuous between stories in accordance with Section R611.6.3, and shall terminate in accordance with Section R611.6.4. Vertical shear reinforcement required by this section is permitted to be used for vertical reinforcement required by Table R611.6(1), R611.6(2), R611.6(3) or R611.6(4), whichever is applicable.

R611.7.2.3 Solid wall segments at corners. At all interior and exterior corners of exterior walls, a solid wall segment shall extend the full height of each wall *story*. The segment shall have the length required to develop the horizontal reinforcement above and below the adjacent opening in tension in accordance with Section R611.5.4.4. For an exterior corner, the limiting dimension is measured on the outside of the wall, and for an interior corner the limiting dimension is measured on the inside of the wall. See Section R611.8.1. The length of a segment contributing to the required length of solid wall shall comply with Section R611.7.2.1.

The end of a solid wall segment complying with the minimum length requirements of Section R611.7.2.1 shall be located no more than 6 feet (1829 mm) from each corner.

TABLE R611.7(1A)
UNREDUCED LENGTH, *UR*, OF SOLID WALL REQUIRED IN EACH EXTERIOR ENDWALL FOR WIND PERPENDICULAR TO RIDGE
ONE STORY OR TOP STORY OF TWO-STORY[a,c,d,e,f,g]

SIDEWALL LENGTH (feet)	ENDWALL LENGTH (feet)	ROOF SLOPE	UNREDUCED LENGTH, *UR*, OF SOLID WALL REQUIRED IN ENDWALLS FOR WIND PERPENDICULAR TO RIDGE (feet)						
			Basic Wind Speed (mph) Exposure						
			85B	90B	100B	110B	120B	130B	
					85C	90C	100C	110C	
						85D	90D	100D	Minimum[b]
15	15	< 1:12	0.90	1.01	1.25	1.51	1.80	2.11	0.98
		5:12	1.25	1.40	1.73	2.09	2.49	2.92	1.43
		7:12	1.75	1.96	2.43	2.93	3.49	4.10	1.64
		12:12	2.80	3.13	3.87	4.68	5.57	6.54	2.21
	30	< 1:12	0.90	1.01	1.25	1.51	1.80	2.11	1.09
		5:12	1.25	1.40	1.73	2.09	2.49	2.92	2.01
		7:12	2.43	2.73	3.37	4.08	4.85	5.69	2.42
		12:12	4.52	5.07	6.27	7.57	9.01	10.58	3.57
	45	< 1:12	0.90	1.01	1.25	1.51	1.80	2.11	1.21
		5:12	1.25	1.40	1.73	2.09	2.49	2.92	2.59
		7:12	3.12	3.49	4.32	5.22	6.21	7.29	3.21
		12:12	6.25	7.00	8.66	10.47	12.45	14.61	4.93
	60	< 1:12	0.90	1.01	1.25	1.51	1.80	2.11	1.33
		5:12	1.25	1.40	1.73	2.09	2.49	2.92	3.16
		7:12	3.80	4.26	5.26	6.36	7.57	8.89	3.99
		12:12	7.97	8.94	11.05	13.36	15.89	18.65	6.29
30	15	< 1:12	1.61	1.80	2.23	2.70	3.21	3.77	1.93
		5:12	2.24	2.51	3.10	3.74	4.45	5.23	2.75
		7:12	3.15	3.53	4.37	5.28	6.28	7.37	3.12
		12:12	4.90	5.49	6.79	8.21	9.77	11.46	4.14
	30	< 1:12	1.61	1.80	2.23	2.70	3.21	3.77	2.14
		5:12	2.24	2.51	3.10	3.74	4.45	5.23	3.78
		7:12	4.30	4.82	5.96	7.20	8.57	10.05	4.52
		12:12	7.79	8.74	10.80	13.06	15.53	18.23	6.57
	45	< 1:12	1.61	1.80	2.23	2.70	3.21	3.77	2.35
		5:12	2.24	2.51	3.10	3.74	4.45	5.23	4.81
		7:12	5.44	6.10	7.54	9.12	10.85	12.73	5.92
		12:12	10.69	11.98	14.81	17.90	21.30	25.00	9.00
	60	< 1:12	1.61	1.80	2.23	2.70	3.21	3.77	2.56
		5:12	2.24	2.51	3.10	3.74	4.45	5.23	5.84
		7:12	6.59	7.39	9.13	11.04	13.14	15.41	7.32
		12:12	13.58	15.22	18.82	22.75	27.07	31.77	11.43

(continued)

TABLE R611.7(1A)—continued
UNREDUCED LENGTH, *UR*, OF SOLID WALL REQUIRED IN EACH EXTERIOR ENDWALL FOR WIND PERPENDICULAR TO RIDGE
ONE STORY OR TOP STORY OF TWO-STORY[a,c,d,e,f,g]

SIDEWALL LENGTH (feet)	ENDWALL LENGTH (feet)	ROOF SLOPE	UNREDUCED LENGTH, *UR*, OF SOLID WALL REQUIRED IN ENDWALLS FOR WIND PERPENDICULAR TO RIDGE (feet)						
			Basic Wind Speed (mph) Exposure						
			85B	90B	100B 85C	110B 90C 85D	120B 100C 90D	130B 110C 100D	Minimum[b]
60	15	< 1:12	2.99	3.35	4.14	5.00	5.95	6.98	3.83
		5:12	4.15	4.65	5.75	6.95	8.27	9.70	5.37
		7:12	5.91	6.63	8.19	9.90	11.78	13.83	6.07
		12:12	9.05	10.14	12.54	15.16	18.03	21.16	8.00
	30	< 1:12	2.99	3.35	4.14	5.00	5.95	6.98	4.23
		5:12	4.15	4.65	5.75	6.95	8.27	9.70	7.31
		7:12	7.97	8.94	11.05	13.36	15.89	18.65	8.71
		12:12	14.25	15.97	19.74	23.86	28.40	33.32	12.57
	45	< 1:12	3.11	3.48	4.30	5.20	6.19	7.26	4.63
		5:12	4.31	4.84	5.98	7.23	8.60	10.09	9.25
		7:12	10.24	11.47	14.19	17.15	20.40	23.84	11.35
		12:12	19.84	22.24	27.49	33.23	39.54	46.40	17.14
	60	< 1:12	3.22	3.61	4.46	5.39	6.42	7.53	5.03
		5:12	4.47	5.01	6.19	7.49	8.91	10.46	11.19
		7:12	12.57	14.09	17.42	21.05	25.05	29.39	13.99
		12:12	25.61	28.70	35.49	42.90	51.04	59.90	21.71

For SI: 1 inch = 25.4 mm; 1 foot = 304.8 mm; 1 mile per hour = 0.447 m/s, 1 pound-force per linear foot = 0.146kN/m, 1 pound per square foot = 47.88 Pa.

a. Tabulated lengths were derived by calculating design wind pressures in accordance with Figure 6-10 of ASCE 7 for a building with a mean roof height of 35 feet (10 668 mm). For wind perpendicular to the ridge, the effects of a 2-foot overhang on each endwall are included. The design pressures were used to calculate forces to be resisted by solid wall segments in each endwall [Table R611.7(1A) or R611.7(1B)] or sidewall (Table R611.7(1C)], as appropriate. The forces to be resisted by each wall line were then divided by the default design strength of 840 pounds per linear foot (12.26 kN/m) of length to determine the required solid wall length. The actual mean roof height of the building shall not exceed the least horizontal dimension of the building.

b. Tabulated lengths in the "minimum" column are based on the requirement of Section 6.1.4.1 of ASCE 7 that the main wind-force resisting system be designed for a minimum service level force of 10 psf multiplied by the area of the building projected onto a vertical plane normal to the assumed wind direction. Tabulated lengths in shaded cells are less than the "minimum" value. Where the minimum controls, it is permitted to be reduced in accordance with Notes c, d and e. See Section R611.7.1.1.

c. For buildings with a mean roof height of less than 35 feet, tabulated lengths are permitted to be reduced by multiplying by the appropriate factor, R_1, from Table R611.7(2). The reduced length shall not be less than the "minimum" value shown in the table.

d. Tabulated lengths for "one story or top story of two-story" are based on a floor-to-ceiling height of 10 feet. Tabulated lengths for "first story of two-story" are based on floor-to-ceiling heights of 10 feet each for the first and second story. For floor-to-ceiling heights less than assumed, use the lengths in Table R611.7(1A), (1B) or (1C), or multiply the value in the table by the reduction factor, R_2, from Table R611.7(3).

e. Tabulated lengths are based on the default design shear strength of 840 pounds per linear foot of solid wall segment. The tabulated lengths are permitted to be reduced by multiplying by the applicable reduction factor for design strength, R_3, from Table R611.7(4).

f. The reduction factors, R_1, R_2, and R_3, in Tables R611.7(2), R611.7(3), and R611.7(4), respectively, are permitted to be compounded, subject to the limitations of Note b. However, the minimum number and minimum length of solid walls segments in each wall line shall comply with Sections R611.7.1 and R611.7.2.1, respectively.

g. For intermediate values of sidewall length, endwall length, roof slope and basic wind speed, use the next higher value, or determine by interpolation.

2009 INTERNATIONAL RESIDENTIAL CODE®

TABLE R611.7(1B)
UNREDUCED LENGTH, *UR*, OF SOLID WALL REQUIRED IN EACH EXTERIOR ENDWALL FOR WIND PERPENDICULAR TO RIDGE
FIRST STORY OF TWO-STORY[a,c,d,e,f,g]

SIDEWALL LENGTH (feet)	ENDWALL LENGTH (feet)	ROOF SLOPE	UNREDUCED LENGTH, *UR*, OF SOLID WALL REQUIRED IN ENDWALLS FOR WIND PERPENDICULAR TO RIDGE (feet)						
			Basic Wind Speed (mph) Exposure						
			85B	90B	100B / 85C	110B / 90C / 85D	120B / 100C / 90D	130B / 110C / 100D	
			Velocity pressure (psf)						
			11.51	12.90	15.95	19.28	22.94	26.92	Minimum[b]
15	15	< 1:12	2.60	2.92	3.61	4.36	5.19	6.09	2.59
		5:12	3.61	4.05	5.00	6.05	7.20	8.45	3.05
		7:12	3.77	4.23	5.23	6.32	7.52	8.82	3.26
		12:12	4.81	5.40	6.67	8.06	9.60	11.26	3.83
	30	< 1:12	2.60	2.92	3.61	4.36	5.19	6.09	2.71
		5:12	3.61	4.05	5.00	6.05	7.20	8.45	3.63
		7:12	4.45	4.99	6.17	7.46	8.88	10.42	4.04
		12:12	6.54	7.33	9.06	10.96	13.04	15.30	5.19
	45	< 1:12	2.60	2.92	3.61	4.36	5.19	6.09	2.83
		5:12	3.61	4.05	5.00	6.05	7.20	8.45	4.20
		7:12	5.14	5.76	7.12	8.60	10.24	12.01	4.83
		12:12	8.27	9.27	11.46	13.85	16.48	19.34	6.55
	60	< 1:12	2.60	2.92	3.61	4.36	5.19	6.09	2.95
		5:12	3.61	4.05	5.00	6.05	7.20	8.45	4.78
		7:12	5.82	6.52	8.06	9.75	11.60	13.61	5.61
		12:12	9.99	11.20	13.85	16.74	19.92	23.37	7.90
30	15	< 1:12	4.65	5.21	6.45	7.79	9.27	10.88	5.16
		5:12	6.46	7.24	8.95	10.82	12.87	15.10	5.98
		7:12	6.94	7.78	9.62	11.62	13.83	16.23	6.35
		12:12	8.69	9.74	12.04	14.55	17.32	20.32	7.38
	30	< 1:12	4.65	5.21	6.45	7.79	9.27	10.88	5.38
		5:12	6.46	7.24	8.95	10.82	12.87	15.10	7.01
		7:12	8.09	9.06	11.21	13.54	16.12	18.91	7.76
		12:12	11.58	12.98	16.05	19.40	23.08	27.09	9.81
	45	< 1:12	4.65	5.21	6.45	7.79	9.27	10.88	5.59
		5:12	6.46	7.24	8.95	10.82	12.87	15.10	8.04
		7:12	9.23	10.35	12.79	15.46	18.40	21.59	9.16
		12:12	14.48	16.22	20.06	24.25	28.85	33.86	12.24
	60	< 1:12	4.65	5.21	6.45	7.79	9.27	10.88	5.80
		5:12	6.46	7.24	8.95	10.82	12.87	15.10	9.08
		7:12	10.38	11.63	14.38	17.38	20.69	24.27	10.56
		12:12	17.37	19.47	24.07	29.10	34.62	40.63	14.67

(continued)

TABLE R611.7(1B)—continued
UNREDUCED LENGTH, *UR*, OF SOLID WALL REQUIRED IN EACH EXTERIOR ENDWALL FOR WIND PERPENDICULAR TO RIDGE
FIRST STORY OF TWO-STORY[a,c,d,e,f,g]

SIDEWALL LENGTH (feet)	ENDWALL LENGTH (feet)	ROOF SLOPE	UNREDUCED LENGTH, *UR*, OF SOLID WALL REQUIRED IN ENDWALLS FOR WIND PERPENDICULAR TO RIDGE (feet)						
			Basic Wind Speed (mph) Exposure						
			85B	90B	100B	110B	120B	130B	
					85C	90C	100C	110C	
						85D	90D	100D	
			Velocity Pressure (psf)						
			11.51	12.90	15.95	19.28	22.94	26.92	Minimum[b]
60	15	< 1:12	8.62	9.67	11.95	14.45	17.19	20.17	10.30
		5:12	11.98	13.43	16.61	20.07	23.88	28.03	11.85
		7:12	13.18	14.78	18.27	22.08	26.28	30.83	12.54
		12:12	16.32	18.29	22.62	27.34	32.53	38.17	14.48
	30	< 1:12	8.62	9.67	11.95	14.45	17.19	20.17	10.70
		5:12	11.98	13.43	16.61	20.07	23.88	28.03	13.79
		7:12	15.25	17.09	21.13	25.54	30.38	35.66	15.18
		12:12	21.52	24.12	29.82	36.05	42.89	50.33	19.05
	45	< 1:12	8.97	10.06	12.43	15.03	17.88	20.99	11.10
		5:12	12.46	13.97	17.27	20.88	24.84	29.15	15.73
		7:12	17.67	19.80	24.48	29.59	35.21	41.32	17.82
		12:12	27.27	30.56	37.79	45.68	54.35	63.78	23.62
	60	< 1:12	9.30	10.43	12.89	15.58	18.54	21.76	11.50
		5:12	12.91	14.47	17.90	21.63	25.74	30.20	17.67
		7:12	20.14	22.58	27.91	33.74	40.15	47.11	20.46
		12:12	33.19	37.19	45.99	55.59	66.14	77.62	28.19

For SI: 1 inch = 25.4 mm; 1 foot = 304.8 mm; 1 mile per hour = 0.447 m/s, 1 pound force per linear foot = 0.146kN/m, 1 pound per square foot = 47.88 Pa.

a. Tabulated lengths were derived by calculating design wind pressures in accordance with Figure 6-10 of ASCE 7 for a building with a mean roof height of 35 feet (10 668 mm). For wind perpendicular to the ridge, the effects of a 2-foot (610 mm) overhang on each endwall are included. The design pressures were used to calculate forces to be resisted by solid wall segments in each endwall [Table R611.7(1A) or Table R611.7(1B)] or sidewall [Table R611.7(1C)], as appropriate. The forces to be resisted by each wall line were then divided by the default design strength of 840 pounds per linear foot (12.26 kN/m) of length to determine the required solid wall length. The actual mean roof height of the building shall not exceed the least horizontal dimension of the building.

b. Tabulated lengths in the "minimum" column are based on the requirement of Section 6.1.4.1 of ASCE 7 that the main wind-force resisting system be designed for a minimum service level force of 10 psf multiplied by the area of the building projected onto a vertical plane normal to the assumed wind direction. Tabulated lengths in shaded cells are less than the "minimum" value. Where the minimum controls, it is permitted to be reduced in accordance with Notes c, d and e. See Section R611.7.1.1.

c. For buildings with a mean roof height of less than 35 feet tabulated lengths are permitted to be reduced by multiplying by the appropriate factor, R_1, from Table R611.7(2). The reduced length shall not be less than the "minimum" value shown in the table.

d. Tabulated lengths for "one story or top story of two-story" are based on a floor-to-ceiling height of 10 feet. Tabulated lengths for "first story of two-story" are based on floor-to-ceiling heights of 10 feet each for the first and second story. For floor-to-ceiling heights less than assumed, use the lengths in Table R611.7(1A), (1B) or (1C), or multiply the value in the table by the reduction factor, R_2, from Table R611.7(3).

e. Tabulated lengths are based on the default design shear strength of 840 pounds per linear foot of solid wall segment. The tabulated lengths are permitted to be reduced by multiplying by the applicable reduction factor for design strength, R_3, from Table R611.7(4).

f. The reduction factors, R_1, R_2, and R_3, in Tables R611.7(2), R611.7(3), and R611.7(4), respectively, are permitted to be compounded, subject to the limitations of Note b. However, the minimum number and minimum length of solid walls segments in each wall line shall comply with Sections R611.7.1 and R611.7.2.1, respectively.

g. For intermediate values of sidewall length, endwall length, roof slope and basic wind speed, use the next higher value, or determine by interpolation.

TABLE R611.7(1C)
UNREDUCED LENGTH, *UR*, OF SOLID WALL REQUIRED IN EACH EXTERIOR SIDEWALL FOR WIND PARALLEL TO RIDGE[a,c,d,e,f,g]

SIDEWALL LENGTH (feet)	ENDWALL LENGTH (feet)	ROOF SLOPE	UNREDUCED LENGTH, *UR*, OF SOLID WALL REQUIRED IN ENDWALLS FOR WIND PERPENDICULAR TO RIDGE (feet)						
			Basic Wind Speed (mph) Exposure						
			85B	90B	100B 85C	110B 90C 85D	120B 100C 90D	130B 110C 100D	Minimum[b]
			One story or top story of two-story						
< 30	15	< 1:12	0.95	1.06	1.31	1.59	1.89	2.22	0.90
		5:12	1.13	1.26	1.56	1.88	2.24	2.63	1.08
		7:12	1.21	1.35	1.67	2.02	2.40	2.82	1.17
		12:12	1.43	1.60	1.98	2.39	2.85	3.34	1.39
	30	< 1:12	1.77	1.98	2.45	2.96	3.53	4.14	1.90
		5:12	2.38	2.67	3.30	3.99	4.75	5.57	2.62
		7:12	2.66	2.98	3.69	4.46	5.31	6.23	2.95
		12:12	3.43	3.85	4.76	5.75	6.84	8.03	3.86
	45	< 1:12	2.65	2.97	3.67	4.43	5.27	6.19	2.99
		5:12	3.98	4.46	5.51	6.66	7.93	9.31	4.62
		7:12	4.58	5.14	6.35	7.68	9.14	10.72	5.36
		12:12	6.25	7.01	8.67	10.48	12.47	14.63	7.39
	60	< 1:12	3.59	4.03	4.98	6.02	7.16	8.40	4.18
		5:12	5.93	6.65	8.22	9.93	11.82	13.87	7.07
		7:12	6.99	7.83	9.69	11.71	13.93	16.35	8.38
		12:12	9.92	11.12	13.75	16.62	19.77	23.21	12.00
60	45	< 1:12	2.77	3.11	3.84	4.65	5.53	6.49	2.99
		5:12	4.15	4.66	5.76	6.96	8.28	9.72	4.62
		7:12	4.78	5.36	6.63	8.01	9.53	11.18	5.36
		12:12	6.51	7.30	9.03	10.91	12.98	15.23	7.39
	60	< 1:12	3.86	4.32	5.35	6.46	7.69	9.02	4.18
		5:12	6.31	7.08	8.75	10.57	12.58	14.76	7.07
		7:12	7.43	8.32	10.29	12.44	14.80	17.37	8.38
		12:12	10.51	11.78	14.56	17.60	20.94	24.57	12.00
			First story of two-story						
< 30	15	< 1:12	2.65	2.97	3.67	4.44	5.28	6.20	2.52
		5:12	2.83	3.17	3.92	4.74	5.64	6.62	2.70
		7:12	2.91	3.26	4.03	4.87	5.80	6.80	2.79
		12:12	3.13	3.51	4.34	5.25	6.24	7.32	3.01
	30	< 1:12	4.81	5.39	6.67	8.06	9.59	11.25	5.14
		5:12	5.42	6.08	7.52	9.09	10.81	12.69	5.86
		7:12	5.70	6.39	7.90	9.55	11.37	13.34	6.19
		12:12	6.47	7.25	8.97	10.84	12.90	15.14	7.10
	45	< 1:12	6.99	7.83	9.69	11.71	13.93	16.35	7.85
		5:12	8.32	9.33	11.53	13.94	16.59	19.47	9.48
		7:12	8.93	10.01	12.37	14.95	17.79	20.88	10.21
		12:12	10.60	11.88	14.69	17.75	21.13	24.79	12.25
	60	< 1:12	9.23	10.35	12.79	15.46	18.40	21.59	10.65
		5:12	11.57	12.97	16.03	19.38	23.06	27.06	13.54
		7:12	12.63	14.15	17.50	21.15	25.17	29.54	14.85
		12:12	15.56	17.44	21.56	26.06	31.01	36.39	18.48

(continued)

TABLE R611.7(1C)—continued
UNREDUCED LENGTH, *UR*, OF SOLID WALL REQUIRED IN EACH EXTERIOR ENDWALL FOR WIND PERPENDICULAR TO RIDGE
FIRST STORY OF TWO-STORY[a,c,d,e,f,g]

SIDEWALL LENGTH (feet)	ENDWALL LENGTH (feet)	ROOF SLOPE	UNREDUCED LENGTH, *UR*, OF SOLID WALL REQUIRED IN ENDWALLS FOR WIND PERPENDICULAR TO RIDGE (feet)						
			Basic Wind Speed (mph) Exposure						
			85B	90B	100B 85C	110B 90C 85D	120B 100C 90D	130B 110C 100D	Minimum[b]
60	45	< 1:12	7.34	8.22	10.17	12.29	14.62	17.16	7.85
		5:12	8.72	9.77	12.08	14.60	17.37	20.39	9.48
		7:12	9.34	10.47	12.95	15.65	18.62	21.85	10.21
		12:12	11.08	12.41	15.35	18.55	22.07	25.90	12.25
	60	< 1:12	9.94	11.14	13.77	16.65	19.81	23.25	10.65
		5:12	12.40	13.89	17.18	20.76	24.70	28.99	13.54
		7:12	13.51	15.14	18.72	22.63	26.92	31.60	14.85
		12:12	16.59	18.59	22.99	27.79	33.06	38.80	18.48

For SI: 1 inch = 25.4 mm, 1 foot = 304.8 mm, 1 mile per hour = 0.447 m/s, 1 pound force per linear foot = 0.146kN/m, 1 pound per square foot = 47.88 Pa.

a. Tabulated lengths were derived by calculating design wind pressures in accordance with Figure 6-10 of ASCE 7 for a building with a mean roof height of 35 feet (10 668 mm). For wind perpendicular to the ridge, the effects of a 2-foot (610 mm) overhang on each endwall are included. The design pressures were used to calculate forces to be resisted by solid wall segments in each endwall [Table R611.7(1A) or R611.7(1B)] or sidewall [(Table R611.7(1C)], as appropriate. The forces to be resisted by each wall line were then divided by the default design strength of 840 pounds per linear foot (12.26 kN/m) of length to determine the required solid wall length. The actual mean roof height of the building shall not exceed the least horizontal dimension of the building.

b. Tabulated lengths in the "minimum" column are based on the requirement of Section 6.1.4.1 of ASCE 7 that the main wind-force resisting system be designed for a minimum service level force of 10 psf multiplied by the area of the building projected onto a vertical plane normal to the assumed wind direction. Tabulated lengths in shaded cells are less than the "minimum" value. Where the minimum controls, it is permitted to be reduced in accordance with Notes c, d and e. See Section R611.7.1.1.

c. For buildings with a mean roof height of less than 35 feet, tabulated lengths are permitted to be reduced by multiplying by the appropriate factor, R_1, from Table R611.7(2). The reduced length shall not be less than the "minimum" value shown in the table.

d. Tabulated lengths for "one story or top story of two-story" are based on a floor-to-ceiling height of 10 feet. Tabulated lengths for "first story of two-story" are based on floor-to-ceiling heights of 10 feet each for the first and second story. For floor-to-ceiling heights less than assumed, use the lengths in Table R611.7(1A), (1B) or (1C), or multiply the value in the table by the reduction factor, R_2, from Table R611.7(3).

e. Tabulated lengths are based on the default design shear strength of 840 pounds per linear foot of solid wall segment. The tabulated lengths are permitted to be reduced by multiplying by the applicable reduction factor for design strength, R_3, from Table R611.7(4).

f. The reduction factors, R_1, R_2, and R_3, in Tables R611.7(2), R611.7(3), and R611.7(4), respectively, are permitted to be compounded, subject to the limitations of Note b. However, the minimum number and minimum length of solid walls segments in each wall line shall comply with Sections R611.7.1 and R611.7.2.1, respectively.

g. For intermediate values of sidewall length, endwall length, roof slope and basic wind speed, use the next higher value, or determine by interpolation.

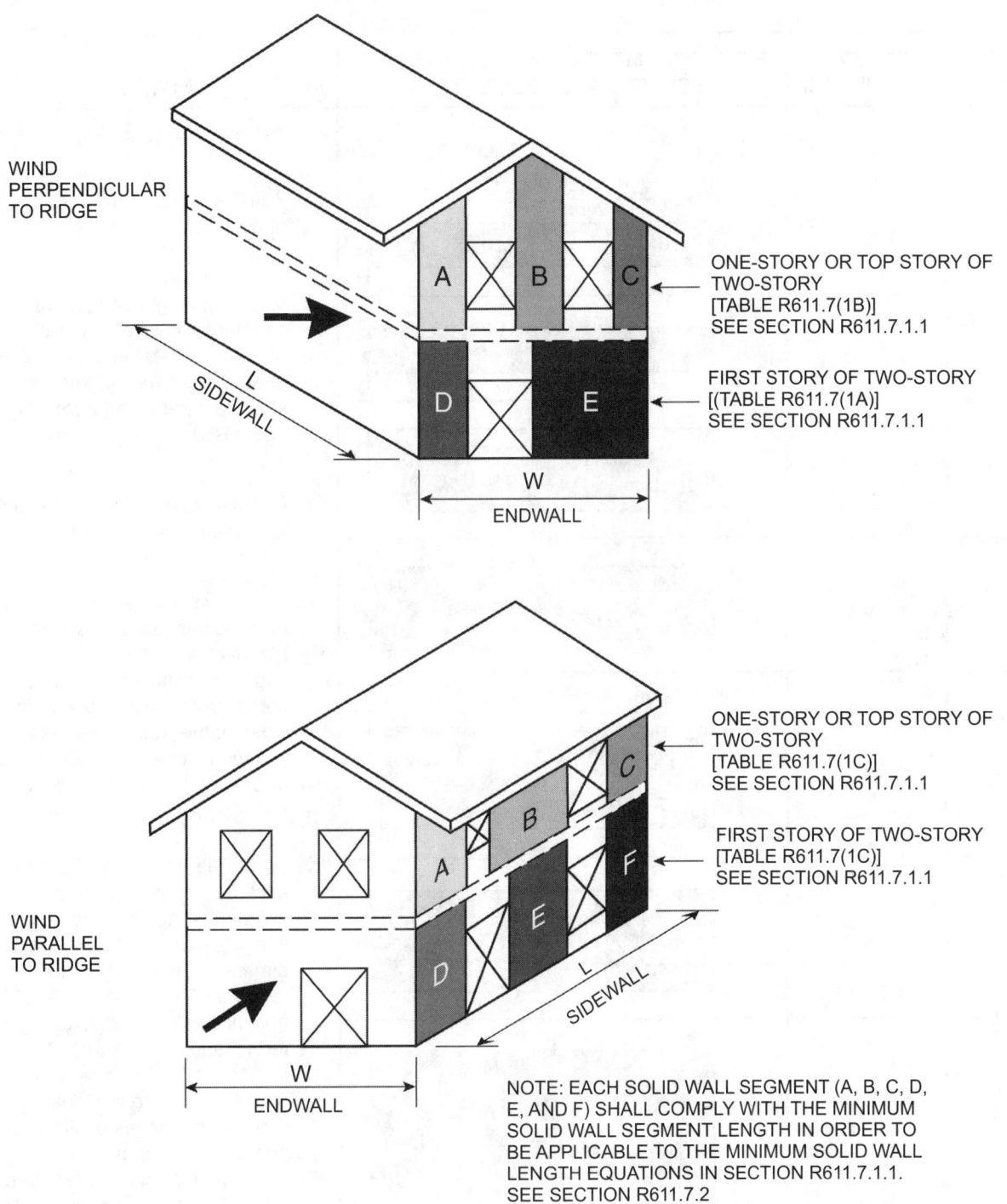

WIND
PERPENDICULAR
TO RIDGE

L
SIDEWALL

A B C

D E

W
ENDWALL

ONE-STORY OR TOP STORY OF
TWO-STORY
[TABLE R611.7(1B)]
SEE SECTION R611.7.1.1

FIRST STORY OF TWO-STORY
[(TABLE R611.7(1A)]
SEE SECTION R611.7.1.1

WIND
PARALLEL
TO RIDGE

C
B
A
F
D E
L
SIDEWALL

W
ENDWALL

ONE-STORY OR TOP STORY OF
TWO-STORY
[TABLE R611.7(1C)]
SEE SECTION R611.7.1.1

FIRST STORY OF TWO-STORY
[TABLE R611.7(1C)]
SEE SECTION R611.7.1.1

NOTE: EACH SOLID WALL SEGMENT (A, B, C, D,
E, AND F) SHALL COMPLY WITH THE MINIMUM
SOLID WALL SEGMENT LENGTH IN ORDER TO
BE APPLICABLE TO THE MINIMUM SOLID WALL
LENGTH EQUATIONS IN SECTION R611.7.1.1.
SEE SECTION R611.7.2

FIGURE R611.7(1)
MINIMUM SOLID WALL LENGTH

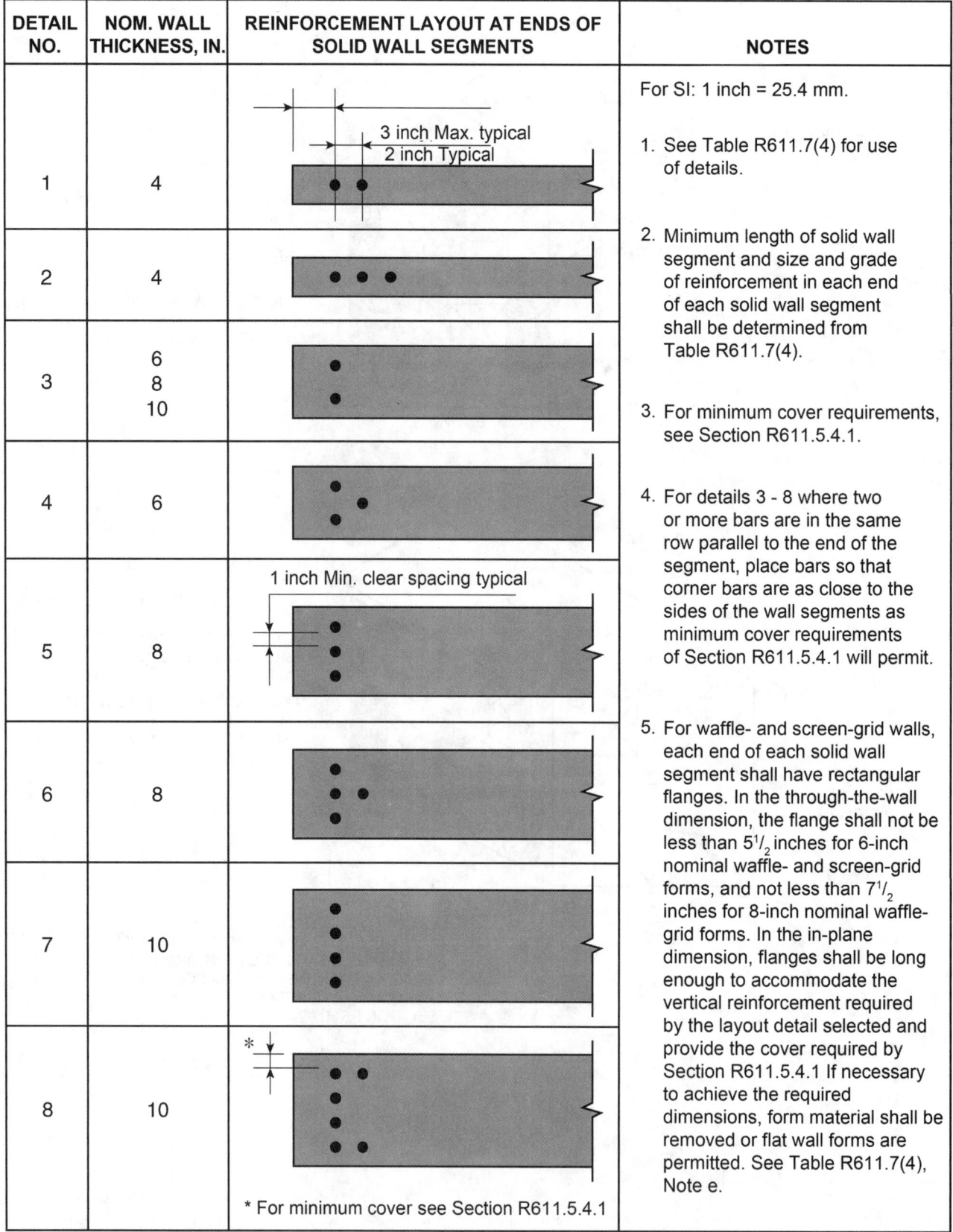

DETAIL NO.	NOM. WALL THICKNESS, IN.	REINFORCEMENT LAYOUT AT ENDS OF SOLID WALL SEGMENTS	NOTES
1	4	3 inch Max. typical / 2 inch Typical	For SI: 1 inch = 25.4 mm. 1. See Table R611.7(4) for use of details.
2	4		2. Minimum length of solid wall segment and size and grade of reinforcement in each end of each solid wall segment shall be determined from Table R611.7(4).
3	6 8 10		3. For minimum cover requirements, see Section R611.5.4.1.
4	6		4. For details 3 - 8 where two or more bars are in the same row parallel to the end of the segment, place bars so that corner bars are as close to the sides of the wall segments as minimum cover requirements of Section R611.5.4.1 will permit.
5	8	1 inch Min. clear spacing typical	5. For waffle- and screen-grid walls, each end of each solid wall segment shall have rectangular flanges. In the through-the-wall dimension, the flange shall not be less than $5\frac{1}{2}$ inches for 6-inch nominal waffle- and screen-grid forms, and not less than $7\frac{1}{2}$ inches for 8-inch nominal waffle-grid forms. In the in-plane dimension, flanges shall be long enough to accommodate the vertical reinforcement required by the layout detail selected and provide the cover required by Section R611.5.4.1 If necessary to achieve the required dimensions, form material shall be removed or flat wall forms are permitted. See Table R611.7(4), Note e.
6	8		
7	10		
8	10	* * For minimum cover see Section R611.5.4.1	

FIGURE R611.7(2)
VERTICAL REINFORCEMENT LAYOUT DETAIL

TABLE R611.7(2)
REDUCTION FACTOR, R_1, FOR BUILDINGS WITH MEAN ROOF HEIGHT LESS THAN 35 FEET[a]

MEAN ROOF HEIGHT[b,c] (feet)	REDUCTION FACTOR R_1, FOR MEAN ROOF HEIGHT		
	Exposure category		
	B	C	D
< 15	0.96	0.84	0.87
20	0.96	0.89	0.91
25	0.96	0.93	0.94
30	0.96	0.97	0.98
35	1.00	1.00	1.00

For SI: 1 foot = 304.8 mm.

a. See Section R611.7.1.1 and note c to Table R611.7(1A) for application of reduction factors in this table. This reduction is not permitted for "minimum" values.

b. For intermediate values of mean roof height, use the factor for the next greater height, or determine by interpolation.

c. Mean roof height is the average of the roof eave height and height of the highest point on the roof surface, except that for roof slopes of less than or equal to $2^1/_8$:12 (10 degrees), the mean roof height is permitted to be taken as the roof eave height.

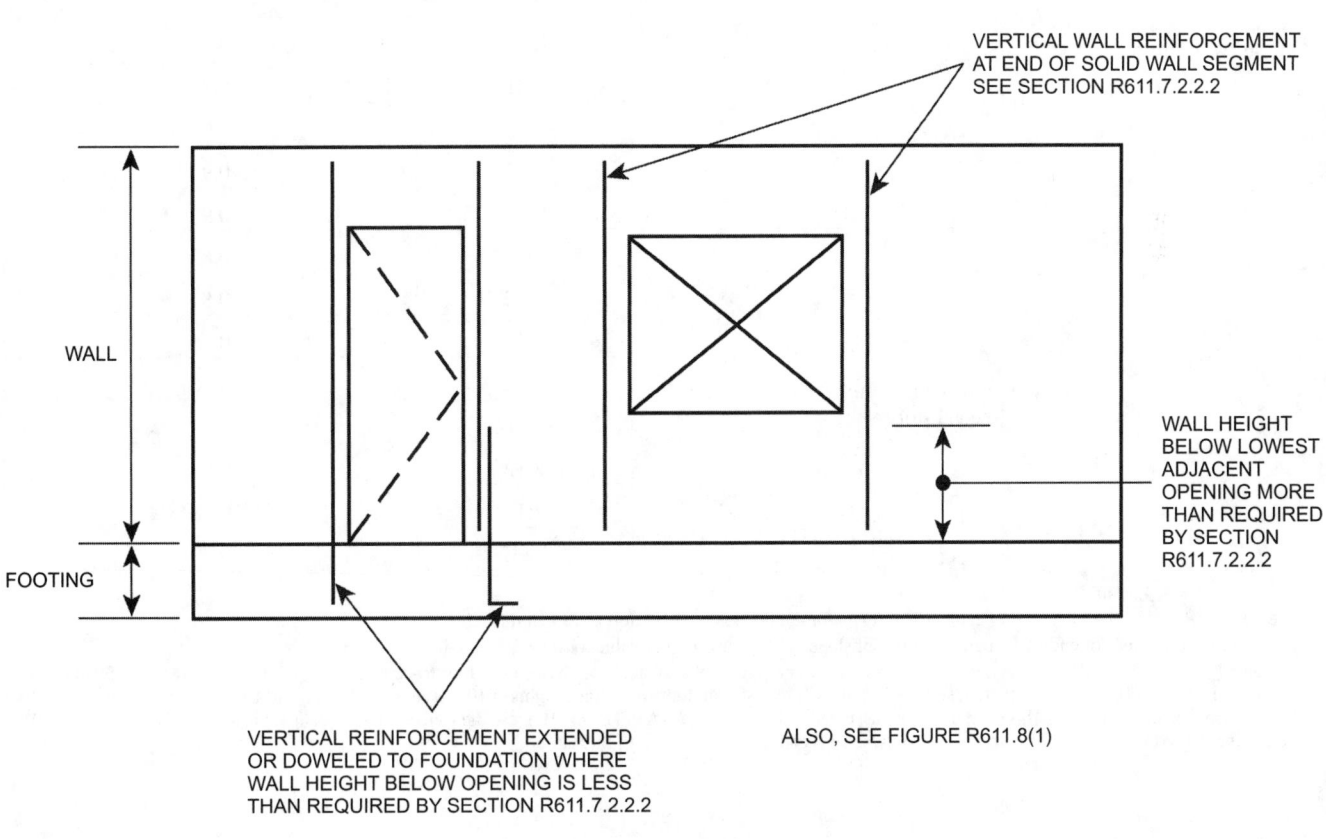

FIGURE R611.7(3)
VERTICAL WALL REINFORCEMENT ADJACENT TO WALL OPENINGS

TABLE R611.7(3)
REDUCTION FACTOR, R_2, FOR FLOOR-TO-CEILING WALL HEIGHTS LESS THAN 10 FEET[a,b]

STORY UNDER CONSIDERATION	FLOOR-TO-CEILING HEIGHT[c] (feet)	ENDWALL LENGTH (feet)	ROOF SLOPE	REDUCTION FACTOR, R_2
Endwalls—for wind perpendicular to ridge				
One story or top story of two-story	8	15	< 5:12	0.83
			7:12	0.90
			12:12	0.94
		60	< 5:12	0.83
			7:12	0.95
			12:12	0.98
First story of two-story	16 combined first and second story	15	< 5:12	0.83
			7:12	0.86
			12:12	0.89
		60	< 5:12	0.83
			7:12	0.91
			12:12	0.95
Sidewalls—for wind parallel to ridge				
One story or top story of two-story	8	15	< 1:12	0.84
			5:12	0.87
			7:12	0.88
			12:12	0.89
		60	< 1:12	0.86
			5:12	0.92
			7:12	0.93
			12:12	0.95
First story of two-story	16 combined first and second story	15	< 1:12	0.83
			5:12	0.84
			7:12	0.85
			12:12	0.86
		60	< 1:12	0.84
			5:12	0.87
			7:12	0.88
			12:12	0.90

For SI: 1 foot = 304.8 mm.

a. See Section R611.7.1.1 and Note d to Table R611.7(1A) for application of reduction factors in this table.

b. For intermediate values of endwall length, and/or roof slope, use the next higher value, or determine by interpolation.

c. Tabulated values in Table R611.7(1A) and (1C) for "one story or top story of two-story" are based on a floor-to-ceiling height of 10 feet (3048 mm). Tabulated values in Table R611.7(1B) and (1C) for "first story of two-story" are based on floor-to-ceiling heights of 10 feet each for the first and second story. For floor to ceiling heights between those shown in this table and those assumed in Table R611.7(1A), (1B) or (1C), use the solid wall lengths in Table R611.7(1A), (1B) or (1C), or determine the reduction factor by interpolating between 1.0 and the factor shown in this table.

TABLE R611.7(4)
REDUCTION FACTOR FOR DESIGN STRENGTH, R_3, FOR FLAT, WAFFLE- AND SCREEN-GRID WALLS[a,c]

NOMINAL THICKNESS OF WALL (inches)	VERTICAL BARS AT EACH END OF SOLID WALL SEGMENT		VERTICAL REINFORCEMENT LAYOUT DETAIL [see Figure R611.7(2)]	REDUCTION FACTOR, R_3, FOR LENGTH OF SOLID WALL			
				Horizontal and vertical shear reinforcement provided			
				No		Yes[d]	
	Number of bars	Bar size		40,000[b]	60,000[b]	40,000[b]	60,000[b]
Flat walls							
4	2	4	1	0.74	0.61	0.74	0.50
	3	4	2	0.61	0.61	0.52	0.27
	2	5	1	0.61	0.61	0.48	0.25
	3	5	2	0.61	0.61	0.26	0.18
6	2	4	3	0.70	0.48	0.70	0.48
	3	4	4	0.49	0.38	0.49	0.33
	2	5	3	0.46	0.38	0.46	0.31
	3	5	4	0.38	0.38	0.32	0.16
8	2	4	3	0.70	0.47	0.70	0.47
	3	4	5	0.47	0.32	0.47	0.32
	2	5	3	0.45	0.31	0.45	0.31
	4	4	6	0.36	0.28	0.36	0.25
	3	5	5	0.31	0.28	0.31	0.16
	4	5	6	0.28	0.28	0.24	0.12
10	2	4	3	0.70	0.47	0.70	0.47
	2	5	3	0.45	0.30	0.45	0.30
	4	4	7	0.36	0.25	0.36	0.25
	6	4	8	0.25	0.22	0.25	0.13
	4	5	7	0.24	0.22	0.24	0.12
	6	5	8	0.22	0.22	0.12	0.08
Waffle-grid walls[e]							
6	2	4	3	0.78	0.78	0.70	0.48
	3	4	4	0.78	0.78	0.49	0.25
	2	5	3	0.78	0.78	0.46	0.23
	3	5	4	0.78	0.78	0.24	0.16
8	2	4	3	0.78	0.78	0.70	0.47
	3	4	5	0.78	0.78	0.47	0.24
	2	5	3	0.78	0.78	0.45	0.23
	4	4	6	0.78	0.78	0.36	0.18
	3	5	5	0.78	0.78	0.23	0.16
	4	5	6	0.78	0.78	0.18	0.13
Screen-grid walls[e]							
6	2	4	3	0.93	0.93	0.70	0.48
	3	4	4	0.93	0.93	0.49	0.25
	2	5	3	0.93	0.93	0.46	0.23
	3	5	4	0.93	0.93	0.24	0.16

For SI: 1 inch = 25.4 mm; 1,000 pounds per square inch = 6.895 MPa.

a. See note e to Table R611.7(1A) for application of adjustment factors in this table.

b. Yield strength in pounds per square inch of vertical wall reinforcement at ends of solid wall segments.

c. Values are based on concrete with a specified compressive strength, f_c', of 2,500 psi. Where concrete with f_c' of not less than 3,000 psi is used, values in shaded cells are permitted to be decreased by multiplying by 0.91.

d. Horizontal and vertical shear reinforcement shall be provided in accordance with Section R611.7.2.2.

e. Each end of each solid wall segment shall have rectangular flanges. In the through-the-wall dimension, the flange shall not be less than $5^1/_2$ inches for 6-inch nominal waffle- and screen-grid walls, and not less than $7^1/_2$ inches for 8-inch nominal waffle-grid walls. In the in-plane dimension, flanges shall be long enough to accommodate the vertical reinforcement required by the layout detail selected from Figure R611.7(2) and provide the cover required by Section R611.5.4.1. If necessary to achieve the required dimensions, form material shall be removed or use of flat wall forms is permitted.

R611.8 Requirements for lintels and reinforcement around openings.

R611.8.1 Reinforcement around openings. Reinforcement shall be provided around openings in walls equal to or greater than 2 feet (610 mm) in width in accordance with this section and Figure R611.8(1), in addition to the minimum wall reinforcement required by Sections R404.1.2, R611.6 and R611.7. Vertical wall reinforcement required by this section is permitted to be used as reinforcement at the ends of solid wall segments required by Section R611.7.2.2.2 provided it is located in accordance with Section R611.8.1.2. Wall openings shall have a minimum depth of concrete over the width of the opening of 8 inches (203 mm) in flat walls and waffle-grid walls, and 12 inches (305 mm) in screen-grid walls. Wall openings in waffle-grid and screen-grid walls shall be located such that not less than one-half of a vertical core occurs along each side of the opening.

R611.8.1.1 Horizontal reinforcement. Lintels complying with Section R611.8.2 shall be provided above wall openings equal to or greater than 2 feet (610 mm) in width.

Exception: Continuous horizontal wall reinforcement placed within 12 inches (305 mm) of the top of the wall *story* as required in Sections R404.1.2.2 and R611.6.2 is permitted in lieu of top or bottom lintel reinforcement required by Section R611.8.2 provided that the continuous horizontal wall reinforcement meets the location requirements specified in Figures R611.8(2), R611.8(3), and R611.8(4) and the size requirements specified in Tables R611.8(2) through R611.8(10).

Openings equal to or greater than 2 feet (610 mm) in width shall have a minimum of one No. 4 bar placed within 12 inches (305 mm) of the bottom of the opening. See Figure R611.8(1).

Horizontal reinforcement placed above and below an opening shall extend beyond the edges of the opening the dimension required to develop the bar in tension in accordance with Section R611.5.4.4.

R611.8.1.2 Vertical reinforcement. Not less than one No. 4 bar [Grade 40 (280 MPa)] shall be provided on each side of openings equal to or greater than 2 feet (610 mm) in width. The vertical reinforcement required by this section shall extend the full height of the wall *story* and shall be located within 12 inches (305 mm) of each side of the opening. The vertical reinforcement required on each side of an opening by this section is permitted to serve as reinforcement at the ends of solid wall segments in accordance with Section R611.7.2.2.2, provided it is located as required by the applicable detail in Figure R611.7(2). Where the vertical reinforcement required by this section is used to satisfy the requirements of Section R611.7.2.2.2 in waffle- and screen-grid walls, a concrete flange shall be created at the ends of the solid wall segments in accordance with Table R611.7(4), note e. In the top-most *story*, the reinforcement shall terminate in accordance with Section R611.6.4.

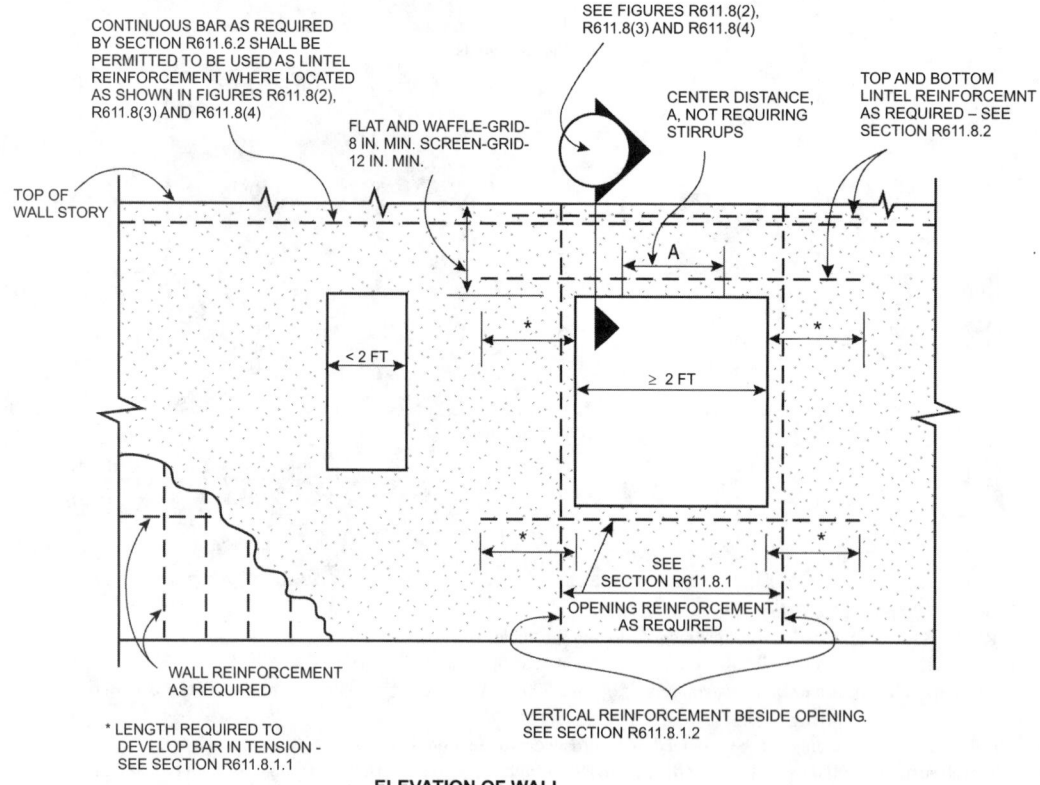

ELEVATION OF WALL

For SI: 1 inch = 25.4 mm, 1 foot = 304.8 mm.

FIGURE R611.8(1)
REINFORCEMENT OF OPENINGS

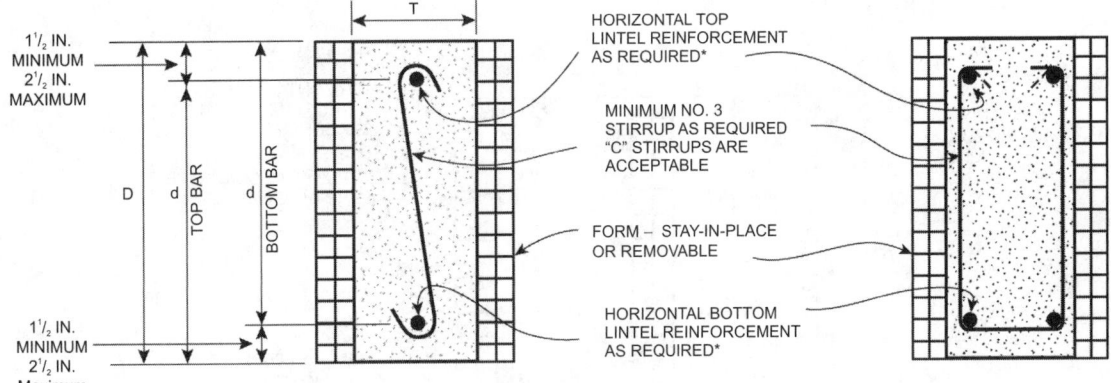

*FOR BUNDLED BARS, SEE SECTION R611.8.2.2.
SECTION CUT THROUGH FLAT WALL LINTEL

For SI: 1 inch = 25.4 mm.

**FIGURE R611.8(2)
LINTEL FOR FLAT WALLS**

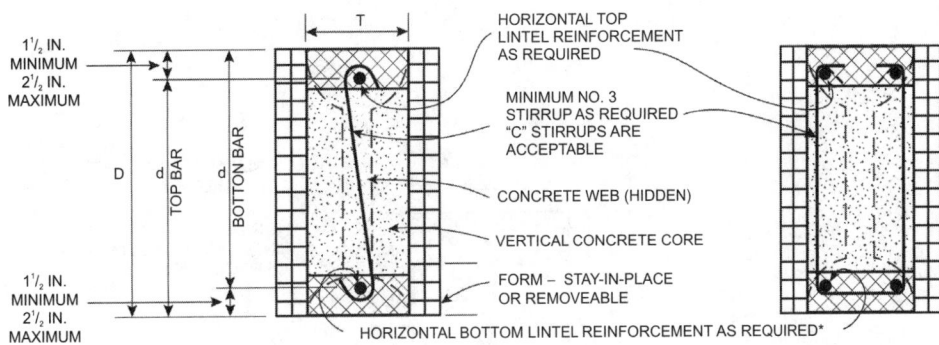

(a) SINGLE FORM HEIGHT SECTION CUT THROUGH VERTICAL CORE OF A WAFFLE-GRID LINTEL

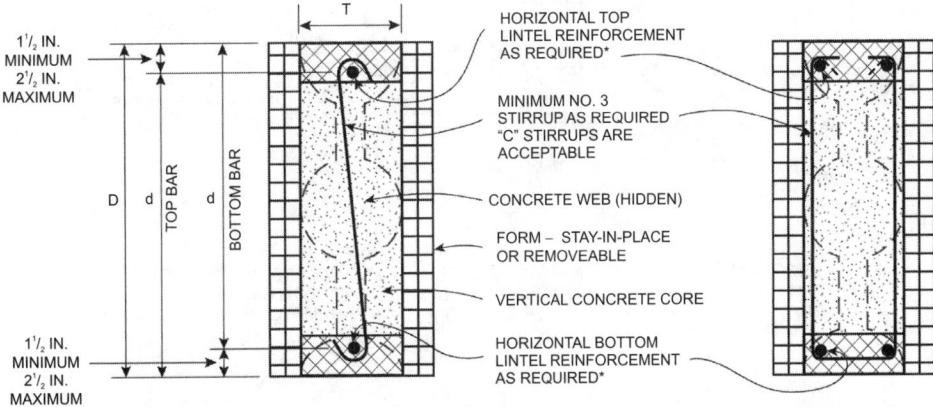

(b) DOUBLE FORM HEIGHT SECTION CUT THROUGH VERTICAL CORE OF A WAFFLE-GRID LINTEL

*FOR BUNDLED BARS, SEE SECTION R611.8.2.2.

NOTE: CROSS-HATCHING REPRESENTS THE AREA IN WHICH FORM MATERIAL SHALL BE REMOVED,
IF NECESSARY, TO CREATE FLANGES CONTINUOUS TO THE LENGTH OF THE LINTEL. FLANGES SHALL
HAVE A MINIMUM THICKNESS OF 3 IN., AND A MINIMUM WIDTH OF 5 IN. AND 7 IN. IN 6 IN. NOMINAL
AND 8 IN. NOMINAL WAFFLE-GRID WALLS, RESPECTIVELY. SEE NOTE a TO TABLES R611.8(6)
AND R611.8(10).

For SI: 1 inch = 25.4 mm.

**FIGURE R611.8(3)
LINTELS FOR WAFFLE-GRID WALLS**

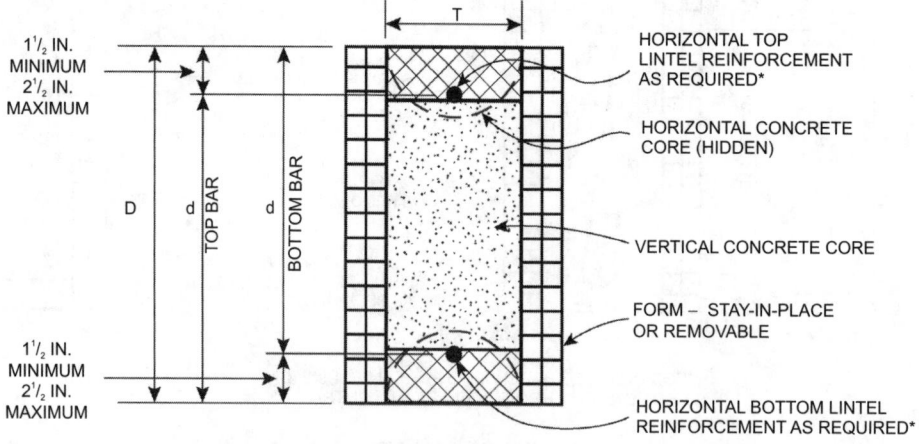

1¹/₂ IN.
MINIMUM
2¹/₂ IN.
MAXIMUM

1¹/₂ IN.
MINIMUM
2¹/₂ IN.
MAXIMUM

D   d   TOP BAR   d   BOTTOM BAR   T

HORIZONTAL TOP
LINTEL REINFORCEMENT
AS REQUIRED*

HORIZONTAL CONCRETE
CORE (HIDDEN)

VERTICAL CONCRETE CORE

FORM – STAY-IN-PLACE
OR REMOVABLE

HORIZONTAL BOTTOM LINTEL
REINFORCEMENT AS REQUIRED*

(a) SINGLE FORM HEIGHT SECTION CUT THROUGH
VERTICAL CORE OF A SCREEN-GRID LINTEL

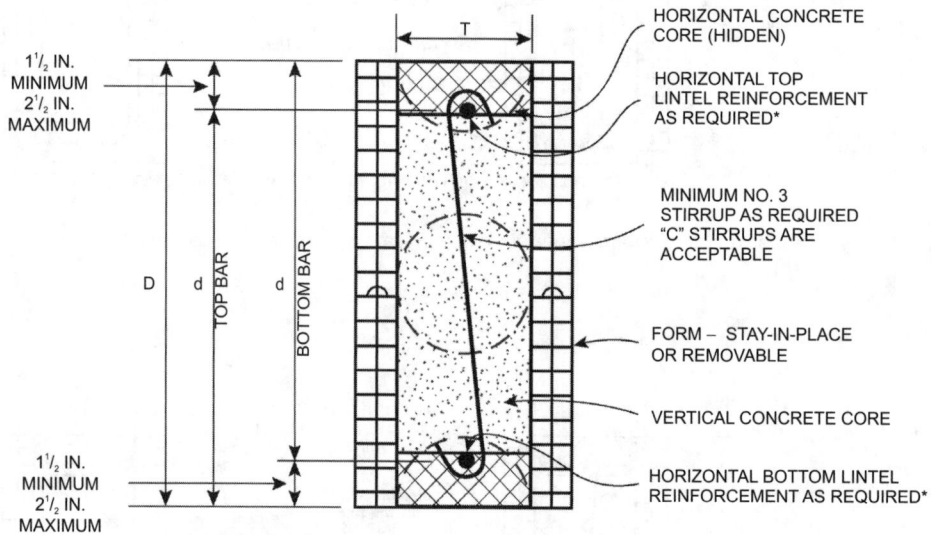

1¹/₂ IN.
MINIMUM
2¹/₂ IN.
MAXIMUM

1¹/₂ IN.
MINIMUM
2¹/₂ IN.
MAXIMUM

D   d   TOP BAR   d   BOTTOM BAR   T

HORIZONTAL CONCRETE
CORE (HIDDEN)

HORIZONTAL TOP
LINTEL REINFORCEMENT
AS REQUIRED*

MINIMUM NO. 3
STIRRUP AS REQUIRED
"C" STIRRUPS ARE
ACCEPTABLE

FORM – STAY-IN-PLACE
OR REMOVABLE

VERTICAL CONCRETE CORE

HORIZONTAL BOTTOM LINTEL
REINFORCEMENT AS REQUIRED*

(b) DOUBLE FORM HEIGHT SECTION CUT THROUGH VERTICAL
CORE OF A SCREEN-GRID LINTEL

*FOR BUNDLED BARS, SEE SECTION R611.8.2.2.

NOTE: CROSS-HATCHING REPRESENTS THE AREA IN WHICH FORM MATERIAL SHALL BE REMOVED,
IF NECESSARY, TO CREATE FLANGES CONTINUOUS THE LENGTH OF THE LINTEL. FLANGES
SHALL HAVE A MINIMUM THICKNESS OF 2.5 IN. AND A MINIMUM WIDTH OF 5 IN. SEE NOTE
a TO TABLES R611.8(8) AND R611.8(10).

For SI: 1 inch = 25.4 mm.

FIGURE R611.8(4)
LINTELS FOR SCREEN-GRID WALLS

R611.8.2 Lintels. Lintels shall be provided over all openings equal to or greater than 2 feet (610 mm) in width. Lintels with uniform loading shall conform to Sections R611.8.2.1, and R611.8.2.2, or Section R611.8.2.3. Lintels supporting concentrated loads, such as from roof or floor beams or girders, shall be designed in accordance with ACI 318.

R611.8.2.1 Lintels designed for gravity load-bearing conditions. Where a lintel will be subjected to gravity load condition 1 through 5 of Table R611.8(1), the clear span of the lintel shall not exceed that permitted by Tables R611.8(2) through R611.8(8). The maximum clear span of lintels with and without stirrups in flat walls shall be determined in accordance with Tables R611.8(2) through R611.8(5), and constructed in accordance with Figure R611.8(2). The maximum clear span of lintels with and without stirrups in waffle-grid walls shall be determined in accordance with Tables R611.8(6) and R611.8(7), and constructed in accordance with Figure R611.8(3). The maximum clear span of lintels with and without stirrups in screen-grid walls shall be determined in accordance with Table R611.8(8), and constructed in accordance with Figure R611.8(4).

Where required by the applicable table, No. 3 stirrups shall be installed in lintels at a maximum spacing of $d/2$ where d equals the depth of the lintel, D, less the cover of the concrete as shown in Figures R611.8(2) through R611.8(4). The smaller value of d computed for the top and bottom bar shall be used to determine the maximum stirrup spacing. Where stirrups are required in a lintel with a single bar or two bundled bars in the top and bottom, they shall be fabricated like the letter "c" or "s" with 135-degree (2.36 rad) standard hooks at each end that comply with Section R611.5.4.5 and Figure R611.5.4(3) and installed as shown in Figures R611.8(2) through R611.8(4). Where two bars are required in the top and bottom of the lintel and the bars are not bundled, the bars shall be separated by a minimum of 1 inch (25 mm). The free end of the stirrups shall be fabricated with 90- or 135-degree (1.57 or 2.36 rad) standard hooks that comply with Section R611.5.4.5 and Figure R611.5.4(3) and installed as shown in Figures R611.8(2) and R611.8(3). For flat, waffle-grid and screen-grid lintels, stirrups are not required in the center distance, A, portion of spans in

accordance with Figure R611.8(1) and Tables R611.8(2) through R611.8(8). See Section R611.8.2.2, item 5, for requirement for stirrups throughout lintels with bundled bars.

R611.8.2.2 Bundled bars in lintels. It is permitted to bundle two bars in contact with each other in lintels if all of the following are observed:

1. Bars no larger than No. 6 are bundled.

2. Where the wall thickness is not sufficient to provide not less than 3 inches (76 mm) of clear space beside bars (total on both sides) oriented horizontally in a bundle, the bundled bars shall be oriented in a vertical plane.

3. Where vertically oriented bundled bars terminate with standard hooks to develop the bars in tension beyond the support (see Section R611.5.4.4), the hook extensions shall be staggered to provide a minimum of one inch (25 mm) clear spacing between the extensions.

4. Bundled bars shall not be lap spliced within the lintel span and the length on each end of the lintel that is required to develop the bars in tension.

5. Bundled bars shall be enclosed within stirrups throughout the length of the lintel. Stirrups and the installation thereof shall comply with Section R611.8.2.1.

R611.8.2.3 Lintels without stirrups designed for nonload-bearing conditions. The maximum clear span of lintels without stirrups designed for nonload-bearing conditions of Table R611.8(1).1 shall be determined in accordance with this section. The maximum clear span of lintels without stirrups in flat walls shall be determined in accordance with Table R611.8(9), and the maximum clear span of lintels without stirrups in walls of waffle-grid or screen-grid construction shall be determined in accordance with Table R611.8(10).

TABLE R611.8(1)
LINTEL DESIGN LOADING CONDITIONS[a, b, d]

DESCRIPTION OF LOADS AND OPENINGS ABOVE INFLUENCING DESIGN OF LINTEL			DESIGN LOAD CONDITION[c]
Opening in wall of top story of two-story building, or first story of one-story building			
Wall supporting loads from roof, including attic floor, if applicable, and	Top of lintel equal to or less than W/2 below top of wall		2
	Top of lintel greater than W/2 below top of wall		NLB
Wall not supporting loads from roof or attic floor			NLB
Opening in wall of first story of two-story building where wall immediately above is of concrete construction, or opening in basement wall of one-story building where wall immediately above is of concrete construction			
LB ledger board mounted to side of wall with bottom of ledger less than or equal to W/2 above top of lintel, and	Top of lintel greater than W/2 below bottom of opening in story above		1
	Top of lintel less than or equal to W/2 below bottom of opening in story above, and	Opening is entirely within the footprint of the opening in the story above	1
		Opening is partially within the footprint of the opening in the story above	4
LB ledger board mounted to side of wall with bottom of ledger more than W/2 above top of lintel			NLB
NLB ledger board mounted to side of wall with bottom of ledger less than or equal to W/2 above top of lintel, or no ledger board, and	Top of lintel greater than W/2 below bottom of opening in story above		NLB
	Top of lintel less than or equal to W/2 below bottom of opening in story above, and	Opening is entirely within the footprint of the opening in the story above	NLB
		Opening is partially within the footprint of the opening in the story above	1
Opening in basement wall of two-story building where walls of two stories above are of concrete construction			
LB ledger board mounted to side of wall with bottom of ledger less than or equal to W/2 above top of lintel, and	Top of lintel greater than W/2 below bottom of opening in story above		1
	Top of lintel less than or equal to W/2 below bottom of opening in story above, and	Opening is entirely within the footprint of the opening in the story above	1
		Opening is partially within the footprint of the opening in the story above	5
LB ledger board mounted to side of wall with bottom of ledger more than W/2 above top of lintel			NLB
NLB ledger board mounted to side of wall with bottom of ledger less than or equal to W/2 above top of lintel, or no ledger board, and	Top of lintel greater than W/2 below bottom of opening in story above		NLB
	Top of lintel less than or equal to W/2 below bottom of opening in story above, and	Opening is entirely within the footprint of the opening in the story above	NLB
		Opening is partially within the footprint of the opening in the story above	1
Opening in wall of first story of two-story building where wall immediately above is of light framed construction, or opening in basement wall of one-story building, where wall immediately above is of light framed construction			
Wall supporting loads from roof, second floor and top-story wall of light-framed construction, and	Top of lintel equal to or less than W/2 below top of wall		3
	Top of lintel greater than W/2 below top of wall		NLB
Wall not supporting loads from roof or second floor			NLB

a. LB means load bearing, NLB means nonload-bearing, and W means width of opening.

b. Footprint is the area of the wall below an opening in the story above, bounded by the bottom of the opening and vertical lines extending downward from the edges of the opening.

c. For design loading condition "NLB" see Tables R611.8(9) and R611.8(10). For all other design loading conditions see Tables R611.8(2) through R611.8(8).

d. A NLB ledger board is a ledger attached to a wall that is parallel to the span of the floor, roof or ceiling framing that supports the edge of the floor, ceiling or roof.

TABLE R611.8(2)
MAXIMUM ALLOWABLE CLEAR SPANS FOR 4-INCH NOMINAL THICK FLAT LINTELS IN LOAD-BEARING WALLS[a, b, c, d, e, f, m]
ROOF CLEAR SPAN 40 FEET AND FLOOR CLEAR SPAN 32 FEET

LINTEL DEPTH, D^g (inches)	NUMBER OF BARS AND BAR SIZE IN TOP AND BOTTOM OF LINTEL	STEEL YIELD STRENGTH[h], f_y (psi)	DESIGN LOADING CONDITION DETERMINED FROM TABLE R611.8(1)							
			1		2		3		40		5	
			30	70	30	70	30	70	30	70	30	70
			Maximum clear span of lintel (feet - inches)									
8	Span without stirrups[i, j]		3-2	3-4	2-4	2-6	2-2	2-1	2-0	2-0	2-0
	1-#4	40,000	5-2	5-5	4-1	4-3	3-10	3-7	3-4	2-9	2-9
		60,000	6-2	6-5	4-11	5-1	4-6	4-2	3-8	2-11	2-10
	1-#5	40,000	6-3	6-7	5-0	5-2	4-6	4-2	3-8	2-11	2-10
		60,000	DR	DR	DR	DR	DR	DR	DR	DR	DR
	Center distance A[k, l]		1-1	1-2	0-8	0-9	0-7	0-6	0-5	0-4	0-4
12	Span without stirrups[i, j]		3-4	3-7	2-9	2-11	2-8	2-6	2-5	2-2	2-2
	1-#4	40,000	6-7	7-0	5-4	5-7	5-0	4-9	4-4	3-8	3-7
		60,000	7-11	8-6	6-6	6-9	6-0	5-9	5-3	4-5	4-4
	1-#5	40,000	8-1	8-8	6-7	6-10	6-2	5-10	5-4	4-6	4-5
		60,000	9-8	10-4	7-11	8-2	7-4	6-11	6-2	4-10	4-8
	2-#4 1-#6	40,000	9-1	9-8	7-4	7-8	6-10	6-6	6-0	4-10	4-8
		60,000	DR	DR	DR	DR	DR	DR	DR	DR	DR
	Center distance A[k, l]		1-8	1-11	1-1	1-3	1-0	0-11	0-9	0-6	0-6
16	Span without stirrups[i, j]		4-7	5-0	3-11	4-0	3-8	3-7	3-4	3-1	3-0
	1-#4	40,000	6-8	7-3	5-6	5-9	5-2	4-11	4-6	3-10	3-8
		60,000	9-3	10-1	7-9	8-0	7-2	6-10	6-3	5-4	5-2
	1-#4	40,000	9-6	10-4	7-10	8-2	7-4	6-11	6-5	5-5	5-3
		60,000	11-5	12-5	9-6	9-10	8-10	8-4	7-9	6-6	6-4
	2-#4 1-#6	40,000	10-7	11-7	8-10	9-2	8-3	7-9	7-2	6-1	5-11
		60,000	12-9	13-10	10-7	11-0	9-10	9-4	8-7	6-9	6-6
	2-#5	40,000	13-0	14-1	10-9	11-2	9-11	9-2	8-2	6-6	6-3
		60,000	DR	DR	DR	DR	DR	DR	DR	DR	DR
	Center distance[k, l]		2-3	2-8	1-7	1-8	1-4	1-3	1-0	0-9	0-8
20	Span without stirrups[i, j]		5-9	6-5	5-0	5-2	4-9	4-7	4-4	3-11	3-11
	1-#4	40,000	7-5	8-2	6-3	6-6	5-10	5-7	5-1	4-4	4-2
		60,000	9-0	10-0	7-8	7-11	7-1	6-9	6-3	5-3	5-1
	1-#5	40,000	9-2	10-2	7-9	8-1	7-3	6-11	6-4	5-4	5-2
		60,000	12-9	14-2	10-10	11-3	10-1	9-7	8-10	7-5	7-3
	2-#4 1-#6	40,000	11-10	13-2	10-1	10-5	9-4	8-11	8-2	6-11	6-9
		60,000	14-4	15-10	12-1	12-7	11-3	10-9	9-11	8-4	8-1
	2-#5	40,000	14-7	16-2	12-4	12-9	11-4	10-6	9-5	7-7	7-3
		60,000	17-5	19-2	14-9	15-3	13-5	12-4	11-0	8-8	8-4
	2-#6	40,000	16-4	18-11	12-7	13-3	11-4	10-6	9-5	7-7	7-3
		60,000	DR	DR	DR	DR	DR	DR	DR	DR	DR
	Center distance A[k, l]		2-9	3-5	2-0	2-2	1-9	1-7	1-4	0-11	0-11

(continued)

TABLE R611.8(2)—continued
MAXIMUM ALLOWABLE CLEAR SPANS FOR 4-INCH NOMINAL THICK FLAT LINTELS IN LOAD-BEARING WALLS[a, b, c, d, e, f, m]
ROOF CLEAR SPAN 40 FEET AND FLOOR CLEAR SPAN 32 FEET

LINTEL DEPTH, D[g] (inches)	NUMBER OF BARS AND BAR SIZE IN TOP AND BOTTOM OF LINTEL		DESIGN LOADING CONDITION DETERMINED FROM TABLE R611.8(1)								
			1	2		3		40		5	
				30	70	30	70	30	70	30	70
			Maximum clear span of lintel (feet - inches)								
24	Span without stirrups[i, j]		6-11	7-9	6-1	6-3	5-9	5-7	5-3	4-9	4-8
	1-#4	40,000	8-0	9-0	6-11	7-2	6-5	6-2	5-8	4-9	4-8
		60,000	9-9	11-0	8-5	8-9	7-10	7-6	6-11	5-10	5-8
	1-#5	40,000	10-0	11-3	8-7	8-11	8-0	7-7	7-0	5-11	5-9
		60,000	13-11	15-8	12-0	12-5	11-2	10-7	9-10	8-3	8-0
	2-#4 1-#6	40,000	12-11	14-6	11-2	11-6	10-5	9-10	9-1	7-8	7-5
		60,000	15-7	17-7	13-6	13-11	12-7	11-11	11-0	9-3	9-0
	2-#5	40,000	15-11	17-11	13-7	14-3	12-8	11-9	10-8	8-7	8-4
		60,000	19-1	21-6	16-5	17-1	15-1	14-0	12-6	9-11	9-7
	2-#6	40,000	17-7	21-1	14-1	14-10	12-8	11-9	10-8	8-7	8-4
		60,000	DR	DR	DR	DR	DR	DR	DR	DR	DR
	Center distance A[k, l]		3-3	4-1	2-5	2-7	2-1	1-11	1-7	1-2	1-1

For SI: 1 inch = 25.4 mm; 1 foot = 304.8 mm; 1 pound per square foot = 0.0479 kPa; Grade 40 = 280 MPa; Grade 60 = 420 MPa.

a. See Table R611.3 for tolerances permitted from nominal thickness.

b. Table values are based on concrete with a minimum specified compressive strength of 2,500 psi. See note j.

c. Table values are based on uniform loading. See Section R611.8.2 for lintels supporting concentrated loads.

d. Deflection criterion is $L/240$, where L is the clear span of the lintel in inches, or $^1/_2$-inch, whichever is less.

e. Linear interpolation is permitted between ground snow loads and between lintel depths.

f. DR indicates design required.

g. Lintel depth, D, is permitted to include the available height of wall located directly above the lintel, provided that the increased lintel depth spans the entire length of the lintel.

h. Stirrups shall be fabricated from reinforcing bars with the same yield strength as that used for the main longitudinal reinforcement.

i. Allowable clear span without stirrups applicable to all lintels of the same depth, D. Top and bottom reinforcement for lintels without stirrups shall not be less than the least amount of reinforcement required for a lintel of the same depth and loading condition with stirrups. All other spans require stirrups spaced at not more than $d/2$.

j. Where concrete with a minimum specified compressive strength of 3,000 psi (20.7 MPa) is used, clear spans for lintels without stirrups shall be permitted to be multiplied by 1.05. If the increased span exceeds the allowable clear span for a lintel of the same depth and loading condition with stirrups, the top and bottom reinforcement shall be equal to or greater than that required for a lintel of the same depth and loading condition that has an allowable clear span that is equal to or greater than that of the lintel without stirrups that has been increased.

k. Center distance, A, is the center portion of the clear span where stirrups are not required. This is applicable to all longitudinal bar sizes and steel yield strengths.

l. Where concrete with a minimum specified compressive strength of 3,000 psi is used, center distance, A, shall be permitted to be multiplied by 1.10.

m. The maximum clear opening width between two solid wall segments shall be 18 feet (5486 mm). See Section R611.7.2.1. Lintel clear spans in the table greater than 18 feet are shown for interpolation and information only.

TABLE R611.8(3)
MAXIMUM ALLOWABLE CLEAR SPANS FOR 6-INCH NOMINAL THICK FLAT LINTELS IN LOAD-BEARING WALLS[a, b, c, d, e, f, m]
ROOF CLEAR SPAN 40 FEET AND FLOOR CLEAR SPAN 32 FEET

LINTEL DEPTH, D^g (inches)	NUMBER OF BARS AND BAR SIZE IN TOP AND BOTTOM OF LINTEL	STEEL YIELD STRENGTH[h], f_y (psi)	DESIGN LOADING CONDITION DETERMINED FROM TABLE R611.8(1)								
			1	2		3		4		5	
			Maximum ground snow load (psf)								
			30	30	70	30	70	30	70	30	70
			Maximum clear span of lintel (feet - inches)								
8	Span without stirrups[i, j]		4-2	4-8	3-1	3-3	2-10	2-6	2-3	2-0	2-0
	1-#4	40,000	5-1	5-5	4-2	4-3	3-10	3-6	3-3	2-8	2-7
		60,000	6-2	6-7	5-0	5-2	4-8	4-2	3-11	3-3	3-2
	1-#5	40,000	6-3	6-8	5-1	5-3	4-9	4-3	4-0	3-3	3-2
		60,000	7-6	8-0	6-1	6-4	5-8	5-1	4-9	3-8	3-6
	2-#4 1-#6	40,000	7-0	7-6	5-8	5-11	5-3	4-9	4-5	3-8	3-6
		60,000	DR	DR	DR	DR	DR	DR	DR	DR	DR
	Center distance A[k, l]		1-7	1-10	1-1	1-2	0-11	0-9	0-8	0-5	0-5
12	Span without stirrups[i, j]		4-2	4-8	3-5	3-6	3-2	2-11	2-9	2-5	2-4
	1-#4	40,000	5-7	6-1	4-8	4-10	4-4	3-11	3-8	3-0	2-11
		60,000	7-9	8-6	6-6	6-9	6-1	5-6	5-1	4-3	4-1
	1-#5	40,000	7-11	8-8	6-8	6-11	6-2	5-7	5-2	4-4	4-2
		60,000	9-7	10-6	8-0	8-4	7-6	6-9	6-3	5-2	5-1
	2-#4 1-#6	40,000	8-11	9-9	7-6	7-9	6-11	6-3	5-10	4-10	4-8
		60,000	10-8	11-9	8-12	9-4	8-4	7-6	7-0	5-10	5-8
	2-#5	40,000	10-11	12-0	9-2	9-6	8-6	7-8	7-2	5-6	5-3
		60,000	12-11	14-3	10-10	11-3	10-1	9-0	8-1	6-1	5-10
	2-#6	40,000	12-9	14-0	10-8	11-1	9-7	8-1	7-3	5-6	5-3
		60,000	DR	DR	DR	DR	DR	DR	DR	DR	DR
	Center distance A[k, l]		2-6	3-0	1-9	1-10	1-6	1-3	1-1	0-9	0-8
16	Span without stirrups[i, j]		5-7	6-5	4-9	4-11	4-5	4-0	3-10	3-4	3-4
	1-#4	40,000	6-5	7-2	5-6	5-9	5-2	4-8	4-4	3-7	3-6
		60,000	7-10	8-9	6-9	7-0	6-3	5-8	5-3	4-4	4-3
	1-#5	40,000	7-11	8-11	6-10	7-1	6-5	5-9	5-4	4-5	4-4
		60,000	11-1	12-6	9-7	9-11	8-11	8-0	7-6	6-2	6-0
	2-#4 1-#6	40,000	10-3	11-7	8-10	9-2	8-3	7-6	6-11	5-9	5-7
		60,000	12-5	14-0	10-9	11-1	10-0	9-0	8-5	7-0	6-9
	2-#5	40,000	12-8	14-3	10-11	11-4	10-2	9-2	8-7	6-9	6-6
		60,000	15-2	17-1	13-1	13-7	12-3	11-0	10-3	7-11	7-7
	2-#6	40,000	14-11	16-9	12-8	13-4	11-4	9-8	8-8	6-9	6-6
		60,000	DR	DR	DR	DR	DR	DR	DR	DR	DR
	Center distance A[k, l]		3-3	4-1	2-5	2-7	2-1	1-9	1-6	1-0	1-0

(continued)

TABLE R611.8(3)—continued
MAXIMUM ALLOWABLE CLEAR SPANS FOR 6-INCH NOMINAL THICK FLAT LINTELS IN LOAD-BEARING WALLS[a, b, c, d, e, f, m]
ROOF CLEAR SPAN 40 FEET AND FLOOR CLEAR SPAN 32 FEET

Design loading condition determined from Table R611.8(1). Maximum ground snow load (psf). Maximum clear span of lintel (feet - inches).

LINTEL DEPTH, D[g] (inches)	NUMBER OF BARS AND BAR SIZE IN TOP AND BOTTOM OF LINTEL	STEEL YIELD STRENGTH[h], f_y (psi)	1 — 30	1 — 70	2 — 30	2 — 70	3 — 30	3 — 70	4 — 30	4 — 70	5 — 30	5 — 70
20	Span without stirrups[i, j]		6-11	8-2	6-1	6-3	5-8	5-2	4-11	4-4	4-3	
	1-#5	40,000	8-9	10-1	7-9	8-0	7-3	6-6	6-1	5-1	4-11	
	1-#5	60,000	10-8	12-3	9-5	9-9	8-10	8-0	7-5	6-2	6-0	
	2-#4 1-#6	40,000	9-11	11-4	8-9	9-1	8-2	7-4	6-10	5-8	5-7	
	2-#4 1-#6	60,000	13-9	15-10	12-2	12-8	11-5	10-3	9-7	7-11	7-9	
	2-#5	40,000	14-0	16-2	12-5	12-11	11-7	10-6	9-9	7-11	7-8	
	2-#5	60,000	16-11	19-6	15-0	15-6	14-0	12-7	11-9	9-1	8-9	
	2-#6	40,000	16-7	19-1	14-7	15-3	13-1	11-3	10-2	7-11	7-8	
	2-#6	60,000	19-11	22-10	17-4	18-3	15-6	13-2	11-10	9-1	8-9	
	Center distance A[k, l]		3-11	5-2	3-1	3-3	2-8	2-2	1-11	1-4	1-3	
24	Span without stirrups[i, j]		8-2	9-10	7-4	7-8	6-11	6-4	5-11	5-3	5-2	
	1-#5	40,000	9-5	11-1	8-7	8-10	8-0	7-3	6-9	5-7	5-5	
	1-#5	60,000	11-6	13-6	10-5	10-9	9-9	8-9	8-2	6-10	6-8	
	2-#4 1-#6	40,000	10-8	12-6	9-8	10-0	9-0	8-2	7-7	6-4	6-2	
	2-#4 1-#6	60,000	12-11	15-2	11-9	12-2	11-0	9-11	9-3	7-8	7-6	
	2-#5	40,000	15-2	17-9	13-9	14-3	12-10	11-7	10-10	9-0	8-9	
	2-#5	60,000	18-4	21-6	16-7	17-3	15-6	14-0	13-1	10-4	10-0	
	2-#6	40,000	18-0	21-1	16-4	16-11	14-10	12-9	11-8	9-2	8-11	
	2-#6	60,000	21-7	25-4	19-2	20-4	17-2	14-9	13-4	10-4	10-0	
	Center distance A[k, l]		4-6	6-2	3-8	4-0	3-3	2-8	2-3	1-7	1-6	

For SI: 1 inch = 25.4 mm; 1 foot = 304.8 mm; 1 psf = 0.0479 kPa; Grade 40 = 280 MPa; Grade 60 = 420 MPa.

a. See Table R611.3 for tolerances permitted from nominal thickness.

b. Table values are based on concrete with a minimum specified compressive strength of 2,500 psi. See Note j.

c. Table values are based on uniform loading. See Section R611.8.2 for lintels supporting concentrated loads.

d. Deflection criterion is $L/240$, where L is the clear span of the lintel in inches, or $1/2$-inch, whichever is less.

e. Linear interpolation is permitted between ground snow loads and between lintel depths.

f. DR indicates design required.

g. Lintel depth, D, is permitted to include the available height of wall located directly above the lintel, provided that the increased lintel depth spans the entire length of the lintel.

h. Stirrups shall be fabricated from reinforcing bars with the same yield strength as that used for the main longitudinal reinforcement.

i. Allowable clear span without stirrups applicable to all lintels of the same depth, D. Top and bottom reinforcement for lintels without stirrups shall not be less than the least amount of reinforcement required for a lintel of the same depth and loading condition with stirrups. All other spans require stirrups spaced at not more than d/2.

j. Where concrete with a minimum specified compressive strength of 3,000 psi is used, clear spans for lintels without stirrups shall be permitted to be multiplied by 1.05. If the increased span exceeds the allowable clear span for a lintel of the same depth and loading condition with stirrups, the top and bottom reinforcement shall be equal to or greater than that required for a lintel of the same depth and loading condition that has an allowable clear span that is equal to or greater than that of the lintel without stirrups that has been increased.

k. Center distance, A, is the center portion of the clear span where stirrups are not required. This is applicable to all longitudinal bar sizes and steel yield strengths.

l. Where concrete with a minimum specified compressive strength of 3,000 psi is used, center distance, A, shall be permitted to be multiplied by 1.10.

m. The maximum clear opening width between two solid wall segments shall be 18 feet (5486 mm). See Section R611.7.2.1. Lintel clear spans in the table greater than 18 feet are shown for interpolation and information only.

TABLE R611.8(4)
MAXIMUM ALLOWABLE CLEAR SPANS FOR 8-INCH NOMINAL THICK FLAT LINTELS IN LOAD-BEARING WALLS[a, b, c, d, e, f, m]
ROOF CLEAR SPAN 40 FEET AND FLOOR CLEAR SPAN 32 FEET

LINTEL DEPTH, D^g (inches)	NUMBER OF BARS AND BAR SIZE IN TOP AND BOTTOM OF LINTEL	STEEL YIELD STRENGTH[h], f_y (psi)	DESIGN LOADING CONDITION DETERMINED FROM TABLE R611.8(1)									
			1		2		3		4		5	
			Maximum ground snow load (psf)									
			30	70	30	70	30	70	30	70	30	70
			Maximum clear span of lintel (feet - inches)									
8	Span without stirrups[i, j]		4-4	4-9	3-7	3-9	3-4	2-10	2-7	2-1	2-0	
	1-#4	40,000	4-4	4-9	3-7	3-9	3-4	2-11	2-9	2-3	2-2	
		60,000	6-1	6-7	5-0	5-3	4-8	4-0	3-9	3-1	3-0	
	1-#5	40,000	6-2	6-9	5-2	5-4	4-9	4-1	3-10	3-2	3-1	
		60,000	7-5	8-1	6-2	6-5	5-9	4-11	4-7	3-9	3-8	
	2-#4 1-#6	40,000	6-11	7-6	5-9	6-0	5-4	4-7	4-4	3-6	3-5	
		60,000	8-3	9-0	6-11	7-2	6-5	5-6	5-2	4-2	4-1	
	2-#5	40,000	8-5	9-2	7-0	7-3	6-6	5-7	5-3	4-2	4-0	
		60,000	DR	DR	DR	DR	DR	DR	DR	DR	DR	
	Center distance A[k, l]		2-1	2-6	1-5	1-6	1-3	0-11	0-10	0-6	0-6	
12	Span without stirrups[i, j]		4-10	5-8	4-0	4-2	3-9	3-2	3-0	2-7	2-6	
	1-#4	40,000	5-5	6-1	4-8	4-10	4-4	3-9	3-6	2-10	2-10	
		60,000	6-7	7-5	5-8	5-11	5-4	4-7	4-3	3-6	3-5	
	1-#5	40,000	6-9	7-7	5-9	6-0	5-5	4-8	4-4	3-7	3-6	
		60,000	9-4	10-6	8-1	8-4	7-6	6-6	6-1	5-0	4-10	
	2-#4 1-#6	40,000	8-8	9-9	7-6	7-9	7-0	6-0	5-8	4-7	4-6	
		60,000	10-6	11-9	9-1	9-5	8-5	7-3	6-10	5-7	5-5	
	2-#5	40,000	10-8	12-0	9-3	9-7	8-7	7-5	6-11	5-6	5-4	
		60,000	12-10	14-5	11-1	11-6	10-4	8-11	8-4	6-7	6-4	
	2-#6	40,000	12-7	14-2	10-10	11-3	10-2	8-3	7-6	5-6	5-4	
		60,000	DR	DR	DR	DR	DR	DR	DR	DR	DR	
	Center distance A[k, l]		3-2	4-0	2-4	2-6	2-0	1-6	1-4	0-11	0-10	
16	Span without stirrups[i, j]		6-5	7-9	5-7	5-10	5-2	4-5	4-2	3-7	3-6	
	1-#4	40,000	6-2	7-1	5-6	5-8	5-1	4-5	4-2	3-5	3-4	
		60,000	7-6	8-8	6-8	6-11	6-3	5-5	5-1	4-2	4-0	
	1-#5	40,000	7-8	8-10	6-10	7-1	6-4	5-6	5-2	4-3	4-1	
		60,000	9-4	10-9	8-4	8-7	7-9	6-8	6-3	5-2	5-0	
	2-#4 1-#6	40,000	8-8	10-0	7-8	8-0	7-2	6-2	5-10	4-9	4-8	
		60,000	12-0	13-11	10-9	11-2	10-0	8-8	8-1	6-8	6-6	
	2-#5	40,000	12-3	14-2	11-0	11-4	10-3	8-10	8-3	6-9	6-7	
		60,000	14-10	17-2	13-3	13-8	12-4	10-8	10-0	7-11	7-8	
	2-#6	40,000	14-6	16-10	13-0	13-5	12-1	10-1	9-2	6-11	6-8	
		60,000	17-5	20-2	15-7	16-1	14-6	11-10	10-8	7-11	7-8	
	Center distance[k, l]		4-1	5-5	3-3	3-6	2-10	2-1	1-10	1-3	1-2	

(continued)

TABLE R611.8(4)—continued
MAXIMUM ALLOWABLE CLEAR SPANS FOR 8-INCH NOMINAL THICK FLAT LINTELS IN LOAD-BEARING WALLS[a, b, c, d, e, f, m]
ROOF CLEAR SPAN 40 FEET AND FLOOR CLEAR SPAN 32 FEET

LINTEL DEPTH, D^g (inches)	NUMBER OF BARS AND BAR SIZE IN TOP AND BOTTOM OF LINTEL	STEEL YIELD STRENGTH[h], f_y (psi)	1 (30)	1 (70)	2 (30)	2 (70)	3 (30)	3 (70)	4 (30)	4 (70)	5 (30)	5 (70)
			\<span\>DESIGN LOADING CONDITION — Maximum ground snow load (psf) — Maximum clear span of lintel (feet - inches)\</span\>									
20	Span without stirrups[i, j]		7-10	9-10	7-1	7-5	6-7	5-8	5-4	4-7	4-6	
	1-#5	40,000	8-4	9-11	7-8	8-0	7-2	6-3	5-10	4-9	4-8	
	1-#5	60,000	10-2	12-1	9-5	9-9	8-9	7-7	7-1	5-10	5-8	
	2-#4 1-#6	40,000	9-5	11-3	8-8	9-0	8-1	7-0	6-7	5-5	5-3	
	2-#4 1-#6	60,000	11-6	13-8	10-7	11-0	9-11	8-7	8-0	6-7	6-5	
	2-#5	40,000	11-9	13-11	10-10	11-2	10-1	8-9	8-2	6-8	6-7	
	2-#5	60,000	16-4	19-5	15-0	15-7	14-0	12-2	11-4	9-3	9-0	
	2-#6	40,000	16-0	19-0	14-9	15-3	13-9	11-10	10-10	8-3	8-0	
	2-#6	60,000	19-3	22-11	17-9	18-5	16-7	13-7	12-4	9-3	9-0	
	Center distance $A^{k, l}$		4-10	6-10	4-1	4-5	3-7	2-8	2-4	1-7	1-6	
24	Span without stirrups[i, j]		9-2	11-9	8-7	8-11	8-0	6-11	6-6	5-7	5-6	
	1-#5	40,000	8-11	10-10	8-6	8-9	7-11	6-10	6-5	5-3	5-2	
	1-#5	60,000	10-11	13-3	10-4	10-8	9-8	8-4	7-10	6-5	6-3	
	2-#4 1-#6	40,000	10-1	12-3	9-7	9-11	8-11	7-9	7-3	6-0	5-10	
	2-#4 1-#6	60,000	12-3	15-0	11-8	12-1	10-11	9-5	8-10	7-3	7-1	
	2-#5	40,000	12-6	15-3	11-11	12-4	11-1	9-7	9-0	7-5	7-3	
	2-#5	60,000	17-6	21-3	16-7	17-2	15-6	13-5	12-7	10-4	10-1	
	2-#6	40,000	17-2	20-11	16-3	16-10	15-3	13-2	12-4	9-7	9-4	
	2-#6	60,000	20-9	25-3	19-8	20-4	18-5	15-4	14-0	10-7	10-3	
	Center distance $A^{k, l}$		5-6	8-1	4-11	5-3	4-4	3-3	2-10	1-11	1-10	

For SI: 1 inch = 25.4 mm; 1 foot = 304.8 mm; 1 psf = 0.0479 kPa; Grade 40 = 280 MPa; Grade 60 = 420 MPa.

Note: Top and bottom reinforcement for lintels without stirrups shown in shaded cells shall be equal to or greater than that required for lintel of the same depth and loading condition that has an allowable clear span that is equal to or greater than that of the lintel without stirrups.

a. See Table R611.3 for tolerances permitted from nominal thickness.

b. Table values are based on concrete with a minimum specified compressive strength of 2,500 psi. See Note j.

c. Table values are based on uniform loading. See Section R611.8.2 for lintels supporting concentrated loads.

d. Deflection criterion is $L/240$, where L is the clear span of the lintel in inches, or $1/_2$-inch, whichever is less.

e. Linear interpolation is permitted between ground snow loads and between lintel depths.

f. DR indicates design required.

g. Lintel depth, D, is permitted to include the available height of wall located directly above the lintel, provided that the increased lintel depth spans the entire length of the lintel.

h. Stirrups shall be fabricated from reinforcing bars with the same yield strength as that used for the main longitudinal reinforcement.

i. Allowable clear span without stirrups applicable to all lintels of the same depth, D. Top and bottom reinforcement for lintels without stirrups shall not be less than the least amount of reinforcement required for a lintel of the same depth and loading condition with stirrups. All other spans require stirrups spaced at not more than d/2.

j. Where concrete with a minimum specified compressive strength of 3,000 psi is used, clear spans for lintels without stirrups shall be permitted to be multiplied by 1.05. If the increased span exceeds the allowable clear span for a lintel of the same depth and loading condition with stirrups, the top and bottom reinforcement shall be equal to or greater than that required for a lintel of the same depth and loading condition that has an allowable clear span that is equal to or greater than that of the lintel without stirrups that has been increased.

k. Center distance, A, is the center portion of the clear span where stirrups are not required. This is applicable to all longitudinal bar sizes and steel yield strengths.

l. Where concrete with a minimum specified compressive strength of 3,000 psi is used, center distance, A, shall be permitted to be multiplied by 1.10.

m. The maximum clear opening width between two solid wall segments shall be 18 feet. See Section R611.7.2.1. Lintel clear spans in the table greater than 18 feet are shown for interpolation and information only.

TABLE R611.8(5)
MAXIMUM ALLOWABLE CLEAR SPANS FOR 10-INCH NOMINAL THICK FLAT LINTELS IN LOAD-BEARING WALLS[a, b, c, d, e, f, m]
ROOF CLEAR SPAN 40 FEET AND FLOOR CLEAR SPAN 32 FEET

LINTEL DEPTH, D^g (inches)	NUMBER OF BARS AND BAR SIZE IN TOP AND BOTTOM OF LINTEL	STEEL YIELD STRENGTH[h], f_y (psi)	DESIGN LOADING CONDITION DETERMINED FROM TABLE R611.8(1)								
			1		2		3		4		5
			\- Maximum ground snow load (psf) -								
			30	70	30	70	30	70	30	70	30
			Maximum clear span of lintel (feet - inches)								
8	Span without stirrups[i, j]		6-0	7-2	4-7	4-10	4-1	3-1	2-11	2-3	2-2
	1-#4	40,000	4-3	4-9	3-7	3-9	3-4	2-9	2-7	2-1	2-1
		60,000	5-11	6-7	5-0	5-3	4-8	3-10	3-8	2-11	2-11
	1-#5	40,000	6-1	6-9	5-2	5-4	4-9	3-11	3-9	3-0	2-11
		60,000	7-4	8-1	6-3	6-5	5-9	4-9	4-6	3-7	3-7
	2-#4 / 1-#6	40,000	6-10	7-6	5-9	6-0	5-5	4-5	4-2	3-4	3-4
		60,000	8-2	9-1	6-11	7-2	6-6	5-4	5-0	4-1	4-0
	2-#5	40,000	8-4	9-3	7-1	7-4	6-7	5-5	5-1	4-1	4-0
		60,000	9-11	11-0	8-5	8-9	7-10	6-6	6-1	4-8	4-6
	2-#6	40,000	9-9	10-10	8-3	8-7	7-9	6-4	5-10	4-1	4-0
		60,000	DR	DR	DR	DR	DR	DR	DR	DR	DR
	Center distance A[k, l]		2-6	3-1	1-10	1-11	1-7	1-1	0-11	0-7	0-7
12	Span without stirrups[i, j]		5-5	6-7	4-7	4-10	4-3	3-5	3-3	2-8	2-8
	1-#4	40,000	5-3	6-0	4-8	4-10	4-4	3-7	3-4	2-9	2-8
		60,000	6-5	7-4	5-8	5-10	5-3	4-4	4-1	3-4	3-3
	1-#5	40,000	6-6	7-6	5-9	6-0	5-5	4-5	4-2	3-5	3-4
		60,000	7-11	9-1	7-0	7-3	6-7	5-5	5-1	4-2	4-0
	2-#4 / 1-#6	40,000	7-4	8-5	6-6	6-9	6-1	5-0	4-9	3-10	3-9
		60,000	10-3	11-9	9-1	9-5	8-6	7-0	6-7	5-4	5-3
	2-#5	40,000	10-5	12-0	9-3	9-7	8-8	7-2	6-9	5-5	5-4
		60,000	12-7	14-5	11-2	11-6	10-5	8-7	8-1	6-6	6-4
	2-#6	40,000	12-4	14-2	10-11	11-4	10-2	8-5	7-8	5-7	5-5
		60,000	14-9	17-0	13-1	13-6	12-2	10-0	9-1	6-6	6-4
	Center distance A[k, l]		3-9	4-11	2-11	3-2	2-7	1-9	1-7	1-0	1-0
16	Span without stirrups[i, j]		7-1	9-0	6-4	6-8	5-10	4-9	4-6	3-9	3-8
	1-#4	40,000	5-11	7-0	5-5	5-8	5-1	4-3	4-0	3-3	3-2
		60,000	7-3	8-7	6-8	6-11	6-3	5-2	4-10	3-11	3-10
	1-#5	40,000	7-4	8-9	6-9	7-0	6-4	5-3	4-11	4-0	3-11
		60,000	9-0	10-8	8-3	8-7	7-9	6-5	6-0	4-11	4-9
	2-#4 / 1-#6	40,000	8-4	9-11	7-8	7-11	7-2	5-11	5-7	4-6	4-5
		60,000	10-2	12-0	9-4	9-8	8-9	7-3	6-10	5-6	5-5
	2-#5	40,000	10-4	12-3	9-6	9-10	8-11	7-4	6-11	5-8	5-6
		60,000	14-4	17-1	13-3	13-8	12-4	10-3	9-8	7-10	7-8
	2-#6	40,000	14-1	16-9	13-0	13-5	12-2	10-1	9-6	7-0	6-10
		60,000	17-0	20-2	15-8	16-2	14-7	12-0	10-11	8-0	7-9
	Center distance[k, l]		4-9	6-8	4-0	4-4	3-6	2-5	2-2	1-5	1-4

(continued)

TABLE R611.8(5)—continued
MAXIMUM ALLOWABLE CLEAR SPANS FOR 10-INCH NOMINAL THICK FLAT LINTELS IN LOAD-BEARING WALLS[a, b, c, d, e, f, m]
ROOF CLEAR SPAN 40 FEET AND FLOOR CLEAR SPAN 32 FEET

LINTEL DEPTH, D^g (inches)	NUMBER OF BARS AND BAR SIZE IN TOP AND BOTTOM OF LINTEL	STEEL YIELD STRENGTH[h], f_y (psi)	DESIGN LOADING CONDITION DETERMINED FROM TABLE R611.8(1)									
			1		2		3		4		5	
			Maximum ground snow load (psf)									
			30	70	30	70	30	70	30	70	30	70
			Maximum clear span of lintel (feet - inches)									
20	Span without stirrups[i, j]		8-7	11-4	8-1	8-5	7-5	6-1	5-9	4-10	4-9	
	1-#4	40,000	6-5	7-10	6-2	6-4	5-9	4-9	4-6	3-8	3-7	
	1-#4	60,000	7-10	9-7	7-6	7-9	7-0	5-10	5-6	4-5	4-4	
	1-#5	40,000	8-0	9-9	7-8	7-11	7-2	5-11	5-7	4-6	4-5	
	1-#5	60,000	9-9	11-11	9-4	9-8	8-9	7-3	6-10	5-6	5-5	
	2-#4 1-#6	40,000	9-0	11-1	8-8	8-11	8-1	6-9	6-4	5-2	5-0	
	2-#4 1-#6	60,000	11-0	13-6	10-6	10-11	9-10	8-2	7-9	6-3	6-2	
	2-#5	40,000	11-3	13-9	10-9	11-1	10-0	8-4	7-10	6-5	6-3	
	2-#5	60,000	15-8	19-2	15-0	15-6	14-0	11-8	11-0	8-11	8-9	
	2-#6	40,000	15-5	18-10	14-8	15-2	13-9	11-5	10-9	8-6	8-3	
	2-#6	60,000	18-7	22-9	17-9	18-5	16-7	13-10	12-9	9-5	9-2	
	Center distance A[k, l]		5-7	8-4	5-1	5-5	4-5	3-1	2-9	1-10	1-9	
24	Span without stirrups[i, j]		9-11	13-7	9-9	10-2	9-0	7-5	7-0	5-10	5-9	
	1-#5	40,000	8-6	10-8	8-5	8-8	7-10	6-6	6-2	5-0	4-11	
	1-#5	60,000	10-5	13-0	10-3	10-7	9-7	8-0	7-6	6-1	6-0	
	2-#4 1-#6	40,000	9-7	12-1	9-6	9-9	8-10	7-5	7-0	5-8	5-6	
	2-#4 1-#6	60,000	11-9	14-9	11-7	11-11	10-10	9-0	8-6	6-11	6-9	
	2-#5	40,000	12-0	15-0	11-9	12-2	11-0	9-2	8-8	7-1	6-11	
	2-#5	60,000	14-7	18-3	14-4	14-10	13-5	11-2	10-7	8-7	8-5	
	2-#6	40,000	14-3	17-11	14-1	14-7	13-2	11-0	10-4	8-5	8-3	
	2-#6	60,000	19-11	25-0	19-7	20-3	18-4	15-3	14-5	10-10	10-7	
	Center distance A[k, l]		6-3	9-11	6-1	6-6	5-4	3-9	3-4	2-2	2-1	

For SI: 1 inch = 25.4 mm; 1 foot = 304.8 mm; 1 pound per square foot = 0.0479 kPa; Grade 40 = 280 MPa; Grade 60 = 420 MPa.

Note: Top and bottom reinforcement for lintels without stirrups shown in shaded cells shall be equal to or greater than that required for lintel of the same depth and loading condition that has an allowable clear span that is equal to or greater than that of the lintel without stirrups.

a. See Table R611.3 for tolerances permitted from nominal thickness.

b. Table values are based on concrete with a minimum specified compressive strength of 2,500 psi. See Note j.

c. Table values are based on uniform loading. See Section R611.8.2 for lintels supporting concentrated loads.

d. Deflection criterion is $L/240$, where L is the clear span of the lintel in inches, or $^1/_2$-inch, whichever is less.

e. Linear interpolation is permitted between ground snow loads and between lintel depths.

f. DR indicates design required.

g. Lintel depth, D, is permitted to include the available height of wall located directly above the lintel, provided that the increased lintel depth spans the entire length of the lintel.

h. Stirrups shall be fabricated from reinforcing bars with the same yield strength as that used for the main longitudinal reinforcement.

i. Allowable clear span without stirrups applicable to all lintels of the same depth, D. Top and bottom reinforcement for lintels without stirrups shall not be less than the least amount of reinforcement required for a lintel of the same depth and loading condition with stirrups. All other spans require stirrups spaced at not more than d/2.

j. Where concrete with a minimum specified compressive strength of 3,000 psi is used, clear spans for lintels without stirrups shall be permitted to be multiplied by 1.05. If the increased span exceeds the allowable clear span for a lintel of the same depth and loading condition with stirrups, the top and bottom reinforcement shall be equal to or greater than that required for a lintel of the same depth and loading condition that has an allowable clear span that is equal to or greater than that of the lintel without stirrups that has been increased.

k. Center distance, A, is the center portion of the clear span where stirrups are not required. This is applicable to all longitudinal bar sizes and steel yield strengths.

l. Where concrete with a minimum specified compressive strength of 3,000 psi is used, center distance, A, shall be permitted to be multiplied by 1.10.

m. The maximum clear opening width between two solid wall segments shall be 18 feet (5486 mm). See Section R611.7.2.1. Lintel clear spans in the table greater than 18 feet are shown for interpolation and information only.

TABLE R611.8(6)
MAXIMUM ALLOWABLE CLEAR SPANS FOR 6-INCH THICK WAFFLE-GRID LINTELS IN LOAD-BEARING WALLS[a, b, c, d, e, f, o]
MAXIMUM ROOF CLEAR SPAN 40 FEET AND MAXIMUM FLOOR SPAN 32 FEET

LINTEL DEPTH, D^g (inches)	NUMBER OF BARS AND BAR SIZE IN TOP AND BOTTOM OF LINTEL	STEEL YIELD STRENGTH[h], f_y (psi)	1 (30)	1 (70)	2 (30)	2 (70)	3 (30)	3 (70)	4 (30)	4 (70)	5 (30)	5 (70)
			— Design loading condition determined from Table R611.8(1); Maximum ground snow load (psf); Maximum clear span of lintel (feet - inches)									
8[i]	Span without stirrups[k, l]		2-7	2-9	2-0	2-1	2-0	2-0	2-0	2-0	2-0	2-0
	1-#4	40,000	5-2	5-5	4-0	4-3	3-7	3-3	2-11	2-11	2-4	2-3
	1-#4	60,000	5-9	6-3	4-0	4-3	3-7	3-3	2-11	2-11	2-4	2-3
	1-#5	40,000	5-9	6-3	4-0	4-3	3-7	3-3	2-11	2-11	2-4	2-3
	1-#5	60,000	5-9	6-3	4-0	4-3	3-7	3-3	2-11	2-11	2-4	2-3
	2-#4 1-#6	40,000	5-9	6-3	4-0	4-3	3-7	3-3	2-11	2-11	2-4	2-3
	2-#4 1-#6	60,000	DR	DR	DR	DR	DR	DR	DR	DR	DR	DR
	Center distance A[m, n]		0-9	0-10	0-6	0-6	0-5	0-5	0-4	0-4	STL	STL
12[i]	Span without stirrups[k, l]		2-11	3-1	2-6	2-7	2-5	2-4	2-3	2-3	2-1	2-0
	1-#4	40,000	5-9	6-2	4-8	4-10	4-4	4-1	3-9	3-9	3-2	3-1
	1-#4	60,000	8-0	8-7	6-6	6-9	6-0	5-5	4-11	4-11	3-11	3-10
	1-#5	40,000	8-1	8-9	6-8	6-11	6-0	5-5	4-11	4-11	3-11	3-10
	1-#5	60,000	9-1	10-3	6-8	7-0	6-0	5-5	4-11	4-11	3-11	3-10
	2-#4 1-#6	40,000	9-1	9-9	6-8	7-0	6-0	5-5	4-11	4-11	3-11	3-10
	Center distance A[m, n]		1-3	1-5	0-10	0-11	0-9	0-8	0-6	0-6	STL	STL
16[i]	Span without stirrups[k, l]		4-0	4-4	3-6	3-7	3-4	3-3	3-1	3-1	2-10	2-10
	1-#4	40,000	6-7	7-3	5-6	5-9	5-2	4-10	4-6	4-6	3-9	3-8
	1-#4	60,000	8-0	8-10	6-9	7-0	6-3	5-11	5-5	5-5	4-7	4-5
	1-#5	40,000	8-2	9-0	6-11	7-2	6-5	6-0	5-7	5-7	4-8	4-6
	1-#5	60,000	11-5	12-6	9-3	9-9	8-4	7-7	6-10	6-10	5-6	5-4
	2-#4 1-#6	40,000	10-7	11-7	8-11	9-3	8-3	7-7	6-10	6-10	5-6	5-4
	2-#4 1-#6	60,000	12-2	14-0	9-3	9-9	8-4	7-7	6-10	6-10	5-6	5-4
	2-#5	40,000	12-2	14-2	9-3	9-9	8-4	7-7	6-10	6-10	5-6	5-4
	2-#5	60,000	DR	DR	DR	DR	DR	DR	DR	DR	DR	DR
	Center distance A[m, n]		1-8	2-0	1-2	1-3	1-0	0-11	0-9	0-9	STL	STL
20[i]	Span without stirrups[k, l]		5-0	5-6	4-6	4-7	4-3	4-1	4-0	4-0	3-8	3-8
	1-#4	40,000	7-2	8-2	6-3	6-6	5-10	5-6	5-1	5-1	4-3	4-2
	1-#4	60,000	8-11	9-11	7-8	7-11	7-1	6-8	6-2	6-2	5-2	5-0
	1-#5	40,000	9-1	10-2	7-9	8-1	7-3	6-10	6-4	6-4	5-4	5-2
	1-#5	60,000	12-8	14-2	10-11	11-3	10-2	9-6	8-9	8-9	7-1	6-10
	2-#4 1-#6	40,000	10-3	11-5	8-9	9-1	8-2	7-8	7-1	7-1	6-0	5-10
	2-#4 1-#6	60,000	14-3	15-11	11-9	12-5	10-8	9-9	8-9	8-9	7-1	6-10
	2-#5	40,000	14-6	16-3	11-6	12-1	10-4	9-6	8-6	8-6	6-11	6-8
	2-#5	60,000	DR	DR	DR	DR	DR	DR	DR	DR	DR	DR
	Center distance A[m, n]		2-0	2-6	1-6	1-7	1-3	1-1	1-0	1-0	STL	STL

(continued)

TABLE R611.8(6)—continued
MAXIMUM ALLOWABLE CLEAR SPANS FOR 6-INCH THICK WAFFLE-GRID LINTELS IN LOAD-BEARING WALLS[a, b, c, d, e, f, o]
MAXIMUM ROOF CLEAR SPAN 40 FEET AND MAXIMUM FLOOR SPAN 32 FEET

LINTEL DEPTH, D^g (inches)	NUMBER OF BARS AND BAR SIZE IN TOP AND BOTTOM OF LINTEL	STEEL YIELD STRENGTH[h], f_y (psi)	DESIGN LOADING CONDITION DETERMINED FROM TABLE R611.8(1)								
			1		2		3		4		5
			Maximum ground snow load (psf)								
			30	70	30	70	30	70	30	70	
										30	70
			Maximum clear span of lintel (feet - inches)								
24w[j]	Span without stirrups[k, l]		6-0	6-8	5-5	5-7	5-3	5-0	4-10	4-6	4-5
	1-#4	40,000	7-11	9-0	6-11	7-2	6-5	6-0	5-7	4-8	4-7
		60,000	9-8	10-11	8-5	8-9	7-10	7-4	6-10	5-9	5-7
	1-#5	40,000	9-10	11-2	8-7	8-11	8-0	7-6	7-0	5-10	5-8
		60,000	12-0	13-7	10-6	10-10	9-9	9-2	8-6	7-2	6-11
	2-#4 1-#6	40,000	11-1	12-7	9-8	10-1	9-1	8-6	7-10	6-7	6-5
		60,000	15-6	17-7	13-6	14-0	12-8	11-10	10-8	8-7	8-4
	2-#5	40,000	15-6	17-11	12-8	13-4	11-6	10-7	9-7	7-10	7-7
		60,000	DR	DR	DR	DR	DR	DR	DR	DR	DR
	Center distance A[m, n]		2-4	3-0	1-9	1-11	1-6	1-4	1-2	STL	STL

For SI: 1 inch = 25.4 mm; 1 pound per square foot = 0.0479 kPa; 1 foot = 304.8 mm; Grade 40 = 280 MPa; Grade 60 = 420 MPa.

a. Where lintels are formed with waffle-grid forms, form material shall be removed, if necessary, to create top and bottom flanges of the lintel that are not less than 3 inches in depth (in the vertical direction), are not less than 5 inches (127 mm) in width for 6-inch nominal waffle-grid forms and not less than 7 inches in width for 8-inch nominal waffle-grid forms. See Figure R611.8(3). Flat form lintels shall be permitted in place of waffle-grid lintels. See Tables R611.8(2) through R611.8(5).

b. See Table R611.3 for tolerances permitted from nominal thicknesses and minimum dimensions and spacing of cores.

c. Table values are based on concrete with a minimum specified compressive strength of 2,500 psi (17.2 MPa). See Notes l and n. Table values are based on uniform loading. See Section R611.8.2 for lintels supporting concentrated loads.

d. Deflection criterion is $L/240$, where L is the clear span of the lintel in inches, or $^1/_2$-inch, whichever is less.

e. Linear interpolation is permitted between ground snow loads.

f. DR indicates design required. STL – stirrups required throughout lintel.

g. Lintel depth, D, is permitted to include the available height of wall located directly above the lintel, provided that the increased lintel depth spans the entire length of the lintel.

h. Stirrups shall be fabricated from reinforcing bars with the same yield strength as that used for the main longitudinal reinforcement.

i. Lintels less than 24 inches in depth with stirrups shall be formed from flat-walls forms [see Tables R611.8(2) through R611.8(5)], or, if necessary, form material shall be removed from waffle-grid forms so as to provide the required cover for stirrups. Allowable spans for lintels formed with flat-wall forms shall be determined from Tables R611.8(2) through R611.8(5).

j. Where stirrups are required for 24-inch (610 mm) deep lintels, the spacing shall not exceed 12 inches (305 mm) on center.

k. Allowable clear span without stirrups applicable to all lintels of the same depth, D. Top and bottom reinforcement for lintels without stirrups shall not be less than the least amount of reinforcement required for a lintel of the same depth and loading condition with stirrups. All other spans require stirrups spaced at not more than $d/2$.

l. Where concrete with a minimum specified compressive strength of 3,000 psi is used, clear spans for lintels without stirrups shall be permitted to be multiplied by 1.05. If the increased span exceeds the allowable clear span for a lintel of the same depth and loading condition with stirrups, the top and bottom reinforcement shall be equal to or greater than that required for a lintel of the same depth and loading condition that has an allowable clear span that is equal to or greater than that of the lintel without stirrups that has been increased.

m. Center distance, A, is the center portion of the span where stirrups are not required. This is applicable to all longitudinal bar sizes and steel yield strengths.

n. Where concrete with a minimum specified compressive strength of 3,000 psi is used, center distance, A, shall be permitted to be multiplied by 1.10.

o. The maximum clear opening width between two solid wall segments shall be 18 feet. See Section R611.7.2.1. Lintel spans in the table greater than 18 feet are shown for interpolation and information only.

TABLE R611.8(7)
MAXIMUM ALLOWABLE CLEAR SPANS FOR 8-INCH THICK WAFFLE-GRID LINTELS IN LOAD-BEARING WALLS[a, b, c, d, e, f, o]
MAXIMUM ROOF CLEAR SPAN 40 FEET AND MAXIMUM FLOOR CLEAR SPAN 32 FEET

LINTEL DEPTH, D^g (inches)	NUMBER OF BARS AND BAR SIZE IN TOP AND BOTTOM OF LINTEL	STEEL YIELD STRENGTH[h], f_y (psi)	1	2		3		4		5	
				Maximum ground snow load (psf)							
				30	70	30	70	30	70	30	70
			Maximum clear span of lintel (feet - inches)								
8[i]	Span with stirrups[k, l]		2-6	2-9	2-0	2-1	2-0	2-0	2-0	2-0	2-0
	1-#4	40,000	4-5	4-9	3-7	3-9	3-4	3-0	2-10	2-3	2-2
		60,000	5-6	6-2	4-0	4-3	3-7	3-1	2-10	2-3	2-2
	1-#5	40,000	5-6	6-2	4-0	4-3	3-7	3-1	2-10	2-3	2-2
	Center distance A[m, n]		0-9	0-10	0-6	0-6	0-5	0-4	0-4	STL	STL
12[i]	Span without stirrups[k, l]		2-10	3-1	2-6	2-7	2-5	2-3	2-2	2-0	2-0
	1-#4	40,000	5-7	6-1	4-8	4-10	4-4	3-11	3-8	3-0	2-11
		60,000	6-9	7-5	5-8	5-11	5-4	4-9	4-5	3-8	3-7
	1-#5	40,000	6-11	7-7	5-10	6-0	5-5	4-10	4-6	3-9	3-7
		60,000	8-8	10-1	6-7	7-0	5-11	5-2	4-8	3-9	3-7
	2-#4 1-#6	40,000	8-8	9-10	6-7	7-0	5-11	5-2	4-8	3-9	3-7
		60,000	8-8	10-1	6-7	7-0	5-11	5-2	4-8	3-9	3-7
	Center distance A[m, n]		1-2	1-5	0-10	0-11	0-9	0-7	0-6	STL	STL
16[i]	Span without stirrups[k, l]		3-10	4-3	3-6	3-7	3-4	3-2	3-0	2-10	2-9
	1-#4	40,000	6-5	7-2	5-6	5-9	5-2	4-8	4-4	3-7	3-6
		60,000	7-9	8-9	6-9	7-0	6-3	5-8	5-3	4-4	4-3
	1-#5	40,000	7-11	8-11	6-10	7-1	6-5	5-9	5-4	4-5	4-4
		60,000	9-8	10-11	8-4	8-8	7-10	7-0	6-6	5-2	5-1
	2-#4 1-#6	40,000	9-0	10-1	7-9	8-0	7-3	6-6	6-1	5-0	4-11
		60,000	11-5	13-10	9-2	9-8	8-3	7-2	6-6	5-2	5-1
	Center distance A[m, n]		1-6	1-11	1-2	1-3	1-0	0-10	0-8	STL	STL
20[i]	Span without stirrups[k, l]		4-10	5-5	4-5	4-7	4-3	4-0	3-11	3-7	3-7
	1-#4	40,000	7-0	8-1	6-3	6-5	5-10	5-3	4-11	4-1	3-11
		60,000	8-7	9-10	7-7	7-10	7-1	6-5	6-0	4-11	4-10
	1-#5	40,000	8-9	10-1	7-9	8-0	7-3	6-6	6-1	5-1	4-11
		60,000	10-8	12-3	9-6	9-10	8-10	8-0	7-5	6-2	6-0
	2-#4 1-#6	40,000	9-10	11-4	8-9	9-1	8-2	7-4	6-10	5-8	5-7
		60,000	12-0	13-10	10-8	11-0	9-11	9-0	8-4	6-8	6-6
	2-#5	40,000	12-3	14-1	10-10	11-3	10-2	8-11	8-1	6-6	6-4
		60,000	14-0	17-6	11-8	12-3	10-6	9-1	8-4	6-8	6-6
	Center distance A[m, n]		1-10	2-5	1-5	1-7	1-3	1-0	0-11	STL	STL
24[j]	Span without stirrups[k, l]		5-9	6-7	5-5	5-6	5-2	4-11	4-9	4-5	4-4
	1-#4	40,000	7-6	8-10	6-10	7-1	6-5	5-9	5-5	4-6	4-4
		60,000	9-2	10-9	8-4	8-8	7-10	7-1	6-7	5-6	5-4
	1-#5	40,000	9-5	11-0	8-6	8-10	8-0	7-2	6-8	5-7	5-5
		60,000	11-5	13-5	10-5	10-9	9-9	8-9	8-2	6-10	6-8
	2-#4 1-#6	40,000	10-7	12-5	9-8	10-0	9-0	8-1	7-7	6-3	6-2
		60,000	12-11	15-2	11-9	12-2	11-0	9-11	9-3	7-8	7-6
	2-#5	40,000	13-2	15-6	12-0	12-5	11-2	9-11	9-2	7-5	7-3
		60,000	16-3	21-0	14-1	14-10	12-9	11-1	10-1	8-1	7-11
	2-#6	40,000	14-4	18-5	12-6	13-2	11-5	9-11	9-2	7-5	7-3
	Center distance A[m, n]		2-1	2-11	1-9	1-10	1-6	1-3	1-1	STL	STL

(continued)

TABLE R611.8(7)—continued
MAXIMUM ALLOWABLE CLEAR SPANS FOR 8-INCH THICK WAFFLE-GRID LINTELS IN LOAD-BEARING WALLS[a, b, c, d, e, f, o]
MAXIMUM ROOF CLEAR SPAN 40 FEET AND MAXIMUM FLOOR CLEAR SPAN 32 FEET

For SI: 1 inch = 25.4 mm; 1 pound per square foot = 0.0479 kPa; 1 foot = 304.8 mm; Grade 40 = 280 MPa; Grade 60 = 420 MPa.

a. Where lintels are formed with waffle-grid forms, form material shall be removed, if necessary, to create top and bottom flanges of the lintel that are not less than 3 inches in depth (in the vertical direction), are not less than 5 inches in width for 6-inch nominal waffle-grid forms and not less than 7 inches in width for 8-inch nominal waffle-grid forms. See Figure R611.8(3). Flat form lintels shall be permitted in lieu of waffle-grid lintels. See Tables R611.8(2) through R611.8(5).

b. See Table R611.3 for tolerances permitted from nominal thicknesses and minimum dimensions and spacing of cores.

c. Table values are based on concrete with a minimum specified compressive strength of 2,500 psi (17.2 MPa). See Notes l and n. Table values are based on uniform loading. See Section R611.8.2 for lintels supporting concentrated loads.

d. Deflection criterion is $L/240$, where L is the clear span of the lintel in inches, or $^1/_2$-inch, whichever is less.

e. Linear interpolation is permitted between ground snow loads.

f. DR indicates design required. STL – stirrups required throughout lintel.

g. Lintel depth, D, is permitted to include the available height of wall located directly above the lintel, provided that the increased lintel depth spans the entire length of the lintel.

h. Stirrups shall be fabricated from reinforcing bars with the same yield strength as that used for the main longitudinal reinforcement.

i. Lintels less than 24 inches in depth with stirrups shall be formed from flat-walls forms [see Tables R611.8(2) through R611.8(5)], or, if necessary, form material shall be removed from waffle-grid forms so as to provide the required cover for stirrups. Allowable spans for lintels formed with flat-wall forms shall be determined from Tables R611.8(2) through R611.8(5).

j. Where stirrups are required for 24-inch (610 mm) deep lintels, the spacing shall not exceed 12 inches on center.

k. Allowable clear span without stirrups applicable to all lintels of the same depth, D. Top and bottom reinforcement for lintels without stirrups shall not be less than the least amount of reinforcement required for a lintel of the same depth and loading condition with stirrups. All other spans require stirrups spaced at not more than $d/2$.

l. Where concrete with a minimum specified compressive strength of 3,000 psi is used, clear spans for lintels without stirrups shall be permitted to be multiplied by 1.05. If the increased span exceeds the allowable clear span for a lintel of the same depth and loading condition with stirrups, the top and bottom reinforcement shall be equal to or greater than that required for a lintel of the same depth and loading condition that has an allowable clear span that is equal to or greater than that of the lintel without stirrups that has been increased.

m. Center distance, A, is the center portion of the span where stirrups are not required. This is applicable to all longitudinal bar sizes and steel yield strengths.

n. Where concrete with a minimum specified compressive strength of 3,000 psi is used, center distance, A, shall be permitted to be multiplied by 1.10.

o. The maximum clear opening width between two solid wall segments shall be 18 feet. See Section R611.7.2.1. Lintel spans in the table greater than 18 feet are shown for interpolation and information only.

TABLE R611.8(8)
MAXIMUM ALLOWABLE CLEAR SPANS FOR 6-INCH THICK SCREEN-GRID LINTELS IN LOAD-BEARING WALLS[a, b, c, d, e, f, p]
ROOF CLEAR SPAN 40 FEET AND FLOOR CLEAR SPAN 32 FEET

LINTEL DEPTH, D[g] (inches)	NUMBER OF BARS AND BAR SIZE IN TOP AND BOTTOM OF LINTEL	STEEL YIELD STRENGTH[h], f_y (psi)	DESIGN LOADING CONDITION DETERMINED FROM TABLE R611.8(1)								
			1	2		3		4		5	
				Maximum ground snow load (psf)							
				30	70	30	70	30	70	30	70
			Maximum clear span of lintel (feet - inches)								
12[i,j]	Span without stirrups		2-9	2-11	2-4	2-5	2-3	2-3	2-2	2-0	2-0
16[i,j]	Span without stirrups		3-9	4-0	3-4	3-5	3-2	3-1	3-0	2-9	2-9
20[i,j]	Span without stirrups		4-9	5-1	4-3	4-4	4-1	4-0	3-10	3-7	3-7
24[k]	Span without stirrups[l, m]		5-8	6-3	5-2	5-3	5-0	4-10	4-8	4-4	4-4
	1-#4	40,000	7-11	9-0	6-11	7-2	6-5	6-1	5-8	4-9	4-7
		60,000	9-9	11-0	8-5	8-9	7-10	7-5	6-10	5-9	5-7
	1-#5	40,000	9-11	11-2	8-7	8-11	8-0	7-7	7-0	5-11	5-9
		60,000	12-1	13-8	10-6	10-10	9-9	9-3	8-6	7-2	7-0
	2-#4 1-#6	40,000	11-2	12-8	9-9	10-1	9-1	8-7	7-11	6-8	6-6
		60,000	15-7	17-7	12-8	13-4	11-6	10-8	9-8	7-11	7-8
	2-#5	40,000	14-11	18-0	12-2	12-10	11-1	10-3	9-4	7-8	7-5
		60,000	DR	DR	DR	DR	DR	DR	DR	DR	DR
	Center distance A[n, o]		2-0	2-6	1-6	1-7	1-4	1-2	1-0	STL	STL

For SI: 1 inch = 25.4 mm; 1 pound per square foot = 0.0479 kPa; 1 foot = 304.8 mm; Grade 40 = 280 MPa; Grade 60 = 420 MPa.

a. Where lintels are formed with screen-grid forms, form material shall be removed if necessary to create top and bottom flanges of the lintel that are not less than 5 inches in width and not less than 2.5 inches in depth (in the vertical direction). See Figure R611.8(4). Flat form lintels shall be permitted in lieu of screen-grid lintels. See Tables R611.8(2) through R611.8(5).

b. See Table R611.3 for tolerances permitted from nominal thickness and minimum dimensions and spacings of cores.

c. Table values are based on concrete with a minimum specified compressive strength of 2,500 psi. See Notes m and o. Table values are based on uniform loading. See Section R611.7.2.1 for lintels supporting concentrated loads.

d. Deflection criterion is L/240, where L is the clear span of the lintel in inches, or $1/2$-inch, whichever is less.

e. Linear interpolation is permitted between ground snow loads.

f. DR indicates design required. STL indicates stirrups required throughout lintel.

g. Lintel depth, D, is permitted to include the available height of wall located directly above the lintel, provided that the increased lintel depth spans the entire length of the lintel.

h. Stirrups shall be fabricated from reinforcing bars with the same yield strength as that used for the main longitudinal reinforcement.

i. Stirrups are not required for lintels less than 24 inches in depth fabricated from screen-grid forms. Top and bottom reinforcement shall consist of a No. 4 bar having a yield strength of 40,000 psi or 60,000 psi.

j. Lintels between 12 and 24 inches in depth with stirrups shall be formed from flat-wall forms [see Tables R611.8(2) through R611.8(5)], or form material shall be removed from screen-grid forms to provide a concrete section comparable to that required for a flat wall. Allowable spans for flat lintels with stirrups shall be determined from Tables R611.8(2) through R6111.8(5).

k. Where stirrups are required for 24-inch deep lintels, the spacing shall not exceed 12 inches on center.

l. Allowable clear span without stirrups applicable to all lintels of the same depth, D. Top and bottom reinforcement for lintels without stirrups shall not be less than the least amount of reinforcement required for a lintel of the same depth and loading condition with stirrups. All other spans require stirrups spaced at not more than 12 inches.

m. Where concrete with a minimum specified compressive strength of 3,000 psi is used, clear spans for lintels without stirrups shall be permitted to be multiplied by 1.05. If the increased span exceeds the allowable clear span for a lintel of the same depth and loading condition with stirrups, the top and bottom reinforcement shall be equal to or greater than that required for a lintel of the same depth and loading condition that has an allowable clear span that is equal to or greater than that of the lintel without stirrups that has been increased.

n. Center distance, A, is the center portion of the span where stirrups are not required. This is applicable to all longitudinal bar sizes and steel yield strengths.

o. Where concrete with a minimum specified compressive strength of 3,000 psi is used, center distance, A, shall be permitted to be multiplied by 1.10.

p. The maximum clear opening width between two solid wall segments shall be 18 feet (5486 mm). See Section R611.7.2.1. Lintel spans in the table greater than 18 feet are shown for interpolation and information only.

TABLE R611.8(9)
MAXIMUM ALLOWABLE CLEAR SPANS FOR FLAT LINTELS WITHOUT STIRRUPS IN NONLOAD-BEARING WALLS[a, b, c, d, e, g, h]

LINTEL DEPTH, D^l (inches)	NUMBER OF BARS AND BAR SIZE	STEEL YIELD STRENGTH, f_y (psi)	NOMINAL WALL THICKNESS (inches)							
			4		6		8		10	
			Lintel Supporting							
			Concrete Wall	Light-framed Gable	Concrete Wall	Light-framed Gable	Concrete Wall	Light-framed Gable	Concrete Wall	Light-framed Gable
			Maximum Clear Span of Lintel (feet - inches)							
8	1-#4	40,000	10-11	11-5	9-7	11-2	7-10	9-5	7-3	9-2
		60,000	12-5	11-7	10-11	13-5	9-11	13-2	9-3	12-10
	1-#5	40,000	12-7	11-7	11-1	13-8	10-1	13-5	9-4	13-1
		60,000	DR	DR	12-7	16-4	11-6	14-7	10-9	14-6
	2-#4 1-#6	40,000	DR	DR	12-0	15-3	10-11	15-0	10-2	14-8
		60,000	DR	DR	DR	DR	12-2	15-3	11-7	15-3
	2-#5	40,000	DR	DR	DR	DR	12-7	16-7	11-9	16-7
		60,000	DR	DR	DR	DR	DR	DR	13-3	16-7
	2-#6	40,000	DR	DR	DR	DR	DR	DR	13-2	17-8
		60,000	DR	DR	DR	DR	DR	DR	DR	DR
12	1-#4	40,000	11-5	9-10	10-6	12-0	9-6	11-6	8-9	11-1
		60,000	11-5	9-10	11-8	13-3	10-11	14-0	10-1	13-6
	1-#5	40,000	11-5	9-10	11-8	13-3	11-1	14-4	10-3	13-9
		60,000	11-5	9-10	11-8	13-3	11-10	16-0	11-9	16-9
	2-#4 1-#6	40,000	DR	DR	11-8	13-3	11-10	16-0	11-2	15-6
		60,000	DR	DR	11-8	13-3	11-10	16-0	11-11	18-4
	2-#5	40,000	DR	DR	11-8	13-3	11-10	16-0	11-11	18-4
		60,000	DR	DR	11-8	13-3	11-10	16-0	11-11	18-4
16	1-#4	40,000	13-6	13-0	11-10	13-8	10-7	12-11	9-11	12-4
		60,000	13-6	13-0	13-8	16-7	12-4	15-9	11-5	15-0
	1-#5	40,000	13-6	13-0	13-10	17-0	12-6	16-1	11-7	15-4
		60,000	13-6	13-0	13-10	17-1	14-0	19-7	13-4	18-8
	2-#4 1-#6	40,000	13-6	13-0	13-10	17-1	13-8	18-2	12-8	17-4
		60,000	13-6	13-0	13-10	17-1	14-0	20-3	14-1	—
	2-#5	40,000	13-6	13-0	13-10	17-1	14-0	20-3	14-1	—
		60,000	DR	DR	13-10	17-1	14-0	20-3	14-1	—
20	1-#4	40,000	14-11	15-10	13-0	14-10	11-9	13-11	10-10	13-2
		60,000	15-3	15-10	14-11	18-1	13-6	17-0	12-6	16-2
	1-#5	40,000	15-3	15-10	15-2	18-6	13-9	17-5	12-8	16-6
		60,000	15-3	15-10	15-8	20-5	15-9	—	14-7	20-1
	2-#4 1-#6	40,000	15-3	15-10	15-8	20-5	14-11	—	13-10	—
		60,000	15-3	15-10	15-8	20-5	15-10	—	15-11	—
	2-#5	40,000	15-3	15-10	15-8	20-5	15-10	—	15-11	—
		60,000	15-3	15-10	15-8	20-5	15-10	—	15-11	—
24	1-#4	40,000	16-1	17-1	13-11	15-10	12-7	14-9	11-8	13-10
		60,000	16-11	18-5	16-1	19-3	14-6	18-0	13-5	17-0
	1-#5	40,000	16-11	18-5	16-3	19-8	14-9	18-5	13-8	17-4
		60,000	16-11	18-5	17-4	—	17-0	—	15-8	—
	2-#4 1-#6	40,000	16-11	18-5	17-4	—	16-1	—	14-10	—
		60,000	16-11	18-5	17-4	—	17-6	—	17-1	—
	2-#5	40,000	16-11	18-5	17-4	—	17-6	—	17-4	—
		60,000	16-11	18-5	17-4	—	17-6	—	17-8	—

(continued)

TABLE R611.8(9)—continued
MAXIMUM ALLOWABLE CLEAR SPANS FOR FLAT LINTELS WITHOUT STIRRUPS IN NONLOAD-BEARING WALLS[a, b, c, d, e, g, h]
ROOF CLEAR SPAN 40 FEET AND FLOOR CLEAR SPAN 32 FEET

For SI: 1 inch = 25.4 mm; 1 foot = 304.8 mm; Grade 40 = 280 MPa; Grade 60 = 420 MPa.

a. See Table R611.3 for tolerances permitted from nominal thickness.

b. Table values are based on concrete with a minimum specified compressive strength of 2,500 psi. See Note e.

c. Deflection criterion is $L/240$, where L is the clear span of the lintel in inches, or $^1/_2$-inch, whichever is less.

d. Linear interpolation between lintels depths, D, is permitted provided the two cells being used to interpolate are shaded.

e. Where concrete with a minimum specified compressive strength of 3,000 psi is used, spans in cells that are shaded shall be permitted to be multiplied by 1.05.

f. Lintel depth, D, is permitted to include the available height of wall located directly above the lintel, provided that the increased lintel depth spans the entire length of the lintel.

g. DR indicates design required.

h. The maximum clear opening width between two solid wall segments shall be 18 feet (5486 mm). See Section R611.7.2.1. Lintel spans in the table greater than 18 feet are shown for interpolation and information purposes only.

TABLE R611.8(10)
MAXIMUM ALLOWABLE CLEAR SPANS FOR WAFFLE-GRID AND SCREEN GRID LINTELS
WITHOUT STIRRUPS IN NONLOAD-BEARING WALLS[c, d, e, f, g]

LINTEL DEPTH[h], D (inches)	FORM TYPE AND NOMINAL WALL THICKNESS (inches)					
	6-inch Waffle-grid[a]		8-inch Waffle-grid[a]		6-inch Screen-grid[b]	
	Lintel supporting					
	Concrete Wall	Light-framed Gable	Concrete Wall	Light-framed Gable	Concrete Wall	Light-framed Gable
	Maximum Clear Span of Lintel (feet - inches)					
8	10-3	8-8	8-8	8-3	—	—
12	9-2	7-6	7-10	7-1	8-8	6-9
16	10-11	10-0	9-4	9-3	—	—
20	12-5	12-2	10-7	11-2	—	—
24	13-9	14-2	11-10	12-11	13-0	12-9

For SI: 1 inch = 25.4 mm; 1 foot = 304.8 mm; Grade 40 = 280 MPa; Grade 60 = 420 MPa

a. Where lintels are formed with waffle-grid forms, form material shall be removed, if necessary, to create top and bottom flanges of the lintel that are not less than 3 inches in depth (in the vertical direction), are not less than 5 inches in width for 6-inch waffle-grid forms and not less than 7 inches in width for 8-inch waffle-grid forms. See Figure R611.8(3). Flat form lintels shall be permitted in lieu of waffle-grid lintels. See Tables R611.8(2) through R611.8(5).

b. Where lintels are formed with screen-grid forms, form material shall be removed if necessary to create top and bottom flanges of the lintel that are not less than 5 inches in width and not less than 2.5 inches in depth (in the vertical direction). See Figure R611.8(4). Flat form lintels shall be permitted in lieu of screen-grid lintels. See Tables R611.8(2) through R611.8(5).

c. See Table R611.3 for tolerances permitted from nominal thickness and minimum dimensions and spacing of cores.

d. Table values are based on concrete with a minimum specified compressive strength of 2,500 psi. See Note g.

e. Deflection criterion is $L/240$, where L is the clear span of the lintel in inches, or $^1/_2$-inch, whichever is less.

f. Top and bottom reinforcement shall consist of a No. 4 bar having a minimum yield strength of 40,000 psi.

g. Where concrete with a minimum specified compressive strength of 3,000 psi is used, spans in shaded cells shall be permitted to be multiplied by 1.05.

h. Lintel depth, D, is permitted to include the available height of wall located directly above the lintel, provided that the increased lintel depth spans the entire length of the lintel.

R611.9 Requirements for connections–general. Concrete walls shall be connected to footings, floors, ceilings and roofs in accordance with this section.

R611.9.1 Connections between concrete walls and light-framed floor, ceiling and roof systems. Connections between concrete walls and light-framed floor, ceiling and roof systems using the prescriptive details of Figures R611.9(1) through R611.9(12) shall comply with this section and Sections R611.9.2 and R611.9.3.

R611.9.1.1 Anchor bolts. Anchor bolts used to connect light-framed floor, ceiling and roof systems to concrete walls in accordance with Figures R611.9(1) through R611.9(12) shall have heads, or shall be rods with threads on both ends with a hex or square nut on the end embedded in the concrete. Bolts and threaded rods shall comply with Section R611.5.2.2. Anchor bolts with J- or L-hooks shall not be used where the connection details in these figures are used.

R611.9.1.2 Removal of stay-in-place form material at bolts. Holes in stay-in-place forms for installing bolts for attaching face-mounted wood ledger boards to the wall shall be a minimum of 4 inches (102 mm) in diameter for forms not greater than $1^1/_2$ inches (38 mm) in thickness, and increased 1 inch (25 mm) in diameter for each $^1/_2$-inch (13 mm) increase in form thickness. Holes in stay-in-place forms for installing bolts for attaching face-mounted cold-formed steel tracks to the wall shall be a minimum of 4 inches (102 mm) square. The wood ledger board or steel track shall be in direct contact with the concrete at each bolt location.

> **Exception:** A vapor retarder or other material less than or equal to $^1/_{16}$-inch (1.6 mm) in thickness is permitted to be installed between the wood ledger or cold-formed track and the concrete.

R611.9.2 Connections between concrete walls and light-framed floor systems. Connections between concrete walls and light-framed floor systems shall be in accordance with one of the following:

1. For floor systems of wood frame construction, the provisions of Section R611.9.1 and the prescriptive details of Figures R611.9(1) through R611.9(4), where permitted by the tables accompanying those figures. Portions of connections of wood-framed floor systems not noted in the figures shall be in accordance with Section R502, or AF&PA/WFCM, if applicable.

2. For floor systems of cold-formed steel construction, the provisions of Section R611.9.1 and the prescriptive details of Figures R611.9(5) through R611.9(8), where permitted by the tables accompanying those figures. Portions of connections of cold-formed-steel framed floor systems not noted in the figures shall be in accordance with Section R505, or AISI S230, if applicable.

3. Proprietary connectors selected to resist loads and load combinations in accordance with Appendix A (ASD) or Appendix B (LRFD) of PCA 100.

4. An engineered design using loads and load combinations in accordance with Appendix A (ASD) or Appendix B (LRFD) of PCA 100.

5. An engineered design using loads and material design provisions in accordance with this code, or in accordance with ASCE 7, ACI 318, and AF&PA/NDS for wood frame construction or AISI S100 for cold-formed steel frame construction.

R611.9.3 Connections between concrete walls and light-framed ceiling and roof systems. Connections between concrete walls and light-framed ceiling and roof systems shall be in accordance with one of the following:

1. For ceiling and roof systems of wood frame construction, the provisions of Section R611.9.1 and the prescriptive details of Figures R611.9(9) and R611.9(10), where permitted by the tables accompanying those figures. Portions of connections of wood-framed ceiling and roof systems not noted in the figures shall be in accordance with Section R802, or AF&PA/WFCM, if applicable.

2. For ceiling and roof systems of cold-formed-steel construction, the provisions of Section R611.9.1 and the prescriptive details of Figures R611.9(11) and R611.9(12), where permitted by the tables accompanying those figures. Portions of connections of cold-formed-steel framed ceiling and roof systems not noted in the figures shall be in accordance with Section R804, or AISI S230, if applicable.

3. Proprietary connectors selected to resist loads and load combinations in accordance with Appendix A (ASD) or Appendix B (LRFD) of PCA 100.

4. An engineered design using loads and load combinations in accordance with Appendix A (ASD) or Appendix B (LRFD) of PCA 100.

5. An engineered design using loads and material design provisions in accordance with this code, or in accordance with ASCE 7, ACI 318, and AF&PA/NDS for wood-frame construction or AISI S100 for cold-formed-steel frame construction.

R611.10 Floor, roof and ceiling diaphragms. Floors and roofs in all buildings with exterior walls of concrete shall be designed and constructed as *diaphragms*. Where gable-end walls occur, ceilings shall also be designed and constructed as *diaphragms*. The design and construction of floors, roofs and ceilings of wood framing or cold-formed-steel framing serving as *diaphragms* shall comply with the applicable requirements of this code, or AF&PA/WFCM or AISI S230, if applicable.

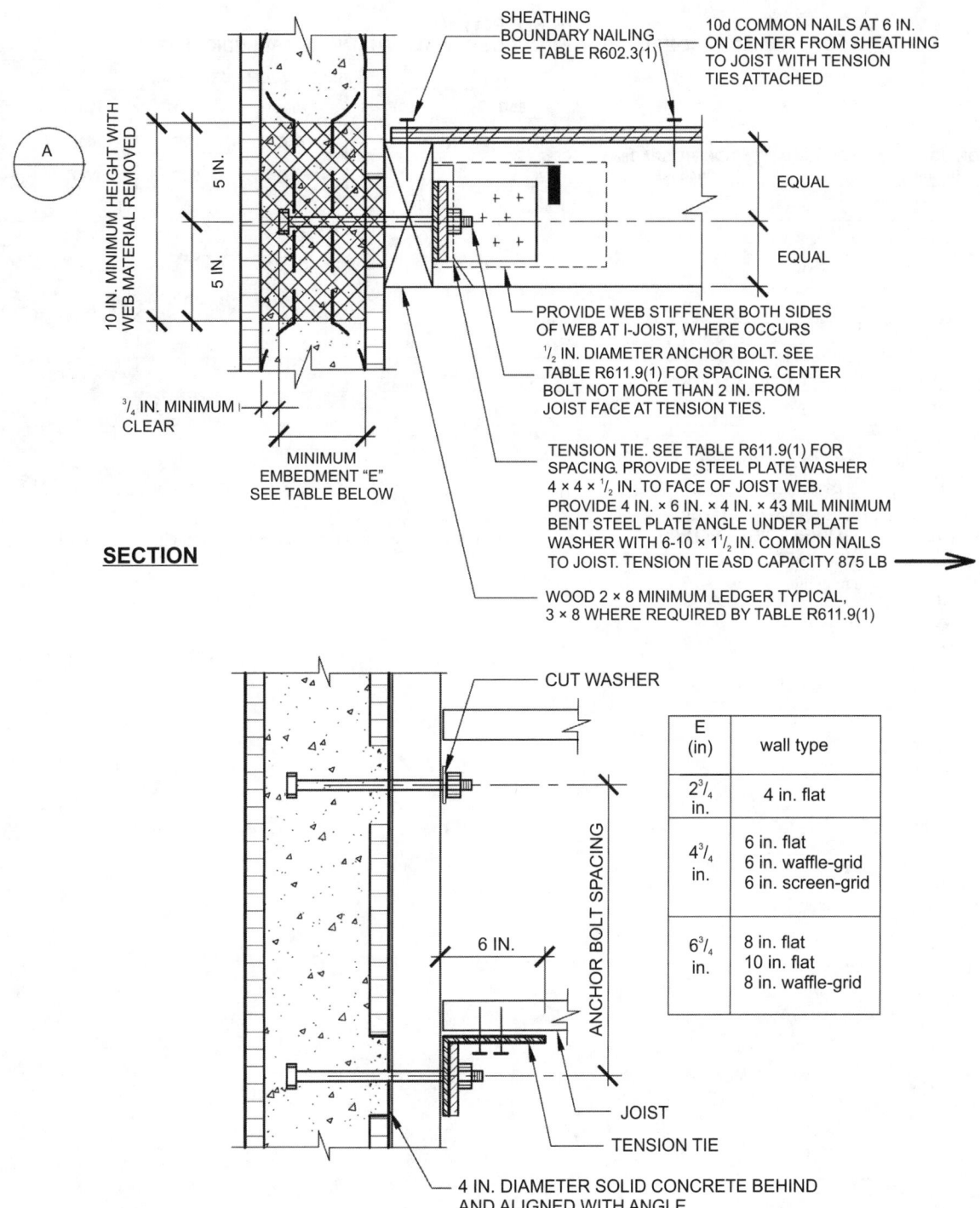

SECTION

DETAIL A – PLAN VIEW

E (in)	wall type
$2^3/_4$ in.	4 in. flat
$4^3/_4$ in.	6 in. flat 6 in. waffle-grid 6 in. screen-grid
$6^3/_4$ in.	8 in. flat 10 in. flat 8 in. waffle-grid

For SI: 1 mil = 0.0254 mm, 1 inch = 25.4 mm, 1 pound-force = 4.448 N.

FIGURE R611.9(1)
WOOD FRAMED FLOOR TO SIDE OF CONCRETE WALL, FRAMING PERPENDICULAR

TABLE R611.9(1)
WOOD FRAMED FLOOR TO SIDE OF CONCRETE WALL, FRAMING PERPENDICULAR[a, b, c]

ANCHOR BOLT SPACING (inches)	TENSION TIE SPACING (inches)	BASIC WIND SPEED (mph)					
		85B	90B	100B / 85C	110B / 90C / 85D	120B / 100C / 90D	130B / 110C / 100D
12	12						
12	24						
12	36				▓	▓	▓
12	48			▓	▓	▓	▓
16	16					A	A
16	32					▓	▓
16	48			▓	▓	▓	▓
19.2	19.2	A	A	A	A	A	▓
19.2	38.4	A	A	A	▓	▓	▓

For SI: 1 inch = 25.4 mm; 1 mile per hour = 0.447 m/s.

a. This table is for use with the detail in Figure R611.9(1). Use of this detail is permitted where a cell is not shaded and prohibited where shaded.

b. Wall design per other provisions of Section R611 is required.

c. Letter "A" indicates that a minimum nominal 3 × 8 ledger is required.

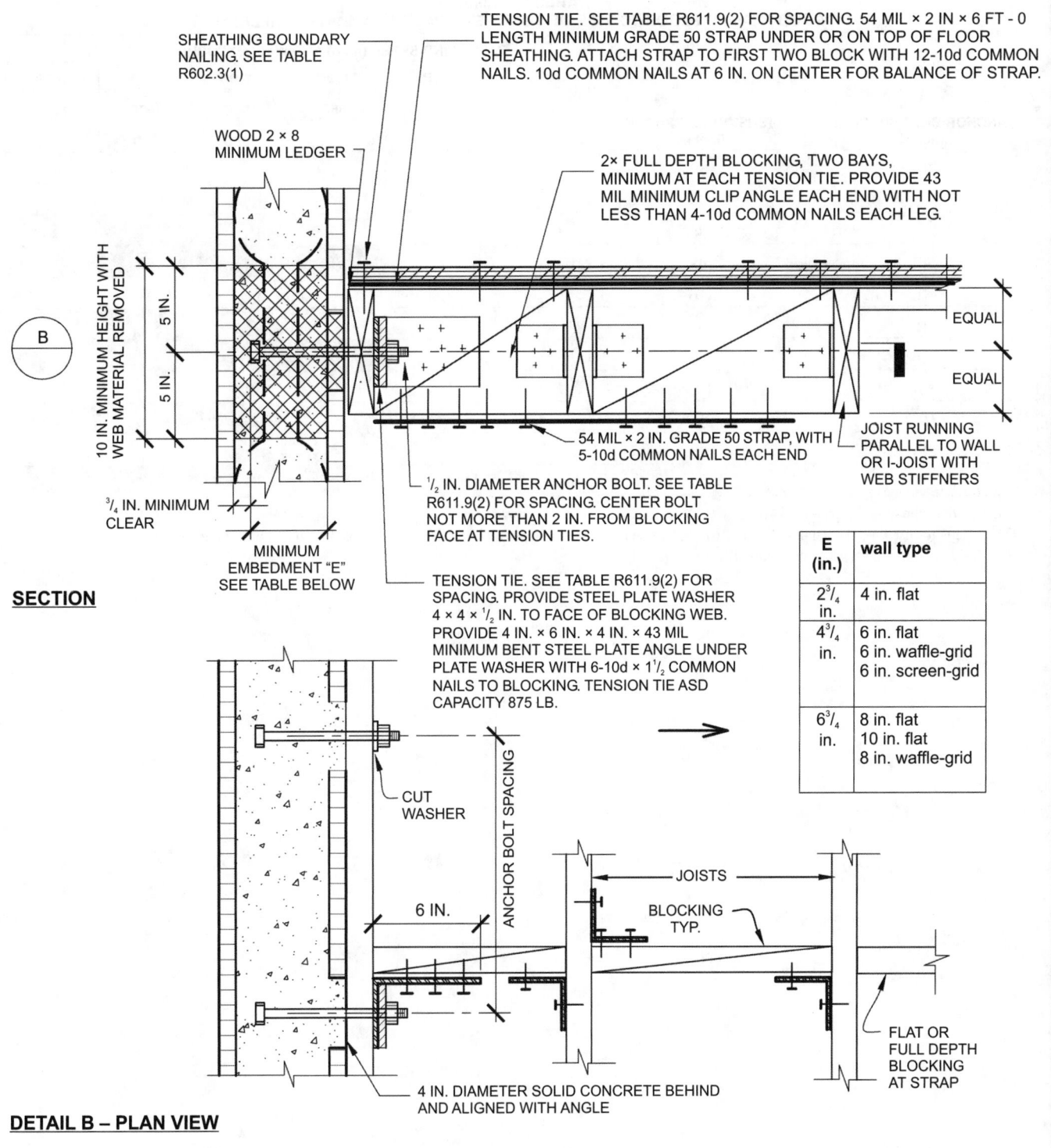

SHEATHING BOUNDARY NAILING. SEE TABLE R602.3(1)

TENSION TIE. SEE TABLE R611.9(2) FOR SPACING. 54 MIL × 2 IN × 6 FT - 0 LENGTH MINIMUM GRADE 50 STRAP UNDER OR ON TOP OF FLOOR SHEATHING. ATTACH STRAP TO FIRST TWO BLOCK WITH 12-10d COMMON NAILS. 10d COMMON NAILS AT 6 IN. ON CENTER FOR BALANCE OF STRAP.

WOOD 2 × 8 MINIMUM LEDGER

2× FULL DEPTH BLOCKING, TWO BAYS, MINIMUM AT EACH TENSION TIE. PROVIDE 43 MIL MINIMUM CLIP ANGLE EACH END WITH NOT LESS THAN 4-10d COMMON NAILS EACH LEG.

10 IN. MINIMUM HEIGHT WITH WEB MATERIAL REMOVED

5 IN.

5 IN.

EQUAL

EQUAL

JOIST RUNNING PARALLEL TO WALL OR I-JOIST WITH WEB STIFFNERS

54 MIL × 2 IN. GRADE 50 STRAP, WITH 5-10d COMMON NAILS EACH END

$^3/_4$ IN. MINIMUM CLEAR

$^1/_2$ IN. DIAMETER ANCHOR BOLT. SEE TABLE R611.9(2) FOR SPACING. CENTER BOLT NOT MORE THAN 2 IN. FROM BLOCKING FACE AT TENSION TIES.

MINIMUM EMBEDMENT "E" SEE TABLE BELOW

TENSION TIE. SEE TABLE R611.9(2) FOR SPACING. PROVIDE STEEL PLATE WASHER 4 × 4 × $^1/_2$ IN. TO FACE OF BLOCKING WEB. PROVIDE 4 IN. × 6 IN. × 4 IN. × 43 MIL MINIMUM BENT STEEL PLATE ANGLE UNDER PLATE WASHER WITH 6-10d × $1^1/_2$ COMMON NAILS TO BLOCKING. TENSION TIE ASD CAPACITY 875 LB.

E (in.)	wall type
$2^3/_4$ in.	4 in. flat
$4^3/_4$ in.	6 in. flat 6 in. waffle-grid 6 in. screen-grid
$6^3/_4$ in.	8 in. flat 10 in. flat 8 in. waffle-grid

SECTION

CUT WASHER

ANCHOR BOLT SPACING

6 IN.

JOISTS

BLOCKING TYP.

4 IN. DIAMETER SOLID CONCRETE BEHIND AND ALIGNED WITH ANGLE

FLAT OR FULL DEPTH BLOCKING AT STRAP

DETAIL B – PLAN VIEW

For SI: 1 mil = 0.0254 mm, 1 inch = 25.4 mm, 1 foot = 304.8 mm, 1 pound-force = 4.448 N.

FIGURE R611.9(2)
WOOD FRAMED FLOOR TO SIDE OF CONCRETE WALL FRAMING PARALLEL

TABLE R611.9(2)
WOOD FRAMED FLOOR TO SIDE OF CONCRETE WALL, FRAMING PARALLEL[a, b]

ANCHOR BOLT SPACING (inches)	TENSION TIE SPACING (inches)	BASIC WIND SPEED (mph) AND WIND EXPOSURE CATEGORY					
		85b	90B	100B / 85C	110B / 90C / 85D	120B / 100C / 90D	130B / 110C / 100D
12	12						
12	24						
12	36					shaded	shaded
12	48				shaded	shaded	shaded
16	16						
16	32						shaded
16	48				shaded	shaded	shaded
19.2	19.2						
19.2	38.4					shaded	shaded
24	24						
24	48				shaded	shaded	shaded

For SI: 1 inch = 25.4 mm; 1 mph = 0.447 m/s.

a. This table is for use with the detail in Figure R611.9(2). Use of this detail is permitted where a cell is not shaded and prohibited where shaded.

b. Wall design per other provisions of Section R611 is required.

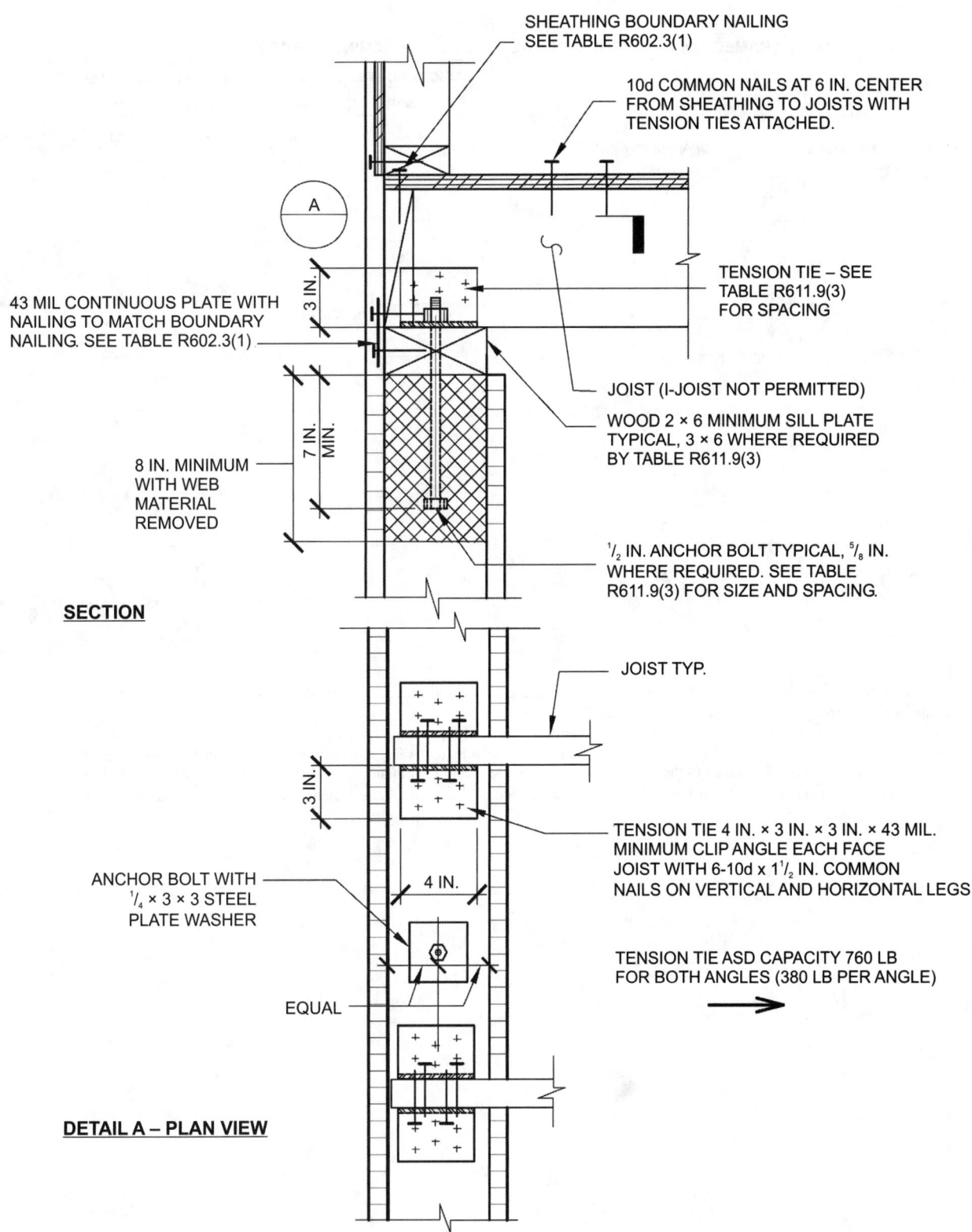

SHEATHING BOUNDARY NAILING
SEE TABLE R602.3(1)

10d COMMON NAILS AT 6 IN. CENTER
FROM SHEATHING TO JOISTS WITH
TENSION TIES ATTACHED.

TENSION TIE – SEE
TABLE R611.9(3)
FOR SPACING

JOIST (I-JOIST NOT PERMITTED)

WOOD 2 × 6 MINIMUM SILL PLATE
TYPICAL, 3 × 6 WHERE REQUIRED
BY TABLE R611.9(3)

$^1/_2$ IN. ANCHOR BOLT TYPICAL, $^5/_8$ IN.
WHERE REQUIRED. SEE TABLE
R611.9(3) FOR SIZE AND SPACING.

43 MIL CONTINUOUS PLATE WITH
NAILING TO MATCH BOUNDARY
NAILING. SEE TABLE R602.3(1)

3 IN.

7 IN. MIN.

8 IN. MINIMUM
WITH WEB
MATERIAL
REMOVED

SECTION

A

JOIST TYP.

3 IN.

TENSION TIE 4 IN. × 3 IN. × 3 IN. × 43 MIL.
MINIMUM CLIP ANGLE EACH FACE
JOIST WITH 6-10d x 1$^1/_2$ IN. COMMON
NAILS ON VERTICAL AND HORIZONTAL LEGS

ANCHOR BOLT WITH
$^1/_4$ × 3 × 3 STEEL
PLATE WASHER

4 IN.

TENSION TIE ASD CAPACITY 760 LB
FOR BOTH ANGLES (380 LB PER ANGLE)

EQUAL

DETAIL A – PLAN VIEW

For SI: 1 mil = 0.0254 mm, 1 inch = 25.4 mm, 1 pound-force = 4.448 N.

FIGURE R611.9(3)
WOOD FRAMED FLOOR TO TOP OF CONCRETE WALL FRAMING PERPENDICULAR

TABLE R611.9(3)
WOOD FRAMED FLOOR TO TOP OF CONCRETE WALL, FRAMING PERPENDICULAR[a, b, c, d, e]

ANCHOR BOLT SPACING (inches)	TENSION TIE SPACING (inches)	BASIC WIND SPEED (mph) AND WIND EXPOSURE CATEGORY					
		85B	90B	100B / 85C	110B / 90C / 85D	120B / 100C / 90D	130B / 110C / 100D
12	12						
12	24						
12	36						(shaded)
12	48				(shaded)	(shaded)	(shaded)
16	16					6 A	6 B
16	32					6 A	6 B
16	48					(shaded)	(shaded)
19.2	19.2				6 A	6 A	6 B
19.2	38.4				6 A	6 A	(shaded)
24	24			6 A	6 B	6 A	
24	48			6 A	(shaded)	(shaded)	(shaded)

For SI: 1 inch = 25.4 mm; 1 mile per hour = 0.447 m/s.

a. This table is for use with the detail in Figure R611.9(3). Use of this detail is permitted where cell is not shaded, prohibited where shaded.

b. Wall design per other provisions in Section R611 is required.

c. For wind design, minimum 4-inch nominal wall is permitted in unshaded cells with no number.

d. Number 6 indicates minimum permitted nominal wall thickness in inches necessary to develop required strength (capacity) of connection. As a minimum, this nominal thickness shall occur in the portion of the wall indicated by the cross-hatching in Figure R611.9(3). For the remainder of the wall, see Note b.

e. Letter "A" indicates that a minimum nominal 3 × 6 sill plate is required. Letter "B" indicates that a $^{5}/_{8}$ inch (16 mm) diameter anchor bolt and a minimal nominal 3 × 6 sill plate are required.

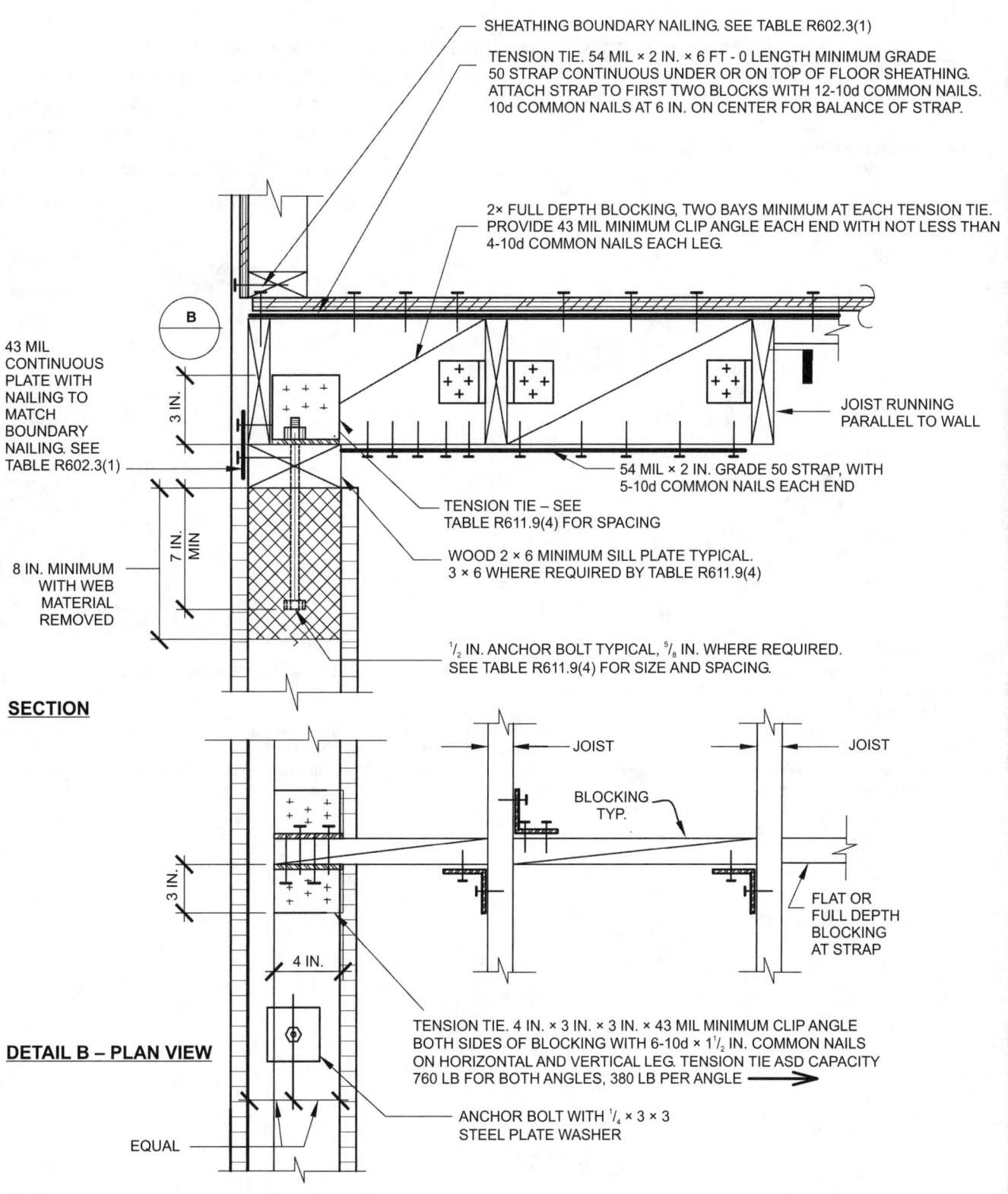

SHEATHING BOUNDARY NAILING. SEE TABLE R602.3(1)

TENSION TIE. 54 MIL × 2 IN. × 6 FT - 0 LENGTH MINIMUM GRADE 50 STRAP CONTINUOUS UNDER OR ON TOP OF FLOOR SHEATHING. ATTACH STRAP TO FIRST TWO BLOCKS WITH 12-10d COMMON NAILS. 10d COMMON NAILS AT 6 IN. ON CENTER FOR BALANCE OF STRAP.

2× FULL DEPTH BLOCKING, TWO BAYS MINIMUM AT EACH TENSION TIE. PROVIDE 43 MIL MINIMUM CLIP ANGLE EACH END WITH NOT LESS THAN 4-10d COMMON NAILS EACH LEG.

43 MIL CONTINUOUS PLATE WITH NAILING TO MATCH BOUNDARY NAILING. SEE TABLE R602.3(1)

3 IN.

JOIST RUNNING PARALLEL TO WALL

54 MIL × 2 IN. GRADE 50 STRAP, WITH 5-10d COMMON NAILS EACH END

TENSION TIE – SEE TABLE R611.9(4) FOR SPACING

7 IN. MIN

8 IN. MINIMUM WITH WEB MATERIAL REMOVED

WOOD 2 × 6 MINIMUM SILL PLATE TYPICAL. 3 × 6 WHERE REQUIRED BY TABLE R611.9(4)

$1/2$ IN. ANCHOR BOLT TYPICAL, $5/8$ IN. WHERE REQUIRED. SEE TABLE R611.9(4) FOR SIZE AND SPACING.

SECTION

DETAIL B – PLAN VIEW

3 IN.

4 IN.

JOIST

JOIST

BLOCKING TYP.

FLAT OR FULL DEPTH BLOCKING AT STRAP

TENSION TIE. 4 IN. × 3 IN. × 3 IN. × 43 MIL MINIMUM CLIP ANGLE BOTH SIDES OF BLOCKING WITH 6-10d × $1^1/2$ IN. COMMON NAILS ON HORIZONTAL AND VERTICAL LEG. TENSION TIE ASD CAPACITY 760 LB FOR BOTH ANGLES, 380 LB PER ANGLE ——→

ANCHOR BOLT WITH $1/4$ × 3 × 3 STEEL PLATE WASHER

EQUAL

For SI: 1 mil = 0.0254 mm, 1 inch = 25.4 mm, 1 foot = 304.8 mm, 1 pound-force = 4.448 N.

FIGURE R611.9(4)
WOOD FRAMED FLOOR TO TOP OF CONCRETE WALL FRAMING PARALLEL

TABLE R611.9(4)
WOOD FRAMED FLOOR TO TOP OF CONCRETE WALL, FRAMING PARALLEL[a, b, c, d, e]

ANCHOR BOLT SPACING (inches)	TENSION TIE SPACING (inches)	85B	90B	100B / 85C	110B / 90C / 85D	120B / 100C / 90D	130B / 110C / 100D
	12						
12	24						
12	36						░
12	48				░	░	░
16	16					6 A	6 B
16	32					6 A	6 B
16	48					░	░
19.2	19.2				6 A	6 A	6 B
19.2	38.4				6 A	6 A	░
24	24			6 A	6 B	6 B	░
24	48			6 A	░	░	░

For SI: 1 inch = 25.4 mm; 1 mile per hour = 0.447 m/s.

a. This table is for use with the detail in Figure R611.9(4). Use of this detail is permitted where a cell is not shaded, prohibited where shaded.

b. Wall design per other provisions of Section R611 is required.

c. For wind design, minimum 4-inch nominal wall is permitted in unshaded cells with no number.

d. Number 6 indicates minimum permitted nominal wall thickness in inches necessary to develop required strength (capacity) of connection. As a minimum, this nominal thickness shall occur in the portion of the wall indicated by the cross-hatching in Figure R611.9(4). For the remainder of the wall, see Note b.

e. Letter "A" indicates that a minimum nominal 3 × 6 sill plate is required. Letter "B" indicates that a $5/_8$ inch diameter anchor bolt and a minimal nominal 3 × 6 sill plate are required.

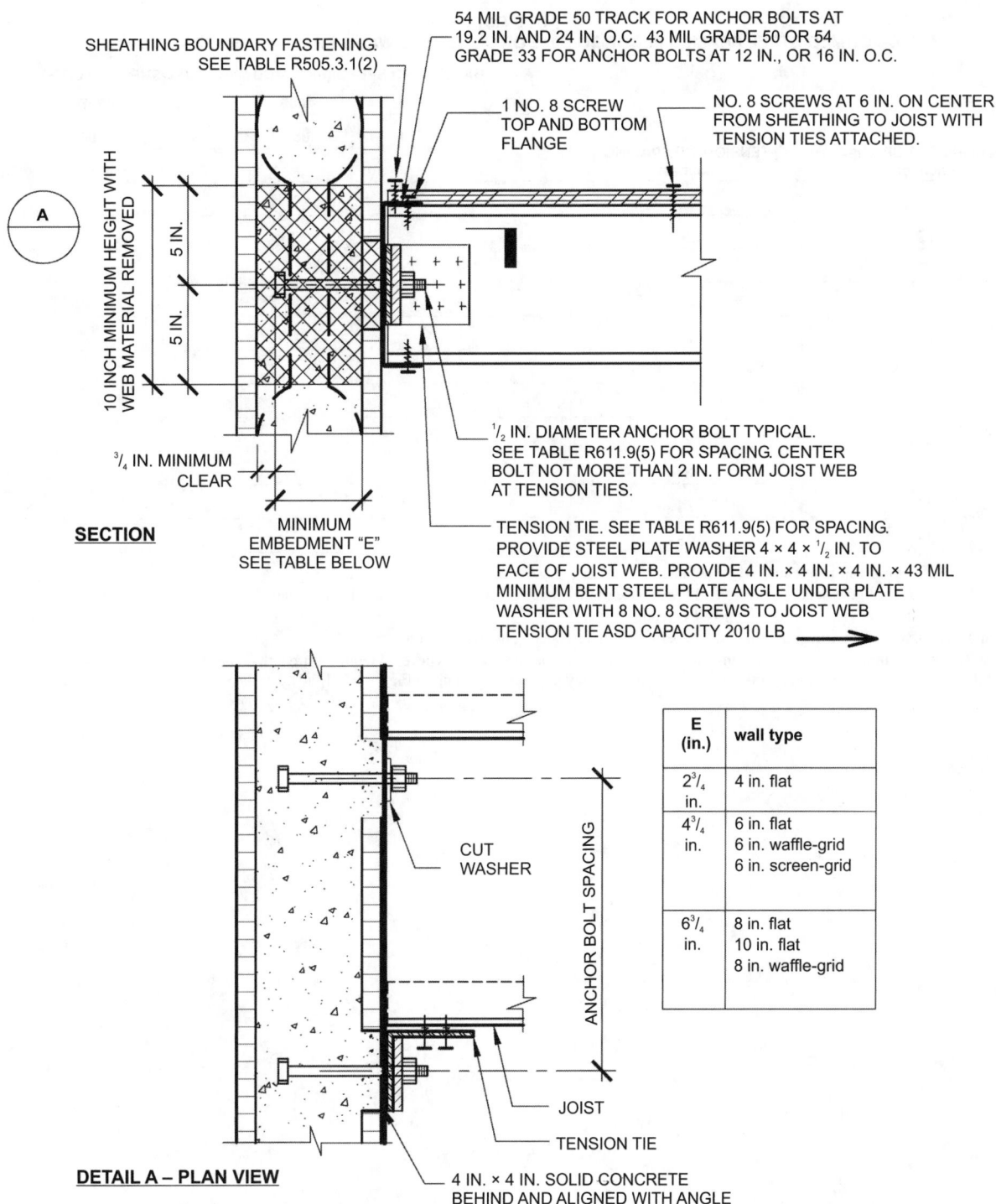

SHEATHING BOUNDARY FASTENING.
SEE TABLE R505.3.1(2)

54 MIL GRADE 50 TRACK FOR ANCHOR BOLTS AT
19.2 IN. AND 24 IN. O.C. 43 MIL GRADE 50 OR 54
GRADE 33 FOR ANCHOR BOLTS AT 12 IN., OR 16 IN. O.C.

1 NO. 8 SCREW
TOP AND BOTTOM
FLANGE

NO. 8 SCREWS AT 6 IN. ON CENTER
FROM SHEATHING TO JOIST WITH
TENSION TIES ATTACHED.

A

10 INCH MINIMUM HEIGHT WITH
WEB MATERIAL REMOVED

5 IN.

5 IN.

5 IN.

³/₄ IN. MINIMUM
CLEAR

SECTION

MINIMUM
EMBEDMENT "E"
SEE TABLE BELOW

¹/₂ IN. DIAMETER ANCHOR BOLT TYPICAL.
SEE TABLE R611.9(5) FOR SPACING. CENTER
BOLT NOT MORE THAN 2 IN. FORM JOIST WEB
AT TENSION TIES.

TENSION TIE. SEE TABLE R611.9(5) FOR SPACING.
PROVIDE STEEL PLATE WASHER 4 × 4 × ¹/₂ IN. TO
FACE OF JOIST WEB. PROVIDE 4 IN. × 4 IN. × 4 IN. × 43 MIL
MINIMUM BENT STEEL PLATE ANGLE UNDER PLATE
WASHER WITH 8 NO. 8 SCREWS TO JOIST WEB
TENSION TIE ASD CAPACITY 2010 LB ⟶

CUT
WASHER

ANCHOR BOLT SPACING

E (in.)	wall type
2³/₄ in.	4 in. flat
4³/₄ in.	6 in. flat 6 in. waffle-grid 6 in. screen-grid
6³/₄ in.	8 in. flat 10 in. flat 8 in. waffle-grid

DETAIL A – PLAN VIEW

JOIST

TENSION TIE

4 IN. × 4 IN. SOLID CONCRETE
BEHIND AND ALIGNED WITH ANGLE

For SI: 1 mil = 0.0254 mm, 1 inch = 25.4 mm, 1 pound-force = 4.448 N.

**FIGURE R611.9(5)
COLD-FORMED STEEL FLOOR TO SIDE OF CONCRETE WALL, FRAMING PERPENDICULAR**

TABLE R611.9(5)
COLD-FORMED STEEL FRAMED FLOOR TO SIDE OF CONCRETE WALL, FRAMING PERPENDICULAR[a, b, c, d]

ANCHOR BOLT SPACING (inches)	TENSION TIE SPACING (inches)	BASIC WIND SPEED (mph) AND WIND EXPOSURE CATEGORY					
		85B	90B	100B / 85C	110B / 90C	120B / 100C / 85D	130B / 110C / 100D
12	12						
12	24						
12	36						6
12	48					6	6
16	16						
16	32						
16	48					6	6
19.2	19.2						
19.2	38.4						6
24	24						
24	48					6	6

For SI: 1 inch = 25.4 mm; 1 mile per hour = 0.4470 m/s.

a. This table is for use with the detail in Figure R611.9(5). Use of this detail is permitted where a cell is not shaded.

b. Wall design per other provisions of Section R611 is required.

c. For wind design, minimum 4-inch nominal wall is permitted in unshaded cells with no number.

d. Number 6 indicates minimum permitted nominal wall thickness in inches necessary to develop required strength (capacity) of connection. As a minimum, this nominal thickness shall occur in the portion of the wall indicated by the cross-hatching in Figure R611.9(5). For the remainder of the wall, see Note b.

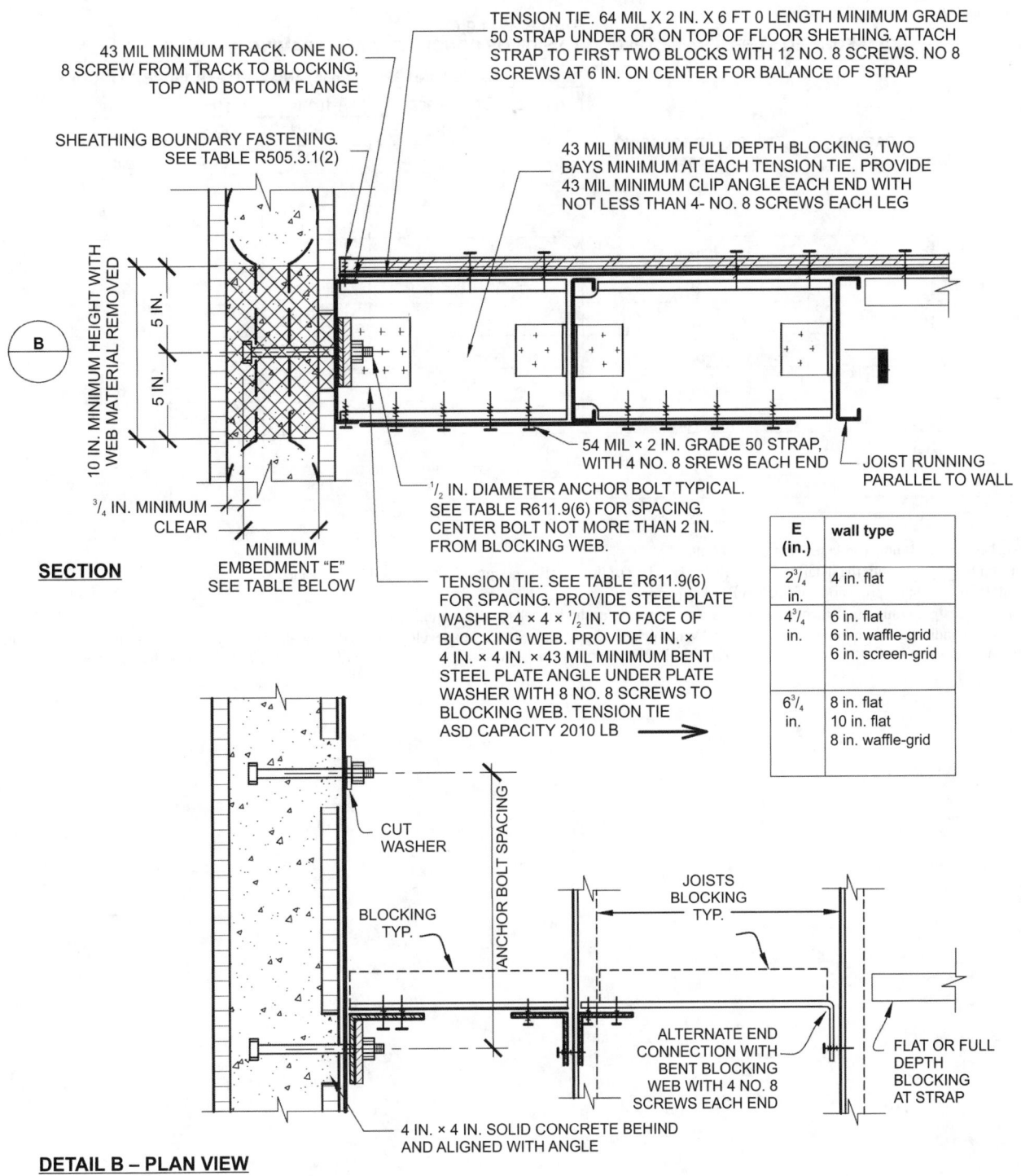

SECTION

43 MIL MINIMUM TRACK. ONE NO. 8 SCREW FROM TRACK TO BLOCKING, TOP AND BOTTOM FLANGE

SHEATHING BOUNDARY FASTENING. SEE TABLE R505.3.1(2)

10 IN. MINIMUM HEIGHT WITH WEB MATERIAL REMOVED

5 IN.

5 IN.

5 IN.

³/₄ IN. MINIMUM CLEAR

MINIMUM EMBEDMENT "E" SEE TABLE BELOW

B

TENSION TIE. 64 MIL X 2 IN. X 6 FT 0 LENGTH MINIMUM GRADE 50 STRAP UNDER OR ON TOP OF FLOOR SHETHING. ATTACH STRAP TO FIRST TWO BLOCKS WITH 12 NO. 8 SCREWS. NO 8 SCREWS AT 6 IN. ON CENTER FOR BALANCE OF STRAP

43 MIL MINIMUM FULL DEPTH BLOCKING, TWO BAYS MINIMUM AT EACH TENSION TIE. PROVIDE 43 MIL MINIMUM CLIP ANGLE EACH END WITH NOT LESS THAN 4- NO. 8 SCREWS EACH LEG

54 MIL × 2 IN. GRADE 50 STRAP, WITH 4 NO. 8 SREWS EACH END

JOIST RUNNING PARALLEL TO WALL

¹/₂ IN. DIAMETER ANCHOR BOLT TYPICAL. SEE TABLE R611.9(6) FOR SPACING. CENTER BOLT NOT MORE THAN 2 IN. FROM BLOCKING WEB.

TENSION TIE. SEE TABLE R611.9(6) FOR SPACING. PROVIDE STEEL PLATE WASHER 4 × 4 × ¹/₂ IN. TO FACE OF BLOCKING WEB. PROVIDE 4 IN. × 4 IN. × 4 IN. × 43 MIL MINIMUM BENT STEEL PLATE ANGLE UNDER PLATE WASHER WITH 8 NO. 8 SCREWS TO BLOCKING WEB. TENSION TIE ASD CAPACITY 2010 LB ➡

E (in.)	wall type
2³/₄ in.	4 in. flat
4³/₄ in.	6 in. flat 6 in. waffle-grid 6 in. screen-grid
6³/₄ in.	8 in. flat 10 in. flat 8 in. waffle-grid

DETAIL B – PLAN VIEW

CUT WASHER

BLOCKING TYP.

ANCHOR BOLT SPACING

JOISTS BLOCKING TYP.

ALTERNATE END CONNECTION WITH BENT BLOCKING WEB WITH 4 NO. 8 SCREWS EACH END

FLAT OR FULL DEPTH BLOCKING AT STRAP

4 IN. × 4 IN. SOLID CONCRETE BEHIND AND ALIGNED WITH ANGLE

For SI: 1 mil = 0.0254 mm, 1 inch = 25.4 mm, 1 pound-force = 4.448 N.

FIGURE R611.9(6)
COLD-FORMED STEEL FLOOR TO SIDE OF CONCRETE WALL, FRAMING PARALLEL

TABLE R611.9(6)
COLD-FORMED STEEL FRAMED FLOOR TO SIDE OF CONCRETE WALL, FRAMING PARALLEL[a, b, c, d]

ANCHOR BOLT SPACING (inches)	TENSION TIE SPACING (inches)	BASIC WIND SPEED (mph) AND WIND EXPOSURE CATEGORY					
		85B	90B	100B 85C	110B 90C 85D	120B 100C 90D	130B 110C 100D
12	12						
12	24						
12	36						6
12	48					6	6
16	16						
16	32						
16	48					6	6
19.2	19.2						
19.2	38.4						6
24	24						
24	48					6	6

For SI: 1 inch = 25.4 mm; 1 mile per hour = 0.447 m/s.

a. This table is for use with the detail in Figure R611.9(6). Use of this detail is permitted where a cell is not shaded.

b. Wall design per other provisions of Section R611 is required.

c. For wind design, minimum 4-inch nominal wall is permitted in unshaded cells with no number.

d. Number 6 indicates minimum permitted nominal wall thickness in inches necessary to develop required strength (capacity) of connection. As a minimum, this nominal thickness shall occur in the portion of the wall indicated by the cross-hatching in Figure R611.9(6). For the remainder of the wall, see Note b.

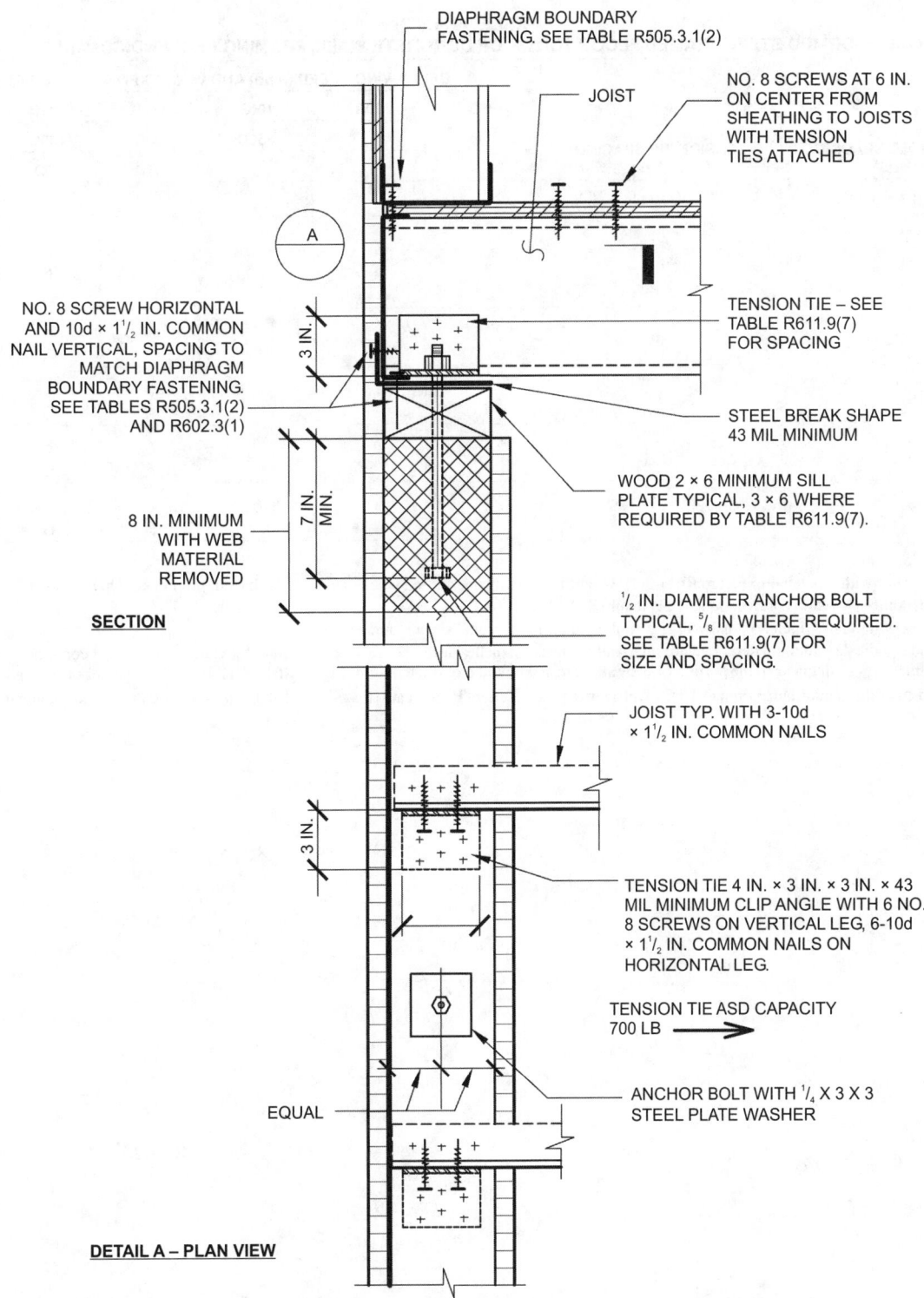

DIAPHRAGM BOUNDARY
FASTENING. SEE TABLE R505.3.1(2)

JOIST

NO. 8 SCREWS AT 6 IN.
ON CENTER FROM
SHEATHING TO JOISTS
WITH TENSION
TIES ATTACHED

A

NO. 8 SCREW HORIZONTAL
AND 10d × 1¹/₂ IN. COMMON
NAIL VERTICAL, SPACING TO
MATCH DIAPHRAGM
BOUNDARY FASTENING.
SEE TABLES R505.3.1(2)
AND R602.3(1)

3 IN.

TENSION TIE – SEE
TABLE R611.9(7)
FOR SPACING

STEEL BREAK SHAPE
43 MIL MINIMUM

7 IN.
MIN.

WOOD 2 × 6 MINIMUM SILL
PLATE TYPICAL, 3 × 6 WHERE
REQUIRED BY TABLE R611.9(7).

8 IN. MINIMUM
WITH WEB
MATERIAL
REMOVED

SECTION

¹/₂ IN. DIAMETER ANCHOR BOLT
TYPICAL, ⁵/₈ IN WHERE REQUIRED.
SEE TABLE R611.9(7) FOR
SIZE AND SPACING.

JOIST TYP. WITH 3-10d
× 1¹/₂ IN. COMMON NAILS

3 IN.

TENSION TIE 4 IN. × 3 IN. × 3 IN. × 43
MIL MINIMUM CLIP ANGLE WITH 6 NO.
8 SCREWS ON VERTICAL LEG, 6-10d
× 1¹/₂ IN. COMMON NAILS ON
HORIZONTAL LEG.

TENSION TIE ASD CAPACITY
700 LB →

EQUAL

ANCHOR BOLT WITH ¹/₄ X 3 X 3
STEEL PLATE WASHER

DETAIL A – PLAN VIEW

For SI: 1 mil = 0.0254 mm, 1 inch = 25.4 mm, 1 pound-force = 4.448 N.

FIGURE R611.9(7)
COLD-FORMED STEEL FLOOR TO TOP OF CONCRETE WALL FRAMING PERPENDICULAR

TABLE R611.9(7)
COLD-FORMED STEEL FRAMED FLOOR TO TOP OF CONCRETE WALL, FRAMING PERPENDICULAR[a, b, c, d, e]

ANCHOR BOLT SPACING (inches)	TENSION TIE SPACING (inches)	BASIC WIND SPEED (mph) AND WIND EXPOSURE CATEGORY					
		85B	90B	100B	110B	120B	130B
				858C	90C	100C	110C
					85D	90D	100D
12	12						
12	24						
16	16					6 A	6 B
16	32					6 A	6 B
19.2	19.2				6 A	8 B	8 B
19.2	38.4				6 A	8 B	8 B
24	24			6 A	8 B	8 B	▓▓

For SI: 1 inch = 25.4 mm; 1 mph = 0.447 m/s.

a. This table is for use with the detail in Figure R611.9(7). Use of this detail is permitted where a cell is not shaded, prohibited where shaded.

b. Wall design per other provisions of Section R611 is required.

c. For wind design, minimum 4-inch nominal wall is permitted in unshaded cells with no number.

d. Numbers 6 and 8 indicate minimum permitted nominal wall thickness in inches necessary to develop required strength (capacity) of connection. As a minimum, this nominal thickness shall occur in the portion of the wall indicated by the cross-hatching in Figure R611.9(7). For the remainder of the wall, see Note b.

e. Letter "A" indicates that a minimum nominal 3 × 6 sill plate is required. Letter "B" indicates that a $^5/_8$ inch diameter anchor bolt and a minimum nominal 3 × 6 sill plate are required.

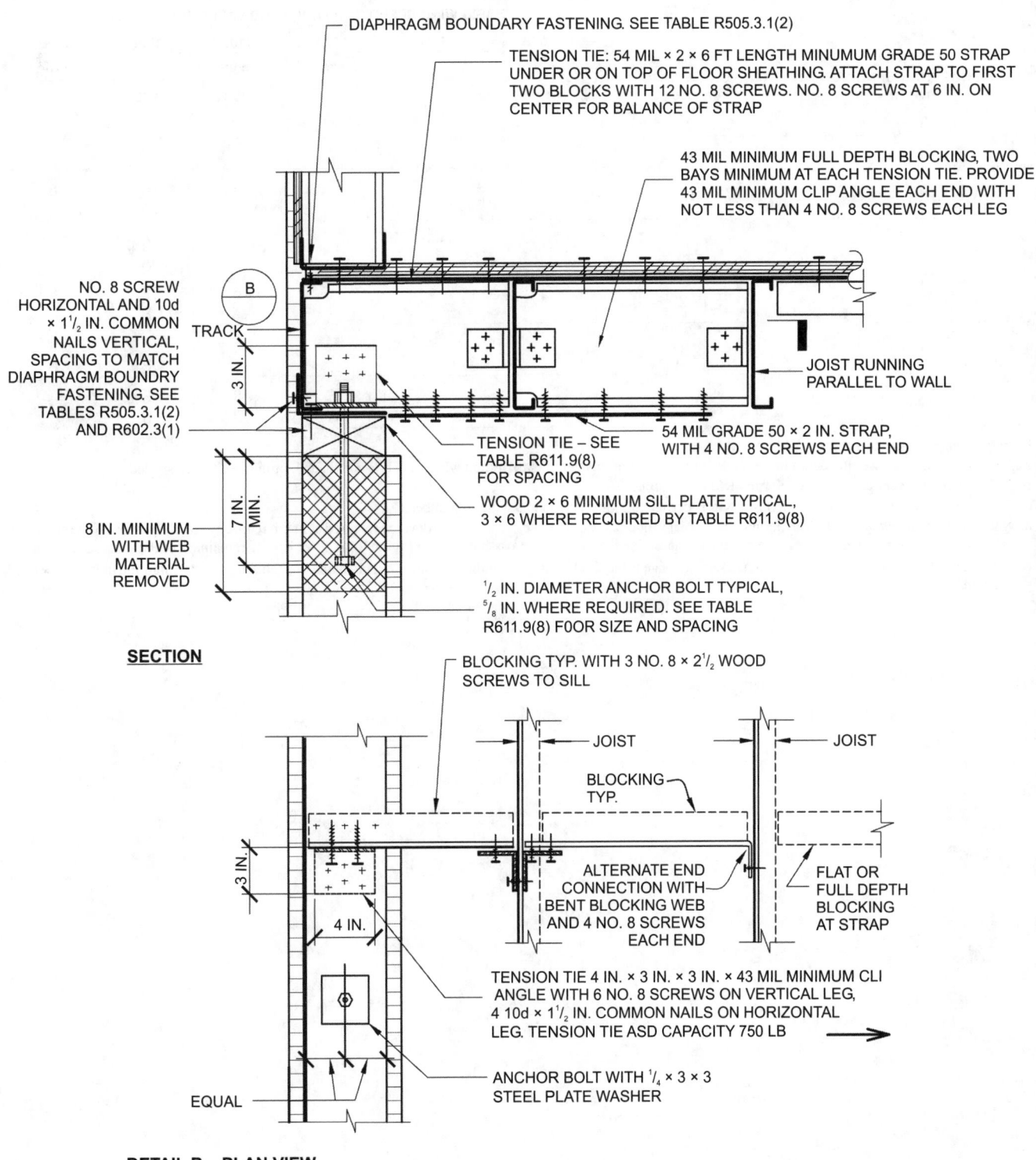

DIAPHRAGM BOUNDARY FASTENING. SEE TABLE R505.3.1(2)

TENSION TIE: 54 MIL × 2 × 6 FT LENGTH MINUMUM GRADE 50 STRAP UNDER OR ON TOP OF FLOOR SHEATHING. ATTACH STRAP TO FIRST TWO BLOCKS WITH 12 NO. 8 SCREWS. NO. 8 SCREWS AT 6 IN. ON CENTER FOR BALANCE OF STRAP

43 MIL MINIMUM FULL DEPTH BLOCKING, TWO BAYS MINIMUM AT EACH TENSION TIE. PROVIDE 43 MIL MINIMUM CLIP ANGLE EACH END WITH NOT LESS THAN 4 NO. 8 SCREWS EACH LEG

NO. 8 SCREW HORIZONTAL AND 10d × 1¹/₂ IN. COMMON NAILS VERTICAL, SPACING TO MATCH DIAPHRAGM BOUNDRY FASTENING. SEE TABLES R505.3.1(2) AND R602.3(1)

TRACK

3 IN.

JOIST RUNNING PARALLEL TO WALL

54 MIL GRADE 50 × 2 IN. STRAP, WITH 4 NO. 8 SCREWS EACH END

TENSION TIE – SEE TABLE R611.9(8) FOR SPACING

WOOD 2 × 6 MINIMUM SILL PLATE TYPICAL, 3 × 6 WHERE REQUIRED BY TABLE R611.9(8)

7 IN. MIN.

8 IN. MINIMUM WITH WEB MATERIAL REMOVED

¹/₂ IN. DIAMETER ANCHOR BOLT TYPICAL, ⁵/₈ IN. WHERE REQUIRED. SEE TABLE R611.9(8) F0OR SIZE AND SPACING

SECTION

BLOCKING TYP. WITH 3 NO. 8 × 2¹/₂ WOOD SCREWS TO SILL

JOIST

JOIST

BLOCKING TYP.

3 IN.

4 IN.

ALTERNATE END CONNECTION WITH BENT BLOCKING WEB AND 4 NO. 8 SCREWS EACH END

FLAT OR FULL DEPTH BLOCKING AT STRAP

TENSION TIE 4 IN. × 3 IN. × 3 IN. × 43 MIL MINIMUM CLI ANGLE WITH 6 NO. 8 SCREWS ON VERTICAL LEG, 4 10d × 1¹/₂ IN. COMMON NAILS ON HORIZONTAL LEG. TENSION TIE ASD CAPACITY 750 LB

EQUAL

ANCHOR BOLT WITH ¹/₄ × 3 × 3 STEEL PLATE WASHER

DETAIL B – PLAN VIEW

For SI: 1 mil = 0.0254 mm, 1 inch = 25.4 mm, 1 pound-force = 4.448 N.

FIGURE R611.9(8)
COLD-FORMED STEEL FLOOR TO TOP OF CONCRETE WALL, FRAMING PARALLEL

TABLE R611.9(8)
COLD-FORMED STEEL FRAMED FLOOR TO TOP OF CONCRETE WALL, FRAMING PARALLEL[a, b, c, d, e]

ANCHOR BOLT SPACING (inches)	TENSION TIE SPACING (inches)	BASIC WIND SPEED (mph) AND WIND EXPOSURE CATEGORY					
		85B	90B	100B 85C	110B 90C 85D	120B 100C 90D	130B 110C 100D
12	12						
12	24						
16	16					6 A	6 B
16	32					6 A	6 B
19.2	19.2				6 A	8 B	8 B
19.2	38.4				6 A	8 B	8 B
24	24			6 A	8 B	8 B	░░░

For SI: 1 inch = 25.4 mm; 1 mph = 0.447 m/s.

a. This table is for use with the detail in Figure R611.9(8). Use of this detail is permitted where a cell is not shaded, prohibited where shaded.

b. Wall design per other provisions of Section R611 is required.

c. For wind design, minimum 4-inch nominal wall is permitted in unshaded cells with no number.

d. Numbers 6 and 8 indicate minimum permitted nominal wall thickness in inches necessary to develop required strength (capacity) of connection. As a minimum, this nominal thickness shall occur in the portion of the wall indicated by the cross-hatching in Figure R611.9(8). For the remainder of the wall, see Note b.

e. Letter "A" indicates that a minimum nominal 3 × 6 sill plate is required. Letter "B" indicates that a $^5/_8$ inch diameter anchor bolt and a minimum nominal 3 × 6 sill plate are required.

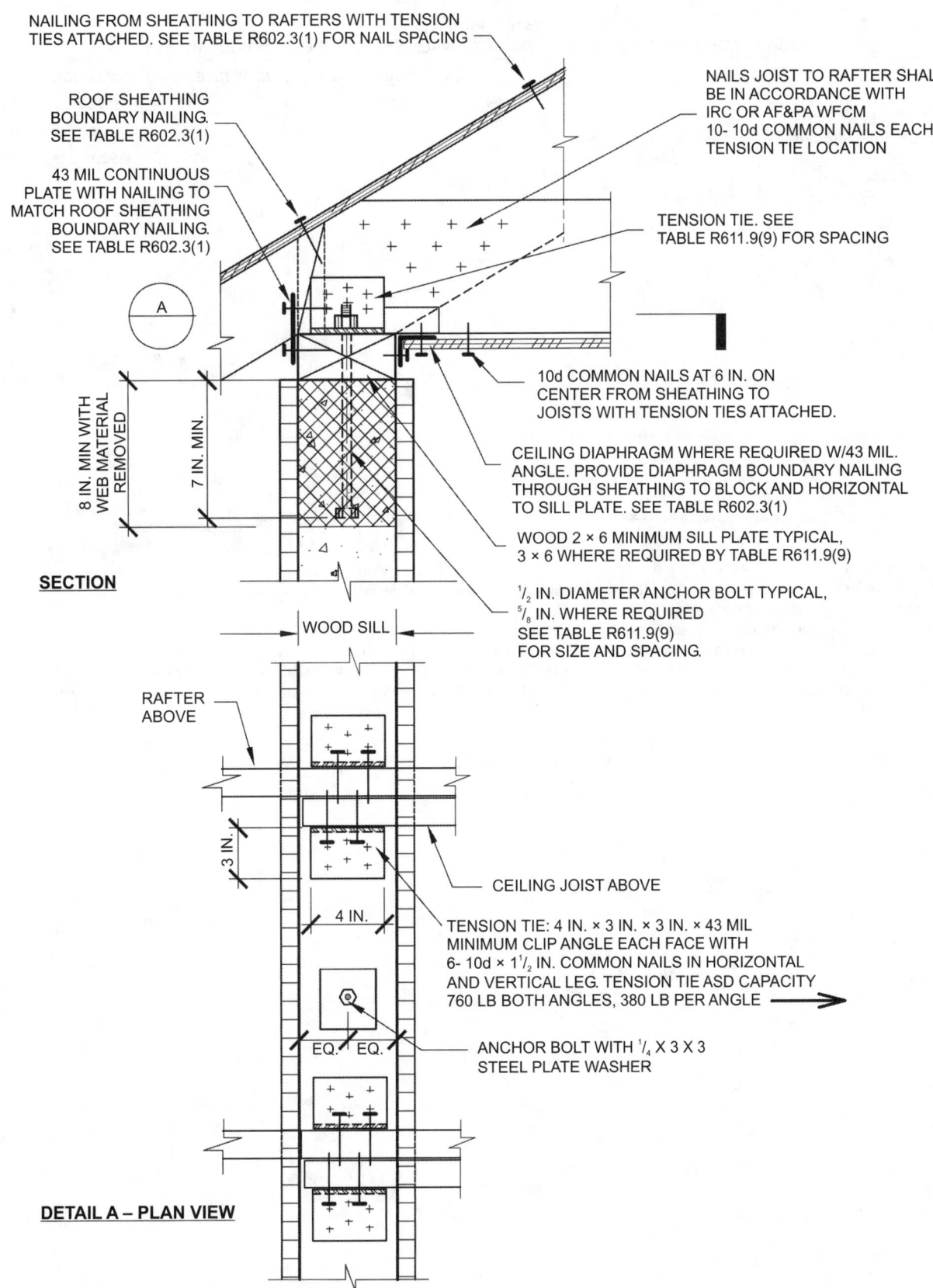

NAILING FROM SHEATHING TO RAFTERS WITH TENSION TIES ATTACHED. SEE TABLE R602.3(1) FOR NAIL SPACING

ROOF SHEATHING BOUNDARY NAILING. SEE TABLE R602.3(1)

43 MIL CONTINUOUS PLATE WITH NAILING TO MATCH ROOF SHEATHING BOUNDARY NAILING. SEE TABLE R602.3(1)

NAILS JOIST TO RAFTER SHALL BE IN ACCORDANCE WITH IRC OR AF&PA WFCM 10- 10d COMMON NAILS EACH TENSION TIE LOCATION

TENSION TIE. SEE TABLE R611.9(9) FOR SPACING

10d COMMON NAILS AT 6 IN. ON CENTER FROM SHEATHING TO JOISTS WITH TENSION TIES ATTACHED.

CEILING DIAPHRAGM WHERE REQUIRED W/43 MIL. ANGLE. PROVIDE DIAPHRAGM BOUNDARY NAILING THROUGH SHEATHING TO BLOCK AND HORIZONTAL TO SILL PLATE. SEE TABLE R602.3(1)

WOOD 2 × 6 MINIMUM SILL PLATE TYPICAL, 3 × 6 WHERE REQUIRED BY TABLE R611.9(9)

$\frac{1}{2}$ IN. DIAMETER ANCHOR BOLT TYPICAL, $\frac{5}{8}$ IN. WHERE REQUIRED SEE TABLE R611.9(9) FOR SIZE AND SPACING.

8 IN. MIN WITH WEB MATERIAL REMOVED

7 IN. MIN.

A

SECTION

WOOD SILL

RAFTER ABOVE

3 IN.

4 IN.

EQ. EQ.

CEILING JOIST ABOVE

TENSION TIE: 4 IN. × 3 IN. × 3 IN. × 43 MIL MINIMUM CLIP ANGLE EACH FACE WITH 6- 10d × 1$\frac{1}{2}$ IN. COMMON NAILS IN HORIZONTAL AND VERTICAL LEG. TENSION TIE ASD CAPACITY 760 LB BOTH ANGLES, 380 LB PER ANGLE

ANCHOR BOLT WITH $\frac{1}{4}$ X 3 X 3 STEEL PLATE WASHER

DETAIL A – PLAN VIEW

For SI: 1 mil = 0.0254 mm, 1 inch = 25.4 mm, 1 pound-force = 4.448 N.

FIGURE R611.9(9)
WOOD FRAMED ROOF TO TOP OF CONCRETE WALL, FRAMING PERPENDICULAR

TABLE R611.9(9)
WOOD FRAMED ROOF TO TOP OF CONCRETE WALL, FRAMING PERPENDICULAR[a, b, c, d, e]

ANCHOR BOLT SPACING (inches)	TENSION TIE SPACING (inches)	BASIC WIND SPEED (mph) AND WIND EXPOSURE CATEGORY					
		85B	90B	100B / 85C	110B / 90C / 85D	120B / 100C / 90D	130B / 110C / 100D
12	12						
12	24						
12	36						(shaded)
12	48				(shaded)		(shaded)
16	16						6
16	32						6
16	48				(shaded)		(shaded)
19.2	19.2					6	6 A
19.2	38.4					6	(shaded)
24	24				6 A	6 A	6 B
24	48				(shaded)	(shaded)	(shaded)

For SI: 1 inch = 25.4 mm; 1 mph = 0.447 m/s.

a. This table is for use with the detail in Figure R611.9(9). Use of this detail is permitted where cell a is not shaded, prohibited where shaded.

b. Wall design per other provisions of Section R611 is required.

c. For wind design, minimum 4-inch nominal wall is permitted in unshaded cells with no number.

d. Number 6 indicates minimum permitted nominal wall thickness in inches necessary to develop required strength (capacity) of connection. As a minimum, this nominal thickness shall occur in the portion of the wall indicated by the cross-hatching in Figure R611.9(9). For the remainder of the wall, see Note b.

e. Letter "A" indicates that a minimum nominal 3 × 6 sill plate is required. Letter "B" indicates that a $^5/_8$ inch diameter anchor bolt and a minimum nominal 3 × 6 sill plate are required.

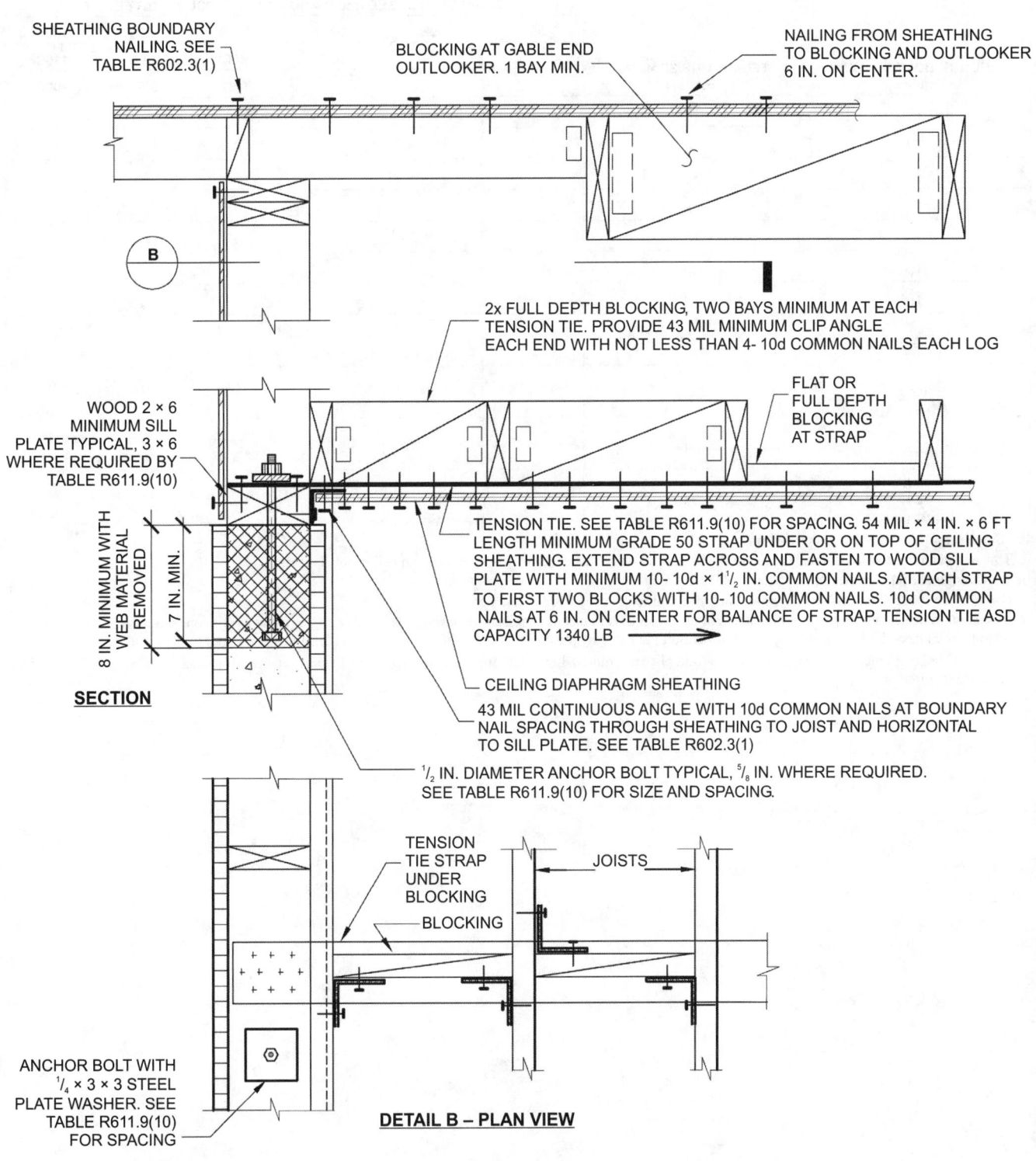

SHEATHING BOUNDARY NAILING. SEE TABLE R602.3(1)

BLOCKING AT GABLE END OUTLOOKER. 1 BAY MIN.

NAILING FROM SHEATHING TO BLOCKING AND OUTLOOKER 6 IN. ON CENTER.

B

2x FULL DEPTH BLOCKING, TWO BAYS MINIMUM AT EACH TENSION TIE. PROVIDE 43 MIL MINIMUM CLIP ANGLE EACH END WITH NOT LESS THAN 4- 10d COMMON NAILS EACH LOG

WOOD 2 × 6 MINIMUM SILL PLATE TYPICAL, 3 × 6 WHERE REQUIRED BY TABLE R611.9(10)

FLAT OR FULL DEPTH BLOCKING AT STRAP

8 IN. MINIMUM WITH WEB MATERIAL REMOVED

7 IN. MIN.

TENSION TIE. SEE TABLE R611.9(10) FOR SPACING. 54 MIL × 4 IN. × 6 FT LENGTH MINIMUM GRADE 50 STRAP UNDER OR ON TOP OF CEILING SHEATHING. EXTEND STRAP ACROSS AND FASTEN TO WOOD SILL PLATE WITH MINIMUM 10- 10d × $1^{1}/_{2}$ IN. COMMON NAILS. ATTACH STRAP TO FIRST TWO BLOCKS WITH 10- 10d COMMON NAILS. 10d COMMON NAILS AT 6 IN. ON CENTER FOR BALANCE OF STRAP. TENSION TIE ASD CAPACITY 1340 LB

SECTION

CEILING DIAPHRAGM SHEATHING

43 MIL CONTINUOUS ANGLE WITH 10d COMMON NAILS AT BOUNDARY NAIL SPACING THROUGH SHEATHING TO JOIST AND HORIZONTAL TO SILL PLATE. SEE TABLE R602.3(1)

$^{1}/_{2}$ IN. DIAMETER ANCHOR BOLT TYPICAL, $^{5}/_{8}$ IN. WHERE REQUIRED. SEE TABLE R611.9(10) FOR SIZE AND SPACING.

TENSION TIE STRAP UNDER BLOCKING

JOISTS

BLOCKING

ANCHOR BOLT WITH $^{1}/_{4}$ × 3 × 3 STEEL PLATE WASHER. SEE TABLE R611.9(10) FOR SPACING

DETAIL B – PLAN VIEW

For SI: 1 mil = 0.0254 mm, 1 inch = 25.4 mm, 1 foot = 304.8 mm, 1 pound-force = 4.448 N.

FIGURE R611.9(10)
WOOD FRAMED ROOF TO TOP OF CONCRETE WALL FRAMING PARALLEL

TABLE R611.9(10)
WOOD FRAMED ROOF TO TOP OF CONCRETE WALL, FRAMING PARALLEL[a, b, c, d, e]

ANCHOR BOLT SPACING (inches)	TENSION TIE SPACING (inches)	BASIC WIND SPEED (mph) AND WIND EXPOSURE CATEGORY					
		85B	90B	100B / 85C	110B / 90C / 85D	120B / 100C / 90D	130B / 110C / 100D
12	12						
12	24						
12	36						
12	48						
16	16					6	6
16	32					6	6
16	48					6	6
19.2	19.2				6	6	6 A
19.2	38.4				6	6	6 A
24	24			6	6 A	6 A	6 B
24	48			6	6 A	6 B	6 B

For SI: 1 inch = 25.4 mm; I mph = 0.447 m/s.

a. This table is for use with the detail in Figure R611.9(10). Use of this detail is permitted where a cell is not shaded.

b. Wall design per other provisions of Section R611 is required.

c. For wind design, minimum 4-inch nominal wall is permitted in cells with no number.

d. Number 6 indicates minimum permitted nominal wall thickness in inches necessary to develop required strength (capacity) of connection. As a minimum, this nominal thickness shall occur in the portion of the wall indicated by the cross-hatching in Figure R611.9(10). For the remainder of the wall, see Note b.

e. Letter "A" indicates that a minimum nominal 3 × 6 sill plate is required. Letter "B" indicates that a $5/_8$ inch diameter anchor bolt and a minimum nominal 3 × 6 sill plate are required.

WHERE CEILING DIAPHRAGM IS NOT PROVIDED, DIAPHRAGM BOUNDARY FASTENING SHALL BE IN ACCORDANCE WITH TABLE R804.3. WHERE CEILING DIAPHRAGM IS PROVIDED, DIAPHRAGM FASTENING SHALL BE IN ACCORDANCE WITH AISI S230

WHERE CEILING DIAPHRAGM IS PROVIDED, CONTINUOUS STRAP SHALL BE IN ACCORDANCE WITH AISI S230

WHERE CEILING DIAPHRAGM NOT PROVIDED, 43 MIL MINIMUM BREAK SHAPE EACH RAFTER BAY. WHERE CEILING DIAPHRAGM IS PROVIDED BREAK SHAPE SHALL BE IN ACCORDANCE WITH AISI S230

WHERE CEILING DIAPHRAGM IS NOT PROVIDED, 10d COMMON NAILS HORIZONTAL, SPACING TO MATCH DIAPHRAGM BOUNDARY FASTENING SHALL BE IN ACCORDANCE WITH TABLE R602.3(1). WHERE CEILING DIAPHRAGM IS PROVIDED, SEE AISI S230

WHERE CEILING DIAPHRAGM IS NOT PROVIDED, NO. 8 SCREWS AT 6 IN. ON CENTER FROM SHEATHING TO RAFTERS WITH TENSION TIES ATTACHED. WHERE CEILING DIAPHRAGM IS PROVIDED, SCREWS SHALL BE IN ACCORDANCE WITH AISI S230.

3 NO. 8 SCREWS MIN. 8 NO. 8 SCREWS EACH TENSION TIE LOCATION WHERE NO CEILING DIAPHRAGM IS PROVIDED. SEE SECTION R611.10

TENSION TIE. SEE TABLE R611.9(11) FOR SPACING.

NO. 8 SCREWS AT 6 IN. ON CENTER FROM SHEATHING TO JOISTS WITH TENSION TIES ATTACHED.

CEILING DIAPHRAGM WHERE REQUIRED W/43 MIL ANGLE, NO. 8 SCREWS TO STEEL, 10d NAILS TO WOOD SILL. SEE TABLE R804.3 FOR DIAPHRAGM BOUNDARY FASTENER SPACING

WOOD 2 × 6 MINIMUM SILL PLATE TYPICAL, 3 × 6 WHERE REQUIRED BY TABLE R611.9(11)

$\frac{1}{2}$ IN. DIAMETER ANCHOR BOLT TYPICAL, $\frac{5}{8}$ IN. WHERE REQUIRED. SEE TABLE R611.9(11) FOR SIZE AND SPACING

CEILING JOIST ABOVE WITH 3- 10d × 1$\frac{1}{2}$ IN. COMMON NAILS TO WOOD SILL

TENSION TIE. 4 IN. × 3 IN. × 3 IN. × 43 MIL MINIMUM CLIP ANGLE WITH 6 NO. 8 SCREWS VERTICAL LEG AND 6- 10d × 1$\frac{1}{2}$ IN. COMMON NAILS IN HORIZONTAL LEG TENSION TIE ASD CAPACITY 700 LB

ANCHOR BOLT WITH $\frac{1}{4}$ × 3 × 3 STEEL PLATE WASHER

A

8 IN. MIN WITH WEB MATERIAL REMOVED

7 IN. MIN.

SECTION

WOOD SILL

3 IN. MINIMUM

RAFTER ABOVE

4 IN.

EQ. EQ.

DETAIL A – PLAN VIEW

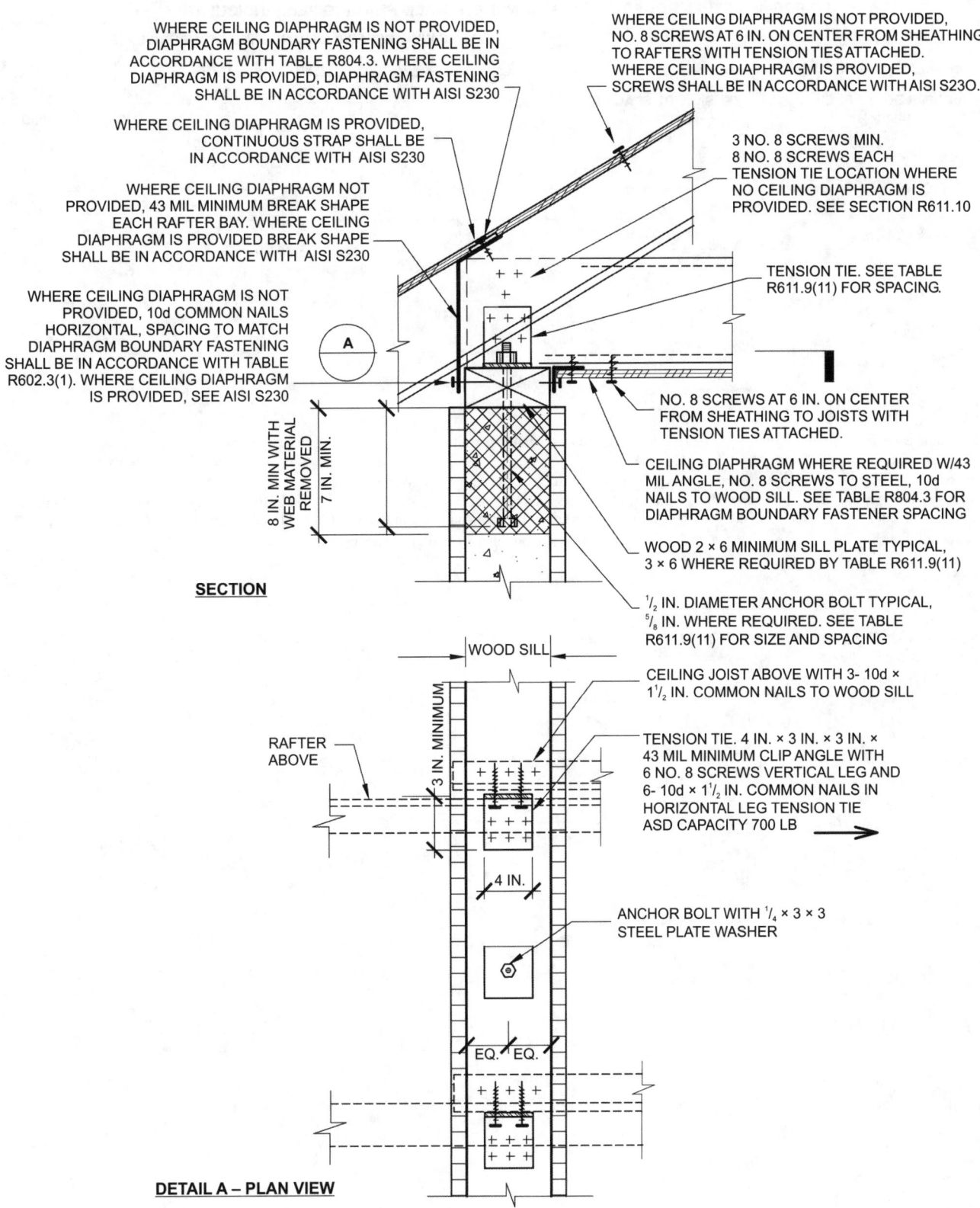

For SI: 1 mil = 0.0254 mm, 1 inch = 25.4 mm, 1 pound-force = 4.448 N.

FIGURE R611.9(11)
COLD-FORMED STEEL ROOF TO TOP OF CONCRETE WALL, FRAMING PERPENDICULAR

TABLE R611.9(11)
COLD-FORMED STEEL ROOF TO TOP OF CONCRETE WALL, FRAMING PERPENDICULAR[a, b, c, d, e]

ANCHOR BOLT SPACING (inches)	TENSION TIE SPACING (inches)	BASIC WIND SPEED (mph) AND WIND EXPOSURE CATEGORY					
		85B	90B	100B / 85C	110B / 90C / 85D	120B / 100C / 90D	130B / 110C / 100D
12	12						
12	24						
16	16					6	6
16	32					6	6
19.2	19.2				6	6	8 B
19.2	38.4				6	6	8 B
24	24			6	6	8 B	(shaded)

For SI: 1 inch = 25.4 mm; 1 mile per hour = 0.447 m/s.

a. This table is for use with the detail in Figure R611.9(11). Use of this detail is permitted where a cell is not shaded, prohibited where shaded.

b. Wall design per other provisions of Section R611 is required.

c. For wind design, minimum 4-inch nominal wall is permitted in unshaded cells with no number.

d. Numbers 6 and 8 indicate minimum permitted nominal wall thickness in inches necessary to develop required strength (capacity) of connection. As a minimum, this nominal thickness shall occur in the portion of the wall indicated by the cross-hatching in Figure R611.9(11). For the remainder of the wall, see Note b.

e. Letter "B" indicates that a $^5/_8$ inch diameter anchor bolt and a minimum nominal 3 × 6 sill plate are required.

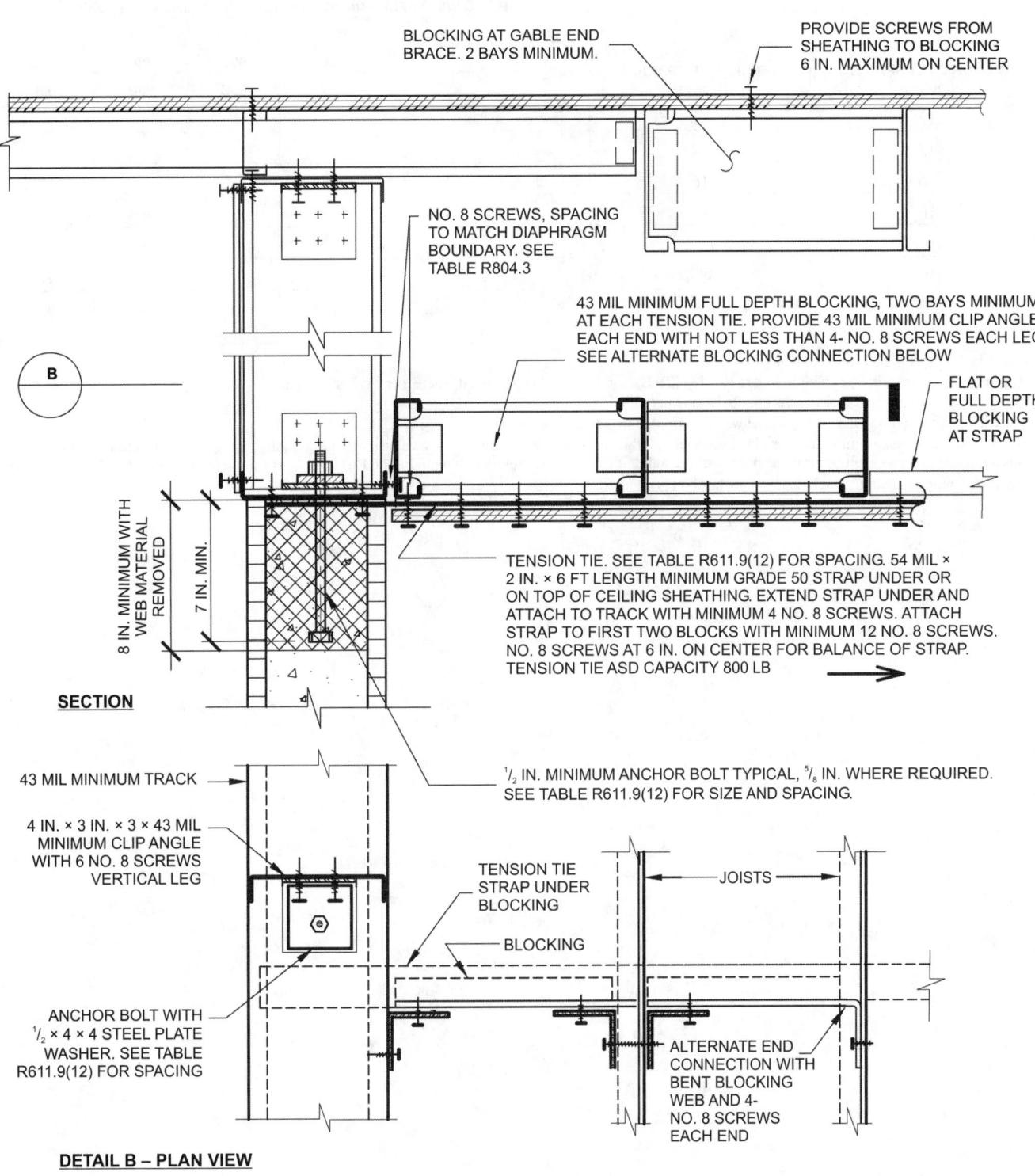

BLOCKING AT GABLE END BRACE. 2 BAYS MINIMUM.

PROVIDE SCREWS FROM SHEATHING TO BLOCKING 6 IN. MAXIMUM ON CENTER

NO. 8 SCREWS, SPACING TO MATCH DIAPHRAGM BOUNDARY. SEE TABLE R804.3

43 MIL MINIMUM FULL DEPTH BLOCKING, TWO BAYS MINIMUM AT EACH TENSION TIE. PROVIDE 43 MIL MINIMUM CLIP ANGLE EACH END WITH NOT LESS THAN 4- NO. 8 SCREWS EACH LEG. SEE ALTERNATE BLOCKING CONNECTION BELOW

FLAT OR FULL DEPTH BLOCKING AT STRAP

B

8 IN. MINIMUM WITH WEB MATERIAL REMOVED

7 IN. MIN.

TENSION TIE. SEE TABLE R611.9(12) FOR SPACING. 54 MIL × 2 IN. × 6 FT LENGTH MINIMUM GRADE 50 STRAP UNDER OR ON TOP OF CEILING SHEATHING. EXTEND STRAP UNDER AND ATTACH TO TRACK WITH MINIMUM 4 NO. 8 SCREWS. ATTACH STRAP TO FIRST TWO BLOCKS WITH MINIMUM 12 NO. 8 SCREWS. NO. 8 SCREWS AT 6 IN. ON CENTER FOR BALANCE OF STRAP. TENSION TIE ASD CAPACITY 800 LB

SECTION

43 MIL MINIMUM TRACK

$\frac{1}{2}$ IN. MINIMUM ANCHOR BOLT TYPICAL, $\frac{5}{8}$ IN. WHERE REQUIRED. SEE TABLE R611.9(12) FOR SIZE AND SPACING.

4 IN. × 3 IN. × 3 × 43 MIL MINIMUM CLIP ANGLE WITH 6 NO. 8 SCREWS VERTICAL LEG

TENSION TIE STRAP UNDER BLOCKING

JOISTS

BLOCKING

ANCHOR BOLT WITH $\frac{1}{2}$ × 4 × 4 STEEL PLATE WASHER. SEE TABLE R611.9(12) FOR SPACING

ALTERNATE END CONNECTION WITH BENT BLOCKING WEB AND 4- NO. 8 SCREWS EACH END

DETAIL B – PLAN VIEW

For SI: 1 mil = 0.0254 mm, 1 inch = 25.4 mm, 1 foot = 304.8 mm, 1 pound-force = 4.448 N.

FIGURE R611.9(12)
COLD-FORMED STEEL ROOF TO TOP OF CONCRETE WALL, FRAMING PARALLEL

TABLE R611.9(12)
COLD-FORMED STEEL ROOF TO TOP OF CONCRETE WALL, FRAMING PARALLEL[a, b, c, d, e]

ANCHOR BOLT SPACING (inches)	TENSION TIE SPACING (inches)	BASIC WIND SPEED (mph) AND WIND EXPOSURE CATEGORY					
		85B	90B	100B / 85C	110B / 90C / 85D	120B / 100C / 90D	130B / 110C / 100D
12	12						
12	24						
16	16						
16	32						
19.2	19.2					6	6
19.2	38.4					6	6
24	24			6	6	8 B	8 B

For SI: 1 inch = 25.4 mm; 1 mile per hour = 0.447 m/s.

a. This table is for use with the detail in Figure R611.9(12). Use of this detail is permitted where a cell is not shaded.

b. Wall design per other provisions of Section R611 is required.

c. For wind design, minimum 4-inch nominal wall is permitted in cells with no number.

d. Numbers 6 and 8 indicate minimum permitted nominal wall thickness in inches necessary to develop required strength (capacity) of connection. As a minimum, this nominal thickness shall occur in the portion of the wall indicated by the cross-hatching in Figure R611.9(12). For the remainder of the wall, see Note b.

e. Letter "B" indicates that a $^5/_8$ inch diameter anchor bolt is required.

SECTION R612
EXTERIOR WINDOWS AND DOORS

R612.1 General. This section prescribes performance and construction requirements for exterior window and door installed in wall. Windows and doors shall be installed and flashed in accordance with the fenestration manufacturer's written installation instructions. Window and door openings shall be flashed in accordance with Section R703.8. Written installation instructions shall be provided by the fenestration manufacturer for each window or door.

R612.2 Window sills. In *dwelling* units, where the opening of an operable window is located more than 72 inches (1829 mm) above the finished *grade* or surface below, the lowest part of the clear opening of the window shall be a minimum of 24 inches (610 mm) above the finished floor of the room in which the window is located. Operable sections of windows shall not permit openings that allow passage of a 4 inch (102 mm) diameter sphere where such openings are located within 24 inches (610 mm) of the finished floor.

Exceptions:

1. Windows whose openings will not allow a 4-inch-diameter (102 mm) sphere to pass through the opening when the opening is in its largest opened position.

2. Openings that are provided with window fall prevention devices that comply with Section R612.3.

3. Openings that are provided with fall prevention devices that comply with ASTM F 2090.

4. Windows that are provided with opening limiting devices that comply with Section R612.4.

R612.3 Window fall prevention devices. Window fall prevention devices and window guards, where provided, shall comply with the requirements of ASTM F 2090.

R612.4 Window opening limiting devices. When required elsewhere in this code, window opening limiting devices shall comply with the provisions of this section.

R612.4.1 General requirements. Window opening limiting devices shall be self acting and shall be positioned to prohibit the free passage of a 4-in. (102-mm) diameter rigid sphere through the window opening when the window opening limiting device is installed in accordance with the manufacturer's instructions.

R612.4.2 Operation for emergency escape. Window opening limiting devices shall be designed with release mechanisms to allow for emergency escape through the window opening without the need for keys, tools or special knowledge. Window opening limiting devices shall comply with all of the following:

1. Release of the window opening-limiting device shall require no more than 15 pounds (66 N) of force.

2. The window opening limiting device release mechanism shall operate properly in all types of weather.

3. Window opening limiting devices shall have their release mechanisms clearly identified for proper use in an emergency.

4. The window opening limiting device shall not reduce the minimum net clear opening area of the window unit below what is required by Section R310.1.1 of the code.

R612.5 Performance. Exterior windows and doors shall be designed to resist the design wind loads specified in Table R301.2(2) adjusted for height and exposure per Table R301.2(3).

R612.6 Testing and labeling. Exterior windows and sliding doors shall be tested by an *approved* independent laboratory, and bear a *label* identifying manufacturer, performance characteristics and *approved* inspection agency to indicate compliance with AAMA/WDMA/CSA 101/I.S.2/A440. Exterior side-hinged doors shall be tested and *labeled* as conforming to AAMA/WDMA/CSA 101/I.S.2/A440 or comply with Section R612.8.

Exception: Decorative glazed openings.

R612.6.1 Comparative analysis. Structural wind load design pressures for window and door units smaller than the size tested in accordance with Section R612.6 shall be permitted to be higher than the design value of the tested unit provided such higher pressures are determined by accepted engineering analysis. All components of the small unit shall be the same as those of the tested unit. Where such calculated design pressures are used, they shall be validated by an additional test of the window or door unit having the highest allowable design pressure.

R612.7 Vehicular access doors. Vehicular access doors shall be tested in accordance with either ASTM E 330 or ANSI/DASMA 108, and shall meet the acceptance criteria of ANSI/DASMA 108.

R612.8 Other exterior window and door assemblies. Exterior windows and door assemblies not included within the scope of Section R612.6 or Section R612.7 shall be tested in accordance with ASTM E 330. Glass in assemblies covered by this exception shall comply with Section R308.5.

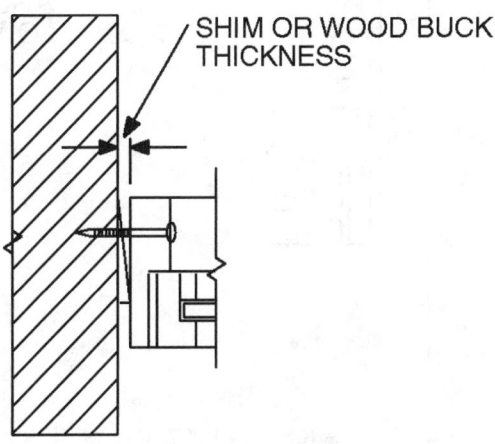

SHIM OR WOOD BUCK THICKNESS

FIGURE R612.8(1)
THROUGH THE FRAME

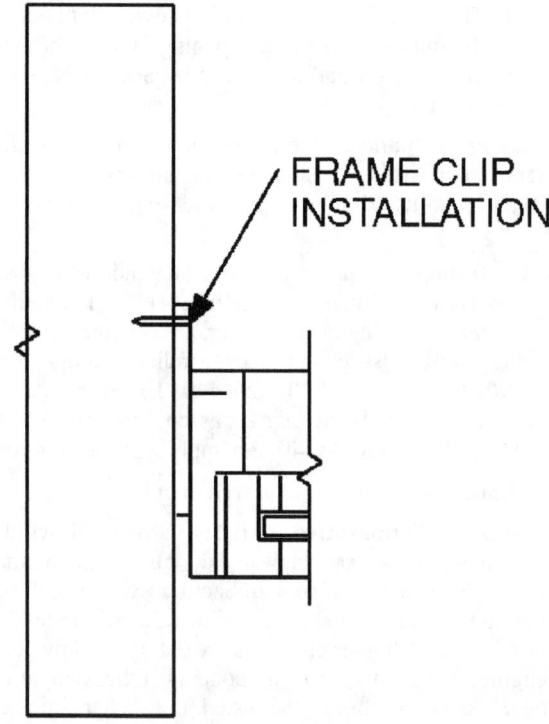

APPLY FRAME CLIP TO WINDOW OR DOOR IN ACCORDANCE WITH PUBLISHED MANUFACTURER'S RECOMMENDATIONS.

FIGURE R612.8(2)
FRAME CLIP

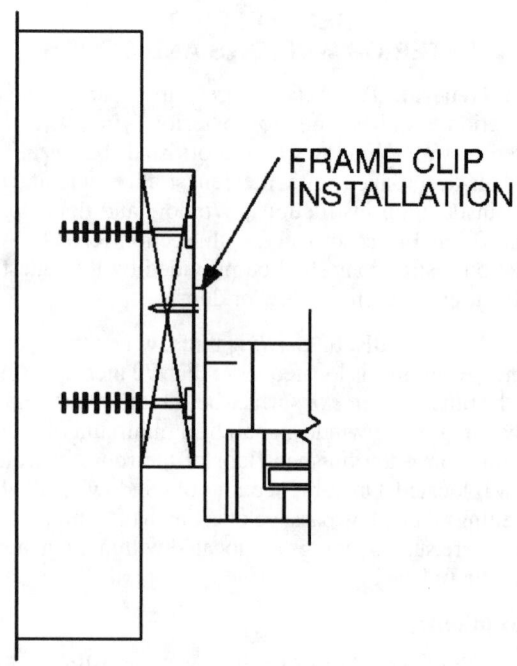

APPLY FRAME CLIP TO WINDOW OR DOOR FRAME IN ACCORDANCE WITH PUBLISHED MANUFACTURER'S RECOMMENDATIONS. ANCHORS SHALL BE PROVIDED TO TRANSFER LOAD FROM THE FRAME CLIP INTO THE ROUGH OPENING SUBSTRATE.

FIGURE R612.8(4)
FRAME CLIP

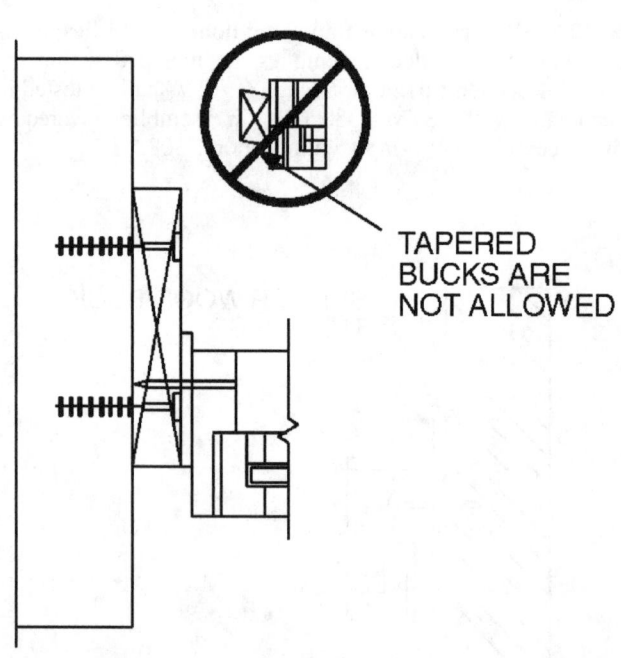

THROUGH THE FRAME ANCHORING METHOD. ANCHORS SHALL BE PROVIDED TO TRANSFER LOAD FROM THE WINDOW OR DOOR FRAME INTO THE ROUGH OPENING SUBSTRATE.

FIGURE R612.8(3)
THROUGH THE FRAME

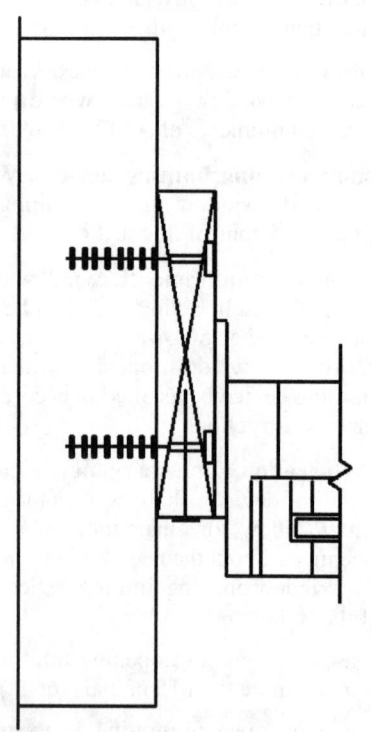

APPLY ANCHORS THROUGH FLANGE IN ACCORDANCE WITH PUBLISHED MANUFACTURER'S RECOMMENDATIONS.

FIGURE R612.8(5)
THROUGH THE FLANGE

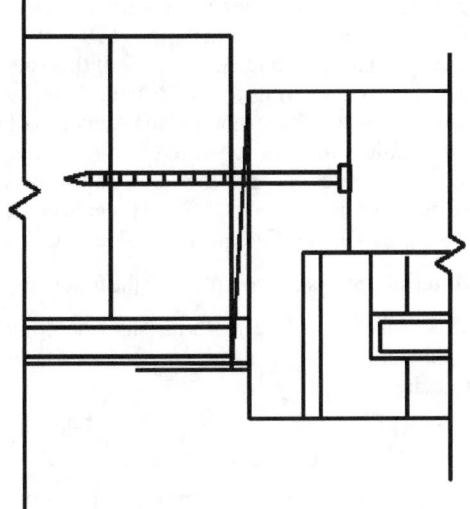

FIGURE R612.8(6)
THROUGH THE FLANGE

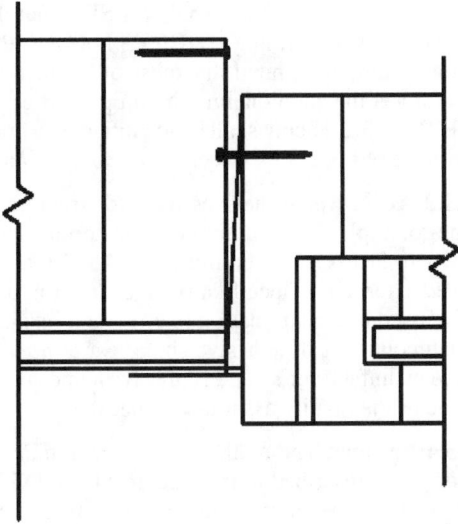

FIGURE R612.8(7)
FRAME CLIP

R612.9 Wind-borne debris protection. Protection of exterior windows and glass doors in buildings located in wind-borne debris regions shall be in accordance with Section R301.2.1.2.

R612.9.1 Fenestration testing and labeling. Fenestration shall be tested by an *approved* independent laboratory, listed by an *approved* entity, and bear a *label* identifying manufacturer, performance characteristics, and *approved* inspection agency to indicate compliance with the requirements of the following specification:

1. ASTM E 1886 and ASTM E 1996; or

2. AAMA 506.

R612.10 Anchorage methods. The methods cited in this section apply only to anchorage of window and glass door assemblies to the main force-resisting system.

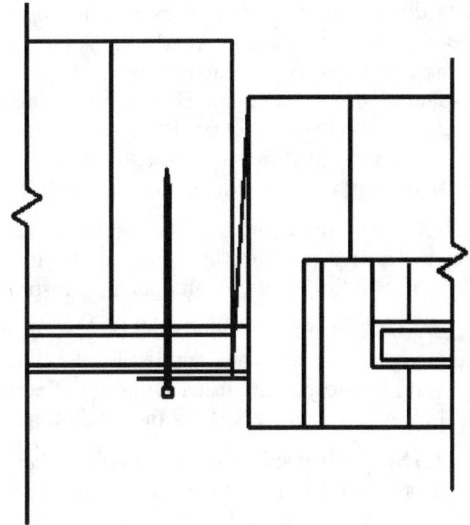

FIGURE R612.8(8)
THROUGH THE FLANGE

R612.10.1 Anchoring requirements. Window and glass door assemblies shall be anchored in accordance with the published manufacturer's recommendations to achieve the design pressure specified. Substitute anchoring systems used for substrates not specified by the fenestration manufacturer shall provide equal or greater anchoring performance as demonstrated by accepted engineering practice.

R612.10.2 Anchorage details. Products shall be anchored in accordance with the minimum requirements illustrated in Figures R612.8(1), R612.8(2), R612.8(3), R612.8(4), R612.8(5), R612.8(6), R612.8(7) and R612.8(8).

R612.10.2.1 Masonry, concrete or other structural substrate. Where the wood shim or buck thickness is less than $1^{1}/_{2}$ inches (38 mm), window and glass door assemblies shall be anchored through the jamb, or by jamb clip and anchors shall be embedded directly into the masonry, concrete or other substantial substrate material. Anchors shall adequately transfer load from the window or door frame into the rough opening substrate [see Figures R612.8(1) and R612.8(2).]

Where the wood shim or buck thickness is $1^{1}/_{2}$ inches (38 mm) or more, the buck is securely fastened to the masonry, concrete or other substantial substrate, and the buck extends beyond the interior face of the window or door frame, window and glass door assemblies shall be anchored through the jamb, or by jamb clip, or through the flange to the secured wood buck. Anchors shall be embedded into the secured wood buck to adequately transfer load from the window or door frame assembly [Figures R612.8(3), R612.8(4) and R612.8(5)].

R612.10.2.2 Wood or other approved framing material. Where the framing material is wood or other *approved* framing material, window and glass door assemblies shall be anchored through the frame, or by frame clip, or through the flange. Anchors shall be embedded into the frame construction to adequately transfer load [Figures R612.8(6), R612.8(7) and R612.8(8)].

R612.11 Mullions. Mullions shall be tested by an *approved* testing laboratory in accordance with AAMA 450, or be engineered in accordance with accepted engineering practice. Mullions tested as stand-alone units or qualified by engineering shall use performance criteria cited in Sections R612.11.1, R612.11.2 and R612.11.3. Mullions qualified by an actual test of an entire assembly shall comply with Sections R612.11.1 and R612.11.3.

R612.11.1 Load transfer. Mullions shall be designed to transfer the design pressure loads applied by the window and door assemblies to the rough opening substrate.

R612.11.2 Deflection. Mullions shall be capable of resisting the design pressure loads applied by the window and door assemblies to be supported without deflecting more than $L/175$, where L is the span of the mullion in inches.

R612.11.3 Structural safety factor. Mullions shall be capable of resisting a load of 1.5 times the design pressure loads applied by the window and door assemblies to be supported without exceeding the appropriate material stress levels. If tested by an *approved* laboratory, the 1.5 times the design pressure load shall be sustained for 10 seconds, and the permanent deformation shall not exceed 0.4 percent of the mullion span after the 1.5 times design pressure load is removed.

SECTION R613
STRUCTURAL INSULATED PANEL WALL CONSTRUCTION

R613.1 General. Structural insulated panel (SIP) walls shall be designed in accordance with the provisions of this section. When the provisions of this section are used to design structural insulated panel walls, project drawings, typical details and specifications are not required to bear the seal of the architect or engineer responsible for design, unless otherwise required by the state law of the *jurisdiction* having authority.

R613.2 Applicability limits. The provisions of this section shall control the construction of exterior structural insulated panel walls and interior load-bearing structural insulated panel walls for buildings not greater than 60 feet (18 288 mm) in length perpendicular to the joist or truss span, not greater than 40 feet (12 192 mm) in width parallel to the joist or truss span and not greater than two stories in height with each wall not greater than 10 feet (3048 mm) high. All exterior walls installed in accordance with the provisions of this section shall be considered as load-bearing walls. Structural insulated panel walls constructed in accordance with the provisions of this section shall be limited to sites subjected to a maximum design wind speed of 130 miles per hour (58 m/s), Exposure A, B or C, and a maximum ground snow load of 70 pounds per foot (3.35 kPa), and Seismic Design Categories A, B, and C.

R613.3 Materials. SIPs shall comply with the following criteria:

R613.3.1 Core. The core material shall be composed of foam plastic insulation meeting one of the following requirements:

1. ASTM C 578 and have a minimum density of 0.90 pounds per cubic feet (14.4 kg/m³); or

2. Polyurethane meeting the physical properties shown in Table R613.3.1, or;

3. An *approved* alternative.

All cores shall meet the requirements of Section R316.

R613.3.2 Facing. Facing materials for SIPs shall be wood structural panels conforming to DOC PS 1 or DOC PS 2, each having a minimum nominal thickness of $^7/_{16}$ inch (11 mm) and shall meet the additional minimum properties specified in Table R613.3.2. Facing shall be identified by a grade mark or certificate of inspection issued by an *approved* agency.

R613.3.3 Adhesive. Adhesives used to structurally laminate the foam plastic insulation core material to the structural wood facers shall conform to ASTM D 2559 or *approved* alternative specifically intended for use as an adhesive used in the lamination of structural insulated panels. Each container of adhesive shall bear a *label* with the adhesive manufacturer's name, adhesive name and type and the name of the quality assurance agency.

R613.3.4 Lumber. The minimum lumber framing material used for SIPs prescribed in this document is NLGA graded No. 2 Spruce-pine-fir. Substitution of other wood species/grades that meet or exceed the mechanical properties and specific gravity of No. 2 Spruce-pine-fir shall be permitted.

TABLE R613.3.1
MINIMUM PROPERTIES FOR POLYURETHANE INSULATION USED AS SIPS CORE

PHYSICAL PROPERTY	POLYURETHANE
Density, core nominal. (ASTM D 1622)	2.2 lb/ft³
Compressive resistance at yield or 10% deformation, whichever occurs first. (ASTM D 1621)	19 psi (perpendicular to rise)
Flexural strength, min. (ASTM C 203)	30 psi
Tensile strength, min. (ASTM D 1623)	35 psi
Shear strength, min. (ASTM C 273)	25 psi
Substrate adhesion, min. (ASTM D 1623)	22 psi
Water vapor permeance of 1.00-in. thickness, max. (ASTM E 96)	2.3 perm
Water absorption by total immersion, max. (ASTM C 272)	4.3% (volume)
Dimensional stability (change in dimensions), max. [ASTM D2126 (7 days at 158°F/100% humidity and 7 days at -20°F)]	2%

For SI: 1 pound per cubic foot = 16.02 kg/m³, 1 pound per square inch = 6.895 kPa, °C = [(°F) - 32]1.8.

TABLE R613.3.2
MINIMUM PROPERTIES[a] FOR WOOD STRUCTURAL PANEL FACING MATERIAL USED IN SIP WALLS

THICKNESS (inch)	PRODUCT	FLATWISE STIFFNESS[b] (lbf-in²/ft)		FLATWISE STRENGTH[c] (lbf-in/ft)		TENSION[c] (lbf/ft)		DENSITY[b, d] (pcf)
		Along	Across	Along	Across	Along	Across	
$^7/_{16}$	Sheathing	54,700	27,100	950	870	6,800	6,500	35

For SI: 1 inch = 25.4 mm, 1 lbf-in²/ft = 9.415 × 10⁻⁶ kPa/m, 1 lbf-in/ft = 3.707 × 10⁻⁴ kN/m, 1 lbf/ft = 0.0146 N/mm, 1 pound per cubic foot = 16.018 kg/m³.
a. Values listed in Table R613.3.2 are qualification test values and are not to be used for design purposes.
b. Mean test value shall be in accordance with Section 7.6 of DOC PS 2.
c. Characteristic test value (5th percent with 75% confidence).
d. Density shall be based on oven-dry weight and oven-dry volume.

R613.3.5 SIP screws. Screws used for the erection of SIPs as specified in Section R613.5 shall be fabricated from steel, shall be provided by the SIPs manufacturer and shall be sized to penetrate the wood member to which the assembly is being attached by a minimum of 1 inch (25 mm). The screws shall be corrosion resistant and have a minimum shank diameter of 0.188 inch (4.7 mm) and a minimum head diameter of 0.620 inch (15.5 mm).

R613.3.6 Nails. Nails specified in Section R613 shall be common or galvanized box unless otherwise stated.

R613.4 SIP wall panels. SIPs shall comply with Figure R613.4 and shall have minimum panel thickness in accordance with Tables R613.5(1) and R613.5(2) for above-grade walls. All SIPs shall be identified by grade mark or certificate of inspection issued by an *approved* agency.

R613.4.1 Labeling. All panels shall be identified by grade mark or certificate of inspection issued by an *approved* agency. Each (SIP) shall bear a stamp or *label* with the following minimum information:

1. Manufacturer name/logo.

2. Identification of the assembly.

3. Quality assurance agency.

R613.5 Wall construction. Exterior walls of SIP construction shall be designed and constructed in accordance with the provisions of this section and Tables R613.5(1) and R613.5(2) and Figures R613.5(1) through R613.5(5). SIP walls shall be fastened to other wood building components in accordance with Tables R602.3(1) through R602.3(4).

Framing shall be attached in accordance with Section R602.3(1) unless otherwise provided for in Section R613.

R613.5.1 Top plate connection. SIP walls shall be capped with a double top plate installed to provide overlapping at corner, intersections and splines in accordance with Figure R613.5.1. The double top plates shall be made up of a single 2 by top plate having a width equal to the width of the panel core, and shall be recessed into the SIP below. Over this top plate a cap plate shall be placed. The cap plate width shall match the SIP thickness and overlap the facers on both sides of the panel. End joints in top plates shall be offset at least 24 inches (610 mm).

R613.5.2 Bottom (sole) plate connection. SIP walls shall have full bearing on a sole plate having a width equal to the nominal width of the foam core. When SIP walls are sup-ported directly on continuous foundations, the wall wood sill plate shall be anchored to the foundation in accordance with Figure R613.5.2 and Section R403.1.

R613.5.3 Wall bracing. SIP walls shall be braced in accordance with Section R602.10. SIP walls shall be considered continuous wood structural panel sheathing for purposes of computing required bracing. SIP walls shall meet the requirements of Section R602.10.4 except that SIPs corners shall be fabricated as shown in Figure R613.9. When SIP walls are used for wall bracing, the SIP bottom plate shall be attached to wood framing below in accordance with Table R602.3(1).

R613.6 Interior load-bearing walls. Interior load-bearing walls shall be constructed as specified for exterior walls.

R613.7 Drilling and notching. The maximum vertical chase penetration in SIPs shall have a maximum side dimension of 2 inches (51 mm) centered in the panel core. Vertical chases shall have a minimum spacing of 24-inches (610 mm) on center. Maximum of two horizontal chases shall be permitted in each wall panel, one at 14 inches (360 mm) from the bottom of the panel and one at mid-height of the wall panel. The maximum allowable penetration size in a wall panel shall be circular or rectangular with a maximum dimension of 12 inches (305 mm). Overcutting of holes in facing panels shall not be permitted.

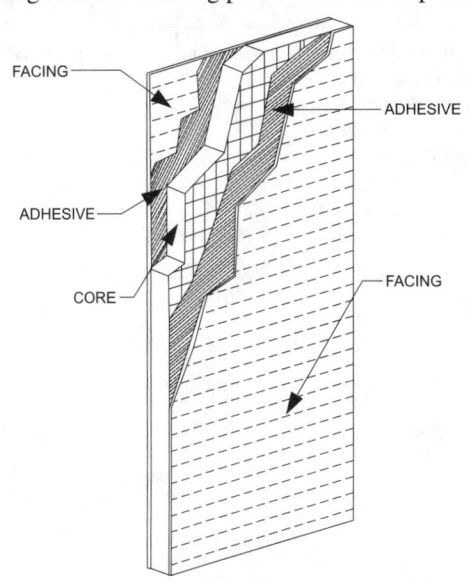

FACING

ADHESIVE

ADHESIVE

CORE

FACING

FIGURE R613.4
SIP WALL PANEL

TABLE R613.5(1)
MINIMUM THICKNESS FOR SIP WALL SUPPORTING SIP LIGHT-FRAME ROOF ONLY (inches)

WIND SPEED (3-second gust)		SNOW LOAD (psf)	BUILDING WIDTH (feet)														
			24			28			32			36			40		
			Wall Height (ft)			Wall Height (ft)			Wall Height (ft)			Wall Height (ft)			Wall Height (ft)		
Exp. A/B	Exp. C		8	9	10	8	9	10	8	9	10	8	9	10	8	9	10
85	—	20	4.5	4.5	4.5	4.5	4.5	4.5	4.5	4.5	4.5	4.5	4.5	4.5	4.5	4.5	4.5
		30	4.5	4.5	4.5	4.5	4.5	4.5	4.5	4.5	4.5	4.5	4.5	4.5	4.5	4.5	4.5
		50	4.5	4.5	4.5	4.5	4.5	4.5	4.5	4.5	4.5	4.5	4.5	4.5	4.5	4.5	4.5
		70	4.5	4.5	4.5	4.5	4.5	4.5	4.5	4.5	4.5	4.5	4.5	4.5	4.5	4.5	4.5
100	85	20	4.5	4.5	4.5	4.5	4.5	4.5	4.5	4.5	4.5	4.5	4.5	4.5	4.5	4.5	4.5
		30	4.5	4.5	4.5	4.5	4.5	4.5	4.5	4.5	4.5	4.5	4.5	4.5	4.5	4.5	4.5
		50	4.5	4.5	4.5	4.5	4.5	4.5	4.5	4.5	4.5	4.5	4.5	4.5	4.5	4.5	4.5
		70	4.5	4.5	4.5	4.5	4.5	4.5	4.5	4.5	4.5	4.5	4.5	4.5	4.5	4.5	4.5
110	100	20	4.5	4.5	4.5	4.5	4.5	4.5	4.5	4.5	4.5	4.5	4.5	4.5	4.5	4.5	4.5
		30	4.5	4.5	4.5	4.5	4.5	4.5	4.5	4.5	4.5	4.5	4.5	4.5	4.5	4.5	4.5
		50	4.5	4.5	4.5	4.5	4.5	4.5	4.5	4.5	4.5	4.5	4.5	4.5	4.5	4.5	4.5
		70	4.5	4.5	4.5	4.5	4.5	4.5	4.5	4.5	4.5	4.5	4.5	4.5	4.5	4.5	4.5
120	110	20	4.5	4.5	4.5	4.5	4.5	4.5	4.5	4.5	4.5	4.5	4.5	4.5	4.5	4.5	4.5
		30	4.5	4.5	4.5	4.5	4.5	4.5	4.5	4.5	4.5	4.5	4.5	4.5	4.5	4.5	4.5
		50	4.5	4.5	4.5	4.5	4.5	4.5	4.5	4.5	4.5	4.5	4.5	4.5	4.5	4.5	4.5
		70	4.5	4.5	4.5	4.5	4.5	4.5	4.5	4.5	4.5	4.5	4.5	6.5	4.5	4.5	6.5
130	120	20	4.5	4.5	4.5	4.5	4.5	4.5	4.5	4.5	4.5	4.5	4.5	4.5	4.5	4.5	4.5
		30	4.5	4.5	4.5	4.5	4.5	4.5	4.5	4.5	4.5	4.5	4.5	4.5	4.5	4.5	4.5
		50	4.5	4.5	4.5	4.5	4.5	4.5	4.5	4.5	6.5	4.5	4.5	6.5	4.5	4.5	6.5
		70	4.5	4.5	4.5	4.5	4.5	6.5	4.5	4.5	6.5	4.5	6.5	N/A	4.5	6.5	N/A
—	130	20	4.5	4.5	6.5	4.5	4.5	N/A	4.5	4.5	N/A	4.5	4.5	N/A	4.5	6.5	N/A
		30	4.5	4.5	N/A	4.5	4.5	N/A	4.5	4.5	N/A	4.5	6.5	N/A	4.5	6.5	N/A
		50	4.5	6.5	N/A	4.5	6.5	N/A	4.5	N/A	N/A	6.5	N/A	N/A	6.5	N/A	N/A
		70	4.5	N/A	N/A	6.5	N/A	N/A	6.5	N/A	N/A	N/A	N/A	N/A	N/A	N/A	N/A

For SI: 1 inch = 25.4 mm; 1 foot = 304.8 mm; 1 pound per square foot = 0.0479 kPa.
Maximum deflection criterion: L/240.
Maximum roof dead load: 10 psf.
Maximum roof live load: 70 psf.
Maximum ceiling dead load: 5 psf.
Maximum ceiling live load: 20 psf.
Wind loads based on Table R301.2 (2).
N/A indicates not applicable.

TABLE R613.5(2)
MINIMUM THICKNESS FOR SIP WALLS SUPPORTING SIP OR LIGHT-FRAME ONE STORY AND ROOF (inches)

WIND SPEED (3-second gust)		SNOW LOAD (psf)	BUILDING WIDTH (feet)														
			24			28			32			36			40		
			Wall Height (feet)			Wall Height (feet)			Wall Height (feet)			Wall Height (feet)			Wall Height (feet)		
Exp. A/B	Exp. C		8	9	10	8	9	10	8	9	10	8	9	10	8	9	10
85	—	20	4.5	4.5	4.5	4.5	4.5	4.5	4.5	4.5	4.5	4.5	4.5	4.5	4.5	4.5	4.5
		30	4.5	4.5	4.5	4.5	4.5	4.5	4.5	4.5	4.5	4.5	4.5	4.5	4.5	4.5	4.5
		50	4.5	4.5	4.5	4.5	4.5	4.5	4.5	4.5	4.5	4.5	4.5	4.5	4.5	4.5	4.5
		70	4.5	4.5	4.5	4.5	4.5	4.5	4.5	4.5	4.5	4.5	4.5	6.5	6.5	6.5	6.5
100	85	20	4.5	4.5	4.5	4.5	4.5	4.5	4.5	4.5	4.5	4.5	4.5	4.5	4.5	4.5	4.5
		30	4.5	4.5	4.5	4.5	4.5	4.5	4.5	4.5	4.5	4.5	4.5	4.5	4.5	4.5	6.5
		50	4.5	4.5	4.5	4.5	4.5	4.5	4.5	4.5	4.5	4.5	4.5	6.5	4.5	6.5	6.5
		70	4.5	4.5	4.5	4.5	4.5	4.5	4.5	4.5	6.5	6.5	6.5	6.5	6.5	N/A	N/A
110	100	20	4.5	4.5	4.5	4.5	4.5	4.5	4.5	4.5	4.5	4.5	4.5	4.5	4.5	4.5	6.5
		30	4.5	4.5	4.5	4.5	4.5	4.5	4.5	4.5	4.5	4.5	4.5	6.5	4.5	6.5	6.5
		50	4.5	4.5	4.5	4.5	4.5	4.5	4.5	4.5	6.5	4.5	6.5	6.5	6.5	6.5	N/A
		70	4.5	4.5	4.5	4.5	4.5	6.5	6.5	6.5	N/A	6.5	N/A	N/A	N/A	N/A	N/A
120	110	20	4.5	4.5	4.5	4.5	4.5	4.5	4.5	4.5	6.5	4.5	4.5	6.5	4.5	6.5	N/A
		30	4.5	4.5	4.5	4.5	4.5	6.5	4.5	4.5	6.5	4.5	6.5	N/A	6.5	6.5	N/A
		50	4.5	4.5	6.5	4.5	4.5	6.5	4.5	6.5	N/A	6.5	N/A	N/A	N/A	N/A	N/A
		70	4.5	4.5	6.5	4.5	6.5	N/A	6.5	N/A	N/A	N/A	N/A	N/A	N/A	N/A	N/A
130	120	20	4.5	4.5	6.5	4.5	4.5	6.5	4.5	6.5	N/A	4.5	6.5	N/A	6.5	N/A	N/A
		30	4.5	4.5	6.5	4.5	4.5	N/A	4.5	6.5	N/A	6.5	N/A	N/A	6.5	N/A	N/A
		50	4.5	6.5	N/A	4.5	6.5	N/A	6.5	N/A	N/A	N/A	N/A	N/A	N/A	N/A	N/A
		70	4.5	6.5	N/A	6.5	N/A	N/A	N/A	N/A	N/A	N/A	N/A	N/A	N/A	N/A	N/A
—	130	20	6.5	N/A	N/A	6.5	N/A	N/A	N/A	N/A	N/A	N/A	N/A	N/A	N/A	N/A	N/A
		30	6.5	N/A	N/A	N/A	N/A	N/A	N/A	N/A	N/A	N/A	N/A	N/A	N/A	N/A	N/A
		50	N/A	N/A	N/A	N/A	N/A	N/A	N/A	N/A	N/A	N/A	N/A	N/A	N/A	N/A	N/A
		70	N/A	N/A	N/A	N/A	N/A	N/A	N/A	N/A	N/A	N/A	N/A	N/A	N/A	N/A	N/A

For SI: 1 inch = 25.4 mm; 1 foot = 304.8 mm; 1 pound per square foot = 0.0479 kPa.
   Maximum deflection criterion: $L/240$.
   Maximum roof dead load: 10 psf.
   Maximum roof live load: 70 psf.
   Maximum ceiling dead load: 5 psf.
   Maximum ceiling live load: 20 psf.
   Maximum second floor live load: 30 psf.
   Maximum second floor dead load: 10 psf.
   Maximum second floor dead load from walls: 10 psf.
   Maximum first floor live load: 40 psf.
   Maximum first floor dead load: 10 psf.
   Wind loads based on Table R301.2 (2).
   N/A indicates not applicable.

R613.8 Connection. SIPs shall be connected at vertical in-plane joints in accordance with Figure R613.8 or by other *approved* methods.

R613.9 Corner framing. Corner framing of SIP walls shall be constructed in accordance with Figure R613.9.

R613.10 Headers. SIP headers shall be designed and constructed in accordance with Table R613.10 and Figure R613.5.1. SIPs headers shall be continuous sections without splines. Headers shall be at least $11^7/_8$ inches (302 mm) deep. Headers longer than 4 feet (1219 mm) shall be constructed in accordance with Section R602.7.

R613.10.1 Wood structural panel box headers. Wood structural panel box headers shall be allowed where SIP headers are not applicable. Wood structural panel box headers shall be constructed in accordance with Figure R602.7.2 and Table R602.7.2.

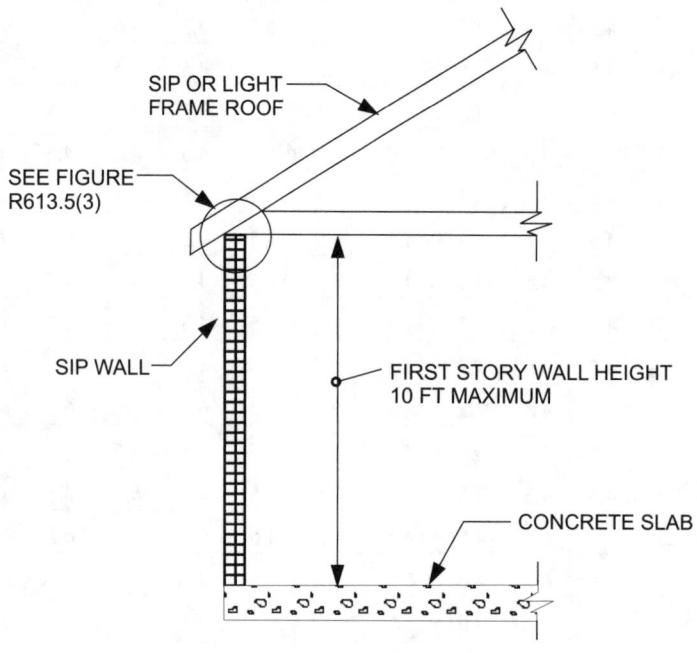

For SI: 1 foot = 304.8 mm.

FIGURE R613.5(1)
MAXIMUM ALLOWABLE HEIGHT OF SIP WALLS

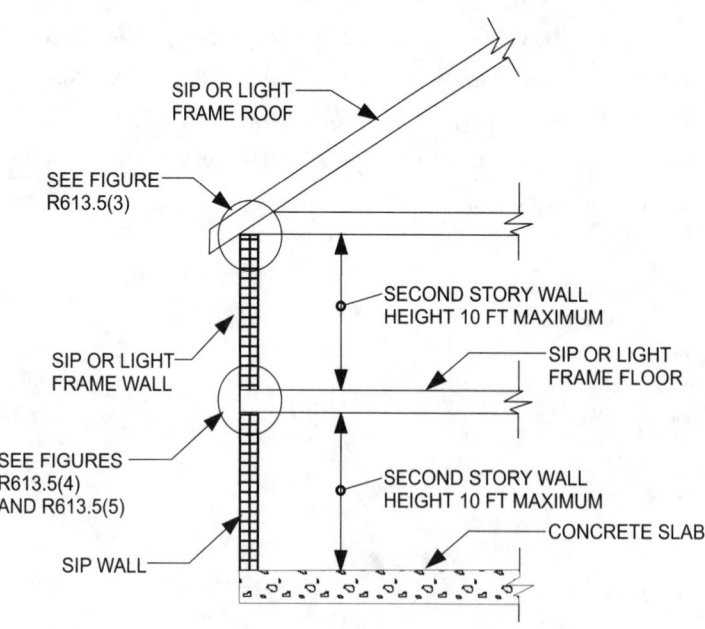

For SI: 1 foot = 304.8 mm.

FIGURE R613.5(2)
MAXIMUM ALLOWABLE HEIGHT OF SIP WALLS

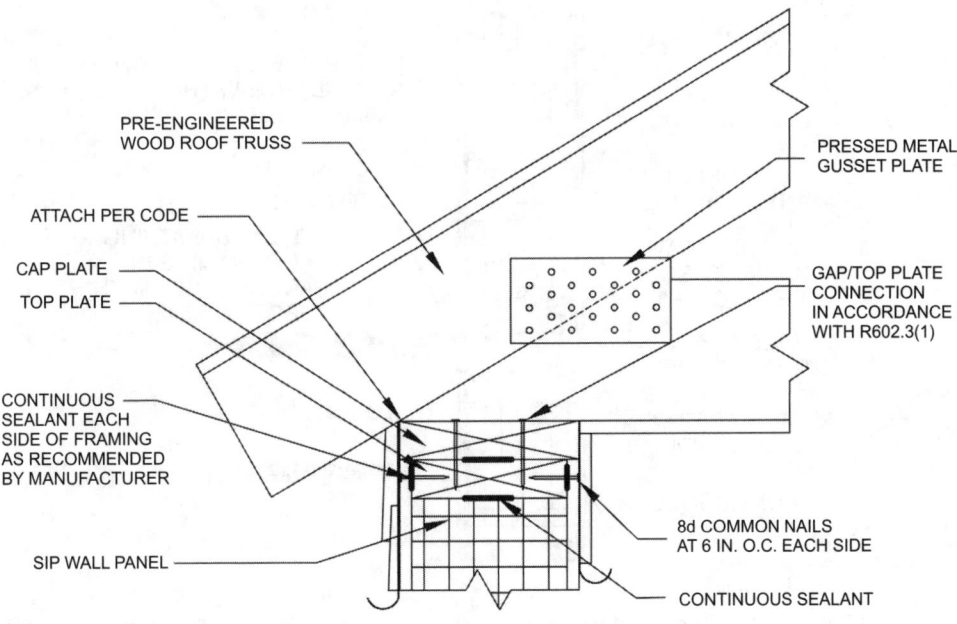

For SI: 1 inch = 25.4 mm.

FIGURE R613.5(3)
TRUSSED ROOF TO TOP PLATE CONNECTION

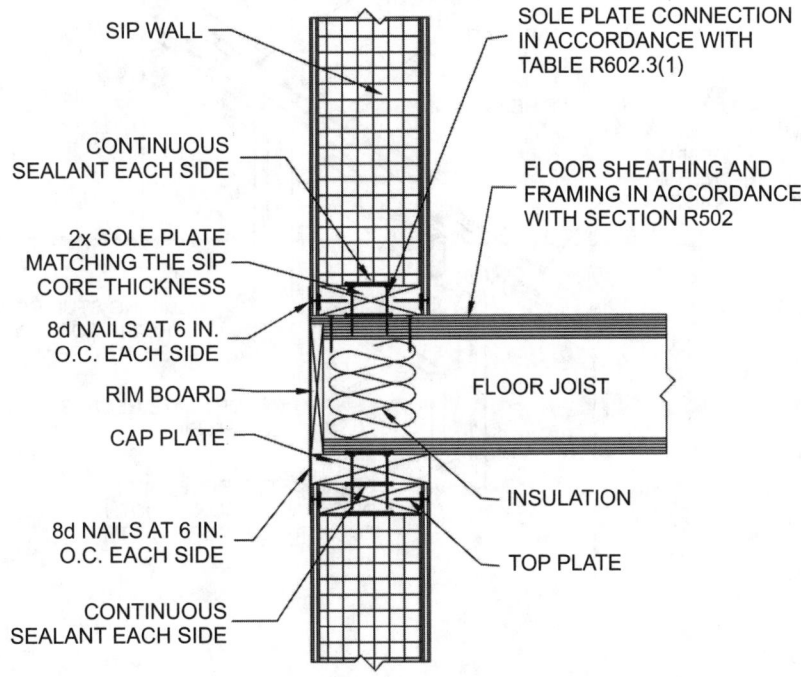

For SI: 1 inch = 25.4 mm.

Note: Figures illustrate SIP-specific attachment requirements. Other connections shall be made in accordance with Table R602.3(1) and (2) as appropriate.

FIGURE R613.5(4)
SIP WALL TO WALL PLATFORM FRAME CONNECTION

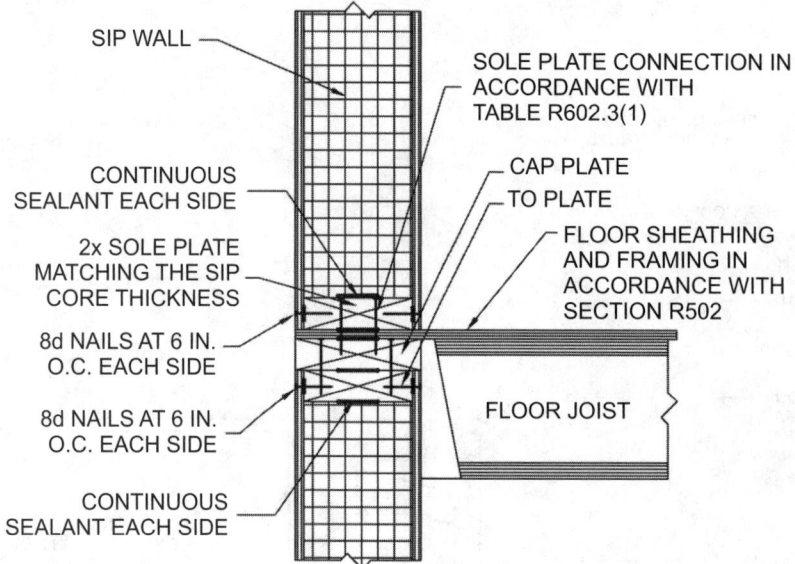

For SI: 1 inch = 25.4 mm.

Note: Figures illustrate SIP-specific attachment requirements. Other connections shall be made in accordance with Tables R602.3(1) and (2), as appropriate.

FIGURE R613.5(5)
SIP WALL TO WALL BALLOON FRAME CONNECTION
(I-Joist floor shown for Illustration only)

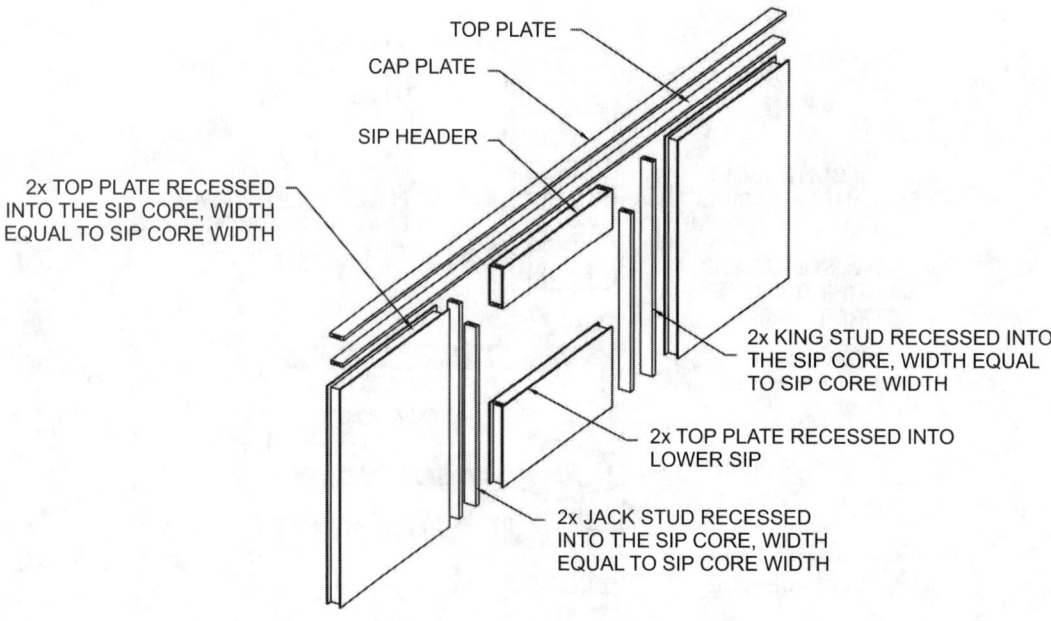

For SI: 1 inch = 25.4 mm.

Notes:

1. Top plates shall be continuous over header.
2. Lower 2x top plate shall have a width equal to the SIP core width and shall be recessed into the top edge of the panel. Cap plate shall be placed over the recessed top plate and shall have a width equal to the SIPs width.
3. SIP facing surfaces shall be nailed to framing and cripples with 8d common or galvanized box nails spaced 6 inches on center.
4. Galvanized nails shall be hot-dipped or tumbled. Framing shall be attached in accordance to Section R602.3(1) unless otherwise provide for in Section R613.

FIGURE R613.5.1
SIP WALL FRAMING CONFIGURATION

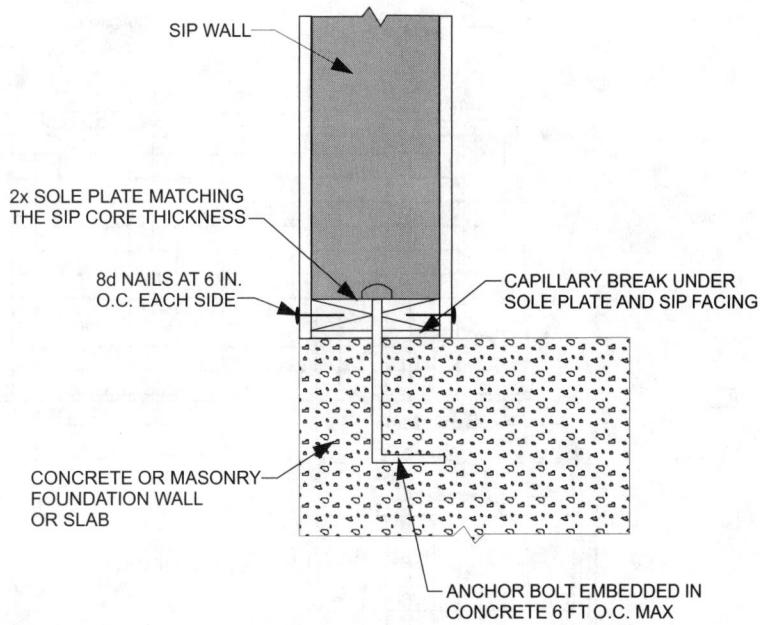

For SI: 1 inch = 25.4 mm, 1 foot = 304.8 mm.

FIGURE R613.5.2
SIP WALL TO CONCRETE SLAB FOR FOUNDATION WALL ATTACHMENT

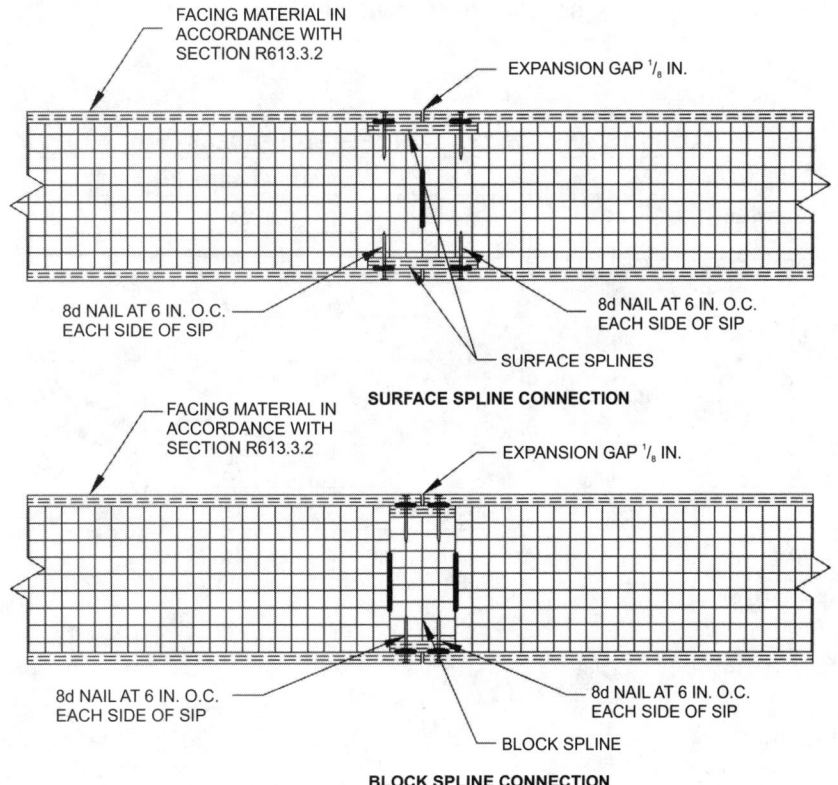

For SI: 1 inch = 25.4 mm.

FIGURE R613.8
TYPICAL SIP CONNECTION DETAILS FOR VERTICAL IN-PLANE JOINTS

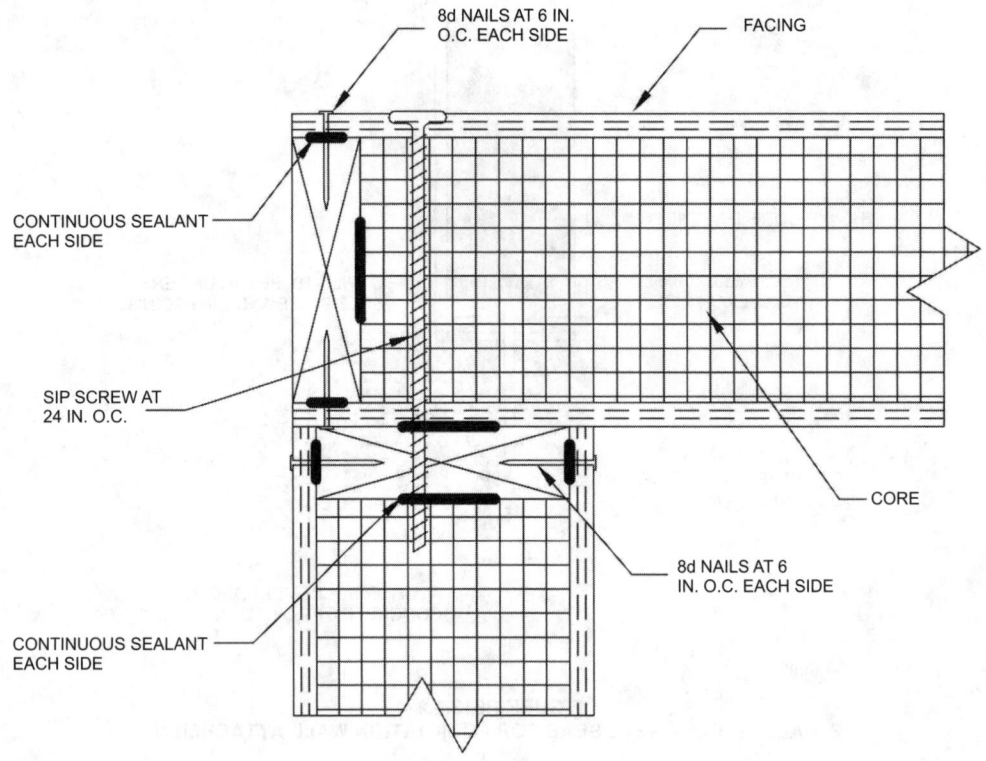

For SI: 1 inch = 25.4 mm.

FIGURE R613.9
SIP CORNER FRAMING DETAIL

TABLE R614.10
MAXIMUM SPANS FOR 11$^7/_8$ INCH DEEP SIP HEADERS (feet)

LOAD CONDITION	SNOW LOAD (psf)	BUILDING WIDTH (feet)				
		24	28	32	36	40
Supporting roof only	20	4	4	4	4	2
	30	4	4	4	2	2
	50	2	2	2	2	2
	70	2	2	2	N/A	N/A
Supporting roof and one-story	20	2	2	N/A	N/A	N/A
	30	2	2	N/A	N/A	N/A
	50	2	N/A	N/A	N/A	N/A
	70	N/A	N/A	N/A	N/A	N/A

For SI: 1 inch = 25.4 mm, 1 foot = 304.8 mm.

Maximum deflection criterion: $L/360$.

Maximum roof dead load: 10 psf.

Maximum ceiling load: 5 psf.

Maximum second floor live load: 30 psf.

Maximum second floor dead load: 10 psf.

Maximum second floor dead load from walls: 10 psf.

N/A indicates not applicable.

CHAPTER 7
WALL COVERING

SECTION R701
GENERAL

R701.1 Application. The provisions of this chapter shall control the design and construction of the interior and exterior wall covering for all buildings.

R701.2 Installation. Products sensitive to adverse weather shall not be installed until adequate weather protection for the installation is provided. Exterior sheathing shall be dry before applying exterior cover.

SECTION R702
INTERIOR COVERING

R702.1 General. Interior coverings or wall finishes shall be installed in accordance with this chapter and Table R702.1(1), Table R702.1(2), Table R702.1(3) and Table R702.3.5. Interior masonry veneer shall comply with the requirements of Section R703.7.1 for support and Section R703.7.4 for anchorage, except an air space is not required. Interior finishes and materials shall conform to the flame spread and smoke-development requirements of Section R302.9.

TABLE R702.1(1)
THICKNESS OF PLASTER

PLASTER BASE	FINISHED THICKNESS OF PLASTER FROM FACE OF LATH, MASONRY, CONCRETE (inches)	
	Gypsum Plaster	Cement Plaster
Expanded metal lath	$5/8$, minimum[a]	$5/8$, minimum[a]
Wire lath	$5/8$, minimum[a]	$3/4$, minimum (interior)[b] $7/8$, minimum (exterior)[b]
Gypsum lath[g]	$1/2$, minimum	$3/4$, minimum (interior)[b]
Masonry walls[c]	$1/2$, minimum	$1/2$, minimum
Monolithic concrete walls[c, d]	$5/8$, maximum	$7/8$, maximum
Monolithic concrete ceilings[c, d]	$3/8$, maximum[e]	$1/2$, maximum
Gypsum veneer base[f, g]	$1/16$, minimum	$3/4$, minimum (interior)[b]
Gypsum sheathing[g]	—	$3/4$, minimum (interior)[b] $7/8$, minimum (exterior)[b]

For SI: 1 inch = 25.4 mm.

a. When measured from back plane of expanded metal lath, exclusive of ribs, or self-furring lath, plaster thickness shall be $3/4$ inch minimum.
b. When measured from face of support or backing.
c. Because masonry and concrete surfaces may vary in plane, thickness of plaster need not be uniform.
d. When applied over a liquid bonding agent, finish coat may be applied directly to concrete surface.
e. Approved acoustical plaster may be applied directly to concrete or over base coat plaster, beyond the maximum plaster thickness shown.
f. Attachment shall be in accordance with Table R702.3.5.
g. Where gypsum board is used as a base for cement plaster, a water-resistive barrier complying with Section R703.2 shall be provided.

TABLE R702.1(2)
GYPSUM PLASTER PROPORTIONS[a]

NUMBER	COAT	PLASTER BASE OR LATH	MAXIMUM VOLUME AGGREGATE PER 100 POUNDS NEAT PLASTER[b] (cubic feet)	
			Damp Loose Sand[a]	Perlite or Vermiculite[c]
Two-coat work	Base coat	Gypsum lath	2.5	2
	Base coat	Masonry	3	3
Three-coat work	First coat	Lath	2[d]	2
	Second coat	Lath	3[d]	2[e]
	First and second coats	Masonry	3	3

For SI: 1 inch = 25.4 mm, 1 cubic foot = 0.0283 m³, 1 pound = 0.454 kg.

a. Wood-fibered gypsum plaster may be mixed in the proportions of 100 pounds of gypsum to not more than 1 cubic foot of sand where applied on masonry or concrete.
b. When determining the amount of aggregate in set plaster, a tolerance of 10 percent shall be allowed.
c. Combinations of sand and lightweight aggregate may be used, provided the volume and weight relationship of the combined aggregate to gypsum plaster is maintained.
d. If used for both first and second coats, the volume of aggregate may be 2.5 cubic feet.
e. Where plaster is 1 inch or more in total thickness, the proportions for the second coat may be increased to 3 cubic feet.

TABLE R702.1(3)
CEMENT PLASTER PROPORTIONS, PARTS BY VOLUME

| COAT | CEMENT PLASTER TYPE | CEMENTITIOUS MATERIALS | | | | VOLUME OF AGGREGATE PER SUM OF SEPARATE VOLUMES OF CEMENTITIOUS MATERIALS[b] |
		Portland Cement Type I, II or III or Blended Cement Type IP, I (PM), IS or I (SM)	Plastic Cement	Masonry Cement Type M, S or N	Lime	
First	Portland or blended	1			$^3/_4$ - $1^1/_2$[a]	$2^1/_2$ - 4
	Masonry				1	$2^1/_2$ - 4
	Plastic		1			$2^1/_2$ - 4
Second	Portland or blended	1			$^3/_4$ - $1^1/_2$	3 - 5
	Masonry			1		3 - 5
	Plastic		1			3 - 5
Finish	Portland or blended	1			$^3/_4$ - 2	$1^1/_2$ - 3
	Masonry			1		$1^1/_2$ - 3
	Plastic		1			$1^1/_2$ - 3

For SI: 1 inch = 25.4 mm, 1 pound = 0.545 kg.

a. Lime by volume of 0 to $^3/_4$ shall be used when the plaster will be placed over low-absorption surfaces such as dense clay tile or brick.

b. The same or greater sand proportion shall be used in the second coat than used in the first coat.

TABLE R702.3.5
MINIMUM THICKNESS AND APPLICATION OF GYPSUM BOARD

| THICKNESS OF GYPSUM BOARD (inches) | APPLICATION | ORIENTATION OF GYPSUM BOARD TO FRAMING | MAXIMUM SPACING OF FRAMING MEMBERS (inches o.c.) | MAXIMUM SPACING OF FASTENERS (inches) | | SIZE OF NAILS FOR APPLICATION TO WOOD FRAMING[c] |
				Nails[a]	Screws[b]	
Application without adhesive						
$^3/_8$	Ceiling[d]	Perpendicular	16	7	12	13 gage, $1^1/_4$″ long, $^{19}/_{64}$″ head; 0.098″ diameter, $1^1/_4$″ long, annular-ringed; or 4d cooler nail, 0.080″ diameter, $1^3/_8$″ long, $^7/_{32}$″ head.
	Wall	Either direction	16	8	16	
$^1/_2$	Ceiling	Either direction	16	7	12	13 gage, $1^3/_8$″ long, $^{19}/_{64}$″ head; 0.098″ diameter, $1^1/_4$″ long, annular-ringed; 5d cooler nail, 0.086″ diameter, $1^5/_8$″ long, $^{15}/_{64}$″ head; or gypsum board nail, 0.086″ diameter, $1^5/_8$″ long, $^9/_{32}$″ head.
	Ceiling[d]	Perpendicular	24	7	12	
	Wall	Either direction	24	8	12	
	Wall	Either direction	16	8	16	
$^5/_8$	Ceiling	Either direction	16	7	12	13 gage, $1^5/_8$″ long, $^{19}/_{64}$″ head; 0.098″ diameter, $1^3/_8$″ long, annular-ringed; 6d cooler nail, 0.092″ diameter, $1^7/_8$″ long, $^1/_4$″ head; or gypsum board nail, 0.0915″ diameter, $1^7/_8$″ long, $^{19}/_{64}$″ head.
	Ceiling[e]	Perpendicular	24	7	12	
	Wall	Either direction	24	8	12	
	Wall	Either direction	16	8	16	
Application with adhesive						
$^3/_8$	Ceiling[d]	Perpendicular	16	16	16	Same as above for $^3/_8$″ gypsum board
	Wall	Either direction	16	16	24	
$^1/_2$ or $^5/_8$	Ceiling	Either direction	16	16	16	Same as above for $^1/_2$″ and $^5/_8$″ gypsum board, respectively
	Ceiling[d]	Perpendicular	24	12	16	
	Wall	Either direction	24	16	24	
Two $^3/_8$ layers	Ceiling	Perpendicular	16	16	16	Base ply nailed as above for $^1/_2$″ gypsum board; face ply installed with adhesive
	Wall	Either direction	24	24	24	

For SI: 1 inch = 25.4 mm.

a. For application without adhesive, a pair of nails spaced not less than 2 inches apart or more than $2^1/_2$ inches apart may be used with the pair of nails spaced 12 inches on center.

b. Screws shall be in accordance with Section R702.3.6. Screws for attaching gypsum board to structural insulated panels shall penetrate the wood structural panel facing not less than $^7/_{16}$ inch.

c. Where cold-formed steel framing is used with a clinching design to receive nails by two edges of metal, the nails shall be not less than $^5/_8$ inch longer than the gypsum board thickness and shall have ringed shanks. Where the cold-formed steel framing has a nailing groove formed to receive the nails, the nails shall have barbed shanks or be 5d, $13^1/_2$ gage, $1^5/_8$ inches long, $^{15}/_{64}$-inch head for $^1/_2$-inch gypsum board; and 6d, 13 gage, $1^7/_8$ inches long, $^{15}/_{64}$-inch head for $^5/_8$-inch gypsum board.

d. Three-eighths-inch-thick single-ply gypsum board shall not be used on a ceiling where a water-based textured finish is to be applied, or where it will be required to support insulation above a ceiling. On ceiling applications to receive a water-based texture material, either hand or spray applied, the gypsum board shall be applied perpendicular to framing. When applying a water-based texture material, the minimum gypsum board thickness shall be increased from $^3/_8$ inch to $^1/_2$ inch for 16-inch on center framing, and from $^1/_2$ inch to $^5/_8$ inch for 24-inch on center framing or $^1/_2$-inch sag-resistant gypsum ceiling board shall be used.

e. Type X gypsum board for garage ceilings beneath habitable rooms shall be installed perpendicular to the ceiling framing and shall be fastened at maximum 6 inches o.c. by minimum $1^7/_8$ inches 6d coated nails or equivalent drywall screws.

2009 INTERNATIONAL RESIDENTIAL CODE®

R702.2 Interior plaster.

R702.2.1 Gypsum plaster. Gypsum plaster materials shall conform to ASTM C 5, C 28, C 35, C 37, C 59, C 61, C 587, C 588, C 631, C 847, C 933, C 1032 and C 1047, and shall be installed or applied in conformance with ASTM C 843 and C 844. Plaster shall not be less than three coats when applied over metal lath and not less than two coats when applied over other bases permitted by this section, except that veneer plaster may be applied in one coat not to exceed $^3/_{16}$ inch (4.76 mm) thickness, provided the total thickness is in accordance with Table R702.1(1).

R702.2.2 Cement plaster. Cement plaster materials shall conform to ASTM C 37, C 91 (Type M, S or N), C 150 (Type I, II and III), C 588, C 595 [Type IP, I (PM), IS and I (SM), C 847, C 897, C 926, C 933, C 1032, C 1047 and C 1328, and shall be installed or applied in conformance with ASTM C 1063. Plaster shall not be less than three coats when applied over metal lath and not less than two coats when applied over other bases permitted by this section, except that veneer plaster may be applied in one coat not to exceed $^3/_{16}$ inch (4.76 mm) thickness, provided the total thickness is in accordance with Table R702.1(1).

R702.2.2.1 Application. Each coat shall be kept in a moist condition for at least 24 hours prior to application of the next coat.

Exception: Applications installed in accordance with ASTM C 926.

R702.2.2.2 Curing. The finish coat for two-coat cement plaster shall not be applied sooner than 48 hours after application of the first coat. For three coat cement plaster the second coat shall not be applied sooner than 24 hours after application of the first coat. The finish coat for three-coat cement plaster shall not be applied sooner than 48 hours after application of the second coat.

R702.2.3 Support. Support spacing for gypsum or metal lath on walls or ceilings shall not exceed 16 inches (406 mm) for $^3/_8$ inch thick (9.5 mm) or 24 inches (610 mm) for $^1/_2$-inch-thick (12.7 mm) plain gypsum lath. Gypsum lath shall be installed at right angles to support framing with end joints in adjacent courses staggered by at least one framing space.

R702.3 Gypsum board.

R702.3.1 Materials. All gypsum board materials and accessories shall conform to ASTM C 36, C 79, C 475, C 514, C 630, C 931, C 960, C 1002, C 1047, C 1177, C 1178, C 1278, C 1395, C 1396 or C 1658 and shall be installed in accordance with the provisions of this section. Adhesives for the installation of gypsum board shall conform to ASTM C 557.

R702.3.2 Wood framing. Wood framing supporting gypsum board shall not be less than 2 inches (51 mm) nominal thickness in the least dimension except that wood furring strips not less than 1-inch-by-2 inch (25 mm by 51 mm) nominal dimension may be used over solid backing or framing spaced not more than 24 inches (610 mm) on center.

R702.3.3 Cold-formed steel framing. Cold-formed steel framing supporting gypsum board shall not be less than 1$^1/_4$ inches (32 mm) wide in the least dimension. Nonload-bearing cold-formed steel framing shall comply with ASTM C 645. Load-bearing cold-formed steel framing and all cold-formed steel framing from 0.033 inch to 0.112 inch (1 mm to 3 mm) thick shall comply with ASTM C 955.

R702.3.4 Insulating concrete form walls. Foam plastics for insulating concrete form walls constructed in accordance with Sections R404.1.2 and R611 on the interior of *habitable spaces* shall be protected in accordance with Section R316.4. Use of adhesives in conjunction with mechanical fasteners is permitted. Adhesives used for interior and exterior finishes shall be compatible with the insulating form materials.

R702.3.5 Application. Maximum spacing of supports and the size and spacing of fasteners used to attach gypsum board shall comply with Table R702.3.5. Gypsum sheathing shall be attached to exterior walls in accordance with Table R602.3(1). Gypsum board shall be applied at right angles or parallel to framing members. All edges and ends of gypsum board shall occur on the framing members, except those edges and ends that are perpendicular to the framing members. Interior gypsum board shall not be installed where it is directly exposed to the weather or to water.

R702.3.6 Fastening. Screws for attaching gypsum board to wood framing shall be Type W or Type S in accordance with ASTM C 1002 and shall penetrate the wood not less than $^5/_8$ inch (16 mm). Gypsum board shall be attached to cold-formed steel framing with minimum No. 6 screws. Screws for attaching gypsum board to cold-formed steel framing less than 0.033 inch (1 mm) thick shall be Type S in accordance with ASTM C 1002 or bugle head style in accordance with ASTM C1513 and shall penetrate the steel not less than $^3/_8$ inch (9.5 mm). Screws for attaching gypsum board to cold-formed steel framing 0.033 inch to 0.112 inch (1 mm to 3 mm) thick shall be in accordance with ASTM C 954 or bugle head style in accordance with ASTM C1513. Screws for attaching gypsum board to structural insulated panels shall penetrate the wood structural panel facing not less than $^7/_{16}$ inch (11 mm).

R702.3.7 Horizontal gypsum board diaphragm ceilings. Use of gypsum board shall be permitted on wood joists to create a horizontal *diaphragm* in accordance with Table R702.3.7. Gypsum board shall be installed perpendicular to ceiling framing members. End joints of adjacent courses of board shall not occur on the same joist. The maximum allowable *diaphragm* proportions shall be 1$^1/_2$:1 between shear resisting elements. Rotation or cantilever conditions shall not be permitted. Gypsum board shall not be used in *diaphragm* ceilings to resist lateral forces imposed by masonry or concrete construction. All perimeter edges shall be blocked using wood members not less than 2-inch (51 mm) by 6-inch (152 mm) nominal dimension. Blocking material shall be installed flat over the top plate of the wall to provide a nailing surface not less than 2 inches (51 mm) in width for the attachment of the gypsum board.

TABLE R702.3.7
SHEAR CAPACITY FOR HORIZONTAL WOOD-FRAMED
GYPSUM BOARD DIAPHRAGM CEILING ASSEMBLIES

MATERIAL	THICKNESS OF MATERIAL (min.) (in.)	SPACING OF FRAMING MEMBERS (max.) (in.)	SHEAR VALUE[a, b] (plf of ceiling)	MINIMUM FASTENER SIZE[c, d]
Gypsum board	$^1/_2$	16 o.c.	90	5d cooler or wallboard nail; $1^5/_8$-inch long; 0.086- inch shank; $^{15}/_{64}$-inch head
Gypsum board	$^1/_2$	24 o.c.	70	5d cooler or wallboard nail; $1^5/_8$-inch long; 0.086- inch shank; $^{15}/_{64}$-inch head

For SI: 1 inch = 25.4 mm, 1 pound per linear foot = 1.488 kg/m.

a. Values are not cumulative with other horizontal diaphragm values and are for short-term loading caused by wind or seismic loading. Values shall be reduced 25 percent for normal loading.

b. Values shall be reduced 50 percent in Seismic Design Categories D_0, D_1, D_2 and E.

c. $1^1/_4''$, #6 Type S or W screws may be substituted for the listed nails.

d. Fasteners shall be spaced not more than 7 inches on center at all supports, including perimeter blocking, and not less than $^3/_8$ inch from the edges and ends of the gypsum board.

R702.3.8 Water-resistant gypsum backing board. Gypsum board used as the base or backer for adhesive application of ceramic tile or other required nonabsorbent finish material shall conform to ASTM C 1396, C 1178 or C1278. Use of water-resistant gypsum backing board shall be permitted on ceilings where framing spacing does not exceed 12 inches (305 mm) on center for $^1/_2$-inch-thick (12.7 mm) or 16 inches (406 mm) for $^5/_8$-inch-thick (16 mm) gypsum board. Water-resistant gypsum board shall not be installed over a Class I or II vapor retarder in a shower or tub compartment. Cut or exposed edges, including those at wall intersections, shall be sealed as recommended by the manufacturer.

R702.3.8.1 Limitations. Water resistant gypsum backing board shall not be used where there will be direct exposure to water, or in areas subject to continuous high humidity.

R702.4 Ceramic tile.

R702.4.1 General. Ceramic tile surfaces shall be installed in accordance with ANSI A108.1, A108.4, A108.5, A108.6, A108.11, A118.1, A118.3, A136.1 and A137.1.

R702.4.2 Fiber-cement, fiber-mat reinforced cement, glass mat gypsum backers and fiber-reinforced gypsum backers. Fiber-cement, fiber-mat reinforced cement, glass mat gypsum backers or fiber-reinforced gypsum backers in compliance with ASTM C 1288, C 1325, C 1178 or C 1278, respectively, and installed in accordance with manufacturers' recommendations shall be used as backers for wall tile in tub and shower areas and wall panels in shower areas.

R702.5 Other finishes. Wood veneer paneling and hardboard paneling shall be placed on wood or cold-formed steel framing spaced not more than 16 inches (406 mm) on center. Wood veneer and hard board paneling less than $^1/_4$ inch (6 mm) nominal thickness shall not have less than a $^3/_8$-inch (10 mm) gypsum board backer. Wood veneer paneling not less than $^1/_4$-inch (6 mm) nominal thickness shall conform to ANSI/

HPVA HP-1. Hardboard paneling shall conform to CPA/ANSI A135.5.

R702.6 Wood shakes and shingles. Wood shakes and shingles shall conform to CSSB *Grading Rules for Wood Shakes and Shingles* and shall be permitted to be installed directly to the studs with maximum 24 inches (610 mm) on-center spacing.

R702.6.1 Attachment. Nails, staples or glue are permitted for attaching shakes or shingles to the wall, and attachment of the shakes or shingles directly to the surface shall be permitted provided the fasteners are appropriate for the type of wall surface material. When nails or staples are used, two fasteners shall be provided and shall be placed so that they are covered by the course above.

R702.6.2 Furring strips. Where furring strips are used, they shall be 1 inch by 2 inches or 1 inch by 3 inches (25 mm by 51 mm or 25 mm by 76 mm), spaced a distance on center equal to the desired exposure, and shall be attached to the wall by nailing through other wall material into the studs.

SECTION R703
EXTERIOR COVERING

R703.1 General. Exterior walls shall provide the building with a weather-resistant exterior wall envelope. The exterior wall envelope shall include flashing as described in Section R703.8.

R703.1.1 Water resistance. The exterior wall envelope shall be designed and constructed in a manner that prevents the accumulation of water within the wall assembly by providing a water-resistant barrier behind the exterior veneer as required by Section R703.2 and a means of draining to the exterior water that enters the assembly. Protection against condensation in the exterior wall assembly shall be provided in accordance with Section R601.3 of this code.

Exceptions:

1. A weather-resistant exterior wall envelope shall not be required over concrete or masonry walls

designed in accordance with Chapter 6 and flashed according to Section R703.7 or R703.8.

2. Compliance with the requirements for a means of drainage, and the requirements of Section R703.2 and Section R703.8, shall not be required for an exterior wall envelope that has been demonstrated to resist wind-driven rain through testing of the exterior wall envelope, including joints, penetrations and intersections with dissimilar materials, in accordance with ASTM E 331 under the following conditions:

2.1. Exterior wall envelope test assemblies shall include at least one opening, one control joint, one wall/eave interface and one wall sill. All tested openings and penetrations shall be representative of the intended end-use configuration.

2.2. Exterior wall envelope test assemblies shall be at least 4 feet (1219 mm) by 8 feet (2438 mm) in size.

2.3. Exterior wall assemblies shall be tested at a minimum differential pressure of 6.24 pounds per square foot (299 Pa).

2.4. Exterior wall envelope assemblies shall be subjected to the minimum test exposure for a minimum of 2 hours.

The exterior wall envelope design shall be considered to resist wind-driven rain where the results of testing indicate that water did not penetrate control joints in the exterior wall envelope, joints at the perimeter of openings penetration or intersections of terminations with dissimilar materials.

703.1.2 Wind resistance. Wall coverings, backing materials and their attachments shall be capable of resisting wind loads in accordance with Tables R301.2(2) and R301.2(3). Wind-pressure resistance of the siding and backing materials shall be determined by ASTM E 330 or other applicable standard test methods. Where wind-pressure resistance is determined by design analysis, data from approved design standards and analysis conforming to generally accepted engineering practice shall be used to evaluate the siding and backing material and its fastening. All applicable failure modes including bending rupture of siding, fastener withdrawal and fastener head pull-through shall be considered in the testing or design analysis. Where the wall covering and the backing material resist wind load as an assembly, use of the design capacity of the assembly shall be permitted.

R703.2 Water-resistive barrier. One layer of No. 15 asphalt felt, free from holes and breaks, complying with ASTM D 226 for Type 1 felt or other approved water-resistive barrier shall be applied over studs or sheathing of all exterior walls. Such felt or material shall be applied horizontally, with the upper layer lapped over the lower layer not less than 2 inches (51 mm). Where joints occur, felt shall be lapped not less than 6 inches (152 mm). The felt or other approved material shall be continuous to the top of walls and terminated at penetrations and build-

ing appendages in a manner to meet the requirements of the exterior wall envelope as described in Section R703.1.

Exception: Omission of the water-resistive barrier is permitted in the following situations:

1. In detached accessory buildings.

2. Under exterior wall finish materials as permitted in Table R703.4.

3. Under paperbacked stucco lath when the paper backing is an approved water-resistive barrier.

R703.3 Wood, hardboard and wood structural panel siding.

R703.3.1 Panel siding. Joints in wood, hardboard or wood structural panel siding shall be made as follows unless otherwise approved. Vertical joints in panel siding shall occur over framing members, unless wood or wood structural panel sheathing is used, and shall be shiplapped or covered with a batten. Horizontal joints in panel siding shall be lapped a minimum of 1 inch (25 mm) or shall be shiplapped or shall be flashed with Z-flashing and occur over solid blocking, wood or wood structural panel sheathing.

R703.3.2 Horizontal siding. Horizontal lap siding shall be installed in accordance with the manufacturer's recommendations. Where there are no recommendations the siding shall be lapped a minimum of 1 inch (25 mm), or $^1/_2$ inch (13 mm) if rabbeted, and shall have the ends caulked, covered with a batten or sealed and installed over a strip of flashing.

R703.4 Attachments. Unless specified otherwise, all wall coverings shall be securely fastened in accordance with Table R703.4 or with other *approved* aluminum, stainless steel, zinc-coated or other *approved* corrosion-resistive fasteners. Where the basic wind speed per Figure R301.2(4) is 110 miles per hour (49 m/s) or higher, the attachment of wall coverings shall be designed to resist the component and cladding loads specified in Table R301.2(2), adjusted for height and exposure in accordance with Table R301.2(3).

R703.5 Wood shakes and shingles. Wood shakes and shingles shall conform to CSSB *Grading Rules for Wood Shakes and Shingles.*

R703.5.1 Application. Wood shakes or shingles shall be applied either single-course or double-course over nominal $^1/_2$-inch (13 mm) wood-based sheathing or to furring strips over $^1/_2$-inch (13 mm) nominal nonwood sheathing . A permeable water-resistive barrier shall be provided over all sheathing, with horizontal overlaps in the membrane of not less than 2 inches (51mm) and vertical overlaps of not less than 6 inches (152 mm). Where furring strips are used, they shall be 1 inch by 3 inches or 1 inch by 4 inches (25 mm by 76 mm or 25 mm by 102 mm) and shall be fastened horizontally to the studs with 7d or 8d box nails and shall be spaced a distance on center equal to the actual weather exposure of the shakes or shingles, not to exceed the maximum exposure specified in Table R703.5.2. The spacing between adjacent shingles to allow for expansion shall not exceed $^1/_4$ inch (6 mm), and between adjacent shakes, it shall not exceed $^1/_2$ inch (13 mm). The offset spacing between joints in adjacent courses shall be a minimum of $1^1/_2$ inches (38 mm).

TABLE R703.4
WEATHER–RESISTANT SIDING ATTACHMENT AND MINIMUM THICKNESS

SIDING MATERIAL		NOMINAL THICKNESS[a] (inches)	JOINT TREATMENT	WATER-RESISTIVE BARRIER REQUIRED	TYPE OF SUPPORTS FOR THE SIDING MATERIAL AND FASTENERS[b, c, d]					Number or spacing of fasteners
					Wood or wood structural panel sheathing	Fiberboard sheathing into stud	Gypsum sheathing into stud	Foam plastic sheathing into stud	Direct to studs	
Horizontal aluminum[e]	Without insulation	0.019[f]	Lap	Yes	0.120 nail 1^1/$_2$″ long	0.120 nail 2″ long	0.120 nail 2″ long	0.120 nail[y]	Not allowed	Same as stud spacing
		0.024	Lap	Yes	0.120 nail 1^1/$_2$″ long	0.120 nail 2″ long	0.120 nail 2″ long	0.120 nail[y]	Not allowed	
	With insulation	0.019	Lap	Yes	0.120 nail 1^1/$_2$″ long	0.120 nail 2^1/$_2$″ long	0.120 nail 2^1/$_2$″ long	0.120 nail[y]	0.120 nail 1^1/$_2$″ long	
Anchored veneer: brick, concrete, masonry or stone		2	Section R703	Yes	See Section R703 and Figure R703.7[g]					
Adhered veneer: concrete, stone or masonry[w]		—	Section R703	Yes Note w	See Section R703.6.1[g] or in accordance with the manufacturer's instructions.					
Hardboard[k] Panel siding-vertical		^{7}/$_{16}$	—	Yes	Note m	Note m	Note m	Note m	Note m	6″ panel edges 12″ inter. sup.[n]
Hardboard[k] Lap-siding-horizontal		^{7}/$_{16}$	Note p	Yes	Note o	Note o	Note o	Note o	Note o	Same as stud spacing 2 per bearing
Steel[h]		29 ga.	Lap	Yes	0.113 nail 1^3/$_4$″ Staple-1^3/$_4$″	0.113 nail 2^3/$_4$″ Staple-2^1/$_2$″	0.113 nail 2^1/$_2$″ Staple-2^1/$_4$″	0.113 nail[v] Staple[v]	Not allowed	Same as stud spacing
Particleboard panels		^{3}/$_8$ – ^{1}/$_2$	—	Yes	6d box nail (2″ × 0.099″)	6d box nail (2″ × 0.099″)	6d box nail (2″ × 0.099″)	box nail[v]	6d box nail (2″ × 0.099″), ^{3}/$_8$ not allowed	6″ panel edge, 12″ inter. sup.
		^{5}/$_8$	—	Yes	6d box nail (2″ × 0.099″)	8d box nail (2^1/$_2$″ × 0.113″)	8d box nail (2^1/$_2$″ × 0.113″)	box nail[v]	6d box nail (2″ × 0.099″)	
Wood structural panel siding[i] (exterior grade)		^{3}/$_8$ – ^{1}/$_2$	Note p	Yes	0.099 nail–2″	0.113 nail–2^1/$_2$″	0.113 nail–2^1/$_2$″	0.113 nail[v]	0.099 nail–2″	6″ panel edges, 12″ inter. sup.
Wood structural panel lapsiding		^{3}/$_8$ – ^{1}/$_2$	Note p Note x	Yes	0.099 nail–2″	0.113 nail–2^1/$_2$″	0.113 nail–2^1/$_2$″	0.113 nail[x]	0.099 nail–2″	8″ along bottom edge
Vinyl siding[l]		0.035	Lap	Yes	0.120 nail (shank) with a 0.313 head or 16 gauge staple with ^{3}/$_8$ to ^{1}/$_2$-inch crown[y, z]	0.120 nail (shank) with a 0.313 head or 16 gage staple with ^{3}/$_8$ to ^{1}/$_2$-inch crown[y]	0.120 nail (shank) with a 0.313 head or 16 gage staple with ^{3}/$_8$ to ^{1}/$_2$-inch crown[y]	0.120 nail (shank) with a 0.313 head per Section R703.11.2	Not allowed	16 inches on center or specified by the manufacturer instructions or test report
Wood[j] rustic, drop		^{3}/$_8$ Min	Lap	Yes	Fastener penetration into stud–1″				0.113 nail–2^1/$_2$″ Staple–2″	Face nailing up to 6″ widths, 1 nail per bearing; 8″ widths and over, 2 nails per bearing
Shiplap		^{19}/$_{32}$ Average	Lap	Yes						
Bevel		^{7}/$_{16}$								
Butt tip		^{3}/$_{16}$	Lap	Yes						
Fiber cement panel siding[q]		^{5}/$_{16}$	Note q	Yes Note u	6d common corrosion-resistant nail[r]	6d common corrosion-resistant nail[r]	6d common corrosion-resistant nail[r]	6d common corrosion resistant (12″ × 0.113″) nail[r, v]	4d common corrosion resistant nail[r]	6″ o.c. on edges, 12″ o.c. on intermed. studs
Fiber cement lap siding[s]		^{5}/$_{16}$	Note s	Yes Note u	6d common corrosion-resistant nail[r]	6d common corrosion-resistant nail[r]	6d common corrosion-resistant nail[r]	6d common corrosion-resistant (12″ × 0.113″) nail[r, v]	6d common corrosion-resistant nail or 11 gage roofing nail[r]	Note t

For SI: 1 inch = 25.4 mm.

a. Based on stud spacing of 16 inches on center where studs are spaced 24 inches, siding shall be applied to sheathing approved for that spacing.

b. Nail is a general description and shall be T-head, modified round head, or round head with smooth or deformed shanks.

c. Staples shall have a minimum crown width of ^{7}/$_{16}$-inch outside diameter and be manufactured of minimum 16 gage wire.

d. Nails or staples shall be aluminum, galvanized, or rust-preventative coated and shall be driven into the studs for fiberboard or gypsum backing.

e. Aluminum nails shall be used to attach aluminum siding.

f. Aluminum (0.019 inch) shall be unbacked only when the maximum panel width is 10 inches and the maximum flat area is 8 inches. The tolerance for aluminum siding shall be +0.002 inch of the nominal dimension.

g. All attachments shall be coated with a corrosion-resistant coating.

h. Shall be of approved type.

i. Three-eighths-inch plywood shall not be applied directly to studs spaced more than 16 inches on center when long dimension is parallel to studs. Plywood ^{1}/$_2$-inch or thinner shall not be applied directly to studs spaced more than 24 inches on center. The stud spacing shall not exceed the panel span rating provided by the manufacturer unless the panels are installed with the face grain perpendicular to the studs or over sheathing approved for that stud spacing.

j. Wood board sidings applied vertically shall be nailed to horizontal nailing strips or blocking set 24 inches on center. Nails shall penetrate 1^1/$_2$ inches into studs, studs and wood sheathing combined or blocking.

(continued)

TABLE R703.4—continued
WEATHER–RESISTANT SIDING ATTACHMENT AND MINIMUM THICKNESS

k. Hardboard siding shall comply with CPA/ANSI A135.6.
l. Vinyl siding shall comply with ASTM D 3679.
m. Minimum shank diameter of 0.092 inch, minimum head diameter of 0.225 inch, and nail length must accommodate sheathing and penetrate framing $1^1/_2$ inches.
n. When used to resist shear forces, the spacing must be 4 inches at panel edges and 8 inches on interior supports.
o. Minimum shank diameter of 0.099 inch, minimum head diameter of 0.240 inch, and nail length must accommodate sheathing and penetrate framing $1^1/_2$ inches.
p. Vertical end joints shall occur at studs and shall be covered with a joint cover or shall be caulked.
q. See Section R703.10.1.
r. Fasteners shall comply with the nominal dimensions in ASTM F 1667.
s. See Section R703.10.2.
t. Face nailing: one 6d common nail through the overlapping planks at each stud. Concealed nailing: one 11 gage $1^1/_2$ inch long galv. roofing nail through the top edge of each plank at each stud.
u. See Section R703.2 exceptions.
v. Minimum nail length must accommodate sheathing and penetrate framing $1^1/_2$ inches.
w. Adhered masonry veneer shall comply with the requirements of Section R703.6.3 and shall comply with the requirements in Sections 6.1 and 6.3 of ACI 530/ASCE 5/TMS-402.
x. Vertical joints, if staggered shall be permitted to be away from studs if applied over wood structural panel sheathing.
y. Minimum fastener length must accommodate sheathing and penetrate framing .75 inches or in accordance with the manufacturer's installation instructions.
z. Where approved by the manufacturer's instructions or test report siding shall be permitted to be installed with fasteners penetrating not less than .75 inches through wood or wood structural sheathing with or without penetration into the framing.

R703.5.2 Weather exposure. The maximum weather exposure for shakes and shingles shall not exceed that specified in Table R703.5.2.

R703.5.3 Attachment. Each shake or shingle shall be held in place by two hot-dipped zinc-coated, stainless steel, or aluminum nails or staples. The fasteners shall be long enough to penetrate the sheathing or furring strips by a minimum of $^1/_2$ inch (13 mm) and shall not be overdriven.

R703.5.3.1 Staple attachment. Staples shall not be less than 16 gage and shall have a crown width of not less than $^7/_{16}$ inch (11 mm), and the crown of the staples shall be parallel with the butt of the shake or shingle. In single-course application, the fasteners shall be concealed by the course above and shall be driven approximately 1 inch (25 mm) above the butt line of the succeeding course and $^3/_4$ inch (19 mm) from the edge. In double-course applications, the exposed shake or shingle shall be face-nailed with two casing nails, driven approximately 2 inches (51 mm) above the butt line and $^3/_4$ inch (19 mm) from each edge. In all applications, staples shall be concealed by the course above. With shingles wider than 8 inches (203 mm) two additional nails shall be required and shall be nailed approximately 1 inch (25 mm) apart near the center of the shingle.

R703.5.4 Bottom courses. The bottom courses shall be doubled.

R703.6 Exterior plaster. Installation of these materials shall be in compliance with ASTM C 926 and ASTM C 1063 and the provisions of this code.

R703.6.1 Lath. All lath and lath attachments shall be of corrosion-resistant materials. Expanded metal or woven wire lath shall be attached with $1^1/_2$-inch-long (38 mm), 11 gage nails having a $^7/_{16}$-inch (11.1 mm) head, or $^7/_8$-inch-long (22.2 mm), 16 gage staples, spaced at no more than 6 inches (152 mm), or as otherwise *approved*.

R703.6.2 Plaster. Plastering with portland cement plaster shall be not less than three coats when applied over metal lath or wire lath and shall be not less than two coats when applied over masonry, concrete, pressure-preservative treated wood or decay-resistant wood as specified in Section R317.1 or gypsum backing. If the plaster surface is completely covered by veneer or other facing material or is completely concealed, plaster application need be only two coats, provided the total thickness is as set forth in Table R702.1(1).

On wood-frame construction with an on-grade floor slab system, exterior plaster shall be applied to cover, but not extend below, lath, paper and screed.

TABLE R703.5.2
MAXIMUM WEATHER EXPOSURE FOR WOOD SHAKES AND SHINGLES ON EXTERIOR WALLS[a, b, c]
(Dimensions are in inches)

LENGTH	EXPOSURE FOR SINGLE COURSE	EXPOSURE FOR DOUBLE COURSE
Shingles[a]		
16	$7^1/_2$	12[b]
18	$8^1/_2$	14[c]
24	$11^1/_2$	16
Shakes[a]		
18	$8^1/_2$	14
24	$11^1/_2$	18

For SI: 1 inch = 25.4 mm.

a. Dimensions given are for No. 1 grade.
b. A maximum 10-inch exposure is permitted for No. 2 grade.
c. A maximum 11-inch exposure is permitted for No. 2 grade.

The proportion of aggregate to cementitious materials shall be as set forth in Table R702.1(3).

R703.6.2.1 Weep screeds. A minimum 0.019-inch (0.5 mm) (No. 26 galvanized sheet gage), corrosion-resistant weep screed or plastic weep screed, with a minimum vertical attachment flange of $3^1/_2$ inches (89 mm) shall be provided at or below the foundation plate line on exterior stud walls in accordance with ASTM C 926. The weep screed shall be placed a minimum of 4 inches (102 mm) above the earth or 2 inches (51 mm) above paved areas and shall be of a type that will allow trapped water to drain to the exterior of the building. The weather-resistant barrier shall lap the attachment flange. The exterior lath shall cover and terminate on the attachment flange of the weep screed.

R703.6.3 Water-resistive barriers. Water-resistive barriers shall be installed as required in Section R703.2 and, where applied over wood-based sheathing, shall include a water-resistive vapor-permeable barrier with a performance at least equivalent to two layers of Grade D paper.

Exception: Where the water-resistive barrier that is applied over wood-based sheathing has a water resistance equal to or greater than that of 60 minute Grade D paper and is separated from the stucco by an intervening, substantially nonwater-absorbing layer or designed drainage space.

R703.6.4 Application. Each coat shall be kept in a moist condition for at least 48 hours prior to application of the next coat.

Exception: Applications installed in accordance with ASTM C 926.

R703.6.5 Curing. The finish coat for two-coat cement plaster shall not be applied sooner than seven days after application of the first coat. For three-coat cement plaster, the second coat shall not be applied sooner than 48 hours after application of the first coat. The finish coat for three-coat cement plaster shall not be applied sooner than seven days after application of the second coat.

R703.7 Stone and masonry veneer, general. Stone and masonry veneer shall be installed in accordance with this chapter, Table R703.4 and Figure R703.7. These veneers installed over a backing of wood or cold-formed steel shall be limited to the first *story* above-grade and shall not exceed 5 inches (127 mm) in thickness. See Section R602.12 for wall bracing requirements for masonry veneer for wood framed construction and Section R603.9.5 for wall bracing requirements for masonry veneer for cold-formed steel construction.

Exceptions:

1. For all buildings in Seismic Design Categories A, B and C, exterior stone or masonry veneer, as specified in Table R703.7(1), with a backing of wood or steel framing shall be permitted to the height specified in Table R703.7(1) above a noncombustible foundation.

2. For detached one- or two-family *dwellings* in Seismic Design Categories D_0, D_1 and D_2, exterior stone or masonry veneer, as specified in Table R703.7(2), with a backing of wood framing shall be permitted to the height specified in Table R703.7(2) above a noncombustible foundation.

R703.7.1 Interior veneer support. Veneers used as interior wall finishes shall be permitted to be supported on wood or cold-formed steel floors that are designed to support the loads imposed.

R703.7.2 Exterior veneer support. Except in Seismic Design Categories D_0, D_1 and D_2, exterior masonry veneers having an installed weight of 40 pounds per square foot (195 kg/m²) or less shall be permitted to be supported on wood or cold-formed steel construction. When masonry veneer supported by wood or cold-formed steel construction adjoins masonry veneer supported by the foundation, there shall be a movement joint between the veneer supported by the wood or cold-formed steel construction and the veneer supported by the foundation. The wood or cold-formed steel construction supporting the masonry veneer shall be designed to limit the deflection to $1/_{600}$ of the span for the supporting members. The design of the wood or cold-formed steel construction shall consider the weight of the veneer and any other loads.

R703.7.2.1 Support by steel angle. A minimum 6 inches by 4 inches by $5/_{16}$ inch (152 mm by 102 mm by 8 mm) steel angle, with the long leg placed vertically, shall be anchored to double 2 inches by 4 inches (51 mm by 102 mm) wood studs at a maximum on-center spacing of 16 inches (406 mm). Anchorage of the steel angle at every double stud spacing shall be a minimum of two $7/_{16}$ inch (11 mm) diameter by 4 inch (102 mm) lag screws. The steel angle shall have a minimum clearance to underlying construction of $1/_{16}$ inch (2 mm). A minimum of two-thirds the width of the masonry veneer thickness shall bear on the steel angle. Flashing and weep holes shall be located in the masonry veneer wythe in accordance with Figure R703.7.2.1. The maximum height of masonry veneer above the steel angle support shall be 12 feet, 8 inches (3861 mm). The air space separating the masonry veneer from the wood backing shall be in accordance with Sections R703.7.4 and R703.7.4.2. The method of support for the masonry veneer on wood construction shall be constructed in accordance with Figure R703.7.2.1.

The maximum slope of the roof construction without stops shall be 7:12. Roof construction with slopes greater than 7:12 but not more than 12:12 shall have stops of a minimum 3 inch × 3 inch × $1/_4$ inch (76 mm × 76 mm × 6 mm) steel plate welded to the angle at 24 inches (610 mm) on center along the angle or as *approved* by the *building official*.

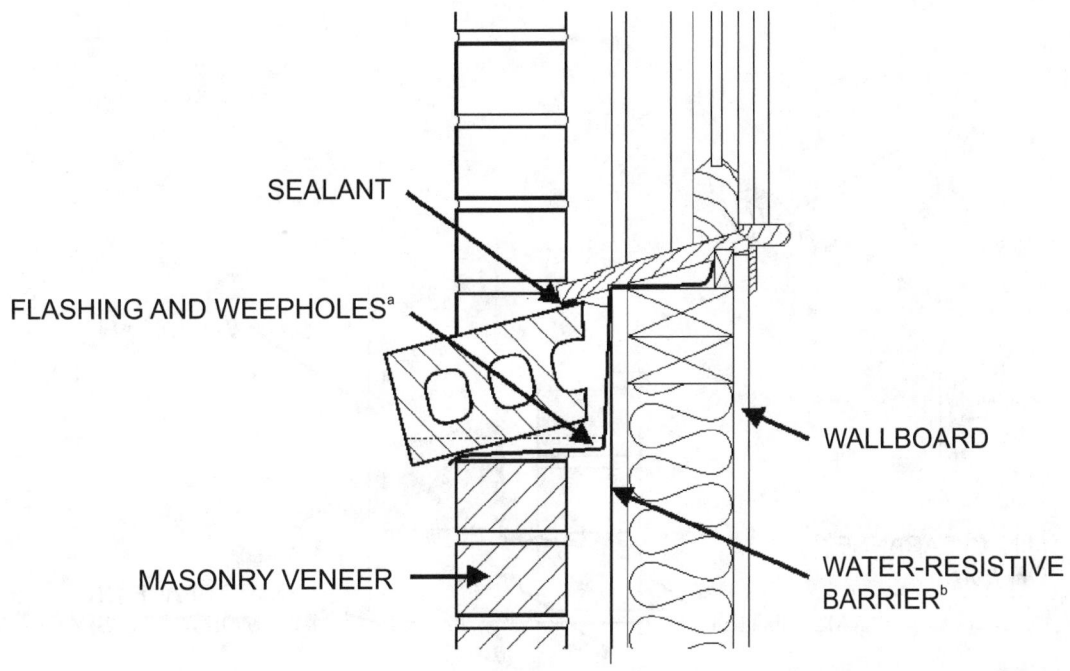

SEALANT

FLASHING AND WEEPHOLES[a]

MASONRY VENEER

WALLBOARD

WATER-RESISTIVE BARRIER[b]

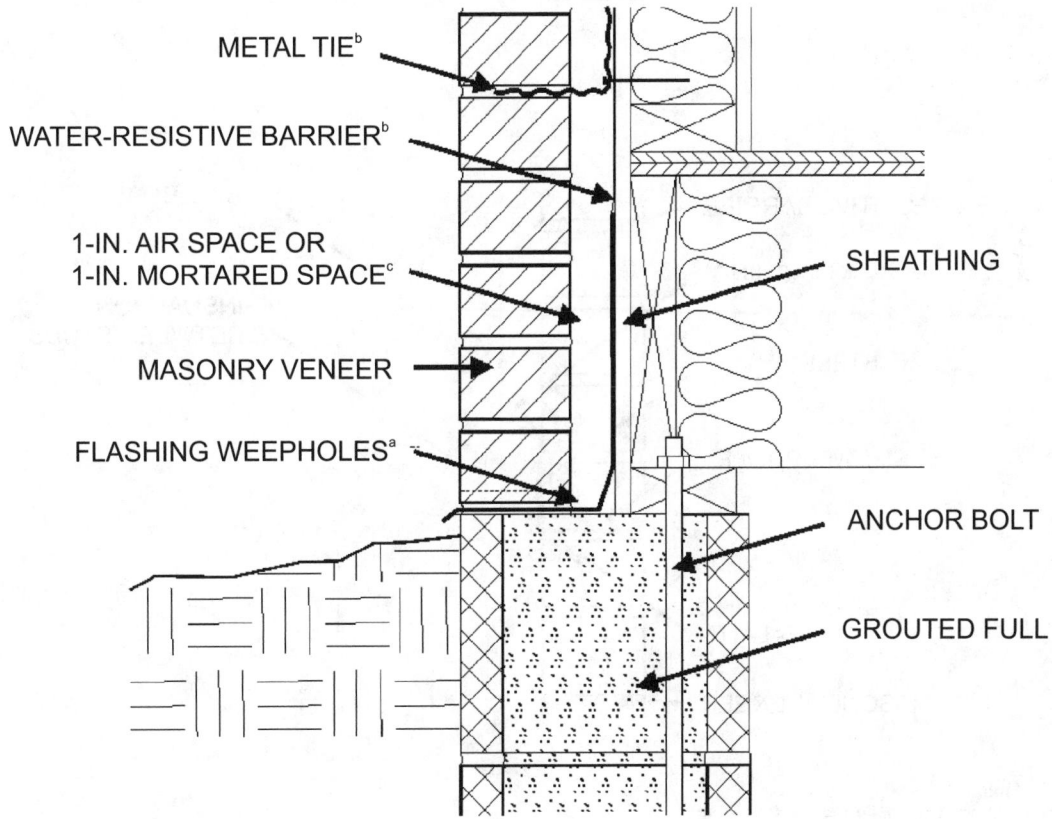

METAL TIE[b]

WATER-RESISTIVE BARRIER[b]

1-IN. AIR SPACE OR
1-IN. MORTARED SPACE[c]

MASONRY VENEER

FLASHING WEEPHOLES[a]

SHEATHING

ANCHOR BOLT

GROUTED FULL

For SI: 1 inch = 25.4 mm.

FIGURE R703.7
MASONRY VENEER WALL DETAILS

(continued)

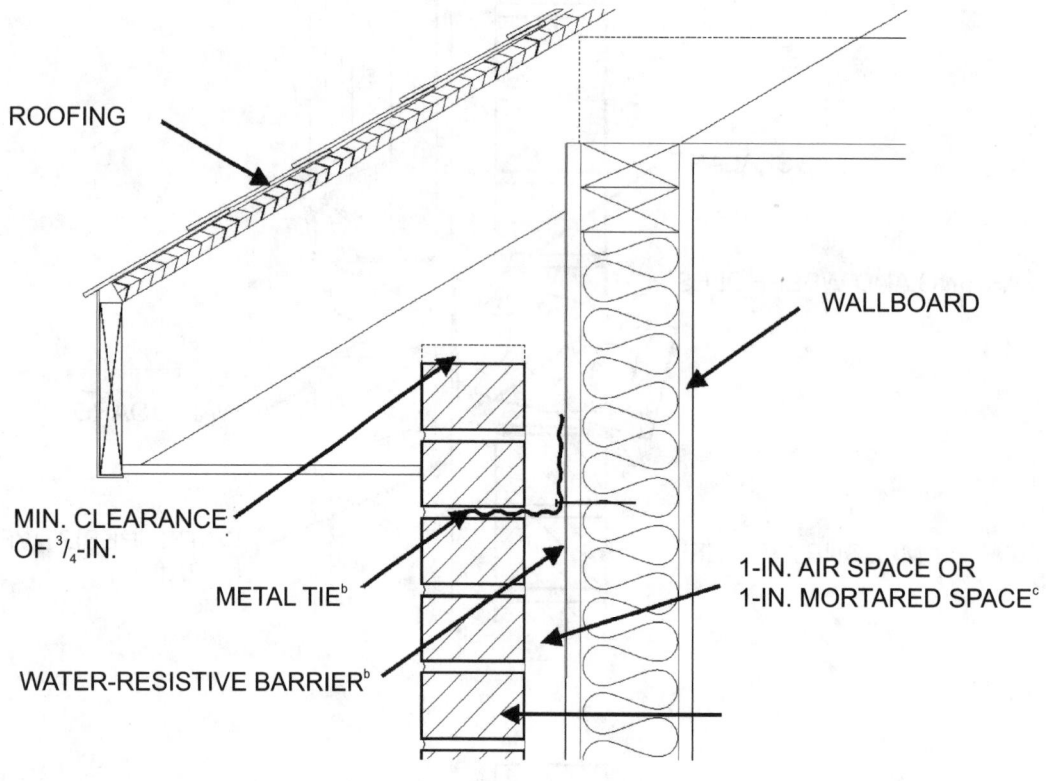

ROOFING

WALLBOARD

MIN. CLEARANCE OF $^3/_4$-IN.

METAL TIE[b]

WATER-RESISTIVE BARRIER[b]

1-IN. AIR SPACE OR 1-IN. MORTARED SPACE[c]

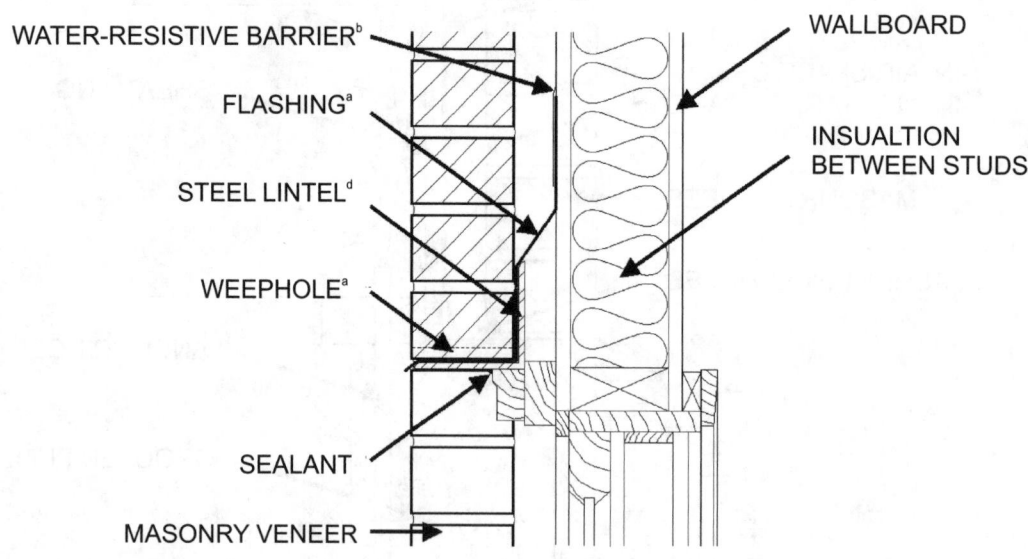

WATER-RESISTIVE BARRIER[b]

FLASHING[a]

STEEL LINTEL[d]

WEEPHOLE[a]

SEALANT

MASONRY VENEER

WALLBOARD

INSUALTION BETWEEN STUDS

For SI: 1 inch = 25.4 mm.

a. See Sections R703.7.5, R703.7.6 and R703.8.
b. See Sections R703.2 and R703.7.4.
c. See Sections R703.7.4.2 and R703.7.4.3.
d. See Section R703.7.3.

FIGURE R703.7—continued
MASONRY VENEER WALL DETAILS

TABLE R703.7(1)
STONE OR MASONRY VENEER LIMITATIONS AND REQUIREMENTS, WOOD
OR STEEL FRAMING, SEISMIC DESIGN CATEGORIES A, B AND C

SEISMIC DESIGN CATEGORY	NUMBER OF WOOD OR STEEL FRAMED STORIES	MAXIMUM HEIGHT OF VENEER ABOVE NONCOMBUSTIBLE FOUNDATION[a] (feet)	MAXIMUM NOMINAL THICKNESS OF VENEER (inches)	MAXIMUM WEIGHT OF VENEER (psf)[b]	WOOD OR STEEL FRAMED STORY
A or B	Steel: 1 or 2 Wood: 1, 2 or 3	30	5	50	all
C	1	30	5	50	1 only
	2	30	5	50	top
					bottom
	Wood only: 3	30	5	50	top
					middle
					bottom

For SI: 1 inch = 25.4 mm, 1 foot = 304.8 mm, 1 pound per square foot = 0.479 kPa.

a. An Additional 8 feet is permitted for gable end walls. See also story height limitations of Section R301.3.

b. Maximum weight is installed weight and includes weight of mortar, grout, lath and other materials used for installation. Where veneer is placed on both faces of a wall, the combined weight shall not exceed that specified in this table.

TABLE R703.7(2)
STONE OR MASONRY VENEER LIMITATIONS AND REQUIREMENTS, ONE- AND TWO-FAMILY DETACHED DWELLINGS,
WOOD FRAMING, SEISMIC DESIGN CATEGORIES D_0, D_1 AND D_2

SEISMIC DESIGN CATEGORY	NUMBER OF WOOD FRAMED STORIES[a]	MAXIMUM HEIGHT OF VENEER ABOVE NONCOMBUSTIBLE FOUNDATION OR FOUNDATION WALL (feet)	MAXIMUM NOMINAL THICKNESS OF VENEER (inches)	MAXIMUM WEIGHT OF VENEER (psf)[b]
D_0	1	20[c]	4	40
	2	20[c]	4	40
	3	30[d]	4	40
D_1	1	20[c]	4	40
	2	20[c]	4	40
	3	20[c]	4	40
D_2	1	20[c]	3	30
	2	20[c]	3	30

For SI: 1 inch = 25.4 mm, 1 foot = 304.8 mm, 1 pound per square foot = 0.479 kPa, 1 pound-force = 4.448 N.

a. Cripple walls are not permitted in Seismic Design Categories D_0, D_1 and D_2.

b. Maximum weight is installed weight and includes weight of mortar, grout and lath, and other materials used for installation.

c. The veneer shall not exceed 20 feet in height above a noncombustible foundation, with an additional 8 feet permitted for gable end walls, or 30 feet in height with an additional 8 feet for gable end walls where the lower 10 feet has a backing of concrete or masonry wall. See also story height limitations of Section R301.3.

d. The veneer shall not exceed 30 feet in height above a noncombustible foundation, with an additional 8 feet permitted for gable end walls. See also story height limitations of Section R301.3.

R703.7.2.2 Support by roof construction. A steel angle shall be placed directly on top of the roof construction. The roof supporting construction for the steel angle shall consist of a minimum of three 2-inch by 6-inch (51 mm by 152 mm) wood members. The wood member abutting the vertical wall stud construction shall be anchored with a minimum of three $^5/_8$-inch (16 mm) diameter by 5-inch (127 mm) lag screws to every wood stud spacing. Each additional roof member shall be anchored by the use of two 10d nails at every wood stud spacing. A minimum of two-thirds the width of the masonry veneer thickness shall bear on the steel angle. Flashing and weep holes shall be located in the masonry veneer wythe in accordance with Figure R703.7.2.2. The maximum height of the masonry veneer above the steel angle support shall be 12 feet, 8 inches (3861 mm). The air space separating the masonry veneer from the wood backing shall be in accordance with Sections R703.7.4 and R703.7.4.2. The support for the masonry veneer on wood construction shall be constructed in accordance with Figure R703.7.2.2.

The maximum slope of the roof construction without stops shall be 7:12. Roof construction with slopes greater than 7:12 but not more than 12:12 shall have stops of a minimum 3 inch × 3 inch × $^1/_4$ inch (76 mm × 76 mm × 6 mm) steel plate welded to the angle at 24 inches (610 mm) on center along the angle or as *approved* by the *building official.*

R703.7.3 Lintels. Masonry veneer shall not support any vertical load other than the dead load of the veneer above. Veneer above openings shall be supported on lintels of noncombustible materials. The lintels shall have a length of bearing not less than 4 inches (102 mm). Steel lintels shall be shop coated with a rust-inhibitive paint, except for lintels made of corrosion-resistant steel or steel treated with coatings to provide corrosion resistance. Construction of openings shall comply with either Section R703.7.3.1 or 703.7.3.2.

R703.7.3.1 The allowable span shall not exceed the values set forth in Table R703.7.3.1.

R703.7.3.2 The allowable span shall not exceed 18 feet 3 inches (5562 mm) and shall be constructed to comply with Figure R703.7.3.2 and the following:

1. Provide a minimum length of 18 inches (457 mm) of masonry veneer on each side of opening as shown in Figure R703.7.3.2.

2. Provide a minimum 5 inch by $3^1/_2$ inch by $^5/_{16}$ inch (127 mm by 89 mm by 7.9 mm) steel angle above the opening and shore for a minimum of 7 days after installation.

3. Provide double-wire joint reinforcement extending 12 inches (305 mm) beyond each side of the opening. Lap splices of joint reinforcement a minimum of 12 inches (305 mm). Comply with one of the following:

   3.1. Double-wire joint reinforcement shall be $^3/_{16}$ inch (4.8 mm) diameter and shall be

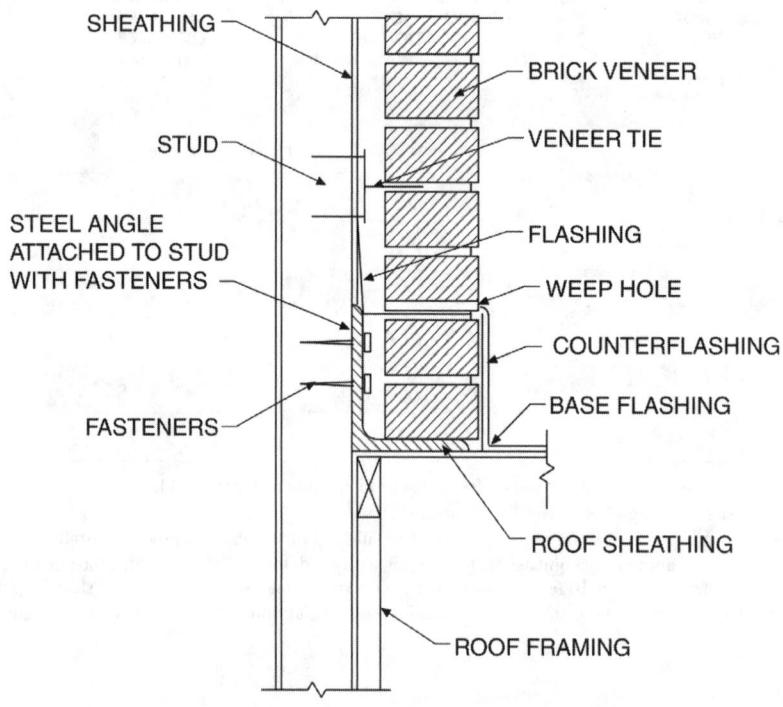

SUPPORT BY STEEL ANGLE

FIGURE R703.7.2.1
EXTERIOR MASONRY VENEER SUPPORT BY STEEL ANGLES

placed in the first two bed joints above the opening.

   3.2. Double-wire joint reinforcement shall be 9 gauge (0.144 inch or 3.66 mm diameter) and shall be placed in the first three bed joints above the opening.

R703.7.4 Anchorage. Masonry veneer shall be anchored to the supporting wall with corrosion-resistant metal ties embedded in mortar or grout and extending into the veneer a minimum of $1^1/_2$ inches (38 mm), with not less than $^5/_8$ inch (15.9 mm) mortar or grout cover to outside face. Where veneer is anchored to wood backings by corrugated sheet metal ties, the distance separating the veneer from the sheathing material shall be a maximum of a nominal 1 inch (25 mm). Where the veneer is anchored to wood backings using metal strand wire ties, the distance separating the veneer from the sheathing material shall be a maximum of $4^1/_2$ inches (114 mm). Where the veneer is anchored to cold-formed steel backings, adjustable metal strand wire ties shall be used. Where veneer is anchored to cold-formed steel backings, the distance separating the veneer from the sheathing material shall be a maximum of $4^1/_2$ inches (114 mm).

   R703.7.4.1 Size and spacing. Veneer ties, if strand wire, shall not be less in thickness than No. 9 U.S. gage [(0.148 in.) (4 mm)] wire and shall have a hook embedded in the mortar joint, or if sheet metal, shall be not less than No. 22 U.S. gage by [(0.0299 in.)(0.76 mm)] $^7/_8$ inch (22 mm) corrugated. Each tie shall be spaced not more than 24 inches (610 mm) on center horizontally and vertically and shall support not more than 2.67 square feet (0.25 m²) of wall area.

   Exception: In Seismic Design Category D_0, D_1 or D_2 or townhouses in Seismic Design Category C or in wind areas of more than 30 pounds per square foot pressure (1.44 kPa), each tie shall support not more than 2 square feet (0.2 m²) of wall area.

   R703.7.4.1.1 Veneer ties around wall openings. Veneer ties around wall openings. Additional metal ties shall be provided around all wall openings greater than 16 inches (406 mm) in either dimension. Metal ties around the perimeter of openings shall be spaced not more than 3 feet (9144 mm) on center and placed within 12 inches (305 mm) of the wall opening.

R703.7.4.2 Air space. The veneer shall be separated from the sheathing by an air space of a minimum of a nominal 1 inch (25 mm) but not more than $4^1/_2$ inches (114 mm).

R703.7.4. 3 Mortar or grout fill. As an alternate to the air space required by Section R703.7.4.2, mortar or grout shall be permitted to fill the air space .When the air space is filled with mortar, a water-resistive barrier is required over studs or sheathing. When filling the air space, replacing the sheathing and water-resistive barrier with a wire mesh and *approved* water-resistive barrier or an *approved* water-resistive barrier-backed reinforcement attached directly to the studs is permitted.

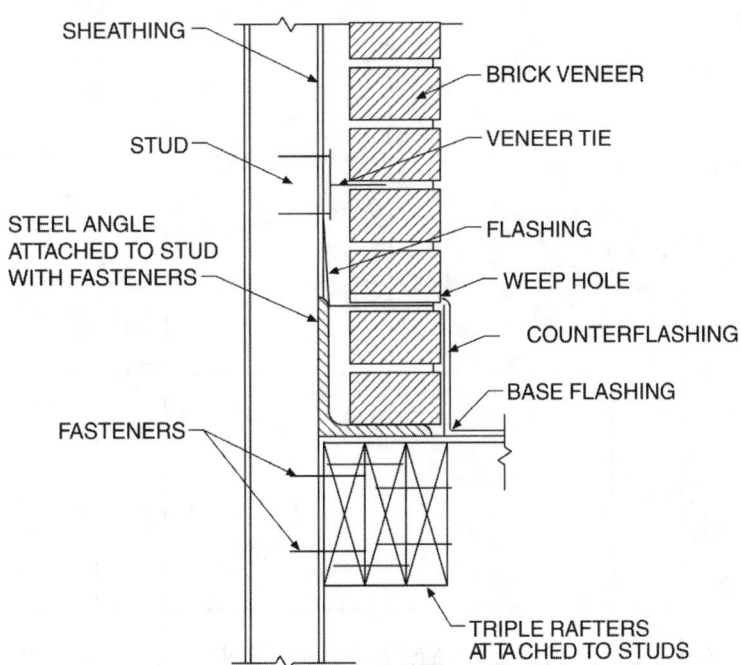

SUPPORT BY ROOF MEMBERS

FIGURE R703.7.2.2
EXTERIOR MASONRY VENEER SUPPORT BY ROOF MEMBERS

R703.7.5 Flashing. Flashing shall be located beneath the first course of masonry above finished ground level above the foundation wall or slab and at other points of support, including structural floors, shelf angles and lintels when masonry veneers are designed in accordance with Section R703.7. See Section R703.8 for additional requirements.

R703.7.6 Weepholes. Weepholes shall be provided in the outside wythe of masonry walls at a maximum spacing of 33 inches (838 mm) on center. Weepholes shall not be less than $^3/_{16}$ inch (5 mm) in diameter. Weepholes shall be located immediately above the flashing.

R703.8 Flashing. *Approved* corrosion-resistant flashing shall be applied shingle-fashion in a manner to prevent entry of water into the wall cavity or penetration of water to the building structural framing components. Self-adhered membranes used as flashing shall comply with AAMA 711. The flashing shall extend to the surface of the exterior wall finish. *Approved* corrosion-resistant flashings shall be installed at all of the following locations:

1. Exterior window and door openings. Flashing at exterior window and door openings shall extend to the surface of the exterior wall finish or to the water-resistive barrier for subsequent drainage.

TABLE R703.7.3.1
ALLOWABLE SPANS FOR LINTELS SUPPORTING MASONRY VENEER[a, b, c, d]

SIZE OF STEEL ANGLE[a, c, d] (inches)	NO STORY ABOVE	ONE STORY ABOVE	TWO STORIES ABOVE	NO. OF $^1/_2$" OR EQUIVALENT REINFORCING BARS IN REINFORCED LINTEL[b, d]
$3 \times 3 \times ^1/_4$	6'-0"	4'-6"	3'-0"	1
$4 \times 3 \times ^1/_4$	8'-0"	6'-0"	4'-6"	1
$5 \times 3^1/_2 \times ^5/_{16}$	10'-0"	8'-0"	6'-0"	2
$6 \times 3^1/_2 \times ^5/_{16}$	14'-0"	9'-6"	7'-0"	2
$2\text{-}6 \times 3^1/_2 \times ^5/_{16}$	20'-0"	12'-0"	9'-6"	4

For SI: 1 inch = 25.4 mm, 1 foot =304.8 mm.

a. Long leg of the angle shall be placed in a vertical position.

b. Depth of reinforced lintels shall not be less than 8 inches and all cells of hollow masonry lintels shall be grouted solid. Reinforcing bars shall extend not less than 8 inches into the support.

c. Steel members indicated are adequate typical examples; other steel members meeting structural design requirements may be used.

d. Either steel angle or reinforced lintel shall span opening.

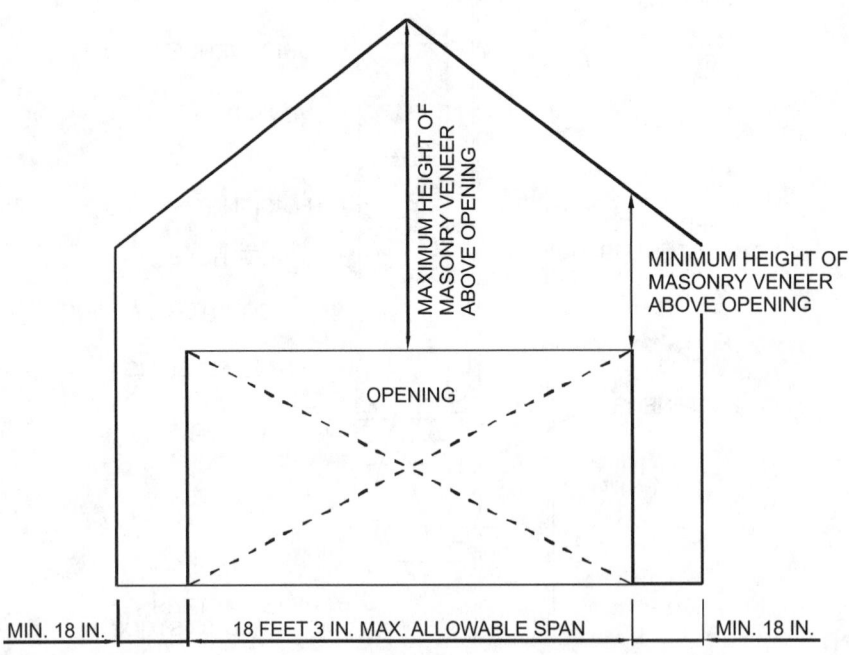

For SI: 1 inch = 25.4 mm, 1 foot = 304.8 mm.

FIGURE R703.7.3.2
MASONRY VENEER OPENING

2. At the intersection of chimneys or other masonry construction with frame or stucco walls, with projecting lips on both sides under stucco copings.

3. Under and at the ends of masonry, wood or metal copings and sills.

4. Continuously above all projecting wood trim.

5. Where exterior porches, decks or stairs attach to a wall or floor assembly of wood-frame construction.

6. At wall and roof intersections.

7. At built-in gutters.

R703.9 Exterior insulation and finish system (EIFS)/EIFS with drainage. Exterior Insulation and Finish System (EIFS) shall comply with this chapter and Sections R703.9.1 and R703.9.3. EIFS with drainage shall comply with this chapter and Sections R703.9.2, R703.9.3 and R703.9.4.

R703.9.1 Exterior insulation and finish system (EIFS). EIFS shall comply with ASTM E 2568.

R703.9.2 Exterior insulation and finish system (EIFS) with drainage. EIFS with drainage shall comply with ASTM E 2568 and shall have an average minimum drainage efficiency of 90 percent when tested in accordance with ASTM E 2273.

R703.9.2.1 Water-resistive barrier. The water-resistive barrier shall comply with Section R703.2 or ASTM E 2570.

R703.9.2.2 Installation. The water-resistive barrier shall be applied between the EIFS and the wall sheathing.

R703.9.3 Flashing, general. Flashing of EIFS shall be provided in accordance with the requirements of Section R703.8.

R703.9.4 EIFS/EIFS with drainage installation. All EIFS shall be installed in accordance with the manufacturer's installation instructions and the requirements of this section.

R703.9.4.1 Terminations. The EIFS shall terminate not less than 6 inches (152 mm) above the finished ground level.

R703.9.4.2 Decorative trim. Decorative trim shall not be face nailed though the EIFS.

R703.10 Fiber cement siding.

R703.10.1 Panel siding. Fiber-cement panels shall comply with the requirements of ASTM C1186, Type A, minimum Grade II. Panels shall be installed with the long dimension either parallel or perpendicular to framing. Vertical and horizontal joints shall occur over framing members and shall be sealed with caulking, covered with battens or shall be designed to comply with Section R703.1. Panel siding shall be installed with fasteners according to Table R703.4 or *approved* manufacturer's installation instructions.

R703.10.2 Lap siding. Fiber-cement lap siding having a maximum width of 12 inches shall comply with the requirements of ASTM C1186, Type A, minimum Grade II. Lap

siding shall be lapped a minimum of 1¼ inches (32 mm) and lap siding not having tongue-and-groove end joints shall have the ends sealed with caulking, installed with an H-section joint cover, located over a strip of flashing or shall be designed to comply with Section R703.1. Lap siding courses may be installed with the fastener heads exposed or concealed, according to Table R703.4 or *approved* manufacturers' installation instructions.

R703.11 Vinyl siding. Vinyl siding shall be certified and *labeled* as conforming to the requirements of ASTM D 3679 by an *approved* quality control agency.

R703.11.1 Installation. Vinyl siding, soffit and accessories shall be installed in accordance with the manufacturer's installation instructions.

R703.11.1.1 Soffit panels shall be individually fastened to a supporting component such as a nailing strip, fascia or subfascia component or as specified by the manufacturer's instructions.

R703.11.2 Foam plastic sheathing. Vinyl siding used with foam plastic sheathing shall be installed in accordance with Section R703.11.2.1, R703.11.2.2, or R703.11.2.3.

Exception: Where the foam plastic sheathing is applied directly over wood structural panels, fiberboard, gypsum sheathing or other *approved* backing capable of independently resisting the design wind pressure, the vinyl siding shall be installed in accordance with Section R703.11.1.

R703.11.2.1 Basic wind speed not exceeding 90 miles per hour and Exposure Category B. Where the basic wind speed does not exceed 90 miles per hour (40 m/s), the Exposure Category is B and gypsum wall board or equivalent is installed on the side of the wall opposite the foam plastic sheathing, the minimum siding fastener penetration into wood framing shall be 1¼ inches (32 mm) using minimum 0.120-inch diameter nail (shank) with a minimum 0.313-inch diameter head, 16 inches on center. The foam plastic sheathing shall be minimum ½-inch-thick (12.7 mm) (nominal) extruded polystyrene per ASTM C578, ½-inch-thick (12.7 mm) (nominal) polyisocyanurate per ASTM C1289, or 1-inch-thick (25 mm) (nominal) expanded polystyrene per ASTM C578.

R703.11.2.2 Basic wind speed exceeding 90 miles per hour or Exposure Categories C and D. Where the basic wind speed exceeds 90 miles per hour (40 m/s) or the Exposure Category is C or D, or all conditions of Section R703.11.2.1 are not met, the adjusted design pressure rating for the assembly shall meet or exceed the loads listed in Tables R301.2(2) adjusted for height and exposure using Section R301.2(3). The design wind pressure rating of the vinyl siding for installation over solid sheathing as provided in the vinyl siding manufacturer's product specifications shall be adjusted for the following wall assembly conditions:

1. For wall assemblies with foam plastic sheathing on the exterior side and gypsum wall board or equivalent on the interior side of the wall, the vinyl sid-

ing's design wind pressure rating shall be multiplied by 0.39.

2. For wall assemblies with foam plastic sheathing on the exterior side and no gypsum wall board or equivalent on the interior side of wall, the vinyl siding's design wind pressure rating shall be multiplied by 0.27.

R703.11.2.3 Manufacturer specification. Where the vinyl siding manufacturer's product specifications provide an *approved* design wind pressure rating for installation over foam plastic sheathing, use of this design wind pressure rating shall be permitted and the siding shall be installed in accordance with the manufacturer's installation instructions.

R703.12 Adhered masonry veneer installation. Adhered masonry veneer shall be installed in accordance with the manufacturer's instructions.

CHAPTER 8

ROOF-CEILING CONSTRUCTION

SECTION R801
GENERAL

R801.1 Application. The provisions of this chapter shall control the design and construction of the roof-ceiling system for all buildings.

R801.2 Requirements. Roof and ceiling construction shall be capable of accommodating all loads imposed according to Section R301 and of transmitting the resulting loads to the supporting structural elements.

R801.3 Roof drainage. In areas where expansive or collapsible soils are known to exist, all *dwellings* shall have a controlled method of water disposal from roofs that will collect and discharge roof drainage to the ground surface at least 5 feet (1524 mm) from foundation walls or to an *approved* drainage system.

SECTION R802
WOOD ROOF FRAMING

R802.1 Identification. Load-bearing dimension lumber for rafters, trusses and ceiling joists shall be identified by a grade mark of a lumber grading or inspection agency that has been approved by an accreditation body that complies with DOC PS 20. In lieu of a grade mark, a certificate of inspection issued by a lumber grading or inspection agency meeting the requirements of this section shall be accepted.

R802.1.1 Blocking. Blocking shall be a minimum of utility grade lumber.

R802.1.2 End-jointed lumber. *Approved* end-jointed lumber identified by a grade mark conforming to Section R802.1 may be used interchangeably with solid-sawn members of the same species and grade.

R802.1.3 Fire-retardant-treated wood. Fire-retardant-treated wood (FRTW) is any wood product which, when impregnated with chemicals by a pressure process or other means during manufacture, shall have, when tested in accordance with ASTM E 84, a listed flame spread index of 25 or less and shows no evidence of significant progressive combustion when the test is continued for an additional 20-minute period. In addition, the flame front shall not progress more than 10.5 feet (3200 mm) beyond the center line of the burners at any time during the test.

R802.1.3.1 Pressure process. For wood products impregnated with chemicals by a pressure process, the process shall be performed in closed vessels under pressures not less than 50 pounds per square inch gauge (psig) (344.7 kPa).

R802.1.3.2 Other means during manufacture. For wood products produced by other means during manufacture the treatment shall be an integral part of the manufacturing process of the wood product. The treatment shall provide permanent protection to all surfaces of the wood product.

R802.1.3.3 Testing. For wood products produced by other means during manufacture, other than a pressure process, all sides of the wood product shall be tested in accordance with and produce the results required in Section R802.1.3. Testing of only the front and back faces of wood structural panels shall be permitted.

R802.1.3.4 Labeling. Fire-retardant-treated lumber and wood structural panels shall be *labeled*. The *label* shall contain:

1. The identification *mark* of an *approved agency* in accordance with Section 1703.5 of the *International Building Code*.

2. Identification of the treating manufacturer.

3. The name of the fire-retardant treatment.

4. The species of wood treated.

5. Flame spread index and smoke-developed index.

6. Method of drying after treatment.

7. Conformance to applicable standards in accordance with Sections R802.1.3.5 through R802.1.3.8.

8. For FRTW exposed to weather, or a damp or wet location, the words "No increase in the listed classification when subjected to the Standard Rain Test" (ASTM D 2898).

R802.1.3.5 Strength adjustments. Design values for untreated lumber and wood structural panels as specified in Section R802.1 shall be adjusted for fire-retardant-treated wood. Adjustments to design values shall be based upon an *approved* method of investigation which takes into consideration the effects of the anticipated temperature and humidity to which the fire-retardant-treated wood will be subjected, the type of treatment and redrying procedures.

R802.1.3.5.1 Wood structural panels. The effect of treatment and the method of redrying after treatment, and exposure to high temperatures and high humidities on the flexure properties of fire-retardant-treated softwood plywood shall be determined in accordance with ASTM D 5516. The test data developed by ASTM D 5516 shall be used to develop adjustment factors, maximum loads and spans, or both for untreated plywood design values in accordance with ASTM D 6305. Each manufacturer shall publish the allowable maximum loads and spans for service as floor and roof sheathing for their treatment.

R802.1.3.5.2 Lumber. For each species of wood treated, the effect of the treatment and the method of redrying after treatment and exposure to high temperatures and high humidities on the allowable design properties of fire-retardant-treated lumber shall be determined in accordance with ASTM D 5664. The test data developed by ASTM D 5664 shall be used to develop modification factors for use at or near room temperature and at elevated temperatures and humidity in accordance with ASTM D 6841. Each manufacturer shall publish the modification factors for service at temperatures of not less than 80°F (27°C) and for roof framing. The roof framing modification factors shall take into consideration the climatological location.

R802.1.3.6 Exposure to weather. Where fire-retardant-treated wood is exposed to weather or damp or wet locations, it shall be identified as "Exterior" to indicate there is no increase in the listed flame spread index as defined in Section R802.1.3 when subjected to ASTM D 2898.

R802.1.3.7 Interior applications. Interior fire-retardant-treated wood shall have a moisture content of not over 28 percent when tested in accordance with ASTM D 3201 procedures at 92 percent relative humidity. Interior fire-retardant-treated wood shall be tested in accordance with Section R802.1.3.5.1 or R802.1.3.5.2. Interior fire-retardant-treated wood designated as Type A shall be tested in accordance with the provisions of this section.

R802.1.3.8 Moisture content. Fire-retardant-treated wood shall be dried to a moisture content of 19 percent or less for lumber and 15 percent or less for wood structural panels before use. For wood kiln dried after treatment (KDAT) the kiln temperatures shall not exceed those used in kiln drying the lumber and plywood submitted for the tests described in Section R802.1.3.5.1 for plywood and R802.1.3.5.2 for lumber.

R802.1.4 Structural glued laminated timbers. Glued laminated timbers shall be manufactured and identified as required in ANSI/AITC A190.1 and ASTM D 3737.

R802.1.5 Structural log members. Stress grading of structural log members of nonrectangular shape, as typically used in log buildings, shall be in accordance with ASTM D 3957. Such structural log members shall be identified by the grade mark of an *approved* lumber grading or inspection agency. In lieu of a grade mark on the material, a certificate of inspection as to species and grade issued by a lumber-grading or inspection agency meeting the requirements of this section shall be permitted to be accepted.

R802.2 Design and construction. The framing details required in Section R802 apply to roofs having a minimum slope of three units vertical in 12 units horizontal (25-percent slope) or greater. Roof-ceilings shall be designed and constructed in accordance with the provisions of this chapter and Figures R606.11(1), R606.11(2) and R606.11(3) or in accordance with AFPA/NDS. Components of roof-ceilings shall be fastened in accordance with Table R602.3(1).

R802.3 Framing details. Rafters shall be framed to ridge board or to each other with a gusset plate as a tie. Ridge board shall be at least 1-inch (25 mm) nominal thickness and not less in depth than the cut end of the rafter. At all valleys and hips there shall be a valley or hip rafter not less than 2-inch (51 mm) nominal thickness and not less in depth than the cut end of the rafter. Hip and valley rafters shall be supported at the ridge by a brace to a bearing partition or be designed to carry and distribute the specific load at that point. Where the roof pitch is less than three units vertical in 12 units horizontal (25-percent slope), structural members that support rafters and ceiling joists, such as ridge beams, hips and valleys, shall be designed as beams.

R802.3.1 Ceiling joist and rafter connections. Ceiling joists and rafters shall be nailed to each other in accordance with Table R802.5.1(9), and the rafter shall be nailed to the top wall plate in accordance with Table R602.3(1). Ceiling joists shall be continuous or securely joined in accordance with Table R802.5.1(9) where they meet over interior partitions and are nailed to adjacent rafters to provide a continuous tie across the building when such joists are parallel to the rafters.

Where ceiling joists are not connected to the rafters at the top wall plate, joists connected higher in the *attic* shall be installed as rafter ties, or rafter ties shall be installed to provide a continuous tie. Where ceiling joists are not parallel to rafters, rafter ties shall be installed. Rafter ties shall be a minimum of 2-inch by 4-inch (51 mm by 102 mm) (nominal), installed in accordance with the connection requirements in Table R802.5.1(9), or connections of equivalent capacities shall be provided. Where ceiling joists or rafter ties are not provided, the ridge formed by these rafters shall be supported by a wall or girder designed in accordance with accepted engineering practice.

Collar ties or ridge straps to resist wind uplift shall be connected in the upper third of the *attic* space in accordance with Table R602.3(1).

Collar ties shall be a minimum of 1-inch by 4-inch (25 mm by 102 mm) (nominal), spaced not more than 4 feet (1219 mm) on center.

R802.3.2 Ceiling joists lapped. Ends of ceiling joists shall be lapped a minimum of 3 inches (76 mm) or butted over bearing partitions or beams and toenailed to the bearing member. When ceiling joists are used to provide resistance to rafter thrust, lapped joists shall be nailed together in accordance with Table R602.3(1) and butted joists shall be tied together in a manner to resist such thrust.

R802.4 Allowable ceiling joist spans. Spans for ceiling joists shall be in accordance with Tables R802.4(1) and R802.4(2). For other *grades and species and for other loading conditions, refer to the AF&PA Span Tables for Joists and Rafters.*

R802.5 Allowable rafter spans. Spans for rafters shall be in accordance with Tables R802.5.1(1) through R802.5.1(8). For other *grades and species and for other loading conditions, refer to the AF&PA Span Tables for Joists and Rafters. The span of each rafter shall be measured along the horizontal projection of the rafter.*

R802.5.1 Purlins. Installation of purlins to reduce the span of rafters is permitted as shown in Figure R802.5.1. Purlins shall be sized no less than the required size of the rafters that they support. Purlins shall be continuous and shall be supported by 2-inch by 4-inch (51 mm by 102 mm) braces installed to bearing walls at a slope not less than 45 degrees from the horizontal. The braces shall be spaced not more than 4 feet (1219 mm) on center and the unbraced length of braces shall not exceed 8 feet (2438 mm).

R802.6 Bearing. The ends of each rafter or ceiling joist shall have not less than $1^1/_2$ inches (38 mm) of bearing on wood or metal and not less than 3 inches (76 mm) on masonry or concrete.

R802.6.1 Finished ceiling material. If the finished ceiling material is installed on the ceiling prior to the attachment of the ceiling to the walls, such as in construction at a factory, a compression strip of the same thickness as the finish ceiling material shall be installed directly above the top plate of bearing walls if the compressive strength of the finish ceiling material is less than the loads it will be required to withstand. The compression strip shall cover the entire length of such top plate and shall be at least one-half the width of the top plate. It shall be of material capable of transmitting the loads transferred through it.

R802.7 Cutting and notching. Structural roof members shall not be cut, bored or notched in excess of the limitations specified in this section.

R802.7.1 Sawn lumber. Notches in solid lumber joists, rafters, blocking and beams shall not exceed one-sixth of the depth of the member, shall not be longer than one-third of the depth of the member and shall not be located in the middle one-third of the span. Notches at the ends of the member shall not exceed one-fourth the depth of the member. The tension side of members 4 inches (102 mm) or greater in nominal thickness shall not be notched except at the ends of the members. The diameter of the holes bored or cut into members shall not exceed one-third the depth of the member. Holes shall not be closer than 2 inches (51 mm) to the top or bottom of the member, or to any other hole located in the member. Where the member is also notched, the hole shall not be closer than 2 inches (51 mm) to the notch.

Exception: Notches on cantilevered portions of rafters are permitted provided the dimension of the remaining portion of the rafter is not less than 4-inch nominal (102 mm) and the length of the cantilever does not exceed 24 inches (610 mm).

R802.7.2 Engineered wood products. Cuts, notches and holes bored in trusses, structural composite lumber, structural glue-laminated members or I-joists are prohibited except where permitted by the manufacturer's recommendations or where the effects of such *alterations* are specifically considered in the design of the member by a registered *design professional*.

R802.8 Lateral support. Roof framing members and ceiling joists having a depth-to-thickness ratio exceeding 5 to 1 based on nominal dimensions shall be provided with lateral support at points of bearing to prevent rotation. For roof rafters with ceiling joists attached per Table R602.3(1), the depth-thickness ratio for the total assembly shall be determined using the combined thickness of the rafter plus the attached ceiling joist.

Exception: Roof trusses shall be braced in accordance with Section R802.10.3.

R802.8.1 Bridging. Rafters and ceiling joists having a depth-to-thickness ratio exceeding 6 to 1 based on nominal dimensions shall be supported laterally by solid blocking, diagonal bridging (wood or metal) or a continuous 1-inch by 3-inch (25 mm by 76 mm) wood strip nailed across the rafters or ceiling joists at intervals not exceeding 8 feet (2438 mm).

R802.9 Framing of openings. Openings in roof and ceiling framing shall be framed with header and trimmer joists. When the header joist span does not exceed 4 feet (1219 mm), the header joist may be a single member the same size as the ceiling joist or rafter. Single trimmer joists may be used to carry a single header joist that is located within 3 feet (914 mm) of the trimmer joist bearing. When the header joist span exceeds 4 feet (1219 mm), the trimmer joists and the header joist shall be doubled and of sufficient cross section to support the ceiling joists or rafter framing into the header. *Approved* hangers shall be used for the header joist to trimmer joist connections when the header joist span exceeds 6 feet (1829 mm). Tail joists over 12 feet (3658 mm) long shall be supported at the header by framing anchors or on ledger strips not less than 2 inches by 2 inches (51 mm by 51 mm).

R802.10 Wood trusses.

R802.10.1 Truss design drawings. Truss design drawings, prepared in conformance to Section R802.10.1, shall be provided to the *building official* and *approved* prior to installation. Truss design drawings shall include, at a minimum, the information specified below. Truss design drawing shall be provided with the shipment of trusses delivered to the jobsite.

1. Slope or depth, span and spacing.

2. Location of all joints.

3. Required bearing widths.

4. Design loads as applicable.

    4.1. Top chord live load (as determined from Section R301.6).

    4.2. Top chord dead load.

    4.3. Bottom chord live load.

    4.4. Bottom chord dead load.

    4.5. Concentrated loads and their points of application.

    4.6. Controlling wind and earthquake loads.

5. Adjustments to lumber and joint connector design values for conditions of use.

6. Each reaction force and direction.

7. Joint connector type and description (e.g., size, thickness or gage) and the dimensioned location of each joint connector except where symmetrically located relative to the joint interface.

8. Lumber size, species and *grade for each member.*

9. Connection requirements for:

    9.1. Truss to girder-truss.

    9.2. Truss ply to ply.

    9.3. Field splices.

10. Calculated deflection ratio and/or maximum description for live and total load.

11. Maximum axial compression forces in the truss members to enable the building designer to design the size, connections and anchorage of the perma-

nent continuous lateral bracing. Forces shall be shown on the truss design drawing or on supplemental documents.

12. Required permanent truss member bracing location.

R802.10.2 Design. Wood trusses shall be designed in accordance with accepted engineering practice. The design and manufacture of metal-plate-connected wood trusses shall comply with ANSI/TPI 1. The truss design drawings shall be prepared by a registered professional where required by the statutes of the *jurisdiction* in which the project is to be constructed in accordance with Section R106.1.

R802.10.2.1 Applicability limits. The provisions of this section shall control the design of truss roof framing when snow controls for buildings not greater than 60 feet (18 288 mm) in length perpendicular to the joist, rafter or truss span, not greater than 36 feet (10 973 mm) in width parallel to the joist, rafter or truss span, not greater than two stories in height with each *story* not greater than 10 feet (3048 mm) high, and roof slopes not smaller than 3:12 (25-percent slope) or greater than 12:12 (100-percent slope). Truss roof framing constructed in accordance with the provisions of this section shall be limited to sites subjected to a maximum design wind speed of 110 miles per hour (49 m/s), Exposure A, B or C, and a maximum ground snow load of 70 psf (3352 Pa). For consistent loading of all truss types, roof snow load is to be computed as: 0.7 p_g.

R802.10.3 Bracing. Trusses shall be braced to prevent rotation and provide lateral stability in accordance with the requirements specified in the *construction documents* for the building and on the individual truss design drawings. In the absence of specific bracing requirements, trusses shall be braced in accordance with the Building Component Safety Information (BCSI 1-03) Guide to Good Practice for Handling, Installing & Bracing of Metal Plate Connected Wood Trusses.

R802.10.4 Alterations to trusses. Truss members shall not be cut, notched, drilled, spliced or otherwise altered in any way without the approval of a registered *design professional*. Alterations resulting in the addition of load (e.g., HVAC equipment, water heater) that exceeds the design load for the truss shall not be permitted without verification that the truss is capable of supporting such additional loading.

R802.10.5 Truss to wall connection. Trusses shall be connected to wall plates by the use of *approved* connectors having a resistance to uplift of not less than 175 pounds (779 N) and shall be installed in accordance with the manufacturer's specifications. For roof assemblies subject to wind uplift pressures of 20 pounds per square foot (960 Pa) or greater, as established in Table R301.2(2), adjusted for height and exposure per Table R301.2(3), see section R802.11.

R802.11 Roof tie-down.

R802.11.1 Uplift resistance. Roof assemblies which are subject to wind uplift pressures of 20 pounds per square foot (960 Pa) or greater shall have roof rafters or trusses attached to their supporting wall assemblies by connections capable of providing the resistance required in Table R802.11. Wind uplift pressures shall be determined using an effective wind area of 100 square feet (9.3 m²) and Zone 1 in Table R301.2(2), as adjusted for height and exposure per Table R301.2(3).

A continuous load path shall be designed to transmit the uplift forces from the rafter or truss ties to the foundation.

TABLE R802.4(1)
CEILING JOIST SPANS FOR COMMON LUMBER SPECIES
(Uninhabitable attics without storage, live load = 10 psf, L/Δ = 240)

CEILING JOIST SPACING (inches)	SPECIES AND GRADE		DEAD LOAD = 5 psf			
			2 × 4	2 × 6	2 × 8	2 × 10
			Maximum ceiling joist spans			
			(feet - inches)	(feet - inches)	(feet - inches)	(feet - inches)
12	Douglas fir-larch	SS	13-2	20-8	Note a	Note a
	Douglas fir-larch	#1	12-8	19-11	Note a	Note a
	Douglas fir-larch	#2	12-5	19-6	25-8	Note a
	Douglas fir-larch	#3	10-10	15-10	20-1	24-6
	Hem-fir	SS	12-5	19-6	25-8	Note a
	Hem-fir	#1	12-2	19-1	25-2	Note a
	Hem-fir	#2	11-7	18-2	24-0	Note a
	Hem-fir	#3	10-10	15-10	20-1	24-6
	Southern pine	SS	12-11	20-3	Note a	Note a
	Southern pine	#1	12-8	19-11	Note a	Note a
	Southern pine	#2	12-5	19-6	25-8	Note a
	Southern pine	#3	11-6	17-0	21-8	25-7
	Spruce-pine-fir	SS	12-2	19-1	25-2	Note a
	Spruce-pine-fir	#1	11-10	18-8	24-7	Note a
	Spruce-pine-fir	#2	11-10	18-8	24-7	Note a
	Spruce-pine-fir	#3	10-10	15-10	20-1	24-6
16	Douglas fir-larch	SS	11-11	18-9	24-8	Note a
	Douglas fir-larch	#1	11-6	18-1	23-10	Note a
	Douglas fir-larch	#2	11-3	17-8	23-0	Note a
	Douglas fir-larch	#3	9-5	13-9	17-5	21-3
	Hem-fir	SS	11-3	17-8	23-4	Note a
	Hem-fir	#1	11-0	17-4	22-10	Note a
	Hem-fir	#2	10-6	16-6	21-9	Note a
	Hem-fir	#3	9-5	13-9	17-5	21-3
	Southern pine	SS	11-9	18-5	24-3	Note a
	Southern pine	#1	11-6	18-1	23-1	Note a
	Southern pine	#2	11-3	17-8	23-4	Note a
	Southern pine	#3	10-0	14-9	18-9	22-2
	Spruce-pine-fir	SS	11-0	17-4	22-10	Note a
	Spruce-pine-fir	#1	10-9	16-11	22-4	Note a
	Spruce-pine-fir	#2	10-9	16-11	22-4	Note a
	Spruce-pine-fir	#3	9-5	13-9	17-5	21-3
19.2	Douglas fir-larch	SS	11-3	17-8	23-3	Note a
	Douglas fir-larch	#1	10-10	17-0	22-5	Note a
	Douglas fir-larch	#2	10-7	16-7	21-0	25-8
	Douglas fir-larch	#3	8-7	12-6	15-10	19-5
	Hem-fir	SS	10-7	16-8	21-11	Note a
	Hem-fir	#1	10-4	16-4	21-6	Note a
	Hem-fir	#2	9-11	15-7	20-6	25-3
	Hem-fir	#3	8-7	12-6	15-10	19-5
	Southern -pine	SS	11-0	17-4	22-10	Note a
	Southern pine	#1	10-10	17-0	22-5	Note a
	Southern pine	#2	10-7	16-8	21-11	Note a
	Southern pine	#3	9-1	13-6	17-2	20-3
	Spruce-pine-fir	SS	10-4	16-4	21-6	Note a
	Spruce-pine-fir	#1	10-2	15-11	21-0	25-8
	Spruce-pine-fir	#2	10-2	15-11	21-0	25-8
	Spruce-pine-fir	#3	8-7	12-6	15-10	19-5

(continued)

TABLE R802.4(1)—continued
CEILING JOIST SPANS FOR COMMON LUMBER SPECIES
(Uninhabitable attics without storage, live load = 10 psf, L/Δ = 240)

CEILING JOIST SPACING (inches)	SPECIES AND GRADE		DEAD LOAD = 5 psf			
			2 × 4	2 × 6	2 × 8	2 × 10
			Maximum ceiling joist spans			
			(feet - inches)	(feet - inches)	(feet - inches)	(feet - inches)
24	Douglas fir-larch	SS	10-5	16-4	21-7	Note a
	Douglas fir-larch	#1	10-0	15-9	20-1	24-6
	Douglas fir-larch	#2	9-10	14-10	18-9	22-11
	Douglas fir-larch	#3	7-8	11-2	14-2	17-4
	Hem-fir	SS	9-10	15-6	20-5	Note a
	Hem-fir	#1	9-8	15-2	19-7	23-11
	Hem-fir	#2	9-2	14-5	18-6	22-7
	Hem-fir	#3	7-8	11-2	14-2	17-4
	Southern pine	SS	10-3	16-1	21-2	Note a
	Southern pine	#1	10-0	15-9	20-10	Note a
	Southern pine	#2	9-10	15-6	20-1	23-11
	Southern pine	#3	8-2	12-0	15-4	18-1
	Spruce-pine-fir	SS	9-8	15-2	19-11	25-5
	Spruce-pine-fir	#1	9-5	14-9	18-9	22-11
	Spruce-pine-fir	#2	9-5	14-9	18-9	22-11
	Spruce-pine-fir	#3	7-8	11-2	14-2	17-4

Check sources for availability of lumber in lengths greater than 20 feet.

For SI: 1 inch = 25.4 mm, 1 foot = 304.8 mm, 1 pound per square foot = 0.0479 kPa.

a. Span exceeds 26 feet in length.

TABLE R802.4(2)
CEILING JOIST SPANS FOR COMMON LUMBER SPECIES
(Uninhabitable attics with limited storage, live load = 20 psf, L/Δ = 240)

CEILING JOIST SPACING (inches)	SPECIES AND GRADE		DEAD LOAD = 10 psf			
			2 × 4	2 × 6	2 × 8	2 × 10
			Maximum ceiling joist spans			
			(feet - inches)	(feet - inches)	(feet - inches)	(feet - inches)
12	Douglas fir-larch	SS	10-5	16-4	21-7	Note a
	Douglas fir-larch	#1	10-0	15-9	20-1	24-6
	Douglas fir-larch	#2	9-10	14-10	18-9	22-11
	Douglas fir-larch	#3	7-8	11-2	14-2	17-4
	Hem-fir	SS	9-10	15-6	20-5	Note a
	Hem-fir	#1	9-8	15-2	19-7	23-11
	Hem-fir	#2	9-2	14-5	18-6	22-7
	Hem-fir	#3	7-8	11-2	14-2	17-4
	Southern pine	SS	10-3	16-1	21-2	Note a
	Southern pine	#1	10-0	15-9	20-10	Note a
	Southern pine	#2	9-10	15-6	20-1	23-11
	Southern pine	#3	8-2	12-0	15-4	18-1
	Spruce-pine-fir	SS	9-8	15-2	19-11	25-5
	Spruce-pine-fir	#1	9-5	14-9	18-9	22-11
	Spruce-pine-fir	#2	9-5	14-9	18-9	22-11
	Spruce-pine-fir	#3	7-8	11-2	14-2	17-4
16	Douglas fir-larch	SS	9-6	14-11	19-7	25-0
	Douglas fir-larch	#1	9-1	13-9	17-5	21-3
	Douglas fir-larch	#2	8-9	12-10	16-3	19-10
	Douglas fir-larch	#3	6-8	9-8	12-4	15-0
	Hem-fir	SS	8-11	14-1	18-6	23-8
	Hem-fir	#1	8-9	13-5	16-10	20-8
	Hem-fir	#2	8-4	12-8	16-0	19-7
	Hem-fir	#3	6-8	9-8	12-4	15-0
	Southern pine	SS	9-4	14-7	19-3	24-7
	Southern pine	#1	9-1	14-4	18-11	23-1
	Southern pine	#2	8-11	13-6	17-5	20-9
	Southern pine	#3	7-1	10-5	13-3	15-8
	Spruce-pine-fir	SS	8-9	13-9	18-1	23-1
	Spruce-pine-fir	#1	8-7	12-10	16-3	19-10
	Spruce-pine-fir	#2	8-7	12-10	16-3	19-10
	Spruce-pine-fir	#3	6-8	9-8	12-4	15-0
19.2	Douglas fir-larch	SS	8-11	14-0	18-5	23-4
	Douglas fir-larch	#1	8-7	12-6	15-10	19-5
	Douglas fir-larch	#2	8-0	11-9	14-10	18-2
	Douglas fir-larch	#3	6-1	8-10	11-3	13-8
	Hem-fir	SS	8-5	13-3	17-5	22-3
	Hem-fir	#1	8-3	12-3	15-6	18-11
	Hem-fir	#2	7-10	11-7	14-8	17-10
	Hem-fir	#3	6-1	8-10	11-3	13-8
	Southern pine	SS	8-9	13-9	18-1	23-1
	Southern pine	#1	8-7	13-6	17-9	21-1
	Southern pine	#2	8-5	12-3	15-10	18-11
	Southern pine	#3	6-5	9-6	12-1	14-4
	Spruce-pine-fir	SS	8-3	12-11	17-1	21-8
	Spruce-pine-fir	#1	8-0	11-9	14-10	18-2
	Spruce-pine-fir	#2	8-0	11-9	14-10	18-2
	Spruce-pine-fir	#3	6-1	8-10	11-3	13-8

(continued)

TABLE R802.4(2)—continued
CEILING JOIST SPANS FOR COMMON LUMBER SPECIES
(Uninhabitable attics with limited storage, live load = 20 psf, L/Δ = 240)

CEILING JOIST SPACING (inches)	SPECIES AND GRADE		DEAD LOAD = 10 psf			
			2 × 4	2 × 6	2 × 8	2 × 10
			Maximum ceiling joist spans			
			(feet - inches)	(feet - inches)	(feet - inches)	(feet - inches)
24	Douglas fir-larch	SS	8-3	13-0	17-1	20-11
	Douglas fir-larch	#1	7-8	11-2	14-2	17-4
	Douglas fir-larch	#2	7-2	10-6	13-3	16-3
	Douglas fir-larch	#3	5-5	7-11	10-0	12-3
	Hem-fir	SS	7-10	12-3	16-2	20-6
	Hem-fir	#1	7-6	10-11	13-10	16-11
	Hem-fir	#2	7-1	10-4	13-1	16-0
	Hem-fir	#3	5-5	7-11	10-0	12-3
	Southern pine	SS	8-1	12-9	16-10	21-6
	Southern pine	#1	8-0	12-6	15-10	18-10
	Southern pine	#2	7-8	11-0	14-2	16-11
	Southern pine	#3	5-9	8-6	10-10	12-10
	Spruce-pine-fir	SS	7-8	12-0	15-10	19-5
	Spruce-pine-fir	#1	7-2	10-6	13-3	16-3
	Spruce-pine-fir	#2	7-2	10-6	13-3	16-3
	Spruce-pine-fir	#3	5-5	7-11	10-0	12-3

Check sources for availability of lumber in lengths greater than 20 feet.

For SI: 1 inch = 25.4 mm, 1 foot = 304.8 mm, 1 pound per square foot = 0.0479 kPa.

a. Span exceeds 26 feet in length.

TABLE R802.5.1(1)
RAFTER SPANS FOR COMMON LUMBER SPECIES
(Roof live load=20 psf, ceiling not attached to rafters, L/Δ = 180)

RAFTER SPACING (inches)	SPECIES AND GRADE		DEAD LOAD = 10 psf					DEAD LOAD = 20 psf				
			2 × 4	2 × 6	2 × 8	2 × 10	2 × 12	2 × 4	2 × 6	2 × 8	2 × 10	2 × 12
			Maximum rafter spans[a]									
			(feet - inches)	(feet - inches)	(feet - inches)	(feet - inches)	(feet - inches)	(feet - inches)	(feet - inches)	(feet - inches)	(feet - inches)	(feet - inches)
12	Douglas fir-larch	SS	11-6	18-0	23-9	Note b	Note b	11-6	18-0	23-5	Note b	Note b
	Douglas fir-larch	#1	11-1	17-4	22-5	Note b	Note b	10-6	15-4	19-5	23-9	Note b
	Douglas fir-larch	#2	10-10	16-7	21-0	25-8	Note b	9-10	14-4	18-2	22-3	25-9
	Douglas fir-larch	#3	8-7	12-6	15-10	19-5	22-6	7-5	10-10	13-9	16-9	19-6
	Hem-fir	SS	10-10	17-0	22-5	Note b	Note b	10-10	17-0	22-5	Note b	Note b
	Hem-fir	#1	10 -7	16-8	21-10	Note b	Note b	10-3	14-11	18-11	23-2	Note b
	Hem-fir	#2	10-1	15-11	20-8	25-3	Note b	9-8	14-2	17-11	21-11	25-5
	Hem-fir	#3	8-7	12-6	15-10	19-5	22-6	7-5	10-10	13-9	16-9	19-6
	Southern pine	SS	11-3	17-8	23-4	Note b	Note b	11-3	17-8	23-4	Note b	Note b
	Southern pine	#1	11-1	17-4	22-11	Note b	Note b	11-1	17-3	21-9	25-10	Note b
	Southern pine	#2	10-10	17-0	22-5	Note b	Note b	10-6	15-1	19-5	23-2	Note b
	Southern pine	#3	9-1	13-6	17-2	20-3	24-1	7-11	11-8	14-10	17-6	20-11
	Spruce-pine-fir	SS	10-7	16-8	21-11	Note b	Note b	10-7	16-8	21-9	Note b	Note b
	Spruce-pine-fir	#1	10-4	16-3	21-0	25-8	Note b	9-10	14-4	18-2	22-3	25-9
	Spruce-pine-fir	#2	10-4	16-3	21-0	25-8	Note b	9-10	14-4	18-2	22-3	25-9
	Spruce-pine-fir	#3	8-7	12-6	15-10	19-5	22-6	7-5	10-10	13-9	16-9	19-6
16	Douglas fir-larch	SS	10-5	16-4	21-7	Note b	Note b	10-5	16-0	20-3	24-9	Note b
	Douglas fir-larch	#1	10-0	15-4	19-5	23-9	Note b	9-1	13-3	16-10	20-7	23-10
	Douglas fir-larch	#2	9-10	14-4	18-2	22-3	25-9	8-6	12-5	15-9	19-3	22-4
	Douglas fir-larch	#3	7-5	10-10	13-9	16-9	19-6	6-5	9-5	11-11	14-6	16-10
	Hem-fir	SS	9-10	15-6	20-5	Note b	Note b	9-10	15-6	19-11	24-4	Note b
	Hem-fir	#1	9-8	14-11	18-11	23-2	Note b	8-10	12-11	16-5	20-0	23-3
	Hem-fir	#2	9-2	14-2	17-11	21-11	25-5	8-5	12-3	15-6	18-11	22-0
	Hem-fir	#3	7-5	10-10	13-9	16-9	19-6	6-5	9-5	11-11	14-6	16-10
	Southern pine	SS	10-3	16-1	21-2	Note b	Note b	10-3	16-1	21-2	Note b	Note b
	Southern pine	#1	10-0	15-9	20-10	25-10	Note b	10-0	15-0	18-10	22-4	Note b
	Southern pine	#2	9-10	15-1	19-5	23-2	Note b	9-1	13-0	16-10	20-1	23-7
	Southern pine	#3	7-11	11-8	14-10	17-6	20-11	6-10	10-1	12-10	15-2	18-1
	Spruce-pine-fir	SS	9-8	15-2	19-11	25-5	Note b	9-8	14-10	18-10	23-0	Note b
	Spruce-pine-fir	#1	9-5	14-4	18-2	22-3	25-9	8-6	12-5	15-9	19-3	22-4
	Spruce-pine-fir	#2	9-5	14-4	18-2	22-3	25-9	8-6	12-5	15-9	19-3	22-4
	Spruce-pine-fir	#3	7-5	10-10	13-9	16-9	19-6	6-5	9-5	11-11	14-6	16-10
19.2	Douglas fir-larch	SS	9-10	15-5	20-4	25-11	Note b	9-10	14-7	18-6	22-7	Note b
	Douglas fir-larch	#1	9-5	14-0	17-9	21-8	25-2	8-4	12-2	15-4	18-9	21-9
	Douglas fir-larch	#2	8-11	13-1	16-7	20-3	23-6	7-9	11-4	14-4	17-7	20-4
	Douglas fir-larch	#3	6-9	9-11	12-7	15-4	17-9	5-10	8-7	10-10	13-3	15-5
	Hem-fir	SS	9-3	14-7	19-2	24-6	Note b	9-3	14-4	18-2	22-3	25-9
	Hem-fir	#1	9-1	13-8	17-4	21-1	24-6	8-1	11-10	15-0	18-4	21-3
	Hem-fir	#2	8-8	12-11	16-4	20-0	23-2	7-8	11-2	14-2	17-4	20-1
	Hem-fir	#3	6-9	9-11	12-7	15-4	17-9	5-10	8-7	10-10	13-3	15-5
	Southern pine	SS	9-8	15-2	19-11	25-5	Note b	9-8	15-2	19-11	25-5	Note b
	Southern pine	#1	9-5	14-10	19-7	23-7	Note b	9-3	13-8	17-2	20-5	24-4
	Southern pine	#2	9-3	13-9	17-9	21-2	24-10	8-4	11-11	15-4	18-4	21-6
	Southern pine	#3	7-3	10-8	13-7	16-0	19-1	6-3	9-3	11-9	13-10	16-6
	Spruce-pine-fir	SS	9-1	14-3	18-9	23-11	Note b	9-1	13-7	17-2	21-0	24-4
	Spruce-pine-fir	#1	8-10	13-1	16-7	20-3	23-6	7-9	11-4	14-4	17-7	20-4
	Spruce-pine-fir	#2	8-10	13-1	16-7	20-3	23-6	7-9	11-4	14-4	17-7	20-4
	Spruce-pine-fir	#3	6-9	9-11	12-7	15-4	17-9	5-10	8-7	10-10	13-3	15-5

(continued)

TABLE R802.5.1(1)—continued
RAFTER SPANS FOR COMMON LUMBER SPECIES
(Roof live load=20 psf, ceiling not attached to rafters, L/Δ = 180)

RAFTER SPACING (inches)	SPECIES AND GRADE		DEAD LOAD = 10 psf					DEAD LOAD = 20 psf				
			2 × 4	2 × 6	2 × 8	2 × 10	2 × 12	2 × 4	2 × 6	2 × 8	2 × 10	2 × 12
			Maximum rafter spans[a]									
			(feet - inches)	(feet - inches)	(feet - inches)	(feet - inches)	(feet - inches)	(feet - inches)	(feet - inches)	(feet - inches)	(feet - inches)	(feet - inches)
24	Douglas fir-larch	SS	9-1	14-4	18-10	23-4	Note b	8-11	13-1	16-7	20-3	23-5
	Douglas fir-larch	#1	8-7	12-6	15-10	19-5	22-6	7-5	10-10	13-9	16-9	19-6
	Douglas fir-larch	#2	8-0	11-9	14-10	18-2	21-0	6-11	10-2	12-10	15-8	18-3
	Douglas fir-larch	#3	6-1	8-10	11-3	13-8	15-11	5-3	7-8	9-9	11-10	13-9
	Hem-fir	SS	8-7	13-6	17-10	22-9	Note b	8-7	12-10	16-3	19-10	23-0
	Hem-fir	#1	8-4	12-3	15-6	18-11	21-11	7-3	10-7	13-5	16-4	19-0
	Hem-fir	#2	7-11	11-7	14-8	17-10	20-9	6-10	10-0	12-8	15-6	17-11
	Hem-fir	#3	6-1	8-10	11-3	13-8	15-11	5-3	7-8	9-9	11-10	13-9
	Southern pine	SS	8-11	14-1	18-6	23-8	Note b	8-11	14-1	18-6	22-11	Note b
	Southern pine	#1	8-9	13-9	17-9	21-1	25-2	8-3	12-3	15-4	18-3	21-9
	Southern pine	#2	8-7	12-3	15-10	18-11	22-2	7-5	10-8	13-9	16-5	19-3
	Southern pine	#3	6-5	9-6	12-1	14-4	17-1	5-7	8-3	10-6	12-5	14-9
	Spruce-pine-fir	SS	8-5	13-3	17-5	21-8	25-2	8-4	12-2	15-4	18-9	21-9
	Spruce-pine-fir	#1	8-0	11-9	14-10	18-2	21-0	6-11	10-2	12-10	15-8	18-3
	Spruce-pine-fir	#2	8-0	11-9	14-10	18-2	21-0	6-11	10-2	12-10	15-8	18-3
	Spruce-pine-fir	#3	6-1	8-10	11-3	13-8	15-11	5-3	7-8	9-9	11-10	13-9

Check sources for availability of lumber in lengths greater than 20 feet.

For SI: 1 inch = 25.4 mm, 1 foot = 304.8 mm, 1 pound per square foot = 0.0479 kPa.

a. The tabulated rafter spans assume that ceiling joists are located at the bottom of the attic space or that some other method of resisting the outward push of the rafters on the bearing walls, such as rafter ties, is provided at that location. When ceiling joists or rafter ties are located higher in the attic space, the rafter spans shall be multiplied by the factors given below:

H_C/H_R	Rafter Span Adjustment Factor
1/3	0.67
1/4	0.76
1/5	0.83
1/6	0.90
1/7.5 or less	1.00

where:

H_C = Height of ceiling joists or rafter ties measured vertically above the top of the rafter support walls.

H_R = Height of roof ridge measured vertically above the top of the rafter support walls.

b. Span exceeds 26 feet in length.

TABLE R802.5.1(2)
RAFTER SPANS FOR COMMON LUMBER SPECIES
(Roof live load=20 psf, ceiling attached to rafters, L/Δ = 240)

RAFTER SPACING (inches)	SPECIES AND GRADE		DEAD LOAD = 10 psf					DEAD LOAD = 20 psf				
			2 × 4	2 × 6	2 × 8	2 × 10	2 × 12	2 × 4	2 × 6	2 × 8	2 × 10	2 × 12
			Maximum rafter spans[a]									
			(feet - inches)	(feet - inches)	(feet - inches)	(feet - inches)	(feet - inches)	(feet - inches)	(feet - inches)	(feet - inches)	(feet - inches)	(feet - inches)
12	Douglas fir-larch	SS	10-5	16-4	21-7	Note b	Note b	10-5	16-4	21-7	Note b	Note b
	Douglas fir-larch	#1	10-0	15-9	20-10	Note b	Note b	10-0	15-4	19-5	23-9	Note b
	Douglas fir-larch	#2	9-10	15-6	20-5	25-8	Note b	9-10	14-4	18-2	22-3	25-9
	Douglas fir-larch	#3	8-7	12-6	15-10	19-5	22-6	7-5	10-10	13-9	16-9	19-6
	Hem-fir	SS	9-10	15-6	20-5	Note b	Note b	9-10	15-6	20-5	Note b	Note b
	Hem-fir	#1	9-8	15-2	19-11	25-5	Note b	9-8	14-11	18-11	23-2	Note b
	Hem-fir	#2	9-2	14-5	19-0	24-3	Note b	9-2	14-2	17-11	21-11	25-5
	Hem-fir	#3	8-7	12-6	15-10	19-5	22-6	7-5	10-10	13-9	16-9	19-6
	Southern pine	SS	10-3	16-1	21-2	Note b	Note b	10-3	16-1	21-2	Note b	Note b
	Southern pine	#1	10-0	15-9	20-10	Note b	Note b	10-0	15-9	20-10	25-10	Note b
	Southern pine	#2	9-10	15-6	20-5	Note b	Note b	9-10	15-1	19-5	23-2	Note b
	Southern pine	#3	9-1	13-6	17-2	20-3	24-1	7-11	11-8	14-10	17-6	20-11
	Spruce-pine-fir	SS	9-8	15-2	19-11	25-5	Note b	9-8	15-2	19-11	25-5	Note b
	Spruce-pine-fir	#1	9-5	14-9	19-6	24-10	Note b	9-5	14-4	18-2	22-3	25-9
	Spruce-pine-fir	#2	9-5	14-9	19-6	24-10	Note b	9-5	14-4	18-2	22-3	25-9
	Spruce-pine-fir	#3	8-7	12-6	15-10	19-5	22-6	7-5	10-10	13-9	16-9	19-6
16	Douglas fir-larch	SS	9-6	14-11	19-7	25-0	Note b	9-6	14-11	19-7	24-9	Note b
	Douglas fir-larch	#1	9-1	14-4	18-11	23-9	Note b	9-1	13-3	16-10	20-7	23-10
	Douglas fir-larch	#2	8-11	14-1	18-2	22-3	25-9	8-6	12-5	15-9	19-3	22-4
	Douglas fir-larch	#3	7-5	10-10	13-9	16-9	19-6	6-5	9-5	11-11	14-6	16-10
	Hem-fir	SS	8-11	14-1	18-6	23-8	Note b	8-11	14-1	18-6	23-8	Note b
	Hem-fir	#1	8-9	13-9	18-1	23-1	Note b	8-9	12-11	16-5	20-0	23-3
	Hem-fir	#2	8-4	13-1	17-3	21-11	25-5	8-4	12-3	15-6	18-11	22-0
	Hem-fir	#3	7-5	10-10	13-9	16-9	19-6	6-5	9-5	11-11	14-6	16-10
	Southern pine	SS	9-4	14-7	19-3	24-7	Note b	9-4	14-7	19-3	24-7	Note b
	Southern pine	#1	9-1	14-4	18-11	24-1	Note b	9-1	14-4	18-10	22-4	Note b
	Southern pine	#2	8-11	14-1	18-6	23-2	Note b	8-11	13-0	16-10	20-1	23-7
	Southern pine	#3	7-11	11-8	14-10	17-6	20-11	6-10	10-1	12-10	15-2	18-1
	Spruce-pine-fir	SS	8-9	13-9	18-1	23-1	Note b	8-9	13-9	18-1	23-0	Note b
	Spruce-pine-fir	#1	8-7	13-5	17-9	22-3	25-9	8-6	12-5	15-9	19-3	22-4
	Spruce-pine-fir	#2	8-7	13-5	17-9	22-3	25-9	8-6	12-5	15-9	19-3	22-4
	Spruce-pine-fir	#3	7-5	10-10	13-9	16-9	19-6	6-5	9-5	11-11	14-6	16-10
19.2	Douglas fir-larch	SS	8-11	14-0	18-5	23-7	Note b	8-11	14-0	18-5	22-7	Note b
	Douglas fir-larch	#1	8-7	13-6	17-9	21-8	25-2	8-4	12-2	15-4	18-9	21-9
	Douglas fir-larch	#2	8-5	13-1	16-7	20-3	23-6	7-9	11-4	14-4	17-7	20-4
	Douglas fir-larch	#3	6-9	9-11	12-7	15-4	17-9	5-10	8-7	10-10	13-3	15-5
	Hem-fir	SS	8-5	13-3	17-5	22-3	Note b	8-5	13-3	17-5	22-3	25-9
	Hem-fir	#1	8-3	12-11	17-1	21-1	24-6	8-1	11-10	15-0	18-4	21-3
	Hem-fir	#2	7-10	12-4	16-3	20-0	23-2	7-8	11-2	14-2	17-4	20-1
	Hem-fir	#3	6-9	9-11	12-7	15-4	17-9	5-10	8-7	10-10	13-3	15-5
	Southern pine	SS	8-9	13-9	18-1	23-1	Note b	8-9	13-9	18-1	23-1	Note b
	Southern pine	#1	8-7	13-6	17-9	22-8	Note b	8-7	13-6	17-2	20-5	24-4
	Southern pine	#2	8-5	13-3	17-5	21-2	24-10	8-4	11-11	15-4	18-4	21-6
	Southern pine	#3	7-3	10-8	13-7	16-0	19-1	6-3	9-3	11-9	13-10	16-6
	Spruce-pine-fir	SS	8-3	12-11	17-1	21-9	Note b	8-3	12-11	17-1	21-0	24-4
	Spruce-pine-fir	#1	8-1	12-8	16-7	20-3	23-6	7-9	11-4	14-4	17-7	20-4
	Spruce-pine-fir	#2	8-1	12-8	16-7	20-3	23-6	7-9	11-4	14-4	17-7	20-4
	Spruce-pine-fir	#3	6-9	9-11	12-7	15-4	17-9	5-10	8-7	10-10	13-3	15-5

(continued)

TABLE R802.5.1(2)—continued
RAFTER SPANS FOR COMMON LUMBER SPECIES
(Roof live load=20 psf, ceiling attached to rafters, L/Δ = 240)

RAFTER SPACING (inches)	SPECIES AND GRADE		DEAD LOAD = 10 psf					DEAD LOAD = 20 psf				
			2 × 4	2 × 6	2 × 8	2 × 10	2 × 12	2 × 4	2 × 6	2 × 8	2 × 10	2 × 12
			Maximum rafter spans[a]									
			(feet - inches)	(feet - inches)	(feet - inches)	(feet - inches)	(feet - inches)	(feet - inches)	(feet - inches)	(feet - inches)	(feet - inches)	(feet - inches)
24	Douglas fir-larch	SS	8-3	13-0	17-2	21-10	Note b	8-3	13-0	16-7	20-3	23-5
	Douglas fir-larch	#1	8-0	12-6	15-10	19-5	22-6	7-5	10-10	13-9	16-9	19-6
	Douglas fir-larch	#2	7-10	11-9	14-10	18-2	21-0	6-11	10-2	12-10	15-8	18-3
	Douglas fir-larch	#3	6-1	8-10	11-3	13-8	15-11	5-3	7-8	9-9	11-10	13-9
	Hem-fir	SS	7-10	12-3	16-2	20-8	25-1	7-10	12-3	16-2	19-10	23-0
	Hem-fir	#1	7-8	12-0	15-6	18-11	21-11	7-3	10-7	13-5	16-4	19-0
	Hem-fir	#2	7-3	11-5	14-8	17-10	20-9	6-10	10-0	12-8	15-6	17-11
	Hem-fir	#3	6-1	8-10	11-3	13-8	15-11	5-3	7-8	9-9	11-10	13-9
	Southern pine	SS	8-1	12-9	16-10	21-6	Note b	8-1	12-9	16-10	21-6	Note b
	Southern pine	#1	8-0	12-6	16-6	21-1	25-2	8-0	12-3	15-4	18-3	21-9
	Southern pine	#2	7-10	12-3	15-10	18-11	22-2	7-5	10-8	13-9	16-5	19-3
	Southern pine	#3	6-5	9-6	12-1	14-4	17-1	5-7	8-3	10-6	12-5	14-9
	Spruce-pine-fir	SS	7-8	12-0	15-10	20-2	24-7	7-8	12-0	15-4	18-9	21-9
	Spruce-pine-fir	#1	7-6	11-9	14-10	18-2	21-0	6-11	10-2	12-10	15-8	18-3
	Spruce-pine-fir	#2	7-6	11-9	14-10	18-2	21-0	6-11	10-2	12-10	15-8	18-3
	Spruce-pine-fir	#3	6-1	8-10	11-3	13-8	15-11	5-3	7-8	9-9	11-10	13-9

Check sources for availability of lumber in lengths greater than 20 feet.

For SI: 1 inch = 25.4 mm, 1 foot = 304.8 mm, 1 pound per square foot = 0.0479 kPa.

a. The tabulated rafter spans assume that ceiling joists are located at the bottom of the attic space or that some other method of resisting the outward push of the rafters on the bearing walls, such as rafter ties, is provided at that location. When ceiling joists or rafter ties are located higher in the attic space, the rafter spans shall be multiplied by the factors given below:

H_C/H_R	Rafter Span Adjustment Factor
1/3	0.67
1/4	0.76
1/5	0.83
1/6	0.90
1/7.5 or less	1.00

where:

H_C = Height of ceiling joists or rafter ties measured vertically above the top of the rafter support walls.

H_R = Height of roof ridge measured vertically above the top of the rafter support walls.

b. Span exceeds 26 feet in length.

TABLE R802.5.1(3)
RAFTER SPANS FOR COMMON LUMBER SPECIES
(Ground snow load=30 psf, ceiling not attached to rafters, L/Δ = 180)

RAFTER SPACING (inches)	SPECIES AND GRADE		DEAD LOAD = 10 psf					DEAD LOAD = 20 psf				
			2 × 4	2 × 6	2 × 8	2 × 10	2 × 12	2 × 4	2 × 6	2 × 8	2 × 10	2 × 12
			Maximum rafter spans[a]									
			(feet - inches)	(feet - inches)	(feet - inches)	(feet - inches)	(feet - inches)	(feet - inches)	(feet - inches)	(feet - inches)	(feet - inches)	(feet - inches)
12	Douglas fir-larch	SS	10-0	15-9	20-9	Note b	Note b	10-0	15-9	20-1	24-6	Note b
	Douglas fir-larch	#1	9-8	14-9	18-8	22-9	Note b	9-0	13-2	16-8	20-4	23-7
	Douglas fir-larch	#2	9-5	13-9	17-5	21-4	24-8	8-5	12-4	15-7	19-1	22-1
	Douglas fir-larch	#3	7-1	10-5	13-2	16-1	18-8	6-4	9-4	11-9	14-5	16-8
	Hem-fir	SS	9-6	14-10	19-7	25-0	Note b	9-6	14-10	19-7	24-1	Note b
	Hem-fir	#1	9-3	14-4	18-2	22-2	25-9	8-9	12-10	16-3	19-10	23-0
	Hem-fir	#2	8-10	13-7	17-2	21-0	24-4	8-4	12-2	15-4	18-9	21-9
	Hem-fir	#3	7-1	10-5	13-2	16-1	18-8	6-4	9-4	11-9	14-5	16-8
	Southern pine	SS	9-10	15-6	20-5	Note b	Note b	9-10	15-6	20-5	Note b	Note b
	Southern pine	#1	9-8	15-2	20-0	24-9	Note b	9-8	14-10	18-8	22-2	Note b
	Southern pine	#2	9-6	14-5	18-8	22-3	Note b	9-0	12-11	16-8	19-11	23-4
	Southern pine	#3	7-7	11-2	14-3	16-10	20-0	6-9	10-0	12-9	15-1	17-11
	Spruce-pine-fir	SS	9-3	14-7	19-2	24-6	Note b	9-3	14-7	18-8	22-9	Note b
	Spruce-pine-fir	#1	9-1	13-9	17-5	21-4	24-8	8-5	12-4	15-7	19-1	22-1
	Spruce-pine-fir	#2	9-1	13-9	17-5	21-4	24-8	8-5	12-4	15-7	19-1	22-1
	Spruce-pine-fir	#3	7-1	10-5	13-2	16-1	18-8	6-4	9-4	11-9	14-5	16-8
16	Douglas fir-larch	SS	9-1	14-4	18-10	23-9	Note b	9-1	13-9	17-5	21-3	24-8
	Douglas fir-larch	#1	8-9	12-9	16-2	19-9	22-10	7-10	11-5	14-5	17-8	20-5
	Douglas fir-larch	#2	8-2	11-11	15-1	18-5	21-5	7-3	10-8	13-6	16-6	19-2
	Douglas fir-larch	#3	6-2	9-0	11-5	13-11	16-2	5-6	8-1	10-3	12-6	14-6
	Hem-fir	SS	8-7	13-6	17-10	22-9	Note b	8-7	13-6	17-1	20-10	24-2
	Hem-fir	#1	8-5	12-5	15-9	19-3	22-3	7-7	11-1	14-1	17-2	19-11
	Hem-fir	#2	8-0	11-9	14-11	18-2	21-1	7-2	10-6	13-4	16-3	18-10
	Hem-fir	#3	6-2	9-0	11-5	13-11	16-2	5-6	8-1	10-3	12-6	14-6
	Southern pine	SS	8-11	14-1	18-6	23-8	Note b	8-11	14-1	18-6	23-8	Note b
	Southern pine	#1	8-9	13-9	18-1	21-5	25-7	8-8	12-10	16-2	19-2	22-10
	Southern pine	#2	8-7	12-6	16-2	19-3	22-7	7-10	11-2	14-5	17-3	20-2
	Southern pine	#3	6-7	9-8	12-4	14-7	17-4	5-10	8-8	11-0	13-0	15-6
	Spruce-pine-fir	SS	8-5	13-3	17-5	22-1	25-7	8-5	12-9	16-2	19-9	22-10
	Spruce-pine-fir	#1	8-2	11-11	15-1	18-5	21-5	7-3	10-8	13-6	16-6	19-2
	Spruce-pine-fir	#2	8-2	11-11	15-1	18-5	21-5	7-3	10-8	13-6	16-6	19-2
	Spruce-pine-fir	#3	6-2	9-0	11-5	13-11	16-2	5-6	8-1	10-3	12-6	14-6
19.2	Douglas fir-larch	SS	8-7	13-6	17-9	21-8	25-2	8-7	12-6	15-10	19-5	22-6
	Douglas fir-larch	#1	7-11	11-8	14-9	18-0	20-11	7-1	10-5	13-2	16-1	18-8
	Douglas fir-larch	#2	7-5	10-11	13-9	16-10	19-6	6-8	9-9	12-4	15-1	17-6
	Douglas fir-larch	#3	5-7	8-3	10-5	12-9	14-9	5-0	7-4	9-4	11-5	13-2
	Hem-fir	SS	8-1	12-9	16-9	21-4	24-8	8-1	12-4	15-7	19-1	22-1
	Hem-fir	#1	7-9	11-4	14-4	17-7	20-4	6-11	10-2	12-10	15-8	18-2
	Hem-fir	#2	7-4	10-9	13-7	16-7	19-3	6-7	9-7	12-2	14-10	17-3
	Hem-fir	#3	5-7	8-3	10-5	12-9	14-9	5-0	7-4	9-4	11-5	13-2
	Southern pine	SS	8-5	13-3	17-5	22-3	Note b	8-5	13-3	17-5	22-0	25-9
	Southern pine	#1	8-3	13-0	16-6	19-7	23-4	7-11	11-9	14-9	17-6	20-11
	Southern pine	#2	7-11	11-5	14-9	17-7	20-7	7-1	10-2	13-2	15-9	18-5
	Southern pine	#3	6-0	8-10	11-3	13-4	15-10	5-4	7-11	10-1	11-11	14-2
	Spruce-pine-fir	SS	7-11	12-5	16-5	20-2	23-4	7-11	11-8	14-9	18-0	20-11
	Spruce-pine-fir	#1	7-5	10-11	13-9	16-10	19-6	6-8	9-9	12-4	15-1	17-6
	Spruce-pine-fir	#2	7-5	10-11	13-9	16-10	19-6	6-8	9-9	12-4	15-1	17-6
	Spruce-pine-fir	#3	5-7	8-3	10-5	12-9	14-9	5-0	7-4	9-4	11-5	13-2

(continued)

RAFTER SPANS FOR COMMON LUMBER SPECIES
(Ground snow load=30 psf, ceiling not attached to rafters, L/Δ = 180)

RAFTER SPACING (inches)	SPECIES AND GRADE		DEAD LOAD = 10 psf					DEAD LOAD = 20 psf				
			2 × 4	2 × 6	2 × 8	2 × 10	2 × 12	2 × 4	2 × 6	2 × 8	2 × 10	2 × 12
			(feet-inches)	(feet-inches)	(feet-inches)	(feet-inches)	(feet-inches)	(feet-inches)	(feet-inches)	(feet-inches)	(feet-inches)	(feet-inches)
24	Douglas fir-larch	SS	7-11	12-6	15-10	19-5	22-6	7-8	11-3	14-2	17-4	20-1
	Douglas fir-larch	#1	7-1	10-5	13-2	16-1	18-8	6-4	9-4	11-9	14-5	16-8
	Douglas fir-larch	#2	6-8	9-9	12-4	15-1	17-6	5-11	8-8	11-0	13-6	15-7
	Douglas fir-larch	#3	5-0	7-4	9-4	11-5	13-2	4-6	6-7	8-4	10-2	11-10
	Hem-fir	SS	7-6	11-10	15-7	19-1	22-1	7-6	11-0	13-11	17-0	19-9
	Hem-fir	#1	6-11	10-2	12-10	15-8	18-2	6-2	9-1	11-6	14-0	16-3
	Hem-fir	#2	6-7	9-7	12-2	14-10	17-3	5-10	8-7	10-10	13-3	15-5
	Hem-fir	#3	5-0	7-4	9-4	11-5	13-2	4-6	6-7	8-4	10-2	11-10
	Southern pine	SS	7-10	12-3	16-2	20-8	25-1	7-10	12-3	16-2	19-8	23-0
	Southern pine	#1	7-8	11-9	14-9	17-6	20-11	7-1	10-6	13-2	15-8	18-8
	Southern pine	#2	7-1	10-2	13-2	15-9	18-5	6-4	9-2	11-9	14-1	16-6
	Southern pine	#3	5-4	7-11	10-1	11-11	14-2	4-9	7-1	9-0	10-8	12-8
	Spruce-pine-fir	SS	7-4	11-7	14-9	18-0	20-11	7-1	10-5	13-2	16-1	18-8
	Spruce-pine-fir	#1	6-8	9-9	12-4	15-1	17-6	5-11	8-8	11-0	13-6	15-7
	Spruce-pine-fir	#2	6-8	9-9	12-4	15-1	17-6	5-11	8-8	11-0	13-6	15-7
	Spruce-pine-fir	#3	5-0	7-4	9-4	11-5	13-2	4-6	6-7	8-4	10-2	11-10

Check sources for availability of lumber in lengths greater than 20 feet.

For SI: 1 inch = 25.4 mm, 1 foot = 304.8 mm, 1 pound per square foot = 0.0479 kPa.

a. The tabulated rafter spans assume that ceiling joists are located at the bottom of the attic space or that some other method of resisting the outward push of the rafters on the bearing walls, such as rafter ties, is provided at that location. When ceiling joists or rafter ties are located higher in the attic space, the rafter spans shall be multiplied by the factors given below:

H_C/H_R	Rafter Span Adjustment Factor
1/3	0.67
1/4	0.76
1/5	0.83
1/6	0.90
1/7.5 or less	1.00

where:

H_C = Height of ceiling joists or rafter ties measured vertically above the top of the rafter support walls.

H_R = Height of roof ridge measured vertically above the top of the rafter support walls.

b. Span exceeds 26 feet in length.

TABLE R802.5.1(4)
RAFTER SPANS FOR COMMON LUMBER SPECIES
(Ground snow load=50 psf, ceiling not attached to rafters, L/Δ = 180)

RAFTER SPACING (inches)	SPECIES AND GRADE		DEAD LOAD = 10 psf					DEAD LOAD = 20 psf				
			2 × 4	2 × 6	2 × 8	2 × 10	2 × 12	2 × 4	2 × 6	2 × 8	2 × 10	2 × 12
			Maximum rafter spans[a]									
			(feet - inches)	(feet - inches)	(feet - inches)	(feet - inches)	(feet - inches)	(feet - inches)	(feet - inches)	(feet - inches)	(feet - inches)	(feet - inches)
12	Douglas fir-larch	SS	8-5	13-3	17-6	22-4	26-0	8-5	13-3	17-0	20-9	24-0
	Douglas fir-larch	#1	8-2	12-0	15-3	18-7	21-7	7-7	11-2	14-1	17-3	20-0
	Douglas fir-larch	#2	7-8	11-3	14-3	17-5	20-2	7-1	10-5	13-2	16-1	18-8
	Douglas fir-larch	#3	5-10	8-6	10-9	13-2	15-3	5-5	7-10	10-0	12-2	14-1
	Hem-fir	SS	8-0	12-6	16-6	21-1	25-6	8-0	12-6	16-6	20-4	23-7
	Hem-fir	#1	7-10	11-9	14-10	18-1	21-0	7-5	10-10	13-9	16-9	19-5
	Hem-fir	#2	7-5	11-1	14-0	17-2	19-11	7-0	10-3	13-0	15-10	18-5
	Hem-fir	#3	5-10	8-6	10-9	13-2	15-3	5-5	7-10	10-0	12-2	14-1
	Southern pine	SS	8-4	13-0	17-2	21-11	Note b	8-4	13-0	17-2	21-11	Note b
	Southern pine	#1	8-2	12-10	16-10	20-3	24-1	8-2	12-6	15-9	18-9	22-4
	Southern pine	#2	8-0	11-9	15-3	18-2	21-3	7-7	10-11	14-1	16-10	19-9
	Southern pine	#3	6-2	9-2	11-8	13-9	16-4	5-9	8-5	10-9	12-9	15-2
	Spruce-pine-fir	SS	7-10	12-3	16-2	20-8	24-1	7-10	12-3	15-9	19-3	22-4
	Spruce-pine-fir	#1	7-8	11-3	14-3	17-5	20-2	7-1	10-5	13-2	16-1	18-8
	Spruce-pine-fir	#2	7-8	11-3	14-3	17-5	20-2	7-1	10-5	13-2	16-1	18-8
	Spruce-pine-fir	#3	5-10	8-6	10-9	13-2	15-3	5-5	7-10	10-0	12-2	14-1
16	Douglas fir-larch	SS	7-8	12-1	15-10	19-5	22-6	7-8	11-7	14-8	17-11	20-10
	Douglas fir-larch	#1	7-1	10-5	13-2	16-1	18-8	6-7	9-8	12-2	14-11	17-3
	Douglas fir-larch	#2	6-8	9-9	12-4	15-1	17-6	6-2	9-0	11-5	13-11	16-2
	Douglas fir-larch	#3	5-0	7-4	9-4	11-5	13-2	4-8	6-10	8-8	10-6	12-3
	Hem-fir	SS	7-3	11-5	15-0	19-1	22-1	7-3	11-5	14-5	17-8	20-5
	Hem-fir	#1	6-11	10-2	12-10	15-8	18-2	6-5	9-5	11-11	14-6	16-10
	Hem-fir	#2	6-7	9-7	12-2	14-10	17-3	6-1	8-11	11-3	13-9	15-11
	Hem-fir	#3	5-0	7-4	9-4	11-5	13-2	4-8	6-10	8-8	10-6	12-3
	Southern pine	SS	7-6	11-10	15-7	19-11	24-3	7-6	11-10	15-7	19-11	23-10
	Southern pine	#1	7-5	11-7	14-9	17-6	20-11	7-4	10-10	13-8	16-2	19-4
	Southern pine	#2	7-1	10-2	13-2	15-9	18-5	6-7	9-5	12-2	14-7	17-1
	Southern pine	#3	5-4	7-11	10-1	11-11	14-2	4-11	7-4	9-4	11-0	13-1
	Spruce-pine-fir	SS	7-1	11-2	14-8	18-0	20-11	7-1	10-9	13-8	15-11	19-4
	Spruce-pine-fir	#1	6-8	9-9	12-4	15-1	17-6	6-2	9-0	11-5	13-11	16-2
	Spruce-pine-fir	#2	6-8	9-9	12-4	15-1	17-6	6-2	9-0	11-5	13-11	16-2
	Spruce-pine-fir	#3	5-0	7-4	9-4	11-5	13-2	4-8	6-10	8-8	10-6	12-3
19.2	Douglas fir-larch	SS	7-3	11-4	14-6	17-8	20-6	7-3	10-7	13-5	16-5	19-0
	Douglas fir-larch	#1	6-6	9-6	12-0	14-8	17-1	6-0	8-10	11-2	13-7	15-9
	Douglas fir-larch	#2	6-1	8-11	11-3	13-9	15-11	5-7	8-3	10-5	12-9	14-9
	Douglas fir-larch	#3	4-7	6-9	8-6	10-5	12-1	4-3	6-3	7-11	9-7	11-2
	Hem-fir	SS	6-10	10-9	14-2	17-5	20-2	6-10	10-5	13-2	16-1	18-8
	Hem-fir	#1	6-4	9-3	11-9	14-4	16-7	5-10	8-7	10-10	13-3	15-5
	Hem-fir	#2	6-0	8-9	11-1	13-7	15-9	5-7	8-1	10-3	12-7	14-7
	Hem-fir	#3	4-7	6-9	8-6	10-5	12-1	4-3	6-3	7-11	9-7	11-2
	Southern pine	SS	7-1	11-2	14-8	18-9	22-10	7-1	11-2	14-8	18 7	21-9
	Southern pine	#1	7-0	10-8	13-5	16-0	19-1	6-8	9-11	12-5	14-10	17-8
	Southern pine	#2	6-6	9-4	12-0	14-4	16-10	6-0	8-8	11-2	13-4	15-7
	Southern pine	#3	4-11	7-3	9-2	10-10	12-11	4-6	6-8	8-6	10-1	12-0
	Spruce-pine-fir	SS	6-8	10-6	13-5	16-5	19-1	6-8	9-10	12-5	15-3	17-8
	Spruce-pine-fir	#1	6-1	8-11	11-3	13-9	15-11	5-7	8-3	10-5	12-9	14-9
	Spruce-pine-fir	#2	6-1	8-11	11-3	13-9	15-11	5-7	8-3	10-5	12-9	14-9
	Spruce-pine-fir	#3	4-7	6-9	8-6	10-5	12-1	4-3	6-3	7-11	9-7	11-2

(continued)

TABLE R802.5.1(4)—continued
RAFTER SPANS FOR COMMON LUMBER SPECIES
(Ground snow load=50 psf, ceiling not attached to rafters, L/Δ = 180)

RAFTER SPACING (inches)	SPECIES AND GRADE		DEAD LOAD = 10 psf					DEAD LOAD = 20 psf				
			2 × 4	2 × 6	2 × 8	2 × 10	2 × 12	2 × 4	2 × 6	2 × 8	2 × 10	2 × 12
			Maximum rafter spans[a]									
			(feet - inches)	(feet - inches)	(feet - inches)	(feet - inches)	(feet - inches)	(feet - inches)	(feet - inches)	(feet - inches)	(feet - inches)	(feet - inches)
24	Douglas fir-larch	SS	6-8	10-	13-0	15-10	18-4	6-6	9-6	12-0	14-8	17-0
	Douglas fir-larch	#1	5-10	8-6	10-9	13-2	15-3	5-5	7-10	10-0	12-2	14-1
	Douglas fir-larch	#2	5-5	7-11	10-1	12-4	14-3	5-0	7-4	9-4	11-5	13-2
	Douglas fir-larch	#3	4-1	6-0	7-7	9-4	10-9	3-10	5-7	7-1	8-7	10-0
	Hem-fir	SS	6-4	9-11	12-9	15-7	18-0	6-4	9-4	11-9	14-5	16-8
	Hem-fir	#1	5-8	8-3	10-6	12-10	14-10	5-3	7-8	9-9	11-10	13-9
	Hem-fir	#2	5-4	7-10	9-11	12-1	14-1	4-11	7-3	9-2	11-3	13-0
	Hem-fir	#3	4-1	6-0	7-7	9-4	10-9	3-10	5-7	7-1	8-7	10-0
	Southern pine	SS	6-7	10-4	13-8	17-5	21-0	6-7	10-4	13-8	16-7	19-5
	Southern pine	#1	6-5	9-7	12-0	14-4	17-1	6-0	8-10	11-2	13-3	15-9
	Southern pine	#2	5-10	8-4	10-9	12-10	15-1	5-5	7-9	10-0	11-11	13-11
	Southern pine	#3	4-4	6-5	8-3	9-9	11-7	4-1	6-0	7-7	9-0	10-8
	Spruce-pine-fir	SS	6-2	9-6	12-0	14-8	17-1	6-0	8-10	11-2	13-7	15-9
	Spruce-pine-fir	#1	5-5	7-11	10-1	12-4	14-3	5-0	7-4	9-4	11-5	13-2
	Spruce-pine-fir	#2	5-5	7-11	10-1	12-4	14-3	5-0	7-4	9-4	11-5	13-2
	Spruce-pine-fir	#3	4-1	6-0	7-7	9-4	10-9	3-10	5-7	7-1	8-7	10-0

Check sources for availability of lumber in lengths greater than 20 feet.

For SI: 1 inch = 25.4 mm, 1 foot = 304.8 mm, 1 pound per square foot = 0.0479 kPa.

a. The tabulated rafter spans assume that ceiling joists are located at the bottom of the attic space or that some other method of resisting the outward push of the rafters on the bearing walls, such as rafter ties, is provided at that location. When ceiling joists or rafter ties are located higher in the attic space, the rafter spans shall be multiplied by the factors given below:

H_C/H_R	Rafter Span Adjustment Factor
1/3	0.67
1/4	0.76
1/5	0.83
1/6	0.90
1/7.5 or less	1.00

where:

H_C = Height of ceiling joists or rafter ties measured vertically above the top of the rafter support walls.

H_R = Height of roof ridge measured vertically above the top of the rafter support walls.

b. Span exceeds 26 feet in length.

TABLE R802.5.1(5)
RAFTER SPANS FOR COMMON LUMBER SPECIES
(Ground snow load=30 psf, ceiling attached to rafters, L/Δ = 240)

RAFTER SPACING (inches)	SPECIES AND GRADE		DEAD LOAD = 10 psf					DEAD LOAD = 20 psf				
			2 × 4	2 × 6	2 × 8	2 × 10	2 × 12	2 × 4	2 × 6	2 × 8	2 × 10	2 × 12
			Maximum rafter spans[a]									
			(feet - inches)	(feet - inches)	(feet - inches)	(feet - inches)	(feet - inches)	(feet - inches)	(feet - inches)	(feet - inches)	(feet - inches)	(feet - inches)
12	Douglas fir-larch	SS	9-1	14-4	18-10	24-1	Note b	9-1	14-4	18-10	24-1	Note b
	Douglas fir-larch	#1	8-9	13-9	18-2	22-9	Note b	8-9	13-2	16-8	20-4	23-7
	Douglas fir-larch	#2	8-7	13-6	17-5	21-4	24-8	8-5	12-4	15-7	19-1	22-1
	Douglas fir-larch	#3	7-1	10-5	13-2	16-1	18-8	6-4	9-4	11-9	14-5	16-8
	Hem-fir	SS	8-7	13-6	17-10	22-9	Note b	8-7	13-6	17-10	22-9	Note b
	Hem-fir	#1	8-5	13-3	17-5	22-2	25-9	8-5	12-10	16-3	19-10	23-0
	Hem-fir	#2	8-0	12-7	16-7	21-0	24-4	8-0	12-2	15-4	18-9	21-9
	Hem-fir	#3	7-1	10-5	13-2	16-1	18-8	6-4	9-4	11-9	14-5	16-8
	Southern pine	SS	8-11	14-1	18-6	23-8	Note b	8-11	14-1	18-6	23-8	Note b
	Southern pine	#1	8-9	13-9	18-2	23-2	Note b	8-9	13-9	18-2	22-2	Note b
	Southern pine	#2	8-7	13-6	17-10	22-3	Note b	8-7	12-11	16-8	19-11	23-4
	Southern pine	#3	7-7	11-2	14-3	16-10	20-0	6-9	10-0	12-9	15-1	17-11
	Spruce-pine-fir	SS	8-5	13-3	17-5	22-3	Note b	8-5	13-3	17-5	22-3	Note b
	Spruce-pine-fir	#1	8-3	12-11	17-0	21-4	24-8	8-3	12-4	15-7	19-1	22-1
	Spruce-pine-fir	#2	8-3	12-11	17-0	21-4	24-8	8-3	12-4	15-7	19-1	22-1
	Spruce-pine-fir	#3	7-1	10-5	13-2	16-1	18-8	6-4	9-4	11-9	14-5	16-8
16	Douglas fir-larch	SS	8-3	13-0	17-2	21-10	Note b	8-3	13-0	17-2	21-3	24-8
	Douglas fir-larch	#1	8-0	12-6	16-2	19-9	22-10	7-10	11-5	14-5	17-8	20-5
	Douglas fir-larch	#2	7-10	11-11	15-1	18-5	21-5	7-3	10-8	13-6	16-6	19-2
	Douglas fir-larch	#3	6-2	9-0	11-5	13-11	16-2	5-6	8-1	10-3	12-6	14-6
	Hem-fir	SS	7-10	12-3	16-2	20-8	25-1	7-10	12-3	16-2	20-8	24-2
	Hem-fir	#1	7-8	12-0	15-9	19-3	22-3	7-7	11-1	14-1	17-2	19-11
	Hem-fir	#2	7-3	11-5	14-11	18-2	21-1	7-2	10-6	13-4	16-3	18-10
	Hem-fir	#3	6-2	9-0	11-5	13-11	16-2	5-6	8-1	10-3	12-6	14-6
	Southern pine	SS	8-1	12-9	16-10	21-6	Note b	8-1	12-9	16-10	21-6	Note b
	Southern pine	#1	8-0	12-6	16-6	21-1	25-7	8-0	12-6	16-2	19-2	22-10
	Southern pine	#2	7-10	12-3	16-2	19-3	22-7	7-10	11-2	14-5	17-3	20-2
	Southern pine	#3	6-7	9-8	12-4	14-7	17-4	5-10	8-8	11-0	13-0	15-6
	Spruce-pine-fir	SS	7-8	12-0	15-10	20-2	24-7	7-8	12-0	15-10	19-9	22-10
	Spruce-pine-fir	#1	7-6	11-9	15-1	18-5	21-5	7-3	10-8	13-6	16-6	19-2
	Spruce-pine-fir	#2	7-6	11-9	15-1	18-5	21-5	7-3	10-8	13-6	16-6	19-2
	Spruce-pine-fir	#3	6-2	9-0	11-5	13-11	16-2	5-6	8-1	10-3	12-6	14-6
19.2	Douglas fir-larch	SS	7-9	12-3	16-1	20-7	25-0	7-9	12-3	15-10	19-5	22-6
	Douglas fir-larch	#1	7-6	11-8	14-9	18-0	20-11	7-1	10-5	13-2	16-1	18-8
	Douglas fir-larch	#2	7-4	10-11	13-9	16-10	19-6	6-8	9-9	12-4	15-1	17-6
	Douglas fir-larch	#3	5-7	8-3	10-5	12-9	14-9	5-0	7-4	9-4	11-5	13-2
	Hem-fir	SS	7-4	11-7	15-3	19-5	23-7	7-4	11-7	15-3	19-1	22-1
	Hem-fir	#1	7-2	11-4	14-4	17-7	20-4	6-11	10-2	12-10	15-8	18-2
	Hem-fir	#2	6-10	10-9	13-7	16-7	19-3	6-7	9-7	12-2	14-10	17-3
	Hem-fir	#3	5-7	8-3	10-5	12-9	14-9	5-0	7-4	9-4	11-5	13-2
	Southern pine	SS	7-8	12-0	15-10	20-2	24-7	7-8	12-0	15-10	20-2	24-7
	Southern pine	#1	7-6	11-9	15-6	19-7	23-4	7-6	11-9	14-9	17-6	20-11
	Southern pine	#2	7-4	11-5	14-9	17-7	20-7	7-1	10-2	13-2	15-9	18-5
	Southern pine	#3	6-0	8-10	11-3	13-4	15-10	5-4	7-11	10-1	11-11	14-2
	Spruce-pine-fir	SS	7-2	11-4	14-11	19-0	23-1	7-2	11-4	14-9	18-0	20-11
	Spruce-pine-fir	#1	7-0	10-11	13-9	16-10	19-6	6-8	9-9	12-4	15-1	17-6
	Spruce-pine-fir	#2	7-0	10-11	13-9	16-10	19-6	6-8	9-9	12-4	15-1	17-6
	Spruce-pine-fir	#3	5-7	8-3	10-5	12-9	14-9	5-0	7-4	9-4	11-5	13-2

(continued)

TABLE R802.5.1(5)—continued
RAFTER SPANS FOR COMMON LUMBER SPECIES
(Ground snow load=30 psf, ceiling attached to rafters, L/Δ = 240)

RAFTER SPACING (inches)	SPECIES AND GRADE		DEAD LOAD = 10 psf					DEAD LOAD = 20 psf				
			2 × 4	2 × 6	2 × 8	2 × 10	2 × 12	2 × 4	2 × 6	2 × 8	2 × 10	2 × 12
			Maximum rafter spans[a]									
			(feet-inches)	(feet-inches)	(feet-inches)	(feet-inches)	(feet-inches)	(feet-inches)	(feet-inches)	(feet-inches)	(feet-inches)	(feet-inches)
24	Douglas fir-larch	SS	7-3	11-4	15-0	19-1	22-6	7-3	11-3	14-2	17-4	20-1
	Douglas fir-larch	#1	7-0	10-5	13-2	16-1	18-8	6-4	9-4	11-9	14-5	16-8
	Douglas fir-larch	#2	6-8	9-9	12-4	15-1	17-6	5-11	8-8	11-0	13-6	15-7
	Douglas fir-larch	#3	5-0	7-4	9-4	11-5	13-2	4-6	6-7	8-4	10-2	11-10
	Hem-fir	SS	6-10	10-9	14-2	18-0	21-11	6-10	10-9	13-11	17-0	19-9
	Hem-fir	#1	6-8	10-2	12-10	15-8	18-2	6-2	9-1	11-6	14-0	16-3
	Hem-fir	#2	6-4	9-7	12-2	14-10	17-3	5-10	8-7	10-10	13-3	15-5
	Hem-fir	#3	5-0	7-4	9-4	11-5	13-2	4-6	6-7	8-4	10-2	11-10
	Southern pine	SS	7-1	11-2	14-8	18-9	22-10	7-1	11-2	14-8	18-9	22-10
	Southern pine	#1	7-0	10-11	14-5	17-6	20-11	7-0	10-6	13-2	15-8	18-8
	Southern pine	#2	6-10	10-2	13-2	15-9	18-5	6-4	9-2	11-9	14-1	16-6
	Southern pine	#3	5-4	7-11	10-1	11-11	14-2	4-9	7-1	9-0	10-8	12-8
	Spruce-pine-fir	SS	6-8	10-6	13-10	17-8	20-11	6-8	10-5	13-2	16-1	18-8
	Spruce-pine-fir	#1	6-6	9-9	12-4	15-1	17-6	5-11	8-8	11-0	13-6	15-7
	Spruce-pine-fir	#2	6-6	9-9	12-4	15-1	17-6	5-11	8-8	11-0	13-6	15-7
	Spruce-pine-fir	#3	5-0	7-4	9-4	11-5	13-2	4-6	6-7	8-4	10-2	11-10

Check sources for availability of lumber in lengths greater than 20 feet.

For SI: 1 inch = 25.4 mm, 1 foot = 304.8 mm, 1 pound per square foot = 0.0479 kPa.

a. The tabulated rafter spans assume that ceiling joists are located at the bottom of the attic space or that some other method of resisting the outward push of the rafters on the bearing walls, such as rafter ties, is provided at that location. When ceiling joists or rafter ties are located higher in the attic space, the rafter spans shall be multiplied by the factors given below:

H_C/H_R	Rafter Span Adjustment Factor
1/3	0.67
1/4	0.76
1/5	0.83
1/6	0.90
1/7.5 or less	1.00

where:

H_C = Height of ceiling joists or rafter ties measured vertically above the top of the rafter support walls.

H_R = Height of roof ridge measured vertically above the top of the rafter support walls.

b. Span exceeds 26 feet in length.

TABLE R802.5.1(6)
RAFTER SPANS FOR COMMON LUMBER SPECIES
(Ground snow load=50 psf, ceiling attached to rafters, L/Δ = 240)

RAFTER SPACING (inches)	SPECIES AND GRADE		DEAD LOAD = 10 psf					DEAD LOAD = 20 psf				
			2 × 4	2 × 6	2 × 8	2 × 10	2 × 12	2 × 4	2 × 6	2 × 8	2 × 10	2 × 12
			Maximum rafter spans[a]									
			(feet-inches)	(feet-inches)	(feet-inches)	(feet-inches)	(feet-inches)	(feet-inches)	(feet-inches)	(feet-inches)	(feet-inches)	(feet-inches)
12	Douglas fir-larch	SS	7-8	12-1	15-11	20-3	24-8	7-8	12-1	15-11	20-3	24-0
	Douglas fir-larch	#1	7-5	11-7	15-3	18-7	21-7	7-5	11-2	14-1	17-3	20-0
	Douglas fir-larch	#2	7-3	11-3	14-3	17-5	20-2	7-1	10-5	13-2	16-1	18-8
	Douglas fir-larch	#3	5-10	8-6	10-9	13-2	15-3	5-5	7-10	10-0	12-2	14-1
	Hem-fir	SS	7-3	11-5	15-0	19-2	23-4	7-3	11-5	15-0	19-2	23-4
	Hem-fir	#1	7-1	11-2	14-8	18-1	21-0	7-1	10-10	13-9	16-9	19-5
	Hem-fir	#2	6-9	10-8	14-0	17-2	19-11	6-9	10-3	13-0	15-10	18-5
	Hem-fir	#3	5-10	8-6	10-9	13-2	15-3	5-5	7-10	10-0	12-2	14-1
	Southern pine	SS	7-6	11-10	15-7	19-11	24-3	7-6	11-10	15-7	19-11	24-3
	Southern pine	#1	7-5	11-7	15-4	19-7	23-9	7-5	11-7	15-4	18-9	22-4
	Southern pine	#2	7-3	11-5	15-0	18-2	21-3	7-3	10-11	14-1	16-10	19-9
	Southern pine	#3	6-2	9-2	11-8	13-9	16-4	5-9	8-5	10-9	12-9	15-2
	Spruce-pine-fir	SS	7-1	11-2	14-8	18-9	22-10	7-1	11-2	14-8	18-9	22-4
	Spruce-pine-fir	#1	6-11	10-11	14-3	17-5	20-2	6-11	10-5	13-2	16-1	18-8
	Spruce-pine-fir	#2	6-11	10-11	14-3	17-5	20-2	6-11	10-5	13-2	16-1	18-8
	Spruce-pine-fir	#3	5-10	8-6	10-9	13-2	15-3	5-5	7-10	10-0	12-2	14-1
16	Douglas fir-larch	SS	7-0	11-0	14-5	18-5	22-5	7-0	11-0	14-5	17-11	20-10
	Douglas fir-larch	#1	6-9	10-5	13-2	16-1	18-8	6-7	9-8	12-2	14-11	17-3
	Douglas fir-larch	#2	6-7	9-9	12-4	15-1	17-6	6-2	9-0	11-5	13-11	16-2
	Douglas fir-larch	#3	5-0	7-4	9-4	11-5	13-2	4-8	6-10	8-8	10-6	12-3
	Hem-fir	SS	6-7	10-4	13-8	17-5	21-2	6-7	10-4	13-8	17-5	20-5
	Hem-fir	#1	6-5	10-2	12-10	15-8	18-2	6-5	9-5	11-11	14-6	16-10
	Hem-fir	#2	6-2	9-7	12-2	14-10	17-3	6-1	8-11	11-3	13-9	15-11
	Hem-fir	#3	5-0	7-4	9-4	11-5	13-2	4-8	6-10	8-8	10-6	12-3
	Southern pine	SS	6-10	10-9	14-2	18-1	22-0	6-10	10-9	14-2	18-1	22-0
	Southern pine	#1	6-9	10-7	13-11	17-6	20-11	6-9	10-7	13-8	16-2	19-4
	Southern pine	#2	6-7	10-2	13-2	15-9	18-5	6-7	9-5	12-2	14-7	17-1
	Southern pine	#3	5-4	7-11	10-1	11-11	14-2	4-11	7-4	9-4	11-0	13-1
	Spruce-pine-fir	SS	6-5	10-2	13-4	17-0	20-9	6-5	10-2	13-4	16-8	19-4
	Spruce-pine-fir	#1	6-4	9-9	12-4	15-1	17-6	6-2	9-0	11-5	13-11	16-2
	Spruce-pine-fir	#2	6-4	9-9	12-4	15-1	17-6	6-2	9-0	11-5	13-11	16-2
	Spruce-pine-fir	#3	5-0	7-4	9-4	11-5	13-2	4-8	6-10	8-8	10-6	12-3
19.2	Douglas fir-larch	SS	6-7	10-4	13-7	17-4	20-6	6-7	10-4	13-5	16-5	19-0
	Douglas fir-larch	#1	6-4	9-6	12-0	14-8	17-1	6-0	8-10	11-2	13-7	15-9
	Douglas fir-larch	#2	6-1	8-11	11-3	13-9	15-11	5-7	8-3	10-5	12-9	14-9
	Douglas fir-larch	#3	4-7	6-9	8-6	10-5	12-1	4-3	6-3	7-11	9-7	11-2
	Hem-fir	SS	6-2	9-9	12-10	16-5	19-11	6-2	9-9	12-10	16-1	18-8
	Hem-fir	#1	6-1	9-3	11-9	14-4	16-7	5-10	8-7	10-10	13-3	15-5
	Hem-fir	#2	5-9	8-9	11-1	13-7	15-9	5-7	8-1	10-3	12-7	14-7
	Hem-fir	#3	4-7	6-9	8-6	10-5	12-1	4-3	6-3	7-11	9-7	11-2
	Southern pine	SS	6-5	10-2	13-4	17-0	20-9	6-5	10-2	13-4	17-0	20-9
	Southern pine	#1	6-4	9-11	13-1	16-0	19-1	6-4	9-11	12-5	14-10	17-8
	Southern pine	#2	6-2	9-4	12-0	14-4	16-10	6-0	8-8	11-2	13-4	15-7
	Southern pine	#3	4-11	7-3	9-2	10-10	12-11	4-6	6-8	8-6	10-1	12-0
	Spruce-pine-fir	SS	6-1	9-6	12-7	16-0	19-1	6-1	9-6	12-5	15-3	17-8
	Spruce-pine-fir	#1	5-11	8-11	11-3	13-9	15-11	5-7	8-3	10-5	12-9	14-9
	Spruce-pine-fir	#2	5-11	8-11	11-3	13-9	15-11	5-7	8-3	10-5	12-9	14-9
	Spruce-pine-fir	#3	4-7	6-9	8-6	10-5	12-1	4-3	6-3	7-11	9-7	11-2

(continued)

TABLE R802.5.1(6)—continued
RAFTER SPANS FOR COMMON LUMBER SPECIES
(Ground snow load=50 psf, ceiling attached to rafters, L/Δ = 240)

RAFTER SPACING (inches)	SPECIES AND GRADE		DEAD LOAD = 10 psf					DEAD LOAD = 20 psf				
			2 × 4	2 × 6	2 × 8	2 × 10	2 × 12	2 × 4	2 × 6	2 × 8	2 × 10	2 × 12
			Maximum rafter spans[a]									
			(feet-inches)	(feet-inches)	(feet-inches)	(feet-inches)	(feet-inches)	(feet-inches)	(feet-inches)	(feet-inches)	(feet-inches)	(feet-inches)
24	Douglas fir-larch	SS	6-1	9-7	12-7	15-10	18-4	6-1	9-6	12-0	14-8	17-0
	Douglas fir-larch	#1	5-10	8-6	10-9	13-2	15-3	5-5	7-10	10-0	12-2	14-1
	Douglas fir-larch	#2	5-5	7-11	10-1	12-4	14-3	5-0	7-4	9-4	11-5	13-2
	Douglas fir-larch	#3	4-1	6-0	7-7	9-4	10-9	3-10	5-7	7-1	8-7	10-0
	Hem-fir	SS	5-9	9-1	11-11	15-2	18-0	5-9	9-1	11-9	14-5	15-11
	Hem-fir	#1	5-8	8-3	10-6	12-10	14-10	5-3	7-8	9-9	11-10	13-9
	Hem-fir	#2	5-4	7-10	9-11	12-1	14-1	4-11	7-3	9-2	11-3	13-0
	Hem-fir	#3	4-1	6-0	7-7	9-4	10-9	3-10	5-7	7-1	8-7	10-0
	Southern pine	SS	6-0	9-5	12-5	15-10	19-3	6-0	9-5	12-5	15-10	19-3
	Southern pine	#1	5-10	9-3	12-0	14-4	17-1	5-10	8-10	11-2	13-3	15-9
	Southern pine	#2	5-9	8-4	10-9	12-10	15-1	5-5	7-9	10-0	11-11	13-11
	Southern pine	#3	4-4	6-5	8-3	9-9	11-7	4-1	6-0	7-7	9-0	10-8
	Spruce-pine-fir	SS	5-8	8-10	11-8	14-8	17-1	5-8	8-10	11-2	13-7	15-9
	Spruce-pine-fir	#1	5-5	7-11	10-1	12-4	14-3	5-0	7-4	9-4	11-5	13-2
	Spruce-pine-fir	#2	5-5	7-11	10-1	12-4	14-3	5-0	7-4	9-4	11-5	13-2
	Spruce-pine-fir	#3	4-1	6-0	7-7	9-4	10-9	3-10	5-7	7-1	8-7	10-0

Check sources for availability of lumber in lengths greater than 20 feet.

For SI: 1 inch = 25.4 mm, 1 foot = 304.8 mm, 1 pound per square foot = 0.0479 kPa.

a. The tabulated rafter spans assume that ceiling joists are located at the bottom of the attic space or that some other method of resisting the outward push of the rafters on the bearing walls, such as rafter ties, is provided at that location. When ceiling joists or rafter ties are located higher in the attic space, the rafter spans shall be multiplied by the factors given below:

H_C/H_R	Rafter Span Adjustment Factor
1/3	0.67
1/4	0.76
1/5	0.83
1/6	0.90
1/7.5 or less	1.00

where:

H_C = Height of ceiling joists or rafter ties measured vertically above the top of the rafter support walls.

H_R = Height of roof ridge measured vertically above the top of the rafter support walls.

TABLE R802.5.1(7)
RAFTER SPANS FOR 70 PSF GROUND SNOW LOAD
(Ceiling not attached to rafters, L/Δ = 180)

RAFTER SPACING (inches)	SPECIES AND GRADE		DEAD LOAD = 10 psf					DEAD LOAD = 20 psf				
			2 × 4	2 × 6	2 × 8	2 × 10	2 × 12	2 × 4	2 × 6	2 × 8	2 × 10	2 × 12
			Maximum Rafter Spans[a]									
			(feet-inches)	(feet-inches)	(feet-inches)	(feet-inches)	(feet-inches)	(feet-inches)	(feet-inches)	(feet-inches)	(feet-inches)	(feet-inches)
12	Douglas fir-larch	SS	7-7	11-10	15-8	19-5	22-6	7-7	11-10	15-0	18-3	21-2
	Douglas fir-larch	#1	7-1	10-5	13-2	16-1	18-8	6-8	9-10	12-5	15-2	17-7
	Douglas fir-larch	#2	6-8	9-9	12-4	15-1	17-6	6-3	9-2	11-8	14-2	16-6
	Douglas fir-larch	#3	5-0	7-4	9-4	11-5	13-2	4-9	6-11	8-9	10-9	12-5
	Hem-fir	SS	7-2	11-3	14-9	18-10	22-1	7-2	11-3	14-8	18-0	20-10
	Hem-fir	#1	6-11	10-2	12-10	15-8	18-2	6-6	9-7	12-1	14-10	17-2
	Hem-fir	#2	6-7	9-7	12-2	14-10	17-3	6-2	9-1	11-5	14-0	16-3
	Hem-fir	#3	5-0	7-4	9-4	11-5	13-2	4-9	6-11	8-9	10-9	12-5
	Southern pine	SS	7-5	11-8	15-4	19-7	23-10	7-5	11-8	15-4	19-7	23-10
	Southern pine	#1	7-3	11-5	14-9	17-6	20-11	7-3	11-1	13-11	16-6	19-8
	Southern pine	#2	7-1	10-2	13-2	15-9	18-5	6-8	9-7	12-5	14-10	17-5
	Southern pine	#3	5-4	7-11	10-1	11-11	14-2	5-1	7-5	9-6	11-3	13-4
	Spruce-pine-fir	SS	7-0	11-0	14-6	18-0	20-11	7-0	11-0	13-11	17-0	19-8
	Spruce-pine-fir	#1	6-8	9-9	12-4	15-1	17-6	6-3	9-2	11-8	14-2	16-6
	Spruce-pine-fir	#2	6-8	9-9	12-4	15-1	17-6	6-3	9-2	11-8	14-2	16-6
	Spruce-pine-fir	#3	5-0	7-4	9-4	11-5	13-2	4-9	6-11	8-9	10-9	12-5
16	Douglas fir-larch	SS	6-10	10-9	13-9	16-10	19-6	6-10	10-3	13-0	15-10	18-4
	Douglas fir-larch	#1	6-2	9-0	11-5	13-11	16-2	5-10	8-6	10-9	13-2	15-3
	Douglas fir-larch	#2	5-9	8-5	10-8	13-1	15-2	5-5	7-11	10-1	12-4	14-3
	Douglas fir-larch	#3	4-4	6-4	8-1	9-10	11-5	4-1	6-0	7-7	9-4	10-9
	Hem-fir	SS	6-6	10-2	13-5	16-6	19-2	6-6	10-1	12-9	15-7	18-0
	Hem-fir	#1	6-0	8-9	11-2	13-7	15-9	5-8	8-3	10-6	12-10	14-10
	Hem-fir	#2	5-8	8-4	10-6	12-10	14-11	5-4	7-10	9-11	12-1	14-1
	Hem-fir	#3	4-4	6-4	8-1	9-10	11-5	4-1	6-0	7-7	9-4	10-9
	Southern pine	SS	6-9	10-7	14-0	17-10	21-8	6-9	10-7	14-0	17-10	21-0
	Southern pine	#1	6-7	10-2	12-9	15-2	18-1	6-5	9-7	12-0	14-4	17-1
	Southern pine	#2	6-2	8-10	11-5	13-7	16-0	5-10	8-4	10-9	12-10	15-1
	Southern pine	#3	4-8	6-10	8-9	10-4	12-3	4-4	6-5	8-3	9-9	11-7
	Spruce-pine-fir	SS	6-4	10-0	12-9	15-7	18-1	6-4	9-6	12-0	14-8	17-1
	Spruce-pine-fir	#1	5-9	8-5	10-8	13-1	15-2	5-5	7-11	10-1	12-4	14-3
	Spruce-pine-fir	#2	5-9	8-5	10-8	13-1	15-2	5-5	7-11	10-1	12-4	14-3
	Spruce-pine-fir	#3	4-4	6-4	8-1	9-10	11-5	4-1	6-0	7-7	9-4	10-9
19.2	Douglas fir-larch	SS	6-5	9-11	12-7	15-4	17-9	6-5	9-4	11-10	14-5	16-9
	Douglas fir-larch	#1	5-7	8-3	10-5	12-9	14-9	5-4	7-9	9-10	12-0	13-11
	Douglas fir-larch	#2	5-3	7-8	9-9	11-11	13-10	5-0	7-3	9-2	11-3	13-0
	Douglas fir-larch	#3	4-0	5-10	7-4	9-0	10-5	3-9	5-6	6-11	8-6	9-10
	Hem-fir	SS	6-1	9-7	12-4	15-1	17-4	6-1	9-2	11-8	14-2	15-5
	Hem-fir	#1	5-6	8-0	10-2	12-5	14-5	5-2	7-7	9-7	11-8	13-7
	Hem-fir	#2	5-2	7-7	9-7	11-9	13-7	4-11	7-2	9-1	11-1	12-10
	Hem-fir	#3	4-0	5-10	7-4	9-0	10-5	3-9	5-6	6-11	8-6	9-10
	Southern pine	SS	6-4	10-0	13-2	16-9	20-4	6-4	10-0	13-2	16-5	19-2
	Southern pine	#1	6-3	9-3	11-8	13-10	16-6	5-11	8-9	11-0	13-1	15-7
	Southern pine	#2	5-7	8-1	10-5	12-5	14-7	5-4	7-7	9-10	11-9	13-9
	Southern pine	#3	4-3	6-3	8-0	9-5	11-2	4-0	5-11	7-6	8-10	10-7
	Spruce-pine-fir	SS	6-0	9-2	11-8	14-3	16-6	5-11	8-8	11-0	13-5	15-7
	Spruce-pine-fir	#1	5-3	7-8	9-9	11-11	13-10	5-0	7-3	9-2	11-3	13-0
	Spruce-pine-fir	#2	5-3	7-8	9-9	11-11	13-10	5-0	7-3	9-2	11-3	13-0
	Spruce-pine-fir	#3	4-0	5-10	7-4	9-0	10-5	3-9	5-6	6-11	8-6	9-10

(continued)

TABLE R802.5.1(7)—continued
RAFTER SPANS FOR 70 PSF GROUND SNOW LOAD
(Ceiling not attached to rafters, L/Δ = 180)

RAFTER SPACING (inches)	SPECIES AND GRADE		DEAD LOAD = 10 psf					DEAD LOAD = 20 psf				
			2 × 4	2 × 6	2 × 8	2 × 10	2 × 12	2 × 4	2 × 6	2 × 8	2 × 10	2 × 12
			Maximum rafter spans[a]									
			(feet-inches)	(feet-inches)	(feet-inches)	(feet-inches)	(feet-inches)	(feet-inches)	(feet-inches)	(feet-inches)	(feet-inches)	(feet-inches)
24	Douglas fir-larch	SS	6-0	8-10	11-3	13-9	15-11	5-9	8-4	10-7	12-11	15-0
	Douglas fir-larch	#1	5-0	7-4	9-4	11-5	13-2	4-9	6-11	8-9	10-9	12-5
	Douglas fir-larch	#2	4-8	6-11	8-9	10-8	12-4	4-5	6-6	8-3	10-0	11-8
	Douglas fir-larch	#3	3-7	5-2	6-7	8-1	9-4	3-4	4-11	6-3	7-7	8-10
	Hem-fir	SS	5-8	8-8	11-0	13-6	13-11	5-7	8-3	10-5	12-4	12-4
	Hem-fir	#1	4-11	7-2	9-1	11-1	12-10	4-7	6-9	8-7	10-6	12-2
	Hem-fir	#2	4-8	6-9	8-7	10-6	12-2	4-4	6-5	8-1	9-11	11-6
	Hem-fir	#3	3-7	5-2	6-7	8-1	9-4	3-4	4-11	6-3	7-7	8-10
	Southern pine	SS	5-11	9-3	12-2	15-7	18-2	5-11	9-3	12-2	14-8	17-2
	Southern pine	#1	5-7	8-3	10-5	12-5	14-9	5-3	7-10	9-10	11-8	13-11
	Southern pine	#2	5-0	7-3	9-4	11-1	13-0	4-9	6-10	8-9	10-6	12-4
	Southern pine	#3	3-9	5-7	7-1	8-5	10-0	3-7	5-3	6-9	7-11	9-5
	Spruce-pine-fir	SS	5-6	8-3	10-5	12-9	14-9	5-4	7-9	9-10	12-0	12-11
	Spruce-pine-fir	#1	4-8	6-11	8-9	10-8	12-4	4-5	6-6	8-3	10-0	11-8
	Spruce-pine-fir	#2	4-8	6-11	8-9	10-8	12-4	4-5	6-6	8-3	10-0	11-8
	Spruce-pine-fir	#3	3-7	5-2	6-7	8-1	9-4	3-4	4-11	6-3	7-7	8-10

Check sources for availability of lumber in lengths greater than 20 feet.

For SI: 1 inch = 25.4 mm, 1 foot = 304.8 mm, 1 pound per square foot = 0.0479 kPa.

a. The tabulated rafter spans assume that ceiling joists are located at the bottom of the attic space or that some other method of resisting the outward push of the rafters on the bearing walls, such as rafter ties, is provided at that location. When ceiling joists or rafter ties are located higher in the attic space, the rafter spans shall be multiplied by the factors given below:

H_C/H_R	Rafter Span Adjustment Factor
1/3	0.67
1/4	0.76
1/5	0.83
1/6	0.90
1/7.5 or less	1.00

where:

H_C = Height of ceiling joists or rafter ties measured vertically above the top of the rafter support walls.

H_R = Height of roof ridge measured vertically above the top of the rafter support walls.

TABLE R802.5.1(8)
RAFTER SPANS FOR 70 PSF GROUND SNOW LOAD
(Ceiling attached to rafters, L/Δ = 240)

RAFTER SPACING (inches)	SPECIES AND GRADE		DEAD LOAD = 10 psf					DEAD LOAD = 20 psf				
			2 × 4	2 × 6	2 × 8	2 × 10	2 × 12	2 × 4	2 × 6	2 × 8	2 × 10	2 × 12
			Maximum rafter spans[a]									
			(feet - inches)	(feet - inches)	(feet - inches)	(feet - inches)	(feet - inches)	(feet - inches)	(feet - inches)	(feet - inches)	(feet - inches)	(feet - inches)
12	Douglas fir-larch	SS	6-10	10-9	14-3	18-2	22-1	6-10	10-9	14-3	18-2	21-2
	Douglas fir-larch	#1	6-7	10-5	13-2	16-1	18-8	6-7	9-10	12-5	15-2	17-7
	Douglas fir-larch	#2	6-6	9-9	12-4	15-1	17-6	6-3	9-2	11-8	14-2	16-6
	Douglas fir-larch	#3	5-0	7-4	9-4	11-5	13-2	4-9	6-11	8-9	10-9	12-5
	Hem-fir	SS	6-6	10-2	13-5	17-2	20-10	6-6	10-2	13-5	17-2	20-10
	Hem-fir	#1	6-4	10-0	12-10	15-8	18-2	6-4	9-7	12-1	14-10	17-2
	Hem-fir	#2	6-1	9-6	12-2	14-10	17-3	6-1	9-1	11-5	14-0	16-3
	Hem-fir	#3	5-0	7-4	9-4	11-5	13-2	4-9	6-11	8-9	10-9	12-5
	Southern pine	SS	6-9	10-7	14-0	17-10	21-8	6-9	10-7	14-0	17-10	21-8
	Southern pine	#1	6-7	10-5	13-8	17-6	20-11	6-7	10-5	13-8	16-6	19-8
	Southern pine	#2	6-6	10-2	13-2	15-9	18-5	6-6	9-7	12-5	14-10	17-5
	Southern pine	#3	5-4	7-11	10-1	11-11	14-2	5-1	7-5	9-6	11-3	13-4
	Spruce-pine-fir	SS	6-4	10-0	13-2	16-9	20-5	6-4	10-0	13-2	16-9	19-8
	Spruce-pine-fir	#1	6-2	9-9	12-4	15-1	17-6	6-2	9-2	11-8	14-2	16-6
	Spruce-pine-fir	#2	6-2	9-9	12-4	15-1	17-6	6-2	9-2	11-8	14-2	16-6
	Spruce-pine-fir	#3	5-0	7-4	9-4	11-5	13-2	4-9	6-11	8-9	10-9	12-5
16	Douglas fir-larch	SS	6-3	9-10	12-11	16-6	19-6	6-3	9-10	12-11	15-10	18-4
	Douglas fir-larch	#1	6-0	9-0	11-5	13-11	16-2	5-10	8-6	10-9	13-2	15-3
	Douglas fir-larch	#2	5-9	8-5	10-8	13-1	15-2	5-5	7-11	10-1	12-4	14-3
	Douglas fir-larch	#3	4-4	6-4	8-1	9-10	11-5	4-1	6-0	7-7	9-4	10-9
	Hem-fir	SS	5-11	9-3	12-2	15-7	18-11	5-11	9-3	12-2	15-7	18-0
	Hem-fir	#1	5-9	8-9	11-2	13-7	15-9	5-8	8-3	10-6	12-10	14-10
	Hem-fir	#2	5-6	8-4	10-6	12-10	14-11	5-4	7-10	9-11	12-1	14-1
	Hem-fir	#3	4-4	6-4	8-1	9-10	11-5	4-1	6-0	7-7	9-4	10-9
	Southern pine	SS	6-1	9-7	12-8	16-2	19-8	6-1	9-7	12-8	16-2	19-8
	Southern pine	#1	6-0	9-5	12-5	15-2	18-1	6-0	9-5	12-0	14-4	17-1
	Southern pine	#2	5-11	8-10	11-5	13-7	16-0	5-10	8-4	10-9	12-10	15-1
	Southern pine	#3	4-8	6-10	8-9	10-4	12-3	4-4	6-5	8-3	9-9	11-7
	Spruce-pine-fir	SS	5-9	9-1	11-11	15-3	18-1	5-9	9-1	11-11	14-8	17-1
	Spruce-pine-fir	#1	5-8	8-5	10-8	13-1	15-2	5-5	7-11	10-1	12-4	14-3
	Spruce-pine-fir	#2	5-8	8-5	10-8	13-1	15-2	5-5	7-11	10-1	12-4	14-3
	Spruce-pine-fir	#3	4-4	6-4	8-1	9-10	11-5	4-1	6-0	7-7	9-4	10-9
19.2	Douglas fir-larch	SS	5-10	9-3	12-2	15-4	17-9	5-10	9-3	11-10	14-5	16-9
	Douglas fir-larch	#1	5-7	8-3	10-5	12-9	14-9	5-4	7-9	9-10	12-0	13-11
	Douglas fir-larch	#2	5-3	7-8	9-9	11-11	13-10	5-0	7-3	9-2	11-3	13-0
	Douglas fir-larch	#3	4-0	5-10	7-4	9-0	10-5	3-9	5-6	6-11	8-6	9-10
	Hem-fir	SS	5-6	8-8	11-6	14-8	17-4	5-6	8-8	11-6	14-2	15-5
	Hem-fir	#1	5-5	8-0	10-2	12-5	14-5	5-2	7-7	9-7	11-8	13-7
	Hem-fir	#2	5-2	7-7	9-7	11-9	13-7	4-11	7-2	9-1	11-1	12-10
	Hem-fir	#3	4-0	5-10	7-4	9-0	10-5	3-9	5-6	6-11	8-6	9-10
	Southern pine	SS	5-9	9-1	11-11	15-3	18-6	5-9	9-1	11-11	15-3	18-6
	Southern pine	#1	5-8	8-11	11-8	13-10	16-6	5-8	8-9	11-0	13-1	15-7
	Southern pine	#2	5-6	8-1	10-5	12-5	14-7	5-4	7-7	9-10	11-9	13-9
	Southern pine	#3	4-3	6-3	8-0	9-5	11-2	4-0	5-11	7-6	8-10	10-7
	Spruce-pine-fir	SS	5-5	8-6	11-3	14-3	16-6	5-5	8-6	11-0	13-5	15-7
	Spruce-pine-fir	#1	5-3	7-8	9-9	11-11	13-10	5-0	7-3	9-2	11-3	13-0
	Spruce-pine-fir	#2	5-3	7-8	9-9	11-11	13-10	5-0	7-3	9-2	11-3	13-0
	Spruce-pine-fir	#3	4-0	5-10	7-4	9-0	10-5	3-9	5-6	6-11	8-6	9-10

(continued)

TABLE R802.5.1(8)—continued
RAFTER SPANS FOR 70 PSF GROUND SNOW LOAD[a]
(Ceiling attached to rafters, L/Δ = 240)

RAFTER SPACING (inches)	SPECIES AND GRADE		DEAD LOAD = 10 psf					DEAD LOAD = 20 psf				
			2 × 4	2 × 6	2 × 8	2 × 10	2 × 12	2 × 4	2 × 6	2 × 8	2 × 10	2 × 12
			Maximum rafter spans[a]									
			(feet - inches)	(feet - inches)	(feet - inches)	(feet - inches)	(feet - inches)	(feet - inches)	(feet - inches)	(feet - inches)	(feet - inches)	(feet - inches)
24	Douglas fir-larch	SS	5-5	8-7	11-3	13-9	15-11	5-5	8-4	10-7	12-11	15-0
	Douglas fir-larch	#1	5-0	7-4	9-4	11-5	13-2	4-9	6-11	8-9	10-9	12-5
	Douglas fir-larch	#2	4-8	6-11	8-9	10-8	12-4	4-5	6-6	8-3	10-0	11-8
	Douglas fir-larch	#3	3-7	5-2	6-7	8-1	9-4	3-4	4-11	6-3	7-7	8-10
	Hem-fir	SS	5-2	8-1	10-8	13-6	13-11	5-2	8-1	10-5	12-4	12-4
	Hem-fir	#1	4-11	7-2	9-1	11-1	12-10	4-7	6-9	8-7	10-6	12-2
	Hem-fir	#2	4-8	6-9	8-7	10-6	12-2	4-4	6-5	8-1	9-11	11-6
	Hem-fir	#3	3-7	5-2	6-7	8-1	9-4	3-4	4-11	6-3	7-7	8-10
	Southern pine	SS	5-4	8-5	11-1	14-2	17-2	5-4	8-5	11-1	14-2	17-2
	Southern pine	#1	5-3	8-3	10-5	12-5	14-9	5-3	7-10	9-10	11-8	13-11
	Southern pine	#2	5-0	7-3	9-4	11-1	13-0	4-9	6-10	8-9	10-6	12-4
	Southern pine	#3	3-9	5-7	7-1	8-5	10-0	3-7	5-3	6-9	7-11	9-5
	Spruce-pine-fir	SS	5-0	7-11	10-5	12-9	14-9	5-0	7-9	9-10	12-0	12-11
	Spruce-pine-fir	#1	4-8	6-11	8-9	10-8	12-4	4-5	6-6	8-3	10-0	11-8
	Spruce-pine-fir	#2	4-8	6-11	8-9	10-8	12-4	4-5	6-6	8-3	10-0	11-8
	Spruce-pine-fir	#3	3-7	5-2	6-7	8-1	9-4	3-4	4-11	6-3	7-7	8-10

Check sources for availability of lumber in lengths greater than 20 feet.

For SI: 1 inch = 25.4 mm, 1 foot = 304.8 mm, 1 pound per square foot = 0.0479 kPa.

a. The tabulated rafter spans assume that ceiling joists are located at the bottom of the attic space or that some other method of resisting the outward push of the rafters on the bearing walls, such as rafter ties, is provided at that location. When ceiling joists or rafter ties are located higher in the attic space, the rafter spans shall be multiplied by the factors given below:

H_C/H_R	Rafter Span Adjustment Factor
1/3	0.67
1/4	0.76
1/5	0.83
1/6	0.90
1/7.5 or less	1.00

where:

H_C = Height of ceiling joists or rafter ties measured vertically above the top of the rafter support walls.

H_R = Height of roof ridge measured vertically above the top of the rafter support walls.

TABLE R802.5.1(9)
RAFTER/CEILING JOIST HEEL JOINT CONNECTIONS[a, b, c, d, e, f, h]

RAFTER SLOPE	RAFTER SPACING (inches)	GROUND SNOW LOAD (psf)															
		20[g]				30				50				70			
		Roof span (feet)															
		12	20	28	36	12	20	28	36	12	20	28	36	12	20	28	36
		Required number of 16d common nails[a, b] per heel joint splices[c, d, e, f]															
3:12	12	4	6	8	10	4	6	8	11	5	8	12	15	6	11	15	20
	16	5	8	10	13	5	8	11	14	6	11	15	20	8	14	20	26
	24	7	11	15	19	7	11	16	21	9	16	23	30	12	21	30	39
4:12	12	3	5	6	8	3	5	6	8	4	6	9	11	5	8	12	15
	16	4	6	8	10	4	6	8	11	5	8	12	15	6	11	15	20
	24	5	8	12	15	5	9	12	16	7	12	17	22	9	16	23	29
5:12	12	3	4	5	6	3	4	5	7	3	5	7	9	4	7	9	12
	16	3	5	6	8	3	5	7	9	4	7	9	12	5	9	12	16
	24	4	7	9	12	4	7	10	13	6	10	14	18	7	13	18	23
7:12	12	3	4	4	5	3	3	4	5	3	4	5	7	3	5	7	9
	16	3	4	5	6	3	4	5	6	3	5	7	9	4	6	9	11
	24	3	5	7	9	3	5	7	9	4	7	10	13	5	9	13	17
9:12	12	3	3	4	4	3	3	3	4	3	3	4	5	3	4	5	7
	16	3	4	4	5	3	3	4	5	3	4	5	7	3	5	7	9
	24	3	4	6	7	3	4	6	7	3	6	8	10	4	7	10	13
12:12	12	3	3	3	3	3	3	3	3	3	3	3	4	3	3	4	5
	16	3	3	4	4	3	3	3	4	3	3	4	5	3	4	5	7
	24	3	4	4	5	3	3	4	6	3	4	6	8	3	6	8	10

For SI: 1 inch = 25.4 mm, 1 foot = 304.8 mm, 1 pound per square foot = 0.0479 kPa.

a. 40d box nails shall be permitted to be substituted for 16d common nails.

b. Nailing requirements shall be permitted to be reduced 25 percent if nails are clinched.

c. Heel joint connections are not required when the ridge is supported by a load-bearing wall, header or ridge beam.

d. When intermediate support of the rafter is provided by vertical struts or purlins to a loadbearing wall, the tabulated heel joint connection requirements shall be permitted to be reduced proportionally to the reduction in span.

e. Equivalent nailing patterns are required for ceiling joist to ceiling joist lap splices.

f. When rafter ties are substituted for ceiling joists, the heel joint connection requirement shall be taken as the tabulated heel joint connection requirement for two-thirds of the actual rafter-slope.

g. Applies to roof live load of 20 psf or less.

h. Tabulated heel joint connection requirements assume that ceiling joists or rafter ties are located at the bottom of the attic space. When ceiling joists or rafter ties are located higher in the attic, heel joint connection requirements shall be increased by the following factors:

H_C/H_R	Heel Joint Connection Adjustment Factor
1/3	1.5
1/4	1.33
1/5	1.25
1/6	1.2
1/10 or less	1.11

where:

H_C = Height of ceiling joists or rafter ties measured vertically above the top of the rafter support walls.

H_R = Height of roof ridge measured vertically above the top of the rafter support walls.

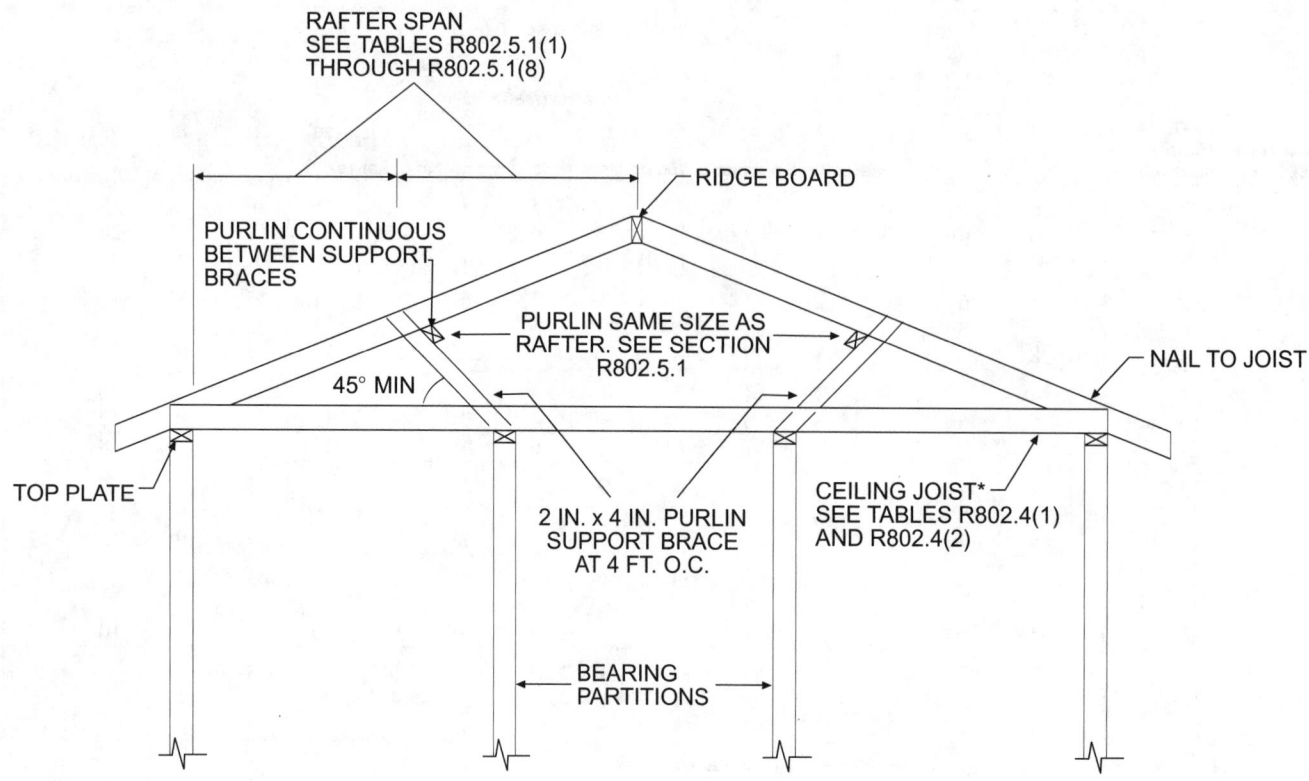

For SI: 1 inch = 25.4 mm, 1 foot = 305 mm, 1 degree = 0.018 rad.

Note: Where ceiling joints run perpendicular to the rafters, rafter ties shall be nailed to each rafter near the top of the ceiling joist.

FIGURE R802.5.1
BRACED RAFTER CONSTRUCTION

TABLE R802.11
REQUIRED STRENGTH OF TRUSS OR RAFTER CONNECTIONS TO RESIST WIND UPLIFT FORCES[a, b, c, e, f]
(Pounds per connection)

BASIC WIND SPEED (mph) (3–second gust)	ROOF SPAN (feet)							OVERHANGS[d] (pounds/foot)
	12	20	24	28	32	36	40	
85	-72	-120	-145	-169	-193	-217	-241	-38.55
90	-91	-151	-181	-212	-242	-272	-302	-43.22
100	-131	-218	-262	-305	-349	-393	-436	-53.36
110	-175	-292	-351	-409	-467	-526	-584	-64.56

For SI: 1 inch = 25.4 mm, 1 foot = 305 mm, 1 mph = 0.447 m/s, 1 pound/foot = 14.5939 N/m, 1 pound = 0.454 kg.

a. The uplift connection requirements are based on a 30 foot mean roof height located in Exposure B. For Exposures C and D and for other mean roof heights, multiply the above loads by the Adjustment Coefficients in Table R301.2(3).

b. The uplift connection requirements are based on the framing being spaced 24 inches on center. Multiply by 0.67 for framing spaced 16 inches on center and multiply by 0.5 for framing spaced 12 inches on center.

c. The uplift connection requirements include an allowance for 10 pounds of dead load.

d. The uplift connection requirements do not account for the effects of overhangs. The magnitude of the above loads shall be increased by adding the overhang loads found in the table. The overhang loads are also based on framing spaced 24 inches on center. The overhang loads given shall be multiplied by the overhang projection and added to the roof uplift value in the table.

e. The uplift connection requirements are based on wind loading on end zones as defined in Figure 6-2 of ASCE 7. Connection loads for connections located a distance of 20% of the least horizontal dimension of the building from the corner of the building are permitted to be reduced by multiplying the table connection value by 0.7 and multiplying the overhang load by 0.8.

f. For wall-to-wall and wall-to-foundation connections, the capacity of the uplift connector is permitted to be reduced by 100 pounds for each full wall above. (For example, if a 600-pound rated connector is used on the roof framing, a 500-pound rated connector is permitted at the next floor level down).

SECTION R803
ROOF SHEATHING

R803.1 Lumber sheathing. Allowable spans for lumber used as roof sheathing shall conform to Table R803.1. Spaced lumber sheathing for wood shingle and shake roofing shall conform to the requirements of Sections R905.7 and R905.8. Spaced lumber sheathing is not allowed in Seismic Design Category D_2.

TABLE R803.1
MINIMUM THICKNESS OF LUMBER ROOF SHEATHING

RAFTER OR BEAM SPACING (inches)	MINIMUM NET THICKNESS (inches)
24	$^5/_8$
48[a]	
60[b]	$1^1/_2$ T & G
72[c]	

For SI: 1 inch = 25.4 mm.

a. Minimum 270 F_b, 340,000 E.

b. Minimum 420 F_b, 660,000 E.

c. Minimum 600 F_b, 1,150,000 E.

R803.2 Wood structural panel sheathing.

R803.2.1 Identification and grade. *Wood structural panels shall conform to DOC PS 1, DOC PS 2 or, when manufactured in Canada, CSA O437 or CSA O325, and shall be identified by a grade mark* or certificate of inspection issued by an *approved* agency. Wood structural panels shall comply with the *grades specified in Table R503.2.1.1(1).*

R803.2.1.1 Exposure durability. All wood structural panels, when designed to be permanently exposed in outdoor applications, shall be of an exterior exposure durability. Wood structural panel roof sheathing exposed to the underside may be of interior type bonded with exterior glue, identified as Exposure 1.

R803.2.1.2 Fire-retardant-treated plywood. The allowable unit stresses for fire-retardant-treated plywood, including fastener values, shall be developed from an *approved* method of investigation that considers the effects of anticipated temperature and humidity to which the fire-retardant-treated plywood will be subjected, the type of treatment and redrying process. The fire-retardant- treated plywood shall be graded by an *approved agency.*

R803.2.2 Allowable spans. The maximum allowable spans for wood structural panel roof sheathing shall not exceed the values set forth in Table R503.2.1.1(1), or APA E30.

R803.2.3 Installation. Wood structural panel used as roof sheathing shall be installed with joints staggered or not staggered in accordance with Table R602.3(1), or APA E30 for wood roof framing or with Table R804.3 for steel roof framing.

SECTION R804
STEEL ROOF FRAMING

R804.1 General. Elements shall be straight and free of any defects that would significantly affect their structural performance. Cold-formed steel roof framing members shall comply with the requirements of this section.

R804.1.1 Applicability limits. The provisions of this section shall control the construction of cold-formed steel roof framing for buildings not greater than 60 feet (18 288 mm) perpendicular to the joist, rafter or truss span, not greater than 40 feet (12 192 mm) in width parallel to the joist span or truss, less than or equal to three stories above *grade* plane and with roof slopes not less than 3:12 (25-percent slope) or greater than 12:12 (100 percent slope). Cold-formed steel roof framing constructed in accordance with the provisions of this section shall be limited to sites subjected to a maximum design wind speed of 110 miles per hour (49 m/s), Exposure B or C, and a maximum ground snow load of 70 pounds per square foot (3350 Pa).

R804.1.2 In-line framing. Cold-formed steel roof framing constructed in accordance with Section R804 shall be located in line with load-bearing studs in accordance with Figure R804.1.2 and the tolerances specified as follows:

1. The maximum tolerance shall be $^3/_4$ inch (19.1 mm) between the centerline of the horizontal framing member and the centerline of the vertical framing member.

2. Where the centerline of the horizontal framing member and bearing stiffener are located to one side of the center line of the vertical framing member, the maximum tolerance shall be $^1/_8$ inch (3 mm) between the web of the horizontal framing member and the edge of the vertical framing member.

R804.2 Structural framing. Load-bearing cold-formed steel roof framing members shall comply with Figure R804.2(1) and with the dimensional and minimum thickness requirements specified in Tables R804.2(1) and R804.2(2). Tracks shall comply with Figure R804.2(2) and shall have a minimum flange width of $1^1/_4$ inches (32 mm). The maximum inside bend radius for members shall be the greater of $^3/_{32}$ inch (2.4 mm) minus half the base steel thickness or 1.5 times the base steel thickness.

R804.2.1 Material. Load-bearing cold-formed steel framing members shall be cold-formed to shape from structural quality sheet steel complying with the requirements of one of the following:

1. ASTM A 653: *Grades* 33 and 50 (Class 1 and 3).

2. ASTM A 792: *Grades* 33 and 50A.

3. ASTM A 1003: Structural *Grades* 33 Type H and 50 Type H.

R804.2.2 Identification. Load-bearing cold-formed steel framing members shall have a legible *label*, stencil, stamp or embossment with the following information as a minimum:

1. Manufacturer's identification.

2. Minimum base steel thickness in inches (mm).

3. Minimum coating designation.

4. Minimum yield strength, in kips per square inch (ksi) (MPa).

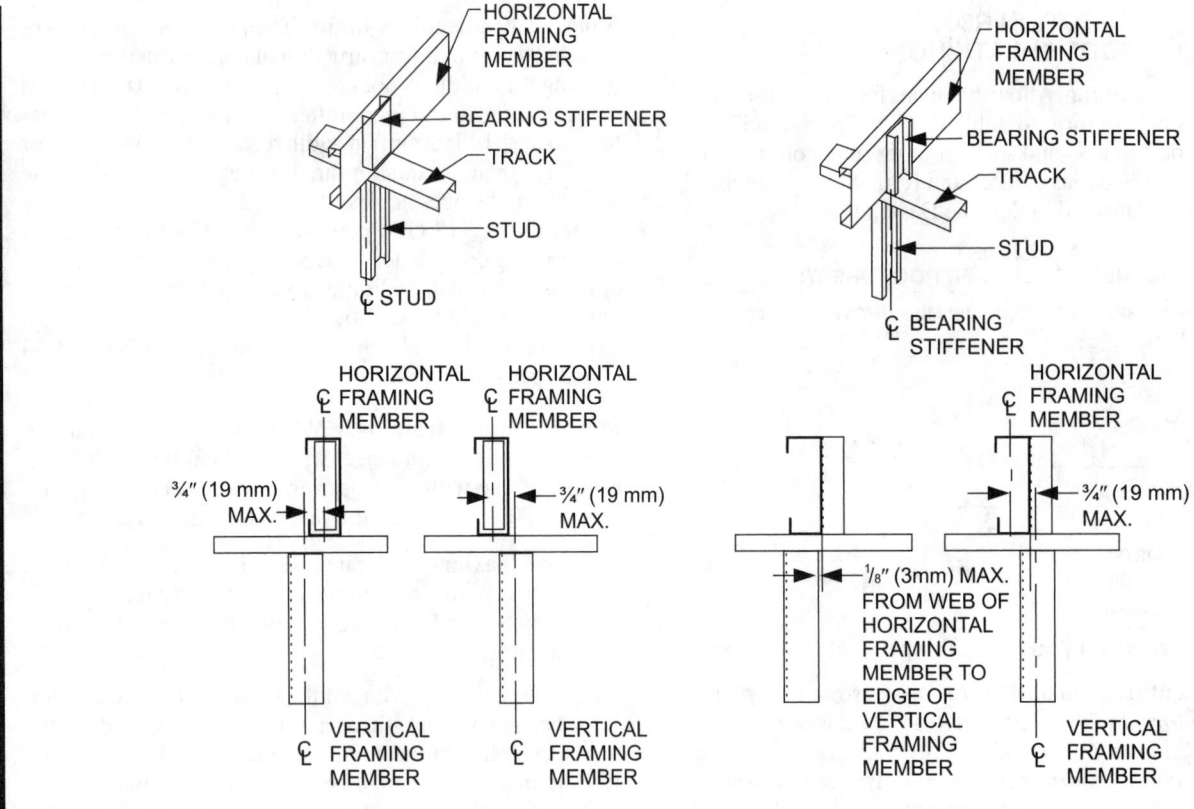

For SI: 1 inch = 25.4 mm.

FIGURE R804.1.2
IN-LINE FRAMING

TABLE R804.2(1)
LOAD-BEARING COLD-FORMED STEEL MEMBER SIZES

NOMINAL MEMBER SIZE MEMBER DESIGNATION[a]	WEB DEPTH (inches)	MINIMUM FLANGE WIDTH (inches)	MAXIMUM FLANGE WIDTH (inches)	MINIMUM LIP SIZE (inches)
350S162-t	3.5	1.625	2	0.5
550S162-t	5.5	1.625	2	0.5
800S162-t	8	1.625	2	0.5
1000S162-t	10	1.625	2	0.5
1200S162-t	12	1.625	2	0.5

For SI: 1 inch = 25.4 mm.

a. The member designation is defined by the first number representing the member depth in hundredths of an inch, the letter "s" representing a stud or joist member, the second number representing the flange width in hundredths of an inch, and the letter "t" shall be a number representing the minimum base metal thickness in mils [see Table R804.2(2)].

TABLE R804.2(2)
MINIMUM THICKNESS OF COLD-FORMED STEEL MEMBERS

DESIGNATION THICKNESS (mils)	MINIMUM BASE STEEL THICKNESS (inches)
33	0.0329
43	0.0428
54	0.0538
68	0.0677
97	0.0966

For SI: 1 inch = 25.4 mm, 1 mil = 0.0254 mm.

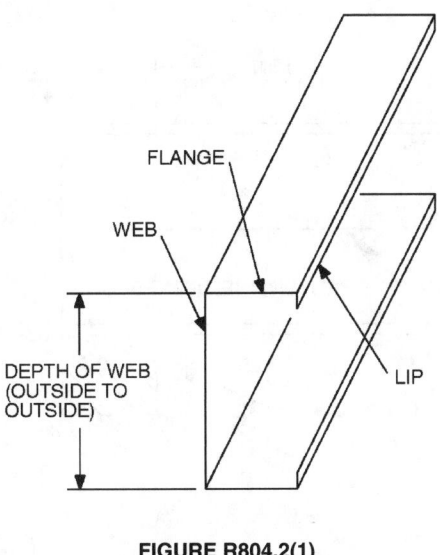

FIGURE R804.2(1)
C-SHAPED SECTION

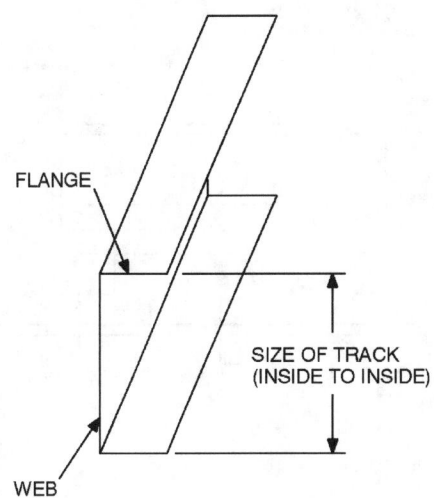

FIGURE R804.2(2)
TRACK SECTION

R804.2.3 Corrosion protection. Load-bearing cold-formed steel framing shall have a metallic coating complying with ASTM A 1003 and one of the following:

1. A minimum of G 60 in accordance with ASTM A 653.

2. A minimum of AZ 50 in accordance with ASTM A 792.

R804.2.4 Fastening requirements. Screws for steel-to-steel connections shall be installed with a minimum edge distance and center-to-center spacing of $^1/_2$ inch (13 mm), shall be self-drilling tapping, and shall conform to ASTM C 1513. Structural sheathing shall be attached to cold-formed steel roof rafters with minimum No. 8 self-drilling tapping screws that conform to ASTM C 1513. Screws for attaching structural sheathing to cold-formed steel roof framing shall have a minimum head diameter of 0.292 inch (7.4 mm) with countersunk heads and shall be installed with a minimum edge distance of $^3/_8$ inch (10 mm). Gypsum board ceilings shall be attached to cold-formed steel joists with minimum No. 6 screws conforming to ASTM C 954 or ASTM C 1513 with a bugle head style and shall be installed in accordance with Section R805. For all connections, screws shall extend through the steel a minimum of three exposed threads. All fasteners shall have rust inhibitive coating suitable for the installation in which they are being used, or be manufactured from material not susceptible to corrosion.

Where No. 8 screws are specified in a steel-to-steel connection, reduction of the required number of screws in the connection is permitted in accordance with the reduction factors in Table R804.2.4 when larger screws are used or when one of the sheets of steel being connected is thicker than 33 mils (0.84 mm). When applying the reduction factor, the resulting number of screws shall be rounded up.

TABLE R804.2.4
SCREW SUBSTITUTION FACTOR

	THINNEST CONNECTED STEEL SHEET (mils)	
SCREW SIZE	33	43
#8	1.0	0.67
#10	0.93	0.62
#12	0.86	0.56

For SI: 1 mil = 0.0254 mm.

R804.2.5 Web holes, web hole reinforcing and web hole patching. Web holes, web hole reinforcing, and web hole patching shall be in accordance with this section.

R804.2.5.1 Web holes. Web holes in roof framing members shall comply with all of the following conditions:

1. Holes shall conform to Figure R804.2.5.1;

2. Holes shall be permitted only along the centerline of the web of the framing member;

3. Center-to-center spacing of holes shall not be less than 24 inches (610 mm);

4. The web hole width shall not be greater than one-half the member depth, or $2^1/_2$ inches (64.5 mm);

5. Holes shall have a web hole length not exceeding $4^1/_2$ inches (114 mm); and

6. The minimum distance between the edge of the bearing surface and the edge of the web hole shall not be less than 10 inches (254 mm).

Framing members with web holes not conforming to the above requirements shall be reinforced in accordance with Section R804.2.5.2, patched in accordance with

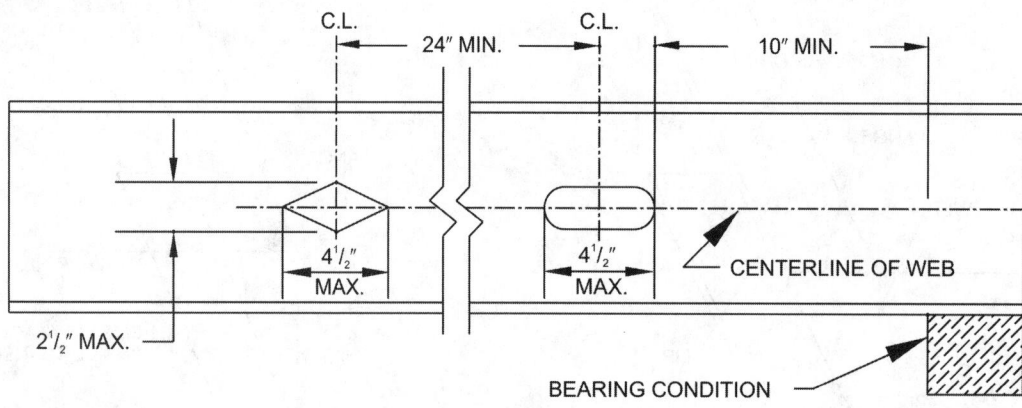

For SI: 1 inch = 25.4 mm.

FIGURE R804.2.5.1
WEB HOLES

Section R804.2.5.3 or designed in accordance with accepted engineering practices.

R804.2.5.2 Web hole reinforcing. Reinforcement of web holes in ceiling joists not conforming to the requirements of Section R804.2.5.1 shall be permitted if the hole is located fully within the center 40 percent of the span and the depth and length of the hole does not exceed 65 percent of the flat width of the web. The reinforcing shall be a steel plate or C-shape section with a hole that does not exceed the web hole size limitations of Section R804.2.5.1 for the member being reinforced. The steel reinforcing shall be the same thickness as the receiving member and shall extend at least 1 inch (25.4 mm) beyond all edges of the hole. The steel reinforcing shall be fastened to the web of the receiving member with No.8 screws spaced no greater than 1 inch (25.4 mm) center-to-center along the edges of the patch with minimum edge distance of $^1/_2$ inch (13 mm).

R804.2.5.3 Hole patching. Patching of web holes in roof framing members not conforming to the requirements in Section R804.2.5.1 shall be permitted in accordance with either of the following methods:

1. Framing members shall be replaced or designed in accordance with accepted engineering practices where web holes exceed the following size limits:

    1.1. The depth of the hole, measured across the web, exceeds 70 percent of the flat width of the web; or

    1.2. The length of the hole measured along the web, exceeds 10 inches (254 mm) or the depth of the web, whichever is greater.

2. Web holes not exceeding the dimensional requirements in Section R804.2.5.3, Item 1, shall be patched with a solid steel plate, stud section or track section in accordance with Figure R804.2.5.3. The steel patch shall, as a minimum, be the same thickness as the receiving member and shall extend at least 1 inch (25 mm) beyond all

edges of the hole. The steel patch shall be fastened to the web of the receiving member with No.8 screws spaced no greater than 1 inch (25 mm) center-to-center along the edges of the patch with minimum edge distance of $^1/_2$ inch (13 mm).

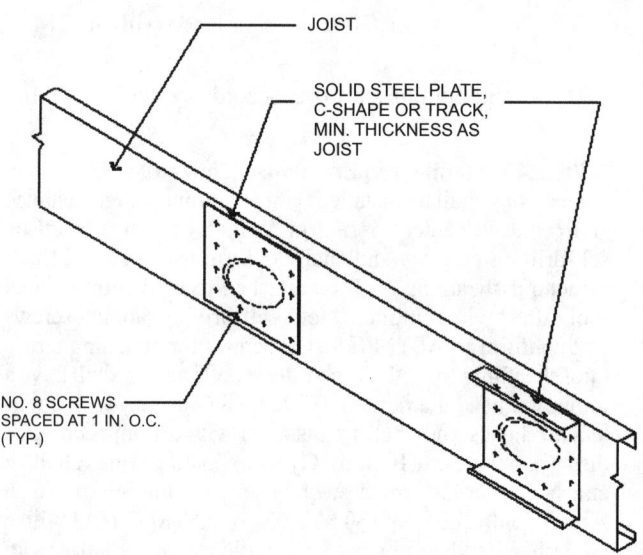

For SI: 1 inch = 25.4 mm.

FIGURE R804.2.5.3
WEB HOLE PATCH

R804.3 Roof construction. Cold-formed steel roof systems constructed in accordance with the provisions of this section shall consist of both ceiling joists and rafters in accordance with Figure R804.3 and fastened in accordance with Table R804.3, and hip framing in accordance with Section R804.3.3.

R804.3.1 Ceiling joists. Cold-formed steel ceiling joists shall be in accordance with this section.

R804.3.1.1 Minimum ceiling joist size. Ceiling joist size and thickness shall be determined in accordance with the limits set forth in Tables R804.3.1.1(1) through R804.3.1.1(8). When determining the size of ceiling joists, the lateral support of the top flange shall be classified as unbraced, braced at mid-span or braced at third points in accordance with Section R804.3.1.4. Where sheathing material is attached to the top flange of ceiling joists or where the bracing is spaced closer than third

point of the joists, the "third point" values from Tables R804.3.1.1(1) through R804.3.1.1(8) shall be used.

Ceiling joists shall have a bearing support length of not less than $1^{1}/_{2}$ inches (38 mm) and shall be connected to roof rafters (heel joint) with No. 10 screws in accordance with Figures R804.3.1.1(1) and R804.3.1.1(2) and Table 804.3.1.1(9).

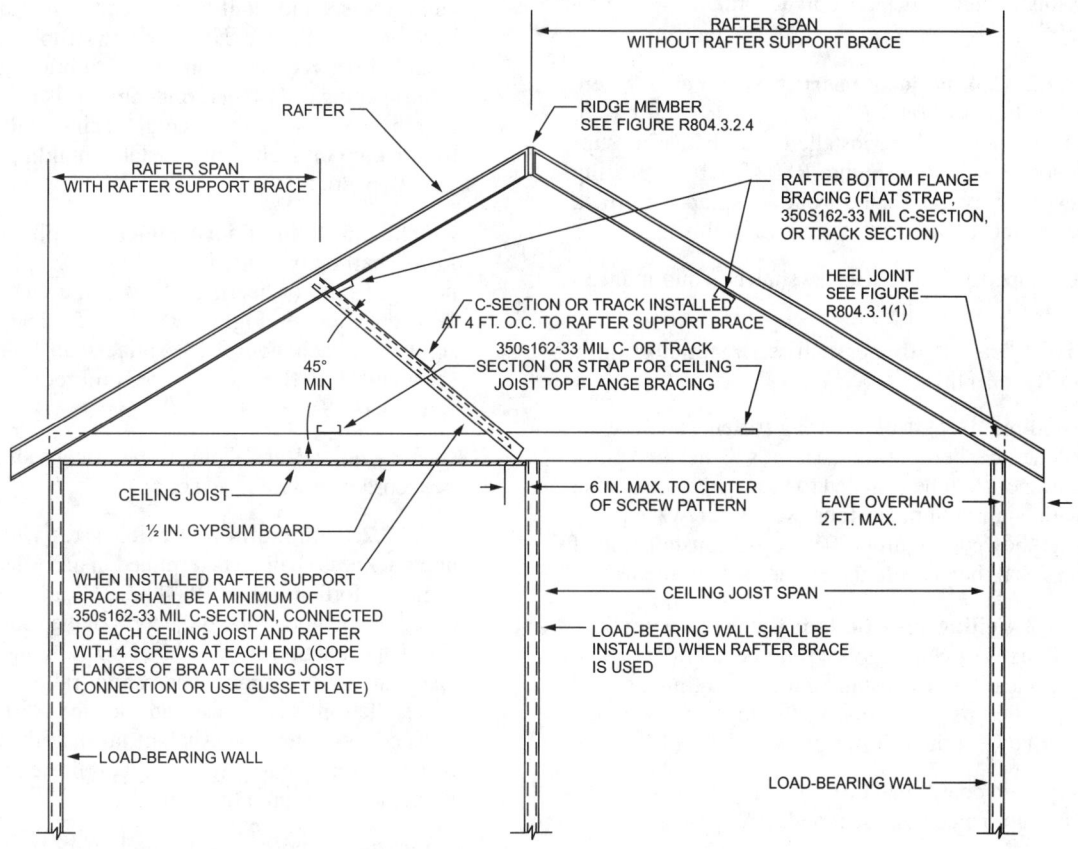

For SI: 1 inch = 25.4 mm, 1 foot = 304.8 mm, 1 mil = 0.0254 mm.

FIGURE R804.3
STEEL ROOF CONSTRUCTION

TABLE R804.3
ROOF FRAMING FASTENING SCHEDULE[a, b]

DESCRIPTION OF BUILDING ELEMENTS	NUMBER AND SIZE OF FASTENERS	SPACING OF FASTENERS
Ceiling joist to top track of load-bearing wall	2 No. 10 screws	Each joist
Roof sheathing (oriented strand board or plywood) to rafters	No. 8 screws	6″ o.c. on edges and 12″ o.c. at interior supports. 6″ o.c. at gable end truss
Truss to bearing wall[a]	2 No. 10 screws	Each truss
Gable end truss to endwall top track	No. 10 screws	12″ o.c.
Rafter to ceiling joist	Minimum No. 10 screws, per Table R804.3.1	Evenly spaced, not less than $^{1}/_{2}$″ from all edges.

For SI: 1 inch = 25.4 mm, 1 foot = 304.8 mm, 1 pound per square foot = 0.0479 kPa, 1 mil = 0.0254 mm.

a. Screws shall be applied through the flanges of the truss or ceiling joist or a 54 mil clip angle shall be used with two No. 10 screws in each leg. See Section R804.3.9 for additional requirements to resist uplift forces.

b. Spacing of fasteners on roof sheathing panel edges applies to panel edges supported by framing members and at all roof plane perimeters. Blocking of roof sheathing panel edges perpendicular to the framing members shall not be required except at the intersection of adjacent roof planes. Roof perimeter shall be supported by framing members or cold-formed blocking of the same depth and gage as the floor members.

When continuous joists are framed across interior bearing supports, the interior bearing supports shall be located within 24 inches (610 mm) of midspan of the ceiling joist, and the individual spans shall not exceed the applicable spans in Tables R804.3.1.1(2), R804.3.1.1(4), R804.3.1.1(6) and R804.3.1.1(8).

When the *attic* is to be used as an *occupied space*, the ceiling joists shall be designed in accordance with Section R505.

R804.3.1.2 Ceiling joist bearing stiffeners. Where required in Tables R804.3.1.1(1) through R804.3.1.1(8), bearing stiffeners shall be installed at each bearing support in accordance with Figure R804.3.1.1(2). Bearing stiffeners shall be fabricated from a C-shaped or track member in accordance with the one of following:

1. C-shaped bearing stiffeners shall be a minimum 33 mils (0.84 mm) thick.

2. Track bearing stiffener shall be a minimum 43 mils (1.09 mm) thick.

The minimum length of a bearing stiffener shall be the depth of member being stiffened minus $^3/_8$ inch (9.5 mm). Each stiffener shall be fastened to the web of the ceiling joist with a minimum of four No. 8 screws equally spaced as shown in Figure R804.3.1.1(2). Installation of stiffeners shall be permitted on either side of the web.

R804.3.1.3 Ceiling joist bottom flange bracing. The bottom flanges of ceiling joists shall be laterally braced by the application of gypsum board or continuous steel straps installed perpendicular to the joist run in accordance with one of the following:

1. Gypsum board shall be fastened with No. 6 screws in accordance with Section R702.

2. Steel straps with a minimum size of $1^1/_2$ inches × 33 mils (38 mm × 0.84 mm) shall be installed at a maximum spacing of 4 feet (1219 mm). Straps shall be fastened to the bottom flange at each joist with one No.8 screw and shall be fastened to blocking with two No.8 screws. Blocking shall be installed between joists at a maximum spacing of 12 feet (3658 mm) measured along a line of continuous strapping (perpendicular to the joist run). Blocking shall also be located at the termination of all straps.

R804.3.1.4 Ceiling joist top flange bracing. The top flanges of ceiling joists shall be laterally braced as required by Tables R804.3.1.1(1) through R804.3.1.1(8), in accordance with one of the following:

1. Minimum 33-mil (0.84 mm) C-shaped member in accordance with Figure R804.3.1.4(1).

2. Minimum 33-mil (0.84 mm) track section in accordance with Figure R804.3.1.4(1).

3. Minimum 33-mil (0.84 mm) hat section in accordance with Figure R804.3.1.4(1).

4. Minimum 54-mil (1.37 mm) $1^1/_2$ inch cold-rolled channel section in accordance with Figure R804.3.1.4(1).

5. Minimum $1^1/_2$ inch by 33 mil (38 mm by 0.84 mm) continuous steel strap in accordance with Figure R804.3.1.4(2).

Lateral bracing shall be installed perpendicular to the ceiling joists and shall be fastened to the top flange of each joist with one No. 8 screw. Blocking shall be installed between joists in line with bracing at a maximum spacing of 12 feet (3658 mm) measured perpendicular to the joists. Ends of lateral bracing shall be attached to blocking or anchored to a stable building component with two No. 8 screws.

R804.3.1.5 Ceiling joist splicing. Splices in ceiling joists shall be permitted, if ceiling joist splices are supported at interior bearing points and are constructed in accordance with Figure R804.3.1.5. The number of screws on each side of the splice shall be the same as required for the heel joint connection in Table R804.3.1.1(9).

R804.3.2 Roof rafters. Cold-formed steel roof rafters shall be in accordance with this section.

R804.3.2.1 Minimum roof rafter sizes. Roof rafter size and thickness shall be determined in accordance with the limits set forth in Tables R804.3.2.1(1) and R804.3.2.1(2) based on the horizontal projection of the roof rafter span. For determination of roof rafter sizes, reduction of roof spans shall be permitted when a roof rafter support brace is installed in accordance with Section R804.3.2.2. The reduced roof rafter span shall be taken as the larger of the distance from the roof rafter support brace to the ridge or to the heel measured horizontally.

For the purpose of determining roof rafter sizes in Tables R804.3.2.1(1) and R804.3.2.1(2), wind speeds shall be converted to equivalent ground snow loads in accordance with Table R804.3.2.1(3). Roof rafter sizes shall be based on the higher of the ground snow load or the equivalent snow load converted from the wind speed.

R804.3.2.1.1 Eave overhang. Eave overhangs shall not exceed 24 inches (610 mm) measured horizontally.

R804.3.2.1.2 Rake overhangs. Rake overhangs shall not exceed 12 inches (305 mm) measured horizontally. Outlookers at gable endwalls shall be installed in accordance with Figure R804.3.2.1.2.

R804.3.2.2 Roof rafter support brace. When used to reduce roof rafter spans in determining roof rafter sizes, a roof rafter support brace shall meet all of the following conditions:

1. Minimum 350S162-33 C-shaped brace member with maximum length of 8 feet (2438 mm).

2. Minimum brace member slope of 45 degrees (0.785 rad) to the horizontal.

3. Minimum connection of brace to a roof rafter and ceiling joist with four No.10 screws at each end.

4. Maximum 6 inches (152 mm) between brace/ceiling joist connection and load-bearing wall below.

5. Each roof rafter support brace greater than 4 feet (1219 mm) in length, shall be braced with a supplemental brace having a minimum size of 350S162-33 or 350T162-33 such that the maximum unsupported length of the roof rafter support brace is 4 feet (1219 mm). The supplemental brace shall be continuous and shall be connected to each roof rafter support brace using two No.8 screws.

R804.3.2.3 Roof rafter splice. Roof rafters shall not be spliced.

R804.3.2.4 Roof rafter to ceiling joist and ridge member connection. Roof rafters shall be connected to a parallel ceiling joist to form a continuous tie between exterior walls in accordance with Figures R804.3.1.1(1) or R804.3.1.1(2) and Table R804.3.1.1(9). Ceiling joists shall be connected to the top track of the load-bearing wall in accordance with Table R804.3, either with two No.10 screws applied through the flange of the ceiling joist or by using a 54 mil (1.37 mm) clip angle with two No.10 screws in each leg. Roof rafters shall be connected to a ridge member with a minimum 2-inch by 2-inch (51 mm by 51 mm) clip angle fastened with No. 10 screws to the ridge member in accordance with Figure R804.3.2.4 and Table R804.3.2.4. The clip angle shall have a steel thickness equivalent to or greater than the roof rafter thickness and shall extend the depth of the roof rafter member to the extent possible. The ridge member shall be fabricated from a C-shaped member and a track section, which shall have a minimum size and steel thickness equivalent to or greater than that of adjacent roof rafters and shall be installed in accordance with Figure R804.3.2.4. The ridge member shall extend the full depth of the sloped roof rafter cut.

R804.3.2.5 Roof rafter bottom flange bracing. The bottom flanges of roof rafters shall be continuously braced, at a maximum spacing of 8 feet (2440 mm) as measured parallel to the roof rafters, with one of the following members:

1. Minimum 33-mil (0.84 mm) C-shaped member.

2. Minimum 33-mil (0.84 mm) track section.

3. Minimum $1^{1}/_{2}$-inch by 33-mil (38 mm by 0.84 mm) steel strap.

The bracing element shall be fastened to the bottom flange of each roof rafter with one No.8 screw and shall be fastened to blocking with two No.8 screws. Blocking shall be installed between roof rafters in-line with the continuous bracing at a maximum spacing of 12 feet (3658 mm) measured perpendicular to the roof rafters. The ends of continuous bracing shall be fastened to blocking or anchored to a stable building component with two No.8 screws.

R804.3.3 Hip framing. Hip framing shall consist of jack-rafters, hip members, hip support columns and connections in accordance with this section, or shall be in accordance with an *approved* design. The provisions of this section for hip members and hip support columns shall apply only where the jack rafter slope is greater than or equal to the roof slope. For the purposes of determining member sizes in this section, wind speeds shall be converted to equivalent ground snow load in accordance with Table R804.3.2.1(3).

R804.3.3.1 Jack rafters. Jack rafters shall meet the requirements for roof rafters in accordance with Section R804.3.2, except that the requirements in Section R804.3.2.4 shall not apply.

R804.3.3.2 Hip members. Hip members shall be fabricated from C-shape members and track section, which shall have minimum sizes determined in accordance with Table R804.3.3.2. The C-shape member and track section shall be connected at a maximum spacing of 24 inches (610 mm) using No. 10 screws through top and bottom flanges in accordance with Figure R804.3.2.4. The depth of the hip member shall match that of the roof rafters and jack rafters, or shall be based on an *approved* design for a beam pocket at the corner of the supporting wall.

R804.3.3.3 Hip support columns. Hip support columns shall be used to support hip members at the ridge. A hip support column shall consist of a pair of C-shape members, with a minimum size determined in accordance with Table R804.3.3.3. The C-shape members shall be connected at a maximum spacing of 24 inches (610 mm) on center to form a box using minimum 3-inch (76 mm) × 33-mil (0.84 mm) strap connected to each of the flanges of the C-shape members with three-No. 10 screws. Hip support columns shall have a continuous load path to the foundation and shall be supported at the ceiling line by an interior wall or by an *approved* design for a supporting element.

TABLE R804.3.1.1(1)
CEILING JOIST SPANS
SINGLE SPANS WITH BEARING STIFFENERS
10 lb per sq ft LIVE LOAD (NO ATTIC STORAGE)[a, b, c] 33 ksi STEEL

MEMBER DESIGNATION	ALLOWABLE SPAN (feet-inches)					
	Lateral Support of Top (Compression) Flange					
	Unbraced		Mid-Span Bracing		Third-Point Bracing	
	Ceiling Joist Spacing (inches)					
	16	24	16	24	16	24
350S162-33	9'-5"	8'-6"	12'-2"	10'-4"	12'-2"	10'-7"
350S162-43	10'-3"	9'-2"	12'-10"	11'-2"	12'-10"	11'-2"
350S162-54	11'-1"	9'-11"	13'-9"	12'-0"	13'-9"	12'-0"
350S162-68	12'-1"	10'-9"	14'-8"	12'-10"	14'-8"	12'-10"
350S162-97	14'-4"	12'-7"	16'-4"	14'-3"	16'-4"	14'-3"
550S162-33	10'-7"	9'-6"	14'-10"	12'-10"	15'-11"	13'-4"
550S162-43	11'-8"	10'-6"	16'-4"	14'-3"	17'-10"	15'-3"
550S162-54	12'-6"	11'-2"	17'-7"	15'-7"	19'-5"	16'-10"
550S162-68	13'-6"	12'-1"	19'-2"	17'-1"	21'-0"	18'-4"
550S162-97	15'-9"	13'-11"	21'-8"	19'-3"	23'-5"	20'-5"
800S162-33	12'-2"	10'-11"	17'-8"	15'-10"	19'-10"	17'-1"
800S162-43	13'-0"	11'-9"	18'-10"	17'-0"	21'-6"	19'-1"
800S162-54	13'-10"	12'-5"	20'-0"	18'-0"	22'-9"	20'-4"
800S162-68	14'-11"	13'-4"	21'-3"	19'-1"	24'-1"	21'-8"
800S162-97	17'-1"	15'-2"	23'-10"	21'-3"	26'-7"	23'-10"
1000S162-43	13'-11"	12'-6"	20'-2"	18'-3"	23'-1"	20'-9"
1000S162-54	14'-9"	13'-3"	21'-4"	19'-3"	24'-4"	22'-0"
1000S162-68	15'-10"	14'-2"	22'-8"	20'-5"	25'-9"	23'-2"
1000S162-97	18'-0"	16'-0"	25'-3"	22'-7"	28'-3"	25'-4"
1200S162-43	14'-8"	13'-3"	21'-4"	19'-3"	24'-5"	21'-8"
1200S162-54	15'-7"	14'-0"	22'-6"	20'-4"	25'-9"	23'-2"
1200S162-68	16'-8"	14'-11"	23'-11"	21'-6"	27'-2"	24'-6"
1000S162-97	18'-9"	16'-9"	26'-6"	23'-8"	29'-9"	26'-9"

For SI: 1 inch = 25.4 mm, 1 foot = 304.8 mm, 1 pound per square foot = 0.0479 kPa.

a. Deflection criterion: L/240 for total loads.

b. Ceiling dead load = 5 psf.

c. Bearing stiffeners are required at all bearing points and concentrated load locations.

TABLE R804.3.1.1(2)
CEILING JOIST SPANS
TWO EQUAL SPANS WITH BEARING STIFFENERS
10 lb per sq ft LIVE LOAD (NO ATTIC STORAGE)[a, b, c] 33 ksi STEEL

MEMBER DESIGNATION	ALLOWABLE SPAN (feet-inches)					
	Lateral Support of Top (Compression) Flange					
	Unbraced		Mid-Span Bracing		Third-Point Bracing	
	Ceiling Joist Spacing (inches)					
	16	24	16	24	16	24
350S162-33	12'-11"	10'-11"	13'-5"	10'-11"	13'-5"	10'-11"
350S162-43	14'-2"	12'-8"	15'-10"	12'-11"	15'-10"	12'-11"
350S162-54	15'-6"	13'-10"	17'-1"	14'-6"	17'-9"	14'-6"
350S162-68	17'-3"	15'-3"	18'-6"	16'-1"	19'-8"	16'-1"
350S162-97	20'-10"	18'-4"	21'-5"	18'-10"	21'-11"	18'-10"
550S162-33	14'-4"	12'-11"	16'-7"	14'-1"	17'-3"	14'-1"
550S162-43	16'-0"	14'-1"	17'-11"	16'-1"	20'-7"	16'-10"
550S162-54	17'-4"	15'-6"	19'-5"	17'-6"	23'-2"	19'-0"
550S162-68	19'-1"	16'-11"	20'-10"	18'-8"	25'-2"	21'-5"
550S162-97	22'-8"	19'-9"	23'-6"	20'-11"	27'-11"	25'-1"
800S162-33	16'-5"	14'-10"	19'-2"	17'-3"	23'-1"	18'-3"
800S162-43	17'-9"	15'-11"	20'-6"	18'-5"	25'-0"	22'-6"
800S162-54	19'-1"	17'-1"	21'-8"	19'-6"	26'-4"	23'-9"
800S162-68	20'-9"	18'-6"	23'-1"	20'-9"	28'-0"	25'-2"
800S162-97	24'-5"	21'-6"	26'-0"	23'-2"	31'-1"	27'-9"
1000S162-43	18'-11"	17'-0"	21'-11"	19'-9"	26'-8"	24'-1"
1000S162-54	20'-3"	18'-2"	23'-2"	20'-10"	28'-2"	25'-5"
1000S162-68	21'-11"	19'-7"	24'-7"	22'-2"	29'-10"	26'-11"
1000S162-97	25'-7"	22'-7"	27'-6"	24'-6"	33'-0"	29'-7"
1200S162-43	19'-11"	17'-11"	23'-1"	20'-10"	28'-3"	25'-6"
1200S162-54	21'-3"	19'-1"	24'-5"	22'-0"	29'-9"	26'-10"
1200S162-68	23'-0"	20'-7"	25'-11"	23'-4"	31'-6"	28'-4"
1000S162-97	26'-7"	23'-6"	28'-9"	25'-10"	34'-8"	31'-1"

For SI: 1 inch = 25.4 mm, 1 foot = 304.8 mm, 1 pound per square foot = 0.0479 kPa.

a. Deflection criterion: L/240 for total loads.

b. Ceiling dead load = 5 psf.

c. Bearing stiffeners are required at all bearing points and concentrated load locations.

TABLE R804.3.1.1(3)
CEILING JOIST SPANS
SINGLE SPANS WITH BEARING STIFFENERS
20 lb per sq ft LIVE LOAD (LIMITED ATTIC STORAGE)[a, b, c] 33 ksi STEEL

MEMBER DESIGNATION	ALLOWABLE SPAN (feet-inches)					
	Lateral Support of Top (Compression) Flange					
	Unbraced		Mid-Span Bracing		Third-Point Bracing	
	Ceiling Joist Spacing (inches)					
	16	24	16	24	16	24
350S162-33	8'-2"	7'-2"	9'-9"	8'-1"	9'-11"	8'-1"
350S162-43	8'-10"	7'-10"	11'-0"	9'-5"	11'-0"	9'-7"
350S162-54	9'-6"	8'-6"	11'-9"	10'-3"	11'-9"	10'-3"
350S162-68	10'-4"	9'-2"	12'-7"	11'-0"	12'-7"	11'-0"
350S162-97	12'-1"	10'-8"	14'-0"	12'-0"	14'-0"	12'-0"
550S162-33	9'-2"	8'-3"	12'-2"	10'-2"	12'-6"	10'-5"
550S162-43	10'-1"	9'-1"	13'-7"	11'-7"	14'-5"	12'-2"
550S162-54	10'-9"	9'-8"	14'-10"	12'-10"	15'-11"	13'-6"
550S162-68	11'-7"	10'-4"	16'-4"	14'-0"	17'-5"	14'-11"
550S162-97	13'-4"	11'-10"	18'-5"	16'-2"	20'-1"	17'-1"
800S162-33	10'-7"	9'-6"	15'-1"	13'-0"	16'-2"	13'-7"
800S162-43	11'-4"	10'-2"	16'-5"	14'-6"	18'-2"	15'-9"
800S162-54	12'-0"	10'-9"	17'-4"	15'-6"	19'-6"	17'-0"
800S162-68	12'-10"	11'-6"	18'-5"	16'-6"	20'-10"	18'-3"
800S162-97	14'-7"	12'-11"	20'-5"	18'-3"	22'-11"	20'-5"
1000S162-43	12'-1"	10'-11"	17'-7"	15'-10"	19'-11"	17'-3"
1000S162-54	12'-10"	11'-6"	18'-7"	16'-9"	21'-2"	18'-10"
1000S162-68	13'-8"	12'-3"	19'-8"	17'-8"	22'-4"	20'-1"
1000S162-97	15'-4"	13'-8"	21'-8"	19'-5"	24'-5"	21'-11"
1200S162-43	12'-9"	11'-6"	18'-7"	16'-6"	20'-9"	18'-2"
1200S162-54	13'-6"	12'-2"	19'-7"	17'-8"	22'-5"	20'-2"
1200S162-68	14'-4"	12'-11"	20'-9"	18'-8"	23'-7"	21'-3"
1000S162-97	16'-1"	14'-4"	22'-10"	20'-6"	25'-9"	23'-2"

For SI: 1 inch = 25.4 mm, 1 foot = 304.8 mm, 1 pound per square foot = 0.0479 kPa.

a. Deflection criterion: $L/240$ for total loads.

b. Ceiling dead load = 5 psf.

c. Bearing stiffeners are required at all bearing points and concentrated load locations.

TABLE R804.3.1.1(4)
CEILING JOIST SPANS
TWO EQUAL SPANS WITH BEARING STIFFENERS
20 lb per sq ft LIVE LOAD (LIMITED ATTIC STORAGE)[a, b, c] 33 ksi STEEL

MEMBER DESIGNATION	ALLOWABLE SPAN (feet-inches)					
	Lateral Support of Top (Compression) Flange					
	Unbraced		Mid-Span Bracing		Third-Point Bracing	
	Ceiling Joist Spacing (inches)					
	16	24	16	24	16	24
350S162-33	10'-2"	8'-4"	10'-2"	8'-4"	10'-2"	8'-4"
350S162-43	12'-1"	9'-10"	12'-1"	9'-10"	12'-1"	9'-10"
350S162-54	13'-3"	11'-0"	13'-6"	11'-0"	13'-6"	11'-0"
350S162-68	14'-7"	12'-3"	15'-0"	12'-3"	15'-0"	12'-3"
350S162-97	17'-6"	14'-3"	17'-6"	14'-3"	17'-6"	14'-3"
550S162-33	12'-5"	10'-9"	13'-2"	10'-9"	13'-2"	10'-9"
550S162-43	13'-7"	12'-1"	15'-6"	12'-9"	15'-8"	12'-9"
550S162-54	14'-11"	13'-4"	16'-10"	14'-5"	17'-9"	14'-5"
550S162-68	16'-3"	14'-5"	18'-0"	16'-1"	20'-0"	16'-4"
550S162-97	19'-1"	16'-10"	20'-3"	18'-0"	23'-10"	19'-5"
800S162-33	14'-3"	12'-4"	16'-7"	12'-4"	16'-7"	12'-4"
800S162-43	15'-4"	13'-10"	17'-9"	16'-0"	21'-8"	17'-9"
800S162-54	16'-5"	14'-9"	18'-10"	16'-11"	22'-11"	20'-6"
800S162-68	17'-9"	15'-11"	20'-0"	18'-0"	24'-3"	21'-10"
800S162-97	20'-8"	18'-3"	22'-3"	19'-11"	26'-9"	24'-0"
1000S162-43	16'-5"	14'-9"	19'-0"	17'-2"	23'-3"	18'-11"
1000S162-54	17'-6"	15'-8"	20'-1"	18'-1"	24'-6"	22'-1"
1000S162-68	18'-10"	16'-10"	21'-4"	19'-2"	25'-11"	23'-4"
1000S162-97	21'-8"	19'-3"	23'-7"	21'-2"	28'-5"	25'-6"
1200S162-43	17'-3"	15'-7"	20'-1"	18'-2"	24'-6"	18'-3"
1200S162-54	18'-5"	16'-6"	21'-3"	19'-2"	25'-11"	23'-5"
1200S162-68	19'-9"	17'-8"	22'-6"	20'-3"	27'-4"	24'-8"
1000S162-97	22'-7"	20'-1"	24'-10"	22'-3"	29'-11"	26'-11"

For SI: 1 inch = 25.4 mm, 1 foot = 304.8 mm, 1 pound per square foot = 0.0479 kPa.

a. Deflection criterion: $L/240$ for total loads.

b. Ceiling dead load = 5 psf.

c. Bearing stiffeners are required at all bearing points and concentrated load locations.

TABLE R804.3.1.1(5)
CEILING JOIST SPANS
SINGLE SPANS WITHOUT BEARING STIFFENERS
10 lb per sq ft LIVE LOAD (NO ATTIC STORAGE)[a, b] 33 ksi STEEL

MEMBER DESIGNATION	ALLOWABLE SPAN (feet-inches)					
	Lateral Support of Top (Compression) Flange					
	Unbraced		Mid-Span Bracing		Third-Point Bracing	
	Ceiling Joist Spacing (inches)					
	16	24	16	24	16	24
350S162-33	9'-5"	8'-6"	12'-2"	10'-4"	12'-2"	10'-7"
350S162-43	10'-3"	9'-12"	13'-2"	11'-6"	13'-2"	11'-6"
350S162-54	11'-1"	9'-11"	13'-9"	12'-0"	13'-9"	12'-0"
350S162-68	12'-1"	10'-9"	14'-8"	12'-10"	14'-8"	12'-10"
350S162-97	14'-4"	12'-7"	16'-10"	14'-3"	16'-4"	14'-3"
550S162-33	10'-7"	9'-6"	14'-10"	12'-10"	15'-11"	13'-4"
550S162-43	11'-8"	10'-6"	16'-4"	14'-3"	17'-10"	15'-3"
550S162-54	12'-6"	11'-2"	17'-7"	15'-7"	19'-5"	16'-10"
550S162-68	13'-6"	12'-1"	19'-2"	17'-0"	21'-0"	18'-4"
550S162-97	15'-9"	13'-11"	21'-8"	19'-3"	23'-5"	20'-5"
800S162-33	—	—	—	—	—	—
800S162-43	13'-0"	11'-9"	18'-10"	17'-0"	21'-6"	19'-0"
800S162-54	13'-10"	12'-5"	20'-0"	18'-0"	22'-9"	20'-4"
800S162-68	14'-11"	13'-4"	21'-3"	19'-1"	24'-1"	21'-8"
800S162-97	17'-1"	15'-2"	23'-10"	21'-3"	26'-7"	23'-10"
1000S162-43	—	—	—	—	—	—
1000S162-54	14'-9"	13'-3"	21'-4"	19'-3"	24'-4"	22'-0"
1000S162-68	15'-10"	14'-2"	22'-8"	20'-5"	25'-9"	23'-2"
1000S162-97	18'-0"	16'-0"	25'-3"	22'-7"	28'-3"	25'-4"
1200S162-43	—	—	—	—	—	—
1200S162-54	—	—	—	—	—	—
1200S162-68	16'-8"	14'-11"	23'-11"	21'-6"	27'-2"	24'-6"
1000S162-97	18'-9"	16'-9"	26'-6"	23'-8"	29'-9"	26'-9"

For SI: 1 inch = 25.4 mm, 1 foot = 304.8 mm, 1 pound per square foot = 0.0479 kPa.
a. Deflection criterion: L/240 for total loads.
b. Ceiling dead load = 5 psf.

TABLE R804.3.1.1(6)
CEILING JOIST SPANS
TWO EQUAL SPANS WITHOUT BEARING STIFFENERS
10 lb per sq ft LIVE LOAD (NO ATTIC STORAGE)[a, b] 33 ksi STEEL

MEMBER DESIGNATION	ALLOWABLE SPAN (feet-inches)					
	Lateral Support of Top (Compression) Flange					
	Unbraced		Mid-Span Bracing		Third-Point Bracing	
	Ceiling Joist Spacing (inches)					
	16	24	16	24	16	24
350S162-33	11'-9"	8'-11"	11'-9"	8'-11"	11'-9"	8'-11"
350S162-43	14'-2"	11'-7"	14'-11"	11'-7"	14'-11"	11'-7"
350S162-54	15'-6"	13'-10"	17'-1"	13'-10"	17'-7"	13'-10"
350S162-68	17'-3"	15'-3"	18'-6"	16'-1"	19'-8"	16'-1"
350S162-97	20'-10"	18'-4"	21'-5"	18'-9"	21'-11"	18'-9"
550S162-33	13'-4"	9'-11"	13'-4"	9'-11"	13'-4"	9'-11"
550S162-43	16'-0"	13'-6"	17'-9"	13'-6"	17'-9"	13'-6"
550S162-54	17'-4"	15'-6"	19'-5"	16'-10"	21'-9"	16'-10"
550S162-68	19'-1"	16'-11"	20'-10"	18'-8"	24'-11"	20'-6"
550S162-97	22'-8"	20'-0"	23'-9"	21'-1"	28'-2"	25'-1"
800S162-33	—	—	—	—	—	—
800S162-43	17'-9"	15'-7"	20'-6"	15'-7"	21'-0"	15'-7"
800S162-54	19'-1"	17'-1"	21'-8"	19'-6"	26'-4"	23'-10"
800S162-68	20'-9"	18'-6"	23'-1"	20'-9"	28'-0"	25'-2"
800S162-97	24'-5"	21'-6"	26'-0"	23'-2"	31'-1"	27'-9"
1000S162-43	—	—	—	—	—	—
1000S162-54	20'-3"	18'-2"	23'-2"	20'-10"	28'-2"	21'-2"
1000S162-68	21'-11"	19'-7"	24'-7"	22'-2"	29'-10"	26'-11"
1000S162-97	25'-7"	22'-7"	27'-6"	24'-6"	33'-0"	29'-7"
1200S162-43	—	—	—	—	—	—
1200S162-54	—	—	—	—	—	—
1200S162-68	23'-0"	20'-7"	25'-11"	23'-4"	31'-6"	28'-4"
1000S162-97	26'-7"	23'-6"	28'-9"	25'-10"	34'-8"	31'-1"

For SI: 1 inch = 25.4 mm, 1 foot = 304.8 mm, 1 pound per square foot = 0.0479 kPa.

a. Deflection criterion: *L*/240 for total loads.

b. Ceiling dead load = 5 psf.

TABLE R804.3.1.1(7)
CEILING JOIST SPANS
SINGLE SPANS WITHOUT BEARING STIFFENERS
20 lb per sq ft LIVE LOAD (LIMITED ATTIC STORAGE)[a, b] 33 ksi STEEL

MEMBER DESIGNATION	ALLOWABLE SPAN (feet-inches)					
	Lateral Support of Top (Compression) Flange					
	Unbraced		Mid-Span Bracing		Third-Point Bracing	
	Ceiling Joist Spacing (inches)					
	16	24	16	24	16	24
350S162-33	8'-2"	6'-10"	9'-9"	6'-10"	9'-11"	6'-10"
350S162-43	8'-10"	7'-10"	11'-0"	9'-5"	11'-0"	9'-7"
350S162-54	9'-6"	8'-6"	11'-9"	10'-3"	11'-9"	10'-3"
350S162-68	10'-4"	9'-2"	12'-7"	11'-0"	12'-7"	11'-0"
350S162-97	12'-10"	10'-8"	13'-9"	12'-0"	13'-9"	12'-0"
550S162-33	9'-2"	8'-3"	12'-2"	8'-5"	12'-6"	8'-5"
550S162-43	10'-1"	9'-1"	13'-7"	11'-8"	14'-5"	12'-2"
550S162-54	10'-9"	9'-8"	14'-10"	12'-10"	15'-11"	13'-6"
550S162-68	11'-7"	10'-4"	16'-4"	14'-0"	17'-5"	14'-11"
550S162-97	13'-4"	11'-10"	18'-5"	16'-2"	20'-1"	17'-4"
800S162-33	—	—	—	—	—	—
800S162-43	11'-4"	10'-1"	16'-5"	13'-6"	18'-1"	13'-6"
800S162-54	20'-0"	10'-9"	17'-4"	15'-6"	19'-6"	27'-0"
800S162-68	12'-10"	11'-6"	18'-5"	16'-6"	20'-10"	18'-3"
800S162-97	14'-7"	12'-11"	20'-5"	18'-3"	22'-11"	20'-5"
1000S162-43	—	—	—	—	—	—
1000S162-54	12'-10"	11'-6"	18'-7"	16'-9"	21'-2"	15'-5"
1000S162-68	13'-8"	12'-3"	19'-8"	17'-8"	22'-4"	20'-1"
1000S162-97	15'-4"	13'-8"	21'-8"	19'-5"	24'-5"	21'-11"
1200S162-43	—	—	—	—	—	—
1200S162-54	—	—	—	—	—	—
1200S162-68	14'-4"	12'-11"	20'-9"	18'-8"	23'-7"	21'-3"
1000S162-97	16'-1"	14'-4"	22'-10"	20'-6"	25'-9"	23'-2"

For SI: 1 inch = 25.4 mm, 1 foot = 304.8 mm, 1 pound per square foot = 0.0479 kPa.
a. Deflection criterion: L/240 for total loads.
b. Ceiling dead load = 5 psf.

TABLE R804.3.1.1(8)
CEILING JOIST SPANS
TWO EQUAL SPANS WITHOUT BEARING STIFFENERS
20 lb per sq ft LIVE LOAD (LIMITED ATTIC STORAGE)[a, b] 33 ksi STEEL

MEMBER DESIGNATION	ALLOWABLE SPAN (feet-inches)					
	Lateral Support of Top (Compression) Flange					
	Unbraced		Mid-Span Bracing		Third-Point Bracing	
	Ceiling Joist Spacing (inches)					
	16	24	16	24	16	24
350S162-33	8'-1"	6'-1"	8'-1"	6'-1"	8'-1"	6'-1"
350S162-43	10'-7"	8'-1"	10'-7"	8'-1"	10'-7"	8'-1"
350S162-54	12'-8"	9'-10"	12'-8"	9'-10"	12'-8"	9'-10"
350S162-68	14'-7"	11'-10"	14'-11"	11'-10"	14'-11"	11'-10"
350S162-97	17'-6"	14'-3"	17'-6"	14'-3"	17'-6"	14'-3"
550S162-33	8'-11"	6'-8"	8'-11"	6'-8"	8'-11"	6'-8"
550S162-43	12'-3"	9'-2"	12'-3"	9'-2"	12'-3"	9'-2"
550S162-54	14'-11"	11'-8"	15'-4"	11'-8"	15'-4"	11'-8"
550S162-68	16'-3"	14'-5"	18'-0"	15'-8"	18'-10"	14'-7"
550S162-97	19'-1"	16'-10"	20'-3"	18'-0"	23'-9"	19'-5"
800S162-33	—	—	—	—	—	—
800S162-43	13'-11"	9'-10"	13'-11"	9'-10"	13'-11"	9'-10"
800S162-54	16'-5"	13'-9"	18'-8"	13'-9"	18'-8"	13'-9"
800S162-68	17'-9"	15'-11"	20'-0"	18'-0"	24'-1"	18'-3"
800S162-97	20'-8"	18'-3"	22'-3"	19'-11"	26'-9"	24'-0"
1000S162-43	—	—	—	—	—	—
1000S162-54	17'-6"	13'-11"	19'-1"	13'-11"	19'-1"	13'-11"
1000S162-68	18'-10"	16'-10"	21'-4"	19'-2"	25'-11"	19'-7"
1000S162-97	21'-8"	19'-3"	23'-7"	21'-2"	28'-5"	25'-6"
1200S162-43	—	—	—	—	—	—
1200S162-54	—	—	—	—	—	—
1200S162-68	19'-9"	17'-8"	22'-6"	19'-8"	26'-8"	19'-8"
1000S162-97	22'-7"	20'-1"	24'-10"	22'-3"	29'-11"	26'-11"

For SI: 1 inch = 25.4 mm, 1 foot = 304.8 mm, 1 pound per square foot = 0.0479 kPa.

a. Deflection criterion: $L/240$ for total loads.

b. Ceiling dead load = 5 psf.

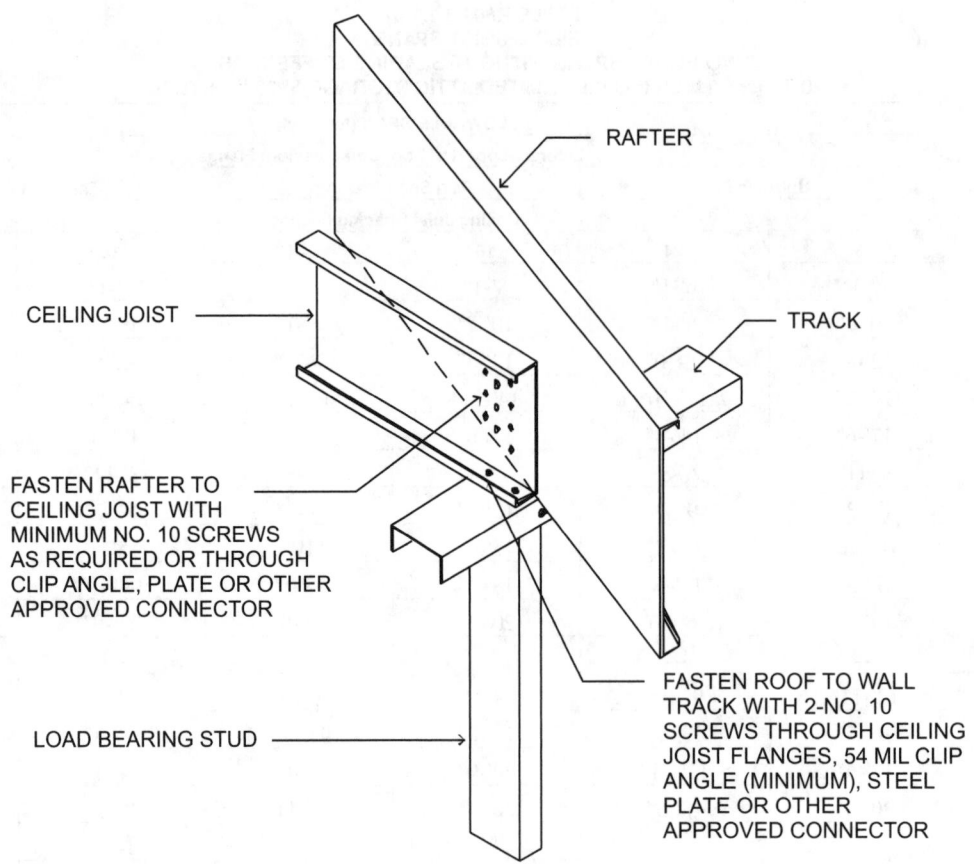

RAFTER

CEILING JOIST

TRACK

FASTEN RAFTER TO
CEILING JOIST WITH
MINIMUM NO. 10 SCREWS
AS REQUIRED OR THROUGH
CLIP ANGLE, PLATE OR OTHER
APPROVED CONNECTOR

FASTEN ROOF TO WALL
TRACK WITH 2-NO. 10
SCREWS THROUGH CEILING
JOIST FLANGES, 54 MIL CLIP
ANGLE (MINIMUM), STEEL
PLATE OR OTHER
APPROVED CONNECTOR

LOAD BEARING STUD

For SI: 1 mil = 0.0254 mm.

FIGURE R804.3.1.1(1)
JOIST TO RAFTER CONNECTION

TABLE R804.3.1.1(9)
NUMBER OF SCREWS REQUIRED FOR CEILING JOIST TO ROOF RAFTER CONNECTION[a]

ROOF SLOPE	NUMBER OF SCREWS																			
	Building width (feet)																			
	24				28				32				36				40			
	Ground snow load (psf)																			
	20	30	50	70	20	30	50	70	20	30	50	70	20	30	50	70	20	30	50	70
3/12	5	6	9	11	5	7	10	13	6	8	11	15	7	8	13	17	8	9	14	19
4/12	4	5	7	9	4	5	8	10	5	6	9	12	5	7	10	13	6	7	11	14
5/12	3	4	6	7	4	4	6	8	4	5	7	10	5	5	8	11	5	6	9	12
6/12	3	3	5	6	3	4	6	7	4	4	6	8	4	5	7	9	4	5	8	10
7/12	3	3	4	6	3	3	5	7	3	4	6	7	4	4	6	8	4	5	7	9
8/12	2	3	4	5	3	3	5	6	3	4	5	7	3	4	6	8	4	4	6	8
9/12	2	3	4	5	3	3	4	6	3	3	5	6	3	4	5	7	3	4	6	8
10/12	2	2	4	5	2	3	4	5	3	3	5	6	3	3	5	7	3	4	6	7
11/12	2	2	3	4	2	3	4	5	3	3	4	6	3	3	5	6	3	4	5	7
12/12	2	2	3	4	2	3	4	5	2	3	4	5	3	3	5	6	3	4	5	7

For SI: 1 inch = 25.4 mm, 1 foot = 304.8 mm, 1 pound per square foot = 0.0479 kPa.
a. Screws shall be No. 10.

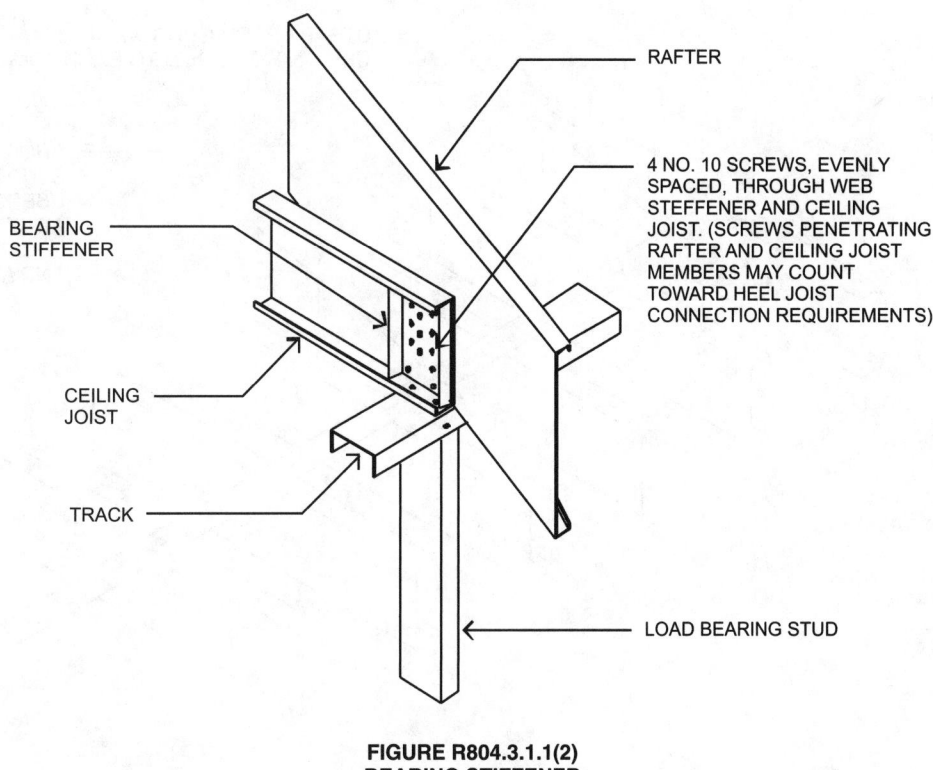

RAFTER

4 NO. 10 SCREWS, EVENLY SPACED, THROUGH WEB STEFFENER AND CEILING JOIST. (SCREWS PENETRATING RAFTER AND CEILING JOIST MEMBERS MAY COUNT TOWARD HEEL JOIST CONNECTION REQUIREMENTS)

BEARING STIFFENER

CEILING JOIST

TRACK

LOAD BEARING STUD

FIGURE R804.3.1.1(2)
BEARING STIFFENER

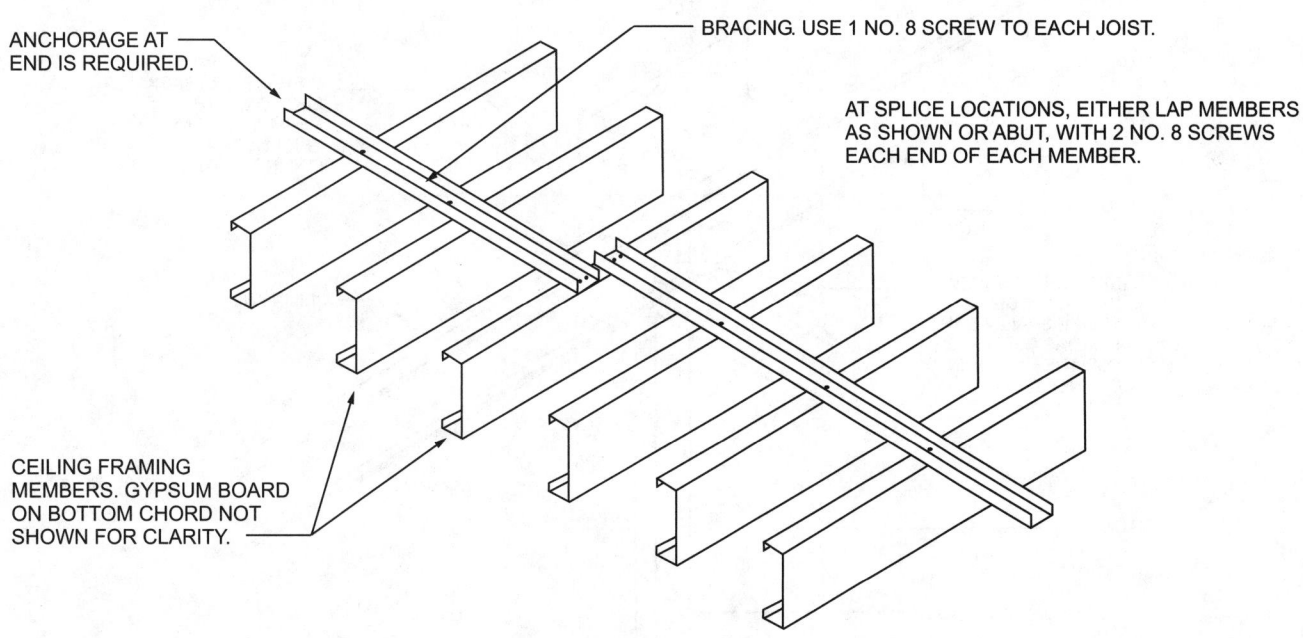

ANCHORAGE AT END IS REQUIRED.

BRACING. USE 1 NO. 8 SCREW TO EACH JOIST.

AT SPLICE LOCATIONS, EITHER LAP MEMBERS AS SHOWN OR ABUT, WITH 2 NO. 8 SCREWS EACH END OF EACH MEMBER.

CEILING FRAMING MEMBERS. GYPSUM BOARD ON BOTTOM CHORD NOT SHOWN FOR CLARITY.

FIGURE R804.3.1.4(1)
CEILING JOIST TOP FLANGE BRACING WITH C-SHAPE, TRACK OR COLD-ROLLED CHANNEL

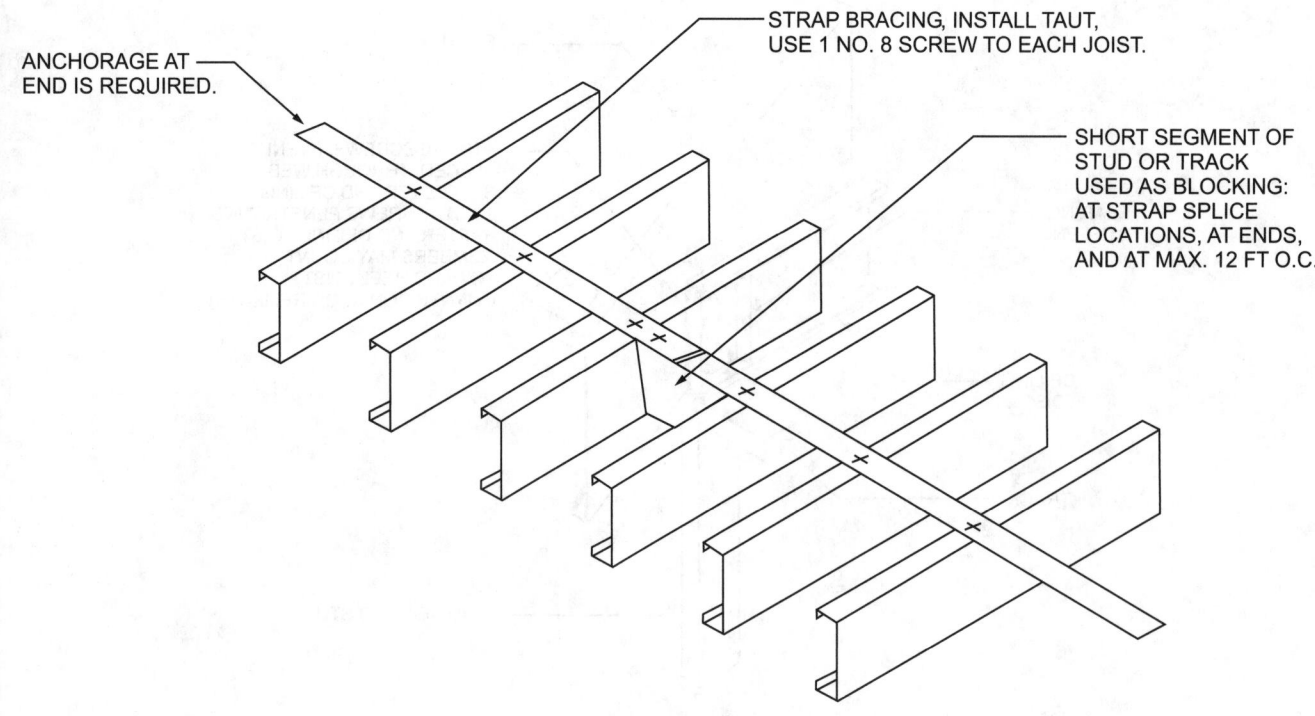

ANCHORAGE AT
END IS REQUIRED.

STRAP BRACING, INSTALL TAUT,
USE 1 NO. 8 SCREW TO EACH JOIST.

SHORT SEGMENT OF
STUD OR TRACK
USED AS BLOCKING:
AT STRAP SPLICE
LOCATIONS, AT ENDS,
AND AT MAX. 12 FT O.C.

For SI: 1 foot = 304.8 mm.

FIGURE R804.3.1.4(2)
CEILING JOIST TOP FLANGE BRACING WITH CONTINUOUS STEEL STRAP AND BLOCKING

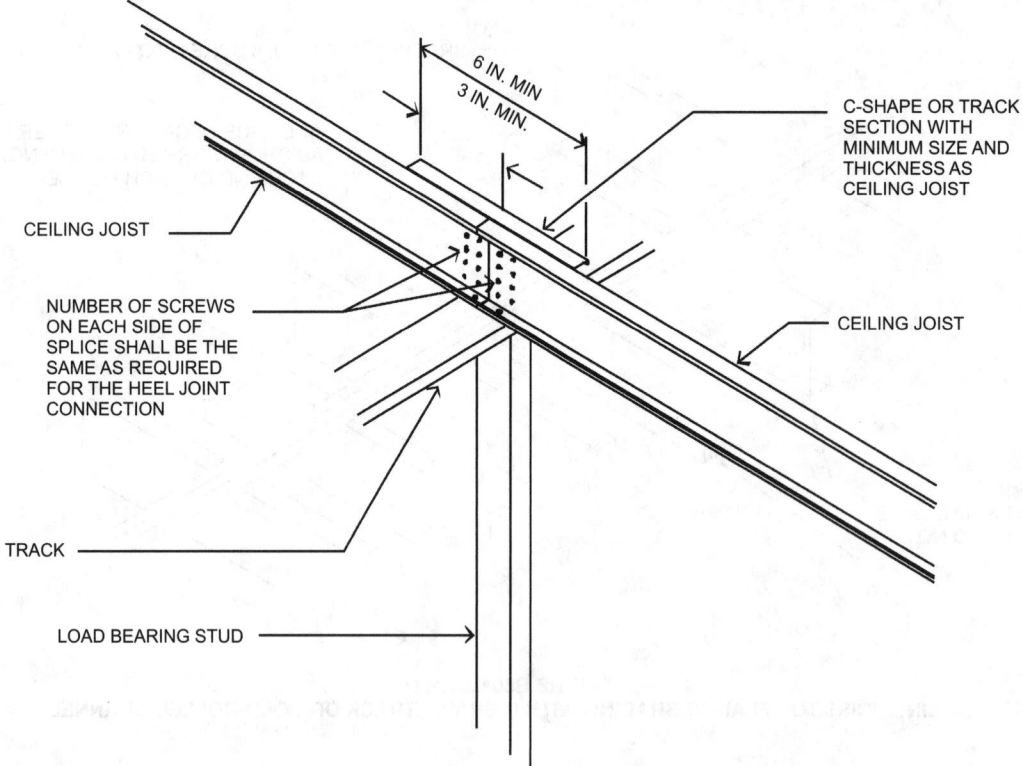

6 IN. MIN

3 IN. MIN.

C-SHAPE OR TRACK
SECTION WITH
MINIMUM SIZE AND
THICKNESS AS
CEILING JOIST

CEILING JOIST

NUMBER OF SCREWS
ON EACH SIDE OF
SPLICE SHALL BE THE
SAME AS REQUIRED
FOR THE HEEL JOINT
CONNECTION

CEILING JOIST

TRACK

LOAD BEARING STUD

For SI: 1 inch = 25.4 mm.

FIGURE R804.3.1.5
SPLICED CEILING JOISTS

TABLE R804.3.2.1(1)
ROOF RAFTER SPANS[a, b, c]
33 ksi STEEL

MEMBER DESIGNATION	ALLOWABLE SPAN MEASURED HORIZONTALLY (feet-inches)							
	Ground snow load (psf)							
	20		30		50		70	
	Rafter spacing (inches)							
	16	24	16	24	16	24	16	24
550S162-33	14'-0"	11'-6"	11'-11"	9'-7"	9'-6"	7'-9"	8'-2"	6'-8"
550S162-43	16'-8"	13'-11"	14'-5"	11'-9"	11'-6"	9'-5"	9'-10"	8'-0"
550S162-54	17'-11"	15'-7"	15'-7"	13'-3"	12'-11"	10'-7"	11'-1"	9'-1"
550S162-68	19'-2"	16'-9"	16'-9"	14'-7"	14'-1"	11'-10"	12'-6"	10'-2"
550S162-97	21'-3"	18'-6"	18'-6"	16'-2"	15'-8"	13'-8"	14'-0"	12'-2"
800S162-33	16'-5"	13'-5"	13'-11"	11'-4"	11'-1"	8'-2"	9'-0"	6'-0"
800S162-43	19'-9"	16'-1"	16'-8"	13'-7"	13'-4"	10'-10"	11'-5"	9'-4"
800S162-54	22'-8"	18'-6"	19'-2"	15'-8"	15'-4"	12'-6"	13'-1"	10'-8"
800S162-68	25'-10"	21'-2"	21'-11"	17'-10"	17'-6"	14'-4"	15'-0"	12'-3"
800S162-97	21'-3"	18'-6"	18'-6"	16'-2"	15'-8"	13'-8"	14'-0"	12'-2"
1000S162-43	22'-3"	18'-2"	18'-9"	15'-8"	15'-0"	12'-3"	12'-10"	10'-6"
1000S162-54	25'-8"	20'-11"	21'-8"	17'-9"	17'-4"	14'-2"	14'-10"	12'-1"
1000S162-68	29'-7"	24'-2"	25'-0"	20'-5"	20'-0"	16'-4"	17'-2"	14'-0"
1000S162-97	34'-8"	30'-4"	30'-4"	25'-10"	25'-3"	20'-8"	21'-8"	17'-8"
1200S162-54	28'-3"	23'-1"	23'-11"	19'-7"	19'-2"	15'-7"	16'-5"	13'-5"
1200S162-68	32'-10"	26'-10"	27'-9"	22'-8"	22'-2"	18'-1"	19'-0"	15'-6"
1200S162-97	40'-6"	33'-5"	34'-6"	28'-3"	27'-7"	22'-7"	23'-8"	19'-4"

For SI: 1 inch = 25.4 mm, 1 foot = 304.8 mm, 1 pound per square foot = 0.0479 kPa.

a. Table provides maximum horizontal rafter spans in feet and inches for slopes between 3:12 and 12:12.

b. Deflection criterion: $L/240$ for live loads and $L/180$ for total loads.

c. Roof dead load = 12 psf.

TABLE R804.3.2.1(2)
ROOF RAFTER SPANS[a, b, c]
50 ksi STEEL

MEMBER DESIGNATION	ALLOWABLE SPAN MEASURED HORIZONTALLY (feet-inches)							
	Equivalent ground snow load (psf)							
	20		30		50		70	
	Rafter spacing (inches)							
	16	24	16	24	16	24	16	24
550S162-33	15'-4"	12'-11"	13'-4"	10"-11"	10'-9"	8'-9"	9'-2"	7'-6"
550S162-43	16'-8"	14'-7"	14'-7"	12'-9"	12'-3"	10'-6"	11'-0"	9'-0"
550S162-54	17'-11"	15'-7"	15'-7"	13'-8"	13'-2"	11'-6"	11'-9"	10'-3"
550S162-68	19'-2"	16'-9"	16'-9"	14'-7"	14'-1"	12'-4"	12'-7"	11'-0"
550S162-97	21'-3"	18'-6"	18'-6"	16'-2"	15'-8"	13'-8"	14'-0"	12'-3"
800S162-33	18'-10"	15'-5"	15'-11"	12'-9"	12'-3"	8'-2"	9'-0"	6'-0"
800S162-43	22'-3"	18'-2"	18'-10"	15'-5"	15'-1"	12'-3"	12'-11"	10'-6"
800S162-54	24'-2"	21'-2"	21'-1"	18'-5"	17'-10"	14'-8"	15'-5"	12'-7"
800S162-68	25'-11"	22'-8"	22'-8"	19'-9"	19'-1"	16'-8"	17'-1"	14'-9"
800S162-97	28'-10"	25'-2"	25'-2"	22'-0"	21'-2"	18'-6"	19'-0"	16'-7"
1000S162-43	25'-2"	20'-7"	21'-4"	17'-5"	17'-0"	13'-11"	14'-7"	10'-7"
1000S162-54	29'-0"	24'-6"	25'-4"	20'-9"	20'-3"	16'-7"	17'-5"	14'-2"
1000S162-68	31'-2"	27'-3"	27'-3"	23'-9"	20'-0"	19'-6"	20'-6"	16'-8"
1000S162-97	34'-8"	30'-4"	30'-4"	26'-5"	25'-7"	22'-4"	22'-10"	20'-0"
1200S162-54	33'-2"	27'-1"	28'-1"	22'-11"	22'-5"	18'-4"	19'-3"	15'-8"
1200S162-68	36'-4"	31'-9"	31'-9"	27'-0"	26'-5"	21'-6"	22'-6"	18'-6"
1200S162-97	40'-6"	35'-4"	35'-4"	30'-11"	29'-10"	26'-1"	26'-8"	23'-1"

For SI: 1 inch = 25.4 mm, 1 foot = 304.8 mm, 1 pound per square foot = 0.0479 kPa.

a. Table provides maximum horizontal rafter spans in feet and inches for slopes between 3:12 and 12:12.

b. Deflection criterion: $L/240$ for live loads and $L/180$ for total loads.

c. Roof dead load = 12 psf.

TABLE R804.3.2.1(3)
BASIC WIND SPEED TO EQUIVALENT SNOW LOAD CONVERSION

BASIC WIND SPEED AND EXPOSURE		EQUIVALENT GROUND SNOW LOAD (psf)									
		Roof slope									
Exp. B	Exp. C	3:12	4:12	5:12	6:12	7:12	8:12	9:12	10:12	11:12	12:12
85 mph	—	20	20	20	20	20	20	30	30	30	30
100 mph	85 mph	20	20	20	20	30	30	30	30	50	50
110 mph	100 mph	20	20	20	20	30	50	50	50	50	50
—	110 mph	30	30	30	50	50	50	70	70	70	—

For SI: 1 mile per hour = 0.447 m/s, 1 pound per square foot = 0.0479 kPa.

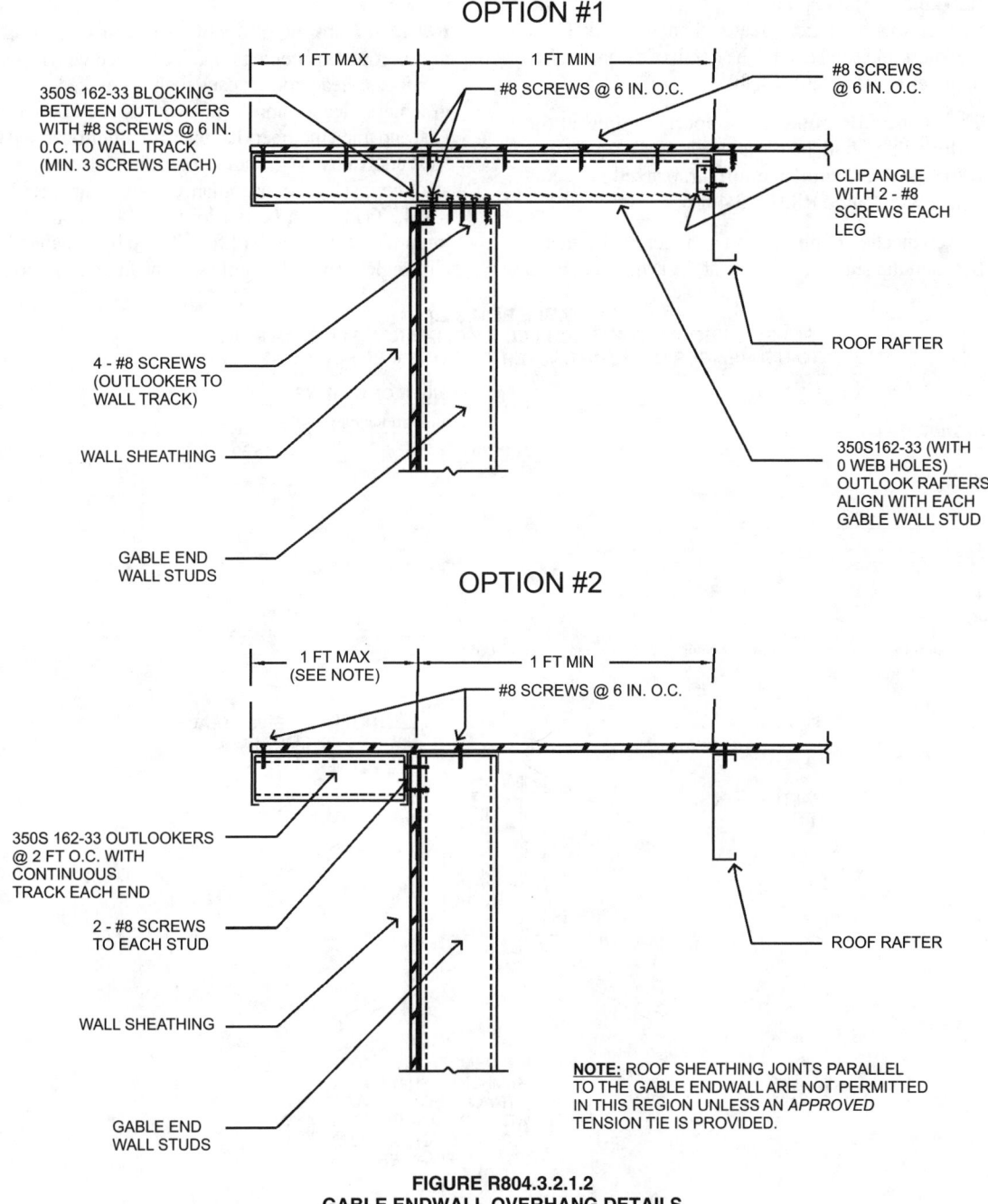

OPTION #1

1 FT MAX — 1 FT MIN

350S 162-33 BLOCKING BETWEEN OUTLOOKERS WITH #8 SCREWS @ 6 IN. O.C. TO WALL TRACK (MIN. 3 SCREWS EACH)

#8 SCREWS @ 6 IN. O.C.

#8 SCREWS @ 6 IN. O.C.

CLIP ANGLE WITH 2 - #8 SCREWS EACH LEG

4 - #8 SCREWS (OUTLOOKER TO WALL TRACK)

ROOF RAFTER

WALL SHEATHING

350S162-33 (WITH 0 WEB HOLES) OUTLOOK RAFTERS ALIGN WITH EACH GABLE WALL STUD

GABLE END WALL STUDS

OPTION #2

1 FT MAX (SEE NOTE) — 1 FT MIN

#8 SCREWS @ 6 IN. O.C.

350S 162-33 OUTLOOKERS @ 2 FT O.C. WITH CONTINUOUS TRACK EACH END

2 - #8 SCREWS TO EACH STUD

ROOF RAFTER

WALL SHEATHING

GABLE END WALL STUDS

NOTE: ROOF SHEATHING JOINTS PARALLEL TO THE GABLE ENDWALL ARE NOT PERMITTED IN THIS REGION UNLESS AN *APPROVED* TENSION TIE IS PROVIDED.

FIGURE R804.3.2.1.2
GABLE ENDWALL OVERHANG DETAILS

R804.3.3.4 Hip framing connections. Hip rafter framing connections shall be installed in accordance with the following:

1. Jack rafters shall be connected at the eave to a parallel C-shape blocking member in accordance with Figure R804.3.3.4(1). The C-shape blocking member shall be attached to the supporting wall track with minimum two No. 10 screws.

2. Jack rafters shall be connected to a hip member with a minimum 2 inch × 2 inch (51 mm × 51 mm) clip angle fastened with No. 10 screws to the hip member in accordance with Figure R804.3.2.1.2 and Table R804.3.2.4. The clip angle shall have a steel thickness equivalent to or greater than the jack rafter thickness and shall extend the depth of the jack rafter member to the extent possible.

3. The connection of the hip support columns at the ceiling line shall be in accordance with Figure R804.3.3.4(2), with an uplift strap sized in accordance with Table R804.3.3.4(1).

4. The connection of hip support members, ridge members and hip support columns at the ridge shall be in accordance with Figures R804.3.3.4(3) and R804.3.3.4(4) and Table R804.3.3.4(2).

5. The connection of hip members to the wall corner shall be in accordance with Figure R804.3.3.4(5) and Table R804.3.3.4(3).

R804.3.4 Cutting and notching. Flanges and lips of load-bearing cold-formed steel roof framing members shall not be cut or notched.

R804.3.5 Headers. Roof-ceiling framing above wall openings shall be supported on headers. The allowable spans for headers in load-bearing walls shall not exceed the values set forth in Section R603.6 and Tables R603.6(1) through R603.6(24).

R804.3.6 Framing of openings in roofs and ceilings. Openings in roofs and ceilings shall be framed with header and trimmer joists. Header joist spans shall not exceed 4 feet (1219 mm) in length. Header and trimmer joists shall be fabricated from joist and track members having a minimum size and thickness at least equivalent to the adjacent ceiling joists or roof rafters and shall be installed in accordance with Figures R804.3.6(1) and R804.3.6(2). Each header joist shall be connected to trimmer joists with a minimum of four 2-inch by 2-inch (51 by 51 mm) clip angles. Each clip angle shall be fastened to both the header

TABLE R804.3.2.4
SCREWS REQUIRED AT EACH LEG OF CLIP ANGLE FOR HIP RAFTER
TO HIP MEMBER OR ROOF RAFTER TO RIDGE MEMBER CONNECTION[a]

BUILDING WIDTH (feet)	NUMBER OF SCREWS			
	Ground snow load (psf)			
	0 to 20	21 to 30	31 to 50	51 to 70
24	2	2	3	4
28	2	3	4	5
32	2	3	4	5
36	3	3	5	6
40	3	4	5	7

For SI: 1 inch = 25.4 mm, 1 foot = 304.8 mm, 1 pound per square foot = 0.0479 kPa.
a. Screws shall be No. 10 minimum.

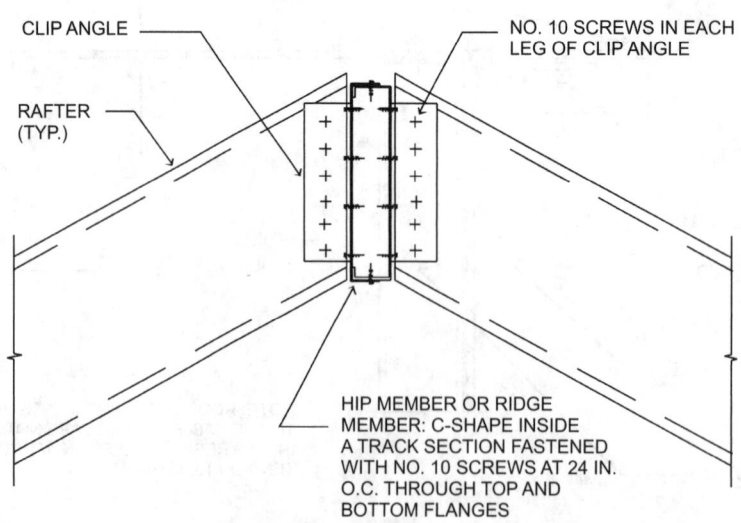

FIGURE R804.3.2.4
HIP MEMBER OR RIDGE MEMBER CONNECTION

and trimmer joists with four No. 8 screws, evenly spaced, through each leg of the clip angle. The steel thickness of the clip angles shall be not less than that of the ceiling joist or roof rafter. Each track section for a built-up header or trimmer joist shall extend the full length of the joist (continuous).

R804.3.7 Roof trusses. Cold-formed steel trusses shall be designed and installed in accordance with AISI S100, Section D4. Trusses shall be connected to the top track of the load-bearing wall in accordance with Table R804.3, either with two No.10 screws applied through the flange of the truss or by using a 54 mil (1.37 mm) clip angle with two No.10 screws in each leg.

R804.3.8 Ceiling and roof diaphragms. Ceiling and roof diaphragms shall be in accordance with this section.

R804.3.8.1 At gable endwalls a ceiling *diaphragm* shall be provided by attaching a minimum $^1/_2$-inch (12.7 mm) gypsum board in accordance with Tables R804.3.8(1) and R804.3.8(2) or a minimum $^3/_8$-inch (9.5 mm) wood structural panel sheathing, which complies with Section R803, in accordance with Table R804.6(3) to the bottom of ceiling joists or roof trusses and connected to wall framing in accordance with Figures R804.3.8(1) and R804.3.8(2), unless studs are designed as full height without bracing at the ceiling. Flat blocking shall consist of C-shape or track section with a minimum thickness of 33 mils (0.84 mm).

The ceiling *diaphragm* shall be secured with screws spaced at a maximum 6 inches (152 mm) o.c. at panel edges and a maximum 12 inches (305 mm) o.c. in the field. Multiplying the required lengths in Tables R804.3.8(1) and R804.3.8(2) for gypsum board sheathed ceiling diaphragms shall be permitted to be multiplied by 0.35 shall be permitted if all panel edges are blocked. Multiplying the required lengths in Tables R804.3.8(1) and R804.3.8(2) for gypsum board sheathed ceiling diaphragms by 0.9 shall be permitted if all panel edges are secured with screws spaced at 4 inches (102 mm) o.c.

R804.3.8.2 Roof diaphragm. A roof *diaphragm* shall be provided by attaching a minimum of $^3/_8$ inch (9.5 mm) wood structural panel which complies with Section R803 to roof rafters or truss top chords in accordance with Table R804.3. Buildings with 3:1 or larger plan *aspect ratio* and with roof rafter slope (pitch) of 9:12 or larger shall have the roof rafters and ceiling joists blocked in accordance with Figure R804.3.8(3).

R804.3.9 Roof tie-down. Roof assemblies subject to wind uplift pressures of 20 pounds per square foot (0.96 kPa) or greater, as established in Table R301.2(2), shall have rafter-to-bearing wall ties provided in accordance with Table R802.11.

TABLE R804.3.3.2
HIP MEMBER SIZES, 33 ksi STEEL

| BUILDING WIDTH (feet) | HIP MEMBER DESIGNATION[a] | | | |
| | Equivalent ground snow load (psf) | | | |
	0 to 20	21 to 30	31 to 50	51 to 70
24	800S162-68 800T150-68	800S162-68 800T150-68	800S162-97 800T150-97	1000S162-97 1000T150-97
28	1000S162-68 1000T150-68	1000S162-68 1000T150-68	1000S162-97 1000T150-97	1200S162-97 1200T150-97
32	1000S162-97 1000T150-97	1000S162-97 1000T150-97	1200S162-97 1200T150-97	—
36	1200S162-97 1200T150-97	—	—	—
40	—	—	—	—

For SI: 1 foot = 304.8 mm, 1 pound per square foot = 0.0479 kPa.

a. The web depth of the roof rafters and jack rafters is to match at the hip or they shall be installed in accordance with an approved design.

TABLE R804.3.3.3
HIP SUPPORT COLUMN SIZES

| BUILDING WIDTH (feet) | HIP SUPPORT COLUMN DESIGNATION[a, b] | | | |
| | Equivalent ground snow load (psf) | | | |
	0 to 20	21 to 30	31 to 50	51 to 70
24	2-350S162-33	2-350S162-33	2-350S162-43	2-350S162-54
28	2-350S162-54	2-550S162-54	2-550S162-68	2-550S162-68
32	2-550S162-68	2-550S162-68	2-550S162-97	—
36	2-550S162-97	—	—	—
40	—	—	—	—

For SI: 1 foot = 304,8 mm, 1 pound per square foot = 0.0479 kPa.

a. Box shape column only in accordance with Figure R804.3.3.4(2).

b. 33 ksi steel for 33 and 43 mil material; 50 ksi steel for thicker material.

TABLE R804.3.3.4(1)
UPLIFT STRAP CONNECTION REQUIREMENTS
HIP SUPPORT COLUMN AT CEILING LINE

BUILDING WIDTH (feet)	BASIC WIND SPEED (mph) EXPOSURE B				
	85	100	110	—	—
	BASIC WIND SPEED (mph) EXPOSURE C				
	—	85	—	100	110
	Number of No. 10 screws in each end of each 3 inch by 54-mil steel strap[a, b, c]				
24	3	4	4	6	7
28	4	6	6	8	10
32	5	8	8	11	13
36	7	10	11	14	17
40	—	—	—	—	—

For SI: 1 foot = 304.8 mm, 1 pound per square foot = 0.0479 kPa, 1 mil = 0.0254 mm.

a. Two straps are required, one each side of the column.
b. Space screws at $^3/_4$ inch on-center and provide $^3/_4$ inch end distance.
c. 50 ksi steel strap.

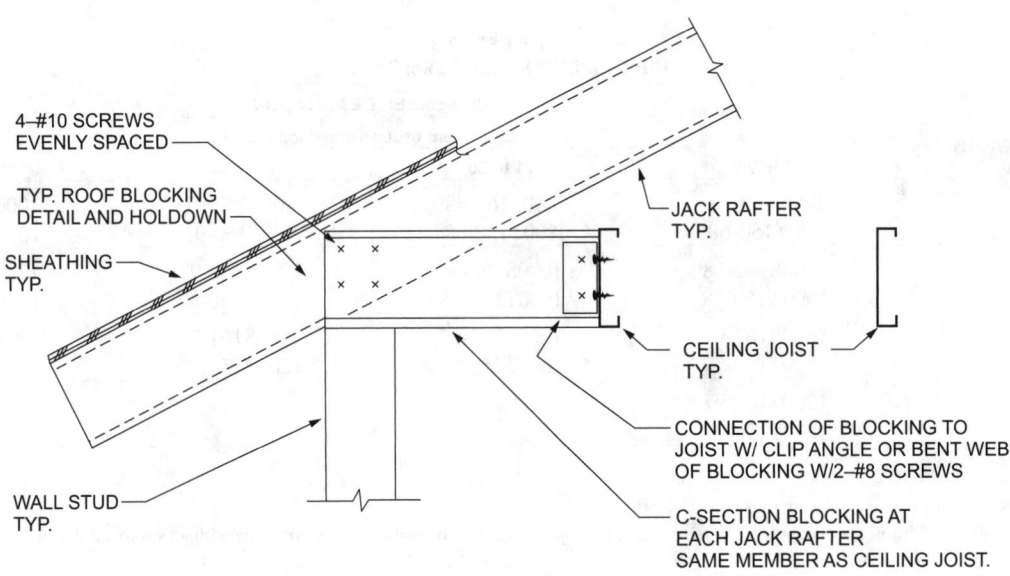

FIGURE R804.3.3.4(1)
JACK RAFTER CONNECTION AT EAVE

TABLE R804.3.3.4(2)
CONNECTION REQUIREMENTS
HIP MEMBER TO HIP SUPPORT COLUMN

BUILDING WIDTH (feet)	NUMBER OF NO. 10 SCREWS IN EACH FRAMING ANGLE[a, b, c]			
	Equivalent ground snow load (psf)			
	0 to 20	21 to 30	31 to 50	51 to 70
24	10	10	10	12
28	10	10	14	18
32	10	12	—	—
36	14	—	—	—
40	—	—	—	—

For SI: 1 foot = 304.8 mm, 1 pound per square foot = 0.0479 kPa.

a. Screws to be divided equally between the connection to the hip member and the column. Refer to Figures R804.3.3.4(3) and R804.3.3.4(4).

b. The number of screws required in each framing angle is not to be less than shown in Table R804.3.3.4(1).

c. 50 ksi steel from the framing angle.

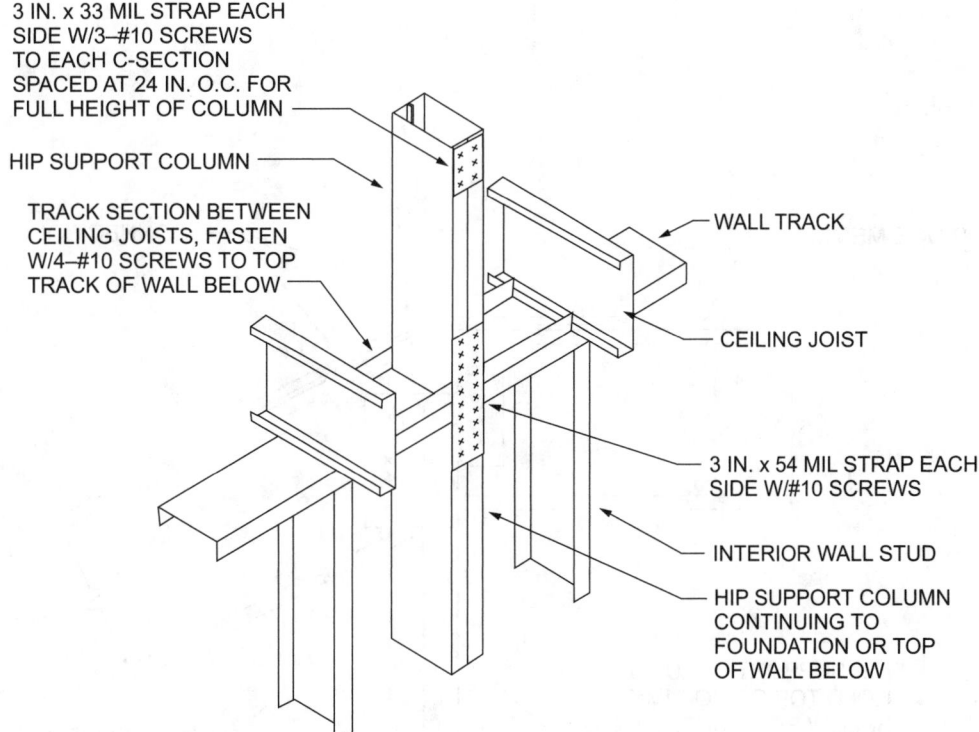

3 IN. x 33 MIL STRAP EACH SIDE W/3–#10 SCREWS TO EACH C-SECTION SPACED AT 24 IN. O.C. FOR FULL HEIGHT OF COLUMN

HIP SUPPORT COLUMN

TRACK SECTION BETWEEN CEILING JOISTS, FASTEN W/4–#10 SCREWS TO TOP TRACK OF WALL BELOW

WALL TRACK

CEILING JOIST

3 IN. x 54 MIL STRAP EACH SIDE W/#10 SCREWS

INTERIOR WALL STUD

HIP SUPPORT COLUMN CONTINUING TO FOUNDATION OR TOP OF WALL BELOW

For SI: 1 inch = 25.4 mm, 1 mil = 0.0254 mm.

FIGURE R804.3.3.4(2)
HIP SUPPORT COLUMN

TABLE R804.3.3.4(3)
UPLIFT STRAP CONNECTION REQUIREMENTS
HIP MEMBER TO WALL

BUILDING WIDTH (feet)	BASIC WIND SPEED (mph) EXPOSURE B				
	85	100	110	—	—
	BASIC WIND SPEED (mph) EXPOSURE C				
	—	85	—	100	110
	Number of No. 10 screws in each end of each 3 inch by 54-mil Steel strap[a, b, c]				
24	2	2	3	3	4
28	2	3	3	4	5
32	3	4	4	6	7
36	3	5	5	7	8
40	—	—	—	—	—

For SI: 1 foot = 304.8 mm, 1 pound per square foot = 0.0479 kPa.

a. Two straps are required, one each side of the column.

b. Space screws at $^3/_4$ inches on-center and provide $^3/_4$ inch end distance.

c. 50 ksi steel strap.

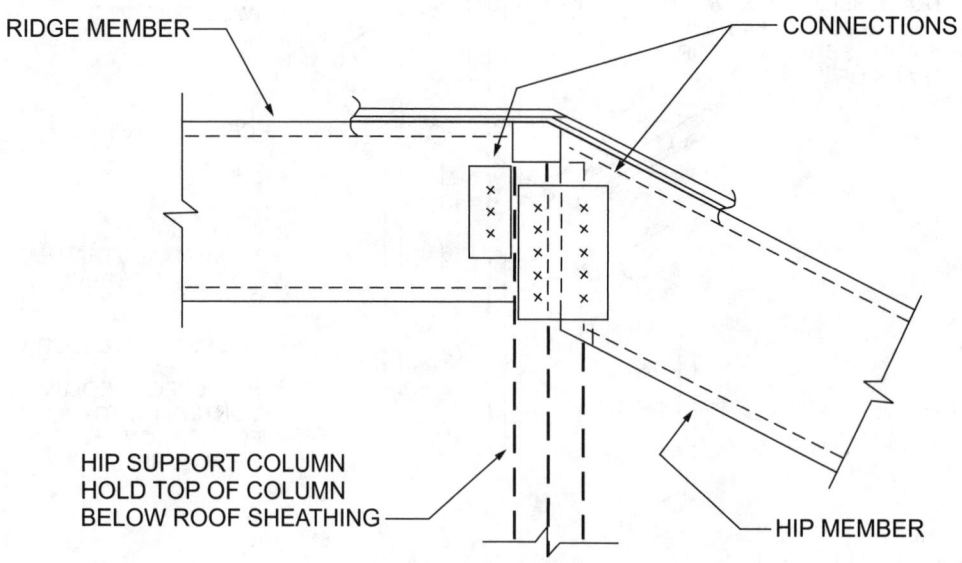

FIGURE R804.3.3.4(3)
HIP CONNECTIONS AT RIDGE

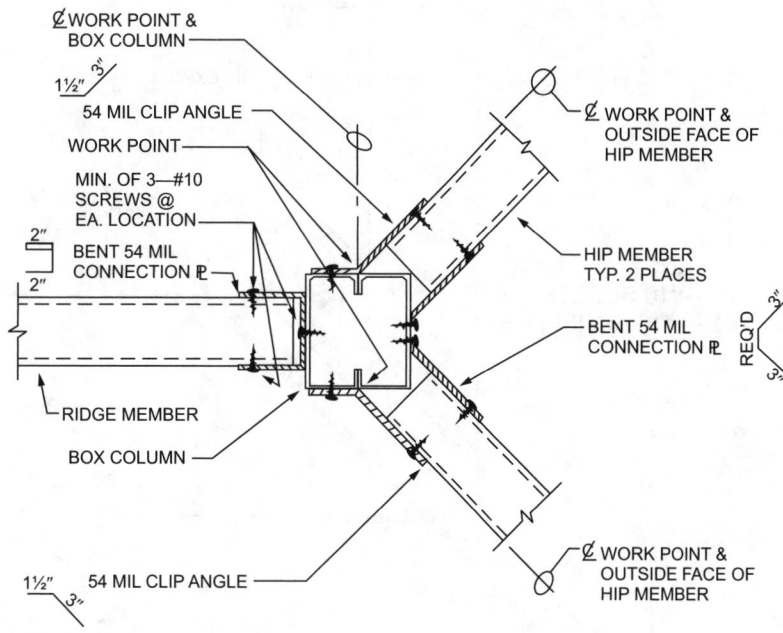

NOTE: RAFTERS NOT SHOWN FOR CLARITY

CONNECTION @ 3½″ BOX COLUMN

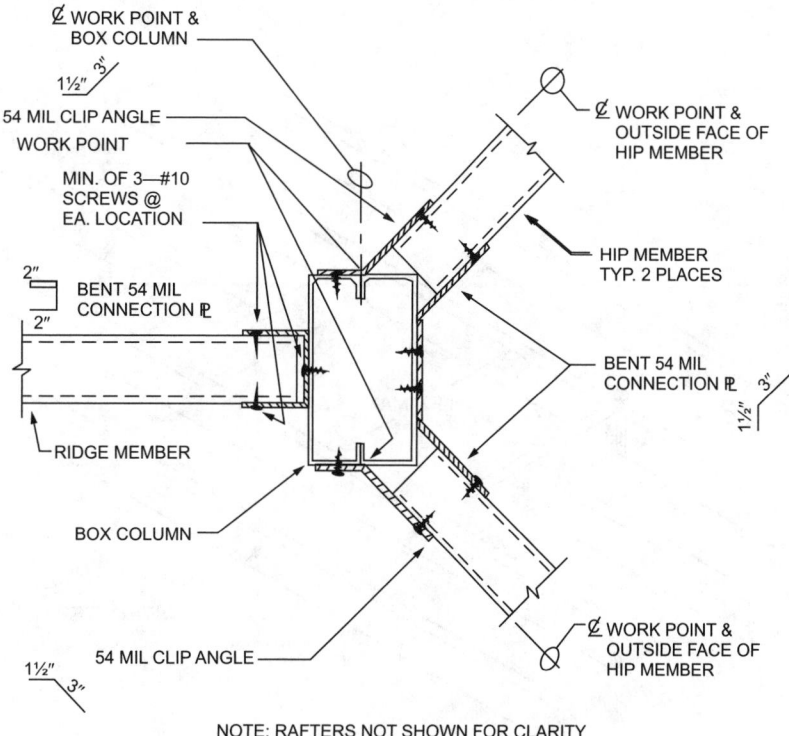

NOTE: RAFTERS NOT SHOWN FOR CLARITY

CONNECTION @ 5½″ BOX COLUMN

For SI: 1 inch = 25.4 mm, 1 mil = 0.0254 mm.

FIGURE R804.3.3.4(4)
HIP CONNECTIONS AT RIDGE AND BOX COLUMN

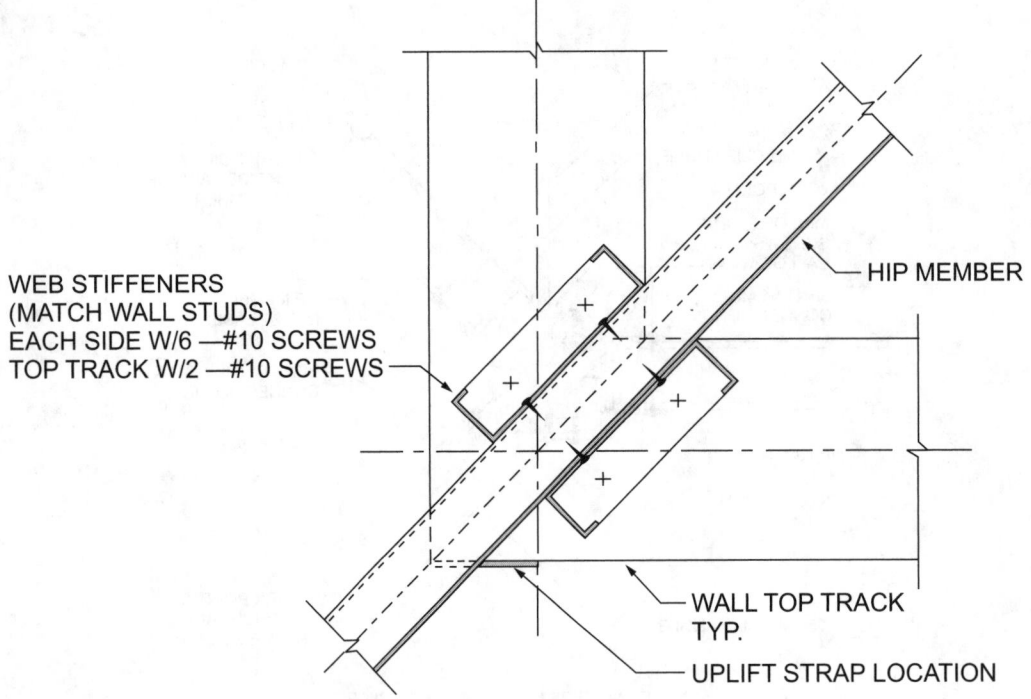

WEB STIFFENERS
(MATCH WALL STUDS)
EACH SIDE W/6 —#10 SCREWS
TOP TRACK W/2 —#10 SCREWS

HIP MEMBER

WALL TOP TRACK
TYP.

UPLIFT STRAP LOCATION

FIGURE R804.3.3.4(5)
HIP MEMBER CONNECTION AT WALL CORNER

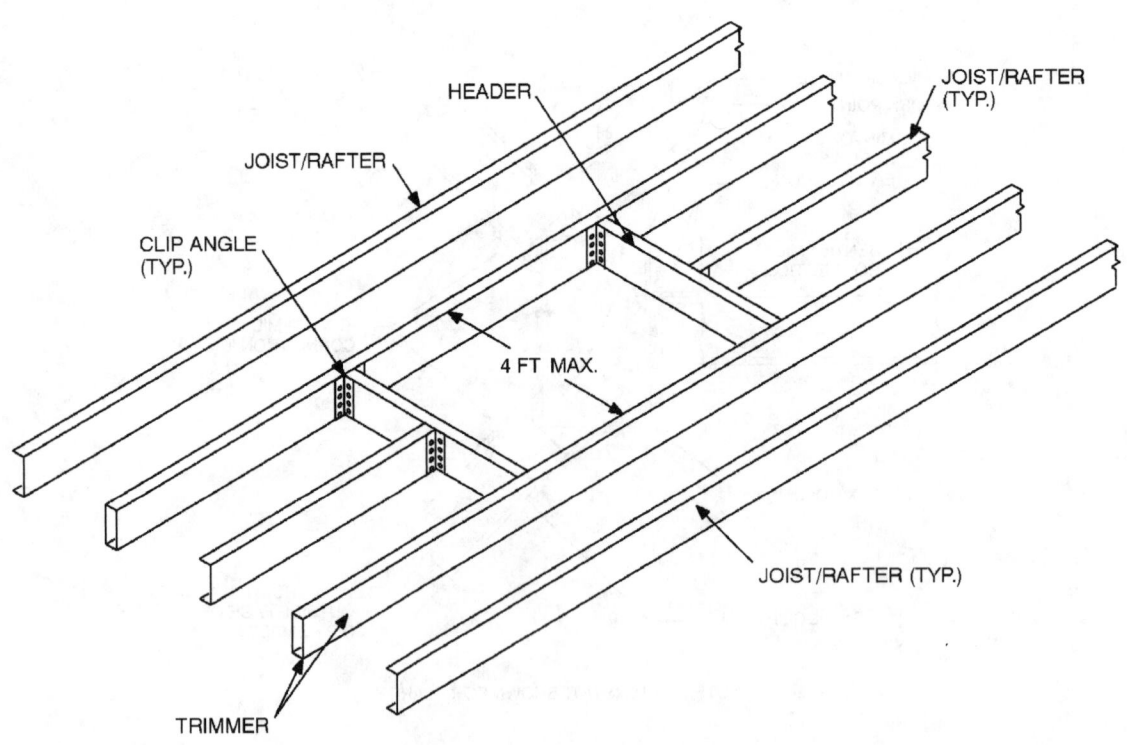

HEADER

JOIST/RAFTER
(TYP.)

JOIST/RAFTER

CLIP ANGLE
(TYP.)

4 FT MAX.

JOIST/RAFTER (TYP.)

TRIMMER

For SI: 1 foot = 304.8 mm.

FIGURE R804.3.6(1)
ROOF OR CEILING OPENING

2009 INTERNATIONAL RESIDENTIAL CODE®

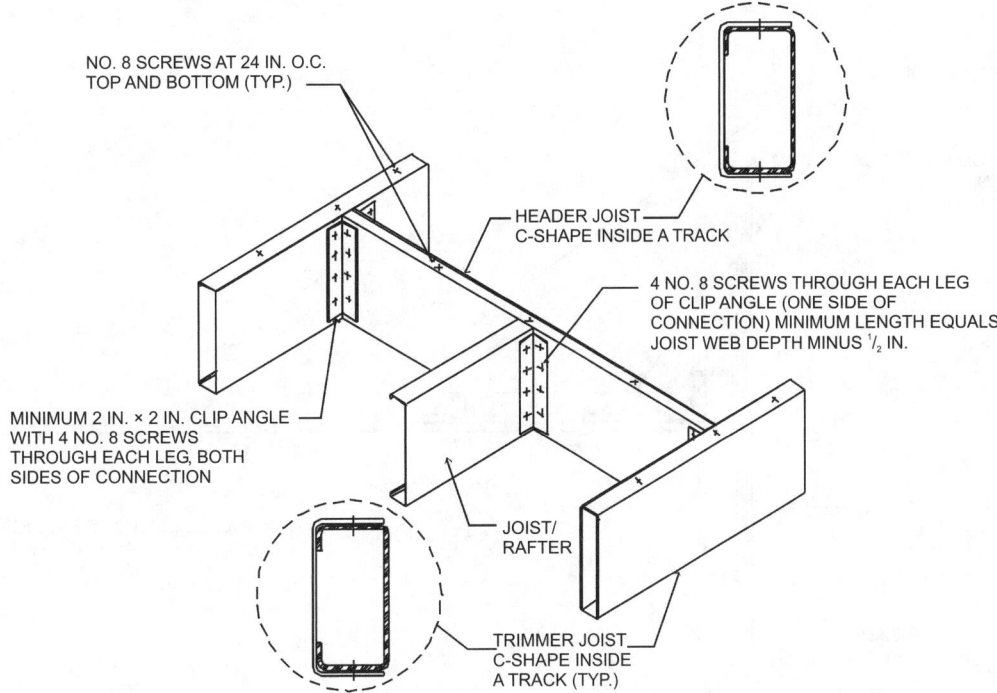

NO. 8 SCREWS AT 24 IN. O.C.
TOP AND BOTTOM (TYP.)

HEADER JOIST
C-SHAPE INSIDE A TRACK

4 NO. 8 SCREWS THROUGH EACH LEG
OF CLIP ANGLE (ONE SIDE OF
CONNECTION) MINIMUM LENGTH EQUALS
JOIST WEB DEPTH MINUS $1/2$ IN.

MINIMUM 2 IN. × 2 IN. CLIP ANGLE
WITH 4 NO. 8 SCREWS
THROUGH EACH LEG, BOTH
SIDES OF CONNECTION

JOIST/
RAFTER

TRIMMER JOIST
C-SHAPE INSIDE
A TRACK (TYP.)

For SI: 1 inch = 25.4 mm.

FIGURE R804.3.6(2)
HEADER TO TRIMMER CONNECTION

TABLE R804.3.8(1)
REQUIRED LENGTHS FOR CEILING DIAPHRAGMS AT GABLE ENDWALLS
GYPSUM BOARD SHEATHED, CEILING HEIGHT = 8 FT [a, b, c, d, e, f]

		BASIC WIND SPEED (mph)				
Exposure B		85	100	110	—	—
Exposure C		—	85	—	100	110
Roof pitch	**Building endwall width (feet)**	Minimum diaphragm length (feet)				
3:12 to 6:12	24 - 28	14	20	22	28	32
	28 - 32	16	22	28	32	38
	32 - 36	20	26	32	38	44
	36 - 40	22	30	36	44	50
6:12 to 9:12	24 - 28	16	22	26	32	36
	28 - 32	20	26	32	38	44
	32 - 36	22	32	38	44	52
	36 - 40	26	36	44	52	60
9:12 to 12:12	24 - 28	18	26	30	36	42
	28 - 32	22	30	36	42	50
	32 - 36	26	36	42	50	60
	36 - 40	30	42	50	60	70

For SI: 1 inch = 25.4 mm, 1 pound per square foot = 0.0479 kPa, 1 mile per hour = 0.447 m/s, 1 foot = 304.8 mm, 1 mil = 0.0254 mm.

a. Ceiling diaphragm is composed of $1/2$ inch gypsum board (min. thickness) secured with screws spaced at 6 inches o.c. at panel edges and 12 inches o.c. in field. Use No. 8 screws (min.) when framing members have a designation thickness of 54 mils or less and No. 10 screws (min.) when framing members have a designation thickness greater than 54 mils.

b. Maximum aspect ratio (length/width) of diaphragms is 2:1.

c. Building width is in the direction of horizontal framing members supported by the wall studs.

d. Required diaphragm lengths are to be provided at each end of the structure.

e. Multiplying required diaphragm lengths by 0.35 is permitted if all panel edges are blocked.

f. Multiplying required diaphragm lengths by 0.9 is permitted if all panel edges are secured with screws spaced at 4 inches o.c.

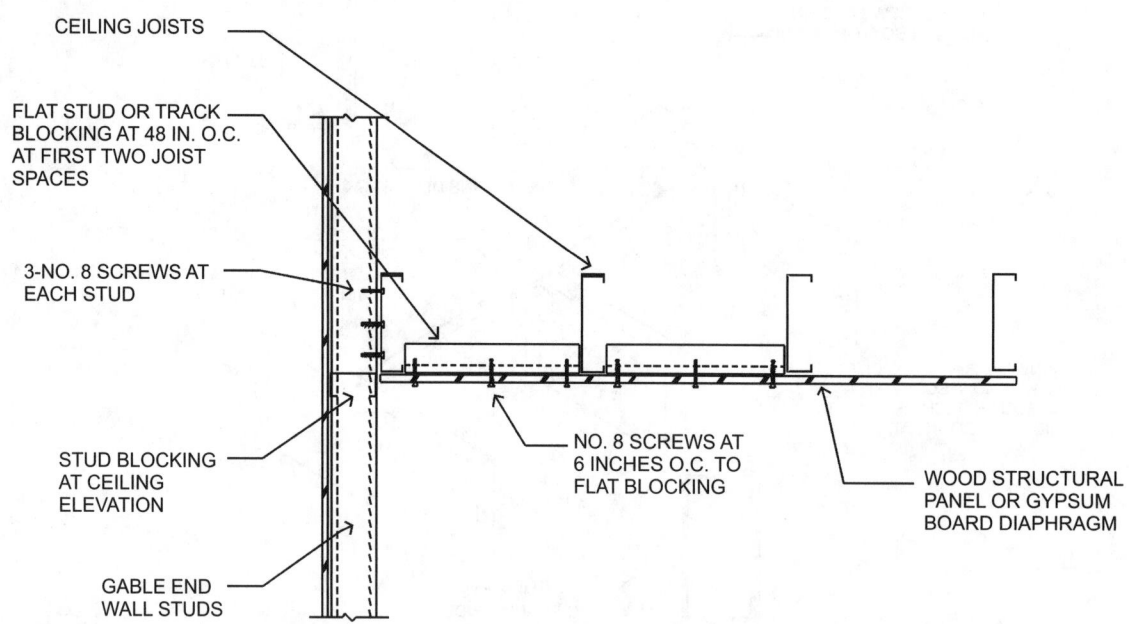

For SI: 1 inch = 25.4 mm.

FIGURE R804.3.8(1)
CEILING DIAPHRAGM TO GABLE ENDWALL DETAIL

TABLE R804.3.8(2)
REQUIRED LENGTHS FOR CEILING DIAPHRAGMS AT GABLE ENDWALLS
GYPSUM BOARD SHEATHED
CEILING HEIGHT = 9 OR 10 FT[a, b, c, d, e, f]

		BASIC WIND SPEED (mph)				
Exposure B		85	100	110	—	—
Exposure C		—	85	—	100	110
Roof pitch	**Building endwall width (feet)**	Minimum diaphragm length (feet)				
3:12 to 6:12	24 - 28	16	22	26	32	38
	28 - 32	20	26	32	38	44
	32 - 36	22	30	36	44	50
	36 - 40	26	36	42	50	58
6:12 to 9:12	24 - 28	18	26	30	36	42
	28 - 32	22	30	36	42	50
	32 - 36	26	36	42	50	58
	36 - 40	30	42	48	58	68
9:12 to 12:12	24 - 28	20	28	34	40	46
	28 - 32	24	34	40	48	56
	32 - 36	28	40	48	56	66
	36 - 40	34	46	56	66	78

For SI: 1 inch = 25.4 mm, 1 pound per square foot = 0.0479 kPa, 1 mph = 0.447 m/s, 1 foot = 304.8 mm, 1 mil = 0.0254 mm.

a. Ceiling diaphragm is composed of $^1/_2$ inch gypsum board (min. thickness) secured with screws spaced at 6 inches o.c. at panel edges and 12 inches o.c. in field. Use No. 8 screws (min.) when framing members have a designation thickness of 54 mils or less and No. 10 screws (min.) when framing members have a designation thickness greater than 54 mils.

b. Maximum aspect ratio (length/width) of diaphragms is 2:1.

c. Building width is in the direction of horizontal framing members supported by the wall studs.

d. Required diaphragm lengths are to be provided at each end of the structure.

e. Required diaphragm lengths are permitted to be multiplied by 0.35 if all panel edges are blocked.

f. Required diaphragm lengths are permitted to be multiplied by 0.9 if all panel edges are secured with screws spaced at 4 inches o.c.

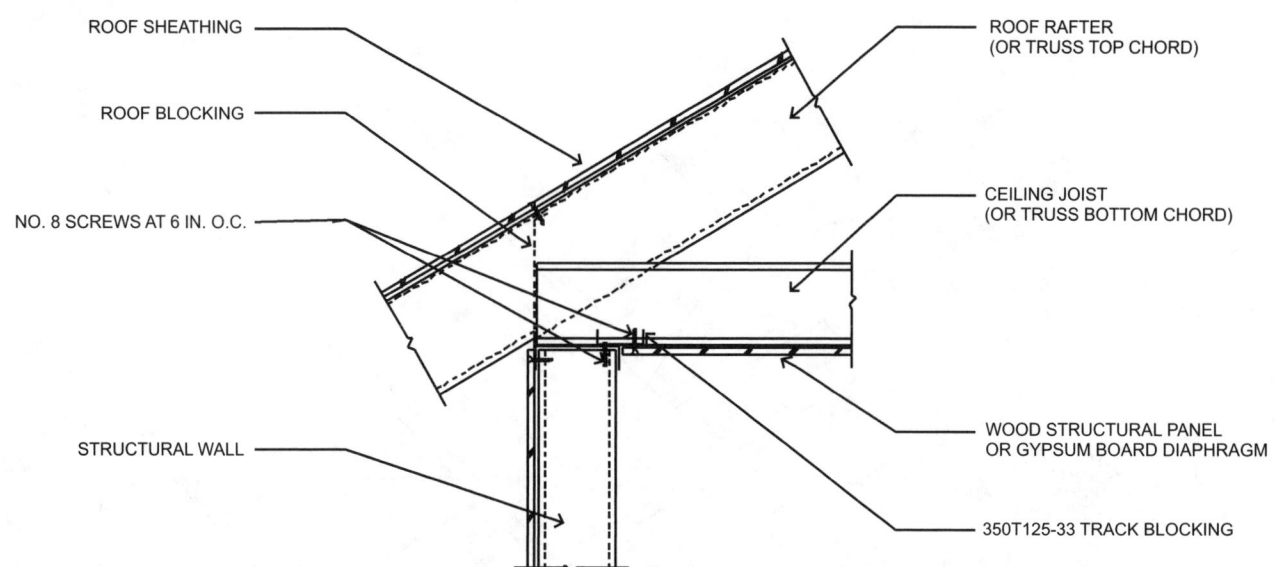

For SI: 1 inch = 25.4 mm.

FIGURE R804.3.8(2)
CEILING DIAPHRAGM TO SIDEWALL DETAIL

TABLE R804.3.8(3)
REQUIRED LENGTHS FOR CEILING DIAPHRAGMS AT GABLE ENDWALLS
WOOD STRUCTURAL PANEL SHEATHED
CEILING HEIGHT = 8, 9 OR 10 FT[a, b, c, d]

		BASIC WIND SPEED (mph)				
Exposure B		85	100	110	—	—
Exposure C		—	85	—	100	110
Roof pitch	**Building endwall width (feet)**	Minimum diaphragm length (feet)				
3:12 to 6:12	24 - 28	10	10	10	10	10
	28 - 32	12	12	12	12	12
	32 - 36	12	12	12	12	12
	36 - 40	14	14	14	14	14
6:12 to 9:12	24 - 28	10	10	10	10	10
	28 - 32	12	12	12	12	12
	32 - 36	12	12	12	12	12
	36 - 40	14	14	14	14	14
9:12 to 12:12	24 - 28	10	10	10	10	10
	28 - 32	12	12	12	12	12
	32 - 36	12	12	12	12	12
	36 - 40	14	14	14	14	14

For SI: 1 inch = 25.4 mm, 1 pound per square foot = 0.0479 kPa, 1 mile per hour = 0.447 m/s, 1 foot = 304.8 mm, 1 mil = 0.0254 mm.

a. Ceiling diaphragm is composed of $^3/_8$ inch wood structural panel sheathing (min. thickness) secured with screws spaced at 6 inches o.c. at panel edges and in field. Use No. 8 screws (min.) when framing members have a designation thickness of 54 mils or less and No. 10 screws (min.) when framing members have a designation thickness greater than 54 mils.

b. Maximum aspect ratio (length/width) of diaphragms is 3:1.

c. Building width is in the direction of horizontal framing members supported by the wall studs.

d. Required diaphragm lengths are to be provided at each end of the structure.

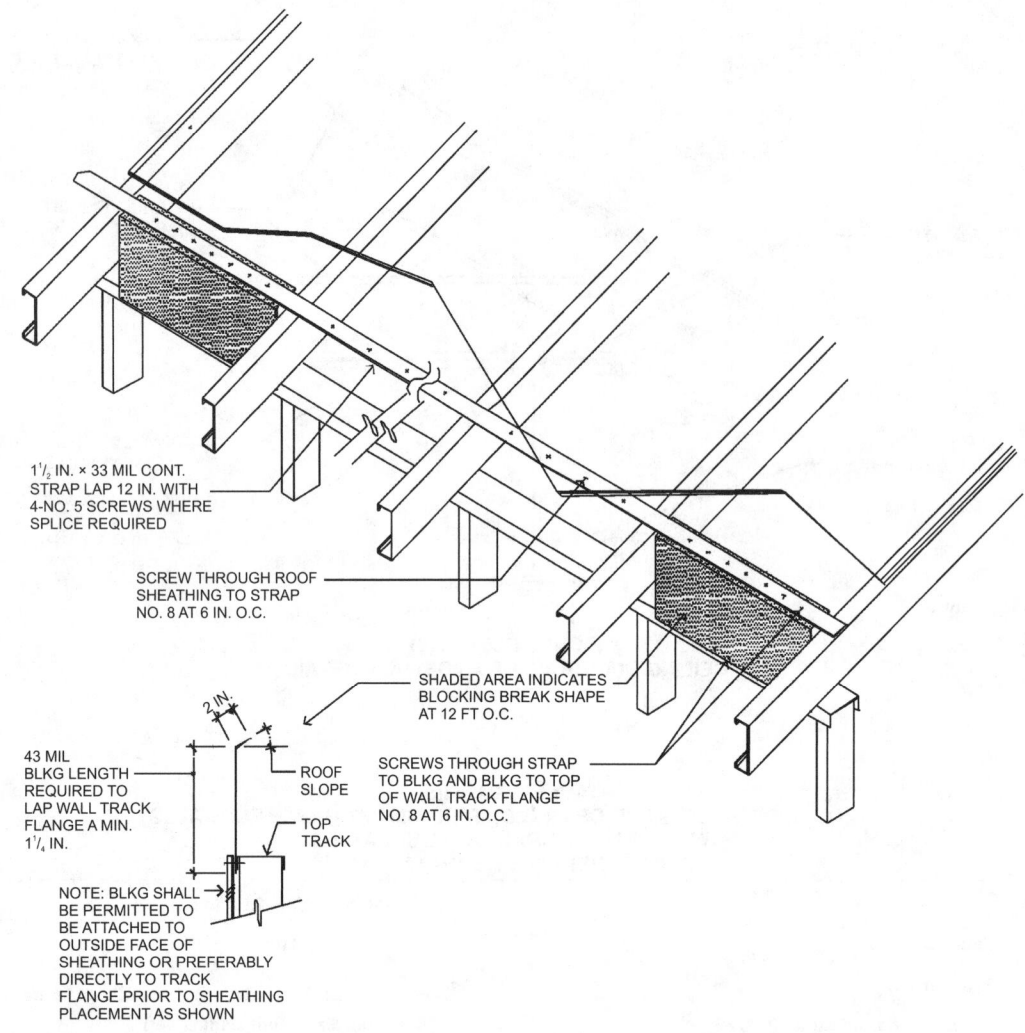

1¹/₂ IN. × 33 MIL CONT.
STRAP LAP 12 IN. WITH
4-NO. 5 SCREWS WHERE
SPLICE REQUIRED

SCREW THROUGH ROOF
SHEATHING TO STRAP
NO. 8 AT 6 IN. O.C.

SHADED AREA INDICATES
BLOCKING BREAK SHAPE
AT 12 FT O.C.

2 IN.

43 MIL
BLKG LENGTH
REQUIRED TO
LAP WALL TRACK
FLANGE A MIN.
1¹/₄ IN.

ROOF
SLOPE

TOP
TRACK

SCREWS THROUGH STRAP
TO BLKG AND BLKG TO TOP
OF WALL TRACK FLANGE
NO. 8 AT 6 IN. O.C.

NOTE: BLKG SHALL
BE PERMITTED TO
BE ATTACHED TO
OUTSIDE FACE OF
SHEATHING OR PREFERABLY
DIRECTLY TO TRACK
FLANGE PRIOR TO SHEATHING
PLACEMENT AS SHOWN

For SI: 1 mil = 0.0254 mm, 1 inch = 25.4 mm.

FIGURE R804.3.8(3)
ROOF BLOCKING DETAIL

SECTION R805
CEILING FINISHES

R805.1 Ceiling installation. Ceilings shall be installed in accordance with the requirements for interior wall finishes as provided in Section R702.

SECTION R806
ROOF VENTILATION

R806.1 Ventilation required. Enclosed *attics* and enclosed rafter spaces formed where ceilings are applied directly to the underside of roof rafters shall have cross ventilation for each separate space by ventilating openings protected against the entrance of rain or snow. Ventilation openings shall have a least dimension of ¹/₁₆ inch (1.6 mm) minimum and ¹/₄ inch (6.4 mm) maximum. Ventilation openings having a least dimension larger than ¹/₄ inch (6.4 mm) shall be provided with corrosion-resistant wire cloth screening, hardware cloth, or similar material with openings having a least dimension of ¹/₁₆ inch (1.6 mm) mini-

mum and ¹/₄ inch (6.4 mm) maximum. Openings in roof framing members shall conform to the requirements of Section R802.7.

R806.2 Minimum area. The total net free ventilating area shall not be less than ¹/₁₅₀ of the area of the space ventilated except that reduction of the total area to ¹/₃₀₀ is permitted provided that at least 50 percent and not more than 80 percent of the required ventilating area is provided by ventilators located in the upper portion of the space to be ventilated at least 3 feet (914 mm) above the eave or cornice vents with the balance of the required ventilation provided by eave or cornice vents. As an alternative, the net free cross-ventilation area may be reduced to ¹/₃₀₀ when a Class I or II vapor barrier is installed on the warm-in-winter side of the ceiling.

R806.3 Vent and insulation clearance. Where eave or cornice vents are installed, insulation shall not block the free flow of air. A minimum of a 1-inch (25 mm) space shall be provided between the insulation and the roof sheathing and at the location of the vent.

R806.4 Unvented attic assemblies. Unvented *attic* assemblies (spaces between the ceiling joists of the top *story* and the roof rafters) shall be permitted if all the following conditions are met:

1. The unvented *attic* space is completely contained within the *building thermal envelope*.

2. No interior vapor retarders are installed on the ceiling side (*attic* floor) of the unvented *attic* assembly.

3. Where wood shingles or shakes are used, a minimum $^1/_4$ inch (6 mm) vented air space separates the shingles or shakes and the roofing underlayment above the structural sheathing.

4. In climate zones 5, 6, 7 and 8, any *air-impermeable insulation* shall be a vapor retarder, or shall have a vapor retarder coating or covering in direct contact with the underside of the insulation.

5. Either Items 5.1, 5.2 or 5.3 shall be met, depending on the air permeability of the insulation directly under the structural roof sheathing.

   5.1. *Air-impermeable insulation* only. Insulation shall be applied in direct contact with the underside of the structural roof sheathing.

   5.2. Air-permeable insulation only. In addition to the air-permeable installed directly below the structural sheathing, rigid board or sheet insulation shall be installed directly above the structural roof sheathing as specified in Table R806.4 for condensation control.

   5.3. Air-impermeable and air-permeable insulation. The *air-impermeable insulation* shall be applied in direct contact with the underside of the structural roof sheathing as specified in Table R806.4 for condensation control. The air-permeable insulation shall be installed directly under the *air-impermeable insulation*.

SECTION R807
ATTIC ACCESS

R807.1 Attic access. Buildings with combustible ceiling or roof construction shall have an *attic* access opening to *attic* areas that exceed 30 square feet (2.8 m²) and have a vertical height of 30 inches (762 mm) or greater. The vertical height shall be measured from the top of the ceiling framing members to the underside of the roof framing members.

The rough-framed opening shall not be less than 22 inches by 30 inches (559 mm by 762 mm) and shall be located in a hallway or other readily accessible location. When located in a wall, the opening shall be a minimum of 22 inches wide by 30 inches high. When the access is located in a ceiling, minimum unobstructed headroom in the *attic* space shall be 30 inches (762 mm) at some point above the access measured vertically from the bottom of ceiling framing members. See Section M1305.1.3 for access requirements where mechanical *equipment* is located in *attics*.

TABLE R806.4
INSULATION FOR CONDENSATION CONTROL

CLIMATE ZONE	MINIMUM RIGID BOARD ON AIR-IMPERMEABLE INSULATION *R*-VALUE[a]
2B and 3B tile roof only	0 (none required)
1, 2A, 2B, 3A, 3B, 3C	R-5
4C	R-10
4A, 4B	R-15
5	R-20
6	R-25
7	R-30
8	R-35

a. Contributes to but does not supersede Chapter 11 energy requirements.

CHAPTER 9

ROOF ASSEMBLIES

SECTION R901
GENERAL

R901.1 Scope. The provisions of this chapter shall govern the design, materials, construction and quality of roof assemblies.

SECTION R902
ROOF CLASSIFICATION

R902.1 Roofing covering materials. Roofs shall be covered with materials as set forth in Sections R904 and R905. Class A, B or C roofing shall be installed in areas designated by law as requiring their use or when the edge of the roof is less than 3 feet (914 mm) from a property line. Classes A, B and C roofing required by this section to be listed shall be tested in accordance with UL 790 or ASTM E 108.

Exceptions:

1. Class A roof assemblies include those with coverings of brick, masonry and exposed concrete roof deck.

2. Class A roof assemblies also include ferrous or copper shingles or sheets, metal sheets and shingles, clay or concrete roof tile, or slate installed on noncombustible decks.

R902.2 Fire-retardant-treated shingles and shakes. Fire-retardant-treated wood shakes and shingles shall be treated by impregnation with chemicals by the full-cell vacuum-pressure process, in accordance with AWPA C1. Each bundle shall be marked to identify the manufactured unit and the manufacturer, and shall also be *labeled* to identify the classification of the material in accordance with the testing required in Section R902.1, the treating company and the quality control agency.

SECTION R903
WEATHER PROTECTION

R903.1 General. Roof decks shall be covered with *approved* roof coverings secured to the building or structure in accordance with the provisions of this chapter. Roof assemblies shall be designed and installed in accordance with this code and the *approved* manufacturer's installation instructions such that the roof assembly shall serve to protect the building or structure.

R903.2 Flashing. Flashings shall be installed in a manner that prevents moisture from entering the wall and roof through joints in copings, through moisture permeable materials and at intersections with parapet walls and other penetrations through the roof plane.

R903.2.1 Locations. Flashings shall be installed at wall and roof intersections, wherever there is a change in roof slope or direction and around roof openings. Where flashing is of metal, the metal shall be corrosion resistant with a thickness of not less than 0.019 inch (0.5 mm) (No. 26 galvanized sheet).

R903.2.2 Crickets and saddles. A cricket or saddle shall be installed on the ridge side of any chimney or penetration more than 30 inches (762 mm) wide as measured perpendicular to the slope. Cricket or saddle coverings shall be sheet metal or of the same material as the roof covering.

R903.3 Coping. Parapet walls shall be properly coped with noncombustible, weatherproof materials of a width no less than the thickness of the parapet wall.

R903.4 Roof drainage. Unless roofs are sloped to drain over roof edges, roof drains shall be installed at each low point of the roof. Where required for roof drainage, scuppers shall be placed level with the roof surface in a wall or parapet. The scupper shall be located as determined by the roof slope and contributing roof area.

R903.4.1 Overflow drains and scuppers. Where roof drains are required, overflow drains having the same size as the roof drains shall be installed with the inlet flow line located 2 inches (51 mm) above the low point of the roof, or overflow scuppers having three times the size of the roof drains and having a minimum opening height of 4 inches (102 mm) shall be installed in the adjacent parapet walls with the inlet flow located 2 inches (51 mm) above the low point of the roof served. The installation and sizing of overflow drains, leaders and conductors shall comply with the *International Plumbing Code*.

Overflow drains shall discharge to an *approved* location and shall not be connected to roof drain lines.

R903.5 Hail exposure. Hail exposure, as specified in Sections R903.5.1 and R903.5.2, shall be determined using Figure R903.5.

R903.5.1 Moderate hail exposure. One or more hail days with hail diameters larger than 1.5 inches (38 mm) in a 20-year period.

R903.5.2 Severe hail exposure. One or more hail days with hail diameters larger than or equal to 2.0 inches (51 mm) in a 20-year period.

SECTION R904
MATERIALS

R904.1 Scope. The requirements set forth in this section shall apply to the application of roof covering materials specified herein. Roof assemblies shall be applied in accordance with this chapter and the manufacturer's installation instructions. Installation of roof assemblies shall comply with the applicable provisions of Section R905.

R904.2 Compatibility of materials. Roof assemblies shall be of materials that are compatible with each other and with the building or structure to which the materials are applied.

R904.3 Material specifications and physical characteristics. Roof covering materials shall conform to the applicable standards listed in this chapter. In the absence of applicable

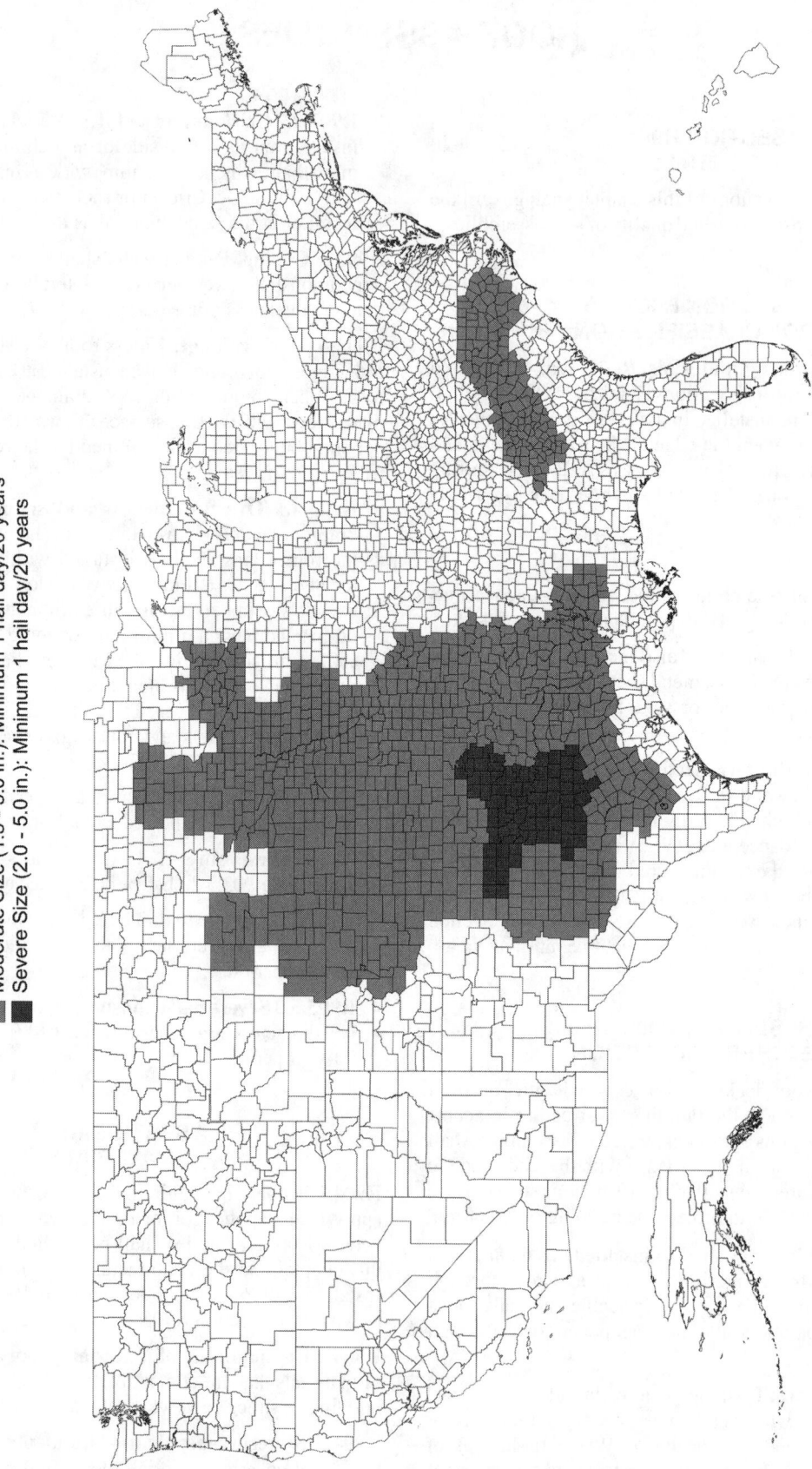

Moderate Size (1.5 - 5.0 in.): Minimum 1 hail day/20 years
Severe Size (2.0 - 5.0 in.): Minimum 1 hail day/20 years

**FIGURE R903.5
HAIL EXPOSURE MAP**

standards or where materials are of questionable suitability, testing by an *approved* testing agency shall be required by the *building official* to determine the character, quality and limitations of application of the materials.

R904.4 Product identification. Roof covering materials shall be delivered in packages bearing the manufacturer's identifying marks and *approved* testing agency *labels* when required. Bulk shipments of materials shall be accompanied by the same information issued in the form of a certificate or on a bill of lading by the manufacturer.

SECTION R905
REQUIREMENTS FOR ROOF COVERINGS

R905.1 Roof covering application. Roof coverings shall be applied in accordance with the applicable provisions of this section and the manufacturer's installation instructions. Unless otherwise specified in this section, roof coverings shall be installed to resist the component and cladding loads specified in Table R301.2(2), adjusted for height and exposure in accordance with Table R301.2(3).

R905.2 Asphalt shingles. The installation of asphalt shingles shall comply with the provisions of this section.

R905.2.1 Sheathing requirements. Asphalt shingles shall be fastened to solidly sheathed decks.

R905.2.2 Slope. Asphalt shingles shall be used only on roof slopes of two units vertical in 12 units horizontal (2:12) or greater. For roof slopes from two units vertical in 12 units horizontal (2:12) up to four units vertical in 12 units horizontal (4:12), double underlayment application is required in accordance with Section R905.2.7.

R905.2.3 Underlayment. Unless otherwise noted, required underlayment shall conform to ASTM D 226 Type I, ASTM D 4869 Type I, or ASTM D 6757.

Self-adhering polymer modified bitumen sheet shall comply with ASTM D 1970.

R905.2.4 Asphalt shingles. Asphalt shingles shall comply with ASTM D 225 or D 3462.

R905.2.4.1 Wind resistance of asphalt shingles. Asphalt shingles shall be tested in accordance with ASTM D 7158. Asphalt shingles shall meet the classification requirements of Table R905.2.4.1(1) for the appropriate maximum basic wind speed. Asphalt shingle packaging shall bear a *label* to indicate compliance with ASTM D 7158 and the required classification in Table R905.2.4.1(1).

Exception: Asphalt shingles not included in the scope of ASTM D 7158 shall be tested and *labeled* to indicate compliance with ASTM D 3161 and the required classification in Table R905.2.4.1(2).

TABLE R905.2.4.1(1)
CLASSIFICATION OF ASPHALT ROOF SHINGLES PER ASTM D 7158

MAXIMUM BASIC WIND SPEED FROM FIGURE 301.2(4) (mph)	CLASSIFICATION REQUIREMENT
85	D, G or H
90	D, G or H
100	G or H
110	G or H
120	G or H
130	H
140	H
150	H

For SI: 1 mile per hour = 0.447 m/s.

TABLE R905.2.4.1(2)
CLASSIFICATION OF ASPHALT SHINGLES PER ASTM D 3161

MAXIMUM BASIC WIND SPEED FROM FIGURE 301.2(4) (mph)	CLASSIFICATION REQUIREMENT
85	A, D or F
90	A, D or F
100	A, D or F
110	F
120	F
130	F
140	F
150	F

For SI: 1 mile per hour = 0.447 m/s.

R905.2.5 Fasteners. Fasteners for asphalt shingles shall be galvanized steel, stainless steel, aluminum or copper roofing nails, minimum 12 gage [0.105 inch (3 mm)] shank with a minimum $^3/_8$-inch (10 mm) diameter head, ASTM F 1667, of a length to penetrate through the roofing materials and a minimum of $^3/_4$ inch (19 mm) into the roof sheathing. Where the roof sheathing is less than $^3/_4$ inch (19 mm) thick, the fasteners shall penetrate through the sheathing. Fasteners shall comply with ASTM F 1667.

R905.2.6 Attachment. Asphalt shingles shall have the minimum number of fasteners required by the manufacturer, but not less than four fasteners per strip shingle or two fasteners per individual shingle. Where the roof slope exceeds 21 units vertical in 12 units horizontal (21:12, 175 percent slope), shingles shall be installed as required by the manufacturer.

R905.2.7 Underlayment application. For roof slopes from two units vertical in 12 units horizontal (17-percent slope), up to four units vertical in 12 units horizontal (33-percent slope), underlayment shall be two layers applied in the following manner. Apply a 19-inch (483 mm) strip of underlayment felt parallel to and starting at the eaves, fastened sufficiently to hold in place. Starting at the eave, apply 36-inch-wide (914 mm) sheets of underlayment, overlapping successive sheets 19 inches (483 mm), and fastened sufficiently to hold in place. Distortions in the underlayment shall not interfere with the ability of the shingles to seal. For roof slopes of four units vertical in 12 units horizontal (33-percent slope) or greater, underlayment shall be one layer applied in the following manner. Underlayment shall be applied shingle fashion, parallel to and starting from the eave and lapped 2 inches (51 mm), fastened sufficiently to hold in place. Distortions in the underlayment shall not interfere with the ability of the shingles to seal. End laps shall be offset by 6 feet (1829 mm).

R905.2.7.1 Ice barrier. In areas where there has been a history of ice forming along the eaves causing a backup of water as designated in Table R301.2(1), an ice barrier that consists of a least two layers of underlayment cemented together or of a self-adhering polymer modified bitumen sheet, shall be used in lieu of normal underlayment and extend from the lowest edges of all roof surfaces to a point at least 24 inches (610 mm) inside the exterior wall line of the building.

Exception: Detached *accessory structures* that contain no *conditioned floor area*.

R905.2.7.2 Underlayment and high wind. Underlayment applied in areas subject to high winds [above 110 mph (49 m/s) per Figure R301.2(4)] shall be applied with corrosion-resistant fasteners in accordance with manufacturer's installation instructions. Fasteners are to be applied along the overlap not farther apart than 36 inches (914 mm) on center.

R905.2.8 Flashing. Flashing for asphalt shingles shall comply with this section.

R905.2.8.1 Base and cap flashing. Base and cap flashing shall be installed in accordance with manufacturer's installation instructions. Base flashing shall be of either corrosion-resistant metal of minimum nominal 0.019-inch (0.5 mm) thickness or mineral surface roll roofing weighing a minimum of 77 pounds per 100 square feet (4 kg/m^2). Cap flashing shall be corrosion-resistant metal of minimum nominal 0.019-inch (0.5 mm) thickness.

R905.2.8.2 Valleys. Valley linings shall be installed in accordance with the manufacturer's installation instructions before applying shingles. Valley linings of the following types shall be permitted:

1. For open valleys (valley lining exposed) lined with metal, the valley lining shall be at least 24 inches (610 mm) wide and of any of the corrosion-resistant metals in Table R905.2.8.2.

2. For open valleys, valley lining of two plies of mineral surfaced roll roofing, complying with ASTM D 3909 or ASTM D 6380 Class M, shall be permitted. The bottom layer shall be 18 inches (457 mm) and the top layer a minimum of 36 inches (914 mm) wide.

3. For closed valleys (valley covered with shingles), valley lining of one ply of smooth roll roofing complying with ASTM D 6380 and at least 36 inches wide (914 mm) or valley lining as described in Item 1 or 2 above shall be permitted. Self-adhering polymer modified bitumen underlayment complying with ASTM D 1970 shall be permitted in lieu of the lining material.

TABLE R905.2.8.2
VALLEY LINING MATERIAL

MATERIAL	MINIMUM THICKNESS (inches)	GAGE	WEIGHT (pounds)
Cold-rolled copper	0.0216 nominal	—	ASTM B 370, 16 oz. per square foot
Lead-coated copper	0.0216 nominal	—	ASTM B 101, 16 oz. per square foot
High-yield copper	0.0162 nominal	—	ASTM B 370, 12 oz. per square foot
Lead-coated high-yield copper	0.0162 nominal	—	ASTM B 101, 12 oz. per square foot
Aluminum	0.024	—	—
Stainless steel	—	28	—
Galvanized steel	0.0179	26 (zinc coated G90)	—
Zinc alloy	0.027	—	—
Lead	—	—	$2^1/_2$
Painted terne	—	—	20

For SI: 1 inch = 25.4 mm, 1 pound = 0.454 kg.

R905.2.8.3 Sidewall flashing. Flashing against a vertical sidewall shall be by the step-flashing method. The flashing shall be a minimum of 4 inches (102 mm) high and 4 inches (102 mm) wide. At the end of the vertical sidewall the step flashing shall be turned out in a manner that directs water away from the wall and onto the roof and/or gutter.

R905.2.8.4 Other flashing. Flashing against a vertical front wall, as well as soil stack, vent pipe and chimney flashing, shall be applied according to the asphalt shingle manufacturer's printed instructions.

R905.3 Clay and concrete tile. The installation of clay and concrete tile shall comply with the provisions of this section.

R905.3.1 Deck requirements. Concrete and clay tile shall be installed only over solid sheathing or spaced structural sheathing boards.

R905.3.2 Deck slope. Clay and concrete roof tile shall be installed on roof slopes of two and one-half units vertical in 12 units horizontal ($2^1/_2$:12) or greater. For roof slopes from two and one-half units vertical in 12 units horizontal ($2^1/_2$:12) to four units vertical in 12 units horizontal (4:12), double underlayment application is required in accordance with Section R905.3.3.

R905.3.3 Underlayment. Unless otherwise noted, required underlayment shall conform to ASTM D 226 Type II; ASTM D 2626 Type I; or ASTM D 6380 Class M mineral surfaced roll roofing.

R905.3.3.1 Low slope roofs. For roof slopes from two and one-half units vertical in 12 units horizontal ($2^1/_2$:12), up to four units vertical in 12 units horizontal (4:12), underlayment shall be a minimum of two layers underlayment applied as follows:

1. Starting at the eave, a 19-inch (483 mm) strip of underlayment shall be applied parallel with the eave and fastened sufficiently in place.

2. Starting at the eave, 36-inch-wide (914 mm) strips of underlayment felt shall be applied, overlapping successive sheets 19 inches (483 mm), and fastened sufficiently in place.

R905.3.3.2 High slope roofs. For roof slopes of four units vertical in 12 units horizontal (4:12) or greater, underlayment shall be a minimum of one layer of underlayment felt applied shingle fashion, parallel to and starting from the eaves and lapped 2 inches (51 mm), fastened sufficiently in place.

R905.3.3.3 Underlayment and high wind. Underlayment applied in areas subject to high wind [over 110 miles per hour (49 m/s) per Figure R301.2(4)] shall be applied with corrosion-resistant fasteners in accordance with manufacturer's installation instructions. Fasteners are to be applied along the overlap not farther apart than 36 inches (914 mm) on center.

R905.3.4 Clay tile. Clay roof tile shall comply with ASTM C 1167.

R905.3.5 Concrete tile. Concrete roof tile shall comply with ASTM C 1492.

R905.3.6 Fasteners. Nails shall be corrosion resistant and not less than 11 gage, $^5/_{16}$-inch (11 mm) head, and of sufficient length to penetrate the deck a minimum of $^3/_4$ inch (19 mm) or through the thickness of the deck, whichever is less. Attaching wire for clay or concrete tile shall not be smaller than 0.083 inch (2 mm). Perimeter fastening areas include three tile courses but not less than 36 inches (914 mm) from either side of hips or ridges and edges of eaves and gable rakes.

R905.3.7 Application. Tile shall be applied in accordance with this chapter and the manufacturer's installation instructions, based on the following:

1. Climatic conditions.

2. Roof slope.

3. Underlayment system.

4. Type of tile being installed.

Clay and concrete roof tiles shall be fastened in accordance with this section and the manufacturer's installation instructions. Perimeter tiles shall be fastened with a minimum of one fastener per tile. Tiles with installed weight less than 9 pounds per square foot (0.4 kg/m²) require a minimum of one fastener per tile regardless of roof slope. Clay and concrete roof tile attachment shall be in accordance with the manufacturer's installation instructions where applied in areas where the wind speed exceeds 100 miles per hour (45 m/s) and on buildings where the roof is located more than 40 feet (12 192 mm) above *grade*. In areas subject to snow, a minimum of two fasteners per tile is required. In all other areas, clay and concrete roof tiles shall be attached in accordance with Table R905.3.7.

TABLE R905.3.7
CLAY AND CONCRETE TILE ATTACHMENT

SHEATHING	ROOF SLOPE	NUMBER OF FASTENERS
Solid without battens	All	One per tile
Spaced or solid with battens and slope < 5:12	Fasteners not required	—
Spaced sheathing without battens	5:12 ≤ slope < 12:12	One per tile/every other row
	12:12 ≤ slope < 24:12	One per tile

R905.3.8 Flashing. At the juncture of roof vertical surfaces, flashing and counterflashing shall be provided in accordance with this chapter and the manufacturer's installation instructions and, where of metal, shall not be less than 0.019 inch (0.5 mm) (No. 26 galvanized sheet gage) corrosion-resistant metal. The valley flashing shall extend at least 11 inches (279 mm) from the centerline each way and have a splash diverter rib not less than 1 inch (25 mm) high at the flow line formed as part of the flashing. Sections of flashing shall have an end lap of not less than 4 inches (102 mm). For roof slopes of three units vertical in 12 units horizontal (25-percent slope) and greater, valley flashing shall have a 36-inch-wide (914 mm) underlayment of one layer of Type I underlayment running the full length of the valley, in addition to other required underlayment. In areas where the average daily temperature in January is 25°F (-4°C) or less, metal valley flashing underlayment shall be solid-cemented to the roofing underlayment for slopes less than seven units vertical in 12 units horizontal (58-percent slope) or be of self-adhering polymer modified bitumen sheet.

R905.4 Metal roof shingles. The installation of metal roof shingles shall comply with the provisions of this section.

R905.4.1 Deck requirements. Metal roof shingles shall be applied to a solid or closely fitted deck, except where the roof covering is specifically designed to be applied to spaced sheathing.

R905.4.2 Deck slope. Metal roof shingles shall not be installed on roof slopes below three units vertical in 12 units horizontal (25-percent slope).

R905.4.3 Underlayment. Underlayment shall comply with ASTM D 226, Type I or Type II, ASTM D 4869, Type I or Type II, or ASTM D 1970. Underlayment shall be installed in accordance with the manufacturer's installation instructions.

R905.4.3.1 Ice barrier. In areas where there has been a history of ice forming along the eaves causing a backup of water as designated in Table R301.2(1), an ice barrier that consists of at least two layers of underlayment cemented together or a self-adhering polymer modified bitumen sheet shall be used in place of normal underlayment and extend from the lowest edges of all roof surfaces to a point at least 24 inches (610 mm) inside the exterior wall line of the building.

Exception: Detached *accessory structures* that contain no *conditioned floor area*.

R905.4.4 Material standards. Metal roof shingle roof coverings shall comply with Table R905.10.3(1). The materials used for metal roof shingle roof coverings shall be naturally corrosion resistant or be made corrosion resistant in accordance with the standards and minimum thicknesses listed in Table R905.10.3(2).

R905.4.5 Application. Metal roof shingles shall be secured to the roof in accordance with this chapter and the *approved* manufacturer's installation instructions.

R905.4.6 Flashing. Roof valley flashing shall be of corrosion-resistant metal of the same material as the roof covering or shall comply with the standards in Table R905.10.3(1). The valley flashing shall extend at least 8 inches (203 mm) from the center line each way and shall have a splash diverter rib not less than $^3/_4$ inch (19 mm) high at the flow line formed as part of the flashing. Sections of flashing shall have an end lap of not less than 4 inches (102 mm). The metal valley flashing shall have a 36-inch-wide (914 mm) underlayment directly under it consisting of one layer of underlayment running the full length of the valley, in addition to underlayment required for metal roof shingles. In areas where the average daily temperature in January is 25°F (-4°C) or less, the metal valley flashing underlayment shall be solid cemented to the roofing underlayment for roof slopes under seven units vertical in 12 units horizontal (58-percent slope) or self-adhering polymer modified bitumen sheet.

R905.5 Mineral-surfaced roll roofing. The installation of mineral-surfaced roll roofing shall comply with this section.

R905.5.1 Deck requirements. Mineral-surfaced roll roofing shall be fastened to solidly sheathed roofs.

R905.5.2 Deck slope. Mineral-surfaced roll roofing shall not be applied on roof slopes below one unit vertical in 12 units horizontal (8-percent slope).

R905.5.3 Underlayment. Underlayment shall comply with ASTM D 226, Type I or ASTM D 4869, Type I or II.

R905.5.3.1 Ice barrier. In areas where there has been a history of ice forming along the eaves causing a backup of water as designated in Table R301.2(1), an ice barrier that consists of at least two layers of underlayment cemented together or a self-adhering polymer modified bitumen sheet shall be used in place of normal underlayment and extend from the lowest edges of all roof surfaces to a point at least 24 inches (610 mm) inside the exterior wall line of the building.

Exception: Detached *accessory structures* that contain no *conditioned floor area*.

R905.5.4 Material standards. Mineral-surfaced roll roofing shall conform to ASTM D 3909 or ASTM D 6380, Class M.

R905.5.5 Application. Mineral-surfaced roll roofing shall be installed in accordance with this chapter and the manufacturer's installation instructions.

R905.6 Slate and slate-type shingles. The installation of slate and slate-type shingles shall comply with the provisions of this section.

R905.6.1 Deck requirements. Slate shingles shall be fastened to solidly sheathed roofs.

R905.6.2 Deck slope. Slate shingles shall be used only on slopes of four units vertical in 12 units horizontal (33-percent slope) or greater.

R905.6.3 Underlayment. Underlayment shall comply with ASTM D 226, Type I, or ASTM D 4869, Type I or II. Underlayment shall be installed in accordance with the manufacturer's installation instructions.

R905.6.3.1 Ice barrier. In areas where there has been a history of ice forming along the eaves causing a backup of water as designated in Table R301.2(1), an ice barrier that consists of at least two layers of underlayment cemented together or a self-adhering polymer modified bitumen sheet shall be used in lieu of normal underlayment and extend from the lowest edges of all roof surfaces to a point at least 24 inches (610 mm) inside the exterior wall line of the building.

Exception: Detached *accessory structures* that contain no *conditioned floor area*.

R905.6.4 Material standards. Slate shingles shall comply with ASTM C 406.

R905.6.5 Application. Minimum headlap for slate shingles shall be in accordance with Table R905.6.5. Slate shingles shall be secured to the roof with two fasteners per slate. Slate shingles shall be installed in accordance with this chapter and the manufacturer's installation instructions.

TABLE R905.6.5
SLATE SHINGLE HEADLAP

SLOPE	HEADLAP (inches)
4:12 ≤ slope < 8:12	4
8:12 ≤ slope < 20:12	3
Slope ≤ 20:12	2

For SI: 1 inch = 25.4 mm.

R905.6.6 Flashing. Flashing and counterflashing shall be made with sheet metal. Valley flashing shall be a minimum of 15 inches (381 mm) wide. Valley and flashing metal shall be a minimum uncoated thickness of 0.0179-inch (0.5 mm) zinc coated G90. Chimneys, stucco or brick walls shall have a minimum of two plies of felt for a cap flashing consisting of a 4-inch-wide (102 mm) strip of felt set in plastic cement and extending 1 inch (25 mm) above the first felt and a top coating of plastic cement. The felt shall extend over the base flashing 2 inches (51 mm).

R905.7 Wood shingles. The installation of wood shingles shall comply with the provisions of this section.

R905.7.1 Deck requirements. Wood shingles shall be installed on solid or spaced sheathing. Where spaced sheathing is used, sheathing boards shall not be less than 1-inch by 4-inch (25.4 mm by 102 mm) nominal dimensions and shall be spaced on centers equal to the weather exposure to coincide with the placement of fasteners.

R905.7.1.1 Solid sheathing required. In areas where the average daily temperature in January is 25°F (-4°C) or less, solid sheathing is required on that portion of the roof requiring the application of an ice barrier.

R905.7.2 Deck slope. Wood shingles shall be installed on slopes of three units vertical in 12 units horizontal (25-percent slope) or greater.

R905.7.3 Underlayment. Underlayment shall comply with ASTM D 226, Type I or ASTM D 4869, Type I or II.

R905.7.3.1 Ice barrier. In areas where there has been a history of ice forming along the eaves causing a backup of water as designated in Table R301.2(1), an ice barrier that consists of at least two layers of underlayment cemented together or a self-adhering polymer modified bitumen sheet shall be used in lieu of normal underlayment and extend from the lowest edges of all roof surfaces to a point at least 24 inches (610 mm) inside the exterior wall line of the building.

Exception: Detached *accessory structures* that contain no *conditioned floor area*.

R905.7.4 Material standards. Wood shingles shall be of naturally durable wood and comply with the requirements of Table R905.7.4.

TABLE R905.7.4
WOOD SHINGLE MATERIAL REQUIREMENTS

MATERIAL	MINIMUM GRADES	APPLICABLE GRADING RULES
Wood shingles of naturally durable wood	1, 2 or 3	Cedar Shake and Shingle Bureau

R905.7.5 Application. Wood shingles shall be installed according to this chapter and the manufacturer's installation instructions. Wood shingles shall be laid with a side lap not less than 1¹/₂ inches (38 mm) between joints in courses, and no two joints in any three adjacent courses shall be in direct alignment. Spacing between shingles shall not be less than ¹/₄ inch to ³/₈ inch (6 mm to 10 mm). Weather exposure for wood shingles shall not exceed those set in Table R905.7.5. Fasteners for wood shingles shall be corrosion resistant with a minimum penetration of ¹/₂ inch (13 mm) into the sheathing. For sheathing less than ¹/₂ inch (13 mm) in thickness, the fasteners shall extend through the sheathing. Wood shingles shall be attached to the roof with two fasteners per shingle, positioned no more than ³/₄ inch (19 mm) from each edge and no more than 1 inch (25 mm) above the exposure line.

TABLE R905.7.5
WOOD SHINGLE WEATHER EXPOSURE AND ROOF SLOPE

ROOFING MATERIAL	LENGTH (inches)	GRADE	EXPOSURE (inches)	
			3:12 pitch to < 4:12	4:12 pitch or steeper
Shingles of naturally durable wood	16	No. 1	3³/₄	5
		No. 2	3¹/₂	4
		No. 3	3	3¹/₂
	18	No. 1	4¹/₄	5¹/₂
		No. 2	4	4¹/₂
		No. 3	3¹/₂	4
	24	No. 1	5³/₄	7¹/₂
		No. 2	5¹/₂	6¹/₂
		No. 3	5	5¹/₂

For SI: 1 inch = 25.4 mm.

R905.7.6 Valley flashing. Roof flashing shall be not less than No. 26 gage [0.019 inches (0.5 mm)] corrosion-resistant sheet metal and shall extend 10 inches (254 mm) from the centerline each way for roofs having slopes less than 12 units vertical in 12 units horizontal (100-percent slope), and 7 inches (178 mm) from the centerline each way for slopes of 12 units vertical in 12 units horizontal and greater. Sections of flashing shall have an end lap of not less than 4 inches (102 mm).

R905.7.7 Label required. Each bundle of shingles shall be identified by a *label* of an *approved* grading or inspection bureau or agency.

R905.8 Wood shakes. The installation of wood shakes shall comply with the provisions of this section.

R905.8.1 Deck requirements. Wood shakes shall be used only on solid or spaced sheathing. Where spaced sheathing is used, sheathing boards shall not be less than 1-inch by 4-inch (25 mm by 102 mm) nominal dimensions and shall be spaced on centers equal to the weather exposure to coincide with the placement of fasteners. Where 1-inch by 4-inch (25 mm by 102 mm) spaced sheathing is installed at 10 inches (254 mm) on center, additional 1-inch by 4-inch (25 mm by 102 mm) boards shall be installed between the sheathing boards.

R905.8.1.1 Solid sheathing required. In areas where the average daily temperature in January is 25°F (-4°C) or less, solid sheathing is required on that portion of the roof requiring an ice barrier.

R905.8.2 Deck slope. Wood shakes shall only be used on slopes of three units vertical in 12 units horizontal (25-percent slope) or greater.

R905.8.3 Underlayment. Underlayment shall comply with ASTM D 226, Type I or ASTM D 4869, Type I or II.

R905.8.3.1 Ice barrier. In areas where there has been a history of ice forming along the eaves causing a backup of water as designated in Table R301.2(1), an ice barrier that consists of at least two layers of underlayment cemented together or a self-adhering polymer modified bitumen sheet shall be used in place of normal underlayment and extend from the lowest edges of all roof surfaces to a point at least 24 inches (610 mm) inside the exterior wall line of the building.

Exception: Detached *accessory structures* that contain no *conditioned floor area*.

R905.8.4 Interlayment. Interlayment shall comply with ASTM D 226, Type I.

R905.8.5 Material standards. Wood shakes shall comply with the requirements of Table R905.8.5.

TABLE R905.8.5
WOOD SHAKE MATERIAL REQUIREMENTS

MATERIAL	MINIMUM GRADES	APPLICABLE GRADING RULES
Wood shakes of naturally durable wood	1	Cedar Shake and Shingle Bureau
Taper sawn shakes of naturally durable wood	1 or 2	Cedar Shake and Shingle Bureau
Preservative-treated shakes and shingles of naturally durable wood	1	Cedar Shake and Shingle Bureau
Fire-retardant-treated shakes and shingles of naturally durable wood	1	Cedar Shake and Shingle Bureau
Preservative-treated taper sawn shakes of Southern pine treated in accordance with AWPA Standard U1 (Commodity Specification A, Use Category 3B and Section 5.6)	1 or 2	Forest Products Laboratory of the Texas Forest Services

R905.8.6 Application. Wood shakes shall be installed according to this chapter and the manufacturer's installation instructions. Wood shakes shall be laid with a side lap not less than $1^1/_2$ inches (38 mm) between joints in adjacent courses. Spacing between shakes in the same course shall be $^3/_8$ inch to $^5/_8$ inch (9.5 mm to 15.9 mm) for shakes and tapersawn shakes of naturally durable wood and shall be $^3/_8$ inch to $^5/_8$ inch (9.5 mm to 15.9 mm) for preservative-treated taper sawn shakes. Weather exposure for wood shakes shall not exceed those set forth in Table R905.8.6. Fasteners for wood shakes shall be corrosion-resistant, with a minimum

penetration of $^1/_2$ inch (12.7 mm) into the sheathing. For sheathing less than $^1/_2$ inch (12.7 mm) thick, the fasteners shall extend through the sheathing. Wood shakes shall be attached to the roof with two fasteners per shake, positioned no more than 1 inch (25 mm) from each edge and no more than 2 inches (51 mm) above the exposure line.

R905.8.7 Shake placement. The starter course at the eaves shall be doubled and the bottom layer shall be either 15-inch (381 mm), 18-inch (457 mm) or 24-inch (610 mm) wood shakes or wood shingles. Fifteen-inch (381 mm) or 18-inch (457 mm) wood shakes may be used for the final course at the ridge. Shakes shall be interlaid with 18-inch-wide (457 mm) strips of not less than No. 30 felt shingled between each course in such a manner that no felt is exposed to the weather by positioning the lower edge of each felt strip above the butt end of the shake it covers a distance equal to twice the weather exposure.

TABLE R905.8.6
WOOD SHAKE WEATHER EXPOSURE AND ROOF SLOPE

ROOFING MATERIAL	LENGTH (inches)	GRADE	EXPOSURE (inches) 4:12 pitch or steeper
Shakes of naturally durable wood	18	No. 1	$7^1/_2$
	24	No. 1	10[a]
Preservative-treated taper sawn shakes of Southern Yellow Pine	18	No. 1	$7^1/_2$
	24	No. 1	10
	18	No. 2	$5^1/_2$
	24	No. 2	$7^1/_2$
Taper-sawn shakes of naturally durable wood	18	No. 1	$7^1/_2$
	24	No. 1	10
	18	No. 2	$5^1/_2$
	24	No. 2	$7^1/_2$

For SI: 1 inch = 25.4 mm.

a. For 24-inch by $^3/_8$-inch handsplit shakes, the maximum exposure is $7^1/_2$ inches.

R905.8.8 Valley flashing. Roof valley flashing shall not be less than No. 26 gage [0.019 inch (0.5 mm)] corrosion-resistant sheet metal and shall extend at least 11 inches (279 mm) from the centerline each way. Sections of flashing shall have an end lap of not less than 4 inches (102 mm).

R905.8.9 Label required. Each bundle of shakes shall be identified by a *label* of an *approved* grading or inspection bureau or agency.

R905.9 Built-up roofs. The installation of built-up roofs shall comply with the provisions of this section.

R905.9.1 Slope. Built-up roofs shall have a design slope of a minimum of one-fourth unit vertical in 12 units horizontal (2-percent slope) for drainage, except for coal-tar built-up roofs, which shall have a design slope of a minimum one-eighth unit vertical in 12 units horizontal (1-percent slope).

R905.9.2 Material standards. Built-up roof covering materials shall comply with the standards in Table R905.9.2.

R905.9.3 Application. Built-up roofs shall be installed according to this chapter and the manufacturer's installation instructions.

TABLE R905.9.2
BUILT-UP ROOFING MATERIAL STANDARDS

MATERIAL STANDARD	STANDARD
Acrylic coatings used in roofing	ASTM D 6083
Aggregate surfacing	ASTM D 1863
Asphalt adhesive used in roofing	ASTM D 3747
Asphalt cements used in roofing	ASTM D 3019; D 2822; D 4586
Asphalt-coated glass fiber base sheet	ASTM D 4601
Asphalt coatings used in roofing	ASTM D 1227; D 2823; D 2824; D 4479
Asphalt glass felt	ASTM D 2178
Asphalt primer used in roofing	ASTM D 41
Asphalt-saturated and asphalt-coated organic felt base sheet	ASTM D 2626
Asphalt-saturated organic felt (perforated)	ASTM D 226
Asphalt used in roofing	ASTM D 312
Coal-tar cements used in roofing	ASTM D 4022; D 5643
Coal-tar primer used in roofing, dampproofing and waterproofing	ASTM D 43
Coal-tar saturated organic felt	ASTM D 227
Coal-tar used in roofing	ASTM D 450, Types I or II
Glass mat, coal tar	ASTM D 4990
Glass mat, venting type	ASTM D 4897
Mineral-surfaced inorganic cap sheet	ASTM D 3909
Thermoplastic fabrics used in roofing	ASTM D 5665; D 5726

R905.10 Metal roof panels. The installation of metal roof panels shall comply with the provisions of this section.

R905.10.1 Deck requirements. Metal roof panel roof coverings shall be applied to solid or spaced sheathing, except where the roof covering is specifically designed to be applied to spaced supports.

R905.10.2 Slope. Minimum slopes for metal roof panels shall comply with the following:

1. The minimum slope for lapped, nonsoldered-seam metal roofs without applied lap sealant shall be three units vertical in 12 units horizontal (25-percent slope).

2. The minimum slope for lapped, nonsoldered-seam metal roofs with applied lap sealant shall be one-half vertical unit in 12 units horizontal (4-percent slope). Lap sealants shall be applied in accordance with the *approved* manufacturer's installation instructions.

3. The minimum slope for standing-seam roof systems shall be one-quarter unit vertical in 12 units horizontal (2-percent slope).

R905.10.3 Material standards. Metal-sheet roof covering systems that incorporate supporting structural members shall be designed in accordance with the *International Building Code*. Metal-sheet roof coverings installed over structural decking shall comply with Table R905.10.3(1). The materials used for metal-sheet roof coverings shall be naturally corrosion resistant or provided with corrosion resistance in accordance with the standards and minimum thicknesses shown in Table R905.10.3(2).

R905.10.4 Attachment. Metal roof panels shall be secured to the supports in accordance with this chapter and the manufacturer's installation instructions. In the absence of manufacturer's installation instructions, the following fasteners shall be used:

1. Galvanized fasteners shall be used for steel roofs.

2. Copper, brass, bronze, copper alloy and Three hundred series stainless steel fasteners shall be used for copper roofs.

3. Stainless steel fasteners are acceptable for metal roofs.

R905.10.5 Underlayment. Underlayment shall be installed in accordance with the manufacturer's installation instructions.

TABLE R905.10.3(1)
METAL ROOF COVERINGS STANDARDS

ROOF COVERING TYPE	STANDARD APPLICATION RATE/THICKNESS
Galvanized steel	ASTM A 653 G90 Zinc coated
Stainless steel	ASTM A 240, 300 Series alloys
Steel	ASTM A 924
Lead-coated copper	ASTM B 101
Cold rolled copper	ASTM B 370 minimum 16 oz/square ft and 12 oz/square ft high yield copper for metal-sheet roof-covering systems; 12 oz/square ft for preformed metal shingle systems.
Hard lead	2 lb/sq ft
Soft lead	3 lb/sq ft
Aluminum	ASTM B 209, 0.024 minimum thickness for rollformed panels and 0.019 inch minimum thickness for pressformed shingles.
Terne (tin) and terne-coated stainless	Terne coating of 40 lb per double base box, field painted where applicable in accordance with manufacturer's installation instructions.
Zinc	0.027 inch minimum thickness: 99.995% electrolytic high grade zinc with alloy additives of copper (0.08 - 0.20%), titanium (0.07% - 0.12%) and aluminum (0.015%).

For SI: 1 ounce per square foot = 0.305 kg/m^2, 1 pound per square foot = 4.214 kg/m^2, 1 inch = 25.4 mm, 1 pound = 0.454 kg.

TABLE R905.10.3(2)
MINIMUM CORROSION RESISTANCE

55% aluminum-zinc alloy coated steel	ASTM A 792 AZ 50
5% aluminum alloy-coated steel	ASTM A 875 GF60
Aluminum-coated steel	ASTM A 463 T2 65
Galvanized steel	ASTM A 653 G-90
Prepainted steel	ASTM A 755[a]

a. Paint systems in accordance with ASTM A 755 shall be applied over steel products with corrosion-resistant coatings complying with ASTM A 792, ASTM A 875, ASTM A 463, or ASTM A 653.

R905.11 Modified bitumen roofing. The installation of modified bitumen roofing shall comply with the provisions of this section.

R905.11.1 Slope. Modified bitumen membrane roofs shall have a design slope of a minimum of one-fourth unit vertical in 12 units horizontal (2-percent slope) for drainage.

R905.11.2 Material standards. Modified bitumen roof coverings shall comply with the standards in Table R905.11.2.

TABLE R905.11.2
MODIFIED BITUMEN ROOFING MATERIAL STANDARDS

MATERIAL	STANDARD
Acrylic coating	ASTM D 6083
Asphalt adhesive	ASTM D 3747
Asphalt cement	ASTM D 3019
Asphalt coating	ASTM D 1227; D 2824
Asphalt primer	ASTM D 41
Modified bitumen roof membrane	ASTM D 6162; D 6163; D 6164; D 6222; D 6223; D 6298; CGSB 37–GP–56M

R905.11.3 Application. Modified bitumen roofs shall be installed according to this chapter and the manufacturer's installation instructions.

R905.12 Thermoset single-ply roofing. The installation of thermoset single-ply roofing shall comply with the provisions of this section.

R905.12.1 Slope. Thermoset single-ply membrane roofs shall have a design slope of a minimum of one-fourth unit vertical in 12 units horizontal (2-percent slope) for drainage.

R905.12.2 Material standards. Thermoset single-ply roof coverings shall comply with ASTM D 4637, ASTM D 5019 or CGSB 37-GP-52M.

R905.12.3 Application. Thermoset single-ply roofs shall be installed according to this chapter and the manufacturer's installation instructions.

R905.13 Thermoplastic single-ply roofing. The installation of thermoplastic single-ply roofing shall comply with the provisions of this section.

R905.13.1 Slope. Thermoplastic single-ply membrane roofs shall have a design slope of a minimum of one-fourth unit vertical in 12 units horizontal (2-percent slope).

R905.13.2 Material standards. Thermoplastic single-ply roof coverings shall comply with ASTM D 4434, ASTM D 6754, ASTM D 6878, or CGSB CAN/CGSB 37.54.

R905.13.3 Application. Thermoplastic single-ply roofs shall be installed according to this chapter and the manufacturer's installation instructions.

R905.14 Sprayed polyurethane foam roofing. The installation of sprayed polyurethane foam roofing shall comply with the provisions of this section.

R905.14.1 Slope. Sprayed polyurethane foam roofs shall have a design slope of a minimum of one-fourth unit vertical in 12 units horizontal (2-percent slope) for drainage.

R905.14.2 Material standards. Spray-applied polyurethane foam insulation shall comply with ASTM C 1029, Type III or IV.

R905.14.3 Application. Foamed-in-place roof insulation shall be installed in accordance with this chapter and the manufacturer's installation instructions. A liquid-applied protective coating that complies with Section R905.15 shall be applied no less– than 2 hours nor more than 72 hours following the application of the foam.

R905.14.4 Foam plastics. Foam plastic materials and installation shall comply with Section R314.

R905.15 Liquid-applied coatings. The installation of liquid-applied coatings shall comply with the provisions of this section.

R905.15.1 Slope. Liquid-applied roofs shall have a design slope of a minimum of one-fourth unit vertical in 12 units horizontal (2-percent slope).

R905.15.2 Material standards. Liquid-applied roof coatings shall comply with ASTM C 836, C 957, D 1227, D 3468, D 6083, D 6694 or D 6947.

R905.15.3 Application. Liquid-applied roof coatings shall be installed according to this chapter and the manufacturer's installation instructions.

SECTION R906
ROOF INSULATION

R906.1 General. The use of above-deck thermal insulation shall be permitted provided such insulation is covered with an *approved* roof covering and passes FM 4450 or UL 1256.

R906.2 Material standards. Above-deck thermal insulation board shall comply with the standards in Table R906.2.

TABLE R906.2
MATERIAL STANDARDS FOR ROOF INSULATION

Cellular glass board	ASTM C 552
Composite boards	ASTM C 1289, Type III, IV, V or VI
Expanded polystyrene	ASTM C 578
Extruded polystyrene board	ASTM C 578
Perlite board	ASTM C 728
Polyisocyanurate board	ASTM C 1289, Type I or Type II
Wood fiberboard	ASTM C 208

SECTION R907
REROOFING

R907.1 General. Materials and methods of application used for re-covering or replacing an existing roof covering shall comply with the requirements of Chapter 9.

Exception: Reroofing shall not be required to meet the minimum design slope requirement of one-quarter unit vertical in 12 units horizontal (2-percent slope) in Section R905 for roofs that provide positive roof drainage.

R907.2 Structural and construction loads. The structural roof components shall be capable of supporting the roof covering system and the material and equipment loads that will be encountered during installation of the roof covering system.

R907.3 Recovering versus replacement. New roof coverings shall not be installed without first removing all existing layers of roof coverings where any of the following conditions exist:

1. Where the existing roof or roof covering is water-soaked or has deteriorated to the point that the existing roof or roof covering is not adequate as a base for additional roofing.

2. Where the existing roof covering is wood shake, slate, clay, cement or asbestos-cement tile.

3. Where the existing roof has two or more applications of any type of roof covering.

4. For asphalt shingles, when the building is located in an area subject to moderate or severe hail exposure according to Figure R903.5.

Exceptions:

1. Complete and separate roofing systems, such as standing-seam metal roof systems, that are designed to transmit the roof loads directly to the building's structural system and that do not rely on existing roofs and roof coverings for support, shall not require the removal of existing roof coverings.

2. Installation of metal panel, metal shingle and concrete and clay tile roof coverings over existing wood shake roofs shall be permitted when the application is in accordance with Section R907.4.

3. The application of new protective coating over existing spray polyurethane foam roofing systems shall be permitted without tear-off of existing roof coverings.

R907.4 Roof recovering. Where the application of a new roof covering over wood shingle or shake roofs creates a combustible concealed space, the entire existing surface shall be covered with gypsum board, mineral fiber, glass fiber or other *approved* materials securely fastened in place.

R907.5 Reinstallation of materials. Existing slate, clay or cement tile shall be permitted for reinstallation, except that damaged, cracked or broken slate or tile shall not be reinstalled. Existing vent flashing, metal edgings, drain outlets, collars and metal counterflashings shall not be reinstalled where rusted, damaged or deteriorated. Aggregate surfacing materials shall not be reinstalled.

R907.6 Flashings. Flashings shall be reconstructed in accordance with *approved* manufacturer's installation instructions. Metal flashing to which bituminous materials are to be adhered shall be primed prior to installation.

CHAPTER 10

CHIMNEYS AND FIREPLACES

SECTION R1001
MASONRY FIREPLACES

R1001.1 General. Masonry fireplaces shall be constructed in accordance with this section and the applicable provisions of Chapters 3 and 4.

R1001.2 Footings and foundations. Footings for masonry fireplaces and their chimneys shall be constructed of concrete or *solid masonry* at least 12 inches (305 mm) thick and shall extend at least 6 inches (152 mm) beyond the face of the fireplace or foundation wall on all sides. Footings shall be founded on natural, undisturbed earth or engineered fill below frost depth. In areas not subjected to freezing, footings shall be at least 12 inches (305 mm) below finished *grade*.

R1001.2.1 Ash dump cleanout. Cleanout openings located within foundation walls below fireboxes, when provided, shall be equipped with ferrous metal or masonry doors and frames constructed to remain tightly closed except when in use. Cleanouts shall be accessible and located so that ash removal will not create a hazard to combustible materials.

R1001.3 Seismic reinforcing. Masonry or concrete chimneys in Seismic Design Category D_0, D_1 or D_2 shall be reinforced. Reinforcing shall conform to the requirements set forth in Table R1001.1 and Section R609, Grouted Masonry.

R1001.3.1 Vertical reinforcing. For chimneys up to 40 inches (1016 mm) wide, four No. 4 continuous vertical bars shall be placed between wythes of *solid masonry* or within the cells of hollow unit masonry and grouted in accordance with Section R609. Grout shall be prevented from bonding with the flue liner so that the flue liner is free to move with thermal expansion. For chimneys more than 40 inches (1016 mm) wide, two additional No. 4 vertical bars shall be provided for each additional flue incorporated into the chimney or for each additional 40 inches (1016 mm) in width or fraction thereof.

R1001.3.2 Horizontal reinforcing. Vertical reinforcement shall be placed within $^1/_4$-inch (6 mm) ties, or other reinforcing of equivalent net cross-sectional area, placed in the bed joints according to Section R607 at a minimum of every 18 inches (457 mm) of vertical height. Two such ties shall be installed at each bend in the vertical bars.

R1001.4 Seismic anchorage. Masonry or concrete chimneys in Seismic Design Categories D_0, D_1 or D_2 shall be anchored at each floor, ceiling or roof line more than 6 feet (1829 mm) above *grade*, except where constructed completely within the exterior walls. Anchorage shall conform to the requirements of Section R1001.4.1.

R1001.4.1 Anchorage. Two $^3/_{16}$-inch by 1-inch (5 mm by 25 mm) straps shall be embedded a minimum of 12 inches (305 mm) into the chimney. Straps shall be hooked around the outer bars and extend 6 inches (152 mm) beyond the bend. Each strap shall be fastened to a minimum of four floor ceiling or floor joists or rafters with two $^1/_2$-inch (13 mm) bolts.

R1001.5 Firebox walls. Masonry fireboxes shall be constructed of *solid masonry* units, hollow masonry units grouted solid, stone or concrete. When a lining of firebrick at least 2 inches (51 mm) thick or other *approved* lining is provided, the minimum thickness of back and side walls shall each be 8 inches (203 mm) of *solid masonry*, including the lining. The width of joints between firebricks shall not be greater than $^1/_4$ inch (6 mm). When no lining is provided, the total minimum thickness of back and side walls shall be 10 inches (254 mm) of *solid masonry*. Firebrick shall conform to ASTM C 27 or C 1261 and shall be laid with medium duty refractory mortar conforming to ASTM C 199.

R1001.5.1 Steel fireplace units. Installation of steel fireplace units with *solid masonry* to form a masonry fireplace is permitted when installed either according to the requirements of their listing or according to the requirements of this section. Steel fireplace units incorporating a steel firebox lining, shall be constructed with steel not less than $^1/_4$ inch (6 mm) thick, and an air circulating chamber which is ducted to the interior of the building. The firebox lining shall be encased with *solid masonry* to provide a total thickness at the back and sides of not less than 8 inches (203 mm), of which not less than 4 inches (102 mm) shall be of *solid masonry* or concrete. Circulating air ducts used with steel fireplace units shall be constructed of metal or masonry.

R1001.6 Firebox dimensions. The firebox of a concrete or masonry fireplace shall have a minimum depth of 20 inches (508 mm). The throat shall not be less than 8 inches (203 mm) above the fireplace opening. The throat opening shall not be less than 4 inches (102 mm) deep. The cross-sectional area of the passageway above the firebox, including the throat, damper and smoke chamber, shall not be less than the cross-sectional area of the flue.

Exception: Rumford fireplaces shall be permitted provided that the depth of the fireplace is at least 12 inches (305 mm) and at least one-third of the width of the fireplace opening, that the throat is at least 12 inches (305 mm) above the lintel and is at least $^1/_{20}$ the cross-sectional area of the fireplace opening.

R1001.7 Lintel and throat. Masonry over a fireplace opening shall be supported by a lintel of noncombustible material. The minimum required bearing length on each end of the fireplace opening shall be 4 inches (102 mm). The fireplace throat or damper shall be located a minimum of 8 inches (203 mm) above the lintel.

R1001.7.1 Damper. Masonry fireplaces shall be equipped with a ferrous metal damper located at least 8 inches (203 mm) above the top of the fireplace opening. Dampers shall be installed in the fireplace or the chimney venting the fire-

TABLE R1001.1
SUMMARY OF REQUIREMENTS FOR MASONRY FIREPLACES AND CHIMNEYS

ITEM	LETTER[a]	REQUIREMENTS
Hearth slab thickness	A	4″
Hearth extension (each side of opening)	B	8″ fireplace opening < 6 square foot. 12″ fireplace opening ≥ 6 square foot.
Hearth extension (front of opening)	C	16″ fireplace opening < 6 square foot. 20″ fireplace opening ≥ 6 square foot.
Hearth slab reinforcing	D	Reinforced to carry its own weight and all imposed loads.
Thickness of wall of firebox	E	10″ solid brick or 8″ where a firebrick lining is used. Joints in firebrick $^1/_4$″ maximum.
Distance from top of opening to throat	F	8″
Smoke chamber wall thickness Unlined walls	G	6″ 8″
Chimney Vertical reinforcing[b]	H	Four No. 4 full-length bars for chimney up to 40″ wide. Add two No. 4 bars for each additional 40″ or fraction of width or each additional flue.
Horizontal reinforcing	J	$^1/_4$″ ties at 18″ and two ties at each bend in vertical steel.
Bond beams	K	No specified requirements.
Fireplace lintel	L	Noncombustible material.
Chimney walls with flue lining	M	Solid masonry units or hollow masonry units grouted solid with at least 4 inch nominal thickness.
Distances between adjacent flues	—	See Section R1003.13.
Effective flue area (based on area of fireplace opening)	P	See Section R1003.15.

Clearances:
    Combustible material
    Mantel and trim
    Above roof
	R	See Sections R1001.11 and R1003.18.
		See Section R1001.11, Exception 4.
		3′ at roofline and 2′ at 10′.

Anchorage[b]
    Strap
    Number
    Embedment into chimney
Fasten to
Bolts
	S	$^3/_{16}$″ × 1″
		Two
		12″ hooked around outer bar with 6″ extension.
		4 joists
		Two $^1/_2$″ diameter.

Footing
    Thickness
    Width
	T	12″ min.
		6″ each side of fireplace wall.

For SI: 1 inch = 25.4 mm, 1 foot = 304.8 mm, 1 square foot = 0.0929 m².

Note: This table provides a summary of major requirements for the construction of masonry chimneys and fireplaces. Letter references are to Figure R1001.1, which shows examples of typical construction. This table does not cover all requirements, nor does it cover all aspects of the indicated requirements. For the actual mandatory requirements of the code, see the indicated section of text.

a. The letters refer to Figure R1001.1.

b. Not required in Seismic Design Category A, B or C.

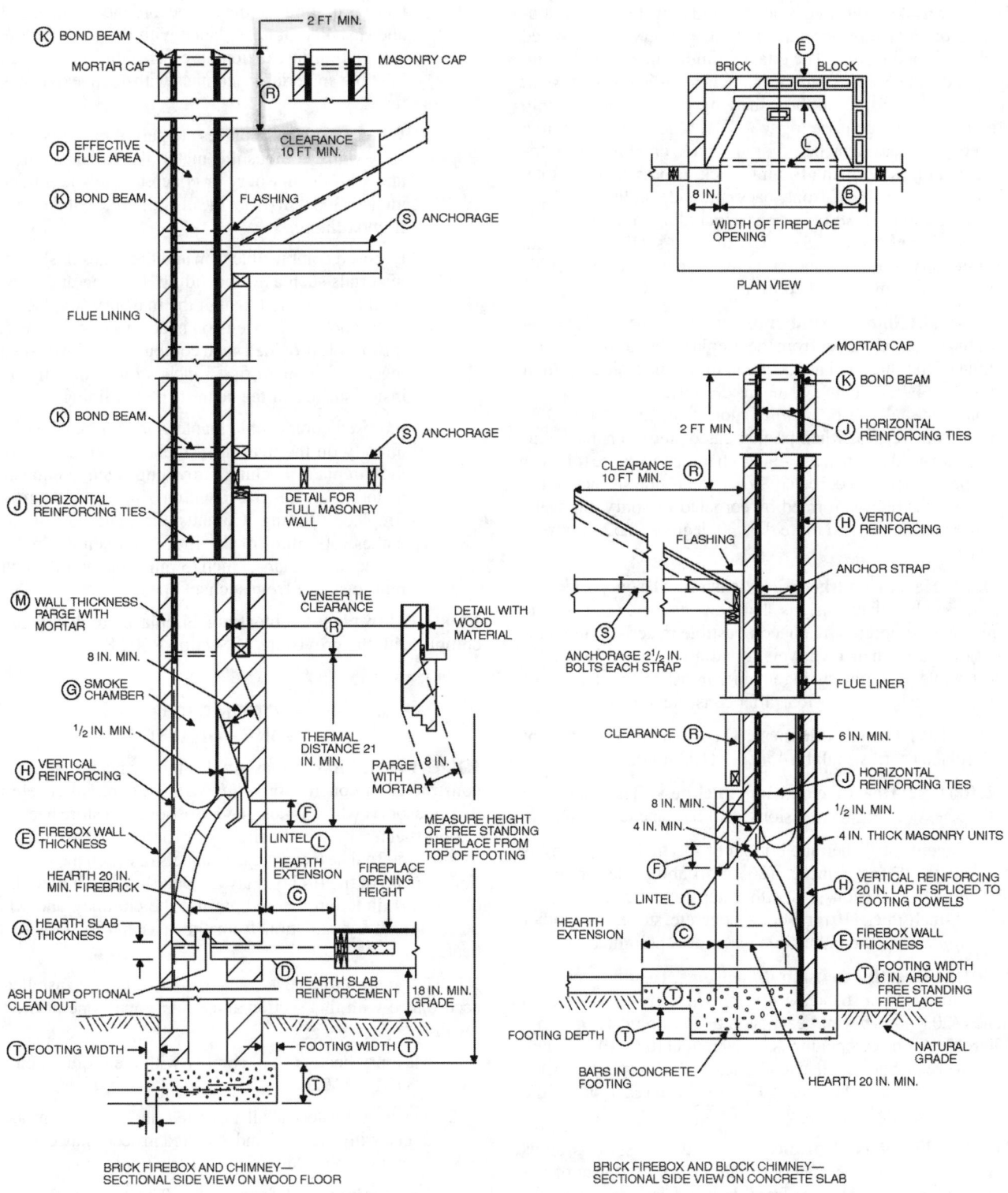

FIGURE R1001.1
FIREPLACE AND CHIMNEY DETAILS

For SI: 1 inch = 25.4 mm, 1 foot = 304.8 mm.

place, and shall be operable from the room containing the fireplace.

R1001.8 Smoke chamber. Smoke chamber walls shall be constructed of *solid masonry* units, hollow masonry units grouted solid, stone or concrete. The total minimum thickness of front, back and side walls shall be 8 inches (203 mm) of *solid masonry*. The inside surface shall be parged smooth with refractory mortar conforming to ASTM C 199. When a lining of firebrick at least 2 inches (51 mm) thick, or a lining of vitrified clay at least $^5/_8$ inch (16 mm) thick, is provided, the total minimum thickness of front, back and side walls shall be 6 inches (152 mm) of *solid masonry*, including the lining. Firebrick shall conform to ASTM C 1261 and shall be laid with medium duty refractory mortar conforming to ASTM C 199. Vitrified clay linings shall conform to ASTM C 315.

R1001.8.1 Smoke chamber dimensions. The inside height of the smoke chamber from the fireplace throat to the beginning of the flue shall not be greater than the inside width of the fireplace opening. The inside surface of the smoke chamber shall not be inclined more than 45 degrees (0.79 rad) from vertical when prefabricated smoke chamber linings are used or when the smoke chamber walls are rolled or sloped rather than corbeled. When the inside surface of the smoke chamber is formed by corbeled masonry, the walls shall not be corbeled more than 30 degrees (0.52 rad) from vertical.

R1001.9 Hearth and hearth extension. Masonry fireplace hearths and hearth extensions shall be constructed of concrete or masonry, supported by noncombustible materials, and reinforced to carry their own weight and all imposed loads. No combustible material shall remain against the underside of hearths and hearth extensions after construction.

R1001.9.1 Hearth thickness. The minimum thickness of fireplace hearths shall be 4 inches (102 mm).

R1001.9.2 Hearth extension thickness. The minimum thickness of hearth extensions shall be 2 inches (51 mm).

Exception: When the bottom of the firebox opening is raised at least 8 inches (203 mm) above the top of the hearth extension, a hearth extension of not less than $^3/_8$-inch-thick (10 mm) brick, concrete, stone, tile or other *approved* noncombustible material is permitted.

R1001.10 Hearth extension dimensions. Hearth extensions shall extend at least 16 inches (406 mm) in front of and at least 8 inches (203 mm) beyond each side of the fireplace opening. Where the fireplace opening is 6 square feet (0.6 m²) or larger, the hearth extension shall extend at least 20 inches (508 mm) in front of and at least 12 inches (305 mm) beyond each side of the fireplace opening.

R1001.11 Fireplace clearance. All wood beams, joists, studs and other combustible material shall have a clearance of not less than 2 inches (51 mm) from the front faces and sides of masonry fireplaces and not less than 4 inches (102 mm) from the back faces of masonry fireplaces. The air space shall not be filled, except to provide fire blocking in accordance with Section R1001.12.

Exceptions:

1. Masonry fireplaces *listed* and *labeled* for use in contact with combustibles in accordance with UL 127 and installed in accordance with the manufacturer's installation instructions are permitted to have combustible material in contact with their exterior surfaces.

2. When masonry fireplaces are part of masonry or concrete walls, combustible materials shall not be in contact with the masonry or concrete walls less than 12 inches (306 mm) from the inside surface of the nearest firebox lining.

3. Exposed combustible trim and the edges of sheathing materials such as wood siding, flooring and drywall shall be permitted to abut the masonry fireplace side walls and hearth extension in accordance with Figure R1001.11, provided such combustible trim or sheathing is a minimum of 12 inches (305 mm) from the inside surface of the nearest firebox lining.

4. Exposed combustible mantels or trim may be placed directly on the masonry fireplace front surrounding the fireplace opening providing such combustible materials are not placed within 6 inches (152 mm) of a fireplace opening. Combustible material within 12 inches (306 mm) of the fireplace opening shall not project more than $^1/_8$ inch (3 mm) for each 1-inch (25 mm) distance from such an opening.

R1001.12 Fireplace fireblocking. Fireplace fireblocking shall comply with the provisions of Section R602.8.

SECTION R1002
MASONRY HEATERS

R1002.1 Definition. A masonry heater is a heating *appliance* constructed of concrete or *solid masonry*, hereinafter referred to as masonry, which is designed to absorb and store heat from a solid-fuel fire built in the firebox by routing the exhaust gases through internal heat exchange channels in which the flow path downstream of the firebox may include flow in a horizontal or downward direction before entering the chimney and which delivers heat by radiation from the masonry surface of the heater.

R1002.2 Installation. Masonry heaters shall be installed in accordance with this section and comply with one of the following:

1. Masonry heaters shall comply with the requirements of ASTM E 1602; or

2. Masonry heaters shall be *listed* and *labeled* in accordance with UL 1482 and installed in accordance with the manufacturer's installation instructions.

R1002.3 Footings and foundation. The firebox floor of a masonry heater shall be a minimum thickness of 4 inches (102 mm) of noncombustible material and be supported on a noncombustible footing and foundation in accordance with Section R1003.2.

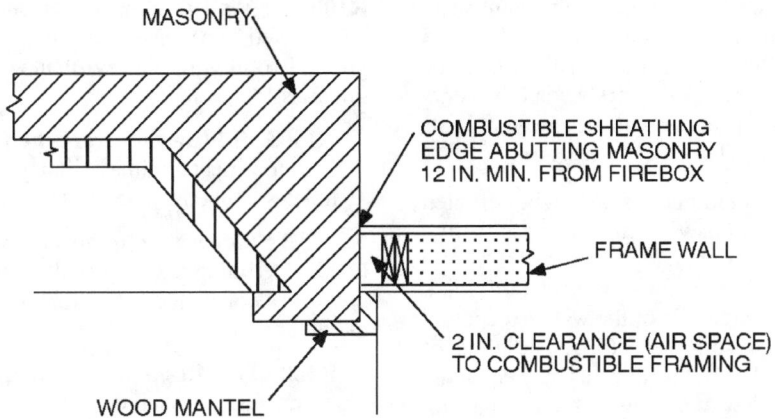

For SI: 1 inch = 25.4 mm.

FIGURE R1001.11
CLEARANCE FROM COMBUSTIBLES

R1002.4 Seismic reinforcing. In Seismic Design Categories D_0, D_1 and D_2, masonry heaters shall be anchored to the masonry foundation in accordance with Section R1003.3. Seismic reinforcing shall not be required within the body of a masonry heater whose height is equal to or less than 3.5 times it's body width and where the masonry chimney serving the heater is not supported by the body of the heater. Where the masonry chimney shares a common wall with the facing of the masonry heater, the chimney portion of the structure shall be reinforced in accordance with Section R1003.

R1002.5 Masonry heater clearance. Combustible materials shall not be placed within 36 inches (914 mm) of the outside surface of a masonry heater in accordance with NFPA 211 Section 8-7 (clearances for solid-fuel-burning *appliances*), and the required space between the heater and combustible material shall be fully vented to permit the free flow of air around all heater surfaces.

Exceptions:

1. When the masonry heater wall is at least 8 inches (203 mm) thick of *solid masonry* and the wall of the heat exchange channels is at least 5 inches (127 mm) thick of *solid masonry*, combustible materials shall not be placed within 4 inches (102 mm) of the outside surface of a masonry heater. A clearance of at least 8 inches (203 mm) shall be provided between the gas-tight capping slab of the heater and a combustible ceiling.

2. Masonry heaters tested and listed by an American National Standards Association (ANSI)-accredited laboratory to the requirements of UL1482 may be installed in accordance with the listing specifications and the manufacturer's written instructions.

SECTION R1003
MASONRY CHIMNEYS

R1003.1 Definition. A masonry chimney is a chimney constructed of *solid masonry* units, hollow masonry units grouted solid, stone or concrete, hereinafter referred to as masonry. Masonry chimneys shall be constructed, anchored, supported and reinforced as required in this chapter.

R1003.2 Footings and foundations. Footings for masonry chimneys shall be constructed of concrete or *solid masonry* at least 12 inches (305 mm) thick and shall extend at least 6 inches (152 mm) beyond the face of the foundation or support wall on all sides. Footings shall be founded on natural undisturbed earth or engineered fill below frost depth. In areas not subjected to freezing, footings shall be at least 12 inches (305 mm) below finished *grade*.

R1003.3 Seismic reinforcing. Masonry or concrete chimneys shall be constructed, anchored, supported and reinforced as required in this chapter. In Seismic Design Category D_0, D_1 or D_2 masonry and concrete chimneys shall be reinforced and anchored as detailed in Section R1003.3.1, R1003.3.2 and R1003.4. In Seismic Design Category A, B or C, reinforcement and seismic anchorage is not required.

R1003.3.1 Vertical reinforcing. For chimneys up to 40 inches (1016 mm) wide, four No. 4 continuous vertical bars, anchored in the foundation, shall be placed in the concrete, or between wythes of *solid masonry*, or within the cells of hollow unit masonry, and grouted in accordance with Section R609.1.1. Grout shall be prevented from bonding with the flue liner so that the flue liner is free to move with thermal expansion. For chimneys more than 40 inches (1016 mm) wide, two additional No. 4 vertical bars shall be installed for each additional 40 inches (1016 mm) in width or fraction thereof.

R1003.3.2 Horizontal reinforcing. Vertical reinforcement shall be placed enclosed within $^1/_4$-inch (6 mm) ties, or other reinforcing of equivalent net cross-sectional area, spaced not to exceed 18 inches (457 mm) on center in concrete, or placed in the bed joints of unit masonry, at a minimum of every 18 inches (457 mm) of vertical height. Two such ties shall be installed at each bend in the vertical bars.

R1003.4 Seismic anchorage. Masonry and concrete chimneys and foundations in Seismic Design Category D_0, D_1 or D_2 shall be anchored at each floor, ceiling or roof line more than 6 feet (1829 mm) above *grade*, except where constructed completely within the exterior walls. Anchorage shall conform to the requirements in Section R1003.4.1.

R1003.4.1 Anchorage. Two $^3/_{16}$-inch by 1-inch (5 mm by 25 mm) straps shall be embedded a minimum of 12 inches (305 mm) into the chimney. Straps shall be hooked around the outer bars and extend 6 inches (152 mm) beyond the bend. Each strap shall be fastened to a minimum of four floor joists with two $^1/_2$-inch (13 mm) bolts.

R1003.5 Corbeling. Masonry chimneys shall not be corbeled more than one-half of the chimney's wall thickness from a wall or foundation, nor shall a chimney be corbeled from a wall or foundation that is less than 12 inches (305 mm) thick unless it projects equally on each side of the wall, except that on the second *story* of a two-story *dwelling*, corbeling of chimneys on the exterior of the enclosing walls may equal the wall thickness. The projection of a single course shall not exceed one-half the unit height or one-third of the unit bed depth, whichever is less.

R1003.6 Changes in dimension. The chimney wall or chimney flue lining shall not change in size or shape within 6 inches (152 mm) above or below where the chimney passes through floor components, ceiling components or roof components.

R1003.7 Offsets. Where a masonry chimney is constructed with a fireclay flue liner surrounded by one wythe of masonry, the maximum offset shall be such that the centerline of the flue above the offset does not extend beyond the center of the chimney wall below the offset. Where the chimney offset is supported by masonry below the offset in an *approved* manner, the maximum offset limitations shall not apply. Each individual corbeled masonry course of the offset shall not exceed the projection limitations specified in Section R1003.5.

R1003.8 Additional load. Chimneys shall not support loads other than their own weight unless they are designed and constructed to support the additional load. Construction of masonry chimneys as part of the masonry walls or reinforced concrete walls of the building shall be permitted.

R1003.9 Termination. Chimneys shall extend at least 2 feet (610 mm) higher than any portion of a building within 10 feet (3048 mm), but shall not be less than 3 feet (914 mm) above the highest point where the chimney passes through the roof.

R1003.9.1 Spark arrestors. Where a spark arrestor is installed on a masonry chimney, the spark arrestor shall meet all of the following requirements:

1. The net free area of the arrestor shall not be less than four times the net free area of the outlet of the chimney flue it serves.

2. The arrestor screen shall have heat and corrosion resistance equivalent to 19-gage galvanized steel or 24-gage stainless steel.

3. Openings shall not permit the passage of spheres having a diameter greater than $^1/_2$ inch (13 mm) nor block the passage of spheres having a diameter less than $^3/_8$ inch (10 mm).

4. The spark arrestor shall be accessible for cleaning and the screen or chimney cap shall be removable to allow for cleaning of the chimney flue.

R1003.10 Wall thickness. Masonry chimney walls shall be constructed of *solid masonry* units or hollow masonry units grouted solid with not less than a 4-inch (102 mm) nominal thickness.

R1003.10.1 Masonry veneer chimneys. Where masonry is used to veneer a frame chimney, through-flashing and weep holes shall be installed as required by Section R703.

R1003.11 Flue lining (material). Masonry chimneys shall be lined. The lining material shall be appropriate for the type of *appliance* connected, according to the terms of the *appliance* listing and manufacturer's instructions.

R1003.11.1 Residential-type appliances (general). Flue lining systems shall comply with one of the following:

1. Clay flue lining complying with the requirements of ASTM C 315.

2. Listed chimney lining systems complying with UL 1777.

3. Factory-built chimneys or chimney units listed for installation within masonry chimneys.

4. Other *approved* materials that will resist corrosion, erosion, softening or cracking from flue gases and condensate at temperatures up to 1,800°F (982°C).

R1003.11.2 Flue linings for specific appliances. Flue linings other than these covered in Section R1003.11.1, intended for use with specific types of *appliances*, shall comply with Sections R1003.11.3 through R1003.11.6.

R1003.11.3 Gas appliances. Flue lining systems for gas *appliances* shall be in accordance with Chapter 24.

R1003.11.4 Pellet fuel-burning appliances. Flue lining and vent systems for use in masonry chimneys with pellet fuel-burning *appliances* shall be limited to the following:

1. Flue lining systems complying with Section R1003.11.1.

2. Pellet vents listed for installation within masonry chimneys. (See Section R1003.11.6 for marking.)

R1003.11.5 Oil-fired appliances approved for use with Type L vent. Flue lining and vent systems for use in masonry chimneys with oil-fired *appliances approved* for use with Type L vent shall be limited to the following:

1. Flue lining systems complying with Section R1003.11.1.

2. Listed chimney liners complying with UL 641. (See Section R1003.11.6 for marking.)

R1003.11.6 Notice of usage. When a flue is relined with a material not complying with Section R1003.11.1, the chimney shall be plainly and permanently identified by a *label* attached to a wall, ceiling or other conspicuous location adjacent to where the connector enters the chimney. The *label* shall include the following message or equivalent language:

THIS CHIMNEY FLUE IS FOR USE ONLY WITH [TYPE OR CATEGORY OF *APPLIANCE*] *APPLIANCES* THAT BURN [TYPE OF FUEL]. DO NOT CONNECT OTHER TYPES OF *APPLIANCES*.

R1003.12 Clay flue lining (installation). Clay flue liners shall be installed in accordance with ASTM C 1283 and extend from a point not less than 8 inches (203 mm) below the lowest inlet or, in the case of fireplaces, from the top of the smoke chamber to a point above the enclosing walls. The lining shall be carried up vertically, with a maximum slope no greater than 30 degrees (0.52 rad) from the vertical.

Clay flue liners shall be laid in medium-duty water insoluble refractory mortar conforming to ASTM C 199 with tight mortar joints left smooth on the inside and installed to maintain an air space or insulation not to exceed the thickness of the flue liner separating the flue liners from the interior face of the chimney masonry walls. Flue liners shall be supported on all sides. Only enough mortar shall be placed to make the joint and hold the liners in position.

R1003.12.1 Listed materials. *Listed* materials used as flue linings shall be installed in accordance with the terms of their listings and manufacturer's instructions.

R1003.12.2 Space around lining. The space surrounding a chimney lining system or vent installed within a masonry chimney shall not be used to vent any other *appliance*.

Exception: This shall not prevent the installation of a separate flue lining in accordance with the manufacturer's installation instructions.

R1003.13 Multiple flues. When two or more flues are located in the same chimney, masonry wythes shall be built between adjacent flue linings. The masonry wythes shall be at least 4 inches (102 mm) thick and bonded into the walls of the chimney.

Exception: When venting only one *appliance*, two flues may adjoin each other in the same chimney with only the flue lining separation between them. The joints of the adjacent flue linings shall be staggered at least 4 inches (102 mm).

R1003.14 Flue area (appliance). Chimney flues shall not be smaller in area than that of the area of the connector from the *appliance* [see Tables R1003.14(1) and R1003.14(2)]. The sizing of a chimney flue to which multiple *appliance* venting systems are connected shall be in accordance with Section M1805.3.

R1003.15 Flue area (masonry fireplace). Flue sizing for chimneys serving fireplaces shall be in accordance with Section R1003.15.1 or Section R1003.15.2.

R1003.15.1 Option 1. Round chimney flues shall have a minimum net cross-sectional area of at least $^1/_{12}$ of the fireplace opening. Square chimney flues shall have a minimum net cross-sectional area of $^1/_{10}$ of the fireplace opening. Rectangular chimney flues with an *aspect ratio* less than 2 to 1 shall have a minimum net cross-sectional area of $^1/_{10}$ of the fireplace opening. Rectangular chimney flues with an *aspect ratio* of 2 to 1 or more shall have a minimum net cross-sectional area of $^1/_8$ of the fireplace opening. Cross-sectional areas of clay flue linings are shown in Tables R1001.14(1) and R1001.14(2) or as provided by the manufacturer or as measured in the field.

R1003.15.2 Option 2. The minimum net cross-sectional area of the chimney flue shall be determined in accordance with Figure R1003.15.2. A flue size providing at least the equiva-

lent net cross-sectional area shall be used. Cross-sectional areas of clay flue linings are shown in Tables R1003.14(1) and R1003.14(2) or as provided by the manufacturer or as measured in the field. The height of the chimney shall be measured from the firebox floor to the top of the chimney flue.

TABLE R1003.14(1)
NET CROSS–SECTIONAL AREA OF ROUND FLUE SIZES[a]

FLUE SIZE, INSIDE DIAMETER (inches)	CROSS–SECTIONAL AREA (square inches)
6	28
7	38
8	50
10	78
10$^3/_4$	90
12	113
15	176
18	254

For SI: 1 inch = 25.4 mm, 1 square inch = 645.16 mm².
a. Flue sizes are based on ASTM C 315.

TABLE R1003.14(2)
NET CROSS–SECTIONAL AREA OF SQUARE AND RECTANGULAR FLUE SIZES

FLUE SIZE, OUTSIDE NOMINAL DIMENSIONS (inches)	CROSS–SECTIONAL AREA (square inches)
4.5 × 8.5	23
4.5 × 13	34
8 × 8	42
8.5 × 8.5	49
8 × 12	67
8.5 × 13	76
12 × 12	102
8.5 × 18	101
13 × 13	127
12 × 16	131
13 × 18	173
16 × 16	181
16 × 20	222
18 × 18	233
20 × 20	298
20 × 24	335
24 × 24	431

For SI: 1 inch = 25.4 mm, 1 square inch = 645.16 mm².

R1003.16 Inlet. Inlets to masonry chimneys shall enter from the side. Inlets shall have a thimble of fireclay, rigid refractory material or metal that will prevent the connector from pulling out of the inlet or from extending beyond the wall of the liner.

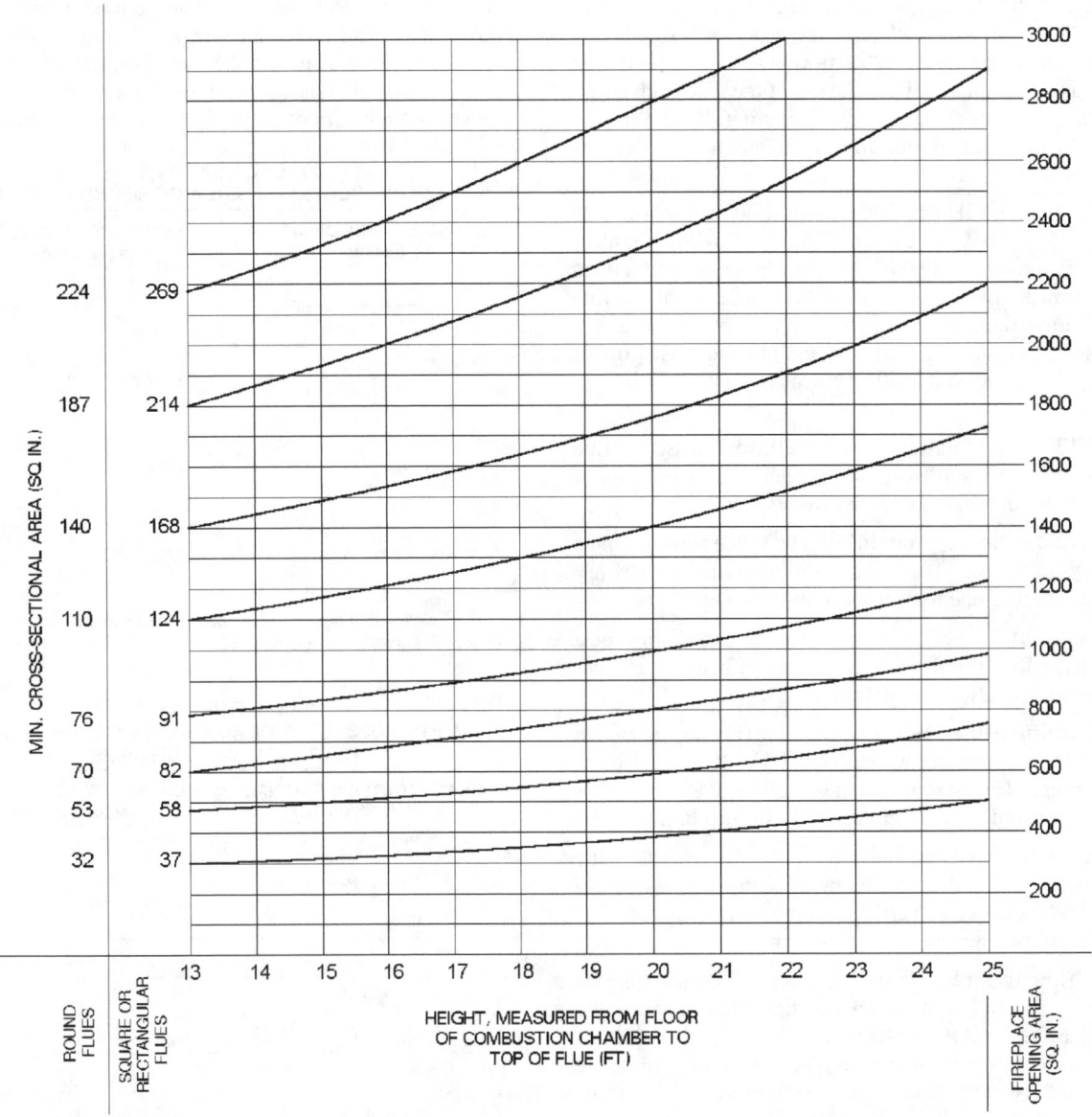

For SI: 1 foot = 304.8 mm, 1 square inch = 645.16 mm².

FIGURE R1003.15.2
FLUE SIZES FOR MASONRY CHIMNEYS

R1003.17 Masonry chimney cleanout openings. Cleanout openings shall be provided within 6 inches (152 mm) of the base of each flue within every masonry chimney. The upper edge of the cleanout shall be located at least 6 inches (152 mm) below the lowest chimney inlet opening. The height of the opening shall be at least 6 inches (152 mm). The cleanout shall be provided with a noncombustible cover.

Exception: Chimney flues serving masonry fireplaces where cleaning is possible through the fireplace opening.

R1003.18 Chimney clearances. Any portion of a masonry chimney located in the interior of the building or within the exterior wall of the building shall have a minimum air space clearance to combustibles of 2 inches (51 mm). Chimneys located entirely outside the exterior walls of the building, including chimneys that pass through the soffit or cornice, shall

have a minimum air space clearance of 1 inch (25 mm). The air space shall not be filled, except to provide fire blocking in accordance with Section R1003.19.

Exceptions:

1. Masonry chimneys equipped with a chimney lining system listed and *labeled* for use in chimneys in contact with combustibles in accordance with UL 1777 and installed in accordance with the manufacturer's installation instructions are permitted to have combustible material in contact with their exterior surfaces.

2. When masonry chimneys are constructed as part of masonry or concrete walls, combustible materials shall not be in contact with the masonry or concrete

wall less than 12 inches (305 mm) from the inside surface of the nearest flue lining.

3. Exposed combustible trim and the edges of sheathing materials, such as wood siding and flooring, shall be permitted to abut the masonry chimney side walls, in accordance with Figure R1003.18, provided such combustible trim or sheathing is a minimum of 12 inches (305 mm) from the inside surface of the nearest flue lining. Combustible material and trim shall not overlap the corners of the chimney by more than 1 inch (25 mm).

R1003.19 Chimney fireblocking. All spaces between chimneys and floors and ceilings through which chimneys pass shall be fireblocked with noncombustible material securely fastened in place. The fireblocking of spaces between chimneys and wood joists, beams or headers shall be self-supporting or be placed on strips of metal or metal lath laid across the spaces between combustible material and the chimney.

R1003.20 Chimney crickets. Chimneys shall be provided with crickets when the dimension parallel to the ridgeline is greater than 30 inches (762 mm) and does not intersect the ridgeline. The intersection of the cricket and the chimney shall be flashed and counterflashed in the same manner as normal roof-chimney intersections. Crickets shall be constructed in compliance with Figure R1003.20 and Table R1003.20.

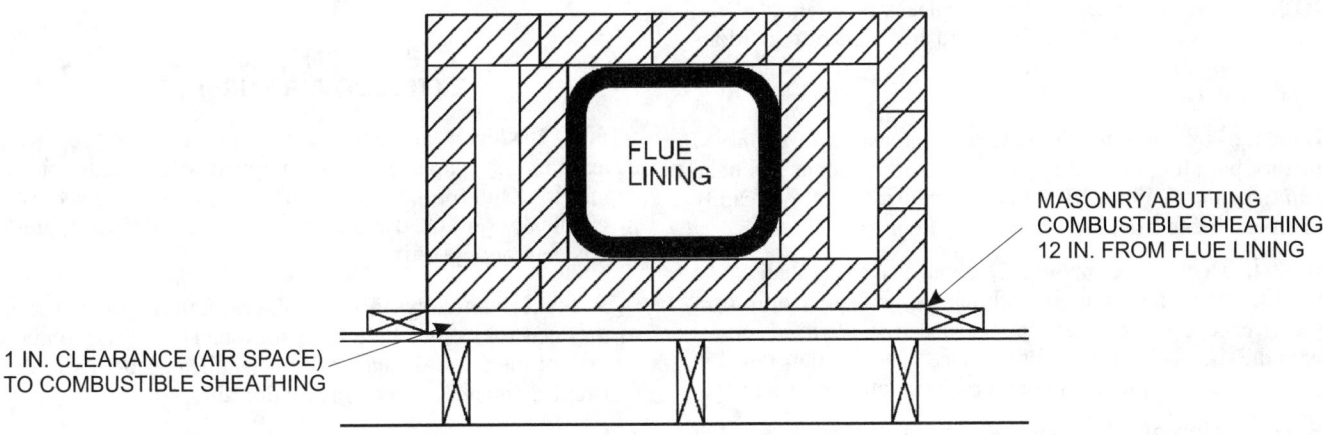

For SI: 1 inch = 25.4 mm.

FIGURE R1003.18
CLEARANCE FROM COMBUSTIBLES

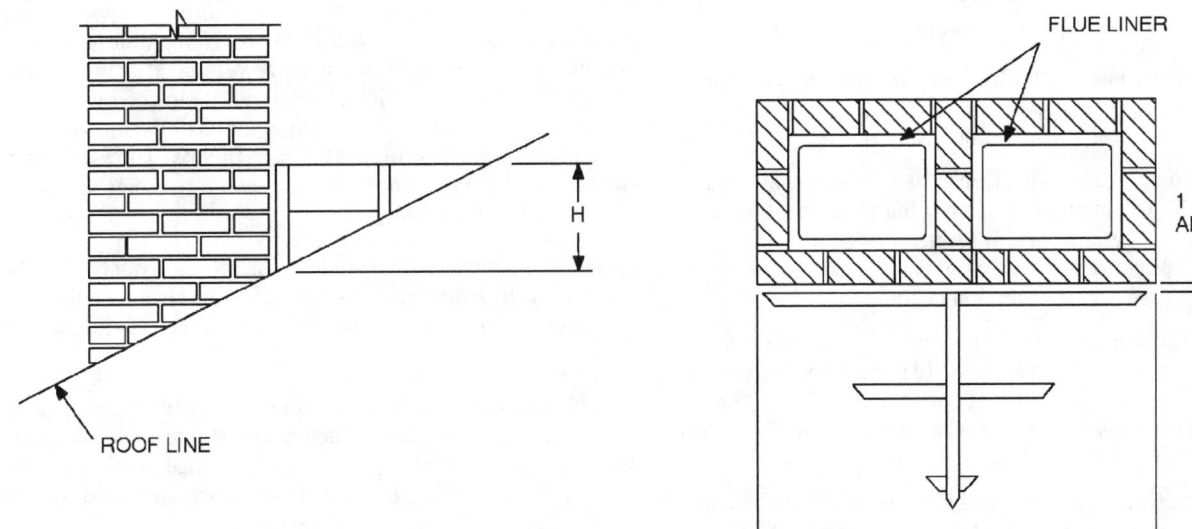

For SI: 1 inch = 25.4 mm.

FIGURE R1003.20
CHIMNEY CRICKET

TABLE R1003.20
CRICKET DIMENSIONS

ROOF SLOPE	H
12 - 12	$^1/_2$ of W
8 - 12	$^1/_3$ of W
6 - 12	$^1/_4$ of W
4 - 12	$^1/_6$ of W
3 - 12	$^1/_8$ of W

SECTION R1004
FACTORY-BUILT FIREPLACES

R1004.1 General. Factory-built fireplaces shall be *listed* and *labeled* and shall be installed in accordance with the conditions of the *listing*. Factory-built fireplaces shall be tested in accordance with UL 127.

R1004.2 Hearth extensions. Hearth extensions of *approved* factory-built fireplaces shall be installed in accordance with the *listing* of the fireplace. The hearth extension shall be readily distinguishable from the surrounding floor area.

R1004.3 Decorative shrouds. Decorative shrouds shall not be installed at the termination of chimneys for factory-built fireplaces except where the shrouds are listed and *labeled* for use with the specific factory-built fireplace system and installed in accordance with the manufacturer's installation instructions.

R1004.4 Unvented gas log heaters. An unvented gas log heater shall not be installed in a factory-built fireplace unless the fireplace system has been specifically tested, *listed* and *labeled* for such use in accordance with UL 127.

SECTION R1005
FACTORY-BUILT CHIMNEYS

R1005.1 Listing. Factory-built chimneys shall be *listed* and *labeled* and shall be installed and terminated in accordance with the manufacturer's installation instructions.

R1005.2 Decorative shrouds. Decorative shrouds shall not be installed at the termination of factory-built chimneys except where the shrouds are *listed* and *labeled* for use with the specific factory-built chimney system and installed in accordance with the manufacturer's installation instructions.

R1005.3 Solid-fuel appliances. Factory-built chimneys installed in *dwelling units* with solid-fuel-burning *appliances* shall comply with the Type HT requirements of UL 103 and shall be marked "Type HT and "Residential Type and Building Heating *Appliance* Chimney."

> **Exception:** Chimneys for use with open combustion chamber fireplaces shall comply with the requirements of UL 103 and shall be marked "Residential Type and Building Heating *Appliance* Chimney."

Chimneys for use with open combustion chamber *appliances* installed in buildings other than *dwelling units* shall comply with the requirements of UL 103 and shall be marked

"Building Heating *Appliance* Chimney" or "Residential Type and Building Heating *Appliance* Chimney."

R1005.4 Factory-built fireplaces. Chimneys for use with factory-built fireplaces shall comply with the requirements of UL 127.

R1005.5 Support. Where factory-built chimneys are supported by structural members, such as joists and rafters, those members shall be designed to support the additional load.

R1005.6 Medium-heat appliances. Factory-built chimneys for medium-heat *appliances* producing flue gases having a temperature above 1,000°F (538°C), measured at the entrance to the chimney shall comply with UL 959.

SECTION R1006
EXTERIOR AIR SUPPLY

R1006.1 Exterior air. Factory-built or masonry fireplaces covered in this chapter shall be equipped with an exterior air supply to assure proper fuel combustion unless the room is mechanically ventilated and controlled so that the indoor pressure is neutral or positive.

R1006.1.1 Factory-built fireplaces. Exterior *combustion air* ducts for factory-built fireplaces shall be a *listed* component of the fireplace and shall be installed according to the fireplace manufacturer's instructions.

R1006.1.2 Masonry fireplaces. *Listed combustion air* ducts for masonry fireplaces shall be installed according to the terms of their *listing* and the manufacturer's instructions.

R1006.2 Exterior air intake. The exterior air intake shall be capable of supplying all *combustion air* from the exterior of the *dwelling* or from spaces within the *dwelling* ventilated with outside air such as nonmechanically ventilated crawl or *attic* spaces. The exterior air intake shall not be located within the garage or *basement* of the *dwelling* nor shall the air intake be located at an elevation higher than the firebox. The exterior air intake shall be covered with a corrosion-resistant screen of $^1/_4$-inch (6 mm) mesh.

R1006.3 Clearance. Unlisted *combustion air* ducts shall be installed with a minimum 1-inch (25 mm) clearance to combustibles for all parts of the duct within 5 feet (1524 mm) of the duct outlet.

R1006.4 Passageway. The *combustion air* passageway shall be a minimum of 6 square inches (3870 mm²) and not more than 55 square inches (0.035 m²), except that *combustion air* systems for listed fireplaces shall be constructed according to the fireplace manufacturer's instructions.

R1006.5 Outlet. Locating the exterior air outlet in the back or sides of the firebox chamber or within 24 inches (610 mm) of the firebox opening on or near the floor is permitted. The outlet shall be closable and designed to prevent burning material from dropping into concealed combustible spaces.

Part IV—Energy Conservation

CHAPTER 11

ENERGY EFFICIENCY

SECTION N1101
GENERAL

N1101.1 Scope. This chapter regulates the energy efficiency for the design and construction of buildings regulated by this code.

Exception: Portions of the building envelope that do not enclose *conditioned space*.

N1101.2 Compliance. Compliance shall be demonstrated by either meeting the requirements of the *International Energy Conservation Code* or meeting the requirements of this chapter. Climate zones from Figure N1101.2 or Table N1101.2 shall be used in determining the applicable requirements from this chapter.

N1101.2.1 Warm humid counties. Warm humid counties are identified in Table N1101.2 by an asterisk.

N1101.3 Identification. Materials, systems and *equipment* shall be identified in a manner that will allow a determination of compliance with the applicable provisions of this chapter.

N1101.4 Building thermal envelope insulation. An *R*-value identification *mark* shall be applied by the manufacturer to each piece of *building thermal envelope* insulation 12 inches (305 mm) or more wide. Alternately, the insulation installers shall provide a certification listing the type, manufacturer and *R*-value of insulation installed in each element of the *building thermal envelope*. For blown or sprayed insulation (fiberglass and cellulose), the initial installed thickness, settled thickness, settled *R*-value, installed density, coverage area and number of bags installed shall be listed on the certification. For sprayed polyurethane foam (SPF) insulation, the installed thickness of the area covered and *R*-value of installed thickness shall be listed on the certificate. The insulation installer shall sign, date and post the certificate in a conspicuous location on the job site.

N1101.4.1 Blown or sprayed roof/ceiling insulation. The thickness of blown in or sprayed roof/ceiling insulation (fiberglass or cellulose) shall be written in inches (mm) on markers that are installed at least one for every 300 ft^2 (28 m^2) throughout the *attic* space. The markers shall be affixed to the trusses or joists and marked with the minimum initial installed thickness with numbers a minimum of 1 inch (25 mm) high. Each marker shall face the *attic* access opening. Spray polyurethane foam thickness and installed *R*-value shall be listed on the certificate provided by the insulation installer.

N1101.4.2 Insulation mark installation. Insulating materials shall be installed such that the manufacturer's *R*-value *mark* is readily observable upon inspection.

N1101.5 Fenestration product rating. *U*-factors of fenestration products (windows, doors and skylights) shall be determined in accordance with NFRC 100 by an accredited, independent laboratory, and *labeled* and certified by the manu-

facturer. Products lacking such a *labeled U*-factor shall be assigned a default *U*-factor from Tables N1101.5(1) and N1101.5(2). The solar heat gain coefficient (SHGC) of glazed fenestration products (windows, glazed doors and skylights) shall be determined in accordance with NFRC 200 by an accredited, independent laboratory, and *labeled* and certified by the manufacturer. Products lacking such a *labeled* SHGC shall be assigned a default SHGC from Table N1101.5(3).

N1101.6 Insulation product rating. The thermal resistance (*R*-value) of insulation shall be determined in accordance with the CFR Title 16, Part 460, in units of h · ft^2 ·°F/Btu at a mean temperature of 75°F (24°C).

N1101.7 Installation. All materials, systems and *equipment* shall be installed in accordance with the manufacturer's installation instructions and the provisions of this code.

N1101.7.1 Protection of exposed foundation insulation. Insulation applied to the exterior of *basement* walls, crawl space walls, and the perimeter of slab-on-grade floors shall have a rigid, opaque and weather-resistant protective covering to prevent the degradation of the insulation's thermal performance. The protective covering shall cover the exposed exterior insulation and extend a minimum of 6 inches (152 mm) below *grade*.

N1101.8 Above code programs. The *building official* or other authority having *jurisdiction* shall be permitted to deem a national, state or local energy efficiency program to exceed the energy efficiency required by this chapter. Buildings *approved* in writing by such an energy efficiency program shall be considered in compliance with this chapter.

N1101.9 Certificate. A permanent certificate shall be posted on or in the electrical distribution panel. The certificate shall not cover or obstruct the visibility of the circuit directory *label*, service disconnect *label* or other required *labels*. The certificate shall be completed by the builder or registered *design professional*. The certificate shall list the predominant *R*-values of insulation installed in or on ceiling/roof, walls, foundation (slab, *basement wall*, crawlspace wall and/or floor) and ducts outside *conditioned spaces*; *U*-factors for fenestration; and the solar heat gain coefficient (SHGC) of fenestration. Where there is more than one value for each component, the certificate shall list the value covering the largest area. The certificate shall list the types and efficiencies of heating, cooling and service water heating *equipment*. Where a gas-fired unvented room heater, electric furnace and/or baseboard electric heater is installed in the residence, the certificate shall list "gas-fired unvented room heater," "electric furnace" or "baseboard electric heater," as appropriate. An efficiency shall not be listed for gas-fired unvented room heaters, electric furnaces or electric base board heaters.

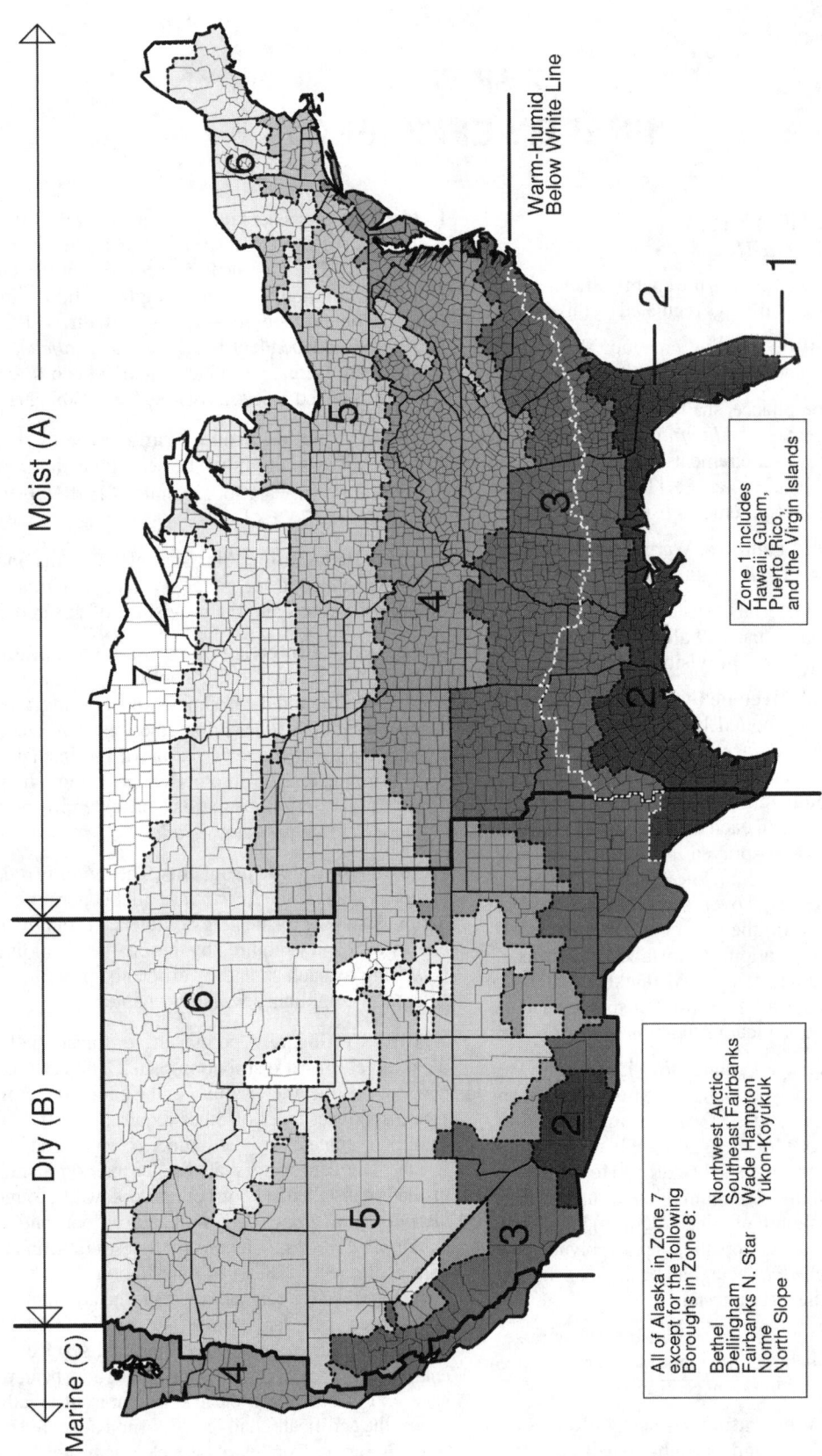

FIGURE N1101.2
CLIMATE ZONES

Moist (A)

Dry (B)

Marine (C)

Warm-Humid
Below White Line

Zone 1 includes
Hawaii, Guam,
Puerto Rico,
and the Virgin Islands

All of Alaska in Zone 7
except for the following
Boroughs in Zone 8:

Bethel   Northwest Arctic
Dellingham   Southeast Fairbanks
Fairbanks N. Star   Wade Hampton
Nome   Yukon-Koyukuk
North Slope

TABLE N1101.2
CLIMATE ZONES, MOISTURE REGIMES AND WARM-HUMID DESIGNATIONS BY STATE, COUNTY AND TERRITORY

Key:

A—Moist, B—Dry, C—Marine, Absence of moisture designation indicates moisture regime is irrelevant. Asterisk (*) indicates a warm-humid location.

UNITED STATES

Alabama

3A	Autauga*
2A	Baldwin*
3A	Barbour*
3A	Bibb
3A	Blount
3A	Bullock*
3A	Butler*
3A	Calhoun
3A	Chambers
3A	Cherokee
3A	Chilton
3A	Choctaw*
3A	Clarke*
3A	Clay
3A	Cleburne
3A	Coffee*
3A	Colbert
3A	Conecuh*
3A	Coosa
3A	Covington*
3A	Crenshaw*
3A	Cullman
3A	Dale*
3A	Dallas*
3A	Dekalb
3A	Elmore*
3A	Escambia*
3A	Etowah
3A	Fayette
3A	Franklin
3A	Geneva*
3A	Greene
3A	Hale
3A	Henry*
3A	Houston*
3A	Jackson
3A	Jefferson
3A	Lamar
3A	Lauderdale
3A	Lawrence
3A	Lee
3A	Limestone
3A	Lowndes*
3A	Macon*
3A	Madison
3A	Marengo*
3A	Marion
3A	Marshall
2A	Mobile*
3A	Monroe*
3A	Montgomery*
3A	Morgan
3A	Perry*

3A	Pickens
3A	Pike
3A	Randolph
3A	Russell*
3A	Shelby
3A	St. Clair
3A	Sumter
3A	Talladega
3A	Tallapoosa
3A	Tuscaloosa
3A	Walker
3A	Washington*
3A	Wilcox*
3A	Winston

Alaska

7	Aleutians East
7	Aleutians West
7	Anchorage
8	Bethel
7	Bristol Bay
7	Denali
8	Dillingham
8	Fairbanks North Star
7	Haines
7	Juneau
7	Kenai Peninsula
7	Ketchikan Gateway
7	Kodiak Island
7	Lake and Peninsula
7	Matanuska-Susitna
8	Nome
8	North Slope
8	Northwest Arctic
7	Prince of Wales-Outer ketchikan
7	Sitka
7	Skagway-Hoonah-Angoon
8	Southeast Fairbanks
7	Valdez-Cordova
8	Wade Hampton
7	Wrangell-Petersburg
7	Yakutat
8	Yukon-Koyukuk

Arizona

5B	Apache
3B	Cochise
5B	Coconino
4B	Gila

3B	Graham
3B	Greenlee
2B	La Paz
2B	Maricopa
3B	Mohave
5B	Navajo
2B	Pima
2B	Pinal
3B	Santa Cruz
4B	Yavapai
2B	Yuma

Arkansas

3A	Arkansas
3A	Ashley
4A	Baxter
4A	Benton
4A	Boone
3A	Bradley
3A	Calhoun
4A	Carroll
3A	Chicot
3A	Clark
3A	Clay
3A	Cleburne
3A	Cleveland
3A	Columbia*
3A	Conway
3A	Craighead
3A	Crawford
3A	Crittenden
3A	Cross
3A	Dallas
3A	Desha
3A	Drew
3A	Faulkner
3A	Franklin
4A	Fulton
3A	Garland
3A	Grant
3A	Greene
3A	Hempstead*
3A	Hot Spring
3A	Howard
3A	Independence
4A	Izard
3A	Jackson
3A	Jefferson
3A	Johnson
3A	Lafayette*
3A	Lawrence
3A	Lee
3A	Lincoln
3A	Little River*
3A	Logan

3A	Lonoke
4A	Madison
4A	Marion
3A	Miller*
3A	Mississippi
3A	Monroe
3A	Montgomery
3A	Nevada
4A	Newton
3A	Ouachita
3A	Perry
3A	Phillips
3A	Pike
3A	Poinsett
3A	Polk
3A	Pope
3A	Prairie
3A	Pulaski
3A	Randolph
3A	Saline
3A	Scott
4A	Searcy
3A	Sebastian
3A	Sevier*
3A	Sharp
3A	St. Francis
4A	Stone
3A	Union*
3A	Van Buren
4A	Washington
3A	White
3A	Woodruff
3A	Yell

California

3C	Alameda
6B	Alpine
4B	Amador
3B	Butte
4B	Calaveras
3B	Colusa
3B	Contra Costa
4C	Del Norte
4B	El Dorado
3B	Fresno
3B	Glenn
4C	Humboldt
2B	Imperial
4B	Inyo
3B	Kern
3B	Kings
4B	Lake
5B	Lassen
3B	Los Angeles
3B	Madera

3C	Marin
4B	Mariposa
3C	Mendocino
3B	Merced
5B	Modoc
6B	Mono
3C	Monterey
3C	Napa
5B	Nevada
3B	Orange
3B	Placer
5B	Plumas
3B	Riverside
3B	Sacramento
3C	San Benito
3B	San Bernardino
3B	San Diego
3C	San Francisco
3B	San Joaquin
3C	San Luis Obispo
3C	San Mateo
3C	Santa Barbara
3C	Santa Clara
3C	Santa Cruz
3B	Shasta
5B	Sierra
5B	Siskiyou
3B	Solano
3C	Sonoma
3B	Stanislaus
3B	Sutter
3B	Tehama
4B	Trinity
3B	Tulare
4B	Tuolumne
3C	Ventura
3B	Yolo
3B	Yuba

Colorado

5B	Adams
6B	Alamosa
5B	Arapahoe
6B	Archuleta
4B	Baca
5B	Bent
5B	Boulder
6B	Chaffee
5B	Cheyenne
7	Clear Creek
6B	Conejos
6B	Costilla
5B	Crowley
6B	Custer
5B	Delta

(continued)

TABLE N1101.2—continued
CLIMATE ZONES, MOISTURE REGIMES AND WARM-HUMID DESIGNATIONS BY STATE, COUNTY AND TERRITORY

Key:

A—Moist, B—Dry, C—Marine, Absence of moisture designation indicates moisture regime is irrelevant. Asterisk (*) indicates a warm-humid location.

5B	Denver	**District of Columbia**		2A	Pinellas*	3A	Coweta	4A	Lumpkin

5B Denver
6B Dolores
5B Douglas
6B Eagle
5B Elbert
5B El Paso
5B Fremont
5B Garfield
5B Gilpin
7 Grand
7 Gunnison
7 Hinsdale
5B Huerfano
7 Jackson
5B Jefferson
5B Kiowa
5B Kit Carson
7 Lake
5B La Plata
5B Larimer
4B Las Animas
5B Lincoln
5B Logan
5B Mesa
7 Mineral
6B Moffat
5B Montezuma
5B Montrose
5B Morgan
4B Otero
6B Ouray
7 Park
5B Phillips
7 Pitkin
5B Prowers
5B Pueblo
6B Rio Blanco
7 Rio Grande
7 Routt
6B Saguache
7 San Juan
6B San Miguel
5B Sedgwick
7 Summit
5B Teller
5B Washington
5B Weld
5B Yuma

Connecticut
5A (all)

Delaware
4A (all)

District of Columbia
4A (all)

Florida
2A Alachua*
2A Baker*
2A Bay*
2A Bradford*
2A Brevard*
1A Broward*
2A Calhoun*
2A Charlotte*
2A Citrus*
2A Clay*
2A Collier*
2A Columbia*
2A DeSoto*
2A Dixie*
2A Duval*
2A Escambia*
2A Flagler*
2A Franklin*
2A Gadsden*
2A Gilchrist*
2A Glades*
2A Gulf*
2A Hamilton*
2A Hardee*
2A Hendry*
2A Hernando*
2A Highlands*
2A Hillsborough*
2A Holmes*
2A Indian River*
2A Jackson*
2A Jefferson*
2A Lafayette*
2A Lake*
2A Lee*
2A Leon*
2A Levy*
2A Liberty*
2A Madison*
2A Manatee*
2A Marion*
2A Martin*
1A Miami-Dade*
1A Monroe*
2A Nassau*
2A Okaloosa*
2A Okeechobee*
2A Orange*
2A Osceola*
2A Palm Beach*
2A Pasco*

2A Pinellas*
2A Polk*
2A Putnam*
2A Santa Rosa*
2A Sarasota*
2A Seminole*
2A St. Johns*
2A St. Lucie*
2A Sumter*
2a Suwannee*
2A Taylor*
2A Union*
2A Volusia*
2A Wakulla*
2A Walton
2A Washington*

Georgia
2A Appling*
2A Atkinson*
2A Bacon*
2A Baker*
3A Baldwin
4A Banks
3A Barrow
3A Bartow
3A Ben Hill*
2A Berrien*
3A Bibb
3A Bleckley*
2A Brantley*
2A Brooks*
2A Bryan*
3A Bulloch*
3A Burke
3A Butts
3A Calhoun*
2A Camden*
3A Candler*
3A Carroll
4A Catoosa
2A Charlton*
2A Chatham*
3A Chattahoochee*
4A Chattooga
3A Cherokee
3A Clarke
3A Clay*
3A Clayton
2A Clinch*
3A Cobb
3A Coffee*
2A Colquitt*
3A Columbia
2A Cook*

3A Coweta
3A Crawford
3A Crisp
4A Dade
4A Dawson
2A Decatur*
3A Dekalb
3A Dodge*
3A Dooly*
3A Dougherty*
3A Douglas
2A Early*
2A Echols*
2A Effingham*
3A Elbert
3A Emanuel*
2A Evans*
4A Fannin
3A Fayette
4A Floyd
3A Forsyth
4A Franklin
3A Fulton
4A Gilmer
3A Glascock
2A Glynn*
4A Gordon
2A Grady*
3A Greene
3A Gwinnett
4A Habersham
4A Hall
3A Hancock
3A Haralson
3A Harris
3A Hart
3A Heard
3A Henry
3A Houston*
3A Irwin*
3A Jackson
3A Jasper
2A Jeff Davis*
3A Jefferson
3A Jenkins*
3A Johnson*
3A Jones
3A Lamar
2A Lanier*
3A Laurens*
3A Lee*
2A Liberty*
3A Lincoln
2A Long*
2A Lowndes*

4A Lumpkin
3A Macon*
3A Madison
3A Marion*
3A McDuffie
2A McIntosh*
3A Meriwether
2A Miller*
2A Mitchell*
3A Monroe
3A Montgomery*
3A Morgan
4A Murray
3A Muscogee
3A Newton
3A Oconee
3A Oglethorpe
3A Paulding
3A Peach*
4A Pickens
2A Pierce*
3A Pike
3A Polk
3A Pulaski*
3A Putnam
3A Quitman*
4A Rabun
3A Randolph*
3A Richmond
3A Rockdale
3A Schley*
3A Screven*
2A Seminole*
3A Spalding
4A Stephens
3A Stewart*
3A Sumter*
3A Talbot
3A Taliaferro
2A Tattnall*
3A Taylor*
3A Telfair*
3A Terrell*
2A Thomas*
3A Tift*
2A Toombs*
4A Towns
3A Treutlen*
3A Troup
3A Turner*
3A Twiggs*
4A Union
3A Upson
4A Walker
3A Walton
2A Ware*

(continued)

TABLE N1101.2—continued
CLIMATE ZONES, MOISTURE REGIMES AND WARM-HUMID DESIGNATIONS BY STATE, COUNTY AND TERRITORY

Key:

A—Moist, B—Dry, C—Marine, Absence of moisture designation indicates moisture regime is irrelevant. Asterisk (*) indicates a warm-humid location.

3A	Warren	6B	Teton	4A	Lawrence	5A	Allen	5A	Noble
3A	Washington	5B	Twin Falls	5A	Lee	5A	Bartholomew	4A	Ohio
2A	Wayne*	6B	Valley	5A	Livingston	5A	Benton	4A	Orange
3A	Webster*	5B	Washington	5A	Logan	5A	Blackford	5A	Owen
3A	Wheeler*			5A	Macon	5A	Boone	5A	Parke
4A	White		**Illinois**	4A	Macoupin	4A	Brown	4A	Perry
4A	Whitfield	5A	Adams	4A	Madison	5A	Carroll	4A	Pike
3A	Wilcox*	4A	Alexander	4A	Marion	5A	Cass	5A	Porter
3A	Wilkes	4A	Bond	5A	Marshall	4A	Clark	4A	Posey
3A	Wilkinson	5A	Boone	5A	Mason	5A	Clay	5a	Pulaski
3A	Worth*	5A	Brown	4A	Massac	5A	Clinton	5A	Putnam
		5A	Bureau	5A	McDonough	4A	Crawford	5A	Randolph
	Hawaii	5A	Calhoun	5A	McHenry	4A	Daviess	4A	Ripley
1A	(all)*	5A	Carroll	5A	McLean	4A	Dearborn	5A	Rush
		5A	Cass	5A	Menard	5A	Decatur	4A	Scott
	Idaho	5A	Champaign	5A	Mercer	5A	De Kalb	5A	Shelby
5B	Ada	4A	Christian	4A	Monroe	5A	Delaware	4A	Spencer
6B	Adams	5A	Clark	4A	Montgomery	4A	Dubois	5A	Starke
6B	Bannock	4A	Clay	5A	Morgan	5A	Elkhart	5A	Steuben
6B	Bear Lake	4A	Clinton	5A	Moultrie	5A	Fayette	5A	St. Joseph
5B	Benewah	5A	Coles	5A	Ogle	4A	Floyd	4A	Sullivan
6B	Bingham	5A	Cook	5A	Peoria	5A	Fountain	4A	Switzerland
6B	Blaine	4A	Crawford	4A	Perry	5A	Franklin	5A	Tippecanoe
6B	Boise	5A	Cumberland	5A	Piatt	5A	Fulton	5A	Tipton
6B	Bonner	5A	Dekalb	5A	Pike	4A	Gibson	5A	Union
6B	Bonneville	5A	De Witt	4A	Pope	5A	Grant	4A	Vanderburgh
6B	Boundary	5A	Douglas	4A	Pulaski	4A	Greene	5A	Vermillion
6B	Butte	5A	DuPage	5A	Putnam	5A	Hamilton	5A	Vigo
6B	Camas	5A	Edgar	4A	Randolph	5A	Hancock	5A	Wabash
5B	Canyon	4A	Edwards	4A	Richland	5A	Hendricks	5A	Warren
6B	Caribou	4A	Effingham	5A	Rock Island	5A	Henry	4A	Warrick
5B	Cassia	4A	Fayette	4A	Saline	5A	Howard	4A	Washington
6B	Clark	5A	Ford	5A	Sangamon	5A	Huntington	5A	Wayne
5B	Clearwater	4A	Franklin	5A	Schuyler	4A	Jackson	5A	Wells
6B	Custer	5A	Fulton	5A	Scott	5A	Jasper	5A	White
5B	Elmore	4A	Gallatin	4A	Shelby	5A	Jay	5A	Whitley
6B	Franklin	5A	Greene	5A	Stark	4A	Jefferson		
6B	Fremont	5A	Grundy	4A	St. Clair	4A	Jennings		**Iowa**
5B	Gem	4A	Hamilton	5A	Stephenson	5A	Johnson	5A	Adair
5B	Gooding	5A	Hancock	5A	Tazewell	4A	Knox	5A	Adams
6B	Idaho	4A	Hardin	4A	Union	5A	Kosciusko	6A	Allamakee
6B	Jefferson	5A	Henderson	5A	Vermilion	5A	Lagrange	5A	Appanoose
5B	Jerome	5A	Henry	4A	Wabash	5A	Lake	5A	Audubon
5B	Kootenai	5A	Iroquois	5A	Warren	5A	La Porte	5A	Benton
5B	Latah	4A	Jackson	4A	Washington	4A	Lawrence	6A	Black Hawk
6B	Lemhi	4A	Jasper	4A	Wayne	5A	Madison	5A	Boone
5B	Lewis	4A	Jefferson	4A	White	5A	Marion	6A	Bremer
5B	Lincoln	5A	Jersey	5A	Whiteside	5A	Marshall	6A	Buchanan
6B	Madison	5A	Jo Daviess	5A	Will	4A	Martin	6A	Buena Vista
5B	Minidoka	4A	Johnson	4A	Williamson	5A	Miami	6A	Butler
5B	Nez Perce	5A	Kane	5A	Winnebago	4A	Monroe	6A	Calhoun
6B	Oneida	5A	Kankakee	5A	Woodford	5A	Montgomery	5A	Carroll
5B	Owyhee	5A	Kendall			5A	Morgan	5A	Cass
5B	Payette	5A	Knox		**Indiana**	5A	Newton	5A	Cedar
5B	Power	5A	Lake	5A	Adams			6A	Cerro Gordo
5B	Shoshone	5A	La Salle						

(continued)

TABLE N1101.2—continued
CLIMATE ZONES, MOISTURE REGIMES AND WARM-HUMID DESIGNATIONS BY STATE, COUNTY AND TERRITORY

Key:

A—Moist, B—Dry, C—Marine, Absence of moisture designation indicates moisture regime is irrelevant. Asterisk (*) indicates a warm-humid location.

6A Cherokee	5A Page	4A Ellsworth	5A Rooks	2A Jefferson
6A Chickasaw	6A Palo Alto	4A Finney	4A Rush	2A Jefferson Davis*
5A Clarke	6A Plymouth	4A Ford	4A Russell	2A Lafayette*
6A Clay	6A Pocahontas	4A Franklin	4A Saline	2A Lafourche*
6A Clayton	5A Polk	4A Geary	5A Scott	3A La Salle*
6A Clinton	5A Pottawattamie	5A Gove	4A Sedgwick	3A Lincoln*
5A Crawford	5A Poweshiek	5A Graham	4A Seward	2A Livingston*
5A Dallas	5A Ringgold	4A Grant	4A Shawnee	3A Madison*
5A Davis	6A Sac	4A Gray	5A Sheridan	3A Morehouse*
5A Decatur	5A Scott	5A Greeley	5A Sherman	3A Natchitoches*
6A Delaware	5A Shelby	4A Greenwood	5A Smith	2A Orleans*
5A Des Moines	6A Sioux	5A Hamilton	4A Stafford	3A Ouachita*
6A Dickinson	5A Story	4A Harper	4A Stanton	2A Plaquemines*
5A Dubuque	5A Tama	4A Harvey	4A Stevens	2A Pointe Coupee*
6A Emmet	5A Taylor	4A Haskell	4A Sumner	2A Rapides*
6A Fayette	5a Union	4A Hodgeman	5A Thomas	3A Red River*
6A Floyd	5A Van Buren	4A Jackson	5A Trego	3A Richland*
6A Franklin	5A Wapello	4A Jefferson	5A Wabaunsee	3A Sabine*
5A Fremont	5A Warren	5A Jewell	5A Wallace	2A St. Bernard*
5A Greene	5A Washington	4A Johnson	4A Washington	2A St. Charles*
6A Grundy	5A Wayne	4A Kearny	5A Wichita	2A St. Helena*
5A Guthrie	6A Webster	4A Kingman	4A Wilson	2A St. James*
6A Hanilton	6A Winnebago	4A Kiowa	4A Woodson	2A St. John the
6A Hancock	6A Winneshiek	4A Labette	4A Wyandotte	Baptist*
6A Hardin	5A Woodbury	5A Lane		2A St. Landry*
5A Harrison	6A Worth	4A Leavenworth	**Kentucky**	2A St. Martin*
5A Henry	6A Wright	4A Lincoln	4A (all)	2A St. Mary*
6A Howard		4A Linn		2A St. Tammany*
6A Humboldt	**Kansas**	5A Logan	**Louisiana**	2A Tangipahoa*
6A Ida	4A Allen	4A Lyon	2A Acadia*	3A Tensas*
5A Iowa	4A Anderson	4A Marion	2A Allen*	2A Terrebonne*
5A Jackson	4A Atchison	4A Marshall	2A Ascension*	3A Union*
5A Jasper	4A Barber	4A McPherson	2A Assumption*	2A Vermilion*
5A Jefferson	4A Barton	4a Meade	2A Avoyelles*	3A Vernon*
5A Johnson	4A Bourbon	4A Miami	2A Beauregard*	2A Washington*
5A Jones	4A Brown	5A Mitchell	3A Bienville*	3A Webster*
5A Keokuk	4A Butler	4A Montgomery	3A Bossier*	2A West Baton
6A Kossuth	4A Chase	4A Morris	3A Caddo*	Rouge*
5A Lee	4A Chautauqua	4A Morton	2A Calcasieu*	3A West Carroll
5A Linn	4A Cherokee	4A Nemaha	3A Caldwell*	2A West Feliciana*
5A Louisa	5A Cheyenne	4A Neosho	2A Cameron*	3A Winn*
5A Lucas	4A Clark	5A Ness	3A Catahoula*	
6A Lyon	5A Clay	5A Norton	3A Claiborne*	**Maine**
5A Madison	5A Cloud	4A Osage	3A Concordia*	6A Androscoggin
5A Mahaska	4A Coffey	5A Osborne	3A De Soto*	7 Aroostook
5A Marion	4A Comanche	4A Ottawa	2A East Baton	6A Cumberland
5A Marshall	4A Cowley	4A Pawnee	Rouge*	6A Franklin
5A Mills	4A Crawford	5A Phillips	3A East Carroll	6A Hancock
6A Mitchell	5A Decatur	4A Pottawatomie	2A East Feliciana*	6A Kennebec
5A Monona	4A Dickinson	4A Pratt	2A Evangeline*	6A Knox
5A Monroe	4A Doniphan	5A Rawlins	3A Franklin*	6A Lincoln
5A Montgomery	4A Douglas	4A Reno	3A Grant*	6A Oxford
5A Muscatine	4A Edwards	5A Republic	2A Iberia*	6A Penobscot
5A O'Brien	4A Elk	4A Rice	2A Iberville*	6A Piscataquis
6A Osceola	5A Ellis	4A Riley	3A Jackson*	6A Sagadahoc

(continued)

TABLE N1101.2—continued
CLIMATE ZONES, MOISTURE REGIMES AND WARM-HUMID DESIGNATIONS BY STATE, COUNTY AND TERRITORY

Key:
A—Moist, B—Dry, C—Marine, Absence of moisture designation indicates moisture regime is irrelevant. Asterisk (*) indicates a warm-humid location.

6A	Somerset	6A	Dickinson	5A	St. Clair	6A	Meeker	3A	Clay
6A	Waldo	5A	Eaton	5A	St. Joseph	7	Mille Lacs	3A	Coahoma
6A	Washington	6A	Emmet	5A	Tuscola	6A	Morrison	3A	Copiah*
6A	York	5A	Genesee	5A	Van Buren	6A	Mower	3A	Covington*
		6A	Gladwin	5A	Washtenaw	6A	Murray	3A	DeSoto
	Maryland	7	Gogebic	5A	Wayne	6A	Nicollet	3A	Forrest*
4A	Allegany	6A	Grand Traverse	6A	Wexford	6A	Nobles	3A	Franklin*
4A	Anne Arundel	5A	Gratiot			7	Norman	3A	George*
4A	Baltimore	5A	Hillsdale		**Minnesota**	6A	Olmsted	3A	Greene*
4A	Baltimore (city)	7	Houghton	7	Aitkin	7	Otter Tail	3A	Grenada
4A	Calvert	6A	Huron	6A	Anoka	7	Pennington	2A	Hancock*
4A	Caroline	5A	Ingham	7	Becker	7	Pine	2A	Harrison*
4A	Carroll	5A	Ionia	7	Beltrami	6A	Pipestone	3A	Hinds*
4A	Cecil	6A	Iosco	6A	Benton	7	Polk	3A	Holmes
4A	Charles	7	Iron	6A	Big Stone	6A	Pope	3A	Humphreys
4A	Dorchester	6A	Isabella	6A	Blue Earth	6A	Ramsey	3A	Issaquena
4A	Frederick	5A	Jackson	6A	Brown	7	Red Lake	3A	Itawamba
5A	Garrett	5A	Kalamazoo	7	Carlton	6A	Redwood	2A	Jackson*
4A	Harford	6A	Kalkaska	6A	Carver	6A	Renville	3A	Jasper
4A	Howard	5A	Kent	7	Cass	6A	Rice	3A	Jefferson*
4A	Kent	7	Keweenaw	6A	Chippewa	6A	Rock	3A	Jefferson Davis*
4A	Montgomery	6A	Lake	6A	Chisago	7	Roseau	3A	Jones*
4A	Prince George's	5A	Lapeer	7	Clay	6A	Scott	3A	Kemper
4A	Queen Anne's	6A	Leelanau	7	Clearwater	6A	Sherburne	3A	Lafayette
4A	Somerset	5A	Lenawee	7	Cook	6A	Sibley	3A	Lamar*
4A	St. Mary's	5A	Livingston	6A	Cottonwood	6A	Stearns	3A	Lauderdale
4A	Talbot	7	Luce	7	Crow Wing	6A	Steele	3A	Lawrence*
4A	Washington	7	Mackinac	6A	Dakota	6A	Stevens	3A	Leake
4A	Wicomico	5A	Macomb	6A	Dodge	7	St. Louis	3A	Lee
4A	Worcester	6A	Manistee	6A	Douglas	6	Swift	3A	Leflore
		6A	Marquette	6A	Faribault	6A	Todd	3A	Lincoln*
	Massachusetts	6A	Mason	6A	Fillmore	6A	Traverse	3A	Lowndes
5A	(all)	6A	Mecosta	6A	Freeborn	6A	Wabasha	3A	Madison
		6A	Menominee	6A	Goodhue	7	Wadena	3A	Marion*
	Michigan	5A	Midland	7	Grant	6A	Waseca	3A	Marshall
6A	Alcona	6A	Missaukee	6A	Hennepin	6A	Washington	3A	Monroe
6A	Alger	5A	Monroe	6A	Houston	6A	Watonwan	3A	Montgomery
5A	Allegan	5A	Montcalm	7	Hubbard	7	Wilkin	3A	Neshoba
6A	Alpena	6A	Montmorency	6A	Isanti	6A	Winona	3A	Newton
6A	Antrim	5A	Muskegon	7	Itasca	6A	Wright	3A	Noxubee
6A	Arenac	6A	Newaygo	6A	Jackson	6A	Yellow Medicine	3A	Oktibbeha
7	Baraga	5A	Oakland	7	Kanabec			3A	Panola
5A	Barry	6A	Oceana	6A	Kandiyohi		**Mississippi**	2A	Pearl River*
5A	Bay	6A	Ogemaw	7	Kittson	3A	Adams*	3A	Perry*
6A	Benzie	7	Ontonagon	7	Koochiching	3A	Alcorn	3A	Pike*
5A	Berrien	6A	Osceola	6A	Lac qui Parle	3A	Amite*	3A	Pontotoc
5A	Branch	6A	Oscoda	7	Lake	3A	Attala	3A	Prentiss
5A	Calhoun	6A	Otsego	7	Lake of the Woods	3A	Benton	3A	Quitman
5A	Cass	5A	Ottawa	6A	Le Sueur	3A	Bolivar	3A	Rankin*
6A	Charlevoix	6A	Presque Isle	6A	Lincoln	3A	Calhoun	3A	Scott
6A	Cheboygan	6A	Roscommon	6A	Lyon	3A	Carroll	3A	Sharkey
7	Chippewa	5A	Saginaw	7	Mahnomen	3A	Chickasaw	3A	Simpson*
6A	Clare	6A	Sanilac	7	Marshall	3A	Choctaw	3A	Smith*
5A	Clinton	7	Schoolcraft	6A	Martin	3A	Claiborne*	2A	Stone*
6A	Crawford	5A	Shiawassee	6A	McLeod	3A	Clarke	3A	Sunflower
6A	Delta								

(continued)

TABLE N1101.2—continued
CLIMATE ZONES, MOISTURE REGIMES AND WARM-HUMID DESIGNATIONS BY STATE, COUNTY AND TERRITORY

Key:

A—Moist, B—Dry, C—Marine, Absence of moisture designation indicates moisture regime is irrelevant. Asterisk (*) indicates a warm-humid location.

3A	Tallahatchie	4A	Greene	5A	Scotland	5A	Rockingham	4B	Socorro
3A	Tate	5A	Grundy	4A	Scott	5A	Strafford	5B	Taos
3A	Tippah	5A	Harrison	4a	Shannon	6A	Sullivan	5B	Torrance
3A	Tishomingo	4A	Henry	5A	Shelby			4B	Union
3A	Tunica	4A	Hickory	4A	St. Charles	**New Jersey**		4B	Valencia
3A	Union	5A	Holt	4A	St. Clair	4A	Atlantic		
3A	Walthall*	4A	Howard	4A	Ste. Genevieve	5A	Bergen	**New York**	
3A	Warren*	4A	Howell	4A	St. Francois	4A	Burlington	5A	Albany
3A	Washington	4A	Iron	4A	St. Louis	4A	Camden	6A	Allegany
3A	Wayne*	4A	Jackson	4A	St. Louis (city)	4A	Cape May	4A	Bronx
3A	Webster	4A	Jasper	4A	Stoddard	4A	Cumberland	6A	Broome
3A	Wilkinson*	4A	Jefferson	4A	Stone	4A	Essex	6A	Cattaraugus
3A	Winston	4A	Johnson	5A	Sullivan	4A	Gloucester	5A	Cayuga
3A	Yalobusha	5A	Knox	4A	Taney	4A	Hudson	5A	Chautauga
3A	Yazoo	4A	Laclede	4A	Texas	5A	Hunterdon	5A	Chemung
		4A	Lafayette	4A	Vernon	5A	Mercer	6A	Chenango
Missouri		4A	Lawrence	4A	Warren	4A	Middlesex	6A	Clinton
5A	Adair	5A	Lewis	4A	Washington	4A	Monmouth	5A	Columbia
5A	Andrew	4A	Lincoln	4A	Wayne	5A	Morris	5A	Cortland
5A	Atchison	5A	Linn	4A	Webster	4A	Ocean	6A	Delaware
4A	Audrain	5A	Livingston	5A	Worth	5A	Passaic	5A	Dutchess
4A	Barry	5A	Macon	4A	Wright	4A	Salem	5A	Erie
4A	Barton	4A	Madison			5A	Somerset	6A	Essex
4A	Bates	4A	Maries	**Montana**		5A	Sussex	6A	Franklin
4A	Benton	5A	Marion	6B	(all)	4A	Union	6A	Fulton
4A	Bollinger	4A	McDonald			5A	Warren	5A	Genesee
4A	Boone	5A	Mercer	**Nebraska**				5A	Greene
5A	Buchanan	4A	Miller	5A	(all)	**New Mexico**		6A	Hamilton
4A	Butler	4A	Mississippi			4B	Bernalillo	6A	Herkimer
5A	Caldwell	4A	Moniteau	**Nevada**		5B	Catron	6A	Jefferson
4A	Callaway	4A	Monroe	5B	Carson City (city)	3B	Chaves	4A	Kings
4A	Camden	4A	Montgomery	5B	Churchill	4B	Cibola	6A	Lewis
4A	Cape Girardeau	4A	Morgan	3B	Clark	5B	Colfax	5A	Livingston
4A	Carroll	4A	New Madrid	5B	Douglas	4B	Curry	6A	Madison
4A	Carter	4A	Newton	5B	Elko	4B	DeBaca	5A	Monroe
4A	Cass	5A	Nodaway	5B	Esmeralda	3B	Dona Ana	6A	Montgomery
4A	Cedar	4A	Oregon	5B	Eureka	3B	Eddy	4A	Nassau
5A	Chariton	4A	Osage	5B	Humboldt	4B	Grant	4A	New York
4A	Christian	4A	Ozark	5B	Lander	4B	Guadalupe	5A	Niagara
5A	Clark	4A	Pemiscot	5B	Lincoln	5B	Harding	6A	Oneida
4A	Clay	4A	Perry	5B	Lyon	3B	Hidalgo	5A	Onondaga
5A	Clinton	4A	Pettis	5B	Mineral	3B	Lea	5A	Ontario
4A	Cole	4A	Phelps	5B	Nye	4B	Lincoln	5A	Orange
4a	Cooper	5A	Pike	5B	Pershing	5B	Los Alamos	5A	Orleans
4A	Crawford	4A	Platte	5B	Storey	3B	Luna	5A	Oswego
4A	Dade	4A	Polk	5B	Washoe	5B	McKinley	6A	Otsego
4A	Dallas	4A	Pulaski	5B	White Pine	5B	Mora	5A	Putnam
5A	Daviess	5A	Putnam			3B	Otero	4A	Queens
5A	DeKalb	5A	Ralls	**New Hampshire**		4B	Quay	5A	Rensselaer
4A	Dent	4A	Randolph	6A	Belknap	5B	Rio Arriba	4A	Richmond
4A	Douglas	4A	Ray	6A	Carroll	4B	Roosevelt	5A	Rockland
4A	Dunklin	4A	Reynolds	5A	Cheshire	5B	Sandoval	5A	Saratoga
4A	Franklin	4A	Ripley	6A	Coos	5B	San Juan	5A	Schenectady
4A	Gasconade	4A	Saline	6A	Grafton	5B	San Miguel	6A	Schoharie
5A	Gentry	5A	Schuyler	5A	Hillsborough	5B	Santa Fe	6A	Schuyler
				6A	Merrimack	4B	Sierra		

(continued)

TABLE N1101.2—continued
CLIMATE ZONES, MOISTURE REGIMES AND WARM-HUMID DESIGNATIONS BY STATE, COUNTY AND TERRITORY

Key:

A—Moist, B—Dry, C—Marine, Absence of moisture designation indicates moisture regime is irrelevant. Asterisk (*) indicates a warm-humid location.

5A	Seneca	3A	Greene	5A	Watauga	7	Towner	5A	Lucas
6A	Steuben	4A	Guilford	3A	Wayne	7	Traill	5A	Madison
6A	St. Lawrence	4A	Halifax	4A	Wilkes	7	Walsh	5A	Mahoning
4A	Suffolk	4A	Harnett	3A	Wilson	7	Ward	5A	Marion
6A	Sullivan	4A	Haywood	4A	Yadkin	7	Wells	5A	Medina
5A	Tioga	4A	Henderson	5A	Yancey	7	Williams	5A	Meigs
6A	Tompkins	4A	Hertford					5A	Mercer
6A	Ulster	3A	Hoke		**North Dakota**		**Ohio**	5A	Miami
6A	Warren	3A	Hyde	6A	Adams	4A	Adams	5A	Monroe
5A	Washington	4A	Iredell	7	Barnes	5A	Allen	5A	Montgomery
5A	Wayne	4A	Jackson	7	Benson	5A	Ashland	5A	Morgan
4A	Westchester	3A	Johnston	6A	Billings	5A	Ashtabula	5A	Morrow
6A	Wyoming	3A	Jones	7	Bottineau	5A	Athens	5A	Muskingum
5A	Yates	4A	Lee	6A	Bowman	5A	Auglaize	5A	Noble
		3A	Lenoir	7	Burke	5A	Belmont	5A	Ottawa
	North Carolina	4A	Lincoln	6A	Burleigh	4A	Brown	5A	Paulding
4A	Alamance	4A	Macon	7	Cass	5A	Butler	5A	Perry
4A	Alexander	4A	Madison	7	Cavalier	5A	Carroll	5A	Pickaway
5A	Alleghany	3A	Martin	6A	Dickey	5A	Champaign	4A	Pike
3A	Anson	4A	McDowell	7	Divide	5A	Clark	5A	Portage
5A	Ashe	3A	Mecklenburg	6A	Dunn	4A	Clermont	5A	Preble
5A	Avery	5A	Mitchell	7	Eddy	5A	Clinton	5A	Putnam
3A	Beaufort	3A	Montgomery	6A	Emmons	5A	Columbiana	5A	Richland
4A	Bertie	3A	Moore	7	Foster	5A	Coshocton	5A	Ross
3A	Bladen	4A	Nash	6A	Golden Valley	5A	Crawford	5A	Sandusky
3A	Brunswick*	3A	New Hanover*	7	Grand Forks	5A	Cuyahoga	4A	Scioto
4A	Buncombe	4A	Northampton	6A	Grant	5A	Darke	5A	Seneca
4A	Burke	3A	Onslow*	7	Griggs	5A	Defiance	5A	Shelby
3A	Cabarrus	4A	Orange	6A	Hettinger	5A	Delaware	5A	Stark
4A	Caldwell	3A	Pamlico	7	Kidder	5A	Erie	5A	Summit
3A	Camden	3A	Pasquotank	6A	LaMoure	5A	Fairfield	5A	Trumbull
3A	Carteret*	3A	Pender*	6A	Logan	5A	Fayette	5A	Tuscarawas
4A	Caswell	3A	Perquimans	7	McHenry	5A	Franklin	5A	Union
4A	Catawba	4A	Person	6A	McIntosh	5A	Fulton	5A	Van Wert
4A	Chatham	3A	Pitt	6A	McKenzie	4A	Gallia	5A	Vinton
4A	Cherokee	4A	Polk	7	McLean	5A	Geauga	5A	Warren
3A	Chowan	3A	Randolph	6A	Mercer	5A	Greene	4A	Washington
4A	Clay	3A	Richmond	6A	Morton	5A	Guernsey	5A	Wayne
4A	Cleveland	3A	Robeson	7	Mountrail	4A	Hamilton	5A	Williams
3A	Columbus*	4A	Rockingham	7	Nelson	5A	Hancock	5A	Wood
3A	Craven	3A	Rowan	6A	Oliver	5A	Hardin	5A	Wyandot
3A	Cumberland	4A	Rutherford	7	Pembina	5A	Harrison		
3A	Currituck	3A	Sampson	7	Pierce	5A	Henry		**Oklahoma**
3A	Dare	3A	Scotland	7	Ramsey	5A	Highland	3A	Adair
3A	Davidson	3A	Stanly	6A	Ransom	5A	Hocking	3A	Alfalfa
4A	Davie	4A	Stokes	7	Renville	5A	Holmes	3A	Atoka
3A	Duplin	4A	Surry	6A	Richland	5A	Huron	4B	Beaver
4A	Durham	4A	Swain	7	Rolette	5A	Jackson	3A	Beckham
3A	Edgecombe	4A	Transylvania	6A	Sargent	5A	Jefferson	3A	Blaine
4A	Forsyth	3A	Tyrrell	7	Sheridan	5A	Knox	3A	Bryan
4A	Franklin	3A	Union	6A	Sioux	5A	Lake	3A	Caddo
3A	Gaston	4A	Vance	6A	Slope	4A	Lawrence	3A	Canadian
4A	Gates	4A	Wake	6A	Stark	5A	Licking	3A	Carter
4A	Graham	4A	Warren	7	Steele	5A	Logan	3A	Cherokee
4A	Granville	3A	Washington	7	Stutsman	5A	Lorain	3A	Choctaw

(continued)

TABLE N1101.2—continued
CLIMATE ZONES, MOISTURE REGIMES AND WARM-HUMID DESIGNATIONS BY STATE, COUNTY AND TERRITORY

Key:
A—Moist, B—Dry, C—Marine, Absence of moisture designation indicates moisture regime is irrelevant. Asterisk (*) indicates a warm-humid location.

4B Cimarron	3A Sequoyah	5A Berks	5A Venango	3A Williamsburg
3A Cleveland	3A Stephens	5A Blair	5A Warren	3A York
3A Coal	4B Texas	5A Bradford	5A Washington	
3A Comanche	3A Tillman	4A Bucks	6A Wayne	**South Dakota**
3A Cotton	3A Tulsa	5A Butler	5A Westmoreland	6A Aurora
3A Craig	3A Wagoner	5A Cambria	5A Wyoming	6A Beadle
3A Creek	3A Washington	6A Cameron	4A York	5A Bennett
3A Custer	3A Washita	5A Carbon		5A Bon Homme
3A Delaware	3A Woods	5A Centre	**Rhode Island**	6A Brookings
3A Dewey	3A Woodward	4A Chester	5A (all)	6A Brown
3A Ellis		5A Clarion		6A Brule
3A Garfield	**Oregon**	6A Clearfield	**South Carolina**	6A Buffalo
3A Garvin	5B Baker	5A Clinton	3A Abbeville	6A Butte
3A Grady	4C Benton	5A Columbia	3A Aiken	6A Campbell
3A Grant	4C Clackamas	5A Crawford	3A Allendale*	5A Charles Mix
3A Greer	4C Clatsop	5A Cumberland	3A Anderson	6A Clark
3A Harmon	4C Columbia	5A Dauphin	3A Bamberg*	5A Clay
3A Harper	4C Coos	4A Delaware	3A Barnwell*	6A Codington
3A Haskell	5B Crook	6A Elk	3A Beaufort*	6A Corson
3A Hughes	4C Curry	5A Erie	3A Berkeley*	6A Custer
3A Jackson	5B Deschutes	5A Fayette	3A Calhoun	6A Davison
3A Jefferson	4C Douglas	5A Forest	3A Charleston*	6A Day
3A Johnston	5B Gilliam	5A Franklin	3A Cherokee	6A Deuel
3A Kay	5B Grant	5A Fulton	3A Chester	6A Dewey
3A Kingfisher	5B Harney	5A Greene	3A Chesterfield	5A Douglas
3A Kiowa	5B Hood River	5A Huntingdon	3A Clarendon	6A Edmunds
3A Latimer	4C Jackson	5A Indiana	3A Colleton*	6A Fall River
3A Le Flore	5B Jefferson	5A Jefferson	3A Darlington	6A Faulk
3A Lincoln	4C Josephine	5A Juniata	3A Dillon	6A Grant
3A Logan	5B Klamath	5A Lackawanna	3A Dorchester*	5A Gregory
3A Love	5B Lake	5A Lancaster	3A Edgefield	6A Haakon
3A Major	4C Lane	5A Lawrence	3A Fairfield	6A Hamlin
3A Marshall	4C Lincoln	5A Lebanon	3A Florence	6A Hand
3A Mayes	4C Linn	5A Lehigh	3A Georgetown*	6A Hanson
3A MaClain	5B Malheur	5A Luzerne	3A Greenville	6A Harding
3A McCurtain	4C Marion	5A Lycoming	3A Greenwood	6A Hughes
3A McIntosh	5B Morrow	6A McKean	3A Hampton*	5A Hutchinson
3A Murray	4C Multnomah	5A Mercer	3A Horry*	6A Hyde
3A Muskogee	4C Polk	5A Mifflin	3A Jasper*	5A Jackson
3A Noble	5B Sherman	5A Monroe	3A Kershaw	6A Jerauld
3A Nowata	4C Tillamook	4A Montgomery	3A Lancaster	6A Jones
3A Okfuskee	5B Umatilla	5A Montour	3A Laurens	6A Kingsbury
3A Oklahoma	5B Union	5A Northampton	3A Lee	6A Lake
3A Okmulgee	5B Wallowa	5A Northumberland	3A Lexington	6A Lawrence
3A Osage	5B Wasco	5A Perry	3A Marion	6A Lincoln
3A Ottawa	4C Washington	4A Philadelphia	3A Marlboro	6A Lyman
3A Pawnee	5B Wheeler	5A Pike	3A McCormick	6A Marshall
3A Payne	4C Yamhill	6A Potter	3A Newberry	6A McCook
3A Pittsburg		5A Schuylkill	3A Oconee	6A McPherson
3A Pontotoc	**Pennsylvania**	5A Snyder	3A Orangeburg	6A Meade
3A Pottawatomie	5A Adams	5A Somerset	3A Pickens	5A Mellette
3A Pushmataha	5A Allegheny	5A Sullivan	3A Richland	6A Miner
3A Roger Mills	5A Armstrong	6A Susquehanna	3A Saluda	6A Minnehaha
3A Rogers	5A Beaver	6A Tioga	3A Spartanburg	6A Moody
3A Seminole	5A Bedford	5A Union	3A Sumter	6A Pennington
			3A Union	

(continued)

2009 INTERNATIONAL RESIDENTIAL CODE®

TABLE N1101.2—continued
CLIMATE ZONES, MOISTURE REGIMES AND WARM-HUMID DESIGNATIONS BY STATE, COUNTY AND TERRITORY

Key:
A—Moist, B—Dry, C—Marine, Absence of moisture designation indicates moisture regime is irrelevant. Asterisk (*) indicates a warm-humid location.

6A	Perkins	3A	Henderson	4A	Williamson	3B	Crane	3A	Henderson*
6A	Potter	4A	Henry	4A	Wilson	3B	Crockett	2A	Hidalgo*
6A	Roberts	4A	Hickman			3B	Crosby	2A	Hill*
6A	Sanborn	4A	Houston		**Texas**	3B	Culberson	4B	Hockley
6A	Shannon	4A	Humphreys	2A	Anderson*	4B	Dallam	3A	Hood*
6A	Spink	4A	Jackson	3B	Andrews	3A	Dallas*	3A	Hopkins*
6A	Stanley	4A	Jefferson	2A	Angelina*	3B	Dawson	2A	Houston*
6A	Sully	4A	Johnson	2A	Aransas*	4B	Deaf Smith	3B	Howard
5A	Todd	4A	Knox	3A	Archer	3A	Delta	3B	Hudspeth
5A	Tripp	3A	Lake	4B	Armstrong	3A	Denton*	3A	Hunt*
6A	Turner	3A	Lauderdale	2A	Atascosa*	2A	DeWitt*	4B	Hutchinson
5A	Union	4A	Lawrence	2A	Austin*	3B	Dickens	3B	Irion
6A	Walworth	4A	Lewis	4B	Bailey	2B	Dimmit*	3A	Jack
5A	Yankton	4A	Lincoln	2B	Bandera*	4B	Donley	2A	Jackson*
6A	Ziebach	4A	Loudon	2A	Bastrop	2A	Duval*	2A	Jasper*
		4A	Macon	3B	Baylor	3A	Eastland	3B	Jeff Davis
	Tennessee	3A	Madison	2A	Bee*	3B	Ector	2A	Jefferson*
4A	Anderson	4A	Marion	2A	Bell*	2B	Edwards*	2A	Jim Hogg*
4A	Bedford	4A	Marshall	2A	Bexar*	3A	Ellis*	2A	Jim Wells*
4A	Benton	4A	Maury	3A	Blanco*	3B	El Paso	3A	Johnson*
4A	Bledsoe	4A	McMinn	3B	Borden	3A	Erath*	3B	Jones
4A	Blount	3A	McNairy	2A	Bosque*	2A	Falls*	2A	Karnes*
4A	Bradley	4A	Meigs	3A	Bowie*	3A	Fannin	3A	Kaufman*
4A	Campbell	4A	Monroe	2A	Brazoria*	2A	Fayette*	3A	Kendall*
4A	Cannon	4A	Montgomery	2A	Brazos*	3A	Fisher	2A	Kenedy*
4A	Carroll	4A	Moore	3B	Brewster	4B	Floyd	3B	Kent
4A	Carter	4A	Morgan	4B	Briscoe	3B	Foard	3B	Kerr
4A	Cheatham	4A	Obion	2A	Brooks*	2A	Fort Bend*	3B	Kimble
3A	Chester	4A	Overton	3A	Brown*	3A	Franklin*	3B	King
4A	Claiborne	4A	Perry	2A	Burleson*	2A	Freestone*	2B	Kinney*
4A	Clay	4A	Pickett	3A	Burnet*	2B	Frio*	2A	Kleberg*
4A	Cocke	4A	Polk	2A	Caldwell*	3B	Gaines	3B	Knox
4A	Coffee	4A	Putnam	2A	Calhoun*	2A	Galveston*	3A	Lamar*
3A	Crockett	4A	Rhea	3B	Callahan	3B	Garza	4B	Lamb
4A	Cumberland	4A	Roane	2A	Cameron*	3A	Gillespie*	3A	Lampasas*
4A	Davidson	4A	Robertson	3A	Camp*	3B	Glasscock	2B	La Salle*
4A	Decatur	4A	Rutherford	4B	Carson	2A	Goliad*	2A	Lavaca*
4A	DeKalb	4A	Scott	3A	Cass*	2A	Gonzales*	2A	Lee*
4A	Dickson	4A	Sequatchie	4B	Castro	4B	Gray	2A	Leon*
3A	Dyer	4A	Sevier	2A	Chambers*	3A	Grayson	2A	Liberty*
3A	Fayette	3A	Shelby	2A	Cherokee*	3A	Gregg*	2A	Limestone*
4A	Fentress	4A	Smith	3B	Childress	2A	Grimes*	4B	Lipscomb
4A	Franklin	4A	Stewart	3A	Clay	2A	Guadalupe*	2A	Live Oak*
4A	Gibson	4A	Sullivan	4B	Cochran	4B	Hale	3A	Llano*
4A	Giles	4A	Sumner	3B	Coke	3B	Hall	3B	Loving
4A	Grainger	3A	Tipton	3B	Coleman	3A	Hamilton*	3B	Lubbock
4A	Greene	4A	Trousdale	3A	Collin*	4B	Hansford	3B	Lynn
4A	Grundy	4A	Unicoi	3B	Collingsworth	3B	Hardeman	2A	Madison*
4A	Hamblen	4A	Union	2A	Colorado*	2A	Hardin*	3A	Marion*
4A	Hamilton	4A	Van Buren	2A	Comal*	2A	Harris*	3B	Martin
4A	Hancock	4A	Warren	3A	Comanche*	3A	Harrison*	3B	Mason
3A	Hardeman	4A	Washington	3B	Concho	4B	Hartley	2A	Matagorda*
3A	Hardin	4A	Wayne	3A	Cooke	3B	Haskell	2B	Maverick*
4A	Hawkins	4A	Weakley	2A	Coryell*	2A	Hays*	3B	McCulloch
3A	Haywood	4A	White	3B	Cottle	3B	Hemphill	2A	McLennan*

(continued)

TABLE N1101.2—continued
CLIMATE ZONES, MOISTURE REGIMES AND WARM-HUMID DESIGNATIONS BY STATE, COUNTY AND TERRITORY

Key:

A—Moist, B—Dry, C—Marine, Absence of moisture designation indicates moisture regime is irrelevant. Asterisk (*) indicates a warm-humid location.

2A	McMullen*	3B	Stonewall	6B	Rich	4C	Wahkiakum	5A	Upshur
2A	Medina*	3B	Sutton	5B	Salt Lake	5B	Walla Walla	4A	Wayne
3B	Menard	4B	Swisher	5B	San Juan	4C	Whatcom	5A	Webster
3A	Midland	3A	Tarrant*	5B	Sanpete	5B	Whitman	5A	Wetzel
2A	Milam*	3B	Taylor	5B	Sevier	5B	Yakima	4A	Wirt
3A	Mills*	3B	Terrell	6B	Summit			4A	Wood
3B	Mitchell	3B	Terry	5B	Tooele	**West Virginia**		4A	Wyoming
3A	Montague	3B	Throckmorton	6B	Uintah	5A	Barbour		
2A	Montgomery*	3A	Titus*	5B	Utah	4A	Berkeley	**Wisconsin**	
4A	Moore	3B	Tom Green	6B	Wasatch	4A	Boone	6A	Adams
3A	Morris*	2A	Travis*	3B	Washington	4A	Braxton	7	Ashland
3B	Motley	2A	Trinity*	5B	Wayne	5A	Brooke	6A	Barron
3A	Nacogdoches*	2A	Tyler*	5B	Weber	4A	Cabell	7	Bayfield
3A	Navarro*	3A	Upshur*			4A	Calhoun	6A	Brown
2A	Newton*	3B	Upton	**Vermont**		4A	Clay	6A	Buffalo
3A	Nolan	2B	Uvalde*	6A	(all)	5A	Doddridge	7	Burnett
2A	Nueces*	2B	Val Verde*			5A	Fayette	6A	Calumet
4B	Ochiltree	3A	Van Zandt*	**Virginia**		4A	Gilmer	6A	Chippewa
4B	Oldham	2A	Victoria*	4A	(all)	5A	Grant	6A	Clark
2A	Orange*	2A	Walker*			5A	Greenbrier	6A	Columbia
3A	Palo Pinto*	2A	Waller*	**Washington**		5A	Hamphire	6A	Crawford
3A	Panola*	3B	Ward	5B	Adams	5A	Hancock	6A	Dane
3A	Parker*	2A	Washington*	5B	Asotin	5A	Hardy	6A	Dodge
4B	Parmer	2B	Webb*	5B	Benton	5A	Harrison	6A	Door
3B	Pecos	2A	Wharton*	5B	Chelan	4A	Jackson	7	Douglas
2A	Polk*	3B	Wheeler	4C	Clallam	4A	Jefferson	6A	Dunn
4B	Potter	3A	Wichita	4C	Clark	4A	Kanawha	6A	Eau Claire
3B	Presidio	3B	Wilbarger	5B	Columbia	5A	Lewis	7	Florence
3A	Rains*	2A	Willacy*	4C	Cowlitz	4A	Lincoln	6A	Fond du Lac
4B	Randall	2A	Williamson*	5B	Douglas	4A	Logan	7	Forest
3B	Reagan	2A	Wilson*	6B	Ferry	5A	Marion	6A	Grant
2B	Real*	3B	Winkler	5B	Franklin	5A	Marshall	6A	Green
3A	Red River*	3A	Wise	5B	Garfield	4A	Mason	6A	Green Lake
3B	Reeves	3A	Wood*	5B	Grant	4A	McDowell	6A	Iowa
2A	Refugio*	4B	Yoakum	5C	Grays Harbor	4A	Mercer	7	Iron
4B	Roberts	3A	Young	4C	Island	5A	Mineral	6A	Jackson
2A	Robertson*	2B	Zavala*	4C	Jefferson	4A	Mingo	6A	Jefferson
3A	Rockwall*			4C	King	5A	Monongalia	6A	Juneau
3B	Runnels	**Utah**		4C	Kitsap	4A	Monroe	6A	Kenosha
3A	Rusk*	5B	Beaver	5B	Kittitas	4A	Morgan	6A	Kewaunee
3A	Sabine*	6B	Box Elder	5B	Klickitat	5A	Nicholas	6A	La Crosse
3A	San Augustine*	6B	Cache	4C	Lewis	5A	Ohio	6A	Lafayette
2A	San Jacinto*	6B	Carbon	5B	Lincoln	4A	Pendleton	7	Langlade
2A	San Patricio*	6B	Daggett	4C	Mason	4A	Pleasants	7	Lincoln
3A	San Saba*	5B	Davis	6B	Okanogan	5A	Pocahontas	6A	Manitowoc
3B	Schleicher	6B	Duchesne	4C	Pacific	5A	Preston	6A	Marathon
3B	Scurry	5B	Emery	6B	Pend Oreille	4A	Putnam	6A	Marinette
3B	Shackelford	5B	Garfield	4C	Pierce	5A	Raleigh	6A	Marquette
3A	Shelby*	5B	Grand	4C	San Juan	5A	Randolph	6A	Menominee
4B	Sherman	5B	Iron	4C	Skagit	4A	Ritchie	6A	Milwaukee
3A	Smith*	5B	Juab	5B	Skamania	4A	Roane	6A	Monroe
3A	Somervell*	5B	Kane	4C	Snohomish	5A	Summers	6A	Oconto
2A	Starr*	5B	Millard	5B	Spokane	5A	Taylor	7	Oneida
3A	Stephens	6B	Morgan	6B	Stevens	5A	Tucker	6A	Outagamie
3B	Sterling	5B	Piute	4C	Thurston	4A	Tyler	6A	Ozaukee

(continued)

TABLE N1101.2—continued
CLIMATE ZONES, MOISTURE REGIMES AND WARM-HUMID DESIGNATIONS BY STATE, COUNTY AND TERRITORY

Key:

A—Moist, B—Dry, C—Marine, Absence of moisture designation indicates moisture regime is irrelevant. Asterisk (*) indicates a warm-humid location.

6A Pepin	6A Trempealeau	6B Campbell	7 Sublette	**Northern Mariana Islands**
6A Pierce	6A Vernon	6B Carbon	6B Sweetwater	1A (all)*
6A Polk	7 Vilas	6B Converse	7 Teton	
6A Portage	6A Walworth	6B Crook	6B Uinta	**Puerto Rico**
7 Price	7 Washburn	6B Fremont	6B Washakie	1A (all)*
6A Racine	6A Washington	5B Goshen	6B Weston	
6A Richland	6A Waukesha	6B Hot Springs		**Virgin Islands**
6A Rock	6A Waupaca	6B Johnson		1A (all)*
6A Rusk	6A Waushara	6B Laramie	**US TERRITORIES**	
6A Sauk	6A Winnebago	7 Lincoln		
7 Sawyer	6A Wood	6B Natrona	**American Samoa**	
6A Shawano		6B Niobrara	1A (all)*	
6A Sheboyan	**Wyoming**	6B Park		
6A St. Croix	6B Albany	5B Platte	**Guam**	
7 Taylor	6B Big Horn	6B Sheridan	1A (all)*	

TABLE N1101.5(1)
DEFAULT GLAZED FENESTRATION U-FACTORS

FRAME TYPE	SINGLE PANE	DOUBLE PANE	SKYLIGHT	
			Single	Double
Metal	1.2	0.8	2	1.3
Metal with thermal break	1.1	0.65	1.9	1.1
Nonmetal or metal clad	0.95	0.55	1.75	1.05
Glazed block	0.6			

TABLE N1101.5(2)
DEFAULT DOOR U-FACTORS

DOOR TYPE	U-FACTOR
Uninsulated metal	1.2
Insulated metal	0.6
Wood	0.5
Insulated, nonmetal edge, max 45% glazing, any glazing double pane	0.35

TABLE N1101.5(3)
DEFAULT GLAZED FENESTRATION SHGC

SINGLE GLAZED		DOUBLE GLAZED		GLAZED BLOCK
Clear	Tinted	Clear	Tinted	
0.8	0.7	0.7	0.6	0.6

SECTION N1102
BUILDING THERMAL ENVELOPE

N1102.1 Insulation and fenestration criteria. The *building thermal envelope* shall meet the requirements of Table N1102.1 based on the climate zone specified in Table N1101.2.

N1102.1.1 *R*-value computation. Insulation material used in layers, such as framing cavity insulation and insulating sheathing, shall be summed to compute the component *R*-value. The manufacturer's settled *R*-value shall be used for blown insulation. Computed *R*-values shall not include an *R*-value for other building materials or air films.

N1102.1.2 *U*-factor alternative. An assembly with a *U*-factor equal to or less than that specified in Table

N1102.1.2 shall be permitted as an alternative to the *R*-value in Table N1102.1.

N1102.1.3 Total UA alternative. If the total *building thermal envelope* UA (sum of *U*-factor times assembly area) is less than or equal to the total UA resulting from using the *U*-factors in Table N1102.1.2, (multiplied by the same assembly area as in the proposed building), the building shall be considered in compliance with Table N1102.1. The UA calculation shall be done using a method consistent with the ASHRAE *Handbook of Fundamentals* and shall include the thermal bridging effects of framing materials. The SHGC requirements shall be met in addition to UA compliance.

TABLE N1102.1
INSULATION AND FENESTRATION REQUIREMENTS BY COMPONENT[a]

CLIMATE ZONE	FENESTRATION *U*-FACTOR	SKYLIGHT[b] *U*-FACTOR	GLAZED FENESTRATION SHGC	CEILING *R*-VALUE	WOOD FRAME WALL *R*-VALUE	MASS WALL *R*-VALUE[k]	FLOOR *R*-VALUE	BASEMENT[c] WALL *R*-VALUE	SLAB[d] *R*-VALUE AND DEPTH	CRAWL SPACE[c] WALL *R*-VALUE
1	1.2	0.75	0.35[j]	30	13	3/4	13	0	0	0
2	0.65[i]	0.75	0.35[j]	30	13	4/6	13	0	0	0
3	0.50[i]	0.65	0.35[e, j]	30	13	5/8	19	5/13[f]	0	5/13
4 except Marine	0.35	0.60	NR	38	13	5/10	19	10/13	10, 2 ft	10/13
5 and Marine 4	0.35	0.60	NR	38	20 or 13 + 5[h]	13/17	30[f]	10/13	10, 2 ft	10/13
6	0.35	0.60	NR	49	20 or 13 + 5[h]	15/19	30[g]	10/13	10, 4 ft	10/13
7 and 8	0.35	0.60	NR	49	21	19/21	30[g]	10/13	10, 4 ft	10/13

a. *R*-values are minimums. *U*-factors and solar heat gain coefficient (SHGC) are maximums. R-19 batts compressed in to nominal 2 × 6 framing cavity such that the *R*-value is reduced by R-1 or more shall be marked with the compressed batt *R*-value in addition to the full thickness *R*-value.

b. The fenestration *U*-factor column excludes skylights. The SHGC column applies to all glazed fenestration.

c. The first *R*-value applies to continuous insulation, the second to framing cavity insulation; either insulation meets the requirement.

d. R-5 shall be added to the required slab edge *R*-values for heated slabs. Insulation depth shall be the depth of the footing or 2 feet, whichever is less, in zones 1 through 3 for heated slabs.

e. There are no SHGC requirements in the Marine Zone.

f. Basement wall insulation is not required in warm-humid locations as defined by Figure N1101.2 and Table N1101.2.

g. Or insulation sufficient to fill the framing cavity, R-19 minimum.

h. "13+5" means R-13 cavity insulation plus R-5 insulated sheathing. If structural sheathing covers 25% or less of the exterior, R-5 sheathing is not required where structural sheathing is used. If structural sheathing covers more than 25% of exterior, structural sheathing shall be supplemented with insulated sheathing of at least R-2.

i. For impact-rated fenestration complying with Section R301.2.1.2, the maximum *U*-factor shall be 0.75 in zone 2 and 0.65 in zone 3.

j. For impact-resistant fenestration complying with Section R301.2.1.2 of the *International Residential Code*, the maximum SHGC shall be 0.40.

k. The second *R*-value applies when more than half the insulation is on the interior.

N1102.2 Specific insulation requirements.

N1102.2.1 Ceilings with attic spaces. When Section N1102.1 would require R-38 in the ceiling, R-30 shall be deemed to satisfy the requirement for R-38 wherever the full height of uncompressed R-30 insulation extends over the wall top plate at the eaves. Similarly R-38 shall be deemed to satisfy the requirement for R-49 wherever the full height of uncompressed R-38 insulation extends over the wall top plate at the eaves. This reduction shall not apply to the *U*-factor alternative approach in Section N1102.1.2 and the Total UA alternative in Section N1102.1.3.

N1102.2.2 Ceilings without attic spaces. Where Section N1102.1 would require insulation levels above R-30 and the design of the roof/ceiling assembly does not allow sufficient space for the required insulation, the minimum required insulation for such roof/ceiling assemblies shall be R-30. This reduction of insulation from the requirements of Section 402.1.1shall be limited to 500 square feet (46 m²) of ceiling area. This reduction shall not apply to the *U*-factor alternative approach in Section N1102.1.2 and the Total UA alternative in Section N1102.1.3.

N1102.2.3 Access hatches and doors. Access doors from *conditioned spaces* to unconditioned spaces (e.g., attics and crawl spaces) shall be weatherstripped and insulated to a level equivalent to the insulation on the surrounding surfaces. Access shall be provided to all *equipment* which prevents damaging or compressing the insulation. A wood framed or equivalent baffle or retainer is required to be provided when loose fill insulation is installed, the purpose of which is to prevent the loose fill insulation from spilling into the living space when the *attic* access is opened and to provide a permanent means of maintaining the installed *R*-value of the loose fill insulation.

N1102.2.4 Mass walls. Mass walls, for the purposes of this chapter, shall be considered above-grade walls of concrete block, concrete, insulated concrete form (ICF), masonry cavity, brick (other than brick veneer), earth (adobe, compressed earth block, rammed earth) and solid timber/logs.

N1102.2.5 Steel-frame ceilings, walls and floors. Steel-frame ceilings, walls and floors shall meet the insulation requirements of Table N1102.2.5 or shall meet the *U*-factor requirements in Table N1102.1.2. The calculation of the *U*-factor for a steel-frame envelope assembly shall use a series-parallel path calculation method.

> **Exception:** In climate zones 1 and 2, the continuous insulation requirements in Table N1102.2.5 shall be permitted to be reduced to R-3 for steel frame wall assemblies with studs spaced at 24 inches (610 mm) on center.

N1102.2.6 Floors. Floor insulation shall be installed to maintain permanent contact with the underside of the subfloor decking.

N1102.2.7 Basement walls. *Exterior walls* associated with conditioned basements shall be insulated from the top of the *basement wall* down to 10 feet (3048 mm) below *grade* or to the *basement* floor, whichever is less. Walls associated with unconditioned basements shall meet this requirement unless the floor overhead is insulated in accordance with Sections N1102.1 and N1102.2.6.

N1102.2.8 Slab-on-grade floors. Slab-on-grade floors with a floor surface less than 12 inches below *grade* shall be insulated in accordance with Table N1102.1. The insulation shall extend downward from the top of the slab on the outside or inside of the foundation wall. Insulation located below *grade* shall be extended the distance provided in Table N1102.1 by any combination of vertical insulation, insulation extending under the slab or insulation extending out from the building. Insulation extending away from the building shall be protected by pavement or by a minimum of 10 inches (254 mm) of soil. The top edge of the insulation installed between the *exterior wall* and the edge of the interior slab shall be permitted to be cut at a 45-degree (0.79 rad) angle away from the *exterior wall*. Slab-edge insulation is not required in jurisdictions designated by the code official as having a very heavy termite infestation.

TABLE N1102.1.2
EQUIVALENT *U*-FACTORS[a]

CLIMATE ZONE	FENESTRATION *U*-FACTOR	SKYLIGHT *U*-FACTOR	CEILING *U*-FACTOR	FRAME WALL *U*-FACTOR	MASS WALL *U*-FACTOR[b]	FLOOR *U*-FACTOR	BASEMENT WALL *U*-FACTOR	CRAWL SPACE WALL *U*-FACTOR
1	1.20	0.75	0.035	0.082	0.197	0.064	0.360	0.477
2	0.65	0.75	0.035	0.082	0.165	0.064	0.360	0.477
3	0.50	0.65	0.035	0.082	0.141	0.047	0.091[c]	0.136
4 except Marine	0.35	0.60	0.030	0.082	0.141	0.047	0.059	0.065
5 and Marine 4	0.35	0.60	0.030	0.060	0.082	0.033	0.059	0.065
6	0.35	0.60	0.026	0.060	0.060	0.033	0.059	0.065
7 and 8	0.35	0.60	0.026	0.057	0.057	0.033	0.059	0.065

a. Nonfenestration *U*-factors shall be obtained from measurement, calculation or an approved source.

b. When more than half the insulation is on the interior, the mass wall *U*-factors shall be a maximum of 0.17 in zone 1, 0.14 in zone 2, 0.12 in zone 3, 0.10 in zone 4 except Marine and the same as the frame wall *U*-factor in Marine zone 4 and in zones 5 through 8.

c. Basement wall *U*-factor of 0.360 in warm-humid climates as defined by Figure N1101.2 and Table N1101.2.

TABLE N1102.2.5
STEEL-FRAME CEILING, WALL AND FLOOR INSULATION (*R*-VALUE)

WOOD FRAME *R*-VALUE REQUIREMENT	COLD-FORMED STEEL EQUIVALENT *R*-VALUE[a]
Steel Truss Ceilings[a]	
R-30	R-38 or R-30 + 3 or R-26 + 5
R-38	R-49 or R-38 + 3
R-49	R-38 + 5
Steel Joist Ceilings[b]	
R-30	R-38 in 2 × 4 or 2 × 6 or 2 × 8 R-49 in any framing
R-38	R-49 in 2 × 4 or 2 × 6 or 2 × 8 or 2 × 10
Steel Framed Wall	
R-13	R-13 + 5 or R15 + 4 or R-21 + 3 or R-0 + 10
R-19	R-13 + 9 or R-19 + 8 or R-25 + 7
R-21	R-13 + 10 or R-19 + 9 or R-25 + 8
Steel Joist Floor	
R-13	R-19 in 2 × 6 R-19 + R-6 in 2 × 8 or 2 × 10
R-19	R-19 + R-6 in 2 × 6 R-19 + R-12 in 2 × 8 or 2 × 10

For SI: 1 inch = 25.4 mm.
a. Cavity insulation *R*-value is listed first, followed by continuous insulation *R*-value.
b. Insulation exceeding the height of the framing shall cover the framing.

N1102.2.9 Crawl space walls. As an alternative to insulating floors over crawl spaces, insulation of crawl space walls shall be permitted when the crawl space is not vented to the outside. Crawl space wall insulation shall be permanently fastened to the wall and extend downward from the floor to the finished *grade* level and then vertically and/or horizontally for at least an additional 24 inches (610 mm). Exposed earth in unvented crawl space foundations shall be covered with a continuous Class I vapor retarder. All joints of the vapor retarder shall overlap by 6 inches (152 mm) and be sealed or taped. The edges of the vapor retarder shall extend at least 6 inches (152 mm) up the stem wall and shall be attached to the stem wall.

N1102.2.10 Masonry veneer. Insulation shall not be required on the horizontal portion of the foundation that supports a masonry veneer.

N1102.2.11 Thermally isolated sunroom insulation. The minimum ceiling insulation *R*-values shall be R-19 in zones 1 through 4 and R-24 in zones 5 though 8. The minimum wall *R*-value shall be R-13 in all zones. New wall(s) separating the sunroom from *conditioned space* shall meet the *building thermal envelope* requirements.

N1102.3 Fenestration.

N1102.3.1 *U*-factor. An area-weighted average of fenestration products shall be permitted to satisfy the *U*-factor requirements.

N1102.3.2 Glazed fenestration SHGC. An area-weighted average of fenestration products more than 50 percent glazed shall be permitted to satisfy the solar heat gain coefficient (SHGC) requirements.

N1102.3.3 Glazed fenestration exemption. Up to 15 square feet (1.4 m²) of glazed fenestration per *dwelling unit* shall be permitted to be exempt from *U*-factor and SHGC requirements in Section N1102.1. This exemption shall not apply to the *U*-factor alternative approach in Section N1102.1.2 and the Total UA alternative in Section N1102.1.3.

N1102.3.4 Opaque door exemption. One side-hinged opaque door assembly up to 24 square feet (2.22 m²) in area is exempted from the *U*-factor requirement in Section N1102.1.1. This exemption shall not apply to the *U*-factor alternative approach in Section N1102.1.2 and the Total UA alternative in Section N1102.1.3.

N1102.3.5 Thermally isolated sunroom *U*-factor. For zones 4 through 8 the maximum fenestration *U*-factor shall be 0.50 and the maximum skylight *U*-factor shall be 0.75. New windows and doors separating the sunroom from *conditioned space* shall meet the *building thermal envelope* requirements.

N1102.3.6 Replacement fenestration. Where some or all of an existing fenestration unit is replaced with a new fenestration product, including sash and glazing, the replacement fenestration unit shall meet the applicable requirements for *U*-factor and solar heat gain coefficient (SHGC) in Table N1102.1.

N1102.4 Air leakage.

N1102.4.1 Building thermal envelope. The *building thermal envelope* shall be durably sealed to limit infiltration. The sealing methods between dissimilar materials shall allow for differential expansion and contraction. The following shall be caulked, gasketed, weatherstripped or otherwise sealed with an air barrier material, suitable film or solid material.

1. All joints, seams and penetrations.

2. Site-built windows, doors and skylights.

3. Openings between window and door assemblies and their respective jambs and framing.

4. Utility penetrations.

5. Dropped ceilings or chases adjacent to the thermal envelope.

6. Knee walls.

7. Walls and ceilings separating the garage from *conditioned spaces*.

8. Behind tubs and showers on *exterior walls*.

9. Common walls between *dwelling units*.

10. Attic access openings.

11. Rim joists junction.

12. Other sources of infiltration.

N1102.4.2 Air sealing and insulation. Building envelope air tightness and insulation installation shall be demonstrated to comply with one of the following options given by Section N1102.4.2.1 or N1102.4.2.2.

N1102.4.2.1 Testing option. Tested air leakage is less than 7 ACH when tested with a blower door at a pressure of 50 pascals (0.007 psi). Testing shall occur after rough in and after installation of penetrations of the building envelope, including penetrations for utilities, plumbing, electrical, ventilation and combustion appliances.

During testing:

1. Exterior windows and doors, fireplace and stove doors shall be closed, but not sealed;

2. Dampers shall be closed, but not sealed; including exhaust, intake, makeup air, back draft, and flue dampers;

3. Interior doors shall be open;

4. Exterior openings for continuous ventilation systems and heat recovery ventilators shall be closed and sealed;

5. Heating and cooling system(s) shall be turned off;

6. HVAC ducts shall not be sealed; and

7. Supply and return registers shall not be sealed.

N1102.4.2.2 Visual inspection option. The items listed in Table N1102.4.2, applicable to the method of construction, are field verified. Where required by the code official, an *approved* party independent from the installer of the insulation, shall inspect the air barrier and insulation.

N1102.4.3 Fireplaces. New wood-burning fireplaces shall have gasketed doors and outdoor combustion air.

N1102.4.4 Fenestration air leakage. Windows, skylights and sliding glass doors shall have an air infiltration rate of no more than 0.3 cubic foot per minute per square foot [1.5(L/s)/m²], and swinging doors no more than 0.5 cubic foot per minute per square foot [2.5(L/s)/m²], when tested according to NFRC 400 or AAMA/WDMA/CSA 101/I.S.2/A440 by an accredited, independent laboratory, and listed and *labeled* by the manufacturer.

Exception: Site-built windows, skylights and doors.

N1102.4.5 Recessed lighting. Recessed luminaires installed in the *building thermal envelope* shall be sealed to limit air leakage between conditioned and unconditioned spaces. All recessed luminaires shall be IC-rated and *labeled* as meeting ASTM E 283 when tested at 1.57 psi (75 Pa) pressure differential with no more than 2.0 cfm (0.944 L/s) of air movement from the *conditioned space* to the ceiling cavity. All recessed luminaires shall be sealed with a gasket or caulk between the housing and the interior wall or ceiling covering.

SECTION N1103
SYSTEMS

N1103.1 Controls. At least one thermostat shall be installed for each separate heating and cooling system.

N1103.1.1 Programmable thermostat. Where the primary heating system is a forced air furnace, at least one thermostat per *dwelling unit* shall be capable of controlling the heating and cooling system on a daily schedule to maintain different temperature set points at different times of the day. This thermostat shall include the capability to set back or temporarily operate the system to maintain zone temperatures down to 55°F (13°C) or up to 85°F (29°C). The thermostat shall initially be programmed with a heating temperature set point no higher than 70°F (21°C) and a cooling temperature set point no lower than 78°F (26°C).

N1103.1.2 Heat pump supplementary heat. Heat pumps having supplementary electric-resistance heat shall have controls that, except during defrost, prevent supplemental heat operation when the heat pump compressor can meet the heating load.

N1103.2 Ducts.

N1103.2.1 Insulation. Supply ducts in attics shall be insulated to a minimum of R-8. All other ducts shall be insulated to a minimum of R-6.

Exception: Ducts or portions thereof located completely inside the *building thermal envelope*.

N1103.2.2 Sealing. Ducts, air handlers, filter boxes and building cavities used as ducts shall be sealed. Joints and seams shall comply with Section M1601.4. Duct tightness shall be verified by either fo the following:

1. Post-construction test: Leakage to outdoors shall be less than or equal to 8 cfm (3.78 L/s) per 100 ft² (9.29

m²) of conditioned floor area or a total leakage less than or equal to 12 cfm (5.66 L/s) per 100 ft² (9.29 m²) of conditioned floor area when tested at a pressure differential of 0.1 inch w.g. (25 Pa) across the entire system, including the manufacturer's air handler end closure. All register boots shall be taped or otherwise sealed during the test.

2. Rough-in test: Total leakage shall be less than or equal to 6 cfm (2.83 L/s) per 100 ft² (9.29 m²) of conditioned floor area when tested at a pressure differential of 0.1 inch w.g. (25 Pa) across the roughed in system, including the manufacturer's air handler enclosure. All register boots shall be taped or otherwise sealed during the test. If the air handler is not installed at the time of the test, total leakage shall be less than or equal to 4 cfm (1.89 L/s) per 100 ft² (9.29 m²) of conditioned floor area.

Exception: Duct tightness test is not required if the air handler and all ducts are located within *conditioned space.*

N1103.2.3 Building cavities. Building framing cavities shall not be used as supply ducts.

N1103.3 Mechanical system piping insulation. Mechanical system piping capable of carrying fluids above 105°F (40°C) or below 55°F (13°C) shall be insulated to a minimum of R-3.

N1103.4 Circulating hot water systems. All circulating service hot water piping shall be insulated to at least R-2. Circulating hot water systems shall include an automatic or *readily accessible* manual switch that can turn off the hot water circulating pump when the system is not in use.

N1103.5 Mechanical ventilation. Outdoor air intakes and exhausts shall have automatic or gravity dampers that close when the ventilation system is not operating.

TABLE N1102.4.2
AIR BARRIER AND INSULATION INSPECTION

COMPONENT	CRITERIA
Air barrier and thermal barrier	Exterior thermal envelope insulation for framed walls is installed in substantial contact and continuous alignment with building envelope air barrier. Breaks or joints in the air barrier are filled or repaired. Air-permeable insulation is not used as a sealing material.
Ceiling/attic	Air barrier in any dropped ceiling/soffit is substantially aligned with insulation and any gaps are sealed Attic access (except unvented attic), knee wall door, or drop down stair is sealed.
Walls	Corners and headers are insulated. Junction of foundation and sill plate is sealed.
Windows and doors	Space between window/door jambs and framing is sealed.
Rim joists	Rim joists are insulated and include an air barrier.
Floors (including above garage and cantilevered floors)	Insulation is installed to maintain permanent contact with underside of subfloor decking. Air barrier is installed at any exposed edge of floor.
Crawlspace walls	Insulation is permanently attached to walls. Exposed earth in unvented crawlspaces is covered with Class I vapor retarder with overlapping joints taped.
Shafts, penetrations	Duct shafts, utility penetrations, knee walls and flue shafts opening to exterior or unconditioned space are sealed.
Narrow cavities	Batts in narrow cavities are cut to fit, or narrow cavities are filled by sprayed/blown insulation.
Garage separation	Air sealing is provided between the garage and conditioned spaces.
Recessed lighting	Recessed light fixtures are airtight, IC rated and sealed to drywall. Exception—fixtures in conditioned space.
Plumbing and wiring	Insulation is placed between outside and pipes. Batt insulation is cut to fit around wiring and plumbing, or sprayed/blown insulation extends behind piping and wiring.
Shower/tub on exterior wall	Showers and tubs on exterior walls have insulation and an air barrier separating them from the exterior wall.
Electrical/phone box on exterior wall	Air barrier extends behind boxes or air sealed type boxes are installed.
Common wall	Air barrier is installed in common wall between dwelling units.
HVAC register boots	HVAC register boots that penetrate building envelope are sealed to subfloor or drywall.
Fireplace	Fireplace walls include an air barrier.

N1103.6 Equipment sizing. Heating and cooling *equipment* shall be sized as specified in Section M1401.3.

N1103.7 Snow melt system controls. Snow- and ice-melting systems supplied through energy service to the building shall include automatic controls capable of shutting off the system when the pavement temperature is above 50°F (10°C) and no precipitation is falling and an automatic or manual control that will allow shutoff when the outdoor temperature is above 40°F (5°C).

N1103.8 Pools. Pools shall be provided with energy conserving measures in accordance with Sections N1103.8.1 through N1103.8.3.

N1103.8.1 Pool heaters. All pool heaters shall be equipped with a *readily accessible* on-off switch to allow shutting off the heater without adjusting the thermostat setting. Pool heaters fired by natural gas or LPG shall not have continuously burning pilot lights.

N1103.8.2 Time switches. Time switches that can automatically turn off and on heaters and pumps according to a pre-set schedule shall be installed on swimming pool heaters and pumps.

Exceptions:

1. Where public health standards require 24-hour pump operation.

2. Where pumps are required to operate solar- and waste-heat-recovery pool heating systems.

N1103.8.3 Pool covers. Heated pools shall be equipped with a vapor retardant pool cover on or at the water surface. Pools heated to more than 90°F (32°C) shall have a pool cover with a minimum insulation value of R-12.

SECTION N1104
LIGHTING SYSTEMS

N1104.1 Lighting equipment. A minimum of 50 percent of the lamps in permanently installed lighting fixtures shall be *high-efficacy lamps*.

Part V—Mechanical

CHAPTER 12

MECHANICAL ADMINISTRATION

SECTION M1201
GENERAL

M1201.1 Scope. The provisions of Chapters 12 through 24 shall regulate the design, installation, maintenance, *alteration* and inspection of mechanical systems that are permanently installed and used to control environmental conditions within buildings. These chapters shall also regulate those mechanical systems, system components, *equipment* and *appliances* specifically addressed in this code.

M1201.2 Application. In addition to the general administration requirements of Chapter 1, the administrative provisions of this chapter shall also apply to the mechanical requirements of Chapters 13 through 24.

[EB] SECTION M1202
EXISTING MECHANICAL SYSTEMS

M1202.1 Additions, alterations or repairs. *Additions, alterations*, renovations or repairs to a mechanical system shall conform to the requirements for a new mechanical system without requiring the existing mechanical system to comply with all of the requirements of this code. *Additions, alterations* or repairs shall not cause an existing mechanical system to become unsafe, hazardous or overloaded. Minor *additions, alterations* or repairs to existing mechanical systems shall meet the provisions for new construction, unless such work is done in the same manner and arrangement as was in the existing system, is not hazardous, and is *approved*.

M1202.2 Existing installations. Except as otherwise provided for in this code, a provision in this code shall not require the removal, *alteration* or abandonment of, nor prevent the continued use and maintenance of, an existing mechanical system lawfully in existence at the time of the adoption of this code.

M1202.3 Maintenance. Mechanical systems, both existing and new, and parts thereof shall be maintained in proper operating condition in accordance with the original design and in a safe and sanitary condition. Devices or safeguards that are required by this code shall be maintained in compliance with the code edition under which installed. The owner or the owner's designated agent shall be responsible for maintenance of the mechanical systems. To determine compliance with this provision, the *building official* shall have the authority to require a mechanical system to be reinspected.

CHAPTER 13

GENERAL MECHANICAL SYSTEM REQUIREMENTS

SECTION M1301
GENERAL

M1301.1 Scope. The provisions of this chapter shall govern the installation of mechanical systems not specifically covered in other chapters applicable to mechanical systems. Installations of mechanical *appliances*, *equipment* and systems not addressed by this code shall comply with the applicable provisions of the *International Mechanical Code* and the *International Fuel Gas Code*.

M1301.1.1 Flood-resistant installation. In areas prone to flooding as established by Table R301.2(1), mechanical *appliances*, *equipment* and systems shall be located or installed in accordance with Section R322.1.6.

SECTION M1302
APPROVAL

M1302.1 Listed and labeled. *Appliances* regulated by this code shall be *listed* and *labeled* for the application in which they are installed and used, unless otherwise *approved* in accordance with Section R104.11.

SECTION M1303
LABELING OF APPLIANCES

M1303.1 Label information. A permanent factory-applied nameplate(s) shall be affixed to *appliances* on which shall appear, in legible lettering, the manufacturer's name or trademark, the model number, a serial number and the seal or *mark* of the testing agency. A *label* shall also include the following:

1. Electrical *appliances*. Electrical rating in volts, amperes and motor phase; identification of individual electrical components in volts, amperes or watts and motor phase; and in Btu/h (W) output and required clearances.

2. Absorption units. Hourly rating in Btu/h (W), minimum hourly rating for units having step or automatic modulating controls, type of fuel, type of refrigerant, cooling capacity in Btu/h (W) and required clearances.

3. Fuel-burning units. Hourly rating in Btu/h (W), type of fuel *approved* for use with the *appliance* and required clearances.

4. Electric comfort heating *appliances*. Name and trademark of the manufacturer; the model number or equivalent; the electric rating in volts, amperes and phase; Btu/h (W) output rating; individual marking for each electrical component in amperes or watts, volts and phase; required clearances from combustibles and a seal indicating approval of the *appliance* by an *approved agency*.

5. Maintenance instructions. Required regular maintenance actions and title or publication number for the operation and maintenance manual for that particular model and type of product.

SECTION M1304
TYPE OF FUEL

M1304.1 Fuel types. Fuel-fired *appliances* shall be designed for use with the type of fuel to which they will be connected and the altitude at which they are installed. *Appliances* that comprise parts of the building mechanical system shall not be converted for the use of a different fuel, except where *approved* and converted in accordance with the manufacturer's instructions. The fuel input rate shall not be increased or decreased beyond the limit rating for the altitude at which the *appliance* is installed.

SECTION M1305
APPLIANCE ACCESS

M1305.1 Appliance access for inspection service, repair and replacement. *Appliances* shall be accessible for inspection, service, repair and replacement without removing permanent construction, other *appliances*, or any other piping or ducts not connected to the *appliance* being inspected, serviced, repaired or replaced. A level working space at least 30 inches deep and 30 inches wide (762 mm by 762 mm) shall be provided in front of the control side to service an *appliance*. Installation of room heaters shall be permitted with at least an 18-inch (457 mm) working space. A platform shall not be required for room heaters.

M1305.1.1 Furnaces and air handlers. Furnaces and air handlers within compartments or alcoves shall have a minimum working space clearance of 3 inches (76 mm) along the sides, back and top with a total width of the enclosing space being at least 12 inches (305 mm) wider than the furnace or air handler. Furnaces having a firebox open to the atmosphere shall have at least a 6-inch (152 mm) working space along the front combustion chamber side. Combustion air openings at the rear or side of the compartment shall comply with the requirements of Chapter 17.

Exception: This section shall not apply to replacement *appliances* installed in existing compartments and alcoves where the working space clearances are in accordance with the *equipment* or *appliance* manufacturer's installation instructions.

M1305.1.2 Appliances in rooms. *Appliances* installed in a compartment, alcove, *basement* or similar space shall be accessed by an opening or door and an unobstructed passageway measuring not less than 24 inches (610 mm) wide and large enough to allow removal of the largest *appliance* in the space, provided there is a level service space of not less than 30 inches (762 mm) deep and the height of the *appliance*, but not less than 30 inches (762 mm), at the front or service side of the *appliance* with the door open.

M1305.1.3 Appliances in attics. *Attics* containing *appliances* shall be provided with an opening and a clear and unobstructed passageway large enough to allow removal of the largest *appliance*, but not less than 30 inches (762 mm) high and 22 inches (559 mm) wide and not more than 20 feet (6096 mm) long measured along the centerline of the passageway from the opening to the *appliance*. The passageway shall have continuous solid flooring in accordance with Chapter 5 not less than 24 inches (610 mm) wide. A level service space at least 30 inches (762 mm) deep and 30 inches (762 mm) wide shall be present along all sides of the *appliance* where access is required. The clear access opening dimensions shall be a minimum of 20 inches by 30 inches (508 mm by 762 mm), and large enough to allow removal of the largest appliance.

Exceptions:

1. The passageway and level service space are not required where the *appliance* can be serviced and removed through the required opening.

2. Where the passageway is unobstructed and not less than 6 feet (1829 mm) high and 22 inches (559 mm) wide for its entire length, the passageway shall be not more than 50 feet (15 250 mm) long.

M1305.1.3.1 Electrical requirements. A luminaire controlled by a switch located at the required passageway opening and a receptacle outlet shall be installed at or near the *appliance* location in accordance with Chapter 39.

M1305.1.4 Appliances under floors. Underfloor spaces containing *appliances* shall be provided with an unobstructed passageway large enough to remove the largest *appliance*, but not less than 30 inches (762 mm) high and 22 inches (559 mm) wide, nor more than 20 feet (6096 mm) long measured along the centerline of the passageway from the opening to the *appliance*. A level service space at least 30 inches (762 mm) deep and 30 inches (762 mm) wide shall be present at the front or service side of the *appliance*. If the depth of the passageway or the service space exceeds 12 inches (305 mm) below the adjoining grade, the walls of the passageway shall be lined with concrete or masonry extending 4 inches (102 mm) above the adjoining grade in accordance with Chapter 4. The rough-framed access opening dimensions shall be a minimum of 22 inches by 30 inches (559 mm by 762 mm), and large enough to remove the largest *appliance*.

Exceptions:

1. The passageway is not required where the level service space is present when the access is open, and the *appliance* can be serviced and removed through the required opening.

2. Where the passageway is unobstructed and not less than 6 feet high (1929 mm) and 22 inches (559 mm) wide for its entire length, the passageway shall not be limited in length.

M1305.1.4.1 Ground clearance. *Equipment* and *appliances* supported from the ground shall be level and firmly supported on a concrete slab or other *approved* material extending not less than 3 inches (76 mm) above the adjoining ground. Such support shall be in accordance with the manufacturer's installation instructions. *Appliances* suspended from the floor shall have a clearance of not less than 6 inches (152 mm) from the ground.

M1305.1.4.2 Excavations. Excavations for *appliance* installations shall extend to a depth of 6 inches (152 mm) below the *appliance* and 12 inches (305 mm) on all sides, except that the control side shall have a clearance of 30 inches (762 mm).

M1305.1.4.3 Electrical requirements. A luminaire controlled by a switch located at the required passageway opening and a receptacle outlet shall be installed at or near the *appliance* location in accordance with Chapter 39.

SECTION M1306
CLEARANCES FROM COMBUSTIBLE CONSTRUCTION

M1306.1 Appliance clearance. *Appliances* shall be installed with the clearances from unprotected combustible materials as indicated on the *appliance label* and in the manufacturer's installation instructions.

M1306.2 Clearance reduction. Reduction of clearances shall be in accordance with the *appliance* manufacturer's instructions and Table M1306.2. Forms of protection with ventilated air space shall conform to the following requirements:

1. Not less than 1-inch (25 mm) air space shall be provided between the protection and combustible wall surface.

2. Air circulation shall be provided by having edges of the wall protection open at least 1 inch (25 mm).

3. If the wall protection is mounted on a single flat wall away from corners, air circulation shall be provided by having the bottom and top edges, or the side and top edges open at least 1 inch (25 mm).

4. Wall protection covering two walls in a corner shall be open at the bottom and top edges at least 1 inch (25 mm).

M1306.2.1 Solid-fuel appliances. Table M1306.2 shall not be used to reduce the clearance required for solid-fuel *appliances* listed for installation with minimum clearances of 12 inches (305 mm) or less. For *appliances listed* for installation with minimum clearances greater than 12 inches (305 mm), Table M1306.2 shall not be used to reduce the clearance to less than 12 inches (305 mm).

SECTION M1307
APPLIANCE INSTALLATION

M1307.1 General. Installation of *appliances* shall conform to the conditions of their *listing* and *label* and the manufacturer's installation instructions. The manufacturer's operating and installation instructions shall remain attached to the *appliance*.

TABLE M1306.2
REDUCTION OF CLEARANCES WITH SPECIFIED FORMS OF PROTECTION[a, c, d, e, f, g, h, I, j, k, l]

TYPE OF PROTECTION APPLIED TO AND COVERING ALL SURFACES OF COMBUSTIBLE MATERIAL WITHIN THE DISTANCE SPECIFIED AS THE REQUIRED CLEARANCE WITH NO PROTECTION (See Figures M1306.1 and M1306.2)	WHERE THE REQUIRED CLEARANCE WITH NO PROTECTION FROM APPLIANCE, VENT CONNECTOR, OR SINGLE WALL METAL PIPE IS:									
	36 inches		18 inches		12 inches		9 inches		6 inches	
	Allowable clearances with specified protection (Inches)[b]									
	Use column 1 for clearances above an appliance or horizontal connector. Use column 2 for clearances from an appliance, vertical connector and single-wall metal pipe.									
	Above column 1	Sides and rear column 2	Above column 1	Sides and rear column 2	Above column 1	Sides and rear column 2	Above column 1	Sides and rear column 2	Above column 1	Sides and rear column 2
3^1/$_2$-inch thick masonry wall without ventilated air space	—	24	—	12	—	9	—	6	—	5
^{1}/$_2$-in. insulation board over 1-inch glass fiber or mineral wool batts	24	18	12	9	9	6	6	5	4	3
Galvanized sheet steel having a minimum thickness of 0.0236-inch (No. 24 gage) over 1-inch glass fiber or mineral wool batts reinforced with wire or rear face with a ventilated air space	18	12	9	6	6	4	5	3	3	3
3^1/$_2$-inch thick masonry wall with ventilated air space	—	12	—	6	—	6	—	6	—	6
Galvanized sheet steel having a minimum thickness of 0.0236-inch (No. 24 gage) with a ventilated air space 1-inch off the combustible assembly	18	12	9	6	6	4	5	3	3	2
^{1}/$_2$-inch thick insulation board with ventilated air space	18	12	9	6	6	4	5	3	3	3
Galvanized sheet steel having a minimum thickness of 0.0236-inch (No. 24 gage) with ventilated air space over 24 gage sheet steel with a ventilated space	18	12	9	6	6	4	5	3	3	3
1-inch glass fiber or mineral wool batts sandwiched between two sheets of galvanized sheet steel having a minimum thickness of 0.0236-inch (No. 24 gage) with a ventilated air space	18	12	9	6	6	4	5	3	3	3

For SI: 1 inch = 25.4 mm, 1 pound per cubic foot = 16.019 kg/m^3, °C = [(°F)-32/1.8], 1 Btu/(h × ft^2 × °F/in.) = 0.001442299 (W/cm^2 × °C/cm).

a. Reduction of clearances from combustible materials shall not interfere with combustion air, draft hood clearance and relief, and accessibility of servicing.

b. Clearances shall be measured from the surface of the heat producing appliance or equipment to the outer surface of the combustible material or combustible assembly.

c. Spacers and ties shall be of noncombustible material. No spacer or tie shall be used directly opposite appliance or connector.

d. Where all clearance reduction systems use a ventilated air space, adequate provision for air circulation shall be provided as described. (See Figures M1306.1 and M1306.2.)

e. There shall be at least 1 inch between clearance reduction systems and combustible walls and ceilings for reduction systems using ventilated air space.

f. If a wall protector is mounted on a single flat wall away from corners, adequate air circulation shall be permitted to be provided by leaving only the bottom and top edges or only the side and top edges open with at least a 1-inch air gap.

g. Mineral wool and glass fiber batts (blanket or board) shall have a minimum density of 8 pounds per cubic foot and a minimum melting point of 1,500°F.

h. Insulation material used as part of a clearance reduction system shall have a thermal conductivity of 1.0 Btu inch per square foot per hour °F or less. Insulation board shall be formed of noncombustible material.

i. There shall be at least 1 inch between the appliance and the protector. In no case shall the clearance between the appliance and the combustible surface be reduced below that allowed in this table.

j. All clearances and thicknesses are minimum; larger clearances and thicknesses are acceptable.

k. Listed single-wall connectors shall be permitted to be installed in accordance with the terms of their listing and the manufacturer's instructions.

l. For limitations on clearance reduction for solid-fuel-burning appliances see Section M1306.2.1.

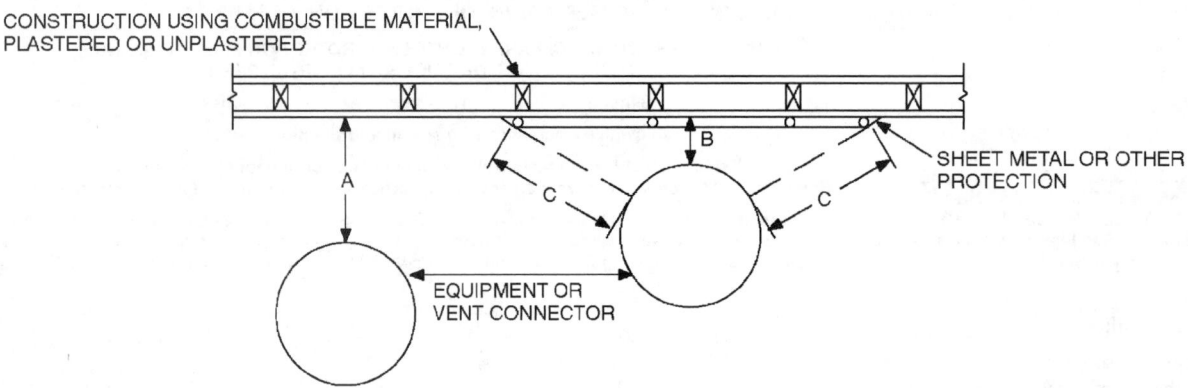

NOTE: "A" equals the required clearance with no protection. "B" equals the reduced clearance permitted in accordance with Table M1306.2. The protection applied to the construction using combustible material shall extend far enough in each direction to make "C" equal to "A."

FIGURE M1306.1
REDUCED CLEARANCE DIAGRAM

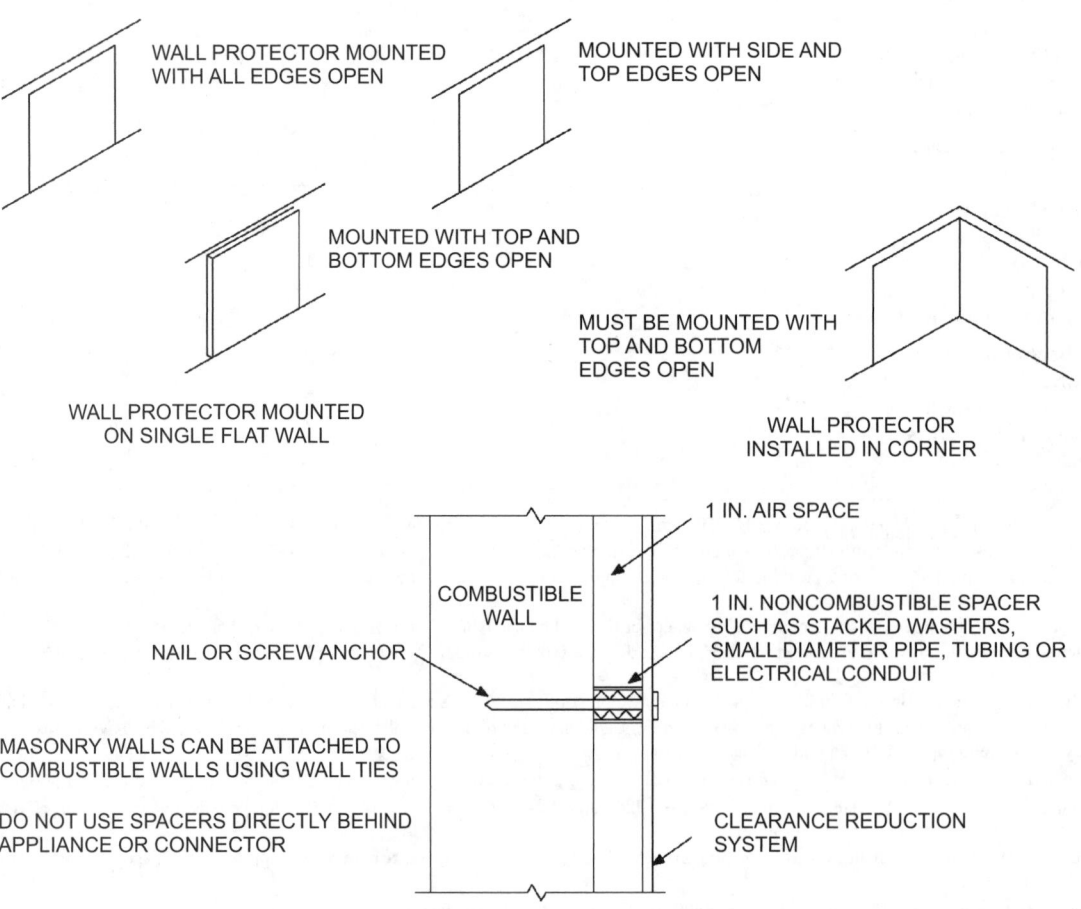

For SI: 1 inch = 25.4 mm.

FIGURE M1306.2
WALL PROTECTOR CLEARANCE REDUCTION SYSTEM

M1307.2 Anchorage of appliances. *Appliances* designed to be fixed in position shall be fastened or anchored in an *approved* manner. In Seismic Design Categories D_1 and D_2, water heaters shall be anchored or strapped to resist horizontal displacement caused by earthquake motion. Strapping shall be at points within the upper one-third and lower one-third of the *appliance's* vertical dimensions. At the lower point, the strapping shall maintain a minimum distance of 4 inches (102 mm) above the controls.

M1307.3 Elevation of ignition source. *Appliances* having an *ignition source* shall be elevated such that the source of ignition is not less than 18 inches (457 mm) above the floor in garages. For the purpose of this section, rooms or spaces that are not part of the living space of a *dwelling unit* and that communicate with a private garage through openings shall be considered to be part of the garage.

> **M1307.3.1 Protection from impact.** *Appliances* shall not be installed in a location subject to vehicle damage except where protected by *approved* barriers.

M1307.4 Hydrogen generating and refueling operations. *Ventilation* shall be required in accordance with Section M1307.4.1, M1307.4.2 or M1307.4.3 in private garages that contain hydrogen-generating *appliances* or refueling systems. For the purpose of this section, rooms or spaces that are not part of the living space of a *dwelling unit* and that communicate directly with a private garage through openings shall be considered to be part of the private garage.

> **M1307.4.1 Natural ventilation.** Indoor locations intended for hydrogen-generating or refueling operations shall be limited to a maximum floor area of 850 square feet (79 m²) and shall communicate with the outdoors in accordance with Sections M1307.4.1.1 and M1307.4.1.2. The maximum rated output capacity of hydrogen generating *appliances* shall not exceed 4 standard cubic feet per minute (1.9 L/s) of hydrogen for each 250 square feet (23 m²) of floor area in such spaces. The minimum cross-sectional dimension of air openings shall be 3 inches (76 mm). Where ducts are used, they shall be of the same cross-sectional area as the free area of the openings to which they connect. In those locations, *equipment* and *appliances* having an *ignition source* shall be located so that the source of ignition is not within 12 inches (305 mm) of the ceiling.

> > **M1307.4.1.1 Two openings.** Two permanent openings shall be constructed within the garage. The upper opening shall be located entirely within 12 inches (305 mm) of the ceiling of the garage. The lower opening shall be located entirely within 12 inches (305 mm) of the floor of the garage. Both openings shall be constructed in the same exterior wall. The openings shall communicate directly with the outdoors and shall have a minimum free area of ¹/₂ square foot per 1,000 cubic feet (1.7 m²/1000 m³) of garage volume.

> > **M1307.4.1.2 Louvers and grilles.** In calculating free area required by Section M1307.4.1, the required size of openings shall be based on the net free area of each opening. If the free area through a design of louver or grille is known, it shall be used in calculating the size opening required to provide the free area specified. If the design

and free area are not known, it shall be assumed that wood louvers will have a 25-percent free area and metal louvers and grilles will have a 75-percent free area. Louvers and grilles shall be fixed in the open position.

> **M1307.4.2 Mechanical ventilation.** Indoor locations intended for hydrogen-generating or refueling operations shall be ventilated in accordance with Section 502.16 of the *International Mechanical Code*. In these locations, *equipment* and *appliances* having an *ignition source* shall be located so that the source of ignition is below the mechanical *ventilation* outlet(s).

> **M1307.4.3 Specially engineered installations.** As an alternative to the provisions of Sections M1307.4.1 and M1307.4.2, the necessary supply of air for *ventilation* and dilution of flammable gases shall be provided by an *approved* engineered system.

M1307.5 Electrical appliances. Electrical *appliances* shall be installed in accordance with Chapters 14, 15, 19, 20 and 34 through 43 of this code.

M1307.6 Plumbing connections. Potable water and drainage system connections to *equipment* and *appliances* regulated by this code shall be in accordance with Chapters 29 and 30.

SECTION M1308
MECHANICAL SYSTEMS INSTALLATION

M1308.1 Drilling and notching. Wood-framed structural members shall be drilled, notched or altered in accordance with the provisions of Sections R502.8, R602.6, R602.6.1 and R802.7. Holes in load-bearing members of cold-formed steel light-frame construction shall be permitted only in accordance with Sections R505.2.5, R603.2.5 and R804.2.5. In accordance with the provisions of Sections R505.3.5, R603.3.4 and R804.3.4, cutting and notching of flanges and lips of load-bearing members of cold-formed steel light frame construction shall not be permitted. Structural insulated panels (SIPs) shall be drilled and notched or altered in accordance with the provisions of Section R612.9.

M1308.2 Protection against physical damage. In concealed locations where piping, other than cast-iron or galvanized steel, is installed through holes or notches in studs, joists, rafters or similar members less than 1.5 inches (38 mm) from the nearest edge of the member, the pipe shall be protected by shield plates. Protective steel shield plates having a minimum thickness of 0.0575-inch (1.463 mm) (No. 16 gage), shall cover the area of the pipe where the member is notched or bored, and shall extend a minimum of 2 inches (51 mm) above sole plates and below top plates.

CHAPTER 14

HEATING AND COOLING EQUIPMENT

SECTION M1401
GENERAL

M1401.1 Installation. Heating and cooling *equipment* and *appliances* shall be installed in accordance with the manufacturer's installation instructions and the requirements of this code.

M1401.2 Access. Heating and cooling *equipment* shall be located with respect to building construction and other *equipment* to permit maintenance, servicing and replacement. Clearances shall be maintained to permit cleaning of heating and cooling surfaces; replacement of filters, blowers, motors, controls and vent connections; lubrication of moving parts; and adjustments.

M1401.3 Sizing. Heating and cooling *equipment* shall be sized in accordance with ACCA Manual S based on building loads calculated in accordance with ACCA Manual J or other *approved* heating and cooling calculation methodologies.

M1401.4 Exterior installations. *Equipment* installed outdoors shall be *listed* and *labeled* for outdoor installation. Supports and foundations shall prevent excessive vibration, settlement or movement of the *equipment*. Supports and foundations shall be level and conform to the manufacturer's installation instructions.

M1401.5 Flood hazard. In areas prone to flooding as established by Table R301.2(1), heating and cooling *equipment* and *appliances* shall be located or installed in accordance with Section R322.1.6.

SECTION M1402
CENTRAL FURNACES

M1402.1 General. Oil-fired central furnaces shall conform to ANSI/UL 727. Electric furnaces shall conform to UL 1995.

M1402.2 Clearances. Clearances shall be provided in accordance with the *listing* and the manufacturer's installation instructions.

M1402.3 Combustion air. *Combustion air* shall be supplied in accordance with Chapter 17. *Combustion air* openings shall be unobstructed for a distance of not less than 6 inches (152 mm) in front of the openings.

SECTION M1403
HEAT PUMP EQUIPMENT

M1403.1 Heat pumps. The minimum unobstructed total area of the outside and return air ducts or openings to a heat pump shall be not less than 6 square inches per 1,000 Btu/h (13 208 mm²/kW) output rating or as indicated by the conditions of the listing of the heat pump. Electric heat pumps shall conform to UL 1995.

M1403.2 Foundations and supports. Supports and foundations for the outdoor unit of a heat pump shall be raised at least 3 inches (76 mm) above the ground to permit free drainage of defrost water, and shall conform to the manufacturer's installation instructions.

SECTION M1404
REFRIGERATION COOLING EQUIPMENT

M1404.1 Compliance. Refrigeration cooling *equipment* shall comply with Section M1411.

SECTION M1405
BASEBOARD CONVECTORS

M1405.1 General. Electric baseboard convectors shall be installed in accordance with the manufacturer's installation instructions and Chapters 34 through 43 of this code.

SECTION M1406
RADIANT HEATING SYSTEMS

M1406.1 General. Electric radiant heating systems shall be installed in accordance with the manufacturer's installation instructions and Chapters 34 through 43 of this code.

M1406.2 Clearances. Clearances for radiant heating panels or elements to any wiring, outlet boxes and junction boxes used for installing electrical devices or mounting luminaires shall comply with Chapters 34 through 43 of this code.

M1406.3 Installation of radiant panels. Radiant panels installed on wood framing shall conform to the following requirements:

1. Heating panels shall be installed parallel to framing members and secured to the surface of framing members or mounted between framing members.

2. Panels shall be nailed or stapled only through the unheated portions provided for this purpose and shall not be fastened at any point closer than $^1/_4$ inch (6.4 mm) to an element.

3. Unless *listed* and *labeled* for field cutting, heating panels shall be installed as complete units.

M1406.4 Installation in concrete or masonry. Radiant heating systems installed in concrete or masonry shall conform to the following requirements:

1. Radiant heating systems shall be identified as being suitable for the installation, and shall be secured in place as specified in the manufacturer's installation instructions.

2. Radiant heating panels or radiant heating panel sets shall not be installed where they bridge expansion joints unless protected from expansion and contraction.

M1406.5 Gypsum panels. Where radiant heating systems are used on gypsum assemblies, operating temperatures shall not exceed 125°F (52°C).

M1406.6 Finish surfaces. Finish materials installed over radiant heating panels or systems shall be installed in accordance with the manufacturer's installation instructions. Surfaces shall be secured so that nails or other fastenings do not pierce the radiant heating elements.

SECTION M1407
DUCT HEATERS

M1407.1 General. Electric duct heaters shall be installed in accordance with the manufacturer's installation instructions and Chapters 34 through 43 of this code. Electric furnaces shall be tested in accordance with UL 1995.

M1407.2 Installation. Electric duct heaters shall be installed so that they will not create a fire hazard. Class 1 ducts, duct coverings and linings shall be interrupted at each heater to provide the clearances specified in the manufacturer's installation instructions. Such interruptions are not required for duct heaters *listed* and *labeled* for zero clearance to combustible materials. Insulation installed in the immediate area of each heater shall be classified for the maximum temperature produced on the duct surface.

M1407.3 Installation with heat pumps and air conditioners. Duct heaters located within 4 feet (1219 mm) of a heat pump or air conditioner shall be *listed* and *labeled* for such installations. The heat pump or air conditioner shall additionally be *listed* and *labeled* for such duct heater installations.

M1407.4 Access. Duct heaters shall be accessible for servicing, and clearance shall be maintained to permit adjustment, servicing and replacement of controls and heating elements.

M1407.5 Fan interlock. The fan circuit shall be provided with an interlock to prevent heater operation when the fan is not operating.

SECTION M1408
VENTED FLOOR FURNACES

M1408.1 General. Vented floor furnaces shall conform to UL 729 and be installed in accordance with their *listing*, the manufacturer's installation instructions and the requirements of this code.

M1408.2 Clearances. Vented floor furnaces shall be installed in accordance with their listing and the manufacturer's installation instructions.

M1408.3 Location. Location of floor furnaces shall conform to the following requirements:

1. Floor registers of floor furnaces shall be installed not less than 6 inches (152 mm) from a wall.

2. Wall registers of floor furnaces shall be installed not less than 6 inches (152 mm) from the adjoining wall at inside corners.

3. The furnace register shall be located not less than 12 inches (305 mm) from doors in any position, draperies or similar combustible objects.

4. The furnace register shall be located at least 5 feet (1524 mm) below any projecting combustible materials.

5. The floor furnace burner assembly shall not project into an occupied under-floor area.

6. The floor furnace shall not be installed in concrete floor construction built on grade.

7. The floor furnace shall not be installed where a door can swing within 12 inches (305 mm) of the grille opening.

M1408.4 Access. An opening in the foundation not less than 18 inches by 24 inches (457 mm by 610 mm), or a trap door not less than 22 inches by 30 inches (559 mm by 762 mm) shall be provided for access to a floor furnace. The opening and passageway shall be large enough to allow replacement of any part of the *equipment*.

M1408.5 Installation. Floor furnace installations shall conform to the following requirements:

1. Thermostats controlling floor furnaces shall be located in the room in which the register of the floor furnace is located.

2. Floor furnaces shall be supported independently of the furnace floor register.

3. Floor furnaces shall be installed not closer than 6 inches (152 mm) to the ground. Clearance may be reduced to 2 inches (51 mm), provided that the lower 6 inches (152 mm) of the furnace is sealed to prevent water entry.

4. Where excavation is required for a floor furnace installation, the excavation shall extend 30 inches (762 mm) beyond the control side of the floor furnace and 12 inches (305 mm) beyond the remaining sides. Excavations shall slope outward from the perimeter of the base of the excavation to the surrounding grade at an angle not exceeding 45 degrees (0.79 rad) from horizontal.

5. Floor furnaces shall not be supported from the ground.

SECTION M1409
VENTED WALL FURNACES

M1409.1 General. Vented wall furnaces shall conform to UL 730 and be installed in accordance with their listing, the manufacturer's installation instructions and the requirements of this code.

M1409.2 Location. The location of vented wall furnaces shall conform to the following requirements:

1. Vented wall furnaces shall be located where they will not cause a fire hazard to walls, floors, combustible furnishings or doors. Vented wall furnaces installed between bathrooms and adjoining rooms shall not circulate air from bathrooms to other parts of the building.

2. Vented wall furnaces shall not be located where a door can swing within 12 inches (305 mm) of the furnace air inlet or outlet measured at right angles to the opening.

Doorstops or door closers shall not be installed to obtain this clearance.

M1409.3 Installation. Vented wall furnace installations shall conform to the following requirements:

1. Required wall thicknesses shall be in accordance with the manufacturer's installation instructions.

2. Ducts shall not be attached to a wall furnace. Casing extensions or boots shall be installed only when listed as part of a *listed* and *labeled appliance*.

3. A manual shut off valve shall be installed ahead of all controls.

M1409.4 Access. Vented wall furnaces shall be provided with access for cleaning of heating surfaces; removal of burners; replacement of sections, motors, controls, filters and other working parts; and for adjustments and lubrication of parts requiring such attention. Panels, grilles and access doors that must be removed for normal servicing operations shall not be attached to the building construction.

SECTION M1410
VENTED ROOM HEATERS

M1410.1 General. Vented room heaters shall be tested in accordance with ASTM E 1509, UL 896 for oil-fired or UL 1482 for solid fuel-fired and installed in accordance with their *listing*, the manufacturer's installation instructions and the requirements of this code.

M1410.2 Floor mounting. Room heaters shall be installed on noncombustible floors or *approved* assemblies constructed of noncombustible materials that extend at least 18 inches (457 mm) beyond the *appliance* on all sides.

Exceptions:

1. *Listed* room heaters shall be installed on noncombustible floors, assemblies constructed of noncombustible materials or *listed* floor protectors with materials and dimensions in accordance with the *appliance* manufacturer's instructions.

2. Room heaters *listed* for installation on combustible floors without floor protection shall be installed in accordance with the *appliance* manufacturer's instructions.

SECTION M1411
HEATING AND COOLING EQUIPMENT

M1411.1 Approved refrigerants. Refrigerants used in direct refrigerating systems shall conform to the applicable provisions of ANSI/ASHRAE 34.

M1411.2 Refrigeration coils in warm-air furnaces. Where a cooling coil is located in the supply plenum of a warm-air furnace, the furnace blower shall be rated at not less than 0.5-inch water column (124 Pa) static pressure unless the furnace is *listed* and *labeled* for use with a cooling coil. Cooling coils shall not be located upstream from heat exchangers unless *listed* and *labeled* for such use. Conversion of existing furnaces for use with cooling coils shall be permitted provided the fur-

nace will operate within the temperature rise specified for the furnace.

M1411.3 Condensate disposal. Condensate from all cooling coils or evaporators shall be conveyed from the drain pan outlet to an *approved* place of disposal. Such piping shall maintain a minimum horizontal slope in the direction of discharge of not less than $^1/_8$ unit vertical in 12 units horizontal (1-percent slope). Condensate shall not discharge into a street, alley or other areas where it would cause a nuisance.

M1411.3.1 Auxiliary and secondary drain systems. In addition to the requirements of Section M1411.3, a secondary drain or auxiliary drain pan shall be required for each cooling or evaporator coil where damage to any building components will occur as a result of overflow from the *equipment* drain pan or stoppage in the condensate drain piping. Such piping shall maintain a minimum horizontal slope in the direction of discharge of not less than $^1/_8$ unit vertical in 12 units horizontal (1-percent slope). Drain piping shall be a minimum of $^3/_4$-inch (19 mm) nominal pipe size. One of the following methods shall be used:

1. An auxiliary drain pan with a separate drain shall be installed under the coils on which condensation will occur. The auxiliary pan drain shall discharge to a conspicuous point of disposal to alert occupants in the event of a stoppage of the primary drain. The pan shall have a minimum depth of 1.5 inches (38 mm), shall not be less than 3 inches (76 mm) larger than the unit or the coil dimensions in width and length and shall be constructed of corrosion-resistant material. Galvanized sheet steel pans shall have a minimum thickness of not less than 0.0236-inch (0.6010 mm) (No. 24 Gage). Nonmetallic pans shall have a minimum thickness of not less than 0.0625 inch (1.6 mm).

2. A separate overflow drain line shall be connected to the drain pan installed with the *equipment*. This overflow drain shall discharge to a conspicuous point of disposal to alert occupants in the event of a stoppage of the primary drain. The overflow drain line shall connect to the drain pan at a higher level than the primary drain connection.

3. An auxiliary drain pan without a separate drain line shall be installed under the coils on which condensation will occur. This pan shall be equipped with a water level detection device conforming to UL 508 that will shut off the *equipment* served prior to overflow of the pan. The pan shall be equipped with a fitting to allow for drainage. The auxiliary drain pan shall be constructed in accordance with Item 1 of this section.

4. A water level detection device conforming to UL 508 shall be installed that will shut off the *equipment* served in the event that the primary drain is blocked. The device shall be installed in the primary drain line, the overflow drain line or the *equipment*-supplied drain pan, located at a point higher than the primary drain line connection and below the overflow rim of such pan.

M1411.3.1.1 Water-level monitoring devices. On down-flow units and all other coils that have no secondary drain or provisions to install a secondary or auxiliary drain pan, a water-level monitoring device shall be installed inside the primary drain pan. This device shall shut off the equipment served in the event that the primary drain becomes restricted. Devices shall not be installed in the drain line.

M1411.3.2 Drain pipe materials and sizes. Components of the condensate disposal system shall be cast iron, galvanized steel, copper, polybutylene, polyethylene, ABS, CPVC or PVC pipe or tubing. All components shall be selected for the pressure and temperature rating of the installation. Joints and connections shall be made in accordance with the materials specified in Chapter 30. Condensate waste and drain line size shall be not less than $^3/_4$-inch (19 mm) internal diameter and shall not decrease in size from the drain pan connection to the place of condensate disposal. Where the drain pipes from more than one unit are manifolded together for condensate drainage, the pipe or tubing shall be sized in accordance with an *approved* method.

M1411.3.3 Appliances, equipment and insulation in pans. Where *appliances, equipment* or insulation are subject to water damage when auxiliary drain pans fill, those portions of the *appliances, equipment* and insulation shall be installed above the flood level rim of the pan. Supports located inside of the pan to support the *appliance* or *equipment* shall be water resistant and *approved*.

M1411.4 Auxiliary drain pan. Category IV condensing *appliances* shall have an auxiliary drain pan where damage to any building component will occur as a result of stoppage in the condensate drainage system. These pans shall be installed in accordance with the applicable provisions of Section M1411.3.

> **Exception:** Fuel-fired *appliances* that automatically shut down operation in the event of a stoppage in the condensate drainage system.

M1411.5 Insulation of refrigerant piping. Piping and fittings for refrigerant vapor (suction) lines shall be insulated with insulation having a thermal resistivity of at least R-4 and having external surface permeance not exceeding 0.05 perm [2.87 ng/(s · m^2 · Pa)] when tested in accordance with ASTM E 96.

M1411.6 Locking access port caps. Refrigerant circuit access ports located outdoors shall be fitted with locking-type tamper-resistant caps.

SECTION M1412
ABSORPTION COOLING EQUIPMENT

M1412.1 Approval of equipment. Absorption systems shall be installed in accordance with the manufacturer's installation instructions.

M1412.2 Condensate disposal. Condensate from the cooling coil shall be disposed of as provided in Section M1411.3.

M1412.3 Insulation of piping. Refrigerant piping, brine piping and fittings within a building shall be insulated to prevent condensation from forming on piping.

M1412.4 Pressure-relief protection. Absorption systems shall be protected by a pressure-relief device. Discharge from the pressure-relief device shall be located where it will not create a hazard to persons or property.

SECTION M1413
EVAPORATIVE COOLING EQUIPMENT

M1413.1 General. Cooling *equipment* that uses evaporation of water for cooling shall be installed in accordance with the manufacturer's installation instructions. Evaporative coolers shall be installed on a level platform or base not less than 3 inches (76 mm) above the adjoining ground and secured to prevent displacement. Openings in exterior walls shall be flashed in accordance with Section R703.8.

M1413.2 Protection of potable water. The potable water system shall be protected from backflow in accordance with the provisions in Section P2902.

SECTION 1414
FIREPLACE STOVES

M1414.1 General. Fireplace stoves shall be *listed*, *labeled* and installed in accordance with the terms of the listing. Fireplace stoves shall be tested in accordance with UL 737.

M1414.2 Hearth extensions. Hearth extensions for fireplace stoves shall be installed in accordance with the *listing* of the fireplace stove. The supporting structure for a hearth extension for a fireplace stove shall be at the same level as the supporting structure for the fireplace unit. The hearth extension shall be readily distinguishable from the surrounding floor area.

SECTION M1415
MASONRY HEATERS

M1415.1 General. Masonry heaters shall be constructed in accordance with Section R1002.

CHAPTER 15

EXHAUST SYSTEMS

SECTION M1501
GENERAL

M1501.1 Outdoor discharge. The air removed by every mechanical exhaust system shall be discharged to the outdoors. Air shall not be exhausted into an *attic*, soffit, ridge vent or crawl space.

> **Exception:** Whole-house *ventilation*-type *attic* fans that discharge into the *attic* space of *dwelling units* having private *attics* shall be permitted.

SECTION M1502
CLOTHES DRYER EXHAUST

M1502.1 General. Clothes dryers shall be exhausted in accordance with the manufacturer's instructions.

M1502.2 Independent exhaust systems. Dryer exhaust systems shall be independent of all other systems and shall convey the moisture to the outdoors.

> **Exception:** This section shall not apply to *listed* and *labeled* condensing (ductless) clothes dryers.

M1502.3 Duct termination. Exhaust ducts shall terminate on the outside of the building. Exhaust duct terminations shall be in accordance with the dryer manufacturer's installation instructions. If the manufacturer's instructions do not specify a termination location, the exhaust duct shall terminate not less than 3 feet (914 mm) in any direction from openings into buildings. Exhaust duct terminations shall be equipped with a backdraft damper. Screens shall not be installed at the duct termination.

M1502.4 Dryer exhaust ducts. Dryer exhaust ducts shall conform to the requirements of Sections M1502.4.1 through M1502.4.6.

> **M1502.4.1 Material and size.** Exhaust ducts shall have a smooth interior finish and shall be constructed of metal a minimum 0.016-inch (0.4 mm) thick. The exhaust duct size shall be 4 inches (102 mm) nominal in diameter.

M1502.4.2 Duct installation. Exhaust ducts shall be supported at 4 foot (1219 mm) intervals and secured in place. The insert end of the duct shall extend into the adjoining duct or fitting in the direction of airflow. Ducts shall not be joined with screws or similar fasteners that protrude into the inside of the duct.

M1502.4.3 Transition duct. Transition ducts used to connect the dryer to the exhaust *duct system* shall be a single length that is *listed* and *labeled* in accordance with UL 2158A. Transition ducts shall be a maximum of 8 feet (2438 mm) in length. Transition ducts shall not be concealed within construction.

M1502.4.4 Duct length. The maximum allowable exhaust duct length shall be determined by one of the methods specified in Section M1502.4.4.1 or M1502.4.4.2.

> **M1502.4.4.1 Specified length.** The maximum length of the exhaust duct shall be 25 feet (7620 mm) from the connection to the transition duct from the dryer to the outlet terminal. Where fittings are used, the maximum length of the exhaust duct shall be reduced in accordance with Table M1502.4.4.1.

> **M1502.4.4.2 Manufacturer's instructions.** The size and maximum length of the exhaust duct shall be determined by the dryer manufacturer's installation instructions. The code official shall be provided with a copy of the installation instructions for the make and model of the dryer at the concealment inspection. In the absence of fitting equivalent length calculations from the clothes dryer manufacturer, Table M1502.4.4.1 shall be used.

M1502.4.5 Length identification. Where the exhaust duct is concealed within the building construction, the equivalent length of the exhaust duct shall be identified on a permanent label or tag. The label or tag shall be located within 6 feet (1829 mm) of the exhaust duct connection.

TABLE M1502.4.4.1
DRYER EXHAUST DUCT FITTING EQUIVALENT LENGTH

DRYER EXHAUST DUCT FITTING TYPE	EQUIVALENT LENGTH
4 inch radius mitered 45 degree elbow	2 feet 6 inches
4 inch radius mitered 90 degree elbow	5 feet
6 inch radius smooth 45 degree elbow	1 foot
6 inch radius smooth 90 degree elbow	1 foot 9 inches
8 inch radius smooth 45 degree elbow	1 foot
8 inch radius smooth 90 degree elbow	1 foot 7 inches
10 inch radius smooth 45 degree elbow	9 inches
10 inch radius smooth 90 degree elbow	1 foot 6 inches

For SI: 1 inch = 25.4 mm, 1 foot = 304.8 mm, 1 degree = 0.0175 rad.

M1502.4.6 Exhaust duct required. Where space for a clothes dryer is provided, an exhaust *duct system* shall be installed. Where the clothes dryer is not installed at the time of occupancy the exhaust duct shall be capped or plugged in the space in which it originates and identified and marked "future use."

> **Exception:** Where a *listed* condensing clothes dryer is installed prior to occupancy of the structure.

M1502.5 Protection required. Protective shield plates shall be placed where nails or screws from finish or other work are likely to penetrate the clothes dryer exhaust duct. Shield plates shall be placed on the finished face of all framing members where there is less than $1^1/_4$ inches (32 mm) between the duct and the finished face of the framing member. Protective shield plates shall be constructed of steel, shall have a minimum thickness of 0.062-inch (1.6 mm) and shall extend a minimum of 2 inches (51 mm) above sole plates and below top plates.

SECTION M1503
RANGE HOODS

M1503.1 General. Range hoods shall discharge to the outdoors through a single-wall duct. The duct serving the hood shall have a smooth interior surface, shall be air tight and shall be equipped with a backdraft damper. Ducts serving range hoods shall not terminate in an *attic* or crawl space or areas inside the building.

> **Exception:** Where installed in accordance with the manufacturer's installation instructions, and where mechanical or natural *ventilation* is otherwise provided, *listed* and *labeled* ductless range hoods shall not be required to discharge to the outdoors.

M1503.2 Duct material. Single-wall ducts serving range hoods shall be constructed of galvanized steel, stainless steel or copper.

> **Exception:** Ducts for domestic kitchen cooking *appliances* equipped with down-draft exhaust systems shall be permitted to be constructed of schedule 40 PVC pipe and fittings provided that the installation complies with all of the following:
>
> 1. The duct is installed under a concrete slab poured on grade; and
>
> 2. The underfloor trench in which the duct is installed is completely backfilled with sand or gravel; and
>
> 3. The PVC duct extends not more than 1 inch (25 mm) above the indoor concrete floor surface; and
>
> 4. The PVC duct extends not more than 1 inch (25 mm) above grade outside of the building; and
>
> 5. The PVC ducts are solvent cemented.

M1503.3 Kitchen exhaust rates. Where domestic kitchen cooking *appliances* are equipped with ducted range hoods or

down-draft exhaust systems, the fans shall be sized in accordance with Section M1507.3.

M1503.4 Makeup air required. Exhaust hood systems capable of exhausting in excess of 400 cubic feet per minute (0.19 m³/s) shall be provided with makeup air at a rate approximately equal to the exhaust air rate. Such makeup air systems shall be equipped with a means of closure and shall be automatically controlled to start and operate simultaneously with the exhaust system.

SECTION M1504
INSTALLATION OF MICROWAVE OVENS

M1504.1 Installation of a microwave oven over a cooking appliance. The installation of a *listed* and *labeled* cooking *appliance* or microwave oven over a *listed* and *labeled* cooking *appliance* shall conform to the terms of the upper *appliance's listing* and *label* and the manufacturer's installation instructions. The microwave oven shall conform to UL 923.

SECTION M1505
OVERHEAD EXHAUST HOODS

M1505.1 General. Domestic open-top broiler units shall have a metal exhaust hood, having a minimum thickness of 0.0157-inch (0.3950 mm) (No. 28 gage) with $^1/_4$ inch (6.4 mm) clearance between the hood and the underside of combustible material or cabinets. A clearance of at least 24 inches (610 mm) shall be maintained between the cooking surface and the combustible material or cabinet. The hood shall be at least as wide as the broiler unit, extend over the entire unit, discharge to the outdoors and be equipped with a backdraft damper or other means to control infiltration/exfiltration when not in operation. Broiler units incorporating an integral exhaust system, and *listed* and *labeled* for use without an exhaust hood, need not have an exhaust hood.

SECTION M1506
EXHAUST DUCTS

M1506.1 Ducts. Where exhaust duct construction is not specified in this chapter, construction shall comply with Chapter 16.

SECTION M1507
MECHANICAL VENTILATION

M1507.1 General. Where toilet rooms and bathrooms are mechanically ventilated, the *ventilation equipment* shall be installed in accordance with this section.

M1507.2 Recirculation of air. Exhaust air from bathrooms and toilet rooms shall not be recirculated within a residence or to another *dwelling unit* and shall be exhausted directly to the outdoors. Exhaust air from bathrooms and toilet rooms shall not discharge into an *attic*, crawl space or other areas inside the building.

M1507.3 Ventilation rate. *Ventilation* systems shall be designed to have the capacity to exhaust the minimum air flow rate determined in accordance with Table M1507.3.

TABLE M1507.3
MINIMUM REQUIRED EXHAUST RATES FOR
ONE- AND TWO-FAMILY DWELLINGS

AREA TO BE VENTILATED	VENTILATION RATES
Kitchens	100 cfm intermittent or 25 cfm continuous
Bathrooms—Toilet Rooms	Mechanical exhaust capacity of 50 cfm intermittent or 20 cfm continuous

For SI: 1 cubic foot per minute = 0.4719 L/s.

CHAPTER 16

DUCT SYSTEMS

SECTION M1601
DUCT CONSTRUCTION

M1601.1 Duct design. *Duct systems* serving heating, cooling and *ventilation equipment* shall be fabricated in accordance with the provisions of this section and ACCA Manual D or other *approved* methods.

M1601.1.1 Above-ground duct systems. Above-ground *duct systems* shall conform to the following:

1. *Equipment* connected to *duct systems* shall be designed to limit discharge air temperature to a maximum of 250°F (121°C).

2. Factory-made air ducts shall be constructed of Class 0 or Class 1 materials as designated in Table M1601.1.1(1).

3. Fibrous duct construction shall conform to the SMACNA *Fibrous Glass Duct Construction Standards* or NAIMA *Fibrous Glass Duct Construction Standards*.

4. Minimum thickness of metal duct material shall be as listed in Table M1601.1.1(2). Galvanized steel shall conform to ASTM A 653.

5. Use of gypsum products to construct return air ducts or plenums is permitted, provided that the air temperature does not exceed 125°F (52°C) and exposed surfaces are not subject to condensation.

6. *Duct systems* shall be constructed of materials having a flame spread index not greater than 200.

7. Stud wall cavities and the spaces between solid floor joists to be used as air plenums shall comply with the following conditions:

    7.1. These cavities or spaces shall not be used as a plenum for supply air.

    7.2. These cavities or spaces shall not be part of a required fire-resistance-rated assembly.

    7.3. Stud wall cavities shall not convey air from more than one floor level.

    7.4. Stud wall cavities and joist-space plenums shall be isolated from adjacent concealed spaces by tight-fitting fire blocking in accordance with Section R602.8.

TABLE M1601.1.1(1)
CLASSIFICATION OF FACTORY-MADE AIR DUCTS

DUCT CLASS	MAXIMUM FLAME-SPREAD RATING
0	0
1	25

M1601.1.2 Underground duct systems. Underground *duct systems* shall be constructed of *approved* concrete, clay, metal or plastic. The maximum duct temperature for plastic ducts shall not be greater than 150°F (66°C). Metal ducts shall be protected from corrosion in an *approved* manner or shall be completely encased in concrete not less than 2 inches (51 mm) thick. Nonmetallic ducts shall be installed in accordance with the manufacturer's installation instructions. Plastic pipe and fitting materials shall conform to cell classification 12454-B of ASTM D 1248 or ASTM D 1784 and external loading properties of ASTM D 2412. All ducts shall slope to an accessible point for drainage. Where encased in concrete, ducts shall be sealed and secured prior to any concrete being poured. Metallic ducts having an *approved* protective coating and nonmetallic ducts shall be installed in accordance with the manufacturer's installation instructions.

M1601.2 Factory-made ducts. Factory-made air ducts or duct material shall be *approved* for the use intended, and shall be installed in accordance with the manufacturer's installation instructions. Each portion of a factory-made air *duct system* shall bear a *listing* and *label* indicating compliance with UL 181 and UL 181A or UL 181B.

TABLE M1601.1.1(2)
GAGES OF METAL DUCTS AND PLENUMS USED FOR HEATING OR COOLING

DUCT SIZE	MINIMUM THICKNESS inches and (mm)	EQUIVALENT GALVANIZED SHEET NO.	MINIMUM THICKNESS (in.)
Round ducts and enclosed rectangular ducts			
14 inches or less	0.0157 (0.3950 mm)	28	0.0175
16 and 18 inches	0.0187 (0.4712 mm)	26	0.018
20 inches and over	0.0236 (0.6010 mm)	24	0.023
Exposed rectangular ducts			
14 inches or	0.0157 (0.3950 mm)	28	0.0175
Over 14[a] inches	0.0187 (0.4712 mm)	26	0.018

For SI: 1 inch = 25.4 mm.

a. For duct gages and reinforcement requirements at static pressures of $^1/_2$ inch, 1 inch and 2 inches w.g., SMACNA *Duct Construction Standard*, Tables 2-1; 2-2 and 2-3 shall apply.

M1601.2.1 Vibration isolators. Vibration isolators installed between mechanical *equipment* and metal ducts shall be fabricated from *approved* materials and shall not exceed 10 inches (254 mm) in length.

M1601.3 Duct insulation materials. Duct insulation materials shall conform to the following requirements:

1. Duct coverings and linings, including adhesives where used, shall have a flame spread index not higher than 25, and a smoke-developed index not over 50 when tested in accordance with ASTM E 84 or UL 723, using the specimen preparation and mounting procedures of ASTM E 2231.

    Exception: Spray application of polyurethane foam to the exterior of ducts in *attics* and crawl spaces shall be permitted subject to all of the following:

    1. The flame spread index is not greater than 25 and the smoke-developed index is not greater than 450 at the specified installed thickness.

    2. The foam plastic is protected in accordance with the ignition barrier requirements of Sections R316.5.3 and R316.5.4.

    3. The foam plastic complies with the requirements of Section R316.

2. Duct coverings and linings shall not flame, glow, smolder or smoke when tested in accordance with ASTM C 411 at the temperature to which they are exposed in service. The test temperature shall not fall below 250°F (121°C).

3. External duct insulation and factory-insulated flexible ducts shall be legibly printed or identified at intervals not longer than 36 inches (914 mm) with the name of the manufacturer, the thermal resistance *R*-value at the specified installed thickness and the flame spread and smoke-developed indexes of the composite materials. Spray polyurethane foam manufacturers shall provide the same product information and properties, at the nominal installed thickness, to the customer in writing at the time of foam application. All duct insulation product *R*-values shall be based on insulation only, excluding air films, vapor retarders or other duct components, and shall be based on tested C-values at 75°F (24°C) mean temperature at the installed thickness, in accordance with recognized industry procedures. The installed thickness of duct insulation used to determine its *R*-value shall be determined as follows:

    3.1. For duct board, duct liner and factory-made rigid ducts not normally subjected to compression, the nominal insulation thickness shall be used.

    3.2. For ductwrap, the installed thickness shall be assumed to be 75 percent (25-percent compression)of nominal thickness.

    3.3. For factory-made flexible air ducts, The installed thickness shall be determined by dividing the difference between the actual outside diameter and nominal inside diameter by two.

    3.4. For spray polyurethane foam, the aged *R*-value per inch measured in accordance with recognized industry standards shall be provided to the customer in writing at the time of foam application. In addition, the total *R*-value for the nominal application thickness shall be provided.

M1601.4 Installation. Duct installation shall comply with Sections M1601.4.1 through M1601.4.7.

M1601.4.1 Joints and seams. Joints of *duct systems* shall be made substantially airtight by means of tapes, mastics, liquid sealants, gasketing or other *approved* closure systems. Closure systems used with rigid fibrous glass ducts shall comply with UL181A and shall be marked 181A-P for pressure-sensitive tape, 181A-M for mastic or 181 A-H for heat-sensitive tape. Closure systems used with flexible air ducts and flexible air connectors shall comply with UL 181B and shall be marked 181B-FX for pressure-sensitive tape or 181B-M for mastic. Duct connections to flanges of air distribution system *equipment* or sheet metal fittings shall be mechanically fastened. Mechanical fasteners for use with flexible nonmetallic air ducts shall comply with UL 181B and shall be marked 181B-C. Crimp joints for round metal ducts shall have a contact lap of at least 1¹/₂ inches (38 mm) and shall be mechanically fastened by means of at least three sheet-metal screws or rivets equally spaced around the joint. Closure systems used to seal metal ductwork shall be installed in accordance with the manufacturer's installation instructions.

Exceptions:

1. Spray polyurethane foam shall be permitted to be applied without additional joint seals.

2. Where a duct connection is made that is partially inaccessible, three screws or rivets shall be equally spaced on the exposed portion of the joint so as to prevent a hinge effect.

3. Continuously welded and locking type longitudinal joints and seams in ducts operating at static pressures less than 2 inches of water column (500 Pa) pressure classification shall not require additional closure systems.

M1601.4.2 Plastic duct joints. Joints between plastic ducts and plastic fittings shall be made in accordance with the manufacturer's installation instructions.

M1601.4.3 Support. Metal ducts shall be supported by ¹/₂-inch (13 mm) wide 18-gage metal straps or 12-gage galvanized wire at intervals not exceeding 10 feet (3048 mm) or other *approved* means. Nonmetallic ducts shall be supported in accordance with the manufacturer's installation instructions.

M1601.4.4 Fireblocking. Duct installations shall be fireblocked in accordance with Section R602.8.

M1601.4.5 Duct insulation. Duct insulation shall be installed in accordance with the following requirements:

1. A vapor retarder having a maximum permeance of 0.05 perm [2.87 ng/(s · m² · Pa)] in accordance with ASTM E 96, or aluminum foil with a minimum thick-

ness of 2 mils (0.05 mm), shall be installed on the exterior of insulation on cooling supply ducts that pass through unconditioned spaces conducive to condensation except where the insulation is spray polyurethane foam with a maximum water vapor permeance of 3 perm per inch [1722 ng/(s · m² ·Pa)] at the installed thickness.

2. Exterior *duct systems* shall be protected against the elements.

3. Duct coverings shall not penetrate a fireblocked wall or floor.

M1601.4.6 Factory-made air ducts. Factory-made air ducts shall not be installed in or on the ground, in tile or metal pipe, or within masonry or concrete.

M 1601.4.7 Duct separation. Ducts shall be installed with at least 4 inches (102 mm) separation from earth except where they meet the requirements of Section M1601.1.2.

M1601.4.8 Ducts located in garages. Ducts in garages shall comply with the requirements of Section R302.5.2.

M1601.4.9 Flood hazard areas. In areas prone to flooding as established by Table R301.2(1), *duct systems* shall be located or installed in accordance with Section R322.1.6.

M1601.5 Under-floor plenums. Under-floor plenums shall be prohibited in new structures. Modification or repairs to under-floor plenums in existing structures shall conform to the requirements of this section.

M1601.5.1 General. The space shall be cleaned of loose combustible materials and scrap, and shall be tightly enclosed. The ground surface of the space shall be covered with a moisture barrier having a minimum thickness of 4 mils (0.1 mm). Plumbing waste cleanouts shall not be located within the space.

Exception: Plumbing waste cleanouts shall be permitted to be located in unvented crawl spaces that receive *conditioned air* in accordance with Section R408.3.

M1601.5.2 Materials. The under-floor space, including the sidewall insulation, shall be formed by materials having flame-spread ratings not greater than 200 when tested in accordance with ASTM E 84.

M1601.5.3 Furnace connections. A duct shall extend from the furnace supply outlet to not less than 6 inches (152 mm) below the combustible framing. This duct shall comply with the provisions of Section M1601.1. A noncombustible receptacle shall be installed below any floor opening into the plenum in accordance with the following requirements:

1. The receptacle shall be securely suspended from the floor members and shall not be more than 18 inches (457 mm) below the floor opening.

2. The area of the receptacle shall extend 3 inches (76 mm) beyond the opening on all sides.

3. The perimeter of the receptacle shall have a vertical lip at least 1 inch (25 mm) high at the open sides.

M1601.5.4 Access. Access to an under-floor plenum shall be provided through an opening in the floor with minimum dimensions of 18 inches by 24 inches (457 mm by 610 mm).

M1601.5.5 Furnace controls. The furnace shall be equipped with an automatic control that will start the air-circulating fan when the air in the furnace bonnet reaches a temperature not higher than 150°F (66°C). The furnace shall additionally be equipped with an *approved* automatic control that limits the outlet air temperature to 200°F (93°C).

M1601.6 Independent garage HVAC systems. Furnaces and air-handling systems that supply air to living spaces shall not supply air to or return air from a garage.

SECTION M1602
RETURN AIR

M1602.1 Return air. Return air shall be taken from inside the *dwelling*. Dilution of return air with outdoor air shall be permitted.

M1602.2 Prohibited sources. Outdoor and return air for a forced-air heating or cooling system shall not be taken from the following locations:

1. Closer than 10 feet (3048 mm) to an *appliance* vent outlet, a vent opening from a plumbing drainage system or the discharge outlet of an exhaust fan, unless the outlet is 3 feet (914 mm) above the outside air inlet.

2. Where flammable vapors are present; or where located less than 10 feet (3048 mm) above the surface of any abutting public way or driveway; or where located at grade level by a sidewalk, street, alley or driveway.

3. A room or space, the volume of which is less than 25 percent of the entire volume served by the system. Where connected by a permanent opening having an area sized in accordance with ACCA Manual D, adjoining rooms or spaces shall be considered as a single room or space for the purpose of determining the volume of the rooms or spaces.

   Exception: The minimum volume requirement shall not apply where the amount of return air taken from a room or space is less than or equal to the amount of supply air delivered to the room or space.

4. A closet, bathroom, toilet room, kitchen, garage, mechanical room, boiler room, furnace room, unconditioned *attic* or other *dwelling unit*.

5. A room or space containing a fuel-burning *appliance* where such room or space serves as the sole source of return air.

   Exceptions:

   1. The fuel-burning *appliance* is a direct-vent *appliance* or an *appliance* not requiring a vent in accordance with Section M1801.1 or Chapter 24.

   2. The room or space complies with the following requirements:

2.1. The return air shall be taken from a room or space having a volume exceeding 1 cubic foot for each 10 Btu/h (9.6 L/W) of combined input rating of all fuel-burning *appliances* therein.

2.2. The volume of supply air discharged back into the same space shall be approximately equal to the volume of return air taken from the space.

2.3. Return-air inlets shall not be located within 10 feet (3048 mm) of any *appliance* firebox or draft hood in the same room or space.

3. Rooms or spaces containing solid-fuel burning *appliances*, if return-air inlets are located not less than 10 feet (3048 mm) from the firebox of those *appliances*.

6. An unconditioned crawl space by means of direct connection to the return side of a forced air system. Transfer openings in the crawl space enclosure shall not be prohibited.

M1602.3 Inlet opening protection. Outdoor air inlets shall be covered with screens having openings that are not less than $^1/_4$ inch (6.4 mm) and not greater than $^1/_2$ inch (12.7 mm).

CHAPTER 17

COMBUSTION AIR

SECTION M1701
GENERAL

M1701.1 Scope. Solid-fuel-burning *appliances* shall be provided with *combustion air* in accordance with the *appliance* manufacturer's installation instructions. Oil-fired *appliances* shall be provided with *combustion air* in accordance with NFPA 31. The methods of providing *combustion air* in this chapter do not apply to fireplaces, fireplace stoves and direct-vent *appliances*. The requirements for combustion and dilution air for gas-fired *appliances* shall be in accordance with Chapter 24.

M1701.2 Opening location. In areas prone to flooding as established in Table R301.2(1), *combustion air* openings shall be located at or above the elevation required in Section R322.2.1 or R322.3.2.

CHAPTER 18

CHIMNEYS AND VENTS

SECTION M1801
GENERAL

M1801.1 Venting required. Fuel-burning *appliances* shall be vented to the outdoors in accordance with their *listing* and *label* and manufacturer's installation instructions except *appliances listed* and *labeled* for unvented use. Venting systems shall consist of *approved* chimneys or vents, or venting assemblies that are integral parts of *labeled appliances*. Gas-fired *appliances* shall be vented in accordance with Chapter 24.

M1801.2 Draft requirements. A venting system shall satisfy the draft requirements of the *appliance* in accordance with the manufacturer's installation instructions, and shall be constructed and installed to develop a positive flow to convey combustion products to the outside atmosphere.

M1801.3 Existing chimneys and vents. Where an *appliance* is permanently disconnected from an existing chimney or vent, or where an *appliance* is connected to an existing chimney or vent during the process of a new installation, the chimney or vent shall comply with Sections M1801.3.1 through M1801.3.4.

M1801.3.1 Size. The chimney or vent shall be resized as necessary to control flue gas condensation in the interior of the chimney or vent and to provide the *appliance*, or *appliances* served, with the required draft. For the venting of oil-fired *appliances* to masonry chimneys, the resizing shall be done in accordance with NFPA 31.

M1801.3.2 Flue passageways. The flue gas passageway shall be free of obstructions and combustible deposits and shall be cleaned if previously used for venting a solid- or liquid-fuel-burning *appliance* or fireplace. The flue liner, chimney inner wall or vent inner wall shall be continuous and free of cracks, gaps, perforations, or other damage or deterioration that would allow the escape of combustion products, including gases, moisture and creosote.

M1801.3.3 Cleanout. Masonry chimneys shall be provided with a cleanout opening complying with Section R1003.17.

M1801.3.4 Clearances. Chimneys and vents shall have airspace clearance to combustibles in accordance with this code and the chimney or vent manufacturer's installation instructions.

Exception: Masonry chimneys equipped with a chimney lining system tested and *listed* for installation in chimneys in contact with combustibles in accordance with UL 1777, and installed in accordance with the manufacturer's instruction, shall not be required to have a clearance between combustible materials and exterior surfaces of the masonry chimney. Noncombustible firestopping shall be provided in accordance with this code.

M1801.4 Space around lining. The space surrounding a flue lining system or other vent installed within a masonry chimney shall not be used to vent any other *appliance*. This shall not pre-

vent the installation of a separate flue lining in accordance with the manufacturer's installation instructions and this code.

M1801.5 Mechanical draft systems. A mechanical draft system shall be used only with *appliances listed* and *labeled* for such use. Provisions shall be made to prevent the flow of fuel to the *equipment* when the draft system is not operating. Forced draft systems and all portions of induced draft systems under positive pressure during operation shall be designed and installed to prevent leakage of flue gases into a building.

M1801.6 Direct-vent appliances. Direct-vent *appliances* shall be installed in accordance with the manufacturer's installation instructions.

M1801.7 Support. Venting systems shall be adequately supported for the weight of the material used.

M1801.8 Duct penetrations. Chimneys, vents and vent connectors shall not extend into or through supply and return air ducts or plenums.

M1801.9 Fireblocking. Vent and chimney installations shall be fireblocked in accordance with Section R602.8.

M1801.10 Unused openings. Unused openings in any venting system shall be closed or capped.

M1801.11 Multiple-appliance venting systems. Two or more *listed* and *labeled appliances* connected to a common natural draft venting system shall comply with the following requirements:

1. *Appliances* that are connected to common venting systems shall be located on the same floor of the *dwelling*.

   Exception: Engineered systems as provided for in Section G2427.

2. Inlets to common venting systems shall be offset such that no portion of an inlet is opposite another inlet.

3. Connectors serving *appliances* operating under a natural draft shall not be connected to any portion of a mechanical draft system operating under positive pressure.

M1801.12 Multiple solid fuel prohibited. A solid-fuel-burning *appliance* or fireplace shall not connect to a chimney passageway venting another *appliance*.

SECTION M1802
VENT COMPONENTS

M1802.1 Draft hoods. Draft hoods shall be located in the same room or space as the *combustion air* openings for the *appliances*.

M1802.2 Vent dampers. Vent dampers shall comply with Sections M1802.2.1 and M1802.2.2.

M1802.2.1 Manually operated. Manually operated dampers shall not be installed except in connectors or chimneys serving solid-fuel-burning *appliances*.

M1802.2.2 Automatically operated. Automatically operated dampers shall conform to UL 17 and be installed in accordance with the terms of their *listing* and *label*. The installation shall prevent firing of the burner when the damper is not opened to a safe position.

M1802.3 Draft regulators. Draft regulators shall be provided for oil-fired *appliances* that must be connected to a chimney. Draft regulators provided for solid-fuel-burning *appliances* to reduce draft intensity shall be installed and set in accordance with the manufacturer's installation instructions.

M1802.3.1 Location. Where required, draft regulators shall be installed in the same room or enclosure as the *appliance* so that no difference in pressure will exist between the air at the regulator and the *combustion air* supply.

SECTION M1803
CHIMNEY AND VENT CONNECTORS

M1803.1 General. Connectors shall be used to connect fuel-burning *appliances* to a vertical chimney or vent except where the chimney or vent is attached directly to the *appliance*.

M1803.2 Connectors for oil and solid fuel appliances. Connectors for oil and solid-fuel-burning *appliances* shall be constructed of factory-built chimney material, Type L vent material or single-wall metal pipe having resistance to corrosion and heat and thickness not less than that of galvanized steel as specified in Table M1803.2.

TABLE M1803.2
THICKNESS FOR SINGLE-WALL METAL PIPE CONNECTORS

DIAMETER OF CONNECTOR (inches)	GALVANIZED SHEET METAL GAGE NUMBER	MINIMUM THICKNESS (inch)
Less than 6	26	0.019
6 to 10	24	0.024
Over 10 through 16	22	0.029

For SI: 1 inch = 25.4 mm.

M1803.3 Installation. Vent and chimney connectors shall be installed in accordance with the manufacturer's installation instructions and within the space where the *appliance* is located. *Appliances* shall be located as close as practical to the vent or chimney. Connectors shall be as short and straight as possible and installed with a slope of not less than $^1/_4$ inch (6 mm) rise per foot of run. Connectors shall be securely supported and joints shall be fastened with sheet metal screws or rivets. Devices that obstruct the flow of flue gases shall not be installed in a connector unless *listed* and *labeled* or *approved* for such installations.

M1803.3.1 Floor, ceiling and wall penetrations. A chimney connector or vent connector shall not pass through any floor or ceiling. A chimney connector or vent connector shall not pass through a wall or partition unless the connector is *listed* and *labeled* for wall pass-through, or is routed through a device *listed* and *labeled* for wall pass-through and is installed in accordance with the conditions of its *listing* and *label*. Connectors for oil-fired *appliances listed* and *labeled* for Type L vents, passing through walls or partitions shall be in accordance with the following:

1. Type L vent material for oil *appliances* shall be installed with not less than *listed* and *labeled* clearances to combustible material.

2. Single-wall metal pipe shall be guarded by a ventilated metal thimble not less than 4 inches (102 mm) larger in diameter than the vent connector. A minimum 6 inches (152 mm) of clearance shall be maintained between the thimble and combustibles.

M1803.3.2 Length. The horizontal run of an uninsulated connector to a natural draft chimney shall not exceed 75 percent of the height of the vertical portion of the chimney above the connector. The horizontal run of a *listed* connector to a natural draft chimney shall not exceed 100 percent of the height of the vertical portion of the chimney above the connector.

M1803.3.3 Size. A connector shall not be smaller than the flue collar of the *appliance*.

Exception: Where installed in accordance with the *appliance* manufacturer's installation instructions.

M1803.3.4 Clearance. Connectors shall be installed with clearance to combustibles as set forth in Table M1803.3.4. Reduced clearances to combustible materials shall be in accordance with Table M1306.2 and Figure M1306.1.

TABLE M1803.3.4
CHIMNEY AND VENT CONNECTOR CLEARANCES TO COMBUSTIBLE MATERIALS[a]

TYPE OF CONNECTOR	MINIMUM CLEARANCE (inches)
Single-wall metal pipe connectors:	
Oil and solid-fuel appliances	18
Oil appliances listed for use with Type L vents	9
Type L vent piping connectors:	
Oil and solid-fuel appliances	9
Oil appliances listed for use with Type L vents	3[b]

For SI: 1 inch = 25.4 mm.

a. These minimum clearances apply to unlisted single-wall chimney and vent connectors. Reduction of required clearances is permitted as in Table M1306.2.

b. When listed Type L vent piping is used, the clearance shall be in accordance with the vent listing.

M1803.3.5 Access. The entire length of a connector shall be accessible for inspection, cleaning and replacement.

M1803.4 Connection to fireplace flue. Connection of *appliances* to chimney flues serving fireplaces shall comply with Sections M1803.4.1 through M1803.4.4.

M1803.4.1 Closure and accessibility. A noncombustible seal shall be provided below the point of connection to prevent entry of room air into the flue. Means shall be provided for access to the flue for inspection and cleaning.

M1803.4.2 Connection to factory-built fireplace flue. A different *appliance* shall not be connected to a flue serving a factory-built fireplace unless the *appliance* is specifically *listed* for such an installation. The connection shall be made in conformance with the *appliance* manufacturer's instructions.

M1803.4.3 Connection to masonry fireplace flue. A connector shall extend from the *appliance* to the flue serving a masonry fireplace to convey the flue gases directly into the flue. The connector shall be accessible or removable for inspection and cleaning of both the connector and the flue. *Listed* direct-connection devices shall be installed in accordance with their *listing*.

M1803.4.4 Size of flue. The size of the fireplace flue shall be in accordance with Section M1805.3.1.

SECTION M1804
VENTS

M1804.1 Type of vent required. *Appliances* shall be provided with a *listed* and *labeled* venting system as set forth in Table M1804.1.

TABLE M1804.1
VENT SELECTION CHART

VENT TYPES	APPLIANCE TYPES
Type L oil vents	Oil-burning appliances listed and labeled for venting with Type L vents
Pellet vents	Pellet fuel-burning appliances listed and labeled for use with pellet vents

M1804.2 Termination. Vent termination shall comply with Sections M1804.2.1 through M1804.2.6.

M1804.2.1 Through the roof. Vents passing through a roof shall extend through flashing and terminate in accordance with the manufacturer's installation requirements.

M1804.2.2 Decorative shrouds. Decorative shrouds shall not be installed at the termination of vents except where the shrouds are *listed* and *labeled* for use with the specific venting system and are installed in accordance with the manufacturer's installation instructions.

M1804.2.3 Natural draft appliances. Vents for natural draft *appliances* shall terminate at least 5 feet (1524 mm) above the highest connected *appliance* outlet, and natural draft gas vents serving wall furnaces shall terminate at an elevation at least 12 feet (3658 mm) above the bottom of the furnace.

M1804.2.4 Type L vent. Type L venting systems shall conform to UL 641 and shall terminate with a *listed* and *labeled* cap in accordance with the vent manufacturer's installation instructions not less than 2 feet (610 mm) above the roof and not less than 2 feet (610 mm) above any portion of the building within 10 feet (3048 mm).

M1804.2.5 Direct vent terminations. Vent terminals for direct-vent *appliances* shall be installed in accordance with the manufacturer's installation instructions.

M1804.2.6 Mechanical draft systems. Mechanical draft systems shall be installed in accordance with their *listing*,

the manufacturer's installation instructions and, except for direct vent *appliances*, the following requirements:

1. The vent terminal shall be located not less than 3 feet (914 mm) above a forced air inlet located within 10 feet (3048 mm).

2. The vent terminal shall be located not less than 4 feet (1219 mm) below, 4 feet (1219 mm) horizontally from, or 1 foot (305 mm) above any door, window or gravity air inlet into a *dwelling*.

3. The vent termination point shall not be located closer than 3 feet (914 mm) to an interior corner formed by two walls perpendicular to each other.

4. The bottom of the vent terminal shall be located at least 12 inches (305 mm) above finished ground level.

5. The vent termination shall not be mounted directly above or within 3 feet (914 mm) horizontally of an oil tank vent or gas meter.

6. Power exhauster terminations shall be located not less than 10 feet (3048 mm) from *lot lines* and adjacent buildings.

7. The discharge shall be directed away from the building.

M1804.3 Installation. Type L and pellet vents shall be installed in accordance with the terms of their *listing* and *label* and the manufacturer's installation instructions.

M1804.3.1 Size of single-appliance venting systems. An individual vent for a single *appliance* shall have a cross-sectional area equal to or greater than the area of the connector to the *appliance*, but not less than 7 square inches (4515 mm^2) except where the vent is an integral part of a *listed* and *labeled appliance*.

SECTION M1805
MASONRY AND FACTORY-BUILT CHIMNEYS

M1805.1 General. Masonry and factory-built chimneys shall be built and installed in accordance with Sections R1003 and R1005, respectively. Flue lining for masonry chimneys shall comply with Section R1003.11.

M1805.2 Masonry chimney connection. A chimney connector shall enter a masonry chimney not less than 6 inches (152 mm) above the bottom of the chimney. Where it is not possible to locate the connector entry at least 6 inches (152 mm) above the bottom of the chimney flue, a cleanout shall be provided by installing a capped tee in the connector next to the chimney. A connector entering a masonry chimney shall extend through, but not beyond, the wall and shall be flush with the inner face of the liner. Connectors, or thimbles where used, shall be firmly cemented into the masonry.

M1805.3 Size of chimney flues. The effective area of a natural draft chimney flue for one *appliance* shall be not less than the area of the connector to the *appliance*. The area of chimney flues connected to more than one *appliance* shall be not less than the area of the largest connector plus 50 percent of the areas of additional chimney connectors.

Exception: Chimney flues serving oil-fired *appliances* sized in accordance with NFPA 31.

M1805.3.1 Size of chimney flue for solid-fuel appliance. Except where otherwise specified in the manufacturer's installation instructions, the cross-sectional area of a flue connected to a solid-fuel-burning *appliance* shall be not less than the area of the flue collar or connector, and not larger than three times the area of the flue collar.

CHAPTER 19

SPECIAL FUEL-BURNING EQUIPMENT

SECTION M1901
RANGES AND OVENS

M1901.1 Clearances. Freestanding or built-in ranges shall have a vertical clearance above the cooking top of not less than 30 inches (762 mm) to unprotected combustible material. Reduced clearances are permitted in accordance with the *listing* and *labeling* of the range hoods or *appliances*.

M1901.2 Cooking appliances. Household cooking *appliances* shall be *listed* and *labeled* and shall be installed in accordance with the manufacturer's installation instructions. The installation shall not interfere with *combustion air* or access for operation and servicing.

SECTION M1902
SAUNA HEATERS

M1902.1 Locations and protection. Sauna heaters shall be protected from accidental contact by persons with a guard of material having a low thermal conductivity, such as wood. The guard shall have no substantial effect on the transfer of heat from the heater to the room.

M1902.2 Installation. Sauna heaters shall be installed in accordance with the manufacturer's installation instructions.

M1902.3 Combustion air. *Combustion air* and venting for a nondirect vent-type heater shall be provided in accordance with Chapters 17 and 18, respectively.

M1902.4 Controls. Sauna heaters shall be equipped with a thermostat that will limit room temperature to not greater than 194°F (90°C). Where the thermostat is not an integral part of the heater, the heat-sensing element shall be located within 6 inches (152 mm) of the ceiling.

SECTION M1903
STATIONARY FUEL CELL POWER PLANTS

M1903.1 General. Stationary fuel cell power plants having a power output not exceeding 1,000 kW, shall be tested in accordance with ANSI Z21.83 and shall be installed in accordance with the manufacturer's installation instructions and NFPA 853.

SECTION M1904
GASEOUS HYDROGEN SYSTEMS

M1904.1 Installation. Gaseous hydrogen systems shall be installed in accordance with the applicable requirements of Sections M1307.4 and M1903.1 and the *International Fuel Gas Code*, the *International Fire Code* and the *International Building Code*.

CHAPTER 20

BOILERS AND WATER HEATERS

SECTION M2001
BOILERS

M2001.1 Installation. In addition to the requirements of this code, the installation of boilers shall conform to the manufacturer's instructions. The manufacturer's rating data, the nameplate and operating instructions of a permanent type shall be attached to the boiler. Boilers shall have all controls set, adjusted and tested by the installer. A complete control diagram together with complete boiler operating instructions shall be furnished by the installer. Solid- and liquid-fuel-burning boilers shall be provided with *combustion air* as required by Chapter 17.

M2001.1.1 Standards. Oil-fired boilers and their control systems shall be listed and *labeled* in accordance with UL 726. Electric boilers and their control systems shall be *listed* in accordance with UL 834. Boilers shall be designed and constructed in accordance with the requirements of ASME CSD-1 and as applicable, the ASME *Boiler and Pressure Vessel Code*, Sections I and IV. Gas-fired boilers shall conform to the requirements listed in Chapter 24.

M2001.2 Clearance. Boilers shall be installed in accordance with their *listing* and *label*.

M2001.3 Valves. Every boiler or modular boiler shall have a shutoff valve in the supply and return piping. For multiple boiler or multiple modular boiler installations, each boiler or modular boiler shall have individual shutoff valves in the supply and return piping.

Exception: Shutoff valves are not required in a system having a single low-pressure steam boiler.

M2001.4 Flood-resistant installation. In areas prone to flooding as established in Table R301.2(1), boilers, water heaters and their control systems shall be located or installed in accordance with Section R322.1.6.

SECTION M2002
OPERATING AND SAFETY CONTROLS

M2002.1 Safety controls. Electrical and mechanical operating and safety controls for boilers shall be *listed* and *labeled*.

M2002.2 Hot water boiler gauges. Every hot water boiler shall have a pressure gauge and a temperature gauge, or combination pressure and temperature gauge. The gauges shall indicate the temperature and pressure within the normal range of the system's operation.

M2002.3 Steam boiler gauges. Every steam boiler shall have a water-gauge glass and a pressure gauge. The pressure gauge shall indicate the pressure within the normal range of the system's operation. The gauge glass shall be installed so that the midpoint is at the normal water level.

M2002.4 Pressure-relief valve. Boilers shall be equipped with pressure-relief valves with minimum rated capacities for the *equipment* served. Pressure-relief valves shall be set at the maximum rating of the boiler. Discharge shall be piped to drains by gravity to within 18 inches (457 mm) of the floor or to an open receptor.

M2002.5 Boiler low-water cutoff. All steam and hot water boilers shall be protected with a low-water cutoff control. The low-water cutoff shall automatically stop the combustion operation of the *appliance* when the water level drops below the lowest safe water level as established by the manufacturer.

SECTION M2003
EXPANSION TANKS

M2003.1 General. Hot water boilers shall be provided with expansion tanks. Nonpressurized expansion tanks shall be securely fastened to the structure or boiler and supported to carry twice the weight of the tank filled with water. Provisions shall be made for draining nonpressurized tanks without emptying the system.

M2003.1.1 Pressurized expansion tanks. Pressurized expansion tanks shall be consistent with the volume and capacity of the system. Tanks shall be capable of withstanding a hydrostatic test pressure of two and one-half times the allowable working pressure of the system.

M2003.2 Minimum capacity. The minimum capacity of expansion tanks shall be determined from Table M2003.2.

SECTION M2004
WATER HEATERS USED FOR SPACE HEATING

M2004.1 General. Water heaters used to supply both potable hot water and hot water for space heating shall be installed in accordance with this chapter, Chapter 24, Chapter 28 and the manufacturer's installation instructions.

SECTION M2005
WATER HEATERS

M2005.1 General. Water heaters shall be installed in accordance with the manufacturer's installation instructions and the requirements of this code. Water heaters installed in an *attic* shall conform to the requirements of Section M1305.1.3. Gas-fired water heaters shall conform to the requirements in Chapter 24. Domestic electric water heaters shall conform to UL 174 or UL 1453. Commercial electric water heaters shall conform to UL 1453. Oiled-fired water heaters shall conform to UL 732.

M2005.2 Prohibited locations. Fuel-fired water heaters shall not be installed in a room used as a storage closet. Water heaters located in a bedroom or bathroom shall be installed in a sealed enclosure so that *combustion air* will not be taken from the living space. Installation of direct-vent water heaters within an enclosure is not required.

TABLE M2003.2
EXPANSION TANK MINIMUM CAPACITY[a] FOR FORCED HOT-WATER SYSTEMS

SYSTEM VOLUME[b] (gallons)	PRESSURIZED DIAPHRAGM TYPE	NONPRESSURIZED TYPE
10	1.0	1.5
20	1.5	3.0
30	2.5	4.5
40	3.0	6.0
50	4.0	7.5
60	5.0	9.0
70	6.0	10.5
80	6.5	12.0
90	7.5	13.5
100	8.0	15.0

For SI: 1 gallon = 3.785 L, 1 pound per square inch gauge = 6.895 kPa, °C = [(°F)-32]/1.8.

a. Based on average water temperature of 195°F, fill pressure of 12 psig and a maximum operating pressure of 30 psig.

b. System volume includes volume of water in boiler, convectors and piping, not including the expansion tank.

M2005.2.1 Water heater access. Access to water heaters that are located in an *attic* or underfloor crawl space is permitted to be through a closet located in a sleeping room or bathroom where *ventilation* of those spaces is in accordance with this code.

M2005.3 Electric water heaters. Electric water heaters shall also be installed in accordance with the applicable provisions of Chapters 34 through 43.

M2005.4 Supplemental water-heating devices. Potable water heating devices that use refrigerant-to-water heat exchangers shall be *approved* and installed in accordance with the manufacturer's installation instructions.

SECTION M2006
POOL HEATERS

M2006.1 General. Pool and spa heaters shall be installed in accordance with the manufacturer's installation instructions. Oil-fired pool heaters shall be tested in accordance with UL 726. Electric pool and spa heaters shall be tested in accordance UL 1261.

M2006.2 Clearances. In no case shall the clearances interfere with *combustion air*, draft hood or flue terminal relief, or accessibility for servicing.

M2006.3 Temperature-limiting devices. Pool heaters shall have temperature-relief valves.

M2006.4 Bypass valves. Where an integral bypass system is not provided as a part of the pool heater, a bypass line and valve shall be installed between the inlet and outlet piping for use in adjusting the flow of water through the heater.

CHAPTER 21

HYDRONIC PIPING

SECTION M2101
HYDRONIC PIPING SYSTEMS INSTALLATION

M2101.1 General. Hydronic piping shall conform to Table M2101.1. *Approved* piping, valves, fittings and connections shall be installed in accordance with the manufacturer's installation instructions. Pipe and fittings shall be rated for use at the operating temperature and pressure of the hydronic system. Used pipe, fittings, valves or other materials shall be free of foreign materials.

M2101.2 System drain down. Hydronic piping systems shall be installed to permit draining of the system. Where the system drains to the plumbing drainage system, the installation shall conform to the requirements of Chapters 25 through 32 of this code.

> **Exception:** The buried portions of systems embedded underground or under floors.

M2101.3 Protection of potable water. The potable water system shall be protected from backflow in accordance with the provisions listed in Section P2902.

M2101.4 Pipe penetrations. Openings through concrete or masonry building elements shall be sleeved.

M2101.5 Contact with building material. A hydronic piping system shall not be in direct contact with any building material that causes the piping material to degrade or corrode.

M2101.6 Drilling and notching. Wood-framed structural members shall be drilled, notched or altered in accordance with the provisions of Sections R502.8, R602.6, R602.6.1 and R802.7. Holes in load bearing members of cold-formed steel light-frame construction shall be permitted only in accordance with Sections R505.2.5, R603.2.5 and R804.2.5. In accordance with the provisions of Sections R505.3.5, R603.3.4 and R804.3.4, cutting and notching of flanges and lips of load-bearing members of cold-formed steel light-frame construction shall not be permitted. Structural insulated panels (SIPs) shall be drilled and notched or altered in accordance with the provisions of Section R614.

M2101.7 Prohibited tee applications. Fluid in the supply side of a hydronic system shall not enter a tee fitting through the branch opening.

M2101.8 Expansion, contraction and settlement. Piping shall be installed so that piping, connections and *equipment* shall not be subjected to excessive strains or stresses. Provisions shall be made to compensate for expansion, contraction, shrinkage and structural settlement.

M2101.9 Piping support. Hangers and supports shall be of material of sufficient strength to support the piping, and shall be fabricated from materials compatible with the piping material. Piping shall be supported at intervals not exceeding the spacing specified in Table M2101.9.

M2101.10 Tests. Hydronic piping shall be tested hydrostatically at a pressure of not less than 100 pounds per square inch (690 kPa) for a duration of not less than 15 minutes.

SECTION M2102
BASEBOARD CONVECTORS

M2102.1 General. Baseboard convectors shall be installed in accordance with the manufacturer's installation instructions. Convectors shall be supported independently of the hydronic piping.

SECTION M2103
FLOOR HEATING SYSTEMS

M2103.1 Piping materials. Piping for embedment in concrete or gypsum materials shall be standard-weight steel pipe, copper tubing, cross-linked polyethylene/aluminum/cross-linked polyethylene (PEX-AL-PEX) pressure pipe, chlorinated polyvinyl chloride (CPVC), polybutylene, cross-linked polyethylene (PEX) tubing or polypropylene (PP) with a minimum rating of 100 psi at 180°F (690 kPa at 82°C).

M2103.2 Thermal barrier required. Radiant floor heating systems shall have a thermal barrier in accordance with Sections M2103.2.1 through M2103.2.4.

> **M2103.2.1 Slab on grade installation.** Radiant piping used in slab-on-grade applications shall have insulating materials having a minimum *R*-value of 5 installed beneath the piping.

> **M2103.2.2 Suspended floor installation.** In suspended floor applications, insulation shall be installed in the joist bay cavity serving the heating space above and shall consist of materials having a minimum *R*-value of 11.

> **M2103.2.3 Thermal break required.** A thermal break consisting of asphalt expansion joint materials or similar insulating materials shall be provided at a point where a heated slab meets a foundation wall or other conductive slab.

> **M2103.2.4 Thermal barrier material marking.** Insulating materials used in thermal barriers shall be installed so that the manufacturer's *R*-value mark is readily observable upon inspection.

> > **Exception:** Insulation shall not be required in engineered systems where it can be demonstrated that the insulation will decrease the efficiency or have a negative effect on the installation.

M2103.3 Piping joints. Piping joints that are embedded shall be installed in accordance with the following requirements:

1. Steel pipe joints shall be welded.

2. Copper tubing shall be joined with brazing material having a melting point exceeding 1,000°F (538°C).

3. Polybutylene pipe and tubing joints shall be installed with socket-type heat-fused polybutylene fittings.

4. CPVC tubing shall be joined using solvent cement joints.

5. Polypropylene pipe and tubing joints shall be installed with socket-type heat-fused polypropylene fittings.

6. Cross-linked polyethylene (PEX) tubing shall be joined using cold expansion, insert or compression fittings.

TABLE M2101.1
HYDRONIC PIPING MATERIALS

MATERIAL	USE CODE[a]	STANDARD[b]	JOINTS	NOTES
Brass pipe	1	ASTM B 43	Brazed, welded, threaded, mechanical and flanged fittings	
Brass tubing	1	ASTM B 135	Brazed, soldered and mechanical fittings	
Chlorinated poly (vinyl chloride) (CPVC) pipe and tubing	1, 2, 3	ASTM D 2846	Solvent cement joints, compression joints and threaded adapters	
Copper pipe	1	ASTM B 42, B 302	Brazed, soldered and mechanical fittings threaded, welded and flanged	
Copper tubing (type K, L or M)	1, 2	ASTM B 75, B 88, B 251, B 306	Brazed, soldered and flared mechanical fittings	Joints embedded in concrete
Cross-linked polyethylene (PEX)	1, 2, 3	ASTM F 876, F 877	(See PEX fittings)	Install in accordance with manufacturer's instructions.
Cross-linked polyethylene/aluminum/ cross-linked polyethylene-(PEX-AL-PEX) pressure pipe	1, 2	ASTM F 1281 or CAN/ CSA B137.10	Mechanical, crimp/insert	Install in accordance with manufacturer's instructions.
PEX Fittings		ASTM F 1807 ASTM F 1960 ASTM F 2098	Copper-crimp/insert fittings, cold expansion fittings, stainless steel clamp, insert fittings	Install in accordance with manufacturer's instructions
Plastic fittings PEX		ASTM F 1807		
Polybutylene (PB) pipe and tubing	1, 2, 3	ASTM D 3309	Heat-fusion, crimp/insert and compression	Joints in concrete shall be heat-fused.
Polyethylene (PE) pipe, tubing and fittings (for ground source heat pump loop systems)	1, 2, 4	ASTM D 2513; ASTM D 3350; ASTM D 2513; ASTM D 3035; ASTM D 2447; ASTM D 2683; ASTM F 1055; ASTM D 2837; ASTM D 3350; ASTM D 1693	Heat-fusion	
Polyethylene/aluminum/polyethylene (PE-AL-PE) pressure pipe	1, 2, 3	ASTM F 1282 CSA B 137.9	Mechanical, crimp/insert	
Polyproplylene (PP)	1, 2, 3	ISO 15874 ASTM F 2389	Heat-fusion joints, mechanical fittings, threaded adapters, compression joints	
Raised temperature polyethylene (PE-RT)	1, 2, 3	ASTM F 2623	Copper crimp/insert fitting stainless steel clamp, insert fittings	
Soldering fluxes	1	ASTM B 813	Copper tube joints	
Steel pipe	1, 2	ASTM A 53, A 106	Brazed, welded, threaded, flanged and mechanical fittings	Joints in concrete shall be welded. Galvanized pipe shall not be welded or brazed.
Steel tubing	1	ASTM A 254	Mechanical fittings, welded	

For SI: °C = [(°F)-32]/1.8.

a. Use code:
   1. Above ground.
   2. Embedded in radiant systems.
   3. Temperatures below 180°F only.
   4. Low temperature (below 130°F) applications only.

b. Standards as listed in Chapter 43.

M2103.4 Testing. Piping or tubing to be embedded shall be tested by applying a hydrostatic pressure of not less than 100 psi (690 kPa). The pressure shall be maintained for 30 minutes, during which all joints shall be visually inspected for leaks.

SECTION M2104
LOW TEMPERATURE PIPING

M2104.1 Piping materials. Low temperature piping for embedment in concrete or gypsum materials shall be as indicated in Table M2101.1.

M2104.2 Piping joints. Piping joints (other than those in Section M2103.2) that are embedded shall comply with the following requirements:

1. Cross-linked polyethylene (PEX) tubing shall be installed in accordance with the manufacturer's instructions.

2. Polyethylene tubing shall be installed with heat fusion joints.

3. Polypropylene (PP) tubing shall be installed in accordance with the manufacturer's instructions.

M2104.2.1 Polyethylene plastic pipe and tubing for ground source heat pump loop systems. Joints between polyethylene plastic pipe and tubing or fittings for ground source heat pump loop systems shall be heat fusion joints conforming to Section M2104.2.1.1, electrofusion joints conforming to Section M2104.2.1.2 or stab-type insertion joints conforming to Section M2104.2.1.3.

M2104.2.1.1 Heat-fusion joints. Joints shall be of the socket-fusion, saddle-fusion or butt-fusion type, fabricated in accordance with the piping manufacturer's instructions. Joint surfaces shall be clean and free of moisture. Joint surfaces shall be heated to melt temperatures and joined. The joint shall be undisturbed until cool. Fittings shall be manufactured in accordance with ASTM D 2683.

M2104.2.1.2 Electrofusion joints. Joint surfaces shall be clean and free of moisture, and scoured to expose virgin resin. Joint surfaces shall be heated to melt temperatures for the period of time specified by the manufacturer. The joint shall be undisturbed until cool. Fittings shall be manufactured in accordance with ASTM F 1055.

M2104.2.1.3 Stab-type insert fittings. Joint surfaces shall be clean and free of moisture. Pipe ends shall be chamfered and inserted into the fitting to full depth. Fittings shall be manufactured in accordance with ASTM D 2513.

M2104.3 Raised temperature polyethylene (PE-RT) plastic tubing. Joints between raised temperature polyethylene tubing and fittings shall conform to Sections M2104.3.1 and M2104.3.2. Mechanical joints shall be installed in accordance with the manufacturer's instructions.

M2104.3.1 Compression-type fittings. Where compression type fittings include inserts and ferrules or O-rings, the fittings shall be installed without omitting such inserts and ferrules or O-rings.

M2104.3.2 PE-RT-to-metal connections. Solder joints in a metal pipe shall not occur within 18 inches (457 mm) of a transition from such metal pipe to PE-RT pipe.

TABLE M2101.9
HANGER SPACING INTERVALS

PIPING MATERIAL	MAXIMUM HORIZONTAL SPACING (feet)	MAXIMUM VERTICAL SPACING (feet)
ABS	4	10
CPVC ≤ 1 inch pipe or tubing	3	5
CPVC ≥ 1¼ inch	4	10
Copper or copper alloy pipe	12	10
Copper or copper alloy tubing	6	10
PB pipe or tubing	2.67	4
PE pipe or tubing	2.67	4
PEX tubing	2.67	4
PP < 1 inch pipe or tubing	2.67	4
PP > 1¼ inch	4	10
PVC	4	10
Steel pipe	12	15
Steel tubing	8	10

For SI: 1 inch = 25.4 mm, 1 foot = 304.8 mm.

M2104.4 Polyethylene/Aluminum/Polyethylene (PE-AL-PE) pressure pipe. Joints between polyethylene/aluminum/polyethylene pressure pipe and fittings shall conform to Sections M2104.4.1 and M2104.4.2. Mechanical joints shall be installed in accordance with the manufacturer's instructions.

M2104.4.1 Compression-type fittings. Where compression type fittings include inserts and ferrules or O-rings, the fittings shall be installed without omitting such inserts and ferrules or O-rings.

M2104.4.2 PE-AL-PE to metal connections. Solder joints in a metal pipe shall not occur within 18 inches (457 mm) of a transition from such metal pipe to PE-AL-PE pipe.

SECTION M2105
GROUND SOURCE HEAT PUMP SYSTEM LOOP PIPING

M2105.1 Testing. The assembled loop system shall be pressure tested with water at 100 psi (690 kPa) for 30 minutes with no observed leaks before connection (header) trenches are backfilled. Flow rates and pressure drops shall be compared to calculated values. If actual flow rate or pressure drop figures differ from calculated values by more than 10 percent, the problem shall be identified and corrected.

CHAPTER 22

SPECIAL PIPING AND STORAGE SYSTEMS

SECTION M2201
OIL TANKS

M2201.1 Materials. Supply tanks shall be *listed* and *labeled* and shall conform to UL 58 for underground tanks and UL 80 for indoor tanks.

M2201.2 Above-ground tanks. The maximum amount of fuel oil stored above ground or inside of a building shall be 660 gallons (2498 L). The supply tank shall be supported on rigid noncombustible supports to prevent settling or shifting.

> **Exception:** The storage of fuel oil, used for space or water heating, above ground or inside buildings in quantities exceeding 660 gallons (2498 L) shall comply with NFPA 31.

M2201.2.1 Tanks within buildings. Supply tanks for use inside of buildings shall be of such size and shape to permit installation and removal from *dwellings* as whole units. Supply tanks larger than 10 gallons (38 L) shall be placed not less than 5 feet (1524 mm) from any fire or flame either within or external to any fuel-burning *appliance*.

M2201.2.2 Outside above-ground tanks. Tanks installed outside above ground shall be a minimum of 5 feet (1524 mm) from an adjoining property line. Such tanks shall be suitably protected from the weather and from physical damage.

M2201.3 Underground tanks. Excavations for underground tanks shall not undermine the foundations of existing structures. The clearance from the tank to the nearest wall of a *basement*, pit or property line shall not be less than 1 foot (305 mm). Tanks shall be set on and surrounded with noncorrosive inert materials such as clean earth, sand or gravel well tamped in place. Tanks shall be covered with not less than 1 foot (305 mm) of earth. Corrosion protection shall be provided in accordance with Section M2203.7.

M2201.4 Multiple tanks. Cross connection of two supply tanks shall be permitted in accordance with Section M2203.6.

M2201.5 Oil gauges. Inside tanks shall be provided with a device to indicate when the oil in the tank has reached a predetermined safe level. Glass gauges or a gauge subject to breakage that could result in the escape of oil from the tank shall not be used.

M2201.6 Flood-resistant installation. In areas prone to flooding as established by Table R301.2(1), tanks shall be installed at or above the elevation required in Section R322.2.1 or R322.3.2 or shall be anchored to prevent flotation, collapse and lateral movement under conditions of the design flood.

M2201.7 Tanks abandoned or removed. Exterior above-grade fill piping shall be removed when tanks are abandoned or removed. Tank abandonment and removal shall be in accordance with the *International Fire Code*.

SECTION M2202
OIL PIPING, FITTING AND CONNECTIONS

M2202.1 Materials. Piping shall consist of steel pipe, copper tubing or steel tubing conforming to ASTM A 539. Aluminum tubing shall not be used between the fuel-oil tank and the burner units.

M2202.2 Joints and fittings. Piping shall be connected with standard fittings compatible with the piping material. Cast iron fittings shall not be used for oil piping. Unions requiring gaskets or packings, right or left couplings, and sweat fittings employing solder having a melting point less than 1,000°F (538°C) shall not be used for oil piping. Threaded joints and connections shall be made tight with a lubricant or pipe thread compound.

M2202.3 Flexible connectors. Flexible metallic hoses shall be *listed* and *labeled* in accordance with UL 536 and shall be installed in accordance with their *listing* and *labeling* and the manufacturer's installation instructions. Connectors made from combustible materials shall not be used inside of buildings or above ground outside of buildings.

SECTION M2203
INSTALLATION

M2203.1 General. Piping shall be installed in a manner to avoid placing stresses on the piping, and to accommodate expansion and contraction of the piping system.

M2203.2 Supply piping. Supply piping used in the installation of oil burners and *appliances* shall be not smaller than $^3/_8$-inch (9 mm) pipe or $^3/_8$-inch (9 mm) outside diameter tubing. Copper tubing and fittings shall be a minimum of Type L.

M2203.3 Fill piping. Fill piping shall terminate outside of buildings at a point at least 2 feet (610 mm) from any building opening at the same or lower level. Fill openings shall be equipped with a tight metal cover.

M2203.4 Vent piping. Vent piping shall be not smaller than $1^1/_4$-inch (32 mm) pipe. Vent piping shall be laid to drain toward the tank without sags or traps in which the liquid can collect. Vent pipes shall not be cross connected with fill pipes, lines from burners or overflow lines from auxiliary tanks. The lower end of a vent pipe shall enter the tank through the top and shall extend into the tank not more than 1 inch (25 mm).

M2203.5 Vent termination. Vent piping shall terminate outside of buildings at a point not less than 2 feet (610 mm), measured vertically or horizontally, from any building opening. Outer ends of vent piping shall terminate in a weather-proof cap or fitting having an unobstructed area at least equal to the cross-sectional area of the vent pipe, and shall be located sufficiently above the ground to avoid being obstructed by snow and ice.

M2203.6 Cross connection of tanks. Cross connection of two supply tanks, not exceeding 660 gallons (2498 L) aggregate capacity, with gravity flow from one tank to another, shall be acceptable providing that the two tanks are on the same horizontal plane.

M2203.7 Corrosion protection. Underground tanks and buried piping shall be protected by corrosion-resistant coatings or special alloys or fiberglass-reinforced plastic.

SECTION M2204
OIL PUMPS AND VALVES

M2204.1 Pumps. Oil pumps shall be positive displacement types that automatically shut off the oil supply when stopped. Automatic pumps shall be *listed* and *labeled* in accordance with UL 343 and shall be installed in accordance with their *listing*.

M2204.2 Shutoff valves. A *readily accessible* manual shutoff valve shall be installed between the oil supply tank and the burner. Where the shutoff valve is installed in the discharge line of an oil pump, a pressure-relief valve shall be incorporated to bypass or return surplus oil.

M2204.3 Maximum pressure. Pressure at the oil supply inlet to an *appliance* shall be not greater than 3 pounds per square inch (20.7 kPa).

M2204.4 Relief valves. Fuel-oil lines incorporating heaters shall be provided with relief valves that will discharge to a return line when excess pressure exists.

CHAPTER 23

SOLAR SYSTEMS

SECTION M2301
SOLAR ENERGY SYSTEMS

M2301.1 General. This section provides for the design, construction, installation, *alteration* and repair of *equipment* and systems using solar energy to provide space heating or cooling, hot water heating and swimming pool heating.

M2301.2 Installation. Installation of solar energy systems shall comply with Sections M2301.2.1 through M2301.2.9.

M2301.2.1 Access. Solar energy collectors, controls, dampers, fans, blowers and pumps shall be accessible for inspection, maintenance, repair and replacement.

M2301.2.2 Roof-mounted collectors. The roof shall be constructed to support the loads imposed by roof-mounted solar collectors. Roof-mounted solar collectors that serve as a roof covering shall conform to the requirements for roof coverings in Chapter 9 of this code. Where mounted on or above the roof coverings, the collectors and supporting structure shall be constructed of noncombustible materials or fire-retardant-treated wood equivalent to that required for the roof construction.

M2301.2.3 Pressure and temperature relief. System components containing fluids shall be protected with pressure- and temperature-relief valves. Relief devices shall be installed in sections of the system so that a section cannot be valved off or isolated from a relief device.

M2301.2.4 Vacuum relief. System components that might be subjected to pressure drops below atmospheric pressure during operation or shutdown shall be protected by a vacuum-relief valve.

M2301.2.5 Protection from freezing. System components shall be protected from damage resulting from freezing of heat-transfer liquids at the winter design temperature provided in Table R301.2(1). Freeze protection shall be provided by heating, insulation, thermal mass and heat transfer fluids with freeze points lower than the winter design temperature, heat tape or other *approved* methods, or combinations thereof.

> **Exception:** Where the winter design temperature is greater than 32°F (0°C).

M2301.2.6 Expansion tanks. Expansion tanks in solar energy systems shall be installed in accordance with Section M2003 in closed fluid loops that contain heat transfer fluid.

M2301.2.7 Roof and wall penetrations. Roof and wall penetrations shall be flashed and sealed in accordance with Chapter 9 of this code to prevent entry of water, rodents and insects.

M2301.2.8 Solar loop isolation. Valves shall be installed to allow the solar collectors to be isolated from the remainder of the system. Each isolation valve shall be labeled with the open and closed position.

M2301.2.9 Maximum temperature limitation. Systems shall be equipped with means to limit the maximum water temperature of the system fluid entering or exchanging heat with any pressurized vessel inside the *dwelling* to 180°F (82°C). This protection is in addition to the required temperature- and pressure-relief valves required by Section M2301.2.3.

M2301.3 Labeling. *Labeling* shall comply with Sections M2301.3.1 and M2301.3.2.

M2301.3.1 Collectors. Collectors shall be *listed* and *labeled* to show the manufacturer's name, model number, serial number, collector weight, collector maximum allowable temperatures and pressures, and the type of heat transfer fluids that are compatible with the collector. The *label* shall clarify that these specifications apply only to the collector.

M2301.3.2 Thermal storage units. Pressurized thermal storage units shall be *listed* and *labeled* to show the manufacturer's name, model number, serial number, storage unit maximum and minimum allowable operating temperatures and pressures, and the type of heat transfer fluids that are compatible with the storage unit. The *label* shall clarify that these specifications apply only to the thermal storage unit.

M2301.4 Prohibited heat transfer fluids. Flammable gases and liquids shall not be used as heat transfer fluids.

M2301.5 Backflow protection. Connections from the potable water supply to solar systems shall comply with Section P2902.4.5.

Part VI—Fuel Gas

CHAPTER 24

FUEL GAS

The text of this chapter is extracted from the 2009 edition of the *International Fuel Gas Code* and has been modified where necessary to conform to the scope of application of the *International Residential Code for One- and Two-Family Dwellings*. The section numbers appearing in parentheses after each section number are the section numbers of the corresponding text in the *International Fuel Gas Code*.

SECTION G2401 (101)
GENERAL

G2401.1 (101.2) Application. This chapter covers those *fuel gas piping systems*, fuel-gas *appliances* and related accessories, *venting systems* and *combustion air* configurations most commonly encountered in the construction of one- and two-family dwellings and structures regulated by this *code*.

Coverage of *piping systems* shall extend from the *point of delivery* to the outlet of the *appliance* shutoff *valves* (see definition of *"Point of delivery"*). *Piping systems* requirements shall include design, materials, components, fabrication, assembly, installation, testing, inspection, operation and maintenance. Requirements for gas *appliances* and related accessories shall include installation, *combustion* and ventilation air and venting and connections to *piping systems*.

The omission from this chapter of any material or method of installation provided for in the *International Fuel Gas Code* shall not be construed as prohibiting the use of such material or method of installation. *Fuel-gas piping systems*, fuel-gas *appliances* and related accessories, *venting systems* and *combustion air* configurations not specifically covered in these chapters shall comply with the applicable provisions of the *International Fuel Gas Code*.

Gaseous hydrogen systems shall be regulated by Chapter 7 of the *International Fuel Gas Code*.

This chapter shall not apply to the following:

1. Liquified natural gas (LNG) installations.

2. Temporary LP-*gas piping* for buildings under construction or renovation that is not to become part of the permanent *piping system*.

3. Except as provided in Section G2412.1.1, *gas piping, meters*, gas *pressure regulators*, and other appurtenances used by the serving gas supplier in the distribution of gas, other than undiluted LP-gas.

4. Portable LP-gas *appliances* and *equipment* of all types that is not connected to a fixed fuel *piping system*.

5. Portable fuel cell *appliances* that are neither connected to a fixed *piping system* nor interconnected to a power grid.

6. Installation of hydrogen gas, LP-gas and compressed natural gas (CNG) systems on vehicles.

SECTION G2402 (201)
GENERAL

G2402.1 (201.1) Scope. Unless otherwise expressly stated, the following words and terms shall, for the purposes of this chapter, have the meanings indicated in this chapter.

G2402.2 (201.2) Interchangeability. Words used in the present tense include the future; words in the masculine gender include the feminine and neuter; the singular number includes the plural and the plural, the singular.

G2402.3 (201.3) Terms defined in other codes. Where terms are not defined in this *code* and are defined in the *International Building Code, International Fire Code, International Mechanical Code* or *International Plumbing Code*, such terms shall have meanings ascribed to them as in those *codes*.

SECTION G2403 (202)
GENERAL DEFINITIONS

AIR CONDITIONING, GAS FIRED. A gas-burning, automatically operated *appliance* for supplying cooled and/or dehumidified air or chilled liquid.

AIR, EXHAUST. Air being removed from any space or piece of *equipment* or *appliance* and conveyed directly to the atmosphere by means of openings or ducts.

AIR-HANDLING UNIT. A blower or fan used for the purpose of distributing supply air to a room, space or area.

AIR, MAKEUP. Air that is provided to replace air being exhausted.

ALTERATION. A change in a system that involves an extension, addition or change to the arrangement, type or purpose of the original installation.

ANODELESS RISER. A transition assembly in which plastic *piping* is installed and terminated above ground outside of a building.

APPLIANCE. Any apparatus or device that uses gas as a fuel or raw material to produce light, heat, power, refrigeration or air conditioning.

APPLIANCE, FAN-ASSISTED COMBUSTION. An *appliance* equipped with an integral mechanical means to either draw or force products of *combustion* through the *combustion* chamber or heat exchanger.

APPLIANCE, AUTOMATICALLY CONTROLLED. *Appliances* equipped with an automatic *burner* ignition and safety shut-off device and other automatic devices, which accomplish complete turn-on and shut-off of the gas to the *main burner* or *burners*, and graduate the gas supply to the *burner* or *burners*, but do not affect complete shut-off of the gas.

APPLIANCE, UNVENTED. An *appliance* designed or installed in such a manner that the products of *combustion* are not conveyed by a vent or *chimney* directly to the outside atmosphere.

APPLIANCE, VENTED. An *appliance* designed and installed in such a manner that all of the products of *combustion* are conveyed directly from the *appliance* to the outside atmosphere through an *approved chimney* or vent system.

APPROVED. Acceptable to the *code official* or other authority having jurisdiction.

ATMOSPHERIC PRESSURE. The pressure of the weight of air and water vapor on the surface of the earth, approximately 14.7 pounds per square inch (psia) (101 kPa absolute) at sea level.

AUTOMATIC IGNITION. Ignition of gas at the *burner(s)* when the gas controlling device is turned on, including reignition if the flames on the *burner(s)* have been extinguished by means other than by the closing of the gas controlling device.

BAROMETRIC DRAFT REGULATOR. A balanced *damper* device attached to a *chimney,* vent *connector,* breeching or flue gas manifold to protect *combustion appliances* by controlling *chimney draft.* A double-acting *barometric draft regulator* is one whose balancing *damper* is free to move in either direction to protect *combustion appliances* from both excessive *draft* and backdraft.

BOILER, LOW-PRESSURE. A self-contained gas-fired *appliance* for supplying steam or hot water.

Hot water heating boiler. A boiler in which no steam is generated, from which hot water is circulated for heating purposes and then returned to the boiler, and that operates at water pressures not exceeding 160 psig (1100 kPa gauge) and at water temperatures not exceeding 250°F (121°C) at or near the boiler outlet.

Hot water supply boiler. A boiler, completely filled with water, which furnishes hot water to be used externally to itself, and that operates at water pressures not exceeding 160 psig (1100 kPa gauge) and at water temperatures not exceeding 250°F (121°C) at or near the boiler outlet.

Steam heating boiler. A boiler in which steam is generated and that operates at a steam pressure not exceeding 15 psig (100 kPa gauge).

BONDING JUMPER. A conductor installed to electrically connect metallic *gas piping* to the grounding electrode system.

BRAZING. A metal joining process wherein coalescence is produced by the use of a nonferrous filler metal having a melting point above 1,000°F (538°C), but lower than that of the base metal being joined. The filler material is distributed between the closely fitted surfaces of the joint by capillary action.

BTU. Abbreviation for British thermal unit, which is the quantity of heat required to raise the temperature of 1 pound (454 g) of water 1°F (0.56°C) (1 *Btu* = 1055 J).

BURNER. A device for the final conveyance of the gas, or a mixture of gas and air, to the *combustion* zone.

Induced-draft. A *burner* that depends on *draft* induced by a fan that is an integral part of the *appliance* and is located downstream from the *burner.*

Power. A *burner* in which gas, air or both are supplied at pressures exceeding, for gas, the line pressure, and for air, *atmospheric pressure,* with this added pressure being applied at the *burner.*

CHIMNEY. A primarily vertical structure containing one or more flues, for the purpose of carrying gaseous products of *combustion* and air from an *appliance* to the outside atmosphere.

Factory-built chimney. A listed and labeled *chimney* composed of factory-made components, assembled in the field in accordance with manufacturer's instructions and the conditions of the listing.

Masonry chimney. A field-constructed *chimney* composed of solid masonry units, bricks, stones or concrete.

CLEARANCE. The minimum distance through air measured between the heat-producing surface of the mechanical *appliance,* device or *equipment* and the surface of the combustible material or assembly.

CLOTHES DRYER. An *appliance* used to dry wet laundry by means of heated air.

Type 1. Factory-built package, multiple production. Primarily used in the family living environment. Usually the smallest unit physically and in function output.

CODE. These regulations, subsequent amendments thereto, or any emergency rule or regulation that the administrative authority having jurisdiction has lawfully adopted.

CODE OFFICIAL. The officer or other designated authority charged with the administration and enforcement of this *code,* or a duly authorized representative.

COMBUSTION. In the context of this *code,* refers to the rapid oxidation of fuel accompanied by the production of heat or heat and light.

COMBUSTION AIR. Air necessary for complete *combustion* of a fuel, including theoretical air and excess air.

COMBUSTION CHAMBER. The portion of an *appliance* within which *combustion* occurs.

COMBUSTION PRODUCTS. Constituents resulting from the *combustion* of a fuel with the oxygen of the air, including the inert gases, but excluding excess air.

CONCEALED LOCATION. A location that cannot be accessed without damaging permanent parts of the building structure or finish surface. Spaces above, below or behind readily removable panels or doors shall not be considered as concealed.

CONCEALED PIPING. *Piping* that is located in a *concealed location* (see *"Concealed location"*).

CONDENSATE. The liquid that condenses from a gas (including flue gas) caused by a reduction in temperature or increase in pressure.

CONNECTOR, APPLIANCE (Fuel). Rigid metallic *pipe* and fittings, semirigid metallic *tubing* and fittings or a listed and labeled device that connects an *appliance* to the *gas piping system*.

CONNECTOR, CHIMNEY OR VENT. The *pipe* that connects an *appliance* to a *chimney* or vent.

CONTROL. A manual or automatic device designed to regulate the gas, air, water or electrical supply to, or operation of, a mechanical system.

CONVERSION BURNER. A unit consisting of a *burner* and its *controls* for installation in an *appliance* originally utilizing another fuel.

CUBIC FOOT. The amount of gas that occupies 1 *cubic foot* (0.02832 m³) when at a temperature of 60°F (16°C), saturated with water vapor and under a pressure equivalent to that of 30 inches of mercury (101 kPa).

DAMPER. A manually or automatically controlled device to regulate *draft* or the rate of flow of air or *combustion* gases.

DECORATIVE GAS APPLIANCE, VENTED. A *vented appliance* wherein the primary function lies in the aesthetic effect of the flames.

DECORATIVE GAS APPLIANCES FOR INSTALLATION IN VENTED FIREPLACES. A *vented appliance* designed for installation within the fire chamber of a vented *fireplace*, wherein the primary function lies in the aesthetic effect of the flames.

DEMAND. The maximum amount of gas input required per unit of time, usually expressed in cubic feet per hour, or *Btu*/h (1 *Btu*/h = 0.2931 W).

DESIGN FLOOD ELEVATION. The elevation of the "design flood," including wave height, relative to the datum specified on the community's legally designated flood hazard map.

DILUTION AIR. Air that is introduced into a *draft hood* and is mixed with the *flue gases*.

DIRECT-VENT APPLIANCES. *Appliances* that are constructed and installed so that all air for *combustion* is derived directly from the outside atmosphere and all *flue gases* are discharged directly to the outside atmosphere.

DRAFT. The pressure difference existing between the *appliance* or any component part and the atmosphere, that causes a continuous flow of air and products of *combustion* through the gas passages of the *appliance* to the atmosphere.

> **Mechanical or induced draft.** The pressure difference created by the action of a fan, blower or ejector that is located between the *appliance* and the *chimney* or vent termination.

> **Natural draft.** The pressure difference created by a vent or *chimney* because of its height, and the temperature difference between the *flue gases* and the atmosphere.

DRAFT HOOD. A nonadjustable device built into an *appliance*, or made as part of the vent *connector* from an *appliance*, that is designed to (1) provide for ready escape of the *flue gases* from the *appliance* in the event of no *draft*, backdraft, or stoppage beyond the *draft hood*, (2) prevent a backdraft from entering the *appliance*, and (3) neutralize the effect of stack action of the *chimney* or gas vent upon operation of the *appliance*.

DRAFT REGULATOR. A device that functions to maintain a desired *draft* in the *appliance* by automatically reducing the *draft* to the desired value.

DRIP. The container placed at a low point in a system of *piping* to collect *condensate* and from which the *condensate* is removable.

DUCT FURNACE. A warm-air *furnace* normally installed in an air-distribution duct to supply warm air for heating. This definition shall apply only to a warm-air heating *appliance* that depends for air circulation on a blower not furnished as part of the *furnace*.

DWELLING UNIT. A *single* unit providing complete, independent living facilities for one or more persons, including permanent provisions for living, sleeping, eating, cooking and sanitation.

EQUIPMENT. Apparatus and devices other than *appliances*.

EXTERIOR MASONRY CHIMNEYS. *Masonry chimneys* exposed to the outdoors on one or more sides below the roof line.

FIREPLACE. A fire chamber and hearth constructed of noncombustible material for use with solid fuels and provided with a *chimney*.

> **Masonry fireplace.** A hearth and fire chamber of solid masonry units such as bricks, stones, listed masonry units or reinforced concrete, provided with a suitable *chimney*.

> **Factory-built fireplace.** A *fireplace* composed of listed factory-built components assembled in accordance with the terms of listing to form the completed *fireplace*.

FLAME SAFEGUARD. A device that will automatically shut off the fuel supply to a *main burner* or group of *burners* when the means of ignition of such *burners* becomes inoperative, and when flame failure occurs on the *burner* or group of *burners*.

FLOOD HAZARD AREA. The greater of the following two areas:

1. The area within a floodplain subject to a 1 percent or greater chance of flooding in any given year.

2. This area designated as a *flood hazard area* on a community's flood hazard map, or otherwise legally designated.

FLOOR FURNACE. A completely self-contained *furnace* suspended from the floor of the space being heated, taking air for *combustion* from outside such space and with means for observing flames and lighting the *appliance* from such space.

FLUE, APPLIANCE. The passage(s) within an *appliance* through which *combustion products* pass from the *combustion chamber* of the *appliance* to the *draft hood* inlet opening on an *appliance* equipped with a *draft hood* or to the outlet of the *appliance* on an *appliance* not equipped with a *draft hood*.

FLUE COLLAR. That portion of an *appliance* designed for the attachment of a *draft hood*, *vent connector* or venting system.

FLUE GASES. Products of *combustion* plus excess air in *appliance flues* or heat exchangers.

FLUE LINER (LINING). A system or material used to form the inside surface of a flue in a *chimney* or vent, for the purpose of protecting the surrounding structure from the effects of *combustion products* and for conveying *combustion products* without leakage to the atmosphere.

FUEL GAS. A natural gas, manufactured gas, *liquefied petroleum gas* or mixtures of these gases.

FUEL GAS UTILIZATION EQUIPMENT. See *"Appliance."*

FURNACE. A completely self-contained heating unit that is designed to supply heated air to spaces remote from or adjacent to the *appliance* location.

FURNACE, CENTRAL FURNACE. A self-contained *appliance* for heating air by transfer of heat of *combustion* through metal to the air, and designed to supply heated air through ducts to spaces remote from or adjacent to the *appliance* location.

FURNACE PLENUM. An air compartment or chamber to which one or more ducts are connected and which forms part of an air distribution system.

GAS CONVENIENCE OUTLET. A permanently mounted, manually operated device that provides the means for connecting an *appliance* to, and disconnecting an *appliance* from, the gas supply *piping*. The device includes an integral, manually operated *valve* with a nondisplaceable *valve* member and is designed so that disconnection of an *appliance* only occurs when the manually operated *valve* is in the closed position.

GAS PIPING. An installation of *pipe*, *valves* or fittings installed on a premises or in a building and utilized to convey *fuel gas*.

HAZARDOUS LOCATION. Any location considered to be a fire hazard for flammable vapors, dust, combustible fibers or other highly combustible substances. The location is not necessarily categorized in the *International Building Code* as a high-hazard use group classification.

HOUSE PIPING. See *"Piping system."*

IGNITION PILOT. A *pilot* that operates during the lighting cycle and discontinues during *main burner* operation.

IGNITION SOURCE. A flame spark or hot surface capable of igniting flammable vapors or fumes. Such sources include *appliance burners*, *burner* ignitors and electrical switching devices.

INFRARED RADIANT HEATER. A heater which directs a substantial amount of its energy output in the form of infrared radiant energy into the area to be heated. Such heaters are of either the vented or unvented type.

JOINT, FLARED. A metal-to-metal compression joint in which a conical spread is made on the end of a tube that is compressed by a flare nut against a mating flare.

JOINT, MECHANICAL. A general form of gas-tight joints obtained by the joining of metal parts through a positive-holding mechanical construction, such as flanged joint, threaded joint, *flared joint* or compression joint.

JOINT, PLASTIC ADHESIVE. A joint made in thermoset *plastic piping* by the use of an adhesive substance which forms a continuous bond between the mating surfaces without dissolving either one of them.

LEAK CHECK. An operation performed on a *gas piping system* to verify that the system does not leak.

LIQUEFIED PETROLEUM GAS or LPG (LP-GAS). *Liquefied petroleum gas* composed predominately of propane, propylene, butanes or butylenes, or mixtures thereof that is gaseous under normal atmospheric conditions, but is capable of being liquefied under moderate pressure at normal temperatures.

LIVING SPACE. Space within a *dwelling unit* utilized for living, sleeping, eating, cooking, bathing, washing and sanitation purposes.

LOG LIGHTER, GAS-FIRED. A manually operated solid-fuel ignition *appliance* for installation in a vented solid-fuel-burning *fireplace*.

MAIN BURNER. A device or group of devices essentially forming an integral unit for the final conveyance of gas or a mixture of gas and air to the *combustion* zone, and on which *combustion* takes place to accomplish the function for which the *appliance* is designed.

METER. The instrument installed to measure the volume of gas delivered through it.

MODULATING. Modulating or throttling is the action of a *control* from its maximum to minimum position in either predetermined steps or increments of movement as caused by its actuating medium.

OFFSET (VENT). A combination of *approved* bends that make two changes in direction bringing one section of the vent out of line, but into a line parallel with the other section.

OUTLET. The point at which a gas-fired *appliance* connects to the *gas piping system*.

OXYGEN DEPLETION SAFETY SHUTOFF SYSTEM (ODS). A system designed to act to shut off the gas supply to the main and *pilot burners* if the oxygen in the surrounding atmosphere is reduced below a predetermined level.

PILOT. A small flame that is utilized to ignite the gas at the *main burner* or *burners*.

PIPING. Where used in this *code*, *"piping"* refers to either *pipe* or *tubing*, or both.

    Pipe. A rigid conduit of iron, steel, copper, brass or plastic.

    Tubing. Semirigid conduit of copper, aluminum, plastic or steel.

PIPING SYSTEM. All fuel *piping, valves* and fittings from the outlet of the *point of delivery* to the outlets of the *appliance* shutoff valves.

PLASTIC, THERMOPLASTIC. A plastic that is capable of being repeatedly softened by increase of temperature and hardened by decrease of temperature.

POINT OF DELIVERY. For natural gas systems, the *point of delivery* is the outlet of the service *meter* assembly or the outlet of the service *regulator* or *service shutoff valve* where a *meter* is not provided. Where a *valve* is provided at the outlet of the service *meter* assembly, such *valve* shall be considered to be downstream of the *point of delivery*. For undiluted *liquefied petroleum gas* systems, the *point of delivery* shall be considered to be the outlet of the first *regulator* that reduces pressure to 2 psig (13.8 kPa) or less.

PRESSURE DROP. The loss in pressure due to friction or obstruction in pipes, *valves*, fittings, *regulators* and *burners*.

PRESSURE TEST. An operation performed to verify the gas-tight integrity of *gas piping* following its installation or modification.

READY ACCESS (TO). That which enables a device, *appliance* or *equipment* to be directly reached, without requiring the removal or movement of any panel, door or similar obstruction. (See "Access.")

REGULATOR. A device for controlling and maintaining a uniform gas supply pressure, either pounds-to-inches water column (MP *regulator*) or inches-to-inches water column (*appliance regulator*).

REGULATOR, GAS APPLIANCE. A *pressure regulator* for controlling pressure to the manifold of the gas *appliance*.

REGULATOR, LINE GAS PRESSURE. A device placed in a gas line between the *service pressure regulator* and the *appliance* for controlling, maintaining or reducing the pressure in that portion of the *piping system* downstream of the device.

REGULATOR, MEDIUM-PRESSURE (MP Regulator). A line *pressure regulator* that reduces gas pressure from the range of greater than 0.5 psig (3.4 kPa) and less than or equal to 5 psig (34.5 kPa) to a lower pressure.

REGULATOR, PRESSURE. A device placed in a gas line for reducing, controlling and maintaining the pressure in that portion of the *piping system* downstream of the device.

REGULATOR, SERVICE PRESSURE. A device installed by the serving gas supplier to reduce and limit the service line gas pressure to delivery pressure.

RELIEF OPENING. The opening provided in a *draft hood* to permit the ready escape to the atmosphere of the flue products from the *draft hood* in the event of no *draft*, backdraft or stoppage beyond the *draft hood*, and to permit air into the *draft hood* in the event of a strong *chimney* updraft.

RELIEF VALVE (DEVICE). A safety *valve* designed to forestall the development of a dangerous condition by relieving either pressure, temperature or vacuum in the hot water supply system.

RELIEF VALVE, PRESSURE. An *automatic valve* which opens and closes a *relief vent*, depending on whether the pressure is above or below a predetermined value.

RELIEF VALVE, TEMPERATURE.

Manual reset type. A *valve* which automatically opens a *relief* vent at a predetermined temperature and which must be manually returned to the closed position.

Reseating or self-closing type. An *automatic valve* which opens and closes a *relief* vent, depending on whether the temperature is above or below a predetermined value.

RELIEF VALVE, VACUUM. A *valve* that automatically opens and closes a vent for relieving a vacuum within the hot water supply system, depending on whether the vacuum is above or below a predetermined value.

RISER, GAS. A vertical *pipe* supplying *fuel gas*.

ROOM HEATER, UNVENTED. See "*Unvented room heater.*"

ROOM HEATER, VENTED. A free-standing gas-fired heating unit used for direct heating of the space in and adjacent to that in which the unit is located. (See also "*Vented room heater.*")

SAFETY SHUTOFF DEVICE. See "*Flame safeguard.*"

SHAFT. An enclosed space extending through one or more stories of a building, connecting vertical openings in successive floors, or floors and the roof.

SPECIFIC GRAVITY. As applied to gas, *specific gravity* is the ratio of the weight of a given volume to that of the same volume of air, both measured under the same condition.

THERMOSTAT.

Electric switch type. A device that senses changes in temperature and controls electrically, by means of separate components, the flow of gas to the *burner(s)* to maintain selected temperatures.

Integral gas valve type. An automatic device, actuated by temperature changes, designed to control the gas supply to the *burner(s)* in order to maintain temperatures between predetermined limits, and in which the thermal actuating element is an integral part of the device.

1. Graduating thermostat. A *thermostat* in which the motion of the *valve* is approximately in direct proportion to the effective motion of the thermal element induced by temperature change.

2. Snap-acting thermostat. A *thermostat* in which the thermostatic valve travels instantly from the closed to the open position, and vice versa.

TRANSITION FITTINGS, PLASTIC TO STEEL. An adapter for joining plastic *pipe* to steel *pipe*. The purpose of this fitting is to provide a permanent, pressure-tight connection between two materials that cannot be joined directly one to another.

UNIT HEATER.

High-static pressure type. A self-contained, automatically controlled, *vented appliance* having integral means for circulation of air against 0.2 inch w.c. (50 Pa) or greater static pressure. Such *appliance* is equipped with provisions for attaching an outlet air duct and, where the *appliance* is for indoor installation remote from the space to be heated, is also equipped with provisions for attaching an inlet air duct.

Low-static pressure type. A self-contained, automatically controlled, *vented appliance*, intended for installation in the space to be heated without the use of ducts, having integral means for circulation of air. Such units are allowed to be equipped with louvers or face extensions made in accordance with the manufacturer's specifications.

UNVENTED ROOM HEATER. An unvented heating *appliance* designed for stationary installation and utilized to provide comfort heating. Such *appliances* provide radiant heat or convection heat by gravity or fan circulation directly from the heater and do not utilize ducts.

VALVE. A device used in *piping* to control the gas supply to any section of a system of *piping* or to an *appliance*.

Automatic. An automatic or semiautomatic device consisting essentially of a *valve* and an operator that control the gas supply to the *burner(s)* during operation of an *appliance*. The operator shall be actuated by application of gas pressure on a flexible diaphragm, by electrical means, by mechanical means or by other *approved* means.

Appliance shutoff. A *valve* located in the *piping system*, used to isolate individual *appliances* for purposes such as service or replacement.

Automatic gas shutoff. A *valve* used in conjunction with an automatic gas shutoff device to shut off the gas supply to a water heating system. It shall be constructed integrally with the gas shutoff device or shall be a separate assembly.

Individual main burner. A *valve* that controls the gas supply to an individual *main burner*.

Main burner control. A *valve* that controls the gas supply to the *main burner* manifold.

Manual main gas-control. A manually operated *valve* in the gas line for the purpose of completely turning on or shutting off the gas supply to the *appliance*, except to a *pilot* or pilots that have independent shutoff.

Manual reset. An automatic shutoff *valve* installed in the gas supply *piping* and set to shut off when unsafe conditions occur. The device remains closed until manually reopened.

Service shutoff. A *valve*, installed by the serving gas supplier between the service *meter* or source of supply and the customer *piping system*, to shut off the entire *piping system*.

VENT. A *pipe* or other conduit composed of factory-made components, containing a passageway for conveying *combustion products* and air to the atmosphere, listed and labeled for use with a specific type or class of *appliance*.

Special gas vent. A vent listed and labeled for use with listed Category II, III and IV gas *appliances*.

Type B vent. A vent listed and labeled for use with *appliances* with *draft hoods* and other Category I *appliances* that are listed for use with Type B vents.

Type BW vent. A vent listed and labeled for use with wall *furnaces*.

Type L vent. A vent listed and labeled for use with *appliances* that are listed for use with Type L or Type B vents.

VENT CONNECTOR. See "Connector."

VENT PIPING.

Breather. *Piping* run from a pressure-regulating device to the outdoors, designed to provide a reference to *atmospheric pressure*. If the device incorporates an integral pressure *relief* mechanism, a breather vent can also serve as a *relief* vent.

Relief. *Piping* run from a pressure-regulating or pressure-limiting device to the outdoors, designed to provide for the safe venting of gas in the event of excessive pressure in the *gas piping system*.

VENTED GAS APPLIANCE CATEGORIES. *Appliances* that are categorized for the purpose of vent selection are classified into the following four categories:

Category I. An *appliance* that operates with a nonpositive vent static pressure and with a vent gas temperature that avoids excessive *condensate* production in the vent.

Category II. An *appliance* that operates with a nonpositive *vent* static pressure and with a vent gas temperature that is capable of causing excessive *condensate* production in the vent.

Category III. An *appliance* that operates with a positive vent static pressure and with a vent gas temperature that avoids excessive *condensate* production in the vent.

Category IV. An *appliance* that operates with a positive vent static pressure and with a vent gas temperature that is capable of causing excessive *condensate* production in the vent.

VENTED ROOM HEATER. A vented self-contained, free-standing, nonrecessed *appliance* for furnishing warm air to the space in which it is installed, directly from the heater without duct connections.

VENTED WALL FURNACE. A self-contained *vented appliance* complete with grilles or equivalent, designed for incorporation in or permanent attachment to the structure of a building, mobile home or travel trailer, and furnishing heated air circulated by gravity or by a fan directly into the space to be heated through openings in the casing. This definition shall exclude *floor furnaces, unit heaters* and *central furnaces* as herein defined.

VENTING SYSTEM. A continuous open passageway from the *flue collar* or *draft hood* of an *appliance* to the outside atmosphere for the purpose of removing flue or vent gases. A venting system is usually composed of a vent or a *chimney* and *vent connector*, if used, assembled to form the open passageway.

WALL HEATER, UNVENTED TYPE. A room heater of the type designed for insertion in or attachment to a wall or partition. Such heater does not incorporate concealed venting arrangements in its construction and discharges all products of *combustion* through the front into the room being heated.

WATER HEATER. Any heating *appliance* or *equipment* that heats potable water and supplies such water to the potable hot water distribution system.

SECTION G2404 (301)
GENERAL

G2404.1 (301.1) Scope. This section shall govern the approval and installation of all *equipment* and *appliances* that comprise parts of the installations regulated by this *code* in accordance with Section G2401.

G2404.2 (301.1.1) Other fuels. The requirements for *combustion* and *dilution air* for gas-fired *appliances* shall be governed by Section G2407. The requirements for *combustion* and *dilution air* for *appliances* operating with fuels other than fuel gas shall be regulated by Chapter 17.

G2404.3 (301.3) Listed and labeled. *Appliances* regulated by this *code* shall be listed and labeled for the application in which they are used unless otherwise *approved* in accordance with Section R104.11. The approval of unlisted *appliances* in accordance with Section R104.11 shall be based upon *approved* engineering evaluation.

G2404.4 (301.8) Vibration isolation. Where means for isolation of vibration of an *appliance* is installed, an *approved* means for support and restraint of that *appliance* shall be provided.

G2404.5 (301.9) Repair. Defective material or parts shall be replaced or repaired in such a manner so as to preserve the original approval or listing.

G2404.6 (301.10) Wind resistance. *Appliances* and supports that are exposed to wind shall be designed and installed to resist the wind pressures determined in accordance with this *code*.

G2404.7 (301.11) Flood hazard. For structures located in *flood hazard areas*, the *appliance*, *equipment* and system installations regulated by this *code* shall be located at or above the *design flood elevation* and shall comply with the flood-resistant construction requirements of Section R322.

> **Exception:** The *appliance, equipment* and system installations regulated by this *code* are permitted to be located below the *design flood elevation* provided that they are designed and installed to prevent water from entering or accumulating within the components and to resist hydrostatic and hydrodynamic loads and stresses, including the effects of buoyancy, during the occurrence of flooding to the *design flood elevation* and shall comply with the flood-resistant construction requirements of Section R322.

G2404.8 (301.12) Seismic resistance. When earthquake loads are applicable in accordance with this *code*, the supports shall be designed and installed for the seismic forces in accordance with this *code*.

G2404.9 (301.14) Rodentproofing. Buildings or structures and the walls enclosing habitable or occupiable rooms and spaces in which persons live, sleep or work, or in which feed, food or foodstuffs are stored, prepared, processed, served or sold, shall be constructed to protect against the entry of rodents.

G2404.10 (307.5) Auxiliary drain pan. Category IV condensing *appliances* shall be provided with an auxiliary drain pan where damage to any building component will occur as a result of stoppage in the *condensate* drainage system. Such pan shall be installed in accordance with the applicable provisions of Section M1411.

> **Exception:** An auxiliary drain pan shall not be required for *appliances* that automatically shut down operation in the event of a stoppage in the *condensate* drainage system.

SECTION G2405 (302)
STRUCTURAL SAFETY

G2405.1 (302.1) Structural safety. The building shall not be weakened by the installation of any *gas piping*. In the process of installing or repairing any *gas piping*, the finished floors, walls, ceilings, tile work or any other part of the building or premises which are required to be changed or replaced shall be left in a safe structural condition in accordance with the requirements of this *code*.

G2405.2 (302.4) Alterations to trusses. Truss members and components shall not be cut, drilled, notched, spliced or otherwise altered in any way without the written concurrence and approval of a registered design professional. *Alterations* resulting in the addition of loads to any member (e.g., HVAC *equipment, water heaters*) shall not be permitted without verification that the truss is capable of supporting such additional loading.

G2405.3 (302.3.1) Engineered wood products. Cuts, notches and holes bored in trusses, structural composite lumber, structural glued-laminated members and I-joists are prohibited except where permitted by the manufacturer's recommendations or where the effects of such *alterations* are specifically considered in the design of the member by a registered design professional.

SECTION G2406 (303)
APPLIANCE LOCATION

G2406.1 (303.1) General. *Appliances* shall be located as required by this section, specific requirements elsewhere in this *code* and the conditions of the *equipment* and *appliance* listing.

G2406.2 (303.3) Prohibited locations. *Appliances* shall not be located in sleeping rooms, bathrooms, toilet rooms, storage closets or surgical rooms, or in a space that opens only into such rooms or spaces, except where the installation complies with one of the following:

1. The *appliance* is a direct-vent *appliance* installed in accordance with the conditions of the listing and the manufacturer's instructions.

2. *Vented room heaters*, wall *furnaces*, vented decorative *appliances*, vented gas *fireplaces*, vented gas *fireplace* heaters and decorative *appliances* for installation in vented solid fuel-burning *fireplaces* are installed in rooms that meet the required volume criteria of Section G2407.5.

3. A single wall-mounted *unvented room heater* is installed in a bathroom and such *unvented room heater* is equipped as specified in Section G2445.6 and has an input rating not greater than 6,000 *Btu*/h (1.76 kW). The bathroom shall meet the required volume criteria of Section G2407.5.

4. A single wall-mounted *unvented room heater* is installed in a bedroom and such *unvented room heater* is equipped

as specified in Section G2445.6 and has an input rating not greater than 10,000 *Btu*/h (2.93 kW). The bedroom shall meet the required volume criteria of Section G2407.5.

5. The *appliance* is installed in a room or space that opens only into a bedroom or bathroom, and such room or space is used for no other purpose and is provided with a solid weather-stripped door equipped with an *approved* self-closing device. All *combustion air* shall be taken directly from the outdoors in accordance with Section G2407.6.

G2406.3 (303.6) Outdoor locations. *Appliances* installed in outdoor locations shall be either listed for outdoor installation or provided with protection from outdoor environmental factors that influence the operability, durability and safety of the *appliance.*

SECTION G2407 (304)
COMBUSTION, VENTILATION AND DILUTION AIR

G2407.1 (304.1) General. Air for *combustion*, ventilation and dilution of *flue gases* for *appliances* installed in buildings shall be provided by application of one of the methods prescribed in Sections G2407.5 through G2407.9. Where the requirements of Section G2407.5 are not met, outdoor air shall be introduced in accordance with one of the methods prescribed in Sections G2407.6 through G2407.9. *Direct-vent appliances*, gas *appliances* of other than *natural draft* design and vented gas *appliances* other than Category I shall be provided with *combustion*, ventilation and *dilution air* in accordance with the *appliance* manufacturer's instructions.

> **Exception:** *Type 1 clothes dryers* that are provided with *makeup air* in accordance with Section G2439.4.

G2407.2 (304.2) Appliance location. *Appliances* shall be located so as not to interfere with proper circulation of *combustion*, ventilation and *dilution air.*

G2407.3 (304.3) Draft hood/regulator location. Where used, a *draft hood* or a *barometric draft regulator* shall be installed in the same room or enclosure as the *appliance* served so as to prevent any difference in pressure between the hood or *regulator* and the *combustion air* supply.

G2407.4 (304.4) Makeup air provisions. Where exhaust fans, *clothes dryers* and kitchen ventilation systems interfere with the operation of *appliances*, *makeup air* shall be provided.

G2407.5 (304.5) Indoor combustion air. The required volume of indoor air shall be determined in accordance with Section G2407.5.1 or G2407.5.2, except that where the air infiltration rate is known to be less than 0.40 air changes per hour (ACH), Section G2407.5.2 shall be used. The total required volume shall be the sum of the required volume calculated for all *appliances* located within the space. Rooms communicating directly with the space in which the *appliances* are installed through openings not furnished with doors, and through *combustion air* openings sized and located in accordance with Section G2407.5.3, are considered to be part of the required volume.

G2407.5.1 (304.5.1) Standard method. The minimum required volume shall be 50 cubic feet per 1,000 *Btu*/h (4.8 m³/kW).

G2407.5.2 (304.5.2) Known air-infiltration-rate method. Where the air infiltration rate of a structure is known, the minimum required volume shall be determined as follows:

For *appliances* other than fan assisted, calculate volume using Equation 24-1.

$$\text{Required Volume}_{other} \geq \frac{21\,\text{ft}^3}{ACH}\left(\frac{I_{other}}{1,000\,\text{Btu}/\text{hr}}\right)$$

(Equation 24-1)

For fan-assisted *appliances*, calculate volume using Equation 24-2.

$$\text{Required Volume}_{fan} \geq \frac{15\,\text{ft}^3}{ACH}\left(\frac{I_{fan}}{1,000\,\text{Btu}/\text{hr}}\right)$$

(Equation 24-2)

where:

I_{other} = All *appliances* other than fan assisted (input in *Btu*/h).

I_{fan} = Fan-assisted *appliance* (input in *Btu*/h).

ACH = Air change per hour (percent of volume of space exchanged per hour, expressed as a decimal).

For purposes of this calculation, an infiltration rate greater than 0.60 ACH shall not be used in Equations 24-1 and 24-2.

G2407.5.3 (304.5.3) Indoor opening size and location. Openings used to connect indoor spaces shall be sized and located in accordance with Sections G2407.5.3.1 and G2407.5.3.2 (see Figure G2407.5.3).

G2407.5.3.1 (304.5.3.1) Combining spaces on the same story. Each opening shall have a minimum free area of 1 square inch per 1,000 *Btu*/h (2,200 mm²/kW) of the total input rating of all *appliances* in the space, but not less than 100 square inches (0.06 m²). One opening shall commence within 12 inches (305 mm) of the top and one opening shall commence within 12 inches (305 mm) of the bottom of the enclosure. The minimum dimension of air openings shall be not less than 3 inches (76 mm).

G2407.5.3.2 (304.5.3.2) Combining spaces in different stories. The volumes of spaces in different stories shall be considered as communicating spaces where such spaces are connected by one or more openings in doors or floors having a total minimum free area of 2 square inches per 1,000 *Btu*/h (4402 mm²/kW) of total input rating of all *appliances*.

G2407.6 (304.6) Outdoor combustion air. Outdoor *combustion* air shall be provided through opening(s) to the outdoors in accordance with Section G2407.6.1 or G2407.6.2. The minimum dimension of air openings shall be not less than 3 inches (76 mm).

G2407.6.1 (304.6.1) Two-permanent-openings method. Two permanent openings, one commencing within 12 inches (305 mm) of the top and one commencing within 12 inches

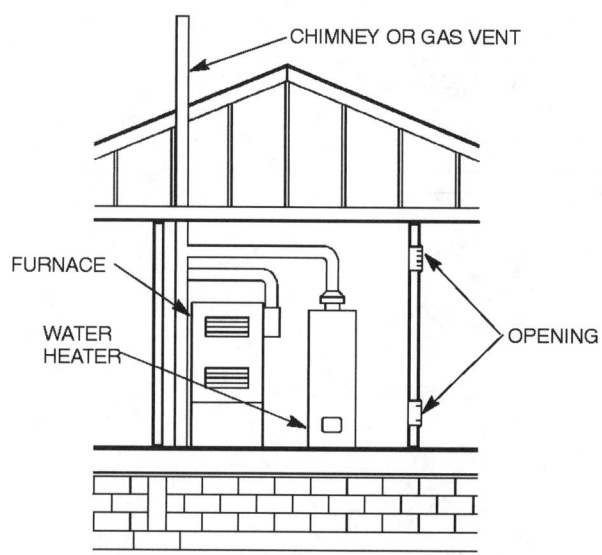

FIGURE G2407.5.3 (304.5.3)
ALL AIR FROM INSIDE THE BUILDING
(see Section 2407.5.3)

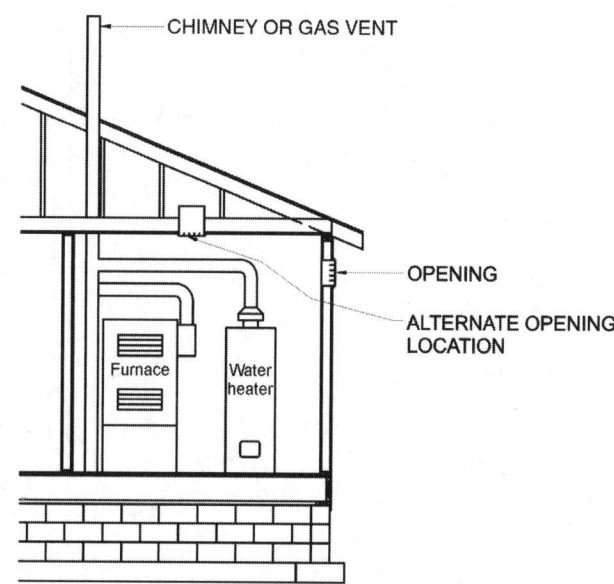

FIGURE G2407.6.2 (304.6.2)
SINGLE COMBUSTION AIR OPENING,
ALL AIR FROM OUTDOORS
(see Section 2407.6.2)

(305 mm) of the bottom of the enclosure, shall be provided. The openings shall communicate directly, or by ducts, with the outdoors or spaces that freely communicate with the outdoors.

Where directly communicating with the outdoors, or where communicating with the outdoors through vertical ducts, each opening shall have a minimum free area of 1 square inch per 4,000 *Btu*/h (550 mm²/kW) of total input rating of all *appliances* in the enclosure [see Figures G2407.6.1(1) and G2407.6.1(2)].

Where communicating with the outdoors through horizontal ducts, each opening shall have a minimum free area of not less than 1 square inch per 2,000 *Btu*/h (1,100 mm²/kW) of total input rating of all *appliances* in the enclosure [see Figure G2407.6.1(3)].

G2407.6.2 (304.6.2) One-permanent-opening method. One permanent opening, commencing within 12 inches (305 mm) of the top of the enclosure, shall be provided. The *appliance* shall have *clearances* of at least 1 inch (25 mm) from the sides and back and 6 inches (152 mm) from the front of the *appliance*. The opening shall directly communicate with the outdoors or through a vertical or horizontal duct to the outdoors, or spaces that freely communicate with the outdoors (see Figure G2407.6.2) and shall have a minimum free area of 1 square inch per 3,000 *Btu*/h (734 mm²/kW) of the total input rating of all *appliances* located in the enclosure and not less than the sum of the areas of all *vent connectors* in the space.

G2407.7 (304.7) Combination indoor and outdoor combustion air. The use of a combination of indoor and outdoor *combustion air* shall be in accordance with Sections G2407.7.1 through G2407.7.3.

G2407.7.1 (304.7.1) Indoor openings. Where used, openings connecting the interior spaces shall comply with Section G2407.5.3.

G2407.7.2 (304.7.2) Outdoor opening location. Outdoor opening(s) shall be located in accordance with Section G2407.6.

G2407.7.3 (304.7.3) Outdoor opening(s) size. The outdoor opening(s) size shall be calculated in accordance with the following:

1. The ratio of interior spaces shall be the available volume of all communicating spaces divided by the required volume.

2. The outdoor size reduction factor shall be one minus the ratio of interior spaces.

3. The minimum size of outdoor opening(s) shall be the full size of outdoor opening(s) calculated in accordance with Section G2407.6, multiplied by the reduction factor. The minimum dimension of air openings shall be not less than 3 inches (76 mm).

G2407.8 (304.8) Engineered installations. Engineered *combustion air* installations shall provide an adequate supply of *combustion*, ventilation and *dilution air* and shall be *approved*.

G2407.9 (304.9) Mechanical combustion air supply. Where all *combustion air* is provided by a mechanical air supply system, the *combustion air* shall be supplied from the outdoors at a rate not less than 0.35 cubic feet per minute per 1,000 *Btu*/h (0.034 m³/min per kW) of total input rating of all *appliances* located within the space.

G2407.9.1 (304.9.1) Makeup air. Where exhaust fans are installed, *makeup air* shall be provided to replace the exhausted air.

G2407.9.2 (304.9.2) Appliance interlock. Each of the *appliances* served shall be interlocked with the mechanical air supply system to prevent *main burner* operation when the mechanical air supply system is not in operation.

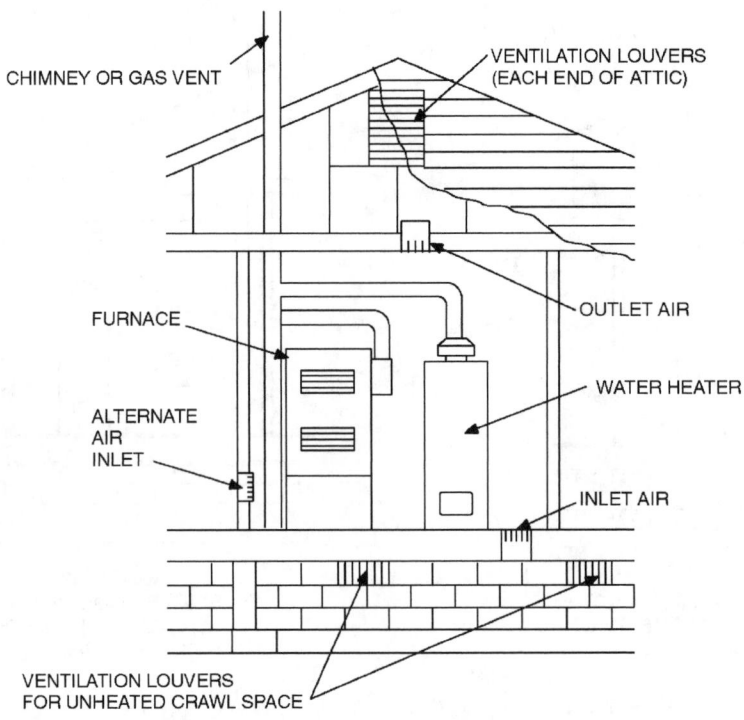

FIGURE G2407.6.1(1) [304.6.1(1)]
ALL AIR FROM OUTDOOR-INLET AIR FROM VENTILATED
CRAWL SPACE AND OUTLET AIR TO VENTILATED ATTIC (see Section G2407.6.1)

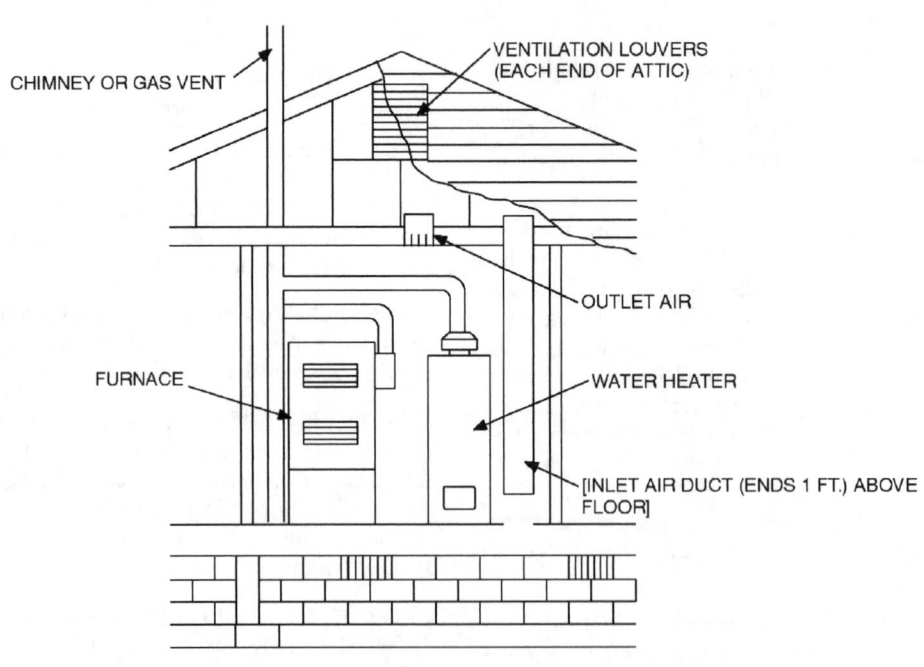

For SI: 1 foot = 304.8 mm.

FIGURE G2407.6.1(2) [304.6.1(2)]
ALL AIR FROM OUTDOORS THROUGH VENTILATED ATTIC
(see Section G2407.6.1)

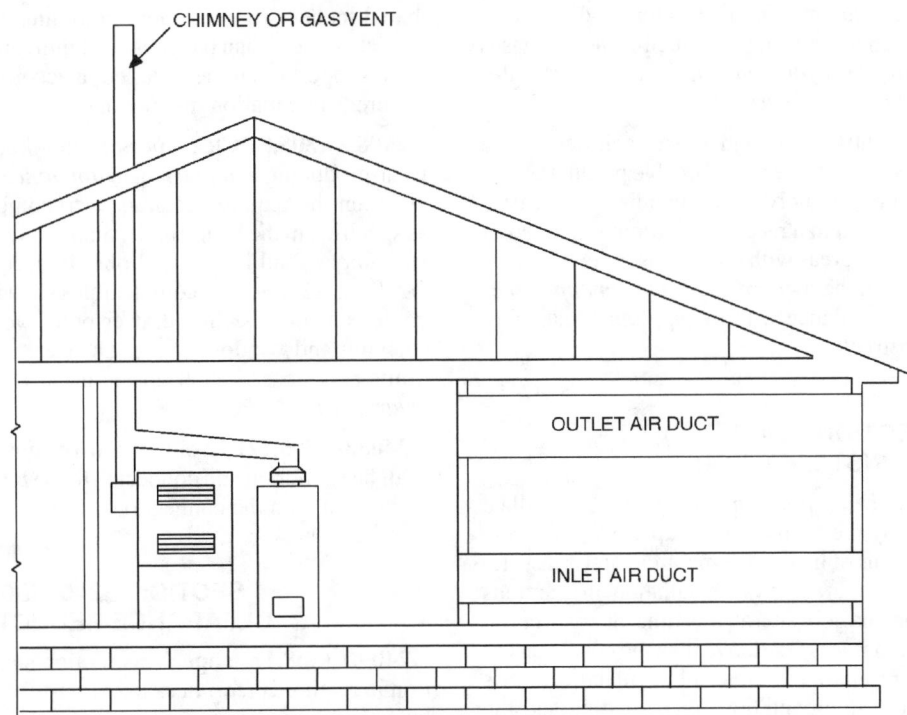

FIGURE G2407.6.1(3) [304.6.1(3)]
ALL AIR FROM OUTDOORS
(see Section G2407.6.1)

G2407.9.3 (304.9.3) Combined combustion air and ventilation air system. Where *combustion air* is provided by the building's mechanical ventilation system, the system shall provide the specified *combustion air* rate in addition to the required ventilation air.

G2407.10 (304.10) Louvers and grilles. The required size of openings for *combustion*, ventilation and *dilution air* shall be based on the net free area of each opening. Where the free area through a design of louver, grille or screen is known, it shall be used in calculating the size opening required to provide the free area specified. Where the design and free area of louvers and grilles are not known, it shall be assumed that wood louvers will have 25-percent free area and metal louvers and grilles will have 75-percent free area. Screens shall have a mesh size not smaller than $^1/_4$ inch (6.4 mm). Nonmotorized louvers and grilles shall be fixed in the open position. Motorized louvers shall be interlocked with the *appliance* so that they are proven to be in the full open position prior to *main burner* ignition and during *main burner* operation. Means shall be provided to prevent the *main burner* from igniting if the louvers fail to open during *burner* start-up and to shut down the *main burner* if the louvers close during operation.

G2407.11 (304.11) Combustion air ducts. *Combustion air* ducts shall comply with all of the following:

1. Ducts shall be constructed of galvanized steel complying with Chapter 16 or of a material having equivalent corrosion resistance, strength and rigidity.

   Exception: Within dwellings units, unobstructed stud and joist spaces shall not be prohibited from con-

veying *combustion air*, provided that not more than one required fireblock is removed.

2. Ducts shall terminate in an unobstructed space allowing free movement of *combustion air* to the *appliances*.

3. Ducts shall serve a single enclosure.

4. Ducts shall not serve both upper and lower *combustion air* openings where both such openings are used. The separation between ducts serving upper and lower *combustion air* openings shall be maintained to the source of *combustion air*.

5. Ducts shall not be screened where terminating in an attic space.

6. Horizontal upper *combustion air* ducts shall not slope downward toward the source of *combustion air*.

7. The remaining space surrounding a *chimney* liner, gas vent, special gas vent or plastic *piping* installed within a masonry, metal or factory-built *chimney* shall not be used to supply *combustion air*.

   Exception: Direct-vent gas-fired *appliances* designed for installation in a solid fuel-burning *fireplace* where installed in accordance with the manufacturer's instructions.

8. *Combustion air* intake openings located on the exterior of a building shall have the lowest side of such openings located not less than 12 inches (305 mm) vertically from the adjoining finished ground level.

G2407.12 (304.12) Protection from fumes and gases. Where corrosive or flammable process fumes or gases, other than products of *combustion*, are present, means for the disposal of such fumes or gases shall be provided. Such fumes or gases include carbon monoxide, hydrogen sulfide, ammonia, chlorine and halogenated hydrocarbons.

In barbershops, beauty shops and other facilities where chemicals that generate corrosive or flammable products, such as aerosol sprays, are routinely used, nondirect vent-type *appliances* shall be located in a mechanical room separated or partitioned off from other areas with provisions for *combustion air* and *dilution air* from the outdoors. *Direct-vent appliances* shall be installed in accordance with the *appliance* manufacturer's installation instructions.

SECTION G2408 (305)
INSTALLATION

G2408.1 (305.1) General. *Equipment* and *appliances* shall be installed as required by the terms of their approval, in accordance with the conditions of listing, the manufacturer's instructions and this *code*. Manufacturers' installation instructions shall be available on the job site at the time of inspection. Where a *code* provision is less restrictive than the conditions of the listing of the *equipment* or *appliance* or the manufacturer's installation instructions, the conditions of the listing and the manufacturer's installation instructions shall apply.

Unlisted *appliances approved* in accordance with Section G2404.3 shall be limited to uses recommended by the manufacturer and shall be installed in accordance with the manufacturer's instructions, the provisions of this *code* and the requirements determined by the *code official*.

G2408.2 (305.3) Elevation of ignition source. *Equipment* and *appliances* having an *ignition source* shall be elevated such that the source of ignition is not less than 18 inches (457 mm) above the floor in *hazardous locations* and public garages, private garages, repair garages, motor fuel-dispensing facilities and parking garages. For the purpose of this section, rooms or spaces that are not part of the *living space* of a *dwelling unit* and that communicate directly with a private garage through openings shall be considered to be part of the private garage.

Exception: Elevation of the *ignition source* is not required for *appliances* that are listed as flammable vapor ignition resistant.

G2408.2.1 (305.3.1) Installation in residential garages. In residential garages where *appliances* are installed in a separate, enclosed space having access only from outside of the garage, such *appliances* shall be permitted to be installed at floor level, provided that the required *combustion air* is taken from the exterior of the garage.

G2408.3 (305.5) Private garages. *Appliances* located in private garages shall be installed with a minimum *clearance* of 6 feet (1829 mm) above the floor.

Exception: The requirements of this section shall not apply where the *appliances* are protected from motor vehicle impact and installed in accordance with Section G2408.2.

G2408.4 (305.7) Clearances from grade. *Equipment* and *appliances* installed at grade level shall be supported on a level concrete slab or other *approved* material extending not less than 3 inches (76 mm) above adjoining grade or shall be suspended not less than 6 inches (152 mm) above adjoining grade. Such supports shall be installed in accordance with the manufacturer's installation instructions.

G2408.5 (305.8) Clearances to combustible construction. Heat-producing *equipment* and *appliances* shall be installed to maintain the required clearances to combustible construction as specified in the listing and manufacturer's instructions. Such *clearances* shall be reduced only in accordance with Section G2409. *Clearances* to combustibles shall include such considerations as door swing, drawer pull, overhead projections or shelving and window swing. Devices, such as door stops or limits and closers, shall not be used to provide the required *clearances*.

G2408.6 (305.12) Avoid strain on gas piping. *Appliances* shall be supported and connected to the *piping* so as not to exert undue strain on the connections.

SECTION G2409 (308)
CLEARANCE REDUCTION

G2409.1 (308.1) Scope. This section shall govern the reduction in required *clearances* to combustible materials and combustible assemblies for *chimneys*, vents, *appliances*, devices and *equipment*.

G2409.2 (308.2) Reduction table. The allowable *clearance* reduction shall be based on one of the methods specified in Table G2409.2 or shall utilize an assembly listed for such application. Where required *clearances* are not listed in Table G2409.2, the reduced *clearances* shall be determined by linear interpolation between the distances listed in the table. Reduced *clearances* shall not be derived by extrapolation below the range of the table. The reduction of the required *clearances* to combustibles for listed and labeled *appliances* and *equipment* shall be in accordance with the requirements of this section except that such *clearances* shall not be reduced where reduction is specifically prohibited by the terms of the *appliance* or *equipment* listing [see Figures G2409.2(1), G2409.2(2) and G2409.2(3)].

G2409.3 (308.3) Clearances for indoor air-conditioning appliances. *Clearance* requirements for indoor air-conditioning *appliances* shall comply with Sections G2409.3.1 through G2409.3.5.

G2409.3.1 (308.3.1) Appliances installed in rooms that are large in comparison with the size of the appliances. Air-conditioning *appliances* installed in rooms that are large in comparison with the size of the *appliance* shall be installed with *clearances* in accordance with the manufacturer's instructions.

G2409.3.2 (308.3.2) Appliances installed in rooms that are not large in comparison with the size of the appliances. Air-conditioning *appliances* installed in rooms that are not large in comparison with the size of the *appliance*, such as alcoves and closets, shall be listed for such installations and installed in accordance with the manufacturer's instructions. Listed *clearances* shall not be reduced by the protection methods described in Table G2409.2, regardless of whether the enclosure is of combustible or noncombustible material.

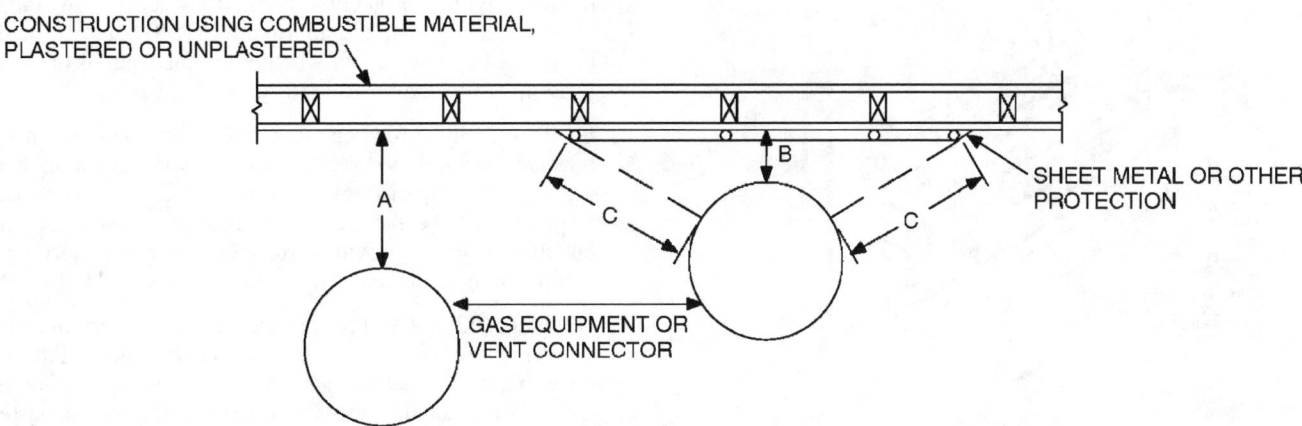

CONSTRUCTION USING COMBUSTIBLE MATERIAL, PLASTERED OR UNPLASTERED

SHEET METAL OR OTHER PROTECTION

GAS EQUIPMENT OR VENT CONNECTOR

NOTES:
"A" equals the clearance with no protection.
"B" equals the reduced clearance permitted in accordance with Table G2409.2. The protection applied to the construction using combustible material shall extend far enough in each direction to make "C" equal to "A."

FIGURE G2409.2(1) [308.2(1)]
EXTENT OF PROTECTION NECESSARY TO REDUCE CLEARANCES FROM GAS EQUIPMENT OR VENT CONNECTORS

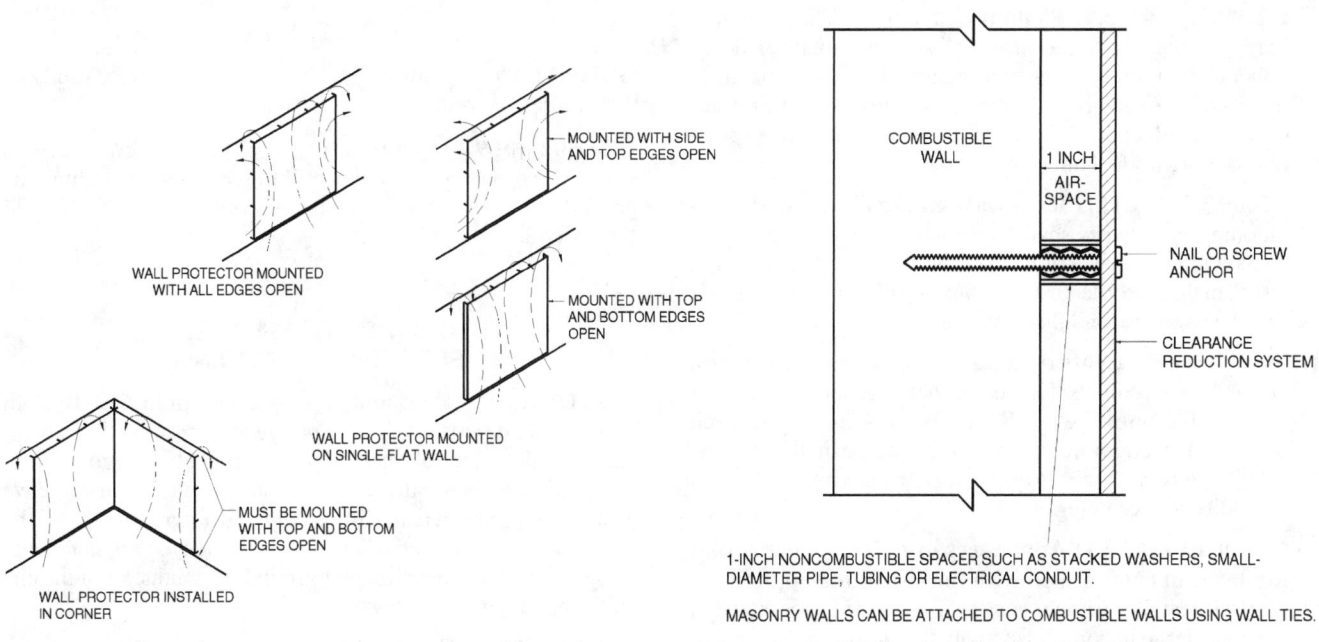

WALL PROTECTOR MOUNTED WITH ALL EDGES OPEN

MOUNTED WITH SIDE AND TOP EDGES OPEN

MOUNTED WITH TOP AND BOTTOM EDGES OPEN

WALL PROTECTOR MOUNTED ON SINGLE FLAT WALL

MUST BE MOUNTED WITH TOP AND BOTTOM EDGES OPEN

WALL PROTECTOR INSTALLED IN CORNER

COMBUSTIBLE WALL

1 INCH AIR-SPACE

NAIL OR SCREW ANCHOR

CLEARANCE REDUCTION SYSTEM

1-INCH NONCOMBUSTIBLE SPACER SUCH AS STACKED WASHERS, SMALL-DIAMETER PIPE, TUBING OR ELECTRICAL CONDUIT.

MASONRY WALLS CAN BE ATTACHED TO COMBUSTIBLE WALLS USING WALL TIES.

DO NOT USE SPACERS DIRECTLY BEHIND APPLIANCE OR CONNECTOR.

For SI: 1 inch = 25.4 mm.

FIGURE G2409.2(2) [308.2(2)]
WALL PROTECTOR CLEARANCE REDUCTION SYSTEM

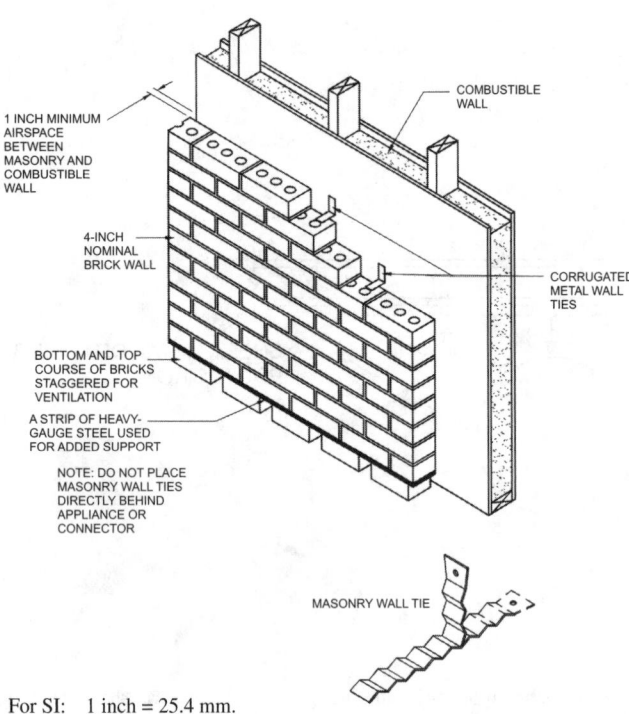

1 INCH MINIMUM
AIRSPACE
BETWEEN
MASONRY AND
COMBUSTIBLE
WALL

4-INCH
NOMINAL
BRICK WALL

BOTTOM AND TOP
COURSE OF BRICKS
STAGGERED FOR
VENTILATION

A STRIP OF HEAVY-
GAUGE STEEL USED
FOR ADDED SUPPORT

NOTE: DO NOT PLACE
MASONRY WALL TIES
DIRECTLY BEHIND
APPLIANCE OR
CONNECTOR

COMBUSTIBLE
WALL

CORRUGATED
METAL WALL
TIES

MASONRY WALL TIE

For SI: 1 inch = 25.4 mm.

FIGURE G2409.2(3) [308.2(3)]
MASONRY CLEARANCE REDUCTION SYSTEM

G2409.3.3 (308.3.3) Clearance reduction. Air-conditioning *appliances* installed in rooms that are large in comparison with the size of the *appliance* shall be permitted to be installed with reduced clearances to combustible material, provided that the combustible material or *appliance* is protected as described in Table G2409.2.

G2409.3.4 (308.3.4) Plenum clearances. Where the *furnace plenum* is adjacent to plaster on metal lath or noncombustible material attached to combustible material, the *clearance* shall be measured to the surface of the plaster or other noncombustible finish where the *clearance* specified is 2 inches (51 mm) or less.

G2409.3.5 (308.3.5) Clearance from supply ducts. Air-conditioning *appliances* shall have the *clearance* from supply ducts within 3 feet (914 mm) of the *furnace plenum* be not less than that specified from the *furnace plenum*. *Clearance* is not necessary beyond this distance.

G2409.4 (308.4) Central heating boilers and furnaces. *Clearance* requirements for central-heating boilers and *furnaces* shall comply with Sections G2409.4.1 through G2409.4.6. The *clearance* to these *appliances* shall not interfere with *combustion air*; *draft hood clearance* and *relief*; and accessibility for servicing.

> **G2409.4.1 (308.4.1) Appliances installed in rooms that are large in comparison with the size of the appliances.** Central-heating *furnaces* and *low-pressure boilers* installed in rooms large in comparison with the size of the *appliance* shall be installed with *clearances* in accordance with the manufacturer's instructions.

> **G2409.4.2 (308.4.2) Appliances installed in rooms that are not large in comparison with the size of the appli-**

ances. Central-heating *furnaces* and *low-pressure boilers* installed in rooms that are not large in comparison with the size of the appliance, such as alcoves and closets, shall be listed for such installations. Listed *clearances* shall not be reduced by the protection methods described in Table G2409.2 and illustrated in Figures G2409.2(1) through G2409.2(3), regardless of whether the enclosure is of combustible or noncombustible material.

G2409.4.3 (308.4.3) Clearance reduction. Central heating *furnaces* and *low-pressure boilers* installed in rooms that are large in comparison with the size of the *appliance* shall be permitted to be installed with reduced *clearances* to combustible material provided the combustible material or equipment is protected as described in Table G2409.2.

G2409.4.4 (308.4.5) Plenum clearances. Where the *furnace plenum* is adjacent to plaster on metal lath or noncombustible material attached to combustible material, the *clearance* shall be measured to the surface of the plaster or other noncombustible finish where the *clearance* specified is 2 inches (51 mm) or less.

G2409.4.5 (308.4.6) Clearance from supply ducts. Central-heating *furnaces* shall have the *clearance* from supply ducts within 3 feet (914 mm) of the *furnace plenum* be not less than that specified from the *furnace plenum*. No *clearance* is necessary beyond this distance.

G2409.4.6 (308.4.4) Clearance for servicing appliances. Front *clearance* shall be sufficient for servicing the *burner* and the *furnace* or boiler.

SECTION G2410 (309)
ELECTRICAL

G2410.1 (309.1) Grounding. *Gas piping* shall not be used as a *grounding electrode.*

G2410.2 (309.2) Connections. Electrical connections between *appliances* and the building wiring, including the grounding of the *appliances,* shall conform to Chapters 34 through 43.

SECTION G2411 (310)
ELECTRICAL BONDING

G2411.1 (310.1) Pipe and *tubing* other than CSST. Each above-ground portion of a *gas piping system* other than corrugated stainless steel tubing (CSST), that is likely to become energized shall be electrically continuous and bonded to an effective ground-fault current path. *Gas piping*, other than CSST, shall be considered to be bonded where it is connected to *appliances* that are connected to the equipment grounding conductor of the circuit supplying that *appliance.*

> **G2411.1.1 (310.1.1) CSST.** Corrugated stainless steel tubing (CSST) *gas piping systems* shall be bonded to the electrical service grounding electrode system at the point where the gas service enters the building. The *bonding jumper* shall be not smaller than 6 AWG copper wire or equivalent.

TABLE G2409.2 (308.2)[a through k]
REDUCTION OF CLEARANCES WITH SPECIFIED FORMS OF PROTECTION

TYPE OF PROTECTION APPLIED TO AND COVERING ALL SURFACES OF COMBUSTIBLE MATERIAL WITHIN THE DISTANCE SPECIFIED AS THE REQUIRED CLEARANCE WITH NO PROTECTION [see Figures G2409.2(1), G2409.2(2), and G2409.2(3)]	WHERE THE REQUIRED CLEARANCE WITH NO PROTECTION FROM APPLIANCE, VENT CONNECTOR, OR SINGLE-WALL METAL PIPE IS: (inches)									
	36		18		12		9		6	
	Allowable clearances with specified protection (inches)									
	Use Column 1 for clearances above appliance or horizontal connector. Use Column 2 for clearances from appliance, vertical connector and single-wall metal pipe.									
	Above Col. 1	Sides and rear Col. 2	Above Col. 1	Sides and rear Col. 2	Above Col. 1	Sides and rear Col. 2	Above Col. 1	Sides and rear Col. 2	Above Col. 1	Sides and rear Col. 2
1. 3½-inch-thick masonry wall without ventilated airspace	—	24	—	12	—	9	—	6	—	5
2. ½-inch insulation board over 1-inch glass fiber or mineral wool batts	24	18	12	9	9	6	6	5	4	3
3. 0.024-inch (nominal 24 gage) sheet metal over 1-inch glass fiber or mineral wool batts reinforced with wire on rear face with ventilated airspace	18	12	9	6	6	4	5	3	3	3
4. 3½-inch-thick masonry wall with ventilated airspace	—	12	—	6	—	6	—	6	—	6
5. 0.024-inch (nominal 24 gage) sheet metal with ventilated airspace	18	12	9	6	6	4	5	3	3	2
6. ½-inch-thick insulation board with ventilated airspace	18	12	9	6	6	4	5	3	3	3
7. 0.024-inch (nominal 24 gage) sheet metal with ventilated airspace over 0.024-inch (nominal 24 gage) sheet metal with ventilated airspace	18	12	9	6	6	4	5	3	3	3
8. 1-inch glass fiber or mineral wool batts sandwiched between two sheets 0.024-inch (nominal 24 gage) sheet metal with ventilated airspace	18	12	9	6	6	4	5	3	3	3

For SI: 1 inch = 25.4 mm, °C = [(°F - 32)/1.8], 1 pound per cubic foot = 16.02 kg/m³, 1 Btu per inch per square foot per hour per °F = 0.144 W/m² · K.

a. Reduction of clearances from combustible materials shall not interfere with combustion air, draft hood clearance and relief, and accessibility of servicing.

b. All clearances shall be measured from the outer surface of the combustible material to the nearest point on the surface of the appliance, disregarding any intervening protection applied to the combustible material.

c. Spacers and ties shall be of noncombustible material. No spacer or tie shall be used directly opposite an appliance or connector.

d. For all clearance reduction systems using a ventilated airspace, adequate provision for air circulation shall be provided as described [see Figures G2409.2(2) and G2409.2(3)].

e. There shall be at least 1 inch between clearance reduction systems and combustible walls and ceilings for reduction systems using ventilated airspace.

f. Where a wall protector is mounted on a single flat wall away from corners, it shall have a minimum 1-inch air gap. To provide air circulation, the bottom and top edges, or only the side and top edges, or all edges shall be left open.

g. Mineral wool batts (blanket or board) shall have a minimum density of 8 pounds per cubic foot and a minimum melting point of 1500°F.

h. Insulation material used as part of a clearance reduction system shall have a thermal conductivity of 1.0 Btu per inch per square foot per hour per °F or less.

i. There shall be at least 1 inch between the appliance and the protector. In no case shall the clearance between the appliance and the combustible surface be reduced below that allowed in this table.

j. All clearances and thicknesses are minimum; larger clearances and thicknesses are acceptable.

k. Listed single-wall connectors shall be installed in accordance with the manufacturer's installation instructions.

SECTION G2412 (401)
GENERAL

G2412.1 (401.1) Scope. This section shall govern the design, installation, modification and maintenance of *piping systems*. The applicability of this *code* to *piping systems* extends from the *point of delivery* to the connections with the *appliances* and includes the design, materials, components, fabrication, assembly, installation, testing, inspection, operation and maintenance of such *piping systems*.

G2412.1.1 (401.1.1) Utility piping systems located within buildings. Utility service *piping* located within buildings shall be installed in accordance with the structural safety and fire protection provisions of this *code*.

G2412.2 (401.2) Liquefied petroleum gas storage. The storage system for *liquefied petroleum gas* shall be designed and installed in accordance with the *International Fire Code* and NFPA 58.

G2412.3 (401.3) Modifications to existing systems. In modifying or adding to existing *piping systems*, sizes shall be maintained in accordance with this chapter.

G2412.4 (401.4) Additional appliances. Where an additional *appliance* is to be served, the existing *piping* shall be checked to determine if it has adequate capacity for all *appliances* served. If inadequate, the existing system shall be enlarged as required or separate *piping* of adequate capacity shall be provided.

G2412.5 (401.5) Identification. For other than steel *pipe*, exposed *piping* shall be identified by a yellow label marked "Gas" in black letters. The marking shall be spaced at intervals not exceeding 5 feet (1524 mm). The marking shall not be required on *pipe* located in the same room as the *appliance* served.

G2412.6 (401.6) Interconnections. Where two or more *meters* are installed on the same premises, but supply separate consumers, the *piping systems* shall not be interconnected on the outlet side of the *meters*.

G2412.7 (401.7) Piping meter identification. *Piping* from multiple *meter* installations shall be marked with an *approved* permanent identification by the installer so that the *piping system* supplied by each *meter* is readily identifiable.

G2412.8 (401.8) Minimum sizes. All *pipe* utilized for the installation, extension and *alteration* of any *piping system* shall be sized to supply the full number of outlets for the intended purpose and shall be sized in accordance with Section G2413.

SECTION G2413 (402)
PIPE SIZING

G2413.1 (402.1) General considerations. *Piping systems* shall be of such size and so installed as to provide a supply of gas sufficient to meet the maximum *demand* and supply gas to each *appliance* inlet at not less than the minimum supply pressure required by the *appliance*.

G2413.2 (402.2) Maximum gas demand. The volume of gas to be provided, in cubic feet per hour, shall be determined directly from the manufacturer's input ratings of the *appliances* served. Where an input rating is not indicated, the gas

supplier, *appliance* manufacturer or a qualified agency shall be contacted, or the rating from Table G2413.2 shall be used for estimating the volume of gas to be supplied.

The total connected hourly load shall be used as the basis for *pipe* sizing, assuming that all *appliances* could be operating at full capacity simultaneously. Where a diversity of load can be established, *pipe* sizing shall be permitted to be based on such loads.

TABLE G2413.2 (402.2)
APPROXIMATE GAS INPUT FOR TYPICAL APPLIANCES

APPLIANCE	INPUT BTU/H (Approx.)
Space Heating Units	
Hydronic boiler	
Single family	100,000
Multifamily, per unit	60,000
Warm-air furnace	
Single family	100,000
Multifamily, per unit	60,000
Space and Water Heating Units	
Hydronic boiler	
Single family	120,000
Multifamily, per unit	75,000
Water Heating Appliances	
Water heater, automatic instantaneous	
Capacity at 2 gal./minute	142,800
Capacity at 4 gal./minute	285,000
Capacity at 6 gal./minute	428,400
Water heater, automatic storage, 30- to 40-gal. tank	35,000
Water heater, automatic storage, 50-gal. tank	50,000
Water heater, domestic, circulating or side-arm	35,000
Cooking Appliances	
Built-in oven or broiler unit, domestic	25,000
Built-in top unit, domestic	40,000
Range, free-standing, domestic	65,000
Other Appliances	
Barbecue	40,000
Clothes dryer, Type 1 (domestic)	35,000
Gas fireplace, direct-vent	40,000
Gas light	2,500
Gas log	80,000
Refrigerator	3,000

For SI: 1 British thermal unit per hour = 0.293 W, 1 gallon = 3.785 L, 1 gallon per minute = 3.785 L/m.

G2413.3 (402.3) Sizing. *Gas piping* shall be sized in accordance with one of the following:

1. *Pipe* sizing tables or sizing equations in accordance with Section G2413.4.

2. The sizing tables included in a listed *piping* system's manufacturer's installation instructions.

3. Other *approved* engineering methods.

G2413.4 (402.4) Sizing tables and equations. Where Tables G2413.4(1) through G2413.4(21) are used to size *piping* or *tubing*, the *pipe* length shall be determined in accordance with Section G2413.4.1, G2413.4.2 or G2413.4.3.

Where Equations 24-3 and 24-4 are used to size *piping* or *tubing*, the *pipe* or *tubing* shall have smooth inside walls and the *pipe* length shall be determined in accordance with Section G2413.4.1, G2413.4.2 or G2413.4.3.

1. Low-pressure gas equation [Less than 1.5 pounds per square inch (psi) (10.3 kPa)]:

$$D = \frac{Q^{0.381}}{19.17 \left(\dfrac{\Delta H}{C_r \times L} \right)^{0.206}}$$

(Equation 24-3)

2. High-pressure gas equation [1.5 psi (10.3 kPa) and above]:

$$D = \frac{Q^{0.381}}{18.93 \left[\dfrac{\left(P_1^{\,2} - P_2^{\,2} \right) \times Y}{C_r \times L} \right]^{0.206}}$$

(Equation 24-4)

where:

D = Inside diameter of *pipe*, inches (mm).

Q = Input rate *appliance(s)*, cubic feet per hour at 60°F (16°C) and 30-inch mercury column.

P_1 = Upstream pressure, psia (P_1 + 14.7).

P_2 = Downstream pressure, psia (P_2 + 14.7).

L = Equivalent length of *pipe*, feet.

ΔH = *Pressure drop*, inch water column (27.7 inch water column = 1 psi).

TABLE G2413.4 (402.4)
C_r AND Y VALUES FOR NATURAL GAS AND UNDILUTED PROPANE AT STANDARD CONDITIONS

GAS	EQUATION FACTORS	
	C_r	Y
Natural gas	0.6094	0.9992
Undiluted propane	1.2462	0.9910

For SI: 1 cubic foot = 0.028 m³, 1 foot = 305 mm, 1 inch water column = 0.249 kPa, 1 pound per square inch = 6.895 kPa, 1 British thermal unit per hour = 0.293 W.

G2413.4.1 (402.4.1) Longest length method. The *pipe* size of each section of *gas piping* shall be determined using the longest length of *piping* from the *point of delivery* to the most remote *outlet* and the load of the section.

G2413.4.2 (402.4.2) Branch length method. *Pipe* shall be sized as follows:

1. *Pipe* size of each section of the longest *pipe* run from the *point of delivery* to the most remote *outlet* shall be determined using the longest run of *piping* and the load of the section.

2. The *pipe* size of each section of branch *piping* not previously sized shall be determined using the length of *piping* from the *point of delivery* to the most remote *outlet* in each branch and the load of the section.

G2413.4.3 (402.4.3) Hybrid pressure. The *pipe* size for each section of higher pressure *gas piping* shall be determined using the longest length of *piping* from the *point of delivery* to the most remote line *pressure regulator*. The *pipe* size from the line *pressure regulator* to each *outlet* shall be determined using the length of *piping* from the *regulator* to the most remote outlet served by the *regulator*.

G2413.5 (402.5) Allowable pressure drop. The design pressure loss in any *piping system* under maximum probable flow conditions, from the *point of delivery* to the inlet connection of the *appliance*, shall be such that the supply pressure at the *appliance* is greater than or equal to the minimum pressure required by the *appliance*.

G2413.6 (402.6) Maximum design operating pressure. The maximum design operating pressure for *piping systems* located inside buildings shall not exceed 5 pounds per square inch gauge (psig) (34 kPa gauge) except where one or more of the following conditions are met:

1. The *piping system* is welded.

2. The *piping* is located in a ventilated chase or otherwise enclosed for protection against accidental gas accumulation.

3. The *piping* is a temporary installation for buildings under construction.

G2413.6.1 (402.6.1) Liquefied petroleum gas systems. LP-gas systems designed to operate below -5°F (-21°C) or with butane or a propane-butane mix shall be designed to either accommodate liquid LP-gas or prevent LP-gas vapor from condensing into a liquid.

TABLE G2413.4(1) [402.4(2)]
SCHEDULE 40 METALLIC PIPE

Gas	Natural
Inlet Pressure	Less than 2 psi
Pressure Drop	0.5 in. w.c.
Specific Gravity	0.60

	PIPE SIZE (inch)													
Nominal	$^1/_2$	$^3/_4$	1	$1^1/_4$	$1^1/_2$	2	$2^1/_2$	3	4	5	6	8	10	12
Actual ID	0.622	0.824	1.049	1.380	1.610	2.067	2.469	3.068	4.026	5.047	6.065	7.981	10.020	11.938
Length (ft)	Capacity in Cubic Feet of Gas per Hour													
10	172	360	678	1,390	2,090	4,020	6,400	11,300	23,100	41,800	67,600	139,000	252,000	399,000
20	118	247	466	957	1,430	2,760	4,400	7,780	15,900	28,700	46,500	95,500	173,000	275,000
30	95	199	374	768	1,150	2,220	3,530	6,250	12,700	23,000	37,300	76,700	139,000	220,000
40	81	170	320	657	985	1,900	3,020	5,350	10,900	19,700	31,900	65,600	119,000	189,000
50	72	151	284	583	873	1,680	2,680	4,740	9,660	17,500	28,300	58,200	106,000	167,000
60	65	137	257	528	791	1,520	2,430	4,290	8,760	15,800	25,600	52,700	95,700	152,000
70	60	126	237	486	728	1,400	2,230	3,950	8,050	14,600	23,600	48,500	88,100	139,000
80	56	117	220	452	677	1,300	2,080	3,670	7,490	13,600	22,000	45,100	81,900	130,000
90	52	110	207	424	635	1,220	1,950	3,450	7,030	12,700	20,600	42,300	76,900	122,000
100	50	104	195	400	600	1,160	1,840	3,260	6,640	12,000	19,500	40,000	72,600	115,000
125	44	92	173	355	532	1,020	1,630	2,890	5,890	10,600	17,200	35,400	64,300	102,000
150	40	83	157	322	482	928	1,480	2,610	5,330	9,650	15,600	32,100	58,300	92,300
175	37	77	144	296	443	854	1,360	2,410	4,910	8,880	14,400	29,500	53,600	84,900
200	34	71	134	275	412	794	1,270	2,240	4,560	8,260	13,400	27,500	49,900	79,000
250	30	63	119	244	366	704	1,120	1,980	4,050	7,320	11,900	24,300	44,200	70,000
300	27	57	108	221	331	638	1,020	1,800	3,670	6,630	10,700	22,100	40,100	63,400
350	25	53	99	203	305	587	935	1,650	3,370	6,100	9,880	20,300	36,900	58,400
400	23	49	92	189	283	546	870	1,540	3,140	5,680	9,190	18,900	34,300	54,300
450	22	46	86	177	266	512	816	1,440	2,940	5,330	8,620	17,700	32,200	50,900
500	21	43	82	168	251	484	771	1,360	2,780	5,030	8,150	16,700	30,400	48,100
550	20	41	78	159	239	459	732	1,290	2,640	4,780	7,740	15,900	28,900	45,700
600	19	39	74	152	228	438	699	1,240	2,520	4,560	7,380	15,200	27,500	43,600
650	18	38	71	145	218	420	669	1,180	2,410	4,360	7,070	14,500	26,400	41,800
700	17	36	68	140	209	403	643	1,140	2,320	4,190	6,790	14,000	25,300	40,100
750	17	35	66	135	202	389	619	1,090	2,230	4,040	6,540	13,400	24,400	38,600
800	16	34	63	130	195	375	598	1,060	2,160	3,900	6,320	13,000	23,600	37,300
850	16	33	61	126	189	363	579	1,020	2,090	3,780	6,110	12,600	22,800	36,100
900	15	32	59	122	183	352	561	992	2,020	3,660	5,930	12,200	22,100	35,000
950	15	31	58	118	178	342	545	963	1,960	3,550	5,760	11,800	21,500	34,000
1,000	14	30	56	115	173	333	530	937	1,910	3,460	5,600	11,500	20,900	33,100
1,100	14	28	53	109	164	316	503	890	1,810	3,280	5,320	10,900	19,800	31,400
1,200	13	27	51	104	156	301	480	849	1,730	3,130	5,070	10,400	18,900	30,000
1,300	12	26	49	100	150	289	460	813	1,660	3,000	4,860	9,980	18,100	28,700
1,400	12	25	47	96	144	277	442	781	1,590	2,880	4,670	9,590	17,400	27,600
1,500	11	24	45	93	139	267	426	752	1,530	2,780	4,500	9,240	16,800	26,600
1,600	11	23	44	89	134	258	411	727	1,480	2,680	4,340	8,920	16,200	25,600
1,700	11	22	42	86	130	250	398	703	1,430	2,590	4,200	8,630	15,700	24,800
1,800	10	22	41	84	126	242	386	682	1,390	2,520	4,070	8,370	15,200	24,100
1,900	10	21	40	81	122	235	375	662	1,350	2,440	3,960	8,130	14,800	23,400
2,000	NA	20	39	79	119	229	364	644	1,310	2,380	3,850	7,910	14,400	22,700

For SI: 1 inch = 25.4 mm, 1 foot = 304.8 mm, 1 pound per square inch = 6.895 kPa, 1-inch water column = 0.2488 kPa,
1 British thermal unit per hour = 0.2931 W, 1 cubic foot per hour = 0.0283 m³/h, 1 degree = 0.01745 rad.

Notes:
1. NA means a flow of less than 10 cfh.
2. All table entries have been rounded to three significant digits.

TABLE G2413.4(2) [402.4(3)]
SCHEDULE 40 METALLIC PIPE

Gas	Natural
Inlet Pressure	2.0 psi
Pressure Drop	1.0 psi
Specific Gravity	0.60

PIPE SIZE (inch)									
Nominal	$^1/_2$	$^3/_4$	1	$1^1/_4$	$1^1/_2$	2	$2^1/_2$	3	4
Actual ID	0.622	0.824	1.049	1.380	1.610	2.067	2.469	3.068	4.026
Length (ft)	Capacity in Cubic Feet of Gas per Hour								
10	1,510	3,040	5,560	11,400	17,100	32,900	52,500	92,800	189,000
20	1,070	2,150	3,930	8,070	12,100	23,300	37,100	65,600	134,000
30	869	1,760	3,210	6,590	9,880	19,000	30,300	53,600	109,000
40	753	1,520	2,780	5,710	8,550	16,500	26,300	46,400	94,700
50	673	1,360	2,490	5,110	7,650	14,700	23,500	41,500	84,700
60	615	1,240	2,270	4,660	6,980	13,500	21,400	37,900	77,300
70	569	1,150	2,100	4,320	6,470	12,500	19,900	35,100	71,600
80	532	1,080	1,970	4,040	6,050	11,700	18,600	32,800	67,000
90	502	1,010	1,850	3,810	5,700	11,000	17,500	30,900	63,100
100	462	934	1,710	3,510	5,260	10,100	16,100	28,500	58,200
125	414	836	1,530	3,140	4,700	9,060	14,400	25,500	52,100
150	372	751	1,370	2,820	4,220	8,130	13,000	22,900	46,700
175	344	695	1,270	2,601	3,910	7,530	12,000	21,200	43,300
200	318	642	1,170	2,410	3,610	6,960	11,100	19,600	40,000
250	279	583	1,040	2,140	3,210	6,180	9,850	17,400	35,500
300	253	528	945	1,940	2,910	5,600	8,920	15,800	32,200
350	232	486	869	1,790	2,670	5,150	8,210	14,500	29,600
400	216	452	809	1,660	2,490	4,790	7,640	13,500	27,500
450	203	424	759	1,560	2,330	4,500	7,170	12,700	25,800
500	192	401	717	1,470	2,210	4,250	6,770	12,000	24,400
550	182	381	681	1,400	2,090	4,030	6,430	11,400	23,200
600	174	363	650	1,330	2,000	3,850	6,130	10,800	22,100
650	166	348	622	1,280	1,910	3,680	5,870	10,400	21,200
700	160	334	598	1,230	1,840	3,540	5,640	9,970	20,300
750	154	322	576	1,180	1,770	3,410	5,440	9,610	19,600
800	149	311	556	1,140	1,710	3,290	5,250	9,280	18,900
850	144	301	538	1,100	1,650	3,190	5,080	8,980	18,300
900	139	292	522	1,070	1,600	3,090	4,930	8,710	17,800
950	135	283	507	1,040	1,560	3,000	4,780	8,460	17,200
1,000	132	275	493	1,010	1,520	2,920	4,650	8,220	16,800
1,100	125	262	468	960	1,440	2,770	4,420	7,810	15,900
1,200	119	250	446	917	1,370	2,640	4,220	7,450	15,200
1,300	114	239	427	878	1,320	2,530	4,040	7,140	14,600
1,400	110	230	411	843	1,260	2,430	3,880	6,860	14,000
1,500	106	221	396	812	1,220	2,340	3,740	6,600	13,500
1,600	102	214	382	784	1,180	2,260	3,610	6,380	13,000
1,700	99	207	370	759	1,140	2,190	3,490	6,170	12,600
1,800	96	200	358	736	1,100	2,120	3,390	5,980	12,200
1,900	93	195	348	715	1,070	2,060	3,290	5,810	11,900
2,000	91	189	339	695	1,040	2,010	3,200	5,650	11,500

For SI: 1 inch = 25.4 mm, 1 foot = 304.8 mm, 1 pound per square inch = 6.895 kPa, 1-inch water column = 0.2488 kPa,
1 British thermal unit per hour = 0.2931 W, 1 cubic foot per hour = 0.0283 m³/h, 1 degree = 0.01745 rad.

Note: All table entries have been rounded to three significant digits.

TABLE G2413.4(3) [402.4(7)]
SEMIRIGID COPPER TUBING

Gas	Natural
Inlet Pressure	Less than 2 psi
Pressure Drop	0.5 in. w.c.
Specific Gravity	0.60

		\(^1/_4\)	\(^3/_8\)	\(^1/_2\)	\(^5/_8\)	\(^3/_4\)	1	\(1^1/_4\)	\(1^1/_2\)	2
Nominal	K & L									
	ACR	\(^3/_8\)	\(^1/_2\)	\(^5/_8\)	\(^3/_4\)	\(^7/_8\)	\(1^1/_8\)	\(1^3/_8\)	—	—
Outside		0.375	0.500	0.625	0.750	0.875	1.125	1.375	1.625	2.125
Inside		0.305	0.402	0.527	0.652	0.745	0.995	1.245	1.481	1.959
Length (ft)	Capacity in Cubic Feet of Gas per Hour									
10		27	55	111	195	276	590	1,060	1,680	3,490
20		18	38	77	134	190	406	730	1,150	2,400
30		15	30	61	107	152	326	586	925	1,930
40		13	26	53	92	131	279	502	791	1,650
50		11	23	47	82	116	247	445	701	1,460
60		10	21	42	74	105	224	403	635	1,320
70		NA	19	39	68	96	206	371	585	1,220
80		NA	18	36	63	90	192	345	544	1,130
90		NA	17	34	59	84	180	324	510	1,060
100		NA	16	32	56	79	170	306	482	1,000
125		NA	14	28	50	70	151	271	427	890
150		NA	13	26	45	64	136	245	387	806
175		NA	12	24	41	59	125	226	356	742
200		NA	11	22	39	55	117	210	331	690
250		NA	NA	20	34	48	103	186	294	612
300		NA	NA	18	31	44	94	169	266	554
350		NA	NA	16	28	40	86	155	245	510
400		NA	NA	15	26	38	80	144	228	474
450		NA	NA	14	25	35	75	135	214	445
500		NA	NA	13	23	33	71	128	202	420
550		NA	NA	13	22	32	68	122	192	399
600		NA	NA	12	21	30	64	116	183	381
650		NA	NA	12	20	29	62	111	175	365
700		NA	NA	11	20	28	59	107	168	350
750		NA	NA	11	19	27	57	103	162	338
800		NA	NA	10	18	26	55	99	156	326
850		NA	NA	10	18	25	53	96	151	315
900		NA	NA	NA	17	24	52	93	147	306
950		NA	NA	NA	17	24	50	90	143	297
1,000		NA	NA	NA	16	23	49	88	139	289
1,100		NA	NA	NA	15	22	46	84	132	274
1,200		NA	NA	NA	15	21	44	80	126	262
1,300		NA	NA	NA	14	20	42	76	120	251
1,400		NA	NA	NA	13	19	41	73	116	241
1,500		NA	NA	NA	13	18	39	71	111	232
1,600		NA	NA	NA	13	18	38	68	108	224
1,700		NA	NA	NA	12	17	37	66	104	217
1,800		NA	NA	NA	12	17	36	64	101	210
1,900		NA	NA	NA	11	16	35	62	98	204
2,000		NA	NA	NA	11	16	34	60	95	199

For SI: 1 inch = 25.4 mm, 1 foot = 304.8 mm, 1 pound per square inch = 6.895 kPa, 1-inch water column = 0.2488 kPa,
1 British thermal unit per hour = 0.2931 W, 1 cubic foot per hour = 0.0283 m³/h, 1 degree = 0.01745 rad.

Notes:
1. Table capacities are based on Type K copper tubing inside diameter (shown), which has the smallest inside diameter of the copper tubing products.
2. NA means a flow of less than 10 cfh.
3. All table entries have been rounded to three significant digits.

2009 INTERNATIONAL RESIDENTIAL CODE®

TABLE G2413.4(4) [402.4(10)]
SEMIRIGID COPPER TUBING

Gas	Natural
Inlet Pressure	2.0 psi
Pressure Drop	1.0 psi
Specific Gravity	0.60

		\(^1/_4\)	\(^3/_8\)	\(^1/_2\)	\(^5/_8\)	\(^3/_4\)	1	\(1^1/_4\)	\(1^1/_2\)	2
	K & L	\(^1/_4\)	\(^3/_8\)	\(^1/_2\)	\(^5/_8\)	\(^3/_4\)	1	\(1^1/_4\)	\(1^1/_2\)	2
Nominal	**ACR**	\(^3/_8\)	\(^1/_2\)	\(^5/_8\)	\(^3/_4\)	\(^7/_8\)	\(1^1/_8\)	\(1^3/_8\)	—	—
Outside		0.375	0.500	0.625	0.750	0.875	1.125	1.375	1.625	2.125
Inside		0.305	0.402	0.527	0.652	0.745	0.995	1.245	1.481	1.959
Length (ft)		Capacity in Cubic Feet of Gas per Hour								
10		245	506	1,030	1,800	2,550	5,450	9,820	15,500	32,200
20		169	348	708	1,240	1,760	3,750	6,750	10,600	22,200
30		135	279	568	993	1,410	3,010	5,420	8,550	17,800
40		116	239	486	850	1,210	2,580	4,640	7,310	15,200
50		103	212	431	754	1,070	2,280	4,110	6,480	13,500
60		93	192	391	683	969	2,070	3,730	5,870	12,200
70		86	177	359	628	891	1,900	3,430	5,400	11,300
80		80	164	334	584	829	1,770	3,190	5,030	10,500
90		75	154	314	548	778	1,660	2,990	4,720	9,820
100		71	146	296	518	735	1,570	2,830	4,450	9,280
125		63	129	263	459	651	1,390	2,500	3,950	8,220
150		57	117	238	416	590	1,260	2,270	3,580	7,450
175		52	108	219	383	543	1,160	2,090	3,290	6,850
200		49	100	204	356	505	1,080	1,940	3,060	6,380
250		43	89	181	315	448	956	1,720	2,710	5,650
300		39	80	164	286	406	866	1,560	2,460	5,120
350		36	74	150	263	373	797	1,430	2,260	4,710
400		33	69	140	245	347	741	1,330	2,100	4,380
450		31	65	131	230	326	696	1,250	1,970	4,110
500		30	61	124	217	308	657	1,180	1,870	3,880
550		28	58	118	206	292	624	1,120	1,770	3,690
600		27	55	112	196	279	595	1,070	1,690	3,520
650		26	53	108	188	267	570	1,030	1,620	3,370
700		25	51	103	181	256	548	986	1,550	3,240
750		24	49	100	174	247	528	950	1,500	3,120
800		23	47	96	168	239	510	917	1,450	3,010
850		22	46	93	163	231	493	888	1,400	2,920
900		22	44	90	158	224	478	861	1,360	2,830
950		21	43	88	153	217	464	836	1,320	2,740
1,000		20	42	85	149	211	452	813	1,280	2,670
1,100		19	40	81	142	201	429	772	1,220	2,540
1,200		18	38	77	135	192	409	737	1,160	2,420
1,300		18	36	74	129	183	392	705	1,110	2,320
1,400		17	35	71	124	176	376	678	1,070	2,230
1,500		16	34	68	120	170	363	653	1,030	2,140
1,600		16	33	66	116	164	350	630	994	2,070
1,700		15	31	64	112	159	339	610	962	2,000
1,800		15	30	62	108	154	329	592	933	1,940
1,900		14	30	60	105	149	319	575	906	1,890
2,000		14	29	59	102	145	310	559	881	1,830

For SI: 1 inch = 25.4 mm, 1 foot = 304.8 mm, 1 pound per square inch = 6.895 kPa, 1-inch water column = 0.2488 kPa,
1 British thermal unit per hour = 0.2931 W, 1 cubic foot per hour = 0.0283 m³/h, 1 degree = 0.01745 rad.

Notes:

1. Table capacities are based on Type K copper tubing inside diameter (shown), which has the smallest inside diameter of the copper tubing products.
2. All table entries have been rounded to three significant digits.

TABLE G2413.4(5) [402.4(13)]
CORRUGATED STAINLESS STEEL TUBING (CSST)

Gas	Natural
Inlet Pressure	Less than 2 psi
Pressure Drop	0.5 in. w.c.
Specific Gravity	0.60

	TUBE SIZE (EHD)													
Flow Designation	13	15	18	19	23	25	30	31	37	39	46	48	60	62
Length (ft)	Capacity in Cubic Feet of Gas per Hour													
5	46	63	115	134	225	270	471	546	895	1,037	1,790	2,070	3,660	4,140
10	32	44	82	95	161	192	330	383	639	746	1,260	1,470	2,600	2,930
15	25	35	66	77	132	157	267	310	524	615	1,030	1,200	2,140	2,400
20	22	31	58	67	116	137	231	269	456	536	888	1,050	1,850	2,080
25	19	27	52	60	104	122	206	240	409	482	793	936	1,660	1,860
30	18	25	47	55	96	112	188	218	374	442	723	856	1,520	1,700
40	15	21	41	47	83	97	162	188	325	386	625	742	1,320	1,470
50	13	19	37	42	75	87	144	168	292	347	559	665	1,180	1,320
60	12	17	34	38	68	80	131	153	267	318	509	608	1,080	1,200
70	11	16	31	36	63	74	121	141	248	295	471	563	1,000	1,110
80	10	15	29	33	60	69	113	132	232	277	440	527	940	1,040
90	10	14	28	32	57	65	107	125	219	262	415	498	887	983
100	9	13	26	30	54	62	101	118	208	249	393	472	843	933
150	7	10	20	23	42	48	78	91	171	205	320	387	691	762
200	6	9	18	21	38	44	71	82	148	179	277	336	600	661
250	5	8	16	19	34	39	63	74	133	161	247	301	538	591
300	5	7	15	17	32	36	57	67	95	148	226	275	492	540

For SI: 1 inch = 25.4 mm, 1 foot = 304.8 mm, 1 pound per square inch = 6.895 kPa, 1-inch water column = 0.2488 kPa, 1 British thermal unit per hour = 0.2931 W, 1 cubic foot per hour = 0.0283 m^3/h, 1 degree = 0.01745 rad.

Notes:

1. Table includes losses for four 90-degree bends and two end fittings. Tubing runs with larger numbers of bends and/or fittings shall be increased by an equivalent length of tubing to the following equation: $L = 1.3n$, where L is additional length (feet) of tubing and n is the number of additional fittings and/or bends.

2. EHD—Equivalent Hydraulic Diameter, which is a measure of the relative hydraulic efficiency between different tubing sizes. The greater the value of EHD, the greater the gas capacity of the tubing.

3. All table entries have been rounded to three significant digits.

TABLE G2413.4(6) [402.4(16)]
CORRUGATED STAINLESS STEEL TUBING (CSST)

Gas	Natural
Inlet Pressure	2.0 psi
Pressure Drop	1.0 psi
Specific Gravity	0.60

	TUBE SIZE (EHD)													
Flow Designation	13	15	18	19	23	25	30	31	37	39	46	48	60	62
Length (ft)	Capacity in Cubic Feet of Gas Per Hour													
10	270	353	587	700	1,100	1,370	2,590	2,990	4,510	5,037	9,600	10,700	18,600	21,600
25	166	220	374	444	709	876	1,620	1,870	2,890	3,258	6,040	6,780	11,900	13,700
30	151	200	342	405	650	801	1,480	1,700	2,640	2,987	5,510	6,200	10,900	12,500
40	129	172	297	351	567	696	1,270	1,470	2,300	2,605	4,760	5,380	9,440	10,900
50	115	154	266	314	510	624	1,140	1,310	2,060	2,343	4,260	4,820	8,470	9,720
75	93	124	218	257	420	512	922	1,070	1,690	1,932	3,470	3,950	6,940	7,940
80	89	120	211	249	407	496	892	1,030	1,640	1,874	3,360	3,820	6,730	7,690
100	79	107	189	222	366	445	795	920	1,470	1,685	3,000	3,420	6,030	6,880
150	64	87	155	182	302	364	646	748	1,210	1,389	2,440	2,800	4,940	5,620
200	55	75	135	157	263	317	557	645	1,050	1,212	2,110	2,430	4,290	4,870
250	49	67	121	141	236	284	497	576	941	1,090	1,890	2,180	3,850	4,360
300	44	61	110	129	217	260	453	525	862	999	1,720	1,990	3,520	3,980
400	38	52	96	111	189	225	390	453	749	871	1,490	1,730	3,060	3,450
500	34	46	86	100	170	202	348	404	552	783	1,330	1,550	2,740	3,090

For SI: 1 inch = 25.4 mm, 1 foot = 304.8 mm, 1 pound per square inch = 6.895 kPa, 1-inch water column = 0.2488 kPa,
1 British thermal unit per hour = 0.2931 W, 1 cubic foot per hour = 0.0283 m³/h, 1 degree = 0.01745 rad.

Notes:

1. Table does not include effect of pressure drop across the line regulator. Where regulator loss exceeds $^3/_4$ psi, DO NOT USE THIS TABLE. Consult with the regulator manufacturer for pressure drops and capacity factors. Pressure drops across a regulator can vary with flow rate.
2. CAUTION: Capacities shown in the table might exceed maximum capacity for a selected regulator. Consult with the regulator or tubing manufacturer for guidance.
3. Table includes losses for four 90-degree bends and two end fittings. Tubing runs with larger numbers of bends and/or fittings shall be increased by an equivalent length of tubing to the following equation: $L = 1.3n$ where L is additional length (feet) of tubing and n is the number of additional fittings and/or bends.
4. EHD—Equivalent Hydraulic Diameter, which is a measure of the relative hydraulic efficiency between different tubing sizes. The greater the value of EHD, the greater the gas capacity of the tubing.
5. All table entries have been rounded to three significant digits.

TABLE G2413.4(7) [402.4(19)]
POLYETHYLENE PLASTIC PIPE

Gas	Natural
Inlet Pressure	Less than 2 psi
Pressure Drop	0.5 in. w.c.
Specific Gravity	0.60

PIPE SIZE (in.)						
Nominal OD	$^1/_2$	$^3/_4$	1	$1^1/_4$	$1^1/_2$	2
Designation	SDR 9.33	SDR 11.0	SDR 11.00	SDR 10.00	SDR 11.00	SDR 11.00
Actual ID	0.660	0.860	1.077	1.328	1.554	1.943
Length (ft)	Capacity in Cubic Feet of Gas per Hour					
10	201	403	726	1,260	1,900	3,410
20	138	277	499	865	1,310	2,350
30	111	222	401	695	1,050	1,880
40	95	190	343	594	898	1,610
50	84	169	304	527	796	1,430
60	76	153	276	477	721	1,300
70	70	140	254	439	663	1,190
80	65	131	236	409	617	1,110
90	61	123	221	383	579	1,040
100	58	116	209	362	547	983
125	51	103	185	321	485	871
150	46	93	168	291	439	789
175	43	86	154	268	404	726
200	40	80	144	249	376	675
250	35	71	127	221	333	598
300	32	64	115	200	302	542
350	29	59	106	184	278	499
400	27	55	99	171	258	464
450	26	51	93	160	242	435
500	24	48	88	152	229	411

For SI: 1 inch = 25.4 mm, 1 foot = 304.8 mm, 1 pound per square inch = 6.895 kPa, 1-inch water column = 0.2488 kPa,
    1 British thermal unit per hour = 0.2931 W, 1 cubic foot per hour = 0.0283 m³/h, 1 degree = 0.01745 rad.

Note: All table entries have been rounded to three significant digits.

TABLE G2413.4(8) [402.4(20)]
POLYETHYLENE PLASTIC PIPE

Gas	Natural
Inlet Pressure	2.0 psi
Pressure Drop	1.0 psi
Specific Gravity	0.60

	PIPE SIZE (in.)					
Nominal OD	$^1/_2$	$^3/_4$	1	$1^1/_4$	$1^1/_2$	2
Designation	SDR 9.33	SDR 11.0	SDR 11.00	SDR 10.00	SDR 11.00	SDR 11.00
Actual ID	0.660	0.860	1.077	1.328	1.554	1.943
Length (ft)	Capacity in Cubic Feet of Gas per Hour					
10	1,860	3,720	6,710	11,600	17,600	31,600
20	1,280	2,560	4,610	7,990	12,100	21,700
30	1,030	2,050	3,710	6,420	9,690	17,400
40	878	1,760	3,170	5,490	8,300	14,900
50	778	1,560	2,810	4,870	7,350	13,200
60	705	1,410	2,550	4,410	6,660	12,000
70	649	1,300	2,340	4,060	6,130	11,000
80	603	1,210	2,180	3,780	5,700	10,200
90	566	1,130	2,050	3,540	5,350	9,610
100	535	1,070	1,930	3,350	5,050	9,080
125	474	949	1,710	2,970	4,480	8,050
150	429	860	1,550	2,690	4,060	7,290
175	395	791	1,430	2,470	3,730	6,710
200	368	736	1,330	2,300	3,470	6,240
250	326	652	1,180	2,040	3,080	5,530
300	295	591	1,070	1,850	2,790	5,010
350	272	544	981	1,700	2,570	4,610
400	253	506	913	1,580	2,390	4,290
450	237	475	856	1,480	2,240	4,020
500	224	448	809	1,400	2,120	3,800
550	213	426	768	1,330	2,010	3,610
600	203	406	733	1,270	1,920	3,440
650	194	389	702	1,220	1,840	3,300
700	187	374	674	1,170	1,760	3,170
750	180	360	649	1,130	1,700	3,050
800	174	348	627	1,090	1,640	2,950
850	168	336	607	1,050	1,590	2,850
900	163	326	588	1,020	1,540	2,770
950	158	317	572	990	1,500	2,690
1,000	154	308	556	963	1,450	2,610
1,100	146	293	528	915	1,380	2,480
1,200	139	279	504	873	1,320	2,370
1,300	134	267	482	836	1,260	2,270
1,400	128	257	463	803	1,210	2,180
1,500	124	247	446	773	1,170	2,100
1,600	119	239	431	747	1,130	2,030
1,700	115	231	417	723	1,090	1,960
1,800	112	224	404	701	1,060	1,900
1,900	109	218	393	680	1,030	1,850
2,000	106	212	382	662	1,000	1,800

For SI: 1 inch = 25.4 mm, 1 foot = 304.8 mm, 1 pound per square inch = 6.895 kPa, 1-inch water column = 0.2488 kPa,
   1 British thermal unit per hour = 0.2931 W, 1 cubic foot per hour = 0.0283 m³/h, 1 degree = 0.01745 rad.

Note: All table entries have been rounded to three significant digits.

TABLE G2413.4(9) [402.4(23)]
SCHEDULE 40 METALLIC PIPE

Gas	Undiluted Propane
Inlet Pressure	10.0 psi
Pressure Drop	1.0 psi
Specific Gravity	1.50

INTENDED USE	Pipe sizing between first stage (high-pressure regulator) and second stage (low-pressure regulator).								
	PIPE SIZE (in.)								
Nominal	$^1/_2$	$^3/_4$	1	$1^1/_4$	$1^1/_2$	2	$2^1/_2$	3	4
Actual ID	0.622	0.824	1.049	1.380	1.610	2.067	2.469	3.068	4.026
Length (ft)	Capacity in Thousands of Btu per Hour								
10	3,320	6,950	13,100	26,900	40,300	77,600	124,000	219,000	446,000
20	2,280	4,780	9,000	18,500	27,700	53,300	85,000	150,000	306,000
30	1,830	3,840	7,220	14,800	22,200	42,800	68,200	121,000	246,000
40	1,570	3,280	6,180	12,700	19,000	36,600	58,400	103,000	211,000
50	1,390	2,910	5,480	11,300	16,900	32,500	51,700	91,500	187,000
60	1,260	2,640	4,970	10,200	15,300	29,400	46,900	82,900	169,000
70	1,160	2,430	4,570	9,380	14,100	27,100	43,100	76,300	156,000
80	1,080	2,260	4,250	8,730	13,100	25,200	40,100	70,900	145,000
90	1,010	2,120	3,990	8,190	12,300	23,600	37,700	66,600	136,000
100	956	2,000	3,770	7,730	11,600	22,300	35,600	62,900	128,000
125	848	1,770	3,340	6,850	10,300	19,800	31,500	55,700	114,000
150	768	1,610	3,020	6,210	9,300	17,900	28,600	50,500	103,000
175	706	1,480	2,780	5,710	8,560	16,500	26,300	46,500	94,700
200	657	1,370	2,590	5,320	7,960	15,300	24,400	43,200	88,100
250	582	1,220	2,290	4,710	7,060	13,600	21,700	38,300	78,100
300	528	1,100	2,080	4,270	6,400	12,300	19,600	34,700	70,800
350	486	1,020	1,910	3,930	5,880	11,300	18,100	31,900	65,100
400	452	945	1,780	3,650	5,470	10,500	16,800	29,700	60,600
450	424	886	1,670	3,430	5,140	9,890	15,800	27,900	56,800
500	400	837	1,580	3,240	4,850	9,340	14,900	26,300	53,700
550	380	795	1,500	3,070	4,610	8,870	14,100	25,000	51,000
600	363	759	1,430	2,930	4,400	8,460	13,500	23,900	48,600
650	347	726	1,370	2,810	4,210	8,110	12,900	22,800	46,600
700	334	698	1,310	2,700	4,040	7,790	12,400	21,900	44,800
750	321	672	1,270	2,600	3,900	7,500	12,000	21,100	43,100
800	310	649	1,220	2,510	3,760	7,240	11,500	20,400	41,600
850	300	628	1,180	2,430	3,640	7,010	11,200	19,800	40,300
900	291	609	1,150	2,360	3,530	6,800	10,800	19,200	39,100
950	283	592	1,110	2,290	3,430	6,600	10,500	18,600	37,900
1,000	275	575	1,080	2,230	3,330	6,420	10,200	18,100	36,900
1,100	261	546	1,030	2,110	3,170	6,100	9,720	17,200	35,000
1,200	249	521	982	2,020	3,020	5,820	9,270	16,400	33,400
1,300	239	499	940	1,930	2,890	5,570	8,880	15,700	32,000
1,400	229	480	903	1,850	2,780	5,350	8,530	15,100	30,800
1,500	221	462	870	1,790	2,680	5,160	8,220	14,500	29,600
1,600	213	446	840	1,730	2,590	4,980	7,940	14,000	28,600
1,700	206	432	813	1,670	2,500	4,820	7,680	13,600	27,700
1,800	200	419	789	1,620	2,430	4,670	7,450	13,200	26,900
1,900	194	407	766	1,570	2,360	4,540	7,230	12,800	26,100
2,000	189	395	745	1,530	2,290	4,410	7,030	12,400	25,400

For SI: 1 inch = 25.4 mm, 1 foot = 304.8 mm, 1 pound per square inch = 6.895 kPa, 1-inch water column = 0.2488 kPa,
1 British thermal unit per hour = 0.2931 W, 1 cubic foot per hour = 0.0283 m³/h, 1 degree = 0.01745 rad.
Note: All table entries have been rounded to three significant digits.

2009 INTERNATIONAL RESIDENTIAL CODE®

TABLE G2413.4(10) [402.4(24)]
SCHEDULE 40 METALLIC PIPE

Gas	Undiluted Propane
Inlet Pressure	10.0 psi
Pressure Drop	3.0 psi
Specific Gravity	1.50

INTENDED USE	Pipe sizing between first stage (high-pressure regulator) and second stage (low-pressure regulator).								
PIPE SIZE (in)									
Nominal	$^1/_2$	$^3/_4$	1	$1^1/_4$	$1^1/_2$	2	$2^1/_2$	3	4
Actual ID	0.622	0.824	1.049	1.380	1.610	2.067	2.469	3.068	4.026
Length (ft)	Capacity in Thousands of Btu per Hour								
10	5,890	12,300	23,200	47,600	71,300	137,000	219,000	387,000	789,000
20	4,050	8,460	15,900	32,700	49,000	94,400	150,000	266,000	543,000
30	3,250	6,790	12,800	26,300	39,400	75,800	121,000	214,000	436,000
40	2,780	5,810	11,000	22,500	33,700	64,900	103,000	183,000	373,000
50	2,460	5,150	9,710	19,900	29,900	57,500	91,600	162,000	330,000
60	2,230	4,670	8,790	18,100	27,100	52,100	83,000	147,000	299,000
70	2,050	4,300	8,090	16,600	24,900	47,900	76,400	135,000	275,000
80	1,910	4,000	7,530	15,500	23,200	44,600	71,100	126,000	256,000
90	1,790	3,750	7,060	14,500	21,700	41,800	66,700	118,000	240,000
100	1,690	3,540	6,670	13,700	20,500	39,500	63,000	111,000	227,000
125	1,500	3,140	5,910	12,100	18,200	35,000	55,800	98,700	201,000
150	1,360	2,840	5,360	11,000	16,500	31,700	50,600	89,400	182,000
175	1,250	2,620	4,930	10,100	15,200	29,200	46,500	82,300	167,800
200	1,160	2,430	4,580	9,410	14,100	27,200	43,300	76,500	156,100
250	1,030	2,160	4,060	8,340	12,500	24,100	38,400	67,800	138,400
300	935	1,950	3,680	7,560	11,300	21,800	34,800	61,500	125,400
350	860	1,800	3,390	6,950	10,400	20,100	32,000	56,500	115,300
400	800	1,670	3,150	6,470	9,690	18,700	29,800	52,600	107,300
450	751	1,570	2,960	6,070	9,090	17,500	27,900	49,400	100,700
500	709	1,480	2,790	5,730	8,590	16,500	26,400	46,600	95,100
550	673	1,410	2,650	5,450	8,160	15,700	25,000	44,300	90,300
600	642	1,340	2,530	5,200	7,780	15,000	23,900	42,200	86,200
650	615	1,290	2,420	4,980	7,450	14,400	22,900	40,500	82,500
700	591	1,240	2,330	4,780	7,160	13,800	22,000	38,900	79,300
750	569	1,190	2,240	4,600	6,900	13,300	21,200	37,400	76,400
800	550	1,150	2,170	4,450	6,660	12,800	20,500	36,200	73,700
850	532	1,110	2,100	4,300	6,450	12,400	19,800	35,000	71,400
900	516	1,080	2,030	4,170	6,250	12,000	19,200	33,900	69,200
950	501	1,050	1,970	4,050	6,070	11,700	18,600	32,900	67,200
1,000	487	1,020	1,920	3,940	5,900	11,400	18,100	32,000	65,400
1,100	463	968	1,820	3,740	5,610	10,800	17,200	30,400	62,100
1,200	442	923	1,740	3,570	5,350	10,300	16,400	29,000	59,200
1,300	423	884	1,670	3,420	5,120	9,870	15,700	27,800	56,700
1,400	406	849	1,600	3,280	4,920	9,480	15,100	26,700	54,500
1,500	391	818	1,540	3,160	4,740	9,130	14,600	25,700	52,500
1,600	378	790	1,490	3,060	4,580	8,820	14,100	24,800	50,700
1,700	366	765	1,440	2,960	4,430	8,530	13,600	24,000	49,000
1,800	355	741	1,400	2,870	4,300	8,270	13,200	23,300	47,600
1,900	344	720	1,360	2,780	4,170	8,040	12,800	22,600	46,200
2,000	335	700	1,320	2,710	4,060	7,820	12,500	22,000	44,900

For SI: 1 inch = 25.4 mm, 1 foot = 304.8 mm, 1 pound per square inch = 6.895 kPa, 1-inch water column = 0.2488 kPa,
1 British thermal unit per hour = 0.2931 W, 1 cubic foot per hour = 0.0283 m³/h, 1 degree = 0.01745 rad.

Note: All table entries have been rounded to three significant digits.

TABLE G2413.4(11) [402.4(25)]
SCHEDULE 40 METALLIC PIPE

Gas	Undiluted Propane
Inlet Pressure	2.0 psi
Pressure Drop	1.0 psi
Specific Gravity	1.50

INTENDED USE	Pipe sizing between 2 psig service and line pressure regulator.								
	PIPE SIZE (in.)								
Nominal	$^1/_2$	$^3/_4$	1	$1^1/_4$	$1^1/_2$	2	$2^1/_2$	3	4
Actual ID	0.622	0.824	1.049	1.380	1.610	2.067	2.469	3.068	4.026
Length (ft)	Capacity in Thousands of Btu per Hour								
10	2,680	5,590	10,500	21,600	32,400	62,400	99,500	176,000	359,000
20	1,840	3,850	7,240	14,900	22,300	42,900	68,400	121,000	247,000
30	1,480	3,090	5,820	11,900	17,900	34,500	54,900	97,100	198,000
40	1,260	2,640	4,980	10,200	15,300	29,500	47,000	83,100	170,000
50	1,120	2,340	4,410	9,060	13,600	26,100	41,700	73,700	150,000
60	1,010	2,120	4,000	8,210	12,300	23,700	37,700	66,700	136,000
70	934	1,950	3,680	7,550	11,300	21,800	34,700	61,400	125,000
80	869	1,820	3,420	7,020	10,500	20,300	32,300	57,100	116,000
90	815	1,700	3,210	6,590	9,880	19,000	30,300	53,600	109,000
100	770	1,610	3,030	6,230	9,330	18,000	28,600	50,600	103,000
125	682	1,430	2,690	5,520	8,270	15,900	25,400	44,900	91,500
150	618	1,290	2,440	5,000	7,490	14,400	23,000	40,700	82,900
175	569	1,190	2,240	4,600	6,890	13,300	21,200	37,400	76,300
200	529	1,110	2,080	4,280	6,410	12,300	19,700	34,800	71,000
250	469	981	1,850	3,790	5,680	10,900	17,400	30,800	62,900
300	425	889	1,670	3,440	5,150	9,920	15,800	27,900	57,000
350	391	817	1,540	3,160	4,740	9,120	14,500	25,700	52,400
400	364	760	1,430	2,940	4,410	8,490	13,500	23,900	48,800
450	341	714	1,340	2,760	4,130	7,960	12,700	22,400	45,800
500	322	674	1,270	2,610	3,910	7,520	12,000	21,200	43,200
550	306	640	1,210	2,480	3,710	7,140	11,400	20,100	41,100
600	292	611	1,150	2,360	3,540	6,820	10,900	19,200	39,200
650	280	585	1,100	2,260	3,390	6,530	10,400	18,400	37,500
700	269	562	1,060	2,170	3,260	6,270	9,990	17,700	36,000
750	259	541	1,020	2,090	3,140	6,040	9,630	17,000	34,700
800	250	523	985	2,020	3,030	5,830	9,300	16,400	33,500
850	242	506	953	1,960	2,930	5,640	9,000	15,900	32,400
900	235	490	924	1,900	2,840	5,470	8,720	15,400	31,500
950	228	476	897	1,840	2,760	5,310	8,470	15,000	30,500
1,000	222	463	873	1,790	2,680	5,170	8,240	14,600	29,700
1,100	210	440	829	1,700	2,550	4,910	7,830	13,800	28,200
1,200	201	420	791	1,620	2,430	4,680	7,470	13,200	26,900
1,300	192	402	757	1,550	2,330	4,490	7,150	12,600	25,800
1,400	185	386	727	1,490	2,240	4,310	6,870	12,100	24,800
1,500	178	372	701	1,440	2,160	4,150	6,620	11,700	23,900
1,600	172	359	677	1,390	2,080	4,010	6,390	11,300	23,000
1,700	166	348	655	1,340	2,010	3,880	6,180	10,900	22,300
1,800	161	337	635	1,300	1,950	3,760	6,000	10,600	21,600
1,900	157	327	617	1,270	1,900	3,650	5,820	10,300	21,000
2,000	152	318	600	1,230	1,840	3,550	5,660	10,000	20,400

For SI: 1 inch = 25.4 mm, 1 foot = 304.8 mm, 1 pound per square inch = 6.895 kPa, 1-inch water column = 0.2488 kPa,
1 British thermal unit per hour = 0.2931 W, 1 cubic foot per hour = 0.0283 m³/h, 1 degree = 0.01745 rad.

Note: All table entries have been rounded to three significant digits.

TABLE G2413.4(12) [402.4(26)]
SCHEDULE 40 METALLIC PIPE

Gas	Undiluted Propane
Inlet Pressure	11.0 in. w.c.
Pressure Drop	0.5 in. w.c.
Specific Gravity	1.50

INTENDED USE	Pipe sizing between single- or second-stage (low pressure) regulator and appliance.							
	PIPE SIZE (in.)							
Nominal	$^1/_2$	$^3/_4$	1	$1^1/_4$	$1^1/_2$	2	$2^1/_2$	3	4
Actual ID	0.622	0.824	1.049	1.380	1.610	2.067	2.469	3.068	4.026
Length (ft)	Capacity in Thousands of Btu per Hour								
10	291	608	1,150	2,350	3,520	6,790	10,800	19,100	39,000
20	200	418	787	1,620	2,420	4,660	7,430	13,100	26,800
30	160	336	632	1,300	1,940	3,750	5,970	10,600	21,500
40	137	287	541	1,110	1,660	3,210	5,110	9,030	18,400
50	122	255	480	985	1,480	2,840	4,530	8,000	16,300
60	110	231	434	892	1,340	2,570	4,100	7,250	14,800
80	101	212	400	821	1,230	2,370	3,770	6,670	13,600
100	94	197	372	763	1,140	2,200	3,510	6,210	12,700
125	89	185	349	716	1,070	2,070	3,290	5,820	11,900
150	84	175	330	677	1,010	1,950	3,110	5,500	11,200
175	74	155	292	600	899	1,730	2,760	4,880	9,950
200	67	140	265	543	814	1,570	2,500	4,420	9,010
250	62	129	243	500	749	1,440	2,300	4,060	8,290
300	58	120	227	465	697	1,340	2,140	3,780	7,710
350	51	107	201	412	618	1,190	1,900	3,350	6,840
400	46	97	182	373	560	1,080	1,720	3,040	6,190
450	42	89	167	344	515	991	1,580	2,790	5,700
500	40	83	156	320	479	922	1,470	2,600	5,300
550	37	78	146	300	449	865	1,380	2,440	4,970
600	35	73	138	283	424	817	1,300	2,300	4,700
650	33	70	131	269	403	776	1,240	2,190	4,460
700	32	66	125	257	385	741	1,180	2,090	4,260
750	30	64	120	246	368	709	1,130	2,000	4,080
800	29	61	115	236	354	681	1,090	1,920	3,920
850	28	59	111	227	341	656	1,050	1,850	3,770
900	27	57	107	220	329	634	1,010	1,790	3,640
950	26	55	104	213	319	613	978	1,730	3,530
1,000	25	53	100	206	309	595	948	1,680	3,420
1,100	25	52	97	200	300	578	921	1,630	3,320
1,200	24	50	95	195	292	562	895	1,580	3,230
1,300	23	48	90	185	277	534	850	1,500	3,070
1,400	22	46	86	176	264	509	811	1,430	2,930
1,500	21	44	82	169	253	487	777	1,370	2,800
1,600	20	42	79	162	243	468	746	1,320	2,690
1,700	19	40	76	156	234	451	719	1,270	2,590
1,800	19	39	74	151	226	436	694	1,230	2,500
1,900	18	38	71	146	219	422	672	1,190	2,420
2,000	18	37	69	142	212	409	652	1,150	2,350

For SI: 1 inch = 25.4 mm, 1 foot = 304.8 mm, 1 pound per square inch = 6.895 kPa, 1-inch water column = 0.2488 kPa,
1 British thermal unit per hour = 0.2931 W, 1 cubic foot per hour = 0.0283 m³/h, 1 degree = 0.01745 rad.

Note: All table entries have been rounded to three significant digits.

TABLE G2413.4(13) [402.4(27)]
SEMIRIGID COPPER TUBING

Gas	Undiluted Propane
Inlet Pressure	10.0 psi
Pressure Drop	1.0 psi
Specific Gravity	1.50

INTENDED USE		Sizing between first stage (high-pressure regulator) and second stage (low-pressure regulator).								
		TUBE SIZE (in.)								
Nominal	K & L	$^1/_4$	$^3/_8$	$^1/_2$	$^5/_8$	$^3/_4$	1	$1^1/_4$	$1^1/_2$	2
	ACR	$^3/_8$	$^1/_2$	$^5/_8$	$^3/_4$	$^7/_8$	$1^1/_8$	$1^3/_8$	—	—
Outside		0.375	0.500	0.625	0.750	0.875	1.125	1.375	1.625	2.125
Inside		0.305	0.402	0.527	0.652	0.745	0.995	1.245	1.481	1.959
Length (ft)		Capacity in Thousands of Btu per Hour								
10		513	1,060	2,150	3,760	5,330	11,400	20,500	32,300	67,400
20		352	727	1,480	2,580	3,670	7,830	14,100	22,200	46,300
30		283	584	1,190	2,080	2,940	6,290	11,300	17,900	37,200
40		242	500	1,020	1,780	2,520	5,380	9,690	15,300	31,800
50		215	443	901	1,570	2,230	4,770	8,590	13,500	28,200
60		194	401	816	1,430	2,020	4,320	7,780	12,300	25,600
70		179	369	751	1,310	1,860	3,980	7,160	11,300	23,500
80		166	343	699	1,220	1,730	3,700	6,660	10,500	21,900
90		156	322	655	1,150	1,630	3,470	6,250	9,850	20,500
100		147	304	619	1,080	1,540	3,280	5,900	9,310	19,400
125		131	270	549	959	1,360	2,910	5,230	8,250	17,200
150		118	244	497	869	1,230	2,630	4,740	7,470	15,600
175		109	225	457	799	1,130	2,420	4,360	6,880	14,300
200		101	209	426	744	1,060	2,250	4,060	6,400	13,300
250		90	185	377	659	935	2,000	3,600	5,670	11,800
300		81	168	342	597	847	1,810	3,260	5,140	10,700
350		75	155	314	549	779	1,660	3,000	4,730	9,840
400		70	144	292	511	725	1,550	2,790	4,400	9,160
450		65	135	274	480	680	1,450	2,620	4,130	8,590
500		62	127	259	453	643	1,370	2,470	3,900	8,120
550		59	121	246	430	610	1,300	2,350	3,700	7,710
600		56	115	235	410	582	1,240	2,240	3,530	7,350
650		54	111	225	393	558	1,190	2,140	3,380	7,040
700		51	106	216	378	536	1,140	2,060	3,250	6,770
750		50	102	208	364	516	1,100	1,980	3,130	6,520
800		48	99	201	351	498	1,060	1,920	3,020	6,290
850		46	96	195	340	482	1,030	1,850	2,920	6,090
900		45	93	189	330	468	1,000	1,800	2,840	5,910
950		44	90	183	320	454	970	1,750	2,750	5,730
1,000		42	88	178	311	442	944	1,700	2,680	5,580
1,100		40	83	169	296	420	896	1,610	2,540	5,300
1,200		38	79	161	282	400	855	1,540	2,430	5,050
1,300		37	76	155	270	383	819	1,470	2,320	4,840
1,400		35	73	148	260	368	787	1,420	2,230	4,650
1,500		34	70	143	250	355	758	1,360	2,150	4,480
1,600		33	68	138	241	343	732	1,320	2,080	4,330
1,700		32	66	134	234	331	708	1,270	2,010	4,190
1,800		31	64	130	227	321	687	1,240	1,950	4,060
1,900		30	62	126	220	312	667	1,200	1,890	3,940
2,000		29	60	122	214	304	648	1,170	1,840	3,830

For SI: 1 inch = 25.4 mm, 1 foot = 304.8 mm, 1 pound per square inch = 6.895 kPa, 1-inch water column = 0.2488 kPa,
     1 British thermal unit per hour = 0.2931 W, 1 cubic foot per hour = 0.0283 m³/h, 1 degree = 0.01745 rad.

Notes:
1. Table capacities are based on Type K copper tubing inside diameter (shown), which has the smallest inside diameter of the copper tubing products.
2. All table entries have been rounded to three significant digits.

TABLE G2413.4(14) [402.4(28)]
SEMIRIGID COPPER TUBING

Gas	Undiluted Propane
Inlet Pressure	11.0 in. w.c.
Pressure Drop	0.5 in. w.c.
Specific Gravity	1.50

INTENDED USE		Sizing between single- or second-stage (low-pressure regulator) and appliance.							
TUBE SIZE (in.)									
Nominal	K & L	$1/4$	$3/8$	$1/2$	$5/8$	$3/4$	1	$1 1/4$	$1 1/2$	2
	ACR	$3/8$	$1/2$	$5/8$	$3/4$	$7/8$	$1 1/8$	$1 3/8$	—	—
Outside		0.375	0.500	0.625	0.750	0.875	1.125	1.375	1.625	2.125
Inside		0.305	0.402	0.527	0.652	0.745	0.995	1.245	1.481	1.959
Length (ft)		**Capacity in Thousands of Btu per Hour**								
10		45	93	188	329	467	997	1,800	2,830	5,890
20		31	64	129	226	321	685	1,230	1,950	4,050
30		25	51	104	182	258	550	991	1,560	3,250
40		21	44	89	155	220	471	848	1,340	2,780
50		19	39	79	138	195	417	752	1,180	2,470
60		17	35	71	125	177	378	681	1,070	2,240
70		16	32	66	115	163	348	626	988	2,060
80		15	30	61	107	152	324	583	919	1,910
90		14	28	57	100	142	304	547	862	1,800
100		13	27	54	95	134	287	517	814	1,700
125		11	24	48	84	119	254	458	722	1,500
150		10	21	44	76	108	230	415	654	1,360
175		NA	20	40	70	99	212	382	602	1,250
200		NA	18	37	65	92	197	355	560	1,170
250		NA	16	33	58	82	175	315	496	1,030
300		NA	15	30	52	74	158	285	449	936
350		NA	14	28	48	68	146	262	414	861
400		NA	13	26	45	63	136	244	385	801
450		NA	12	24	42	60	127	229	361	752
500		NA	11	23	40	56	120	216	341	710
550		NA	11	22	38	53	114	205	324	674
600		NA	10	21	36	51	109	196	309	643
650		NA	NA	20	34	49	104	188	296	616
700		NA	NA	19	33	47	100	180	284	592
750		NA	NA	18	32	45	96	174	274	570
800		NA	NA	18	31	44	93	168	264	551
850		NA	NA	17	30	42	90	162	256	533
900		NA	NA	17	29	41	87	157	248	517
950		NA	NA	16	28	40	85	153	241	502
1,000		NA	NA	16	27	39	83	149	234	488
1,100		NA	NA	15	26	37	78	141	223	464
1,200		NA	NA	14	25	35	75	135	212	442
1,300		NA	NA	14	24	34	72	129	203	423
1,400		NA	NA	13	23	32	69	124	195	407
1,500		NA	NA	13	22	31	66	119	188	392
1,600		NA	NA	12	21	30	64	115	182	378
1,700		NA	NA	12	20	29	62	112	176	366
1,800		NA	NA	11	20	28	60	108	170	355
1,900		NA	NA	11	19	27	58	105	166	345
2,000		NA	NA	11	19	27	57	102	161	335

For SI: 1 inch = 25.4 mm, 1 foot = 304.8 mm, 1 pound per square inch = 6.895 kPa, 1-inch water column = 0.2488 kPa, 1 British thermal unit per hour = 0.2931 W, 1 cubic foot per hour = 0.0283 m³/h, 1 degree = 0.01745 rad.

Notes:
1. Table capacities are based on Type K copper tubing inside diameter (shown), which has the smallest inside diameter of the copper tubing products.
2. NA means a flow of less than 10,000 Btu/hr.
3. All table entries have been rounded to three significant digits.

TABLE G2413.4(15) [402.4(29)]
SEMIRIGID COPPER TUBING

Gas	Undiluted Propane
Inlet Pressure	2.0 psi
Pressure Drop	1.0 psi
Specific Gravity	1.50

INTENDED USE		Tube sizing between 2 psig service and line pressure regulator.								
		TUBE SIZE (in.)								
Nominal	K & L	1/4	3/8	1/2	5/8	3/4	1	1 1/4	1 1/2	2
	ACR	3/8	1/2	5/8	3/4	7/8	1 1/8	1 3/8	—	—
Outside		0.375	0.500	0.625	0.750	0.875	1.125	1.375	1.625	2.125
Inside		0.305	0.402	0.527	0.652	0.745	0.995	1.245	1.481	1.959
Length (ft)		Capacity in Thousands of Btu per Hour								
10		413	852	1,730	3,030	4,300	9,170	16,500	26,000	54,200
20		284	585	1,190	2,080	2,950	6,310	11,400	17,900	37,300
30		228	470	956	1,670	2,370	5,060	9,120	14,400	29,900
40		195	402	818	1,430	2,030	4,330	7,800	12,300	25,600
50		173	356	725	1,270	1,800	3,840	6,920	10,900	22,700
60		157	323	657	1,150	1,630	3,480	6,270	9,880	20,600
70		144	297	605	1,060	1,500	3,200	5,760	9,090	18,900
80		134	276	562	983	1,390	2,980	5,360	8,450	17,600
90		126	259	528	922	1,310	2,790	5,030	7,930	16,500
100		119	245	498	871	1,240	2,640	4,750	7,490	15,600
125		105	217	442	772	1,100	2,340	4,210	6,640	13,800
150		95	197	400	700	992	2,120	3,820	6,020	12,500
175		88	181	368	644	913	1,950	3,510	5,540	11,500
200		82	168	343	599	849	1,810	3,270	5,150	10,700
250		72	149	304	531	753	1,610	2,900	4,560	9,510
300		66	135	275	481	682	1,460	2,620	4,140	8,610
350		60	124	253	442	628	1,340	2,410	3,800	7,920
400		56	116	235	411	584	1,250	2,250	3,540	7,370
450		53	109	221	386	548	1,170	2,110	3,320	6,920
500		50	103	209	365	517	1,110	1,990	3,140	6,530
550		47	97	198	346	491	1,050	1,890	2,980	6,210
600		45	93	189	330	469	1,000	1,800	2,840	5,920
650		43	89	181	316	449	959	1,730	2,720	5,670
700		41	86	174	304	431	921	1,660	2,620	5,450
750		40	82	168	293	415	888	1,600	2,520	5,250
800		39	80	162	283	401	857	1,540	2,430	5,070
850		37	77	157	274	388	829	1,490	2,350	4,900
900		36	75	152	265	376	804	1,450	2,280	4,750
950		35	72	147	258	366	781	1,410	2,220	4,620
1,000		34	71	143	251	356	760	1,370	2,160	4,490
1,100		32	67	136	238	338	721	1,300	2,050	4,270
1,200		31	64	130	227	322	688	1,240	1,950	4,070
1,300		30	61	124	217	309	659	1,190	1,870	3,900
1,400		28	59	120	209	296	633	1,140	1,800	3,740
1,500		27	57	115	201	286	610	1,100	1,730	3,610
1,600		26	55	111	194	276	589	1,060	1,670	3,480
1,700		26	53	108	188	267	570	1,030	1,620	3,370
1,800		25	51	104	182	259	553	1,000	1,570	3,270
1,900		24	50	101	177	251	537	966	1,520	3,170
2,000		23	48	99	172	244	522	940	1,480	3,090

For SI: 1 inch = 25.4 mm, 1 foot = 304.8 mm, 1 pound per square inch = 6.895 kPa, 1-inch water column = 0.2488 kPa,
1 British thermal unit per hour = 0.2931 W, 1 cubic foot per hour = 0.0283 m³/h, 1 degree = 0.01745 rad.

Notes:

1. Table capacities are based on Type K copper tubing inside diameter (shown), which has the smallest inside diameter of the copper tubing products.
2. All table entries have been rounded to three significant digits.

TABLE G2413.4(16) [402.4(30)]
CORRUGATED STAINLESS STEEL TUBING (CSST)

Gas	Undiluted Propane
Inlet Pressure	11.0 in. w.c.
Pressure Drop	0.5 in. w.c.
Specific Gravity	1.50

INTENDED USE	Sizing between single or second stage (low pressure) regulator and the appliance shutoff valve.													
	TUBE SIZE (EHD)													
Flow Designation	13	15	18	19	23	25	30	31	37	39	46	48	60	62
Length (ft)	**Capacity in Thousands of Btu per Hour**													
5	72	99	181	211	355	426	744	863	1,420	1,638	2,830	3,270	5,780	6,550
10	50	69	129	150	254	303	521	605	971	1,179	1,990	2,320	4,110	4,640
15	39	55	104	121	208	248	422	490	775	972	1,620	1,900	3,370	3,790
20	34	49	91	106	183	216	365	425	661	847	1,400	1,650	2,930	3,290
25	30	42	82	94	164	192	325	379	583	762	1,250	1,480	2,630	2,940
30	28	39	74	87	151	177	297	344	528	698	1,140	1,350	2,400	2,680
40	23	33	64	74	131	153	256	297	449	610	988	1,170	2,090	2,330
50	20	30	58	66	118	137	227	265	397	548	884	1,050	1,870	2,080
60	19	26	53	60	107	126	207	241	359	502	805	961	1,710	1,900
70	17	25	49	57	99	117	191	222	330	466	745	890	1,590	1,760
80	15	23	45	52	94	109	178	208	307	438	696	833	1,490	1,650
90	15	22	44	50	90	102	169	197	286	414	656	787	1,400	1,550
100	14	20	41	47	85	98	159	186	270	393	621	746	1,330	1,480
150	11	15	31	36	66	75	123	143	217	324	506	611	1,090	1,210
200	9	14	28	33	60	69	112	129	183	283	438	531	948	1,050
250	8	12	25	30	53	61	99	117	163	254	390	476	850	934
300	8	11	23	26	50	57	90	107	147	234	357	434	777	854

For SI: 1 inch = 25.4 mm, 1 foot = 304.8 mm, 1 pound per square inch = 6.895 kPa, 1-inch water column = 0.2488 kPa,
1 British thermal unit per hour = 0.2931 W, 1 cubic foot per hour = 0.0283 m³/h, 1 degree = 0.01745 rad.

Notes:

1. Table includes losses for four 90-degree bends and two end fittings. Tubing runs with larger numbers of bends and/or fittings shall be increased by an equivalent length of tubing to the following equation: $L = 1.3n$ where L is additional length (feet) of tubing and n is the number of additional fittings and/or bends.

2. EHD—Equivalent Hydraulic Diameter, which is a measure of the relative hydraulic efficiency between different tubing sizes. The greater the value of EHD, the greater the gas capacity of the tubing.

3. All table entries have been rounded to three significant digits.

TABLE G2413.4(17) [402.4(31)]
CORRUGATED STAINLESS STEEL TUBING (CSST)

Gas	Undiluted Propane
Inlet Pressure	2.0 psi
Pressure Drop	1.0 psi
Specific Gravity	1.50

INTENDED USE	Sizing between 2 psi service and the line pressure regulator.													
TUBE SIZE (EHD)														
Flow Designation	13	15	18	19	23	25	30	31	37	39	46	48	60	62
Length (ft)	Capacity in Thousands of Btu per Hour													
10	426	558	927	1,110	1,740	2,170	4,100	4,720	7,130	7,958	15,200	16,800	29,400	34,200
25	262	347	591	701	1,120	1,380	2,560	2,950	4,560	5,147	9,550	10,700	18,800	21,700
30	238	316	540	640	1,030	1,270	2,330	2,690	4,180	4,719	8,710	9,790	17,200	19,800
40	203	271	469	554	896	1,100	2,010	2,320	3,630	4,116	7,530	8,500	14,900	17,200
50	181	243	420	496	806	986	1,790	2,070	3,260	3,702	6,730	7,610	13,400	15,400
75	147	196	344	406	663	809	1,460	1,690	2,680	3,053	5,480	6,230	11,000	12,600
80	140	189	333	393	643	768	1,410	1,630	2,590	2,961	5,300	6,040	10,600	12,200
100	124	169	298	350	578	703	1,260	1,450	2,330	2,662	4,740	5,410	9,530	10,900
150	101	137	245	287	477	575	1,020	1,180	1,910	2,195	3,860	4,430	7,810	8,890
200	86	118	213	248	415	501	880	1,020	1,660	1,915	3,340	3,840	6,780	7,710
250	77	105	191	222	373	448	785	910	1,490	1,722	2,980	3,440	6,080	6,900
300	69	96	173	203	343	411	716	829	1,360	1,578	2,720	3,150	5,560	6,300
400	60	82	151	175	298	355	616	716	1,160	1,376	2,350	2,730	4,830	5,460
500	53	72	135	158	268	319	550	638	1,030	1,237	2,100	2,450	4,330	4,880

For SI: 1 inch = 25.4 mm, 1 foot = 304.8 mm, 1 pound per square inch = 6.895 kPa, 1-inch water column = 0.2488 kPa,
1 British thermal unit per hour = 0.2931 W, 1 cubic foot per hour = 0.0283 m³/h, 1 degree = 0.01745 rad.

Notes:

1. Table does not include effect of pressure drop across the line regulator. Where regulator loss exceeds $^1/_2$ psi (based on 13 in. w.c. outlet pressure), DO NOT USE THIS TABLE. Consult with the regulator manufacturer for pressure drops and capacity factors. Pressure drops across a regulator can vary with flow rate.

2. CAUTION: Capacities shown in the table might exceed maximum capacity for a selected regulator. Consult with the regulator or tubing manufacturer for guidance.

3. Table includes losses for four 90-degree bends and two end fittings. Tubing runs with larger numbers of bends and/or fittings shall be increased by an equivalent length of tubing to the following equation: $L = 1.3n$ where L is additional length (feet) of tubing and n is the number of additional fittings and/or bends.

4. EHD—Equivalent Hydraulic Diameter, which is a measure of the relative hydraulic efficiency between different tubing sizes. The greater the value of EHD, the greater the gas capacity of the tubing.

5. All table entries have been rounded to three significant digits.

TABLE G2413.4(18) [402.4(32)]
CORRUGATED STAINLESS STEEL TUBING (CSST)

Gas	Undiluted Propane
Inlet Pressure	5.0 psi
Pressure Drop	3.5 psi
Specific Gravity	1.50

	TUBE SIZE (EHD)													
Flow Designation	13	15	18	19	23	25	30	31	37	39	46	48	60	62
Length (ft)	Capacity in Thousands of Btu per Hour													
10	826	1,070	1,710	2,060	3,150	4,000	7,830	8,950	13,100	14,441	28,600	31,200	54,400	63,800
25	509	664	1,090	1,310	2,040	2,550	4,860	5,600	8,400	9,339	18,000	19,900	34,700	40,400
30	461	603	999	1,190	1,870	2,340	4,430	5,100	7,680	8,564	16,400	18,200	31,700	36,900
40	396	520	867	1,030	1,630	2,030	3,820	4,400	6,680	7,469	14,200	15,800	27,600	32,000
50	352	463	777	926	1,460	1,820	3,410	3,930	5,990	6,717	12,700	14,100	24,700	28,600
75	284	376	637	757	1,210	1,490	2,770	3,190	4,920	5,539	10,300	11,600	20,300	23,400
80	275	363	618	731	1,170	1,450	2,680	3,090	4,770	5,372	9,990	11,200	19,600	22,700
100	243	324	553	656	1,050	1,300	2,390	2,760	4,280	4,830	8,930	10,000	17,600	20,300
150	196	262	453	535	866	1,060	1,940	2,240	3,510	3,983	7,270	8,210	14,400	16,600
200	169	226	393	464	755	923	1,680	1,930	3,050	3,474	6,290	7,130	12,500	14,400
250	150	202	352	415	679	828	1,490	1,730	2,740	3,124	5,620	6,390	11,200	12,900
300	136	183	322	379	622	757	1,360	1,570	2,510	2,865	5,120	5,840	10,300	11,700
400	117	158	279	328	542	657	1,170	1,360	2,180	2,498	4,430	5,070	8,920	10,200
500	104	140	251	294	488	589	1,050	1,210	1,950	2,247	3,960	4,540	8,000	9,110

For SI: 1 inch = 25.4 mm, 1 foot = 304.8 mm, 1 pound per square inch = 6.895 kPa, 1-inch water column = 0.2488 kPa,
1 British thermal unit per hour = 0.2931 W, 1 cubic foot per hour = 0.0283 m³/h, 1 degree = 0.01745 rad.

Notes:

1. Table does not include effect of pressure drop across line regulator. Where regulator loss exceeds 1 psi, DO NOT USE THIS TABLE. Consult with the regulator manufacturer for pressure drops and capacity factors. Pressure drop across regulator can vary with the flow rate.

2. CAUTION: Capacities shown in the table might exceed maximum capacity of selected regulator. Consult with the tubing manufacturer for guidance.

3. Table includes losses for four 90-degree bends and two end fittings. Tubing runs with larger numbers of bends and/or fittings shall be increased by an equivalent length of tubing to the following equation: $L = 1.3n$ where L is additional length (feet) of tubing and n is the number of additional fittings and/or bends.

4. EHD— Equivalent Hydraulic Diameter, which is a measure of the relative hydraulic efficiency between different tubing sizes. The greater the value of EHD, the greater the gas capacity of the tubing.

5. All table entries have been rounded to three significant digits.

TABLE G2413.4(19) [402.4(33)]
POLYETHYLENE PLASTIC PIPE

Gas	Undiluted Propane
Inlet Pressure	11.0 in. w.c.
Pressure Drop	0.5 in. w.c.
Specific Gravity	1.50

INTENDED USE	PE pipe sizing between integral 2-stage regulator at tank or second stage (low pressure regulator) and building.					
	PIPE SIZE (in.)					
Nominal OD	$^1/_2$	$^3/_4$	1	$1^1/_4$	$1^1/_2$	2
Designation	SDR 9.33	SDR 11.0	SDR 11.00	SDR 10.00	SDR 11.00	SDR 11.00
Actual ID	0.660	0.860	1.077	1.328	1.554	1.943
Length (ft)	**Capacity in Thousands of Btu per Hour**					
10	340	680	1,230	2,130	3,210	5,770
20	233	468	844	1,460	2,210	3,970
30	187	375	677	1,170	1,770	3,180
40	160	321	580	1,000	1,520	2,730
50	142	285	514	890	1,340	2,420
60	129	258	466	807	1,220	2,190
70	119	237	428	742	1,120	2,010
80	110	221	398	690	1,040	1,870
90	103	207	374	648	978	1,760
100	98	196	353	612	924	1,660
125	87	173	313	542	819	1,470
150	78	157	284	491	742	1,330
175	72	145	261	452	683	1,230
200	67	135	243	420	635	1,140
250	60	119	215	373	563	1,010
300	54	108	195	338	510	916
350	50	99	179	311	469	843
400	46	92	167	289	436	784
450	43	87	157	271	409	736
500	41	82	148	256	387	695

For SI: 1 inch = 25.4 mm, 1 foot = 304.8 mm, 1 pound per square inch = 6.895 kPa, 1-inch water column = 0.2488 kPa,
   1 British thermal unit per hour = 0.2931 W, 1 cubic foot per hour = 0.0283 m³/h, 1 degree = 0.01745 rad.

Note: All table entries have been rounded to three significant digits.

**TABLE G2413.4(20) [402.4(34)]
POLYETHYLENE PLASTIC PIPE**

Gas	Undiluted Propane
Inlet Pressure	2.0 psi
Pressure Drop	1.0 psi
Specific Gravity	1.50

INTENDED USE	PE pipe sizing between 2 psig service regulator and line pressure regulator.					
	PIPE SIZE (in.)					
Nominal OD	$^1/_2$	$^3/_4$	1	$1^1/_4$	$1^1/_2$	2
Designation	SDR 9.33	SDR 11.0	SDR 11.00	SDR 10.00	SDR 11.00	SDR 11.00
Actual ID	0.660	0.860	1.077	1.328	1.554	1.943
Length (ft)	**Capacity in Thousands of Btu per Hour**					
10	3,130	6,260	11,300	19,600	29,500	53,100
20	2,150	4,300	7,760	13,400	20,300	36,500
30	1,730	3,450	6,230	10,800	16,300	29,300
40	1,480	2,960	5,330	9,240	14,000	25,100
50	1,310	2,620	4,730	8,190	12,400	22,200
60	1,190	2,370	4,280	7,420	11,200	20,100
70	1,090	2,180	3,940	6,830	10,300	18,500
80	1,010	2,030	3,670	6,350	9,590	17,200
90	952	1,910	3,440	5,960	9,000	16,200
100	899	1,800	3,250	5,630	8,500	15,300
125	797	1,600	2,880	4,990	7,530	13,500
150	722	1,450	2,610	4,520	6,830	12,300
175	664	1,330	2,400	4,160	6,280	11,300
200	618	1,240	2,230	3,870	5,840	10,500
250	548	1,100	1,980	3,430	5,180	9,300
300	496	994	1,790	3,110	4,690	8,430
350	457	914	1,650	2,860	4,320	7,760
400	425	851	1,530	2,660	4,020	7,220
450	399	798	1,440	2,500	3,770	6,770
500	377	754	1,360	2,360	3,560	6,390
550	358	716	1,290	2,240	3,380	6,070
600	341	683	1,230	2,140	3,220	5,790
650	327	654	1,180	2,040	3,090	5,550
700	314	628	1,130	1,960	2,970	5,330
750	302	605	1,090	1,890	2,860	5,140
800	292	585	1,050	1,830	2,760	4,960
850	283	566	1,020	1,770	2,670	4,800
900	274	549	990	1,710	2,590	4,650
950	266	533	961	1,670	2,520	4,520
1,000	259	518	935	1,620	2,450	4,400
1,100	246	492	888	1,540	2,320	4,170
1,200	234	470	847	1,470	2,220	3,980
1,300	225	450	811	1,410	2,120	3,810
1,400	216	432	779	1,350	2,040	3,660
1,500	208	416	751	1,300	1,960	3,530
1,600	201	402	725	1,260	1,900	3,410
1,700	194	389	702	1,220	1,840	3,300
1,800	188	377	680	1,180	1,780	3,200
1,900	183	366	661	1,140	1,730	3,110
2,000	178	356	643	1,110	1,680	3,020

For SI: 1 inch = 25.4 mm, 1 foot = 304.8 mm, 1 pound per square inch = 6.895 kPa, 1-inch water column = 0.2488 kPa,
1 British thermal unit per hour = 0.2931 W, 1 cubic foot per hour = 0.0283 m³/h, 1 degree = 0.01745 rad.

Note: All table entries have been rounded to three significant digits.

**TABLE G2413.4(21) [402.4(35)]
POLYETHYLENE PLASTIC TUBING**

Gas	Undiluted Propane	
Inlet Pressure	11.0 in. w.c.	
Pressure Drop	0.5 in. w.c.	
Specific Gravity	1.50	

INTENDED USE	PE pipe sizing between integral 2-stage regulator at tank or second stage (low pressure regulator) and building.	
	Plastic Tubing Size (CTS) (in.)	
Nominal OD	$^1/_2$	1
Designation	SDR 7.00	SDR 11.00
Actual ID	0.445	0.927
Length (ft)	**Capacity in Cubic Feet of Gas per Hour**	
10	121	828
20	83	569
30	67	457
40	57	391
50	51	347
60	46	314
70	42	289
80	39	269
90	37	252
100	35	238
125	31	211
150	28	191
175	26	176
200	24	164
225	22	154
250	21	145
275	20	138
300	19	132
350	18	121
400	16	113
450	15	106
500	15	100

For SI: 1 inch = 25.4 mm, 1 foot = 304.8 mm, 1 pound per square inch = 6.895 kPa, 1-inch water column = 0.2488 kPa, 1 British thermal unit per hour = 0.2931 W, 1 cubic foot per hour = 0.0283 m³/h, 1 degree = 0.01745 rad.

Note: All table entries have been rounded to three significant digits.

SECTION G2414 (403)
PIPING MATERIALS

G2414.1 (403.1) General. Materials used for piping systems shall comply with the requirements of this chapter or shall be *approved*.

G2414.2 (403.2) Used materials. *Pipe*, fittings, *valves* or other materials shall not be used again unless they are free of foreign

materials and have been ascertained to be adequate for the service intended.

G2414.3 (403.3) Other materials. Material not covered by the standards specifications listed herein shall be investigated and tested to determine that it is safe and suitable for the proposed service, and, in addition, shall be recommended for that service by the manufacturer and shall be *approved* by the *code official*.

G2414.4 (403.4) Metallic pipe. Metallic *pipe* shall comply with Sections G2414.4.1 and G2414.4.2.

G2414.4.1 (403.4.1) Cast iron. Cast-iron *pipe* shall not be used.

G2414.4.2 (403.4.2) Steel. Steel and wrought-iron *pipe* shall be at least of standard weight (Schedule 40) and shall comply with one of the following:

1. ASME B 36.10, 10M;

2. ASTM A 53/A 53M; or

3. ASTM A 106.

G2414.5 (403.5) Metallic tubing. Seamless copper, aluminum alloy or steel *tubing* shall be permitted to be used with gases not corrosive to such material.

G2414.5.1 (403.5.1) Steel tubing. Steel *tubing* shall comply with ASTM A 254.

G2414.5.2 (403.5.2) Copper tubing. Copper *tubing* shall comply with standard Type K or L of ASTM B 88 or ASTM B 280.

Copper and brass *tubing* shall not be used if the gas contains more than an average of 0.3 grains of hydrogen sulfide per 100 standard cubic feet of gas (0.7 milligrams per 100 liters).

G2414.5.3 (403.5.4) Corrugated stainless steel tubing. Corrugated stainless steel *tubing* shall be listed in accordance with ANSI LC 1/CSA 6.26.

G2414.6 (403.6) Plastic pipe, tubing and fittings. *Plastic pipe*, *tubing* and fittings used to supply *fuel gas* shall conform to ASTM D 2513. *Pipe* shall be marked "Gas" and "ASTM D 2513."

G2414.6.1 (403.6.1) Anodeless risers. *Anodeless risers* shall comply with the following:

1. Factory-assembled *anodeless risers* shall be recommended by the manufacturer for the gas used and shall be leak-tested by the manufacturer in accordance with written procedures.

2. Service head adapters and field-assembled *anodeless risers* incorporating service head adapters shall be recommended by the manufacturer for the gas used by the manufacturer and shall be designed certified to meet the requirements of Category I of ASTM D 2513, and U.S. Department of Transportation, Code of Federal Regulations, Title 49, Part 192.281(e). The manufacturer shall provide the user qualified installation instructions as prescribed by the U.S. Department of Transportation, Code of Federal Regulations, Title 49, Part 192.283(b).

G2414.6.2 (403.6.2) LP-gas systems. The use of plastic *pipe, tubing* and fittings in undiluted *liquefied petroleum gas piping systems* shall be in accordance with NFPA 58.

G2414.6.3 (403.6.3) Regulator vent piping. Plastic *pipe, tubing* and fittings used to connect *regulator* vents to remote vent terminations shall be of PVC conforming to ANSI/UL 651. PVC vent *piping* shall not be installed indoors.

G2414.7 (403.7) Workmanship and defects. *Pipe* or *tubing* and fittings shall be clear and free from cutting burrs and defects in structure or threading, and shall be thoroughly brushed, and chip and scale blown.

Defects in *pipe* or *tubing* or fittings shall not be repaired. Defective *pipe, tubing* or fittings shall be replaced. (See Section G2417.1.2.)

G2414.8 (403.8) Protective coating. Where in contact with material or atmosphere exerting a corrosive action, metallic *piping* and fittings coated with a corrosion-resistant material shall be used. External or internal coatings or linings used on *piping* or components shall not be considered as adding strength.

G2414.9 (403.9) Metallic pipe threads. Metallic *pipe* and fitting threads shall be taper *pipe* threads and shall comply with ASME B1.20.1.

G2414.9.1 (403.9.1) Damaged threads. *Pipe* with threads that are stripped, chipped, corroded or otherwise damaged shall not be used. If a weld opens during the operation of cutting or threading, that portion of the *pipe* shall not be used.

G2414.9.2 (403.9.2) Number of threads. Field threading of metallic *pipe* shall be in accordance with Table G2414.9.2.

TABLE G2414.9.2 (403.9.2)
SPECIFICATIONS FOR THREADING METALLIC PIPE

IRON PIPE SIZE (inches)	APPROXIMATE LENGTH OF THREADED PORTION (inches)	APPROXIMATE NO. OF THREADS TO BE CUT
$^1/_2$	$^3/_4$	10
$^3/_4$	$^3/_4$	10
1	$^7/_8$	10
$1^1/_4$	1	11
$1^1/_2$	1	11

For SI: 1 inch = 25.4 mm.

G2414.9.3 (403.9.3) Thread compounds. Thread (joint) compounds (*pipe* dope) shall be resistant to the action of *liquefied petroleum gas* or to any other chemical constituents of the gases to be conducted through the *piping*.

G2414.10 (403.10) Metallic piping joints and fittings. The type of *piping* joint used shall be suitable for the pressure-temperature conditions and shall be selected giving consideration to joint tightness and mechanical strength under the service conditions. The joint shall be able to sustain the maximum end force due to the internal pressure and any additional forces due to temperature expansion or contraction, vibration, fatigue, or to the weight of the *pipe* and its contents.

G2414.10.1 (403.10.1) Pipe joints. *Pipe* joints shall be threaded, flanged, brazed or welded. Where nonferrous *pipe* is brazed, the *brazing* materials shall have a melting point in excess of 1,000°F (538°C). *Brazing* alloys shall not contain more than 0.05-percent phosphorus.

G2414.10.2 (403.10.2) Tubing joints. *Tubing* joints shall be made with *approved gas tubing* fittings or be brazed with a material having a melting point in excess of 1,000°F (538°C) or made with press-connect fittings complying with ANSI LC-4. *Brazing alloys* shall not contain more than 0.05-percent phosphorus.

G2414.10.3 (403.10.3) Flared joints. *Flared joints* shall be used only in systems constructed from nonferrous *pipe* and *tubing* where experience or tests have demonstrated that the joint is suitable for the conditions and where provisions are made in the design to prevent separation of the joints.

G2414.10.4 (403.10.4) Metallic fittings. Metallic fittings, including *valves*, strainers and filters shall comply with the following:

1. Fittings used with steel or wrought-iron *pipe* shall be steel, brass, bronze, malleable iron, ductile iron or cast iron.

2. Fittings used with copper or brass *pipe* shall be copper, brass or bronze.

3. Cast-iron bushings shall be prohibited.

4. Special fittings. Fittings such as couplings, proprietary-type joints, saddle tees, gland-type compression fittings, and flared, flareless or compression-type *tubing* fittings shall be: used within the fitting manufacturer's pressure-temperature recommendations; used within the service conditions anticipated with respect to vibration, fatigue, thermal expansion or contraction; installed or braced to prevent separation of the joint by gas pressure or external physical damage; and shall be *approved*.

G2414.11 (403.11) Plastic piping, joints and fittings. Plastic *pipe, tubing* and fittings shall be joined in accordance with the manufacturers' instructions. Such joints shall comply with the following:

1. The joints shall be designed and installed so that the longitudinal pull-out resistance of the joints will be at least equal to the tensile strength of the plastic *piping* material.

2. Heat-fusion joints shall be made in accordance with qualified procedures that have been established and proven by test to produce gas-tight joints at least as strong as the *pipe* or *tubing* being joined. Joints shall be made with the joining method recommended by the *pipe* manufacturer. Heat fusion fittings shall be marked "ASTM D 2513."

3. Where compression-type *mechanical joints* are used, the gasket material in the fitting shall be compatible with the plastic *piping* and with the gas distributed by the system. An internal tubular rigid stiffener shall be used in conjunction with the fitting. The stiffener shall be flush with the end of the *pipe* or *tubing* and shall extend at least to the outside end of the compression fitting when installed.

The stiffener shall be free of rough or sharp edges and shall not be a force fit in the plastic. Split tubular stiffeners shall not be used.

4. Plastic *piping* joints and fittings for use in *liquefied petroleum gas piping systems* shall be in accordance with NFPA 58.

SECTION G2415 (404)
PIPING SYSTEM INSTALLATION

G2415.1 (404.1) Prohibited locations. *Piping* shall not be installed in or through a ducted supply, return or exhaust, or a clothes chute, *chimney* or gas vent, dumbwaiter or elevator *shaft*. *Piping* installed downstream of the *point of delivery* shall not extend through any townhouse unit other than the unit served by such *piping*.

G2415.2 (404.2) Piping in solid partitions and walls. *Concealed piping* shall not be located in solid partitions and solid walls, unless installed in a chase or casing.

G2415.3 (404.3) Piping in concealed locations. Portions of a *piping system* installed in *concealed locations* shall not have unions, *tubing* fittings, right and left couplings, bushings, compression couplings, and swing joints made by combinations of fittings.

Exceptions:

1. *Tubing* joined by *brazing*.

2. Fittings listed for use in *concealed locations*.

G2415.4 (404.4) Underground penetrations prohibited. *Gas piping* shall not penetrate building foundation walls at any point below grade. *Gas piping* shall enter and exit a building at a point above grade and the annular space between the *pipe* and the wall shall be sealed.

G2415.5 (404.5) Protection against physical damage. In *concealed locations*, where *piping* other than black or galvanized steel is installed through holes or notches in wood studs, joists, rafters or similar members less than $1^1/_2$ inches (38 mm) from the nearest edge of the member, the *pipe* shall be protected by shield plates. Protective steel shield plates having a minimum thickness of 0.0575-inch (1.463 mm) (No. 16 Gage) shall cover the area of the *pipe* where the member is notched or bored and shall extend a minimum of 4 inches (102 mm) above sole plates, below top plates and to each side of a stud, joist or rafter.

G2415.6 (404.6) Piping in solid floors. *Piping* in solid floors shall be laid in channels in the floor and covered in a manner that will allow access to the *piping* with a minimum amount of damage to the building. Where such *piping* is subject to exposure to excessive moisture or corrosive substances, the *piping* shall be protected in an *approved* manner. As an alternative to installation in channels, the *piping* shall be installed in a conduit of Schedule 40 steel, wrought iron, PVC or ABS *pipe* in accordance with Section G2415.6.1 or G2415.6.2.

G2415.6.1 (404.6.1) Conduit with one end terminating outdoors. The conduit shall extend into an occupiable portion of the building and, at the point where the conduit terminates in the building, the space between the conduit and the *gas piping* shall be sealed to prevent the possible entrance of any gas leakage. The conduit shall extend not less than 2 inches (51 mm) beyond the point where the *pipe* emerges from the floor. If the end sealing is capable of withstanding the full pressure of the gas *pipe*, the conduit shall be designed for the same pressure as the *pipe*. Such conduit shall extend not less than 4 inches (102 mm) outside of the building, shall be vented above grade to the outdoors and shall be installed to prevent the entrance of water and insects.

G2415.6.2 (404.6.2) Conduit with both ends terminating indoors. Where the conduit originates and terminates within the same building, the conduit shall originate and terminate in an accessible portion of the building and shall not be sealed. The conduit shall extend not less than 2 inches (51 mm) beyond the point where the *pipe* emerges from the floor.

G2415.7 (404.7) Above-ground piping outdoors. All *piping* installed outdoors shall be elevated not less than $3^1/_2$ inches (152 mm) above ground and where installed across roof surfaces, shall be elevated not less than $3^1/_2$ inches (152 mm) above the roof surface. *Piping* installed above ground, outdoors, and installed across the surface of roofs shall be securely supported and located where it will be protected from physical damage. Where passing through an outside wall, the *piping* shall also be protected against corrosion by coating or wrapping with an inert material. Where *piping* is encased in a protective *pipe* sleeve, the annular space between the *piping* and the sleeve shall be sealed.

G2415.8 (404.8) Isolation. Metallic *piping* and metallic *tubing* that conveys *fuel gas* from an LP-gas storage container shall be provided with an *approved* dielectric fitting to electrically isolate the underground portion of the *pipe* or tube from the above ground portion that enters a building. Such dielectric fitting shall be installed aboveground outdoors.

G2415.9 (404.9) Protection against corrosion. Metallic *pipe* or *tubing* exposed to corrosive action, such as soil condition or moisture, shall be protected in an *approved* manner. Zinc coatings (galvanizing) shall not be deemed adequate protection for *gas piping* underground. Where dissimilar metals are joined underground, an insulating coupling or fitting shall be used. *Piping* shall not be laid in contact with cinders.

G2415.9.1 (404.9.1) Prohibited use. Uncoated threaded or socket welded joints shall not be used in *piping* in contact with soil or where internal or external crevice corrosion is known to occur.

G2415.9.2 (404.9.2) Protective coatings and wrapping. *Pipe* protective coatings and wrappings shall be *approved* for the application and shall be factory applied.

Exception: Where installed in accordance with the manufacturer's installation instructions, field application of coatings and wrappings shall be permitted for *pipe* nipples, fittings and locations where the factory coating or wrapping has been damaged or necessarily removed at joints.

G2415.10 (404.10) Minimum burial depth. Underground *piping systems* shall be installed a minimum depth of 12 inches (305 mm) below grade, except as provided for in Section G2415.10.1.

G2415.10.1 (404.10.1) Individual outside appliances. Individual lines to outside lights, grills or other *appliances* shall be installed a minimum of 8 inches (203 mm) below finished grade, provided that such installation is *approved* and is installed in locations not susceptible to physical damage.

G2415.11 (404.11) Trenches. The trench shall be graded so that the *pipe* has a firm, substantially continuous bearing on the bottom of the trench.

G2415.12 (404.12) Piping underground beneath buildings. *Piping* installed underground beneath buildings is prohibited except where the *piping* is encased in a conduit of wrought iron, plastic *pipe*, steel *pipe* or other *approved* conduit material designed to withstand the superimposed loads. The conduit shall be protected from corrosion in accordance with Section G2415.9 and shall be installed in accordance with Section G2415.12.1 or G2415.12.2.

G2415.12.1 (404.12.1) Conduit with one end terminating outdoors. The conduit shall extend into an occupiable portion of the building and, at the point where the conduit terminates in the building, the space between the conduit and the *gas piping* shall be sealed to prevent the possible entrance of any gas leakage. The conduit shall extend not less than 2 inches (51 mm) beyond the point where the *pipe* emerges from the floor. Where the end sealing is capable of withstanding the full pressure of the gas *pipe*, the conduit shall be designed for the same pressure as the *pipe*. Such conduit shall extend not less than 4 inches (102 mm) outside the building, shall be vented above grade to the outdoors and shall be installed so as to prevent the entrance of water and insects.

G2415.12.2 (404.12.2) Conduit with both ends terminating indoors. Where the conduit originates and terminates within the same building, the conduit shall originate and terminate in an accessible portion of the building and shall not be sealed. The conduit shall extend not less than 2 inches (51 mm) beyond the point where the *pipe* emerges from the floor.

G2415.13 (404.13) Outlet closures. Gas *outlets* that do not connect to *appliances* shall be capped gas tight.

Exception: Listed and labeled flush-mounted-type quick-disconnect devices and listed and labeled *gas convenience outlets* shall be installed in accordance with the manufacturer's installation instructions.

G2415.14 (404.14) Location of outlets. The unthreaded portion of *piping outlets* shall extend not less than l inch (25 mm) through finished ceilings and walls and where extending through floors, outdoor patios and slabs, shall not be less than 2 inches (51 mm) above them. The *outlet* fitting or *piping* shall be securely supported. *Outlets* shall not be placed behind doors. *Outlets* shall be located in the room or space where the *appliance* is installed.

Exception: Listed and labeled flush-mounted-type quick-disconnect devices and listed and labeled *gas convenience outlets* shall be installed in accordance with the manufacturer's installation instructions.

G2415.15 (404.15) Plastic pipe. The installation of plastic *pipe* shall comply with Sections G2415.15.1 through G2415.15.3.

G2415.15.1 (404.15.1) Limitations. Plastic *pipe* shall be installed outdoors underground only. Plastic *pipe* shall not be used within or under any building or slab or be operated at pressures greater than 100 psig (689 kPa) for natural gas or 30 psig (207 kPa) for LP-gas.

Exceptions:

1. Plastic *pipe* shall be permitted to terminate above ground outside of buildings where installed in premanufactured *anodeless risers* or service head adapter risers that are installed in accordance with the manufacturer's installation instructions.

2. Plastic *pipe* shall be permitted to terminate with a wall head adapter within buildings where the plastic *pipe* is inserted in a *piping* material for *fuel gas* use in buildings.

3. Plastic pipe shall be permitted under outdoor patio, walkway and driveway slabs provided that the burial depth complies with Section G2415.10.

G2415.15.2 (404.15.2) Connections. Connections outdoors and underground between metallic and plastic *piping* shall be made only with transition fittings conforming to ASTM D 2513 Category I or ASTM F 1973.

G2415.15.3 (404.15.3) Tracer. A yellow insulated copper tracer wire or other *approved* conductor shall be installed adjacent to underground nonmetallic *piping*. Access shall be provided to the tracer wire or the tracer wire shall terminate above ground at each end of the nonmetallic *piping*. The tracer wire size shall not be less than 18 AWG and the insulation type shall be suitable for direct burial.

G2415.16 (404.16) Prohibited devices. A device shall not be placed inside the *piping* or fittings that will reduce the cross-sectional area or otherwise obstruct the free flow of gas.

Exception: *Approved* gas filters.

G2415.17 (404.17) Testing of piping. Before any system of *piping* is put in service or concealed, it shall be tested to ensure that it is gas tight. Testing, inspection and purging of *piping systems* shall comply with Section G2417.

SECTION G2416 (405)
PIPING BENDS AND CHANGES IN DIRECTION

G2416.1 (405.1) General. Changes in direction of *pipe* shall be permitted to be made by the use of fittings, factory bends or field bends.

G2416.2 (405.2) Metallic pipe. Metallic *pipe* bends shall comply with the following:

1. Bends shall be made only with bending tools and procedures intended for that purpose.

2. All bends shall be smooth and free from buckling, cracks or other evidence of mechanical damage.

3. The longitudinal weld of the *pipe* shall be near the neutral axis of the bend.

4. *Pipe* shall not be bent through an arc of more than 90 degrees (1.6 rad).

5. The inside radius of a bend shall be not less than six times the outside diameter of the *pipe*.

G2416.3 (405.3) Plastic pipe. Plastic *pipe* bends shall comply with the following:

1. The *pipe* shall not be damaged and the internal diameter of the *pipe* shall not be effectively reduced.

2. Joints shall not be located in *pipe* bends.

3. The radius of the inner curve of such bends shall not be less than 25 times the inside diameter of the *pipe*.

4. Where the *piping* manufacturer specifies the use of special bending tools or procedures, such tools or procedures shall be used.

SECTION G2417 (406)
INSPECTION, TESTING AND PURGING

G2417.1 (406.1) General. Prior to acceptance and initial operation, all *piping* installations shall be inspected and *pressure tested* to determine that the materials, design, fabrication, and installation practices comply with the requirements of this *code*.

G2417.1.1 (406.1.1) Inspections. Inspection shall consist of visual examination, during or after manufacture, fabrication, assembly or *pressure tests* as appropriate.

G2417.1.2 (406.1.2) Repairs and additions. In the event repairs or additions are made after the *pressure test*, the affected *piping* shall be tested.

Minor repairs and additions are not required to be *pressure tested* provided that the work is inspected and connections are tested with a noncorrosive leak-detecting fluid or other *approved* leak-detecting methods.

G2417.1.3 (406.1.3) New branches. Where new branches are installed to new *appliances*, only the newly installed branches shall be required to be *pressure tested*. Connections between the new *piping* and the existing *piping* shall be tested with a noncorrosive leak-detecting fluid or other *approved* leak-detecting methods.

G2417.1.4 (406.1.4) Section testing. A *piping system* shall be permitted to be tested as a complete unit or in sections. Under no circumstances shall a *valve* in a line be used as a bulkhead between gas in one section of the *piping system* and test medium in an adjacent section, unless two *valves* are installed in series with a valved "tell-tale" located between these *valves*. A valve shall not be subjected to the test pressure unless it can be determined that the valve, including the valve closing mechanism, is designed to safely withstand the test pressure.

G2417.1.5 (406.1.5) Regulators and valve assemblies. *Regulator* and valve assemblies fabricated independently of the *piping system* in which they are to be installed shall be permitted to be tested with inert gas or air at the time of fabrication.

G2417.2 (406.2) Test medium. The test medium shall be air, nitrogen, carbon dioxide or an inert gas. Oxygen shall not be used.

G2417.3 (406.3) Test preparation. *Pipe* joints, including welds, shall be left exposed for examination during the test.

> **Exception:** Covered or *concealed pipe* end joints that have been previously tested in accordance with this *code*.

G2417.3.1 (406.3.1) Expansion joints. Expansion joints shall be provided with temporary restraints, if required, for the additional thrust load under test.

G2417.3.2 (406.3.2) Equipment isolation. *Equipment* that is not to be included in the test shall be either disconnected from the *piping* or isolated by blanks, blind flanges or caps.

G2417.3.3 (406.3.3) Appliance and equipment disconnection. Where the *piping system* is connected to *appliances* or *equipment* designed for operating pressures of less than the test pressure, such *appliances* or *equipment* shall be isolated from the *piping system* by disconnecting them and capping the *outlet(s)*.

G2417.3.4 (406.3.4) Valve isolation. Where the *piping system* is connected to *appliances* or *equipment* designed for operating pressures equal to or greater than the test pressure, such *appliances* or *equipment* shall be isolated from the *piping system* by closing the individual *appliance* or *equipment* shutoff valve(s).

G2417.3.5 (406.3.5) Testing precautions. All testing of *piping systems* shall be done with due regard for the safety of employees and the public during the test. Prior to testing, the interior of the *pipe* shall be cleared of all foreign material.

G2417.4 (406.4) Test pressure measurement. Test pressure shall be measured with a manometer or with a pressure-measuring device designed and calibrated to read, record, or indicate a pressure loss caused by leakage during the *pressure test* period. The source of pressure shall be isolated before the *pressure tests* are made. Mechanical gauges used to measure test pressures shall have a range such that the highest end of the scale is not greater than five times the test pressure.

G2417.4.1 (406.4.1) Test pressure. The test pressure to be used shall be not less than one and one-half times the proposed maximum working pressure, but not less than 3 psig (20 kPa gauge), irrespective of design pressure. Where the test pressure exceeds 125 psig (862 kPa gauge), the test pressure shall not exceed a value that produces a hoop stress in the *piping* greater than 50 percent of the specified minimum yield strength of the *pipe*.

G2417.4.2 (406.4.2) Test duration. The test duration shall be not less than 10 minutes.

G2417.5 (406.5) Detection of leaks and defects. The *piping system* shall withstand the test pressure specified without showing any evidence of leakage or other defects. Any reduction of test pressures as indicated by pressure gauges shall be deemed to indicate the presence of a leak unless such reduction can be readily attributed to some other cause.

G2417.5.1 (406.5.1) Detection methods. The leakage shall be located by means of an *approved* combustible gas detector, a noncorrosive leak detection fluid or an equivalent nonflammable solution. Matches, candles, open flames or other methods that could provide a source of ignition shall not be used.

G2417.5.2 (406.5.2) Corrections. Where leakage or other defects are located, the affected portion of the *piping system* shall be repaired or replaced and retested.

G2417.6 (406.6) Piping system and equipment leakage check. Leakage checking of systems and *equipment* shall be in accordance with Sections G2417.6.1 through G2417.6.4.

G2417.6.1 (406.6.1) Test gases. *Fuel gas* shall be permitted to be used for *leak checks* in *piping systems* that have been tested in accordance with Section G2417.

G2417.6.2 (406.6.2) Turning gas on. During the process of turning gas on into a system of new *gas piping*, the entire system shall be inspected to determine that there are no open fittings or ends and that all *valves* at unused outlets are closed and plugged or capped.

G2417.6.3 (406.6.3) Leak check. Immediately after the gas is turned on into a new system or into a system that has been initially restored after an interruption of service, the *piping system* shall be checked for leakage. Where leakage is indicated, the gas supply shall be shut off until the necessary repairs have been made.

G2417.6.4 (406.6.4) Placing appliances and equipment in operation. *Appliances* and *equipment* shall not be placed in operation until after the *piping system* has been checked for leakage and determined to be free of leakage and purged in accordance with Section G2417.7.2.

G2417.7 (406.7) Purging. Purging of *piping* shall comply with Sections G2417.7.1 through G2417.7.4.

G2417.7.1 (406.7.1) Removal from service. When *gas piping* is to be opened for servicing, addition or modification, the section to be worked on shall be turned off from the gas supply at the nearest convenient point, and the line pressure vented to the outdoors, or to ventilated areas of sufficient size to prevent accumulation of flammable mixtures.

G2417.7.2 (406.7.2) Placing in operation. When *piping* full of air is placed in operation, the air in the *piping* shall be displaced with *fuel gas*. The air can be safely displaced with *fuel gas* provided that a moderately rapid and continuous flow of *fuel gas* is introduced at one end of the line and air is vented out at the other end. The *fuel gas* flow should be continued without interruption until the vented gas is free of air. The point of discharge shall not be left unattended during purging. After purging, the vent shall then be closed.

G2417.7.3 (406.7.3) Discharge of purged gases. The open end of *piping systems* being purged shall not discharge into confined spaces or areas where there are sources of ignition unless precautions are taken to perform this operation in a safe manner by ventilation of the space, control or purging rate, and elimination of all hazardous conditions.

G2417.7.4 (406.7.4) Placing appliances and equipment in operation. After the *piping system* has been placed in operation, all *appliances* and *equipment* shall be purged and then placed in operation, as necessary.

SECTION G2418 (407)
PIPING SUPPORT

G2418.1 (407.1) General. *Piping* shall be provided with support in accordance with Section G2418.2.

G2418.2 (407.2) Design and installation. *Piping* shall be supported with metal *pipe* hooks, metal *pipe* straps, metal bands, metal brackets, metal hangers or building structural components suitable for the size of *piping*, of adequate strength and quality, and located at intervals so as to prevent or damp out excessive vibration. *Piping* shall be anchored to prevent undue strains on connected *appliances* and shall not be supported by other *piping*. *Pipe* hangers and supports shall conform to the requirements of MSS SP-58 and shall be spaced in accordance with Section G2424. Supports, hangers and anchors shall be installed so as not to interfere with the free expansion and contraction of the *piping* between anchors. All parts of the supporting *equipment* shall be designed and installed so that they will not be disengaged by movement of the supported *piping*.

SECTION G2419 (408)
DRIPS AND SLOPED PIPING

G2419.1 (408.1) Slopes. *Piping* for other than dry gas conditions shall be sloped not less than 0.25 inch in 15 feet (6.4 mm in 4572 mm) to prevent traps.

G2419.2 (408.2) Drips. Where wet gas exists, a *drip* shall be provided at any point in the line of *pipe* where *condensate* could collect. A *drip* shall also be provided at the outlet of the *meter* and shall be installed so as to constitute a trap wherein an accumulation of *condensate* will shut off the flow of gas before the *condensate* will run back into the *meter*.

G2419.3 (408.3) Location of drips. *Drips* shall be provided with *ready access* to permit cleaning or emptying. A *drip* shall not be located where the *condensate* is subject to freezing.

G2419.4 (408.4) Sediment trap. Where a sediment trap is not incorporated as part of the *appliance,* a sediment trap shall be installed downstream of the *appliance shutoff valve* as close to the inlet of the *appliance* as practical. The sediment trap shall be either a tee fitting having a capped nipple of any length installed vertically in the bottom-most opening of the tee or other device *approved* as an effective sediment trap. Illuminating *appliances*, ranges, *clothes dryers* and outdoor grills need not be so equipped.

SECTION G2420 (409)
GAS SHUTOFF VALVES

G2420.1 (409.1) General. *Piping systems* shall be provided with shutoff *valves* in accordance with this section.

G2420.1.1 (409.1.1) Valve approval. Shutoff *valves* shall be of an *approved* type; shall be constructed of materials compatible with the *piping*; and shall comply with the standard that is applicable for the pressure and application, in accordance with Table G2420.1.1.

G2420.1.2 (409.1.2) Prohibited locations. Shutoff *valves* shall be prohibited in *concealed locations* and *furnace plenums*.

G2420.1.3 (409.1.3) Access to shutoff valves. Shutoff *valves* shall be located in places so as to provide access for operation and shall be installed so as to be protected from damage.

G2420.2 (409.2) Meter valve. Every *meter* shall be equipped with a shutoff *valve* located on the supply side of the *meter*.

G2420.3 (409.3.2) Individual buildings. In a common system serving more than one building, shutoff *valves* shall be installed outdoors at each building.

G2420.4 (409.4) MP regulator valves. A listed shutoff valve shall be installed immediately ahead of each MP *regulator*.

G2420.5 (409.5) Appliance shutoff valve. Each *appliance* shall be provided with a shutoff *valve* in accordance with Section G2420.5.1, G2420.5.2 or G2420.5.3.

G2420.5.1 (409.5.1) Located within same room. The shutoff *valve* shall be located in the same room as the *appliance*. The shutoff *valve* shall be within 6 feet (1829 mm) of the *appliance*, and shall be installed upstream of the union, connector or quick disconnect device it serves. Such shutoff *valves* shall be provided with access. *Appliance shutoff valves* located in the firebox of a *fireplace* shall be installed in accordance with the *appliance* manufacturer's instructions.

G2420.5.2 (409.5.2) Vented decorative appliances and room heaters. Shutoff *valves* for vented decorative *appliances*, room heaters and decorative *appliances* for installation in vented fireplaces shall be permitted to be installed in an area remote from the *appliances* where such *valves* are provided with *ready access*. Such *valves* shall be permanently identified and shall serve no other *appliance*. The *piping* from the shutoff *valve* to within 6 feet (1829 mm) of the *appliance* shall be designed, sized and installed in accordance with Sections G2412 through G2419.

G2420.5.3 (409.5.3) Located at manifold. Where the *appliance shutoff valve* is installed at a manifold, such shutoff valve shall be located within 50 feet (15 240 mm) of the

appliance served and shall be readily accessible and permanently identified. The *piping* from the manifold to within 6 feet (1829 mm) of the *appliance* shall be designed, sized and installed in accordance with Sections G2412 through G2419.

SECTION G2421 (410)
FLOW CONTROLS

G2421.1 (410.1) Pressure regulators. A line *pressure regulator* shall be installed where the *appliance* is designed to operate at a lower pressure than the supply pressure. *Line gas pressure regulators* shall be listed as complying with ANSI Z21.80. Access shall be provided to *pressure regulators*. *Pressure regulators* shall be protected from physical damage. *Regulators* installed on the exterior of the building shall be *approved* for outdoor installation.

G2421.2 (410.2) MP regulators. MP *pressure regulators* shall comply with the following:

1. The MP *regulator* shall be *approved* and shall be suitable for the inlet and *outlet* gas pressures for the application.

2. The MP *regulator* shall maintain a reduced *outlet* pressure under lockup (no-flow) conditions.

3. The capacity of the MP *regulator*, determined by published ratings of its manufacturer, shall be adequate to supply the *appliances* served.

4. The MP *pressure regulator* shall be provided with access. Where located indoors, the *regulator* shall be vented to the outdoors or shall be equipped with a leak-limiting device, in either case complying with Section G2421.3.

5. A tee fitting with one opening capped or plugged shall be installed between the MP *regulator* and its upstream shutoff *valve*. Such tee fitting shall be positioned to allow connection of a pressure measuring instrument and to serve as a sediment trap.

6. A tee fitting with one opening capped or plugged shall be installed not less than 10 *pipe* diameters downstream of the MP *regulator* outlet. Such tee fitting shall be positioned to allow connection of a pressure measuring instrument.

TABLE G2420.1.1
MANUAL GAS VALVE STANDARDS

VALVE STANDARDS	APPLIANCE SHUTOFF VALVE APPLICATION UP TO $^1/_2$ psig PRESSURE	OTHER VALVE APPLICATIONS			
		UP TO $^1/_2$ psig PRESSURE	UP TO 2 psig PRESSURE	UP TO 5 psig PRESSURE	UP TO 125 psig PRESSURE
ANSI Z21.15	X	—	—	—	—
CSA Requirement 3-88	X	X	X[a]	X[b]	—
ASME B16.44	X	X	X[a]	X[b]	—
ASME B16.33	X	X	X	X	X

For SI: 1 pound per square inch gauge = 6.895 kPa.
a. If labeled 2G.
b. If labeled 5G.

G2421.3 (410.3) Venting of regulators. *Pressure regulators* that require a vent shall be vented directly to the outdoors. The vent shall be designed to prevent the entry of insects, water and foreign objects.

Exception: A vent to the outdoors is not required for *regulators* equipped with and labeled for utilization with an *approved* vent-limiting device installed in accordance with the manufacturer's instructions.

G2421.3.1 (410.3.1) Vent piping. Vent *piping* for *relief* vents and *breather* vents shall be constructed of materials allowed for *gas piping* in accordance with Section G2414. Vent *piping* shall be not smaller than the vent connection on the pressure regulating device. Vent *piping* serving *relief* vents and combination relief and *breather* vents shall be run independently to the outdoors and shall serve only a single device vent. Vent *piping* serving only *breather* vents is permitted to be connected in a manifold arrangement where sized in accordance with an *approved* design that minimizes back pressure in the event of diaphragm rupture. *Regulator* vent *piping* shall not exceed the length specified in the *regulator* manufacturer's installation instructions.

SECTION G2422 (411)
APPLIANCE CONNECTIONS

G2422.1 (411.1) Connecting appliances. *Appliances* shall be connected to the *piping system* by one of the following:

1. Rigid metallic *pipe* and fittings.

2. Corrugated stainless steel *tubing* (CSST) where installed in accordance with the manufacturer's instructions.

3. Listed and labeled *appliance connectors* in compliance with ANSI Z21.24 and installed in accordance with the manufacturer's installation instructions and located entirely in the same room as the *appliance*.

4. Listed and labeled quick-disconnect devices used in conjunction with listed and labeled *appliance connectors*.

5. Listed and labeled convenience outlets used in conjunction with listed and labeled *appliance connectors*.

6. Listed and labeled outdoor *appliance connectors* in compliance with ANSI Z21.75/CSA 6.27 and installed in accordance with the manufacturer's installation instructions.

G2422.1.1 (411.1.2) Protection from damage. Connectors and *tubing* shall be installed so as to be protected against physical damage.

G2422.1.2 (411.1.3) Connector installation. *Appliance* fuel connectors shall be installed in accordance with the manufacturer's instructions and Sections G24221.2.1 through G2422.1.2.4.

G2422.1.2.1 (411.1.3.1) Maximum length. Connectors shall not exceed 6 feet (1829 mm) in overall length. Measurement shall be made along the centerline of the connector. Only one connector shall be used for each *appliance*.

Exception: Rigid metallic *piping* used to connect an *appliance* to the *piping system* shall be permitted to have a total length greater than 6 feet (1829 mm) provided that the connecting *pipe* is sized as part of the *piping system* in accordance with Section G2413 and the location of the *appliance shutoff valve* complies with Section G2420.5.

G2422.1.2.2 (411.1.3.2) Minimum size. Connectors shall have the capacity for the total *demand* of the connected *appliance*.

G2422.1.2.3 (411.1.3.3) Prohibited locations and penetrations. Connectors shall not be concealed within, or extended through, walls, floors, partitions, ceilings or *appliance* housings.

Exceptions:

1. Connectors constructed of materials allowed for *piping systems* in accordance with Section G2414 shall be permitted to pass through walls, floors, partitions and ceilings where installed in accordance with Section G2420.5.2 or G2420.5.3.

2. Rigid steel *pipe* connectors shall be permitted to extend through openings in *appliance* housings.

3. *Fireplace* inserts that are factory equipped with grommets, sleeves or other means of protection in accordance with the listing of the *appliance*.

4. Semirigid *tubing* and listed connectors shall be permitted to extend through an opening in an *appliance* housing, cabinet or casing where the tubing or connector is protected against damage.

G2422.1.2.4 (411.1.3.4) Shutoff valve. A shutoff *valve* not less than the nominal size of the connector shall be installed ahead of the connector in accordance with Section G2420.5.

G2422.1.3 (411.1.5) Connection of gas engine-powered air conditioners. Internal *combustion* engines shall not be rigidly connected to the gas supply *piping*.

G2422.1.4 (411.1.6) Unions. A union fitting shall be provided for *appliances* connected by rigid metallic *pipe*. Such unions shall be accessible and located within 6 feet (1829 mm) of the *appliance*.

G2422.1.5 (411.1.4) Movable appliances. Where *appliances* are equipped with casters or are otherwise subject to periodic movement or relocation for purposes such as routine cleaning and maintenance, such *appliances* shall be connected to the supply system *piping* by means of an *approved* flexible connector designed and labeled for the application. Such flexible connectors shall be installed and protected against physical damage in accordance with the manufacturer's installation instructions.

G2422.2 (411.3) Suspended low-intensity infrared tube heaters. Suspended low-intensity infrared tube heaters shall be connected to the building *piping system* with a connector listed for the application complying with ANSI Z21.24/CGA 6.10. The connector shall be installed as specified by the tube heater manufacturer's instructions.

SECTION G2423 (413)
CNG GAS-DISPENSING SYSTEMS

G2423.1 (413.1) General. Motor fuel-dispensing facilities for CNG fuel shall be in accordance with Section 413 of the *International Fuel Gas Code.*

SECTION G2424 (415)
PIPING SUPPORT INTERVALS

G2424.1 (415.1) Interval of support. *Piping* shall be supported at intervals not exceeding the spacing specified in Table G2424.1. Spacing of supports for CSST shall be in accordance with the CSST manufacturer's instructions.

TABLE G2424.1
SUPPORT OF PIPING

STEEL PIPE, NOMINAL SIZE OF PIPE (inches)	SPACING OF SUPPORTS (feet)	NOMINAL SIZE OF TUBING SMOOTH-WALL (inch O.D.)	SPACING OF SUPPORTS (feet)
$^1/_2$	6	$^1/_2$	4
$^3/_4$ or 1	8	$^5/_8$ or $^3/_4$	6
$1^1/_4$ or larger (horizontal)	10	$^7/_8$ or 1 (horizontal)	8
$1^1/_4$ or larger (vertical)	Every floor level	1 or larger (vertical)	Every floor level

For SI: 1 inch = 25.4 mm, 1 foot = 304.8 mm.

SECTION G2425 (501)
GENERAL

G2425.1 (501.1) Scope. This section shall govern the installation, maintenance, repair and approval of factory-built and *masonry chimneys, chimney* liners, vents and connectors serving gas-fired *appliances.*

G2425.2 (501.2) General. Every *appliance* shall discharge the products of *combustion* to the outdoors, except for *appliances* exempted by Section G2425.8.

G2425.3 (501.3) Masonry chimneys. *Masonry chimneys* shall be constructed in accordance with Section G2427.5 and Chapter 10.

G2425.4 (501.4) Minimum size of chimney or vent. *Chimneys* and vents shall be sized in accordance with Sections G2427 and G2428.

G2425.5 (501.5) Abandoned inlet openings. Abandoned inlet openings in *chimneys* and vents shall be closed by an *approved* method.

G2425.6 (501.6) Positive pressure. Where an *appliance* equipped with a mechanical forced *draft* system creates a positive pressure in the venting system, the venting system shall be designed for positive pressure applications.

G2425.7 (501.7) Connection to fireplace. Connection of *appliances* to *chimney* flues serving *fireplaces* shall be in accordance with Sections G2425.7.1 through G2425.7.3.

G2425.7.1 (501.7.1) Closure and access. A noncombustible seal shall be provided below the point of connection to prevent entry of room air into the flue. Means shall be provided for access to the flue for inspection and cleaning.

G2425.7.2 (501.7.2) Connection to factory-built fireplace flue. An *appliance* shall not be connected to a flue serving a *factory-built fireplace* unless the *appliance* is specifically listed for such installation. The connection shall be made in accordance with the *appliance* manufacturer's installation instructions.

G2425.7.3 (501.7.3) Connection to masonry fireplace flue. A connector shall extend from the *appliance* to the flue serving a *masonry fireplace* such that the *flue gases* are exhausted directly into the flue. The connector shall be accessible or removable for inspection and cleaning of both the connector and the flue. Listed direct connection devices shall be installed in accordance with their listing.

G2425.8 (501.8) Appliances not required to be vented. The following *appliances* shall not be required to be vented:

1. Ranges.

2. Built-in domestic cooking units listed and marked for optional venting.

3. Hot plates and laundry stoves.

4. *Type 1 clothes dryers* (*Type 1 clothes dryers* shall be exhausted in accordance with the requirements of Section G2439).

5. Refrigerators.

6. Counter *appliances.*

7. Room heaters listed for unvented use.

Where the *appliances* listed in Items 5 through 7 above are installed so that the aggregate input rating exceeds 20 *Btu* per hour per *cubic foot* (207 W/m^3) of volume of the room or space in which such *appliances* are installed, one or more shall be provided with venting *systems* or other *approved* means for conveying the *vent gases* to the outdoor atmosphere so that the aggregate input rating of the remaining *unvented appliances* does not exceed 20 *Btu* per hour per *cubic foot* (207 W/m^3). Where the room or space in which the *appliance* is installed is directly connected to another room or space by a doorway, archway or other opening of comparable size that cannot be closed, the volume of such adjacent room or space shall be permitted to be included in the calculations.

G2425.9 (501.9) Chimney entrance. Connectors shall connect to a *masonry chimney* flue at a point not less than 12 inches (305 mm) above the lowest portion of the interior of the *chimney* flue.

G2425.10 (501.10) Connections to exhauster. *Appliance* connections to a *chimney* or vent equipped with a power exhauster shall be made on the inlet side of the exhauster. Joints on the positive pressure side of the exhauster shall be sealed to prevent flue-gas leakage as specified by the manufacturer's installation instructions for the exhauster.

G2425.11 (501.11) Masonry chimneys. *Masonry chimneys* utilized to vent *appliances* shall be located, constructed and sized as specified in the manufacturer's installation instructions for the *appliances* being vented and Section G2427.

G2425.12 (501.12) Residential and low-heat appliances flue lining systems. *Flue lining* systems for use with residential-type and low-heat *appliances* shall be limited to the following:

1. Clay *flue lining* complying with the requirements of ASTM C 315 or equivalent. Clay *flue lining* shall be installed in accordance with Chapter 10.

2. Listed *chimney* lining systems complying with UL 1777.

3. Other *approved* materials that will resist, without cracking, softening or corrosion, *flue gases* and *condensate* at temperatures up to 1,800°F (982°C).

G2425.13 (501.13) Category I appliance flue lining systems. *Flue lining* systems for use with Category I *appliances* shall be limited to the following:

1. *Flue lining* systems complying with Section G2425.12.

2. *Chimney* lining systems listed and labeled for use with *appliances* with *draft hoods* and other Category I gas *appliances* listed and labeled for use with Type B vents.

G2425.14 (501.14) Category II, III and IV appliance venting systems. The design, sizing and installation of vents for Category II, III and IV *appliances* shall be in accordance with the *appliance* manufacturer's installation instructions.

G2425.15 (501.15) Existing chimneys and vents. Where an *appliance* is permanently disconnected from an existing *chimney* or vent, or where an *appliance* is connected to an existing *chimney* or vent during the process of a new installation, the *chimney* or vent shall comply with Sections G2425.15.1 through G2425.15.4.

G2425.15.1 (501.15.1) Size. The *chimney* or vent shall be resized as necessary to control flue gas condensation in the interior of the *chimney* or vent and to provide the *appliance* or *appliances* served with the required *draft*. For Category I *appliances*, the resizing shall be in accordance with Section G2426.

G2425.15.2 (501.15.2) Flue passageways. The flue gas passageway shall be free of obstructions and combustible deposits and shall be cleaned if previously used for venting a solid or liquid fuel-burning appliance or *fireplace*. The *flue liner*, *chimney* inner wall or vent inner wall shall be continuous and shall be free of cracks, gaps, perforations, or other damage or deterioration that would allow the escape of *combustion products*, including gases, moisture and creosote.

G2425.15.3 (501.15.3) Cleanout. *Masonry chimney* flues shall be provided with a cleanout opening having a minimum height of 6 inches (152 mm). The upper edge of the opening shall be located not less than 6 inches (152 mm) below the lowest *chimney* inlet opening. The cleanout shall be provided with a tight-fitting, noncombustible cover.

G2425.15.4 (501.15.4) Clearances. *Chimneys* and vents shall have airspace *clearance* to combustibles in accordance

with Chapter 10 and the *chimney* or vent manufacturer's installation instructions.

> **Exception:** *Masonry chimneys* without the required air-space *clearances* shall be permitted to be used if lined or relined with a *chimney* lining system listed for use in *chimneys* with reduced *clearances* in accordance with UL 1777. The *chimney clearance* shall be not less than that permitted by the terms of the *chimney* liner listing and the manufacturer's instructions.

G2425.15.4.1 (501.15.4.1) Fireblocking. Noncombustible fireblocking shall be provided in accordance with Chapter 10.

SECTION G2426 (502)
VENTS

G2426.1 (502.1) General. All vents, except as provided in Section G2427.7, shall be listed and labeled. Type B and BW vents shall be tested in accordance with UL 441. Type L vents shall be tested in accordance with UL 641. Vents for Category II and III *appliances* shall be tested in accordance with UL 1738. Plastic vents for Category IV *appliances* shall not be required to be listed and labeled where such vents are as specified by the *appliance* manufacturer and are installed in accordance with the *appliance* manufacturer's installation instructions.

G2426.2 (502.2) Connectors required. Connectors shall be used to connect *appliances* to the vertical *chimney* or vent, except where the *chimney* or vent is attached directly to the *appliance*. Vent *connector* size, material, construction and installation shall be in accordance with Section G2427.

G2426.3 (502.3) Vent application. The application of vents shall be in accordance with Table G2427.4.

G2426.4 (502.4) Insulation shield. Where vents pass through insulated assemblies, an insulation shield constructed of steel having a minimum thickness of 0.0187 inch (0.4712 mm) (26 gage) shall be installed to provide *clearance* between the vent and the insulation material. The *clearance* shall not be less than the *clearance* to combustibles specified by the vent manufacturer's installation instructions. Where vents pass through attic space, the shield shall terminate not less than 2 inches (51 mm) above the insulation materials and shall be secured in place to prevent displacement. Insulation shields provided as part of a listed vent system shall be installed in accordance with the manufacturer's installation instructions.

G2426.5 (502.5) Installation. Vent systems shall be sized, installed and terminated in accordance with the vent and *appliance* manufacturer's installation instructions and Section G2427.

G2426.6 (502.6) Support of vents. All portions of vents shall be adequately supported for the design and weight of the materials employed.

G2426.7 (502.7) Protection against physical damage. In *concealed locations*, where a vent is installed through holes or notches in studs, joists, rafters or similar members less than 1¹/₂ inches (38 mm) from the nearest edge of the member, the vent shall be protected by shield plates. Protective steel shield plates having a minimum thickness of 0.0575-inch (1.463 mm) (16 gage) shall cover the area of the vent where the member is notched or bored and shall extend a minimum of 4 inches (102 mm) above sole plates, below top plates and to each side of a stud, joist or rafter.

SECTION G2427 (503)
VENTING OF APPLIANCES

G2427.1 (503.1) General. This section recognizes that the choice of venting materials and the methods of installation of *venting systems* are dependent on the operating characteristics of the *appliance* being vented. The operating characteristics of *vented appliances* can be categorized with respect to: (1) positive or negative pressure within the venting system; and (2) whether or not the *appliance* generates flue or *vent gases* that might condense in the venting system. See Section G2403 for the definitions of these *vented appliance* categories.

G2427.2 (503.2) Venting systems required. Except as permitted in Sections G2427.2.1, G2427.2.2 and G2425.8, all *appliances* shall be connected to *venting systems*.

G2427.2.1 (503.2.3) Direct-vent appliances. Listed *direct*-vent *appliances* shall be installed in accordance with the manufacturer's instructions and Section G2427.8, Item 3.

G2427.2.2 (503.2.4) Appliances with integral vents. *Appliances* incorporating integral venting means shall be considered properly vented where installed in accordance with the manufacturer's instructions and Section G2427.8, Items 1 and 2.

G2427.3 (503.3) Design and construction. A venting system shall be designed and constructed so as to develop a positive flow adequate to convey flue or *vent gases* to the outdoors.

G2427.3.1 (503.3.1) Appliance draft requirements. A venting system shall satisfy the *draft* requirements of the *appliance* in accordance with the manufacturer's instructions.

G2427.3.2 (503.3.2) Design and construction. *Appliances* required to be vented shall be connected to a venting system designed and installed in accordance with the provisions of Sections G2427.4 through G2427.16.

G2427.3.3 (503.3.3) Mechanical draft systems. *Mechanical draft* systems shall comply with the following:

1. *Mechanical draft* systems shall be listed and shall be installed in accordance with the manufacturer's installation instructions for both the *appliance* and the *mechanical draft* system.

2. *Appliances*, except incinerators, requiring venting shall be permitted to be vented by means of *mechanical draft* systems of either forced or *induced draft* design.

3. Forced *draft* systems and all portions of *induced draft* systems under positive pressure during operation shall be designed and installed so as to prevent leakage of flue or *vent gases* into a building.

4. *Vent connectors* serving *appliances* vented by *natural draft* shall not be connected into any portion of

mechanical draft systems operating under positive pressure.

5. Where a *mechanical draft* system is employed, provisions shall be made to prevent the flow of gas to the *main burners* when the *draft* system is not performing so as to satisfy the operating requirements of the *appliance* for safe performance.

6. The exit terminals of *mechanical draft* systems shall be not less than 7 feet (2134 mm) above finished ground level where located adjacent to public walkways and shall be located as specified in Section G2427.8, Items 1 and 2.

G2427.3.4 (503.3.5) Air ducts and furnace plenums. *Venting systems* shall not extend into or pass through any fabricated air duct or *furnace plenum*.

G2427.3.5 (503.3.6) Above-ceiling air-handling spaces. Where a venting system passes through an above-ceiling air-handling space or other nonducted portion of an air-handling system, the venting system shall conform to one of the following requirements:

1. The venting system shall be a listed special gas vent; other venting system serving a Category III or Category IV *appliance*; or other positive pressure vent, with joints sealed in accordance with the *appliance* or vent manufacturer's instructions.

2. The venting system shall be installed such that fittings and joints between sections are not installed in the above-ceiling space.

3. The venting system shall be installed in a conduit or enclosure with sealed joints separating the interior of the conduit or enclosure from the ceiling space.

G2427.4 (503.4) Type of venting system to be used. The type of venting system to be used shall be in accordance with Table G2427.4.

G2427.4.1 (503.4.1) Plastic piping. Plastic *piping* used for venting *appliances* listed for use with such venting materials shall be *approved*.

G2427.4.1.1 (503.4.1.1) (IFGS) Plastic vent joints. Plastic *pipe* and fittings used to vent *appliances* shall be installed in accordance with the *appliance* manufacturer's installation instructions. Where a primer is required, it shall be of a contrasting color.

G2427.4.2 (503.4.2) Special gas vent. *Special gas vent* shall be listed and installed in accordance with the *special gas vent* manufacturer's installation instructions.

G2427.5 (503.5) Masonry, metal and factory-built chimneys. Masonry, metal and factory-built *chimneys* shall comply with Sections G2427.5.1 through G2427.5.9.

G2427.5.1 (503.5.1) Factory-built chimneys. Factory-built *chimneys* shall be installed in accordance with the manufacturer's installation instructions. Factory-built *chimneys* used to vent *appliances* that operate at a positive vent pressure shall be listed for such application.

G2427.5.2 (503.5.3) Masonry chimneys. Masonry *chimneys* shall be built and installed in accordance with NFPA

TABLE G2427.4
TYPE OF VENTING SYSTEM TO BE USED

APPLIANCES	TYPE OF VENTING SYSTEM
Listed Category I appliances Listed appliances equipped with draft hood Appliances listed for use with Type B gas vent	Type B gas vent (Section G2427.6) Chimney (Section G2427.5) Single-wall metal pipe (Section G2427.7) Listed chimney lining system for gas venting (Section G2427.5.2) Special gas vent listed for these appliances (Section G2427.4.2)
Listed vented wall furnaces	Type B-W gas vent (Sections G2427.6, G2436)
Category II appliances	As specified or furnished by manufacturers of listed appliances (Sections G2427.4.1, G2427.4.2)
Category III appliances	As specified or furnished by manufacturers of listed appliances (Sections G2427.4.1, G2427.4.2)
Category IV appliances	As specified or furnished by manufacturers of listed appliances (Sections G2427.4.1, G2427.4.2)
Unlisted appliances	Chimney (Section G2427.5)
Decorative appliances in vented fireplaces	Chimney
Direct-vent appliances	See Section G2427.2.1
Appliances with integral vent	See Section G2427.2.2

211 and shall be lined with *approved* clay *flue lining*, a listed *chimney* lining system or other *approved* material that will resist corrosion, erosion, softening or cracking from vent gases at temperatures up to 1,800°F (982°C).

Exception: Masonry *chimney* flues serving listed gas *appliances* with *draft hoods*, Category I *appliances* and other gas *appliances* listed for use with Type B vents shall be permitted to be lined with a *chimney* lining system specifically listed for use only with such *appliances*. The liner shall be installed in accordance with the liner manufacturer's installation instructions. A permanent identifying label shall be attached at the point where the connection is to be made to the liner. The label shall read: "This *chimney* liner is for *appliances* that burn gas only. Do not connect to solid or liquid fuel-burning appliances or incinerators."

G2427.5.3 (503.5.4) Chimney termination. *Chimneys* for residential-type or low-heat *appliances* shall extend at least 3 feet (914 mm) above the highest point where they pass through a roof of a building and at least 2 feet (610 mm) higher than any portion of a building within a horizontal distance of 10 feet (3048 mm) (see Figure G2427.5.3). *Chimneys* for medium-heat *appliances* shall extend at least 10 feet (3048 mm) higher than any portion of any building within 25 feet (7620 mm). *Chimneys* shall extend at least 5 feet (1524 mm) above the highest connected *appliance draft hood* outlet or *flue collar*. Decorative shrouds shall not be installed at the termination of factory-built *chimneys* except where such shrouds are listed and labeled for use with the specific factory-built *chimney* system and are installed in accordance with the manufacturer's installation instructions.

G2427.5.4 (503.5.5) Size of chimneys. The effective area of a *chimney* venting system serving listed *appliances* with *draft hoods*, Category I *appliances*, and other *appliances*

listed for use with Type B vents shall be determined in accordance with one of the following methods:

1. The provisions of Section G2428.

2. For sizing an individual *chimney* venting system for a single *appliance* with a *draft hood*, the effective areas of the *vent connector* and *chimney* flue shall be not less than the area of the *appliance flue collar* or *draft hood* outlet, nor greater than seven times the *draft hood* outlet area.

3. For sizing a *chimney* venting system connected to two *appliances* with *draft hoods*, the effective area of the *chimney* flue shall be not less than the area of the larger *draft hood* outlet plus 50 percent of the area of the smaller *draft hood* outlet, nor greater than seven times the smallest *draft hood* outlet area.

4. *Chimney venting systems* using *mechanical draft* shall be sized in accordance with *approved* engineering methods.

5. Other *approved* engineering methods.

G2427.5.5 (503.5.6) Inspection of chimneys. Before replacing an existing *appliance* or connecting a vent *connector* to a *chimney*, the *chimney* passageway shall be examined to ascertain that it is clear and free of obstructions and it shall be cleaned if previously used for venting solid or liquid fuel-burning appliances or *fireplaces*.

G2427.5.5.1 (503.5.6.1) Chimney lining. *Chimneys* shall be lined in accordance with NFPA 211.

Exception: Where an existing chimney complies with Sections G2427.5.5 through G2427.5.5.3 and its sizing is in accordance with Section G2427.5.4, its continued use shall be allowed where the *appliance* vented by that *chimney* is replaced by an *appliance* of similar type, input rating and efficiency.

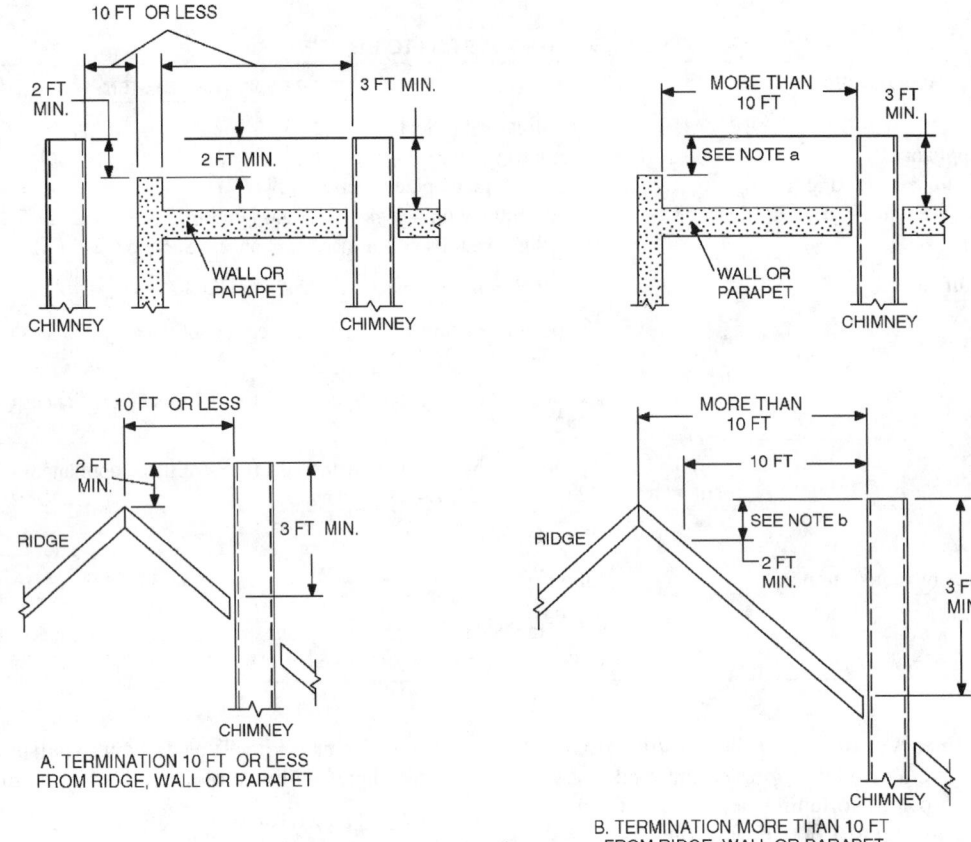

For SI: 1 inch = 25.4 mm, 1 foot = 304.8 mm.

NOTES:

a. No height above parapet required when distance from walls or parapet is more than 10 feet.

b. Height above any roof surface within 10 feet horizontally.

FIGURE G2427.5.3 (503.5.4)
TYPICAL TERMINATION LOCATIONS FOR CHIMNEYS AND SINGLE-WALL METAL PIPES
SERVING RESIDENTIAL-TYPE AND LOW-HEAT APPLIANCES

G2427.5.5.2 (503.5.6.2) Cleanouts. Cleanouts shall be examined to determine that they will remain tightly closed when not in use.

G2427.5.5.3 (503.5.6.3) Unsafe chimneys. Where inspection reveals that an existing *chimney* is not safe for the intended application, it shall be repaired, rebuilt, lined, relined or replaced with a vent or *chimney* to conform to NFPA 211 and it shall be suitable for the *appliances* to be vented.

G2427.5.6 (503.5.7) Chimneys serving appliances burning other fuels. *Chimneys* serving *appliances* burning other fuels shall comply with Sections G2427.5.6.1 through G2427.5.6.4.

G2427.5.6.1 (503.5.7.1) Solid fuel-burning appliances. An *appliance* shall not be connected to a *chimney* flue serving a separate appliance designed to burn solid fuel.

G2427.5.6.2 (503.5.7.2) Liquid fuel-burning appliances. Where one *chimney* flue serves gas *appliances* and liquid fuel-burning appliances, the appliances shall be connected through separate openings or shall be connected through a single opening where joined by a suitable fitting located as close as practical to the *chimney*. Where two or more openings are provided into one *chimney* flue, they shall be at different levels. Where the appliances are automatically controlled, they shall be equipped with *safety shutoff devices*.

G2427.5.6.3 (503.5.7.3) Combination gas- and solid fuel-burning appliances. A combination gas- and solid fuel-burning *appliance* equipped with a manual reset device to shut off gas to the *main burner* in the event of sustained backdraft or flue gas spillage shall be permitted to be connected to a single *chimney* flue. The *chimney* flue shall be sized to properly vent the *appliance*.

G2427.5.6.4 (503.5.7.4) Combination gas- and oil fuel-burning appliances. A listed combination gas- and oil fuel-burning *appliance* shall be permitted to be connected to a single *chimney* flue. The *chimney* flue shall be sized to properly vent the *appliance*.

G2427.5.7 (503.5.8) Support of chimneys. All portions of *chimneys* shall be supported for the design and weight of the materials employed. Factory-built *chimneys* shall be supported and spaced in accordance with the manufacturer's installation instructions.

G2427.5.8 (503.5.9) Cleanouts. Where a *chimney* that formerly carried flue products from liquid or solid fuel-burning appliances is used with an *appliance* using *fuel gas*, an accessible cleanout shall be provided. The cleanout shall have a tight-fitting cover and be installed so its upper edge is at least 6 inches (152 mm) below the lower edge of the lowest *chimney* inlet opening.

G2427.5.9 (503.5.10) Space surrounding lining or vent. The remaining space surrounding a *chimney* liner, gas vent, *special gas vent* or plastic *piping* installed within a *masonry chimney* flue shall not be used to vent another *appliance*. The insertion of another liner or vent within the *chimney* as provided in this *code* and the liner or vent manufacturer's instructions shall not be prohibited.

The remaining space surrounding a *chimney* liner, gas vent, special gas vent or plastic *piping* installed within a masonry, metal or factory-built *chimney* shall not be used to supply *combustion air*. Such space shall not be prohibited from supplying *combustion air* to *direct-vent appliances* designed for installation in a solid fuel-burning *fireplace* and installed in accordance with the manufacturer's installation instructions.

G2427.6 (503.6) Gas vents. Gas vents shall comply with Sections G2427.6.1 through G2427.6.11. (See Section G2403, Definitions.)

G2427.6.1 (503.6.1) Installation, general. Gas vents shall be installed in accordance with the terms of their listings and the manufacturer's instructions.

G2427.6.2 (503.6.2) Type B-W vent capacity. A Type B-W gas vent shall have a listed capacity not less than that of the listed *vented wall furnace* to which it is connected.

G2427.6.3 (503.6.4) Gas vent termination. A gas vent shall terminate in accordance with one of the following:

1. Gas vents that are 12 inches (305 mm) or less in size and located not less than 8 feet (2438 mm) from a vertical wall or similar obstruction shall terminate above the roof in accordance with Figure G2427.6.3.

2. Gas vents that are over 12 inches (305 mm) in size or are located less than 8 feet (2438 mm) from a vertical wall or similar obstruction shall terminate not less than 2 feet (610 mm) above the highest point where they pass through the roof and not less than 2 feet (610 mm) above any portion of a building within 10 feet (3048 mm) horizontally.

3. As provided for direct-vent systems in Section G2427.2.1.

4. As provided for *appliances* with integral vents in Section G2427.2.2.

5. As provided for *mechanical draft* systems in Section G2427.3.3.

G2427.6.3.1 (503.6.4.1) Decorative shrouds. Decorative shrouds shall not be installed at the termination of

gas vents except where such shrouds are listed for use with the specific gas venting system and are installed in accordance with manufacturer's installation instructions.

G2427.6.4 (503.6.5) Minimum height. A Type B or L gas vent shall terminate at least 5 feet (1524 mm) in vertical height above the highest connected *appliance draft hood* or *flue collar*. A Type B-W gas vent shall terminate at least 12 feet (3658 mm) in vertical height above the bottom of the wall *furnace*.

G2427.6.5 (503.6.6) Roof terminations. Gas vents shall extend through the roof flashing, roof jack or roof thimble and terminate with a listed cap or listed roof assembly.

G2427.6.6 (503.6.7) Forced air inlets. Gas vents shall terminate not less than 3 feet (914 mm) above any forced air inlet located within 10 feet (3048 mm).

G2427.6.7 (503.6.8) Exterior wall penetrations. A gas *vent* extending through an exterior wall shall not terminate adjacent to the wall or below eaves or parapets, except as provided in Sections G2427.2.1 and G2427.3.3.

G2427.6.8 (503.6.9) Size of gas vents. *Venting systems* shall be sized and constructed in accordance with Section G2428 or other *approved* engineering methods and the gas vent and *appliance* manufacturer's installation instructions.

G2427.6.8.1 (503.6.9.1) Category I appliances. The sizing of *natural draft venting systems* serving one or more listed *appliances* equipped with a *draft hood* or *appliances* listed for use with Type B gas vent, installed in a single story of a building, shall be in accordance with one of the following methods:

1. The provisions of Section G2428.

2. For sizing an individual gas vent for a single, draft-hood-equipped *appliance*, the effective area of the vent *connector* and the gas vent shall be not less than the area of the *appliance draft hood* outlet, nor greater than seven times the *draft hood* outlet area.

3. For sizing a gas vent connected to two *appliances* with *draft hoods*, the effective area of the vent shall be not less than the area of the larger *draft hood* outlet plus 50 percent of the area of the smaller *draft hood* outlet, nor greater than seven times the smaller *draft hood* outlet area.

4. *Approved* engineering practices.

G2427.6.8.2 (503.6.9.2) Vent offsets. Type B and L vents sized in accordance with Item 2 or 3 of Section G2427.6.8.1 shall extend in a generally vertical direction with offsets not exceeding 45 degrees (0.79 rad), except that a vent system having not more than one 60-degree (1.04 rad) *offset* shall be permitted. Any angle greater than 45 degrees (0.79 rad) from the vertical is considered horizontal. The total horizontal distance of a vent plus the horizontal vent *connector* serving *draft hood*-equipped *appliances* shall be not greater than 75 percent of the vertical height of the vent.

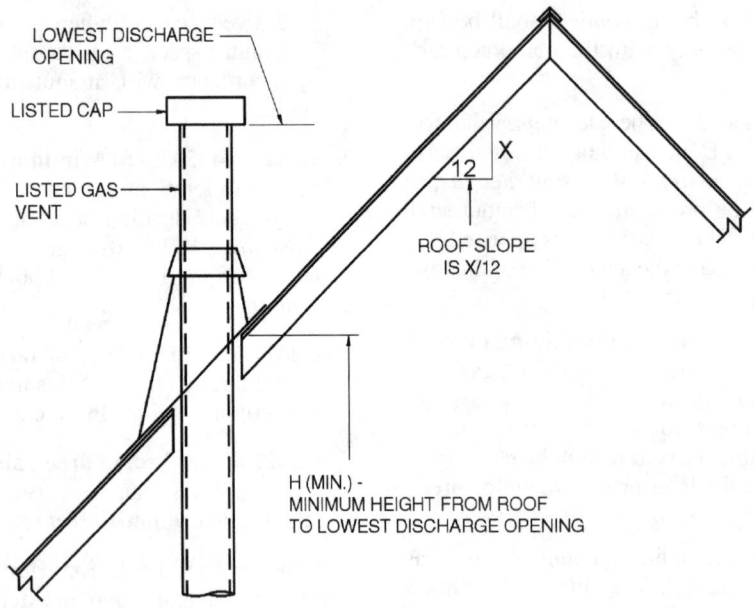

ROOF SLOPE	H (minimum) ft
Flat to $^6/_{12}$	1.0
Over $^6/_{12}$ to $^7/_{12}$	1.25
Over $^7/_{12}$ to $^8/_{12}$	1.5
Over $^8/_{12}$ to $^9/_{12}$	2.0
Over $^9/_{12}$ to $^{10}/_{12}$	2.5
Over $^{10}/_{12}$ to $^{11}/_{12}$	3.25
Over $^{11}/_{12}$ to $^{12}/_{12}$	4.0
Over $^{12}/_{12}$ to $^{14}/_{12}$	5.0
Over $^{14}/_{12}$ to $^{16}/_{12}$	6.0
Over $^{16}/_{12}$ to $^{18}/_{12}$	7.0
Over $^{18}/_{12}$ to $^{20}/_{12}$	7.5
Over $^{20}/_{12}$ to $^{21}/_{12}$	8.0

For SI: 1 foot = 304.8 mm.

FIGURE G2427.6.3 (503.6.4)
GAS VENT TERMINATION LOCATIONS FOR LISTED CAPS 12 INCHES
OR LESS IN SIZE AT LEAST 8 FEET FROM A VERTICAL WALL

G2427.6.8.3 (503.6.9.3) Category II, III and IV appliances. The sizing of gas vents for Category II, III and IV appliances shall be in accordance with the appliance manufacturer's instructions.

G2427.6.8.4 (503.6.9.4) Mechanical draft. *Chimney venting systems* using *mechanical draft* shall be sized in accordance with *approved* engineering methods.

G2427.6.9 (503.6.11) Support of gas vents. Gas vents shall be supported and spaced in accordance with the manufacturer's installation instructions.

G2427.6.10 (503.6.12) Marking. In those localities where solid and liquid fuels are used extensively, gas vents shall be permanently identified by a label attached to the wall or ceiling at a point where the *vent connector* enters the gas vent. The determination of where such localities exist shall be made by the *code official*. The label shall read:

"This gas vent is for *appliances* that burn gas. Do not connect to solid or liquid fuel-burning appliances or incinerators."

G2427.6.11 (503.6.13) Fastener penetrations. Screws, rivets and other fasteners shall not penetrate the inner wall of double-wall gas vents, except at the transition from an *appliance draft hood* outlet, a *flue collar* or a single-wall metal connector to a double-wall vent.

G2427.7 (503.7) Single-wall metal pipe. Single-wall metal *pipe* vents shall comply with Sections G2427.7.1 through G2427.7.13.

G2427.7.1 (503.7.1) Construction. Single-wall metal pipe shall be constructed of galvanized sheet steel not less than 0.0304 inch (0.7 mm) thick, or other *approved*, noncombustible, corrosion-resistant material.

G2427.7.2 (503.7.2) Cold climate. Uninsulated single-wall metal pipe shall not be used outdoors for venting *appliances* in regions where the 99-percent winter design temperature is below 32°F (0°C).

G2427.7.3 (503.7.3) Termination. Single-wall metal pipe shall terminate at least 5 feet (1524 mm) in vertical height above the highest connected *appliance draft hood* outlet or *flue collar*. Single-wall metal pipe shall extend at least 2 feet (610 mm) above the highest point where it passes through a roof of a building and at least 2 feet (610 mm) higher than any portion of a building within a horizontal distance of 10 feet (3048 mm) (see Figure G2427.5.3). An *approved* cap or roof assembly shall be attached to the terminus of a single-wall metal pipe (see also Section G2427.7.9, Item 3).

G2427.7.4 (503.7.4) Limitations of use. Single-wall metal pipe shall be used only for runs directly from the space in which the *appliance* is located through the roof or exterior wall to the outdoor atmosphere.

G2427.7.5 (503.7.5) Roof penetrations. A pipe passing through a roof shall extend without interruption through the roof flashing, roof jack, or roof thimble. Where a single-wall metal pipe passes through a roof constructed of combustible material, a noncombustible, nonventilating thimble shall be used at the point of passage. The thimble shall extend at least 18 inches (457 mm) above and 6 inches (152 mm) below the roof with the annular space open at the bottom and closed only at the top. The thimble shall be sized in accordance with Section G2427.7.7.

G2427.7.6 (503.7.6) Installation. Single-wall metal pipe shall not originate in any unoccupied attic or concealed space and shall not pass through any attic, inside wall, concealed space, or floor. The installation of a single-wall metal pipe through an exterior combustible wall shall comply with Section G2427.7.7. Single-wall metal pipe used for venting an incinerator shall be exposed and readily examinable for its full length and shall have suitable *clearances* maintained.

G2427.7.7 (503.7.7) Single-wall penetrations of combustible walls. Single-wall metal pipe shall not pass through a combustible exterior wall unless guarded at the point of passage by a ventilated metal thimble not smaller than the following:

1. For listed *appliances* equipped with *draft hoods* and *appliances* listed for use with Type B gas vents, the thimble shall be not less than 4 inches (102 mm) larger in diameter than the metal pipe. Where there is a run of not less than 6 feet (1829 mm) of metal pipe in the open between the *draft hood* outlet and the thimble, the thimble shall be permitted to be not less than 2 inches (51 mm) larger in diameter than the metal pipe.

2. For unlisted *appliances* having *draft hoods*, the thimble shall be not less than 6 inches (152 mm) larger in diameter than the metal pipe.

3. For residential and low-heat *appliances*, the thimble shall be not less than 12 inches (305 mm) larger in diameter than the metal pipe.

Exception: In lieu of thimble protection, all combustible material in the wall shall be removed a sufficient distance from the metal pipe to provide the specified *clearance* from such metal pipe to combustible material. Any material used to close up such opening shall be noncombustible.

G2427.7.8 (503.7.8) Clearances. Minimum *clearances* from single-wall metal pipe to combustible material shall be in accordance with Table G2427.10.5. The *clearance* from single-wall metal pipe to combustible material shall be permitted to be reduced where the combustible material is protected as specified for *vent connectors* in Table G2409.2.

G2427.7.9 (503.7.8) Size of single-wall metal pipe. A venting system constructed of single-wall metal pipe shall be sized in accordance with one of the following methods and the *appliance* manufacturer's instructions:

1. For a draft-hood-equipped *appliance*, in accordance with Section G2428.

2. For a venting system for a single *appliance* with a *draft hood*, the areas of the connector and the pipe each shall be not less than the area of the *appliance flue collar* or *draft hood* outlet, whichever is smaller. The vent area shall not be greater than seven times the *draft hood* outlet area.

3. Other *approved* engineering methods.

G2427.7.10 (503.7.9) Pipe geometry. Any shaped single-wall metal pipe shall be permitted to be used, provided that its equivalent effective area is equal to the effective area of the round pipe for which it is substituted, and provided that the minimum internal dimension of the pipe is not less than 2 inches (51 mm).

G2427.7.11 (503.7.10) Termination capacity. The vent cap or a roof assembly shall have a venting capacity not less than that of the pipe to which it is attached.

G2427.7.12 (503.7.11) Support of single-wall metal pipe. All portions of single-wall metal pipe shall be supported for the design and weight of the material employed.

G2427.7.13 (503.7.12) Marking. Single-wall metal pipe shall comply with the marking provisions of Section G2427.6.10.

G2427.8 (503.8) Venting system termination location. The location of venting system terminations shall comply with the following (see Appendix C):

1. A *mechanical draft* venting system shall terminate at least 3 feet (914 mm) above any forced-air inlet located within 10 feet (3048 mm).

Exceptions:

1. This provision shall not apply to the *combustion air* intake of a direct-vent *appliance*.

2. This provision shall not apply to the separation of the integral outdoor air inlet and flue gas discharge of listed outdoor *appliances*.

2. A *mechanical draft* venting system, excluding *direct*-vent *appliances*, shall terminate at least 4 feet (1219 mm) below, 4 feet (1219 mm) horizontally from, or 1 foot (305 mm) above any door, operable window, or gravity air inlet into any building. The bottom of the vent terminal shall be located at least 12 inches (305 mm) above finished ground level.

3. The vent terminal of a *direct*-vent *appliance* with an input of 10,000 *Btu* per hour (3 kW) or less shall be located at least 6 inches (152 mm) from any air opening into a building, and such an *appliance* with an input over 10,000 *Btu* per hour (3 kW) but not over 50,000 *Btu* per hour (14.7 kW) shall be installed with a 9-inch (230 mm) vent termination *clearance*, and an *appliance* with an input over 50,000 *Btu*/h (14.7 kW) shall have at least a 12-inch (305 mm) vent termination *clearance*. The bottom of the vent terminal and the air intake shall be located at least 12 inches (305 mm) above grade finished ground level.

4. Through-the-wall vents for Category II and IV *appliances* and noncategorized condensing *appliances* shall not terminate over public walkways or over an area where *condensate* or vapor could create a nuisance or hazard or could be detrimental to the operation of *regulators, relief valves,* or other *equipment*. Where local experience indicates that *condensate* is a problem with Category I and III *appliances*, this provision shall also apply. Drains for *condensate* shall be installed in accordance with the manufacturer's installation instructions.

G2427.9 (503.9) Condensation drainage. Provisions shall be made to collect and dispose of *condensate* from *venting systems* serving Category II and IV *appliances* and noncategorized condensing *appliances* in accordance with Section G2427.8, Item 4. Where local experience indicates that condensation is a problem, provision shall be made to drain off and dispose of *condensate* from *venting systems* serving Category I and III *appliances* in accordance with Section G2427.8, Item 4.

G2427.10 (503.10) Vent connectors for Category I appliances. Vent *connectors* for Category I *appliances* shall comply with Sections G2427.10.1 through G2427.10.14.

G2427.10.1 (503.10.1) Where required. A vent *connector* shall be used to connect an *appliance* to a gas vent, *chimney* or single-wall metal pipe, except where the gas vent, *chimney* or single-wall metal pipe is directly connected to the *appliance*.

G2427.10.2 (503.10.2) Materials. *Vent connectors* shall be constructed in accordance with Sections G2427.10.2.1 through G2427.10.2.4.

G2427.10.2.1 (503.10.2.1) General. A *vent connector* shall be made of noncombustible corrosion-resistant material capable of withstanding the vent gas temperature produced by the *appliance* and of sufficient thickness to withstand physical damage.

G2427.10.2.2 (503.10.2.2) Vent connectors located in unconditioned areas. Where the *vent connector* used for an *appliance* having a *draft hood* or a Category I

appliance is located in or passes through attics, crawl spaces or other unconditioned spaces, that portion of the *vent connector* shall be listed Type B, Type L or listed vent material having equivalent insulation properties.

Exception: Single-wall metal pipe located within the exterior walls of the building in areas having a local 99-percent winter design temperature of 5°F (-15°C) or higher shall be permitted to be used in unconditioned spaces other than attics and crawl spaces.

G2427.10.2.3 (503.10.2.3) Residential-type appliance connectors. Where *vent connectors* for residential-type *appliances* are not installed in attics or other unconditioned spaces, connectors for listed *appliances* having *draft hoods, appliances* having *draft hoods* and equipped with listed *conversion burners* and Category I *appliances* shall be one of the following:

1. Type B or L vent material;

2. Galvanized sheet steel not less than 0.018 inch (0.46 mm) thick;

3. Aluminum (1100 or 3003 alloy or equivalent) sheet not less than 0.027 inch (0.69 mm) thick;

4. Stainless steel sheet not less than 0.012 inch (0.31 mm) thick;

5. Smooth interior wall metal pipe having resistance to heat and corrosion equal to or greater than that of Item 2, 3 or 4 above; or

6. A listed vent *connector*.

Vent connectors shall not be covered with insulation.

Exception: Listed insulated *vent connectors* shall be installed in accordance with the manufacturer's installation instructions.

G2427.10.2.4 (503.10.2.4) Low-heat appliance. A *vent connector* for a nonresidential, low-heat *appliance* shall be a factory-built *chimney* section or steel *pipe* having resistance to heat and corrosion equivalent to that for the appropriate galvanized pipe as specified in Table G2427.10.2.4. Factory-built *chimney* sections shall be joined together in accordance with the *chimney* manufacturer's instructions.

TABLE G2427.10.2.4 (503.10.2.4)
MINIMUM THICKNESS FOR GALVANIZED STEEL VENT CONNECTORS FOR LOW-HEAT APPLIANCES

DIAMETER OF CONNECTOR (inches)	MINIMUM THICKNESS (inch)
Less than 6	0.019
6 to less than 10	0.023
10 to 12 inclusive	0.029
14 to 16 inclusive	0.034
Over 16	0.056

For SI: 1 inch = 25.4 mm.

G2427.10.3 (503.10.3) Size of vent connector. *Vent connectors* shall be sized in accordance with Sections G2427.10.3.1 through G2427.3.5.

G2427.10.3.1 (503.10.3.1) Single draft hood and fan-assisted. A *vent connector* for an *appliance* with a single *draft hood* or for a Category I fan-assisted *combustion* system *appliance* shall be sized and installed in accordance with Section G2428 or other *approved* engineering methods.

G2427.10.3.2 (503.10.3.2) Multiple draft hood. For a single *appliance* having more than one *draft hood* outlet or *flue collar*, the manifold shall be constructed according to the instructions of the *appliance* manufacturer. Where there are no instructions, the manifold shall be designed and constructed in accordance with *approved* engineering practices. As an alternate method, the effective area of the manifold shall equal the combined area of the *flue collars* or *draft hood* outlets and the *vent connectors* shall have a minimum 1-foot (305 mm) rise.

G2427.10.3.3 (503.10.3.3) Multiple appliances. Where two or more *appliances* are connected to a common *vent* or *chimney*, each *vent connector* shall be sized in accordance with Section G2428 or other *approved* engineering methods.

As an alternative method applicable only when all of the *appliances* are *draft hood* equipped, each *vent connector* shall have an effective area not less than the area of the *draft hood* outlet of the *appliance* to which it is connected.

G2427.10.3.4 (503.10.3.4) Common connector/manifold. Where two or more *appliances* are vented through a common *vent connector* or vent manifold, the common *vent connector* or vent manifold shall be located at the highest level consistent with available headroom and the required *clearance* to combustible materials and shall be sized in accordance with Section G2428 or other *approved* engineering methods.

As an alternate method applicable only where there are two *draft hood*-equipped *appliances*, the effective area of the common *vent connector* or vent manifold and all junction fittings shall be not less than the area of the larger *vent connector* plus 50 percent of the area of the smaller *flue collar* outlet.

G2427.10.3.5 (503.10.3.5) Size increase. Where the size of a *vent connector* is increased to overcome installation limitations and obtain connector capacity equal to the *appliance* input, the size increase shall be made at the *appliance draft hood* outlet.

G2427.10.4 (503.10.4) Two or more appliances connected to a single vent or chimney. Where two or more *vent connectors* enter a common gas vent, *chimney* flue, or single-wall metal pipe, the smaller connector shall enter at the highest level consistent with the available headroom or *clearance* to combustible material. *Vent connectors* serving Category I *appliances* shall not be connected to any portion of a *mechanical draft* system operating under positive static pressure, such as those serving Category III or IV *appliances*.

G2427.10.4.1 (503.10.4.1) Two or more openings. Where two or more openings are provided into one *chimney* flue or vent, the openings shall be at different levels, or the connectors shall be attached to the vertical portion of the *chimney* or vent at an angle of 45 degrees (0.79 rad) or less relative to the vertical.

G2427.10.5 (503.10.5) Clearance. Minimum *clearances* from *vent connectors* to combustible material shall be in accordance with Table G2427.10.5.

Exception: The *clearance* between a *vent connector* and combustible material shall be permitted to be reduced where the combustible material is protected as specified for *vent connectors* in Table G2409.2.

G2427.10.6 (503.10.6) Flow resistance. A *vent connector* shall be installed so as to avoid turns or other construction features that create excessive resistance to flow of vent gases.

TABLE G2427.10.5 (503.10.5)[a]
CLEARANCES FOR CONNECTORS

APPLIANCE	MINIMUM DISTANCE FROM COMBUSTIBLE MATERIAL			
	Listed Type B gas vent material	Listed Type L vent material	Single-wall metal pipe	Factory-built chimney sections
Listed appliances with draft hoods and appliances listed for use with Type B gas vents	As listed	As listed	6 inches	As listed
Residential boilers and furnaces with listed gas conversion burner and with draft hood	6 inches	6 inches	9 inches	As listed
Residential appliances listed for use with Type L vents	Not permitted	As listed	9 inches	As listed
Listed gas-fired toilets	Not permitted	As listed	As listed	As listed
Unlisted residential appliances with draft hood	Not permitted	6 inches	9 inches	As listed
Residential and low-heat appliances other than above	Not permitted	9 inches	18 inches	As listed
Medium-heat appliances	Not permitted	Not permitted	36 inches	As listed

For SI: 1 inch = 25.4 mm.

a. These clearances shall apply unless the manufacturer's installation instructions for a listed appliance or connector specify different clearances, in which case the listed clearances shall apply.

G2427.10.7 (503.10.7) Joints. Joints between sections of connector piping and connections to *flue collars* and *draft hood* outlets shall be fastened by one of the following methods:

1. Sheet metal screws.

2. *Vent connectors* of listed vent material assembled and connected to *flue collars* or *draft hood* outlets in accordance with the manufacturers' instructions.

3. Other *approved* means.

G2427.10.8 (503.10.8) Slope. A *vent connector* shall be installed without dips or sags and shall slope upward toward the vent or *chimney* at least $^1/_4$ inch per foot (21 mm/m).

> **Exception:** *Vent connectors* attached to a *mechanical draft* system installed in accordance with the *appliance* and *draft* system manufacturers' instructions.

G2427.10.9 (503.10.9) Length of vent connector. A *vent connector* shall be as short as practical and the *appliance* located as close as practical to the *chimney* or vent. The maximum horizontal length of a single-wall connector shall be 75 percent of the height of the *chimney* or vent except for engineered systems. The maximum horizontal length of a Type B double-wall connector shall be 100 percent of the height of the *chimney* or vent except for engineered systems.

G2427.10.10 (503.10.10) Support. A *vent connector* shall be supported for the design and weight of the material employed to maintain *clearances* and prevent physical damage and separation of joints.

G2427.10.11 (503.10.11) Chimney connection. Where entering a flue in a masonry or metal *chimney*, the *vent connector* shall be installed above the extreme bottom to avoid stoppage. Where a thimble or slip joint is used to facilitate removal of the connector, the connector shall be firmly attached to or inserted into the thimble or slip joint to prevent the connector from falling out. Means shall be employed to prevent the connector from entering so far as to restrict the space between its end and the opposite wall of the *chimney* flue (see Section G2425.9).

G2427.10.12 (503.10.12) Inspection. The entire length of a *vent connector* shall be provided with *ready access* for inspection, cleaning, and replacement.

G2427.10.13 (503.10.13) Fireplaces. A *vent connector* shall not be connected to a *chimney* flue serving a *fireplace* unless the *fireplace* flue opening is permanently sealed.

G2427.10.14 (503.10.14) Passage through ceilings, floors or walls. Single-wall metal pipe connectors shall not pass through any wall, floor or ceiling except as permitted by Section G2427.7.4.

G2427.11 (503.11) Vent connectors for Category II, III and IV appliances. *Vent connectors* for Category II, III and IV *appliances* shall be as specified for the *venting systems* in accordance with Section G2427.4.

G2427.12 (503.12) Draft hoods and draft controls. The installation of *draft hoods* and *draft controls* shall comply with Sections G2427.12.1 through G2427.12.7.

G2427.12.1 (503.12.1) Appliances requiring draft hoods. *Vented appliances* shall be installed with *draft hoods*.

> **Exception:** Dual oven-type combination ranges; incinerators; *direct*-vent *appliances*; fan-assisted *combustion* system *appliances*; *appliances* requiring *chimney draft* for operation; single firebox boilers equipped with *conversion burners* with inputs greater than 400,000 *Btu* per hour (117 kW); *appliances* equipped with blast, power or pressure *burners* that are not listed for use with *draft hoods*; and *appliances* designed for forced venting.

G2427.12.2 (503.12.2) Installation. A *draft hood* supplied with or forming a part of a listed *vented appliance* shall be installed without *alteration*, exactly as furnished and specified by the *appliance* manufacturer.

G2427.12.2.1 (503.12.2.1) Draft hood required. If a *draft hood* is not supplied by the *appliance* manufacturer where one is required, a *draft hood* shall be installed, shall be of a listed or *approved* type and, in the absence of other instructions, shall be of the same size as the *appliance flue* collar. Where a *draft hood* is required with a *conversion burner*, it shall be of a listed or *approved* type.

G2427.12.2.2 (503.12.2.2) Special design draft hood. Where it is determined that a *draft hood* of special design is needed or preferable for a particular installation, the installation shall be in accordance with the recommendations of the *appliance* manufacturer and shall be *approved*.

G2427.12.3 (503.12.3) Draft control devices. Where a *draft control* device is part of the *appliance* or is supplied by the *appliance* manufacturer, it shall be installed in accordance with the manufacturer's instructions. In the absence of manufacturer's instructions, the device shall be attached to the *flue collar* of the *appliance* or as near to the *appliance* as practical.

G2427.12.4 (503.12.4) Additional devices. *Appliances* (except incinerators) requiring a controlled *chimney draft* shall be permitted to be equipped with a listed double-acting barometric-*draft regulator* installed and adjusted in accordance with the manufacturer's instructions.

G2427.12.5 (503.12.5) Location. *Draft hoods* and *barometric draft regulators* shall be installed in the same room or enclosure as the *appliance* in such a manner as to prevent any difference in pressure between the hood or *regulator* and the *combustion air* supply.

G2427.12.6 (503.12.6) Positioning. *Draft hoods* and *draft regulators* shall be installed in the position for which they were designed with reference to the horizontal and vertical planes and shall be located so that the *relief opening* is not obstructed by any part of the *appliance* or adjacent construction. The *appliance* and its *draft hood* shall be located so that the *relief opening* is accessible for checking *vent* operation.

G2427.12.7 (503.12.7) Clearance. A *draft hood* shall be located so its *relief opening* is not less than 6 inches (152 mm) from any surface except that of the *appliance* it serves and the venting system to which the *draft hood* is connected. Where a greater or lesser *clearance* is indicated on the *appli-*

ance label, the *clearance* shall be not less than that specified on the label. Such *clearances* shall not be reduced.

G2427.13 (503.13) Manually operated dampers. A manually operated *damper* shall not be placed in the vent *connector* for any *appliance*. Fixed baffles shall not be classified as manually operated *dampers*.

G2427.14 (503.14) Automatically operated vent dampers. An automatically operated vent damper shall be of a listed type.

G2427.15 (503.15) Obstructions. Devices that retard the flow of *vent gases* shall not be installed in a *vent connector, chimney,* or vent. The following shall not be considered as obstructions:

1. *Draft regulators* and safety *controls* specifically listed for installation in *venting systems* and installed in accordance with the manufacturer's installation instructions.

2. *Approved draft regulators* and safety *controls* that are designed and installed in accordance with *approved* engineering methods.

3. Listed heat reclaimers and automatically operated vent dampers installed in accordance with the manufacturer's installation instructions.

4. *Approved* economizers, heat reclaimers, and recuperators installed in *venting systems* of *appliances* not required to be equipped with *draft hoods*, provided that the *appliance* manufacturer's instructions cover the installation of such a device in the venting system and performance in accordance with Sections G2427.3 and G2427.3.1 is obtained.

5. Vent dampers serving listed *appliances* installed in accordance with Sections G2428.2.1 and G2428.3.1 or other *approved* engineering methods.

G2427.16 (503.16) (IFGS) Outside wall penetrations. Where vents, including those for *direct-vent appliances*, penetrate outside walls of buildings, the annular spaces around such penetrations shall be permanently sealed using *approved* materials to prevent entry of *combustion products* into the building.

SECTION G2428 (504)
SIZING OF CATEGORY I APPLIANCE
VENTING SYSTEMS

G2428.1 (504.1) Definitions. The following definitions apply to tables in this section.

APPLIANCE CATEGORIZED VENT DIAMETER/AREA. The minimum vent area/diameter permissible for Category I *appliances* to maintain a nonpositive vent static pressure when tested in accordance with nationally recognized standards.

FAN-ASSISTED COMBUSTION SYSTEM. An *appliance* equipped with an integral mechanical means to either draw or force products of *combustion* through the *combustion chamber* or heat exchanger.

FAN MIN. The minimum input rating of a Category I fan-assisted *appliance* attached to a vent or connector.

FAN MAX. The maximum input rating of a Category I fan-assisted *appliance* attached to a vent or connector.

NAT MAX. The maximum input rating of a Category I draft-hood-equipped *appliance* attached to a vent or connector.

FAN + FAN. The maximum combined *appliance* input rating of two or more Category I fan-assisted *appliances* attached to the common vent.

FAN + NAT. The maximum combined *appliance* input rating of one or more Category I fan-assisted *appliances* and one or more Category I draft-hood-equipped *appliances* attached to the common vent.

NA. Vent configuration is not permitted due to potential for *condensate* formation or pressurization of the venting system, or not applicable due to physical or geometric restraints.

NAT + NAT. The maximum combined *appliance* input rating of two or more Category I draft-hood-equipped *appliances* attached to the common vent.

G2428.2 (504.2) Application of single appliance vent Tables G2428.2(1) and G2428.2(2). The application of Tables G2428.2(1) and G2428.2(2) shall be subject to the requirements of Sections G2428.2.1 through G2428.2.16.

G2428.2.1 (504.2.1) Vent obstructions. These venting tables shall not be used where obstructions, as described in Section G2427.15, are installed in the venting system. The installation of vents serving listed *appliances* with vent dampers shall be in accordance with the *appliance* manufacturer's instructions or in accordance with the following:

1. The maximum capacity of the vent system shall be determined using the "NAT Max" column.

2. The minimum capacity shall be determined as if the *appliance* were a fan-assisted *appliance*, using the "FAN Min" column to determine the minimum capacity of the vent system. Where the corresponding "FAN Min" is "NA," the vent configuration shall not be permitted and an alternative venting configuration shall be utilized.

G2428.2.2 (504.2.2) Minimum size. Where the vent size determined from the tables is smaller than the *appliance draft hood* outlet or *flue collar*, the smaller size shall be permitted to be used provided all of the following are met:

1. The total vent height (H) is at least 10 feet (3048 mm).

2. Vents for *appliance draft hood* outlets or *flue collars* 12 inches (305 mm) in diameter or smaller are not reduced more than one table size.

3. Vents for *appliance draft hood* outlets or *flue collars* larger than 12 inches (305 mm) in diameter are not reduced more than two table sizes.

4. The maximum capacity listed in the tables for a fan-assisted *appliance* is reduced by 10 percent (0.90 by maximum table capacity).

5. The *draft hood* outlet is greater than 4 inches (102 mm) in diameter. Do not connect a 3-inch-diameter (76 mm) vent to a 4-inch-diameter (102 mm) *draft hood* outlet. This provision shall not apply to fan-assisted *appliances*.

TABLE G2428.2(1) [504.2(1)]
TYPE B DOUBLE-WALL GAS VENT

Number of Appliances	Single
Appliance Type	Category I
Appliance Vent Connection	Connected directly to vent

VENT DIAMETER—(D) inches

APPLIANCE INPUT RATING IN THOUSANDS OF BTU/H

HEIGHT (H) (feet)	LATERAL (L) (feet)	3 FAN Min	3 FAN Max	3 NAT Max	4 FAN Min	4 FAN Max	4 NAT Max	5 FAN Min	5 FAN Max	5 NAT Max	6 FAN Min	6 FAN Max	6 NAT Max	7 FAN Min	7 FAN Max	7 NAT Max	8 FAN Min	8 FAN Max	8 NAT Max	9 FAN Min	9 FAN Max	9 NAT Max
6	0	0	78	46	0	152	86	0	251	141	0	375	205	0	524	285	0	698	370	0	897	470
	2	13	51	36	18	97	67	27	157	105	32	232	157	44	321	217	53	425	285	63	543	370
	4	21	49	34	30	94	64	39	153	103	50	227	153	66	316	211	79	419	279	93	536	362
	6	25	46	32	36	91	61	47	149	100	59	223	149	78	310	205	93	413	273	110	530	354
8	0	0	84	50	0	165	94	0	276	155	0	415	235	0	583	320	0	780	415	0	1,006	537
	2	12	57	40	16	109	75	25	178	120	28	263	180	42	365	247	50	483	322	60	619	418
	5	23	53	38	32	103	71	42	171	115	53	255	173	70	356	237	83	473	313	99	607	407
	8	28	49	35	39	98	66	51	164	109	64	247	165	84	347	227	99	463	303	117	596	396
10	0	0	88	53	0	175	100	0	295	166	0	447	255	0	631	345	0	847	450	0	1,096	585
	2	12	61	42	17	118	81	23	194	129	26	289	195	40	402	273	48	533	355	57	684	457
	5	23	57	40	32	113	77	41	187	124	52	280	188	68	392	263	81	522	346	95	671	446
	10	30	51	36	41	104	70	54	176	115	67	267	175	88	376	245	104	504	330	122	651	427
15	0	0	94	58	0	191	112	0	327	187	0	502	285	0	716	390	0	970	525	0	1,263	682
	2	11	69	48	15	136	93	20	226	150	22	339	225	38	475	316	45	633	414	53	815	544
	5	22	65	45	30	130	87	39	219	142	49	330	217	64	463	300	76	620	403	90	800	529
	10	29	59	41	40	121	82	51	206	135	64	315	208	84	445	288	99	600	386	116	777	507
	15	35	53	37	48	112	76	61	195	128	76	301	198	98	429	275	115	580	373	134	755	491
20	0	0	97	61	0	202	119	0	349	202	0	540	307	0	776	430	0	1,057	575	0	1,384	752
	2	10	75	51	14	149	100	18	250	166	20	377	249	33	531	346	41	711	470	50	917	612
	5	21	71	48	29	143	96	38	242	160	47	367	241	62	519	337	73	697	460	86	902	599
	10	28	64	44	38	133	89	50	229	150	62	351	228	81	499	321	95	675	443	112	877	576
	15	34	58	40	46	124	84	59	217	142	73	337	217	94	481	308	111	654	427	129	853	557
	20	48	52	35	55	116	78	69	206	134	84	322	206	107	464	295	125	634	410	145	830	537

(continued)

TABLE G2428.2(1) [504.2(1)]—continued
TYPE B DOUBLE-WALL GAS VENT

Number of Appliances	Single
Appliance Type	Category I
Appliance Vent Connection	Connected directly to vent

VENT DIAMETER—(D) inches

APPLIANCE INPUT RATING IN THOUSANDS OF BTU/H

HEIGHT (H) (feet)	LATERAL (L) (feet)	3 FAN Min	3 FAN Max	3 NAT Max	4 FAN Min	4 FAN Max	4 NAT Max	5 FAN Min	5 FAN Max	5 NAT Max	6 FAN Min	6 FAN Max	6 NAT Max	7 FAN Min	7 FAN Max	7 NAT Max	8 FAN Min	8 FAN Max	8 NAT Max	9 FAN Min	9 FAN Max	9 NAT Max
30	0	0	100	64	0	213	128	0	374	220	0	587	336	0	853	475	0	1,173	650	0	1,548	855
	2	9	81	56	13	166	112	14	283	185	18	432	280	27	613	394	33	826	535	42	1,072	700
	5	21	77	54	28	160	108	36	275	176	45	421	273	58	600	385	69	811	524	82	1,055	688
	10	27	70	50	37	150	102	48	262	171	59	405	261	77	580	371	91	788	507	107	1,028	668
	15	33	64	NA	44	141	96	57	249	163	70	389	249	90	560	357	105	765	490	124	1,002	648
	20	56	58	NA	53	132	90	66	237	154	80	374	237	102	542	343	119	743	473	139	977	628
	30	NA	NA	NA	73	113	NA	88	214	NA	104	346	219	131	507	321	149	702	444	171	929	594
50	0	0	101	67	0	216	134	0	397	232	0	633	363	0	932	518	0	1,297	708	0	1,730	952
	2	8	86	61	11	183	122	14	320	206	15	497	314	22	715	445	26	975	615	33	1,276	813
	5	20	82	NA	27	177	119	35	312	200	43	487	308	55	702	438	65	960	605	77	1,259	798
	10	26	76	NA	35	168	114	45	299	190	56	471	298	73	681	426	86	935	589	101	1,230	773
	15	59	70	NA	42	158	NA	54	287	180	66	455	288	85	662	413	100	911	572	117	1,203	747
	20	NA	NA	NA	50	149	NA	63	275	169	76	440	278	97	642	401	113	888	556	131	1,176	722
	30	NA	NA	NA	69	131	NA	84	250	NA	99	410	259	123	605	376	141	844	522	161	1,125	670

For SI: 1 inch = 25.4 mm, 1 foot = 304.8 mm, 1 British thermal unit per hour = 0.2931 W.

TABLE G2428.2(2) [504.2(2)]
TYPE B DOUBLE-WALL GAS VENT

Number of Appliances	Single
Appliance Type	Category I
Appliance Vent Connection	Single-wall metal connector

APPLIANCE INPUT RATING IN THOUSANDS OF BTU/H

HEIGHT (H) (feet)	LATERAL (L) (feet)	3" FAN Min	3" FAN Max	3" NAT Max	4" FAN Min	4" FAN Max	4" NAT Max	5" FAN Min	5" FAN Max	5" NAT Max	6" FAN Min	6" FAN Max	6" NAT Max	7" FAN Min	7" FAN Max	7" NAT Max	8" FAN Min	8" FAN Max	8" NAT Max	9" FAN Min	9" FAN Max	9" NAT Max	10" FAN Min	10" FAN Max	10" NAT Max	12" FAN Min	12" FAN Max	12" NAT Max
6	0	38	77	45	59	151	85	85	249	140	126	373	204	165	522	284	211	695	369	267	894	469	371	1,118	569	537	1,639	849
6	2	39	51	36	60	96	66	85	156	104	123	231	156	159	320	213	201	423	284	251	541	368	347	673	453	498	979	648
6	4	NA	NA	33	74	92	63	102	152	102	146	225	152	187	313	208	237	416	277	295	533	360	409	664	443	584	971	638
6	6	NA	NA	31	83	89	60	114	147	99	163	220	148	207	307	203	263	409	271	327	526	352	449	656	433	638	962	627
8	0	37	83	50	58	164	93	83	273	154	123	412	234	161	580	319	206	777	414	258	1,002	536	360	1,257	658	521	1,852	967
8	2	39	56	39	59	108	75	83	176	119	121	261	179	155	363	246	197	482	321	246	617	417	339	768	513	486	1,120	743
8	5	NA	NA	37	77	102	69	107	168	114	151	252	171	193	352	235	245	470	311	305	604	404	418	754	500	598	1,104	730
8	8	NA	NA	33	90	95	64	122	161	107	175	243	163	223	342	225	280	458	300	344	591	392	470	740	486	665	1,089	715
10	0	37	87	53	57	174	99	82	293	165	120	444	254	158	628	344	202	844	449	253	1,093	584	351	1,373	718	507	2,031	1,057
10	2	39	61	41	59	117	80	82	193	128	119	287	194	153	400	272	193	531	354	242	681	456	332	849	559	475	1,242	848
10	5	52	56	39	76	111	76	105	185	122	148	277	186	190	388	261	241	518	344	299	667	443	409	834	544	584	1,224	825
10	10	NA	NA	34	97	100	68	132	171	112	188	261	171	237	369	241	296	497	325	363	643	423	492	808	520	688	1,194	788
15	0	36	93	57	56	190	111	80	325	186	116	499	283	153	713	388	195	966	523	244	1,259	681	336	1,591	838	488	2,374	1,237
15	2	38	69	47	57	136	93	80	225	149	115	337	224	148	473	314	187	631	413	232	812	543	319	1,015	673	457	1,491	983
15	5	51	63	44	75	128	86	102	216	140	144	326	217	182	459	298	231	616	400	287	795	526	392	997	657	562	1,469	963
15	10	NA	NA	39	95	116	79	128	201	131	182	308	203	228	438	284	284	592	381	349	768	501	470	966	628	664	1,433	928
15	15	NA	NA	NA	NA	NA	72	158	186	124	220	290	192	272	418	269	334	568	367	404	742	484	540	937	601	750	1,399	894
20	0	35	96	60	54	200	118	78	346	201	114	537	306	149	772	428	190	1,053	573	238	1,379	750	326	1,751	927	473	2,631	1,346
20	2	37	74	50	56	148	99	78	248	165	113	375	248	144	528	344	182	708	468	227	914	611	309	1,146	754	443	1,689	1,098
20	5	50	68	47	73	140	94	100	239	158	141	363	239	178	514	334	224	692	457	279	896	596	381	1,126	734	547	1,665	1,074
20	10	NA	NA	41	93	129	86	125	223	146	177	344	224	222	491	316	277	666	437	339	866	570	457	1,092	702	646	1,626	1,037
20	15	NA	NA	NA	NA	NA	80	155	208	136	216	325	210	264	469	301	325	640	419	393	838	549	526	1,060	677	730	1,587	1,005
20	20	NA	NA	NA	NA	NA	NA	186	192	126	254	306	196	309	448	285	374	616	400	448	810	526	592	1,028	651	808	1,550	973

(continued)

TABLE G2428.2(2) [504.2(2)]—continued
TYPE B DOUBLE-WALL GAS VENT

Number of Appliances	Single
Appliance Type	Category I
Appliance Vent Connection	Single-wall metal connector

APPLIANCE INPUT RATING IN THOUSANDS OF BTU/H

HEIGHT (H) (feet)	LATERAL (L) (feet)	VENT DIAMETER—(D) inches																									
		3			4			5			6			7			8			9			10			12		
		FAN		NAT	FAN		NAT	FAN		NAT	FAN		NAT	FAN		NAT	FAN		NAT	FAN		NAT	FAN		NAT	FAN		NAT
		Min	Max	Max	Min	Max	Max	Min	Max	Max	Min	Max	Max	Min	Max	Max	Min	Max	Max	Min	Max	Max	Min	Max	Max	Min	Max	Max
30	0	34	99	63	53	211	127	76	372	219	110	584	334	144	849	472	184	1,168	647	229	1,542	852	312	1,971	1,056	454	2,996	1,545
	2	37	80	56	55	164	111	76	281	183	109	429	279	139	610	392	175	823	533	219	1,069	698	296	1,346	863	424	1,999	1,308
	5	49	74	52	72	157	106	98	271	173	136	417	271	171	595	382	215	806	521	269	1,049	684	366	1,324	846	524	1,971	1,283
	10	NA	NA	NA	91	144	98	122	255	168	171	397	257	213	570	367	265	777	501	327	1,017	662	440	1,287	821	620	1,927	1,234
	15	NA	NA	NA	115	131	NA	151	239	157	208	377	242	255	547	349	312	750	481	379	985	638	507	1,251	794	702	1,884	1,205
	20	NA	NA	NA	NA	NA	NA	181	223	NA	246	357	228	298	524	333	360	723	461	433	955	615	570	1,216	768	780	1,841	1,166
	30	NA	NA	NA	NA	NA	NA	NA	NA	NA	NA	NA	NA	389	477	305	461	670	426	541	895	574	704	1,147	720	937	1,759	1,101
50	0	33	99	66	51	213	133	73	394	230	105	629	361	138	928	515	176	1,292	704	220	1,724	948	295	2,223	1,189	428	3,432	1,818
	2	36	84	61	53	181	121	73	318	205	104	495	312	133	712	443	168	971	613	209	1,273	811	280	1,615	1,007	401	2,426	1,509
	5	48	80	NA	70	174	117	94	308	198	131	482	305	164	696	435	204	953	602	257	1,252	795	347	1,591	991	496	2,396	1,490
	10	NA	NA	NA	89	160	NA	118	292	186	162	461	292	203	671	420	253	923	583	313	1,217	765	418	1,551	963	589	2,347	1,455
	15	NA	NA	NA	112	148	NA	145	275	174	199	441	280	244	646	405	299	894	562	363	1,183	736	481	1,512	934	668	2,299	1,421
	20	NA	NA	NA	NA	NA	NA	176	257	NA	236	420	267	285	622	389	345	866	543	415	1,150	708	544	1,473	906	741	2,251	1,387
	30	NA	NA	NA	NA	NA	NA	NA	NA	NA	315	376	NA	373	573	NA	442	809	502	521	1,086	649	674	1,399	848	892	2,159	1,318

For SI: 1 inch = 25.4 mm, 1 foot = 304.8 mm, 1 British thermal unit per hour = 0.2931 W.

G2428.2.3 (504.2.3) Vent offsets. Single-*appliance* venting configurations with zero (0) lateral lengths in Tables G2428.2(1) and G2428.2(2) shall not have elbows in the *venting system.* Single-*appliance* venting configurations with lateral lengths include two 90-degree (1.57 rad) elbows. For each additional elbow up to and including 45 degrees (0.79 rad), the maximum capacity listed in the venting tables shall be reduced by 5 percent. For each additional elbow greater than 45 degrees (0.79 rad) up to and including 90 degrees (1.57 rad), the maximum capacity listed in the venting tables shall be reduced by 10 percent. Where multiple *offsets* occur in a vent, the total lateral length of all *offsets* combined shall not exceed that specified in Tables G2428.2(1) and G2428.2(2).

G2428.2.4 (504.2.4) Zero lateral. Zero (0) lateral (L) shall apply only to a straight vertical vent attached to a top outlet *draft hood* or *flue collar.*

G2428.2.5 (504.2.5) High altitude installations. Sea level input ratings shall be used when determining maximum capacity for high altitude installation. Actual input, derated for altitude, shall be used for determining minimum capacity for high altitude installation.

G2428.2.6 (504.2.6) Multiple input rate appliances. For *appliances* with more than one input rate, the minimum vent capacity (FAN Min) determined from the tables shall be less than the lowest *appliance* input rating, and the maximum vent capacity (FAN Max/NAT Max) determined from tables shall be greater than the highest *appliance* rating input.

G2428.2.7 (504.2.7) Liner system sizing and connections. Listed corrugated metallic *chimney* liner systems in *masonry chimneys* shall be sized by using Table G2428.2(1) or G2428.2(2) for Type B vents with the maximum capacity reduced by 20 percent (0.80 × maximum capacity) and the minimum capacity as shown in Table G2428.2(1) or G2428.2(2). Corrugated metallic liner systems installed with bends or offsets shall have their maximum capacity further reduced in accordance with Section G2428.2.3. The 20-percent reduction for corrugated metallic *chimney* liner systems includes an allowance for one long-radius 90-degree (1.57 rad) turn at the bottom of the liner.

Connections between *chimney* liners and listed double-wall connectors shall be made with listed adapters designed for such purpose.

G2428.2.8 (504.2.8) Vent area and diameter. Where the vertical vent has a larger diameter than the *vent connector*, the vertical vent diameter shall be used to determine the minimum vent capacity, and the connector diameter shall be used to determine the maximum vent capacity. The flow area of the vertical vent shall not exceed seven times the flow area of the listed *appliance* categorized vent area, *flue collar* area, or *draft hood* outlet area unless designed in accordance with *approved* engineering methods.

G2428.2.9 (504.2.9) Chimney and vent locations. Tables G2428.2(1) and G2428.2(2) shall be used only for *chimneys* and vents not exposed to the outdoors below the roof line. A Type B vent or listed *chimney* lining system passing through an unused *masonry chimney* flue shall not be considered to be exposed to the outdoors. A Type B vent shall not be considered to be exposed to the outdoors where it passes through an unventilated enclosure or chase insulated to a value of not less than R-8.

G2428.2.10 (504.2.10) Corrugated vent connector size. Corrugated *vent connectors* shall be not smaller than the listed *appliance* categorized *vent* diameter, *flue collar* diameter, or *draft hood* outlet diameter.

G2428.2.11 (504.2.11) Vent connector size limitation. *Vent connectors* shall not be increased in size more than two sizes greater than the listed *appliance* categorized vent diameter, *flue collar* diameter or *draft hood* outlet diameter.

G2428.2.12 (504.2.12) Component commingling. In a single run of vent or *vent connector*, different diameters and types of vent and connector components shall be permitted to be used, provided that all such sizes and types are permitted by the tables.

G2428.2.13 (504.2.13) Draft hood conversion accessories. *Draft hood* conversion accessories for use with *masonry chimneys* venting listed Category I fan-assisted *appliances* shall be listed and installed in accordance with the manufacturer's installation instructions for such listed accessories.

G2428.2.14 (504.2.14) Table interpolation. Interpolation shall be permitted in calculating capacities for vent dimensions that fall between the table entries (see Example 3, Appendix B).

G2428.2.15 (504.2.15) Extrapolation prohibited. Extrapolation beyond the table entries shall not be permitted.

G2428.2.16 (504.2.16) Engineering calculations. For *vent* heights less than 6 feet (1829 mm) and greater than shown in the tables, engineering methods shall be used to calculate *vent* capacities.

G2428.3 (504.3) Application of multiple appliance vent Tables G2428.3(1) through G2428.3(4). The application of Tables G2428.3(1) through G2428.3(4) shall be subject to the requirements of Sections G2428.3.1 through G2428.3.23.

TABLE G2428.3(1) [504.3(1)]
TYPE B DOUBLE-WALL VENT

Number of Appliances	Two or more
Appliance Type	Category I
Appliance Vent Connection	Type B double-wall connector

VENT CONNECTOR CAPACITY

VENT HEIGHT (*H*) (feet)	CONNECTOR RISE (*R*) (feet)	3 FAN Min	3 FAN Max	3 NAT Max	4 FAN Min	4 FAN Max	4 NAT Max	5 FAN Min	5 FAN Max	5 NAT Max	6 FAN Min	6 FAN Max	6 NAT Max	7 FAN Min	7 FAN Max	7 NAT Max	8 FAN Min	8 FAN Max	8 NAT Max	9 FAN Min	9 FAN Max	9 NAT Max	10 FAN Min	10 FAN Max	10 NAT Max
6	1	22	37	26	35	66	46	46	106	72	58	164	104	77	225	142	92	296	185	109	376	237	128	466	289
	2	23	41	31	37	75	55	48	121	86	60	183	124	79	253	168	95	333	220	112	424	282	131	526	345
	3	24	44	35	38	81	62	49	132	96	62	199	139	82	275	189	97	363	248	114	463	317	134	575	386
8	1	22	40	27	35	72	48	49	114	76	64	176	109	84	243	148	100	320	194	118	408	248	138	507	303
	2	23	44	32	36	80	57	51	128	90	66	195	129	86	269	175	103	356	230	121	454	294	141	564	358
	3	24	47	36	37	87	64	53	139	101	67	210	145	88	290	198	105	384	258	123	492	330	143	612	402
10	1	22	43	28	34	78	50	49	123	78	65	189	113	89	257	154	106	341	200	125	436	257	146	542	314
	2	23	47	33	36	86	59	51	136	93	67	206	134	91	282	182	109	374	238	128	479	305	149	596	372
	3	24	50	37	37	92	67	52	146	104	69	220	150	94	303	205	111	402	268	131	515	342	152	642	417
15	1	21	50	30	33	89	53	47	142	83	64	220	120	88	298	163	110	389	214	134	493	273	162	609	333
	2	22	53	35	35	96	63	49	153	99	66	235	142	91	320	193	112	419	253	137	532	323	165	658	394
	3	24	55	40	36	102	71	51	163	111	68	248	160	93	339	218	115	445	286	140	565	365	167	700	444
20	1	21	54	31	33	99	56	46	157	87	62	246	125	86	334	171	107	436	224	131	552	285	158	681	347
	2	22	57	37	34	105	66	48	167	104	64	259	149	89	354	202	110	463	265	134	587	339	161	725	414
	3	23	60	42	35	110	74	50	176	116	66	271	168	91	371	228	113	486	300	137	618	383	164	764	466
30	1	20	62	33	31	113	59	45	181	93	60	288	134	83	391	182	103	512	238	125	649	305	151	802	372
	2	21	64	39	33	118	70	47	190	110	62	299	158	85	408	215	105	535	282	129	679	360	155	840	439
	3	22	66	44	34	123	79	48	198	124	64	309	178	88	423	242	108	555	317	132	706	405	158	874	494

COMMON VENT CAPACITY

VENT HEIGHT (*H*) (feet)	4 FAN +FAN	4 FAN +NAT	4 NAT +NAT	5 FAN +FAN	5 FAN +NAT	5 NAT +NAT	6 FAN +FAN	6 FAN +NAT	6 NAT +NAT	7 FAN +FAN	7 FAN +NAT	7 NAT +NAT	8 FAN +FAN	8 FAN +NAT	8 NAT +NAT	9 FAN +FAN	9 FAN +NAT	9 NAT +NAT	10 FAN +FAN	10 FAN +NAT	10 NAT +NAT
6	92	81	65	140	116	103	204	161	147	309	248	200	404	314	260	547	434	335	672	520	410
8	101	90	73	155	129	114	224	178	163	339	275	223	444	348	290	602	480	378	740	577	465
10	110	97	79	169	141	124	243	194	178	367	299	242	477	377	315	649	522	405	800	627	495
15	125	112	91	195	164	144	283	228	206	427	352	280	556	444	365	753	612	465	924	733	565
20	136	123	102	215	183	160	314	255	229	475	394	310	621	499	405	842	688	523	1,035	826	640
30	152	138	118	244	210	185	361	297	266	547	459	360	720	585	470	979	808	605	1,209	975	740
50	167	153	134	279	244	214	421	353	310	641	547	423	854	706	550	1,164	977	705	1,451	1,188	860

For SI: 1 inch = 25.4 mm, 1 foot = 304.8 mm, 1 British thermal unit per hour = 0.2931 W.

TABLE G2428.3(2) [504.3(2)]
TYPE B DOUBLE-WALL VENT

Number of Appliances	Two or more
Appliance Type	Category I
Appliance Vent Connection	Single-wall metal connector

VENT CONNECTOR CAPACITY

		SINGLE-WALL METAL VENT CONNECTOR DIAMETER—(D) inches																						
		3			4			5			6			7			8			9			10		
VENT HEIGHT (H) (feet)	CONNECTOR RISE (R) (feet)	APPLIANCE INPUT RATING LIMITS IN THOUSANDS OF BTU/H																						
		FAN		NAT	FAN		NAT	FAN		NAT	FAN		NAT	FAN		NAT	FAN		NAT	FAN		NAT	FAN		NAT
		Min	Max	Max	Min	Max	Max	Min	Max	Max	Min	Max	Max	Min	Max	Max	Min	Max	Max	Min	Max	Max	Min	Max	Max
6	1	NA	NA	26	NA	NA	46	NA	NA	71	NA	NA	102	207	223	140	262	293	183	325	373	234	447	463	286
	2	NA	NA	31	NA	NA	55	NA	NA	85	168	182	123	215	251	167	271	331	219	334	422	281	458	524	344
	3	NA	NA	34	NA	NA	62	121	131	95	175	198	138	222	273	188	279	361	247	344	462	316	468	574	385
8	1	NA	NA	27	NA	NA	48	NA	NA	75	NA	NA	106	226	240	145	285	316	191	352	403	244	481	502	299
	2	NA	NA	32	NA	NA	57	125	126	89	184	193	127	234	266	173	293	353	228	360	450	292	492	560	355
	3	NA	NA	35	NA	NA	64	130	138	100	191	208	144	241	287	197	302	381	256	370	489	328	501	609	400
10	1	NA	NA	28	NA	NA	50	119	121	77	182	186	110	240	253	150	302	335	196	372	429	252	506	534	308
	2	NA	NA	33	84	85	59	124	134	91	189	203	132	248	278	183	311	369	235	381	473	302	517	589	368
	3	NA	NA	36	89	91	67	129	144	102	197	217	148	257	299	203	320	398	265	391	511	339	528	637	413
15	1	NA	NA	29	79	87	52	116	138	81	177	214	116	238	291	158	312	380	208	397	482	266	556	596	324
	2	NA	NA	34	83	94	62	121	150	97	185	230	138	246	314	189	321	411	248	407	522	317	568	646	387
	3	NA	NA	39	87	100	70	127	160	109	193	243	157	255	333	215	331	438	281	418	557	360	579	690	437
20	1	49	56	30	78	97	54	115	152	84	175	238	120	233	325	165	306	425	217	390	538	276	546	664	336
	2	52	59	36	82	103	64	120	163	101	182	252	144	243	346	197	317	453	259	400	574	331	558	709	403
	3	55	62	40	87	107	72	125	172	113	190	264	164	252	363	223	326	476	294	412	607	375	570	750	457
30	1	47	60	31	77	110	57	112	175	89	169	278	129	226	380	175	296	497	230	378	630	294	528	779	358
	2	51	62	37	81	115	67	117	185	106	177	290	152	236	397	208	307	521	274	389	662	349	541	819	425
	3	54	64	42	85	119	76	122	193	120	185	300	172	244	412	235	316	542	309	400	690	394	555	855	482

COMMON VENT CAPACITY

	TYPE B DOUBLE-WALL COMMON VENT DIAMETER— (D) inches																				
	4			5			6			7			8			9			10		
VENT HEIGHT (H) (feet)	COMBINED APPLIANCE INPUT RATING IN THOUSANDS OF BTU/H																				
	FAN +FAN	FAN +NAT	NAT +NAT	FAN +FAN	FAN +NAT	NAT +NAT	FAN +FAN	FAN +NAT	NAT +NAT	FAN +FAN	FAN +NAT	NAT +NAT	FAN +FAN	FAN +NAT	NAT +NAT	FAN +FAN	FAN +NAT	NAT +NAT	FAN +FAN	FAN +NAT	NAT +NAT
6	NA	78	64	NA	113	99	200	158	144	304	244	196	398	310	257	541	429	332	665	515	407
8	NA	87	71	NA	126	111	218	173	159	331	269	218	436	342	285	592	473	373	730	569	460
10	NA	94	76	163	137	120	237	189	174	357	292	236	467	369	309	638	512	398	787	617	487
15	121	108	88	189	159	140	275	221	200	416	343	274	544	434	357	738	599	456	905	718	553
20	131	118	98	208	177	156	305	247	223	463	383	302	606	487	395	824	673	512	1,013	808	626
30	145	132	113	236	202	180	350	286	257	533	446	349	703	570	459	958	790	593	1,183	952	723
50	159	145	128	268	233	208	406	337	296	622	529	410	833	686	535	1,139	954	689	1,418	1,157	838

For SI: 1 inch = 25.4 mm, 1 foot = 304.8 mm, 1 British thermal unit per hour = 0.2931 W.

TABLE G2428.3(3) [504.3(3)]
MASONRY CHIMNEY

Number of Appliances	Two or more
Appliance Type	Category I
Appliance Vent Connection	Type B double-wall connector

VENT CONNECTOR CAPACITY

		TYPE B DOUBLE-WALL VENT CONNECTOR DIAMETER—(D) inches																							
		3			4			5			6			7			8			9			10		
		APPLIANCE INPUT RATING LIMITS IN THOUSANDS OF BTU/H																							
VENT HEIGHT (H) (feet)	CONNECTOR RISE (R) (feet)	FAN		NAT	FAN		NAT	FAN		NAT	FAN		NAT	FAN		NAT	FAN		NAT	FAN		NAT	FAN		NAT
		Min	Max	Max	Min	Max	Max	Min	Max	Max	Min	Max	Max	Min	Max	Max	Min	Max	Max	Min	Max	Max	Min	Max	Max
6	1	24	33	21	39	62	40	52	106	67	65	194	101	87	274	141	104	370	201	124	479	253	145	599	319
	2	26	43	28	41	79	52	53	133	85	67	230	124	89	324	173	107	436	232	127	562	300	148	694	378
	3	27	49	34	42	92	61	55	155	97	69	262	143	91	369	203	109	491	270	129	633	349	151	795	439
8	1	24	39	22	39	72	41	55	117	69	71	213	105	94	304	148	113	414	210	134	539	267	156	682	335
	2	26	47	29	40	87	53	57	140	86	73	246	127	97	350	179	116	473	240	137	615	311	160	776	394
	3	27	52	34	42	97	62	59	159	98	75	269	145	99	383	206	119	517	276	139	672	358	163	848	452
10	1	24	42	22	38	80	42	55	130	71	74	232	108	101	324	153	120	444	216	142	582	277	165	739	348
	2	26	50	29	40	93	54	57	153	87	76	261	129	103	366	184	123	498	247	145	652	321	168	825	407
	3	27	55	35	41	105	63	58	170	100	78	284	148	106	397	209	126	540	281	147	705	366	171	893	463
15	1	24	48	23	38	93	44	54	154	74	72	277	114	100	384	164	125	511	229	153	658	297	184	824	375
	2	25	55	31	39	105	55	56	174	89	74	299	134	103	419	192	128	558	260	156	718	339	187	900	432
	3	26	59	35	41	115	64	57	189	102	76	319	153	105	448	215	131	597	292	159	760	382	190	960	486
20	1	24	52	24	37	102	46	53	172	77	71	313	119	98	437	173	123	584	239	150	752	312	180	943	397
	2	25	58	31	39	114	56	55	190	91	73	335	138	101	467	199	126	625	270	153	805	354	184	1,011	452
	3	26	63	35	40	123	65	57	204	104	75	353	157	104	493	222	129	661	301	156	851	396	187	1,067	505

COMMON VENT CAPACITY

	MINIMUM INTERNAL AREA OF MASONRY CHIMNEY FLUE (square inches)																							
	12			19			28			38			50			63			78			113		
VENT HEIGHT (H) (feet)	COMBINED APPLIANCE INPUT RATING IN THOUSANDS OF BTU/H																							
	FAN +FAN	FAN +NAT	NAT +NAT	FAN +FAN	FAN +NAT	NAT +NAT	FAN +FAN	FAN +NAT	NAT +NAT	FAN +FAN	FAN +NAT	NAT +NAT	FAN +FAN	FAN +NAT	NAT +NAT	FAN +FAN	FAN +NAT	NAT +NAT	FAN +FAN	FAN +NAT	NAT +NAT	FAN +FAN	FAN +NAT	NAT +NAT
6	NA	74	25	NA	119	46	NA	178	71	NA	257	103	NA	351	143	NA	458	188	NA	582	246	1,041	853	NA
8	NA	80	28	NA	130	53	NA	193	82	NA	279	119	NA	384	163	NA	501	218	724	636	278	1,144	937	408
10	NA	84	31	NA	138	56	NA	207	90	NA	299	131	NA	409	177	606	538	236	776	686	302	1,226	1,010	454
15	NA	NA	36	NA	152	67	NA	233	106	NA	334	152	523	467	212	682	611	283	874	781	365	1,374	1,156	546
20	NA	NA	41	NA	NA	75	NA	250	122	NA	368	172	565	508	243	742	668	325	955	858	419	1,513	1,286	648
30	NA	NA	NA	NA	NA	NA	NA	270	137	NA	404	198	615	564	278	816	747	381	1,062	969	496	1,702	1,473	749
50	NA	NA	NA	NA	NA	NA	NA	NA	NA	NA	NA	NA	NA	620	328	879	831	461	1,165	1,089	606	1,905	1,692	922

For SI: 1 inch = 25.4 mm, 1 square inch = 645.16 mm², 1 foot = 304.8 mm, 1 British thermal unit per hour = 0.2931 W.

Number of Appliances	Two or more
Appliance Type	Category I
Appliance Vent Connection	Single-wall metal connector

TABLE G2428.3(4) [504.3(4)]
MASONRY CHIMNEY

VENT CONNECTOR CAPACITY

VENT HEIGHT (*H*) (feet)	CONNECTOR RISE (*R*) (feet)	SINGLE-WALL METAL VENT CONNECTOR DIAMETER (*D*)—inches																						
		3			4			5			6			7			8			9			10		
		\<APPLIANCE INPUT RATING LIMITS IN THOUSANDS OF BTU/H\>																						
		FAN		NAT	FAN		NAT	FAN		NAT	FAN		NAT	FAN		NAT	FAN		NAT	FAN		NAT	FAN		NAT
		Min	Max	Max	Min	Max	Max	Min	Max	Max	Min	Max	Max	Min	Max	Max	Min	Max	Max	Min	Max	Max	Min	Max	Max
6	1	NA	NA	21	NA	NA	39	NA	NA	66	179	191	100	231	271	140	292	366	200	362	474	252	499	594	316
	2	NA	NA	28	NA	NA	52	NA	NA	84	186	227	123	239	321	172	301	432	231	373	557	299	509	696	376
	3	NA	NA	34	NA	NA	61	134	153	97	193	258	142	247	365	202	309	491	269	381	634	348	519	793	437
8	1	NA	NA	21	NA	NA	40	NA	NA	68	195	208	103	250	298	146	313	407	207	387	530	263	529	672	331
	2	NA	NA	28	NA	NA	52	137	139	85	202	240	125	258	343	177	323	465	238	397	607	309	540	766	391
	3	NA	NA	34	NA	NA	62	143	156	98	210	264	145	266	376	205	332	509	274	407	663	356	551	838	450
10	1	NA	NA	22	NA	NA	41	130	151	70	202	225	106	267	316	151	333	434	213	410	571	273	558	727	343
	2	NA	NA	29	NA	NA	53	136	150	86	210	255	128	276	358	181	343	489	244	420	640	317	569	813	403
	3	NA	NA	34	97	102	62	143	166	99	217	277	147	284	389	207	352	530	279	430	694	363	580	880	459
15	1	NA	NA	23	NA	NA	43	129	151	73	199	271	112	268	376	161	349	502	225	445	646	291	623	808	366
	2	NA	NA	30	92	103	54	135	170	88	207	295	132	277	411	189	359	548	256	456	706	334	634	884	424
	3	NA	NA	34	96	112	63	141	185	101	215	315	151	286	439	213	368	586	289	466	755	378	646	945	479
20	1	NA	NA	23	87	99	45	128	167	76	197	303	117	265	425	169	345	569	235	439	734	306	614	921	347
	2	NA	NA	30	91	111	55	134	185	90	205	325	136	274	455	195	355	610	266	450	787	348	627	986	443
	3	NA	NA	35	96	119	64	140	199	103	213	343	154	282	481	219	365	644	298	461	831	391	639	1,042	496

COMMON VENT CAPACITY

VENT HEIGHT (*H*) (feet)	MINIMUM INTERNAL AREA OF MASONRY CHIMNEY FLUE (square inches)																							
	12			19			28			38			50			63			78			113		
	\<COMBINED APPLIANCE INPUT RATING IN THOUSANDS OF BTU/H\>																						
	FAN +FAN	FAN +NAT	NAT +NAT	FAN +FAN	FAN +NAT	NAT +NAT	FAN +FAN	FAN +NAT	NAT +NAT	FAN +FAN	FAN +NAT	NAT +NAT	FAN +FAN	FAN +NAT	NAT +NAT	FAN +FAN	FAN +NAT	NAT +NAT	FAN +FAN	FAN +NAT	NAT +NAT	FAN +FAN	FAN +NAT	NAT +NAT
6	NA	NA	25	NA	118	45	NA	176	71	NA	255	102	NA	348	142	NA	455	187	NA	579	245	NA	846	NA
8	NA	NA	28	NA	128	52	NA	190	81	NA	276	118	NA	380	162	NA	497	217	NA	633	277	1,136	928	405
10	NA	NA	31	NA	136	56	NA	205	89	NA	295	129	NA	405	175	NA	532	234	171	680	300	1,216	1,000	450
15	NA	NA	36	NA	NA	66	NA	230	105	NA	335	150	NA	400	210	677	602	280	866	772	360	1,359	1,139	540
20	NA	NA	NA	NA	NA	74	NA	247	120	NA	362	170	NA	503	240	765	661	321	947	849	415	1,495	1,264	640
30	NA	NA	NA	NA	NA	NA	NA	NA	135	NA	398	195	NA	558	275	808	739	377	1,052	957	490	1,682	1,447	740
50	NA	NA	NA	NA	NA	NA	NA	NA	NA	NA	NA	NA	NA	612	325	NA	821	456	1,152	1,076	600	1,879	1,672	910

For SI: 1 inch = 25.4 mm, 1 square inch = 645.16 mm^2, 1 foot = 304.8 mm, 1 British thermal unit per hour = 0.2931 W.

G2428.3.1 (504.3.1) Vent obstructions. These venting tables shall not be used where obstructions, as described in Section G2427.15, are installed in the venting system. The installation of vents serving listed *appliances* with vent dampers shall be in accordance with the *appliance* manufacturer's instructions or in accordance with the following:

1. The maximum capacity of the *vent connector* shall be determined using the NAT Max column.

2. The maximum capacity of the vertical vent or *chimney* shall be determined using the FAN+NAT column when the second *appliance* is a fan-assisted *appliance*, or the NAT+NAT column when the second *appliance* is equipped with a *draft hood*.

3. The minimum capacity shall be determined as if the *appliance* were a fan-assisted *appliance*.

   3.1. The minimum capacity of the *vent connector* shall be determined using the FAN Min column.

   3.2. The FAN+FAN column shall be used when the second *appliance* is a fan-assisted *appliance*, and the FAN+NAT column shall be used when the second *appliance* is equipped with a *draft hood*, to determine whether the vertical vent or *chimney* configuration is not permitted (NA). Where the vent configuration is NA, the vent configuration shall not be permitted and an alternative venting configuration shall be utilized.

G2428.3.2 (504.3.2) Connector length limit. The *vent connector* shall be routed to the vent utilizing the shortest possible route. Except as provided in Section G2428.3.3, the maximum *vent connector* horizontal length shall be 1.5 feet (457 mm) for each inch (18 mm per mm) of connector diameter as shown in Table G2428.3.2.

TABLE G2428.3.2 (504.3.2)
MAXIMUM VENT CONNECTOR LENGTH

CONNECTOR DIAMETER	CONNECTOR HORIZONTAL
Maximum (inches)	Length (feet)
3	4.5
4	6
5	7.5
6	9
7	10.5
8	12
9	13.5

For SI: 1 inch = 25.4 mm, 1 foot = 304.8 mm.

G2428.3.3 (504.3.3) Connectors with longer lengths. Connectors with longer horizontal lengths than those listed in Section G2428.3.2 are permitted under the following conditions:

1. The maximum capacity (FAN Max or NAT Max) of the *vent connector* shall be reduced 10 percent for each additional multiple of the length listed above. For example, the maximum length listed above for a 4-inch (102 mm) connector is 6 feet (1829 mm). With a con-

nector length greater than 6 feet (1829 mm), but not exceeding 12 feet (3658 mm), the maximum capacity must be reduced by 10 percent (0.90 × maximum *vent connector* capacity). With a connector length greater than 12 feet (3658 mm), but not exceeding 18 feet (5486 mm), the maximum capacity must be reduced by 20 percent (0.80 × maximum vent capacity).

2. For a connector serving a fan-assisted *appliance*, the minimum capacity (FAN Min) of the connector shall be determined by referring to the corresponding single *appliance* table. For Type B double-wall connectors, Table G2428.2(1) shall be used. For single-wall connectors, Table G2428.2(2) shall be used. The height (H) and lateral (L) shall be measured according to the procedures for a single *appliance* vent, *as if* the other *appliances* were not present.

G2428.3.4 (504.3.4) Vent connector manifold. Where the *vent connectors* are combined prior to entering the vertical portion of the common vent to form a common vent manifold, the size of the common vent manifold and the common vent shall be determined by applying a 10-percent reduction (0.90 × maximum common vent capacity) to the common vent capacity part of the common vent tables. The length of the common *vent connector* manifold (L_M) shall not exceed $1^1/_2$ feet for each inch (18 mm per mm) of common *vent connector* manifold diameter (D) (see Appendix B Figure B-11).

G2428.3.5 (504.3.5) Common vertical vent offset. Where the common vertical vent is *offset*, the maximum capacity of the common vent shall be reduced in accordance with Section G2428.3.6. The horizontal length of the common vent *offset* (L_o) shall not exceed $1^1/_2$ feet for each inch (18 mm per mm) of common vent diameter (D). Where multiple *offsets* occur in a common vent, the total horizontal length of all *offsets* combined shall not exceed $1^1/_2$ feet for each inch (18 mm/mm per) of the common vent diameter (D).

G2428.3.6 (504.3.6) Elbows in vents. For each elbow up to and including 45 degrees (0.79 rad) in the common vent, the maximum common vent capacity listed in the venting tables shall be reduced by 5 percent. For each elbow greater than 45 degrees (0.79 rad) up to and including 90 degrees (1.57 rad), the maximum common vent capacity listed in the venting tables shall be reduced by 10 percent.

G2428.3.7 (504.3.7) Elbows in connectors. The *vent connector* capacities listed in the common vent sizing tables include allowance for two 90-degree (1.57 rad) elbows. For each additional elbow up to and including 45 degrees (0.79 rad), the maximum *vent connector* capacity listed in the venting tables shall be reduced by 5 percent. For each elbow greater than 45 degrees (0.79 rad) up to and including 90 degrees (1.57 rad), the maximum *vent connector* capacity listed in the venting tables shall be reduced by 10 percent.

G2428.3.8 (504.3.8) Common vent minimum size. The cross-sectional area of the common vent shall be equal to or greater than the cross-sectional area of the largest connector.

G2428.3.9 (504.3.9) Common vent fittings. At the point where tee or wye fittings connect to a common vent, the opening size of the fitting shall be equal to the size of the common vent. Such fittings shall not be prohibited from having reduced-size openings at the point of connection of *appliance vent connectors*.

> **G2428.3.9.1 (504.3.9.1) Tee and wye fittings.** Tee and wye fittings connected to a common gas vent shall be considered as part of the common gas vent and shall be constructed of materials consistent with that of the common gas vent.

G2428.3.10 (504.3.10) High altitude installations. Sea-level input ratings shall be used when determining maximum capacity for high altitude installation. Actual input, derated for altitude, shall be used for determining minimum capacity for high altitude installation.

G2428.3.11 (504.3.11) Connector rise measurement. Connector rise (R) for each *appliance connector* shall be measured from the *draft hood* outlet or *flue collar* to the centerline where the vent gas streams come together.

G2428.3.12 (504.3.12) Vent height measurement. For multiple *appliances* all located on one floor, available total height (H) shall be measured from the highest *draft hood* outlet or *flue collar* up to the level of the outlet of the common vent.

G2428.3.13 (504.3.17) Vertical vent maximum size. Where two or more *appliances* are connected to a vertical vent or *chimney*, the flow area of the largest section of vertical vent or *chimney* shall not exceed seven times the smallest listed *appliance* categorized vent areas, *flue collar* area, or *draft hood* outlet area unless designed in accordance with *approved* engineering methods.

G2428.3.14 (504.3.18) Multiple input rate appliances. For *appliances* with more than one input rate, the minimum *vent connector* capacity (FAN Min) determined from the tables shall be less than the lowest *appliance* input rating, and the maximum *vent connector* capacity (FAN Max or NAT Max) determined from the tables shall be greater than the highest *appliance* input rating.

G2428.3.15 (504.3.19) Liner system sizing and connections. Listed, corrugated metallic *chimney* liner systems in *masonry chimneys* shall be sized by using Table G2428.3(1) or G2428.3(2) for Type B vents, with the maximum capacity reduced by 20 percent (0.80 × maximum capacity) and the minimum capacity as shown in Table G2428.3(1) or G2428.3(2). Corrugated metallic liner systems installed with bends or offsets shall have their maximum capacity further reduced in accordance with Sections G2428.3.5 and G2428.3.6. The 20-percent reduction for corrugated metallic *chimney* liner systems includes an allowance for one long-radius 90-degree (1.57 rad) turn at the bottom of the liner. Where double-wall connectors are required, tee and wye fittings used to connect to the common vent *chimney* liner shall be listed double-wall fittings. Connections between *chimney* liners and listed double-wall fittings shall be made with listed adapter fittings designed for such purpose.

G2428.3.16 (504.3.20) Chimney and vent location. Tables G2428.3(1), G2428.3(2), G2428.3(3) and G2428.3(4) shall be used only for *chimneys* and vents not exposed to the outdoors below the roof line. A Type B vent or listed *chimney* lining system passing through an unused masonry *chimney* flue shall not be considered to be exposed to the outdoors. A Type B vent shall not be considered to be exposed to the outdoors where it passes through an unventilated enclosure or chase insulated to a value of not less than R-8.

G2428.3.17 (504.3.21) Connector maximum and minimum size. *Vent connectors* shall not be increased in size more than two sizes greater than the listed *appliance* categorized vent diameter, *flue collar* diameter, or *draft hood* outlet diameter. *Vent connectors* for draft-hood-equipped *appliances* shall not be smaller than the *draft hood* outlet diameter. Where a *vent connector* size(s) determined from the tables for a fan-assisted *appliance(s)* is smaller than the *flue collar* diameter, the use of the smaller size(s) shall be permitted provided that the installation complies with all of the following conditions:

1. *Vent connectors* for fan-assisted *appliance flue collars* 12 inches (305 mm) in diameter or smaller are not reduced by more than one table size [e.g., 12 inches to 10 inches (305 mm to 254 mm) is a one-size reduction] and those larger than 12 inches (305 mm) in diameter are not reduced more than two table sizes [e.g., 24 inches to 20 inches (610 mm to 508 mm) is a two-size reduction].

2. The fan-assisted *appliance(s)* is common vented with a draft-hood-equipped *appliance(s)*.

3. The vent *connector* has a smooth interior wall.

G2428.3.18 (504.3.22) Component commingling. All combinations of pipe sizes, single-wall, and double-wall metal pipe shall be allowed within any connector run(s) or within the common vent, provided all of the appropriate tables permit all of the desired sizes and types of pipe, as if they were used for the entire length of the subject connector or vent. Where single-wall and Type B double-wall metal pipes are used for *vent connectors* within the same venting system, the common vent must be sized using Table G2428.3(2) or G2428.3(4), as appropriate.

G2428.3.19 (504.3.23) Draft hood conversion accessories. *Draft hood* conversion accessories for use with *masonry chimneys* venting listed Category I fan-assisted *appliances* shall be listed and installed in accordance with the manufacturer's installation instructions for such listed accessories.

G2428.3.20 (504.3.24) Multiple sizes permitted. Where a table permits more than one diameter of pipe to be used for a connector or vent, all the permitted sizes shall be permitted to be used.

G2428.3.21 (504.3.25) Table interpolation. Interpolation shall be permitted in calculating capacities for vent dimensions that fall between table entries. (See Example 3, Appendix B.)

G2428.3.22 (504.3.26) Extrapolation prohibited. Extrapolation beyond the table entries shall not be permitted.

G2428.3.23 (504.3.27) Engineering calculations. For vent heights less than 6 feet (1829 mm) and greater than shown in the tables, engineering methods shall be used to calculate vent capacities.

SECTION G2429 (505)
DIRECT-VENT, INTEGRAL VENT, MECHANICAL VENT AND VENTILATION/EXHAUST HOOD VENTING

G2429.1 (505.1) General. The installation of direct-vent and integral vent *appliances* shall be in accordance with Section G2427. Mechanical *venting systems* shall be designed and installed in accordance with Section G2427.

SECTION G2430 (506)
FACTORY-BUILT CHIMNEYS

G2430.1 (506.1) Listing. Factory-built *chimneys* for building heating *appliances* producing *flue gases* having a temperature not greater than 1,000°F (538°C), measured at the entrance to the *chimney*, shall be listed and labeled in accordance with UL 103 and shall be installed and terminated in accordance with the manufacturer's installation instructions.

G2430.2 (506.2) Support. Where factory-built *chimneys* are supported by structural members, such as joists and rafters, such members shall be designed to support the additional load.

SECTION G2431 (601)
GENERAL

G2431.1 (601.1) Scope. Sections G2432 through G2453 shall govern the approval, design, installation, construction, maintenance, *alteration* and repair of the *appliances* and *equipment* specifically identified herein.

SECTION G2432 (602)
DECORATIVE APPLIANCES FOR INSTALLATION IN FIREPLACES

G2432.1 (602.1) General. Decorative *appliances* for installation in *approved* solid fuel burning *fireplaces* shall be tested in accordance with ANSI Z21.60 and shall be installed in accordance with the manufacturer's installation instructions. Manually lighted natural gas decorative *appliances* shall be tested in accordance with ANSI Z21.84.

G2432.2 (602.2) Flame safeguard device. Decorative *appliances* for installation in *approved* solid fuel-burning *fireplaces*, with the exception of those tested in accordance with ANSI Z21.84, shall utilize a direct ignition device, an ignitor or a *pilot* flame to ignite the fuel at the *main burner*, and shall be equipped with a *flame safeguard* device. The *flame safeguard* device shall automatically shut off the fuel supply to a *main burner* or group of *burners* when the means of ignition of such *burners* becomes inoperative.

G2432.3 (602.3) Prohibited installations. Decorative *appliances* for installation in *fireplaces* shall not be installed where prohibited by Section G2406.2.

SECTION G2433 (603)
LOG LIGHTERS

G2433.1 (603.1) General. Log lighters shall be tested in accordance with CSA 8 and shall be installed in accordance with the manufacturer's installation instructions.

SECTION G2434 (604)
VENTED GAS FIREPLACES (DECORATIVE APPLIANCES)

G2434.1 (604.1) General. Vented gas *fireplaces* shall be tested in accordance with ANSI Z21.50, shall be installed in accordance with the manufacturer's installation instructions and shall be designed and equipped as specified in Section G2432.2.

G2434.2 (604.2) Access. Panels, grilles, and access doors that are required to be removed for normal servicing operations shall not be attached to the building.

SECTION G2435 (605)
VENTED GAS FIREPLACE HEATERS

G2435.1 (605.1) General. Vented gas *fireplace* heaters shall be installed in accordance with the manufacturer's installation instructions, shall be tested in accordance with ANSI Z21.88 and shall be designed and equipped as specified in Section G2432.2.

SECTION G2436 (608)
VENTED WALL FURNACES

G2436.1 (608.1) General. *Vented wall furnaces* shall be tested in accordance with ANSI Z21.86/CSA 2.32 and shall be installed in accordance with the manufacturer's installation instructions.

G2436.2 (608.2) Venting. *Vented wall furnaces* shall be vented in accordance with Section G2427.

G2436.3 (608.3) Location. *Vented wall furnaces* shall be located so as not to cause a fire hazard to walls, floors, combustible furnishings or doors. *Vented wall furnaces* installed between bathrooms and adjoining rooms shall not circulate air from bathrooms to other parts of the building.

G2436.4 (608.4) Door swing. *Vented wall furnaces* shall be located so that a door cannot swing within 12 inches (305 mm) of an air inlet or air outlet of such *furnace* measured at right angles to the opening. Doorstops or door closers shall not be installed to obtain this *clearance*.

G2436.5 (608.5) Ducts prohibited. Ducts shall not be attached to wall *furnaces*. Casing extension boots shall not be installed unless listed as part of the *appliance*.

G2436.6 (608.6) Access. *Vented wall furnaces* shall be provided with access for cleaning of heating surfaces, removal of *burners*, replacement of sections, motors, *controls*, filters and other working parts, and for adjustments and lubrication of parts requiring such attention. Panels, grilles and access doors that are required to be removed for normal servicing operations shall not be attached to the building construction.

SECTION G2437 (609)
FLOOR FURNACES

G2437.1 (609.1) General. *Floor furnaces* shall be tested in accordance with ANSI Z21.86/CSA 2.32 and shall be installed in accordance with the manufacturer's installation instructions.

G2437.2 (609.2) Placement. The following provisions apply to *floor furnaces*:

1. Floors. *Floor furnaces* shall not be installed in the floor of any doorway, stairway landing, aisle or passageway of any enclosure, public or private, or in an exitway from any such room or space.

2. Walls and corners. The register of a *floor furnace* with a horizontal warm air outlet shall not be placed closer than 6 inches (152 mm) to the nearest wall. A distance of at least 18 inches (457 mm) from two adjoining sides of the *floor furnace* register to walls shall be provided to eliminate the necessity of occupants walking over the warm air discharge. The remaining sides shall be permitted to be placed not closer than 6 inches (152 mm) to a wall. Wall-register models shall not be placed closer than 6 inches (152 mm) to a corner.

3. Draperies. The *furnace* shall be placed so that a door, drapery, or similar object cannot be nearer than 12 inches (305 mm) to any portion of the register of the *furnace*.

4. Floor construction. *Floor furnaces* shall not be installed in concrete floor construction built on grade.

5. *Thermostat*. The controlling *thermostat* for a *floor furnace* shall be located within the same room or space as the *floor furnace* or shall be located in an adjacent room or space that is permanently open to the room or space containing the *floor furnace*.

G2437.3 (609.3) Bracing. The floor around the *furnace* shall be braced and headed with a support framework designed in accordance with Chapter 5.

G2437.4 (609.4) Clearance. The lowest portion of the *floor furnace* shall have not less than a 6-inch (152 mm) *clearance* from the grade level; except where the lower 6-inch (152 mm) portion of the *floor furnace* is sealed by the manufacturer to prevent entrance of water, the minimum *clearance* shall be reduced to not less than 2 inches (51 mm). Where these *clearances* cannot be provided, the ground below and to the sides shall be excavated to form a pit under the *furnace* so that the required *clearance* is provided beneath the lowest portion of the *furnace*. A 12-inch (305 mm) minimum clearance shall be provided on all sides except the *control* side, which shall have an 18-inch (457 mm) minimum *clearance*.

G2437.5 (609.5) First floor installation. Where the basement story level below the floor in which a *floor furnace* is installed is utilized as habitable space, such *floor furnaces* shall be enclosed as specified in Section G2437.6 and shall project into a nonhabitable space.

G2437.6 (609.6) Upper floor installations. *Floor furnaces* installed in upper stories of buildings shall project below into nonhabitable space and shall be separated from the nonhabitable space by an enclosure constructed of noncombustible materials. The *floor furnace* shall be provided with access, *clearance* to all sides and bottom of not less than 6 inches (152 mm) and *combustion air* in accordance with Section G2407.

SECTION G2438 (613)
CLOTHES DRYERS

G2438.1 (613.1) General. *Clothes dryers* shall be tested in accordance with ANSI Z21.5.1 and shall be installed in accordance with the manufacturer's installation instructions.

SECTION G2439 (614)
CLOTHES DRYER EXHAUST

G2439.1 (614.1) Installation. *Clothes dryers* shall be exhausted in accordance with the manufacturer's instructions. Dryer exhaust systems shall be independent of all other systems and shall convey the moisture and any products of *combustion* to the outside of the building.

G2439.2 (614.2) Duct penetrations. Ducts that exhaust *clothes dryers* shall not penetrate or be located within any fireblocking, draftstopping or any wall, floor/ceiling or other assembly required by this *code* to be fire-resistance rated, unless such duct is constructed of galvanized steel or aluminum of the thickness specified in the mechanical provisions of this *code* and the fire-resistance rating is maintained in accordance with this *code*. Fire dampers shall not be installed in *clothes dryer* exhaust duct systems.

G2439.3 (614.4) Exhaust installation. Dryer exhaust ducts for *clothes dryers* shall terminate on the outside of the building and shall be equipped with a backdraft *damper*. Screens shall not be installed at the duct termination. Ducts shall not be connected or installed with sheet metal screws or other fasteners that will obstruct the flow. *Clothes dryer* exhaust ducts shall not be connected to a *vent connector*, vent or *chimney*. *Clothes dryer* exhaust ducts shall not extend into or through ducts or plenums.

G2439.4 (614.5) Makeup air. Installations exhausting more than 200 cfm (0.09 m³/s) shall be provided with *makeup air*. Where a closet is designed for the installation of a *clothes dryer*, an opening having an area of not less than 100 square inches (0.0645 m²) for *makeup air* shall be provided in the closet enclosure, or *makeup air* shall be provided by other *approved* means.

G2439.5 (614.6) Domestic clothes dryer exhaust ducts. Exhaust ducts for domestic *clothes dryers* shall conform to the requirements of Sections G2429.5.1 through G2429.5.7.

G2439.5.1 (614.6.1) Material and size. Exhaust ducts shall have a smooth interior finish and shall be constructed of metal a minimum 0.016-inch (0.4 mm) thick. The exhaust duct size shall be 4 inches (102 mm) nominal in diameter.

G2439.5.2 (614.6.2) Duct installation. Exhaust ducts shall be supported at 4 foot (1219 mm) intervals and secured in place. The insert end of the duct shall extend into the adjoining duct or fitting in the direction of airflow. Ducts shall not be joined with screws or similar fasteners that protrude into the inside of the duct.

G2439.5.3 (614.6.3) Protection required. Protective shield plates shall be placed where nails or screws from finish or other work are likely to penetrate the *clothes dryer* exhaust duct. Shield plates shall be placed on the finished face of all framing members where there is less than 1¹/₄ inches (32 mm) between the duct and the finished face of the framing member. Protective shield plates shall be constructed of steel, shall have a minimum thickness of 0.062 inch (1.6 mm) and shall extend a minimum of 2 inches (51 mm) above sole plates and below top plates.

G2439.5.4 (614.6.4) Transition ducts. Transition ducts used to connect the dryer to the exhaust duct system shall be a single length that is listed and labeled in accordance with UL 2158A. Transition ducts shall be a maximum of 8 feet (2438 mm) in length and shall not be concealed within construction.

G2439.5.5 (614.6.5) Duct length. The maximum allowable exhaust duct length shall be determined by one of the methods specified in Section G2439.5.5.1 or G2439.5.5.2.

G2439.5.5.1 (614.6.5.1) Specified length. The maximum length of the exhaust duct shall be 35 feet (10 668 mm) from the connection to the transition duct from the dryer to the outlet terminal. Where fittings are used, the maximum length of the exhaust duct shall be reduced in accordance with Table G2439.5.5.1.

G2439.5.5.2 (614.6.5.2) Manufacturer's instructions. The maximum length of the exhaust duct shall be determined by the dryer manufacturer's installation instructions. The *code official* shall be provided with a copy of the installation instructions for the make and model of the dryer. Where the exhaust duct is to be concealed, the installation instructions shall be provided to the *code official* prior to the concealment inspection. In the absence of fitting equivalent length calculations from the clothes dryer manufacturer, Table G2439.5.5.1 shall be used.

G2439.5.6 (614.6.5) Length identification. Where the exhaust duct is concealed within the building construction, the equivalent length of the exhaust duct shall be identified on a permanent label or tag. The label or tag shall be located within 6 feet (1829 mm) of the exhaust duct connection.

G2439.5.7 (614.6.6) Exhaust duct required. Where space for a *clothes dryer* is provided, an exhaust duct system shall be installed. Where the *clothes dryer* is not installed at the time of occupancy, the exhaust duct shall be capped at location of the future dryer.

> **Exception:** Where a listed condensing *clothes dryer* is installed prior to occupancy of the structure.

SECTION G2440 (615)
SAUNA HEATERS

G2440.1 (615.1) General. Sauna heaters shall be installed in accordance with the manufacturer's installation instructions.

G2440.2 (615.2) Location and protection. Sauna heaters shall be located so as to minimize the possibility of accidental contact by a person in the room.

G2440.2.1 (615.2.1) Guards. Sauna heaters shall be protected from accidental contact by an *approved* guard or barrier of material having a low coefficient of thermal conductivity. The guard shall not substantially affect the transfer of heat from the heater to the room.

G2440.3 (615.3) Access. Panels, grilles and access doors that are required to be removed for normal servicing operations, shall not be attached to the building.

G2440.4 (615.4) Combustion and dilution air intakes. Sauna heaters of other than the direct-vent type shall be installed with the *draft hood* and *combustion air* intake located outside the sauna room. Where the *combustion air* inlet and the *draft hood* are in a dressing room adjacent to the sauna room, there shall be provisions to prevent physically blocking the *combustion air* inlet and the *draft hood* inlet, and to prevent physical contact with the *draft hood* and vent assembly, or warning notices shall be posted to avoid such contact. Any warning notice shall be easily readable, shall contrast with its background, and the wording shall be in letters not less than 0.25 inch (6.4 mm) high.

TABLE G2439.5.5.1 (TABLE 614.6.5.1)
DRYER EXHAUST DUCT FITTING EQUIVALENT LENGTH

DRYER EXHAUST DUCT FITTING TYPE	EQUIVALENT LENGTH
4 inch radius mitered 45 degree elbow	2 feet 6 inches
4 inch radius mitered 90 degree elbow	5 feet
6 inch radius smooth 45 degree elbow	1 foot
6 inch radius smooth 90 degree elbow	1 foot 9 inches
8 inch radius smooth 45 degree elbow	1 foot
8 inch radius smooth 90 degree elbow	1 foot 7 inches
10 inch radius smooth 45 degree elbow	9 inches
10 inch radius smooth 90 degree elbow	1 foot 6 inches

For SI: 1 inch = 25.4 mm, 1 foot = 304.8 mm, 1 degree = 0.0175 rad.

G2440.5 (615.5) Combustion and ventilation air. Combustion air shall not be taken from inside the sauna room. *Combustion* and ventilation air for a sauna heater not of the direct-vent type shall be provided to the area in which the *combustion air* inlet and *draft hood* are located in accordance with Section G2407.

G2440.6 (615.6) Heat and time controls. Sauna heaters shall be equipped with a *thermostat* which will limit room temperature to 194°F (90°C). If the *thermostat* is not an integral part of the sauna heater, the heat-sensing element shall be located within 6 inches (152 mm) of the ceiling. If the heat-sensing element is a capillary tube and bulb, the assembly shall be attached to the wall or other support, and shall be protected against physical damage.

G2440.6.1 (615.6.1) Timers. A timer, if provided to *control main burner* operation, shall have a maximum operating time of 1 hour. The *control* for the timer shall be located outside the sauna room.

G2440.7 (615.7) Sauna room. A ventilation opening into the sauna room shall be provided. The opening shall be not less than 4 inches by 8 inches (102 mm by 203 mm) located near the top of the door into the sauna room.

SECTION G2441 (617)
POOL AND SPA HEATERS

G2441.1 (617.1) General. Pool and spa heaters shall be tested in accordance with ANSI Z21.56 and shall be installed in accordance with the manufacturer's installation instructions.

SECTION G2442 (618)
FORCED-AIR WARM-AIR FURNACES

G2442.1 (618.1) General. Forced-air warm-air *furnaces* shall be tested in accordance with ANSI Z21.47 or UL 795 and shall be installed in accordance with the manufacturer's installation instructions.

G2442.2 (618.2) Forced-air furnaces. The minimum unobstructed total area of the outside and return air ducts or openings to a forced-air warm-air *furnace* shall be not less than 2 square inches for each 1,000 *Btu*/h (4402 mm²/W) output rating capacity of the *furnace* and not less than that specified in the *furnace* manufacturer's installation instructions. The minimum unobstructed total area of supply ducts from a forced-air warm-air *furnace* shall be not less than 2 square inches for each 1,000 *Btu*/h (4402 mm²/W) output rating capacity of the *furnace* and not less than that specified in the *furnace* manufacturer's installation instructions.

Exception: The total area of the supply air ducts and outside and return air ducts shall not be required to be larger than the minimum size required by the *furnace* manufacturer's installation instructions.

G2442.3 (618.3) Dampers. Volume dampers shall not be placed in the air inlet to a *furnace* in a manner that will reduce the required air to the *furnace*.

G2442.4 (618.4) Circulating air ducts for forced-air warm-air furnaces. Circulating air for forced-air-type, warm-air *furnaces* shall be conducted into the blower housing from outside the *furnace* enclosure by continuous air-tight ducts.

G2442.5 (618.5) Prohibited sources. Outside or return air for a forced-air heating system shall not be taken from the following locations:

1. Closer than 10 feet (3048 mm) from an *appliance* vent outlet, a vent opening from a plumbing drainage system or the discharge outlet of an exhaust fan, unless the outlet is 3 feet (914 mm) above the outside air inlet.

2. Where objectionable odors, fumes or flammable vapors are present; or where located less than 10 feet (3048 mm) above the surface of any abutting public way or driveway; or where located at grade level by a sidewalk, street, alley or driveway.

3. A hazardous or insanitary location or a refrigeration machinery room as defined in the *International Mechanical Code*.

4. A room or space, the volume of which is less than 25 percent of the entire volume served by such system. Where connected by a permanent opening having an area sized in accordance with Section G2442.2, adjoining rooms or spaces shall be considered as a single room or space for the purpose of determining the volume of such rooms or spaces.

   Exception: The minimum volume requirement shall not apply where the amount of return air taken from a room or space is less than or equal to the amount of supply air delivered to that room or space.

5. A room or space containing an *appliance* where such a room or space serves as the sole source of return air.

   Exception: This shall not apply where:

   1. The *appliance* is a direct-vent *appliance* or an *appliance* not requiring a vent in accordance with Section G2425.8.

   2. The room or space complies with the following requirements:

      2.1. The return air shall be taken from a room or space having a volume exceeding 1 *cubic foot* for each 10 *Btu*/h (9.6 L/W) of combined input rating of all fuel-burning *appliances* therein.

      2.2. The volume of supply air discharged back into the same space shall be approximately equal to the volume of return air taken from the space.

      2.3. Return-air inlets shall not be located within 10 feet (3048 mm) of any *appliance* firebox or *draft hood* in the same room or space.

3. Rooms or spaces containing solid-fuel-burning *appliances*, provided that return-air inlets are located not less than 10 feet (3048 mm) from the firebox of such *appliances*.

6. A closet, bathroom, toilet room, kitchen, garage, mechanical room, boiler room, *furnace* room or attic.

   Exception: Where return air intakes are located not less than 10 feet (3048 mm) from cooking *appliances*, and serve only the kitchen area, taking return air from a kitchen area shall not be prohibited.

7. A crawl space by means of direct connection to the return side of a forced air system. Transfer openings in the crawl space enclosure shall not be prohibited.

G2442.6 (618.6) Screen. Required outdoor air inlets shall be covered with a screen having $^1/_4$-inch (6.4 mm) openings. Required outdoor air inlets serving a nonresidential portion of a building shall be covered with screen having openings larger than $^1/_4$ inch (6.4 mm) and not larger than 1 inch (25 mm).

G2442.7 (618.7) Return-air limitation. Return air from one *dwelling unit* shall not be discharged into another *dwelling unit*.

G2442.8 (618.8) Furnace plenums and air ducts. Where a *furnace* is installed so that supply ducts carry air circulated by the *furnace* to areas outside of the space containing the *furnace*, the return air shall also be handled by a duct(s) sealed to the *furnace* casing and terminating outside of the space containing the *furnace*.

SECTION G2443 (619)
CONVERSION BURNERS

G2443.1 (619.1) Conversion burners. The installation of *conversion burners* shall conform to ANSI Z21.8.

SECTION G2444 (620)
UNIT HEATERS

G2444.1 (620.1) General. *Unit heaters* shall be tested in accordance with ANSI Z83.8 and shall be installed in accordance with the manufacturer's installation instructions.

G2444.2 (620.2) Support. Suspended-type *unit heaters* shall be supported by elements that are designed and constructed to accommodate the weight and dynamic loads. Hangers and brackets shall be of noncombustible material.

G2444.3 (620.3) Ductwork. Ducts shall not be connected to a unit heater unless the heater is listed for such installation.

G2444.4 (620.4) Clearance. Suspended-type *unit heaters* shall be installed with *clearances* to combustible materials of not less than 18 inches (457 mm) at the sides, 12 inches (305 mm) at the bottom and 6 inches (152 mm) above the top where the unit heater has an internal *draft hood* or 1 inch (25 mm) above the top of the sloping side of the vertical *draft hood*.

Floor-mounted-type *unit heaters* shall be installed with *clearances* to combustible materials at the back and one side only of not less than 6 inches (152 mm). Where the *flue gases* are vented horizontally, the 6-inch (152 mm) *clearance* shall be measured from the *draft hood* or *vent* instead of the rear wall of the unit heater. Floor-mounted-type *unit heaters* shall not be installed on combustible floors unless listed for such installation.

Clearance for servicing all *unit heaters* shall be in accordance with the manufacturer's installation instructions.

Exception: *Unit heaters* listed for reduced *clearance* shall be permitted to be installed with such *clearances* in accordance with their listing and the manufacturer's instructions.

SECTION G2445 (621)
UNVENTED ROOM HEATERS

G2445.1 (621.1) General. *Unvented room heaters* shall be tested in accordance with ANSI Z21.11.2 and shall be installed in accordance with the conditions of the listing and the manufacturer's installation instructions.

G2445.2 (621.2) Prohibited use. One or more *unvented room heaters* shall not be used as the sole source of comfort heating in a *dwelling unit*.

G2445.3 (621.3) Input rating. *Unvented room heaters* shall not have an input rating in excess of 40,000 *Btu*/h (11.7 kW).

G2445.4 (621.4) Prohibited locations. The location of *unvented room heaters* shall comply with Section G2406.2.

G2445.5 (621.5) Room or space volume. The aggregate input rating of all *unvented appliances* installed in a room or space shall not exceed 20 *Btu*/h per *cubic foot* (0.21 kW/m³) of volume of such room or space. Where the room or space in which the *appliance* is installed is directly connected to another room or space by a doorway, archway or other opening of comparable size that cannot be closed, the volume of such adjacent room or space shall be permitted to be included in the calculations.

G2445.6 (621.6) Oxygen-depletion safety system. *Unvented room heaters* shall be equipped with an oxygen-depletion-sensitive safety shutoff system. The system shall shut off the gas supply to the main and *pilot burners* when the oxygen in the surrounding atmosphere is depleted to the percent concentration specified by the manufacturer, but not lower than 18 percent. The system shall not incorporate field adjustment means capable of changing the set point at which the system acts to shut off the gas supply to the room heater.

G2445.7 (621.7) Unvented decorative room heaters. An unvented decorative room heater shall not be installed in a *factory-built fireplace* unless the *fireplace* system has been specifically tested, listed and labeled for such use in accordance with UL 127.

G2445.7.1 (621.7.1) Ventless firebox enclosures. Ventless firebox enclosures used with unvented decorative room heaters shall be listed as complying with ANSI Z21.91.

SECTION G2446 (622)
VENTED ROOM HEATERS

G2446.1 (622.1) General. *Vented room heaters* shall be tested in accordance with ANSI Z21.86/CSA 2.32, shall be designed and equipped as specified in Section G2432.2 and shall be installed in accordance with the manufacturer's installation instructions.

SECTION G2447 (623)
COOKING APPLIANCES

G2447.1 (623.1) Cooking appliances. Cooking *appliances* that are designed for permanent installation, including ranges, ovens, stoves, broilers, grills, fryers, griddles, hot plates and barbecues, shall be tested in accordance with ANSI Z21.1 or ANSI Z21.58 and shall be installed in accordance with the manufacturer's installation instructions.

G2447.2 (623.2) Prohibited location. Cooking *appliances* designed, tested, listed and labeled for use in commercial occupancies shall not be installed within *dwelling units* or within any area where domestic cooking operations occur.

G2447.3 (623.3) Domestic appliances. Cooking *appliances* installed within *dwelling units* and within areas where domestic cooking operations occur shall be listed and labeled as household-type *appliances* for domestic use.

G2447.4 (623.4) Range installation. Ranges installed on combustible floors shall be set on their own bases or legs and shall be installed with *clearances* of not less than that shown on the label.

G2447.5 (623.7) Vertical clearance above cooking top. Household cooking *appliances* shall have a vertical *clearance* above the cooking top of not less than 30 inches (760 mm) to combustible material and metal cabinets. A minimum *clearance* of 24 inches (610 mm) is permitted where one of the following is installed:

1. The underside of the combustible material or metal cabinet above the cooking top is protected with not less than $^1/_4$ inch (6 mm) thick insulating millboard covered with sheet metal not less than 0.0122 inch (0.3 mm) thick.

2. A metal ventilating hood constructed of sheet metal not less than 0.0122 inch (0.3 mm) thick is installed above the cooking top with a *clearance* of not less than $^1/_4$ inch (6 mm) between the hood and the underside of the combustible material or metal cabinet. The hood shall have a width not less than the width of the *appliance* and shall be centered over the *appliance*.

3. A listed cooking *appliance* or microwave oven is installed over a listed cooking *appliance* and in compliance with the terms of the manufacturer's installation instructions for the upper *appliance*.

SECTION G2448 (624)
WATER HEATERS

G2448.1 (624.1) General. *Water heaters* shall be tested in accordance with ANSI Z 21.10.1 and ANSI Z 21.10.3 and shall be installed in accordance with the manufacturer's installation instructions.

G2448.1.1 (624.1.1) Installation requirements. The requirements for *water heaters* relative to sizing, *relief valves*, drain pans and scald protection shall be in accordance with this *code*.

G2448.2 (624.2) Water heaters utilized for space heating. *Water heaters* utilized both to supply potable hot water and provide hot water for space-heating applications shall be listed and labeled for such applications by the manufacturer and shall be installed in accordance with the manufacturer's installation instructions and this *code*.

SECTION G2449 (627)
AIR CONDITIONING APPLIANCES

G2449.1 (627.1) General. Air conditioning *appliances* shall be tested in accordance with ANSI Z21.40.1 or ANSI Z21.40.2 and shall be installed in accordance with the manufacturer's installation instructions.

G2449.2 (627.2) Independent piping. *Gas piping* serving heating *appliances* shall be permitted to also serve cooling *appliances* where such heating and cooling *appliances* cannot be operated simultaneously. (See Section G2413.)

G2449.3 (627.3) Connection of gas engine-powered air conditioners. To protect against the effects of normal vibration in service, gas engines shall not be rigidly connected to the gas supply *piping*.

G2449.4 (627.6) Installation. Air conditioning *appliances* shall be installed in accordance with the manufacturer's instructions. Unless the *appliance* is listed for installation on a combustible surface such as a floor or roof, or unless the surface is protected in an *approved* manner, the *appliance* shall be installed on a surface of noncombustible construction with noncombustible material and surface finish and with no combustible material against the underside thereof.

SECTION G2450 (628)
ILLUMINATING APPLIANCES

G2450.1 (628.1) General. Illuminating *appliances* shall be tested in accordance with ANSI Z21.42 and shall be installed in accordance with the manufacturer's installation instructions.

G2450.2 (628.2) Mounting on buildings. Illuminating *appliances* designed for wall or ceiling mounting shall be securely attached to substantial structures in such a manner that they are not dependent on the *gas piping* for support.

G2450.3 (628.3) Mounting on posts. Illuminating *appliances* designed for post mounting shall be securely and rigidly attached to a post. Posts shall be rigidly mounted. The strength and rigidity of posts greater than 3 feet (914 mm) in height shall be at least equivalent to that of a 2.5-inch-diameter (64 mm) post constructed of 0.064-inch-thick (1.6 mm) steel or a 1-inch (25 mm) Schedule 40 steel *pipe*. Posts 3 feet (914 mm) or less in height shall not be smaller than $^3/_4$-inch (19.1 mm) Schedule 40 steel *pipe*. Drain openings shall be provided near the base of posts where there is a possibility of water collecting inside them.

G2450.4 (628.4) Appliance pressure regulators. Where an *appliance pressure regulator* is not supplied with an illuminating *appliance* and the service line is not equipped with a *service pressure regulator*, an *appliance pressure regulator* shall be installed in the line to the illuminating *appliance*. For multiple installations, one *regulator* of adequate capacity shall be permitted to serve more than one illuminating *appliance*.

SECTION G2451 (630)
INFRARED RADIANT HEATERS

G2451.1 (630.1) General. *Infrared radiant heaters* shall be tested in accordance with ANSI Z 83.6 and shall be installed in accordance with the manufacturer's installation instructions.

G2451.2 (630.2) Support. *Infrared radiant heaters* shall be fixed in a position independent of gas and electric supply lines. Hangers and brackets shall be of noncombustible material.

SECTION G2452 (631)
BOILERS

G2452.1 (631.1) Standards. Boilers shall be listed in accordance with the requirements of ANSI Z21.13 or UL 795. If applicable, the boiler shall be designed and constructed in accordance with the requirements of ASME CSD-1 and as applicable, the ASME *Boiler and Pressure Vessel Code*, Sections I, II, IV, V and IX and NFPA 85.

G2452.2 (631.2) Installation. In addition to the requirements of this *code*, the installation of boilers shall be in accordance with the manufacturer's instructions and this *code*. Operating instructions of a permanent type shall be attached to the boiler. Boilers shall have all *controls* set, adjusted and tested by the installer. A complete *control* diagram together with complete boiler operating instructions shall be furnished by the installer. The manufacturer's rating data and the nameplate shall be attached to the boiler.

G2452.3 (631.3) Clearance to combustible material. *Clearances* to combustible materials shall be in accordance with Section G2409.4.

SECTION G2453 (634)
CHIMNEY DAMPER OPENING AREA

G2453.1 (634.1) Free opening area of chimney dampers. Where an unlisted decorative *appliance* for installation in a vented *fireplace* is installed, the *fireplace damper* shall have a permanent free opening equal to or greater than specified in Table G2453.1.

TABLE G2453.1 (634.1)
FREE OPENING AREA OF CHIMNEY DAMPER FOR VENTING FLUE GASES
FROM UNLISTED DECORATIVE APPLIANCES FOR INSTALLATION IN VENTED FIREPLACES

CHIMNEY HEIGHT (feet)	MINIMUM PERMANENT FREE OPENING (square inches)[a]						
	8	13	20	29	39	51	64
	Appliance input rating (Btu per hour)						
6	7,800	14,000	23,200	34,000	46,400	62,400	80,000
8	8,400	15,200	25,200	37,000	50,400	68,000	86,000
10	9,000	16,800	27,600	40,400	55,800	74,400	96,400
15	9,800	18,200	30,200	44,600	62,400	84,000	108,800
20	10,600	20,200	32,600	50,400	68,400	94,000	122,200
30	11,200	21,600	36,600	55,200	76,800	105,800	138,600

For SI: 1 inch = 25.4 mm, 1 foot = 304.8 mm, 1 square inch = 645.16 mm², 1,000 Btu per hour = 0.293 kW.

a. The first six minimum permanent free openings (8 square inches to 51 square inches) correspond approximately to the cross-sectional areas of chimneys having diameters of 3 inches through 8 inches, respectively. The 64-square inch opening corresponds to the cross-sectional area of standard 8-inch by 8-inch chimney tile.

Part VII—Plumbing

CHAPTER 25

PLUMBING ADMINISTRATION

SECTION P2501
GENERAL

P2501.1 Scope. The provisions of this chapter shall establish the general administrative requirements applicable to plumbing systems and inspection requirements of this code.

P2501.2 Application. In addition to the general administration requirements of Chapter 1, the administrative provisions of this chapter shall also apply to the plumbing requirements of Chapters 25 through 32.

SECTION P2502
EXISTING PLUMBING SYSTEMS

P2502.1 Existing building sewers and drains. Existing *building sewers* and drains shall be used in connection with new systems when found by examination and/or test to conform to the requirements prescribed by this document.

P2502.2 Additions, alterations or repairs. Additions, *alterations*, renovations or repairs to any plumbing system shall conform to that required for a new plumbing system without requiring the existing plumbing system to comply with all the requirements of this code. Additions, *alterations* or repairs shall not cause an existing system to become unsafe, insanitary or overloaded.

Minor additions, *alterations*, renovations and repairs to existing plumbing systems shall be permitted in the same manner and arrangement as in the existing system, provided that such repairs or replacement are not hazardous and are *approved*.

SECTION P2503
INSPECTION AND TESTS

P2503.1 Inspection required. New plumbing work and parts of existing systems affected by new work or *alterations* shall be inspected by the *building official* to ensure compliance with the requirements of this code.

P2503.2 Concealment. A plumbing or drainage system, or part thereof, shall not be covered, concealed or put into use until it has been tested, inspected and *approved* by the *building official*.

P2503.3 Responsibility of permittee. Test equipment, materials and labor shall be furnished by the permittee.

P2503.4 Building sewer testing. The *building sewer* shall be tested by insertion of a test plug at the point of connection with the public sewer and filling the *building sewer* with water, testing with not less than a 10-foot (3048 mm) head of water and be able to maintain such pressure for 15 minutes.

P2503.5 DWV systems testing. Rough and finished plumbing installations shall be tested in accordance with Sections P2503.5.1 and P2503.5.2.

P2503.5.1 Rough plumbing. DWV systems shall be tested on completion of the rough piping installation by water or air with no evidence of leakage. Either test shall be applied to the drainage system in its entirety or in sections after rough piping has been installed, as follows:

1. Water test. Each section shall be filled with water to a point not less than 10 feet (3048 mm) above the highest fitting connection in that section, or to the highest point in the completed system. Water shall be held in the section under test for a period of 15 minutes. The system shall prove leak free by visual inspection.

2. Air test. The portion under test shall be maintained at a gauge pressure of 5 pounds per square inch (psi) (34 kPa) or 10 inches of mercury column (34 kPa). This pressure shall be held without introduction of additional air for a period of 15 minutes.

P2503.5.2 Finished plumbing. After the plumbing fixtures have been set and their traps filled with water, their connections shall be tested and proved gas tight and/or water tight as follows:

1. Water tightness. Each fixture shall be filled and then drained. Traps and fixture connections shall be proven water tight by visual inspection.

2. Gas tightness. When required by the local administrative authority, a final test for gas tightness of the DWV system shall be made by the smoke or peppermint test as follows:

   2.1. Smoke test. Introduce a pungent, thick smoke into the system. When the smoke appears at vent terminals, such terminals shall be sealed and a pressure equivalent to a 1-inch water column (249 Pa) shall be applied and maintained for a test period of not less than 15 minutes.

   2.2. Peppermint test. Introduce 2 ounces (59 mL) of oil of peppermint into the system. Add 10 quarts (9464 mL) of hot water and seal all vent terminals. The odor of peppermint shall not be detected at any trap or other point in the system.

P2503.6 Shower liner test. Where shower floors and receptors are made water tight by the application of materials required by Section P2709.2, the completed liner installation shall be tested. The pipe from the shower drain shall be plugged water tight for the test. The floor and receptor area shall be filled with potable water to a depth of not less than 2 inches (51 mm) measured at the threshold. Where a threshold of at least 2 inches high does not exist, a temporary threshold shall be constructed to retain the test water in the lined floor or receptor area to a level not less than 2 inches deep measured at the threshold. The water shall be retained for a test period of not less than 15 minutes and there shall be no evidence of leakage.

P2503.7 Water-supply system testing. Upon completion of the water-supply system or a section of it, the system or portion completed shall be tested and proved tight under a water pressure of not less than the working pressure of the system or, for piping systems other than plastic, by an air test of not less than 50 psi (345 kPa). This pressure shall be held for not less than 15 minutes. The water used for tests shall be obtained from a potable water source.

P2503.8 Inspection and testing of backflow prevention devices. Inspection and testing of backflow prevention devices shall comply with Sections P2503.8.1 and P2503.8.2.

P2503.8.1 Inspections. Inspections shall be made of all backflow prevention assemblies to determine whether they are operable.

P2503.8.2 Testing. Reduced pressure principle backflow preventers, double check valve assemblies, double-detector check valve assemblies and pressure vacuum breaker assemblies shall be tested at the time of installation, immediately after repairs or relocation and at least annually.

P2503.9 Test gauges. Gauges used for testing shall be as follows:

1. Tests requiring a pressure of 10 psi or less shall utilize a testing gauge having increments of 0.10 psi (0.69 kPa) or less.

2. Tests requiring a pressure higher than 10 psi (0.69 kPa) but less than or equal to 100 psi (690 kPa) shall use a testing gauge having increments of 1 psi (6.9 kPa) or less.

3. Tests requiring a pressure higher than 100 psi (690 kPa) shall use a testing gauge having increments of 2 psi (14 kPa) or less.

CHAPTER 26

GENERAL PLUMBING REQUIREMENTS

SECTION P2601
GENERAL

P2601.1 Scope. The provisions of this chapter shall govern the installation of plumbing not specifically covered in other chapters applicable to plumbing systems. The installation of plumbing, *appliances, equipment* and systems not addressed by this code shall comply with the applicable provisions of the *International Plumbing Code.*

P2601.2 Connection. Plumbing fixtures, drains and *appliances* used to receive or discharge liquid wastes or sewage shall be connected to the sanitary drainage system of the building or premises in accordance with the requirements of this code. This section shall not be construed to prevent indirect waste systems.

P2601.3 Flood hazard area. In areas prone to flooding as established by Table R301.2(1), plumbing fixtures, drains, and *appliances* shall be located or installed in accordance with Section R322.1.6.

SECTION P2602
INDIVIDUAL WATER SUPPLY
AND SEWAGE DISPOSAL

P2602.1 General. The water-distribution and drainage system of any building or premises where plumbing fixtures are installed shall be connected to a public water supply or sewer system, respectively, if available. When either a public water-supply or sewer system, or both, are not available, or connection to them is not feasible, an individual water supply or individual (private) sewage-disposal system, or both, shall be provided.

P2602.2 Flood-resistant installation. In areas prone to flooding as established by Table R301.2(1):

1. Water supply systems shall be designed and constructed to prevent infiltration of floodwaters.

2. Pipes for sewage disposal systems shall be designed and constructed to prevent infiltration of floodwaters into the systems and discharges from the systems into floodwaters.

SECTION P2603
STRUCTURAL AND PIPING PROTECTION

P2603.1 General. In the process of installing or repairing any part of a plumbing and drainage installation, the finished floors, walls, ceilings, tile work or any other part of the building or premises that must be changed or replaced shall be left in a safe structural condition in accordance with the requirements of the building portion of this code.

P2603.2 Drilling and notching. Wood-framed structural members shall not be drilled, notched or altered in any manner except as provided in Sections R502.8, R602.5, R602.6, R802.7 and R802.7.1. Holes in load-bearing members of

cold-formed steel light-frame construction shall be permitted only in accordance with Sections R505.3.5, R603.2.5 and R804.2.5. In accordance with the provisions in Sections R505.3.5, R603.3.4 and R804.3.4, cutting and notching of flanges and lips of load-bearing members of cold-formed steel light-frame construction shall not be permitted. Structural insulated panels (SIPs) shall be drilled and notched or altered in accordance with the provisions of Section R613.7.

P2603.2.1 Protection against physical damage. In concealed locations, where piping, other than cast-iron or galvanized steel, is installed through holes or notches in studs, joists, rafters or similar members less than $1^1/_2$ inches (38 mm) from the nearest edge of the member, the pipe shall be protected by steel shield plates. Such shield plates shall have a thickness of not less than 0.0575 inch (1.463 mm) (No. 16 Gage). Such plates shall cover the area of the pipe where the member is notched or bored, and shall extend a minimum of 2 inches (51 mm) above sole plates and below top plates.

P2603.3 Breakage and corrosion. Pipes passing through or under walls shall be protected from breakage. Pipes passing through concrete or cinder walls and floors, cold-formed steel framing or other corrosive material shall be protected against external corrosion by a protective sheathing or wrapping or other means that will withstand any reaction from lime and acid of concrete, cinder or other corrosive material. Sheathing or wrapping shall allow for movement including expansion and contraction of piping. Minimum wall thickness of material shall be 0.025 inch (0.64 mm).

P2603.4 Sleeves. Annular spaces between sleeves and pipes shall be filled or tightly caulked as *approved* by the *building official.* Annular spaces between sleeves and pipes in fire-rated assemblies shall be filled or tightly caulked in accordance with the building portion of this code.

P2603.5 Pipes through footings or foundation walls. Any pipe that passes under a footing or through a foundation wall shall be provided with a relieving arch; or there shall be built into the masonry wall a pipe sleeve two pipe sizes greater than the pipe passing through.

P2603.6 Freezing. In localities having a winter design temperature of 32°F (0°C) or lower as shown in Table R301.2(1) of this code, a water, soil or waste pipe shall not be installed outside of a building, in exterior walls, in *attics* or crawl spaces, or in any other place subjected to freezing temperature unless adequate provision is made to protect it from freezing by insulation or heat or both. Water service pipe shall be installed not less than 12 inches (305 mm) deep and not less than 6 inches (152 mm) below the frost line.

P2603.6.1 Sewer depth. *Building sewers* that connect to private sewage disposal systems shall be a minimum of [NUMBER] inches (mm) below finished *grade* at the point of septic tank connection. *Building sewers* shall be a minimum of [NUMBER] inches (mm) below *grade.*

SECTION P2604
TRENCHING AND BACKFILLING

P2604.1 Trenching and bedding. Where trenches are excavated such that the bottom of the trench forms the bed for the pipe, solid and continuous load-bearing support shall be provided between joints. Where over-excavated, the trench shall be backfilled to the proper grade *with compacted earth, sand, fine gravel or similar granular material. Piping shall not be supported on rocks or blocks at any point. Rocky or unstable soil shall be over-excavated by two or more pipe diameters and brought to the proper* grade with suitable compacted granular material.

P2604.2 Common trench. See Section P2905.4.2.

P2604.3 Backfilling. Backfill shall be free from discarded construction material and debris. Backfill shall be free from rocks, broken concrete and frozen chunks until the pipe is covered by at least 12 inches (305 mm) of tamped earth. Backfill shall be placed evenly on both sides of the pipe and tamped to retain proper alignment. Loose earth shall be carefully placed in the trench in 6-inch (152 mm) layers and tamped in place.

P2604.4 Protection of footings. Trenching installed parallel to footings shall not extend below the 45-degree (0.79 rad) bearing plane of the bottom edge of a wall or footing (see Figure P2604.4).

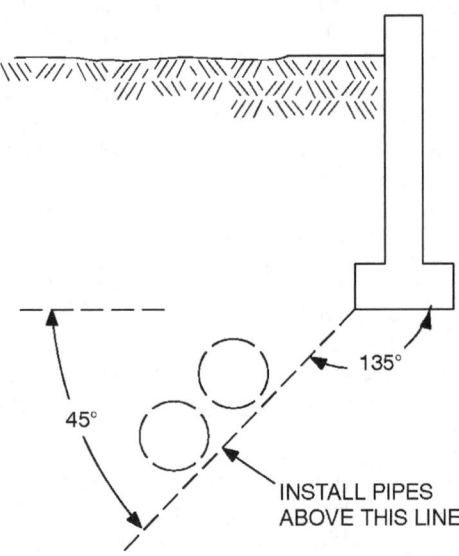

For SI: 1 degree = 0.018 rad.

FIGURE P2604.4
PIPE LOCATION WITH RESPECT TO FOOTINGS

SECTION P2605
SUPPORT

P2605.1 General. Piping shall be supported in accordance with the following:

1. Piping shall be supported to ensure alignment and prevent sagging, and allow movement associated with the expansion and contraction of the piping system.

2. Piping in the ground shall be laid on a firm bed for its entire length, except where support is otherwise provided.

3. Hangers and anchors shall be of sufficient strength to maintain their proportional share of the weight of pipe and contents and of sufficient width to prevent distortion to the pipe. Hangers and strapping shall be of *approved* material that will not promote galvanic action. Rigid support sway bracing shall be provided at changes in direction greater than 45 degrees (0.79 rad) for pipe sizes 4 inches (102 mm) and larger.

4. Piping shall be supported at distances not to exceed those indicated in Table P2605.1.

SECTION P2606
WATERPROOFING OF OPENINGS

P2606.1 General. Roof and exterior wall penetrations shall be made water tight. Joints at the roof, around vent pipes, shall be made water tight by the use of lead, copper or galvanized iron flashings or an *approved* elastomeric material. Counterflashing shall not restrict the required internal cross-sectional area of any vent.

SECTION P2607
WORKMANSHIP

P2607.1 General. Valves, pipes and fittings shall be installed in correct relationship to the direction of the flow. Burred ends shall be reamed to the full bore of the pipe.

SECTION P2608
MATERIALS EVALUATION AND LISTING

P2608.1 Identification. Each length of pipe and each pipe fitting, trap, fixture, material and device used in a plumbing system shall bear the identification of the manufacturer.

P2608.2 Installation of materials. All materials used shall be installed in strict accordance with the standards under which the materials are accepted and *approved*. In the absence of such installation procedures, the manufacturer's installation instructions shall be followed. Where the requirements of referenced standards or manufacturer's installation instructions do not conform to the minimum provisions of this code, the provisions of this code shall apply.

P2608.3 Plastic pipe, fittings and components. All plastic pipe, fittings and components shall be third-party certified as conforming to NSF 14.

P2608.4 Third-party testing and certification. All plumbing products and materials shall comply with the referenced standards, specifications and performance criteria of this code and shall be identified in accordance with Section P2608.1. Where required by Table P2608.4, plumbing products and materials shall either be tested by an *approved* third-party testing agency or certified by an *approved* third-party certification agency.

P2608.5 Water supply systems. Water service pipes, water distribution pipes and the necessary connecting pipes, fittings, control valves, faucets and all appurtenances used to dispense water intended for human ingestion shall be evaluated and listed as conforming to the requirements of NSF 61.

TABLE P2605.1
PIPING SUPPORT

PIPING MATERIAL	MAXIMUM HORIZONTAL SPACING (feet)	MAXIMUM VERTICAL SPACING
ABS pipe	4	10[b]
Aluminum tubing	10	15
Brass pipe	10	10
Cast-iron pipe	5[a]	15
Copper or copper alloy pipe	12	10
Copper or copper alloy tubing ($1^1/_4$ inch diameter and smaller)	6	10
Copper or copper alloy tubing ($1^1/_2$ inch diameter and larger)	10	10
Cross-linked polyethylene (PEX) pipe	2.67 (32 inches)	10[b]
Cross-linked polyethylene/aluminum/cross-linked polyethylene (PEX-AL-PEX) pipe	2.67 (32 inches)	4[b]
CPVC pipe or tubing (1 inch in diameter and smaller)	3	10[b]
CPVC pipe or tubing ($1^1/_4$ inch in diameter and larger)	4	10[b]
Lead pipe	Continuous	4
PB pipe or tubing	2.67 (32 inches)	4
Polyethylene/aluminum/polyethylene (PE-AL-PE) pipe	2.67 (32 inches)	4[b]
Polypropylene (PP) pipe or tubing 1 inch and smaller	2.67 (32 inches)	10[b]
Polypropylene (PP) pipe or tubing, $1^1/_4$ inches and larger	4	10[b]
PVC pipe	4	10[b]
Stainless steel drainage systems	10	10[b]
Steel pipe	12	15

For SI: 1 inch = 25.4 mm, 1 foot = 304.8 mm.

a. The maximum horizontal spacing of cast-iron pipe hangers shall be increased to 10 feet where 10-foot lengths of pipe are installed.

b. Midstory guide for sizes 2 inches and smaller.

TABLE P2608.4
PRODUCTS AND MATERIALS REQUIRING THIRD-PARTY TESTING AND THIRD-PARTY CERTIFICATION

PRODUCT OR MATERIAL	THIRD-PARTY CERTIFIED	THIRD-PARTY TESTED
Backflow prevention devices	Required	—
Plumbing appliance	Required	—
Plumbing fixtures	—	Required
Potable water supply system components and potable water fixture fittings	Required	—
Sanitary drainage and vent system components	Plastic pipe, fittings, and pipe related components	All others
Special waste system components	—	Required
Storm drainage system components	Plastic pipe, fittings, and pipe related components	All others
Subsoil drainage system components	—	Required
Waste fixture fittings	Plastic pipe, fittings, and pipe related components	All others
Water distribution system safety devices	Required	—

CHAPTER 27
PLUMBING FIXTURES

SECTION P2701
FIXTURES, FAUCETS AND FIXTURE FITTINGS

P2701.1 Quality of fixtures. Plumbing fixtures, faucets and fixture fittings shall be constructed of *approved* materials, shall have smooth impervious surfaces, shall be free from defects and concealed fouling surfaces, and shall conform to the standards cited in this code. Plumbing fixtures shall be provided with an adequate supply of potable water to flush and keep the fixtures in a clean and sanitary condition without danger of backflow or cross connection.

SECTION P2702
FIXTURE ACCESSORIES

P2702.1 Plumbing fixtures. Plumbing fixtures, other than water closets, shall be provided with *approved* strainers.

P2702.2 Waste fittings. Waste fittings shall conform to ASME A112.18.2/CSA B125.2, ASTM F 409 or to one of the standards listed in Table P3002.1(1) for above-ground drainage and vent pipe and fittings.

P2702.3 Plastic tubular fittings. Plastic tubular fittings shall conform to ASTM F 409 listed in Table P2701.1.

P2702.4 Carriers for wall-hung water closets. Carriers for wall-hung water closets shall conform to ASME A112.6.1 or ASME A112.6.2.

SECTION P2703
TAIL PIECES

P2703.1 Minimum size. Fixture tail pieces shall be not less than $1^1/_2$ inches (38 mm) in diameter for sinks, dishwashers, laundry tubs, bathtubs and similar fixtures, and not less than $1^1/_4$ inches (32 mm) in diameter for bidets, lavatories and similar fixtures.

SECTION P2704
ACCESS TO CONNECTIONS

P2704.1 General. Slip joints shall be made with an *approved* elastomeric gasket and shall be installed only on the trap outlet, trap inlet and within the trap seal. Fixtures with concealed slip-joint connections shall be provided with an access panel or utility space at least 12 inches (305 mm) in its smallest dimension or other *approved* arrangement so as to provide access to the slip connections for inspection and repair.

SECTION P2705
INSTALLATION

P2705.1 General. The installation of fixtures shall conform to the following:

1. Floor-outlet or floor-mounted fixtures shall be secured to the drainage connection and to the floor, where so designed, by screws, bolts, washers, nuts and similar fasteners of copper, brass or other corrosion-resistant material.

2. Wall-hung fixtures shall be rigidly supported so that strain is not transmitted to the plumbing system.

3. Where fixtures come in contact with walls and floors, the contact area shall be water tight.

4. Plumbing fixtures shall be usable.

5. Water closets, lavatories and bidets. A water closet, lavatory or bidet shall not be set closer than 15 inches (381 mm) from its center to any side wall, partition or vanity or closer than 30 inches (762 mm) center-to-center between adjacent fixtures. There shall be at least a 21-inch (533 mm) clearance in front of the water closet, lavatory or bidet to any wall, fixture or door.

6. The location of piping, fixtures or equipment *shall not interfere with the operation of windows or doors.*

7. In areas prone to flooding as established by Table R301.2(1), plumbing fixtures shall be located or installed in accordance with Section R322.1.7.

8. Integral fixture-fitting mounting surfaces on manufactured plumbing fixtures or plumbing fixtures constructed on site, shall meet the design requirements of ASME A112.19.2 or ASME A 112.19.3.

SECTION P2706
WASTE RECEPTORS

P2706.1 General. Every waste receptor shall be of an *approved* type. Plumbing fixtures or other receptors receiving the discharge of indirect waste pipes shall be shaped and have a capacity to prevent splashing or flooding and shall be *readily accessible* for inspection and cleaning. Waste receptors and standpipes shall be trapped and vented and shall connect to the building drainage system. A removable strainer or basket shall cover the waste outlet of waste receptors. Waste receptors shall be installed in ventilated spaces. Waste receptors shall not be installed in bathrooms or in any inaccessible or unventilated space such as a closet. Ready access shall be provided to waste receptors.

> **Exception:** Open hub waste receptors shall be permitted in the form of a hub or pipe extending not less than 1 inch (25 mm) above a water-impervious floor, and are not required to have a strainer.

P2706.2 Standpipes. Standpipes shall extend a minimum of 18 inches (457 mm) and a maximum of 42 inches (1067 mm) above the trap weir. Access shall be provided to all standpipe traps and drains for rodding.

P2706.2.1 Laundry tray connection. A laundry tray waste line is permitted to connect into a standpipe for the automatic clothes washer drain. The standpipe shall extend not less than 30 inches (762 mm) above the trap weir and shall extend above the flood level rim of the laundry tray. The outlet of the laundry tray shall be a maximum horizontal distance of 30 inches (762 mm) from the standpipe trap.

TABLE P2701.1
PLUMBING FIXTURES, FAUCETS AND FIXTURE FITTINGS

MATERIAL	STANDARD
Air gap fittings for use with plumbing fixtures, appliances and appurtenances	ASME A112.1.3
Bathtub/whirlpool pressure-sealed doors	ASME A112.19.15
Diverters for faucets with hose spray anti-syphon type, residential application	ASSE 1025
Enameled cast-iron plumbing fixtures	ASME A112.19.1M, CSA B45.2
Floor drains	ASME A112.6.3
Floor-affixed supports for off-the-floor plumbing fixtures for public use	ASME A112.6.1M
Framing-affixed supports for off-the-floor water closets with concealed tanks	ASME A112.6.2
Home laundry equipment	ASSE 1007
Hose connection vacuum breaker	ASSE 1052
Hot water dispensers, household storage type, electrical	ASSE 1023
Household dishwashing machines	ASSE 1006
Household disposers	ASSE 1008
Hydraulic performance for water closets and urinals	ASME A112.19.2
Individual pressure balancing valves for individual fixture fittings	ASSE 1066
Individual shower control valves anti-scald	ASSE 1016, CSA B125
Macerating toilet systems and related components	ASME A112.3.4
Nonvitreous ceramic plumbing fixtures	ASME A112.19.9M, CSA B45.1
Plastic bathtub units	ANSI Z124.1, CSA B45.1
Plastic lavatories	ANSI Z124.3, CSA B45.5
Plastic shower receptors and shower stall	ANSI Z124.2, CSA B45.5
Plastic sinks	ANSI Z124.6, CSA B45.5
Plastic water closet bowls and tanks	ANSI Z124.4, CSA B45.5
Plumbing fixture fittings	ASME A112.18.1/CSA B125.1
Plumbing fixture waste fittings	ASME A112.18.2/CSA B125.2, ASTM F 409
Porcelain-enameled formed steel plumbing fixtures	ASME A112.19.4M, CSA B45.3
Pressurized flushing devices for plumbing fixtures	ASSE 1037
Specification for copper sheet and strip for building construction	ASTM B 370
Stainless steel plumbing fixtures (residential)	ASME A112.19.3M, CSA B45.4
Suction fittings for use in swimming pools, wading pools, spas, hot tubs and whirlpool bathtub appliances	ASME A112.19.8M
Temperature-actuated, flow reduction valves to individual fixture fittings	ASSE 1062
Thermoplastic accessible and replaceable plastic tube and tubular fittings	ASTM F 409
Trench drains	ASME A112.6.3
Trim for water closet bowls, tanks and urinals	ASME A112.19.5
Vacuum breaker wall hydrant—frost-resistant, automatic-draining type	ASSE 1019
Vitreous china plumbing fixtures	ASME A112.19.2M
Wall-mounted and pedestal-mounted, adjustable and pivoting lavatory and sink carrier systems	ASME A112.19.12
Water closet flush tank fill valves	ASSE 1002, CSA B125.3
Whirlpool bathtub appliances	ASME A112.19.7M

2009 INTERNATIONAL RESIDENTIAL CODE®

P2706.3 Prohibited waste receptors. Plumbing fixtures that are used for washing or bathing shall not be used to receive the discharge of indirect waste piping.

Exceptions:

1. A kitchen sink trap is acceptable for use as a receptor for a dishwasher.

2. A laundry tray is acceptable for use as a receptor for a clothes washing machine.

SECTION P2707
DIRECTIONAL FITTINGS

P2707.1 Directional fitting required. *Approved* directional-type branch fittings shall be installed in fixture tailpieces receiving the discharge from food waste disposal units or dishwashers.

SECTION P2708
SHOWERS

P2708.1 General. Shower compartments shall have at least 900 square inches (0.6 m²) of interior cross-sectional area. Shower compartments shall be not less than 30 inches (762 mm) in minimum dimension measured from the finished interior dimension of the shower compartment, exclusive of fixture valves, shower heads, soap dishes, and safety grab bars or rails. The minimum required area and dimension shall be measured from the finished interior dimension at a height equal to the top of the threshold and at a point tangent to its centerline and shall be continued to a height of not less than 70 inches (1778 mm) above the shower drain outlet. Hinged shower doors shall open outward. The wall area above built-in tubs having installed shower heads and in shower compartments shall be constructed in accordance with Section R702.4. Such walls shall form a water-tight joint with each other and with either the tub, receptor or shower floor.

Exceptions:

1. Fold-down seats shall be permitted in the shower, provided the required 900-square-inch (0.6 m²) dimension is maintained when the seat is in the folded-up position.

2. Shower compartments having not less than 25 inches (635 mm) in minimum dimension measured from the finished interior dimension of the compartment provided that the shower compartment has a minimum of 1,300 square inches (0.838 m²) of cross-sectional area.

P2708.1.1 Access. The shower compartment access and egress opening shall have a minimum clear and unobstructed finished width of 22 inches (559 mm).

P2708.2 Water supply riser. Water supply risers from the shower valve to the shower head outlet, whether exposed or concealed, shall be attached to the structure using support devices designed for use with the specific piping material or fittings anchored with screws.

P2708.3 Shower control valves. Individual shower and tub/shower combination valves shall be equipped with control valves of the pressure-balance, thermostatic-mixing or combination pressure-balance/thermostatic-mixing valve types with a high limit stop in accordance with ASSE 1016 or CSA B125. The high limit stop shall be set to limit water temperature to a maximum of 120°F (49°C). In-line thermostatic valves shall not be used for compliance with this section.

P2708.4 Hand showers. Hand-held showers shall conform to ASME A112.18.1 or CSA B125.1. Hand-held showers shall be provide backflow protection in accordance with ASME A112.18.1 or CSA B125.1 or shall be protected against backflow by a device complying with ASME A112.18.3.

SECTION P2709
SHOWER RECEPTORS

P2709.1 Construction. Shower receptors shall have a finished curb threshold not less than 1 inch (25 mm) below the sides and back of the receptor. The curb shall be not less than 2 inches (51 mm) and not more than 9 inches (229 mm) deep when measured from the top of the curb to the top of the drain. The finished floor shall slope uniformly toward the drain not less than $^1/_4$ unit vertical in 12 units horizontal (2-percent slope) nor more than $^1/_2$ inch (13 mm), and floor drains shall be flanged to provide a water-tight joint in the floor.

P2709.2 Lining required. The adjoining walls and floor framing enclosing on-site built-up shower receptors shall be lined with one of the following materials:

1. Sheet lead,

2. Sheet copper,

3. Plastic liner material that complies with ASTM D 4068 or ASTM D 4551,

4. Hot mopping in accordance with Section P2709.2.3 or

5. Sheet-applied load-bearing, bonded waterproof membranes that comply with ANSI A118.10.

The lining material shall extend not less than 3 inches (76 mm) beyond or around the rough jambs and not less than 3 inches (76 mm) above finished thresholds. Sheet-applied load bearing, bonded waterproof membranes shall be applied in accordance with the manufacturer's installation instructions.

P2709.2.1 PVC sheets. Plasticized polyvinyl chloride (PVC) sheets shall be a minimum of 0.040 inch (1 mm) thick, and shall meet the requirements of ASTM D 4551. Sheets shall be joined by solvent welding in accordance with the manufacturer's installation instructions.

P2709.2.2 Chlorinated polyethylene (CPE) sheets. Non-plasticized chlorinated polyethylene sheet shall be a minimum of 0.040 inch (1 mm) thick, and shall meet the requirements of ASTM D 4068. The liner shall be joined in accordance with the manufacturer's installation instructions.

P2709.2.3 Hot-mopping. Shower receptors lined by hot mopping shall be built-up with not less than three layers of standard grade Type 15 asphalt-impregnated roofing felt. The bottom layer shall be fitted to the formed subbase and each succeeding layer thoroughly hot-mopped to that below. All corners shall be carefully fitted and shall be made strong and water tight by folding or lapping, and each corner shall be reinforced with suitable webbing hot-mopped in place. All folds, laps and reinforcing webbing shall extend at least 4 inches (102 mm) in all directions from the corner and all webbing shall be of *approved* type and mesh, producing a tensile strength of not less than 50 pounds per inch (893 kg/m) in either direction.

P2709.3 Installation. Lining materials shall be pitched one-fourth unit vertical in 12 units horizontal (2-percent slope) to weep holes in the subdrain by means of a smooth, solidly formed subbase, shall be properly recessed and fastened to *approved* backing so as not to occupy the space required for the wall covering, and shall not be nailed or perforated at any point less than 1 inch (25.4 mm) above the finished threshold.

P2709.3.1 Materials. Lead and copper linings shall be insulated from conducting substances other than the connecting drain by 15-pound (6.80 kg) asphalt felt or its equivalent. Sheet lead liners shall weigh not less than 4 pounds per square foot (19.5 kg/m²). Sheet copper liners shall weigh not less than 12 ounces per square foot (3.7 kg/m²). Joints in lead and copper pans or liners shall be burned or silver brazed, respectively. Joints in plastic liner materials shall be jointed per the manufacturer's recommendations.

P2709.4 Receptor drains. An *approved* flanged drain shall be installed with shower subpans or linings. The flange shall be placed flush with the subbase and be equipped with a clamping ring or other device to make a water-tight connection between the lining and the drain. The flange shall have weep holes into the drain.

SECTION P2710
SHOWER WALLS

P2710.1 Bathtub and shower spaces. Shower walls shall be finished in accordance with Section R307.2.

SECTION P2711
LAVATORIES

P2711.1 Approval. Lavatories shall conform to ANSI Z124.3, ASME A112.19.1, ASME A112.19.2, ASME A112.19.3, ASME A112.19.4, ASME A112.19.9, CSA B45.1, CSA B45.2, CSA B45.3 or CSA B45.4.

P2711.2 Cultured marble lavatories. Cultured marble vanity tops with an integral lavatory shall conform to ANSI Z124.3 or CSA B45.5.

P2711.3 Lavatory waste outlets. Lavatories shall have waste outlets not less than 1¹/₄ inch (32 mm) in diameter. A strainer, pop-up stopper, crossbar or other device shall be provided to restrict the clear opening of the waste outlet.

P2711.4 Movable lavatory systems. Movable lavatory systems shall comply with ASME A112.19.12.

SECTION P2712
WATER CLOSETS

P2712.1 Approval. Water closets shall conform to the water consumption requirements of Section P2903.2 and shall conform to ANSI Z124.4, ASME A112.19.2, CSA B45.1, CSA B45.4 or CSA B45.5. Water closets shall conform to the hydraulic performance requirements of ASME A112.19.6. Water closets tanks shall conform to ANSI Z124.4, ASME A112.19.2, ASME A112.19.9, CSA B45.1, CSA B45.4 or CSA B45.5. Water closets that have an invisible seal and unventilated space or walls that are not thoroughly washed at each discharge shall be prohibited. Water closets that permit backflow of the contents of the bowl into the flush tank shall be prohibited.

P2712.2 Flushing devices required. Water closets shall be provided with a flush tank, flushometer tank or flushometer valve designed and installed to supply water in sufficient quantity and flow to flush the contents of the fixture, to cleanse the fixture and refill the fixture trap in accordance with ASME A112.19.2 and ASME A112.19.6.

P2712.3 Water supply for flushing devices. An adequate quantity of water shall be provided to flush and clean the fixture served. The water supply to flushing devices equipped for manual flushing shall be controlled by a float valve or other automatic device designed to refill the tank after each discharge and to completely shut off the water flow to the tank when the tank is filled to operational capacity. Provision shall be made to automatically supply water to the fixture so as to refill the trap after each flushing.

P2712.4 Flush valves in flush tanks. Flush valve seats in tanks for flushing water closets shall be at least 1 inch (25 mm) above the flood-level rim of the bowl connected thereto, except an *approved* water closet and flush tank combination designed so that when the tank is flushed and the fixture is clogged or partially clogged, the flush valve will close tightly so that water will not spill continuously over the rim of the bowl or backflow from the bowl to the tank.

P2712.5 Overflows in flush tanks. Flush tanks shall be provided with overflows discharging to the water closet connected thereto and such overflow shall be of sufficient size to prevent flooding the tank at the maximum rate at which the tanks are supplied with water according to the manufacturer's design conditions.

P2712.6 Access. All parts in a flush tank shall be accessible for repair and replacement.

P2712.7 Water closet seats. Water closets shall be equipped with seats of smooth, nonabsorbent material and shall be properly sized for the water closet bowl type.

P2712.8 Flush tank lining. Sheet copper used for flush tank linings shall have a minimum weight of 10 ounces per square foot (3 kg/m²).

P2712.9 Electro-hydraulic water closets. Electro-hydraulic water closets shall conform to ASME A112.19.13.

SECTION P2713
BATHTUBS

P2713.1 Bathtub waste outlets and overflows. Bathtubs shall have outlets and overflows at least $1^1/_2$ inches (38 mm) in diameter, and the waste outlet shall be equipped with an *approved* stopper.

P2713.2 Bathtub enclosures. Doors within a bathtub enclosure shall conform to ASME A112.19.15.

P2713.3 Bathtub and whirlpool bathtub valves. The hot water supplied to bathtubs and whirlpool bathtubs shall be limited to a maximum temperature of 120°F (49°C) by a water-temperature-limiting device that conforms to ASSE 1070, except where such protection is otherwise provided by a combination tub/shower valve in accordance with Section P2708.3.

SECTION P2714
SINKS

P2714.1 Sink waste outlets. Sinks shall be provided with waste outlets not less than $1^1/_2$ inches (38 mm) in diameter. A strainer, crossbar or other device shall be provided to restrict the clear opening of the waste outlet.

P2714.2 Movable sink systems. Movable sink systems shall comply with ASME A112.19.12.

SECTION P2715
LAUNDRY TUBS

P2715.1 Laundry tub waste outlet. Each compartment of a laundry tub shall be provided with a waste outlet not less than $1^1/_2$ inches (38 mm) in diameter and a strainer or crossbar to restrict the clear opening of the waste outlet.

SECTION P2716
FOOD WASTE GRINDER

P2716.1 Food waste grinder waste outlets. Food waste grinders shall be connected to a drain of not less than $1^1/_2$ inches (38 mm) in diameter.

P2716.2 Water supply required. Food waste grinders shall be provided with an adequate supply of water at a sufficient flow rate to ensure proper functioning of the unit.

SECTION P2717
DISHWASHING MACHINES

P2717.1 Protection of water supply. The water supply for dishwashers shall be protected by an air gap or integral backflow preventer.

P2717.2 Sink and dishwasher. A sink and dishwasher are permitted to discharge through a single $1^1/_2$-inch (38 mm) trap. The discharge pipe from the dishwasher shall be increased to a minimum of $^3/_4$ inch (19 mm) in diameter and shall be connected with a wye fitting to the sink tailpiece. The dishwasher waste line shall rise and be securely fastened to the underside of the counter before connecting to the sink tailpiece.

P2717.3 Sink, dishwasher and food grinder. The combined discharge from a sink, dishwasher, and waste grinder is permitted to discharge through a single $1^1/_2$ inch (38 mm) trap. The discharge pipe from the dishwasher shall be increased to a minimum of $^3/_4$ inch (19 mm) in diameter and shall connect with a wye fitting between the discharge of the food-waste grinder and the trap inlet or to the head of the food grinder. The dishwasher waste line shall rise and be securely fastened to the underside of the counter before connecting to the sink tail piece or the food grinder.

SECTION P2718
CLOTHES WASHING MACHINE

P2718.1 Waste connection. The discharge from a clothes washing machine shall be through an *air break*.

SECTION P2719
FLOOR DRAINS

P2719.1 Floor drains. Floor drains shall have waste outlets not less than 2 inches (51 mm) in diameter and a removable strainer. The floor drain shall be constructed so that the drain can be cleaned. Access shall be provided to the drain inlet. Floor drains shall not be located under or have their access restricted by permanently installed appliances.

SECTION P2720
WHIRLPOOL BATHTUBS

P2720.1 Access to pump. Access shall be provided to circulation pumps in accordance with the fixture or pump manufacturer's installation instructions. Where the manufacturer's instructions do not specify the location and minimum size of field-fabricated access openings, a 12-inch by 12-inch (305 mm by 305 mm) minimum size opening shall be installed for access to the circulation pump. Where pumps are located more than 2 feet (610 mm) from the access opening, an 18-inch by 18-inch (457 mm by 457 mm) minimum size opening shall be installed. A door or panel shall be permitted to close the opening. In all cases, the access opening shall be unobstructed and be of the size necessary to permit the removal and replacement of the circulation pump.

P2720.2 Piping drainage. The circulation pump shall be accessibly located above the crown weir of the trap. The pump drain line shall be properly graded to ensure minimum water retention in the volute after fixture use. The circulation piping shall be installed to be self-draining.

P2720.3 Leak testing. Leak testing and pump operation shall be performed in accordance with the manufacturer's installation instructions.

P2720.4 Manufacturer's instructions. The product shall be installed in accordance with the manufacturer's installation instructions.

SECTION P2721
BIDET INSTALLATIONS

P2721.1 Water supply. The bidet shall be equipped with either an air-gap-type or vacuum-breaker-type fixture supply fitting.

P2721.2 Bidet water temperature. The discharge water temperature from a bidet fitting shall be limited to a maximum temperature of 110°F (43°C) by a water-temperature-limiting device conforming to ASSE 1070.

SECTION P2722
FIXTURE FITTING

P2722.1 General. Fixture supply valves and faucets shall comply with ASME A112.18.1/ CSA B125.1 as listed in Table P2701.1. Faucets and fixture fittings that supply drinking water for human ingestion shall conform to the requirements of NSF 61, Section 9. Flexible water connectors shall conform to the requirements of Section P2905.7.

P2722.2 Hot water. Fixture fittings and faucets that are supplied with both hot and cold water shall be installed and adjusted so that the left-hand side of the water temperature control represents the flow of hot water when facing the outlet.

> **Exception:** Shower and tub/shower mixing valves conforming to ASSE 1016 or CSA B125, where the water temperature control corresponds to the markings on the device.

P2722.3 Hose-connected outlets. Faucets and fixture fittings with hose-connected outlets shall conform to ASME A112.18.3 or CSA B125.

P2722.4 Individual pressure-balancing in-line valves for individual fixture fittings. Where individual pressure-balancing in-line valves for individual fixture fittings are installed, the valves shall comply with ASSE 1066. Such valves shall be installed in an accessible location and shall not be used alone as a substitute for the balanced pressure, thermostatic or combination shower valves required in Section P2708.3.

SECTION P2723
MACERATING TOILET SYSTEMS

P2723.1 General. Macerating toilet systems shall be installed in accordance with manufacturer's installation instructions.

P2723.2 Drain. The minimum size of the drain from the macerating toilet system shall be $^3/_4$ inch (19 mm) in diameter.

SECTION P2724
SPECIALTY TEMPERATURE CONTROL
DEVICES AND VALVES

P2724.1 Temperature-actuated, flow-reduction devices for individual fixtures. Temperature-actuated, flow-reduction devices, where installed for individual fixture fittings, shall conform to ASSE 1062. Such valves shall not be used alone as a substitute for the balanced pressure, thermostatic or combination shower valves required for showers in Section P2708.3.

CHAPTER 28

WATER HEATERS

SECTION P2801
GENERAL

P2801.1 Required. Each *dwelling* shall have an *approved* automatic water heater or other type of domestic water-heating system sufficient to supply hot water to plumbing fixtures and appliances intended for bathing, washing or culinary purposes. Storaganks shall be constructed of noncorrosive metal or shall be lined with noncorrosive material.

P2801.2 Installation. Water heaters shall be installed in accordance with this chapter and Chapters 20 and 24.

P2801.3 Location. Water heaters and storage tanks shall be installed in accordance with Section M1305 and shall be located and connected to provide access for observation, maintenance, servicing and replacement.

P2801.4 Prohibited locations. Water heaters shall be located in accordance with Chapter 20.

P2801.5 Required pan. Where water heaters or hot water storage tanks are installed in locations where leakage of the tanks or connections will cause damage, the tank or water heater shall be installed in a galvanized steel pan having a material thickness of not less than 0.0236 inch (0.6010 mm) (No. 24 gage), or other pans *approved* for such use. Listed pans shall comply with CSA LC3.

P2801.5.1 Pan size and drain. The pan shall be not less than $1^1/_2$ inches (38 mm) deep and shall be of sufficient size and shape to receive all dripping or condensate from the tank or water heater. The pan shall be drained by an indirect waste pipe having a minimum diameter of $^3/_4$ inch (19 mm). Piping for safety pan drains shall be of those materials listed in Table P2905.5.

P2801.5.2 Pan drain termination. The pan drain shall extend full-size and terminate over a suitably located indirect waste receptor or shall extend to the exterior of the building and terminate not less than 6 inches (152 mm) and not more than 24 inches (610 mm) above the adjacent ground surface.

P2801.6 Water heaters installed in garages. Water heaters having an *ignition source* shall be elevated such that the source of ignition is not less than 18 inches (457 mm) above the garage floor.

P2801.7 Water heater seismic bracing. In Seismic Design Categories D_0, D_1 and D_2 and townhouses in Seismic Design Category C, water heaters shall be anchored or strapped in the upper one-third and in the lower one-third of the appliance to resist a horizontal force equal to one-third of the operating weight of the water heater, acting in any horizontal direction, or in accordance with the appliance manufacturer's recommendations.

SECTION P2802
WATER HEATERS USED FOR SPACE HEATING

P2802.1 Protection of potable water. Piping and components connected to a water heater for space heating applications shall be suitable for use with potable water in accordance with Chapter 29. Water heaters that will be used to supply potable water shall not be connected to a heating system or components previously used with nonpotable-water heating *appliances*. Chemicals for boiler treatment shall not be introduced into the water heater.

P2802.2 Temperature control. Where a combination water heater-space heating system requires water for space heating at temperatures exceeding 140°F (60°C), a master thermostatic mixing valve complying with ASSE 1017 shall be installed to temper the water to a temperature of 140°F (60°C) or less for domestic uses.

SECTION P2803
RELIEF VALVES

P2803.1 Relief valves required. Appliances and equipment used for heating water or storing hot water shall be protected by:

1. A separate pressure-relief valve and a separate temperature-relief valve; or

2. A combination pressure- and temperature-relief valve.

P2803.2 Rating. Relief valves shall have a minimum rated capacity for the equipment served and shall conform to ANSI Z 21.22.

P2803.3 Pressure relief valves. Pressure-relief valves shall have a relief rating adequate to meet the pressure conditions for the appliances or equipment protected. In tanks, they shall be installed directly into a tank tapping or in a water line close to the tank. They shall be set to open at least 25 psi (172 kPa) above the system pressure but not over 150 psi (1034 kPa). The relief-valve setting shall not exceed the tanks rated working pressure.

P2803.4 Temperature relief valves. Temperature-relief valves shall have a relief rating compatible with the temperature conditions of the appliances or equipment protected. The valves shall be installed such that the temperature-sensing element monitors the water within the top 6 inches (152 mm) of the tank. The valve shall be set to open at a maximum temperature of 210°F (99°C).

P2803.5 Combination pressure-/temperature-relief valves. Combination pressure-/temperature-relief valves shall comply with all the requirements for separate pressure- and temperature-relief valves.

P2803.6 Installation of relief valves. A check or shutoff valve shall not be installed in the following locations:

1. Between a relief valve and the termination point of the relief valve discharge pipe;

2. Between a relief valve and a tank; or

3. Between a relief valve and heating appliances or equipment.

P2803.6.1 Requirements for discharge pipe. The discharge piping serving a pressure-relief valve, temperature relief valve or combination valve shall:

1. Not be directly connected to the drainage system.

2. Discharge through an air gap located in the same room as the water heater.

3. Not be smaller than the diameter of the outlet of the valve served and shall discharge full size to the air gap.

4. Serve a single relief device and shall not connect to piping serving any other relief device or equipment.

5. Discharge to the floor, to the pan serving the water heater or storage tank, to a waste receptor or to the outdoors.

6. Discharge in a manner that does not cause personal injury or structural damage.

7. Discharge to a termination point that is readily observable by the building occupants.

8. Not be trapped.

9. Be installed to flow by gravity.

10. Not terminate more than 6 inches (152 mm) above the floor or waste receptor.

11. Not have a threaded connection at the end of the piping.

12. Not have valves or tee fittings.

13. Be constructed of those materials listed in Section P2904.5 or materials tested, rated and *approved* for such use in accordance with ASME A112.4.1.

P2803.7 Vacuum relief valve. Bottom fed tank-type water heaters and bottom fed tanks connected to water heaters shall have a vacuum relief valve installed that complies with ANSI Z21.22.

CHAPTER 29

WATER SUPPLY AND DISTRIBUTION

SECTION P2901
GENERAL

P2901.1 Potable water required. *Dwelling units* shall be supplied with potable water in the amounts and pressures specified in this chapter. In a building where a nonpotable water-distribution system is installed, the nonpotable system shall be identified by color marking, metal tags or other appropriate method. Where color is used for marking, purple shall be used to identify municipally reclaimed water, rain water and gray water distribution systems. Any nonpotable outlet that could inadvertently be used for drinking or domestic purposes shall be posted.

SECTION P2902
PROTECTION OF POTABLE WATER SUPPLY

P2902.1 General. A potable water supply system shall be designed and installed as to prevent contamination from nonpotable liquids, solids or gases being introduced into the potable water supply. Connections shall not be made to a potable water supply in a manner that could contaminate the water supply or provide a cross-connection between the supply and a source of contamination unless an *approved* backflow-prevention device is provided. Cross-connections between an individual water supply and a potable public water supply shall be prohibited.

P2902.2 Plumbing fixtures. The supply lines and fittings for every plumbing fixture shall be installed to prevent backflow. Plumbing fixture fittings shall provide backflow protection in accordance with ASME A112.18.1.

P2902.3 Backflow protection. A means of protection against backflow shall be provided in accordance with Sections P2902.3.1 through P2902.3.6. Backflow prevention applications shall conform to Table P2902.3, except as specifically stated in Sections P2902.4 through P2902.5.5.

P2902.3.1 Air gaps. Air gaps shall comply with ASME A112.1.2 and air gap fittings shall comply with ASME A112.1.3. The minimum air gap shall be measured vertically from the lowest end of a water supply outlet to the flood level rim of the fixture or receptor into which such potable water outlets discharge. The minimum required air gap shall be twice the diameter of the effective opening of the outlet, but in no case less than the values specified in Table P2902.3.1. An air gap is required at the discharge point of a relief valve or piping. Air gap devices shall be incorporated in dishwashing and clothes washing *appliances*.

P2902.3.2 Atmospheric-type vacuum breakers. Pipe-applied atmospheric-type vacuum breakers shall conform to ASSE 1001 or CSA B64.1.1. Hose-connection vacuum breakers shall conform to ASSE 1011, ASSE 1019, ASSE 1035, ASSE 1052, CSA B64.2, CSA B64.2.1, CSA

B64.2.1.1, CSA B64.2.2 or CSA B64.7. These devices shall operate under normal atmospheric pressure when the critical level is installed at the required height.

P2902.3.3 Backflow preventer with intermediate atmospheric vent. Backflow preventers with intermediate atmospheric vents shall conform to ASSE 1012 or CSA CAN/CSA B64.3. These devices shall be permitted to be installed where subject to continuous pressure conditions. The relief opening shall discharge by air gap and shall be prevented from being submerged.

P2902.3.4 Pressure-type vacuum breakers. Pressure-type vacuum breakers shall conform to ASSE 1020 or CSA B64.1.2 and spillproof vacuum breakers shall comply with ASSE 1056. These devices are designed for installation under continuous pressure conditions when the critical level is installed at the required height. Pressure-type vacuum breakers shall not be installed in locations where spillage could cause damage to the structure.

P2902.3.5 Reduced pressure principle backflow preventers. Reduced pressure principle backflow preventers shall conform to ASSE 1013, AWWA C511, CSA B64.4 or CSA B64.4.1. Reduced pressure detector assembly backflow preventers shall conform to ASSE 1047. These devices shall be permitted to be installed where subject to continuous pressure conditions. The relief opening shall discharge by air gap and shall be prevented from being submerged.

P2902.3.6 Double check-valve assemblies. Double check-valve assemblies shall conform to ASSE 1015, CSA B64.5, CSA B64.5.1 or AWWA C510. Double-detector check-valve assemblies shall conform to ASSE 1048. These devices shall be capable of operating under continuous pressure conditions.

P2902.4 Protection of potable water outlets. Potable water openings and outlets shall be protected by an air gap, reduced pressure principle backflow preventer with atmospheric vent, atmospheric-type vacuum breaker, pressure-type vacuum breaker or hose connection backflow preventer.

P2902.4.1 Fill valves. Flush tanks shall be equipped with an antisiphon fill valve conforming to ASSE 1002 or CSA B125.3. The fill valve backflow preventer shall be located at least 1 inch (25 mm) above the full opening of the overflow pipe.

P2902.4.2 Deck-mounted and integral vacuum breakers. *Approved* deck-mounted vacuum breakers and faucets with integral atmospheric or spill-proof vacuum breakers shall be installed in accordance with the manufacturer's installation instructions and the requirements for labeling with the critical level not less than 1 inch (25 mm) above the flood level rim.

TABLE P2902.3
APPLICATION FOR BACKFLOW PREVENTERS

DEVICE	DEGREE OF HAZARD[a]	APPLICATION[b]	APPLICABLE STANDARDS
Air gap	High or low hazard	Backsiphonage or backpressure	ASME A112.1.2
Air gap fittings for use with plumbing fixtures, appliances and appurtenances	High or low hazard	Backsiphonage or backpressure	ASME A112.1.3
Antisiphon-type fill valves for gravity water closet flush tanks	High hazard	Backsiphonage only	ASSE 1002, CSA B125.3
Backflow preventer with intermediate atmospheric vents	Low hazard	Backpressure or backsiphonage Sizes $\frac{1}{4}'' - \frac{3}{4}''$	ASSE 1012, CSA B64.3
Double check backflow prevention assembly and double check fire protection backflow prevention assembly	Low hazard	Backpressure or backsiphonage Sizes $\frac{3}{8}'' - 16''$	ASSE 1015, AWWA C510, CSA B64.5, CSA B64.5.1
Double check detector fire protection backflow prevention assemblies	Low hazard	Backpressure or backsiphonage (Fire sprinkler systems) Sizes $2'' - 16''$	ASSE 1048
Dual-check-valve-type backflow preventer	Low hazard	Backpressure or backsiphonage Sizes $\frac{1}{4}'' - 1''$	ASSE 1024, CSA B64.6
Hose connection backflow preventer	High or low hazard	Low head backpressure, rated working pressure backpressure or backsiphonage Sizes $\frac{1}{2}'' - 1''$	ASSE 1052, CSA B64.2.1.1
Hose-connection vacuum breaker	High or low hazard	Low head backpressure or backsiphonage Sizes $\frac{1}{2}'', \frac{3}{4}'', 1''$	ASSE 1011, CSA B64.2, CSA B64.2.1
Laboratory faucet backflow preventer	High or low hazard	Low head backpressure and backsiphonage	ASSE 1035, CSA B64.7
Pipe-applied atmospheric-type vacuum breaker	High or low hazard	Backsiphonage only Sizes $\frac{1}{4}'' - 4''$	ASSE 1001, CSA B64.1.1
Pressure vacuum breaker assembly	High or low hazard	Backsiphonage only Sizes $\frac{1}{2}'' - 2''$	ASSE 1020, CSA B64.1.2
Reduced pressure detector fire protection backflow prevention assemblies	High or low hazard	Backsiphonage or backpressure (Fire sprinkler systems)	ASSE 1047
Reduced pressure principle backflow preventer and reduced pressure principle fire protection backflow preventer	High or low hazard	Backpressure or backsiphonage Sizes $\frac{3}{8}'' - 16''$	ASSE` 1013, AWWA C511, CSA B64.4, CSA B64.4.1
Spillproof vacuum breaker	High or low hazard	Backsiphonage only Sizes $\frac{1}{4}'' - 2''$	ASSE 1056
Vacuum breaker wall hydrants, frost-resistant, automatic draining type	High or low hazard	Low head backpressure or backsiphonage Sizes $\frac{3}{4}'' - 1''$	ASSE 1019, CSA B64.2.2

For SI: 1 inch = 25.4 mm.

a. Low hazard—See Pollution (Section 202). High hazard—See Contamination (Section 202).

b. See Backpressure (Section 202). See Backpressure, Low Head (Section 202). See Backsiphonage (Section 202).

P2902.4.3 Hose connection. Sillcocks, hose bibbs, wall hydrants and other openings with a hose connection shall be protected by an atmospheric-type or pressure-type vacuum breaker or a permanently attached hose connection vacuum breaker.

Exceptions:

1. This section shall not apply to water heater and boiler drain valves that are provided with hose connection threads and that are intended only for tank or vessel draining.

2. This section shall not apply to water supply valves intended for connection of clothes washing machines where backflow prevention is otherwise provided or is integral with the machine.

P2902.5 Protection of potable water connections. Connections to the potable water shall conform to Sections P2902.5.1 through P2902.5.5.

P2902.5.1 Connections to boilers. The potable supply to the boiler shall be equipped with a backflow preventer with an intermediate atmospheric vent complying with ASSE 1012 or CSA B64.3. Where conditioning chemicals are

TABLE P2902.3.1
MINIMUM AIR GAPS

FIXTURE	MINIMUM AIR GAP	
	Away from a wall[a] (inches)	Close to a wall (inches)
Effective openings greater than 1 inch	Two times the diameter of the effective opening	Three times the diameter of the effective opening
Lavatories and other fixtures with effective opening not greater than $^1/_2$ inch in diameter	1	1.5
Over-rim bath fillers and other fixtures with effective openings not greater than 1 inch in diameter	2	3
Sink, laundry trays, gooseneck back faucets and other fixtures with effective openings not greater than $^3/_4$ inch in diameter	1.5	2.5

For SI: 1 inch = 25.4 mm.

a. Applicable where walls or obstructions are spaced from the nearest inside edge of the spout opening a distance greater than three times the diameter of the effective opening for a single wall, or a distance greater than four times the diameter of the effective opening for two intersecting walls.

introduced into the system, the potable water connection shall be protected by an air gap or a reduced pressure principle backflow preventer complying with ASSE 1013, CSA B64.4 or AWWA C511.

P2902.5.2 Heat exchangers. Heat exchangers using an essentially toxic transfer fluid shall be separated from the potable water by double-wall construction. An air gap open to the atmosphere shall be provided between the two walls. Heat exchangers utilizing an essentially nontoxic transfer fluid shall be permitted to be of single-wall construction.

P2902.5.3 Lawn irrigation systems. The potable water supply to lawn irrigation systems shall be protected against backflow by an atmospheric-type vacuum breaker, a pressure-type vacuum breaker or a reduced pressure principle backflow preventer. A valve shall not be installed downstream from an atmospheric vacuum breaker. Where chemicals are introduced into the system, the potable water supply shall be protected against backflow by a reduced pressure principle backflow preventer.

P2902.5.4 Connections to automatic fire sprinkler systems. The potable water supply to automatic fire sprinkler systems shall be protected against backflow by a double check-valve assembly or a reduced pressure principle backflow preventer.

Exception: Where systems are installed as a portion of the water distribution system in accordance with the requirements of this code and are not provided with a fire department connection, isolation of the water supply system shall not be required.

P2902.5.4.1 Additives or nonpotable source. Where systems contain chemical additives or antifreeze, or where systems are connected to a nonpotable secondary water supply, the potable water supply shall be protected against backflow by a reduced pressure principle backflow preventer. Where chemical additives or anti-freeze is added to only a portion of an automatic fire sprinkler or standpipe system, the reduced pressure principle backflow preventer shall be permitted to be located so as to isolate that portion of the system.

P2902.5.5 Solar systems. The potable water supply to a solar system shall be equipped with a backflow preventer with intermediate atmospheric vent complying with ASSE 1012 or a reduced pressure principle backflow preventer complying with ASSE 1013. Where chemicals are used, the potable water supply shall be protected by a reduced pressure principle backflow preventer.

Exception: Where all solar system piping is a part of the potable water distribution system, in accordance with the requirements of the *International Plumbing Code*, and all components of the piping system are listed for potable water use, cross-connection protection measure shall not be required.

P2902.6 Location of backflow preventers. Access shall be provided to backflow preventers as specified by the manufacturer's installation instructions.

P2902.6.1 Outdoor enclosures for backflow prevention devices. Outdoor enclosures for backflow prevention devices shall comply with ASSE 1060.

P2902.6.2 Protection of backflow preventers. Backflow preventers shall not be located in areas subject to freezing except where they can be removed by means of unions, or are protected by heat, insulation or both.

P2902.6.3 Relief port piping. The termination of the piping from the relief port or air gap fitting of the backflow preventer shall discharge to an *approved* indirect waste receptor or to the outdoors where it will not cause damage or create a nuisance.

SECTION P2903
WATER-SUPPLY SYSTEM

P2903.1 Water supply system design criteria. The water service and water distribution systems shall be designed and pipe sizes shall be selected such that under conditions of peak demand, the capacities at the point of outlet discharge shall not be less than shown in Table P2903.1.

TABLE P2903.1
REQUIRED CAPACITIES AT
POINT OF OUTLET DISCHARGE

FIXTURE AT POINT OF OUTLET	FLOW RATE (gpm)	FLOW PRESSURE (psi)
Bathtub, pressure-balanced or thermostatic mixing valve	4	20
Bidet, thermostatic mixing	2	20
Dishwasher	2.75	8
Laundry tub	4	8
Lavatory	2	8
Shower, pressure-balancing or thermostatic mixing valve	3	20
Shower, temperature controlled	3	20
Sillcock, hose bibb	5	8
Sink	2.5	8
Water closet, flushometer tank	1.6	20
Water closet, tank, close coupled	3	20
Water closet, tank, one-piece	6	20

For SI: 1 gallon per minute = 3.785 L/m,
1 pound per square inch = 6.895 kPa.

P2903.2 Maximum flow and water consumption. The maximum water consumption flow rates and quantities for all plumbing fixtures and fixture fittings shall be in accordance with Table P2903.2.

TABLE P2903.2
MAXIMUM FLOW RATES AND CONSUMPTION FOR
PLUMBING FIXTURES AND FIXTURE FITTINGS[b]

PLUMBING FIXTURE OR FIXTURE FITTING	PLUMBING FIXTURE OR FIXTURE FITTING
Lavatory faucet	2.2 gpm at 60 psi
Shower head[a]	2.5 gpm at 80 psi
Sink faucet	2.2 gpm at 60 psi
Water closet	1.6 gallons per flushing cycle

For SI: 1 gallon per minute = 3.785 L/m,
1 pound per square inch = 6.895 kPa.
a. A handheld shower spray is also a shower head.
b. Consumption tolerances shall be determined from referenced standards.

P2903.3 Minimum pressure. Minimum static pressure (as determined by the local water authority) at the building entrance for either public or private water service shall be 40 psi (276 kPa).

P2903.3.1 Maximum pressure. Maximum static pressure shall be 80 psi (551 kPa). When main pressure exceeds 80 psi (551 kPa), an *approved* pressure-reducing valve conforming to ASSE 1003 shall be installed on the domestic water branch main or riser at the connection to the water-service pipe.

P2903.4 Thermal expansion control. A means for controlling increased pressure caused by thermal expansion shall be installed where required in accordance with Sections P2903.4.1 and P2903.4.2.

P2903.4.1 Pressure-reducing valve. For water service system sizes up to and including 2 inches (51 mm), a device for controlling pressure shall be installed where, because of thermal expansion, the pressure on the downstream side of a pressure-reducing valve exceeds the pressure-reducing valve setting.

P2903.4.2 Backflow prevention device or check valve. Where a backflow prevention device, check valve or other device is installed on a water supply system using storage water heating equipment such that thermal expansion causes an increase in pressure, a device for controlling pressure shall be installed.

P2903.5 Water hammer. The flow velocity of the water distribution system shall be controlled to reduce the possibility of water hammer. Water-hammer arrestors shall be installed in accordance with the manufacturer's installation instructions. Water hammer arrestors shall conform to ASSE 1010.

P2903.6 Determining water-supply fixture units. Supply loads in the building water-distribution system shall be determined by total load on the pipe being sized, in terms of water-supply fixture units (w.s.f.u.), as shown in Table P2903.6, and gallon per minute (gpm) flow rates [see Table P2903.6(1)]. For fixtures not listed, choose a w.s.f.u. value of a fixture with similar flow characteristics.

P2903.7 Size of water-service mains, branch mains and risers. The minimum size water service pipe shall be $^3/_4$ inch (19 mm). The size of water service mains, branch mains and risers shall be determined according to water supply demand [gpm (L/m)], available water pressure [psi (kPa)] and friction loss caused by the water meter and *developed length* of pipe [feet (m)], including *equivalent length* of fittings. The size of each water distribution system shall be determined according to design methods conforming to acceptable engineering practice, such as those methods in Appendix P and shall be *approved* by the code official.

P2903.8 Gridded and parallel water distribution system manifolds. Hot water and cold water manifolds installed with gridded or parallel-connected individual distribution lines to each fixture or fixture fittings shall be designed in accordance with Sections P2903.8.1 through P2903.8.6.

P2903.8.1 Sizing of manifolds. Manifolds shall be sized in accordance with Table P2903.8.1. Total gallons per minute is the demand for all outlets.

P2903.8.2 Minimum size. Where the *developed length* of the distribution line is 60 feet (18 288 mm) or less, and the available pressure at the meter is a minimum of 40 pounds per square inch (276 kPa), the minimum size of individual distri-

TABLE P2903.6
WATER-SUPPLY FIXTURE-UNIT VALUES FOR VARIOUS PLUMBING FIXTURES AND FIXTURE GROUPS

TYPE OF FIXTURES OR GROUP OF FIXTURES	WATER-SUPPLY FIXTURE-UNIT VALUE (w.s.f.u.)		
	Hot	Cold	Combined
Bathtub (with/without overhead shower head)	1.0	1.0	1.4
Clothes washer	1.0	1.0	1.4
Dishwasher	1.4	—	1.4
Full-bath group with bathtub (with/without shower head) or shower stall	1.5	2.7	3.6
Half-bath group (water closet and lavatory)	0.5	2.5	2.6
Hose bibb (sillcock)[a]	—	2.5	2.5
Kitchen group (dishwasher and sink with/without garbage grinder)	1.9	1.0	2.5
Kitchen sink	1.0	1.0	1.4
Laundry group (clothes washer standpipe and laundry tub)	1.8	1.8	2.5
Laundry tub	1.0	1.0	1.4
Lavatory	0.5	0.5	0.7
Shower stall	1.0	1.0	1.4
Water closet (tank type)	—	2.2	2.2

For SI: 1 gallon per minute = 3.785 L/m.

a. The fixture unit value 2.5 assumes a flow demand of 2.5 gpm, such as for an individual lawn sprinkler device. If a hose bibb/sill cock will be required to furnish a greater flow, the equivalent fixture-unit value may be obtained from this table or Table P2903.6(1).

bution lines shall be ³/₈ inch (10 mm). Certain fixtures such as one-piece water closets and whirlpool bathtubs shall require a larger size where specified by the manufacturer. If a water heater is fed from the end of a cold water manifold, the manifold shall be one size larger than the water heater feed.

P2903.8.3 Orientation. Manifolds shall be permitted to be installed in a horizontal or vertical position.

P2903.8.4 Support and protection. Plastic piping bundles shall be secured in accordance with the manufacturer's installation instructions and supported in accordance with Section P2605. Bundles that have a change in direction equal to or greater than 45 degrees (0.79 rad) shall be protected from chafing at the point of contact with framing members by sleeving or wrapping.

P2903.8.5 Valving. Fixture valves, when installed, shall be located either at the fixture or at the manifold. If valves are installed at the manifold, they shall be labeled indicating the fixture served.

P2903.8.6 Hose bibb bleed. A *readily accessible* air bleed shall be installed in hose bibb supplies at the manifold or at the hose bibb exit point.

P2903.9 Valves. Valves shall be installed in accordance with Sections P2903.9.1 through P2903.9.5.

P2903.9.1 Service valve. Each *dwelling unit* shall be provided with an accessible main shutoff valve near the entrance of the water service. The valve shall be of a full-open type having nominal restriction to flow, with provision for drainage such as a bleed orifice or installa-

tion of a separate drain valve. Additionally, the water service shall be valved at the curb or property line in accordance with local requirements.

P2903.9.2 Water heater valve. A *readily accessible* full-open valve shall be installed in the cold-water supply pipe to each water heater at or near the water heater.

P2903.9.3 Fixture valves and access. Valves serving individual fixtures, *appliances*, risers and branches shall be provided with access. An individual shutoff valve shall be required on the fixture supply pipe to each plumbing fixture other than bathtubs and showers.

P2903.9.4 Valve requirements. Valves shall be of an *approved* type and compatible with the type of piping material installed in the system. Ball valves, gate valves, globe valves and plug valves intended to supply drinking water shall meet the requirements of NSF 61.

P2903.9.5 Valves and outlets prohibited below grade. Potable water outlets and combination stop-and-waste valves shall not be installed underground or below grade. Freezeproof yard hydrants that drain the riser into the ground are considered to be stop-and-waste valves.

Exception: Installation of freezeproof yard hydrants that drain the riser into the ground shall be permitted if the potable water supply to such hydrants is protected upstream of the hydrants in accordance with Section P2902 and the hydrants are permanently identified as nonpotable outlets by *approved* signage that reads as follows: "Caution, Nonpotable Water. Do Not Drink."

TABLE P2903.6(1)
CONVERSIONS FROM WATER SUPPLY FIXTURE UNIT TO GALLON PER MINUTE FLOW RATES

SUPPLY SYSTEMS PREDOMINANTLY FOR FLUSH TANKS			SUPPLY SYSTEM PREDOMINANTLY FOR FLUSH VALVES		
Load	Demand		Load	Demand	
(Water supply fixture units)	(Gallons per minute)	(Cubic feet per minute)	(Water supply fixture units)	(Gallons per minute)	(Cubic feet per minute)
1	3.0	0.04104	—	—	—
2	5.0	0.0684	—	—	—
3	6.5	0.86892	—	—	—
4	8.0	1.06944	—	—	—
5	9.4	1.256592	5	15.0	2.0052
6	10.7	1.430376	6	17.4	2.326032
7	11.8	1.577424	7	19.8	2.646364
8	12.8	1.711104	8	22.2	2.967696
9	13.7	1.831416	9	24.6	3.288528
10	14.6	1.951728	10	27.0	3.60936
11	15.4	2.058672	11	27.8	3.716304
12	16.0	2.13888	12	28.6	3.823248
13	16.5	2.20572	13	29.4	3.930192
14	17.0	2.27256	14	30.2	4.037136
15	17.5	2.3394	15	31.0	4.14408
16	18.0	2.90624	16	31.8	4.241024
17	18.4	2.459712	17	32.6	4.357968
18	18.8	2.513184	18	33.4	4.464912
19	19.2	2.566656	19	34.2	4.571856
20	19.6	2.620128	20	35.0	4.6788
25	21.5	2.87412	25	38.0	5.07984
30	23.3	3.114744	30	42.0	5.61356
35	24.9	3.328632	35	44.0	5.88192
40	26.3	3.515784	40	46.0	6.14928
45	27.7	3.702936	45	48.0	6.41664
50	29.1	3.890088	50	50.0	6.684

For SI: 1 gallon per minute = 3.785 L/m, 1 cubic foot per minute = 0.4719 L/s.

TABLE P2903.8.1
MANIFOLD SIZING

PLASTIC		METALLIC	
Nominal Size ID (inches)	Maximum[a] gpm	Nominal Size ID (inches)	Maximum[a] gpm
$^3/_4$	17	$^3/_4$	11
1	29	1	20
$1^1/_4$	46	$1^1/_4$	31
$1^1/_2$	66	$1^1/_2$	44

For SI: 1 inch = 25.4 mm, 1 gallon per minute = 3.785 L/m, 1 foot per second = 0.3048 m/s.

NOTE: See Table P2903.6 for w.s.f.u and Table 2903.6(1) for gallon-per-minute (gpm) flow rates.

a. Based on velocity limitation: plastic—12 fps; metal—8 fps.

P2903.10 Hose bibb. Hose bibbs subject to freezing, including the "frost-proof" type, shall be equipped with an accessible stop-and-waste-type valve inside the building so that they can be controlled and/or drained during cold periods.

Exception: Frostproof hose bibbs installed such that the stem extends through the building insulation into an open heated or semi*conditioned space* need not be separately valved (see Figure P2903.10).

SECTION P2904
DWELLING UNIT FIRE SPRINKLER SYSTEMS

P2904.1 General. Where installed, residential fire sprinkler systems, or portions thereof, shall be in accordance with NFPA 13D or Section P2904, which shall be considered equivalent to NFPA 13D. Section P2904 shall apply to stand-alone and multipurpose wet-pipe sprinkler systems that do not include the use of antifreeze. A multipurpose fire sprinkler system shall supply domestic water to both fire sprinklers and plumbing fixtures. A stand-alone sprinkler system shall be separate and independent from the water distribution system. A backflow flow preventer shall not be required to separate a stand-alone sprinkler system from the water distribution system.

P2904.1.1 Required sprinkler locations. Sprinklers shall be installed to protect all areas of a *dwelling unit*.

Exceptions:

1. Attics, crawl spaces and normally unoccupied concealed spaces that do not contain fuel-fired appliances do not require sprinklers. In *attics*, crawl spaces and normally unoccupied concealed spaces that contain fuel-fired equipment, a sprinkler shall be installed above the equipment; however, sprinklers shall not be required in the remainder of the space.

2. Clothes closets, linen closets and pantries not exceeding 24 square feet (2.2 m²) in area, with the

smallest dimension not greater than 3 feet (915 mm) and having wall and ceiling surfaces of gypsum board.

3. Bathrooms not more than 55 square feet (5.1 m²) in area.

4. Garages; carports; exterior porches; unheated entry areas, such as mud rooms, that are adjacent to an exterior door; and similar areas.

P2904.2 Sprinklers. Sprinklers shall be new listed residential sprinklers and shall be installed in accordance with the sprinkler manufacturer's installation instructions.

P2904.2.1 Temperature rating and separation from heat sources. Except as provided for in Section P2904.2.2, sprinklers shall have a temperature rating of not less than 135°F (57°C) and not more than 170°F (77°C). Sprinklers shall be separated from heat sources as required by the sprinkler manufacturer's installation instructions.

P2904.2.2 Intermediate temperature sprinklers. Sprinklers shall have an intermediate temperature rating not less than 175°F (79°C) and not more than 225°F (107°C) where installed in the following locations:

1. Directly under skylights, where the sprinkler is exposed to direct sunlight.

2. In *attics*.

3. In concealed spaces located directly beneath a roof.

4. Within the distance to a heat source as specified in Table P2904.2.2

P2904.2.3 Freezing areas. Piping shall be protected from freezing as required by Section P2603.6. Where sprinklers are required in areas that are subject to freezing, dry-sidewall or dry-pendent sprinklers extending from a nonfreezing area into a freezing area shall be installed.

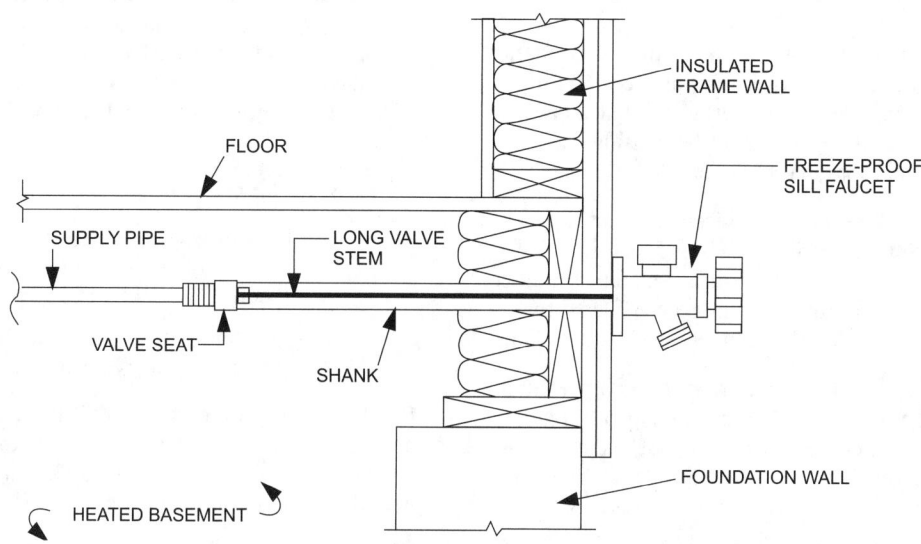

FIGURE P2903.10
TYPICAL FROSTPROOF HOSE BIBB INSTALLATION NOT REQUIRING SEPARATE VALUE

TABLE P2904.2.2
LOCATIONS WHERE INTERMEDIATE TEMPERATURE SPRINKLERS ARE REQUIRED

HEAT SOURCE	RANGE OF DISTANCE FROM HEAT SOURCE WITHIN WHICH INTERMEDIATE TEMPERATURE SPRINKLERS ARE REQUIRED[a,b] (inches)
Fireplace, side of open or recessed fireplace	12 to 36
Fireplace, front of recessed fireplace	36 to 60
Coal and wood burning stove	12 to 42
Kitchen range top	9 to 18
Oven	9 to 18
Vent connector or chimney connector	9 to 18
Heating duct, not insulated	9 to 18
Hot water pipe, not insulated	6 to 12
Side of ceiling or wall warm air register	12 to 24
Front of wall mounted warm air register	18 to 36
Water heater, furnace or boiler	3 to 6
Luminaire up to 250 watts	3 to 6
Luminaire 250 watts up to 499 watts	6 to 12

For SI: 1 inch = 25.4 mm.

a. Sprinklers shall not be located at distances less than the minimum table distance unless the sprinkler listing allows a lesser distance.

b. Distances shall be measured in a straight line from the nearest edge of the heat source to the nearest edge of the sprinkler.

P2904.2.4 Sprinkler coverage. Sprinkler coverage requirements and sprinkler obstruction requirements shall be in accordance with Sections P2904.2.4.1 and P2904.2.4.2.

P2904.2.4.1 Coverage area limit. The area of coverage of a single sprinkler shall not exceed 400 square feet (37 m²) and shall be based on the sprinkler listing and the sprinkler manufacturer's installation instructions.

P2904.2.4.2 Obstructions to coverage. Sprinkler discharge shall not be blocked by obstructions unless additional sprinklers are installed to protect the obstructed area. Sprinkler separation from obstructions shall comply with the minimum distances specified in the sprinkler manufacturer's instructions.

P2904.2.4.2.1 Additional requirements for pendent sprinklers. Pendent sprinklers within 3 feet (915 mm) of the center of a ceiling fan, surface-mounted ceiling luminaire or similar object shall be considered to be obstructed, and additional sprinklers shall be installed.

P2904.2.4.2.2 Additional requirements for sidewall sprinklers. Sidewall sprinklers within 5 feet (1524 mm) of the center of a ceiling fan, surface-mounted ceiling luminaire or similar object shall be considered to be obstructed, and additional sprinklers shall be installed.

P2904.2.5 Sprinkler installation on systems assembled with solvent cement. The solvent cementing of threaded adapter fittings shall be completed and threaded adapters for sprinklers shall be verified as being clear of excess cement prior to the installation of sprinklers on systems assembled with solvent cement.

P2904.2.6 Sprinkler modifications prohibited. Painting, caulking or modifying of sprinklers shall be prohibited.

Sprinklers that have been painted, caulked, modified or damaged shall be replaced with new sprinklers.

P2904.3 Sprinkler piping system. Sprinkler piping shall be supported in accordance with the requirements for cold water distribution piping. Sprinkler piping shall comply with all requirements for cold water distribution piping. For multipurpose piping systems, the sprinkler piping shall connect to and be a part of the cold water distribution piping system.

P2904.3.1 Nonmetallic pipe and tubing. Nonmetallic pipe and tubing, such as CPVC and PEX, shall be listed for use in residential fire sprinkler systems.

P2904.3.1.1 Nonmetallic pipe protection. Nonmetallic pipe and tubing systems shall be protected from exposure to the living space by a layer of not less than $^3/_8$ inch (9.5 mm) thick gypsum wallboard, $^1/_2$ inch thick plywood (13 mm), or other material having a 15 minute fire rating.

Exceptions:

1. Pipe protection shall not be required in areas that do not require protection with sprinklers as specified in Section P2904.1.1.

2. Pipe protection shall not be required where exposed piping is permitted by the pipe listing.

P2904.3.2 Shutoff valves prohibited. With the exception of shutoff valves for the entire water distribution system, valves shall not be installed in any location where the valve would isolate piping serving one or more sprinklers.

P2904.3.3 Single dwelling limit. Piping beyond the service valve located at the beginning of the water distribution system shall not serve more than one *dwelling*.

P2904.3.4 Drain. A means to drain the sprinkler system shall be provided on the system side of the water distribution shutoff valve.

P2904.4 Determining system design flow. The flow for sizing the sprinkler piping system shall be based on the flow rating of each sprinkler in accordance with Section P2904.4.1 and the calculation in accordance with Section P2904.4.2.

P2904.4.1 Determining required flow rate for each sprinkler. The minimum required flow for each sprinkler shall be determined using the sprinkler manufacturer's published data for the specific sprinkler model based on all of the following:

1. The area of coverage.

2. The ceiling configuration.

3. The temperature rating.

4. Any additional conditions specified by the sprinkler manufacturer.

P2904.4.2 System design flow rate. The design flow rate for the system shall be based on the following:

1. The design flow rate for a room having only one sprinkler shall be the flow rate required for that sprinkler, as determined by Section P2904.4.1.

2. The design flow rate for a room having two or more sprinklers a shall be determined by identifying the sprinkler in that room with the highest required flow rate, based on Section P2904.4.1, and multiplying that flow rate by 2.

3. Where the sprinkler manufacturer specifies different criteria for ceiling configurations that are not smooth, flat and horizontal, the required flow rate for that room shall comply with the sprinkler manufacturer's instructions.

4. The design flow rate for the sprinkler system shall be the flow required by the room with the largest flow rate, based on Items 1, 2 and 3.

5. For the purpose of this section, it shall be permissible to reduce the design flow rate for a room by subdividing the space into two or more rooms, where each room is evaluated separately with respect to the required design flow rate. Each room shall be bounded by walls and a ceiling. Openings in walls shall have a lintel not less than 8 inches (203 mm) in depth and each lintel shall form a solid barrier between the ceiling and the top of the opening.

P2904.5 Water supply. The water supply shall provide not less than the required design flow rate for sprinklers in accordance with Section P2904.4.2 at a pressure not less than that used to comply with Section P2904.6.

P2904.5.1 Water supply from individual sources. Where a *dwelling unit* water supply is from a tank system, a private well system or a combination of these, the available water supply shall be based on the minimum pressure control setting for the pump.

P2904.5.2 Required capacity. The water supply shall have the capacity to provide the required design flow rate for sprinklers for a period of time as follows:

1. 7 minutes for *dwelling units* one *story* in height and less than 2,000 square feet (186 m²) in area.

2. 10 minutes for *dwelling units* two or more stories in height or equal to or greater than 2,000 square feet (186 m²) in area.

Where a well system, a water supply tank system or a combination thereof is used, any combination of well capacity and tank storage shall be permitted to meet the capacity requirement.

P2904.6 Pipe sizing. The piping to sprinklers shall be sized for the flow required by Section P2904.4.2. The flow required to supply the plumbing fixtures shall not be required to be added to the sprinkler design flow.

P2904.6.1 Method of sizing pipe. Piping supplying sprinklers shall be sized using the prescriptive method in Section P2904.6.2 or by hydraulic calculation in accordance with NFPA 13D. The minimum pipe size from the water supply source to any sprinkler shall be $^3/_4$ inch (19 mm) nominal. Threaded adapter fittings at the point where sprinklers are attached to the piping shall be a minimum of $^1/_2$ inch (13 mm) nominal.

P2904.6.2 Prescriptive pipe sizing method. Pipe shall be sized by determining the available pressure to offset friction loss in piping and identifying a piping material, diameter and length using the equation in Section P2904.6.2.1 and the procedure in Section P2904.6.2.2.

P2904.6.2.1 Available pressure equation. The pressure available to offset friction loss in the interior piping system (P_t) shall be determined in accordance with the Equation 29-1.

$$P_t = P_{sup} - PL_{svc} - PL_m - PL_d - PL_e - P_{sp} \quad \textbf{(Equation 29-1)}$$

where:

P_t = Pressure used in applying Tables P2904.6.2(4) through P2904.6.2(9).

P_{sup} = Pressure available from the water supply source.

PL_{svc} = Pressure loss in the water-service pipe.

PL_m = Pressure loss in the water meter.

PL_d = Pressure loss from devices other than the water meter.

PL_e = Pressure loss associated with changes in elevation.

P_{sp} = Maximum pressure required by a sprinkler.

2904.6.2.2 Calculation procedure. Determination of the required size for water distribution piping shall be in accordance with the following procedure:

Step 1–Determine P_{sup}

Obtain the static supply pressure that will be available from the water main from the water purveyor, or for an individual source, the available supply pressure shall be in accordance with Section P2904.5.1.

Step 2–Determine PL_{svc}

Use Table P2904.6.2(1) to determine the pressure loss in the water service pipe based on the selected size of the water service.

Step 3–Determine PL_m

Use Table P2904.6.2(2) to determine the pressure loss from the water meter, based on the selected water meter size.

Step 4–Determine PL_d

Determine the pressure loss from devices other than the water meter installed in the piping system supplying sprinklers, such as pressure-reducing valves, backflow preventers, water softeners or water filters. Device pressure losses shall be based on the device manufacturer's specifications. The flow rate used to determine pressure loss shall be the rate from Section P2904.4.2, except that 5 gpm (0.3 L/S) shall be added where the device is installed in a water-service pipe that supplies more than one *dwelling*. As alternative to deducting pressure loss for a device, an automatic bypass valve shall be installed to divert flow around the device when a sprinkler activates.

Step 5–Determine PL_e

Use Table P2904.6.2(3) to determine the pressure loss associated with changes in elevation. The elevation used in applying the table shall be the difference between the elevation where the water source pressure was measured and the elevation of the highest sprinkler.

Step 6–Determine P_{sp}

Determine the maximum pressure required by any individual sprinkler based on the flow rate from Section P2904.4.1. The required pressure is provided in the sprinkler manufacturer's published data for the specific sprinkler model based on the selected flow rate.

Step 7–Calculate P_t

Using Equation 29-1, calculate the pressure available to offset friction loss in water-distribution piping between the service valve and the sprinklers.

Step 8–Determine the maximum allowable pipe length

Use Tables P2904.6.2(4) through P2904.6.2(9) to select a material and size for water distribution piping. The piping material and size shall be acceptable if the *developed length* of pipe between the service valve and the most remote sprinkler does not exceed the maximum allowable length specified by the applicable table. Interpolation of P_t between the tabular values shall be permitted.

The maximum allowable length of piping in Tables P2904.6.2(4) through P2904.6.2(9) incorporates an adjustment for pipe fittings, and no additional consideration of friction losses associated with pipe fittings shall be required.

P2904.7 Instructions and signs. An owner's manual for the fire sprinkler system shall be provided to the owner. A sign or valve tag shall be installed at the main shutoff valve to the water distribution system stating the following: "Warning, the water system for this home supplies fire sprinklers that require certain flows and pressures to fight a fire. Devices that restrict the flow or decrease the pressure or automatically shut off the water to the fire sprinkler system, such as water softeners, filtration systems and automatic shutoff valves, shall not be added to this system without a review of the fire sprinkler system by a fire protection specialist. Do not remove this sign."

P2904.8 Inspections. The water distribution system shall be inspected in accordance with Sections P2904.8.1 and P2904.8.2.

P2904.8.1 Preconcealment inspection. The following items shall be verified prior to the concealment of any sprinkler system piping:

1. Sprinklers are installed in all areas as required by Section P2904.1.1.

2. Where sprinkler water spray patterns are obstructed by construction features, luminaires or ceiling fans, additional sprinklers are installed as required by Section P2904.2.4.2.

3. Sprinklers are the correct temperature rating and are installed at or beyond the required separation distances from heat sources as required by Sections P2904.2.1 and P2904.2.2.

4. The pipe size equals or exceeds the size used in applying Tables P2904.6.2(4) through P2904.6.2(9) or, if the piping system was hydraulically calculated in accordance with Section P2904.6.1, the size used in the hydraulic calculation.

5. The pipe length does not exceed the length permitted by Tables P2904.6.2(4) through P2904.6.2(9) or, if the piping system was hydraulically calculated in accordance with Section P2904.6.1, pipe lengths and fittings do not exceed those used in the hydraulic calculation.

6. Nonmetallic piping that conveys water to sprinklers is listed for use with fire sprinklers.

7. Piping is supported in accordance with the pipe manufacturer's and sprinkler manufacturer's installation instructions.

8. The piping system is tested in accordance with Section P2503.7.

P2904.8.2 Final inspection. The following items shall be verified upon completion of the system:

1. Sprinkler are not painted, damaged or otherwise hindered from operation.

2. Where a pump is required to provide water to the system, the pump starts automatically upon system water demand.

3. Pressure-reducing valves, water softeners, water filters or other impairments to water flow that were not part of the original design have not been installed.

4. The sign or valve tag required by Section P2904.7 is installed and the owner's manual for the system is present.

TABLE P2904.6.2(1)
WATER SERVICE PRESSURE LOSS (PL_{svc})[a,b]

FLOW RATE[c] (gpm)	3/4 INCH WATER SERVICE PRESSURE LOSS (psi)				1 INCH WATER SERVICE PRESSURE LOSS (psi)				1 1/4 INCH WATER SERVICE PRESSURE LOSS (psi)			
	Length of water service pipe (feet)				Length of water service pipe (feet)				Length of water service pipe (feet)			
	40 or less	41 to 75	76 to 100	101 to 150	40 or less	41 to 75	76 to 100	101 to 150	40 or less	41 to 75	76 to 100	101 to 150
8	5.1	8.7	11.8	17.4	1.5	2.5	3.4	5.1	0.6	1.0	1.3	1.9
10	7.7	13.1	17.8	26.3	2.3	3.8	5.2	7.7	0.8	1.4	2.0	2.9
12	10.8	18.4	24.9	NP	3.2	5.4	7.3	10.7	1.2	2.0	2.7	4.0
14	14.4	24.5	NP	NP	4.2	7.1	9.6	14.3	1.6	2.7	3.6	5.4
16	18.4	NP	NP	NP	5.4	9.1	12.4	18.3	2.0	3.4	4.7	6.9
18	22.9	NP	NP	NP	6.7	11.4	15.4	22.7	2.5	4.3	5.8	8.6
20	27.8	NP	NP	NP	8.1	13.8	18.7	27.6	3.1	5.2	7.0	10.4
22	NP	NP	NP	NP	9.7	16.5	22.3	NP	3.7	6.2	8.4	12.4
24	NP	NP	NP	NP	11.4	19.3	26.2	NP	4.3	7.3	9.9	14.6
26	NP	NP	NP	NP	13.2	22.4	NP	NP	5.0	8.5	11.4	16.9
28	NP	NP	NP	NP	15.1	25.7	NP	NP	5.7	9.7	13.1	19.4
30	NP	NP	NP	NP	17.2	NP	NP	NP	6.5	11.0	14.9	22.0
32	NP	NP	NP	NP	19.4	NP	NP	NP	7.3	12.4	16.8	24.8
34	NP	NP	NP	NP	21.7	NP	NP	NP	8.2	13.9	18.8	NP
36	NP	NP	NP	NP	24.1	NP	NP	NP	9.1	15.4	20.9	NP

For SI: 1 inch = 25.4 mm, 1 foot = 304.8 mm, 1 gallon per minute = 0.063 L/s, 1 pound per square inch = 6.895 kPa.

NP - Not permitted. Pressure loss exceeds reasonable limits.

a. Values are applicable for underground piping materials listed in Table P2905.4 and are based on an SDR of 11 and a Hazen Williams C Factor of 150.

b. Values include the following length allowances for fittings: 25% length increase for actual lengths up to 100 feet and 15% length increase for actual lengths over 100 feet.

c. Flow rate from Section P2904.4.2. Add 5 gpm to the flow rate required by Section P2904.4.2 where the water-service pipe supplies more than one dwelling.

TABLE P2904.6.2(2)
MINIMUM WATER METER PRESSURE LOSS (PL_m)[a]

FLOW RATE (gallons per minute, gpm)[b]	$^5/_8$-INCH METER PRESSURE LOSS (pounds per square inch, psi)	$^3/_4$-INCH METER PRESSURE LESS (pounds per square inch, psi)	1-INCH METER PRESSURE LOSS (pounds per square inch, psi)
8	2	1	1
10	3	1	1
12	4	1	1
14	5	2	1
16	7	3	1
18	9	4	1
20	11	4	2
22	NP	5	2
24	NP	5	2
26	NP	6	2
28	NP	6	2
30	NP	7	2
32	NP	7	3
34	NP	8	3
36	NP	8	3

For SI: 1 inch = 25.4 mm, 1 pound per square inch = 6.895 kPa, 1 gallon per minute = 0.063 L/s.

NP - Not permitted unless the actual water meter pressure loss is known.

a. Table 2904.6.2(2) establishes conservative values for water meter pressure loss or installations where the water meter loss is unknown. Where the actual water meter pressure loss is known, P_m shall be the actual loss.

b. Flow rate from Section P2904.4.2. Add 5 gpm to the flow rate required by Section P2904.4.2 where the water-service pipe supplies more than one dwelling.

TABLE P2904.6.2(3)
ELEVATION LOSS (PL_e)

ELEVATION (feet)	PRESSURE LOSS (psi)
5	2.2
10	4.4
15	6.5
20	8.7
25	10.9
30	13
35	15.2
40	17.4

For SI: 1 foot = 304.8 mm, 1 pound per square inch = 6.895 kPa.

TABLE P2904.6.2(4)
ALLOWABLE PIPE LENGTH FOR $^3/_4$-INCH TYPE M COPPER WATER TUBING

SPRINKLER FLOW RATE[a] (gpm)	WATER DISTRIBUTION SIZE (inch)	AVAILABLE PRESSURE - P_t (psi)									
		15	20	25	30	35	40	45	50	55	60
		Allowable length of pipe from service valve to farthest sprinkler (feet)									
8	$^3/_4$	217	289	361	434	506	578	650	723	795	867
9	$^3/_4$	174	232	291	349	407	465	523	581	639	697
10	$^3/_4$	143	191	239	287	335	383	430	478	526	574
11	$^3/_4$	120	160	200	241	281	321	361	401	441	481
12	$^3/_4$	102	137	171	205	239	273	307	341	375	410
13	$^3/_4$	88	118	147	177	206	235	265	294	324	353
14	$^3/_4$	77	103	128	154	180	205	231	257	282	308
15	$^3/_4$	68	90	113	136	158	181	203	226	248	271
16	$^3/_4$	60	80	100	120	140	160	180	200	220	241
17	$^3/_4$	54	72	90	108	125	143	161	179	197	215
18	$^3/_4$	48	64	81	97	113	129	145	161	177	193
19	$^3/_4$	44	58	73	88	102	117	131	146	160	175
20	$^3/_4$	40	53	66	80	93	106	119	133	146	159
21	$^3/_4$	36	48	61	73	85	97	109	121	133	145
22	$^3/_4$	33	44	56	67	78	89	100	111	122	133
23	$^3/_4$	31	41	51	61	72	82	92	102	113	123
24	$^3/_4$	28	38	47	57	66	76	85	95	104	114
25	$^3/_4$	26	35	44	53	61	70	79	88	97	105
26	$^3/_4$	24	33	41	49	57	65	73	82	90	98
27	$^3/_4$	23	30	38	46	53	61	69	76	84	91
28	$^3/_4$	21	28	36	43	50	57	64	71	78	85
29	$^3/_4$	20	27	33	40	47	53	60	67	73	80
30	$^3/_4$	19	25	31	38	44	50	56	63	69	75
31	$^3/_4$	18	24	29	35	41	47	53	59	65	71
32	$^3/_4$	17	22	28	33	39	44	50	56	61	67
33	$^3/_4$	16	21	26	32	37	42	47	53	58	63
34	$^3/_4$	NP	20	25	30	35	40	45	50	55	60
35	$^3/_4$	NP	19	24	28	33	38	42	47	52	57
36	$^3/_4$	NP	18	22	27	31	36	40	45	49	54
37	$^3/_4$	NP	17	21	26	30	34	38	43	47	51
38	$^3/_4$	NP	16	20	24	28	32	36	40	45	49
39	$^3/_4$	NP	15	19	23	27	31	35	39	42	46
40	$^3/_4$	NP	NP	18	22	26	29	33	37	40	44

For SI: 1 inch = 25.4 mm, 1 foot = 304.8 mm, 1 pound per square inch = 6.895 kPa, 1 gallon per minute = 0.963 L/s.
NP - Not permitted
a. Flow rate from Section P2904.4.2.

TABLE P2904.6.2(5)
ALLOWABLE PIPE LENGTH FOR 1-INCH TYPE M COPPER WATER TUBING

SPRINKLER FLOW RATE[a] (gpm)	WATER DISTRIBUTION SIZE (inch)	AVAILABLE PRESSURE - P_t (psi)									
		15	20	25	30	35	40	45	50	55	60
		Allowable length of pipe from service valve to farthest sprinkler (feet)									
8	1	806	1075	1343	1612	1881	2149	2418	2687	2955	3224
9	1	648	864	1080	1296	1512	1728	1945	2161	2377	2593
10	1	533	711	889	1067	1245	1422	1600	1778	1956	2134
11	1	447	586	745	894	1043	1192	1341	1491	1640	1789
12	1	381	508	634	761	888	1015	1142	1269	1396	1523
13	1	328	438	547	657	766	875	985	1094	1204	1313
14	1	286	382	477	572	668	763	859	954	1049	1145
15	1	252	336	420	504	588	672	756	840	924	1008
16	1	224	298	373	447	522	596	671	745	820	894
17	1	200	266	333	400	466	533	600	666	733	799
18	1	180	240	300	360	420	479	539	599	659	719
19	1	163	217	271	325	380	434	488	542	597	651
20	1	148	197	247	296	345	395	444	493	543	592
21	1	135	180	225	270	315	360	406	451	496	541
22	1	124	165	207	248	289	331	372	413	455	496
23	1	114	152	190	228	267	305	343	381	419	457
24	1	106	141	176	211	246	282	317	352	387	422
25	1	98	131	163	196	228	261	294	326	359	392
26	1	91	121	152	182	212	243	273	304	334	364
27	1	85	113	142	170	198	226	255	283	311	340
28	1	79	106	132	159	185	212	238	265	291	318
29	1	74	99	124	149	174	198	223	248	273	298
30	1	70	93	116	140	163	186	210	233	256	280
31	1	66	88	110	132	153	175	197	219	241	263
32	1	62	83	103	124	145	165	186	207	227	248
33	1	59	78	98	117	137	156	176	195	215	234
34	1	55	74	92	111	129	148	166	185	203	222
35	1	53	70	88	105	123	140	158	175	193	210
36	1	50	66	83	100	116	133	150	166	183	199
37	1	47	63	79	95	111	126	142	158	174	190
38	1	45	60	75	90	105	120	135	150	165	181
39	1	43	57	72	86	100	115	129	143	158	172
40	1	41	55	68	82	96	109	123	137	150	164

For SI: 1 inch = 25.4 mm, 1 foot = 304.8 mm, 1 pound per square inch = 6.895 kPa, 1 gallon per minute = 0.963 L/s.

a. Flow rate from Section P2904.4.2.

TABLE P2904.6.2(6)
ALLOWABLE PIPE LENGTH FOR $^3/_4$-INCH CPVC PIPE

SPRINKLER FLOW RATE[a] (gpm)	WATER DISTRIBUTION SIZE (inch)	AVAILABLE PRESSURE - P_t (psi)									
		15	20	25	30	35	40	45	50	55	60
		Allowable length of pipe from service valve to farthest sprinkler (feet)									
8	$^3/_4$	348	465	581	697	813	929	1045	1161	1278	1394
9	$^3/_4$	280	374	467	560	654	747	841	934	1027	1121
10	$^3/_4$	231	307	384	461	538	615	692	769	845	922
11	$^3/_4$	193	258	322	387	451	515	580	644	709	773
12	$^3/_4$	165	219	274	329	384	439	494	549	603	658
13	$^3/_4$	142	189	237	284	331	378	426	473	520	568
14	$^3/_4$	124	165	206	247	289	330	371	412	454	495
15	$^3/_4$	109	145	182	218	254	290	327	363	399	436
16	$^3/_4$	97	129	161	193	226	258	290	322	354	387
17	$^3/_4$	86	115	144	173	202	230	259	288	317	346
18	$^3/_4$	78	104	130	155	181	207	233	259	285	311
19	$^3/_4$	70	94	117	141	164	188	211	234	258	281
20	$^3/_4$	64	85	107	128	149	171	192	213	235	256
21	$^3/_4$	58	78	97	117	136	156	175	195	214	234
22	$^3/_4$	54	71	89	107	125	143	161	179	197	214
23	$^3/_4$	49	66	82	99	115	132	148	165	181	198
24	$^3/_4$	46	61	76	91	107	122	137	152	167	183
25	$^3/_4$	42	56	71	85	99	113	127	141	155	169
26	$^3/_4$	39	52	66	79	92	105	118	131	144	157
27	$^3/_4$	37	49	61	73	86	98	110	122	135	147
28	$^3/_4$	34	46	57	69	80	92	103	114	126	137
29	$^3/_4$	32	43	54	64	75	86	96	107	118	129
30	$^3/_4$	30	40	50	60	70	81	91	101	111	121
31	$^3/_4$	28	38	47	57	66	76	85	95	104	114
32	$^3/_4$	27	36	45	54	63	71	80	89	98	107
33	$^3/_4$	25	34	42	51	59	68	76	84	93	101
34	$^3/_4$	24	32	40	48	56	64	72	80	88	96
35	$^3/_4$	23	30	38	45	53	61	68	76	83	91
36	$^3/_4$	22	29	36	43	50	57	65	72	79	86
37	$^3/_4$	20	27	34	41	48	55	61	68	75	82
38	$^3/_4$	20	26	33	39	46	52	59	65	72	78
39	$^3/_4$	19	25	31	37	43	50	56	62	68	74
40	$^3/_4$	18	24	30	35	41	47	53	59	65	71

For SI: 1 inch = 25.4 mm, 1 foot = 304.8 mm, 1 pound per square inch = 6.895 kPa, 1 gallon per minute = 0.963 L/s.

a. Flow rate from Section P2904.4.2.

TABLE P2904.6.2(7)
ALLOWABLE PIPE LENGTH FOR 1-INCH CPVC PIPE

SPRINKLER FLOW RATE[a] (gpm)	WATER DISTRIBUTION SIZE (inch)	AVAILABLE PRESSURE - P_t (psi)									
		15	20	25	30	35	40	45	50	55	60
		Allowable length of pipe from service valve to farthest sprinkler (feet)									
8	1	1049	1398	1748	2098	2447	2797	3146	3496	3845	4195
9	1	843	1125	1406	1687	1968	2249	2530	2811	3093	3374
10	1	694	925	1157	1388	1619	1851	2082	2314	2545	2776
11	1	582	776	970	1164	1358	1552	1746	1940	2133	2327
12	1	495	660	826	991	1156	1321	1486	1651	1816	1981
13	1	427	570	712	854	997	1139	1281	1424	1566	1709
14	1	372	497	621	745	869	993	1117	1241	1366	1490
15	1	328	437	546	656	765	874	983	1093	1202	1311
16	1	291	388	485	582	679	776	873	970	1067	1164
17	1	260	347	433	520	607	693	780	867	954	1040
18	1	234	312	390	468	546	624	702	780	858	936
19	1	212	282	353	423	494	565	635	706	776	847
20	1	193	257	321	385	449	513	578	642	706	770
21	1	176	235	293	352	410	469	528	586	645	704
22	1	161	215	269	323	377	430	484	538	592	646
23	1	149	198	248	297	347	396	446	496	545	595
24	1	137	183	229	275	321	366	412	458	504	550
25	1	127	170	212	255	297	340	382	425	467	510
26	1	118	158	197	237	276	316	355	395	434	474
27	1	111	147	184	221	258	295	332	368	405	442
28	1	103	138	172	207	241	275	310	344	379	413
29	1	97	129	161	194	226	258	290	323	355	387
30	1	91	121	152	182	212	242	273	303	333	364
31	1	86	114	143	171	200	228	257	285	314	342
32	1	81	108	134	161	188	215	242	269	296	323
33	1	76	102	127	152	178	203	229	254	280	305
34	1	72	96	120	144	168	192	216	240	265	289
35	1	68	91	114	137	160	182	205	228	251	273
36	1	65	87	108	130	151	173	195	216	238	260
37	1	62	82	103	123	144	165	185	206	226	247
38	1	59	78	98	117	137	157	176	196	215	235
39	1	56	75	93	112	131	149	168	187	205	224
40	1	53	71	89	107	125	142	160	178	196	214

For SI: 1 inch = 25.4 mm, 1 foot = 304.8 mm, 1 pound per square inch = 6.895 kPa, 1 gallon per minute = 0.963 L/s.

a. Flow rate from Section P2904.4.2.

TABLE P2904.6.2(8)
ALLOWABLE PIPE LENGTH FOR $^3/_4$-INCH PEX TUBING

SPRINKLER FLOW RATE[a] (gpm)	WATER DISTRIBUTION SIZE (inch)	AVAILABLE PRESSURE - P_t (psi)									
		15	20	25	30	35	40	45	50	55	60
		Allowable length of pipe from service valve to farthest sprinkler (feet)									
8	$^3/_4$	93	123	154	185	216	247	278	309	339	370
9	$^3/_4$	74	99	124	149	174	199	223	248	273	298
10	$^3/_4$	61	82	102	123	143	163	184	204	225	245
11	$^3/_4$	51	68	86	103	120	137	154	171	188	205
12	$^3/_4$	44	58	73	87	102	117	131	146	160	175
13	$^3/_4$	38	50	63	75	88	101	113	126	138	151
14	$^3/_4$	33	44	55	66	77	88	99	110	121	132
15	$^3/_4$	29	39	48	58	68	77	87	96	106	116
16	$^3/_4$	26	34	43	51	60	68	77	86	94	103
17	$^3/_4$	23	31	38	46	54	61	69	77	84	92
18	$^3/_4$	21	28	34	41	48	55	62	69	76	83
19	$^3/_4$	19	25	31	37	44	50	56	62	69	75
20	$^3/_4$	17	23	28	34	40	45	51	57	62	68
21	$^3/_4$	16	21	26	31	36	41	47	52	57	62
22	$^3/_4$	NP	19	24	28	33	38	43	47	52	57
23	$^3/_4$	NP	17	22	26	31	35	39	44	48	52
24	$^3/_4$	NP	16	20	24	28	32	36	40	44	49
25	$^3/_4$	NP	NP	19	22	26	30	34	37	41	45
26	$^3/_4$	NP	NP	17	21	24	28	31	35	38	42
27	$^3/_4$	NP	NP	16	20	23	26	29	33	36	39
28	$^3/_4$	NP	NP	15	18	21	24	27	30	33	36
29	$^3/_4$	NP	NP	NP	17	20	23	26	28	31	34
30	$^3/_4$	NP	NP	NP	16	19	21	24	27	29	32
31	$^3/_4$	NP	NP	NP	15	18	20	23	25	28	30
32	$^3/_4$	NP	NP	NP	NP	17	19	21	24	26	28
33	$^3/_4$	NP	NP	NP	NP	16	18	20	22	25	27
34	$^3/_4$	NP	NP	NP	NP	NP	17	19	21	23	25
35	$^3/_4$	NP	NP	NP	NP	NP	16	18	20	22	24
36	$^3/_4$	NP	NP	NP	NP	NP	15	17	19	21	23
37	$^3/_4$	NP	NP	NP	NP	NP	NP	16	18	20	22
38	$^3/_4$	NP	NP	NP	NP	NP	NP	16	17	19	21
39	$^3/_4$	NP	NP	NP	NP	NP	NP	NP	16	18	20
40	$^3/_4$	NP	NP	NP	NP	NP	NP	NP	16	17	19

For SI: 1 inch = 25.4 mm, 1 foot = 304.8 mm, 1 pound per square inch = 6.895 kPa, 1 gallon per minute = 0.963 L/s.
NP - Not permitted.
a. Flow rate from Section P2904.4.2.

TABLE P2904.6.2(9)
ALLOWABLE PIPE LENGTH FOR 1-INCH PEX TUBING

SPRINKLER FLOW RATE[a] (gpm)	WATER DISTRIBUTION SIZE (inch)	AVAILABLE PRESSURE - P_t (psi)									
		15	20	25	30	35	40	45	50	55	60
		Allowable length of pipe from service valve to farthest sprinkler (feet)									
8	1	314	418	523	628	732	837	941	1046	1151	1255
9	1	252	336	421	505	589	673	757	841	925	1009
10	1	208	277	346	415	485	554	623	692	761	831
11	1	174	232	290	348	406	464	522	580	638	696
12	1	148	198	247	296	346	395	445	494	543	593
13	1	128	170	213	256	298	341	383	426	469	511
14	1	111	149	186	223	260	297	334	371	409	446
15	1	98	131	163	196	229	262	294	327	360	392
16	1	87	116	145	174	203	232	261	290	319	348
17	1	78	104	130	156	182	208	233	259	285	311
18	1	70	93	117	140	163	187	210	233	257	280
19	1	63	84	106	127	148	169	190	211	232	253
20	1	58	77	96	115	134	154	173	192	211	230
21	1	53	70	88	105	123	140	158	175	193	211
22	1	48	64	80	97	113	129	145	161	177	193
23	1	44	59	74	89	104	119	133	148	163	178
24	1	41	55	69	82	96	110	123	137	151	164
25	1	38	51	64	76	89	102	114	127	140	152
26	1	35	47	59	71	83	95	106	118	130	142
27	1	33	44	55	66	77	88	99	110	121	132
28	1	31	41	52	62	72	82	93	103	113	124
29	1	29	39	48	58	68	77	87	97	106	116
30	1	27	36	45	54	63	73	82	91	100	109
31	1	26	34	43	51	60	68	77	85	94	102
32	1	24	32	40	48	56	64	72	80	89	97
33	1	23	30	38	46	53	61	68	76	84	91
34	1	22	29	36	43	50	58	65	72	79	86
35	1	20	27	34	41	48	55	61	68	75	82
36	1	19	26	32	39	45	52	58	65	71	78
37	1	18	25	31	37	43	49	55	62	68	74
38	1	18	23	29	35	41	47	53	59	64	70
39	1	17	22	28	33	39	45	50	56	61	67
40	1	16	21	27	32	37	43	48	53	59	64

For SI: 1 inch = 25.4 mm, 1 foot = 304.8 mm, 1 pound per square inch = 6.895 kPa, 1 gallon per minute = 0.963 L/s.

a. Flow rate from Section P2904.4.2.

SECTION P2905
MATERIALS, JOINTS AND CONNECTIONS

P2905.1 Soil and groundwater. The installation of water service pipe, water distribution pipe, fittings, valves, appurtenances and gaskets shall be prohibited in soil and groundwater that is contaminated with solvents, fuels, organic compounds or other detrimental materials that cause permeation, corrosion, degradation or structural failure of the water service or water distribution piping material.

P2905.1.1 Investigation required. Where detrimental conditions are suspected by or brought to the attention of the *building official*, a chemical analysis of the soil and groundwater conditions shall be required to ascertain the acceptability of the water service material for the specific installation.

P2905.1.2 Detrimental condition. When a detrimental condition exists, *approved* alternate materials or alternate routing shall be required.

P2905.2 Lead content. Pipe and fittings used in the water-supply system shall have a maximum of 8 percent lead.

P2905.3 Polyethylene plastic piping installation. Polyethylene pipe shall be cut square using a cutter designed for plastic pipe. Except where joined by heat fusion, pipe ends shall be chamfered to remove sharp edges. Pipe that has been kinked shall not be installed. For bends, the installed radius of pipe curvature shall be greater than 30 pipe diameters or the coil radius when bending with the coil. Coiled pipe shall not be bent beyond straight. Bends shall not be permitted within 10 pipe diameters of any fitting or valve. Joints between polyethylene plastic pipe and fittings shall comply with Sections P2905.3.1 and P2905.3.2.

P2905.3.1 Heat-fusion joints. Joint surfaces shall be clean and free from moisture. Joint surfaces shall be heated to melting temperature and joined. The joint shall be undisturbed until cool. Joints shall be made in accordance with ASTM D 2657.

P2905.3.2 Mechanical joints. Mechanical joints shall be installed in accordance with the manufacturer's installation instructions.

P2905.4 Water service pipe. Water service pipe shall conform to NSF 61 and shall conform to one of the standards listed in Table P2905.4. Water service pipe or tubing, installed underground and outside of the structure, shall have a minimum working pressure rating of 160 pounds per square inch at 73°F (1103 kPa at 23°C). Where the water pressure exceeds 160 pounds per square inch (1103 kPa), piping material shall have a rated working pressure equal to or greater than the highest available pressure. Water service piping materials not third-party certified for water distribution shall terminate at or before the full open valve located at the entrance to the structure. Ductile iron water service piping shall be cement mortar lined in accordance with AWWA C104.

P2905.4.1 Dual check-valve-type backflow preventer. Where a dual check-valve backflow preventer is installed on the water supply system, it shall comply with ASSE 1024 or CSA B64.6.

P2905.4.2 Water service installation. Trenching, pipe installation and backfilling shall be in accordance with Section P2604. Water-service pipe is permitted to be located in the same trench with a *building sewer* provided such sewer is constructed of materials listed for underground use within a building in Section P3002.1. If the *building sewer* is not constructed of materials listed in Section P3002.1, the water-service pipe shall be separated from the *building sewer* by a minimum of 5 feet (1524 mm), measured horizontally, of undisturbed or compacted earth or placed on a solid ledge at least 12 inches (305 mm) above and to one side of the highest point in the sewer line.

Exception: The required separation distance shall not apply where a water service pipe crosses a sewer pipe, provided that the water service pipe is sleeved to at least 5 feet (1524 mm), horizontally from the sewer pipe centerline, on both sides of the crossing with pipe materials listed in Tables P2905.4, P3002.1(1), P3002.1(2) or P3002.2.

P2905.5 Water-distribution pipe. Water-distribution piping within *dwelling units* shall conform to NSF 61 and shall conform to one of the standards listed in Table P2905.5. All hot-water-distribution pipe and tubing shall have a minimum pressure rating of 100 psi at 180°F (689 kPa at 82°C).

P2905.6 Fittings. Pipe fittings shall be *approved* for installation with the piping material installed and shall comply with the applicable standards listed in Table P2905.6. All pipe fittings used in water supply systems shall also comply with NSF 61.

P2905.7 Flexible water connectors. Flexible water connectors, exposed to continuous pressure, shall conform to ASME A112.18.6. Access shall be provided to all flexible water connectors.

P2905.8 Joint and connection tightness. Joints and connections in the plumbing system shall be gas tight and water tight for the intended use or required test pressure.

P2905.9 Plastic pipe joints. Joints in plastic piping shall be made with *approved* fittings by solvent cementing, heat fusion, corrosion-resistant metal clamps with insert fittings or compression connections. Flared joints for polyethylene pipe are permitted in accordance with Section P2905.3.

P2905.9.1 Solvent cementing. Solvent-cemented joints shall comply with Sections P2905.9.1.1 through P2905.9.1.3.

P2905.9.1.1 ABS plastic pipe. Solvent cement for ABS plastic pipe conforming to ASTM D 2235 shall be applied to all joint surfaces.

P2905.9.1.2 CPVC plastic pipe. Joint surfaces shall be clean and free from moisture and an *approved* primer shall be applied. Solvent cement for CPVC plastic pipe, orange in color and conforming to ASTM F 493, shall be applied to all joint surfaces. The parts shall be joined while the cement is wet and in accordance with ASTM D

2846 or ASTM F 493. Solvent-cement joints shall be permitted above or below ground.

Exception: A primer is not required where all of the following conditions apply:

1. The solvent cement used is third-party certified as conforming to ASTM F 493.

2. The solvent cement used is yellow in color.

3. The solvent cement is used only for joining $1/_2$-inch (13 mm) through 2-inch (51 mm) diameter CPVC pipe and fittings.

4. The CPVC pipe and fittings are manufactured in accordance with ASTM D 2846.

P2905.9.1.3 PVC plastic pipe. A purple primer that conforms to ASTM F 656 shall be applied to PVC solvent cemented joints. Solvent cement for PVC plastic pipe conforming to ASTM D 2564 shall be applied to all joint surfaces.

P2905.9.1.4 Cross-linked polyethylene plastic (PEX). Joints between cross-linked polyethylene plastic tubing or fittings shall comply with Section P2905.9.1.4.1 or Section P2905.9.1.4.2.

P2905.9.1.4.1 Flared joints. Flared pipe ends shall be made by a tool designed for that operation.

P2905.9.1.4.2 Mechanical joints. Mechanical joints shall be installed in accordance with the manufacturer's instructions. Fittings for cross-linked polyethylene (PEX) plastic tubing shall comply with the applicable standards listed in Table P2905.6 and shall be installed in accordance with the manufacturer's installation instructions. PEX tubing shall be factory marked with the applicable standards for the fittings that the PEX manufacturer specifies for use with the tubing.

P2905.10 Polypropylene (PP) plastic. Joints between PP plastic pipe and fittings shall comply with Section P2905.10.1 or P2905.10.2.

P2905.10.1 Heat-fusion joints. Heat fusion joints for polypropylene pipe and tubing joints shall be installed with socket-type heat-fused polypropylene fittings, butt-fusion polypropylene fittings or electrofusion polypropylene fittings. Joint surfaces shall be clean and free from moisture. The joint shall be undisturbed until cool. Joints shall be made in accordance with ASTM F 2389.

P2905.10.2 Mechanical and compression sleeve joints. Mechanical and compression sleeve joints shall be installed in accordance with the manufacturer's installation instructions.

TABLE P2905.4
WATER SERVICE PIPE

MATERIAL	STANDARD
Acrylonitrile butadiene styrene (ABS) plastic pipe	ASTM D 1527; ASTM D 2282
Asbestos-cement pipe	ASTM C 296
Brass pipe	ASTM B 43
Chlorinated polyvinyl chloride (CPVC) plastic pipe	ASTM D 2846; ASTM F 441; ASTM F 442; CSA B137.6
Copper or copper-alloy pipe	ASTM B 42; ASTM B 302
Copper or copper-alloy tubing (Type K, WK, L, WL, M or WM)	ASTM B 75; ASTM B 88; ASTM B 251; ASTM B 447
Cross-linked polyethylene/aluminum/cross-linked polyethylene (PEX-AL-PEX) pipe	ASTM F 1281; ASTM F 2262; CSA B137.10M
Cross-linked polyethylene/aluminum/high-density polyethylene (PEX-AL-HDPE)	ASTM F 1986
Cross-linked polyethylene (PEX) plastic tubing	ASTM F 876; ASTM F 877; CSA B137.5
Ductile iron water pipe	AWWA C151; AWWA C115
Galvanized steel pipe	ASTM A 53
Polyethylene/aluminum/polyethylene (PE-AL-PE) pipe	ASTM F 1282; CSA CAN/CSA-B137.9M
Polyethylene (PE) plastic pipe	ASTM D 2104; ASTM D 2239; CSA-B137.1
Polyethylene (PE) plastic tubing	ASTM D 2737; CSA B137.1
Polypropylene (PP) plastic pipe or tubing	ASTM F 2389; CSA B137.11
Polyvinyl chloride (PVC) plastic pipe	ASTM D 1785; ASTM D 2241; ASTM D 2672; CSA B137.3
Stainless steel (Type 304/304L) pipe	ASTM A 312; ASTM A 778
Stainless steel (Type 316/316L) pipe	ASTM A 312; ASTM A 778

TABLE P2905.5
WATER DISTRIBUTION PIPE

MATERIAL	STANDARD
Brass pipe	ASTM B 43
Chlorinated polyvinyl chloride (CPVC) plastic pipe and tubing	ASTM D 2846; ASTM F 441; ASTM F 442; CSA B137.6
Copper or copper-alloy pipe	ASTM B 42; ASTM B 302
Copper or copper-alloy tubing (Type K, WK, L, WL, M or WM)	ASTM B 75; ASTM B 88; ASTM B 251; ASTM B 447
Cross-linked polyethylene (PEX) plastic tubing	ASTM F 876; ASTM F 877; CSA B137.5
Cross-linked polyethylene/aluminum/cross-linked polyethylene (PEX-AL-PEX) pipe	ASTM F 1281; ASTM F 2262; CSA B137.10M
Cross-linked polyethylene/aluminum/high-density polyethylene (PEX-AL-HDPE)	ASTM F 1986
Galvanized steel pipe	ASTM A 53
Polyethylene/aluminum/polyethylene (PE-AL-PE) composite pipe	ASTM F 1282
Polypropylene (PP) plastic pipe or tubing	ASTM F 2389; CSA B137.11
Stainless steel (Type 304/304L) pipe	ASTM A 312; ASTM A 778

TABLE P2905.6
PIPE FITTINGS

MATERIAL	STANDARD
Acrylonitrile butadiene styrene (ABS) plastic	ASTM D 2468
Brass	ASTM F1974
Cast-iron	ASME B16.4; ASME B16.12
Chlorinated polyvinyl chloride (CPVC) plastic	ASSE 1061; ASTM D 2846; ASTM F 437; ASTM F 438; ASTM F 439; CSA B137.6
Copper or copper alloy	ASSE 1061; ASME B16.15; ASME B16.18; ASME B16.22; ASME B16.23; ASME B16.26; ASME B16.29
Cross-linked polyethylene/aluminum/high-density polyethylene (PEX-AL-HDPE)	ASTM F 1986
Fittings for cross-linked polyethylene (PEX) plastic tubing	ASSE 1061; ASTM F 877; ASTM F 1807; ASTM F 1960; ASTM F 2080; ASTM F 2098; ASTM F 2159; ASTM F 2434; CSA B137.5
Gray iron and ductile iron	AWWA C110; AWWA C153
Malleable iron	ASME B16.3
Insert fittings for Polyethylene/aluminum/polyethylene (PE-AL-PE) and cross-linked polyethylene/aluminum/polyethylene (PEX-AL-PEX)	ASTM F 1974; ASTM F 1281; ASTM F 1282; CSA B137.9; CSA B137.10
Polyethylene (PE) plastic	ASTM D 2609; CSA B137.1
Polypropylene (PP) plastic pipe or tubing	ASTM F 2389; CSA B137.11
Polyvinyl chloride (PVC) plastic	ASTM D 2464; ASTM D 2466; ASTM D 2467; CSA B137.2; CSA B137.3
Stainless steel (Type 304/304L) pipe	ASTM A 312; ASTM A 778
Stainless steel (Type 316/316L) pipe	ASTM A 312; ASTM A 778
Steel	ASME B16.9; ASME B16.11; ASME B16.28

P2905.11 Cross-linked polyethylene/aluminum/cross-linked polyethylene. Joints between polyethylene/aluminum/polyethylene (PE-AL-PE) and cross-linked polyethylene/aluminum/cross-linked polyethylene (PEX-AL-PEX) pipe and fittings shall comply with Section P2905.11.1.

P2905.11.1 Mechanical joints. Mechanical joints shall be installed in accordance with the manufacturer's instructions. Fittings for PE-AL-PE and PEX-AL-PEX as described in ASTM F 1974, ASTM F 1281, ASTM F 1282, CSA B137.9 and CSA B137.10 shall be installed in accordance with the manufacturer's instructions.

P2905.12 Stainless steel. Joints between stainless steel pipe and fittings shall comply with Sections P2905.12.1 and P2905.12.2.

P2905.12.1 Mechanical joints. Mechanical joints shall be installed in accordance with the manufacturer's instructions.

P2905.12.2 Welded joints. Joint surfaces shall be cleaned. The joint shall be welded autogenously or with an *approved* filler metal in accordance with ASTM A 312.

P2905.13 Threaded pipe joints. Threaded joints shall conform to American National Taper Pipe Thread specifications. Pipe ends shall be deburred and chips removed. Pipe joint compound shall be used only on male threads.

P2905.14 Soldered joints. Soldered joints in tubing shall be made with fittings *approved* for water piping and shall conform to ASTM B 828. Surfaces to be soldered shall be cleaned bright. The joints shall be properly fluxed and made with *approved* solder. Solders and fluxes used in potable water-supply systems shall have a maximum of 0.2 percent lead. Fluxes shall conform to ASTM B 813.

P2905.15 Flared joints. Flared joints in water tubing shall be made with *approved* fittings. The tubing shall be reamed and then expanded with a flaring tool.

P2905.16 Above-ground joints. Joints within the building between copper pipe or CPVC tubing, in any combination with compatible outside diameters, are permitted to be made with the use of *approved* push-in mechanical fittings of a pressure-lock design.

P2905.17 Joints between different materials. Joints between different piping materials shall be made in accordance with Sections P2905.17.1, P2905.17.2 and P2905.17.3 or with a mechanical joint of the compression or mechanical sealing type having an elastomeric seal conforming to ASTM D 1869 or ASTM F 477. Joints shall be installed in accordance with the manufacturer's instructions.

P2905.17.1 Copper or copper-alloy tubing to galvanized steel pipe. Joints between copper or copper-alloy tubing and galvanized steel pipe shall be made with a brass fitting or dielectric fitting. The copper tubing shall be joined to the fitting in an *approved* manner, and the fitting shall be screwed to the threaded pipe.

P2904.17.2 Plastic pipe or tubing to other piping material. Joints between different types of plastic pipe or between plastic pipe and other piping material shall be made with an approved adapter fitting.

P2905.17.3 Stainless steel. Joints between stainless steel and different piping materials shall be made with a mechanical joint of the compression or mechanical-sealing type or a dielectric fitting.

P2905.18 Press joints. Press-type mechanical joints in copper tubing shall be made in accordance with the manufacturer's instructions using *approved* tools which affix the copper fitting with integral O-ring to the tubing.

SECTION P2906
CHANGES IN DIRECTION

P2906.1 Bends. Changes in direction in copper tubing are permitted to be made with bends having a radius of not less than four diameters of the tube, providing such bends are made by use of forming equipment that does not deform or create loss in cross-sectional area of the tube.

SECTION P2907
SUPPORT

P2907.1 General. Pipe and tubing support shall conform to Section P2605.

SECTION P2908
DRINKING WATER TREATMENT UNITS

P2908.1 Design. Drinking water treatment units shall meet the requirements of NSF 42, NSF 44 or NSF 53.

P2908.2 Reverse osmosis drinking water treatment units. Point-of-use reverse osmosis drinking water treatment units, designed for residential use, shall meet the requirements of NSF 58. Waste or discharge from reverse osmosis drinking water treatment units shall enter the drainage system through an air gap or an air gap device that meets the requirements of NSF 58.

P2908.3 Connection tubing. The tubing to and from drinking water treatment units shall be of a size and material as recommended by the manufacturer. The tubing shall comply with NSF 14, NSF 42, NSF 44, NSF 53, NSF 58 or NSF 61.

CHAPTER 30

SANITARY DRAINAGE

SECTION P3001
GENERAL

P3001.1 Scope. The provisions of this chapter shall govern the materials, design, construction and installation of sanitary drainage systems. Plumbing materials shall conform to the requirements of this chapter. The drainage, waste and vent (DWV) system shall consist of all piping for conveying wastes from plumbing fixtures, appliances and appurtenances, including fixture traps; above-grade drainage piping; below-grade drains within the building (*building drain*); below- and above-grade venting systems; and piping to the public sewer or private septic system.

P3001.2 Protection from freezing. No portion of the above grade DWV system other than vent terminals shall be located outside of a building, in *attics* or crawl spaces, concealed in outside walls, or in any other place subjected to freezing temperatures unless adequate provision is made to protect them from freezing by insulation or heat or both, except in localities having a winter design temperature above 32°F (0°C) (ASHRAE 97.5 percent column, winter, see Chapter 3).

P3001.3 Flood-resistant installation. In areas prone to flooding as established by Table R301.2(1), drainage, waste and vent systems shall be located and installed to prevent infiltration of floodwaters into the systems and discharges from the systems into floodwaters.

SECTION P3002
MATERIALS

P3002.1 Piping within buildings. Drain, waste and vent (DWV) piping in buildings shall be as shown in Tables P3002.1(1) and P3002.1(2) except that galvanized wrought-iron or galvanized steel pipe shall not be used underground and shall be maintained not less than 6 inches (152 mm) above ground. Allowance shall be made for the thermal expansion and contraction of plastic piping.

P3002.2 Building sewer. *Building sewer* piping shall be as shown in Table P3002.2. Forced main sewer piping shall conform to one of the standards for ABS plastic pipe, copper or copper-alloy tubing, PVC plastic pipe or pressure-rated pipe listed in Table P3002.2.

P3002.3 Fittings. Pipe fittings shall be *approved* for installation with the piping material installed and shall comply with the applicable standards listed in Table P3002.3.

P3002.3.1 Drainage. Drainage fittings shall have a smooth interior waterway of the same diameter as the piping served. All fittings shall conform to the type of pipe used. Drainage fittings shall have no ledges, shoulders or reductions which can retard or obstruct drainage flow in the piping. Threaded drainage pipe fittings shall be of the recessed drainage type, black or galvanized. Drainage fittings shall be designed to maintain one-fourth unit vertical in 12 units horizontal (2-percent slope) grade.

P3002.4 Other materials. Sheet lead, lead bends, lead traps and sheet copper shall comply with Sections P3002.4.1 through P3002.4.3.

P3002.4.1 Sheet lead. Sheet lead for the following uses shall weigh not less than indicated below:

1. Flashing of vent terminals, 3 psf (15 kg/m²).
2. Prefabricated flashing for vent pipes, 2¹/₂ psf (12 kg/m²).

P3002.4.2 Lead bends and traps. Lead bends and lead traps shall not be less than ¹/₈-inch (3 mm) wall thickness.

P3002.4.3 Sheet copper. Sheet copper for the following uses shall weigh not less than indicated below:

1. General use, 12 ounces per square feet (4 kg/m²).
2. Flashing for vent pipes, 8 ounces per square feet (2.5 kg/m²).

SECTION P3003
JOINTS AND CONNECTIONS

P3003.1 Tightness. Joints and connections in the DWV system shall be gas tight and water tight for the intended use or pressure required by test.

P3003.1.1 Threaded joints, general. Pipe and fitting threads shall be tapered.

P3003.2 Prohibited joints. Running threads and bands shall not be used in the drainage system. Drainage and vent piping shall not be drilled, tapped, burned or welded.

The following types of joints and connections shall be prohibited:

1. Cement or concrete.
2. Mastic or hot-pour bituminous joints.
3. Joints made with fittings not *approved* for the specific installation.
4. Joints between different diameter pipes made with elastomeric rolling O-rings.
5. Solvent-cement joints between different types of plastic pipe.
6. Saddle-type fittings.

P3003.3 ABS plastic. Joints between ABS plastic pipe or fittings shall comply with Sections P3003.3.1 through P3003.3.3.

P3003.3.1 Mechanical joints. Mechanical joints on drainage pipes shall be made with an elastomeric seal conforming to ASTM C 1173, ASTM D 3212 or CSA B602. Mechanical joints shall be installed only in underground systems unless otherwise *approved*. Joints shall be installed in accordance with the manufacturer's installation instructions.

TABLE P3002.1(1)
ABOVE-GROUND DRAINAGE AND VENT PIPE

PIPE	STANDARD
Acrylonitrile butadiene styrene (ABS) plastic pipe in IPS diameters, including schedule 40, DR 22 (PS 200) and DR 24 (PS 140); with a solid, cellular core or composite wall	ASTM D 2661; ASTM F 628; ASTM F 1488; CSA B181.1
Brass pipe	ASTM B 43
Cast-iron pipe	ASTM A 74; CISPI 301; ASTM A 888
Copper or copper-alloy pipe	ASTM B 42; ASTM B 302
Copper or copper-alloy tubing (Type K, L, M or DWV)	ASTM B 75; ASTM B 88; ASTM B 251; ASTM B 306
Galvanized steel pipe	ASTM A 53
Polyolefin pipe	CSA B181.3
Polyvinyl chloride (PVC) plastic pipe in IPS diameters, including schedule 40, DR 22 (PS 200) and DR 24 (PS 140); with a solid, cellular core or composite wall	ASTM D 2665; ASTM F 891; CSA B181.2; ASTM F 1488
Polyvinyl chloride (PVC) plastic pipe with a 3.25 inch O.D. and a solid, cellular core or composite wall	ASTM D 2949, ASTM F 1488
Stainless steel drainage systems, Types 304 and 316L	ASME A 112.3.1

For SI: 1 inch = 25.4 mm.

TABLE P3002.1(2)
UNDERGROUND BUILDING DRAINAGE AND VENT PIPE

PIPE	STANDARD
Acrylonitrile butadiene styrene (ABS) plastic pipe in IPS diameters, including schedule 40, DR 22 (PS 200) and DR 24 (PS 140); with a solid, cellular core or composite wall	ASTM D 2661; ASTM F 628; ASTM F 1488; CSA B181.1
Asbestos-cement pipe	ASTM C 428
Cast-iron pipe	ASTM A 74; CISPI 301; ASTM A 888
Copper or copper alloy tubing (Type K, L, M or DWV)	ASTM B 75; ASTM B 88; ASTM B 251; ASTM B 306
Polyolefin pipe	ASTM F 1412; CSA B181.3
Polyvinyl chloride (PVC) plastic pipe in IPS diameters, including schedule 40, DR 22 (PS 200) and DR 24 (PS 140); with a solid, cellular core or composite wall	ASTM D 2665; ASTM F 891; ASTM F 1488; CSA B181.2
Polyvinyl chloride (PVC) plastic pipe with a 3.25 inch O.D. and a solid, cellular core or composite wall	ASTM D 2949; ASTM F 1488
Stainless steel drainage systems, Type 316L	ASME A 112.3.1

For SI: 1 inch = 25.4 mm.

P3003.3.2 Solvent cementing. Joint surfaces shall be clean and free from moisture. Solvent cement that conforms to ASTM D 2235 or CSA B181.1 shall be applied to all joint surfaces. The joint shall be made while the cement is wet. Joints shall be made in accordance with ASTM D 2235, ASTM D 2661, ASTM F 628 or CSA B181.1. Solvent-cement joints shall be permitted above or below ground.

P3003.3.3 Threaded joints. Threads shall conform to ASME B1.20.1. Schedule 80 or heavier pipe shall be permitted to be threaded with dies specifically designed for plastic pipe. *Approved* thread lubricant or tape shall be applied on the male threads only.

P3003.4 Asbestos-cement. Joints between asbestos-cement pipe or fittings shall be made with a sleeve coupling of the same composition as the pipe, sealed with an elastomeric ring conforming to ASTM D 1869.

P3003.5 Brass. Joints between brass pipe or fittings shall comply with Sections P3003.5.1 through P3003.5.3.

P3003.5.1 Brazed joints. All joint surfaces shall be cleaned. An *approved* flux shall be applied where required. The joint shall be brazed with a filler metal conforming to AWS A5.8.

P3003.5.2 Mechanical joints. Mechanical joints shall be installed in accordance with the manufacturer's installation instructions.

TABLE P3002.2
BUILDING SEWER PIPE

MATERIAL	STANDARD
Acrylonitrile butadiene styrene (ABS) plastic pipe in IPS diameters, including schedule 40, DR 22 (PS 200) and DR 24 (PS 140); with a solid, cellular core or composite wall	ASTM D 2661; ASTM F 628; ASTM F 1488
Asbestos-cement pipe	ASTM C 428
Cast-iron pipe	ASTM A 74; ASTM A 888; CISPI 301
Acrylonitrile butadiene styrene (ABS) plastic pipe in sewer and drain diameters, including SDR 42 (PS 20), PS35, SDR 35 (PS 45), PS50, PS100, PS140, SDR 23.5 (PS 150) and PS200; with a solid, cellular core or composite wall	ASTM F 1488; ASTM D 2751
Polyvinyl chloride (PVC) plastic pipe in sewer and drain diameters, including PS 25, SDR 41 (PS 28), PS 35, SDR 35 (PS 46), PS 50, PS 100, SDR 26 (PS 115), PS140 and PS 200; with a solid, cellular core or composite wall	ASTM F 891; ASTM F 1488; ASTM D 3034; CSA B182.2; CSA B182.4
Concrete pipe	ASTM C 14; ASTM C 76; CSA A257.1M; CSA A257.2M
Copper or copper-alloy tubing (Type K or L)	ASTM B 75; ASTM B 88; ASTM B 251
Polyethylene (PE) plastic pipe (SDR-PR)	ASTM F 714
Polyolefin pipe	ASTM F 1412; CSA B181.3
Polyvinyl chloride (PVC) plastic pipe in IPS diameters, including schedule 40, DR 22 (PS 200) and DR 24 (PS 140); with solid, cellular core or composite wall	ASTM D 2665; ASTM D 2949; ASTM D 3034; ASTM F 1412; CSA B182.2; CSA B182.4
Polyvinyl chloride (PVC) plastic pipe with a 3.25 inch O.D. and a solid, cellular core or composite wall	ASTM D 2949, ASTM F 1488
Stainless steel drainage systems, Types 304 and 316L	ASME A 112.3.1
Vitrified clay pipe	ASTM C 425; ASTM C 700

For SI: 1 inch = 25.4 mm.

TABLE P3002.3
PIPE FITTINGS

PIPE MATERIAL	FITTING STANDARD
Acrylonitrile butadiene styrene (ABS) plastic pipe in IPS diameters	ASTM D 2661; ASTM D 3311; ASTM F 628; CSA B181.1
Asbestos cement	ASTM C 428
Cast-iron	ASME B 16.4; ASME B 16.12; ASTM A 74; ASTM A 888; CISPI 301
Acrylonotrile butadiene styrene (ABS) plastic pipe in sewer and drain diameters	ASTM D 2751
Polyvinyl chloride (PVC) plastic pipe in sewer and drain diameters	ASTM D 3034
Copper or copper alloy	ASME B 16.15; ASME B 16.18; ASME B 16.22; ASME B 16.23; ASME B 16.26; ASME B 16.29
Gray iron and ductile iron	AWWA C 110
Polyolefin	ASTM F 1412; CSA B181.3
Polyvinyl chloride (PVC) plastic in IPS diameters	ASTM D 2665; ASTM D 3311; ASTM F 1866
Polyvinyl chloride (PVC) plastic pipe with a 3.25 inch O.D.	ASTM D 2949
PVC fabricated fittings	ASTM F 1866
Stainless steel drainage systems, Types 304 and 316L	ASME A 112.3.1
Vitrified clay	ASTM C 700

For SI: 1 inch = 25.4 mm.

P3003.5.3 Threaded joints. Threads shall conform to ASME B1.20.1. Pipe-joint compound or tape shall be applied on the male threads only.

P3003.6 Cast iron. Joints between cast-iron pipe or fittings shall comply with Sections P3003.6.1 through P3003.6.3.

P3003.6.1 Caulked joints. Joints for hub and spigot pipe shall be firmly packed with oakum or hemp. Molten lead shall be poured in one operation to a depth of not less than 1 inch (25 mm). The lead shall not recede more than $^1/_8$ inch (3 mm) below the rim of the hub and shall be caulked tight. Paint, varnish or other coatings shall not be permitted on the jointing material until after the joint has been tested and *approved*. Lead shall be run in one pouring and shall be caulked tight. Acid-resistant rope and acidproof cement shall be permitted.

P3003.6.2 Compression gasket joints. Compression gaskets for hub and spigot pipe and fittings shall conform to ASTM C 564. Gaskets shall be compressed when the pipe is fully inserted.

P3003.6.3 Mechanical joint coupling. Mechanical joint couplings for hubless pipe and fittings shall comply with CISPI 310 or ASTM C 1277. The elastomeric sealing sleeve shall conform to ASTM C 564 or CSA B602 and shall have a center stop. Mechanical joint couplings shall be installed in accordance with the manufacturer's installation instructions.

P3003.7 Concrete joints. Joints between concrete pipe and fittings shall be made with an elastomeric seal conforming to ASTM C 443, ASTM C 1173, CSA A257.3M or CSA B602.

P3003.8 Coextruded composite ABS pipe. Joints between coextruded composite pipe with an ABS outer layer or ABS fittings shall comply with Sections P3003.8.1 and P3003.8.2.

P3003.8.1 Mechanical joints. Mechanical joints on drainage pipe shall be made with an elastomeric seal conforming to ASTM C 1173, ASTM D 3212 or CSA B602. Mechanical joints shall not be installed in above-ground systems, unless otherwise *approved*. Joints shall be installed in accordance with the manufacturer's installation instructions.

P3003.8.2 Solvent cementing. Joint surfaces shall be clean and free from moisture. Solvent cement that conforms to ASTM D 2235 or CSA B181.1 shall be applied to all joint surfaces. The joint shall be made while the cement is wet. Joints shall be made in accordance with ASTM D 2235, ASTM D 2661, ASTM F 628 or CSA B181.1. Solvent-cement joints shall be permitted above or below ground.

P3003.9 Coextruded composite PVC pipe. Joints between coextruded composite pipe with a PVC outer layer or PVC fittings shall comply with Sections P3003.9.1 and P3003.9.2.

P3003.9.1 Mechanical joints. Mechanical joints on drainage pipe shall be made with an elastomeric seal conforming to ASTM D 3212. Mechanical joints shall not be installed in above-ground systems, unless otherwise *approved*. Joints shall be installed in accordance with the manufacturer's installation instructions.

P3003.9.2 Solvent cementing. Joint surfaces shall be clean and free from moisture. A purple primer that conforms to ASTM F 656 shall be applied. Solvent cement not purple in color and conforming to ASTM D 2564, CSA B137.3 or CSA B181.2 shall be applied to all joint surfaces. The joint shall be made while the cement is wet, and shall be in accordance with ASTM D 2855. Solvent-cement joints shall be permitted above or below ground.

P3003.10 Copper pipe. Joints between copper or copper-alloy pipe or fittings shall comply with Sections P3003.10.1 through P3003.10.4.

P3003.10.1 Brazed joints. All joint surfaces shall be cleaned. An *approved* flux shall be applied where required. The joint shall be brazed with a filler metal conforming to AWS A5.8.

P3003.10.2 Mechanical joints. Mechanical joints shall be installed in accordance with the manufacturer's installation instructions.

P3003.10.3 Soldered joints. Solder joints shall be made in accordance with the methods of ASTM B 828. All cut tube ends shall be reamed to the full inside diameter of the tube end. All joint surfaces shall be cleaned. A flux conforming to ASTM B 813 shall be applied. The joint shall be soldered with a solder conforming to ASTM B 32.

P3003.10.4 Threaded joints. Threads shall conform to ASME B1.20.1. Pipe-joint compound or tape shall be applied on the male threads only.

P3003.11 Copper tubing. Joints between copper or copper-alloy tubing or fittings shall comply with Sections P3003.11.1 through P3003.11.3.

P3003.11.1 Brazed joints. All joint surfaces shall be cleaned. An *approved* flux shall be applied where required. The joint shall be brazed with a filler metal conforming to AWS A5.8.

P3003.11.2 Mechanical joints. Mechanical joints shall be installed in accordance with the manufacturer's installation instructions.

P3003.11.3 Soldered joints. Solder joints shall be made in accordance with the methods of ASTM B 828. Cut tube ends shall be reamed to the full inside diameter of the tube end. All joint surfaces shall be cleaned. A flux conforming to ASTM B 813 shall be applied. The joint shall be soldered with a solder conforming to ASTM B 32.

P3003.12 Steel. Joints between galvanized steel pipe or fittings shall comply with Sections P3003.12.1 and P3003.12.2.

P3003.12.1 Threaded joints. Threads shall conform to ASME B1.20.1. Pipe-joint compound or tape shall be applied on the male threads only.

P3003.12.2 Mechanical joints. Joints shall be made with an *approved* elastomeric seal. Mechanical joints shall be installed in accordance with the manufacturer's installation instructions.

P3003.13 Lead. Joints between lead pipe or fittings shall comply with Sections P3003.13.1 and P3003.13.2.

P3003.13.1 Burned. Burned joints shall be uniformly fused together into one continuous piece. The thickness of the joint shall be at least as thick as the lead being joined. The filler metal shall be of the same material as the pipe.

P3003.13.2 Wiped. Joints shall be fully wiped, with an exposed surface on each side of the joint not less than $^3/_4$ inch (19 mm). The joint shall be at least $^3/_8$ inch (9.5 mm) thick at the thickest point.

P3003.14 PVC plastic. Joints between PVC plastic pipe or fittings shall comply with Sections P3003.14.1 through P3003.14.3.

P3003.14.1 Mechanical joints. Mechanical joints on drainage pipe shall be made with an elastomeric seal conforming to ASTM C 1173, ASTM D 3212 or CSA B602. Mechanical joints shall not be installed in above-ground systems, unless otherwise *approved*. Joints shall be installed in accordance with the manufacturer's installation instructions.

P3003.14.2 Solvent cementing. Joint surfaces shall be clean and free from moisture. A purple primer that conforms to ASTM F 656 shall be applied. Solvent cement not purple in color and conforming to ASTM D 2564, CSA B137.3 or CSA B181.2 shall be applied to all joint surfaces. The joint shall be made while the cement is wet, and shall be in accordance with ASTM D 2855. Solvent-cement joints shall be permitted above or below ground.

P3003.14.3 Threaded joints. Threads shall conform to ASME B1.20.1. Schedule 80 or heavier pipe shall be permitted to be threaded with dies specifically designed for plastic pipe. *Approved* thread lubricant or tape shall be applied on the male threads only.

P3003.15 Vitrified clay. Joints between vitrified clay pipe or fittings shall be made with an elastomeric seal conforming to ASTM C 425, ASTM C 1173 or CSA B602.

P3003.16 Polyolefin plastic. Joints between polyolefin plastic pipe and fittings shall comply with Sections P3003.16.1 and P3003.16.2.

P3003.16.1 Heat-fusion joints. Heat-fusion joints for polyolefin pipe and tubing joints shall be installed with socket-type heat-fused polyolefin fittings or electrofusion polyolefin fittings. Joint surfaces shall be clean and free from moisture. The joint shall be undisturbed until cool. Joints shall be made in accordance with ASTM F 1412 or CSA B181.3.

P3003.16.2 Mechanical and compression sleeve joints. Mechanical and compression sleeve joints shall be installed in accordance with the manufacturer's installation instructions.

P3003.17 Polyethylene plastic pipe. Joints between polyethylene plastic pipe and fittings shall be underground and shall comply with Section P3003.17.1 or P3003.17.2.

P3003.17.1 Heat fusion joints. Joint surfaces shall be clean and free from moisture. All joint surfaces shall be cut, heated to melting temperature and joined using tools specifically designed for the operation. Joints shall be undisturbed until cool. Joints shall be made in accordance with ASTM D 2657 and the manufacturer's installation instructions.

P3003.17.2 Mechanical joints. Mechanical joints in drainage piping shall be made with an elastomeric seal conforming to ASTM C 1173, ASTM D 3212 or CSA B602. Mechanical joints shall be installed in accordance with the manufacturer's installation instructions.

P3003.18 Joints between different materials. Joints between different piping materials shall be made with a mechanical joint of the compression or mechanical-sealing type conforming to ASTM C 1173, ASTM C 1460 or ASTM C 1461. Connectors and adapters shall be *approved* for the application and such joints shall have an elastomeric seal conforming to ASTM C 425, ASTM C 443, ASTM C 564, ASTM C 1440, ASTM D 1869, ASTM F 477, CSA A257.3M or CSA B602, or as required in Sections P3003.18.1 through P3003.18.6. Joints between glass pipe and other types of materials shall be made with adapters having a TFE seal. Joints shall be installed in accordance with the manufacturer's installation instructions.

P3003.18.1 Copper or copper-alloy tubing to cast-iron hub pipe. Joints between copper or copper-alloy tubing and cast-iron hub pipe shall be made with a brass ferrule or compression joint. The copper or copper-alloy tubing shall be soldered to the ferrule in an *approved* manner, and the ferrule shall be joined to the cast-iron hub by a caulked joint or a mechanical compression joint.

P3003.18.2 Copper or copper-alloy tubing to galvanized steel pipe. Joints between copper or copper-alloy tubing and galvanized steel pipe shall be made with a brass converter fitting or dielectric fitting. The copper tubing shall be soldered to the fitting in an *approved* manner, and the fitting shall be screwed to the threaded pipe.

P3003.18.3 Cast-iron pipe to galvanized steel or brass pipe. Joints between cast-iron and galvanized steel or brass pipe shall be made by either caulked or threaded joints or with an *approved* adapter fitting.

P3003.18.4 Plastic pipe or tubing to other piping material. Joints between different types of plastic pipe or between plastic pipe and other piping material shall be made with an *approved* adapter fitting. Joints between plastic pipe and cast-iron hub pipe shall be made by a caulked joint or a mechanical compression joint.

P3003.18.5 Lead pipe to other piping material. Joints between lead pipe and other piping material shall be made by a wiped joint to a caulking ferrule, soldering nipple, or bushing or shall be made with an *approved* adapter fitting.

P3003.18.6 Stainless steel drainage systems to other materials. Joints between stainless steel drainage systems and other piping materials shall be made with *approved* mechanical couplings.

P3003.19 Joints between drainage piping and water closets. Joints between drainage piping and water closets or similar fixtures shall be made by means of a closet flange compatible with the drainage system material, securely fastened to a structurally firm base. The inside diameter of the drainage pipe shall not be used as a socket fitting for a four by three closet flange. The joint shall be bolted, with an *approved* gasket, flange to fixture connection complying with ASME A112.4.3 or setting compound between the fixture and the closet flange.

SECTION P3004
DETERMINING DRAINAGE FIXTURE UNITS

P3004.1 DWV system load. The load on DWV-system piping shall be computed in terms of drainage fixture unit (d.f.u.) values in accordance with Table P3004.1.

SECTION P3005
DRAINAGE SYSTEM

P3005.1 Drainage fittings and connections. Changes in direction in drainage piping shall be made by the appropriate use of sanitary tees, wyes, sweeps, bends or by a combination of these drainage fittings in accordance with Table P3005.1. Change in direction by combination fittings, heel or side inlets or increasers shall be installed in accordance with Table P3005.1 and Sections P3005.1.1 through P3005.1.4. based on the pattern of flow created by the fitting.

TABLE P3004.1
DRAINAGE FIXTURE UNIT (d.f.u.) VALUES FOR VARIOUS PLUMBING FIXTURES

TYPE OF FIXTURE OR GROUP OF FIXTURES	DRAINAGE FIXTURE UNIT VALUE (d.f.u.)[a]
Bar sink	1
Bathtub (with or without shower head and/or whirlpool attachments)	2
Bidet	1
Clothes washer standpipe	2
Dishwasher	2
Floor drain[b]	0
Kitchen sink	2
Lavatory	1
Laundry tub	2
Shower stall	2
Water closet (1.6 gallons per flush)	3
Water closet (greater than 1.6 gallons per flush)	4
Full-bath group with bathtub (with 1.6 gallon per flush water closet, and with or without shower head and/or whirlpool attachment on the bathtub or shower stall)	5
Full-bath group with bathtub (water closet greater than 1.6 gallon per flush, and with or without shower head and/or whirlpool attachment on the bathtub or shower stall)	6
Half-bath group (1.6 gallon per flush water closet plus lavatory)	4
Half-bath group (water closet greater than 1.6 gallon per flush plus lavatory)	5
Kitchen group (dishwasher and sink with or without garbage grinder)	2
Laundry group (clothes washer standpipe and laundry tub)	3

Multiple-bath groups[c]:
  1.5 baths
  2 baths
  2.5 baths
  3 baths
  3.5 baths
	7
	8
	9
	10
	11

For SI: 1 gallon = 3.785 L.

a. For a continuous or semicontinuous flow into a drainage system, such as from a pump or similar device, 1.5 fixture units shall be allowed per gpm of flow. For a fixture not listed, use the highest d.f.u. value for a similar listed fixture.

b. A floor drain itself adds no hydraulic load. However, where used as a receptor, the fixture unit value of the fixture discharging into the receptor shall be applicable.

c. Add 2 d.f.u. for each additional full bath.

TABLE P3005.1
FITTINGS FOR CHANGE IN DIRECTION

TYPE OF FITTING PATTERN	CHANGE IN DIRECTION		
	Horizontal to vertical[c]	Vertical to horizontal	Horizontal to horizontal
Sixteenth bend	X	X	X
Eighth bend	X	X	X
Sixth bend	X	X	X
Quarter bend	X	X[a]	X[a]
Short sweep	X	X[a,b]	X[a]
Long sweep	X	X	X
Sanitary tee	X[c]	—	—
Wye	X	X	X
Combination wye and eighth bend	X	X	X

For SI: 1 inch = 25.4 mm.

a. The fittings shall only be permitted for a 2-inch or smaller fixture drain.

b. Three inches and larger.

c. For a limitation on multiple connection fittings, see Section P3005.1.1.

P3005.1.1 Horizontal to vertical (multiple connection fittings). Double fittings such as double sanitary tees and tee-wyes or *approved* multiple connection fittings and back-to-back fixture arrangements that connect two or more branches at the same level shall be permitted as long as directly opposing connections are the same size and the discharge into directly opposing connections is from similar fixture types or fixture groups. Double sanitary tee patterns shall not receive the discharge of back-to-back water closets and fixtures or appliances with pumping action discharge.

> **Exception:** Back-to-back water closet connections to double sanitary tee patterns shall be permitted where the horizontal *developed length* between the outlet of the water closet and the connection to the double sanitary tee is 18 inches (457 mm) or greater.

P3005.1.2 Heel- or side-inlet quarter bends, drainage. Heel-inlet quarter bends shall be an acceptable means of connection, except where the quarter bends serves a water closet. A low-heel inlet shall not be used as a wet-vented connection. Side-inlet quarter bends shall be an acceptable means of connection for both drainage, wet venting and stack venting arrangements.

P3005.1.3 Heel- or side-inlet quarter bends, venting. Heel-inlet or side-inlet quarter bends, or any arrangement of pipe and fittings producing a similar effect, shall be acceptable as a dry vent where the inlet is placed in a vertical position. The inlet is permitted to be placed in a horizontal position only where the entire fitting is part of a dry vent arrangement.

P3005.1.4 Water closet connection between flange and pipe. One-quarter bends 3 inches (76 mm) in diameter shall be acceptable for water closet or similar connections, provided a 4-inch by 3-inch (102 mm by 76 mm) flange is installed to receive the closet fixture horn. Alternately, a 4-inch by 3-inch (102 mm by 76 mm) elbow shall be acceptable with a 4-inch (102 mm) flange.

P3005.1.5 Dead ends. Dead ends shall be prohibited except where necessary to extend a cleanout or as an *approved* part of a rough-in more than 2 feet (610 mm) in length.

P3005.1.6 Provisions for future fixtures. Where drainage has been roughed-in for future fixtures, the drainage unit values of the future fixtures shall be considered in determining the required drain sizes. Such future installations shall be terminated with an accessible permanent plug or cap fitting.

P3005.1.7 Change in size. The size of the drainage piping shall not be reduced in size in the direction of the flow. A 4-inch by 3-inch (102 mm by 76 mm) water closet connection shall not be considered as a reduction in size.

P3005.2 Drainage pipe cleanouts. Drainage pipe cleanouts shall comply with Sections P3005.2.1 through P3005.2.11.

Exception: These provisions shall not apply to pressurized *building drains* and *building sewers* that convey the discharge of automatic pumping equipment to a gravity drainage system.

P3005.2.1 Materials. Cleanouts shall be liquid and gas tight. Cleanout plugs shall be brass or plastic.

P3005.2.2 Spacing. Cleanouts shall be installed not more than 100 feet (30 480 mm) apart in horizontal drainage lines measured from the upstream entrance of the cleanout.

P3005.2.3 Underground drainage cleanouts. When installed in underground drains, cleanouts shall be extended vertically to or above finished grade either inside or outside the building.

P3005.2.4 Change of direction. Cleanouts shall be installed at each fitting with a change of direction more than 45 degrees (0.79 rad) in the *building sewer, building drain* and horizontal waste or soil lines. Where more than one change of direction occurs in a run of piping, only one cleanout shall be required in each 40 feet (12 192 mm) of *developed length* of the drainage piping.

P3005.2.5 Accessibility. Cleanouts shall be accessible. Minimum clearance in front of cleanouts shall be 18 inches (457 mm) on 3-inch (76 mm) and larger pipes, and 12 inches (305 mm) on smaller pipes. Concealed cleanouts shall be provided with access of sufficient size to permit removal of the cleanout plug and rodding of the system. Cleanout plugs shall not be concealed by permanent finishing material.

P3005.2.6 Base of stacks. A cleanout shall be provided at the base of each waste or soil stack.

P3005.2.7 Building drain and building sewer junction. There shall be a cleanout near the junction of the *building drain* and *building sewer*. This cleanout shall be either inside or outside the building wall, provided that it is brought up to finish grade or to the lowest floor level. An *approved* two-way cleanout shall be permitted to serve as the required cleanout for both the *building drain* and the *building sewer*. The cleanout at the junction of the *building drain* and *building sewer* shall not be required where a cleanout on a 3-inch (76 mm) or larger diameter soil stack is located within a *developed length* of 10 feet (3048 mm) of the *building drain* and *building sewer* junction.

P3005.2.8 Direction of flow. Cleanouts shall be installed so that the cleanout opens to allow cleaning in the direction of the flow of the drainage line.

P3005.2.9 Cleanout size. Cleanouts shall be the same nominal size as the pipe they serve up to 4 inches (102 mm). For pipes larger than 4 inches (102 mm) nominal size, the minimum size of the cleanout shall be 4 inches (102 mm).

Exceptions:

1. "P" trap connections with slip joints or ground joint connections, or stack cleanouts that are not more than one pipe diameter smaller than the drain served, shall be permitted.

2. Cast-iron cleanouts sized in accordance with the referenced standards in Table P3002.3, ASTM A 74 for hub and spigot fittings or ASTM A 888 or CISPI 301 for hubless fittings.

P3005.2.10 Cleanout equivalent. A fixture trap or a fixture with integral trap, readily removable without disturbing concealed piping shall be acceptable as a cleanout equivalent.

P3005.2.11 Connections to cleanouts prohibited. Cleanout openings shall not be used for the installation of new fixtures except where *approved* and an acceptable alternate cleanout is provided.

P3005.3 Horizontal drainage piping slope. Horizontal drainage piping shall be installed in uniform alignment at uniform slopes not less than $^1/_4$ unit vertical in 12 units horizontal (2-percent slope) for $2^1/_2$-inch (64 mm) diameter and less, and not less than $^1/_8$ unit vertical in 12 units horizontal (1-percent slope) for diameters of 3 inches (76 mm) or more.

P3005.4 Drain pipe sizing. Drain pipes shall be sized according to drainage fixture unit (d.f.u.) loads. The size of the drainage piping shall not be reduced in size in the direction of flow. The following general procedure is permitted to be used:

1. Draw an isometric layout or riser diagram denoting fixtures on the layout.

2. Assign d.f.u. values to each fixture group plus individual fixtures using Table P3004.1.

3. Starting with the top floor or most remote fixtures, work downstream toward the *building drain* accumulating d.f.u. values for fixture groups plus individual fixtures for each branch. Where multiple bath groups are being added, use the reduced d.f.u. values in Table P3004.1, which take into account probability factors of simultaneous use.

4. Size branches and stacks by equating the assigned d.f.u. values to pipe sizes shown in Table P3005.4.1.

5. Determine the pipe diameter and slope of the *building drain* and *building sewer* based on the accumulated d.f.u. values, using Table P3005.4.2.

P3005.4.1 Branch and stack sizing. Branches and stacks shall be sized in accordance with Table P3005.4.1. Below grade drain pipes shall be not less than $1^1/_2$ inches (38 mm)

in diameter. Drain stacks shall be not smaller than the largest horizontal branch connected.

Exceptions:

1. A 4-inch by 3-inch (102 mm by 76 mm) closet bend or flange.

2. A 4-inch (102 mm) closet bend connected to a 3-inch (76 mm) stack tee shall not be prohibited.

TABLE P3005.4.1
MAXIMUM FIXTURE UNITS ALLOWED
TO BE CONNECTED TO BRANCHES AND STACKS

NOMINAL PIPE SIZE (inches)	ANY HORIZONTAL FIXTURE BRANCH	ANY ONE VERTICAL STACK OR DRAIN
$1^1/_4$ [a]	—	—
$1^1/_2$ [b]	3	4
2 [b]	6	10
$2^1/_2$ [b]	12	20
3	20	48
4	160	240

For SI: 1 inch = 25.4 mm.

a. $1^1/_4$-inch pipe size limited to a single–fixture drain or trap arm. See Table P3201.7.

b. No water closets.

P3005.4.2 Building drain and sewer size and slope. Pipe sizes and slope shall be determined from Table P3005.4.2 on the basis of drainage load in fixture units (d.f.u.) computed from Table P3004.1.

TABLE P3005.4.2
MAXIMUM NUMBER OF FIXTURE UNITS ALLOWED
TO BE CONNECTED TO THE BUILDING DRAIN,
BUILDING DRAIN BRANCHES OR THE BUILDING SEWER

DIAMETER OF PIPE (inches)	SLOPE PER FOOT		
	$^1/_8$ inch	$^1/_4$ inch	$^1/_2$ inch
$1^1/_2$ [a,b]	—	Note a	Note a
2 [b]	—	21	27
$2^1/_2$ [b]	—	24	31
3	36	42	50
4	180	216	250

For SI: 1 inch = 25.4 mm, 1 foot = 304.8 mm.

a. $1^1/_2$-inch pipe size limited to a building drain branch serving not more than two waste fixtures, or not more than one waste fixture if serving a pumped discharge fixture or garbage grinder discharge.

b. No water closets.

P3005.5 Connections to offsets and bases of stacks. Horizontal branches shall connect to the bases of stacks at a point located not less than 10 times the diameter of the drainage stack downstream from the stack. Horizontal branches shall connect to horizontal stack offsets at a point located not less than 10 times the diameter of the drainage stack downstream from the upper stack.

SECTION P3006
SIZING OF DRAIN PIPE OFFSETS

P3006.1 Vertical offsets. An offset in a vertical drain, with a change of direction of 45 degrees (0.79 rad) or less from the vertical, shall be sized as a straight vertical drain.

P3006.2 Horizontal offsets above the lowest branch. A stack with an offset of more than 45 degrees (0.79 rad) from the vertical shall be sized as follows:

1. The portion of the stack above the offset shall be sized as for a regular stack based on the total number of fixture units above the offset.

2. The offset shall be sized as for a *building drain* in accordance with Table P3005.4.2.

3. The portion of the stack below the offset shall be sized as for the offset or based on the total number of fixture units on the entire stack, whichever is larger.

P3006.3 Horizontal offsets below the lowest branch. In soil or waste stacks below the lowest horizontal branch, there shall be no change in diameter required if the offset is made at an angle not greater than 45 degrees (0.79 rad) from the vertical. If an offset greater than 45 degrees (0.79 rad) from the vertical is made, the offset and stack below it shall be sized as a *building drain* (see Table P3005.4.2).

SECTION P3007
SUMPS AND EJECTORS

P3007.1 Building subdrains. Building subdrains that cannot be discharged to the sewer by gravity flow shall be discharged into a tightly covered and vented sump from which the liquid shall be lifted and discharged into the building gravity drainage system by automatic pumping equipment or other *approved* method. In other than existing structures, the sump shall not receive drainage from any piping within the building capable of being discharged by gravity to the *building sewer*.

P3007.2 Valves required. A check valve and a full open valve located on the discharge side of the check valve shall be installed in the pump or ejector discharge piping between the pump or ejector and the gravity drainage system. Access shall be provided to such valves. Such valves shall be located above the sump cover required by Section P3007.3.2 or, where the discharge pipe from the ejector is below grade, the valves shall be accessibly located outside the sump below grade in an access pit with a removable access cover.

P3007.3 Sump design. The sump pump, pit and discharge piping shall conform to the requirements of Sections P3007.3.1 through P3007.3.5.

P3007.3.1 Sump pump. The sump pump capacity and head shall be appropriate to anticipated use requirements.

P3007.3.2 Sump pit. The sump pit shall be not less than 18 inches (457 mm) in diameter and 24 inches (610 mm) deep, unless otherwise *approved*. The pit shall be accessible and located so that all drainage flows into the pit by gravity. The sump pit shall be constructed of tile, concrete, steel, plastic or other *approved* materials. The pit bottom shall be solid and provide permanent support for the pump. The sump pit shall be fitted with a gastight removable cover adequate to support anticipated loads in the area of use. The sump pit shall be vented in accordance with Chapter 31.

P3007.3.3 Discharge piping. Discharge piping shall meet the requirements of Section P3007.2.

P3007.3.4 Maximum effluent level. The effluent level control shall be adjusted and maintained to at all times prevent the effluent in the sump from rising to within 2 inches (51 mm) of the invert of the gravity drain inlet into the sump.

P3007.3.5 Ejector connection to the drainage system. Pumps connected to the drainage system shall connect to the *building sewer* or shall connect to a wye fitting in the *building drain* a minimum of 10 feet (3048 mm) from the base of any soil stack, waste stack or *fixture drain*. Where the discharge line connects into horizontal drainage piping, the connection shall be made through a wye fitting into the top of the drainage piping.

P3007.4 Sewage pumps and sewage ejectors. A sewage pump or sewage ejector shall automatically discharge the contents of the sump to the building drainage system.

P3007.5 Macerating toilet systems. Macerating toilet systems shall comply with CSA B45.9 or ASME A112.3.4 and shall be installed in accordance with the manufacturer's installation instructions.

P3007.6 Capacity. A sewage pump or sewage ejector shall have the capacity and head for the application requirements. Pumps or ejectors that receive the discharge of water closets shall be capable of handling spherical solids with a diameter of up to and including 2 inches (51 mm). Other pumps or ejectors shall be capable of handling spherical solids with a diameter of up to and including 1 inch (25.4 mm). The minimum capacity of a pump or ejector based on the diameter of the discharge pipe shall be in accordance with Table 3007.6.

Exceptions:

1. Grinder pumps or grinder ejectors that receive the discharge of water closets shall have a minimum discharge opening of $1^1/_4$ inches (32 mm).

2. Macerating toilet assemblies that serve single water closets shall have a minimum discharge opening of $^3/_4$ inch (19 mm).

TABLE 3007.6
MINIMUM CAPACITY OF SEWAGE PUMP OR SEWAGE EJECTOR

DIAMETER OF THE DISCHARGE PIPE (inches)	CAPACITY OF PUMP OR EJECTOR (gpm)
2	21
$2^1/_2$	30
3	46

For SI: 1 inch = 25.4 mm, 1 gallon per minute = 3.785 L/m.

SECTION P3008
BACKWATER VALVES

P3008.1 Sewage backflow. Where the flood level rims of plumbing fixtures are below the elevation of the manhole cover of the next upstream manhole in the public sewer, the fixtures shall be protected by a backwater valve installed in the *building drain*, branch of the *building drain* or horizontal branch serving such fixtures. Plumbing fixtures having flood level rims above the elevation of the manhole cover of the next upstream manhole in the public sewer shall not discharge through a backwater valve.

P3008.2 Material. All bearing parts of backwater valves shall be of corrosion-resistant material. Backwater valves shall comply with ASME A112.14.1, CSA B181.1 or CSA B181.2.

P3008.3 Seal. Backwater valves shall be constructed to provide a mechanical seal against backflow.

P3008.4 Diameter. Backwater valves, when fully opened, shall have a capacity not less than that of the pipes in which they are installed.

P3008.5 Location. Backwater valves shall be installed so that access is provided to the working parts for service and repair.

CHAPTER 31

VENTS

SECTION P3101
VENT SYSTEMS

P3101.1 General. This chapter shall govern the selection and installation of piping, tubing and fittings for vent systems. This chapter shall control the minimum diameter of vent pipes, circuit vents, branch vents and individual vents, and the size and length of vents and various aspects of vent stacks and stack vents. Additionally, this chapter regulates vent grades and connections, height above fixtures and relief vents for stacks and fixture traps, and the venting of sumps and sewers.

P3101.2 Trap seal protection. The plumbing system shall be provided with a system of vent piping that will permit the admission or emission of air so that the seal of any fixture trap shall not be subjected to a pneumatic pressure differential of more than 1 inch of water column (249 Pa).

> **P3101.2.1 Venting required.** Every trap and trapped fixture shall be vented in accordance with one of the venting methods specified in this chapter.

P3101.3 Use limitations. The plumbing vent system shall not be used for purposes other than the venting of the plumbing system.

P3101.4 Extension outside a structure. In climates where the 97.5-percent value for outside design temperature is 0°F (-18°C) or less (ASHRAE 97.5-percent column, winter, see Chapter 3), vent pipes installed on the exterior of the structure shall be protected against freezing by insulation, heat or both. Vent terminals shall be protected from frost closure in accordance with Section P3103.2.

P3101.5 Flood resistance. In areas prone to floodings as established by Table R301.2(1), vents shall be located at or above the elevation required in Section R322.1 (flood hazard areas including A Zones) or R322.2 (coastal high-hazard areas including V Zones).

SECTION P3102
VENT STACKS AND STACK VENTS

P3102.1 Required vent extension. The vent system serving each *building drain* shall have at least one vent pipe that extends to the outdoors.

P3102.2 Installation. The required vent shall be a dry vent that connects to the *building drain* or an extension of a drain that connects to the *building drain*. Such vent shall not be an island fixture vent as permitted by Section P3112.

P3102.3 Size. The required vent shall be sized in accordance with Section P3113.1 based on the required size of the *building drain*.

SECTION P3103
VENT TERMINALS

P3103.1 Roof extension. Open vent pipes that extend through a roof shall be terminated at least 6 inches (152 mm) above the roof or 6 inches (152 mm) above the anticipated snow accumulation, whichever is greater, except that where a roof is to be used for any purpose other than weather protection, the vent extension shall be run at least 7 feet (2134 mm) above the roof.

P3103.2 Frost closure. Where the 97.5-percent value for outside design temperature is 0°F (-18°C) or less, every vent extension through a roof or wall shall be a minimum of 3 inches (76 mm) in diameter. Any increase in the size of the vent shall be made inside the structure a minimum of 1 foot (305 mm) below the roof or inside the wall.

P3103.3 Flashings and sealing. The juncture of each vent pipe with the roof line shall be made water tight by an *approved* flashing. Vent extensions in walls and soffits shall be made weather tight by caulking.

P3103.4 Prohibited use. Vent terminals shall not be used as a flag pole or to support flag poles, TV aerials, or similar items, except when the piping has been anchored in an *approved* manner.

P3103.5 Location of vent terminal. An open vent terminal from a drainage system shall not be located less than 4 feet (1219 mm) directly beneath any door, openable window, or other air intake opening of the building or of an adjacent building, nor shall any such vent terminal be within 10 feet (3048 mm) horizontally of such an opening unless it is at least 2 feet (610 mm) above the top of such opening.

P3103.6 Extension through the wall. Vent terminals extending through the wall shall terminate a minimum of 10 feet (3048 mm) from the *lot line* and 10 feet (3048 mm) above the highest adjacent *grade* within 10 feet (3048 mm) horizontally of the vent terminal. Vent terminals shall not terminate under the overhang of a structure with soffit vents. Side wall vent terminals shall be protected to prevent birds or rodents from entering or blocking the vent opening.

SECTION P3104
VENT CONNECTIONS AND GRADES

3104.1 Connection. All individual branch and circuit vents shall connect to a vent stack, stack vent or extend to the open air.

> **Exception:** Individual, branch and circuit vents shall be permitted to terminate at an *air admittance valve* in accordance with Section P3114.

P3104.2 Grade. Vent and branch vent pipes shall be graded, connected and supported to allow moisture and condensate to drain back to the soil or waste pipe by gravity.

P3104.3 Vent connection to drainage system. Every dry vent connecting to a horizontal drain shall connect above the center-line of the horizontal drain pipe.

P3104.4 Vertical rise of vent. Every dry vent shall rise vertically to a minimum of 6 inches (152 mm) above the flood level rim of the highest trap or trapped fixture being vented.

P3104.5 Height above fixtures. A connection between a vent pipe and a vent stack or stack vent shall be made at least 6 inches (152 mm) above the flood level rim of the highest fixture served by the vent. Horizontal vent pipes forming branch vents shall be at least 6 inches (152 mm) above the flood level rim of the highest fixture served.

P3104.6 Vent for future fixtures. Where the drainage piping has been roughed-in for future fixtures, a rough-in connection for a vent shall be installed a minimum of one-half the diameter of the drain. The vent rough-in shall connect to the vent system or shall be vented by other means as provided in this chapter. The connection shall be identified to indicate that the connection is a vent.

SECTION P3105
FIXTURE VENTS

P3105.1 Distance of trap from vent. Each fixture trap shall have a protecting vent located so that the slope and the *developed length* in the *fixture drain* from the trap weir to the vent fitting are within the requirements set forth in Table P3105.1.

> **Exception:** The *developed length* of the *fixture drain* from the trap weir to the vent fitting for self-siphoning fixtures, such as water closets, shall not be limited.

TABLE P3105.1
MAXIMUM DISTANCE OF FIXTURE TRAP FROM VENT

SIZE OF TRAP (inches)	SLOPE (inch per foot)	DISTANCE FROM TRAP (feet)
$1^1/_4$	$^1/_4$	5
$1^1/_2$	$^1/_4$	6
2	$^1/_4$	8
3	$^1/_8$	12
4	$^1/_8$	16

For SI: 1 inch = 25.4 mm, 1 foot = 304.8 mm,
1 inch per foot = 83.3 mm/m.

P3105.2 Fixture drains. The total fall in a *fixture drain* resulting from pipe slope shall not exceed one pipe diameter, nor shall the vent pipe connection to a *fixture drain*, except for water closets, be below the weir of the trap.

P3105.3 Crown vent. A vent shall not be installed within two pipe diameters of the trap weir.

SECTION P3106
INDIVIDUAL VENT

P3106.1 Individual vent permitted. Each trap and trapped fixture is permitted to be provided with an individual vent. The individual vent shall connect to the *fixture drain* of the trap or trapped fixture being vented.

SECTION P3107
COMMON VENT

P3107.1 Individual vent as common vent. An individual vent is permitted to vent two traps or trapped fixtures as a common vent. The traps or trapped fixtures being common vented shall be located on the same floor level.

P3107.2 Connection at the same level. Where the *fixture drains* being common vented connect at the same level, the vent connection shall be at the interconnection of the *fixture drains* or downstream of the interconnection.

P3107.3 Connection at different levels. Where the *fixture drains* connect at different levels, the vent shall connect as a vertical extension of the vertical drain. The vertical drain pipe connecting the two *fixture drains* shall be considered the vent for the lower *fixture drain*, and shall be sized in accordance with Table P3107.3. The upper fixture shall not be a water closet.

TABLE P3107.3
COMMON VENT SIZES

PIPE SIZE (inches)	MAXIMUM DISCHARGE FROM UPPER FIXTURE DRAIN (d.f.u.)
$1^1/_2$	1
2	4
$2^1/_2$ to 3	6

For SI: 1 inch = 25.4 mm.

SECTION P3108
WET VENTING

P3108.1 Horizontal wet vent permitted. Any combination of fixtures within two *bathroom groups* located on the same floor level are permitted to be vented by a horizontal wet vent. The wet vent shall be considered the vent for the fixtures and shall extend from the connection of the dry vent along the direction of the flow in the drain pipe to the most downstream *fixture drain* connection. Each *fixture drain* shall connect horizontally to the horizontal branch being wet vented or shall have a dry vent. Each wet-vented *fixture drain* shall connect independently to the horizontal wet vent. Only the fixtures within the *bathroom groups* shall connect to the wet-vented horizontal branch drain. Any additional fixtures shall discharge downstream of the horizontal wet vent.

P3108.2 Dry vent connection. The required dry-vent connection for wet-vented systems shall comply with Sections P3108.2.1 and P3108.2.2.

> **P3108.2.1 Horizontal wet vent.** The dry-vent connection for a horizontal wet-vent system shall be an individual vent or a common vent for any *bathroom group* fixture, except an emergency floor drain. Where the dry vent connects to a water closet *fixture drain*, the drain shall connect horizontally to the horizontal wet vent system. Not more than one wet-vented *fixture drain* shall discharge upstream of the dry-vented *fixture drain* connection.

> **P3108.2.2 Vertical wet vent.** The dry-vent connection for a vertical wet-vent system shall be an individual vent or common vent for the most upstream *fixture drain*.

P3108.3 Size. Horizontal and vertical wet vents shall be of a minimum size as specified in Table P3108.3, based on the fixture unit discharge to the wet vent. The dry vent serving the wet vent shall be sized based on the largest required diameter of pipe within the wet-vent system served by the dry vent.

TABLE P3108.3
WET VENT SIZE

WET VENT PIPE SIZE (inches)	FIXTURE UNIT LOAD (d.f.u.)
$1^1/_2$	1
2	4
$2^1/_2$	6
3	12
4	32

For SI: 1 inch = 25.4 mm.

P3108.4 Vertical wet vent permitted. A combination of fixtures located on the same floor level are permitted to be vented by a vertical wet vent. The vertical wet vent shall be considered the vent for the fixtures and shall extend from the connection of the dry vent down to the lowest *fixture drain* connection. Each wet-vented fixture shall connect independently to the vertical wet vent. All water closet drains shall connect at the same elevation. Other *fixture drains* shall connect above or at the same elevation as the water closet *fixture drains*. The dry vent connection to the vertical wet vent shall be an individual or common vent serving one or two fixtures.

P3108.5 Trap weir to wet vent distances. The maximum *developed length* of wet-vented *fixture drains* shall comply with Table P3105.1.

SECTION P3109
WASTE STACK VENT

P3109.1 Waste stack vent permitted. A waste stack shall be considered a vent for all of the fixtures discharging to the stack where installed in accordance with the requirements of this section.

P3109.2 Stack installation. The waste stack shall be vertical, and both horizontal and vertical offsets shall be prohibited between the lowest *fixture drain* connection and the highest *fixture drain* connection to the stack. Every *fixture drain* shall connect separately to the waste stack. The stack shall not receive the discharge of water closets or urinals.

P3109.3 Stack vent. A stack vent shall be installed for the waste stack. The size of the stack vent shall be not less than the size of the waste stack. Offsets shall be permitted in the stack vent and shall be located at least 6 inches (152 mm) above the flood level of the highest fixture, and shall be in accordance with Section P3104.5. The stack vent shall be permitted to connect with other stack vents and vent stacks in accordance with Section P3113.3.

P3109.4 Waste stack size. The waste stack shall be sized based on the total discharge to the stack and the discharge within a *branch interval* in accordance with Table P3109.4. The waste stack shall be the same size throughout the length of the waste stack.

TABLE P3109.4
WASTE STACK VENT SIZE

STACK SIZE (inches)	MAXIMUM NUMBER OF FIXTURE UNITS (d.f.u.)	
	Total discharge into one branch interval	Total discharge for stack
$1^1/_2$	1	2
2	2	4
$2^1/_2$	No limit	8
3	No limit	24
4	No limit	50

For SI: 1 inch = 25.4 mm.

SECTION P3110
CIRCUIT VENTING

P3110.1 Circuit vent permitted. A maximum of eight fixtures connected to a horizontal branch drain shall be permitted to be circuit vented. Each *fixture drain* shall connect horizontally to the horizontal branch being circuit vented. The horizontal branch drain shall be classified as a vent from the most downstream *fixture drain* connection to the most upstream *fixture drain* connection to the horizontal branch.

P3110.2 Vent connection. The circuit vent connection shall be located between the two most upstream *fixture drains*. The vent shall connect to the horizontal branch and shall be installed in accordance with Section P3104. The circuit vent pipe shall not receive the discharge of any soil or waste.

P3110.3 Slope and size of horizontal branch. The maximum slope of the vent section of the horizontal branch drain shall be one unit vertical in 12 units horizontal (8-percent slope). The entire length of the vent section of the horizontal branch drain shall be sized for the total drainage discharge to the branch in accordance with Table P3005.4.1.

P3110.4 Additional fixtures. Fixtures, other than the circuit vented fixtures are permitted to discharge, to the horizontal branch drain. Such fixtures shall be located on the same floor as the circuit vented fixtures and shall be either individually or common vented.

SECTION P3111
COMBINATION WASTE AND VENT SYSTEM

P3111.1 Type of fixtures. A combination waste and vent system shall not serve fixtures other than floor drains, sinks and lavatories. A combination waste and vent system shall not receive the discharge of a food waste grinder.

P3111.2 Installation. The only vertical pipe of a combination drain and vent system shall be the connection between the *fixture drain* and the horizontal combination waste and vent pipe. The maximum vertical distance shall be 8 feet (2438 mm).

P3111.2.1 Slope. The horizontal combination waste and vent pipe shall have a maximum slope of $^1/_2$ unit vertical in 12 units horizontal (4-percent slope). The minimum slope shall be in accordance with Section P3005.3.

P3111.2.2 Connection. The combination waste and vent pipe shall connect to a horizontal drain that is vented or a vent shall connect to the combination waste and vent. The vent connecting to the combination waste and vent pipe shall extend vertically a minimum of 6 inches (152 mm) above the flood level rim of the highest fixture being vented before offsetting horizontally.

P3111.2.3 Vent size. The vent shall be sized for the total fixture unit load in accordance with Section P3113.1.

P3111.2.4 Fixture branch or drain. The fixture branch or *fixture drain* shall connect to the combination waste and vent within a distance specified in Table P3105.1. The combination waste and vent pipe shall be considered the vent for the fixture.

P3111.3 Size. The minimum size of a combination waste and vent pipe shall be in accordance with Table P3111.3.

TABLE P3111.3
SIZE OF COMBINATION WASTE AND VENT PIPE

DIAMETER PIPE (inches)	MAXIMUM NUMBER OF FIXTURE UNITS (d.f.u.)	
	Connecting to a horizontal branch or stack	Connecting to a building drain or building subdrain
2	3	4
$2^1/_2$	6	26
3	12	31
4	20	50

For SI: 1 inch = 25.4 mm.

SECTION P3112
ISLAND FIXTURE VENTING

P3112.1 Limitation. Island fixture venting shall not be permitted for fixtures other than sinks and lavatories. Kitchen sinks with a dishwasher waste connection, a food waste grinder, or both, in combination with the kitchen sink waste, shall be permitted to be vented in accordance with this section.

P3112.2 Vent connection. The island fixture vent shall connect to the *fixture drain* as required for an individual or common vent. The vent shall rise vertically to above the drainage outlet of the fixture being vented before offsetting horizontally or vertically downward. The vent or branch vent for multiple island fixture vents shall extend to a minimum of 6 inches (152 mm) above the highest island fixture being vented before connecting to the outside vent terminal.

P3112.3 Vent installation below the fixture flood level rim. The vent located below the flood level rim of the fixture being vented shall be installed as required for drainage piping in accordance with Chapter 30, except for sizing. The vent shall be sized in accordance with Section P3113.1. The lowest point of the island fixture vent shall connect full size to the drainage system. The connection shall be to a vertical drain pipe or to the top half of a horizontal drain pipe. Cleanouts shall be provided in the island fixture vent to permit rodding of all vent piping located below the flood level rim of the fixtures. Rodding in both directions shall be permitted through a cleanout.

SECTION P3113
VENT PIPE SIZING

P3113.1 Size of vents. The minimum required diameter of individual vents, branch vents, circuit vents, vent stacks and stack vents shall be at least one-half the required diameter of the drain served. The required size of the drain shall be determined in accordance with Chapter 30. Vent pipes shall be not less than $1^1/_4$ inches (32 mm) in diameter. Vents exceeding 40 feet (12 192 mm) in *developed length* shall be increased by one nominal pipe size for the entire *developed length* of the vent pipe.

P3113.2 Developed length. The *developed length* of individual, branch, and circuit vents shall be measured from the farthest point of vent connection to the drainage system, to the point of connection to the vent stack, stack vent or termination outside of the building.

P3113.3 Branch vents. Where branch vents are connected to a common branch vent, the common branch vent shall be sized in accordance with this section, based on the size of the common horizontal drainage branch that is or would be required to serve the total drainage fixture unit (dfu) load being vented.

P3113.4 Sump vents. Sump vent sizes shall be determined in accordance with Sections P3113.4.1 and P3113.4.2.

P3113.4.1 Sewage pumps and sewage ejectors other than pneumatic. Drainage piping below sewer level shall be vented in a manner similar to that of a gravity system. Building sump vent sizes for sumps with sewage pumps or sewage ejectors, other than pneumatic, shall be determined in accordance with Table P3113.4.1.

P3113.4.2 Pneumatic sewage ejectors. The air pressure relief pipe from a pneumatic sewage ejector shall be connected to an independent vent stack terminating as required for vent extensions through the roof. The relief pipe shall be sized to relieve air pressure inside the ejector to atmospheric pressure, but shall not be less than $1^1/_4$ inches (32 mm) in size.

SECTION P3114
AIR ADMITTANCE VALVES

P3114.1 General. Vent systems using *air admittance valves* shall comply with this section. Individual and branch-type air admittance valves shall conform to ASSE 1051. Stack-type air admittance valves shall conform to ASSE 1050.

P3114.2 Installation. The valves shall be installed in accordance with the requirements of this section and the manufacturer's installation instructions. *Air admittance valves* shall be installed after the DWV testing required by Section P2503.5.1 or P2503.5.2 has been performed.

P3114.3 Where permitted. Individual vents, branch vents, circuit vents and stack vents shall be permitted to terminate with a connection to an *air admittance valve*. Individual and branch type air admittance valves shall vent only fixtures that are on the same floor level and connect to a horizontal branch drain.

P3114.4 Location. Individual and branch *air admittance valves* shall be located a minimum of 4 inches (102 mm) above the horizontal branch drain or *fixture drain* being vented. Stack-type air admittance valves shall be located a minimum of 6 inches (152 mm) above the flood level rim of the highest fixture being vented. The *air admittance valve* shall be located within the maximum *developed length* permitted for the vent. The *air admittance valve* shall be installed a minimum of 6 inches (152 mm) above insulation materials where installed in *attics*.

P3114.5 Access and ventilation. Access shall be provided to all *air admittance valves*. The valve shall be located within a ventilated space that allows air to enter the valve.

P3114.6 Size. The *air admittance valve* shall be rated for the size of the vent to which the valve is connected.

P3114.7 Vent required. Within each plumbing system, a minimum of one stack vent or a vent stack shall extend outdoors to the open air.

P3114.8 Prohibited installations. *Air admittance valves* without an engineered design shall not be used to vent sumps or tanks of any type.

TABLE P3113.4.1
SIZE AND LENGTH OF SUMP VENTS

| DISCHARGE CAPACITY OF PUMP (gpm) | MAXIMUM DEVELOPED LENGTH OF VENT (feet)[a] | | | | |
| | Diameter of vent (inches) | | | | |
	$1^1/_4$	$1^1/_2$	2	$2^1/_2$	3
10	No limit[b]	No limit	No limit	No limit	No limit
20	270	No limit	No limit	No limit	No limit
40	72	160	No limit	No limit	No limit
60	31	75	270	No limit	No limit

For SI: 1 inch = 25.4 mm, 1 foot = 304.8 mm, 1 gallon per minute (gpm) = 3.785 L/m.

a. Developed length plus an appropriate allowance for entrance losses and friction caused by fittings, changes in direction and diameter. Suggested allowances shall be obtained from NBS Monograph 31 or other approved sources. An allowance of 50 percent of the developed length shall be assumed if a more precise value is not available.

b. Actual values greater than 500 feet.

CHAPTER 32

TRAPS

SECTION P3201
FIXTURE TRAPS

P3201.1 Design of traps. Traps shall be of standard design, shall have smooth uniform internal waterways, shall be self-cleaning and shall not have interior partitions except where integral with the fixture. Traps shall be constructed of lead, cast iron, cast or drawn brass or *approved* plastic. Tubular brass traps shall be not less than No. 20 gage (0.8 mm) thickness. Solid connections, slip joints and couplings are permitted to be used on the trap inlet, trap outlet, or within the trap seal. Slip joints shall be accessible.

P3201.2 Trap seals and trap seal protection. Traps shall have a liquid seal not less than 2 inches (51 mm) and not more than 4 inches (102 mm). Traps for floor drains shall be fitted with a trap primer or shall be of the deep seal design. Trap seal primer valves shall connect to the trap at a point above the level of the trap seal.

P3201.3 Trap setting and protection. Traps shall be set level with respect to their water seals and shall be protected from freezing. Trap seals shall be protected from siphonage, aspiration or back pressure by an *approved* system of venting (see Section P3101).

P3201.4 Building traps. Building traps shall not be installed, except in special cases where sewer gases are extremely corrosive or noxious, as directed by the *building official*.

P3201.5 Prohibited trap designs. The following types of traps are prohibited:

1. Bell traps.

2. Separate fixture traps with interior partitions, except those lavatory traps made of plastic, stainless steel or other corrosion-resistant material.

3. "S" traps.

4. Drum traps.

5. Trap designs with moving parts.

P3201.6 Number of fixtures per trap. Each plumbing fixture shall be separately trapped by a water seal trap. The vertical distance from the fixture outlet to the trap weir shall not exceed 24 inches (610 mm) and the horizontal distance shall not exceed 30 inches (762 mm) measured from the center line of the fixture outlet to the centerline of the inlet of the trap. The height of a clothes washer standpipe above a trap shall conform to Section P2706.2. Fixtures shall not be double trapped.

Exceptions:

1. Fixtures that have integral traps.

2. A single trap shall be permitted to serve two or three like fixtures limited to kitchen sinks, laundry tubs and lavatories. Such fixtures shall be adjacent to each other and located in the same room with a continuous waste arrangement. The trap shall be installed at the center fixture where three fixtures are installed. Common trapped fixture outlets shall be not more than 30 inches (762 mm) apart.

3. Connection of a laundry tray waste line into a standpipe for the automatic clothes-washer drain is permitted in accordance with Section P2706.2.1.

P3201.7 Size of fixture traps. Fixture trap size shall be sufficient to drain the fixture rapidly and not less than the size indicated in Table P3201.7. A trap shall not be larger than the drainage pipe into which the trap discharges.

TABLE P3201.7
SIZE OF TRAPS AND TRAP ARMS FOR PLUMBING FIXTURES

PLUMBING FIXTURE	TRAP SIZE MINIMUM (inches)
Bathtub (with or without shower head and/or whirlpool attachments)	$1^{1}/_{2}$
Bidet	$1^{1}/_{4}$
Clothes washer standpipe	2
Dishwasher (on separate trap)	$1^{1}/_{2}$
Floor drain	2
Kitchen sink (one or two traps, with or without dishwasher and garbage grinder)	$1^{1}/_{2}$
Laundry tub (one or more compartments)	$1^{1}/_{2}$
Lavatory	$1^{1}/_{4}$
Shower (based on the total flow rate through showerheads and bodysprays) Flow rate: 5.7 gpm and less / More than 5.7 gpm up to 12.3 gpm / More than 12.3 gpm up to 25.8 gpm / More than 25.8 gpm up to 55.6 gpm	$1^{1}/_{2}$ 2 3 4
Water closet	Note a

For SI: 1 inch = 25.4 mm.

a. Consult fixture standards for trap dimensions of specific bowls.

CHAPTER 33

STORM DRAINAGE

SECTION P3301
GENERAL

P3301.1 Scope. The provisions of this chapter shall govern the materials, design, construction and installation of storm drainage.

SECTION P3302
SUBSOIL DRAINS

P3302.1 Subsoil drains. Subsoil drains shall be open-jointed, horizontally split or perforated pipe conforming to one of the standards listed in Table P3302.1 Such drains shall not be less than 4 inches (102 mm) in diameter. Where the building is subject to backwater, the subsoil drain shall be protected by an accessibly located backwater valve. Subsoil drains shall discharge to a trapped area drain, sump, dry well or *approved* location above ground. The subsoil sump shall not be required to have either a gas-tight cover or a vent. The sump and pumping system shall comply with Section P3303.

SECTION P3303
SUMPS AND PUMPING SYSTEMS

P3303.1 Pumping system. The sump pump, pit and discharge piping shall conform to Sections P3303.1.1 through P3303.1.4.

P3303.1.1 Pump capacity and head. The sump pump shall be of a capacity and head appropriate to anticipated use requirements.

P3303.1.2 Sump pit. The sump pit shall not be less than 18 inches (457 mm) in diameter and 24 inches (610 mm) deep, unless otherwise *approved*. The pit shall be accessible and located so that all drainage flows into the pit by gravity. The sump pit shall be constructed of tile, steel, plastic, cast-iron, concrete or other *approved* material, with a removable cover adequate to support anticipated loads in the area of use. The pit floor shall be solid and provide permanent support for the pump.

P3303.1.3 Electrical. Electrical outlets shall meet the requirements of Chapters 34 through 43.

P3303.1.4 Piping. Discharge piping shall meet the requirements of Sections P3002.1, P3002.2, P3002.3 and P3003. Discharge piping shall include an accessible full flow check valve. Pipe and fittings shall be the same size as, or larger than, pump discharge tapping.

TABLE P3302.1
SUBSOIL DRAIN PIPE

MATERIAL	STANDARD
Asbestos-cement pipe	ASTM C 508
Cast-iron pipe	ASTM A 74; ASTM A 888; CISPI 301
Polyethylene (PE) plastic pipe	ASTM F 405; CSA B182.1; CSA B182.6; CSA B182.8
Polyvinyl chloride (PVC) Plastic pipe (type sewer pipe, PS25, PS50 or PS100)	ASTM D 2729; ASTM F 891; CSA B182.2; CSA B182.4
Stainless steel drainage systems, Type 316L	ASME A112.3.1
Vitrified clay pipe	ASTM C 4; ASTM C 700

CHAPTER 34

GENERAL REQUIREMENTS

This Electrical Part (Chapters 34 through 43) is produced and copyrighted by the National Fire Protection Association (NFPA) and is based on the 2008 *National Electrical Code®* (NEC®) (NFPA 70-2008), copyright 2007 National Fire Protection Association, all rights reserved. Use of the Electrical Part is pursuant to license with the NFPA.

The title *National Electrical Code®* and the acronym NEC® are registered trademarks of the National Fire Protection Association, Quincy, Massachusetts. See Appendix Q, *International Residential Code* Electrical Provisions/National Electrical Code Cross Reference.

IMPORTANT NOTICE AND DISCLAIMER CONCERNING THE NEC AND THIS ELECTRICAL PART.
This Electrical Part is a compilation of provisions extracted from the 2008 edition of the NEC. The NEC, like all NFPA codes and standards, is developed through a consensus standards development process approved by the American National Standards Institute. This process brings together volunteers representing varied viewpoints and interests to achieve consensus on fire and other safety issues. While the NFPA administers the process and establishes rules to promote fairness in the development of consensus, it does not independently test, evaluate or verify the accuracy of any information or the soundness of any judgments contained in its codes and standards.

The NFPA disclaims liability for any personal injury, property or other damages of any nature whatsoever, whether special, indirect, consequential or compensatory, directly or indirectly resulting from the publication, use of, or reliance on the NEC or this Electrical Part. The NFPA also makes no guaranty or warranty as to the accuracy or completeness of any information published in these documents.

In issuing and making the NEC and this Electrical Part available, the NFPA is not undertaking to render professional or other services for or on behalf of any person or entity. Nor is the NFPA undertaking to perform any duty owed by any person or entity to someone else. Anyone using these documents should rely on his or her own independent judgment or, as appropriate, seek the advice of a competent professional in determining the exercise of reasonable care in any given circumstances.

The NFPA has no power, nor does it undertake, to police or enforce compliance with the contents of the NEC and this Electrical Part. Nor does the NFPA list, certify, test, or inspect products, designs, or installations for compliance with these documents. Any certification or other statement of compliance with the requirements of these documents shall not be attributable to the NFPA and is solely the responsibility of the certifier or maker of the statement.

For additional notices and disclaimers concerning NFPA codes and standards see www.nfpa.org/disclaimers.

SECTION E3401
GENERAL

E3401.1 Applicability. The provisions of Chapters 34 through 43 shall establish the general scope of the electrical system and equipment requirements of this code. Chapters 34 through 43 cover those wiring methods and materials most commonly encountered in the construction of one- and two-family dwellings and structures regulated by this code. Other wiring methods, materials and subject matter covered in the NFPA 70 are also allowed by this code.

E3401.2 Scope. Chapters 34 through 43 shall cover the installation of electrical systems, equipment and components indoors and outdoors that are within the scope of this code, including services, power distribution systems, fixtures, appliances, devices and appurtenances. Services within the scope of this code shall be limited to 120/240-volt, 0- to 400-ampere, single-phase systems. These chapters specifically cover the equipment, fixtures, appliances, wiring methods and materials that are most commonly used in the construction or alteration of one- and two-family dwellings and accessory structures regulated by this code. The omission from these chapters of any

material or method of construction provided for in the referenced standard NFPA 70 shall not be construed as prohibiting the use of such material or method of construction. Electrical systems, equipment or components not specifically covered in these chapters shall comply with the applicable provisions of the NFPA 70.

E3401.3 Not covered. Chapters 34 through 43 do not cover the following:

1. Installations, including associated lighting, under the exclusive control of communications utilities and electric utilities.

2. Services over 400 amperes.

E3401.4 Additions and alterations. Any addition or alteration to an existing electrical system shall be made in conformity with the provisions of Chapters 34 through 43. Where additions subject portions of existing systems to loads exceeding those permitted herein, such portions shall be made to comply with Chapters 34 through 43.

SECTION E3402
BUILDING STRUCTURE PROTECTION

E3402.1 Drilling and notching. Wood-framed structural members shall not be drilled, notched or altered in any manner except as provided for in this code.

E3402.2 Penetrations of fire-resistance-rated assemblies. Electrical installations in hollow spaces, vertical shafts and ventilation or air-handling ducts shall be made so that the possible spread of fire or products of combustion will not be substantially increased. Electrical penetrations through fire-resistance-rated walls, partitions, floors or ceilings shall be protected by approved methods to maintain the fire-resistance rating of the element penetrated. Penetrations of fire-resistance-rated walls shall be limited as specified in Section R317.3.

E3402.3 Penetrations of firestops and draftstops. Penetrations through fire blocking and draftstopping shall be protected in an approved manner to maintain the integrity of the element penetrated.

SECTION E3403
INSPECTION AND APPROVAL

E3403.1 Approval. Electrical materials, components and equipment shall be approved.

E3403.2 Inspection required. New electrical work and parts of existing systems affected by new work or alterations shall be inspected by the building official to ensure compliance with the requirements of Chapters 34 through 43.

E3403.3 Listing and labeling. Electrical materials, components, devices, fixtures and equipment shall be listed for the application, shall bear the label of an approved agency and shall be installed, and used, or both, in accordance with the manufacturer's installation instructions.

SECTION E3404
GENERAL EQUIPMENT REQUIREMENTS

E3404.1 Voltages. Throughout Chapters 34 through 43, the voltage considered shall be that at which the circuit operates.

E3404.2 Interrupting rating. Equipment intended to interrupt current at fault levels shall have a minimum interrupting rating of 10,000 amperes. Equipment intended to interrupt current at levels other than fault levels shall have an interrupting rating at nominal circuit voltage sufficient for the current that must be interrupted.

E3404.3 Circuit characteristics. The overcurrent protective devices, total impedance, component short-circuit current ratings and other characteristics of the circuit to be protected shall be so selected and coordinated as to permit the circuit protective devices that are used to clear a fault to do so without extensive damage to the electrical components of the circuit. This fault shall be assumed to be either between two or more of the circuit conductors or between any circuit conductor and the grounding conductor or enclosing metal raceway. Listed products applied in accordance with their listing shall be considered to meet the requirements of this section.

E3404.4 Enclosure types. Enclosures, other than surrounding fences or walls, of panelboards, meter sockets, and motor controllers, rated not over 600 volts nominal and intended for such locations, shall be marked with an enclosure-type number as shown in Table E3404.4.

Table E3404.4 shall be used for selecting these enclosures for use in specific locations other than hazardous (classified) locations. The enclosures are not intended to protect against conditions such as condensation, icing, corrosion, or contamination that might occur within the enclosure or enter through the conduit or unsealed openings.

E3404.5 Protection of equipment. Equipment not identified for outdoor use and equipment identified only for indoor use, such as "dry locations," "indoor use only" "damp locations," or enclosure Type 1, 2, 5, 12, 12K and/or 13, shall be protected against permanent damage from the weather during building construction.

E3404.6 Unused openings. Unused openings, other than those intended for the operation of equipment, those intended for the operation of equipment, those intended for mounting purposes, and those permitted as part of the design for listed equipment, shall be closed to afford protection substantially equivalent to the wall of the equipment. Where metallic plugs or plates are used with nonmetallic enclosures they shall be recessed at least $^1/_4$ inch (6.4 mm) from the outer surface of the enclosure.

E3404.7 Integrity of electrical equipment. Internal parts of electrical equipment, including busbars, wiring terminals, insulators and other surfaces, shall not be damaged or contaminated by foreign materials such as paint, plaster, cleaners or abrasives, and corrosive residues. There shall not be any damaged parts that might adversely affect safe operation or mechanical strength of the equipment such as parts that are broken; bent; cut; deteriorated by corrosion, chemical action, or overheating. Foreign debris shall be removed from equipment.

E3404.8 Mounting. Electrical equipment shall be firmly secured to the surface on which it is mounted. Wooden plugs driven into masonry, concrete, plaster, or similar materials shall not be used.

E3404.9 Energized parts guarded against accidental contact. Approved enclosures shall guard energized parts that are operating at 50 volts or more against accidental contact.

E3404.10 Prevent physical damage. In locations where electrical equipment is likely to be exposed to physical damage, enclosures or guards shall be so arranged and of such strength as to prevent such damage.

E3404.11 Equipment identification. The manufacturer's name, trademark or other descriptive marking by which the organization responsible for the product can be identified shall be placed on all electric equipment. Other markings shall be provided that indicate voltage, current, wattage or other ratings as specified elsewhere in Chapters 34 through 43. The marking shall have the durability to withstand the environment involved.

E3404.12 Identification of disconnecting means. Each disconnecting means shall be legibly marked to indicate its purpose, except where located and arranged so that the purpose is evident. The marking shall have the durability to withstand the environment involved.

TABLE E3404.4
ENCLOSURE SELECTION

PROVIDES A DEGREE OF PROTECTION AGAINST THE FOLLOWING ENVIRONMENTAL CONDITIONS	FOR OUTDOOR USE									
	Enclosure-type Number									
	3	3R	3S	3X	3RX	3SX	4	4X	6	6P
Incidental contact with the enclosed equipment	X	X	X	X	X	X	X	X	X	X
Rain, snow and sleet	X	X	X	X	X	X	X	X	X	X
Sleet[a]	—	—	X	—	—	X	—	—	—	—
Windblown dust	X	—	X	X	—	X	X	X	X	X
Hosedown	—	—	—	—	—	—	X	X	X	X
Corrosive agents	—	—	—	X	X	X	—	X	—	X
Temporary submersion	—	—	—	—	—	—	—	—	X	X
Prolonged submersion	—	—	—	—	—	—	—	—	—	X

PROVIDES A DEGREE OF PROTECTION AGAINST THE FOLLOWING ENVIRONMENTAL CONDITIONS	FOR INDOOR USE									
	Enclosure-type Number									
	1	2	4	4X	5	6	6P	12	12K	13
Incidental contact with the enclosed equipment	X	X	X	X	X	X	X	X	X	X
Falling dirt	X	X	X	X	X	X	X	X	X	X
Falling liquids and light splashing	—	X	X	X	X	X	X	X	X	X
Circulating dust, lint, fibers and flyings	—	—	X	X	—	X	X	X	X	X
Settling airborne dust, lint, fibers and flings	—	—	X	X	X	X	X	X	X	X
Hosedown and splashing water	—	—	X	X	—	X	X	—	—	—
Oil and coolant seepage	—	—	—	—	—	—	—	X	X	X
Oil or coolant spraying and splashing	—	—	—	—	—	—	—	—	—	X
Corrosive agents	—	—	—	X	—	—	X	—	—	—
Temporary submersion	—	—	—	—	—	X	X	—	—	—
Prolonged submersion	—	—	—	—	—	—	X	—	—	—

a. Mechanism shall be operable when ice covered.

Note: The term raintight is typically used in conjunction with Enclosure Types 3, 3S, 3SX, 3X, 4, 4X, 6 and 6P. The term rainproof is typically used in conjunction with Enclosure Types 3R and 3RX. The term watertight is typically used in conjunction with Enclosure Types 4, 4X, 6 and 6P. The term driptight is typically used in conjunction with Enclosure Types 2, 5, 12, 12K and 13. The term dusttight is typically used in conjunction with Enclosure Types 3, 3S, 3SX, 3X, 5, 12, 12K and 13.

SECTION E3405
EQUIPMENT LOCATION AND CLEARANCES

E3405.1 Working space and clearances. Sufficient access and working space shall be provided and maintained around all electrical equipment to permit ready and safe operation and maintenance of such equipment in accordance with this section and Figure E3405.1.

E3405.2 Working clearances for energized equipment and panelboards. Except as otherwise specified in Chapters 34 through 43, the dimension of the working space in the direction of access to panelboards and live parts likely to require examination, adjustment, servicing or maintenance while energized shall be not less than 36 inches (914 mm) in depth. Distances shall be measured from the energized parts where such parts are exposed or from the enclosure front or opening where such parts are enclosed. In addition to the 36-inch dimension (914 mm), the work space shall not be less than 30 inches (762 mm) wide in front of the electrical equipment and not less than the width of such equipment. The work space shall be clear and shall extend from the floor or platform to a height of 6.5 feet (1981 mm). In all cases, the work space shall allow at least a 90-degree (1.57 rad) opening of equipment doors or hinged panels. Equipment associated with the electrical installation located above or below the electrical equipment shall be permitted to extend not more than 6 inches (152 mm) beyond the front of the electrical equipment.

E3405.3 Dedicated panelboard space. The space equal to the width and depth of the panelboard and extending from the floor to a height of 6 feet (1829 mm) above the panelboard, or to the structural ceiling, whichever is lower, shall be dedicated to the electrical installation. Piping, ducts, leak protection apparatus and other equipment foreign to the electrical installation shall not be installed in such dedicated space. The area above the dedicated space shall be permitted to contain foreign systems, provided that protection is installed to avoid damage to the electrical equipment from condensation, leaks and breaks in such foreign systems (see Figure E3405.1).

> **Exception:** Suspended ceilings with removable panels shall be permitted within the 6-foot (1829 mm) dedicated space.

E3405.4 Location of working spaces and equipment. Required working space shall not be designated for storage. Panelboards and overcurrent protection devices shall not be located in clothes closets, in bathrooms, or over the steps of a stairway.

E3405.5 Access and entrance to working space. Access shall be provided to the required working space.

E3405.6 Illumination. Artificial illumination shall be provided for all working spaces for service equipment and panelboards installed indoors.

E3405.7 Headroom. The minimum headroom for working spaces for service equipment and panelboards shall be 6.5 feet (1981 mm).

SECTION E3406
ELECTRICAL CONDUCTORS AND CONNECTIONS

E3406.1 General. This section provides general requirements for conductors, connections and splices. These requirements do not apply to conductors that form an integral part of equipment, such as motors, appliances and similar equipment, or to conductors specifically provided for elsewhere in Chapters 34 through 43.

E3406.2 Conductor material. Conductors used to conduct current shall be of copper except as otherwise provided in Chapters 34 through 43. Where the conductor material is not specified, the material and the sizes given in these chapters shall apply to copper conductors. Where other materials are used, the conductor sizes shall be changed accordingly.

E3406.3 Minimum size of conductors. The minimum size of conductors for feeders and branch circuits shall be 14 AWG copper and 12 AWG aluminum. The minimum size of service conductors shall be as specified in Chapter 36. The minimum size of Class 2 remote control, signaling and power-limited circuits conductors shall be as specified in Chapter 43.

E3406.4 Stranded conductors. Where installed in raceways, conductors of size 8 AWG and larger shall be stranded. A solid 8 AWG conductor shall be permitted to be installed in a raceway only to meet the requirements of Sections E3610.2 and E4204.

E3406.5 Individual conductor insulation. Except where otherwise permitted in Sections E3605.1 and E3908.9, and E4303, current-carrying conductors shall be insulated. Insulated conductors shall have insulation types identified as RHH, RHW, RHW-2, THHN, THHW, THW, THW-2, THWN, THWN-2, TW, UF, USE, USE-2, XHHW or XHHW-2. Insulation types shall be approved for the application.

E3406.6 Conductors in parallel. Circuit conductors that are connected in parallel shall be limited to sizes 1/0 AWG and larger. Conductors in parallel shall be of the same length, same conductor material, same circular mil area and same insulation type. Conductors in parallel shall be terminated in the same manner. Where run in separate raceways or cables, the raceway or cables shall have the same physical characteristics. Where conductors are in separate raceways or cables, the same number of conductors shall be used in each raceway or cable.

E3406.7 Conductors of the same circuit. All conductors of the same circuit and, where used, the grounded conductor and all equipment grounding conductors and bonding conductors shall be contained within the same raceway, cable or cord.

E3406.8 Aluminum and copper connections. Terminals and splicing connectors shall be identified for the material of the conductors joined. Conductors of dissimilar metals shall not be joined in a terminal or splicing connector where physical contact occurs between dissimilar conductors such as copper and aluminum, copper and copper-clad aluminum, or aluminum and copper-clad aluminum, except where the device is listed for the purpose and conditions of application. Materials such as inhibitors and compounds shall be suitable for the application and shall be of a type that will not adversely affect the conductors, installation or equipment.

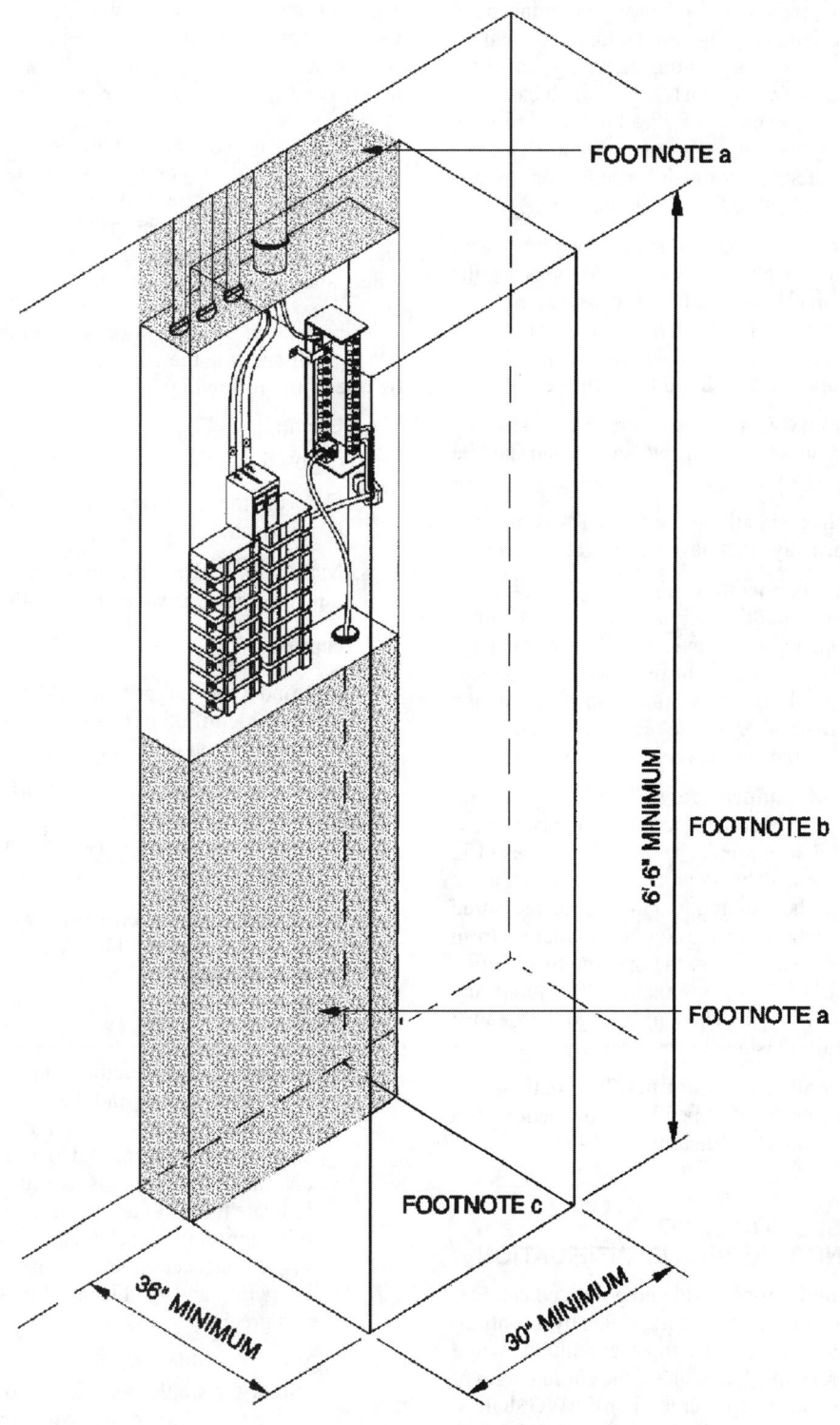

FIGURE E3405.1[a, b, c, d, e]
WORKING SPACE AND CLEARANCES

For SI: 1 inch = 25.4 mm, 1 foot = 304.8 mm.

a. Equipment, piping and ducts foreign to the electrical installation shall not be placed in the shaded areas extending from the floor to a height of 6 feet above the panelboard enclosure, or to the structural ceiling, whichever is lower.

b. The working space shall be clear and unobstructed from the floor to a height of 6.5 feet.

c. The working space shall not be designated for storage.

d. Panelboards, service equipment and similar enclosures shall not be located in bathrooms, toilet rooms, clothes closets or over the steps of a stairway.

e. Such work spaces shall be provided with artificial lighting where located indoors.

E3406.9 Terminals. Connection of conductors to terminal parts shall be made without damaging the conductors and shall be made by means of pressure connectors, including set-screw type, by means of splices to flexible leads, or for conductor sizes of 10 AWG and smaller, by means of wire binding screws or studs and nuts having upturned lugs or the equivalent. Terminals for more than one conductor and terminals for connecting aluminum conductors shall be identified for the application.

E3406.10 Splices. Conductors shall be spliced or joined with splicing devices listed for the purpose. Splices and joints and the free ends of conductors shall be covered with an insulation equivalent to that of the conductors or with an insulating device listed for the purpose. Wire connectors or splicing means installed on conductors for direct burial shall be listed for such use.

E3406.10.1 Continuity. Conductors in raceways shall be continuous between outlets, boxes, and devices and shall be without splices or taps in the raceway.

> **Exception:** Splices shall be permitted within surface-mounted raceways that have a removable cover.

E3406.10.2 Device connections. The continuity of a grounded conductor in multiwire branch circuits shall not be dependent on connection to devices such as receptacles and lampholders. The arrangement of grounding connections shall be such that the disconnection or the removal of a receptacle, luminaire or other device fed from the box does not interfere with or interrupt the grounding continuity.

E3406.10.3 Length of conductor for splice or termination. Where conductors are to be spliced, terminated or connected to fixtures or devices, a minimum length of 6 inches (152 mm) of free conductor shall be provided at each outlet, junction or switch point. The required length shall be measured from the point in the box where the conductor emerges from its raceway or cable sheath. Where the opening to an outlet, junction or switch point is less than 8 inches (200 mm) in any dimension, each conductor shall be long enough to extend at least 3 inches (75 mm) outside of such opening.

E3406.11 Grounded conductor continuity. The continuity of a grounded conductor shall not depend on connection to a metallic enclosure, raceway or cable armor.

SECTION E3407
CONDUCTOR AND TERMINAL IDENTIFICATION

E3407.1 Grounded conductors. Insulated grounded conductors of sizes 6 AWG or smaller shall be identified by a continuous white or gray outer finish or by three continuous white stripes on other than green insulation along the entire length of the conductors. Conductors of sizes larger than 6 AWG shall be identified either by a continuous white or gray outer finish or by three continuous white stripes on other than green insulation along its entire length or at the time of installation by a distinctive white or gray marking at its terminations. This marking shall encircle the conductor or insulation.

E3407.2 Equipment grounding conductors. Equipment grounding conductors of sizes 6 AWG and smaller shall be identified by a continuous green color or a continuous green color with one or more yellow stripes on the insulation or cov-ering, except where bare. Conductors with insulation or individual covering that is green, green with one or more yellow stripes, or otherwise identified as permitted by this section shall not be used for ungrounded or grounded circuit conductors.

Equipment grounding conductors larger than 6 AWG that are not identified as required for conductors of sizes 6 AWG and smaller shall, at the time of installation, be permanently identified as an equipment grounding conductor at each end and at every point where the conductor is accessible, except where such conductors are bare.

The required identification for conductors larger than 6 AWG shall encircle the conductor and shall be accomplished by one of the following:

1. Stripping the insulation or covering from the entire exposed length.

2. Coloring the exposed insulation or covering green at the termination.

3. Marking the exposed insulation or covering with green tape or green adhesive labels at the termination.

Exceptions:

> 1. Conductors larger than 6 AWG shall not be required to be identified in conduit bodies that do not contain splices or unused hubs.

> 2. Power-limited, Class 2 or Class 3 circuit cables containing only circuits operating at less than 50 volts shall be permitted to use a conductor with green insulation for other than equipment grounding purposes.

E3407.3 Ungrounded conductors. Insulation on the ungrounded conductors shall be a continuous color other than white, gray and green.

Exceptions:

> 1. An insulated conductor that is part of a cable or flexible cord assembly and that has a white or gray finish or a finish marking with three continuous white stripes shall be permitted to be used as an ungrounded conductor where it is permanently reidentified to indicate its use as an ungrounded conductor at all terminations and at each location where the conductor is visible and accessible. Identification shall encircle the insulation and shall be a color other than white, gray, and green.

> 2. Where a cable assembly contains an insulated conductor for single-pole, 3-way or 4-way switch loops and the conductor with white or gray insulation or a marking of three continuous white stripes is used for the supply to the switch but not as a return conductor from the switch to the switched outlet. In these applications, the conductor with white or gray insulation or with three continuous white stripes shall be permanently reidentified to indicate its use by painting or other effective means at its terminations and at each location where the conductor is visible and accessible.

E3407.4 Identification of terminals. Terminals for attachment to conductors shall be identified in accordance with Sections E3407.4.1 and E3407.4.2.

E3407.4.1 Device terminals. All devices excluding panelboards, provided with terminals for the attachment of conductors and intended for connection to more than one side of the circuit shall have terminals properly marked for identification, except where the terminal intended to be connected to the grounded conductor is clearly evident.

Exception: Terminal identification shall not be required for devices that have a normal current rating of over 30 amperes, other than polarized attachment caps and polarized receptacles for attachment caps as required in Section E3407.4.2.

E3407.4.2 Receptacles, plugs and connectors. Receptacles, polarized attachment plugs and cord connectors for plugs and polarized plugs shall have the terminal intended for connection to the grounded (white) conductor identified. Identification shall be by a metal or metal coating substantially white in color or by the word "white" or the letter "W" located adjacent to the identified terminal. Where the terminal is not visible, the conductor entrance hole for the connection shall be colored white or marked with the word "white" or the letter "W."

CHAPTER 35

ELECTRICAL DEFINITIONS

SECTION E3501
GENERAL

E3501.1 Scope. This chapter contains definitions that shall apply only to the electrical requirements of Chapters 34 through 43. Unless otherwise expressly stated, the following terms shall, for the purpose of this code, have the meanings indicated in this chapter. Words used in the present tense include the future; the singular number includes the plural and the plural the singular. Where terms are not defined in this section and are defined in Section R202 of this code, such terms shall have the meanings ascribed to them in that section. Where terms are not defined in these sections, they shall have their ordinarily accepted meanings or such as the context implies.

ACCESSIBLE. (As applied to equipment.) Admitting close approach; not guarded by locked doors, elevation or other effective means.

ACCESSIBLE. (As applied to wiring methods.) Capable of being removed or exposed without damaging the building structure or finish, or not permanently closed in by the structure or finish of the building.

ACCESSIBLE, READILY. Capable of being reached quickly for operation, renewal or inspections, without requiring those to whom ready access is requisite to climb over or remove obstacles or to resort to portable ladders, etc.

AMPACITY. The current in amperes that a conductor can carry continuously under the conditions of use without exceeding its temperature rating.

APPLIANCE. Utilization equipment, normally built in standardized sizes or types, that is installed or connected as a unit to perform one or more functions such as clothes washing, air conditioning, food mixing, deep frying, etc.

APPROVED. Acceptable to the authority having jurisdiction.

ARC-FAULT CIRCUIT INTERRUPTER. A device intended to provide protection from the effects of arc-faults by recognizing characteristics unique to arcing and by functioning to de-energize the circuit when an arc-fault is detected.

ATTACHMENT PLUG (PLUG CAP) (PLUG). A device that, by insertion into a receptacle, establishes connection between the conductors of the attached flexible cord and the conductors connected permanently to the receptacle.

AUTOMATIC. Self-acting, operating by its own mechanism when actuated by some impersonal influence, as, for example, a change in current, pressure, temperature or mechanical configuration.

BATHROOM. An area, including a basin, with one or more of the following: a toilet, a tub or a shower.

BONDED (BONDING). Connected to establish electrical continuity and conductivity.

BONDING JUMPER. A reliable conductor to ensure the required electrical conductivity between metal parts required to be electrically connected.

BONDING JUMPER (EQUIPMENT). The connection between two or more portions of the equipment grounding conductor.

BONDING JUMPER, MAIN. The connection between the grounded circuit conductor and the equipment grounding conductor at the service.

BRANCH CIRCUIT. The circuit conductors between the final overcurrent device protecting the circuit and the outlet(s).

BRANCH CIRCUIT, APPLIANCE. A branch circuit that supplies energy to one or more outlets to which appliances are to be connected, and that has no permanently connected luminaires that are not a part of an appliance.

BRANCH CIRCUIT, GENERAL PURPOSE. A branch circuit that supplies two or more receptacle outlets or outlets for lighting and appliances.

BRANCH CIRCUIT, INDIVIDUAL. A branch circuit that supplies only one utilization equipment.

BRANCH CIRCUIT, MULTIWIRE. A branch circuit consisting of two or more ungrounded conductors having voltage difference between them, and a grounded conductor having equal voltage difference between it and each ungrounded conductor of the circuit, and that is connected to the neutral or grounded conductor of the system.

CABINET. An enclosure designed either for surface or flush mounting and provided with a frame, mat or trim in which a swinging door or doors are or may be hung.

CIRCUIT BREAKER. A device designed to open and close a circuit by nonautomatic means and to open the circuit automatically on a predetermined overcurrent without damage to itself when properly applied within its rating.

CLOTHES CLOSET. A nonhabitable room or space intended primarily for storage of garments and apparel.

CONCEALED. Rendered inaccessible by the structure or finish of the building. Wires in concealed raceways are considered to be concealed, even though they become accessible upon withdrawing them [see "Accessible (As applied to wiring methods)"].

CONDUCTOR

Bare. A conductor having no covering or electrical insulation whatsoever.

Covered. A conductor encased within material of composition or thickness that is not recognized by this code as electrical insulation.

Insulated. A conductor encased within material of composition and thickness that is recognized by this code as electrical insulation.

CONDUIT BODY. A separate portion of a conduit or tubing system that provides access through a removable cover(s) to the interior of the system at a junction of two or more sections of the system or at a terminal point of the system. Boxes such as FS and FD or larger cast or sheet metal boxes are not classified as conduit bodies.

CONNECTOR, PRESSURE (SOLDERLESS). A device that establishes a connection between two or more conductors or between one or more conductors and a terminal by means of mechanical pressure and without the use of solder.

CONTINUOUS LOAD. A load where the maximum current is expected to continue for 3 hours or more.

COOKING UNIT, COUNTER-MOUNTED. A cooking appliance designed for mounting in or on a counter and consisting of one or more heating elements, internal wiring and built-in or separately mountable controls.

COPPER-CLAD ALUMINUM CONDUCTORS. Conductors drawn from a copper-clad aluminum rod with the copper metallurgically bonded to an aluminum core. The copper forms a minimum of 10 percent of the cross-sectional area of a solid conductor or each strand of a stranded conductor.

CUTOUT BOX. An enclosure designed for surface mounting and having swinging doors or covers secured directly to and telescoping with the walls of the box proper (see "Cabinet").

DEAD FRONT. Without live parts exposed to a person on the operating side of the equipment.

DEMAND FACTOR. The ratio of the maximum demand of a system, or part of a system, to the total connected load of a system or the part of the system under consideration.

DEVICE. A unit of an electrical system that carries or controls electrical energy as it principal function.

DISCONNECTING MEANS. A device, or group of devices, or other means by which the conductors of a circuit can be disconnected from their source of supply.

DWELLING

>   **Dwelling unit.** A single unit, providing complete and independent living facilities for one or more persons, including permanent provisions for living, sleeping, cooking and sanitation.

>   **One-family dwelling.** A building consisting solely of one dwelling unit.

>   **Two-family dwelling.** A building consisting solely of two dwelling units.

ENCLOSED. Surrounded by a case, housing, fence or walls that will prevent persons from accidentally contacting energized parts.

ENCLOSURE. The case or housing of apparatus, or the fence or walls surrounding an installation, to prevent personnel from accidentally contacting energized parts or to protect the equipment from physical damage.

ENERGIZED. Electrically connected to, or is, a source of voltage.

EQUIPMENT. A general term including material, fittings, devices, appliances, luminaires, apparatus, machinery and the like used as a part of, or in connection with, an electrical installation.

EXPOSED. (As applied to live parts.) Capable of being inadvertently touched or approached nearer than a safe distance by a person. It is applied to parts not suitably guarded, isolated or insulated.

EXPOSED. (As applied to wiring methods.) On or attached to the surface or behind panels designed to allow access.

EXTERNALLY OPERABLE. Capable of being operated without exposing the operator to contact with live parts.

FEEDER. All circuit conductors between the service equipment, or the source of a separately derived system, or other power supply source and the final branch-circuit overcurrent device.

FITTING. An accessory such as a locknut, bushing or other part of a wiring system that is intended primarily to perform a mechanical rather than an electrical function.

GROUND. The earth.

GROUNDED (GROUNDING). Connected (connecting) to ground or to a conductive body that extends the ground connection.

GROUNDED, EFFECTIVELY. Intentionally connected to earth through a ground connection or connections of sufficiently low impedance and having sufficient current-carrying capacity to prevent the buildup of voltages that may result in undue hazards to connected equipment or to persons.

GROUNDED CONDUCTOR. A system or circuit conductor that is intentionally grounded.

GROUNDING CONDUCTOR. A conductor used to connect equipment or the grounded circuit of a wiring system to a grounding electrode or electrodes.

GROUNDING CONDUCTOR, EQUIPMENT (EGC). The conductive path installed to connect normally noncurrent-carrying metal parts of equipment together and, to the system grounded conductor, the grounding electrode conductor or both.

GROUNDING ELECTRODE. A conducting object through which a direct connection to earth is established.

GROUNDING ELECTRODE CONDUCTOR. A conductor used to connect the system grounded conductor or the equipment to a grounding electrode or to a point on the grounding electrode system.

GROUND-FAULT CIRCUIT-INTERRUPTER. A device intended for the protection of personnel that functions to de-energize a circuit or portion thereof within an established period of time when a current to ground exceeds the value for a Class A device.

GUARDED. Covered, shielded, fenced, enclosed or otherwise protected by means of suitable covers, casings, barriers, rails, screens, mats or platforms to remove the likelihood of approach or contact by persons or objects to a point of danger.

IDENTIFIED. (As applied to equipment.) Recognizable as suitable for the specific purpose, function, use, environment, application, etc., where described in a particular code requirement.

INTERRUPTING RATING. The highest current at rated voltage that a device is intended to interrupt under standard test conditions.

INTERSYSTEM BONDING TERMINATION. A device that provides a means for connecting communications system(s) grounding conductor(s) and bonding conductor(s) at the service equipment or at the disconnecting means for buildings or structures supplied by a feeder or branch.

ISOLATED. (As applied to location.) Not readily accessible to persons unless special means for access are used.

KITCHEN. An area with a sink and permanent facilities for food preparation.

LABELED. Equipment or materials to which has been attached a label, symbol or other identifying mark of an organization acceptable to the authority having jurisdiction and concerned with product evaluation that maintains periodic inspection of production of labeled equipment or materials and by whose labeling the manufacturer indicates compliance with appropriate standards or performance in a specified manner.

LIGHTING OUTLET. An outlet intended for the direct connection of a lampholder or luminaire.

LISTED. Equipment, materials or services included in a list published by an organization that is acceptable to the authority having jurisdiction and concerned with evaluation of products or services, that maintains periodic inspection of production of listed equipment or materials or periodic evaluation of services, and whose listing states either that the equipment, material or services meets identified standards or has been tested and found suitable for a specified purpose.

LIVE PARTS. Energized conductive components.

LOCATION, DAMP. Location protected from weather and not subject to saturation with water or other liquids but subject to moderate degrees of moisture. Examples of such locations include partially protected locations under canopies, marquees, roofed open porches and like locations, and interior locations subject to moderate degrees of moisture, such as some basements, some barns and some cold-storage warehouses.

LOCATION, DRY. A location not normally subject to dampness or wetness. A location classified as dry may be temporarily subject to dampness or wetness, as in the case of a building under construction.

LOCATION, WET. Installations underground or in concrete slabs or masonry in direct contact with the earth and locations subject to saturation with water or other liquids, such as vehicle-washing areas, and locations exposed to weather.

LUMINAIRE. A complete lighting unit consisting of a light source such as a lamp or lamps together with the parts designed to position the light source and connect it to the power supply. A luminaire can include parts to protect the light source or the ballast or to distribute the light. A lampholder itself is not a luminaire.

MULTIOUTLET ASSEMBLY. A type of surface, or flush, or freestanding raceway; designed to hold conductors and receptacles, assembled in the field or at the factory.

NEUTRAL CONDUCTOR. The conductor connected to the neutral point of a system that is intended to carry current under normal conditions.

NEUTRAL POINT. The common point on a wye-connection in a polyphase system or midpoint on a single-phase, 3-wire system, or midpoint of a single-phase portion of a 3-phase delta system, or a midpoint of a 3-wire, direct-current system.

OUTLET. A point on the wiring system at which current is taken to supply utilization equipment.

OVERCURRENT. Any current in excess of the rated current of equipment or the ampacity of a conductor. Such current might result from overload, short circuit or ground fault.

OVERLOAD. Operation of equipment in excess of normal, full-load rating, or of a conductor in excess of rated ampacity that, when it persists for a sufficient length of time, would cause damage or dangerous overheating. A fault, such as a short circuit or ground fault, is not an overload.

PANELBOARD. A single panel or group of panel units designed for assembly in the form of a single panel, including buses and automatic overcurrent devices, and equipped with or without switches for the control of light, heat or power circuits, designed to be placed in a cabinet or cutout box placed in or against a wall, partition or other support and accessible only from the front.

PLENUM. A compartment or chamber to which one or more air ducts are connected and that forms part of the air distribution system.

POWER OUTLET. An enclosed assembly that may include receptacles, circuit breakers, fuseholders, fused switches, buses and watt-hour meter mounting means, intended to supply and control power to mobile homes, recreational vehicles or boats, or to serve as a means for distributing power required to operate mobile or temporarily installed equipment.

PREMISES WIRING (SYSTEM). Interior and exterior wiring, including power, lighting, control and signal circuit wiring together with all of their associated hardware, fittings and wiring devices, both permanently and temporarily installed. This includes wiring from the service point or power source to the outlets and wiring from and including the power source to the outlets where there is no service point. Such wiring does not include wiring internal to appliances, luminaires, motors, controllers, and similar equipment.

QUALIFIED PERSON. One who has the skills and knowledge related to the construction and operation of the electrical equipment and installations and has received safety training to recognize and avoid the hazards involved.

RACEWAY. An enclosed channel of metal or nonmetallic materials designed expressly for holding wires, cables, or busbars, with additional functions as permitted in this code. Raceways include, but are not limited to, rigid metal conduit, rigid nonmetallic conduit, intermediate metal conduit, liquid-tight flexible conduit, flexible metallic tubing, flexible metal conduit, electrical nonmetallic tubing, electrical metallic tubing, underfloor raceways, cellular concrete floor raceways, cellular metal floor raceways, surface raceways, wireways and busways.

RAINPROOF. Constructed, protected or treated so as to prevent rain from interfering with the successful operation of the apparatus under specified test conditions.

RAIN TIGHT. Constructed or protected so that exposure to a beating rain will not result in the entrance of water under specified test conditions.

RECEPTACLE. A receptacle is a contact device installed at the outlet for the connection of an attachment plug. A single receptacle is a single contact device with no other contact device on the same yoke. A multiple receptacle is two or more contact devices on the same yoke.

RECEPTACLE OUTLET. An outlet where one or more receptacles are installed.

SERVICE. The conductors and equipment for delivering energy from the serving utility to the wiring system of the premises served.

SERVICE CABLE. Service conductors made up in the form of a cable.

SERVICE CONDUCTORS. The conductors from the service point to the service disconnecting means.

SERVICE DROP. The overhead service conductors from the last pole or other aerial support to and including the splices, if any, connecting to the service-entrance conductors at the building or other structure.

SERVICE-ENTRANCE CONDUCTORS, OVERHEAD SYSTEM. The service conductors between the terminals of the service equipment and a point usually outside the building, clear of building walls, where joined by tap or splice to the service drop.

SERVICE-ENTRANCE CONDUCTORS, UNDERGROUND SYSTEM. The service conductors between the terminals of the service equipment and the point of connection to the service lateral.

SERVICE EQUIPMENT. The necessary equipment, usually consisting of a circuit breaker(s) or switch(es) and fuse(s), and their accessories, connected to the load end of the service conductors to a building or other structure, or an otherwise designated area, and intended to constitute the main control and cutoff of the supply.

SERVICE LATERAL. The underground service conductors between the street main, including any risers at a pole or other structure or from transformers, and the first point of connection to the service-entrance conductors in a terminal box or meter or other enclosure, inside or outside the building wall. Where

there is no terminal box, meter or other enclosure with adequate space, the point of connection shall be considered to be the point of entrance of the service conductors into the building.

SERVICE POINT. Service point is the point of connection between the facilities of the serving utility and the premises wiring.

STRUCTURE. That which is built or constructed.

SWITCHES

    General-use switch. A switch intended for use in general distribution and branch circuits. It is rated in amperes and is capable of interrupting its rated current at its rated voltage.

    General-use snap switch. A form of general-use switch constructed so that it can be installed in device boxes or on box covers or otherwise used in conjunction with wiring systems recognized by this code.

    Isolating switch. A switch intended for isolating an electric circuit from the source of power. It has no interrupting rating and is intended to be operated only after the circuit has been opened by some other means.

    Motor-circuit switch. A switch, rated in horsepower that is capable of interrupting the maximum operating overload current of a motor of the same horsepower rating as the switch at the rated voltage.

UNGROUNDED. Not connected to ground or to a conductive body that extends the ground connection.

UTILIZATION EQUIPMENT. Equipment that utilizes electric energy for electronic, electromechanical, chemical, heating, lighting or similar purposes.

VENTILATED. Provided with a means to permit circulation of air sufficient to remove an excess of heat, fumes or vapors.

VOLTAGE (OF A CIRCUIT). The greatest root-mean-square (rms) (effective) difference of potential between any two conductors of the circuit concerned.

VOLTAGE, NOMINAL. A nominal value assigned to a circuit or system for the purpose of conveniently designating its voltage class (e.g., 120/240). The actual voltage at which a circuit operates can vary from the nominal within a range that permits satisfactory operation of equipment.

VOLTAGE TO GROUND. For grounded circuits, the voltage between the given conductor and that point or conductor of the circuit that is grounded. For ungrounded circuits, the greatest voltage between the given conductor and any other conductor of the circuit.

WATERTIGHT. Constructed so that moisture will not enter the enclosure under specified test conditions.

WEATHERPROOF. Constructed or protected so that exposure to the weather will not interfere with successful operation.

CHAPTER 36

SERVICES

SECTION E3601
GENERAL SERVICES

E3601.1 Scope. This chapter covers service conductors and equipment for the control and protection of services and their installation requirements.

E3601.2 Number of services. One- and two-family dwellings shall be supplied by only one service.

E3601.3 One building or other structure not to be supplied through another. Service conductors supplying a building or other structure shall not pass through the interior of another building or other structure.

E3601.4 Other conductors in raceway or cable. Conductors other than service conductors shall not be installed in the same service raceway or service cable.

Exceptions:

1. Grounding conductors and bonding jumpers.

2. Load management control conductors having overcurrent protection.

E3601.5 Raceway seal. Where a service raceway enters from an underground distribution system, it shall be sealed in accordance with Section E3803.6.

E3601.6 Service disconnect required. Means shall be provided to disconnect all conductors in a building or other structure from the service entrance conductors.

E3601.6.1 Marking of service equipment and disconnects. Service disconnects shall be permanently marked as a service disconnect. Service equipment shall be listed for the purpose. Individual meter socket enclosures shall not be considered service equipment.

E3601.6.2 Service disconnect location. The service disconnecting means shall be installed at a readily accessible location either outside of a building or inside nearest the point of entrance of the service conductors. Service disconnecting means shall not be installed in bathrooms. Each occupant shall have access to the disconnect serving the dwelling unit in which they reside.

E3601.7 Maximum number of disconnects. The service disconnecting means shall consist of not more than six switches or six circuit breakers mounted in a single enclosure or in a group of separate enclosures.

SECTION E3602
SERVICE SIZE AND RATING

E3602.1 Ampacity of ungrounded conductors. Ungrounded service conductors shall have an ampacity of not less than the load served. For one-family dwellings, the ampacity of the ungrounded conductors shall be not less than 100 amperes, 3 wire. For all other installations, the ampacity of the ungrounded conductors shall be not less than 60 amperes.

E3602.2 Service load. The minimum load for ungrounded service conductors and service devices that serve 100 percent of the dwelling unit load shall be computed in accordance with Table E3602.2. Ungrounded service conductors and service devices that serve less than 100 percent of the dwelling unit load shall be computed as required for feeders in accordance with Chapter 37.

TABLE E3602.2
MINIMUM SERVICE LOAD CALCULATION

LOADS AND PROCEDURE
3 volt-amperes per square foot of floor area for general lighting and general use receptacle outlets.
Plus
1,500 volt-amperes multiplied by total number of 20-ampere-rated small appliance and laundry circuits.
Plus
The nameplate volt-ampere rating of all fastened-in-place, permanently connected or dedicated circuit-supplied appliances such as ranges, ovens, cooking units, clothes dryers not connected to the laundry branch circuit and water heaters.
Apply the following demand factors to the above subtotal:
The minimum subtotal for the loads above shall be 100 percent of the first 10,000 volt-amperes of the sum of the above loads plus 40 percent of any portion of the sum that is in excess of 10,000 volt-amperes.
Plus the largest of the following:
One-hundred percent of the nameplate rating(s) of the air-conditioning and cooling equipment.
One hundred percent of the nameplate rating(s) of the heat pump where a heat pump is used without any supplemental electric heating.
One-hundred percent of the nameplate rating of the electric thermal storage and other heating systems where the usual load is expected to be continuous at the full nameplate value. Systems qualifying under this selection shall not be figured under any other category in this table.
One-hundred percent of nameplate rating of the heat pump compressor and sixty-five percent of the supplemental electric heating load for central electric space-heating systems. If the heat pump compressor is prevented from operating at the same time as the supplementary heat, the compressor load does not need to be added to the supplementary heat load for the total central electric space-heating load.
Sixty-five percent of nameplate rating(s) of electric space-heating units if less than four separately controlled units.
Forty percent of nameplate rating(s) of electric space-heating units of four or more separately controlled units.
The minimum total load in amperes shall be the volt-ampere sum calculated above divided by 240 volts.

E3602.2.1 Services under 100 amperes. Services that are not required to be 100 amperes shall be sized in accordance with Chapter 37.

E3602.3 Rating of service disconnect. The combined rating of all individual service disconnects serving a single dwelling unit shall not be less than the load determined from Table E3602.2 and shall not be less than as specified in Section E3602.1.

E3602.4 Voltage rating. Systems shall be three-wire, 120/240-volt, single-phase with a grounded neutral.

SECTION E3603
SERVICE, FEEDER AND GROUNDING ELECTRODE CONDUCTOR SIZING

E3603.1 Grounded and ungrounded service conductor size. Conductors used as ungrounded service entrance conductors, service lateral conductors, and feeder conductors that serve as the main power feeder to a dwelling unit shall be those listed in Table E3603.1. The main power feeder shall be the feeder(s) between the main disconnect and the panelboard that supplies, either by branch circuits or by feeders, or both, all loads that are part of or are associated with the dwelling unit. The feeder conductors to a dwelling unit shall not be required to have an allowable ampacity greater than that of the service-entrance conductors that supply them. Ungrounded service conductors shall have a minimum size in accordance with Table E3603.1. The grounded conductor ampacity shall be not less than the maximum unbalance of the load and its size shall be not smaller than the required minimum grounding electrode conductor size specified in Table E3603.1.

E3603.2 Ungrounded service conductors for accessory buildings and structures. Ungrounded conductors for other than dwelling units shall have an ampacity of not less than 60 amperes and shall be sized as required for feeders in Chapter 37.

Exceptions:

1. For limited loads of a single branch circuit, the service conductors shall have an ampacity of not less than 15 amperes.

2. For loads consisting of not more than two two-wire branch circuits, the service conductors shall have an ampacity of not less than 30 amperes.

TABLE E3603.1
SERVICE CONDUCTOR AND GROUNDING ELECTRODE CONDUCTOR SIZING

CONDUCTOR TYPES AND SIZES—THHN, THHW, THW, THWN, USE, RHH, RHW, XHHW, RHW-2, THW-2, THWN-2, XHHW-2, SE, USE-2 (Parallel sets of 1/0 and larger conductors are permitted in either a single raceway or in separate raceways)		SERVICE OR FEEDER RATING (AMPERES)	MINIMUM GROUNDING ELECTRODE CONDUCTOR SIZE[a]	
Copper (AWG)	Aluminum and copper–clad aluminum (AWG)	Maximum load (amps)	Copper (AWG)	Aluminum (AWG)
4	2	100	8[b]	6[c]
3	1	110	8[b]	6[c]
2	1/0	125	8[b]	6[c]
1	2/0	150	6[c]	4
1/0	3/0	175	6[c]	4
2/0	4/0 or two sets of 1/0	200	4[d]	2[d]
3/0	250 kcmil or two sets of 2/0	225	4[d]	2[d]
4/0 or two sets of 1/0	300 kcmil or two sets of 3/0	250	2[d]	1/0[d]
250 kcmil or two sets of 2/0	350 kcmil or two sets of 4/0	300	2[d]	1/0[d]
350 kcmil or two sets of 3/0	500 kcmil or two sets of 250 kcmil	350	2[d]	1/0[d]
400 kcmil or two sets of 4/0	600 kcmil or two sets of 300 kcmil	400	1/0[d]	3/0[d]

For SI: 1 inch = 25.4 mm.

a. Where protected by a ferrous metal raceway, grounding electrode conductors shall be electrically bonded to the ferrous metal raceway at both ends.

b. An 8 AWG grounding electrode conductor shall be protected with metal conduit, nonmetallic conduit, electrical metallic tubing or cable armor

c. Where not protected, 6 AWG grounding electrode conductor shall closely follow a structural surface for physical protection. The supports shall be spaced not more than 24 inches on center and shall be within 12 inches of any enclosure or termination.

d. Where the sole grounding electrode system is a ground rod or pipe as covered in Section E3608.2, the grounding electrode conductor shall not be required to be larger than 6 AWG copper or 4 AWG aluminum. Where the sole grounding electrode system is the footing steel as covered in Section E3608.1.2, the grounding electrode conductor shall not be required to be larger than 4 AWG copper conductor.

E3603.3 Overload protection. Each ungrounded service conductor shall have overload protection.

E3603.3.1 Ungrounded conductor. Overload protection shall be provided by an overcurrent device installed in series with each ungrounded service conductor. The overcurrent device shall have a rating or setting not higher than the allowable service or feeder rating specified in Table E3603.1. A set of fuses shall be considered all the fuses required to protect all of the ungrounded conductors of a circuit. Single pole circuit breakers, grouped in accordance with Section E3601.7, shall be considered as one protective device.

Exception: Two to six circuit breakers or sets of fuses shall be permitted as the overcurrent device to provide the overload protection. The sum of the ratings of the circuit breakers or fuses shall be permitted to exceed the ampacity of the service conductors, provided that the calculated load does not exceed the ampacity of the service conductors.

E3603.3.2 Not in grounded conductor. Overcurrent devices shall not be connected in series with a grounded service conductor except where a circuit breaker is used that simultaneously opens all conductors of the circuit.

E3603.3.3 Location. The service overcurrent device shall be an integral part of the service disconnecting means or shall be located immediately adjacent thereto.

E3603.4 Grounding electrode conductor size. The grounding electrode conductors shall be sized based on the size of the service entrance conductors as required in Table E3603.1.

E3603.5 Temperature limitations. Except where the equipment is marked otherwise, conductor ampacities used in determining equipment termination provisions shall be based on Table E3603.1.

SECTION E3604
OVERHEAD SERVICE-DROP AND SERVICE CONDUCTOR INSTALLATION

E3604.1 Clearances on buildings. Open conductors and multiconductor cables without an overall outer jacket shall have a clearance of not less than 3 feet (914 mm) from the sides of doors, porches, decks, stairs, ladders, fire escapes and balconies, and from the sides and bottom of windows that open. See Figure E3604.1.

E3604.2 Vertical clearances. Service-drop conductors shall not have ready access and shall comply with Sections E3604.2.1 and E3604.2.2.

E3604.2.1 Above roofs. Conductors shall have a vertical clearance of not less than 8 feet (2438 mm) above the roof surface. The vertical clearance above the roof level shall be maintained for a distance of not less than 3 feet (914 mm)

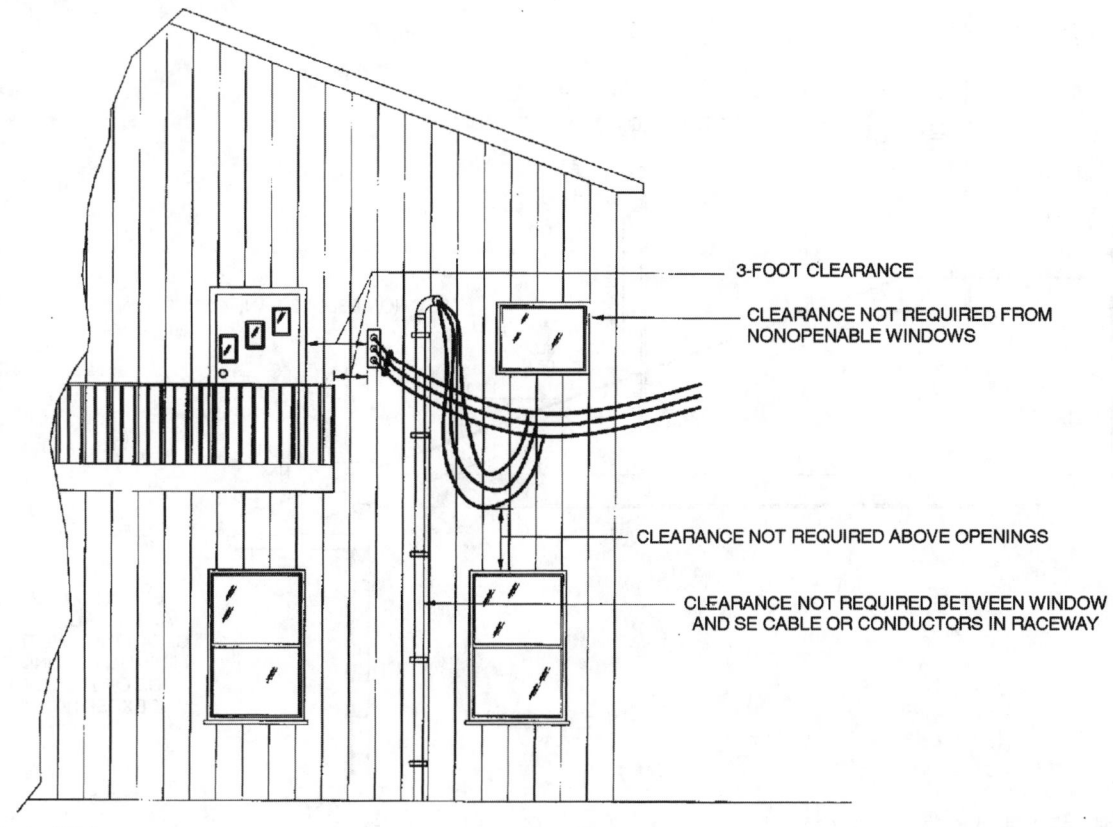

3-FOOT CLEARANCE

CLEARANCE NOT REQUIRED FROM NONOPENABLE WINDOWS

CLEARANCE NOT REQUIRED ABOVE OPENINGS

CLEARANCE NOT REQUIRED BETWEEN WINDOW AND SE CABLE OR CONDUCTORS IN RACEWAY

For SI: 1 foot = 304.8 mm.

FIGURE E3604.1
CLEARANCES FROM BUILDING OPENINGS

in all directions from the edge of the roof. See Figure E3604.2.1.

Exceptions:

1. Conductors above a roof surface subject to pedestrian traffic shall have a vertical clearance from the roof surface in accordance with Section E3604.2.2.

2. Where the roof has a slope of 4 inches (102 mm) in 12 inches (305 mm), or greater, the minimum clearance shall be 3 feet (914 mm).

3. The minimum clearance above only the overhanging portion of the roof shall not be less than 18 inches (457 mm) where not more than 6 feet (1829 mm) of conductor length passes over 4 feet (1219 mm) or less of roof surface measured horizontally and such conductors are terminated at a through-the-roof raceway or approved support.

4. The requirement for maintaining the vertical clearance for a distance of 3 feet (914 mm) from the edge of the roof shall not apply to the final conductor span where the service drop is attached to the side of a building.

E3604.2.2 Vertical clearance from grade. Service-drop conductors shall have the following minimum clearances from final grade:

1. For service-drop cables supported on and cabled together with a grounded bare messenger wire, the minimum vertical clearance shall be 10 feet (3048 mm) at the electric service entrance to buildings, at the lowest point of the drip loop of the building electric entrance, and above areas or sidewalks accessed by pedestrians only. Such clearance shall be measured from final grade or other accessible surfaces.

2. Twelve feet (3658 mm)—over residential property and driveways.

3. Eighteen feet (5486 mm)—over public streets, alleys, roads or parking areas subject to truck traffic.

E3604.3 Point of attachment. The point of attachment of the service-drop conductors to a building or other structure shall provide the minimum clearances as specified in Sections E3604.1 through E3604.2.2. In no case shall the point of attachment be less than 10 feet (3048 mm) above finished grade.

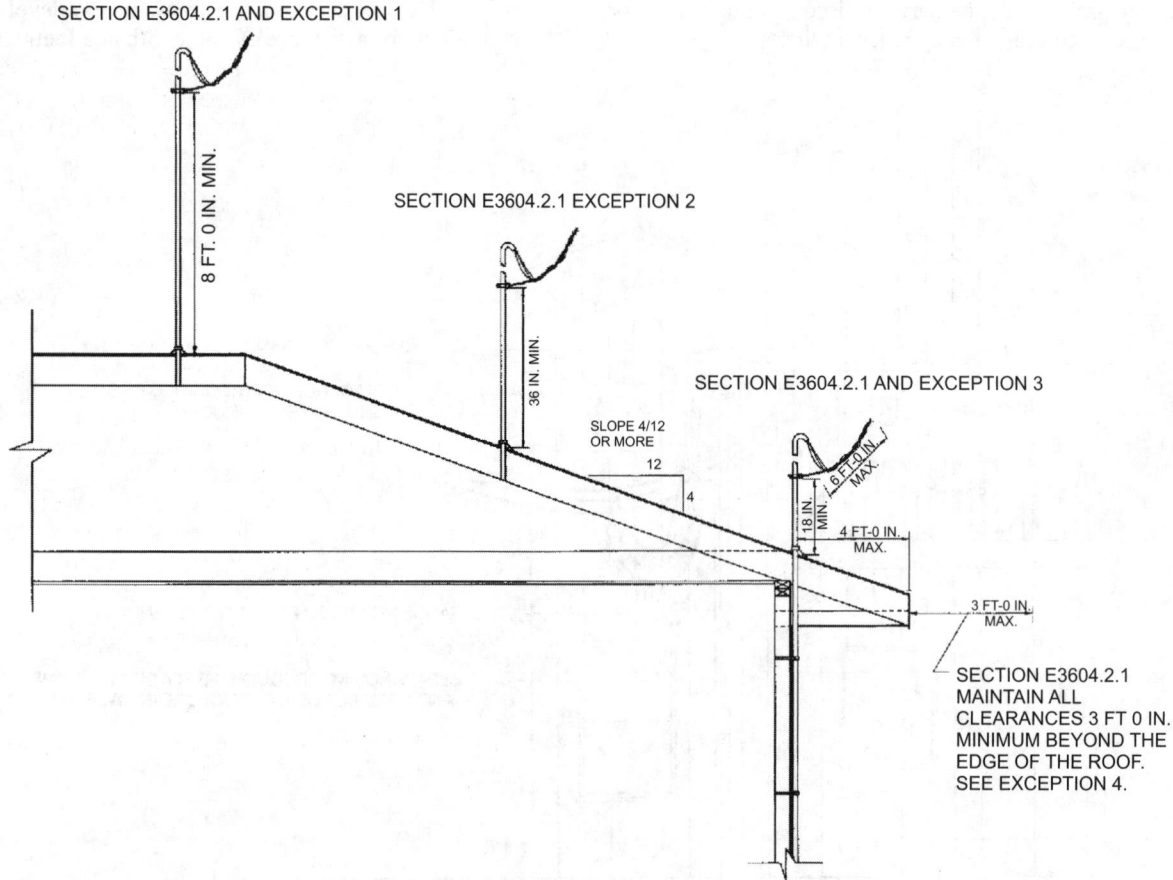

For SI: 1 inch = 25.4 mm, 1 foot = 304.8 mm.

FIGURE E3604.2.1
CLEARANCES FROM ROOFS

E3604.4 Means of attachment. Multiconductor cables used for service drops shall be attached to buildings or other structures by fittings approved for the purpose.

E3604.5 Service masts as supports. Where a service mast is used for the support of service-drop conductors, it shall be of adequate strength or be supported by braces or guys to withstand the strain imposed by the service drop. Where raceway-type service masts are used, all equipment shall be approved. Only power service drop conductors shall be permitted to be attached to a service mast.

E3604.6 Supports over buildings. Service-drop conductors passing over a roof shall be securely supported. Where practicable, such supports shall be independent of the building.

SECTION E3605
SERVICE-ENTRANCE CONDUCTORS

E3605.1 Insulation of service-entrance conductors. Service-entrance conductors entering or on the exterior of buildings or other structures shall be insulated in accordance with Section E3406.5.

Exceptions:

1. A copper grounded conductor shall not be required to be insulated where it is:

   1.1. In a raceway or part of a service cable assembly,

   1.2. Directly buried in soil of suitable condition, or

   1.3. Part of a cable assembly listed for direct burial without regard to soil conditions.

2. An aluminum or copper-clad aluminum grounded conductor shall not be required to be insulated where part of a cable or where identified for direct burial or utilization in underground raceways.

E3605.2 Wiring methods for services. Service-entrance wiring methods shall be installed in accordance with the applicable requirements in Chapter 38.

E3605.3 Spliced conductors. Service-entrance conductors shall be permitted to be spliced or tapped. Splices shall be made in enclosures or, if directly buried, with listed underground splice kits. Conductor splices shall be made in accordance with Chapters 34, 37, 38 and 39.

E3605.4 Protection against physical damage. Underground service-entrance conductors shall be protected against physical damage in accordance with Chapter 38.

E3605.5 Protection of service cables against damage. Above-ground service-entrance cables, where subject to physical damage, shall be protected by one or more of the following: rigid metal conduit, intermediate metal conduit, Schedule 80 PVC conduit, electrical metallic tubing or other approved means.

E3605.6 Locations exposed to direct sunlight. Insulated conductors and cables used where exposed to direct rays of the sun shall comply with one of the following:

1. The conductors and cables shall be listed, or listed and marked, as being sunlight resistant.

2. The conductors and cables are covered with insulating material, such as tape or sleeving, that is listed, or listed and marked, as being sunlight resistant.

E3605.7 Mounting supports. Service cables shall be supported by straps or other approved means within 12 inches (305 mm) of every service head, gooseneck or connection to a raceway or enclosure and at intervals not exceeding 30 inches (762 mm).

E3605.8 Raceways to drain. Where exposed to the weather, raceways enclosing service-entrance conductors shall be suitable for use in wet locations and arranged to drain. Where embedded in masonry, raceways shall be arranged to drain.

E3605.9 Overhead service locations. Connections at service heads shall be in accordance with Sections E3605.9.1 through E3605.9.7.

E3605.9.1 Rain-tight service head. Service raceways shall be equipped with a rain-tight service head at the point of connection to service-drop conductors. The service head shall comply with the requirements for fittings in Section E3905.12.

E3605.9.2 Service cable, service head or gooseneck. Service cable shall be equipped with a rain-tight service head or shall be formed into a gooseneck in an approved manner. The service head shall comply with the requirements for fittings in Section E3905.12.

E3605.9.3 Service head location. Service heads, and goosenecks in service-entrance cables, shall be located above the point of attachment of the service-drop conductors to the building or other structure.

Exception: Where it is impracticable to locate the service head or gooseneck above the point of attachment, the service head or gooseneck location shall be not more than 24 inches (610 mm) from the point of attachment.

E3605.9.4 Separately bushed openings. Service heads shall have conductors of different potential brought out through separately bushed openings.

E3605.9.5 Drip loops. Drip loops shall be formed on individual conductors. To prevent the entrance of moisture, service-entrance conductors shall be connected to the service-drop conductors either below the level of the service head or below the level of the termination of the service-entrance cable sheath.

E3605.9.6 Conductor arrangement. Service-drop conductors and service-entrance conductors shall be arranged so that water will not enter service raceways or equipment.

E3605.9.7 Secured. Service cables shall be held securely in place.

SECTION E3606
SERVICE EQUIPMENT—GENERAL

E3606.1 Service equipment enclosures. Energized parts of service equipment shall be enclosed.

E3606.2 Working space. In no case shall the working space in the vicinity of service equipment be less than that specified in Chapter 34.

E3606.3 Available short-circuit current. Service equipment shall be suitable for the maximum fault current available at its supply terminals, but not less than 10,000 amperes.

E3606.4 Marking. Service equipment shall be marked to identify it as being suitable for use as service equipment. Individual meter socket enclosures shall not be considered service equipment.

SECTION E3607
SYSTEM GROUNDING

E3607.1 System service ground. The premises wiring system shall be grounded at the service with a grounding electrode conductor connected to a grounding electrode system as required by this code. Grounding electrode conductors shall be sized in accordance with Table E3603.1.

E3607.2 Location of grounding electrode conductor connection. The grounding electrode conductor shall be connected to the grounded service conductor at any accessible point from the load end of the service drop or service lateral to and including the terminal or bus to which the grounded service conductor is connected at the service disconnecting means. A grounding connection shall not be made to any grounded circuit conductor on the load side of the service disconnecting means, except as provided in Section E3607.3.2.

E3607.3 Buildings or structures supplied by feeder(s) or branch circuit(s). Buildings or structures supplied by feeder(s) or branch circuit(s) shall have a grounding electrode or grounding electrode system installed in accordance with Section E3608. The grounding electrode conductor(s) shall be connected in a manner specified in Section E3607.3.1 or, for existing premises wiring systems only, Section E3607.3.2. Where there is no existing grounding electrode, the grounding electrode(s) required in Section E3608 shall be installed.

> **Exception:** A grounding electrode shall not be required where only one branch circuit, including a multiwire branch circuit, supplies the building or structure and the branch circuit includes an equipment grounding conductor for grounding the noncurrent-carrying parts of all equipment. For the purposes of this section, a multiwire branch circuit shall be considered as a single branch circuit.

E3607.3.1 Equipment grounding conductor. An equipment grounding conductor as described in Section E3908 shall be run with the supply conductors and connected to the building or structure disconnecting means and to the grounding electrode(s). The equipment grounding conductor shall be used for grounding or bonding of equipment, structures or frames required to be grounded or bonded. The equipment grounding conductor shall be sized in accordance with Section E3908.12. Any installed grounded conductor shall not be connected to the equipment grounding conductor or to the grounding electrode(s).

E3607.3.2 Grounded conductor, existing premises. This section shall apply only to existing premises wiring systems. Where an equipment grounding conductor is not run with the supply conductors to the building or structure, there are no continuous metallic paths bonded to the grounding system in both buildings or structures involved, and ground-fault protection of equipment has not been installed on the supply side of the feeder(s), the grounded conductor run with the supply to the buildings or structure shall be connected to the building or structure disconnecting means and to the grounding electrode(s) and shall be used for grounding or bonding of equipment, structures, or frames required to be grounded or bonded. Where used for grounding in accordance with this provision, the grounded conductor shall be not smaller than the larger of:

1. That required by Section E3704.3.

2. That required by Section E3908.12.

E3607.4 Grounding electrode conductor. A grounding electrode conductor shall be used to connect the equipment grounding conductors, the service equipment enclosures, and the grounded service conductor to the grounding electrode(s). This conductor shall be sized in accordance with Table E3603.1.

E3607.5 Main bonding jumper. An unspliced main bonding jumper shall be used to connect the equipment grounding conductor(s) and the service-disconnect enclosure to the grounded conductor of the system within the enclosure for each service disconnect.

E3607.6 Common grounding electrode. Where an ac system is connected to a grounding electrode in or at a building or structure, the same electrode shall be used to ground conductor enclosures and equipment in or on that building or structure. Where separate services, feeders or branch circuits supply a building and are required to be connected to a grounding electrode(s), the same grounding electrode(s) shall be used. Two or more grounding electrodes that are effectively bonded together shall be considered as a single grounding electrode system.

SECTION E3608
GROUNDING ELECTRODE SYSTEM

E3608.1 Grounding electrode system. All electrodes specified in Sections E3608.1.1, E3608.1.2, E3608.1.3, E3608.1.4 E3608.1.5 and E3608.1.6 that are present at each building or structure served shall be bonded together to form the grounding electrode system. Where none of these electrodes are present, one or more of the electrodes specified in Sections E3608.1.3, E3608.1.4, E3608.1.5 and E3608.1.6 shall be installed and used.

> **Exception:** Concrete-encased electrodes of existing buildings or structures shall not be required to be part of the grounding electrode system where the steel reinforcing bars or rods are not accessible for use without disturbing the concrete.

E3608.1.1 Metal underground water pipe. A metal underground water pipe that is in direct contact with the earth for 10 feet (3048 mm) or more, including any well casing effectively bonded to the pipe and that is electrically continuous, or made electrically continuous by bonding around insulating joints or insulating pipe to the points of connection of the grounding electrode conductor and the bonding conductors, shall be considered as a grounding electrode (see Section E3608.1). Interior metal water piping located more than 5 feet (1524 mm) from the entrance to the building shall not be used as part of the grounding electrode system or as a conductor to interconnect electrodes that are part of the grounding electrode system.

E3608.1.1.1 Installation. Continuity of the grounding path or the bonding connection to interior piping shall not rely on water meters, filtering devices and similar equipment. A metal underground water pipe shall be supplemented by an additional electrode of a type specified in Sections E3608.1.2 through E3608.1.6. The supplemental electrode shall be bonded to the grounding electrode conductor, the grounded service entrance conductor, a nonflexible grounded service raceway or any grounded service enclosure. Where the supplemental electrode is a rod, pipe or plate electrode in accordance with Section E3608.1.4 or E3608.1.5, it shall comply with Section E3608.4.

Where the supplemental electrode is a rod, pipe or plate electrode in accordance with Section E3608.1.4 or E3608.1.5, that portion of the bonding jumper that is the sole connection to the supplemental grounding electrode shall not be required to be larger than 6 AWG copper or 4 AWG aluminum wire.

E3608.1.2 Concrete-encased electrode. An electrode encased by at least 2 inches (51 mm) of concrete, located horizontally near the bottom or vertically and within that portion of a concrete foundation or footing that is in direct contact with the earth, consisting of at least 20 feet (6096 mm) of one or more bare or zinc-galvanized or other electrically conductive coated steel reinforcing bars or rods of not less than $^1/_2$ inch (12.7 mm) diameter, or consisting of at least 20 feet (6096 mm) of bare copper conductor not smaller than 4 AWG shall be considered as a grounding electrode. Reinforcing bars shall be permitted to be bonded together by the usual steel tie wires or other effective means. Where multiple concrete-encased electrodes are present at a building or structure, only one shall be required to be bonded into the grounding electrode system.

E3608.1.3 Ground rings. A ground ring encircling the building or structure, in direct contact with the earth at a depth below the earth's surface of not less than 30 inches (762 mm), consisting of at least 20 feet (6096 mm) of bare copper conductor not smaller than 2 AWG shall be considered as a grounding electrode.

E3608.1.4 Rod and pipe electrodes. Rod and pipe electrodes not less than 8 feet (2438 mm) in length and consisting of the following materials shall be considered as a grounding electrode:

1. Grounding electrodes of pipe or conduit shall not be smaller than trade size $^3/_4$ (metric designator 21) and, where of iron or steel, shall have the outer surface galvanized or otherwise metal-coated for corrosion protection.

2. Grounding electrodes of rods of stainless steel and copper or zinc-coated steel shall be at least $^5/_8$ inch (15.9 mm) in diameter. Stainless steel rods less than $^5/_8$ inch (15.9 mm) in diameter, nonferrous rods or their equivalent shall be listed and shall be not less than $^1/_2$ inch (12.7 mm) in diameter.

E3608.1.4.1 Installation. The rod and pipe electrodes shall be installed such that at least 8 feet (2438 mm) of length is in contact with the soil. They shall be driven to a depth of not less than 8 feet (2438 mm) except that, where rock bottom is encountered, electrodes shall be driven at an oblique angle not to exceed 45 degrees from the vertical or shall be buried in a trench that is at least 30 inches (762 mm) deep. The upper end of the electrodes shall be flush with or below ground level except where the aboveground end and the grounding electrode conductor attachment are protected against physical damage.

E3608.1.5 Plate electrodes. A plate electrode that exposes not less than 2 square feet (0.186 m²) of surface to exterior soil shall be considered as a grounding electrode. Electrodes of iron or steel plates shall be at least $^1/_4$ inch (6.4 mm) in thickness. Electrodes of nonferrous metal shall be at least 0.06 inch (1.5 mm) in thickness. Plate electrodes shall be installed not less than 30 inches (762 mm) below the surface of the earth.

E3608.1.6 Other electrodes. In addition to the grounding electrodes specified in Sections E3608.1.1 through E3608.1.5, other listed grounding electrodes shall be permitted.

E3608.2 Bonding jumper. The bonding jumper(s) used to connect the grounding electrodes together to form the grounding electrode system shall be installed in accordance with Sections E3610.2, and E3610.3, shall be sized in accordance with Section E3603.4, and shall be connected in the manner specified in Section E3611.1.

E3608.3 Rod, pipe and plate electrode requirements. Where practicable, rod, pipe and plate electrodes shall be embedded below permanent moisture level. Such electrodes shall be free from nonconductive coatings such as paint or enamel. Where more than one such electrode is used, each electrode of one grounding system shall be not less than 6 feet (1829 mm) from any other electrode of another grounding system. Two or more grounding electrodes that are effectively bonded together shall be considered as a single grounding electrode system. That portion of a bonding jumper that is the sole connection to a rod, pipe or plate electrode shall not be required to be larger than 6 AWG copper or 4 AWG aluminum wire.

E3608.4 Resistance of rod, pipe and plate electrodes. A single electrode consisting of a rod, pipe or plate that does not have a resistance to ground of 25 ohms or less shall be augmented by one additional electrode of any of the types specified in Sections E3608.1.2 through E3608.1.6. Where multiple listed electrodes or rod, pipe or plate electrodes are installed to meet the requirements of this section, they shall be not less than 6 feet (1829 mm) apart.

E3608.5 Aluminum electrodes. Aluminum electrodes shall not be permitted.

E3608.6 Metal underground gas piping system. A metal underground gas piping system shall not be used as a grounding electrode.

SECTION E3609
BONDING

E3609.1 General. Bonding shall be provided where necessary to ensure electrical continuity and the capacity to conduct safely any fault current likely to be imposed.

E3609.2 Bonding of services. The noncurrent-carrying metal parts of the following equipment shall be effectively bonded together:

1. The service raceways or service cable armor.

2. All service enclosures containing service conductors, including meter fittings, and boxes, interposed in the service raceway or armor.

E3609.3 Bonding for other systems. An intersystem bonding termination for connecting intersystem bonding and grounding conductors required for other systems shall be provided external to enclosures at the service equipment and at the disconnecting means for any additional buildings or structures. The intersystem bonding termination shall be accessible for connection and inspection. The intersystem bonding termination shall have the capacity for connection of not less than three intersystem bonding conductors. The intersystem bonding termination device shall not interfere with the opening of a service or metering equipment enclosure. The intersystem bonding termination shall be one of the following:

1. A set of terminals securely mounted to the meter enclosure and electrically connected to the meter enclosure. The terminals shall be listed as grounding and bonding equipment.

2. A bonding bar near the service equipment enclosure, meter enclosure, or raceway for service conductors. The bonding bar shall be connected with a minimum 6 AWG copper conductor to an equipment grounding conductor(s) in the service equipment enclosure, to a meter enclosure, or to an exposed nonflexible metallic raceway.

3. A bonding bar near the grounding electrode conductor. The bonding bar shall be connected to the grounding electrode conductor with a minimum 6 AWG copper conductor.

E3609.4 Method of bonding at the service. Electrical continuity at service equipment, service raceways and service conductor enclosures shall be ensured by one or more of the methods specified in Sections E3609.4.1 through E3609.4.4.

Bonding jumpers meeting the other requirements of this code shall be used around concentric or eccentric knockouts that are punched or otherwise formed so as to impair the electrical connection to ground. Standard locknuts or bushings shall not be the sole means for the bonding required by this section.

E3609.4.1 Grounded service conductor. Equipment shall be bonded to the grounded service conductor in a manner provided in this code.

E3609.4.2 Threaded connections. Equipment shall be bonded by connections using threaded couplings or threaded bosses on enclosures. Such connections shall be made wrench tight.

E3609.4.3 Threadless couplings and connectors. Equipment shall be bonded by threadless couplings and connectors for metal raceways and metal-clad cables. Such couplings and connectors shall be made wrench tight. Standard locknuts or bushings shall not be used for the bonding required by this section.

E3609.4.4 Other devices. Equipment shall be bonded by other listed devices, such as bonding-type locknuts, bushings and bushings with bonding jumpers.

E3609.5 Sizing bonding jumper on supply side of service and main bonding jumper. The bonding jumper shall not be smaller than the sizes shown in Table E3603.1 for grounding electrode conductors. Where the service-entrance conductors are paralleled in two or more raceways or cables, the equipment bonding jumper, where routed with the raceways or cables, shall be run in parallel. The size of the bonding jumper for each raceway or cable shall be based on the size of the service-entrance conductors in each raceway or cable.

E3609.6 Metal water piping bonding. The metal water piping system shall be bonded to the service equipment enclosure, the grounded conductor at the service, the grounding electrode conductor where of sufficient size, or to the one or more grounding electrodes used. The bonding jumper shall be sized in accordance with Table E3603.1. The points of attachment of the bonding jumper(s) shall be accessible.

E3609.7 Bonding other metal piping. Where installed in or attached to a building or structure, metal piping systems, including gas piping, capable of becoming energized shall be bonded to the service equipment enclosure, the grounded conductor at the service, the grounding electrode conductor where of sufficient size, or to the one or more grounding electrodes used. The bonding jumper shall be sized in accordance with Table E3908.12 using the rating of the circuit capable of energizing the piping. The equipment grounding conductor for the circuit that is capable of energizing the piping shall be permitted to serve as the bonding means. The points of attachment of the bonding jumper(s) shall be accessible.

SECTION E3610
GROUNDING ELECTRODE CONDUCTORS

E3610.1 Continuous. The grounding electrode conductor shall be unspliced and shall run to any convenient grounding electrode available in the grounding electrode system where the other electrode(s), if any, are connected by bonding jumpers in accordance with Section E3608.2, or to one or more grounding electrode(s) individually. The grounding electrode conductor shall be sized for the largest grounding electrode conductor required among all of the electrodes connected to it.

Exception: Splicing of the grounding electrode conductor by irreversible compression-type connectors listed as grounding and bonding equipment or by the exothermic welding process shall not be prohibited.

E3610.2 Securing and protection against physical damage. Where exposed, a grounding electrode conductor or its enclosure shall be securely fastened to the surface on which it is carried. A 4 AWG or larger conductor shall be protected where exposed to physical damage. A 6 AWG grounding conductor that is free from exposure to physical damage shall be permitted to be run along the surface of the building construction without metal covering or protection where it is and securely fastened to the construction; otherwise, it shall be in rigid metal conduit, intermediate metal conduit, rigid nonmetallic conduit, electrical metallic tubing or cable armor. Grounding electrode conductors smaller than 6 AWG shall be in rigid metal conduit, intermediate metal conduit, rigid nonmetallic conduit, electrical metallic tubing or cable armor.

Bare aluminum or copper-clad aluminum grounding conductors shall not be used where in direct contact with masonry or the earth or where subject to corrosive conditions. Where used outside, aluminum or copper-clad aluminum grounding conductors shall not be installed within 18 inches (457 mm) of the earth.

E3610.3 Enclosures for grounding electrode conductors. Ferrous metal enclosures for grounding electrode conductors shall be electrically continuous from the point of attachment to cabinets or equipment to the grounding electrode, and shall be securely fastened to the ground clamp or fitting. Nonferrous metal enclosures shall not be required to be electrically continuous. Ferrous metal enclosures that are not physically continuous from cabinet or equipment to the grounding electrode shall be made electrically continuous by bonding each end to the grounding conductor. The bonding jumper for a grounding electrode conductor raceway shall be the same size or larger than the required enclosed grounding electrode conductor.

Where a raceway is used as protection for a grounding conductor, the installation shall comply with the requirements of Chapter 38.

SECTION E3611
GROUNDING ELECTRODE CONDUCTOR
CONNECTION TO THE GROUNDING ELECTRODES

E3611.1 Methods of grounding conductor connection to electrodes. The grounding or bonding conductor shall be connected to the grounding electrode by exothermic welding, listed lugs, listed pressure connectors, listed clamps or other listed means. Connections depending on solder shall not be used. Ground clamps shall be listed for the materials of the grounding electrode and the grounding electrode conductor and, where used on pipe, rod or other buried electrodes, shall also be listed for direct soil burial or concrete encasement. Not more than one conductor shall be connected to the grounding electrode by a single clamp or fitting unless the clamp or fitting is listed for multiple conductors. One of the methods indicated in the following items shall be used:

1. A pipe fitting, pipe plug or other approved device screwed into a pipe or pipe fitting.

2. A listed bolted clamp of cast bronze or brass, or plain or malleable iron.

3. For indoor telecommunications purposes only, a listed sheet metal strap-type ground clamp having a rigid metal base that seats on the electrode and having a strap of such material and dimensions that it is not likely to stretch during or after installation.

4. Other equally substantial approved means.

E3611.2 Accessibility. All mechanical elements used to terminate a grounding electrode conductor or bonding jumper to the grounding electrodes that are not buried or concrete encased shall be accessible.

E3611.3 Effective grounding path. The connection of the grounding electrode conductor or bonding jumper shall be made in a manner that will ensure a permanent and effective grounding path. Where necessary to ensure effective grounding for a metal piping system used as a grounding electrode, effective bonding shall be provided around insulated joints and sections and around any equipment that is likely to be disconnected for repairs or replacement. Bonding jumpers shall be of sufficient length to permit removal of such equipment while retaining the integrity of the grounding path.

E3611.4 Protection of ground clamps and fittings. Ground clamps or other fittings shall be approved for applications without protection or shall be protected from physical damage by installing them where they are not likely to be damaged or by enclosing them in metal, wood or equivalent protective coverings.

E3611.5 Clean surfaces. Nonconductive coatings (such as paint, enamel and lacquer) on equipment to be grounded shall be removed from threads and other contact surfaces to ensure good electrical continuity or shall be connected by fittings that make such removal unnecessary.

CHAPTER 37

BRANCH CIRCUIT AND FEEDER REQUIREMENTS

SECTION E3701
GENERAL

E3701.1 Scope. This chapter covers branch circuits and feeders and specifies the minimum required branch circuits, the allowable loads and the required overcurrent protection for branch circuits and feeders that serve less than 100 percent of the total dwelling unit load. Feeder circuits that serve 100 percent of the dwelling unit load shall be sized in accordance with the procedures in Chapter 36.

E3701.2 Branch-circuit and feeder ampacity. Branch-circuit and feeder conductors shall have ampacities not less than the maximum load to be served. Where a branch circuit or a feeder supplies continuous loads or any combination of continuous and noncontinuous loads, the minimum branch-circuit or feeder conductor size, before the application of any adjustment or correction factors, shall have an allowable ampacity equal to or greater than the noncontinuous load plus 125 percent of the continuous load.

> **Exception:** The grounded conductors of branch circuits and feeders that are not connected to an overcurrent device shall be permitted to be sized at 100 percent of the continuous and noncontinuous load.

E3701.3 Selection of ampacity. Where more than one calculated or tabulated ampacity could apply for a given circuit length, the lowest value shall be used.

> **Exception:** Where two different ampacities apply to adjacent portions of a circuit, the higher ampacity shall be permitted to be used beyond the point of transition, a distance equal to 10 feet (3048 mm) or 10 percent of the circuit length figured at the higher ampacity, whichever is less.

E3701.4 Multi-outlet branch circuits. Conductors of multi-outlet branch circuits supplying more than one receptacle for cord-and-plug-connected portable loads shall have ampacities of not less than the rating of the branch circuit.

E3701.5 Multiwire branch circuits. All conductors for multiwire branch circuits shall originate from the same panelboard or similar distribution equipment. Except where all ungrounded conductors are opened simultaneously by the branch-circuit overcurrent device, multiwire branch circuits shall supply only line-to-neutral loads or only one appliance.

E3701.5.1 Disconnecting means. Each multiwire branch circuit shall be provided with a means that will simultaneously disconnect all ungrounded conductors at the point where the branch circuit originates.

E3701.5.2 Grouping. The ungrounded and grounded conductors of each multiwire branch circuit shall be grouped by wire ties or similar means in at least one location within the panelboard or other point of origination.

> **Exception:** Grouping shall not be required where the circuit conductors enter from a cable or raceway unique to the circuit, thereby making the grouping obvious.

SECTION E3702
BRANCH CIRCUIT RATINGS

E3702.1 Branch-circuit voltage limitations. The voltage ratings of branch circuits that supply luminaires or receptacles for cord-and-plug-connected loads of up to 1,400 volt-amperes or of less than $1/4$ horsepower shall be limited to a maximum rating of 120 volts, nominal, between conductors.

Branch circuits that supply cord-and-plug-connected or permanently connected utilization equipment and appliances rated at over 1,440 volt-amperes or $1/4$ horsepower (0.186 kW) and greater shall be rated at 120 volts or 240 volts, nominal.

E3702.2 Branch-circuit ampere rating. Branch circuits shall be rated in accordance with the maximum allowable ampere rating or setting of the overcurrent protection device. The rating for other than individual branch circuits shall be 15, 20, 30, 40 and 50 amperes. Where conductors of higher ampacity are used, the ampere rating or setting of the specified over-current device shall determine the circuit rating.

E3702.3 Fifteen- and 20-ampere branch circuits. A 15- or 20-ampere branch circuit shall be permitted to supply lighting units, or other utilization equipment, or a combination of both. The rating of any one cord-and-plug-connected utilization equipment not fastened in place shall not exceed 80 percent of the branch-circuit ampere rating. The total rating of utilization equipment fastened in place, other than luminaires, shall not exceed 50 percent of the branch-circuit ampere rating where lighting units, cord-and-plug-connected utilization equipment not fastened in place, or both, are also supplied.

E3702.4 Thirty-ampere branch circuits. A 30-ampere branch circuit shall be permitted to supply fixed utilization equipment. A rating of any one cord-and-plug-connected utilization equipment shall not exceed 80 percent of the branch-circuit ampere rating.

E3702.5 Branch circuits serving multiple loads or outlets. General-purpose branch circuits shall supply lighting outlets, appliances, equipment or receptacle outlets, and combinations of such. Multi-outlet branch circuits serving lighting or receptacles shall be limited to a maximum branch-circuit rating of 20 amperes.

E3702.6 Branch circuits serving a single motor. Branch-circuit conductors supplying a single motor shall have an ampacity not less than 125 percent of the motor full-load current rating.

E3702.7 Branch circuits serving motor-operated and combination loads. For circuits supplying loads consisting of motor-operated utilization equipment that is fastened in place and that has a motor larger than $1/8$ horsepower (0.093 kW) in combination with other loads, the total calculated load shall be based on 125 percent of the largest motor load plus the sum of the other loads.

E3702.8 Branch-circuit inductive lighting loads. For circuits supplying luminaires having ballasts, the calculated load shall be based on the total ampere ratings of such units and not on the total watts of the lamps.

E3702.9 Branch-circuit load for ranges and cooking appliances. It shall be permissible to calculate the branch-circuit load for one range in accordance with Table E3704.2(2). The branch-circuit load for one wall-mounted oven or one counter-mounted cooking unit shall be the nameplate rating of the appliance. The branch-circuit load for a counter-mounted cooking unit and not more than two wall-mounted ovens all supplied from a single branch circuit and located in the same room shall be calculated by adding the nameplate ratings of the individual appliances and treating the total as equivalent to one range.

E3702.9.1 Minimum branch circuit for ranges. Ranges with a rating of 8.75 kVA or more shall be supplied by a branch circuit having a minimum rating of 40 amperes.

E3702.10 Branch circuits serving heating loads. Electric space-heating and water-heating appliances shall be considered continuous loads. Branch circuits supplying two or more outlets for fixed electric space-heating equipment shall be rated 15, 20, 25 or 30 amperes.

E3702.11 Branch circuits for air-conditioning and heat pump equipment. The ampacity of the conductors supplying multimotor and combination load equipment shall not be less than the minimum circuit ampacity marked on the equipment. The branch-circuit overcurrent device rating shall be the size and type marked on the appliance.

E3702.12 Branch circuits serving room air conditioners. A room air conditioner shall be considered as a single motor unit in determining its branch-circuit requirements where all the following conditions are met:

1. It is cord- and attachment plug-connected.

2. The rating is not more than 40 amperes and 250 volts; single phase.

3. Total rated-load current is shown on the room air-conditioner nameplate rather than individual motor currents.

4. The rating of the branch-circuit short-circuit and ground-fault protective device does not exceed the ampacity of the branch-circuit conductors, or the rating of the branch-circuit conductors, or the rating of the receptacle, whichever is less.

E3702.12.1 Where no other loads are supplied. The total marked rating of a cord- and attachment plug-connected room air conditioner shall not exceed 80 percent of the rating of a branch circuit where no other appliances are also supplied.

E3702.12.2 Where lighting units or other appliances are also supplied. The total marked rating of a cord- and attachment plug-connected room air conditioner shall not exceed 50 percent of the rating of a branch circuit where lighting or other appliances are also supplied. Where the circuitry is interlocked to prevent simultaneous operation of the room air conditioner and energization of other outlets on the same branch circuit, a cord- and attachment-plug-connected room air conditioner shall not exceed 80 percent of the branch-circuit rating.

E3702.13 Branch-circuit requirement—summary. The requirements for circuits having two or more outlets, or receptacles, other than the receptacle circuits of Sections E3703.2 and E3703.3, are summarized in Table E3702.13. Branch circuits in dwelling units shall supply only loads within that dwelling unit or loads associated only with that dwelling unit. Branch circuits required for the purpose of lighting, central alarm, signal, communications or other needs for public or common areas of a two-family dwelling shall not be supplied from equipment that supplies an individual dwelling unit.

TABLE E3702.13
BRANCH-CIRCUIT REQUIREMENTS—SUMMARY[a,b]

	CIRCUIT RATING		
	15 amp	20 amp	30 amp

Conductors:
   Minimum size (AWG)
   circuit conductors
	14	12	10

Maximum overcurrent-
   protection device rating
   Ampere rating
	15	20	30

Outlet devices:
   Lampholders permitted
   Receptacle rating (amperes)
	Any type
	15 maximum
		Any type
		15 or 20
			N/A
			30

Maximum load (amperes)	15	20	30

a. These gages are for copper conductors.
b. N/A means not allowed.

SECTION E3703
REQUIRED BRANCH CIRCUITS

E3703.1 Branch circuits for heating. Central heating equipment other than fixed electric space heating shall be supplied by an individual branch circuit. Permanently connected air-conditioning equipment, and auxiliary equipment directly associated with the central heating equipment such as pumps, motorized valves, humidifiers and electrostatic air cleaners, shall not be prohibited from connecting to the same branch circuit as the central heating equipment.

E3703.2 Kitchen and dining area receptacles. A minimum of two 20-ampere-rated branch circuits shall be provided to serve all wall and floor receptacle outlets located in the kitchen, pantry, breakfast area, dining area or similar area of a dwelling. The kitchen countertop receptacles shall be served by a minimum of two 20-ampere-rated branch circuits, either or both of which shall also be permitted to supply other receptacle outlets in the same kitchen, pantry, breakfast and dining area including receptacle outlets for refrigeration appliances.

Exception: The receptacle outlet for refrigeration appliances shall be permitted to be supplied from an individual branch circuit rated 15 amperes or greater.

E3703.3 Laundry circuit. A minimum of one 20-ampere-rated branch circuit shall be provided for receptacles located in the laundry area and shall serve only receptacle outlets located in the laundry area.

E3703.4 Bathroom branch circuits. A minimum of one 20-ampere branch circuit shall be provided to supply bathroom receptacle outlet(s). Such circuits shall have no other outlets.

Exception: Where the 20-ampere circuit supplies a single bathroom, outlets for other equipment within the same bathroom shall be permitted to be supplied in accordance with Section E3702.

E3703.5 Number of branch circuits. The minimum number of branch circuits shall be determined from the total calculated load and the size or rating of the circuits used. The number of circuits shall be sufficient to supply the load served. In no case shall the load on any circuit exceed the maximum specified by Section E3702.

E3703.6 Branch-circuit load proportioning. Where the branch-circuit load is calculated on a volt-amperes-per-square-foot (m²) basis, the wiring system, up to and including the branch-circuit panelboard(s), shall have the capacity to serve not less than the calculated load. This load shall be evenly proportioned among multioutlet branch circuits within the panelboard(s). Branch-circuit overcurrent devices and circuits shall only be required to be installed to serve the connected load.

SECTION E3704
FEEDER REQUIREMENTS

E3704.1 Conductor size. Feeder conductors that do not serve 100 percent of the dwelling unit load and branch-circuit conductors shall be of a size sufficient to carry the load as determined by this chapter. Feeder conductors shall not be required to be larger than the service-entrance conductors that supply the dwelling unit. The load for feeder conductors that serve as the main power feeder to a dwelling unit shall be determined as specified in Chapter 36 for services.

E3704.2 Feeder loads. The minimum load in volt-amperes shall be calculated in accordance with the load calculation procedure prescribed in Table E3704.2(1). The associated table demand factors shall be applied to the actual load to determine the minimum load for feeders.

E3704.3 Feeder neutral load. The feeder neutral load shall be the maximum unbalance of the load determined in accordance with this chapter. The maximum unbalanced load shall be the maximum net calculated load between the neutral and any one ungrounded conductor. For a feeder or service supplying electric ranges, wall-mounted ovens, counter-mounted cooking units and electric dryers, the maximum unbalanced load shall be considered as 70 percent of the load on the ungrounded conductors.

E3704.4 Lighting and general use receptacle load. A unit load of not less than 3 volt-amperes shall constitute the minimum lighting and general use receptacle load for each square foot of floor area (33 VA for each square meter of floor area). The floor area for each floor shall be calculated from the outside dimensions of the building. The calculated floor area shall not include open porches, garages, or unused or unfinished spaces not adaptable for future use.

E3704.5 Ampacity and calculated loads. The calculated load of a feeder shall be not less than the sum of the loads on the branch circuits supplied, as determined by Section E3704, after any applicable demand factors permitted by Section E3704 have been applied.

E3704.6 Equipment grounding conductor. Where a feeder supplies branch circuits in which equipment grounding conductors are required, the feeder shall include or provide an

TABLE E3704.2(1)
FEEDER LOAD CALCULATION

LOAD CALCULATION PROCEDURE	APPLIED DEMAND FACTOR
Lighting and receptacles: A unit load of not less than 3 VA per square foot of total floor area shall constitute the lighting and 120-volt, 15- and 20-ampere general use receptacle load. 1,500 VA shall be added for each 20-ampere branch circuit serving receptacles in the kitchen, dining room, pantry, breakfast area and laundry area.	100 percent of first 3,000 VA or less and 35 percent of that in excess of 3,000 VA.
Plus	
Appliances and motors: The nameplate rating load of all fastened-in-place appliances other than dryers, ranges, air-conditioning and space-heating equipment.	100 percent of load for three or less appliances. 75 percent of load for four or more appliances.
Plus	
Fixed motors: Full-load current of motors plus 25 percent of the full load current of the largest motor.	
Plus	
Electric clothes dryer: The dryer load shall be 5,000 VA for each dryer circuit or the nameplate rating load of each dryer, whichever is greater.	
Plus	
Cooking appliances: The nameplate rating of ranges, wall-mounted ovens, counter-mounted cooking units and other cooking appliances rated in excess of 1.75 kVA shall be summed.	Demand factors shall be as allowed by Table E3704.2(2).
Plus the largest of either the heating or cooling load	
Largest of the following two selections: 1. 100 percent of the nameplate rating(s) of the air conditioning and cooling, including heat pump compressors. 2. 100 percent of the fixed electric space heating.	

For SI: 1 square foot = 0.0929 m².

equipment grounding conductor that is one or more or a combination of the types specified in Section E3908.8, to which the equipment grounding conductors of the branch circuits shall be connected. Where the feeder supplies a separate building or structure, the requirements of Section E3607.3.1 shall apply.

SECTION E3705
CONDUCTOR SIZING AND OVERCURRENT PROTECTION

E3705.1 General. Ampacities for conductors shall be determined based in accordance with Table E3705.1 and Sections E3705.2 and E3705.3.

E3705.2 Correction factor for ambient temperatures. For ambient temperatures other than 30°C (86°F), multiply the allowable ampacities specified in Table E3705.1 by the appropriate correction factor shown in Table E3705.2.

E3705.3 Adjustment factor for conductor proximity. Where the number of current-carrying conductors in a raceway or cable exceeds three, or where single conductors or multiconductor cables are stacked or bundled for distances greater than 24 inches (610 mm) without maintaining spacing and are not installed in raceways, the allowable ampacity of each conductor shall be reduced as shown in Table E3705.3.

Exceptions:

1. Adjustment factors shall not apply to conductors in nipples having a length not exceeding 24 inches (610 mm).

2. Adjustment factors shall not apply to underground conductors entering or leaving an outdoor trench if those conductors have physical protection in the form

TABLE E3704.2(2)
DEMAND LOADS FOR ELECTRIC RANGES, WALL-MOUNTED OVENS, COUNTER-MOUNTED COOKING UNITS AND OTHER COOKING APPLIANCES OVER $1^3/_4$ kVA RATING[a,b]

NUMBER OF APPLIANCES	MAXIMUM DEMAND[b,c] Column A maximum 12 kVA rating	DEMAND FACTORS (percent)[d] Column B less than $3^1/_2$ kVA rating	Column C $3^1/_2$ to $8^3/_4$ kVA rating
1	8 kVA	80	80
2	11 kVA	75	65

a. Column A shall be used in all cases except as provided for in Footnote d.

b. For ranges all having the same rating and individually rated more than 12 kVA but not more than 27 kVA, the maximum demand in Column A shall be increased 5 percent for each additional kVA of rating or major fraction thereof by which the rating of individual ranges exceeds 12 kVA.

c. For ranges of unequal ratings and individually rated more than 8.75 kVA, but none exceeding 27 kVA, an average value of rating shall be computed by adding together the ratings of all ranges to obtain the total connected load (using 12 kVA for any ranges rated less than 12 kVA) and dividing by the total number of ranges; and then the maximum demand in Column A shall be increased 5 percent for each kVA or major fraction thereof by which this average value exceeds 12 kVA.

d. Over 1.75 kVA through 8.75 kVA. As an alternative to the method provided in Column A, the nameplate ratings of all ranges rated more than 1.75 kVA but not more than 8.75 kVA shall be added and the sum shall be multiplied by the demand factor specified in Column B or C for the given number of appliances.

TABLE E3705.1
ALLOWABLE AMPACITIES

CONDUCTOR SIZE AWG kcmil	CONDUCTOR TEMPERATURE RATING						CONDUCTOR SIZE AWG kcmil
	60°C	75°C	90°C	60°C	75°C	90°C	
	Types TW, UF	Types RHW, THHW, THW, THWN, USE, XHHW	Types RHW-2, THHN, THHW, THW-2, THWN-2, XHHW, XHHW-2, USE-2	Types TW, UF	Types RHW, THHW, THW, THWN, USE, XHHW	Types RHW-2, THHN, THHW, THW-2, THWN-2, XHHW, XHHW-2, USE-2	
	Copper			Aluminum or copper-clad aluminum			
18	—	—	14	—	—	—	—
16	—	—	18	—	—	—	—
14	20	20	25	—	—	—	—
12	25	25	30	20	20	25	12
10	30	35	40	25	30	35	10
8	40	50	55	30	40	45	8
6	55	65	75	40	50	60	6
4	70	85	95	55	65	75	4
3	85	100	110	65	75	85	3
2	95	115	130	75	90	100	2
1	110	130	150	85	100	115	1
1/0	125	150	170	100	120	135	1/0
2/0	145	175	195	115	135	150	2/0
3/0	165	200	225	130	155	175	3/0
4/0	195	230	260	150	180	205	4/0

For SI: °C = [(°F) − 32]/1.8.

TABLE E3705.2
AMBIENT TEMPERATURE CORRECTION FACTORS

	FOR AMBIENT TEMPERATURES OTHER THAN 30°C (86°F), MULTIPLY THE ALLOWABLE AMPACITIES SPECIFIED IN TABLE E3705.1 BY THE APPROPRIATE FACTOR SHOWN BELOW						
	CONDUCTOR TEMPERATURE RATING						
	60°C	75°C	90°C	60°C	75°C	90°C	
AMBIENT TEMP. °C	**Types TW, UF**	**Types RHW, THHW, THW, THWN, USE, XHHW**	**Types RHW-2, THHN, THHW, THW-2, THWN-2, XHHW, XHHW-2, USE-2**	**Types TW, UF**	**Types RHW, THHW, THW, THWN, USE, XHHW**	**Types RHW-2, THHN, THHW, THW-2, THWN-2, XHHW, XHHW-2, USE-2**	**AMBIENT TEMP. °F**
	Copper			**Aluminum or copper-clad aluminum**			
21-25	1.08	1.05	1.04	1.08	1.05	1.04	70-77
26-30	1.00	1.00	1.00	1.00	1.00	1.00	78-86
31-35	0.91	0.94	0.96	0.91	0.94	0.96	87-95
36-40	0.82	0.88	0.91	0.82	0.88	0.91	96-104
41-45	0.71	0.82	0.87	0.71	0.82	0.87	105-113
46-50	0.58	0.75	0.82	0.58	0.75	0.82	114-122
51-55	0.41	0.67	0.76	0.41	0.67	0.76	123-131
56-60	—	0.58	0.71	—	0.58	0.71	132-140
61-70	—	0.33	0.58	—	0.33	0.58	141-158
71-80	—	—	0.41	—	—	0.41	159-176

of rigid metal conduit, intermediate metal conduit, or rigid nonmetallic conduit having a length not exceeding 10 feet (3048 mm) and the number of conductors does not exceed four.

3. Adjustment factors shall not apply to type AC cable or to type MC cable without an overall outer jacket meeting all of the following conditions:

   3.1. Each cable has not more than three current-carrying conductors.

   3.2. The conductors are 12 AWG copper.

   3.3. Not more than 20 current-carrying conductors are bundled, stacked or supported on bridle rings. A 60 percent adjustment factor shall be applied where the current-carrying conductors in such cables exceed 20 and the cables are stacked or bundled for distances greater than 24 inches (610 mm) without maintaining spacing.

TABLE E3705.3
CONDUCTOR PROXIMITY ADJUSTMENT FACTORS

NUMBER OF CURRENT-CARRYING CONDUCTORS IN CABLE OR RACEWAY	PERCENT OF VALUES IN TABLE E3705.1
4-6	80
7-9	70
10-20	50
21-30	45
31-40	40
41 and above	35

E3705.4 Temperature limitations. The temperature rating associated with the ampacity of a conductor shall be so selected and coordinated to not exceed the lowest temperature rating of any connected termination, conductor or device. Conductors with temperature ratings higher than specified for terminations

shall be permitted to be used for ampacity adjustment, correction, or both. Except where the equipment is marked otherwise, conductor ampacities used in determining equipment termination provisions shall be based on Table E3705.1.

E3705.4.1 Conductors rated 60°C. Except where the equipment is marked otherwise, termination provisions of equipment for circuits rated 100 amperes or less, or marked for 14 AWG through 1 AWG conductors, shall be used only for one of the following:

1. Conductors rated 60°C (140°F);

2. Conductors with higher temperature ratings, provided that the ampacity of such conductors is determined based on the 60°C (140°F) ampacity of the conductor size used;

3. Conductors with higher temperature ratings where the equipment is listed and identified for use with such conductors; or

4. For motors marked with design letters B, C, or D conductors having an insulation rating of 75°C (167°F) or higher shall be permitted to be used provided that the ampacity of such conductors does not exceed the 75°C (167°F) ampacity.

E3705.4.2 Conductors rated 75°C. Termination provisions of equipment for circuits rated over 100 amperes, or marked for conductors larger than 1 AWG, shall be used only for:

1. Conductors rated 75°C (167°F).

2. Conductors with higher temperature ratings provided that the ampacity of such conductors does not exceed the 75°C (167°F) ampacity of the conductor size used, or provided that the equipment is listed and identified for use with such conductors.

E3705.4.3 Separately installed pressure connectors. Separately installed pressure connectors shall be used with conductors at the ampacities not exceeding the ampacity at the listed and identified temperature rating of the connector.

E3705.4.4 Conductors of Type NM cable. Conductors in NM cable assemblies shall be rated at 90°C (194°F). Types NM, NMC, and NMS cable identified by the markings NM-B, NMC-B, and NMS-B meet this requirement. The ampacity of Types NM, NMC, and NMS cable shall be at 60°C (140°F) conductors and shall comply with Section E3705.1 and Table E3705.5.3. The 90°C (194°F) rating shall be permitted to be used for ampacity correction and adjustment purposes provided that the final corrected or adjusted ampacity does not exceed that for a 60°C (140°F) rated conductor. Where more than two NM cables containing two or more current-carrying conductors are installed, without maintaining spacing between the cables, through the same opening in wood framing that is to be fire- or draft-stopped using thermal insulation, caulk or sealing foam, the allowable ampacity of each conductor shall be adjusted in accordance with Table E3705.3. Where more than two NM cables containing two or more current-carrying conductors are installed in contact with thermal insulation without maintaining spacing between cables, the allowable ampacity of each conductor shall be adjusted in accordance with Table E3705.3.

E3705.5 Overcurrent protection required. All ungrounded branch-circuit and feeder conductors shall be protected against overcurrent by an overcurrent device installed at the point where the conductors receive their supply. Overcurrent devices shall not be connected in series with a grounded conductor. Overcurrent protection and allowable loads for branch circuits and feeders that do not serve as the main power feeder to the dwelling unit load shall be in accordance with this chapter.

Branch-circuit conductors and equipment shall be protected by overcurrent protective devices having a rating or setting not exceeding the allowable ampacity specified in Table E3705.1 and Sections E3705.2, E3705.3 and E3705.4 except where otherwise permitted or required in Sections E3705.5.1 through E3705.5.3.

E3705.5.1 Cords. Cords shall be protected in accordance with Section E3909.2.

E3705.5.2 Overcurrent devices of the next higher rating. The next higher standard overcurrent device rating, above the ampacity of the conductors being protected, shall be permitted to be used, provided that all of the following conditions are met:

1. The conductors being protected are not part of a multioutlet branch circuit supplying receptacles for cord- and plug-connected portable loads.

2. The ampacity of conductors does not correspond with the standard ampere rating of a fuse or a circuit breaker without overload trip adjustments above its rating (but that shall be permitted to have other trip or rating adjustments).

3. The next higher standard device rating does not exceed 400 amperes.

E3705.5.3 Small conductors. Except as specifically permitted by Section E3705.5.4, the rating of overcurrent protection devices shall not exceed the ratings shown in Table E3705.5.3 for the conductors specified therein.

E3705.5.4 Air-conditioning and heat pump equipment. Air-conditioning and heat pump equipment circuit conductors shall be permitted to be protected against overcurrent in accordance with Section E3702.11.

E3705.6 Fuses and fixed trip circuit breakers. The standard ampere ratings for fuses and inverse time circuit breakers shall be considered 15, 20, 25, 30, 35, 40, 45, 50, 60, 70, 80, 90, 100, 110, 125, 150, 175, 200, 225, 250, 300, 350 and 400 amperes.

TABLE E3705.5.3
OVERCURRENT-PROTECTION RATING

COPPER		ALUMINUM OR COPPER-CLAD ALUMINUM	
Size (AWG)	Maximum overcurrent-protection-device rating[a] (amps)	Size (AWG)	Maximum overcurrent-protection-device rating[a] (amps)
14	15	12	15
12	20	10	25
10	30	8	30

a. The maximum overcurrent-protection-device rating shall not exceed the conductor allowable ampacity determined by the application of the correction and adjustment factors in accordance with Sections E3705.2 and E3705.3.

E3705.7 Location of overcurrent devices in or on premises. Overcurrent devices shall:

1. Be readily accessible.

2. Not be located where they will be exposed to physical damage.

3. Not be located where they will be in the vicinity of easily ignitible material such as in clothes closets.

4. Not be located in bathrooms.

5. Not be located over steps of a stairway.

6. Be installed so that the center of the grip of the operating handle of the switch or circuit breaker, when in its highest position, is not more than 6 feet 7 inches (2007 mm) above the floor or working platform.

Exceptions:

1. This section shall not apply to supplementary overcurrent protection that is integral to utilization equipment.

2. Overcurrent devices installed adjacent to the utilization equipment that they supply shall be permitted to be accessible by portable means.

E3705.8 Ready access for occupants. Each occupant shall have ready access to all overcurrent devices protecting the conductors supplying that occupancy.

E3705.9 Enclosures for overcurrent devices. Overcurrent devices shall be enclosed in cabinets or cutout boxes except where an overcurrent device is part of an assembly that provides equivalent protection. The operating handle of a circuit breaker shall be permitted to be accessible without opening a door or cover.

SECTION E3706
PANELBOARDS

E3706.1 Panelboard rating. All panelboards shall have a rating not less than that of the minimum service entrance or feeder capacity required for the calculated load.

E3706.2 Panelboard circuit identification. All circuits and circuit modifications shall be legibly identified as to their clear, evident, and specific purpose or use. The identification shall include sufficient detail to allow each circuit to be distinguished from all others. Spare positions that contain unused overcurrent devices or switches shall be described accordingly. The identification shall be included in a circuit directory located on the face of the panelboard enclosure or inside the panel door. Circuits shall not be described in a manner that depends on transient conditions of occupancy.

E3706.3 Panelboard overcurrent protection. In addition to the requirement of Section E3706.1, a panelboard shall be protected by an overcurrent protective device having a rating not greater than that of the panelboard. Such overcurrent protective device shall be located within or at any point on the supply side of the panelboard.

E3706.4 Grounded conductor terminations. Each grounded conductor shall terminate within the panelboard on an individual terminal that is not also used for another conductor, except that grounded conductors of circuits with parallel conductors shall be permitted to terminate on a single terminal where the terminal is identified for connection of more than one conductor.

E3706.5 Back-fed devices. Plug-in-type overcurrent protection devices or plug-in-type main lug assemblies that are back-fed and used to terminate field-installed ungrounded supply conductors shall be secured in place by an additional fastener that requires other than a pull to release the device from the mounting means on the panel.

CHAPTER 38

WIRING METHODS

SECTION E3801
GENERAL REQUIREMENTS

E3801.1 Scope. This chapter covers the wiring methods for services, feeders and branch circuits for electrical power and distribution.

E3801.2 Allowable wiring methods. The allowable wiring methods for electrical installations shall be those listed in Table E3801.2. Single conductors shall be used only where part of one of the recognized wiring methods listed in Table E3801.2. As used in this code, abbreviations of the wiring-method types shall be as indicated in Table E3801.2.

TABLE E3801.2
ALLOWABLE WIRING METHODS

ALLOWABLE WIRING METHOD	DESIGNATED ABBREVIATION
Armored cable	AC
Electrical metallic tubing	EMT
Electrical nonmetallic tubing	ENT
Flexible metal conduit	FMC
Intermediate metal conduit	IMC
Liquidtight flexible conduit	LFC
Metal-clad cable	MC
Nonmetallic sheathed cable	NM
Rigid nonmetallic conduit	RNC
Rigid metallic conduit	RMC
Service entrance cable	SE
Surface raceways	SR
Underground feeder cable	UF
Underground service cable	USE

E3801.3 Circuit conductors. All conductors of a circuit, including equipment grounding conductors and bonding conductors, shall be contained in the same raceway, trench, cable or cord.

E3801.4 Wiring method applications. Wiring methods shall be applied in accordance with Table E3801.4.

SECTION E3802
ABOVE-GROUND INSTALLATION REQUIREMENTS

E3802.1 Installation and support requirements. Wiring methods shall be installed and supported in accordance with Table E3802.1.

E3802.2 Cables in accessible attics. Cables in attics or roof spaces provided with access shall be installed as specified in Sections E3802.2.1 and E3802.2.2.

E3802.2.1 Across structural members. Where run across the top of floor joists, or run within 7 feet (2134 mm) of floor or floor joists across the face of rafters or studding, in attics and roof spaces that are provided with access, the cable shall be protected by substantial guard strips that are at least as high as the cable. Where such spaces are not provided with access by permanent stairs or ladders, protection shall only be required within 6 feet (1829 mm) of the nearest edge of the attic entrance.

E3802.2.2 Cable installed through or parallel to framing members. Where cables are installed through or parallel to the sides of rafters, studs or floor joists, guard strips and running boards shall not be required, and the installation shall comply with Table E3802.1.

E3802.3 Exposed cable. In exposed work, except as provided for in Sections E3802.2 and E3802.4, cable assemblies shall be installed as specified in Sections E3802.3.1 and E3802.3.2.

E3802.3.1 Surface installation. Cables shall closely follow the surface of the building finish or running boards.

E3802.3.2 Protection from physical damage. Where subject to physical damage, cables shall be protected by rigid metal conduit, intermediate metal conduit, electrical metallic tubing, Schedule 80 PVC rigid nonmetallic conduit, or other approved means. Where passing through a floor, the cable shall be enclosed in rigid metal conduit, intermediate metal conduit, electrical metallic tubing, Schedule 80 PVC rigid nonmetallic conduit or other approved means extending not less than 6 inches (152 mm) above the floor.

E3802.3.3 Locations exposed to direct sunlight. Insulated conductors and cables used where exposed to direct rays of the sun shall be listed or listed and marked, as being "sunlight resistant," or shall be covered with insulating material, such as tape or sleeving, that is listed or listed and marked as being "sunlight resistant."

E3802.4 In unfinished basements and crawl spaces. Where type SE or NM cable is run at angles with joists in unfinished basements and crawl spaces, cable assemblies containing two or more conductors of sizes 6 AWG and larger and assemblies containing three or more conductors of sizes 8 AWG and larger shall not require additional protection where attached directly to the bottom of the joists. Smaller cables shall be run either through bored holes in joists or on running boards. NM cable installed on the wall of an unfinished basement shall be permitted to be installed in a listed conduit or tubing or shall be protected in accordance with Table E3802.1. Conduit or tubing shall be provided with a suitable insulating bushing or adapter at the point the where cable enters the raceway. The NM or SE cable sheath shall extend through the conduit or tubing and into the outlet or device box not less than $^1/_4$ inch (6.4 mm). The cable shall be secured within 12 inches (305 mm) of the point where the cable enters the conduit or tubing. Metal conduit, tubing, and metal outlet boxes shall be connected to an equipment grounding conductor.

TABLE E3801.4
ALLOWABLE APPLICATIONS FOR WIRING METHODS[a, b, c, d, e, f, g, h, i, j, k]

ALLOWABLE APPLICATIONS (application allowed where marked with an "A")	AC	EMT	ENT	FMC	IMC RMC RNC	LFC[a]	MC	NM	SR	SE	UF	USE
Services	—	A	A[h]	A[i]	A	A[i]	A	—	—	A	—	A
Feeders	A	A	A	A	A	A	A	A	—	A[b]	A	A[b]
Branch circuits	A	A	A	A	A	A	A	A	A	A[c]	A	—
Inside a building	A	A	A	A	A	A	A	A	A	A	A	—
Wet locations exposed to sunlight	—	A	A[h]	—	A	A	A	—	—	A	A[e]	A[e]
Damp locations	—	A	A	A[d]	A	A	A	—	—	A	A	A
Embedded in noncinder concrete in dry location	—	A	A	—	A	A[j]	—	—	—	—	—	—
In noncinder concrete in contact with grade	—	A[f]	A	—	A[f]	A[j]	—	—	—	—	—	—
Embedded in plaster not exposed to dampness	A	A	A	A	A	A	A	—	—	A	A	—
Embedded in masonry	—	A	A	—	A[f]	A	A	—	—	—	—	—
In masonry voids and cells exposed to dampness or below grade line	—	A[f]	A	A[d]	A[f]	A	A	—	—	A	A	—
Fished in masonry voids	A	—	—	A	—	A	A	A	—	A	A	—
In masonry voids and cells not exposed to dampness	A	A	A	A	A	A	A	—	—	A	A	—
Run exposed	A	A	A	A	A	A	A	A	A	A	A	—
Run exposed and subject to physical damage	—	—	—	—	A[g]	—	—	—	—	—	—	—
For direct burial	—	A[f]	—	—	A[f]	A	A[f]	—	—	—	A	A

For SI: 1 foot = 304.8 mm.

a. Liquid-tight flexible nonmetallic conduit without integral reinforcement within the conduit wall shall not exceed 6 feet in length.

b. The grounded conductor shall be insulated except where used to supply other buildings on the same premises. Type USE cable shall not be used inside buildings.

c. The grounded conductor shall be insulated.

d. Conductors shall be a type approved for wet locations and the installation shall prevent water from entering other raceways.

e. Shall be listed as "Sunlight Resistant."

f. Metal raceways shall be protected from corrosion and approved for the application. Aluminum RMC requires approved supplementary corrosion protection.

g. RNC shall be Schedule 80.

h. Shall be listed as "Sunlight Resistant" where exposed to the direct rays of the sun.

i. Conduit shall not exceed 6 feet in length.

j. Liquid-tight flexible nonmetallic conduit is permitted to be encased in concrete where listed for direct burial and only straight connectors listed for use with LFNC are used.

k. In wet locations under any of the following conditions:
    a. The metallic covering is impervious to moisture.
    b. A lead sheath or moisture-impervious jacket is provided under the metal covering.
    c. The insulated conductors under the metallic covering are listed for use in wet locations and a corrosion-resistant jacket is provided over the metallic sheath.

TABLE E3802.1
GENERAL INSTALLATION AND SUPPORT REQUIREMENTS FOR WIRING METHODS[a, b, c, d, e, f, g, h, i, j, k]

INSTALLATION REQUIREMENTS (Requirement applicable only to wiring methods marked "A")	AC MC	EMT IMC RMC	ENT	FMC LFC	NM UF	RNC	SE	SR[a]	USE
Where run parallel with the framing member or furring strip, the wiring shall be not less than $1\frac{1}{4}$ inches from the edge of a furring strip or a framing member such as a joist, rafter or stud or shall be physically protected.	A	—	A	A	A	—	A	—	—
Bored holes in framing members for wiring shall be located not less than $1\frac{1}{4}$ inches from the edge of the framing member or shall be protected with a minimum 0.0625-inch steel plate or sleeve, a listed steel plate or other physical protection.	A[k]	—	A[k]	A[k]	A[k]	—	A[k]	—	—
Where installed in grooves, to be covered by wallboard, siding, paneling, carpeting, or similar finish, wiring methods shall be protected by 0.0625-inch-thick steel plate, sleeve, or equivalent, a listed steel plate or by not less than $1\frac{1}{4}$-inch free space for the full length of the groove in which the cable or raceway is installed.	A	—	A	A	A	—	A	A	A
Securely fastened bushings or grommets shall be provided to protect wiring run through openings in metal framing members.	—	—	A[j]	—	A[j]	—	A[j]	—	—
The maximum number of 90-degree bends shall not exceed four between junction boxes.	—	A	A	A	—	A	—	—	—
Bushings shall be provided where entering a box, fitting or enclosure unless the box or fitting is designed to afford equivalent protection.	A	A	A	A	—	A	—	A	—
Ends of raceways shall be reamed to remove rough edges.	—	A	A	A	—	A	—	A	—
Maximum allowable on center support spacing for the wiring method in feet.	4.5[b, c]	10[l]	3[b]	4.5[b]	4.5[i]	3[d, l]	2.5[e]	—	2.5[e]
Maximum support distance in inches from box or other terminations.	12[b, f]	36	36	12[b, g]	12[h, i]	36	12	—	12

For SI: 1 inch = 25.4 mm, 1 foot = 304.8 mm, 1 degree = 0.0175 rad.

a. Installed in accordance with listing requirements.
b. Supports not required in accessible ceiling spaces between light fixtures where lengths do not exceed 6 feet.
c. Six feet for MC cable.
d. Five feet for trade sizes greater than 1 inch.
e. Two and one-half feet where used for service or outdoor feeder and 4.5 feet where used for branch circuit or indoor feeder.
f. Twenty-four inches where flexibility is necessary.
g. Thirty-six inches where flexibility is necessary.
h. Within 8 inches of boxes without cable clamps.
i. Flat cables shall not be stapled on edge.
j. Bushings and grommets shall remain in place and shall be listed for the purpose of cable protection.
k. See Sections R502.8 and R802.7 for additional limitations on the location of bored holes in horizontal framing members.
l. Where oversized, concentric or eccentric knockouts are not encountered, a raceway not greater than 18 inches in length shall not require support where it is a continuous length without couplings. Such raceways shall terminate at an outlet box, junction box, device box, cabinet, or other termination at each end of the raceway.

E3802.5 Bends. Bends shall be made so as not to damage the wiring method or reduce the internal diameter of raceways.

For types NM and SE cable, bends shall be so made, and other handling shall be such that the cable will not be damaged and the radius of the curve of the inner edge of any bend shall be not less than five times the diameter of the cable.

E3802.6 Raceways exposed to different temperatures. Where portions of a cable, raceway or sleeve are known to be subjected to different temperatures and where condensation is known to be a problem, as in cold storage areas of buildings or where passing from the interior to the exterior of a building, the raceway or sleeve shall be filled with an approved material to prevent the circulation of warm air to a colder section of the raceway or sleeve.

E3802.7 Raceways in wet locations above grade. Where raceways are installed in wet locations abovegrade, the interior of such raceways shall be considered to be a wet location. Insu-lated conductors and cables installed in raceways in wet locations abovegrade shall be listed for use in wet locations.

SECTION E3803
UNDERGROUND INSTALLATION REQUIREMENTS

E3803.1 Minimum cover requirements. Direct buried cable or raceways shall be installed in accordance with the minimum cover requirements of Table E3803.1.

E3803.2 Warning ribbon. Underground service conductors that are not encased in concrete and that are buried 18 inches (457 mm) or more below grade shall have their location identi-fied by a warning ribbon that is placed in the trench not less than 12 inches (305 mm) above the underground installation.

E3803.3 Protection from damage. Direct buried conductors and cables emerging from the ground shall be protected by enclosures or raceways extending from the minimum cover

TABLE E3803.1
MINIMUM COVER REQUIREMENTS, BURIAL IN INCHES[a, b, c, d, e]

LOCATION OF WIRING METHOD OR CIRCUIT	TYPE OF WIRING METHOD OR CIRCUIT				
	1 Direct burial cables or conductors	2 Rigid metal conduit or intermediate metal conduit	3 Nonmetallic raceways listed for direct burial without concrete encasement or other approved raceways	4 Residential branch circuits rated 120 volts or less with GFCI protection and maximum overcurrent protection of 20 amperes	5 Circuits for control of irrigation and landscape lighting limited to not more than 30 volts and installed with type UF or in other identified cable or raceway
All locations not specified below	24	6	18	12	6
In trench below 2-inch-thick concrete or equivalent	18	6	12	6	6
Under a building	0 (In raceway only)	0	0	0 (In raceway only)	0 (In raceway only)
Under minimum of 4-inch-thick concrete exterior slab with no vehicular traffic and the slab extending not less than 6 inches beyond the underground installation	18	4	4	6 (Direct burial) 4 (In raceway)	6 (Direct burial) 4 (In raceway)
Under streets, highways, roads, alleys, driveways and parking lots	24	24	24	24	24
One- and two-family dwelling driveways and outdoor parking areas, and used only for dwelling-related purposes	18	18	18	12	18
In solid rock where covered by minimum of 2 inches concrete extending down to rock	2 (In raceway only)	2	2	2 (In raceway only)	2 (In raceway only)

For SI: 1 inch = 25.4 mm.

a. Raceways approved for burial only where encased concrete shall require concrete envelope not less than 2 inches thick.

b. Lesser depths shall be permitted where cables and conductors rise for terminations or splices or where access is otherwise required.

c. Where one of the wiring method types listed in columns 1 to 3 is combined with one of the circuit types in columns 4 and 5, the shallower depth of burial shall be permitted.

d. Where solid rock prevents compliance with the cover depths specified in this table, the wiring shall be installed in metal or nonmetallic raceway permitted for direct burial. The raceways shall be covered by a minimum of 2 inches of concrete extending down to the rock.

e. Cover is defined as the shortest distance in inches (millimeters) measured between a point on the top surface of any direct-buried conductor, cable, conduit or other raceway and the top surface of finished grade, concrete, or similar cover.

distance below grade required by Section E3803.1 to a point at least 8 feet (2438 mm) above finished grade. In no case shall the protection be required to exceed 18 inches (457 mm) below finished grade. Conductors entering a building shall be protected to the point of entrance. Where the enclosure or raceway is subject to physical damage, the conductors shall be installed in rigid metal conduit, intermediate metal conduit, Schedule 80 rigid nonmetallic conduit or the equivalent.

E3803.4 Splices and taps. Direct buried conductors or cables shall be permitted to be spliced or tapped without the use of splice boxes. The splices or taps shall be made by approved methods with materials listed for the application.

E3803.5 Backfill. Backfill containing large rock, paving materials, cinders, large or sharply angular substances, or corrosive material shall not be placed in an excavation where such materials cause damage to raceways, cables or other substructures or prevent adequate compaction of fill or contribute to corrosion of raceways, cables or other substructures. Where necessary to prevent physical damage to the raceway or cable, protection shall be provided in the form of granular or selected material, suitable boards, suitable sleeves or other approved means.

E3803.6 Raceway seals. Conduits or raceways shall be sealed or plugged at either or both ends where moisture will enter and contact live parts.

E3803.7 Bushing. A bushing, or terminal fitting, with an integral bushed opening shall be installed on the end of a conduit or other raceway that terminates underground where the conductors or cables emerge as a direct burial wiring method. A seal incorporating the physical protection characteristics of a bushing shall be considered equivalent to a bushing.

E3803.8 Single conductors. All conductors of the same circuit and, where present, the grounded conductor and all equipment grounding conductors shall be installed in the same raceway or shall be installed in close proximity in the same trench.

> **Exception:** Where conductors are installed in parallel in raceways, each raceway shall contain all conductors of the same circuit including grounding conductors.

E3803.9 Ground movement. Where direct buried conductors, raceways or cables are subject to movement by settlement or frost, direct buried conductors, raceways or cables shall be arranged to prevent damage to the enclosed conductors or to equipment connected to the raceways.

E3803.10 Wet locations. The interior of enclosures or raceways installed underground shall be considered to be a wet location. Insulated conductors and cables installed in such enclosures or raceways in underground installations shall be listed for use in wet locations. Connections or splices in an underground installation shall be approved for wet locations.

E3803.11 Under buildings. Underground cable installed under a building shall be in a raceway.

CHAPTER 39

POWER AND LIGHTING DISTRIBUTION

SECTION E3901
RECEPTACLE OUTLETS

E3901.1 General. Outlets for receptacles rated at 125 volts, 15- and 20-amperes shall be provided in accordance with Sections E3901.2 through E3901.11. Receptacle outlets required by this section shall be in addition to any receptacle that is:

1. Part of a luminaire or appliance;

2. Located within cabinets or cupboards;

3. Controlled by a wall switch in accordance with Section E3903.2, Exception 1; or

4. Located over 5.5 feet (1676 mm) above the floor.

Permanently installed electric baseboard heaters equipped with factory-installed receptacle outlets, or outlets provided as a separate assembly by the baseboard manufacturer shall be permitted as the required outlet or outlets for the wall space utilized by such permanently installed heaters. Such receptacle outlets shall not be connected to the heater circuits.

E3901.2 General purpose receptacle distribution. In every kitchen, family room, dining room, living room, parlor, library, den, sun room, bedroom, recreation room, or similar room or area of dwelling units, receptacle outlets shall be installed in accordance with the general provisions specified in Sections E3901.2.1 through E3901.2.3 (see Figure E3901.2).

E3901.2.1 Spacing. Receptacles shall be installed so that no point measured horizontally along the floor line in any wall space is more than 6 feet 1829 mm, from a receptacle outlet.

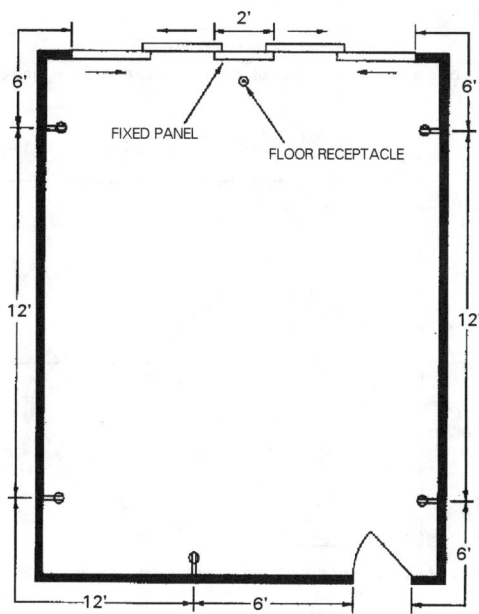

For SI: 1 foot = 304.8 mm.

FIGURE E3901.2
GENERAL USE RECEPTACLE DISTRIBUTION

E3901.2.2 Wall space. As used in this section, a wall space shall include the following:

1. Any space that is 2 feet (610 mm) or more in width, including space measured around corners, and that is unbroken along the floor line by doorways, fireplaces, and similar openings.

2. The space occupied by fixed panels in exterior walls, excluding sliding panels.

3. The space created by fixed room dividers such as railings and freestanding bar-type counters.

E3901.2.3 Floor receptacles. Receptacle outlets in floors shall not be counted as part of the required number of receptacle outlets except where located within 18 inches (457 mm) of the wall.

E3901.3 Small appliance receptacles. In the kitchen, pantry, breakfast room, dining room, or similar area of a dwelling unit, the two or more 20-ampere small-appliance branch circuits required by Section E3703.2, shall serve all wall and floor receptacle outlets covered by Sections E3901.2 and E3901.4 and those receptacle outlets provided for refrigeration appliances.

Exceptions:

1. In addition to the required receptacles specified by Sections E3901.1 and E3901.2, switched receptacles supplied from a general-purpose branch circuit as defined in Section E3903.2, Exception 1 shall be permitted.

2. The receptacle outlet for refrigeration appliances shall be permitted to be supplied from an individual branch circuit rated at 15 amperes or greater.

E3901.3.1 Other outlets prohibited. The two or more small-appliance branch circuits specified in Section E3901.3 shall serve no other outlets.

Exceptions:

1. A receptacle installed solely for the electrical supply to and support of an electric clock in any of the rooms specified in Section E3901.3.

2. Receptacles installed to provide power for supplemental equipment and lighting on gas-fired ranges, ovens, and counter-mounted cooking units.

E3901.3.2 Limitations. Receptacles installed in a kitchen to serve countertop surfaces shall be supplied by not less than two small-appliance branch circuits, either or both of which shall also be permitted to supply receptacle outlets in the same kitchen and in other rooms specified in Section E3901.3. Additional small-appliance branch circuits shall be permitted to supply receptacle outlets in the kitchen and other rooms specified in Section E3901.3. A small-appliance branch circuit shall not serve more than one kitchen.

E3901.4 Countertop receptacles. In kitchens pantries, breakfast rooms, dining rooms and similar areas of dwelling units, receptacle outlets for countertop spaces shall be installed in accordance with Sections E3901.4.1 through E3901.4.5 (see Figure E3901.4). Where a range, counter-mounted cooking unit, or sink is installed in an island or peninsular countertop and the width of the countertop behind the range, counter-mounted cooking unit, or sink is less than 12 inches (305 mm), the range, counter-mounted cooking unit, or sink has divided the countertop space into two separate countertop spaces as defined in Section E3901.4.4. Each separate countertop space shall comply with the applicable requirements of this section.

E3901.4.1 Wall countertop space. A receptacle outlet shall be installed at each wall countertop space 12 inches (305 mm) or wider. Receptacle outlets shall be installed so that no point along the wall line is more than 24 inches (610 mm), measured horizontally from a receptacle outlet in that space.

> **Exception:** Receptacle outlets shall not be required on a wall directly behind a range, counter-mounted cooking unit or sink in the installation described in Figure E3901.4.1.

E3901.4.2 Island countertop spaces. At least one receptacle outlet shall be installed at each island countertop space with a long dimension of 24 inches (610 mm) or greater and a short dimension of 12 inches (305 mm) or greater.

E3901.4.3 Peninsular countertop space. At least one receptacle outlet shall be installed at each peninsular countertop space with a long dimension of 24 inches (610 mm) or greater and a short dimension of 12 inches (305 mm) or greater. A peninsular countertop is measured from the connecting edge.

E3901.4.4 Separate spaces. Countertop spaces separated by range tops, refrigerators, or sinks shall be considered as separate countertop spaces in applying the requirements of Sections E3901.4.1, E3901.4.2 and E3901.4.3.

E3901.4.5 Receptacle outlet location. Receptacle outlets shall be located not more than 20 inches (508 mm) above the countertop. Receptacle outlets shall not be installed in a face-up position in the work surfaces or countertops. Receptacle outlets rendered not readily accessible by appliances fastened in place, appliance garages, sinks or rangetops as addressed in the exception to Section E3901.4.1, or appliances occupying dedicated space shall not be considered as these required outlets.

> **Exception:** Receptacle outlets shall be permitted to be mounted not more than 12 inches (305 mm) below the countertop in construction designed for the physically impaired and for island and peninsular countertops where the countertop is flat across its entire surface and there are no means to mount a receptacle within 20 inches (508 mm)

For SI: 1 foot = 304.8 mm.

FIGURE E3901.4
COUNTERTOP RECEPTACLES

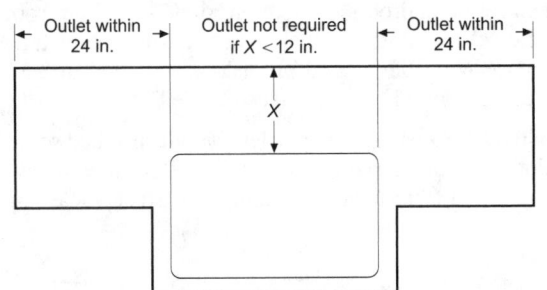

Sink, range or counter-mounted cooking unit extending from face of counter

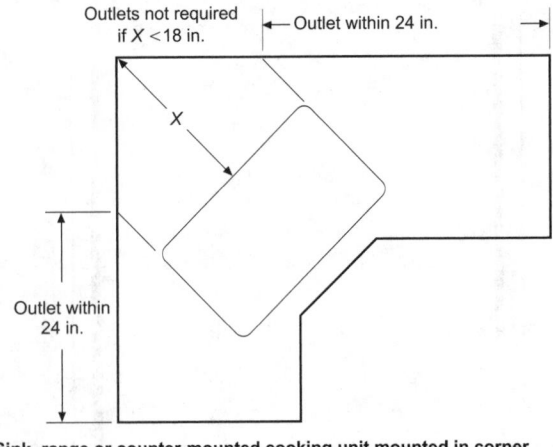

Sink, range or counter-mounted cooking unit mounted in corner

For SI: 1 inch = 25.4 mm.

FIGURE E3901.4.1
DETERMINATION OF AREA BEHIND SINK OR RANGE

2009 INTERNATIONAL RESIDENTIAL CODE®

above the countertop, such as in an overhead cabinet. Receptacles mounted below the countertop in accordance with this exception shall not be located where the countertop extends more than 6 inches (152 mm) beyond its support base.

E3901.5 Appliance receptacle outlets. Appliance receptacle outlets installed for specific appliances, such as laundry equipment, shall be installed within 6 feet (1829 mm) of the intended location of the appliance.

E3901.6 Bathroom. At least one wall receptacle outlet shall be installed in bathrooms and such outlet shall be located within 36 inches (914 mm) of the outside edge of each lavatory basin. The receptacle outlet shall be located on a wall or partition that is adjacent to the lavatory basin location, or installed on the side or face of the basin cabinet not more than 12 inches (305 mm) below the countertop.

Receptacle outlets shall not be installed in a face-up position in the work surfaces or countertops in a bathroom basin location.

E3901.7 Outdoor outlets. At least one receptacle outlet that is accessible while standing at grade level and located not more than 6 feet, 6 inches (1981 mm) above grade, shall be installed outdoors at the front and back of each dwelling unit having direct access to grade. Balconies, decks, and porches that are accessible from inside of the dwelling unit and that have a usable area of 20 square feet (1.86 m²) or greater shall have at least one receptacle outlet installed within the perimeter of the balcony, deck, or porch. The receptacle shall be located not more than 6 feet, 6 inches (1981 mm) above the balcony, deck, or porch surface.

E3901.8 Laundry areas. At least one receptacle outlet shall be installed to serve laundry appliances.

E3901.9 Basements and garages. At least one receptacle outlet, in addition to any provided for specific equipment, shall be installed in each basement and in each attached garage, and in each detached garage that is provided with electrical power. Where a portion of the basement is finished into one or more habitable room(s), each separate unfinished portion shall have a receptacle outlet installed in accordance with this section.

E3901.10 Hallways. Hallways of 10 feet (3048 mm) or more in length shall have at least one receptacle outlet. The hall length shall be considered the length measured along the centerline of the hall without passing through a doorway.

E3901.11 HVAC outlet. A 125-volt, single-phase, 15- or 20-ampere-rated receptacle outlet shall be installed at an accessible location for the servicing of heating, air-conditioning and refrigeration equipment. The receptacle shall be located on the same level and within 25 feet (7620 mm) of the heating, air-conditioning and refrigeration equipment. The receptacle outlet shall not be connected to the load side of the HVAC equipment disconnecting means.

Exception: A receptacle outlet shall not be required for the servicing of evaporative coolers.

SECTION E3902
GROUND-FAULT AND ARC-FAULT
CIRCUIT-INTERRUPTER PROTECTION

E3902.1 Bathroom receptacles. All 125-volt, single-phase, 15- and 20-ampere receptacles installed in bathrooms shall have ground-fault circuit-interrupter protection for personnel.

E3902.2 Garage and accessory building receptacles. All 125-volt, single-phase, 15- or 20-ampere receptacles installed in garages and grade-level portions of unfinished accessory buildings used for storage or work areas shall have ground-fault circuit-interrupter protection for personnel.

E3902.3 Outdoor receptacles. All 125-volt, single-phase, 15- and 20-ampere receptacles installed outdoors shall have ground-fault circuit-interrupter protection for personnel.

Exception: Receptacles as covered in Section E4101.7.

E3902.4 Crawl space receptacles. Where a crawl space is at or below grade level, all 125-volt, single-phase, 15- and 20-ampere receptacles installed in such spaces shall have ground-fault circuit-interrupter protection for personnel.

E3902.5 Unfinished basement receptacles. All 125-volt, single-phase, 15- and 20-ampere receptacles installed in unfinished basements shall have ground-fault circuit-interrupter protection for personnel. For purposes of this section, unfinished basements are defined as portions or areas of the basement not intended as habitable rooms and limited to storage areas, work areas, and the like.

Exception: A receptacle supplying only a permanently installed fire alarm or burglar alarm system.

E3902.6 Kitchen receptacles. All 125-volt, single-phase, 15- and 20-ampere receptacles that serve countertop surfaces shall have ground-fault circuit-interrupter protection for personnel.

E3902.7 Laundry, utility, and bar sink receptacles. All 125-volt, single-phase, 15- and 20-ampere receptacles that are located within 6 feet (1829 mm) of the outside edge of a laundry, utility or wet bar sink shall have ground-fault circuit-interrupter protection for personnel. Receptacle outlets shall not be installed in a face-up position in the work surfaces or countertops.

E3902.8 Boathouse receptacles. All 125-volt, single-phase, 15- or 20-ampere receptacles installed in boathouses shall have ground-fault circuit-interrupter protection for personnel.

E3902.9 Boat hoists. Ground-fault circuit-interrupter protection for personnel shall be provided for 240-volt and less outlets that supply boat hoists.

E3902.10 Electrically heated floors. Ground-fault circuit-interrupter protection for personnel shall be provided for electrically heated floors in bathrooms, and in hydromassage bathtub, spa and hot tub locations.

E3902.11 Arc-fault circuit-interrupter protection. All branch circuits that supply 120-volt, single-phase, 15- and 20-ampere outlets installed in family rooms, dining rooms, living rooms, parlors, libraries, dens, bedrooms, sunrooms, recreations rooms, closets, hallways and similar rooms or areas shall be protected by a combination type arc-fault circuit interrupter installed to provide protection of the branch circuit.

Exception:

1. Where a combination AFCI is installed at the first outlet to provide protection for the remaining portion of the branch circuit, the portion of the branch circuit between the branch-circuit overcurrent device and such outlet shall be wired with metal outlet and junction boxes and RMC, IMC, EMT or steel armored cable, Type AC meeting the requirements of Section E3908.8.

2. AFCI protection is not required for a branch circuit supplying only a fire alarm system where the branch circuit is wired with metal outlet and junction boxes and RMC, IMC, EMT or steel armored cable Type AC meeting the requirements of Section E3908.8.

SECTION E3903
LIGHTING OUTLETS

E3903.1 General. Lighting outlets shall be provided in accordance with Sections E3903.2 through E3903.4.

E3903.2 Habitable rooms. At least one wall switch-controlled lighting outlet shall be installed in every habitable room and bathroom.

Exceptions:

1. In other than kitchens and bathrooms, one or more receptacles controlled by a wall switch shall be considered equivalent to the required lighting outlet.

2. Lighting outlets shall be permitted to be controlled by occupancy sensors that are in addition to wall switches, or that are located at a customary wall switch location and equipped with a manual override that will allow the sensor to function as a wall switch.

E3903.3 Additional locations. At least one wall-switch-controlled lighting outlet shall be installed in hallways, stairways, attached garages, and detached garages with electric power. At least one wall-switch-controlled lighting outlet shall be installed to provide illumination on the exterior side of each outdoor egress door having grade level access, including outdoor egress doors for attached garages and detached garages with electric power. A vehicle door in a garage shall not be considered as an outdoor egress door. Where one or more lighting outlets are installed for interior stairways, there shall be a wall switch at each floor level and landing level that includes an entryway to control the lighting outlets where the stairway between floor levels has six or more risers.

Exception: In hallways, stairways, and at outdoor egress doors, remote, central, or automatic control of lighting shall be permitted.

E3903.4 Storage or equipment spaces. In attics, under-floor spaces, utility rooms and basements, at least one lighting outlet shall be installed where these spaces are used for storage or contain equipment requiring servicing. Such lighting outlet shall be controlled by a wall switch or shall have an integral switch. At least one point of control shall be at the usual point

of entry to these spaces. The lighting outlet shall be provided at or near the equipment requiring servicing.

SECTION E3904
GENERAL INSTALLATION REQUIREMENTS

E3904.1 Electrical continuity of metal raceways and enclosures. Metal raceways, cable armor and other metal enclosures for conductors shall be mechanically joined together into a continuous electric conductor and shall be connected to all boxes, fittings and cabinets so as to provide effective electrical continuity. Raceways and cable assemblies shall be mechanically secured to boxes, fittings cabinets and other enclosures.

Exception: Short sections of raceway used to provide cable assemblies with support or protection against physical damage.

E3904.2 Mechanical continuity—raceways and cables. Metal or nonmetallic raceways, cable armors and cable sheaths shall be continuous between cabinets, boxes, fittings or other enclosures or outlets.

Exception: Short sections of raceway used to provide cable assemblies with support or protection against physical damage.

E3904.3 Securing and supporting. Raceways, cable assemblies, boxes, cabinets and fittings shall be securely fastened in place.

E3904.3.1 Prohibited means of support. Cable wiring methods shall not be used as a means of support for other cables, raceways and nonelectrical equipment.

E3904.4 Raceways as means of support. Raceways shall be used as a means of support for other raceways, cables or nonelectric equipment only under the following conditions:

1. Where the raceway or means of support is identified for the purpose; or

2. Where the raceway contains power supply conductors for electrically controlled equipment and is used to support Class 2 circuit conductors or cables that are solely for the purpose of connection to the control circuits of the equipment served by such raceway; or

3. Where the raceway is used to support boxes or conduit bodies in accordance with Sections E3906.8.4 and E3906.8.5.

E3904.5 Raceway installations. Raceways shall be installed complete between outlet, junction or splicing points prior to the installation of conductors.

Exception: Short sections of raceways used to contain conductors or cable assemblies for protection from physical damage shall not be required to be installed complete between outlet, junction, or splicing points.

E3904.6 Conduit and tubing fill. The maximum number of conductors installed in conduit or tubing shall be in accordance with Tables E3904.6(1) through E3904.6(10).

E3904.7 Air handling—stud cavity and joist spaces. Where wiring methods having a nonmetallic covering pass through stud cavities and joist spaces used for air handling, such wiring shall pass through such spaces perpendicular to the long dimension of the spaces.

TABLE E3904.6(1)
MAXIMUM NUMBER OF CONDUCTORS IN ELECTRICAL METALLIC TUBING (EMT)[a]

TYPE LETTERS	CONDUCTOR SIZE AWG/kcmil	TRADE SIZES (inches)					
		1/2	3/4	1	1 1/4	1 1/2	2
RHW, RHW-2	14	4	7	11	20	27	46
	12	3	6	9	17	23	38
	10	2	5	8	13	18	30
	8	1	2	4	7	9	16
	6	1	1	3	5	8	13
	4	1	1	2	4	6	10
	3	1	1	1	4	5	9
	2	1	1	1	3	4	7
	1	0	1	1	1	3	5
	1/0	0	1	1	1	2	4
	2/0	0	1	1	1	2	4
	3/0	0	0	1	1	1	3
	4/0	0	0	1	1	1	3
TW	14	8	15	25	43	58	96
	12	6	11	19	33	45	74
	10	5	8	14	24	33	55
	8	2	5	8	13	18	30
RHW[a], RHW-2[a], THHW, THW, THW-2	14	6	10	16	28	39	64
	12	4	8	13	23	31	51
	10	3	6	10	18	24	40
	8	1	4	6	10	14	24
RHW[a], RHW-2[a], TW, THW, THHW, THW-2	6	1	3	4	8	11	18
	4	1	1	3	6	8	13
	3	1	1	3	5	7	12
	2	1	1	2	4	6	10
	1	1	1	1	3	4	7
	1/0	0	1	1	2	3	6
	2/0	0	1	1	1	3	5
	3/0	0	1	1	1	2	4
	4/0	0	0	1	1	1	3
THHN, THWN, THWN-2	14	12	22	35	61	84	138
	12	9	16	26	45	61	101
	10	5	10	16	28	38	63
	8	3	6	9	16	22	36
	6	2	4	7	12	16	26
	4	1	2	4	7	10	16
	3	1	1	3	6	8	13
	2	1	1	3	5	7	11
	1	1	1	1	4	5	8
	1/0	1	1	1	3	4	7
	2/0	0	1	1	2	3	6
	3/0	0	1	1	1	3	5
	4/0	0	1	1	1	2	4
XHHW, XHHW-2	14	8	15	25	43	58	96
	12	6	11	19	33	45	74
	10	5	8	14	24	33	55
	8	2	5	8	13	18	30
	6	1	3	6	10	14	22
	4	1	2	4	7	10	16
	3	1	1	3	6	8	14
	2	1	1	3	5	7	11
	1	1	1	1	4	5	8
	1/0	1	1	1	3	4	7
	2/0	0	1	1	2	3	6
	3/0	0	1	1	1	3	5
	4/0	0	1	1	1	2	4

For SI: 1 inch = 25.4 mm.

a. Types RHW, and RHW-2 without outer covering.

TABLE E3904.6(2)
MAXIMUM NUMBER OF CONDUCTORS IN ELECTRICAL NONMETALLIC TUBING (ENT)[a]

TYPE LETTERS	CONDUCTOR SIZE AWG/kcmil	TRADE SIZES (inches)					
		$^1/_2$	$^3/_4$	1	$1^1/_4$	$1^1/_2$	2
RHW, RHW-2	14	3	6	10	19	26	43
	12	2	5	9	16	22	36
	10	1	4	7	13	17	29
	8	1	1	3	6	9	15
	6	1	1	3	5	7	12
	4	1	1	2	4	6	9
	3	1	1	1	3	5	8
	2	0	1	1	3	4	7
	1	0	1	1	1	3	5
	1/0	0	0	1	1	2	4
	2/0	0	0	1	1	1	3
	3/0	0	0	1	1	1	3
	4/0	0	0	1	1	1	2
TW	14	7	13	22	40	55	92
	12	5	10	17	31	42	71
	10	4	7	13	23	32	52
	8	1	4	7	13	17	29
RHW[a], RHW-2[a], THHW, THW, THW-2	14	4	8	15	27	37	61
	12	3	7	12	21	29	49
	10	3	5	9	17	23	38
	8	1	3	5	10	14	23
RHW[a], RHW-2[a], TW, THW, THHW, THW-2	6	1	2	4	7	10	17
	4	1	1	3	5	8	13
	3	1	1	2	5	7	11
	2	1	1	2	4	6	9
	1	0	1	1	3	4	6
	1/0	0	1	1	2	3	5
	2/0	0	1	1	1	3	5
	3/0	0	0	1	1	2	4
	4/0	0	0	1	1	1	3
THHN, THWN, THWN-2	14	10	18	32	58	80	132
	12	7	13	23	42	58	96
	10	4	8	15	26	36	60
	8	2	5	8	15	21	35
	6	1	3	6	11	15	25
	4	1	1	4	7	9	15
	3	1	1	3	5	8	13
	2	1	1	2	5	6	11
	1	1	1	1	3	5	8
	1/0	0	1	1	3	4	7
	2/0	0	1	1	2	3	5
	3/0	0	1	1	1	3	4
	4/0	0	0	1	1	2	4
XHHW, XHHW-2	14	7	13	22	40	55	92
	12	5	10	17	31	42	71
	10	4	7	13	23	32	52
	8	1	4	7	13	17	29
	6	1	3	5	9	13	21
	4	1	1	4	7	9	15
	3	1	1	3	6	8	13
	2	1	1	2	5	6	11
	1	1	1	1	3	5	8
	1/0	0	1	1	3	4	7
	2/0	0	1	1	2	3	6
	3/0	0	1	1	1	3	5
	4/0	0	0	1	1	2	4

For SI: 1 inch = 25.4 mm.

a. Types RHW, and RHW-2 without outer covering.

TABLE E3904.6(3)
MAXIMUM NUMBER OF CONDUCTORS IN FLEXIBLE METALLIC CONDUIT (FMC)[a]

TYPE LETTERS	CONDUCTOR SIZE AWG/kcmil	TRADE SIZES (inches)					
		1/2	3/4	1	1 1/4	1 1/2	2
RHW, RHW-2	14	4	7	11	17	25	44
	12	3	6	9	14	21	37
	10	3	5	7	11	17	30
	8	1	2	4	6	9	15
	6	1	1	3	5	7	12
	4	1	1	2	4	5	10
	3	1	1	1	3	5	7
	2	1	1	1	3	4	7
	1	0	1	1	1	2	5
	1/0	0	1	1	1	2	4
	2/0	0	1	1	1	1	3
	3/0	0	0	1	1	1	3
TW	14	9	15	23	36	53	94
	12	7	11	18	28	41	72
	10	5	8	13	21	30	54
	8	3	5	7	11	17	30
RHW[a], RHW-2[a], THHW, THW, THW-2	14	6	10	15	24	35	62
	12	5	8	12	19	28	50
	10	4	6	10	15	22	39
	8	1	4	6	9	13	23
RHW[a], RHW-2[a], TW, THW, THHW, THW-2	6	1	3	4	7	10	18
	4	1	1	3	5	7	13
	3	1	1	3	4	6	11
	2	1	1	2	4	5	10
	1	1	1	1	2	4	7
	1/0	0	1	1	1	3	6
	2/0	0	1	1	1	3	5
	3/0	0	1	1	1	2	4
	4/0	0	0	1	1	1	3
	4/0	0	0	1	1	1	2
THHN, THWN, THWN-2	14	13	22	33	52	76	134
	12	9	16	24	38	56	98
	10	6	10	15	24	35	62
	8	3	6	9	14	20	35
	6	2	4	6	10	14	25
	4	1	2	4	6	9	16
	3	1	1	3	5	7	13
	2	1	1	3	4	6	11
	1	1	1	1	3	4	8
	1/0	1	1	1	2	4	7
	2/0	0	1	1	1	3	6
	3/0	0	1	1	1	2	5
	4/0	0	1	1	1	1	4
XHHW, XHHW-2	14	9	15	23	36	53	94
	12	7	11	18	28	41	72
	10	5	8	13	21	30	54
	8	3	5	7	11	17	30
	6	1	3	5	8	12	22
	4	1	2	4	6	9	16
	3	1	1	3	5	7	13
	2	1	1	3	4	6	11
	1	1	1	1	3	5	8
	1/0	1	1	1	2	4	7
	2/0	0	1	1	2	3	6
	3/0	0	1	1	1	3	5
	4/0	0	1	1	1	2	4

For SI: 1 inch = 25.4 mm.

a. Types RHW, and RHW-2 without outer covering.

TYPE LETTERS	CONDUCTOR SIZE AWG/kcmil	TRADE SIZES (inches)					
		1/2	3/4	1	1 1/4	1 1/2	2
RHW, RHW-2	14	4	8	13	22	30	49
	12	4	6	11	18	25	41
	10	3	5	8	15	20	33
	8	1	3	4	8	10	17
	6	1	1	3	6	8	14
	4	1	1	3	5	6	11
	3	1	1	2	4	6	9
	2	1	1	1	3	5	8
	1	0	1	1	2	3	5
	1/0	0	1	1	1	3	4
	2/0	0	1	1	1	2	4
	3/0	0	0	1	1	1	3
	4/0	0	0	1	1	1	3
TW	14	10	17	27	47	64	104
	12	7	13	21	36	49	80
	10	5	9	15	27	36	59
	8	3	5	8	15	20	33
RHW[a], RHW-2[a], THHW, THW, THW-2	14	6	11	18	31	42	69
	12	5	9	14	25	34	56
	10	4	7	11	19	26	43
	8	2	4	7	12	16	26
RHW[a], RHW-2[a], TW, THW, THHW, THW-2	6	1	3	5	9	12	20
	4	1	2	4	6	9	15
	3	1	1	3	6	8	13
	2	1	1	3	5	6	11
	1	1	1	1	3	4	7
	1/0	1	1	1	3	4	6
	2/0	0	1	1	2	3	5
	3/0	0	1	1	1	3	4
	4/0	0	1	1	1	2	4
THHN, THWN, THWN-2	14	14	24	39	68	91	149
	12	10	17	29	49	67	109
	10	6	11	18	31	42	68
	8	3	6	10	18	24	39
	6	2	4	7	13	17	28
	4	1	3	4	8	10	17
	3	1	2	4	6	9	15
	2	1	1	3	5	7	12
	1	1	1	2	4	5	9
	1/0	1	1	1	3	4	8
	2/0	1	1	1	3	4	6
	3/0	0	1	1	2	3	5
	4/0	0	1	1	1	2	4
XHHW, XHHW-2	14	10	17	27	47	64	104
	12	7	13	21	36	49	80
	10	5	9	15	27	36	59
	8	3	5	8	15	20	33
	6	1	4	6	11	15	24
	4	1	3	4	8	11	18
	3	1	2	4	7	9	15
	2	1	1	3	5	7	12
	1	1	1	2	4	5	9
	1/0	1	1	1	3	5	8
	2/0	1	1	1	3	4	6
	3/0	0	1	1	2	3	5
	4/0	0	1	1	1	2	4

For SI: 1 inch = 25.4 mm.

a. Types RHW, and RHW-2 without outer covering.

TABLE E3904.6(5)
MAXIMUM NUMBER OF CONDUCTORS IN LIQUID-TIGHT FLEXIBLE NONMETALLIC CONDUIT (FNMC-B)[a]

TYPE LETTERS	CONDUCTOR SIZE AWG/kcmil	TRADE SIZES (inches)						
		3/8	1/2	3/4	1	1 1/4	1 1/2	2
RHW, RHW-2	14	2	4	7	12	21	27	44
	12	1	3	6	10	17	22	36
	10	1	3	5	8	14	18	29
	8	1	1	2	4	7	9	15
	6	1	1	1	3	6	7	12
	4	0	1	1	2	4	6	9
	3	0	1	1	1	4	5	8
	2	0	1	1	1	3	4	7
	1	0	0	1	1	1	3	5
	1/0	0	0	1	1	1	2	4
	2/0	0	0	1	1	1	1	3
	3/0	0	0	0	1	1	1	3
	4/0	0	0	0	1	1	1	2
TW	14	5	9	15	25	44	57	93
	12	4	7	12	19	33	43	71
	10	3	5	9	14	25	32	53
	8	1	3	5	8	14	18	29
RHW[a], RGW-2[a], THHW, THW, THW-2	14	3	6	10	16	29	38	62
	12	3	5	8	13	23	30	50
	10	1	3	6	10	18	23	39
	8	1	1	4	6	11	14	23
RHW[a], RHW-2[a], TW, THW, THHW, THW-2	6	1	1	3	5	8	11	18
	4	1	1	1	3	6	8	13
	3	1	1	1	3	5	7	11
	2	0	1	1	2	4	6	9
	1	0	1	1	1	3	4	7
	1/0	0	0	1	1	2	3	6
	2/0	0	0	1	1	2	3	5
	3/0	0	0	1	1	1	2	4
	4/0	0	0	0	1	1	1	3
THHN, THWN, THWN-2	14	8	13	22	36	63	81	133
	12	5	9	16	26	46	59	97
	10	3	6	10	16	29	37	61
	8	1	3	6	9	16	21	35
	6	1	2	4	7	12	15	25
	4	1	1	2	4	7	9	15
	3	1	1	1	3	6	8	13
	2	1	1	1	3	5	7	11
	1	0	1	1	1	4	5	8
	1/0	0	1	1	1	3	4	7
	2/0	0	0	1	1	2	3	6
	3/0	0	0	1	1	1	3	5
	4/0	0	0	1	1	1	2	4
XHHW, XHHW-2	14	5	9	15	25	44	57	93
	12	4	7	12	19	33	43	71
	10	3	5	9	14	25	32	53
	8	1	3	5	8	14	18	29
	6	1	1	3	6	10	13	22
	4	1	1	2	4	7	9	16
	3	1	1	1	3	6	8	13
	2	1	1	1	3	5	7	11
	1	0	1	1	1	4	5	8
	1/0	0	1	1	1	3	4	7
	2/0	0	0	1	1	2	3	6
	3/0	0	0	1	1	1	3	5
	4/0	0	0	1	1	1	2	4

For SI: 1 inch = 25.4 mm.

a. Types RHW, and RHW-2 without outer covering.

TABLE E3904.6(6)
MAXIMUM NUMBER OF CONDUCTORS IN LIQUID-TIGHT FLEXIBLE NONMETALLIC CONDUIT (FNMC-A)[a]

TYPE LETTERS	CONDUCTOR SIZE AWG/kcmil	TRADE SIZES (inches)						
		3/8	1/2	3/4	1	1 1/4	1 1/2	2
RHW, RHW-2	14	2	4	7	11	20	27	45
	12	1	3	6	9	17	23	38
	10	1	3	5	8	13	18	30
	8	1	1	2	4	7	9	16
	6	1	1	1	3	5	7	13
	4	0	1	1	2	4	6	10
	3	0	1	1	1	4	5	8
	2	0	1	1	1	3	4	7
	1	0	0	1	1	1	3	5
	1/0	0	0	1	1	1	2	4
	2/0	0	0	1	1	1	1	4
	3/0	0	0	0	1	1	1	3
	4/0	0	0	0	1	1	1	3
TW	14	5	9	15	24	43	58	96
	12	4	7	12	19	33	44	74
	10	3	5	9	14	24	33	55
	8	1	3	5	8	13	18	30
RHW[a], RHW-2[a], THHW, THW, THW-2	14	3	6	10	16	28	38	64
	12	3	4	8	13	23	31	51
	10	1	3	6	10	18	24	40
	8	1	1	4	6	10	14	24
RHW[a], RHW-2[a], TW, THW, THHW, THW-2	6	1	1	3	4	8	11	18
	4	1	1	1	3	6	8	13
	3	1	1	1	3	5	7	11
	2	0	1	1	2	4	6	10
	1	0	1	1	1	3	4	7
	1/0	0	0	1	1	2	3	6
	2/0	0	0	1	1	1	3	5
	3/0	0	0	1	1	1	2	4
	4/0	0	0	0	1	1	1	3
THHN, THWN, THWN-2	14	8	13	22	35	62	83	137
	12	5	9	16	25	45	60	100
	10	3	6	10	16	28	38	63
	8	1	3	6	9	16	22	36
	6	1	2	4	6	12	16	26
	4	1	1	2	4	7	9	16
	3	1	1	1	3	6	8	13
	2	1	1	1	3	5	7	11
	1	0	1	1	1	4	5	8
	1/0	0	1	1	1	3	4	7
	2/0	0	0	1	1	2	3	6
	3/0	0	0	1	1	1	3	5
	4/0	0	0	1	1	1	2	4
XHHW, XHHW-2	14	5	9	15	24	43	58	96
	12	4	7	12	19	33	44	74
	10	3	5	9	14	24	33	55
	8	1	3	5	8	13	18	30
	6	1	1	3	5	10	13	22
	4	1	1	2	4	7	10	16
	3	1	1	1	3	6	8	14
	2	1	1	1	3	5	7	11
	1	0	1	1	1	4	5	8
	1/0	0	1	1	1	3	4	7
	2/0	0	0	1	1	2	3	6
	3/0	0	0	1	1	1	3	5
	4/0	0	0	1	1	1	2	4

For SI: 1 inch = 25.4 mm.

a. Types RHW, and RHW-2 without outer covering.

TABLE E3904.6(7)
MAXIMUM NUMBER OF CONDUCTORS IN LIQUID-TIGHT FLEXIBLE METAL CONDUIT (LFMC)[a]

TYPE LETTERS	CONDUCTOR SIZE AWG/kcmil	TRADE SIZES (inches)					
		1/2	3/4	1	1 1/4	1 1/2	2
RHW, RHW-2	14	4	7	12	21	27	44
	12	3	6	10	17	22	36
	10	3	5	8	14	18	29
	8	1	2	4	7	9	15
	6	1	1	3	6	7	12
	4	1	1	2	4	6	9
	3	1	1	1	4	5	8
	2	1	1	1	3	4	7
	1	0	1	1	1	3	5
	1/0	0	1	1	1	2	4
	2/0	0	1	1	1	1	3
	3/0	0	0	1	1	1	3
	4/0	0	0	1	1	1	2
TW	14	9	15	25	44	57	93
	12	7	12	19	33	43	71
	10	5	9	14	25	32	53
	8	3	5	8	14	18	29
RHW[a], RHW-2[a], THHW, THW, THW-2	14	6	10	16	29	38	62
	12	5	8	13	23	30	50
	10	3	6	10	18	23	39
	8	1	4	6	11	14	23
RHW[a], RHW-2[a], TW, THW, THHW, THW-2	6	1	3	5	8	11	18
	4	1	1	3	6	8	13
	3	1	1	3	5	7	11
	2	1	1	2	4	6	9
	1	1	1	1	3	4	7
	1/0	0	1	1	2	3	6
	2/0	0	1	1	2	3	5
	3/0	0	1	1	1	2	4
	4/0	0	0	1	1	1	3
THHN, THWN, THWN-2	14	13	22	36	63	81	133
	12	9	16	26	46	59	97
	10	6	10	16	29	37	61
	8	3	6	9	16	21	35
	6	2	4	7	12	15	25
	4	1	2	4	7	9	15
	3	1	1	3	6	8	13
	2	1	1	3	5	7	11
	1	1	1	1	4	5	8
	1/0	1	1	1	3	4	7
	2/0	0	1	1	2	3	6
	3/0	0	1	1	1	3	5
	4/0	0	1	1	1	2	4
XHHW, XHHW-2	14	9	15	25	44	57	93
	12	7	12	19	33	43	71
	10	5	9	14	25	32	53
	8	3	5	8	14	18	29
	6	1	3	6	10	13	22
	4	1	2	4	7	9	16
	3	1	1	3	6	8	13
	2	1	1	3	5	7	11
	1	1	1	1	4	5	8
	1/0	1	1	1	3	4	7
	2/0	0	1	1	2	3	6
	3/0	0	1	1	1	3	5
	4/0	0	1	1	1	2	4

For SI: 1 inch = 25.4 mm.

a. Types RHW, and RHW-2 without outer covering.

TABLE E3904.6(8)
MAXIMUM NUMBER OF CONDUCTORS IN RIGID METAL CONDUIT (RMC)[a]

TYPE LETTERS	CONDUCTOR SIZE AWG/kcmil	TRADE SIZES (inches)					
		1/2	3/4	1	1 1/4	1 1/2	2
RHW, RHW-2	14	4	7	12	21	28	46
	12	3	6	10	17	23	38
	10	3	5	8	14	19	31
	8	1	2	4	7	10	16
	6	1	1	3	6	8	13
	4	1	1	2	4	6	10
	3	1	1	2	4	5	9
	2	1	1	1	3	4	7
	1	0	1	1	1	3	5
	1/0	0	1	1	1	2	4
	2/0	0	1	1	1	2	4
	3/0	0	0	1	1	1	3
	4/0	0	0	1	1	1	3
TW	14	9	15	25	44	59	98
	12	7	12	19	33	45	75
	10	5	9	14	25	34	56
	8	3	5	8	14	19	31
RHW[a], RHW-2[a], THHW, THW, THW-2	14	6	10	17	29	39	65
	12	5	8	13	23	32	52
	10	3	6	10	18	25	41
	8	1	4	6	11	15	24
RHW[a], RHW-2[a], TW, THW, THHW, THW-2	6	1	3	5	8	11	18
	4	1	1	3	6	8	14
	3	1	1	3	5	7	12
	2	1	1	2	4	6	10
	1	1	1	1	3	4	7
	1/0	0	1	1	2	3	6
	2/0	0	1	1	2	3	5
	3/0	0	1	1	1	2	4
	4/0	0	0	1	1	1	3
THHN, THWN, THWN-2	14	13	22	36	63	85	140
	12	9	16	26	46	62	102
	10	6	10	17	29	39	64
	8	3	6	9	16	22	37
	6	2	4	7	12	16	27
	4	1	2	4	7	10	16
	3	1	1	3	6	8	14
	2	1	1	3	5	7	11
	1	1	1	1	4	5	8
	1/0	1	1	1	3	4	7
	2/0	0	1	1	2	3	6
	3/0	0	1	1	1	3	5
	4/0	0	1	1	1	2	4
XHHW, XHHW-2	14	9	15	25	44	59	98
	12	7	12	19	33	45	75
	10	5	9	14	25	34	56
	8	3	5	8	14	19	31
	6	1	3	6	10	14	23
	4	1	2	4	7	10	16
	3	1	1	3	6	8	14
	2	1	1	3	5	7	12
	1	1	1	1	4	5	9
	1/0	1	1	1	3	4	7
	2/0	0	1	1	2	3	6
	3/0	0	1	1	1	3	5
	4/0	0	1	1	1	2	4

For SI: 1 inch = 25.4 mm.

a. Types RHW, and RHW-2 without outer covering.

TABLE E3904.6(9)
MAXIMUM NUMBER OF CONDUCTORS IN RIGID PVC CONDUIT, SCHEDULE 80 (PVC-80)[a]

TYPE LETTERS	CONDUCTOR SIZE AWG/kcmil	TRADE SIZES (inches)					
		1/2	3/4	1	1 1/4	1 1/2	2
RHW, RHW-2	14	3	5	9	17	23	39
	12	2	4	7	14	19	32
	10	1	3	6	11	15	26
	8	1	1	3	6	8	13
	6	1	1	2	4	6	11
	4	1	1	1	3	5	8
	3	0	1	1	3	4	7
	2	0	1	1	3	4	6
	1	0	1	1	1	2	4
	1/0	0	0	1	1	1	3
	2/0	0	0	1	1	1	3
	3/0	0	0	1	1	1	3
	4/0	0	0	0	1	1	2
TW	14	6	11	20	35	49	82
	12	5	9	15	27	38	63
	10	3	6	11	20	28	47
	8	1	3	6	11	15	26
RHW[a], RHW-2[a], THHW, THW, THW-2	14	4	8	13	23	32	55
	12	3	6	10	19	26	44
	10	2	5	8	15	20	34
	8	1	3	5	9	12	20
RHW[a], RHW-2[a], TW, THW, THHW, THW-2	6	1	1	3	7	9	16
	4	1	1	3	5	7	12
	3	1	1	2	4	6	10
	2	1	1	1	3	5	8
	1	0	1	1	2	3	6
	1/0	0	1	1	1	3	5
	2/0	0	1	1	1	2	4
	3/0	0	0	1	1	1	3
	4/0	0	0	1	1	1	3
THHN, THWN, THWN-2	14	9	17	28	51	70	118
	12	6	12	20	37	51	86
	10	4	7	13	23	32	54
	8	2	4	7	13	18	31
	6	1	3	5	9	13	22
	4	1	1	3	6	8	14
	3	1	1	3	5	7	12
	2	1	1	2	4	6	10
	1	0	1	1	3	4	7
	1/0	0	1	1	2	3	6
	2/0	0	1	1	1	3	5
	3/0	0	1	1	1	2	4
	4/0	0	0	1	1	1	3
XHHW, XHHW-2	14	6	11	20	35	49	82
	12	5	9	15	27	38	63
	10	3	6	11	20	28	47
	8	1	3	6	11	15	26
	6	1	2	4	8	11	19
	4	1	1	3	6	8	14
	3	1	1	3	5	7	12
	2	1	1	2	4	6	10
	1	0	1	1	3	4	7
	1/0	0	1	1	2	3	6
	2/0	0	1	1	1	3	5
	3/0	0	1	1	1	2	4
	4/0	0	0	1	1	1	3

For SI: 1 inch = 25.4 mm.

a. Types RHW, and RHW-2 without outer covering.

TABLE E3904.6(10)
MAXIMUM NUMBER OF CONDUCTORS IN RIGID PVC CONDUIT SCHEDULE 40 (PVC-40)[a]

TYPE LETTERS	CONDUCTOR SIZE AWG/kcmil	TRADE SIZES (inches)					
		1/2	3/4	1	1 1/4	1 1/2	2
RHW, RHW-2	14	4	7	11	20	27	45
	12	3	5	9	16	22	37
	10	2	4	7	13	18	30
	8	1	2	4	7	9	15
	6	1	1	3	5	7	12
	4	1	1	2	4	6	10
	3	1	1	1	4	5	8
	2	1	1	1	3	4	7
	1	0	1	1	1	3	5
	1/0	0	1	1	1	2	4
	2/0	0	0	1	1	1	3
	3/0	0	0	1	1	1	3
	4/0	0	0	1	1	1	2
TW	14	8	14	24	42	57	94
	12	6	11	18	32	44	72
	10	4	8	13	24	32	54
	8	2	4	7	13	18	30
RHW[a], RHW-2[a], THHW, THW, THW-2	14	5	9	16	28	38	63
	12	4	8	12	22	30	50
	10	3	6	10	17	24	39
	8	1	3	6	10	14	23
RHW[a], RHW-2[a], TW, THW, THHW, THW-2	6	1	2	4	8	11	18
	4	1	1	3	6	8	13
	3	1	1	3	5	7	11
	2	1	1	2	4	6	10
	1	0	1	1	3	4	7
	1/0	0	1	1	2	3	6
	2/0	0	1	1	1	3	5
	3/0	0	1	1	1	2	4
	4/0	0	0	1	1	1	3
THHN, THWN, THWN-2	14	11	21	34	60	82	135
	12	8	15	25	43	59	99
	10	5	9	15	27	37	62
	8	3	5	9	16	21	36
	6	1	4	6	11	15	26
	4	1	2	4	7	9	16
	3	1	1	3	6	8	13
	2	1	1	3	5	7	11
	1	1	1	1	3	5	8
	1/0	1	1	1	3	4	7
	2/0	0	1	1	2	3	6
	3/0	0	1	1	1	3	5
	4/0	0	1	1	1	2	4
XHHW, XHHW-2	14	8	14	24	42	57	94
	12	6	11	18	32	44	72
	10	4	8	13	24	32	54
	8	2	4	7	13	18	30
	6	1	3	5	10	13	22
	4	1	2	4	7	9	16
	3	1	1	3	6	8	13
	2	1	1	3	5	7	11
	1	1	1	1	3	5	8
	1/0	1	1	1	3	4	7
	2/0	0	1	1	2	3	6
	3/0	0	1	1	1	3	5
	4/0	0	1	1	1	2	4

For SI: 1 inch = 25.4 mm.

a. Types RHW, and RHW-2 without outer covering.

SECTION E3905
BOXES, CONDUIT BODIES AND FITTINGS

E3905.1 Box, conduit body or fitting—where required. A box or conduit body shall be installed at each conductor splice point, outlet, switch point, junction point and pull point except as otherwise permitted in Sections E3905.1.1 through E3905.1.6.

Fittings and connectors shall be used only with the specific wiring methods for which they are designed and listed.

E3905.1.1 Equipment. An integral junction box or wiring compartment that is part of listed equipment shall be permitted to serve as a box or conduit body.

E3905.1.2 Protection. A box or conduit body shall not be required where cables enter or exit from conduit or tubing that is used to provide cable support or protection against physical damage. A fitting shall be provided on the end(s) of the conduit or tubing to protect the cable from abrasion.

E3905.1.3 Integral enclosure. A wiring device with integral enclosure identified for the use, having brackets that securely fasten the device to walls or ceilings of conventional on-site frame construction, for use with nonmetallic-sheathed cable, shall be permitted in lieu of a box or conduit body.

E3905.1.4 Fitting. A fitting identified for the use shall be permitted in lieu of a box or conduit body where such fitting is accessible after installation and does not contain spliced or terminated conductors.

E3905.1.5 Buried conductors. Splices and taps in buried conductors and cables shall not be required to be enclosed in a box or conduit body where installed in accordance with Section E3803.4.

E3905.1.6 Luminaires. Where a luminaire is listed to be used as a raceway, a box or conduit body shall not be required for wiring installed therein.

E3905.2 Metal boxes. All metal boxes shall be grounded.

E3905.3 Nonmetallic boxes. Nonmetallic boxes shall be used only with cabled wiring methods with entirely nonmetallic sheaths, flexible cords and nonmetallic raceways.

Exceptions:

1. Where internal bonding means are provided between all entries, nonmetallic boxes shall be permitted to be used with metal raceways and metal-armored cables.

2. Where integral bonding means with a provision for attaching an equipment grounding jumper inside the box are provided between all threaded entries in nonmetallic boxes listed for the purpose, nonmetallic boxes shall be permitted to be used with metal raceways and metal-armored cables.

E3905.3.1 Nonmetallic-sheathed cable and nonmetallic boxes. Where nonmetallic-sheathed cable is used, the cable assembly, including the sheath, shall extend into the box not less than $^1/_4$ inch (6.4 mm) through a nonmetallic-sheathed cable knockout opening.

E3905.3.2 Securing to box. All permitted wiring methods shall be secured to the boxes.

Exception: Where nonmetallic-sheathed cable is used with boxes not larger than a nominal size of $2^1/_4$ inches by 4 inches (57 mm by 102 mm) mounted in walls or ceilings, and where the cable is fastened within 8 inches (203 mm) of the box measured along the sheath, and where the sheath extends through a cable knockout not less than $^1/_4$ inch (6.4 mm), securing the cable to the box shall not be required.

E3905.3.3 Conductor rating. Nonmetallic boxes shall be suitable for the lowest temperature-rated conductor entering the box.

E3905.4 Minimum depth of boxes for outlets, devices, and utilization equipment. Outlet and device boxes shall have sufficient depth to allow equipment installed within them to be mounted properly and with sufficient clearance to prevent damage to conductors within the box.

E3905.4.1 Outlet boxes without enclosed devices or utilization equipment. Boxes that do not enclose devices or utilization equipment shall have an internal depth of not less than $^1/_2$ inch (12.7 mm).

E3905.4.2 Outlet and device boxes with enclosed devices. Boxes intended to enclose flush devices shall have an internal depth of not less than $^{15}/_{16}$ inch (23.8 mm).

E3905.4.3 Utilization equipment. Outlet and device boxes that enclose utilization equipment shall have a minimum internal depth that accommodates the rearward projection of the equipment and the size of the conductors that supply the equipment. The internal depth shall include that of any extension boxes, plaster rings, or raised covers. The internal depth shall comply with all of the applicable provisions that follow.

Exception: Utilization equipment that is listed to be installed with specified boxes.

1. Large equipment. Boxes that enclose utilization equipment that projects more than $1^7/_8$ in. (48 mm) rearward from the mounting plane of the box shall have a depth that is not less than the depth of the equipment plus $^1/_4$ in. (6.4 mm).

2. Conductors larger than 4 AWG. Boxes that enclose utilization equipment supplied by conductors larger than 4 AWG shall be identified for their specific function.

3. Conductors 8, 6, or 4 AWG. Boxes that enclose utilization equipment supplied by 8, 6, or 4 AWG conductors shall have an internal depth that is not less than $2^1/_{16}$ in. (52.4 mm).

4. Conductors 12 or 10 AWG. Boxes that enclose utilization equipment supplied by 12 or 10 AWG conductors shall have an internal depth that is not less than $1^3/_{16}$ in. (30.2 mm). Where the equipment projects rearward from the mounting plane of the box by more than 1 in. (25.4 mm), the box shall have a depth that is not less than that of the equipment plus $^1/_4$ in. (6.4 mm).

5. Conductors 14 AWG and smaller. Boxes that enclose equipment supplied by 14 AWG or smaller conductors shall have a depth that is not less than $^{15}/_{16}$ in. (23.8 mm).

E3905.5 Boxes enclosing flush-mounted devices. Boxes enclosing flush-mounted devices shall be of such design that the devices are completely enclosed at the back and all sides and shall provide support for the devices. Screws for supporting the box shall not be used for attachment of the device contained therein.

E3905.6 Boxes at luminaire outlets. Boxes used at luminaire or lampholder outlets in a ceiling shall be designed for the purpose and shall be capable of supporting a luminaire weighing up to 50 pounds (22.7 kg). Boxes used at luminaire or lampholder outlets in a wall shall be designed for the purpose and shall be marked on the interior to indicate the maximum weight of the luminaire that is permitted to be supported by the box in the wall, if other than 50 pounds (22.7 kg). At every outlet used exclusively for lighting, the box shall be designed or installed so that a luminaire can be attached.

> **Exception:** A wall-mounted luminaire weighing not more than 6 pounds (2.7 kg) shall be permitted to be supported on other boxes or plaster rings that are secured to other boxes, provided that the luminaire or its supporting yoke is secured to the box with not fewer than two No. 6 or larger screws.

E3905.7 Maximum luminaire weight. Outlet boxes or fittings designed for the support of luminaires and installed as required by Section E3904.3 shall be permitted to support a luminaire weighing 50 pounds (22.7 kg) or less. A luminaire that weighs more than 50 pounds (22.7 kg) shall be supported independently of the outlet box unless the outlet box is listed and marked for the maximum weight to be supported.

E3905.8 Floor boxes. Where outlet boxes for receptacles are installed in the floor, such boxes shall be listed specifically for that application.

E3905.9 Boxes at fan outlets. Outlet boxes and outlet box systems used as the sole support of ceiling-suspended fans (paddle) shall be marked by their manufacturer as suitable for this purpose and shall not support ceiling-suspended fans (paddle) that weigh more than 70 pounds (31.8 kg). For outlet boxes and outlet box systems designed to support ceiling-suspended fans (paddle) that weigh more than 35 pounds (15.9 kg), the required marking shall include the maximum weight to be supported.

E3905.10 Utilization equipment. Boxes used for the support of utilization equipment other than ceiling-suspended (paddle) fans shall meet the requirements of Sections E3905.6 and E3905.7 for the support of a luminaire that is the same size and weight.

> **Exception:** Utilization equipment weighing not more than 6 pounds (2.7 kg) shall be permitted to be supported on other boxes or plaster rings that are secured to other boxes, provided that the equipment or its supporting yoke is secured to the box with not fewer than two No. 6 or larger screws.

E3905.11 Conduit bodies and junction, pull and outlet boxes to be accessible. Conduit bodies and junction, pull and outlet boxes shall be installed so that the wiring therein can be accessed without removing any part of the building or, in underground circuits, without excavating sidewalks, paving, earth or other substance used to establish the finished grade.

> **Exception:** Boxes covered by gravel, light aggregate or noncohesive granulated soil shall be listed for the applica-

tion, and the box locations shall be effectively identified and access shall be provided for excavation.

E3905.12 Damp or wet locations. In damp or wet locations, boxes, conduit bodies and fittings shall be placed or equipped so as to prevent moisture from entering or accumulating within the box, conduit body or fitting. Boxes, conduit bodies and fittings installed in wet locations shall be listed for use in wet locations.

E3905.13 Number of conductors in outlet, device, and junction boxes, and conduit bodies. Boxes and conduit bodies shall be of sufficient size to provide free space for all enclosed conductors. In no case shall the volume of the box, as calculated in Section E3905.13.1, be less than the box fill calculation as calculated in Section E3905.13.2. The minimum volume for conduit bodies shall be as calculated in Section E3905.13.3. The provisions of this section shall not apply to terminal housings supplied with motors or generators.

E3905.13.1 Box volume calculations. The volume of a wiring enclosure (box) shall be the total volume of the assembled sections, and, where used, the space provided by plaster rings, domed covers, extension rings, etc., that are marked with their volume in cubic inches or are made from boxes the dimensions of which are listed in Table E3905.13.1.

E3905.13.1.1 Standard boxes. The volumes of standard boxes that are not marked with a cubic-inch capacity shall be as given in Table E3905.13.1.

E3905.13.1.2 Other boxes. Boxes 100 cubic inches (1640 cm^3) or less, other than those described in Table E3905.13.1, and nonmetallic boxes shall be durably and legibly marked by the manufacturer with their cubic-inch capacity. Boxes described in Table E3905.13.1 that have a larger cubic inch capacity than is designated in the table shall be permitted to have their cubic-inch capacity marked as required by this section.

E3905.13.2 Box fill calculations. The volumes in Section E3905.13.2.1 through Section E3905.13.2.5, as applicable, shall be added together. No allowance shall be required for small fittings such as locknuts and bushings.

E3905.13.2.1 Conductor fill. Each conductor that originates outside the box and terminates or is spliced within the box shall be counted once, and each conductor that passes through the box without splice or termination shall be counted once. Each loop or coil of unbroken conductor having a length equal to or greater than twice that required for free conductors by Section E3406.10.3, shall be counted twice. The conductor fill, in cubic inches, shall be computed using Table E3905.13.2.1. A conductor, no part of which leaves the box, shall not be counted.

> **Exception:** An equipment grounding conductor or not more than four fixture wires smaller than No. 14, or both, shall be permitted to be omitted from the calculations where such conductors enter a box from a domed fixture or similar canopy and terminate within that box.

TABLE E3905.13.1
MAXIMUM NUMBER OF CONDUCTORS IN METAL BOXES[a]

BOX DIMENSIONS (inches trade size and type)	MAXIMUM CAPACITY (cubic inches)	MAXIMUM NUMBER OF CONDUCTORS[a]						
		18 Awg	16 Awg	14 Awg	12 Awg	10 Awg	8 Awg	6 Awg
$4 \times 1^1/_4$ round or octagonal	12.5	8	7	6	5	5	4	2
$4 \times 1^1/_2$ round or octagonal	15.5	10	8	7	6	6	5	3
$4 \times 2^1/_8$ round or octagonal	21.5	14	12	10	9	8	7	4
$4 \times 1^1/_4$ square	18.0	12	10	9	8	7	6	3
$4 \times 1^1/_2$ square	21.0	14	12	10	9	8	7	4
$4 \times 2^1/_8$ square	30.3	20	17	15	13	12	10	6
$4^{11}/_{16} \times {}^{11}/_4$ square	25.5	17	14	12	11	10	8	5
$4^{11}/_{16} \times {}^{11}/_2$ square	29.5	19	16	14	13	11	9	5
$4^{11}/_{16} \times 2^1/_8$ square	42.0	28	24	21	18	16	14	8
$3 \times 2 \times 1^1/_2$ device	7.5	5	4	3	3	3	2	1
$3 \times 2 \times 2$ device	10.0	6	5	5	4	4	3	2
$3 \times 2 \times 2^1/_4$ device	10.5	7	6	5	4	4	3	2
$3 \times 2 \times 2^1/_2$ device	12.5	8	7	6	5	5	4	2
$3 \times 2 \times 2^3/_4$ device	14.0	9	8	7	6	5	4	2
$3 \times 2 \times 3^1/_2$ device	18.0	12	10	9	8	7	6	3
$4 \times 2^1/_8 \times 1^1/_2$ device	10.3	6	5	5	4	4	3	2
$4 \times 2^1/_8 \times 1^7/_8$ device	13.0	8	7	6	5	5	4	2
$4 \times 2^1/_8 \times 2^1/_8$ device	14.5	9	8	7	6	5	4	2
$3^3/_4 \times 2 \times 2^1/_2$ masonry box/gang	14.0	9	8	7	6	5	4	2
$3^3/_4 \times 2 \times 3^1/_2$ masonry box/gang	21.0	14	12	10	9	8	7	4

For SI: 1 inch = 25.4 mm, 1 cubic inch = 16.4 cm³.

a. Where volume allowances are not required by Sections E3905.13.2.2 through E3905.13.2.5.

TABLE E3905.13.2.1
VOLUME ALLOWANCE REQUIRED PER CONDUCTOR

SIZE OF CONDUCTOR	FREE SPACE WITHIN BOX FOR EACH CONDUCTOR (cubic inches)
18 AWG	1.50
16 AWG	1.75
14 AWG	2.00
12 AWG	2.25
10 AWG	2.50
8 AWG	3.00
6 AWG	5.00

For SI: 1 cubic inch = 16.4 cm³.

E3905.13.2.2 Clamp fill. Where one or more internal cable clamps, whether factory or field supplied, are present in the box, a single volume allowance in accordance with Table E3905.13.2.1 shall be made based on the largest conductor present in the box. No allowance shall be required for a cable connector with its clamping mechanism outside the box.

E3905.13.2.3 Support fittings fill. Where one or more fixture studs or hickeys are present in the box, a single volume allowance in accordance with Table E3905.13.2.1 shall be made for each type of fitting based on the largest conductor present in the box.

E3905.13.2.4 Device or equipment fill. For each yoke or strap containing one or more devices or equipment, a double volume allowance in accordance with Table E3905.13.2.1 shall be made for each yoke or strap based on the largest conductor connected to a device(s) or equipment supported by that yoke or strap. For a device or utilization equipment that is wider than a single 2 in. (51 mm) device box as described in Table E3905.13.1, a double volume allowance shall be made for each ganged portion required for mounting of the device or equipment.

E3905.13.2.5 Equipment grounding conductor fill. Where one or more equipment grounding conductors or equipment bonding jumpers enters a box, a single volume allowance in accordance with Table E3905.13.2.1 shall be made based on the largest equipment grounding conductor or equipment bonding jumper present in the box.

E3905.13.3 Conduit bodies. Conduit bodies enclosing 6 AWG conductors or smaller, other than short radius conduit bodies, shall have a cross-sectional area not less than twice the cross-sectional area of the largest conduit or tubing to which they can be attached. The maximum number of conductors permitted shall be the maximum number permitted by Section E3904.6 for the conduit to which it is attached.

E3905.13.3.1 Splices, taps or devices. Only those conduit bodies that are durably and legibly marked by the manufacturer with their cubic inch capacity shall be permitted to contain splices, taps or devices. The maximum number of conductors shall be calculated using the same procedure for similar conductors in other than standard boxes.

SECTION E3906
INSTALLATION OF BOXES, CONDUIT BODIES AND FITTINGS

E3906.1 Conductors entering boxes, conduit bodies or fittings. Conductors entering boxes, conduit bodies or fittings shall be protected from abrasion.

E3906.1.1 Insulated fittings. Where raceways contain 4 AWG or larger insulated circuit conductors and these conductors enter a cabinet, box enclosure, or raceway, the conductors shall be protected by a substantial fitting providing a smoothly rounded insulating surface, unless the conductors are separated from the fitting or raceway by substantial insulating material securely fastened in place.

Exception: Where threaded hubs or bosses that are an integral part of a cabinet, box enclosure, or raceway provide a smoothly rounded or flared entry for conductors.

Conduit bushings constructed wholly of insulating material shall not be used to secure a fitting or raceway. The insulating fitting or insulating material shall have a temperature rating not less than the insulation temperature rating of the installed conductors.

E3906.2 Openings. Openings through which conductors enter shall be adequately closed.

E3906.3 Metal boxes, conduit bodies and fittings. Where raceway or cable is installed with metal boxes, or conduit bodies, the raceway or cable shall be secured to such boxes and conduit bodies.

E3906.4 Unused openings. Unused openings other than those intended for the operation of equipment, those intended for mounting purposes, or those permitted as part of the design for listed equipment, shall be closed to afford protection substantially equivalent to that of the wall of the equipment. Metal plugs or plates used with nonmetallic boxes or conduit bodies shall be recessed at least $^1/_4$ inch (6.4 mm) from the outer surface of the box or conduit body.

E3906.5 In wall or ceiling. In walls or ceilings of concrete, tile or other noncombustible material, boxes employing a flush-type cover or faceplate shall be installed so that the front edge of the box, plaster ring, extension ring, or listed extender will not be set back from the finished surface more than $^1/_4$ inch (6.4 mm). In walls and ceilings constructed of wood or other combustible material, boxes, plaster rings, extension rings and listed extenders shall be flush with the finished surface or project therefrom.

E3906.6 Plaster, gypsum board and plasterboard. Openings in plaster, gypsum board or plasterboard surfaces that accommodate boxes employing a flush-type cover or faceplate shall be made so that there are no gaps or open spaces greater than $^1/_8$ inch (3.2 mm) around the edge of the box.

E3906.7 Surface extensions. Surface extensions shall be made by mounting and mechanically securing an extension ring over the box.

Exception: A surface extension shall be permitted to be made from the cover of a flush-mounted box where the cover is designed so it is unlikely to fall off, or be removed if its securing means becomes loose. The wiring method shall be flexible for a length sufficient to permit removal of the cover and provide access to the box interior and arranged so that any bonding or grounding continuity is independent of the connection between the box and cover.

E3906.8 Supports. Boxes and enclosures shall be supported in accordance with one or more of the provisions in Sections E3906.8.1 through E3906.8.6.

E3906.8.1 Surface mounting. An enclosure mounted on a building or other surface shall be rigidly and securely fastened in place. If the surface does not provide rigid and secure support, additional support in accordance with other provisions of Section E3906.8 shall be provided.

E3906.8.2 Structural mounting. An enclosure supported from a structural member of a building or from grade shall be rigidly supported either directly, or by using a metal, polymeric or wood brace.

E3906.8.2.1 Nails and screws. Nails and screws, where used as a fastening means, shall be attached by using brackets on the outside of the enclosure, or they shall pass through the interior within $^1/_4$ inch (6.4 mm) of the back or ends of the enclosure. Screws shall not be permitted to pass through the box except where exposed threads in the box are protected by an approved means to avoid abrasion of conductor insulation.

E3906.8.2.2 Braces. Metal braces shall be protected against corrosion and formed from metal that is not less than 0.020 inch (0.508 mm) thick uncoated. Wood braces shall have a cross section not less than nominal 1 inch by 2 inches (25.4 mm by 51 mm). Wood braces in wet locations shall be treated for the conditions. Polymeric braces shall be identified as being suitable for the use.

E3906.8.3 Mounting in finished surfaces. An enclosure mounted in a finished surface shall be rigidly secured there to by clamps, anchors, or fittings identified for the application.

E3906.8.4 Raceway supported enclosures without devices or fixtures. An enclosure that does not contain a device(s), other than splicing devices, or support a luminaire, lampholder or other equipment, and that is supported by entering raceways shall not exceed 100 cubic inches (1640 cm³) in size. The enclosure shall have threaded entries or have hubs identified for the purpose. The enclosure shall be supported by two or more conduits threaded wrenchtight into the enclosure or hubs. Each conduit shall be secured within 3 feet (914 mm) of the enclosure, or within 18 inches (457 mm) of the enclosure if all entries are on the same side of the enclosure.

Exception: Rigid metal, intermediate metal, or rigid nonmetallic conduit or electrical metallic tubing shall be permitted to support a conduit body of any size, provided that the conduit body is not larger in trade size than the largest trade size of the supporting conduit or electrical metallic tubing.

E3906.8.5 Raceway supported enclosures, with devices or luminaire. An enclosure that contains a device(s), other than splicing devices, or supports a luminaire, lampholder or other equipment and is supported by entering raceways shall not exceed 100 cubic inches (1640 cm³) in size. The enclosure shall have threaded entries or have hubs identified for the purpose. The enclosure shall be supported by two or more conduits threaded wrench-tight into the enclosure or hubs. Each conduit shall be secured within 18 inches (457 mm) of the enclosure.

Exceptions:

1. Rigid metal or intermediate metal conduit shall be permitted to support a conduit body of any size, provided that the conduit bodies are not larger in trade size than the largest trade size of the supporting conduit.

2. An unbroken length(s) of rigid or intermediate metal conduit shall be permitted to support a box used for luminaire or lampholder support, or to support a wiring enclosure that is an integral part of a luminaire and used in lieu of a box in accordance with Section E3905.1.1, where all of the following conditions are met:

   2.1. The conduit is securely fastened at a point so that the length of conduit beyond the last point of conduit support does not exceed 3 feet (914 mm).

   2.2. The unbroken conduit length before the last point of conduit support is 12 inches (305 mm) or greater, and that portion of the conduit is securely fastened at some point not less than 12 inches (305 mm) from its last point of support.

   2.3. Where accessible to unqualified persons, the luminaire or lampholder, measured to its lowest point, is not less than 8 feet (2438 mm) above grade or standing area and at least 3 feet (914 mm) measured horizontally to the 8-foot (2438 mm) elevation from windows, doors, porches, fire escapes, or similar locations.

   2.4. A luminaire supported by a single conduit does not exceed 12 inches (305 mm) in any direction from the point of conduit entry.

   2.5. The weight supported by any single conduit does not exceed 20 pounds (9.1 kg).

   2.6. At the luminaire or lampholder end, the conduit(s) is threaded wrenchtight into the box, conduit body, or integral wiring enclosure, or into hubs identified for the purpose. Where a box or conduit body is used for support, the luminaire shall be secured directly to the box or conduit body, or through a threaded conduit nipple not over 3 inches (76 mm) long.

E3906.8.6 Enclosures in concrete or masonry. An enclosure supported by embedment shall be identified as being suitably protected from corrosion and shall be securely embedded in concrete or masonry.

E3906.9 Covers and canopies. Outlet boxes shall be effectively closed with a cover, faceplate or fixture canopy.

E3906.10 Metal covers and plates. Metal covers and plates shall be grounded.

E3906.11 Exposed combustible finish. Combustible wall or ceiling finish exposed between the edge of a fixture canopy or pan and the outlet box shall be covered with noncombustible material.

SECTION E3907
CABINETS AND PANELBOARDS

E3907.1 Enclosures for switches or overcurrent devices. Enclosures for switches or overcurrent devices shall not be used as junction boxes, auxiliary gutters, or raceways for conductors feeding through or tapping off to other switches or overcurrent devices, except where adequate space for this purpose is provided. The conductors shall not fill the wiring space at any cross section to more than 40 percent of the cross-sectional area of the space, and the conductors, splices, and taps shall not fill the wiring space at any cross section to more than 75 percent of the cross-sectional area of that space.

E3907.2 Damp and wet locations. In damp or wet locations, cabinets and panelboards of the surface type shall be placed or equipped so as to prevent moisture or water from entering and accumulating within the cabinet, and shall be mounted to provide an airspace not less than $^1/_4$ inch (6.4 mm) between the enclosure and the wall or other supporting surface. Cabinets installed in wet locations shall be weatherproof. For enclosures in wet locations, raceways and cables entering above the level of uninsulated live parts shall be installed with fittings listed for wet locations.

E3907.3 Position in wall. In walls of concrete, tile or other noncombustible material, cabinets and panelboards shall be installed so that the front edge of the cabinet will not set back of the finished surface more than $^1/_4$ inch (6.4 mm). In walls constructed of wood or other combustible material, cabinets shall be flush with the finished surface or shall project therefrom.

E3907.4 Repairing noncombustible surfaces. Non-combustible surfaces that are broken or incomplete shall be repaired so that there will not be gaps or open spaces greater than $^1/_8$ inch (3.2 mm) at the edge of the cabinet or cutout box employing a flush-type cover.

E3907.5 Unused openings. Unused openings, other than those intended for the operation of equipment, those intended for mounting purposes, and those permitted as part of the design for listed equipment, shall be closed to afford protection substantially equivalent to that of the wall of the equipment. Metal plugs and plates used with nonmetallic cabinets shall be recessed at least $^1/_4$ inch (6.4 mm) from the outer surface. Unused openings for circuit breakers and switches shall be closed using identified closures, or other approved means that provide protection substantially equivalent to the wall of the enclosure.

E3907.6 Conductors entering cabinets. Conductors entering cabinets and panelboards shall be protected from abrasion and shall comply with Section E3906.1.1.

E3907.7 Openings to be closed. Openings through which conductors enter cabinets, panelboards and meter sockets shall be adequately closed.

E3907.8 Cables. Where cables are used, each cable shall be secured to the cabinet, panelboard, cutout box, or meter socket enclosure.

> **Exception:** Cables with entirely nonmetallic sheaths shall be permitted to enter the top of a surface-mounted enclosure through one or more sections of rigid raceway not less than 18 inches (457 mm) nor more than 10 feet (3048 mm) in length, provided all the following conditions are met:
>
> 1. Each cable is fastened within 12 inches (305 mm), measured along the sheath, of the outer end of the raceway.
>
> 2. The raceway extends directly above the enclosure and does not penetrate a structural ceiling.
>
> 3. A fitting is provided on each end of the raceway to protect the cable(s) from abrasion and the fittings remain accessible after installation.
>
> 4. The raceway is sealed or plugged at the outer end using approved means so as to prevent access to the enclosure through the raceway.

5. The cable sheath is continuous through the raceway and extends into the enclosure beyond the fitting not less than $^1/_4$ inch (6.4 mm).

6. The raceway is fastened at its outer end and at other points in accordance with Section E3802.1.

7. The allowable cable fill shall not exceed that permitted by Table E3907.8. A multiconductor cable having two or more conductors shall be treated as a single conductor for calculating the percentage of conduit fill area. For cables that have elliptical cross sections, the cross-sectional area calculation shall be based on the major diameter of the ellipse as a circle diameter.

TABLE E3907.8
PERCENT OF CROSS SECTION
OF CONDUIT AND TUBING FOR CONDUCTORS

NUMBER OF CONDUCTORS	MAXIMUM PERCENT OF CONDUIT AND TUBING AREA FILLED BY CONDUCTORS
1	53
2	31
Over 2	40

SECTION E3908
GROUNDING

E3908.1 Metal enclosures. Metal enclosures of conductors, devices and equipment shall be connected to the equipment grounding conductor.

Exceptions:

1. Short sections of metal enclosures or raceways used to provide cable assemblies with support or protection against physical damage.

2. A metal elbow that is installed in an underground installation of rigid nonmetallic conduit and is isolated from possible contact by a minimum cover of 18 inches (457 mm) to any part of the elbow or that is encased in not less than 2 inches (51 mm) of concrete.

E3908.2 Equipment fastened in place or connected by permanent wiring methods (fixed). Exposed noncurrent- carrying metal parts of fixed equipment likely to become energized shall be connected to the equipment grounding conductor where any of the following conditions apply:

1. Where within 8 feet (2438 mm) vertically or 5 feet (1524 mm) horizontally of earth or grounded metal objects and subject to contact by persons;

2. Where located in a wet or damp location and not isolated; or

3. Where in electrical contact with metal.

E3908.3 Specific equipment fastened in place or connected by permanent wiring methods. Exposed noncurrent-carrying metal parts of the following equipment and enclosures shall be connected to the equipment grounding conductor:

1. Luminaires as provided in Chapter 40.

2. Motor-operated water pumps, including submersible types. Where a submersible pump is used in a metal well casing, the well casing shall be bonded to the pump circuit equipment grounding conductor.

E3908.4 Effective ground-fault current path. Electrical equipment and wiring and other electrically conductive material likely to become energized shall be installed in a manner that creates a low-impedance circuit facilitating the operation of the overcurrent device. Such circuit shall be capable of safely carrying the maximum ground-fault current likely to be imposed on it from any point on the wiring system where a ground fault to the electrical supply source might occur.

E3908.5 Earth as a ground-fault current path. The earth shall not be considered as an effective ground-fault current path.

E3908.6 Load-side grounded conductor neutral. A grounded conductor shall not be connected to normally noncurrent-carrying metal parts of equipment, to equipment grounding conductor(s), or be reconnected to ground on the load side of the service disconnecting means.

E3908.7 Load-side equipment. A grounded circuit conductor shall not be used for grounding noncurrent-carrying metal parts of equipment on the load side of the service disconnecting means.

E3908.8 Types of equipment grounding conductors. The equipment grounding conductor run with or enclosing the circuit conductors shall be one or more or a combination of the following:

1. A copper, aluminum or copper-clad conductor. This conductor shall be solid or stranded; insulated, covered or bare; and in the form of a wire or a busbar of any shape.

2. Rigid metal conduit.

3. Intermediate metal conduit.

4. Electrical metallic tubing.

5. Armor of Type AC cable in accordance with Section E3908.4.

6. Type MC cable where listed and identified for grounding in accordance with the following:

   6.1. The combined metallic sheath and grounding conductor of interlocked metal tape-type MC cable.

   6.2. The metallic sheath or the combined metallic sheath and grounding conductors of the smooth or corrugated tube-type MC cable.

7. Other electrically continuous metal raceways and auxiliary gutters.

8. Surface metal raceways listed for grounding.

E3908.8.1 Flexible metal conduit. Flexible metal conduit shall be permitted as an equipment grounding conductor where all of the following conditions are met:

1. The conduit is terminated in listed fittings.

2. The circuit conductors contained in the conduit are protected by overcurrent devices rated at 20 amperes or less.

3. The combined length of flexible metal conduit and flexible metallic tubing and liquid-tight flexible metal conduit in the same ground return path does not exceed 6 feet (1829 mm).

4. An equipment grounding conductor shall be installed where the conduit is used to connect equipment where flexibility is necessary after installation.

E3908.8.2 Liquid-tight flexible metal conduit. Liquid-tight flexible metal conduit shall be permitted as an equipment grounding conductor where all of the following conditions are met:

1. The conduit is terminated in listed fittings.

2. For trade sizes $^3/_8$ through $^1/_2$ (metric designator 12 through 16), the circuit conductors contained in the conduit are protected by overcurrent devices rated at 20 amperes or less.

3. For trade sizes $^3/_4$ through $1^1/_4$ (metric designator 21 through 35), the circuit conductors contained in the conduit are protected by overcurrent devices rated at not more than 60 amperes and there is no flexible metal conduit, flexible metallic tubing, or liquid-tight flexible metal conduit in trade sizes $^3/_8$ inch or $^1/_2$ inch (9.5 mm through 12.7 mm) in the grounding path.

4. The combined length of flexible metal conduit and flexible metallic tubing and liquid tight flexible metal conduit in the same ground return path does not exceed 6 feet (1829 mm).

5. An equipment grounding conductor shall be installed where the conduit is used to connect equipment where flexibility is necessary after installation.

E3908.8.3 Nonmetallic sheathed cable (Type NM). In addition to the insulated conductors, the cable shall have an insulated or bare equipment grounding conductor. Equipment grounding conductors shall be sized in accordance with Table E3908.12.

E3908.9 Equipment fastened in place or connected by permanent wiring methods. Noncurrent-carrying metal parts of equipment, raceways and other enclosures, where required to be grounded, shall be grounded by one of the following methods:

1. By any of the equipment grounding conductors permitted by Sections E3908.8 through E3908.8.3.

2. By an equipment grounding conductor contained within the same raceway, cable or cord, or otherwise run with the circuit conductors. Equipment grounding conductors shall be identified in accordance with Section E3407.2.

E3908.10 Methods of equipment grounding. Fixtures and equipment shall be considered grounded where mechanically connected to an equipment grounding conductor as specified in Sections E3908.8 through E3908.8.3. Wire type equipment grounding conductors shall be sized in accordance with Section E3908.12.

E3908.11 Equipment grounding conductor installation. Where an equipment grounding conductor consists of a raceway, cable armor or cable sheath or where such conductor is a wire within a raceway or cable, it shall be installed in accordance with the provisions of this chapter and Chapters 34 and 38 using fittings for joints and terminations approved for installation with the type of raceway or cable used. All connections, joints and fittings shall be made tight using suitable tools.

E3908.12 Equipment grounding conductor size. Copper, aluminum and copper-clad aluminum equipment grounding conductors of the wire type shall be not smaller than shown in Table E3908.12, but in no case shall they be required to be larger than the circuit conductors supplying the equipment. Where a raceway or a cable armor or sheath is used as the equipment grounding conductor, as provided in Section E3908.8, it shall comply with Section E3908.4. Where ungrounded connectors are increased in size, equipment grounding conductors shall be increased proportionally according to the circular mil area of the ungrounded conductors.

TABLE E3908.12
EQUIPMENT GROUNDING CONDUCTOR SIZING

RATING OR SETTING OF AUTOMATIC OVERCURRENT DEVICE IN CIRCUIT AHEAD OF EQUIPMENT, CONDUIT, ETC., NOT EXCEEDING THE FOLLOWING RATINGS (amperes)	MINIMUM SIZE	
	Copper wire No. (AWG)	Aluminum or copper-clad aluminum wire No. (AWG)
15	14	12
20	12	10
30	10	8
40	10	8
60	10	8
100	8	6
200	6	4
300	4	2
400	3	1

E3908.12.1 Multiple circuits. Where a single equipment grounding conductor is run with multiple circuits in the same raceway or cable, it shall be sized for the largest overcurrent device protecting conductors in the raceway or cable.

E3908.13 Continuity and attachment of equipment grounding conductors to boxes. Where circuit conductors are spliced within a box or terminated on equipment within or supported by a box, any equipment grounding conductors associated with the circuit conductors shall be connected within the box or to the box with devices suitable for the use. Connections depending solely on solder shall not be used. Splices shall be made in accordance with Section E3406.10 except that insulation shall not be required. The arrangement of grounding connections shall be such that the disconnection or removal of a receptacle, luminaire or other device fed from the box will not interfere with or interrupt the grounding continuity.

E3908.14 Connecting receptacle grounding terminal to box. An equipment bonding jumper, sized in accordance with Table E3908.12 based on the rating of the overcurrent device protecting the circuit conductors, shall be used to connect the grounding terminal of a grounding-type receptacle to a grounded box except where grounded in accordance with one of the following:

1. Surface mounted box. Where the box is mounted on the surface, direct metal-to-metal contact between the device yoke and the box shall be permitted to ground the receptacle to the box. At least one of the insulating washers shall be removed from receptacles that do not have a contact yoke or device designed and listed to be used in conjunction with the supporting screws to establish the grounding circuit between the device yoke and flush-type boxes. This provision shall not apply to cover-mounted receptacles except where the box and cover combination are listed as providing satisfactory ground continuity between the box and the receptacle. A listed exposed work cover shall be considered to be the grounding and bonding means where the device is attached to the cover with at least two fasteners that are permanent, such as a rivet or have a thread locking or screw locking means and where the cover mounting holes are located on a flat non-raised portion of the cover.

2. Contact devices or yokes. Contact devices or yokes designed and listed for the purpose shall be permitted in conjunction with the supporting screws to establish the grounding circuit between the device yoke and flush-type boxes.

3. Floor boxes. The receptacle is installed in a floor box designed for and listed as providing satisfactory ground continuity between the box and the device.

E3908.15 Metal boxes. A connection shall be made between the one or more equipment grounding conductors and a metal box by means of a grounding screw that shall be used for no other purpose, equipment listed for grounding or by means of a listed grounding device. Where screws are used to connect grounding conductors or connection devices to boxes, such screws shall be:

1. Machine screw-type fasteners that engage not less than two threads,

2. Secured with a nut, or

3. Thread-forming machine screws that engage not less than two threads in the enclosure.

E3908.16 Nonmetallic boxes. One or more equipment grounding conductors brought into a nonmetallic outlet box shall be arranged to allow connection to fittings or devices installed in that box.

E3908.17 Clean surfaces. Nonconductive coatings such as paint, lacquer and enamel on equipment to be grounded shall be removed from threads and other contact surfaces to ensure electrical continuity or the equipment shall be connected by means of fittings designed so as to make such removal unnecessary.

E3908.18 Bonding other enclosures. Metal raceways, cable armor, cable sheath, enclosures, frames, fittings and other metal noncurrent-carrying parts that serve as grounding conductors, with or without the use of supplementary equipment grounding conductors, shall be effectively bonded where necessary to ensure electrical continuity and the capacity to conduct safely any fault current likely to be imposed on them. Any nonconductive paint, enamel and similar coating shall be removed at threads, contact points and contact surfaces, or connections shall be made by means of fittings designed so as to make such removal unnecessary.

E3908.19 Size of equipment bonding jumper on load side of service. The equipment bonding jumper on the load side of the service overcurrent devices shall be sized, as a minimum, in accordance with Table E3908.12, but shall not be required to be larger than the circuit conductors supplying the equipment. An equipment bonding conductor shall be not smaller than No. 14 AWG.

A single common continuous equipment bonding jumper shall be permitted to connect two or more raceways or cables where the bonding jumper is sized in accordance with Table E3908.12 for the largest overcurrent device supplying circuits therein.

E3908.20 Installation equipment bonding jumper. The equipment bonding jumper shall be permitted to be installed inside or outside of a raceway or enclosure. Where installed on the outside, the length of the equipment bonding jumper shall not exceed 6 feet (1829 mm) and shall be routed with the raceway or enclosure. Where installed inside of a raceway, the equipment bonding jumper shall comply with the requirements of Sections E3908.9, Item 2; E3908.13; E3908.15; and E3908.16.

Exception: An equipment bonding jumper longer than 6 feet (1829 mm) shall be permitted at outdoor pole locations for the purpose of bonding or grounding isolated sections of metal raceways or elbows installed in exposed risers of metal conduit or other metal raceway.

SECTION E3909
FLEXIBLE CORDS

E3909.1 Where permitted. Flexible cords shall be used only for the connection of appliances where the fastening means and mechanical connections of such appliances are designed to permit ready removal for maintenance, repair or frequent interchange and the appliance is listed for flexible cord connection. Flexible cords shall not be installed as a substitute for the fixed wiring of a structure; shall not be run through holes in walls, structural ceilings, suspended ceilings, dropped ceilings or floors; shall not be concealed behind walls, floors, ceilings or located above suspended or dropped ceilings.

E3909.2 Loading and protection. The ampere load of flexible cords serving fixed appliances shall be in accordance with Table E3909.2. This table shall be used in conjunction with applicable end use product standards to ensure selection of the proper size and type. Where flexible cord is approved for and used with a specific listed appliance, it shall be considered to be protected where applied within the appliance listing requirements.

E3909.3 Splices. Flexible cord shall be used only in continuous lengths without splices or taps.

E3909.4 Attachment plugs. Where used in accordance with Section E3909.1, each flexible cord shall be equipped with an attachment plug and shall be energized from a receptacle outlet.

TABLE E3909.2
MAXIMUM AMPERE LOAD FOR FLEXIBLE CORDS

CORD SIZE (AWG)	CORD TYPES S, SE, SEO, SJ, SJE, SJEO, SJO, SJOO, SJT, SJTO, SJTOO, SO, SOO, SRD, SRDE, SRDT, ST, STD, SV, SVO, SVOO, SVTO, SVTOO	
	Maximum ampere load	
	Three current-carrying conductors	Two current-carrying conductors
18	7	10
16	10	13
14	15	18
12	20	25

CHAPTER 40

DEVICES AND LUMINAIRES

SECTION E4001
SWITCHES

E4001.1 Rating and application of snap switches. General-use snap switches shall be used within their ratings and shall control only the following loads:

1. Resistive and inductive loads, including electric-discharge lamps, not exceeding the ampere rating of the switch at the voltage involved.

2. Tungsten-filament lamp loads not exceeding the ampere rating of the switch at 120 volts.

3. Motor loads not exceeding 80 percent of the ampere rating of the switch at its rated voltage.

E4001.2 CO/ALR snap switches. Snap switches rated 20 amperes or less directly connected to aluminum conductors shall be marked CO/ALR.

E4001.3 Indicating. General-use and motor-circuit switches and circuit breakers shall clearly indicate whether they are in the open OFF or closed ON position. Where single-throw switches or circuit breaker handles are operated vertically rather than rotationally or horizontally, the up position of the handle shall be the ON position.

E4001.4 Time switches and similar devices. Time switches and similar devices shall be of the enclosed type or shall be mounted in cabinets or boxes or equipment enclosures. A barrier shall be used around energized parts to prevent operator exposure when making manual adjustments or switching.

E4001.5 Grounding of enclosures. Metal enclosures for switches or circuit breakers shall be connected to an equipment grounding conductor. Metal enclosures for switches or circuit breakers used as service equipment shall comply with the provisions of Section E3609.4. Where nonmetallic enclosures are used with metal raceways or metal-armored cables, provisions shall be made for connecting the equipment grounding conductor.

Nonmetallic boxes for switches shall be installed with a wiring method that provides or includes an equipment grounding conductor.

E4001.6 Access. All switches and circuit breakers used as switches shall be located to allow operation from a readily accessible location. Such devices shall be installed so that the center of the grip of the operating handle of the switch or circuit breaker, when in its highest position, will not be more than 6 feet 7 inches (2007 mm) above the floor or working platform.

E4001.7 Damp or wet locations. A surface mounted switch or circuit breaker located in a damp or wet location or outside of a building shall be enclosed in a weatherproof enclosure or cabinet. A flush-mounted switch or circuit breaker in a damp or wet location shall be equipped with a weatherproof cover. Switches shall not be installed within wet locations in tub or shower spaces unless installed as part of a listed tub or shower assembly.

E4001.8 Grounded conductors. Switches or circuit breakers shall not disconnect the grounded conductor of a circuit except where the switch or circuit breaker simultaneously disconnects all conductors of the circuit.

E4001.9 Switch connections. Three- and four-way switches shall be wired so that all switching occurs only in the ungrounded circuit conductor. Color coding of switch connection conductors shall comply with Section E3407.3. Where in metal raceways or metal-jacketed cables, wiring between switches and outlets shall be in accordance with Section E3406.7.

Exception: Switch loops do not require a grounded conductor.

E4001.10 Box mounted. Flush-type snap switches mounted in boxes that are recessed from the finished wall surfaces as covered in Section E3906.5 shall be installed so that the extension plaster ears are seated against the surface of the wall. Flush-type snap switches mounted in boxes that are flush with the finished wall surface or project therefrom shall be installed so that the mounting yoke or strap of the switch is seated against the box.

E4001.11 Snap switch faceplates. Faceplates provided for snap switches mounted in boxes and other enclosures shall be installed so as to completely cover the opening and, where the switch is flush mounted, seat against the finished surface.

E4001.11.1 Faceplate grounding. Snap switches, including dimmer and similar control switches, shall be connected to an equipment grounding conductor and shall provide a means to connect metal faceplates to the equipment grounding conductor, whether or not a metal faceplate is installed. Snap switches shall be considered to be part of an effective ground-fault current path if either of the following conditions is met:

1. The switch is mounted with metal screws to a metal box or metal cover that is connected to an equipment grounding conductor or to a nonmetallic box with integral means for connecting to an equipment grounding conductor.

2. An equipment grounding conductor or equipment bonding jumper is connected to an equipment grounding termination of the snap switch.

Exception: Where a means to connect to an equipment grounding conductor does not exist within the snap-switch enclosure or where the wiring method does not include or provide an equipment grounding conductor, a snap switch without a grounding connection to an equipment grounding conductor shall be permitted for replacement purposes only. A snap switch wired under the provisions of this exception and located within reach of earth, grade, conducting floors, or other conducting surfaces shall be provided with a faceplate of nonconducting, noncombustible material or shall be protected by a ground-fault circuit interrupter.

E4001.12 Dimmer switches. General-use dimmer switches shall be used only to control permanently installed incandescent luminaires (lighting fixtures) except where listed for the control of other loads and installed accordingly.

E4001.13 Multipole snap switches. A multipole, general-use snap switch shall not be fed from more than a single circuit unless it is listed and marked as a two-circuit or three-circuit switch, or unless its voltage rating is not less than the nominal line-to-line voltage of the system supplying the circuits.

SECTION E4002
RECEPTACLES

E4002.1 Rating and type. Receptacles and cord connectors shall be rated at not less than 15 amperes, 125 volts, or 15 amperes, 250 volts, and shall not be a lampholder type. Receptacles shall be rated in accordance with this section.

E4002.1.1 Single receptacle. A single receptacle installed on an individual branch circuit shall have an ampere rating not less than that of the branch circuit.

E4002.1.2 Two or more receptacles. Where connected to a branch circuit supplying two or more receptacles or outlets, receptacles shall conform to the values listed in Table E4002.1.2.

TABLE E4002.1.2
RECEPTACLE RATINGS FOR VARIOUS SIZE
MULTI-OUTLET CIRCUITS

CIRCUIT RATING (amperes)	RECEPTACLE RATING (amperes)
15	15
20	15 or 20
30	30
40	40 or 50
50	50

E4002.2 Grounding type. Receptacles installed on 15- and 20-ampere-rated branch circuits shall be of the grounding type.

E4002.3 CO/ALR receptacles. Receptacles rated at 20 amperes or less and directly connected to aluminum conductors shall be marked CO/ALR.

E4002.4 Faceplates. Metal face plates shall be grounded.

E4002.5 Position of receptacle faces. After installation, receptacle faces shall be flush with or project from face plates of insulating material and shall project a minimum of 0.015 inch (0.381 mm) from metal face plates. Faceplates shall be installed so as to completely cover the opening and seat against the mounting surface.

> **Exception:** Listed kits or assemblies encompassing receptacles and nonmetallic faceplates that cover the receptacle face, where the plate cannot be installed on any other receptacle, shall be permitted.

E4002.6 Receptacle mounted in boxes. Receptacles mounted in boxes that are set back from the finished wall surface as permitted by Section E3906.5 shall be installed so that the mounting yoke or strap of the receptacle is held rigidly at the finished surface of the wall. Receptacles mounted in boxes that are flush with the wall surface or project therefrom shall be so installed that the mounting yoke or strap is seated against the box or raised cover.

E4002.7 Receptacles mounted on covers. Receptacles mounted to and supported by a cover shall be held rigidly against the cover by more than one screw or shall be a device assembly or box cover listed and identified for securing by a single screw.

E4002.8 Damp locations. A receptacle installed outdoors in a location protected from the weather or in other damp locations shall have an enclosure for the receptacle that is weatherproof when the receptacle cover(s) is closed and an attachment plug cap is not inserted. An installation suitable for wet locations shall also be considered suitable for damp locations. A receptacle shall be considered to be in a location protected from the weather where located under roofed open porches, canopies and similar structures and not subject to rain or water runoff. Fifteen- and 20-ampere, 125- and 250-volt nonlocking receptacles installed in damp locations shall be listed a weather-resistant type.

E4002.9 Fifteen- and 20-ampere receptacles in wet locations. Where installed in a wet location, 15- and 20-ampere, 125- and 250-volt receptacles shall have an enclosure that is weatherproof whether or not the attachment plug cap is inserted. Fifteen- and 20-ampere, 125- and 250-volt nonlocking receptacles installed in wet locations shall be a listed weather-resistant type.

E4002.10 Other receptacles in wet locations. Where a receptacle other than a 15- or 20-amp, 125- or 250-volt receptacle is installed in a wet location and where the product intended to be plugged into it is not attended while in use, the receptacle shall have an enclosure that is weatherproof both when the attachment plug cap is inserted and when it is removed. Where such receptacle is installed in a wet location and where the product intended to be plugged into it will be attended while in use, the receptacle shall have an enclosure that is weatherproof when the attachment plug cap is removed.

E4002.11 Bathtub and shower space. A receptacle shall not be installed within or directly over a bathtub or shower stall.

E4002.12 Flush mounting with faceplate. In damp or wet locations, the enclosure for a receptacle installed in an outlet box flush-mounted in a finished surface shall be made weatherproof by means of a weatherproof faceplate assembly that provides a water-tight connection between the plate and the finished surface.

E4002.13 Exposed terminals. Receptacles shall be enclosed so that live wiring terminals are not exposed to contact.

E4002.14 Tamper-resistant receptacles. In areas specified in Section E3901.1, 125-volt, 15- and 20-ampere receptacles shall be listed tamper-resistant receptacles.

SECTION E4003
FIXTURES

E4003.1 Energized parts. Luminaires, lampholders, and lamps shall not have energized parts normally exposed to contact.

E4003.2 Luminaires near combustible material. Luminaires shall be installed so that combustible material will not be subjected to temperatures in excess of 90°C (194°F).

E4003.3 Exposed conductive parts. The exposed metal parts of luminaires shall be connected to an equipment grounding conductor or shall be insulated from the equipment grounding conductor and other conducting surfaces. Lamp tie wires, mounting screws, clips and decorative bands on glass spaced at least $1^1/_2$ inches (38 mm) from lamp terminals shall not be required to be grounded.

E4003.4 Screw-shell type. Lampholders of the screw-shell type shall be installed for use as lampholders only.

E4003.5 Recessed incandescent luminaires. Recessed incandescent luminaires shall have thermal protection and shall be listed as thermally protected.

Exceptions:

1. Thermal protection shall not be required in recessed luminaires listed for the purpose and installed in poured concrete.

2. Thermal protection shall not be required in recessed luminaires having design, construction, and thermal performance characteristics equivalent to that of thermally protected luminaires, and such luminaires are identified as inherently protected.

E4003.6 Thermal protection. The ballast of a fluorescent luminaire installed indoors shall have integral thermal protection. Replacement ballasts shall also have thermal protection integral with the ballast. A simple reactance ballast in a fluorescent luminaire with straight tubular lamps shall not be required to be thermally protected.

E4003.7 High-intensity discharge luminaires. Recessed high-intensity luminaires designed to be installed in wall or ceiling cavities shall have thermal protection and be identified as thermally protected. Thermal protection shall not be required in recessed high-intensity luminaires having design, construction and thermal performance characteristics equivalent to that of thermally protected luminaires, and such luminaires are identified as inherently protected. Thermal protection shall not be required in recessed high-intensity discharge luminaires installed in and identified for use in poured concrete. A recessed remote ballast for a high-intensity discharge luminaire shall have thermal protection that is integral with the ballast and shall be identified as thermally protected.

E4003.8 Metal halide lamp containment. Luminaires that use a metal halide lamp other than a thick-glass parabolic reflector lamp (PAR) shall be provided with a containment barrier that encloses the lamp, or shall be provided with a physical means that allows the use of only a lamp that is Type O.

E4003.9 Wet or damp locations. Luminaires installed in wet or damp locations shall be installed so that water cannot enter or accumulate in wiring compartments, lampholders or other electrical parts. All luminaires installed in wet locations shall be marked SUITABLE FOR WET LOCATIONS. All luminaires installed in damp locations shall be marked SUITABLE FOR WET LOCATIONS or SUITABLE FOR DAMP LOCATIONS.

E4003.10 Lampholders in wet or damp locations. Lampholders installed in wet or damp locations shall be of the weatherproof type.

E4003.11 Bathtub and shower areas. Cord-connected luminaires, chain-, cable-, or cord-suspended-luminaires, lighting track, pendants, and ceiling-suspended (paddle) fans shall not have any parts located within a zone measured 3 feet (914 mm) horizontally and 8 feet (2438 mm) vertically from the top of a bathtub rim or shower stall threshold. This zone is all encompassing and includes the space directly over the tub or shower. Luminaires within the actual outside dimension of the bathtub or shower to a height of 8 feet (2438 mm) vertically from the top of the bathtub rim or shower threshold shall be marked for damp locations and where subject to shower spray, shall be marked for wet locations.

E4003.12 Luminaires in clothes closets. For the purposes of this section, storage space shall be defined as a volume bounded by the sides and back closet walls and planes extending from the closet floor vertically to a height of 6 feet (1829 mm) or the highest clothes-hanging rod and parallel to the walls at a horizontal distance of 24 inches (610 mm) from the sides and back of the closet walls respectively, and continuing vertically to the closet ceiling parallel to the walls at a horizontal distance of 12 inches (305 mm) or the width of the shelf, whichever is greater. For a closet that permits access to both sides of a hanging rod, the storage space shall include the volume below the highest rod extending 12 inches (305 mm) on either side of the rod on a plane horizontal to the floor extending the entire length of the rod (see Figure E4003.12).

The types of luminaires installed in clothes closets shall be limited to surface-mounted or recessed incandescent luminaires with completely enclosed lamps, surface-mounted or recessed fluorescent luminaires, and surface-mounted fluorescent or LED luminaires identified as suitable for installation within the storage area. Incandescent luminaires with open or partially enclosed lamps and pendant luminaires or lamp-holders shall be prohibited. The minimum clearance between luminaires installed in clothes closets and the nearest point of a storage area shall be as follows:

1. Surface-mounted incandescent or LED luminaires with a completely enclosed light source shall be installed on the wall above the door or on the ceiling, provided that there is a minimum clearance of 12 inches (305 mm) between the fixture and the nearest point of a storage space.

2. Surface-mounted fluorescent luminaires shall be installed on the wall above the door or on the ceiling, provided that there is a minimum clearance of 6 inches (152 mm).

3. Recessed incandescent luminaires or LED luminaires with a completely enclosed light source shall be installed in the wall or the ceiling provided that there is a minimum clearance of 6 inches (152 mm).

4. Recessed fluorescent luminaires shall be installed in the wall or on the ceiling provided that there is a minimum clearance of 6 inches (152 mm) between the fixture and the nearest point of a storage space.

5. Surface-mounted fluorescent or LED luminaires shall be permitted to be installed within the storage space where identified for this use.

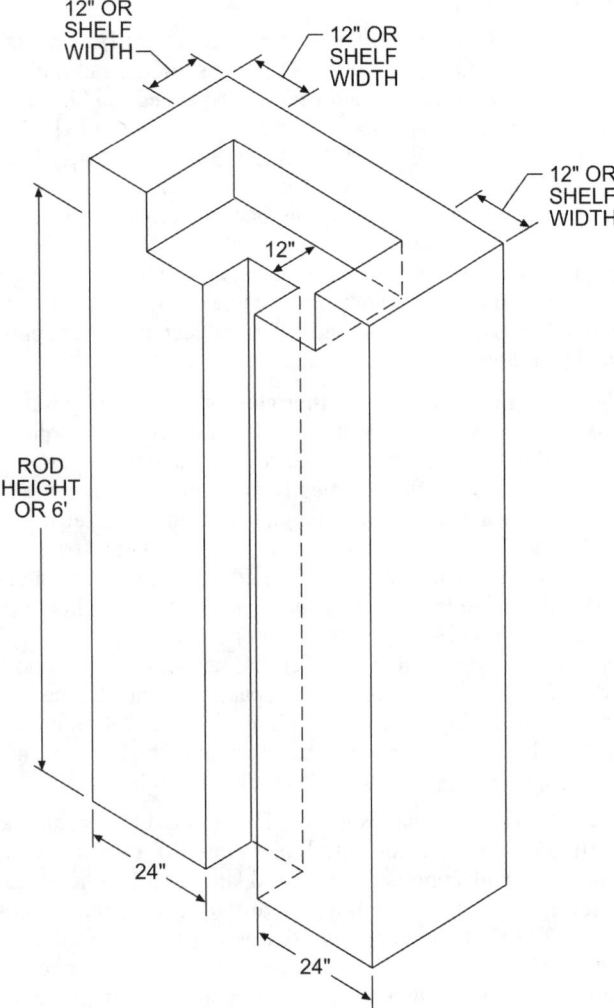

For SI: 1 inch = 25.4 mm, 1 foot = 304.8 mm.

FIGURE E4003.12
CLOSET STORAGE SPACE

E4003.13 Luminaire wiring—general. Wiring on or within luminaires shall be neatly arranged and shall not be exposed to physical damage. Excess wiring shall be avoided. Conductors shall be arranged so that they are not subjected to temperatures above those for which the conductors are rated.

E4003.13.1 Polarization of luminaires. Luminaires shall be wired so that the screw shells of lampholders will be connected to the same luminaire or circuit conductor or terminal. The grounded conductor shall be connected to the screw shell.

E4003.13.2 Luminaires as raceways. Luminaires shall not be used as raceways for circuit conductors except where such luminaires are listed and marked for use as a raceway.

SECTION E4004
LUMINAIRE INSTALLATION

E4004.1 Outlet box covers. In a completed installation, each outlet box shall be provided with a cover except where covered by means of a luminaire canopy, lampholder or device with a faceplate.

E4004.2 Combustible material at outlet boxes. Combustible wall or ceiling finish exposed between the inside edge of a luminaire canopy or pan and the outlet box to which the luminaire connects shall be covered with a noncombustible material.

E4004.3 Access. Luminaires shall be installed so that the connections between the luminaire conductors and the circuit conductors can be accessed without requiring the disconnection of any part of the wiring.

E4004.4 Supports. Luminaires and lampholders shall be securely supported. A luminaire that weighs more than 6 pounds (2.72 kg) or exceeds 16 inches (406 mm) in any dimension shall not be supported by the screw shell of a lampholder.

E4004.5 Means of support. Outlet boxes or fittings installed as required by Sections E3905 and E3906 shall be permitted to support luminaires.

E4004.6 Exposed ballasts. Luminaires having exposed ballasts or transformers shall be installed so that such ballasts or transformers are not in contact with combustible material.

E4004.7 Combustible low-density cellulose fiberboard. Where a surface-mounted luminaire containing a ballast is installed on combustible low-density cellulose fiberboard, the luminaire shall be marked for this purpose or it shall be spaced not less than $1^1/_2$ inches (38 mm) from the surface of the fiberboard. Where such luminaires are partially or wholly recessed, the provisions of Sections E4004.8 and E4004.9 shall apply.

E4004.8 Recessed luminaire clearance. A recessed luminaire that is not identified for contact with insulation shall have all recessed parts spaced at least $^1/_2$ inch (12.7 mm) from combustible materials. The points of support and the finish trim parts at the opening in the ceiling or wall surface shall be permitted to be in contact with combustible materials. A recessed luminaire that is identified for contact with insulation, Type IC, shall be permitted to be in contact with combustible materials at recessed parts, points of support, and portions passing through the building structure and at finish trim parts at the opening in the ceiling or wall.

E4004.9 Recessed luminaire installation. Thermal insulation shall not be installed above a recessed luminaire or within 3 inches (76 mm) of the recessed luminaire's enclosure, wiring compartment or ballast except where such luminaire is identified for contact with insulation, Type IC.

SECTION E4005
TRACK LIGHTING

E4005.1 Installation. Lighting track shall be permanently installed and permanently connected to a branch circuit having a rating not more than that of the track.

E4005.2 Fittings. Fittings identified for use on lighting track shall be designed specifically for the track on which they are to be installed. Fittings shall be securely fastened to the track, shall maintain polarization and connection to the equipment grounding conductor, and shall be designed to be suspended directly from the track. Only lighting track fittings shall be installed on lighting track. Lighting track fittings shall not be equipped with general-purpose receptacles.

E4005.3 Connected load. The connected load on lighting track shall not exceed the rating of the track.

E4005.4 Prohibited locations. Lighting track shall not be installed in the following locations:

1. Where likely to be subjected to physical damage.

2. In wet or damp locations.

3. Where subject to corrosive vapors.

4. In storage battery rooms.

5. In hazardous (classified) locations.

6. Where concealed.

7. Where extended through walls or partitions.

8. Less than 5 feet (1524 mm) above the finished floor except where protected from physical damage or the track operates at less than 30 volts rms open-circuit voltage.

9. Where prohibited by Section E4003.11.

E4005.5 Fastening. Lighting track shall be securely mounted so that each fastening will be suitable for supporting the maximum weight of luminaires that can be installed. Except where identified for supports at greater intervals, a single section 4 feet (1219 mm) or shorter in length shall have two supports and, where installed in a continuous row, each individual section of not more than 4 feet (1219 mm) in length shall have one additional support.

E4005.6 Grounding. Lighting track shall be grounded in accordance with Chapter 39, and the track sections shall be securely coupled to maintain continuity of the circuitry, polarization and grounding throughout.

CHAPTER 41

APPLIANCE INSTALLATION

SECTION E4101
GENERAL

E4101.1 Scope. This section covers installation requirements for appliances and fixed heating equipment.

E4101.2 Installation. Appliances and equipment shall be installed in accordance with the manufacturer's installation instructions. Electrically heated appliances and equipment shall be installed with the required clearances to combustible materials.

E4101.3 Flexible cords. Cord-and-plug-connected appliances shall use cords suitable for the environment and physical conditions likely to be encountered. Flexible cords shall be used only where the appliance is listed to be connected with a flexible cord. The cord shall be identified as suitable for the purpose in the installation instructions of the appliance manufacturer. Receptacles for cord-and-plug-connected appliances shall be accessible and shall be located to avoid physical damage to the flexible cord. Except for a listed appliance marked to indicate that it is protected by a system of double-insulation, the flexible cord supplying an appliance shall terminate in a grounding-type attachment plug. A receptacle for a cord-and-plug-connected range hood shall be supplied by an individual branch circuit. Specific appliances have additional requirements as specified in Table E4101.3 (see Section E3909).

TABLE E4101.3
FLEXIBLE CORD LENGTH

APPLIANCE	MINIMUM CORD LENGTH (inches)	MAXIMUM CORD LENGTH (inches)
Kitchen waste disposal	18	36
Built-in dishwasher	36	48
Trash compactor	36	48
Range hoods	18	36

For SI: 1 inch = 25.4 mm.

E4101.4 Overcurrent protection. Each appliance shall be protected against overcurrent in accordance with the rating of the appliance and its listing.

E4101.4.1 Single nonmotor-operated appliance. The overcurrent protection for a branch circuit that supplies a single nonmotor-operated appliance shall not exceed that marked on the appliance. Where the overcurrent protection rating is not marked and the appliance is rated at over 13.3 amperes, the overcurrent protection shall not exceed 150 percent of the appliance rated current. Where 150 percent of the appliance rating does not correspond to a standard overcurrent device ampere rating, the next higher standard rating shall be permitted. Where the overcurrent protection rating is not marked and the appliance is rated at 13.3 amperes or less, the overcurrent protection shall not exceed 20 amperes.

E4101.5 Disconnecting means. Each appliance shall be provided with a means to disconnect all ungrounded supply conductors. For fixed electric space-heating equipment, means shall be provided to disconnect the heater and any motor controller(s) and supplementary overcurrent-protective devices. Switches and circuit breakers used as a disconnecting means shall be of the indicating type. Disconnecting means shall be as set forth in Table E4101.5.

E4101.6 Support of ceiling-suspended paddle fans. Ceiling-suspended fans (paddle) shall be supported independently of an outlet box or by a listed outlet box or outlet box system identified for the use and installed in accordance with Section E3905.9.

E4101.7 Snow-melting and deicing equipment protection. Outdoor receptacles that are not readily accessible and are supplied from a dedicated branch circuit for electric snow-melting or deicing equipment shall be permitted to be installed without ground-fault circuit-interrupter protection for personnel. However, ground-fault protection of equipment shall be provided for fixed outdoor electric deicing and snow-melting equipment.

TABLE E4101.5
DISCONNECTING MEANS

DESCRIPTION	ALLOWED DISCONNECTING MEANS
Permanently connected appliance rated at not over 300 volt-amperes or $^1/_8$ horsepower.	Branch-circuit overcurrent device.
Permanently connected appliances rated in excess of 300 volt-amperes or $^1/_8$ horsepower.	Branch circuit breaker or switch located within sight of appliance or such devices in any location that are capable of being locked in the open position. The provision for locking or adding a lock to the disconnecting means shall be installed on or at the switch or circuit breaker used as the disconnecting means and shall remain in place with or without the lock installed.
Appliances listed for cord-and-plug connection.	A separable connector or attachment plug and receptacle provided with access.
Permanently installed heating equipment with motors rated at not over $^1/_8$ horsepower with supplementary overcurrent protection.	Disconnect, on the supply side of fuses, in sight from the supplementary overcurrent device, and in sight of the heating equipment or, in any location, if capable of being locked in the open position.
Heating equipment containing motors rated over $^1/_8$ horsepower with supplementary overcurrent protection.	Disconnect permitted to serve as required disconnect for both the heating equipment and the controller where, on the supply side of fuses, and in sight from the supplementary overcurrent devices, if the disconnecting means is also in sight from the controller, or is capable of being locked off and simultaneously disconnects the heater, motor controller(s) and supplementary overcurrent protective devices from all ungrounded conductors. The provision for locking or adding a lock to the disconnecting means shall be installed on or at the switch or circuit breaker used as the disconnecting means and shall remain in place with or without the lock installed. The disconnecting means shall have an ampere rating not less than 125 percent of the total load of the motors and the heaters.
Heating equipment containing no motor rated over $^1/_8$ horsepower without supplementary overcurrent protection.	Branch-circuit switch or circuit breaker where within sight from the heating equipment or capable of being locked off and simultaneously disconnects the heater, motor controller(s) and supplementary overcurrent protective devices from all ungrounded conductors. The provision for locking or adding a lock to the disconnecting means shall be installed on or at the switch or circuit breaker used as the disconnecting means and shall remain in place with or without the lock installed. The disconnecting means shall have an ampere rating not less than 125 percent of the total load of the motors and the heaters.
Heating equipment containing motors rated over $^1/_8$ horsepower without supplementary overcurrent protection.	Disconnecting means in sight from motor controller or as provided for heating equipment with motor rated over $^1/_8$ horsepower with supplementary overcurrent protection and simultaneously disconnects the heater, motor controller(s) and supplementary overcurrent protective devices from all ungrounded conductors. The provision for locking or adding a lock to the disconnecting means shall be installed on or at the switch or circuit breaker used as the disconnecting means and shall remain in place with or without the lock installed. The disconnecting means shall have an ampere rating not less than 125 percent of the total load of the motors and the heaters.
Air-conditioning condensing units and heat pump units.	A readily accessible disconnect within sight from unit as the only allowable means.[a]
Appliances and fixed heating equipment with unit switches having a marked OFF position.	Unit switch where an additional individual switch or circuit breaker serves as a redundant disconnecting means.
Thermostatically controlled fixed heating equipment.	Thermostats with a marked OFF position that directly open all ungrounded conductors, which when manually placed in the OFF position are designed so that the circuit cannot be energized automatically and that are located within sight of the equipment controlled.

For SI: 1 horsepower = 0.746 kW.

a. The disconnecting means shall be permitted to be installed on or within the unit. It shall not be located on panels designed to allow access to the unit or located so as to obscure the air-conditioning equipment nameplate(s).

CHAPTER 42

SWIMMING POOLS

SECTION E4201
GENERAL

E4201.1 Scope. The provisions of this chapter shall apply to the construction and installation of electric wiring and equipment associated with all swimming pools, wading pools, decorative pools, fountains, hot tubs and spas, and hydromassage bathtubs, whether permanently installed or storable, and shall apply to metallic auxiliary equipment, such as pumps, filters and similar equipment. Sections E4202 through E4206 provide general rules for permanent pools, spas and hot tubs. Section E4207 provides specific rules for storable pools. Section E4208 provides specific rules for spas and hot tubs. Section E4209 provides specific rules for hydromassage bathtubs.

E4201.2 Definitions.

CORD-AND-PLUG-CONNECTED LIGHTING ASSEMBLY. A lighting assembly consisting of a cord-and-plug-connected transformer and a luminaire intended for installation in the wall of a spa, hot tub, or storable pool.

DRY-NICHE LUMINAIRE. A luminaire intended for installation in the wall of a pool or fountain in a niche that is sealed against the entry of pool water.

FORMING SHELL. A structure designed to support a wet-niche luminaire assembly and intended for mounting in a pool or fountain structure.

FOUNTAIN. Fountains, ornamental pools, display pools, and reflection pools. The definition does not include drinking fountains.

HYDROMASSAGE BATHTUB. A permanently installed bathtub equipped with a recirculating piping system, pump, and associated equipment. It is designed so it can accept, circulate and discharge water upon each use.

MAXIMUM WATER LEVEL. The highest level that water can reach before it spills out.

NO-NICHE LUMINAIRE. A luminaire intended for installation above or below the water without a niche.

PACKAGED SPA OR HOT TUB EQUIPMENT ASSEMBLY. A factory-fabricated unit consisting of water-circulating, heating and control equipment mounted on a common base, intended to operate a spa or hot tub. Equipment may include pumps, air blowers, heaters, luminaires, controls and sanitizer generators.

PERMANENTLY INSTALLED SWIMMING, WADING, IMMERSION AND THERAPEUTIC POOLS. Those that are constructed in the ground or partially in the ground, and all others capable of holding water with a depth greater than 42 inches (1067 mm), and all pools installed inside of a building, regardless of water depth, whether or not served by electrical circuits of any nature.

POOL. Manufactured or field-constructed equipment designed to contain water on a permanent or semipermanent basis and used for swimming, wading, immersion, or therapeutic purposes.

POOL COVER, ELECTRICALLY OPERATED. Motor-driven equipment designed to cover and uncover the water surface of a pool by means of a flexible sheet or rigid frame.

SELF-CONTAINED SPA OR HOT TUB. A factory-fabricated unit consisting of a spa or hot tub vessel with all water-circulating, heating and control equipment integral to the unit. Equipment may include pumps, air blowers, heaters, luminaires, controls and sanitizer generators.

SPA OR HOT TUB. A hydromassage pool, or tub for recreational or therapeutic use, not located in health care facilities, designed for immersion of users, and usually having a filter, heater, and motor-driven blower. They are installed indoors or outdoors, on the ground or supporting structure, or in the ground or supporting structure. Generally, a spa or hot tub is not designed or intended to have its contents drained or discharged after each use.

STORABLE SWIMMING OR WADING POOL. Those that are constructed on or above the ground and are capable of holding water with a maximum depth of 42 inches (1067 mm), or a pool with nonmetallic, molded polymeric walls or inflatable fabric walls regardless of dimension.

THROUGH-WALL LIGHTING ASSEMBLY. A lighting assembly intended for installation above grade, on or through the wall of a pool, consisting of two interconnected groups of components separated by the pool wall.

WET-NICHE LUMINAIRE. A luminaire intended for installation in a forming shell mounted in a pool or fountain structure where the luminaire will be completely surrounded by water.

SECTION E4202
WIRING METHODS FOR POOLS, SPAS, HOT TUBS AND HYDROMASSAGE BATHTUBS

E4202.1 General. Wiring methods used in conjunction with permanently installed swimming pools, spas, hot tubs or hydromassage bathtubs shall be installed in accordance with Table E4202.1 and Chapter 38 except as otherwise stated in this section. Storable swimming pools shall comply with Section E4207.

E4202.2 Flexible cords. Flexible cords used in conjunction with a pool, spa, hot tub or hydromassage bathtub shall be installed in accordance with the following:

1. For other than underwater luminaires, fixed or stationary equipment shall be permitted to be connected with a flexible cord to facilitate removal or disconnection for maintenance or repair. For other than storable pools, the flexible cord shall not exceed 3 feet (914 mm) in length. Cords that supply swimming pool equipment, shall have a copper

equipment grounding conductor not smaller than 12 AWG and shall be provided with a grounding-type attachment plug.

2. Flexible cord that is supplied as part of a listed underwater swimming pool lighting luminaire shall be permitted to be installed in any of the permitted wiring methods from the luminaire to a deck box or other enclosure. Splices shall not be made within a raceway. The equipment grounding conductor shall be an insulated copper conductor that is not smaller than the supply conductors and not smaller than 16 AWG.

3. A listed packaged spa or hot tub installed outdoors that is GFCI protected shall be permitted to be cord and plug-connected provided that such cord does not exceed 15 feet (4572 mm) in length.

4. A listed packaged spa or hot tub rated at 20 amperes or less and installed indoors shall be permitted to be cord and plug-connected to facilitate maintenance and repair.

5. For other than underwater and storable pool lighting luminaire, the requirements of Item 1 shall apply to any cord-equipped luminaire that is located within 16 feet (4877 mm) radially from any point on the water surface.

E4202.3 Double insulated pool pumps. A listed cord and plug-connected pool pump incorporating an approved system of double insulation that provides a means for grounding only the internal and nonaccessible, noncurrent-carrying metal parts of the pump shall be connected to any wiring method recognized in Chapter 38 that is suitable for the location. Where the bonding grid is connected to the equipment grounding conductor of the motor circuit in accordance with Section E4204.2, Item 6.1, the branch circuit wiring shall comply with Sections E4202.1 and E4205.5.

TABLE E4202.1
ALLOWABLE APPLICATIONS FOR WIRING METHODS[a, b, c, d, e, f, g, h, l]

WIRING LOCATION OR PURPOSE (Application allowed where marked with an "A")	AC, FMC, NM, SR, SE	EMT	ENT	IMC[j], RMC[j], RNC[i]	LFMC	LFNMC	UF	MC[k]	FLEX CORD
Panelboard(s) that supply pool equipment: from service equipment to panelboard	A[b, e] SR not permitted	A[c]	A[b]	A	—	A	A[e]	A[e]	—
Wet-niche and no-niche luminaires: from branch circuit OCPD to deck or junction box	AC[b] only	A[c]	A[b]	A	—	A	—	A[b]	—
Wet-niche and no-niche luminaires: from deck or junction box to forming shell	—	—	—	A[d]	—	A	—	—	A[h]
Dry niche: from branch circuit OCPD to luminaires	AC[b] only	A[c]	A[b]	A	—	A	—	A[b]	—
Pool-associated motors: from branch circuit OCPD to motor	A[b]	A[c]	A[b]	A	A[f]	A[f]	A[b]	A	A[h]
Packaged or self-contained outdoor spas and hot tubs with underwater luminaire: from branch circuit OCPD to spa or hot tub	AC[b] only	A[c]	A[b]	A	A[f]	A[f]	—	A[b]	A[h]
Packaged or self-contained outdoor spas and hot tubs without underwater luminaire: from branch circuit OCPD to spa or hot tub	A[b]	A[c]	A[b]	A	A[f]	A[f]	A[b]	A	A[h]
Indoor spas and hot tubs, hydromassage bathtubs, and other pool, spa or hot tub associated equipment: from branch circuit OCPD to equipment	A[b]	A[c]	A[b]	A	A	A	A	A	A[h]
Connection at pool lighting transformers	AC[b] only	A[c]	A[b]	A	A[g]	A[g]	—	A[b]	—

For SI: 1 foot = 304.8 mm.

a. For all wiring methods, see Section E4205 for equipment grounding conductor requirements.

b. Limited to use within buildings.

c. Limited to use on or within buildings.

d. Metal conduit shall be constructed of brass or other approved corrosion-resistant metal.

e. Permitted only for existing installations in accordance with the exception to Section E4205.6.

f. Limited to use at pool, spa or hot tub equipment where flexibility is necessary. For spas and hot tubs, the maximum length shall be 6 feet.

g. Limited to use in individual lengths not to exceed 6 feet. The total length of all individual runs of LFMC and LFNMC shall not exceed 10 feet. LFNMC Type B shall be limited to lengths not exceeding 10 feet.

h. Flexible cord shall be installed in accordance with Section E4202.2.

i. Nonmetallic conduit shall be rigid polyvinyl chloride conduit Type PVC or reinforced thermosetting resin conduit Type RTRC.

j. Aluminum conduits shall not be permitted in the pool area where subject to corrosion.

k. Where installed as direct burial cable or in wet locations, Type MC cable shall be listed and identified for the location.

l. See Section E4202.3 for listed, double-insulated pool pump motors.

SECTION E4203
EQUIPMENT LOCATION AND CLEARANCES

E4203.1 Receptacle outlets. Receptacles outlets shall be installed and located in accordance with Sections E4203.1.1 through E4203.1.5. Distances shall be measured as the shortest path that an appliance supply cord connected to the receptacle would follow without penetrating a floor, wall, ceiling, doorway with hinged or sliding door, window opening, or other effective permanent barrier.

E4203.1.1 Location. Receptacles that provide power for water-pump motors or other loads directly related to the circulation and sanitation system shall be permitted to be located between 6 feet and 10 feet (1829 mm and 3048 mm) from the inside walls of pools and outdoor spas and hot tubs, and, where so located, shall be single and of the locking and grounding type and shall be protected by ground-fault circuit interrupters.

Other receptacles on the property shall be located not less than 6 feet (1829 mm) from the inside walls of pools and outdoor spas and hot tubs.

E4203.1.2 Where required. At least one 125-volt, 15- or 20-ampere receptacle supplied by a general-purpose branch circuit shall be located a minimum of 6 feet (1829 mm) from and not more than 20 feet (6096 mm) from the inside wall of pools and outdoor spas and hot tubs. This receptacle shall be located not more than 6 feet, 6 inches (1981 mm) above the floor, platform or grade level serving the pool, spa or hot tub.

E4203.1.3 GFCI protection. All 15- and 20-ampere, single phase, 125-volt receptacles located within 20 feet (6096 mm) of the inside walls of pools and outdoor spas and hot tubs shall be protected by a ground-fault circuit-interrupter. Outlets supplying pool pump motors from branch circuits with short-circuit and ground-fault protection rated 15 or 20 amperes, 125 volt or 240 volt, single phase, whether by receptacle or direct connection, shall be provided with ground-fault circuit-interrupter protection for personnel.

E4203.1.4 Indoor locations. Receptacles shall be located not less than 6 feet (1829 mm) from the inside walls of indoor spas and hot tubs. A minimum of one 125-volt receptacle shall be located between 6 feet (1829 mm) and 10 feet (3048 mm) from the inside walls of indoor spas or hot tubs.

E4203.1.5 Indoor GFCI protection. All 125-volt receptacles rated 30 amperes or less and located within 10 feet (3048 mm) of the inside walls of spas and hot tubs installed indoors, shall be protected by ground-fault circuit-interrupters.

E4203.2 Switching devices. Switching devices shall be located not less than 5 feet (1524 mm) horizontally from the inside walls of pools, spas and hot tubs except where separated from the pool, spa or hot tub by a solid fence, wall, or other permanent barrier or the switches are listed for use within 5 feet (1524 mm). Switching devices located in a room or area containing a hydromassage bathtub shall be located in accordance with the general requirements of this code.

E4203.3 Disconnecting means. One or more means to simultaneously disconnect all ungrounded conductors for all utilization equipment, other than lighting, shall be provided. Each of such means shall be readily accessible and within sight from the equipment it serves and shall be located at least 5 feet (1524 mm) horizontally from the inside walls of a pool, spa, or hot tub unless separated from the open water by a permanently installed barrier that provides a 5 foot (1524 mm) or greater reach path. This horizontal distance shall be measured from the water's edge along the shortest path required to reach the disconnect.

E4203.4 Luminaires and ceiling fans. Lighting outlets, luminaires, and ceiling-suspended paddle fans shall be installed and located in accordance with Sections E4203.4.1 through E4203.4.5.

E4203.4.1 Outdoor location. In outdoor pool, outdoor spas and outdoor hot tubs areas, luminaires, lighting outlets, and ceiling-suspended paddle fans shall not be installed over the pool or over the area extending 5 feet (1524 mm) horizontally from the inside walls of a pool except where no part of the luminaire or ceiling-suspended paddle fan is less than 12 feet (3658 mm) above the maximum water level.

E4203.4.2 Indoor locations. In indoor pool areas, the limitations of Section E4203.4.1 shall apply except where the luminaires, lighting outlets and ceiling-suspended paddle fans comply with all of the following conditions:

1. The luminaires are of a totally enclosed type;

2. A ground-fault circuit interrupter is installed in the branch circuit supplying the luminaires or ceiling-suspended (paddle) fans; and

3. The distance from the bottom of the luminaire or ceiling-suspended (paddle) fan to the maximum water level is not less than 7 feet, 6 inches (2286 mm).

E4203.4.3 Existing lighting outlets and luminaires. Existing lighting outlets and luminaires that are located within 5 feet (1524 mm) horizontally from the inside walls of pools and outdoor spas and hot tubs shall be permitted to be located not less than 5 feet (1524 mm) vertically above the maximum water level, provided that such luminaires and outlets are rigidly attached to the existing structure and are protected by a ground-fault circuit-interrupter.

E4203.4.4 Indoor spas and hot tubs.

1. Luminaires, lighting outlets, and ceiling-suspended paddle fans located over the spa or hot tub or within 5 feet (1524 mm) from the inside walls of the spa or hot tub shall be a minimum of 7 feet, 6 inches (2286 mm) above the maximum water level and shall be protected by a ground-fault circuit interrupter.

   Luminaires, lighting outlets, and ceiling-suspended paddle fans that are located 12 feet (3658 mm) or more above the maximum water level shall not require ground-fault circuit interrupter protection.

2. Luminaires protected by a ground-fault circuit interrupter and complying with Item 2.1 or 2.2 shall be permitted to be installed less than 7 feet, 6 inches (2286 mm) over a spa or hot tub.

   2.1. Recessed luminaires shall have a glass or plastic lens and nonmetallic or electrically isolated metal trim, and shall be suitable for use in damp locations.

2.2. Surface-mounted luminaires shall have a glass or plastic globe and a nonmetallic body or a metallic body isolated from contact. Such luminaires shall be suitable for use in damp locations.

E4203.4.5 GFCI protection in adjacent areas. Luminaires and outlets that are installed in the area extending between 5 feet (1524 mm) and 10 feet (3048 mm) from the inside walls of pools and outdoor spas and hot tubs shall be protected by ground-fault circuit-interrupters except where such fixtures and outlets are installed not less than 5 feet (1524 mm) above the maximum water level and are rigidly attached to the structure.

E4203.5 Other outlets. Other outlets such as for remote control, signaling, fire alarm and communications shall be not less than 10 feet (3048 mm) from the inside walls of the pool. Measurements shall be determined in accordance with Section E4203.1.

E4203.6 Overhead conductor clearances. Except where installed with the clearances specified in Table E4203.5, the following parts of pools and outdoor spas and hot tubs shall not be placed under existing service-drop conductors or any other open overhead wiring; nor shall such wiring be installed above the following:

1. Pools and the areas extending 10 feet (3048 mm) horizontally from the inside of the walls of the pool;

2. Diving structures; or

3. Observation stands, towers, and platforms.

Overhead conductors of network-powered broadband communications systems shall comply with the provisions in Table E4203.5 for conductors operating at 0 to 750 volts to ground.

Utility-owned, -operated and -maintained communications conductors, community antenna system coaxial cables and the supporting messengers shall be permitted at a height of not less than 10 feet (3048 mm) above swimming and wading pools, diving structures, and observation stands, towers, and platforms.

E4203.7 Underground wiring. Underground wiring shall not be installed under or within the area extending 5 feet(1524 mm) horizontally from the inside walls of pools and outdoor hot tubs and spas except where the wiring is installed to supply pool, spa or hot tub equipment or where space limitations prevent wiring from being routed 5 feet (1524 mm) or more horizontally from the inside walls. Where installed within 5 feet (1524 mm) of the inside walls, the wiring method shall be a complete raceway system of rigid metal conduit, intermediate metal conduit or a nonmetallic raceway system. Metal conduit shall be corrosion resistant and suitable for the location. The minimum cover depth shall be in accordance with Table E4203.7.

SECTION E4204
BONDING

E4204.1 Performance. The equipotential bonding required by this section shall be installed to reduce voltage gradients in the pool area as prescribed.

TABLE E4203.5
OVERHEAD CONDUCTOR CLEARANCES

	INSULATED SUPPLY OR SERVICE DROP CABLES, 0-750 VOLTS TO GROUND, SUPPORTED ON AND CABLED TOGETHER WITH AN EFFECTIVELY GROUNDED BARE MESSENGER OR EFFECTIVELY GROUNDED NEUTRAL CONDUCTOR (feet)	ALL OTHER SUPPLY OR SERVICE DROP CONDUCTORS (feet)	
		Voltage to ground	
		0-15 kV	Greater than 15 to 50 kV
A. Clearance in any direction to the water level, edge of water surface, base of diving platform, or permanently-anchored raft	22.5	25	27
B. Clearance in any direction to the diving platform	14.5	17	18

For SI: 1 foot = 304.8 mm.

TABLE E4203.7
MINIMUM BURIAL DEPTHS

WIRING METHOD	UNDERGROUND WIRING (inches)
Rigid metal conduit	6
Intermediate metal conduit	6
Nonmetallic raceways listed for direct burial without concrete encasement	18
Other approved raceways[a]	18

For SI: 1 inch = 25.4 mm.

a. Raceways approved for burial only where concrete-encased shall require a concrete envelope not less than 2 inches in thickness.

E4204.2 Bonded parts. The parts of pools, spas, and hot tubs specified in Items 1 through 7 shall be bonded together using insulated, covered or bare solid copper conductors not smaller than 8 AWG or using rigid metal conduit of brass or other identified corrosion-resistant metal. An 8 AWG or larger solid copper bonding conductor provided to reduce voltage gradients in the pool, spa, or hot tub area shall not be required to be extended or attached to remote panelboards, service equipment, or electrodes. Connections shall be made by exothermic welding or by listed pressure connectors or clamps that are labeled as being suitable for the purpose and that are made of stainless steel, brass, copper or copper alloy. Connection devices or fittings that depend solely on solder shall not be used. Sheet metal screws shall not be used to connect bonding conductors or connection devices:

1. Conductive pool shells. Bonding to conductive pool shells shall be provided as specified in Item 1.1 or 1.2. Poured concrete, pneumatically applied or sprayed concrete, and concrete block with painted or plastered coatings shall be considered to be conductive materials because of their water permeability and porosity. Vinyl liners and fiberglass composite shells shall be considered to be nonconductive materials.

   1.1. Structural Reinforcing Steel. Unencapsulated structural reinforcing steel shall be bonded together by steel tie wires or the equivalent. Where structural reinforcing steel is encapsulated in a nonconductive compound, a copper conductor grid shall be installed in accordance with Item 1.2.

   1.2. Copper Conductor Grid. A copper conductor grid shall be provided and shall comply with Items 1.2.1 through 1.2.4:

      1.2.1. It shall be constructed of minimum 8 AWG bare solid copper conductors bonded to each other at all points of crossing.

      1.2.2. It shall conform to the contour of the pool and the pool deck.

      1.2.3. It shall be arranged in a 12 inch (305 mm) by 12 inch (305 mm) network of conductors in a uniformly spaced perpendicular grid pattern with a tolerance of 4 inches (102 mm).

      1.2.4. It shall be secured within or under the pool not more than 6 inches (152 mm) from the outer contour of the pool shell.

2. Perimeter surfaces. The perimeter surface shall extend for 3 feet (914 mm) horizontally beyond the inside walls of the pool and shall include unpaved surfaces, poured concrete and other types of paving. Bonding to perimeter surfaces shall be provided as specified in Item 2.1 or 2.2 and shall be attached to the pool, spa, or hot tub reinforcing steel or copper conductor grid at a minimum of four points uniformly spaced around the perimeter of the pool, spa, or hot tub. For nonconductive pool shells, bonding at four points shall not be required.

   2.1. Structural Reinforcing Steel. Structural reinforcing steel shall be bonded in accordance with Item 1.1.

   2.2. Alternate Means. Where structural reinforcing steel is not available or is encapsulated in a nonconductive compound, a copper conductor(s) shall be used in accordance with Items 2.2.1 through 2.2.5:

      2.2.1. At least one minimum 8 AWG bare solid copper conductor shall be provided.

      2.2.2. The conductors shall follow the contour of the perimeter surface.

      2.2.3. Splices shall be listed.

      2.2.4. The required conductor shall be 18 to 24 inches (457 to 610 mm) from the inside walls of the pool.

      2.2.5. The required conductor shall be secured within or under the perimeter surface 4 to 6 inches (102 mm to 152 mm) below the subgrade.

3. Metallic components. All metallic parts of the pool structure, including reinforcing metal not addressed in Item 1.1, shall be bonded. Where reinforcing steel is encapsulated with a nonconductive compound, the reinforcing steel shall not be required to be bonded.

4. Underwater lighting. All metal forming shells and mounting brackets of no-niche luminaires shall be bonded.

   Exception: Listed low-voltage lighting systems with nonmetallic forming shells shall not require bonding.

5. Metal fittings. All metal fittings within or attached to the pool structure shall be bonded. Isolated parts that are not over 4 inches (102 mm) in any dimension and do not penetrate into the pool structure more than 1 inch (25.4 mm) shall not require bonding.

6. Electrical equipment. Metal parts of electrical equipment associated with the pool water circulating system, including pump motors and metal parts of equipment associated with pool covers, including electric motors, shall be bonded.

   Exception: Metal parts of listed equipment incorporating an approved system of double insulation shall not be bonded.

   6.1. Double-Insulated Water Pump Motors. Where a double-insulated water pump motor is installed under the provisions of this item, a solid 8 AWG copper conductor of sufficient length to make a bonding connection to a replacement motor shall be extended from the bonding grid to an accessible point in the vicinity of the pool pump motor.

Where there is no connection between the swimming pool bonding grid and the equipment grounding system for the premises, this bonding conductor shall be connected to the equipment grounding conductor of the motor circuit.

    6.2. Pool Water Heaters. For pool water heaters rated at more than 50 amperes and having specific instructions regarding bonding and grounding, only those parts designated to be bonded shall be bonded and only those parts designated to be grounded shall be grounded.

7. Metal wiring methods and equipment. Metal-sheathed cables and raceways, metal piping, and all fixed metal parts shall be bonded.

Exceptions:

    1. Those separated from the pool by a permanent barrier shall not be required to be bonded.

    2. Those greater than 5 feet (1524 mm) horizontally from the inside walls of the pool shall not be required to be bonded.

    3. Those greater than 12 feet (3658 mm) measured vertically above the maximum water level of the pool, or as measured vertically above any observation stands, towers, or platforms, or any diving structures, shall not be required to be bonded.

E4204.3 Pool water. The pool water shall be intentionally bonded by means of a conductive surface area not less than 9 square inches (5806 mm²) installed in contact with the pool water. This bond shall be permitted to consist of parts that are required to be bonded in Section E4204.2.

E4204.4 Bonding of outdoor hot tubs and spas. Outdoor hot tubs and spas shall comply with the bonding requirements of Sections E4204.1 through E4204.3. Bonding by metal-to-metal mounting on a common frame or base shall be permitted. The metal bands or hoops used to secure wooden staves shall not be required to be bonded as required in Section E4204.2.

E4204.5 Bonding of indoor hot tubs and spas. The following parts of indoor hot tubs and spas shall be bonded together:

1. All metal fittings within or attached to the hot tub or spa structure.

2. Metal parts of electrical equipment associated with the hot tub or spa water circulating system, including pump motors.

3. Metal raceway and metal piping that are within 5 feet (1524 mm) of the inside walls of the hot tub or spa and that are not separated from the spa or hot tub by a permanent barrier.

4. All metal surfaces that are within 5 feet (1524 mm) of the inside walls of the hot tub or spa and that are not separated from the hot tub or spa area by a permanent barrier.

Exceptions:

    1. Small conductive surfaces not likely to become energized, such as air and water jets and drain fittings, where not connected to metallic piping,

towel bars, mirror frames, and similar nonelectrical equipment, shall not be required to be bonded.

    2. Metal parts of electrical equipment associated with the water circulating system, including pump motors that are part of a listed self-contained hot tub or spa.

5. Electrical devices and controls that are not associated with the hot tubs or spas and that are located less than 5 feet (1524 mm) from such units.

E4204.5.1 Methods. All metal parts associated with the hot tub or spa shall be bonded by any of the following methods:

1. The interconnection of threaded metal piping and fittings.

2. Metal-to-metal mounting on a common frame or base

3. The provision of an insulated, covered or bare solid copper bonding jumper not smaller than 8 AWG. It shall not be the intent to require that the 8 AWG or larger solid copper bonding conductor be extended or attached to any remote panelboard, service equipment, or any electrode, but only that it shall be employed to eliminate voltage gradients in the hot tub or spa area as prescribed.

E4204.5.2 Connections. Connections shall be made by exothermic welding or by listed pressure connectors or clamps that are labeled as being suitable for the purpose and that are made of stainless steel, brass, copper or copper alloy. Connection devices or fittings that depend solely on solder shall not be used. Sheet metal screws shall not be used to connect bonding conductors or connection devices.

SECTION E4205
GROUNDING

E4205.1 Equipment to be grounded. The following equipment shall be grounded:

1. Through-wall lighting assemblies and underwater luminaires other than those low-voltage lighting products listed for the application without a grounding conductor.

2. All electrical equipment located within 5 feet (1524 mm) of the inside wall of the pool, spa or hot tub.

3. All electrical equipment associated with the recirculating system of the pool, spa or hot tub.

4. Junction boxes.

5. Transformer enclosures.

6. Ground-fault circuit-interrupters.

7. Panelboards that are not part of the service equipment and that supply any electrical equipment associated with the pool, spa or hot tub.

E4205.2 Luminaires and related equipment. Through-wall lighting assemblies, wet-niche, dry-niche, or no-niche luminaires shall be connected to an insulated copper equipment grounding conductor sized in accordance with Table

E3908.12 but not smaller than 12 AWG. The equipment grounding conductor between the wiring chamber of the secondary winding of a transformer and a junction box shall be sized in accordance with the overcurrent device in such circuit. The junction box, transformer enclosure, or other enclosure in the supply circuit to a wet-niche or no-niche luminaire and the field-wiring chamber of a dry-niche luminaire shall be grounded to the equipment grounding terminal of the panelboard. The equipment grounding terminal shall be directly connected to the panelboard enclosure. The equipment grounding conductor shall be installed without joint or splice.

Exceptions:

1. Where more than one underwater luminaire is supplied by the same branch circuit, the equipment grounding conductor, installed between the junction boxes, transformer enclosures, or other enclosures in the supply circuit to wet-niche luminaires, or between the field-wiring compartments of dry-niche luminaires, shall be permitted to be terminated on grounding terminals.

2. Where an underwater luminaire is supplied from a transformer, ground-fault circuit-interrupter, clock-operated switch, or a manual snap switch that is located between the panelboard and a junction box connected to the conduit that extends directly to the underwater luminaire, the equipment grounding conductor shall be permitted to terminate on grounding terminals on the transformer, ground-fault circuit-interrupter, clock-operated switch enclosure, or an outlet box used to enclose a snap switch.

E4205.3 Nonmetallic conduit. Where a nonmetallic conduit is installed between a forming shell and a junction box, transformer enclosure, or other enclosure, a 8 AWG insulated copper bonding jumper shall be installed in this conduit except where a listed low-voltage lighting system not requiring grounding is used. The bonding jumper shall be terminated in the forming shell, junction box or transformer enclosure, or ground-fault circuit-interrupter enclosure. The termination of the 8 AWG bonding jumper in the forming shell shall be covered with, or encapsulated in, a listed potting compound to protect such connection from the possible deteriorating effect of pool water.

E4205.4 Flexible cords. Wet-niche luminaires that are supplied by a flexible cord or cable shall have all exposed noncurrent-carrying metal parts grounded by an insulated copper equipment grounding conductor that is an integral part of the cord or cable. This grounding conductor shall be connected to a grounding terminal in the supply junction box, transformer enclosure, or other enclosure. The grounding conductor shall not be smaller than the supply conductors and not smaller than 16 AWG.

E4205.5 Motors. Pool-associated motors shall be connected to an insulated copper equipment grounding conductor sized in accordance with Table E3908.12, but not smaller than 12 AWG. Where the branch circuit supplying the motor is installed in the interior of a one-family dwelling or in the interior of accessory buildings associated with a one-family dwelling, using a cable wiring method permitted by Table E4202.1,

an uninsulated equipment grounding conductor shall be permitted provided that it is enclosed within the outer sheath of the cable assembly.

E4205.6 Feeders. An equipment grounding conductor shall be installed with the feeder conductors between the grounding terminal of the pool equipment panelboard and the grounding terminal of the applicable service equipment or source of a separately derived system. The equipment grounding conductor shall be insulated, shall be sized in accordance with Table E3908.12, and shall be not smaller than 12 AWG.

Exception: An existing feeder between an existing remote panelboard and service equipment shall be permitted to run in flexible metal conduit or an approved cable assembly that includes an equipment grounding conductor within its outer sheath. The equipment grounding conductor shall not be connected to the grounded conductor in the remote panelboard.

E4205.6.1 Separate buildings. A feeder to a separate building or structure shall be permitted to supply swimming pool equipment branch circuits, or feeders supplying swimming pool equipment branch circuits, provided that the grounding arrangements in the separate building meet the requirements of Section E3607.3. Where installed in other than existing feeders covered in the exception to Section E4205.6, a separate equipment grounding conductor shall be an insulated conductor.

E4205.7 Cord-connected equipment. Where fixed or stationary equipment is connected with a flexible cord to facilitate removal or disconnection for maintenance, repair, or storage, as provided in Section E4202.2, the equipment grounding conductors shall be connected to a fixed metal part of the assembly. The removable part shall be mounted on or bonded to the fixed metal part.

E4205.8 Other equipment. Other electrical equipment shall be grounded in accordance with Section E3908.

SECTION E4206
EQUIPMENT INSTALLATION

E4206.1 Transformers. Transformers used for the supply of underwater luminaires, together with the transformer enclosure, shall be listed as a swimming pool and spa transformer. Such transformers shall be of an isolated winding type with an ungrounded secondary that has a grounded metal barrier between the primary and secondary windings.

E4206.2 Ground-fault circuit-interrupters. Ground-fault circuit-interrupters shall be self-contained units, circuit-breaker types, receptacle types or other approved types.

E4206.3 Wiring on load side of ground-fault circuit-interrupters and transformers. For other than grounding conductors, conductors installed on the load side of a ground-fault circuit-interrupter or transformer used to comply with the provisions of Section E4206.4, shall not occupy raceways, boxes, or enclosures containing other conductors except where the other conductors are protected by ground-fault circuit interrupters or are grounding conductors. Supply conductors to a feed-through type ground-fault circuit interrupter shall be permitted in the same enclosure. Ground-fault circuit interrupters shall be permitted in a panelboard that contains circuits protected by other than ground-fault circuit interrupters.

E4206.4 Underwater luminaires. The design of an underwater luminaire supplied from a branch circuit either directly or by way of a transformer meeting the requirements of Section E4206.1, shall be such that, where the fixture is properly installed without a ground-fault circuit-interrupter, there is no shock hazard with any likely combination of fault conditions during normal use (not relamping). In addition, a ground-fault circuit-interrupter shall be installed in the branch circuit supplying luminaires operating at more than 15 volts, so that there is no shock hazard during relamping. The installation of the ground-fault circuit-interrupter shall be such that there is no shock hazard with any likely fault-condition combination that involves a person in a conductive path from any ungrounded part of the branch circuit or the luminaire to ground. Compliance with this requirement shall be obtained by the use of a listed underwater luminaire and by installation of a listed ground-fault circuit-interrupter in the branch circuit. Luminaires that depend on submersion for safe operation shall be inherently protected against the hazards of overheating when not submerged.

E4206.4.1 Maximum voltage. Luminaires shall not be installed for operation on supply circuits over 150 volts between conductors.

E4206.4.2 Luminaire location. Luminaires mounted in walls shall be installed with the top of the fixture lens not less than 18 inches (457 mm) below the normal water level of the pool, except where the luminaire is listed and identified for use at a depth of not less than 4 inches (102 mm) below the normal water level of the pool. A luminaire facing upward shall have the lens adequately guarded to prevent contact by any person or shall be listed for use without a guard.

E4206.5 Wet-niche luminaires. Forming shells shall be installed for the mounting of all wet-niche underwater luminaires and shall be equipped with provisions for conduit entries. Conduit shall extend from the forming shell to a suitable junction box or other enclosure located as provided in Section E4206.9. Metal parts of the luminaire and forming shell in contact with the pool water shall be of brass or other approved corrosion-resistant metal.

The end of flexible-cord jackets and flexible-cord conductor terminations within a luminaire shall be covered with, or encapsulated in, a suitable potting compound to prevent the entry of water into the luminaire through the cord or its conductors. In addition, the grounding connection within a luminaire shall be similarly treated to protect such connection from the deteriorating effect of pool water in the event of water entry into the luminaire.

Luminaires shall be bonded to and secured to the forming shell by a positive locking device that ensures a low-resistance contact and requires a tool to remove the luminaire from the forming shell.

E4206.5.1 Servicing. All wet-niche luminaires shall be removable from the water for inspection, relamping, or other maintenance. The forming shell location and length of cord in the forming shell shall permit personnel to place the removed luminaire on the deck or other dry location for such maintenance. The luminaire maintenance location shall be accessible without entering or going into the pool water.

E4206.6 Dry-niche luminaires. Dry-niche luminaires shall be provided with provisions for drainage of water and means for accommodating one equipment grounding conductor for each conduit entry. Junction boxes shall not be required but, if used, shall not be required to be elevated or located as specified in Section E4206.9 if the luminaire is specifically identified for the purpose.

E4206.7 No-niche luminaires. No-niche luminaires shall be listed for the purpose and shall be installed in accordance with the requirements of Section E4206.5. Where connection to a forming shell is specified, the connection shall be to the mounting bracket.

E4206.8 Through-wall lighting assembly. A through-wall lighting assembly shall be equipped with a threaded entry or hub, or a nonmetallic hub, for the purpose of accommodating the termination of the supply conduit. A through-wall lighting assembly shall meet the construction requirements of Section E4205.4 and be installed in accordance with the requirements of Section E4206.5 Where connection to a forming shell is specified, the connection shall be to the conduit termination point.

E4206.9 Junction boxes and enclosures for transformers or ground-fault circuit interrupters. Junction boxes for underwater luminaires and enclosures for transformers and ground-fault circuit-interrupters that supply underwater luminaires shall comply with the following:

E4206.9.1 Junction boxes. A junction box connected to a conduit that extends directly to a forming shell or mounting bracket of a no-niche luminaire shall be:

1. Listed as a swimming pool junction box;

2. Equipped with threaded entries or hubs or a nonmetallic hub;

3. Constructed of copper, brass, suitable plastic, or other approved corrosion-resistant material;

4. Provided with electrical continuity between every connected metal conduit and the grounding terminals by means of copper, brass, or other approved corrosion-resistant metal that is integral with the box; and

5. Located not less than 4 inches (102 mm), measured from the inside of the bottom of the box, above the ground level, or pool deck, or not less than 8 inches (203 mm) above the maximum pool water level, whichever provides the greatest elevation, and shall be located not less than 4 feet (1219 mm) from the inside wall of the pool, unless separated from the pool by a solid fence, wall or other permanent barrier. Where used on a lighting system operating at 15 volts or less, a flush deck box shall be permitted provided that an approved potting compound is used to fill the box to prevent the entrance of moisture; and the flush deck box is located not less than 4 feet (1219 mm) from the inside wall of the pool.

E4206.9.2 Other enclosures. An enclosure for a transformer, ground-fault circuit-interrupter or a similar device connected to a conduit that extends directly to a forming shell or mounting bracket of a no-niche luminaire shall be:

1. Listed and labeled for the purpose, comprised of copper, brass, suitable plastic, or other approved corrosion-resistant material;

2. Equipped with threaded entries or hubs or a nonmetallic hub;

3. Provided with an approved seal, such as duct seal at the conduit connection, that prevents circulation of air between the conduit and the enclosures;

4. Provided with electrical continuity between every connected metal conduit and the grounding terminals by means of copper, brass or other approved corrosion-resistant metal that is integral with the enclosures; and

5. Located not less than 4 inches (102 mm), measured from the inside bottom of the enclosure, above the ground level or pool deck, or not less than 8 inches (203 mm) above the maximum pool water level, whichever provides the greater elevation, and shall be located not less than 4 feet (1219 mm) from the inside wall of the pool, except where separated from the pool by a solid fence, wall or other permanent barrier.

E4206.9.3 Protection of junction boxes and enclosures. Junction boxes and enclosures mounted above the grade of the finished walkway around the pool shall not be located in the walkway unless afforded additional protection, such as by location under diving boards or adjacent to fixed structures.

E4206.9.4 Grounding terminals. Junction boxes, transformer enclosures, and ground-fault circuit-interrupter enclosures connected to a conduit that extends directly to a forming shell or mounting bracket of a no-niche luminaire shall be provided with grounding terminals in a quantity not less than the number of conduit entries plus one.

E4206.9.5 Strain relief. The termination of a flexible cord of an underwater luminaire within a junction box, transformer enclosure, ground-fault circuit-interrupter, or other enclosure shall be provided with a strain relief.

E4206.10 Underwater audio equipment. Underwater audio equipment shall be identified for the purpose.

E4206.10.1 Speakers. Each speaker shall be mounted in an approved metal forming shell, the front of which is enclosed by a captive metal screen, or equivalent, that is bonded to and secured to the forming shell by a positive locking device that ensures a low-resistance contact and requires a tool to open for installation or servicing of the speaker. The forming shell shall be installed in a recess in the wall or floor of the pool.

E4206.10.2 Wiring methods. Rigid metal conduit or intermediate metal conduit of brass or other identified corrosion-resistant metal, rigid nonmetallic conduit, or liquid tight flexible nonmetallic conduit (LFNC-B) shall extend from the forming shell to a suitable junction box or other

enclosure as provided in Section E4206.9. Where rigid non-metallic conduit or liquid tight flexible nonmetallic conduit is used, an 8 AWG solid or stranded insulated copper bonding jumper shall be installed in this conduit with provisions for terminating in the forming shell and the junction box. The termination of the 8 AWG bonding jumper in the forming shell shall be covered with, or encapsulated in, a suitable potting compound to protect such connection from the possible deteriorating effect of pool water.

E4206.10.3 Forming shell and metal screen. The forming shell and metal screen shall be of brass or other approved corrosion-resistant metal. All forming shells shall include provisions for terminating an 8 AWG copper conductor.

E4206.11 Electrically operated pool covers. The electric motors, controllers, and wiring for pool covers shall be located not less than 5 feet (1524 mm) from the inside wall of the pool except where separated from the pool by a wall, cover, or other permanent barrier. Electric motors installed below grade level shall be of the totally enclosed type. The electric motor and controller shall be connected to a circuit protected by a ground-fault circuit-interrupter. The device that controls the operation of the motor for an electrically operated pool cover shall be located so that the operator has full view of the pool.

E4206.12 Electric pool water heaters. All electric pool water heaters shall have the heating elements subdivided into loads not exceeding 48 amperes and protected at not more than 60 amperes. The ampacity of the branch-circuit conductors and the rating or setting of overcurrent protective devices shall be not less than 125 percent of the total nameplate load rating.

E4206.13 Pool area heating. The provisions of Sections E4206.13.1 through E4206.13.3 shall apply to all pool deck areas, including a covered pool, where electrically operated comfort heating units are installed within 20 feet (6096 mm) of the inside wall of the pool.

E4206.13.1 Unit heaters. Unit heaters shall be rigidly mounted to the structure and shall be of the totally enclosed or guarded types. Unit heaters shall not be mounted over the pool or within the area extending 5 feet (1524 mm) horizontally from the inside walls of a pool.

E4206.13.2 Permanently wired radiant heaters. Electric radiant heaters shall be suitably guarded and securely fastened to their mounting devices. Heaters shall not be installed over a pool or within the area extending 5 feet (1524 mm) horizontally from the inside walls of the pool and shall be mounted not less than 12 feet (3658 mm) vertically above the pool deck.

E4206.13.3 Radiant heating cables prohibited. Radiant heating cables embedded in or below the deck shall be prohibited.

SECTION E4207
STORABLE SWIMMING POOLS

E4207.1 Pumps. A cord and plug-connected pool filter pump for use with storable pools shall incorporate an approved system of double insulation or its equivalent and shall be provided with means for grounding only the internal and nonaccessible noncurrent-carrying metal parts of the appliance.

The means for grounding shall be an equipment grounding conductor run with the power-supply conductors in a flexible cord that is properly terminated in a grounding-type attachment plug having a fixed grounding contact. Cord and plug-connected pool filter pumps shall be provided with a ground-fault circuit interrupter that is an integral part of the attachment plug or located in the power supply cord within 12 inches (305 mm) of the attachment plug.

E4207.2 Ground-fault circuit-interrupters required. Electrical equipment, including power-supply cords, used with storable pools shall be protected by ground-fault circuit-interrupters. All 125-volt receptacles located within 20 feet (6096 mm) of the inside walls of a storable pool shall be protected by a ground-fault circuit interrupter. In determining these dimensions, the distance to be measured shall be the shortest path that the supply cord of an appliance connected to the receptacle would follow without passing through a floor, wall, ceiling, doorway with hinged or sliding door, window opening, or other effective permanent barrier.

E4207.3 Luminaires. Luminaires for storable pools shall not have exposed metal parts and shall be listed for the purpose as an assembly. In addition, luminaires for storable pools shall comply with the requirements of Section E4207.3.1 or E4207.3.2.

> **E4207.3.1 Fifteen volts or less.** A luminaire installed in or on the wall of a storable pool shall be part of a cord and plug-connected lighting assembly. The assembly shall:
>
> 1. Have a luminaire lamp that operates at 15 volts or less;
>
> 2. Have an impact-resistant polymeric lens, luminaire body, and transformer enclosure;
>
> 3. Have a transformer meeting the requirements of section E4206.1 with a primary rating not over 150 volts; and
>
> 4. Have no exposed metal parts.

E4207.3.2 Not over 150 volts. A lighting assembly without a transformer, and with the luminaire lamp(s) operating at not over 150 volts, shall be permitted to be cord and plug-connected where the assembly is listed as an assembly for the purpose and complies with all of the following:

> 1. It has an impact-resistant polymeric lens and luminaire body.
>
> 2. A ground-fault circuit interrupter with open neutral conductor protection is provided as an integral part of the assembly.
>
> 3. The luminaire lamp is permanently connected to the ground-fault circuit interrupter with open-neutral protection.
>
> 4. It complies with the requirements of Section E4206.4.
>
> 5. It has no exposed metal parts.

E4207.4 Receptacle locations. Receptacles shall be located not less than 6 feet (1829 mm) from the inside walls of a pool. In determining these dimensions, the distance to be measured shall be the shortest path that the supply cord of an appliance connected to the receptacle would follow without passing through a floor, wall, ceiling, doorway with hinged or sliding door, window opening, or other effective permanent barrier.

SECTION E4208
SPAS AND HOT TUBS

E4208.1 Ground-fault circuit-interrupters. The outlet(s) that supplies a self-contained spa or hot tub, or a packaged spa or hot tub equipment assembly, or a field-assembled spa or hot tub with a heater load of 50 amperes or less, shall be protected by a ground-fault circuit-interrupter.

A listed self-contained unit or listed packaged equipment assembly marked to indicate that integral ground-fault circuit-interrupter protection is provided for all electrical parts within the unit or assembly, including pumps, air blowers, heaters, luminaires, controls, sanitizer generators and wiring, shall not require that the outlet supply be protected by a ground-fault circuit interrupter.

A combination pool/hot tub or spa assembly commonly bonded need not be protected by a ground-fault circuit interrupter.

E4208.2 Electric water heaters. Electric spa and hot tub water heaters shall be listed and shall have the heating elements subdivided into loads not exceeding 48 amperes and protected at not more than 60 amperes. The ampacity of the branch-circuit conductors, and the rating or setting of overcurrent protective devices, shall be not less than 125 percent of the total nameplate load rating.

E4208.3 Underwater audio equipment. Underwater audio equipment used with spas and hot tubs shall comply with the provisions of Section E4206.10.

E4208.4 Emergency switch for spas and hot tubs. A clearly labeled emergency shutoff or control switch for the purpose of stopping the motor(s) that provides power to the recirculation system and jet system shall be installed at a point that is readily accessible to the users, adjacent to and within sight of the spa or hot tub and not less than 5 feet (1524 mm) away from the spa or hot tub. This requirement shall not apply to single-family dwellings.

SECTION E4209
HYDROMASSAGE BATHTUBS

E4209.1 Ground-fault circuit-interrupters. Hydromassage bathtubs and their associated electrical components shall be supplied by an individual branch circuit(s) and protected by a readily accessible ground-fault circuit-interrupter. All 125-volt, single-phase receptacles not exceeding 30 amperes and located within 6 feet (1829 mm) measured horizontally of the inside walls of a hydromassage tub shall be protected by a ground-fault circuit interrupter(s).

E4209.2 Other electric equipment. Luminaires, switches, receptacles, and other electrical equipment located in the same room, and not directly associated with a hydromassage bathtub, shall be installed in accordance with the requirements of this code relative to the installation of electrical equipment in bathrooms.

E4209.3 Accessibility. Hydromassage bathtub electrical equipment shall be accessible without damaging the building structure or building finish.

E4209.4 Bonding. All metal piping systems and all grounded metal parts in contact with the circulating water shall be bonded together using an insulated, covered or bare solid copper bonding jumper not smaller than 8 AWG. The bonding jumper shall be connected to the terminal on the circulating pump motor that is intended for this purpose. The bonding jumper shall not be required to be connected to a double insualted circulating pump motor. The 8 AWG or larger solid copper bonding jumper shall be required for equipotential bonding in the area of the hydromassage bathtub and shall not be required to be extended or attached to any remote panelboard, service equipment, or any electrode.

CHAPTER 43

CLASS 2 REMOTE-CONTROL, SIGNALING AND POWER-LIMITED CIRCUITS

SECTION E4301
GENERAL

E4301.1 Scope. This chapter contains requirements for power supplies and wiring methods associated with Class 2 remote-control, signaling, and power-limited circuits that are not an integral part of a device or appliance. Other classes of remote-control, signaling and power-limited conductors shall comply with Article 725 of NFPA 70.

E4301.2 Definitions.

CLASS 2 CIRCUIT. That portion of the wiring system between the load side of a Class 2 power source and the connected equipment. Due to its power limitations, a Class 2 circuit considers safety from a fire initiation standpoint and provides acceptable protection from electric shock.

REMOTE-CONTROL CIRCUIT. Any electrical circuit that controls any other circuit through a relay or an equivalent device.

SIGNALING CIRCUIT. Any electrical circuit that energizes signaling equipment.

SECTION E4302
POWER SOURCES

E4302.1 Power sources for Class 2 circuits. The power source for a Class 2 circuit shall be one of the following:

1. A listed Class 2 transformer.

2. A listed Class 2 power supply.

3. Other listed equipment marked to identify the Class 2 power source.

4. Listed information technology (computer) equipment limited power circuits.

5. A dry cell battery provided that the voltage is 30 volts or less and the capacity is equal to or less than that available from series connected No. 6 carbon zinc cells.

E4302.2 Interconnection of power sources. A Class 2 power source shall not have its output connections paralleled or otherwise interconnected with another Class 2 power source except where listed for such interconnection.

SECTION E4303
WIRING METHODS

E4303.1 Wiring methods on supply side of Class 2 power source. Conductors and equipment on the supply side of the power source shall be installed in accordance with the appropriate requirements of Chapters 34 through 41. Transformers or other devices supplied from electric light or power circuits shall be protected by an over current device rated at not over 20 amperes. The input leads of a transformer or other power source supplying Class 2 circuits shall be permitted to be smaller than 14 AWG, if not over 12 inches (305 mm) long and if the conductor insulation is rated at not less than 600 volts. In no case shall such leads be smaller than 18 AWG.

E4303.2 Wiring methods and materials on load side of the Class 2 power source. Class 2 cables installed as wiring within buildings shall be listed as being resistant to the spread of fire and listed as meeting the criteria specified in Sections E4303.2.1 through E4303.2.3. Cables shall be marked in accordance with Section E4303.2.4. Cable substitutions as described in Table E4303.2 and wiring methods covered in Chapter 38 shall also be permitted.

TABLE E4303.2
CABLE USES AND PERMITTED SUBSTITUTIONS

CABLE TYPE	USE	PERMITTED SUBSTITUTIONS[a]
CL2P	Class 2 Plenum Cable	CMP, CL3P
CL2	Class 2 Cable	CMP, CL3P, CL2P, CMR, CL3R, CL2R CMG, CM, CL3
CL2X	Class 2 Cable, Limited Use	CMP, CL3P CL2P, CMR, CL3R, CL2R, CMG, CM, CL3, CL2, CMX, CL3X

a. For identification of cables other than Class 2 cables, see NFPA 70.

E4303.2.1 Type CL2P cables. Cables installed in ducts, plenums and other spaces used to convey environmental air shall be Type CL2P cables listed as being suitable for the use and listed as having adequate fire-resistant and low smoke-producing characteristics.

E4303.2.2 Type CL2 cables. Cables for general-purpose use, shall be listed as being resistant to the spread of fire and listed for the use.

E4303.2.3 Type CL2X cables. Type CL2X limited-use cable shall be listed as being suitable for use in dwellings and for the use and in raceways and shall also be listed as being flame retardant. Cables with a diameter of less than $1/4$ inch (6.4 mm) shall be permitted to be installed without a raceway.

E4303.2.4 Marking. Cables shall be marked in accordance with Table E4303.2. Voltage ratings shall not be marked on cables.

SECTION E4304
INSTALLATION REQUIREMENTS

E4304.1 Separation from other conductors. In cables, compartments, enclosures, outlet boxes, device boxes, and raceways, conductors of Class 2 circuits shall not be placed in any cable, compartment, enclosure, outlet box, device box, raceway, or similar fitting with conductors of electric light, power, Class 1 and nonpower-limited fire alarm circuits.

Exceptions:

1. Where the conductors of the electric light, power, Class 1 and nonpower-limited fire alarm circuits are separated by a barrier from the Class 2 circuits. In enclosures, Class 2 circuits shall be permitted to be installed in a raceway within the enclosure to separate them from Class 1, electric light, power and nonpower-limited fire alarm circuits.

2. Class 2 conductors in compartments, enclosures, device boxes, outlet boxes and similar fittings where electric light, power, Class 1 or nonpower-limited fire alarm circuit conductors are introduced solely to connect to the equipment connected to the Class 2 circuits. The electric light, power, Class 1 and nonpower-limited fire alarm circuit conductors shall be routed to maintain a minimum of $^1/_4$ inch (6.4 mm) separation from the conductors and cables of the Class 2 circuits; or the electric light power, Class 1 and nonpower-limited fire alarm circuit conductors operate at 150 volts or less to ground and the Class 2 circuits are installed using Types CL3, CL3R, or CL3P or permitted substitute cables, and provided that these Class 3 cable conductors extending beyond their jacket are separated by a minimum of $^1/_4$ inch (6.4 mm) or by a nonconductive sleeve or nonconductive barrier from all other conductors.

E4304.2 Other applications. Conductors of Class 2 circuits shall be separated by not less than 2 inches (51 mm) from conductors of any electric light, power, Class 1 or nonpower-limited fire alarm circuits except where one of the following conditions is met:

1. All of the electric light, power, Class 1 and nonpower-limited fire alarm circuit conductors are in raceways or in metal-sheathed, metal-clad, nonmetallic-sheathed or Type UF cables.

2. All of the Class 2 circuit conductors are in raceways or in metal-sheathed, metal-clad, nonmetallic-sheathed or Type UF cables.

E4304.3 Class 2 circuits with communications circuits. Where Class 2 circuit conductors are in the same cable as communications circuits, the Class 2 circuits shall be classified as communications circuits and shall meet the requirements of Article 800 of NFPA 70. The cables shall be listed as communications cables or multipurpose cables.

Cables constructed of individually listed Class 2 and communications cables under a common jacket shall be permitted to be classified as communications cables. The fire-resistance rating of the composite cable shall be determined by the performance of the composite cable.

E4304.4 Class 2 cables with other circuit cables. Jacketed cables of Class 2 circuits shall be permitted in the same enclosure or raceway with jacketed cables of any of the following:

1. Power-limited fire alarm systems in compliance with Article 760 of NFPA 70.

2. Nonconductive and conductive optical fiber cables in compliance with Article 770 of NFPA 70.

3. Communications circuits in compliance with Article 800 of NFPA 70.

4. Community antenna television and radio distribution systems in compliance with Article 820 of NFPA 70.

5. Low-power, network-powered broadband communications in compliance with Article 830 of NFPA 70.

E4304.5 Installation of conductors and cables. Cables and conductors installed exposed on the surface of ceilings and sidewalls shall be supported by the building structure in such a manner that they will not be damaged by normal building use. Such cables shall be supported by straps, staples, hangers, cable ties or similar fittings designed so as to not damage the cable. The installation shall comply with Table E3802.1 regarding cables run parallel with framing members and furring strips. The installation of wires and cables shall not prevent access to equipment nor prevent removal of panels, including suspended ceiling panels. Raceways shall not be used as a means of support for Class 2 circuit conductors, except where the supporting raceway contains conductors supplying power to the functionally associated equipment controlled by the Class 2 conductors.

Part IX—Referenced Standards

CHAPTER 44

REFERENCED STANDARDS

This chapter lists the standards that are referenced in various sections of this document. The standards are listed herein by the promulgating agency of the standard, the standard identification, the effective date and title, and the section or sections of this document that reference the standard. The application of the referenced standards shall be as specified in Section R102.4.

AAMA

American Architectural Manufacturers Association
1827 Walden Office Square, Suite 550
Schaumburg, IL 60173

Standard reference number	Title	Referenced in code section number
AAMA/WDMA/CSA 101/I.S.2/A440—08	North American Fenestration Standards/Specifications for Windows, Doors and Skylights	N1102.4.4, R308.6.9, R613.6
450—06	Voluntary Performance Rating Method for Mulled Fenestration Assemblies	R612.11.1
506—06	Voluntary Specifications for Hurricane Impact and Cycle Testing of Fenestration Products	R612.9.1
711—07	Voluntary Specification for Self Adhering Flashing Used for Installation of Exterior Wall Fenestration Products	R703.8

ACI

American Concrete Institute
38800 Country Club Drive
Farmington Hills, MI 48331

Standard reference number	Title	Referenced in code section number
318—08	Building Code Requirements for Structural Concrete	R301.2.2.2.4, R301.2.2.3.4, R402.2, R404.1.2, Table 404.1.2(5), Table R404.1.2(6), Table R404.1.2(7), Table R404.1.2(8), Table R404.1.2(9), R404.1.2.1, R404.1.2.3, R404.1.2.4, R404.1.4.2, R404.6.1, R611.1, R611.1.1, R611.1.2, R611.2, R611.5.1, R611.8.2, R611.9.2, R611.9.3
332—08	Code Requirements for Residential Concrete Construction	R402.2, R403.1, R404.1.2, R404.1.2.4, R404.1.4.2
530—08	Building Code Requirements for Masonry Structures	R404.1.1, R606.1, R606.1.1, R606.12.1, R606.12.2.2.1, R606.12.2.2.2, R606.12.3.1, Table R703.4
530.1—08	Specification for Masonry Structures	R404.1.1, R606.1, R606.1.1, R606.12.1, R606.12.2.2.1, R606.12.2.2.2, R606.12.3.1, Table R703.4

ACCA

Air Conditioning Contractors of America
2800 Shirlington Road, Suite 300
Arlington, VA 22206

Standard reference number	Title	Referenced in code section number
Manual D—95	Residential Duct Systems	M1601.1, M1602.2
Manual J—02	Residential Load Calculation—Eighth Edition	M1401.3
Manual S—04	Residential Equipment Selection	M1401.3

AFPA

American Forest and Paper Association
1111 19th Street, NW, Suite 800
Washington, DC 20036

Standard reference number	Title	Referenced in code section number
NDS—05	National Design Specification (NDS) for Wood Construction—with 2005 Supplement	R404.2.2, R502.2, Table R503.1, R602.3, Table R602.3.1 R611.9.2, R611.9.3, R802.2,
WFCM—08	Wood Frame Construction Manual for One- and Two-family Dwellings	R301.1.1, R301.2.1.1, R602.10.6.2, R611.9.2, R611.9.3, R611.10
AFPA—93	Span Tables for Joists and Rafters	R502.3, R802.4, R802.5
PWF—07	Permanent Wood Foundation Design Specification	R401.1, R404.2.3

AISI

American Iron and Steel Institute
1140 Connecticut Ave, Suite 705
Washington, DC 20036

Standard reference number	Title	Referenced in code section number
AISI S100—07	North American Specification for the Design of Cold-formed Steel Structural Members	R505.1.3, R603.6, R611.9.2, R611.9.3, R804.3.7
AISI S230—07	Standard for Cold-formed Steel Framing-prescriptive Method for One- and Two-family Dwellings	R301.1.1, R301.2.1.1, R301.2.2.3.1, R301.2.2.3.5, R603.6, R611.9.2, R611.9.3, R611.10

AITC

American Institute of Timber Construction
7012 S. Revere Parkway, Suite 140
Centennial, CO 80112

Standard reference number	Title	Referenced in code section number
ANSI/AITC A 190.1—07	Structural Glued Laminated Timber	R502.1.5, R602.1.2, R802.1.4

ANSI

American National Standards Institute
25 West 43rd Street, Fourth Floor
New York, NY 10036

Standard reference number	Title	Referenced in code section number
A108.1A—99	Installation of Ceramic Tile in the Wet-set Method, with Portland Cement Mortar	R702.4.1
A108.1B—99	Installation of Ceramic Tile, Quarry Tile on a Cured Portland Cement Mortar Setting Bed with Dry-set or Latex-Portland Mortar	R702.4.1
A108.4—99	Installation of Ceramic Tile with Organic Adhesives or Water Cleanable Tile-setting Epoxy Adhesive	R702.4.1
A108.5—99	Installation of Ceramic Tile with Dry-set Portland Cement Mortar or Latex-Portland Cement Mortar	R702.4.1
A108.6—99	Installation of Ceramic Tile with Chemical-resistant, Water-cleanable Tile-setting and -grouting Epoxy	R702.4.1
A108.11—99	Interior Installation of Cementitious Backer Units	R702.4.1
A118.1—99	American National Standard Specifications for Dry-set Portland Cement Mortar	R702.4.1
A118.3—99	American National Standard Specifications for Chemical-resistant, Water-cleanable Tile-setting and Grouting Epoxy and Water-cleanable Tile-setting Epoxy Adhesive	R702.4.1
A118.10—99	Specification for Load Bearing, Bonded, Waterproof Membranes for Thin-set Ceramic Tile and Dimension Stone Installation	P2709.2
A136.1—99	American National Standard Specifications for Organic Adhesives for Installation of Ceramic Tile	R702.4.1
A137.1—88	American National Standard Specifications for Ceramic Tile	R702.4.1
A208.1—99	Particleboard	R503.3.1, R605.1
LC1—97	Interior Fuel Gas Piping Systems Using Corrugated Stainless Steel Tubing —with Addenda LC 1a-1999 and LC 1b-2001	G2414.5.3
LC4—07	Press-connect Copper and Copper Alloy Fittings for use in Fuel Gas Distribution Systems	G2414.10.2
Z21.1—03	Household Cooking Gas Appliances—with Addenda Z21.1a-2003 and Z21.1b-2003	G2447.1
Z21.5.1—02	Gas Clothes Dryers—Volume I—Type I Clothes Dryers—with Addenda Z21.5.1a-2003	G2438.1
Z21.8—94 (R2002)	Installation of Domestic Gas Conversion Burners	G2443.1

ANSI—continued

Z21.10.1—04	Gas Water Heaters—Volume I—Storage Water Heaters with Input Ratings of 75,000 Btu per hour or Less	G2448.1
Z21.10.3—01	Gas Water Heaters—Volume III—Storage Water Heaters with Input Ratings above 75,000 Btu per hour, Circulating and Instantaneous Water Heaters—with Addenda Z21.10.3a-2003 and Z21.10.3b-2004	G2448.1
Z21.11.2—02	Gas-fired Room Heaters—Volume II—Unvented Room Heaters—with Addenda Z21.11.2a-2003	G2445.1
Z21.13—04	Gas-fired Low-Pressure Steam and Hot Water Boilers	G2452.1
Z21.15—97 (R2003)	Manually Operated Gas Valves for Appliances, Appliance Connector Valves and Hose End Valves—with Addenda Z21.15a-2001 (R2003)	Table G2420.1.1
Z21.22—99 (R2003)	Relief Valves for Hot Water Supply Systems—with Addenda Z21.22a-2000 (R2003) and 21.22b-2001 (R2003)	P2803.2, P2803.7
Z21.24-97	Connectors for Gas Appliances	G2422.1
Z21.40.1—96 (R2002)	Gas-fired, Heat-activated Air Conditioning and Heat Pump Appliances—with Z21.40.1a-97 (R2002)	G2449.1
Z21.40.2—96 (R2002)	Gas-fired, Work-activated Air Conditioning and Heat Pump Appliances (Internal Combustion)—with Z21.40.2a-1997 (R2002)	G2449.1
Z21.42—93 (R2002)	Gas-fired Illuminating Appliances	G2450.1
Z21.47—03	Gas-fired Central Furnaces	G2442.1
Z21.50—03	Vented Gas Fireplaces—with Addenda Z21.50a-2003	G2434.1
Z21.56—01	Gas-fired Pool Heaters—with Addenda Z21.56a-2004 and Z21.56b—2004	G2441.1
Z21.58—95 (R2002)	Outdoor Cooking Gas Appliances—with Addenda Z21.58a-1998 (R2002) and Z21.58b-2002	G2447.1
Z21.60—03	Decorative Gas Appliances for Installation in Solid Fuel Burning Fireplaces—with Addenda Z21.60a-2003	G2432.1
Z21.75/CSA 6.27—01	Connectors for Outdoor Gas Appliances	G2422.1
Z21.80—03	Line Pressure Regulators	G2421.1
Z21.83—98	Fuel Cell Power Plants	M1903.1
Z21.84—02	Manually Listed, Natural Gas Decorative Gas Appliances for Installation in Solid Fuel-burning Fireplaces—with Addenda Z21.84a -2003	G2432.1, G2432.2
Z21.86—04	Gas-fired Vented Space Heating Appliances	G2436.1, G2437.1, G2446.1
Z21.88—02	Vented Gas Fireplace Heaters—with Addenda A21.88a-2003 and Z21.88b—2004	G2435.1
Z21.91—01	Ventless Firebox Enclosures for Gas-fired Unvented Decorative Room Heaters	G2445.7.1
Z83.6—90 (R1998)	Gas-fired Infrared Heaters	G2451.1
Z83.8—02	Gas-fired Unit Heaters and Gas-fired Duct Furnaces—with Addenda Z83.8a-2003	G2444.1
Z97.1—04	Safety Glazing Materials Used in Buildings—Safety Performance Specifications and Methods of Test	R308.1.1, R308.3.1
Z124.1—95	Plastic Bathtub Units	Table P2701.1
Z124.2—95	Plastic Shower Receptors and Shower Stalls	Table P2701.1
Z124.3—95	Plastic Lavatories	Table P2701.1, P2711.1, P2711.2
Z124.4—96	Plastic Water Closet Bowls and Tanks	Table P2701.1, P2712.1
Z124.6—97	Plastic Sinks	Table P2701.1

APA

APA–The Engineered Wood Association
7011 South 19th
Tacoma, WA 98466

Standard reference number	Title	Referenced in code section number
APA E30—03	Engineered Wood Construction Guide	Table R503.2.1.1(1), R503.2.2, R803.2.2, R803.2.3

APSP

The Association of Pool & Spa Professionals
2111 Eisenhower Avenue
Alexandria, VA 22314

Standard reference number	Title	Referenced in code section number
ANSI/APSP 7—06	Standard for Suction Entrapment Avoidance in Swimming Pools Wading Pools, Spas, Hot Tubs and Catch Basins	AG106.1
ANSI/NSPI 3—99	Standard for Permanently Installed Residential Spas	AG104.1
ANSI/NSPI 4—99	Standard for Above-ground/On-ground Residential Swimming Pools	AG103.2

APSP—continued

ANSI/NSPI-5—2003	Standard for Residential In-ground Swimming Pools.	AG103.1
ANSI/NSPI 6—99	Standard for Residential Portable Spas	AG104.2

ASCE/SEI

American Society of Civil Engineers
Structural Engineering Institute
1801 Alexander Bell Drive
Reston, VA 20191

Standard reference number	Title	Referenced in code section number
5—08	Building Code Requirements for Masonry Structures.	R404.1.1, R606.1, R606.1.1, R606.12.1, R606.12.2.2.1, R606.12.2.2.2, R606.12.3.1, Table R703.4
6—08	Specification for Masonry Structures.	R404.1.1, R606.1, R606.1.1, R606.12.1, R606.12.2.2.1, R606.12.2.2.2, R606.12.3.1, Table R703.4
7—05	Minimum Design Loads for Buildings and Other Structures	R301.2.1.1, R301.2.1.2, R301.2.1.5, R301.2.1.5.1, R301.2.4.1, Table R611.6(1), Table R611.6(2), Table R611.6(3), Table R611.6(4), Table R611.7(1A), R611.9.2, R611.9.3, Table R802.11, AH107.4.3
24—05	Flood-resistant Design and Construction	R301.2.4, R301.2.4.1, R322.1, R322.1.1, R322.1.6, R322.1.9, R322.2.2, AG103.3
32—01	Design and Construction of Frost-protected Shallow Foundations	R403.1.4.1

ASHRAE

American Society of Heating, Refrigerating
and Air-Conditioning Engineers, Inc.
1791 Tullie Circle, NE
Atlanta, GA 30329

Standard reference number	Title	Referenced in code section number
34—2004	Designation and Safety Classification of Refrigerants	M1411.1
ASHRAE—2005	ASHRAE Fundamentals Handbook—2005	N1102.1.3, P3001.2, P3101.4, P3103.2

ASME

American Society of Mechanical Engineers
Three Park Avenue
New York, NY 10016-5990

Standard reference number	Title	Referenced in code section number
A17.1/CSA B44—2007	Safety Code for Elevators and Escalators.	R321.1
A18.1—2005	Safety Standard for Platforms and Stairway Chair Lifts	R321.2
A112.1.2—2004	Air Gaps in Plumbing Systems.	Table P2902.3, P2902.3.1
A112.1.3—2000 (Reaffirmed 2005)	Air Gap Fittings for Use with Plumbing Fixtures, Appliances and Appurtenances	Table P2701.1, P2902.3.1
A112.3.1—2007	Stainless Steel Drainage Systems for Sanitary, DWV, Storm and Vacuum Applications Above and Below Ground	Table P3002.1(1), Table P3002.1(2), Table P3002.2, Table P3002.3, Table P3302.1
A112.3.4—2000 (R2004)	Macerating Toilet Systems and Related Components	Table P2701.1, P3007.5
A112.4.1—1993 (R2002)	Water Heater Relief Valve Drain Tubes.	P2803.6.2
A112.4.3—1999 (R2004)	Plastic Fittings for Connecting Water Closets to the Sanitary Drainage System	P3003.19
A112.6.1M—1997 (R2002)	Floor Affixed Supports for Off-the-floor Plumbing Fixtures for Public Use	Table P2701.1, P2702.4
A112.6.2—2000 (R2004)	Framing-affixed Supports for Off-the-floor Water Closets with Concealed Tanks	Table P2701.1, P2702.4
A112.6.3—2001 (R2007)	Floor and Trench Drains	Table P2701.1
A112.14.1—03	Backwater Valves	P3008.2
A112.18.1—2005/ CSA B125.1-2005	Plumbing Supply Fittings	Table P2701.1, P2708.4, P2722.1, P2902.2
A112.18.2—2005/ CSA B125.2-2005	Plumbing Waste Fittings	Table P2701.1, P2702.2

ASME—continued

A112.18.3—2002	Performance Requirements for Backflow Protection Devices and Systems in Plumbing Fixture Fittings	P2708.4, P2722.3
A112.18.6—2003	Flexible Water Connectors	P2905.7
A112.19.1M—1994 (R2004)	Enameled Cast Iron Plumbing Fixtures—with 1998 and 2000 Supplements	Table P2701.1, P2711.1
A112.19.2—2003	Vitreous China Plumbing Fixtures—and Hydraulic Requirements for Water Closets and Urinals	Table P2701.1, P2705.1, P2711.1, P2712.1, P2712.2
A112.19.3M—2000 (R2007)	Stainless Steel Plumbing Fixtures (Designed for Residential Use)—with 2002 Supplement	Table P2701.1, P2705.1, P2711.1
A112.19.4M—1994 (R2004)	Porcelain Enameled Formed Steel Plumbing Fixtures—with 1998 and 2000 Supplements	Table P2701.1, P2711.1
A112.19.5—2005	Trim for Water-closet Bowls, Tanks and Urinals	Table P2701.1
A112.19.6—1995	Hydraulic Performance Requirements for Water Closets and Urinals	P2712.1, P2712.2
A112.19.7M—2006	Hydromassage Bathtub Appliances	Table P2701.1
A112.19.8M—1987 (R1996)	Suction Fittings for Use in Swimming Pools, Wading Pools, Spas, Hot Tubs and Whirlpool Bathtub Appliances	Table P2701.1
A112.19.9M—1991 (R2002)	Nonvitreous Ceramic Plumbing Fixtures—with 2002 Supplement	Table P2701.1, P27.11.1, P2712.1
A112.19.12—2006	Wall-mounted and Pedestal-mounted, Adjustable and Pivoting Lavatory and Sink Carrier Systems	Table P2701.1, P2711.4, P2714.2
A112.19.13—2001 (R2007)	Electrohydraulic Water Closets	P2712.9
A112.19.15—2005	Bathtub/Whirlpool Bathtubs with Pressure Sealed Doors	Table P2701.1, P2713.2
B1.20.1—1983 (R2006)	Pipe Threads, General Purpose (Inch)	G2414.9, P3003.3.3, P3003.5.3, P3003.10.4, P3003.12.1, P3003.14.3
B16.3—2006	Malleable-iron-threaded Fittings Classes 150 and 300	Table P2905.6
B16.4—2006	Gray-iron-threaded Fittings Classes 125 and 250	Table P2905.6, Table P3002.3
B16.9—2003	Factory-made Wrought Steel Buttwelding Fittings	Table P2905.6
B16.11—2005	Forged Fittings, Socket-welding and Threaded	Table P2905.6
B16.12—1998	Cast-iron-threaded Drainage Fittings	Table P2905.6, Table P3002.3 (R2006)
B16.15—2006	Cast-bronze-threaded Fittings	Table P2905.6, Table P3002.3
B16.18—2001 (R2005)	Cast Copper Alloy Solder Joint Pressure Fittings	Table P2905.6, Table P3002.3
B16.22—2001(R2005)	Wrought Copper and Copper Alloy Solder Joint Pressure Fittings	Table P2905.6, Table P3002.3
B16.23—2002 (R2006)	Cast Copper Alloy Solder Joint Drainage Fittings (DWV)	Table P2905.6, Table P3002.3
B16.26—2006	Cast Copper Alloy Fittings for Flared Copper Tubes	Table P2905.6, Table P3002.3
B16.28—1994	Wrought Steel Buttwelding Short Radius Elbows and Returns	Table P2905.6
B16.29—2001	Wrought Copper and Wrought Copper Alloy Solder Joint Drainage Fittings (DWV)	Table P2905.6, Table P3002.3
B16.33—2002 (R2006)	Manually Operated Metallic Gas Valves for Use in Gas Piping Systems up to 125 psig (Sizes $1/_2$ through 2)	Table G2420.1.1
B16.44—02	Manually Operated Metallic Gas Valves For Use in Above-ground Piping Systems up to 5 psi	Table G2420.1.1
B36.10M—2004	Welded and Seamless Wrought-steel Pipe	G2414.4.2
BPVC—2004	ASME Boiler and Pressure Vessel Code	G2452.1, M2001.1.1
CSD-1—2004	Controls and Safety Devices for Automatically Fired Boilers	G2452.1, M2001.1.1

ASSE

American Society of Sanitary Engineering
901 Canterbury, Suite A
Westlake, OH 44145

Standard reference number	Title	Referenced in code section number
1001—02	Performance Requirements for Atmospheric-type Vacuum Breakers	Table P2902.3, P2902.3.2
1002—99	Performance Requirements for Antisiphon Fill Valves (Ballcocks) for Gravity Water Closet Flush Tank	Table P2701.1, Table P2902.3, P2902.4.1
1003—01	Performance Requirements for Water-pressure-reducing Valves	P2903.3.1
1006—89	Performance Requirements for Residential Use Dishwashers	Table P2701.1
1007—92	Performance Requirements for Home Laundry Equipment	Table P2701.1
1008—89	Performance Requirements for Household Food Waste Disposer Units	Table P2701.1
1010—04	Performance Requirements for Water Hammer Arresters	P2903.5

ASSE—continued

1011—04	Performance Requirements for Hose Connection Vacuum Breakers	Table P2902.3, P2902.3.2
1012—02	Performance Requirements for Backflow Preventers with Intermediate Atmospheric Vent	Table P2902.3, P2902.3.3, P2902.5.1, P2902.5.5
1013—05	Performance Requirements for Reduced Pressure Principle Backflow Preventers and Reduced Pressure Fire Protection Principle Backflow Preventers	Table P2902.3, P2902.3.5, P2902.5.1, P2902.5.5
1015—05	Performance Requirements For Double Check Backflow Prevention Assemblies and Double Check Fire Protection Backflow Prevention Assemblies	Table P2902.3, P2902.3.6
1016—96	Performance Requirements for Automatic Compensating Valves for Individual Showers and Tub/Shower Combinations	Table P2701.1, P2708.3, P2722.2
1017—03	Performance Requirements for Temperature Actuated Mixing Valves for Hot Water Distribution Systems	P2802.2
1019—04	Performance Requirements for Wall Hydrants, Freeze Resistant, Automatic Draining Types	Table P2701.1, P2902.3
1020—04	Performance Requirements for Pressure Vacuum Breaker Assembly	Table P2902.3, P2902.3.4
1023—79	Performance Requirements for Hot Water Dispensers Household Storage Type-electrical	Table P2701.1
1024—04	Performance Requirements for Dual Check Backflow Preventers	Table P2902.3
1025—78	Performance Requirements for Diverters for Plumbing Faucets with Hose Spray, Anti-siphon Type, Residential Applications	Table P2701.1
1035—02	Performance Requirements for Laboratory Faucet Backflow Preventers	Table P2902.3, P2902.3.2
1037—90	Performance Requirements for Pressurized Flushing Devices (Flushometer) for Plumbing Fixtures	Table P2701.1
1047—05	Performance Requirements for Reduced Pressure Detector Fire Protection Backflow Prevention Assemblies	Table P2902.3, P2902.3.5
1048—05	Performance Requirements for Double Check Detector Fire Protection Backflow Prevention Assemblies	Table P2902.3, P2902.3.6
1050—02	Performance Requirements for Stack Air Admittance Valves for Sanitary Drainage Systems	P3114.1
1051—02	Performance Requirements for Individual and Branch Type Air Admittance Valves for Plumbing Drainage Systems	P3114.1
1052—04	Performance Requirements for Hose Connection Backflow Preventers	Table P2701.1, Table P2902.3, P2902.3.2
1056—01	Performance Requirements for Spill Resistant Vacuum Breakers	Table P2902.3, P2902.3.4
1060—96	Performance Requirements for Outdoor Enclosures for Fluid Conveying Components	P2902.6.1
1061—06	Performance Requirements for Removable and Nonremovable Push Fit Fittings	Table P2905.6
1062—97	Performance Requirements for Temperature Actuated, Flow Reduction (TAFR) Valves for Individual Supply Fittings	Table P2701.1, P2724.1
1066—97	Performance Requirements for Individual Pressure Balancing In-line Valves for Individual Fixture Fittings	Table P2701.1, P2722.4
1070—04	Performance Requirements for Water Temperature Limiting Devices	P2713.3, P2721.2

ASTM

ASTM International
100 Barr Harbor Drive
West Conshohocken, PA 19428

Standard reference number	Title	Referenced in code section number
A 36/A 36M—05	Specification for Carbon Structural Steel	R606.15, R611.5.2.2
A 53/A 53M—06a	Specification for Pipe, Steel, Black and Hot-dipped, Zinc-coated Welded and Seamless	G2414.4.2, Table M2101.1, Table P2905.4, Table P2905.5, Table P3002.1(1)
A 74—06	Specification for Cast Iron Soil Pipe and Fittings	Table P3002.1(1), Table P3002.1(2), Table P3002.2, Table P3002.3, P3005.2.9, Table P3302.1
A 82/A 82M—05a	Specification for Steel Wire, Plain, for Concrete Reinforcement	R606.15
A 106/A 106M—06a	Specification for Seamless Carbon Steel Pipe for High Temperature Service	G2414.4.2, Table M2101.1
A 153/A 153M—05	Specification for Zinc Coating (Hot Dip) on Iron and Steel Hardware	R317.3, Table R606.15.1
A 167—99(2004)	Specification for Stainless and Heat-resisting Chromium-nickel Steel Plate, Sheet and Strip	R606.15, Table R606.15.1
A 240/A 240M—07	Standard Specification for Chromium and Chromium-nickel Stainless Steel Plate, Sheet and Strip for Pressure Vessels and for General Applications	Table R905.10.3(1)
A 254—97(2002)	Specification for Copper Brazed Steel Tubing	G2414.5.1, Table M2101.1
A 307—04e01	Specification for Carbon Steel Bolts and Studs, 6000 psi Tensile Strength	R611.5.2.2
A 312/A 312M—06	Specification for Seamless and Welded Austenitic Stainless Steel Pipes	Table P2905.4, Table P2905.5, Table P2905.6, P2905.12.2

ASTM—continued

A 463/A 463M—05	Standard Specification for Steel Sheet, Aluminum-coated by the Hot-dip Process	Table R905.10.3(2)
A 510—06	Specification for General Requirements for Wire Rods and Coarse Round Wire, Carbon Steel	R606.15
A 539—99	Specification for Electric-resistance-welded Coiled Steel Tubing for Gas and Fuel Oil Lines	M2202.1
A 615/A 615M—04a	Specification for Deformed and Plain Billet-steel Bars for Concrete Reinforcement	R402.3.1, R404.1.2.3.7.1, R611.5.2.1
A 641/A 641M—03	Specification for Zinc-coated (Galvanized) Carbon Steel Wire	Table R606.15.1
A 653/A 653M—07	Specification for Steel Sheet, Zinc-coated (Galvanized) or Zinc-iron Alloy-coated (Galvanized) by the Hot-dip Process	M1601.1.1, R317.3.1, R505.2.1, R505.2.3, R603.2.1, R603.2.3, Table R606.15.1, R611.5.2.3, R804.2.1, R804.2.3, Table R905.10.3(1), Table R905.10.3(2)
A 706/A 706/M—05a	Specification for Low-alloy Steel Deformed and Plain Bars for Concrete Reinforcement	R402.3.1, R404.1.2.3.7.1, R611.5.2.1
A 755/A 755M—07	Specification for Steel Sheet, Metallic Coated by the Hot-dip Process and Prepainted by the Coil-coating Process for Exterior Exposed Building Products	Table R905.10.3(2)
A 778—01	Specification for Welded Unannealed Austenitic Stainless Steel Tubular Products	Table P2904.4, Table P2905.5, Table P2905.6
A 792/A 792M—06a	Specification for Steel Sheet, 55% Aluminum-zinc Alloy-coated by the Hot-dip Process	R505.2.1, R505.2.3, R603.2.1, R603.2.3, R611.5.2.3, R804.2.1, R804.2.3, Table 905.10.3 (2)
A 875/A 875M—06	Specification for Steel Sheet, Zinc-5%, Aluminum Alloy-coated by the Hot-dip Process	R611.5.3.2, Table R905.10.3 (2)
A 888—07a	Specification for Hubless Cast Iron Soil Pipe and Fittings for Sanitary and Storm Drain, Waste and Vent Piping Application	Table P3002.1(1), Table P3002.1(2), Table P3002.2, Table P3002.3, P3005.2.9, Table P3302.1
A 924/A 924M—07	Standard Specification for General Requirements for Steel Sheet, Metallic-coated by the Hot-Dip Process	Table R905.10.3(1)
A 951—06	Specification for Steel Wire Masonry Joint Reinforcement	R606.15
A 996/A 996M—06a	Specifications for Rail-steel and Axel-steel Deformed Bars for Concrete Reinforcement	R404.1.2.3.7, R404.1.2.3.7.1, R611.5.2.1, Table R611.5.4(2)
A 1003/A 1003M—05	Standard Specification for Steel Sheet, Carbon, Metallic and Nonmetallic-coated for Cold-formed Framing Members	R505.2.1, R505.2.3, R603.2.1, R603.2.3, R804.2.1, R804.2.3
B 32—04	Specification for Solder Metal	P3003.10.3, P3003.11.3
B 42—02e01	Specification for Seamless Copper Pipe, Standard Sizes	Table M2101.1, Table P2905.4, Table P2905.5, Table P3002.1(1)
B 43—98 (2004)	Specification for Seamless Red Brass Pipe, Standard Sizes	G2413.5.2, Table M2101.1, Table P2905.4, Table P3002.1(1)
B 75—02	Specification for Seamless Copper Tube	Table M2101.1, Table P2905.4, Table P2905.5, Table P3002.1(1), Table P3002.1(2), Table P3002.2
B 88—03	Specification for Seamless Copper Water Tube	G2414.5.2, Table M2101.1, Table, P2905.4, Table P2905.5, Table P3002.1(1), Table P3002.1(2), Table P3002.2
B 101—02	Specification for Lead-coated Copper Sheet and Strip for Building Construction	Table R905.2.8.2, Table R905.10.3(1)
B 135—02	Specification for Seamless Brass Tube	Table M2101.1
B 209—06	Specification for Aluminum and Aluminum-alloy Sheet and Plate	Table 905.10.3(1)
B 227—04	Specification for Hard-drawn Copper-clad Steel Wire	R606.15
B 251—02e01	Specification for General Requirements for Wrought Seamless Copper and Copper-alloy Tube	Table M2101.1, Table P2905.4, Table P2905.5 Table P3002.1(1), Table P3002.1(2), Table P3002.2
B 302—02	Specification for Threadless Copper Pipe, Standard Sizes	Table M2101.1, Table P2905.4, Table P2905.5, Table P3002.1(1)
B 306—02	Specification for Copper Drainage Tube (DWV)	Table M2101.1, Table P3002.1(1), Table P3002.1(2), Table P3002.2
B 370—03	Specification for Copper Sheet and Strip for Building Construction	Table P2701.1, Table R905.2.8.2, Table R905.10.3(1)
B 447—07	Specification for Welded Copper Tube	Table P2904.4, Table P2905.5
B 695—04	Standard Specification for Coatings of Zinc Mechanically Deposited on Iron and Steel	R317.3.1, R317.3.3, R319.3
B 813—00e01	Specification for Liquid and Paste Fluxes for Soldering Applications of Copper and Copper Alloy Tube	Table M2101.1, P2904.14, P3003.3.4, P3003.10.3, P3003.11.3
B 828—02	Practice for Making Capillary Joints by Soldering of Copper and Copper Alloy Tube and Fittings	P2905.14, P3003.10.3, P3003.11.3
C 4—04e01	Specification for Clay Drain Tile and Perforated Clay Drain Tile	Table P3302.1
C 5—03	Specification for Quicklime for Structural Purposes	R702.2.1
C 14—07	Specification for Concrete Sewer, Storm Drain and Culvert Pipe	Table P3002.2

ASTM—continued

C 836—06	Specification for High Solids Content, Cold Liquid-applied Elastomeric Waterproofing Membrane for Use with Separate Wearing Course	R905.15.2
C 843—99 (2006)	Specification for Application of Gypsum Veneer Plaster	R702.2.1
C 844—04	Specification for Application of Gypsum Base to Receive Gypsum Veneer Plaster	R702.2.1
C 847—06	Specification for Metal Lath	R702.2.1, R702.2.2
C 887—05	Specification for Packaged, Dry, Combined Materials for Surface Bonding Mortar	R406.1
C 897—05	Specification for Aggregate for Job-mixed Portland Cement-based Plasters	R702.2.2
C 920—05	Standard Specification for Elastomeric Joint Sealants	R406.4.1
C 926—98a (2005)	Specification for Application of Portland Cement-based Plaster	R702.2.2, R703.6, R703.6.2, R703.6.4
C 931/C 931M—04	Specification for Exterior Gypsum Soffit Board	R702.3.1
C 933—05	Specification for Welded Wire Lath	R702.2.1, R702.2.2
C 954—04	Specification for Steel Drill Screws for the Application of Gypsum Panel Products or Metal Plaster Bases to Steel Studs from 0.033 in. (0.84 mm) to 0.112 in. (2.84 mm) in Thickness	R505.2.4, R603.2.4, R702.3.6, R804.2.4
C 955—06	Specification for Load-bearing (Transverse and Axial) Steel Studs, Runners (Tracks), and Bracing or Bridging for Screw Application of Gypsum Panel Products and Metal Plaster Bases	R702.3.3
C 957—06	Specification for High-solids Content, Cold Liquid-applied Elastomeric Waterproofing Membrane for Use with Integral Wearing Surface	R905.15.2
C 960—04	Specification for Predecorated Gypsum Board	R702.3.1
C 1002—04	Specification for Steel Drill Screws for the Application of Gypsum Panel Products or Metal Plaster Bases	R702.3.1, R702.3.6
C 1029—05a	Specification for Spray-applied Rigid Cellular Polyurethane Thermal Insulation	R905.14.2
C 1032—06	Specification for Woven Wire Plaster Base	R702.2.1, R702.2.2
C 1047—05	Specification for Accessories for Gypsum Wallboard and Gypsum Veneer Base	R702.2.1, R702.2.2, R702.3.1
C 1063—06	Specification for Installation of Lathing and Furring to Receive Interior and Exterior Portland Cement-based Plaster	R702.2.2, R703.6
C 1107—07	Standard Specification for Packaged Dry, Hydraulic-cement Grout (Nonshrink)	R402.3.1
C 1116—06	Standard Specification for Fiber-reinforced Concrete and Shotcrete	R402.3.1
C 1167—03	Specification for Clay Roof Tiles	R905.3.4
C 1173—06	Specification for Flexible Transition Couplings for Underground Piping Systems	P3003.3, P3003.7, P3003.8.1, P3003.14.1, P3003.15, P3003.17.2, P3003.18
C 1177/C 1177M—06	Specification for Glass Mat Gypsum Substrate for Use as Sheathing	R702.3.1
C 1178/C 1178M—06	Specification for Glass Mat Water-resistant Gypsum Backing Panel	R702.3.1, R702.3.8, R702.4.2
C 1186—07	Specification for Flat Nonasbestos Fiber Cement Sheets	R703.10.1, R703.10.2
C 1261—07	Specification for Firebox Brick for Residential Fireplaces	R1001.5, R1001.8
C 1277—06	Specification for Shielded Couplings Joining Hubless Cast Iron Soil Pipe and Fittings	P3003.6.3
C 1278/C 1278M—06	Specification for Fiber-reinforced Gypsum Panels	R702.3.1, R702.3.8, R702.4.2
C 1283—07	Practice for Installing Clay Flue Lining	R1003.12
C 1288—99(2004)	Standard Specification for Discrete Nonasbestos Fiber-cement Interior Substrate Sheets	R702.4.2
C 1289—07	Standard Specification for Faced Rigid Cellular Polyisocyanurate Thermal Insulation Board	R703.11.2.1, Table R906.2
C 1325—04	Standard Specification for Nonasbestos Fiber-mat Reinforced Cement Interior Substrate Sheets	R702.4.2
C 1328—05	Specification for Plastic (Stucco) Cement	R702.2.2
C 1395/C 1395M—06a	Specification for Gypsum Ceiling Board	R702.3.1
C 1396/C 1396M—06a	Specification for Gypsum Board	Table 602.3(1), R702.3.1, R703.3.8
C 1440—03	Specification for Thermoplastic Elastomeric (TPE) Gasket Materials for Drain, Waste and Vent (DWV), Sewer, Sanitary and Storm Plumbing Systems	P3003.18
C 1460—04	Specification for Shielded Transition Couplings for Use with Dissimilar DWV Pipe and Fittings Above Ground	P3003.18
C 1461—06	Specification for Mechanical Couplings Using Thermoplastic Elastomeric (TPE) Gaskets for Joining Drain, Waste and Vent (DWV) Sewer, Sanitary and Storm Plumbing Systems for Above and Below Ground Use	P3003.18
C 1492—03	Specification for Concrete Roof Tile	R905.3.5
C 1513—04	Standard Specification for Steel Tapping Screws for Cold-formed Steel Framing Connections	R505.2.4, R603.2.4, R702.3.6, R804.2.4
C 1658/C 1658M—06	Standard Specification for Glass Mat Gypsum Panels	R702.3.1
D 41—05	Specification for Asphalt Primer Used in Roofing, Dampproofing and Waterproofing	Table R905.9.2, Table R905.11.2
D 43—00(2006)	Specification for Coal Tar Primer Used in Roofing, Dampproofing and Waterproofing	Table R905.9.2

ASTM—continued

D 225—04	Specification for Asphalt Shingles (Organic Felt) Surfaced with Mineral Granules	R905.2.4
D 226—06	Specification for Asphalt-saturated (Organic Felt) Used in Roofing and Waterproofing	R703.2, R905.2.3, R905.3.3, R905.4.3, R905.5.3, R905.6.3, R905.7.3, R905.8.3, R905.8.4, Table 905.9.2
D 227—03	Specification for Coal Tar Saturated (Organic Felt) Used in Roofing and Waterproofing	Table R905.9.2
D 312—00(2006)	Specification for Asphalt Used in Roofing	Table R905.9.2
D 422—63(2002)e01	Test Method for Particle-size Analysis of Soils	R403.1.8.1
D 449—03	Specification for Asphalt Used in Dampproofing and Waterproofing	R406.2
D 450—07	Specification for Coal-tar Pitch Used in Roofing, Dampproofing and Waterproofing	Table R905.9.2
D 1227—95(2007)	Specification for Emulsified Asphalt Used as a Protective Coating for Roofing	Table R905.9.2, Table R905.11.2, R905.15.2
D 1248—05	Specification for Polyethylene Plastics Extrusion Materials for Wire and Cable	M1601.1.2
D 1527—99(2005)	Specification for Acrylonite-butadiene-styrene (ABS) Plastic Pipe, Schedules 40 and 80	Table P2905.4
D 1622—03	Standard Test Method for Apparent Density of Rigid Cellular Plastics	Table R613.3.1
D 1623—78(1995)	Standard Test Method for Tensile and Tensile Adhesion Properties of Rigid Cellular Plastics	Table R613.3.1
D 1693—07	Test Method for Environmental Stress-cracking of Ethylene Plastics	Table M2101.1
D 1784—06a	Standard Specification for Rigid Poly (Vinyl Chloride) (PVC) Compounds and Chlorinated Poly (Vinyl Chloride) (CPVC) Compounds	M1601.1.2
D 1785—06	Specification for Poly (Vinyl Chloride) (PVC) Plastic Pipe, Schedules 40, 80 and 120	Table P2905.4
D 1863—05	Specification for Mineral Aggregate Used in Built-up Roofs	Table R905.9.2
D 1869—95(2005)	Specification for Rubber Rings for Asbestos-cement Pipe	P2904.17, P3003.4, P3003.18
D 1970—01	Specification for Self-adhering Polymer Modified Bitumen Sheet Materials Used as Steep Roofing Underlayment for Ice Dam Protection	R905.2.3, R905.2.8, R905.4.3
D 2104—03	Specification for Polyethylene (PE) Plastic Pipe, Schedule 40	Table P2905.4
D 2126—04	Standard Test Method for Response of Rigid Cellular Plastics to Thermal and Humid Aging	Table R613.3.1
D 2178—04	Specification for Asphalt Glass Felt Used in Roofing and Waterproofing	Table R905.9.2
D 2235—04	Specification for Solvent Cement for Acrylonitrile-butadiene-styrene (ABS) Plastic Pipe and Fittings	P2905.9.1.1, P3003.3.2, P3003.8.2
D 2239—03	Specification for Polyethylene (PE) Plastic Pipe (SIDR-PR) Based on Controlled Inside Diameter	Table P2905.4
D 2241—05	Specification for Poly (Vinyl Chloride) (PVC) Pressure-rated Pipe (SDR-Series)	Table P2905.4
D 2282—05	Specification for Acrylonitrile-butadiene-styrene (ABS) Plastic Pipe (SDR-PR)	Table P2905.4
D 2412—02	Test Method for Determination of External Loading Characteristics of Plastic Pipe by Parallel-plate Loading	M1601.1.2
D 2447—03	Specification for Polyethylene (PE) Plastic Pipe Schedules 40 and 80, Based on Outside Diameter	Table M2101.1
D 2464—06	Specification for Threaded Poly (Vinyl Chloride) (PVC) Plastic Pipe Fittings, Schedule 80	Table P2905.6
D 2466—06	Specification for Poly (Vinyl Chloride) (PVC) Plastic Pipe Fittings, Schedule 40	Table P2905.6
D 2467—06	Specification for Poly (Vinyl Chloride) (PVC) Plastic Pipe Fittings, Schedule 80	Table P2905.6
D 2468—96a	Specification for Acrylonitrile-butadiene-styrene (ABS) Plastic Pipe Fittings, Schedule 40	Table P2905.6
D 2513—07a	Specification for Thermoplastic Gas Pressure Pipe, Tubing and Fittings	G2414.6, G2414.6.1, G2414.11, G2415.15.2, Table M2101.1, M2104.2.1.3
D 2559—04	Standard Specification for Adhesives for Structural Laminated Wood Products for Use Under Exterior (West Use) Exposure Conditions	R613.3.3
D 2564—04e01	Specification for Solvent Cements for Poly (Vinyl Chloride) (PVC) Plastic Piping Systems	P2905.9.1.3, Table P3002.2, P3003.9.2, P3003.14.2
D 2609—02	Specification for Plastic Insert Fittings for Polyethylene (PE) Plastic Pipe	Table P2905.6
D 2626—04	Specification for Asphalt-saturated and Coated Organic Felt Base Sheet Used in Roofing	R905.3.3, Table R905.9.2
D 2657—07	Standard Practice for Heat Fusion-joining of Polyolefin Pipe Fittings	P2905.3.1, P3003.17.1
D 2661—06	Specification for Acrylonitrile-butadiene-styrene (ABS) Schedule 40 Plastic Drain, Waste, and Vent Pipe and Fittings	Table P3002.1(1), Table P3002.1(2), Table P3002.2, Table P3002.3, P3003.3.2, P3003.8.2
D 2665—07	Specification for Poly (Vinyl Chloride) (PVC) Plastic Drain, Waste and Vent Pipe and Fittings	Table P3002.1(1), Table P3002.1(2), Table P3002.2, Table P3002.3
D 2672—96a(2003)	Specification for Joints for IPS PVC Pipe Using Solvent Cement	Table P2905.4
D 2683—04	Specification for Socket-type Polyethylene Fittings for Outside Diameter-controlled Polyethylene Pipe and Tubing	Table M2101.1, M2104.2.1.1
D 2729—04e01	Specification for Poly (Vinyl Chloride) (PVC) Sewer Pipe and Fittings	P3302.1, Table P3302.1, Table AO103.10
D 2737—03	Specification for Polyethylene (PE) Plastic Tubing	Table P2905.4

ASTM—continued

D 2751—05	Specification for Acrylonitrile-butadiene-styrene (ABS) Sewer Pipe and Fittings	Table P3002.2, Table P3002.3
D 2822—05	Specification for Asphalt Roof Cement	Table R905.9.2
D 2823—05	Specification for Asphalt Roof Coatings	Table R905.9.2
D 2824—06	Specification for Aluminum-pigmented Asphalt Roof Coatings, Nonfibered, Asbestos Fibered and Fibered without Asbestos	Table R905.9.2, Table R905.11.2
D 2837—04e01	Test Method for Obtaining Hydrostatic Design Basis for Thermoplastic Pipe Materials or Pressure Design Basis for Thermoplastic Pipe Products	Table M2101.1
D 2846/D 2846M—06	Specification for Chlorinated Poly (Vinyl Chloride) (CPVC) Plastic Hot- and Cold-water Distribution Systems	Table M2101.1, P2904.9.1.2, Table P2905.4, Table P2905.5, Table P2905.6
D 2855-96 (2002)	Standard Practice for Making Solvent-cemented Joints with Poly (Vinyl Chloride) (PVC) Pipe and Fittings	P3003.9.2, P3003.14.2
D 2898—04	Test Methods for Accelerated Weathering of Fire-retardant-treated Wood for Fire Testing	R802.1.3.4, R802.1.3.6
D 2949—01ae01	Specification for 3.25-in. Outside Diameter Poly (Vinyl Chloride) (PVC) Plastic Drain, Waste and Vent Pipe and Fittings	Table P3002.1(1), Table P3002.1(2), Table P3002.2, Table P3002.3
D 3019—94 (2007)	Specification for Lap Cement Used with Asphalt Roll Roofing, Nonfibered, Asbestos Fibered and Nonasbestos Fibered	Table R905.9.2, Table R905.11.2
D 3034—06	Specification for Type PSM Poly (Vinyl Chloride) (PVC) Sewer Pipe and Fittings	Table P3002.2, Table P3002.3
D 3035—06	Specification for Polyethylene (PE) Plastic Pipe (DR-PR) Based On Controlled Outside Diameter	Table M2101.1
D 3161—06	Test Method for Wind Resistance of Asphalt Shingles (Fan Induced Method)	R905.2.4.1, Table R905.2.4.1(2)
D 3201—07	Test Method for Hygroscopic Properties of Fire-retardant Wood and Wood-base Products	R802.1.3.7
D 3212—96a (2003)e01	Specification for Joints for Drain and Sewer Plastic Pipes Using Flexible Elastomeric Seals	P3003.3.1 P3003.8.1, P3003.9.1, P3003.14.1, P3003.17.2
D 3309—96a (2002)	Specification for Polybutylene (PB) Plastic Hot- and Code-water Distribution System	Table M2101.1
D 3311—06a	Specification for Drain, Waste and Vent (DWV) Plastic Fittings Patters	P3002.3
D 3350—06	Specification for Polyethylene Plastic Pipe and Fitting Materials	Table M2101.1
D 3462—07	Specification for Asphalt Shingles Made From Glass Felt and Surfaced with Mineral Granules	R905.2.4
D 3468—99 (2006)e01	Specification for Liquid-applied Neoprene and Chlorosulfanated Polyethylene Used in Roofing and Waterproofing	R905.15.2
D 3679—06a	Specification for Rigid Poly (Vinyl Chloride) (PVC) Siding	Table R703.4, R703.11
D 3737—07	Practice for Establishing Allowable Properties for Structural Glued Laminated Timber (Glulam)	R502.1.5, R602.1.2, R802.1.4
D 3747—79 (2007)	Specification for Emulsified Asphalt Adhesive for Adhering Roof Insulation	Table R905.9.2, Table R905.11.2
D 3909—97b (2004)e01	Specification for Asphalt Roll Roofing (Glass Felt) Surfaced with Mineral Granules	R905.2.8.2, R905.5.4, Table R905.9.2
D 3957—06	Standard Practices for Establishing Stress Grades for Structural Members Used in Log Buildings	R502.1.6, R602.1.3, R802.1.5
D 4022—07	Specification for Coal Tar Roof Cement, Asbestos Containing	Table R905.9.2
D 4068—01	Specification for Chlorinated Polyethylene (CPE) Sheeting for Concealed Water Containment Membrane	P2709.2, P2709.2.2
D 4318—05	Test Methods for Liquid Limit, Plastic Limit and Plasticity Index of Soils	R403.1.8.1
D 4434—06	Specification for Poly (Vinyl Chloride) Sheet Roofing	R905.13.2
D 4479—07	Specification for Asphalt Roof Coatings-asbestos-free	Table R905.9.2
D 4551—96 (2001)	Specification for Poly (Vinyl) Chloride (PVC) Plastic Flexible Concealed Water-containment Membrane	P2709.2, P2709.2.1
D 4586—00	Specification for Asphalt Roof Cement-asbestos-free	Table R905.9.2
D 4601—04	Specification for Asphalt-coated Glass Fiber Base Sheet Used in Roofing	Table R905.9.2
D 4637—04	Specification for EPDM Sheet Used in Single-ply Roof Membrane	R905.12.2
D 4829—07	Test Method for Expansion Index of Soils	R403.1.8.1
D 4869—05e01	Specification for Asphalt-saturated (Organic Felt) Underlayment Used in Steep Slope Roofing	R905.2.3, R905.4.3, R905.5.3, R905.6.3, R905.7.3, R905.8.3
D 4897—01	Specification for Asphalt Coated Glass-fiber Venting Base Sheet Used in Roofing	Table R905.9.2
D 4990—97a (2005)e01	Specification for Coal Tar Glass Felt Used in Roofing and Waterproofing	Table R905.9.2
D 5019—07	Specification for Reinforced Nonvulcanized Polymeric Sheet Used in Roofing Membrane	R905.12.2
D 5055—05	Specification for Establishing and Monitoring Structural Capacities of Prefabricated Wood I-joists	R502.1.4
D 5516—03	Test Method for Evaluating the Flexural Properties of Fire-retardant-treated Softwood Plywood Exposed to the Elevated Temperatures	R802.1.3.5.1
D 5643—06	Specification for Coal Tar Roof Cement Asbestos-free	Table R905.9.2

ASTM—continued

ASTM—continued

E 2570—07	Standard Test Methods for Evaluating Water-resistive Barrier (WRB) Coatings Used Under Exterior Insulation and Finish Systems (EIFS) or EIFS with Drainage	R703.9.2.1
F 405—05	Specification for Corrugated Polyethylene (PE) Tubing and Fittings	Table P3302.1, Table AO103.10
F 409—02	Specification for Thermoplastic Accessible and Replaceable Plastic Tube and Tubular Fittings	Table P2701.1, P2702.2, P2702.3
F 437—06	Specification for Threaded Chlorinated Poly (Vinyl Chloride) (CPVC) Plastic Pipe Fittings, Schedule 80	Table P2905.6
F 438—04	Specification for Socket-type Chlorinated Poly (Vinyl Chloride) (CPVC) Plastic Pipe Fittings, Schedule 40	Table P2905.6
F 439—06	Specification for Socket-type Chlorinated Poly (Vinyl Chloride) (CPVC) Plastic Pipe Fittings, Schedule 80	Table P2905.6
F 441/F 441M—02	Specification for Chlorinated Poly (Vinyl Chloride) (CPVC) Plastic Pipe, Schedules 40 and 80	Table P2905.4, Table P2905.5
F 442/F 442M—99(2005)	Specification for Chlorinated Poly (Vinyl Chloride) (CPVC) Plastic Pipe (SDR-PR)	Table P2905.4, Table P2905.5
F 477—07	Specification for Elastomeric Seals (Gaskets) for Joining Plastic Pipe	P2905.17, P3003.18
F 493—04	Specification for Solvent Cements for Chlorinated Poly (Vinyl Chloride) (CPVC) Plastic Pipe and Fittings	P2905.9.1.2
F 628—06e01	Specification for Acrylonitrile-butadiene-styrene (ABS) Schedule 40 Plastic Drain, Waste and Vent Pipe with a Cellular Core	Table 3002.1(1), Table P3002.1(2), Table P3002.2, Table P3002.3, P3003.3.2, P3003.8.2
F 656—02	Specification for Primers for Use in Solvent Cement Joints of Poly (Vinyl Chloride) (PVC) Plastic Pipe and Fittings	P2905.9.1.3, P3003.9.2, P3003.14.2
F 714—06a	Specification for Polyethylene (PE) Plastic Pipe (SDR-PR) Based on Outside Diameter	Table P3002.2
F 876—06	Specification for Cross-linked Polyethylene (PEX) Tubing	Table M2101.1, Table P2905.4, Table P2906.5
F 877—07	Specification for Cross-linked Polyethylene (PEX) Plastic Hot- and Cold-water Distribution Systems	Table M2101.1, Table P2905.4, Table P2905.5, Table 2905.6
F 891—04	Specification for Coextruded Poly (Vinyl Chloride) (PVC) Plastic Pipe with a Cellular Core	P2905.6, Table P3002.1(1), Table P3002.1(2), Table P3002.2, Table P3302.1
F 1055—98(2006)	Specification for Electrofusion Type Polyethylene Fittings for Outside Diameter Controlled Polyethylene Pipe and Fittings	Table M2101.1, M2104.2.1.2
F 1281—07	Specification for Cross-linked Polyethylene/Aluminum/Cross-linked Polyethylene (PEX-AL-PEX) Pressure Pipe	Table M2101.1, Table P2905.4, Table P2905.5, Table P2905.6, P2505.11.1
F 1282—06	Specification for Polyethylene/Aluminum/Polyethylene (PE-AL-PE) Composite Pressure Pipe	Table M2101.1, Table P2905.4, Table P2905.5, Table P2905.6, P2905.11.1
F 1346—91(2003)	Performance Specification for Safety Covers and Labeling Requirements for All Covers for Swimming Pools, Spas and Hot Tubs	AG105.2, AG105.5
F 1412—01e01	Specification for Polyolefin Pipe and Fittings for Corrosive Waste Drainage	Table P3002.1(2), Table P3002.2, Table P3002.3, P3003.16.1
F 1488—03	Specification for Coextruded Composite Pipe	Table P3002.1(1), Table P3002.1(2) Table P3002.2, Table AO103.10
F 1554—04e1	Specification for Anchor Bolts, Steel, 36, 55 and 105-ksi Yield Strength	R611.5.2.2
F 1667—05	Specification for Driven Fasteners, Nails, Spikes and Staples	Table R703.4, R905.2.5
F 1807—07	Specification for Metal Insert Fittings Utilizing a Copper Crimp Ring for SDR9 Cross-linked Polyethylene (PEX) Tubing	Table M2101.1, Table P2905.6
F 1866—07	Specification for Poly (Vinyl Chloride) (PVC) Plastic Schedule 40 Drainage and DWV Fabricated Fittings	Table P3002.3
F 1960—07	Specification for Cold Expansion Fittings with PEX Reinforcing Rings for Use with Cross-linked Polyethylene (PEX) Tubing	Table M2101.1, Table P2905.6
F 1973—05	Standard Specification for Factory Assembled Anodeless Risers and Transition Fittings in Polyethylene (PE) and Polyamide 11 (PA 11) Fuel Gas Distribution Systems	G2415.15.2
F 1974—04	Specification for Metal Insert Fittings for Polyethylene/Aluminum/Polyethylene and Cross-linked Polyethylene/Aluminum/Cross-linked Polyethylene Composite Pressure Pipe	P2505.11.1, Table P2905.6
F 1986—01(2006)	Multilayer Pipe Type 2, Compression Joints for Hot and Cold Drinking Water Systems	Table P2905.4, Table P2905.5, Table P2905.6
F 2080—05	Specification for Cold-expansion Fittings with Metal Compression-sleeves for Cross-linked Polyethylene (PEX) Pipe	P2905.6
F 2090—01A(2007)	Specification for Window Fall Prevention Devices—with Emergency Escape (Egress) Release Mechanisms	R612.2, R612.3
F 2098—04e1	Standard Specification for Stainless Steel Clamps for SDR9 PEX Tubing to Metal Insert Fittings	Table M2101.1, Table P2905.6

ASTM—continued

F 2159—05	Standard Specification for Plastic Insert Fittings Utilizing a Copper Crimp Ring for SDR9 Cross-linked Polyethylene (PEX) Tubing	P2905.6
F 2262—05	Standard Specification for Cross-linked Polyethylene /Aluminum/Cross-linked Polyethylene Tubing OD Controlled SDR9	Table P2905.4, Table P2905.5
F 2389—06	Standard for Pressure-rated Polypropylene (PP) Piping Systems	Table M2101.1, Table P2905.4, Table P2905.5, Table P2905.6, P2905.10.1
F 2434—05	Standard Specification for Metal Insert Fittings Utilizing a Copper Crimp Ring for Polyethylene/Aluminum/Cross-linked Polyethylene (PEX-AL-PEX) Tubing	Table P2905.6
F 2623—07	Standard Specification for Polyethylene of Raised Temperature (PE-RT) SDRG Tubing	Table M2101.1

AWPA

American Wood Protection Association
P.O. Box 361784
Birmingham, AL 35236-1784

Standard reference number	Title	Referenced in code section number
C1—03	All Timber Products—Preservative Treatment by Pressure Processes	R902.2
M4—06	Standard for the Care of Preservative-treated Wood Products	R317.1.1, R318.1.2
U1—07	USE CATEGORY SYSTEM: User Specification for Treated Wood Except Section 6 Commodity Specification H	R317.1, R322.1.8, R402.1.2, R504.3, Table R905.8.5

AWS

American Welding Society
550 N. W. LeJeune Road
Miami, FL 33126

Standard reference number	Title	Referenced in code section number
A5.8—04	Specifications for Filler Metals for Brazing and Braze Welding	P3003.5.1, P3003.10.1, P3003.11.1

AWWA

American Water Works Association
6666 West Quincy Avenue
Denver, CO 80235

Standard reference number	Title	Referenced in code section number
C104—98	Standard for Cement-mortar Lining for Ductile-iron Pipe and Fittings for Water	P2905.4
C110/A21.10—03	Standard for Ductile-iron and Gray-iron Fittings, 3 Inches through 48 Inches, for Water	Table P2905.6, Table P3002.3
C115/A21.15—99	Standard for Flanged Ductile-iron Pipe with Ductile-iron or Gray-iron Threaded Flanges	Table P2905.4
C151/A21.51—02	Standard for Ductile-iron Pipe, Centrifugally Cast, for Water	Table P2905.4
C153/A21.53—00	Standard for Ductile-iron Compact Fittings for Water Service	Table P2905.6.1
C510—00	Double Check Valve Backflow Prevention Assembly	Table P2902.3, Table P2902.3.6
C511—00	Reduced-pressure Principle Backflow Prevention Assembly	Table P2902.3, P2902.3.5, P2902.5.1

CGSB

Canadian General Standards Board
Place du Portage 111, 6B1
11 Laurier Street
Gatineau, Quebec, Canada KIA 1G6

Standard reference number	Title	Referenced in code section number
37-GP—52M—(1984)	Roofing and Waterproofing Membrane, Sheet Applied, Elastomeric	R905.12.2
37-GP—56M—(1980)	Membrane, Modified Bituminous, Prefabricated and Reinforced for Roofing —with December 1985 Amendment	Table R905.11.2
CAN/CGSB-37.54—95	Polyvinyl Chloride Roofing and Waterproofing Membrane	R905.13.2

CISPI

Cast Iron Soil Pipe Institute
5959 Shallowford Road, Suite 419
Chattanooga, TN 37421

Standard reference number	Title	Referenced in code section number
301—04a	Standard Specification for Hubless Cast Iron Soil Pipe and Fittings for Sanitary and Storm Drain, Waste and Vent Piping Applications. . . . . Table P3002.1(1), Table P3002.1(2), Table P3002.2, Table P3002.3, P3005.2.9, Table P3302.1	
310—04	Standard Specification for Coupling for Use in Connection with Hubless Cast Iron Soil Pipe and Fittings for Sanitary and Storm Drain, Waste and Vent Piping Applications. P3003.6.3	

CPA

Composite Panel Association
19465 Deerfield Avenue, Suite 306
Leesburg, VA 20176

Standard reference number	Title	Referenced in code section number
ANSI A135.4—04	Basic Hardboard. . . . . Table R602.3(2)	
ANSI A135.5—04	Prefinished Hardboard Paneling. R702.5	
ANSI A135.6—98	Hardboard Siding . . . . Table R703.4	

CPSC

Consumer Product Safety Commission
4330 East West Highway
Bethesda, MD 20814-4408

Standard reference number	Title	Referenced in code section number
16 CFR Part 1201—(1977)	Safety Standard for Architectural Glazing R308.1.1, R308.3.1	
16 CFR Part 1209—(1979)	Interim Safety Standard for Cellulose Insulation R302.10.3	
16 CFR Part 1404—(1979)	Cellulose Insulation. R302.10.3	

CSA

Canadian Standards Association
5060 Spectrum Way
Mississauga, Ontario, Canada L4N 5N6

Standard reference number	Title	Referenced in code section number
CSA Requirement 3—88	Manually Operated Gas Valves for Use in House Piping Systems. . . . . Table G2420.1.1	
CSA 8-93	Requirements for Gas Fired Log Lighters for Wood Burning Fireplaces —with Revisions through January 1999 . . . . G2433.1	
O325—07	Construction Sheathing R503.2.1	
O437-Series—93	Standards on OSB and Waferboard (Reaffirmed 2006) R503.2.1, R803.2.1	
CAN/CSA A 257.1M—92	Circular Concrete Culvert, Storm Drain, Sewer Pipe and Fittings. Table P3002.2	
CAN/CSA A 257.2M—92	Reinforced Circular Concrete Culvert, Storm Drain, Sewer Pipe and Fittings . . . . Table P3002.2	
CAN/CSA A 257.3M—92	Joints for Circular Concrete Sewer and Culvert Pipe, Manhole Sections and Fittings Using Rubber Gaskets P3003.7, P3003.18	
101/I.S.2/A440—08	Specifications for Windows, Doors and Unit Skylights N1102.4.4, R308.6.9, R612.6	
B45.1—02	Ceramic Plumbing Fixtures . . . . Table P2701.1, P2711.1, P2712.1	
B45.2—02	Enameled Cast Iron Plumbing Fixtures. . . . . Table 2701.1, P2711.1	
B45.3—02	Porcelain Enameled Steel Plumbing Fixtures . . . . Table P2701.1, P2711.1	
B45.4—02	Stainless Steel Plumbing Fixtures . . . . Table P2701.1, P2711.1, P2712.1	
B45.5—02	Plastic Plumbing Fixtures. . . . . Table P2701.1, P2711.2, P2712.1	
B45.9—02	Macerating Systems and Related Components. P3007.1, P3007.2.1, P3007.5	
B64.1.2—01	Vacuum Breakers, Pressure Type (PVB) . . . . Table P2902.2, P2902.3.4	
B64.2.1—01	Vacuum Breakers, Hose Connection Type (HCVB) with Manual Draining Feature. . . . . Table P2902.2, P2902.3.2	
B64.2.1.1—01	Vacuum Breakers, Hose Connection Dual Check Type (HCDVB) . . . . Table P2902.2, P2902.3.2	
B64.3—01	Backflow Preventers, Dual Check ValDrain, Wasteve Type with Atmospheric Port (DCAP). . . . . Table P2902.2	

CSA—continued

B64.4.1—01	Backflow Preventers, Reduced Pressure Principle Type for Fire Systems (RPF)	Table P2902.2
B64.5—01	Backflow Preventers, Double Check Valve Type (DCVA)	Table P2902.2, P2902.3.6
B64.5.1—01	Backflow Preventers, Double Check Valve Type for Fire Systems (DCVAF)	Table P2902.2, P2902.3.6
B64.6—01	Backflow Preventers, Dual Check Valve Type (DuC)	Table P2902.3
B64.7—94	Vacuum Breakers, Laboratory Faucet Type (LFVB)	Table P2902.2, P2902.3.2
B125.1—2005/ ASME A112.18.1—2005	Plumbing Supply Fittings	Table P2701.1, P2708.4, P2722.1
B125.1—01	Plumbing Fittings	Table P2701.1, P2708.3, P2722.2, P2722.3
B125.2—2005	Plumbing Waste Fittings	Table P2701.1, P2702.2
B125.3—2005	Plumbing Fittings	Table 2701.1
B137.1—02	Polyethylene Pipe, Tubing and Fittings for Cold Water Pressure Services	Table P2905.4, Table P2905.6
B137.2—02	PVC Injection-moulded Gasketed Fittings for Pressure Applications	Table P2905.6
B137.3—02	Rigid Poly (Vinyl Chloride) (PVC) Pipe for Pressure Applications	Table P2905.4, P3003.9.2, P3003.14.2
B137.5—02	Cross-linked Polyethylene (PEX) Tubing Systems for Pressure Applications	Table P2905.4, Table P2905.5, Table P2905.6
B137.6—02	CPVC Pipe, Tubing and Fittings For Hot- and Cold-water Distribution Systems	Table P2905.4, Table P2905.5, Table 2905.6
B137.11—02	Polypropylene (PP-R) Pipe and Fittings for Pressure Applications	Table P2905.4.1, Table 2905.4, Table P2905.6
B181.1—02	ABS Drain, Waste and Vent Pipe and Pipe Fittings	Table P3002.1(1), Table P3002.1(2), Table P3002.2, Table P3002.3, P3003.3.2, P3003.8.2
B181.2—02	PVC Drain, Waste and Vent Pipe and Pipe Fittings	Table P3002.1(1), Table P3002.1(2), Table P3002.2, Table P3002.3, P3003.9.2, P3003.14.2, P3008.2, Table P3302.1
B181.3—02	Polyolefin Laboratory Drainage Systems	Table P3002.1(1), Table P3002.1(2), Table P3002.2, Table P3002.3, P3003.16.1
B182.2—02	PVC Sewer Pipe and Fittings (PSM Type)	Table P3002.1(1), Table P3002.1(2), Table P3002.2, Table P3002.3, Table P3302.1
B182.4—02	Profile PVC Sewer Pipe & Fittings	Table P3002.2, Table P3002.3, Table P3302.1
B182.6—02	Profile Polyethylene Sewer Pipe and Fittings for Leak-proof Sewer Applications	Table P3302.1
B182.8—02	Profile Polyethylene Storm Sewer and Drainage Pipe and Fittings	Table P3302.1
B602—02	Mechanical Couplings for Drain, Waste and Vent Pipe and Sewer Pipe	P3003.3.1, P3003.6.3, P3003.7, P3003.8.1, P3003.14.1, P3003.15, P3003.17.2
LC3—00	Appliance Stands and Drain Pans	P2801.5
CAN/CSA B64.1.1—01	Vacuum Breakers, Atmospheric Type (AVB)	Table P2902.2, P2902.3.2
CAN/CSA B64.2—01	Vacuum Breakers, Hose Connection Type (HCVP)	Table P2902.2, P2902.3.2
CAN/CSA B64.2.2—01	Vacuum Breakers, Hose Connection Type (HCVP) with Automatic Draining Feature	Table P2902.2, P2902.3.2
CAN/CSA B64.3—01	Backflow Preventers, Dual Check Valve Type with Atmospheric Port (DCAP)	Table P2902.2, P2902.3.3
CAN/CSA B64.4—01	Backflow Preventers, Reduced Pressure Principle Type (RP)	Table P2902.3, P2902.3.5, P2902.5.1,
CAN/CSA B137.9—02	Polyethylene/Aluminum/Polyethylene Composite Pressure Pipe Systems	P2505.11.1, Table P2905.4
CAN/CSA B137.10M—02	Cross-linked Polyethylene/Aluminum/Polyethylene Composite Pressure Pipe Systems	Table M2101.1, P2505.11.1, Table P2905.4, Table P2905.5

CSSB

Cedar Shake & Shingle Bureau
P. O. Box 1178
Sumas, WA 98295-1178

Standard reference number	Title	Referenced in code section number
CSSB—97	Grading and Packing Rules for Western Red Cedar Shakes and Western Red Shingles of the Cedar Shake and Shingle Bureau	R702.6, R703.5, Table R905.7.4, Table R905.8.5

DASMA

Door and Access Systems Manufacturers
Association International
1300 Summer Avenue
Cleveland, OH 44115-2851

Standard reference number	Title	Referenced in code section number
108—05	Standard Method for Testing Garage Doors: Determination of Structural Performance Under Uniform Static Air Pressure Difference	R612.7

DASMA—continued

115—05   Standard Method for Testing Garage Doors: Determination of Structural Performance Under
Missile Impact and Cyclic Wind Pressure R301.2.1.2

DOC

United States Department of Commerce
1401 Constitution Avenue, NW
Washington, DC 20230

Standard reference number	Title	Referenced in code section number
PS 1—07	Structural Plywood . . . . R404.2.1, Table R404.2.3, R503.2.1, R604.1, R613.3.2, R803.2.1	
PS 2—04	Performance Standard for Wood-based Structural-use Panels . . . . R404.2.1, Table R404.2.3, R503.2.1, R604.1, R613.3.2, Table 613.3.2, R803.2.1	
PS 20—05	American Softwood Lumber Standard. R404.2.1, R502.1, R602.1, R802.1	

DOTn

Department of Transportation
1200 New Jersey Avenue SE
East Building, 2nd floor
Washington, DC 20590

Standard reference number	Title	Referenced in code section number
49 CFR, Parts 192.281(e) & 192.283 (b)	Transportation of Natural and Other Gas by Pipeline: Minimum Federal Safety Standards G2414.6.1	

FEMA

Federal Emergency Management Agency
500 C Street, SW
Washington, DC 20472

Standard reference number	Title	Referenced in code section number
TB-2—93	Flood-resistant Materials Requirements R322.1.8	
FIA-TB-11—01	Crawlspace Construction for Buildings Located in Special Flood Hazard Area. R408.7	

FM

Factory Mutual Global Research
Standards Laboratories Department
1301 Atwood Avenue, P. O. Box 7500
Johnson, RI 02919

Standard reference number	Title	Referenced in code section number
4450—(1989)	Approval Standard for Class 1 Insulated Steel Deck Roofs—with Supplements through July 1992. . . . . R906.1	
4880—(2005)	American National Standard for Evaluating Insulated Wall or Wall and Roof/Ceiling Assemblies, Plastic Interior Finish Materials, Plastic Exterior Building Panels, Wall/Ceiling Coating Systems, Interior or Exterior Finish Systems. R316.4, R316.6	

GA

Gypsum Association
810 First Street, Northeast, Suite 510
Washington, DC 20002-4268

Standard reference number	Title	Referenced in code section number
GA-253—07	Application of Gypsum Sheathing. . . . . .Table R602.3(1)	

HPVA

Hardwood Plywood & Veneer Association
1825 Michael Faraday Drive
Reston, Virginia 20190-5350

Standard reference number	Title	Referenced in code section number
HP-1—2004	The American National Standard for Hardwood and Decorative Plywood	R702.5

ICC

International Code Council, Inc.
500 New Jersey Avenue, NW
6th Floor
Washington, DC 20001

Standard reference number	Title	Referenced in code section number
IBC—09	International Building Code®	G2402.3, R101.2, R110.2, R301.1, R301.1.3, R301.2.2.1.1, R301.2.2.1.2, R301.2.2.4, R301.3, R308.5, R320.1, R321.3, R322.1, R403.1.8, R802.1.3.4, R905.10.3, Table AH107.4(1), AH107.4.3
ICC/ANSI A117.1—03	Accessible and Usable Buildings and Facilities	R321.3
ICC 400—06	Standard on the Design and Construction of Log Structures	R301.1.1
ICC 500—08	ICC/NSSA Standard on the Design and Construction of Storm Shelters	R323.1
ICC 600—08	Standard for Residential Construction in High Wind Regions	R301.2.1.1
IECC—09	International Energy Conservation Code®	N1101.2
IFC—09	International Fire Code®	G2402.3, G2412.2, G2423.1, M2201.7, R102.7
IFGC—09	International Fuel Gas Code®	G2401.1, G2423.1
IMC—09	International Mechanical Code®	G2402.3
IPC—09	International Plumbing Code®	G2402.3, Table R301.2(1), R903.4.1, AO102.6
IPMC—09	International Property Maintenance Code®	R102.7
IPSDC—09	International Private Sewage Disposal Code®	R322.1.7, AI101.1

ISO

International Organization for Standardization
1, ch. de la Voie - Creuse
Case postale 56
CH-1211 Geneva 20, Switzerland

Standard reference number	Title	Referenced in code section number
15874—2002	Polypropylene Plastic Piping Systems for Hot and Cold Water Installations	Table M2101.1

MSS

Manufacturers Standardization Society of the Valve and Fittings Industry
127 Park Street, Northeast
Vienna, VA 22180

Standard reference number	Title	Referenced in code section number
SP-58—93	Pipe Hangers and Supports—Materials, Design and Manufacture	G2418.2

NAIMA

North American Insulation Manufacturers Association
44 Canal Center Plaza, Suite 310
Alexandria, VA 22314

Standard reference number	Title	Referenced in code section number
AH 116—02	Fibrous Glass Duct Construction Standards, Fifth Edition	M1601.1.1

NCMA

National Concrete Masonry Association
13750 Sunrise Valley Drive
Herndon, VA 20171-4662

Standard reference number	Title	Referenced in code section number
TR 68-A—75	Design and Construction of Plain and Reinforced Concrete Masonry and Basement and Foundation Walls.	R404.1.1

NFPA

National Fire Protection Association
1 Batterymarch Park
Quincy, MA 02269

Standard reference number	Title	Referenced in code section number
13—07	Installation of Sprinkler Systems	R302.3
13D—07	Standard for the Installation of Sprinkler Systems in One- and Two-family Dwellings and Manufactured Homes.	P2904.1, P2904.2, P2904.6.1, R313.2.1
31—06	Installation of Oil-burning Equipment.	M1801.3.1, M1805.3
58—08	Liquefied Petroleum Gas Code	G2412.2, G2414.6.2
70—08	National Electrical Code	E3401.1, E3401.2, E4301.1, Table E4303.2, E4304.3, E4304.4
72—07	National Fire Alarm Code.	R314.1, R314.2
85—07	Boiler and Construction Systems Hazards Code	G2452.1
211—06	Chimneys, Fireplaces, Vents and Solid Fuel Burning Appliances.	G2427.5.5.1, R1002.5
259—03	Test Method for Potential Heat of Building Materials	R316.5.7, 316.5.8
286—06	Standard Methods of Fire Tests for Evaluating Contribution of Wall and Ceiling Interior Finish to Room Fire Growth.	R302.9.4, R316.4, R316.5.8, R316.6
501—05	Standard on Manufactured Housing.	R202, AE201
853—07	Standard for the Installation of Stationary Fuel Cell Power Systems	M1903.1

NFRC

National Fenestration Rating Council Inc.
8484 Georgia Avenue, Suite 320
Silver Spring, MD 20910

Standard reference number	Title	Referenced section number
100—2004	Procedure for Determining Fenestration Product U-factors	N1101.5
200—2004	Procedure for Determining Fenestration Product Solar Heat Gain Coefficients and Visible Transmittance at Normal Incidence	N1101.5
400—2004	Procedure for Determining Fenestration Product Air Leakage.	N1102.4.4

NSF

NSF International
789 N. Dixboro
Ann Arbor, MI 48105

Standard reference number	Title	Referenced in code section number
14—2007	Plastic Piping System Components and Related Materials.	P2608.3, P2908.3
42—2007e	Drinking Water Treatment Units—Anesthetic Effects	P2908.1, P2908.3
44—2004	Residential Cation Exchange Water Softeners	P2908.1, P2908.3
53—2007	Drinking Water Treatment Units—Health Effects	P2908.1, P2908.3
58—2006	Reverse Osmosis Drinking Water Treatment Systems	P2908.2, P2908.3
61—2007a	Drinking Water System Components—Health Effects	P2608.5, P2722.1, P2903.9.4, P2905.4, P2905.5, P2905.6, P2907.3

PCA

Portland Cement Association
5420 Old Orchard Road
Skokie, IL 60077

Standard reference number	Title	Referenced in code section number
100—07	Prescriptive Design of Exterior Concrete Walls for One- and Two-family Dwellings (Pub. No. EB241) R404.1.2, R404.1.2.2.1, R404.1.2.2.2, R404.1.2.4, R404.1.4.2, R611.1, R611.2, R611.9.2, R611.9.3	

SMACNA

Sheet Metal & Air Conditioning Contractors National Assoc. Inc.
4021 Lafayette Center Road
Chantilly, VA 22021

Standard reference number	Title	Referenced in code section number
SMACNA—03	Fibrous Glass Duct Construction Standards (2003) M1601.1.1	

TMS

The Masonry Society
3970 Broadway, Suite 201-D
Boulder, CO 80304

Standard reference number	Title	Referenced in code section number
302—07	Standard Method for Determining the Sound Transmission Class Rating for Masonry Walls AK102.1.1	
402—05	Building Code Requirements for Masonry Structures...............R404.1.1, R606.1, R606.1.1, R606.11.2.2.2, R606.12.1, R606.12.2.2.1, R606.12.3.1, Table R703.4	
602—05	Specification for Masonry Structures..........................R404.1.1, R606.1, R606.1.1, R606.12.1, R606.12.2.2.1, R606.12.2.2.2, R606.12.3.1, Table R703.4	

TPI

Truss Plate Institute
583 D'Onofrio Drive, Suite 200
Madison, WI 53719

Standard reference number	Title	Referenced in code section number
TPI 1—2002	National Design Standard for Metal-plate-connected Wood Truss Construction R502.11.1, R802.10.2	

UL

Underwriters Laboratories, Inc.
333 Pfingsten Road
Northbrook, IL 60062

Standard reference number	Title	Referenced in code section number
17—94	Vent or Chimney Connector Dampers for Oil-fired Appliances— with Revisions through September 1999 ....M1802.2.2	
58—96	Steel Underground Tanks for Flammable and Combustible Liquids— with Revisions through July 1998..M2201.1	
80—04	Steel Tanks for Oil-burner Fuel M2201.1	
103—01	Factory-built Chimneys for Residential Type and Building Heating Appliances— with Revisions through June 2006..G2430.1, R202, R1005.3	
127—96	Factory-built Fireplaces—with Revisions through November 2006......................................G2445.7, R1001.11, R1004.1, R1004.4, R1005.4	
174—04	Household Electric Storage Tank Water Heaters—with Revisions through November 2005 ....M2005.1	
181—05	Factory-made Air Ducts and Air Connectors—with Revisions through May 2003 ....M1601.2, M1601.4.1	
181A—05	Closure Systems for Use with Rigid Air Ducts and Air Connectors— with Revisions through December 1998 ....M1601.2, M1601.4.1	
181B—05	Closure Systems for Use with Flexible Air Ducts and Air Connectors— with Revisions through August 2003..M1601.2, M1601.4.1	

UL—continued

217—06	Single- and Multiple-station Smoke Alarms—with Revisions through January 2004	R313.1
263—03	Standards for Fire Test of Building Construction and Materials	R302.2, R302.4.1, R316.4
325—02	Standard for Door, Drapery, Gate, Louver and Window Operations and Systems —with Revisions through February 2006	R309.4
343—97	Pumps for Oil-burning Appliances—with Revisions through May 2002	M2204.1
441—96	Gas Vents—with Revisions through August 2006	G2426.1
508—99	Industrial Control Equipment—with Revisions through July 2005	M1411.3.1
536—97	Flexible Metallic Hose—with Revisions through June 2003	M2202.3
641—95	Type L, Low-temperature Venting Systems—with Revisions through August 2005	G2426.1, M1804.2.4, R202, R1003.11.5
651—05	Schedule 40 and Schedule 80 Rigid PVC Conduit and Fittings	G2414.6.3
723—03	Standard for Test for Surface Burning Characteristics of Building Materials— with Revisions through May 2005	M1601.3, R302.9.3, R302.10.1, R302.10.2, R316.3, R316.6
726—95	Oil-fired Boiler Assemblies—with Revisions through March 2006	M2001.1.1, M2006.1
727—06	Oil-fired Central Furnaces	M1402.1
729—03	Oil-fired Floor Furnaces	M1408.1
730—03	Oil-fired Wall Furnaces	M1409.1
732—95	Oil-fired Storage Tank Water Heaters—with Revisions through February 2005	M2005.1
737—96	Fireplaces Stoves—with Revisions through January 2000	M1414.1
790—04	Standard Test Methods for Fire Tests of Roof Coverings	R902.1
795—06	Commercial-industrial Gas Heating Equipment	G2442.1, G2452.1
834—04	Heating, Water Supply and Power Boilers-Electric	M2001.1.1
896—93	Oil-burning Stoves—with Revisions through May 2004	M1410.1
923—02	Microwave Cooking Appliances—with Revisions through February 2006	M1504.1
959—01	Medium Heat Appliance Factory-built Chimneys—with Revisions through September 2006	R1005.6
1040—96	Fire Test of Insulated Wall Construction—with Revisions through June 2001	R316.4, R316.6
1256—02	Fire Test of Roof Deck Construction	R906.1
1261—01	Electric Water Heaters for Pools and Tubs—with Revisions through June 2004	M2006.1
1453—04	Electronic Booster and Commercial Storage Tank Water Heaters	M2005.1
1479—03	Fire Tests of Through-penetration Firestops	R302.4.1.2
1482—98	Solid-fuel-type Room Heaters—with Revisions through January 2000	M1410.1, R1002.2, R1002.5
1715—97	Fire Test of Interior Finish Material—with Revisions through March 2004	R316.4
1738—06	Venting Systems for Gas-burning Appliances, Categories II, III and IV	G2426.1
1777—04	Standard for Chimney Liners	G2425.12, G2425.15.4, M1801.3.4, R1003.11.1, R1003.18
1995—05	Heating and Cooling Equipment	M1402.1, M1403.1, M1407.1
2017—2000	Standard for General-purpose Signaling Devices and Systems—with Revisions through June 2004	AG105.2
2034—2008	Standard for Single- and Multiple-station Carbon Monoxide Alarms	R315.3
2158A—2006	Outline of Investigation for Clothes Dryer Transition Duct	M1502.4.3

ULC

Underwriters' Laboratories of Canada
7 Underwriters Road
Toronto, Ontario, Canada M1R 3B4

Standard reference number	Title	Referenced in code section number
CAN/ULC S 102—1988	Standard Methods for Test for Surface Burning Characteristics of Building Materials and Assemblies—with 2000 Revisions	R302.10.2

US-FTC

United States - Federal Trade Commission
600 Pennsylvania Avenue NW
Washington, DC 20580

Standard reference number	Title	Referenced in code section number
CFR Title 16 Part 460	*R*-value Rule	N1101.6

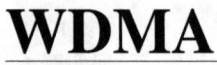

Window & Door Manufacturers Association
1400 East Touhy Avenue, Suite 470
Des Plaines, IL 60018

Standard reference number	Title	Referenced in code section number
AAMA/WDMA/CSA 101/I.S2/A440—08	Specifications for Windows, Doors and Skylights	N1102.4.4, R308.6.9, R613.6

APPENDIX A

SIZING AND CAPACITIES OF GAS PIPING

(This appendix is informative and is not part of the *code*. This appendix is an excerpt from the 2009 *International Fuel Gas Code,* coordinated with the section numbering of the *International Residential Code*.)

A.1 General piping considerations. The first goal of determining the *pipe* sizing for a *fuel gas piping system* is to make sure that there is sufficient gas pressure at the inlet to each *appliance*. The majority of systems are residential and the *appliances* will all have the same, or nearly the same, requirement for minimum gas pressure at the *appliance* inlet. This pressure will be about 5-inch water column (w.c.) (1.25 kPa), which is enough for proper operation of the *appliance regulator* to deliver about 3.5-inches water column (w.c.) (875 kPa) to the *burner* itself. The *pressure drop* in the *piping* is subtracted from the source delivery pressure to verify that the minimum is available at the *appliance*.

There are other systems, however, where the required inlet pressure to the different *appliances* may be quite varied. In such cases, the greatest inlet pressure required must be satisfied, as well as the farthest *appliance*, which is almost always the critical *appliance* in small systems.

There is an additional requirement to be observed besides the capacity of the system at 100-percent flow. That requirement is that at minimum flow, the pressure at the inlet to any *appliance* does not exceed the pressure rating of the *appliance regulator*. This would seldom be of concern in small systems if the source pressure is $^{1}/_{2}$ psi (14-inch w.c.) (3.5 kPa) or less but it should be verified for systems with greater gas pressure at the point of supply.

To determine the size of *piping* used in a *gas piping system*, the following factors must be considered:

(1) Allowable loss in pressure from point of delivery to *equipment*.

(2) Maximum gas *demand*.

(3) Length of *piping* and number of fittings.

(4) *Specific gravity* of the gas.

(5) Diversity factor.

For any *gas piping system*, or special *appliance*, or for conditions other than those covered by the tables provided in this *code*, such as longer runs, greater gas *demands* or greater *pressure drops*, the size of each *gas piping system* should be determined by standard engineering practices acceptable to the *code official*.

A.2 Description of tables

A.2.1 General. The quantity of gas to be provided at each *outlet* should be determined, whenever possible, directly from the manufacturer's gas input *Btu*/h rating of the *appliance* that will be installed. In case the ratings of the appliances to be installed are not known, Table G2413.2 shows the approximate consumption (in *Btu* per hour) of certain types of typical household *appliances*.

To obtain the cubic feet per hour of gas required, divide the total *Btu*/h input of all *appliances* by the average *Btu* heating value per *cubic foot* of the gas. The average *Btu* per *cubic foot* of the gas in the area of the installation can be obtained from the serving gas supplier.

A.2.2 Low pressure natural gas tables. Capacities for gas at low pressure [less than 2.0 psig (13.8 kPa gauge)] in cubic feet per hour of 0.60 *specific gravity* gas for different sizes and lengths are shown in Table G2413.4(1) for iron *pipe* or equivalent rigid *pipe*, in Table G2413.4(3) for smooth wall semi-rigid *tubing*, in Table G2413.4(5) for corrugated stainless steel *tubing* and in Table G2413.4(7) for polyethylene plastic *pipe*. Tables G2413.4(1), G2413.4(3), G2413.4(5) and G2413.4(7) are based upon a *pressure drop* of 0.5-inch w.c. (125 Pa). In using these tables, an allowance (in equivalent length of *pipe*) should be considered for any *piping* run with four or more fittings [see Table A.2.2].

A.2.3 Undiluted liquefied petroleum tables. Capacities in thousands of *Btu* per hour of undiluted liquefied petroleum gases based on a *pressure drop* of 0.5-inch w.c. (125 Pa) for different sizes and lengths are shown in the *International Fuel Gas Code*. See Appendix A of that *code*.

A.2.4 Natural gas specific gravity. *Gas piping systems* that are to be supplied with gas of a *specific gravity* of 0.70 or less can be sized directly from the tables provided in this *code*, unless the *code official* specifies that a gravity factor be applied. Where the *specific gravity* of the gas is greater than 0.70, the gravity factor should be applied.

Application of the gravity factor converts the figures given in the tables provided in this *code* to capacities for another gas of different *specific gravity*. Such application is accomplished by multiplying the capacities given in the tables by the multipliers shown in Table A.2.4. In case the exact *specific gravity* does not appear in the table, choose the next higher value *specific gravity* shown.

TABLE A.2.2
EQUIVALENT LENGTHS OF PIPE FITTINGS AND VALVES

		SCREWED FITTINGS[1]				90° WELDING ELBOWS AND SMOOTH BENDS[2]					
		45°/Ell	90°/Ell	180° close return bends	Tee	R/d = 1	R/d = 1^1/$_3$	R/d = 2	R/d = 4	R/d = 6	R/d = 8
k factor =		0.42	0.90	2.00	1.80	0.48	0.36	0.27	0.21	0.27	0.36
L/d′ ratio[4] n =		14	30	67	60	16	12	9	7	9	12
Nominal pipe size, inches	**Inside diameter d, inches, Schedule 40[6]**	L = Equivalent Length In Feet of Schedule 40 (Standard-Weight) Straight Pipe[6]									
^{1}/$_2$	0.622	0.73	1.55	3.47	3.10	0.83	0.62	0.47	0.36	0.47	0.62
^{3}/$_4$	0.824	0.96	2.06	4.60	4.12	1.10	0.82	0.62	0.48	0.62	0.82
1	1.049	1.22	2.62	5.82	5.24	1.40	1.05	0.79	0.61	0.79	1.05
1^1/$_4$	1.380	1.61	3.45	7.66	6.90	1.84	1.38	1.03	0.81	1.03	1.38
1^1/$_2$	1.610	1.88	4.02	8.95	8.04	2.14	1.61	1.21	0.94	1.21	1.61
2	2.067	2.41	5.17	11.5	10.3	2.76	2.07	1.55	1.21	1.55	2.07
2^1/$_2$	2.469	2.88	6.16	13.7	12.3	3.29	2.47	1.85	1.44	1.85	2.47
3	3.068	3.58	7.67	17.1	15.3	4.09	3.07	2.30	1.79	2.30	3.07
4	4.026	4.70	10.1	22.4	20.2	5.37	4.03	3.02	2.35	3.02	4.03
5	5.047	5.88	12.6	28.0	25.2	6.72	5.05	3.78	2.94	3.78	5.05
6	6.065	7.07	15.2	33.8	30.4	8.09	6.07	4.55	3.54	4.55	6.07
8	7.981	9.31	20.0	44.6	40.0	10.6	7.98	5.98	4.65	5.98	7.98
10	10.02	11.7	25.0	55.7	50.0	13.3	10.0	7.51	5.85	7.51	10.0
12	11.94	13.9	29.8	66.3	59.6	15.9	11.9	8.95	6.96	8.95	11.9
14	13.13	15.3	32.8	73.0	65.6	17.5	13.1	9.85	7.65	9.85	13.1
16	15.00	17.5	37.5	83.5	75.0	20.0	15.0	11.2	8.75	11.2	15.0
18	16.88	19.7	42.1	93.8	84.2	22.5	16.9	12.7	9.85	12.7	16.9
20	18.81	22.0	47.0	105.0	94.0	25.1	18.8	14.1	11.0	14.1	18.8
24	22.63	26.4	56.6	126.0	113.0	30.2	22.6	17.0	13.2	17.0	22.6

(continued)

TABLE A.2.2—continued
EQUIVALENT LENGTHS OF PIPE FITTINGS AND VALVES

		MITER ELBOWS[3] (No. of miters)					WELDING TEES		VALVES (screwed, flanged, or welded)			
		1-45°	1-60°	1-90°	2-90°[5]	3-90°[5]	Forged	Miter[3]	Gate	Globe	Angle	Swing Check
k factor =		0.45	0.90	1.80	0.60	0.45	1.35	1.80	0.21	10	5.0	2.5
L/d' ratio[4] n =		15	30	60	20	15	45	60	7	333	167	83
Nominal pipe size, inches	**Inside diameter d, inches, Schedule 40[6]**	L = Equivalent Length In Feet of Schedule 40 (Standard-Weight) Straight Pipe[6]										
$^1/_2$	0.622	0.78	1.55	3.10	1.04	0.78	2.33	3.10	0.36	17.3	8.65	4.32
$^3/_4$	0.824	1.03	2.06	4.12	1.37	1.03	3.09	4.12	0.48	22.9	11.4	5.72
1	1.049	1.31	2.62	5.24	1.75	1.31	3.93	5.24	0.61	29.1	14.6	7.27
$1^1/_4$	1.380	1.72	3.45	6.90	2.30	1.72	5.17	6.90	0.81	38.3	19.1	9.58
$1^1/_2$	1.610	2.01	4.02	8.04	2.68	2.01	6.04	8.04	0.94	44.7	22.4	11.2
2	2.067	2.58	5.17	10.3	3.45	2.58	7.75	10.3	1.21	57.4	28.7	14.4
$2^1/_2$	2.469	3.08	6.16	12.3	4.11	3.08	9.25	12.3	1.44	68.5	34.3	17.1
3	3.068	3.84	7.67	15.3	5.11	3.84	11.5	15.3	1.79	85.2	42.6	21.3
4	4.026	5.04	10.1	20.2	6.71	5.04	15.1	20.2	2.35	112.0	56.0	28.0
5	5.047	6.30	12.6	25.2	8.40	6.30	18.9	25.2	2.94	140.0	70.0	35.0
6	6.065	7.58	15.2	30.4	10.1	7.58	22.8	30.4	3.54	168.0	84.1	42.1
8	7.981	9.97	20.0	40.0	13.3	9.97	29.9	40.0	4.65	222.0	111.0	55.5
10	10.02	12.5	25.0	50.0	16.7	12.5	37.6	50.0	5.85	278.0	139.0	69.5
12	11.94	14.9	29.8	59.6	19.9	14.9	44.8	59.6	6.96	332.0	166.0	83.0
14	13.13	16.4	32.8	65.6	21.9	16.4	49.2	65.6	7.65	364.0	182.0	91.0
16	15.00	18.8	37.5	75.0	25.0	18.8	56.2	75.0	8.75	417.0	208.0	104.0
18	16.88	21.1	42.1	84.2	28.1	21.1	63.2	84.2	9.85	469.0	234.0	117.0
20	18.81	23.5	47.0	94.0	31.4	23.5	70.6	94.0	11.0	522.0	261.0	131.0
24	22.63	28.3	56.6	113.0	37.8	28.3	85.0	113.0	13.2	629.0	314.0	157.0

For SI: 1 foot = 305 mm, 1 degree = 0.01745 rad.

Note: Values for welded fittings are for conditions where bore is not obstructed by weld spatter or backing rings. If appreciably obstructed, use values for "Screwed Fittings."

1. Flanged fittings have three-fourths the resistance of screwed elbows and tees.

2. Tabular figures give the extra resistance due to curvature alone to which should be added the full length of travel.

3. Small size socket-welding fittings are equivalent to miter elbows and miter tees.

4. Equivalent resistance in number of diameters of straight *pipe* computed for a value of (f - 0.0075) from the relation (n - $k/4f$).

5. For condition of minimum resistance where the centerline length of each miter is between d and $2^1/_2 d$.

6. For *pipe* having other inside diameters, the equivalent resistance may be computed from the above n values.

Source: Crocker, S. *Piping Handbook*, 4th ed., Table XIV, pp. 100-101. Copyright 1945 by McGraw-Hill, Inc. Used by permission of McGraw-Hill Book Company.

TABLE A.2.4
MULTIPLIERS TO BE USED WITH TABLES G2413.4(1)
THROUGH G2413.4(8) WHERE THE SPECIFIC GRAVITY
OF THE GAS IS OTHER THAN 0.60

SPECIFIC GRAVITY	MULTIPLIER	SPECIFIC GRAVITY	MULTIPLIER
0.35	1.31	1.00	0.78
0.40	1.23	1.10	0.74
0.45	1.16	1.20	0.71
0.50	1.10	1.30	0.68
0.55	1.04	1.40	0.66
0.60	1.00	1.50	0.63
0.65	0.96	1.60	0.61
0.70	0.93	1.70	0.59
0.75	0.90	1.80	0.58
0.80	0.87	1.90	0.56
0.85	0.84	2.00	0.55
0.90	0.82	2.10	0.54

A.2.5 Higher pressure natural gas tables. Capacities for gas at pressures of 2.0 psig (13.8 kPa) or greater in cubic feet per hour of 0.60 *specific gravity* gas for different sizes and lengths are shown in Table G2413.4(2) for iron *pipe* or equivalent rigid *pipe*, Table G2413.4(4) for semi-rigid *tubing*, Table G2413.4(6) for corrugated stainless steel *tubing* and Table G2413.4(8) for polyethylene plastic *pipe*.

A.3 Use of capacity tables

A.3.1 Longest length method. This sizing method is conservative in its approach by applying the maximum operating conditions in the system as the norm for the system and by setting the length of *pipe* used to size any given part of the *piping* system to the maximum value.

To determine the size of each section of *gas piping* in a system within the range of the capacity tables, proceed as follows. (also see sample calculations included in this Appendix).

(1) Divide the *piping system* into appropriate segments consistent with the presence of tees, branch lines and main runs. For each segment, determine the gas load (assuming all *appliances* operate simultaneously) and its overall length. An allowance (in equivalent length of *pipe*) as determined from Table A.2.2 shall be considered for *piping* segments that include four or more fittings.

(2) Determine the gas *demand* of each *appliance* to be attached to the *piping system*. Where Tables G2413.4(1) through G2413.4(8) are to be used to select the *piping* size, calculate the gas *demand* in terms of cubic feet per hour for each *piping system outlet*.

(3) Where the *piping system* is for use with other than undiluted liquefied petroleum gases, determine the design system pressure, the allowable loss in pressure (*pressure drop*), and *specific gravity* of the gas to be used in the *piping system*.

(4) Determine the length of *piping* from the point of delivery to the most remote *outlet* in the building/*piping system*.

(5) In the appropriate capacity table, select the row showing the measured length or the next longer length if the table does not give the exact length. This is the only length used in determining the size of any section of *gas piping*. If the gravity factor is to be applied, the values in the selected row of the table are multiplied by the appropriate multiplier from Table A.2.4.

(6) Use this horizontal row to locate ALL gas *demand* figures for this particular system of *piping*.

(7) Starting at the most remote *outlet*, find the gas *demand* for that *outlet* in the horizontal row just selected. If the exact figure of *demand* is not shown, choose the next larger figure left in the row.

(8) Opposite this *demand* figure, in the first row at the top, the correct size of *gas piping* will be found.

(9) Proceed in a similar manner for each *outlet* and each section of *gas piping*. For each section of *piping*, determine the total gas *demand* supplied by that section.

When a large number of *piping* components (such as elbows, tees and *valves*) are installed in a *pipe* run, additional pressure loss can be accounted for by the use of equivalent lengths. Pressure loss across any *piping* component can be equated to the *pressure drop* through a length of *pipe*. The equivalent length of a combination of only four elbows/tees can result in a jump to the next larger length row, resulting in a significant reduction in capacity. The equivalent lengths in feet shown in Table A.2.2 have been computed on a basis that the inside diameter corresponds to that of Schedule 40 (standard-weight) steel *pipe*, which is close enough for most purposes involving other schedules of *pipe*. Where a more specific solution for equivalent length is desired, this may be made by multiplying the actual inside diameter of the *pipe* in inches by $n/12$, or the actual inside diameter in feet by n (n can be read from the table heading). The equivalent length values can be used with reasonable accuracy for copper or brass fittings and bends although the resistance per foot of copper or brass *pipe* is less than that of steel. For copper or brass *valves*, however, the equivalent length of *pipe* should be taken as 45 percent longer than the values in the table, which are for steel *pipe*.

A.3.2 Branch length method. This sizing method reduces the amount of conservatism built into the traditional Longest Length Method. The longest length as measured from the *meter* to the furthest remote *appliance* is only used to size the initial parts of the overall *piping system*. The Branch Length Method is applied in the following manner:

(1) Determine the gas load for each of the connected *appliances*.

(2) Starting from the *meter*, divide the *piping system* into a number of connected segments, and determine the length and amount of gas that each segment would carry assuming that all *appliances* were operated simultaneously. An allowance (in equivalent length of *pipe*) as determined from Table A.2.2

should be considered for *piping* segments that include four or more fittings.

(3) Determine the distance from the outlet of the gas *meter* to the *appliance* furthest removed from the *meter*.

(4) Using the longest distance (found in Step 3), size each *piping* segment from the *meter* to the most remote *appliance outlet*.

(5) For each of these *piping* segments, use the longest length and the calculated gas load for all of the connected *appliances* for the segment and begin the sizing process in Steps 6 through 8.

(6) Referring to the appropriate sizing table (based on operating conditions and *piping* material), find the longest length distance in the first column or the next larger distance if the exact distance is not listed. The use of alternative operating pressures and/or *pressure drops* will require the use of a different sizing table, but will not alter the sizing methodology. In many cases, the use of alternative operating pressures and/or *pressure drops* will require the approval of both the *code official* and the local gas serving utility.

(7) Trace across this row until the gas load is found or the closest larger capacity if the exact capacity is not listed.

(8) Read up the table column and select the appropriate *pipe* size in the top row. Repeat Steps 6, 7 and 8 for each *pipe* segment in the longest run.

(9) Size each remaining section of branch *piping* not previously sized by measuring the distance from the gas *meter* location to the most remote *outlet* in that branch, using the gas load of attached *appliances* and following the procedures of Steps 2 through 8.

A.3.3 Hybrid pressure method. The sizing of a 2 psi (13.8 kPa) *gas piping system* is performed using the traditional Longest Length Method but with modifications. The 2 psi (13.8 kPa) system consists of two independent pressure zones, and each zone is sized separately. The Hybrid Pressure Method is applied as follows.

The sizing of the 2 psi (13.8 kPa) section (from the *meter* to the line *regulator*) is as follows:

(1) Calculate the gas load (by adding up the name plate ratings) from all connected *appliances*. (In certain circumstances the installed gas load may be increased up to 50 percent to accommodate future addition of *appliances*.) Ensure that the line *regulator* capacity is adequate for the calculated gas load and that the required *pressure drop* (across the *regulator*) for that capacity does not exceed $^3/_4$ psi (5.2 kPa) for a 2 psi (13.8 kPa) system. If the *pressure drop* across the *regulator* is too high (for the connected gas load), select a larger *regulator*.

(2) Measure the distance from the *meter* to the line *regulator* located inside the building.

(3) If there are multiple line *regulators*, measure the distance from the *meter* to the *regulator* furthest removed from the *meter*.

(4) The maximum allowable *pressure drop* for the 2 psi (13.8 kPa) section is 1 psi (6.9 kPa).

(5) Referring to the appropriate sizing table (based on *piping* material) for 2 psi (13.8 kPa) systems with a 1 psi (6.9 kPa) *pressure drop*, find this distance in the first column, or the closest larger distance if the exact distance is not listed.

(6) Trace across this row until the gas load is found or the closest larger capacity if the exact capacity is not listed.

(7) Read up the table column to the top row and select the appropriate *pipe* size.

(8) If there are multiple *regulators* in this portion of the *piping system*, each line segment must be sized for its actual gas load, but using the longest length previously determined above.

The low pressure section (all *piping* downstream of the line *regulator*) is sized as follows:

(1) Determine the gas load for each of the connected *appliances*.

(2) Starting from the line *regulator*, divide the *piping system* into a number of connected segments and/or independent parallel *piping* segments, and determine the amount of gas that each segment would carry assuming that all *appliances* were operated simultaneously. An allowance (in equivalent length of *pipe*) as determined from Table A.2.2 should be considered for *piping* segments that include four or more fittings.

(3) For each *piping* segment, use the actual length or longest length (if there are sub-branchlines) and the calculated gas load for that segment and begin the sizing process as follows:

(a) Referring to the appropriate sizing table (based on operating pressure and *piping* material), find the longest length distance in the first column or the closest larger distance if the exact distance is not listed. The use of alternative operating pressures and/or *pressure drops* will require the use of a different sizing table, but will not alter the sizing methodology. In many cases, the use of alternative operating pressures and/or *pressure drops* may require the approval of the *code official*.

(b) Trace across this row until the *appliance* gas load is found or the closest larger capacity if the exact capacity is not listed.

(c) Read up the table column to the top row and select the appropriate *pipe* size.

(d) Repeat this process for each segment of the *piping system*.

A.3.4 Pressure drop per 100 feet method. This sizing method is less conservative than the others, but it allows the designer to immediately see where the largest *pressure drop* occurs in the system. With this information, modifications can be made to bring the total drop to the critical *appliance* within the limitations that are presented to the designer.

Follow the procedures described in the Longest Length Method for Steps (1) through (4) and (9).

For each *piping* segment, calculate the *pressure drop* based on *pipe* size, length as a percentage of 100 feet (30 480 mm), and gas flow. Table A.3.4 shows *pressure drop* per 100 feet (30 480 mm) for *pipe* sizes from $^1/_2$ inch (12.7 mm) through 2 inch (51 mm). The sum of *pressure drops* to the critical *appliance* is subtracted from the supply pressure to verify that sufficient pressure will be available. If not, the layout can be examined to find the high drop section(s) and sizing selections modified.

Note: Other values can be obtained by using the following equation:

$$\text{Desired Value} = MBH \times \sqrt{\frac{\text{Desired Drop}}{\text{Table Drop}}}$$

For example, if it is desired to get flow through $^3/_4$-inch (19.1 mm) *pipe* at 2 inches/100 feet, multiple the capacity of $^3/_4$-inch *pipe* at 1 inch/100 feet by the square root of the pressure ratio:

$$147\, MBH \times \sqrt{\frac{2" w.c.}{1" w.c.}} = 147 \times 1.414 = 208\, MBH$$

$$(MBH = 1000\, Btu/\text{h})$$

A.4 Use of sizing equations. Capacities of smooth wall *pipe* or *tubing* can also be determined by using the following formulae:

(1) High Pressure [1.5 psi (10.3 kPa) and above]:

$$Q = 181.6 \sqrt{\frac{D^5 \cdot \left(P_1^2 - P_2^2\right) \cdot Y}{C_r \cdot fba \cdot L}}$$

$$= 2237\, D^{2.623} \left[\frac{\left(P_1^2 - P_2^2\right) \cdot Y}{C_r \cdot L}\right]^{0.541}$$

(2) Low Pressure [Less than 1.5 psi (10.3 kPa)]:

$$Q = 1873 \sqrt{\frac{D^5 \cdot \Delta H}{C_r \cdot fba \cdot L}}$$

$$= 2313\, D^{2.623} \left(\frac{\Delta H}{C_r \cdot L}\right)^{0.541}$$

where:

Q = Rate, cubic feet per hour at 60°F and 30-inch mercury column

D = Inside diameter of *pipe*, in.

P_1 = Upstream pressure, psia

P_2 = Downstream pressure, psia

Y = Superexpansibility factor = 1/supercompressibility factor

C_r = Factor for viscosity, density and temperature*

$$= 0.00354\, ST \left(\frac{Z}{S}\right)^{0.152}$$

Note: See Table 402.4 for Y and C_r for natural gas and propane.

S = *Specific gravity* of gas at 60°F and 30-inch mercury column (0.60 for natural gas, 1.50 for propane), or = 1488μ

T = Absolute temperature, °F or = $t + 460$

t = Temperature, °F

Z = Viscosity of gas, centipoise (0.012 for natural gas, 0.008 for propane), or = 1488μ

fba = Base friction factor for air at 60°F (CF=1)

L = Length of *pipe*, ft

ΔH = *Pressure drop*, in. w.c. (27.7 in. H$_2$O = 1 psi)

(For SI, see Section G2413.4)

A.5 Pipe and tube diameters. Where the internal diameter is determined by the formulas in Section G2413.4, Tables A.5.1 and A.5.2 can be used to select the nominal or standard *pipe* size based on the calculated internal diameter.

TABLE A.3.4
THOUSANDS OF Btu/h (MBH) OF NATURAL GAS PER 100 FEET OF PIPE AT
VARIOUS PRESSURE DROPS AND PIPE DIAMETERS

PRESSURE DROP PER 100 FEET IN INCHES W.C.	PIPE SIZES (inch)					
	$^1/_2$	$^3/_4$	1	$1^1/_4$	$1^1/_2$	2
0.2	31	64	121	248	372	716
0.3	38	79	148	304	455	877
0.5	50	104	195	400	600	1160
1.0	71	147	276	566	848	1640

For SI: 1 inch = 25.4 mm, 1 foot = 304.8 mm.

TABLE A.5.1
SCHEDULE 40 STEEL PIPE STANDARD SIZES

NOMINAL SIZE (in.)	INTERNAL DIAMETER (in.)	NOMINAL SIZE (in.)	INTERNAL DIAMETER (in.)
$^1/_4$	0.364	$1^1/_2$	1.610
$^3/_8$	0.493	2	2.067
$^1/_2$	0.622	$2^1/_2$	2.469
$^3/_4$	0.824	3	3.068
1	1.049	$3^1/_2$	3.548
$1^1/_4$	1.380	4	4.026

TABLE A.5.2
COPPER TUBE STANDARD SIZES

TUBE TYPE	NOMINAL OR STANDARD SIZE (inches)	INTERNAL DIAMETER (inches)
K	$^1/_4$	0.305
L	$^1/_4$	0.315
ACR (D)	$^3/_8$	0.315
ACR (A)	$^3/_8$	0.311
K	$^3/_8$	0.402
L	$^3/_8$	0.430
ACR (D)	$^1/_2$	0.430
ACR (A)	$^1/_2$	0.436
K	$^1/_2$	0.527
L	$^1/_2$	0.545
ACR (D)	$^5/_8$	0.545
ACR (A)	$^5/_8$	0.555
K	$^5/_8$	0.652
L	$^5/_8$	0.666
ACR (D)	$^3/_4$	0.666
ACR (A)	$^3/_4$	0.680
K	$^3/_4$	0.745
L	$^3/_4$	0.785
ACR	$^7/_8$	0.785
K	1	0.995
L	1	1.025
ACR	$1^1/_8$	1.025
K	$1^1/_4$	1.245
L	$1^1/_4$	1.265
ACR	$1^3/_8$	1.265
K	$1^1/_2$	1.481
L	$1^1/_2$	1.505
ACR	$1^5/_8$	1.505
K	2	1.959
L	2	1.985
ACR	$2^1/_8$	1.985
K	$2^1/_2$	2.435
L	$2^1/_2$	2.465
ACR	$2^5/_8$	2.465
K	3	2.907
L	3	2.945
ACR	$3^1/_8$	2.945

A.6 Use of sizing charts. A third method of sizing *gas piping* is detailed below as an option that is useful when large quantities of *piping* are involved in a job (e.g., an apartment house) and material costs are of concern. If the user is not completely familiar with this method, the resulting *pipe* sizing should be checked by a knowledgeable gas engineer. The sizing charts are applied as follows:

(1) With the layout developed according to Section R106.1.1 of the *code*, indicate in each section the design gas flow under maximum operation conditions. For many layouts, the maximum design flow will be the sum of all connected loads. However, in some cases, certain combinations of *appliances* will not occur simultaneously (e.g., gas heating and air conditioning). For these cases, the design flow is the greatest gas flow that can occur at any one time.

(2) Determine the inlet gas pressure for the system being designed. In most cases, the point of inlet will be the gas *meter* or service *regulator*, but in the case of a system addition, it could be the point of connection to the existing system.

(3) Determine the minimum pressure required at the inlet to the critical *appliance*. Usually, the critical item will be the *appliance* with the highest required pressure for satisfactory operation. If several items have the same required pressure, it will be the one with the greatest length of *piping* from the system inlet.

(4) The difference between the inlet pressure and critical item pressure is the allowable system *pressure drop*. Figures A.6(a) and A.6(b) show the relationship between gas flow, *pipe* size and *pipe* length for natural gas with 0.60 *specific gravity*.

(5) To use Figure A.6(a) (low pressure applications), calculate the *piping* length from the inlet to the critical utilization *equipment*. Increase this length by 50 percent to allow for fittings. Divide the allowable *pressure drop* by the equivalent length (in hundreds of feet) to determine the allowable *pressure drop* per hundred feet. Select the *pipe* size from Figure A.6(a) for the required volume of flow.

(6) To use Figure A.6(b) (high pressure applications), calculate the equivalent length as above. Calculate the index number for Figure A.6(b) by dividing the difference between the squares of the absolute values of inlet and outlet pressures by the equivalent length (in hundreds of feet). Select the *pipe* size from Figure A.6(b) for the gas volume required.

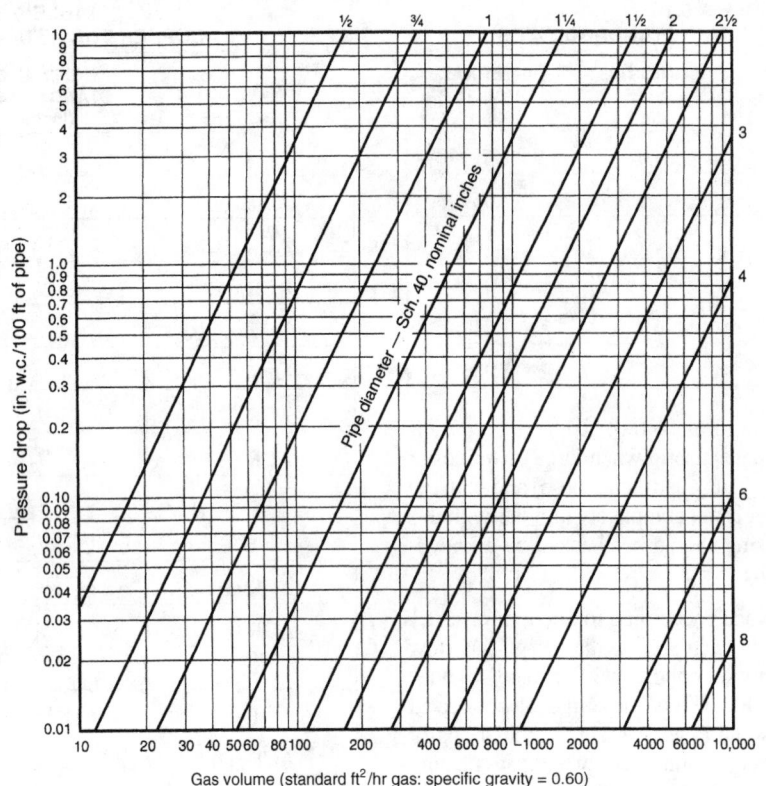

FIGURE A.6(a)
CAPACITY OF NATURAL GAS PIPING, LOW PRESSURE (0.60 WC)

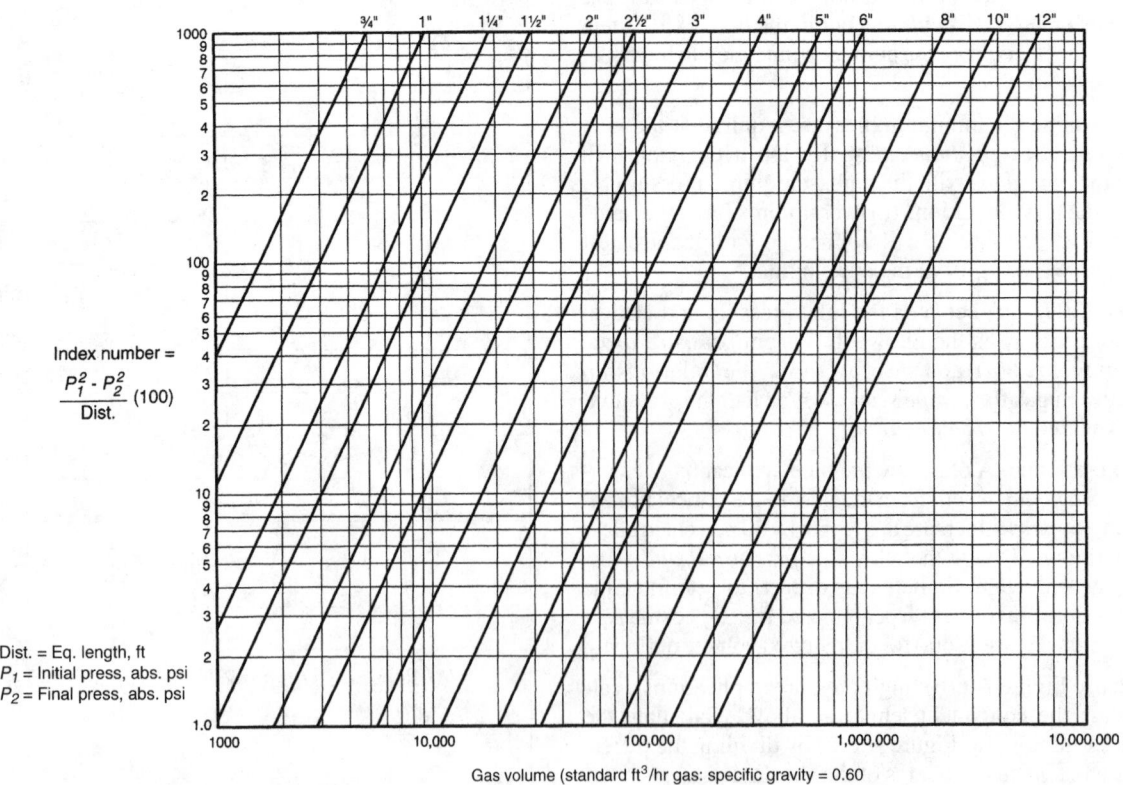

FIGURE A.6 (b)
CAPACITY OF NATURAL GAS PIPING, HIGH PRESSURE (1.5 psi and above)

2009 INTERNATIONAL RESIDENTIAL CODE®

A.7 Examples of piping system design and sizing

A.7.1 Example 1: Longest length method.
Determine the required *pipe* size of each section and *outlet* of the *piping system* shown in Figure A.7.1, with a designated *pressure drop* of 0.5-inch w.c. (125 Pa) using the Longest Length Method. The gas to be used has 0.60 *specific gravity* and a heating value of 1,000 *Btu*/ft³ (37.5 MJ/m³).

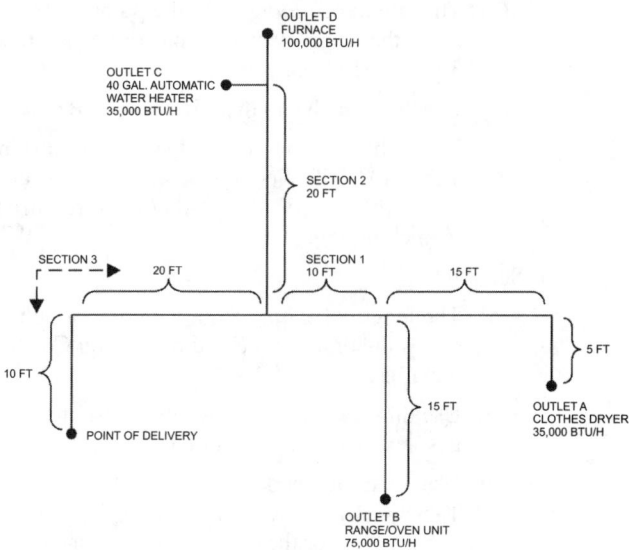

FIGURE A.7.1
PIPING PLAN SHOWING A STEEL PIPING SYSTEM

Solution:

(1) Maximum gas *demand* for *Outlet* A:

$$\frac{\text{Consumption (rating plate input, or Table G 2413.2 if necessary)}}{\text{Btu of gas}} =$$

$$\frac{35,000 \text{ Btu per hour rating}}{1,000 \text{ Btu per cubic foot}} = 35 \text{ cubic feet per hour} = 35 \text{ cfh}$$

Maximum gas *demand* for *Outlet* B:

$$\frac{\text{Consumption}}{\text{Btu of gas}} = \frac{75,000}{1,000} = 75 \text{ cfh}$$

Maximum gas *demand* for *Outlet* C:

$$\frac{\text{Consumption}}{\text{Btu of gas}} = \frac{35,000}{1,000} = 35 \text{ cfh}$$

Maximum gas *demand* for *Outlet* D:

$$\frac{\text{Consumption}}{\text{Btu of gas}} = \frac{100,000}{1,000} = 100 \text{ cfh}$$

(2) The length of *pipe* from the point of delivery to the most remote *outlet* (A) is 60 feet (18 288 mm). This is the only distance used.

(3) Using the row marked 60 feet (18 288 mm) in Table G2413.4(1):

    (a) *Outlet* A, supplying 35 cfh (0.99 m³/hr), requires ³/₈-inch *pipe*.

    (b) *Outlet* B, supplying 75 cfh (2.12 m³/hr), requires ³/₄-inch *pipe*.

    (c) Section 1, supplying *Outlets* A and B, or 110 cfh (3.11 m³/hr), requires ³/₄-inch *pipe*.

    (d) Section 2, supplying *Outlets* C and D, or 135 cfh (3.82 m³/hr), requires ³/₄-inch *pipe*.

    (e) Section 3, supplying *Outlets* A, B, C and D, or 245 cfh (6.94 m³/hr), requires 1-inch *pipe*.

(4) If a different gravity factor is applied to this example, the values in the row marked 60 feet (18 288 mm) of Table G2413.4(1) would be multiplied by the appropriate multiplier from Table A.2.4 and the resulting cubic feet per hour values would be used to size the *piping*.

Section A.7.2 through A7.4 note: These examples are based on tables found in the International Fuel Gas Code.

A.7.2 Example 2: Hybrid or dual pressure systems.
Determine the required CSST size of each section of the *piping system* shown in Figure A.7.2, with a designated *pressure drop* of 1 psi (6.9 kPa) for the 2 psi (13.8 kPa) section and 3-inch w.c. (0.75 kPa) *pressure drop* for the 13-inch w.c. (2.49 kPa) section. The gas to be used has 0.60 *specific gravity* and a heating value of 1,000 *Btu*/ft³ (37.5 MJ/ m³).

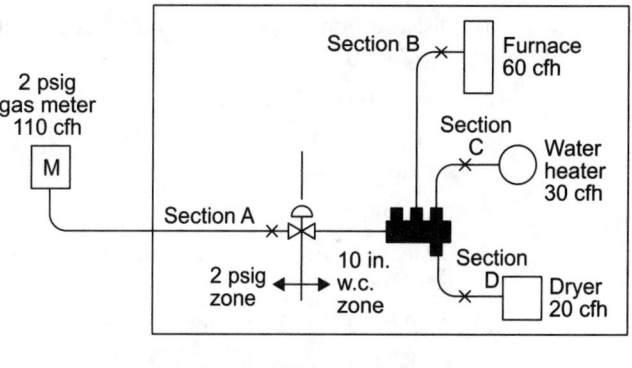

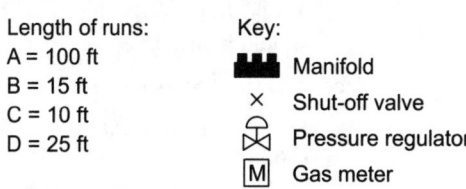

FIGURE A.7.2
PIPING PLAN SHOWING A CSST SYSTEM

Solution

(1) Size 2 psi (13.8 kPa) line using Table 402.4(16).

(2) Size 10-inch w.c. (2.5 kPa) lines using Table 402.4(14).

(3) Using the following, determine if sizing tables can be used.

    (a) Total gas load shown in Figure A.7.2 equals 110 cfh (3.11 m³/hr).

    (b) Determine *pressure drop* across *regulator* [see notes in Table 402.4 (16)].

(c) If *pressure drop* across *regulator* exceeds $^3/_4$ psig (5.2 kPa), Table 402.4 (16) cannot be used. Note: If *pressure drop* exceeds $^3/_4$ psi (5.2 kPa), then a larger *regulator* must be selected or an alternative sizing method must be used.

(d) *Pressure drop* across the line *regulator* [for 110 cfh (3.11 m³/hr)] is 4-inch w.c. (0.99 kPa) based on manufacturer's performance data.

(e) Assume the CSST manufacturer has *tubing* sizes or EHDs of 13, 18, 23 and 30.

(4) Section A [2 psi (13.8 kPa) zone]

(a) Distance from *meter* to *regulator* = 100 feet (30 480 mm).

(b) Total load supplied by A = 110 cfh (3.11 m³/hr) (*furnace + water heater + dryer*).

(c) Table 402.4 (16) shows that EHD size 18 should be used.

Note: It is not unusual to oversize the supply line by 25 to 50 percent of the as-installed load. EHD size 18 has a capacity of 189 cfh (5.35 m³/hr).

(5) Section B (low pressure zone)

(a) Distance from *regulator* to *furnace* is 15 feet (4572 mm).

(b) Load is 60 cfh (1.70 m³/hr).

(c) Table 402.4 (14) shows that EHD size 13 should be used.

(6) Section C (low pressure zone)

(a) Distance from *regulator* to *water heater* is 10 feet (3048 mm).

(b) Load is 30 cfh (0.85 m³/hr).

(c) Table 402.4 (14) shows that EHD size 13 should be used.

(7) Section D (low pressure zone)

(a) Distance from *regulator* to dryer is 25 feet (7620 mm).

(b) Load is 20 cfh (0.57 m³/hr).

(c) Table 402.4(14) shows that EHD size 13 should be used.

A.7.3 Example 3: Branch length method. Determine the required semi-rigid copper *tubing* size of each section of the *piping system* shown in Figure A.7.3, with a designated *pressure drop* of 1-inch w.c. (250 Pa) (using the Branch Length Method). The gas to be used has 0.60 *specific gravity* and a heating value of 1,000 *Btu*/ft³ (37.5 MJ/m³).

Solution

(1) Section A

(a) The length of *tubing* from the point of delivery to the most remote *appliance* is 50 feet (15 240 mm), A + C.

(b) Use this longest length to size Sections A and C.

(c) Using the row marked 50 feet (15 240 mm) in Table 402.4(8), Section A, supplying 220 cfh (6.2 m³/hr) for four *appliances* requires 1-inch *tubing*.

(2) Section B

(a) The length of *tubing* from the point of delivery to the range/oven at the end of Section B is 30 feet (9144 mm), A + B.

(b) Use this branch length to size Section B only.

(c) Using the row marked 30 feet (9144 mm) in Table 402.4(8), Section B, supplying 75 cfh (2.12 m³/hr) for the range/oven requires $^1/_2$-inch *tubing*.

(3) Section C

(a) The length of *tubing* from the point of delivery to the dryer at the end of Section C is 50 feet (15 240 mm), A + C.

(b) Use this branch length (which is also the longest length) to size Section C.

(c) Using the row marked 50 feet (15 240 mm) in Table 402.4(8), Section C, supplying 30 cfh (0.85 m³/hr) for the dryer requires $^3/_8$-inch *tubing*.

(4) Section D

(a) The length of *tubing* from the point of delivery to the *water heater* at the end of Section D is 30 feet (9144 mm), A + D.

(b) Use this branch length to size Section D only.

(c) Using the row marked 30 feet (9144 mm) in Table 402.4(8), Section D, supplying 35 cfh (0.99 m³/hr) for the *water heater* requires $^3/_8$-inch *tubing*.

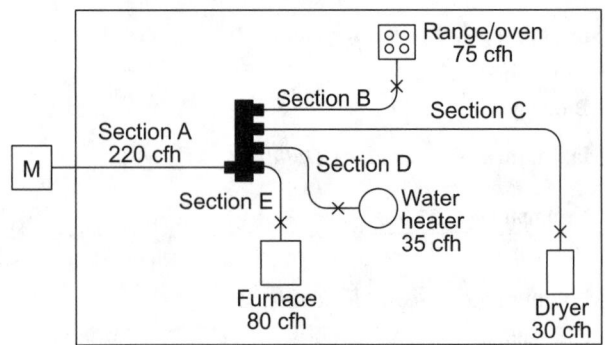

Length of runs:
A = 20 ft
B = 10 ft
C = 30 ft
D = 10 ft
E = 10 ft

Key:
Manifold
× Shut-off valve
M Gas meter
Total gas load = 220 cfh

FIGURE A.7.3
PIPING PLAN SHOWING A COPPER TUBING SYSTEM

(5) Section E

    (a) The length of *tubing* from the point of delivery to the *furnace* at the end of Section E is 30 feet (9144 mm), A + E.

    (b) Use this branch length to size Section E only.

    (c) Using the row marked 30 feet (9144 mm) in Table 402.4(8), Section E, supplying 80 cfh (2.26 m³/hr) for the *furnace* requires ¹/₂-inch *tubing*.

A.7.4 Example 4: Modification to existing piping system.
Determine the required CSST size for Section G (retrofit application) of the *piping system* shown in Figure A.7.4, with a designated *pressure drop* of 0.5-inch w.c. (125 Pa) using the branch length method. The gas to be used has 0.60 *specific gravity* and a heating value of 1,000 *Btu*/ft³ (37.5 MJ/m³).

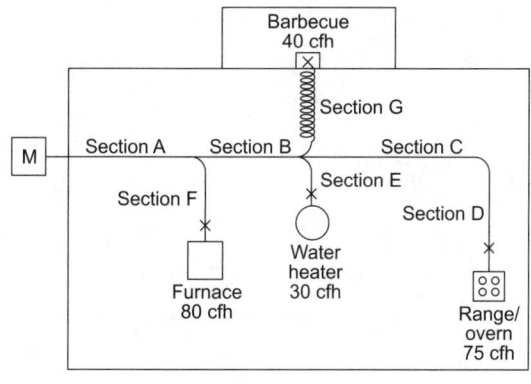

FIGURE A.7.4
PIPING PLAN SHOWING A MODIFICATION
TO EXISTING PIPING SYSTEM

Solution

(1) The length of *pipe* and CSST from the point of delivery to the retrofit *appliance* (barbecue) at the end of Section G is 40 feet (12 192 mm), A + B + G.

(2) Use this branch length to size Section G.

(3) Assume the CSST manufacturer has *tubing* sizes or EHDs of 13, 18, 23 and 30.

(4) Using the row marked 40 feet (12 192 mm) in Table 402.4(13), Section G, supplying 40 cfh (1.13 m³/hr) for the barbecue requires EHD 18 CSST.

(5) The sizing of Sections A, B, F and E must be checked to ensure adequate gas carrying capacity since an *appliance* has been added to the *piping system* (see A.7.1 for details).

A.7.5 Example 5: Calculating pressure drops due to temperature changes.
A test *piping system* is installed on a warm autumn afternoon when the temperature is 70°F (21°C). In accordance with local custom, the new *piping system* is subjected to an air *pressure test* at 20 psig (138 kPa). Overnight, the temperature drops and when the inspector shows up first thing in the morning the temperature is 40°F (4°C).

If the volume of the *piping system* is unchanged, then the formula based on Boyle's and Charles' law for determining the new pressure at a reduced temperature is as follows:

$$\frac{T_1}{T_2} = \frac{P_1}{P_2}$$

where:

T_1 = Initial temperature, absolute (T_1 + 459)

T_2 = Final temperature, absolute (T_2 + 459)

P_1 = Initial pressure, psia (P_1 + 14.7)

P_2 = Final pressure, psia (P_2 + 14.7)

$$\frac{(70+459)}{(40+459)} = \frac{(20+14.7)}{(P_2+14.7)}$$

$$\frac{529}{499} = \frac{34.7}{(P_2+14.7)}$$

$$(P_2+14.7) \times \frac{529}{499} = 34.7$$

$$(P_2+14.7) = \frac{34.7}{1.060}$$

$$P_2 = 32.7 - 14.7$$

$$P_2 = 18 \, psig$$

Therefore, the gauge could be expected to register 18 psig (124 kPa) when the ambient temperature is 40EF (4EC).

A7.6 Example 6: Pressure drop per 100 feet of pipe method.
Using the layout shown in Figure A.7.1 and ΔH = *pressure drop*, in w.c. (27.7 in. H₂O = 1 psi), proceed as follows:

(1) Length to A = 20 feet, with 35,000 *Btu*/hr.

For ¹/₂-inch *pipe*, $\Delta H = {}^{20 \text{ feet}}/_{100 \text{ feet}} \times 0.3$ inch w.c. = 0.06 in. w.c.

(2) Length to B = 15 feet, with 75,000 *Btu*/hr.

For ³/₄-inch *pipe*, $\Delta H = {}^{15 \text{ feet}}/_{100 \text{ feet}} \times 0.3$ inch w.c. = 0.045 in. w.c.

(3) Section 1 = 10 feet, with 110,000 *Btu*/hr. Here there is a choice:

For 1 inch *pipe*: $\Delta H = {}^{10 \text{ feet}}/_{100 \text{ feet}} \times 0.2$ inch w.c. = 0.02 in w.c.

For ³/₄-inch *pipe*: $\Delta H = {}^{10 \text{ feet}}/_{100 \text{ feet}} \times [0.5$ inch w.c. + ${}^{(110,000 \, Btu/hr-104,000 \, Btu/hr)}/_{(147,000 \, Btu/hr-104,000 \, Btu/hr)} \times (1.0$ inches w.c. - 0.5 inch w.c.)] $= 0.1 \times 0.57$ inch w.c. = 0.06 inch w.c.

Note that the pressure drop between 104,000 Btu/hr and 147,000 Btu/hr has been interpolated as 110,000 Btu/hr.

(4) Section 2 = 20 feet, with 135,000 *Btu*/hr. Here there is a choice:

For 1-inch *pipe*: $\Delta H = {}^{20 \text{ feet}}/_{100 \text{ feet}} \times [0.2$ inch w.c. + ${}^{(14,000 \, Btu/hr)}/_{(27,000 \, Btu/hr)} \times 0.1$ inch w.c.)] = 0.05 inch w.c.)]

For $^3/_4$-inch *pipe*: $\Delta H = {^{20\ feet}}/_{100\ feet} \times 1.0$ inch w.c. = 0.2 inch w.c.)

Note that the pressure drop between 121,000 Btu/hr and 148,000 Btu/hr has been interpolated as 135,000 Btu/hr, but interpolation for the ¾-inch pipe (trivial for 104,000 Btu/hr to 147,000 Btu/hr) was not used.

(5) Section 3 = 30 feet, with 245,000 *Btu*/hr. Here there is a choice:

For 1-inch *pipe*: $\Delta H = {^{30\ feet}}/_{100\ feet} \times 1.0$ inches w.c. = 0.3 inch w.c.

For $1^1/_4$-inch *pipe*: $\Delta H = {^{30\ feet}}/_{100\ feet} \times 0.2$ inch w.c. = 0.06 inch w.c.

Note that interpolation for these options is ignored since the table values are close to the 245,000 Btu/hr carried by that section.

(6) The total *pressure drop* is the sum of the section approaching A, Sections 1 and 3, or either of the following, depending on whether an absolute minimum is needed or the larger drop can be accommodated.

Minimum *pressure drop* to farthest *appliance*:

ΔH = 0.06 inch w.c. + 0.02 inch w.c. + 0.06 inch w.c. = 0.14 inch w.c.

Larger *pressure drop* to the farthest *appliance*:

ΔH = 0.06 inch w.c. + 0.06 inch w.c. + 0.3 inch w.c. = 0.42 inch w.c.

Notice that Section 2 and the run to B do not enter into this calculation, provided that the appliances have similar input pressure requirements.

For SI units: 1 *Btu*/hr = 0.293 W, 1 *cubic foot* = 0.028 m³, 1 foot = 0.305 m, 1 inch w.c. = 249 Pa.

APPENDIX B

SIZING OF VENTING SYSTEMS SERVING APPLIANCES EQUIPPED WITH DRAFT HOODS, CATEGORY I APPLIANCES, AND APPLIANCES LISTED FOR USE WITH TYPE B VENTS

(This appendix is informative and is not part of the *code*. This appendix is an excerpt from the 2009 *International Fuel Gas Code,* coordinated with the section numbering of the *International Residential Code.*)

EXAMPLES USING SINGLE APPLIANCE VENTING TABLES

Example 1: Single draft-hood-equipped appliance.

An installer has a 120,000 British thermal unit (*Btu*) per hour input appliance with a 5-inch-diameter *draft hood* outlet that needs to be vented into a 10-foot-high Type B *vent* system. What size vent should be used assuming (a) a 5-foot lateral single-wall metal *vent connector* is used with two 90-degree elbows, or (b) a 5-foot lateral single-wall metal *vent connector* is used with three 90-degree elbows in the vent system?

Solution:

Table G2428.2(2) should be used to solve this problem, because single-wall metal *vent connectors* are being used with a Type B *vent.*

(a) Read down the first column in Table G2428.2(2) until the row associated with a 10-foot height and 5-foot lateral is found. Read across this row until a *vent* capacity greater than 120,000 *Btu* per hour is located in the shaded columns labeled "NAT Max" for *draft*-hood-equipped appliances. In this case, a 5-inch-diameter *vent* has a capacity of 122,000 *Btu* per hour and may be used for this application.

(b) If three 90-degree elbows are used in the vent system, then the maximum vent capacity listed in the tables must be reduced by 10 percent (see Section G2428.2.3 for single appliance vents). This implies that the 5-inch-diameter vent has an adjusted capacity of only 110,000 *Btu* per hour. In this case, the vent system must be increased to 6 inches in diameter (see calculations below).

122,000 (0.90) = 110,000 for 5-inch vent
From Table G2428.2(2), Select 6-inch vent
186,000 (0.90) = 167,000; This is greater than the required 120,000. Therefore, use a 6-inch vent and connector where three elbows are used.

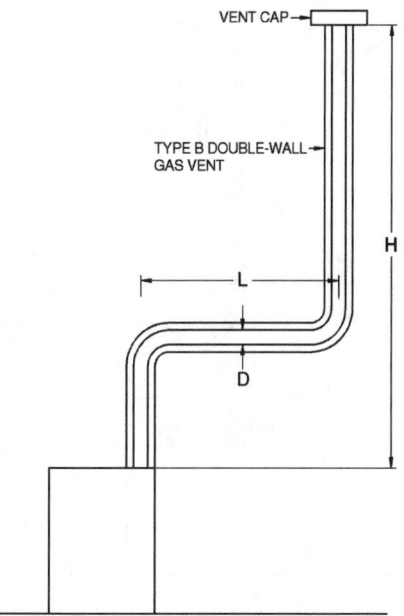

For SI: 1 foot = 304.8 mm, 1 British thermal unit per hour = 0.2931 W.

Table G2428.2(1) is used when sizing Type B double-wall gas vent connected directly to the appliance.

Note: The appliance may be either Category I draft hood equipped or fan-assisted type.

FIGURE B-1
TYPE B DOUBLE-WALL VENT SYSTEM SERVING A SINGLE APPLIANCE WITH A TYPE B DOUBLE-WALL VENT

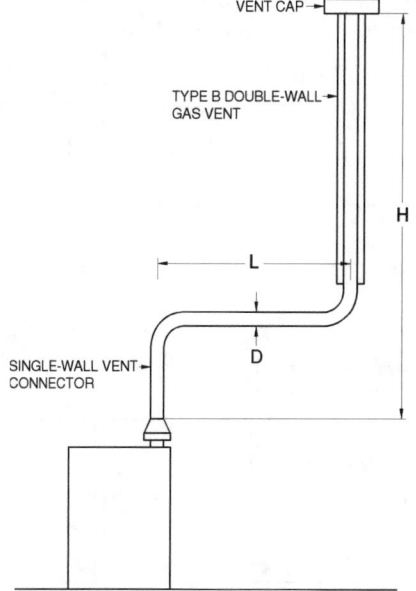

For SI: 1 foot = 304.8 mm, 1 British thermal unit per hour = 0.2931 W.

Table G2428.2(2) is used when sizing a single-wall metal vent connector attached to a Type B double-wall gas vent.

Note: The appliance may be either Category I draft hood equipped or fan-assisted type.

FIGURE B-2
TYPE B DOUBLE-WALL VENT SYSTEM SERVING A SINGLE APPLIANCE WITH A SINGLE-WALL METAL VENT CONNECTOR

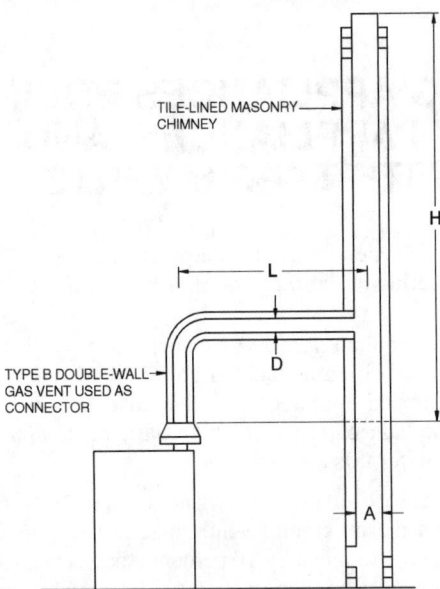

Table 504.2(3) of the *International Fuel Gas Code* is used when sizing a Type B double-wall gas vent connector attached to a tile-lined masonry chimney.

Note: "A" is the equivalent cross-sectional area of the tile liner.

Note: The appliance may be either Category I draft hood equipped or fan-assisted type.

FIGURE B-3
VENT SYSTEM SERVING A SINGLE APPLIANCE
WITH A MASONRY CHIMNEY OF TYPE B
DOUBLE-WALL VENT CONNECTOR

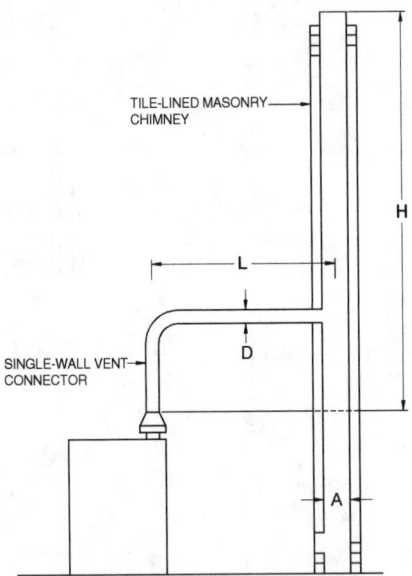

Table 504.2(4) of the *International Fuel Gas Code* is used when sizing a single-wall vent connector attached to a tile-lined masonry chimney.

Note: "A" is the equivalent cross-sectional area of the tile liner.

Note: The appliance may be either Category I draft hood equipped or fan-assisted type.

FIGURE B-4
VENT SYSTEM SERVING A SINGLE APPLIANCE
USING A MASONRY CHIMNEY AND A
SINGLE-WALL METAL VENT CONNECTOR

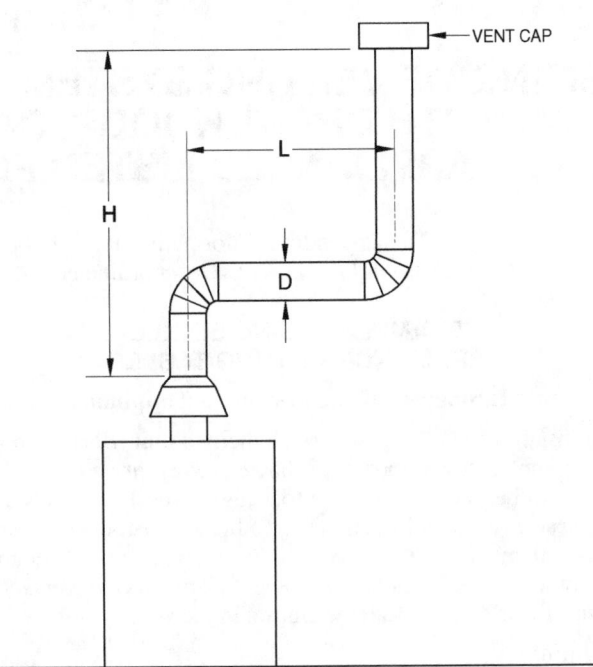

Asbestos cement Type B or single-wall metal vent serving a single draft-hood-equipped appliance [see Table 504.2(5) of the *International Fuel Gas Code*].

FIGURE B-5
ASBESTOS CEMENT TYPE B OR SINGLE-WALL
METAL VENT SYSTEM SERVING A SINGLE
DRAFT-HOOD-EQUIPPED APPLIANCE

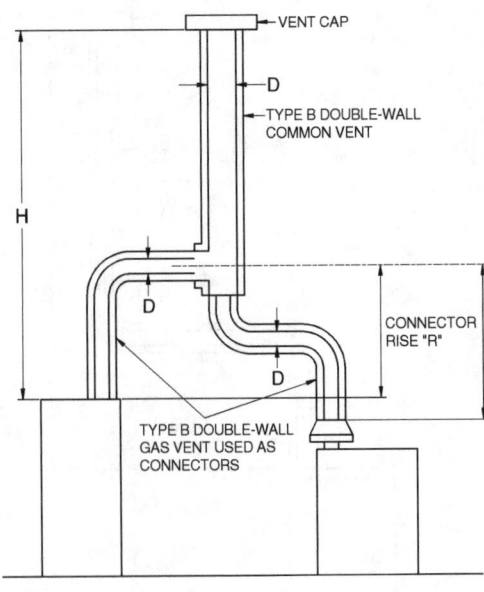

Table G2428.3(1) is used when sizing Type B double-wall vent connectors attached to a Type B double-wall common vent.

Note: Each appliance may be either Category I draft hood equipped or fan-assisted type.

FIGURE B-6
VENT SYSTEM SERVING TWO OR MORE APPLIANCES
WITH TYPE B DOUBLE-WALL VENT AND TYPE B
DOUBLE-WALL VENT CONNECTOR

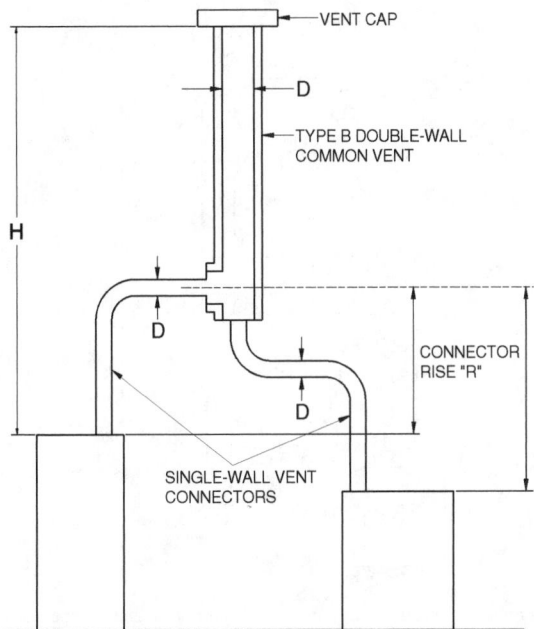

Table G2428.3(2) is used when sizing single-wall vent connectors attached to a Type B double-wall common vent.

Note: Each appliance may be either Category I draft hood equipped or fan-assisted type.

FIGURE B-7
VENT SYSTEM SERVING TWO OR MORE APPLIANCES
WITH TYPE B DOUBLE-WALL VENT AND
SINGLE-WALL METAL VENT CONNECTORS

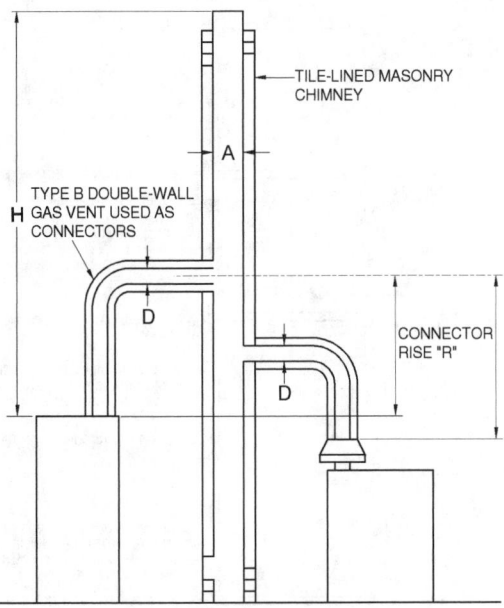

Table G2428.3(3) is used when sizing Type B double-wall vent connectors attached to a tile-lined masonry chimney.

Note: "A" is the equivalent cross-sectional area of the tile liner.

Note: Each appliance may be either Category I draft hood equipped or fan-assisted type.

FIGURE B-8
MASONRY CHIMNEY SERVING TWO OR MORE APPLIANCES
WITH TYPE B DOUBLE-WALL VENT CONNECTOR

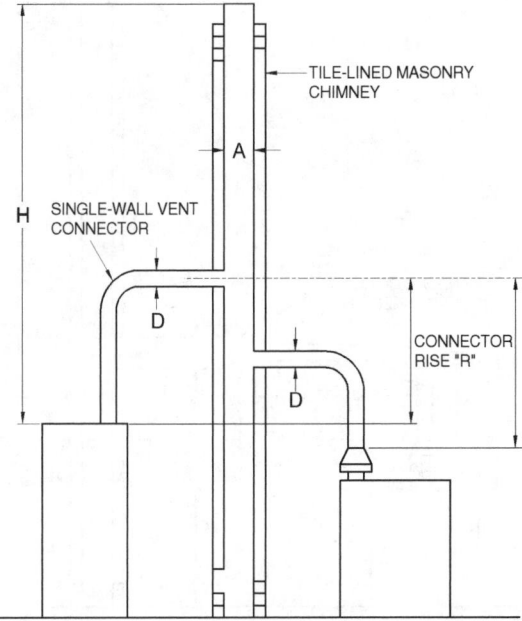

Table G2428.3(4) is used when sizing single-wall metal vent connectors attached to a tile-lined masonry chimney.

Note: "A" is the equivalent cross-sectional area of the tile liner.

Note: Each appliance may be either Category I draft hood equipped or fan-assisted type.

FIGURE B-9
MASONRY CHIMNEY SERVING TWO OR MORE APPLIANCES
WITH SINGLE-WALL METAL VENT CONNECTORS

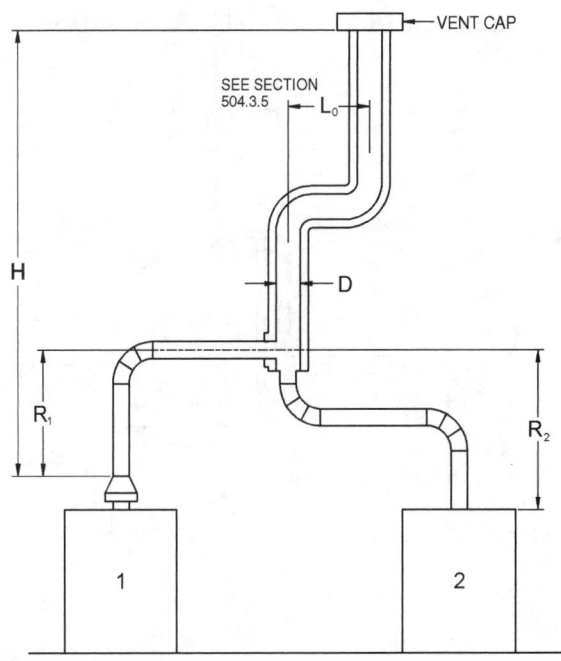

Asbestos cement Type B or single-wall metal pipe vent serving two or more draft-hood-equipped appliances [see Table 504.3(5) of the *International Fuel Gas Code*].

FIGURE B-10
ASBESTOS CEMENT TYPE B OR SINGLE-WALL
METAL VENT SYSTEM SERVING TWO OR MORE
DRAFT-HOOD-EQUIPPED APPLIANCES

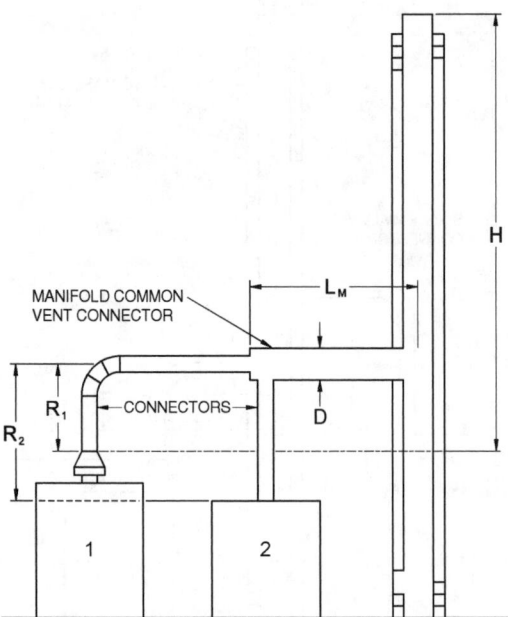

Example: Manifolded Common Vent Connector L_M shall be no greater than 18 times the common vent connector manifold inside diameter; i.e., a 4-inch (102 mm) inside diameter common vent connector manifold shall not exceed 72 inches (1829 mm) in length (see Section G2428.3.4).

Note: This is an illustration of a typical manifolded vent connector. Different appliance, vent connector, or common vent types are possible. Consult Section G2426.3.

FIGURE B-11
USE OF MANIFOLD COMMON VENT CONNECTOR

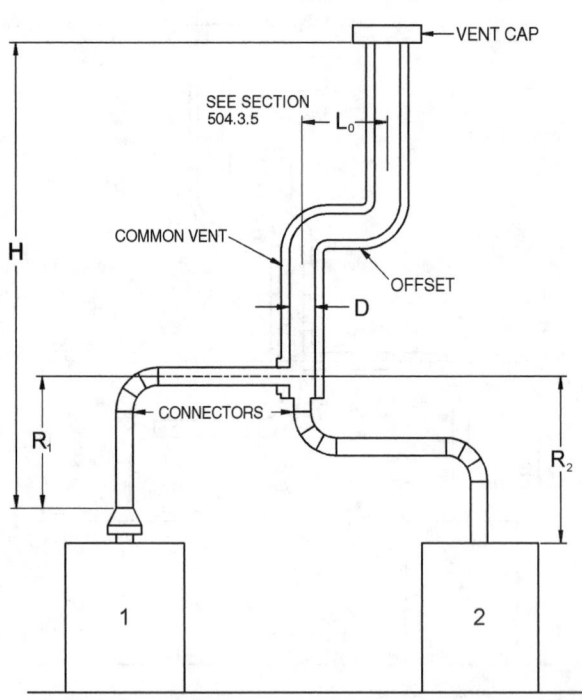

Example: Offset Common Vent

Note: This is an illustration of a typical offset vent. Different appliance, vent connector, or vent types are possible. Consult Sections G2428.2 and G2428.3.

FIGURE B-12
USE OF OFFSET COMMON VENT

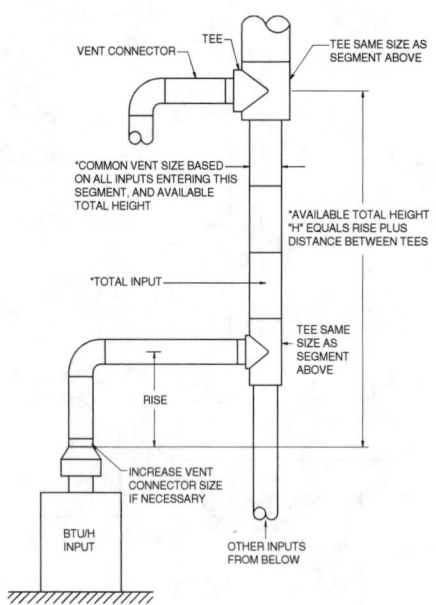

Vent connector size depends on:

• Combined inputs
• Rise
• Available total height "H"
• Table G2428.3(1) connectors

Common vent size depends on:

• Input
• Available total height "H"
• Table G2428.3(1) common vent

FIGURE B-13
MULTISTORY GAS VENT DESIGN PROCEDURE FOR EACH SEGMENT OF SYSTEM

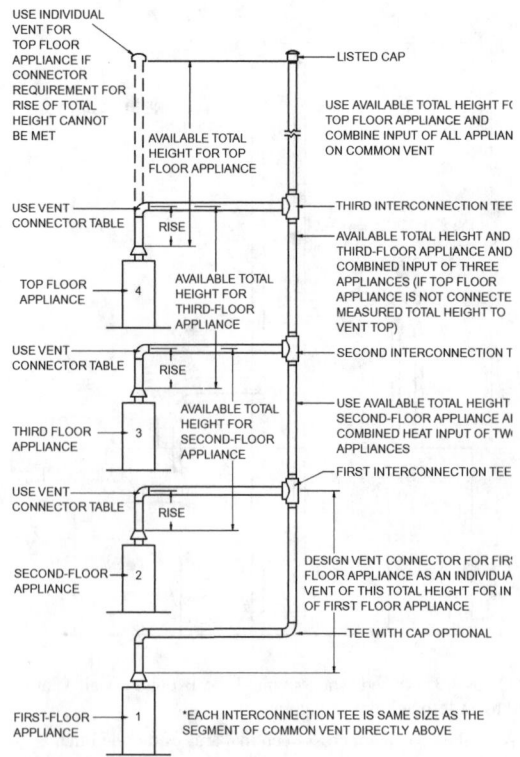

Principles of design of multistory vents using vent connector and common vent design tables (see Sections G2428.3.11 through G2428.3.13).

FIGURE B-14
MULTISTORY VENT SYSTEMS

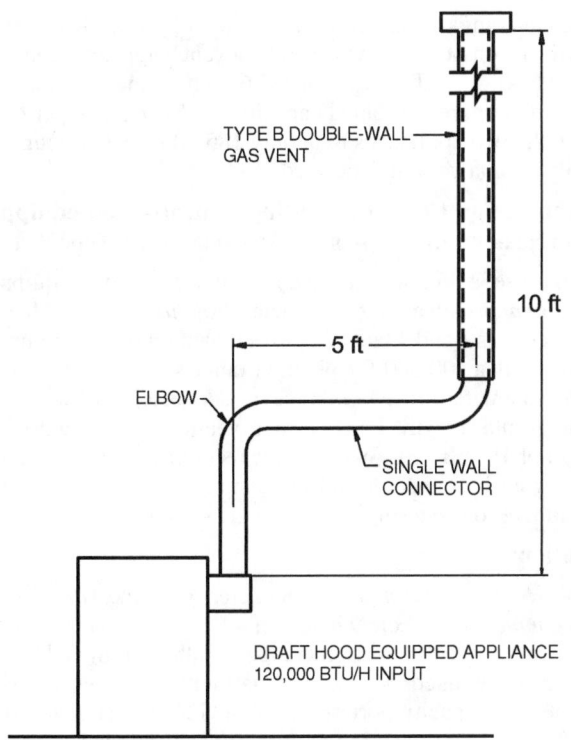

For SI: 1 foot = 304.8 mm, 1 British thermal unit per hour = 0.2931 W.

FIGURE B-15 (EXAMPLE 1)
SINGLE DRAFT-HOOD-EQUIPPED APPLIANCE

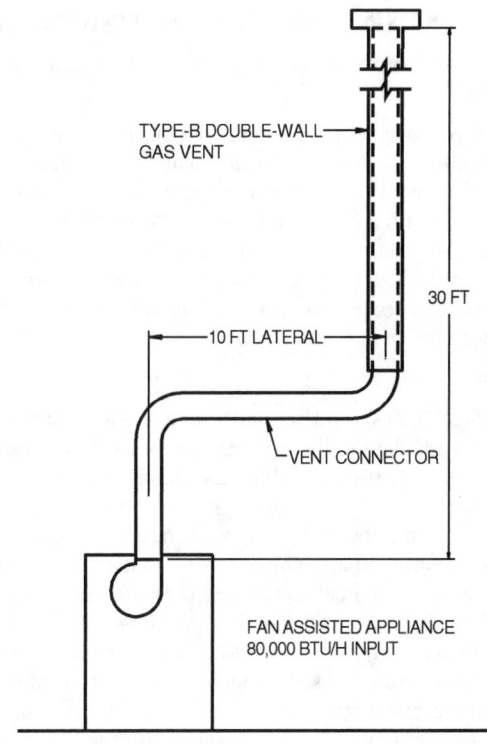

For SI: 1 foot = 304.8 mm, 1 British thermal unit per hour = 0.2931 W.

FIGURE B-16 (EXAMPLE 2)
SINGLE FAN-ASSISTED APPLIANCE

Example 2: Single fan-assisted appliance.

An installer has an 80,000 *Btu* per hour input fan-assisted appliance that must be installed using 10 feet of lateral connector attached to a 30-foot-high Type B *vent*. Two 90-degree elbows are needed for the installation. Can a single-wall metal *vent connector* be used for this application?

Solution:

Table G2428.2(2) refers to the use of single-wall metal *vent connectors* with Type B vent. In the first column find the row associated with a 30-foot height and a 10-foot lateral. Read across this row, looking at the FAN Min and FAN Max columns, to find that a 3-inch-diameter single-wall metal *vent connector* is not recommended. Moving to the next larger size single wall connector (4 inches), note that a 4-inch-diameter single-wall metal connector has a recommended minimum *vent* capacity of 91,000 *Btu* per hour and a recommended maximum *vent* capacity of 144,000 *Btu* per hour. The 80,000 *Btu* per hour fan-assisted appliance is outside this range, so the conclusion is that a single-wall metal *vent connector* cannot be used to *vent* this appliance using 10 feet of lateral for the connector.

However, if the 80,000 *Btu* per hour input appliance could be moved to within 5 feet of the vertical vent, then a 4-inch single-wall metal connector could be used to vent the appliance. Table G2428.2(2) shows the acceptable range of vent capacities for a 4-inch vent with 5 feet of lateral to be between 72,000 *Btu* per hour and 157,000 *Btu* per hour.

If the appliance cannot be moved closer to the vertical vent, then Type B vent could be used as the connector material. In this case, Table G2428.2(1) shows that for a 30-foot-high vent with 10 feet of lateral, the acceptable range of vent capacities for a 4-inch-diameter vent attached to a fan-assisted appliance is between 37,000 *Btu* per hour and 150,000 *Btu* per hour.

Example 3: Interpolating between table values.

An installer has an 80,000 *Btu* per hour input appliance with a 4-inch-diameter *draft hood* outlet that needs to be vented into a 12-foot-high Type B *vent*. The *vent connector* has a 5-foot lateral length and is also Type B. Can this appliance be vented using a 4-inch-diameter vent?

Solution:

Table G2428.2(1) is used in the case of an all Type B *vent* system. However, since there is no entry in Table G2428.2(1) for a height of 12 feet, interpolation must be used. Read down the 4-inch diameter NAT Max column to the row associated with 10-foot height and 5-foot lateral to find the capacity value of 77,000 *Btu* per hour. Read further down to the 15-foot height, 5-foot lateral row to find the capacity value of 87,000 *Btu* per hour. The difference between the 15-foot height capacity value and the 10-foot height capacity value is 10,000 *Btu* per hour. The capacity for a vent system with a 12-foot height is equal to the capacity for a 10-foot height plus $^2/_5$ of the difference between the 10-foot and 15-foot height values, or 77,000 + $^2/_5$ (10,000) = 81,000 *Btu* per hour. Therefore, a 4-inch-diameter *vent* may be used in the installation.

EXAMPLES USING COMMON VENTING TABLES

Example 4: Common venting two draft-hood-equipped appliances.

A 35,000 *Btu* per hour *water heater* is to be common vented with a 150,000 *Btu* per hour *furnace* using a common *vent* with a total height of 30 feet. The connector rise is 2 feet for the *water heater* with a horizontal length of 4 feet. The connector rise for the *furnace* is 3 feet with a horizontal length of 8 feet. Assume single-wall metal connectors will be used with Type B *vent*. What size connectors and combined vent should be used in this installation?

Solution:

Table G2428.3(2) should be used to size single-wall metal *vent connectors* attached to Type B vertical vents. In the *vent connector* capacity portion of Table G2428.3(2), find the row associated with a 30-foot vent height. For a 2-foot rise on the *vent connector* for the *water heater*, read the shaded columns for *draft*-hood-equipped appliances to find that a 3-inch-diameter *vent connector* has a capacity of 37,000 *Btu* per hour. Therefore, a 3-inch single-wall metal *vent connector* may be used with the *water heater*. For a *draft*-hood-equipped *furnace* with a 3-foot rise, read across the appropriate row to find that a 5-inch-diameter *vent connector* has a maximum capacity of 120,000 *Btu* per hour (which is too small for the *furnace*) and a 6-inch-diameter *vent connector* has a maximum vent capacity of 172,000 *Btu* per hour. Therefore, a 6-inch-diameter *vent connector* should be used with the 150,000 *Btu* per hour *furnace*. Since both *vent connector* horizontal lengths are less than the maximum lengths listed in Section G2428.3.2, the table values may be used without adjustments.

In the common vent capacity portion of Table G2428.3(2), find the row associated with a 30-foot vent height and read over to the NAT + NAT portion of the 6-inch-diameter column to find a maximum combined capacity of 257,000 *Btu* per hour. Since the two appliances total only 185,000 *Btu* per hour, a 6-inch common vent may be used.

Example 5a: Common venting a draft-hood-equipped water heater with a fan-assisted furnace into a Type B vent.

In this case, a 35,000 *Btu* per hour input *draft*-hood-equipped *water heater* with a 4-inch-diameter *draft hood* outlet, 2 feet of connector rise, and 4 feet of horizontal length is to be common vented with a 100,000 *Btu* per hour fan-assisted *furnace* with a 4-inch-diameter *flue collar*, 3 feet of connector rise, and 6 feet of horizontal length. The common vent consists of a 30-foot height of Type B vent. What are the recommended vent diameters for each connector and the common vent? The installer would like to use a single-wall metal *vent connector*.

Solution:

Water Heater Vent Connector Diameter. Since the *water heater vent connector* horizontal length of 4 feet is less than the maximum value listed in Section G2428.3.2, the venting table values may be used without adjustments. Using the *Vent Connector* Capacity portion of Table G2428.3(2), read down the Total Vent Height (*H*) column to 30 feet and read across the 2-foot Connector Rise (*R*) row to the first *Btu* per hour rating in the NAT Max column that is equal to or greater than the *water heater* input rating. The table shows that a 3-inch *vent connector* has a maximum input rating of 37,000 *Btu* per hour. Although this is greater than the *water heater* input rating, a 3-inch *vent connector* is prohibited by Section G2428.3.17. A 4-

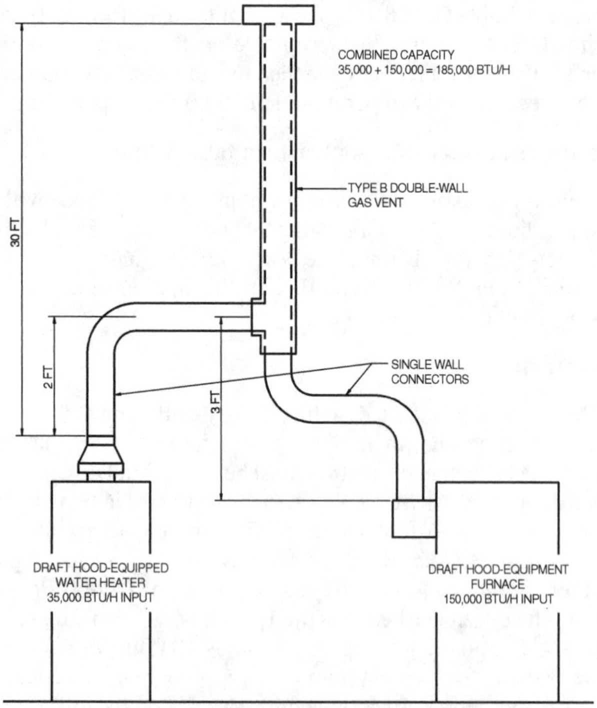

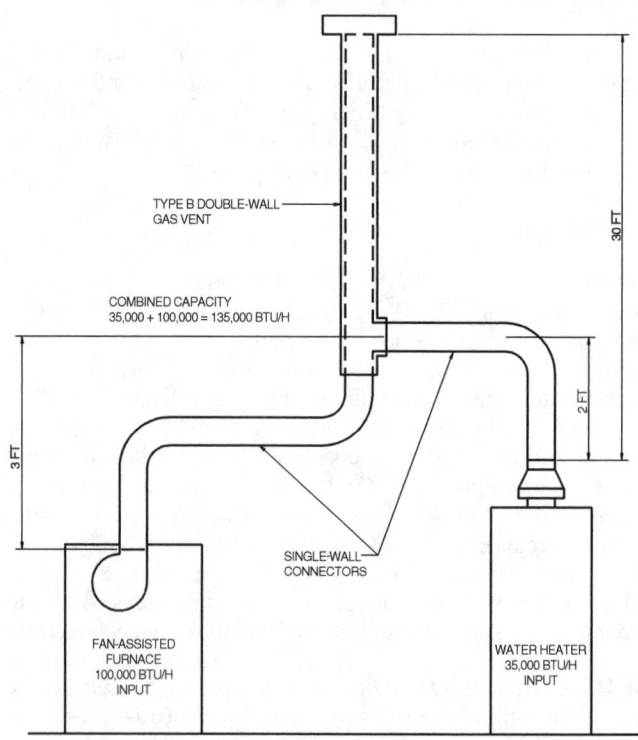

FIGURE B-17 (EXAMPLE 4)
COMMON VENTING TWO DRAFT-HOOD-EQUIPPED APPLIANCES

FIGURE B-18 (EXAMPLE 5A)
COMMON VENTING A DRAFT HOOD WITH A FAN-ASSISTED FURNACE INTO A TYPE B DOUBLE-WALL COMMON VENT

inch *vent connector* has a maximum input rating of 67,000 *Btu* per hour and is equal to the *draft hood* outlet diameter. A 4-inch *vent connector* is selected. Since the *water heater* is equipped with a *draft hood*, there are no minimum input rating restrictions.

Furnace Vent Connector Diameter. Using the *Vent Connector* Capacity portion of Table G2428.3(2), read down the Total *Vent Height* (*H*) column to 30 feet and across the 3-foot Connector Rise (*R*) row. Since the *furnace* has a fan-assisted *combustion* system, find the first FAN Max column with a *Btu* per hour rating greater than the *furnace* input rating. The 4-inch *vent connector* has a maximum input rating of 119,000 *Btu* per hour and a minimum input rating of 85,000 *Btu* per hour. The 100,000 *Btu* per hour *furnace* in this example falls within this range, so a 4-inch connector is adequate. Since the *furnace vent connector* horizontal length of 6 feet does not exceed the maximum value listed in Section G2428.3.2, the venting table values may be used without adjustment. If the *furnace* had an input rating of 80,000 *Btu* per hour, then a Type B *vent connector* [see Table G2428.3(1)] would be needed in order to meet the minimum capacity limit.

Common Vent Diameter. The total input to the common *vent* is 135,000 *Btu* per hour. Using the Common Vent Capacity portion of Table G2428.3(2), read down the Total Vent Height (*H*) column to 30 feet and across this row to find the smallest vent diameter in the FAN + NAT column that has a *Btu* per hour rating equal to or greater than 135,000 *Btu* per hour. The 4-inch common vent has a capacity of 132,000 *Btu* per hour and the 5-inch common vent has a capacity of 202,000 *Btu* per hour. Therefore, the 5-inch common vent should be used in this example.

Summary. In this example, the installer may use a 4-inch-diameter, single-wall metal *vent connector* for the *water heater* and a 4-inch-diameter, single-wall metal *vent connector* for the *furnace*. The common vent should be a 5-inch-diameter Type B vent.

Example 5b: Common venting into a masonry chimney.

In this case, the *water heater* and fan-assisted *furnace* of Example 5a are to be common vented into a clay tile-lined *masonry chimney* with a 30-foot height. The *chimney* is not exposed to the outdoors below the roof line. The internal dimensions of the clay tile liner are nominally 8 inches by 12 inches. Assuming the same *vent connector* heights, laterals, and materials found in Example 5a, what are the recommended *vent connector* diameters, and is this an acceptable installation?

Solution:

Table G2428.3(4) is used to size common venting installations involving single-wall connectors into *masonry chimneys*.

Water Heater Vent Connector Diameter. Using Table G2428.3(4), *Vent Connector* Capacity, read down the Total *Vent Height* (*H*) column to 30 feet, and read across the 2-foot Connector Rise (*R*) row to the first *Btu* per hour rating in the NAT Max column that is equal to or greater than the *water heater* input rating. The table shows that a 3-inch *vent connector* has a maximum input of only 31,000 *Btu* per hour while a 4-inch *vent connector* has a maximum input of 57,000 *Btu* per hour. A 4-inch *vent connector* must therefore be used.

Furnace Vent Connector Diameter. Using the *Vent Connector* Capacity portion of Table G2428.3(4), read down the Total Vent Height (*H*) column to 30 feet and across the 3-foot Connector Rise (*R*) row. Since the *furnace* has a fan-assisted *combustion* system, find the first FAN Max column with a *Btu* per hour rating greater than the *furnace* input rating. The 4-inch *vent connector* has a maximum input rating of 127,000 *Btu* per hour and a minimum input rating of 95,000 *Btu* per hour. The 100,000 *Btu* per hour *furnace* in this example falls within this range, so a 4-inch connector is adequate.

Masonry Chimney. From Table B-1, the equivalent area for a nominal liner size of 8 inches by 12 inches is 63.6 square inches. Using Table G2428.3(4), Common Vent Capacity, read down the FAN + NAT column under the Minimum Internal Area of *Chimney* value of 63 to the row for 30-foot height to find a capacity value of 739,000 *Btu* per hour. The combined input rating of the *furnace* and *water heater*, 135,000 *Btu* per hour, is less than the table value, so this is an acceptable installation.

Section G2428.3.13 requires the common vent area to be no greater than seven times the smallest listed appliance categorized *vent* area, *flue collar* area, or *draft hood* outlet area. Both appliances in this installation have 4-inch-diameter outlets. From Table B-1, the equivalent area for an inside diameter of 4 inches is 12.2 square inches. Seven times 12.2 equals 85.4, which is greater than 63.6, so this configuration is acceptable.

Example 5c: Common venting into an exterior masonry chimney.

In this case, the *water heater* and fan-assisted *furnace* of Examples 5a and 5b are to be common vented into an exterior *masonry chimney*. The *chimney* height, clay tile liner dimensions, and *vent connector* heights and laterals are the same as in Example 5b. This system is being installed in Charlotte, North Carolina. Does this exterior *masonry chimney* need to be relined? If so, what corrugated metallic liner size is recommended? What *vent connector* diameters are recommended?

Solution:

According to Section 504.3.20 of the *International Fuel Gas Code*, Type B *vent connectors* are required to be used with *exterior masonry chimneys*. Use Table 504.3(7) of the *International Fuel Gas Code* to size FAN+NAT common venting installations involving Type-B double wall connectors into *exterior masonry chimneys*.

The local 99-percent winter design temperature needed to use Table 504.3(7) can be found in the ASHRAE *Handbook of Fundamentals*. For Charlotte, North Carolina, this design temperature is 19°F.

Chimney Liner Requirement. As in Example 5b, use the 63 square inch Internal Area columns for this size clay tile liner. Read down the 63 square inch column of Table 504.3(7a) of the *International Fuel Gas Code* to the 30-foot height row to find that the combined appliance maximum input is 747,000 *Btu* per hour. The combined input rating of the appliances in this installation, 135,000 *Btu* per hour, is less than the maximum value, so this criterion is satisfied. Table 504.3(7b), at a 19°F design temperature, and at the same vent height and internal area used above, shows that the minimum allowable input rating of a space-heating appliance is 470,000 *Btu* per hour. The *furnace* input rating of 100,000 *Btu* per hour is less than this minimum value. So this criterion is not satisfied, and an alternative venting design needs to be used, such as a Type B vent shown in Example 5a or a listed *chimney* liner system shown in the remainder of the example.

According to Section G2428.3.15, Table G2428.3(1) or G2428.3(2) is used for sizing corrugated metallic liners in *masonry chimneys*, with the maximum common vent capacities reduced by 20 percent. This example will be continued assuming Type B *vent connectors*.

Water Heater Vent Connector Diameter. Using Table G2428.3(1), *Vent Connector* Capacity, read down the Total *Vent* Height (*H*) column to 30 feet, and read across the 2-foot Connector Rise (*R*) row to the first *Btu*/h rating in the NAT Max column that is equal to or greater than the *water heater* input rating. The table shows that a 3-inch *vent connector* has a maximum capacity of 39,000 *Btu*/h. Although this rating is greater than the *water heater* input rating, a 3-inch *vent connector* is prohibited by Section G2428.3.17. A 4-inch *vent connector* has a maximum input rating of 70,000 *Btu*/h and is equal to the *draft hood* outlet diameter. A 4-inch *vent connector* is selected.

Furnace Vent Connector Diameter. Using Table G2428.3(1), *Vent Connector* Capacity, read down the *Vent* Height (*H*) column to 30 feet, and read across the 3-foot Connector Rise (*R*) row to the first *Btu* per hour rating in the FAN Max column that is equal to or greater than the *furnace* input rating. The 100,000 *Btu* per hour *furnace* in this example falls within this range, so a 4-inch connector is adequate.

Chimney Liner Diameter. The total input to the common vent is 135,000 *Btu* per hour. Using the Common Vent Capacity Portion of Table G2428.3(1), read down the Vent Height (*H*) column to 30 feet and across this row to find the smallest *vent* diameter in the FAN+NAT column that has a *Btu* per hour rating greater than 135,000 *Btu* per hour. The 4-inch common *vent* has a capacity of 138,000 *Btu* per hour. Reducing the maximum capacity by 20 percent (Section G2428.3.15) results in a maximum capacity for a 4-inch corrugated liner of 110,000 *Btu* per hour, less than the total input of 135,000 *Btu* per hour. So a larger liner is needed. The 5-inch common vent capacity listed in Table G2428.3(1) is 210,000 *Btu* per hour, and after reducing by 20 percent is 168,000 *Btu* per hour. Therefore, a 5-inch corrugated metal liner should be used in this example.

Single-Wall Connectors. Once it has been established that relining the *chimney* is necessary, Type B double-wall *vent connectors* are not specifically required. This example could be redone using Table G2428.3(2) for single-wall *vent connectors*. For this case, the *vent connector* and liner diameters would be the same as found above with Type B double-wall connectors.

TABLE B-1
MASONRY CHIMNEY LINER DIMENSIONS
WITH CIRCULAR EQUIVALENTS[a]

NOMINAL LINER SIZE (inches)	INSIDE DIMENSIONS OF LINER (inches)	INSIDE DIAMETER OR EQUIVALENT DIAMETER (inches)	EQUIVALENT AREA (square inches)
4 × 8	$2^1/_2 \times 6^1/_2$	4	12.2
		5	19.6
		6	28.3
		7	38.3
8 × 8	$6^3/_4 \times 6^3/_4$	7.4	42.7
		8	50.3
8 × 12	$6^1/_2 \times 10^1/_2$	9	63.6
		10	78.5
12 × 12	$9^3/_4 \times 9^3/_4$	10.4	83.3
		11	95
12 × 16	$9^1/_2 \times 13^1/_2$	11.8	107.5
		12	113.0
		14	153.9
16 × 16	$13^1/_4 \times 13^1/_4$	14.5	162.9
		15	176.7
16 × 20	13 × 17	16.2	206.1
		18	254.4
20 × 20	$16^3/_4 \times 16^3/_4$	18.2	260.2
		20	314.1
20 × 24	$16^1/_2 \times 20^1/_2$	20.1	314.2
		22	380.1
24 × 24	$20^1/_4 \times 20^1/_4$	22.1	380.1
		24	452.3
24 × 28	$20^1/_4 \times 20^1/_4$	24.1	456.2
28 × 28	$24^1/_4 \times 24^1/_4$	26.4	543.3
		27	572.5
30 × 30	$25^1/_2 \times 25^1/_2$	27.9	607
		30	706.8
30 × 36	$25^1/_2 \times 31^1/_2$	30.9	749.9
		33	855.3
36 × 36	$31^1/_2 \times 31^1/_2$	34.4	929.4
		36	1017.9

For SI: 1 inch = 25.4 mm, 1 square inch = 645.16 mm².

a. Where liner sizes differ dimensionally from those shown in Table B-1, equivalent diameters may be determined from published tables for square and rectangular ducts of equivalent carrying capacity or by other engineering methods.

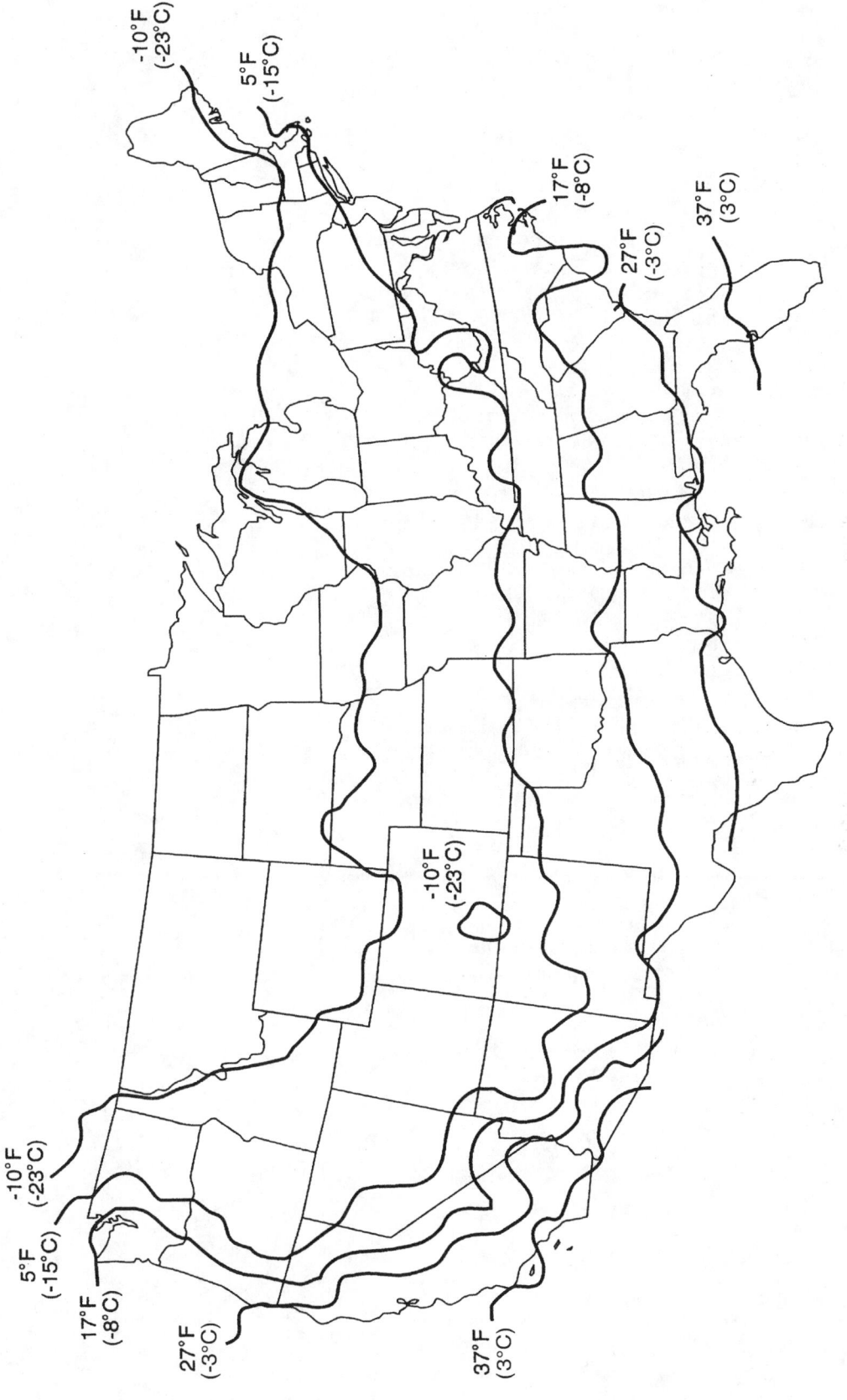

FIGURE B-19

APPENDIX C

EXIT TERMINALS OF MECHANICAL DRAFT
AND DIRECT-VENT VENTING SYSTEMS

(This appendix is informative and is not part of the code. This appendix is an excerpt from the
2009 *International Fuel Gas Code,* coordinated with the section numbering of the *International Residential Code.*)

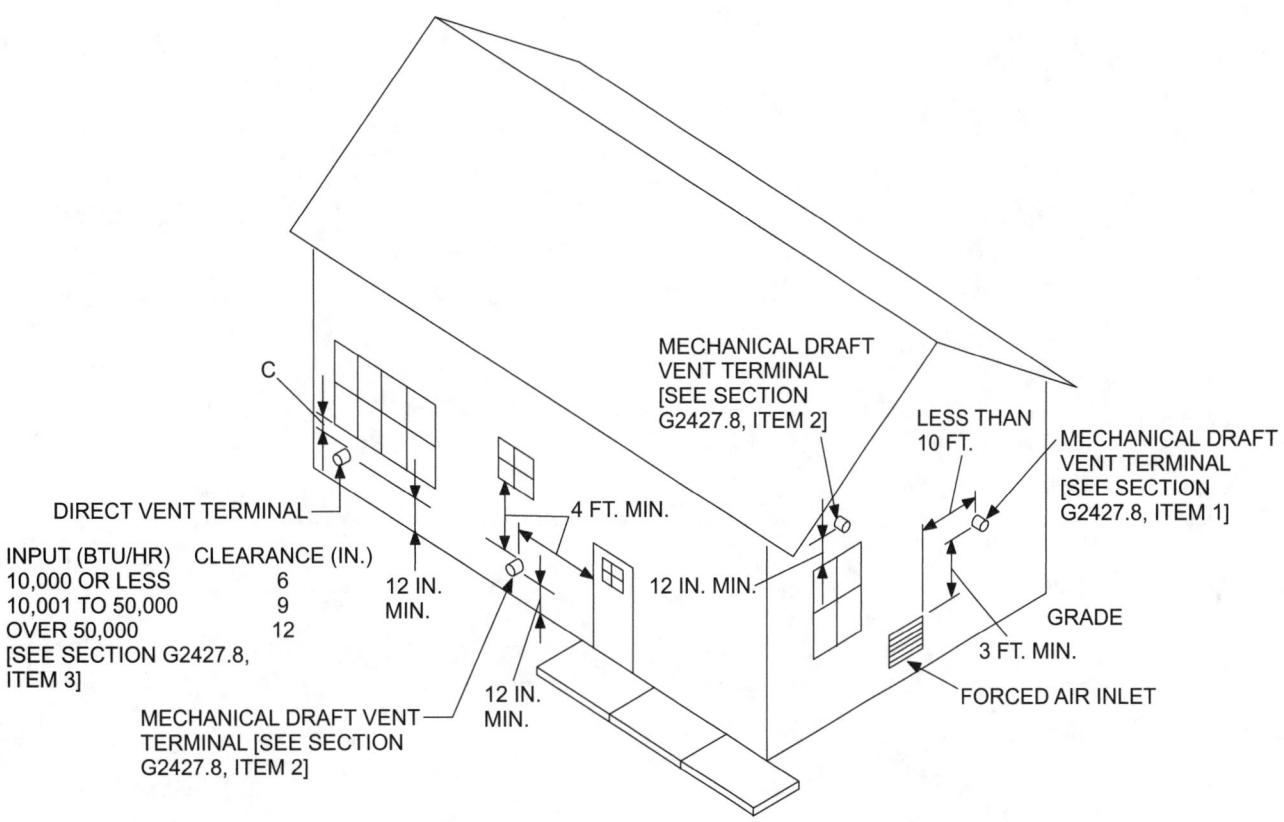

For SI: 1 inch = 25.4 mm, 1 foot = 304.8 mm, 1 British thermal unit per hour = 0.2931 W.

FIGURE C-1
EXIT TERMINALS OF MECHANICAL DRAFT AND DIRECT-VENT VENTING SYSTEMS

APPENDIX D

RECOMMENDED PROCEDURE FOR SAFETY INSPECTION OF AN EXISTING APPLIANCE INSTALLATION

(This appendix is informative and is not part of the *code*. This appendix is an excerpt from the 2009 *International Fuel Gas Code,* coordinated with the section numbering of the *International Residential Code*.)

The following procedure is intended as a guide to aid in determining that an *appliance* is properly installed and is in a safe condition for continuing use.

This procedure is intended for *central furnace* and boiler installations and may not be applicable to all installations.

(a) This procedure should be performed prior to any attempt at modification of the *appliance* or of the installation.

(b) If it is determined that there is a condition that could result in unsafe operation, shut off the *appliance* and advise the owner of the unsafe condition.

The following steps should be followed in making the safety inspection:

1. Conduct a check for gas leakage. (See Section G2417.6.)

2. Visually inspect the *venting system* for proper size and horizontal pitch and determine there is no blockage or restriction, leakage, corrosion and other deficiencies that could cause an unsafe condition.

3. Shut off all gas to the *appliance* and shut off any other fuel-gas-burning *appliance* within the same room. Use the shut-off valve in the supply line to each *appliance*.

4. Inspect *burners* and crossovers for blockage and corrosion.

5. **Furnace installations:** Inspect the heat exchanger for cracks, openings or excessive corrosion.

6. **Boiler installations:** Inspect for evidence of water or *combustion product* leaks.

7. Close all building doors and windows and all doors between the space in which the *appliance* is located and other spaces of the building that can be closed. Turn on any *clothes dryers*. Turn on any exhaust fans, such as range hoods and bathroom exhausts, so they will operate at maximum speed. Do not operate a summer exhaust fan. Close *fireplace dampers*. If, after completing Steps 8 through 13, it is believed sufficient *combustion air* is not available, refer to Section G2407 of this *code*.

8. Place the *appliance* being inspected in operation. Follow the lighting instructions. Adjust the *thermostat* so that the *appliance* will operate continuously.

9. Determine that the *pilot*, where provided, is burning properly and that the *main burner* ignition is satisfactory by interrupting and reestablishing the electrical supply to the *appliance* in any convenient manner. If the *appliance* is equipped with a continuous *pilot*, test all *pilot* safety devices to determine if they are operating properly by extinguishing the *pilot* when the *main burner* is off and determining, after 3 minutes, that the *main burner* gas does not flow upon a call for heat. If the *appliance* is not provided with a *pilot*, test for proper operation of the ignition system in accordance with the *appliance* manufacturer's lighting and operating instructions.

10. Visually determine that the *main burner* gas is burning properly (i.e., no floating, lifting or flashback). Adjust the primary air shutters as required.

If the *appliance* is equipped with high and low flame controlling or flame modulation, check for proper *main burner* operation at low flame.

11. Test for spillage at the *draft hood relief opening* after 5 minutes of *main burner* operation. Use the flame of a match or candle or smoke.

12. Turn on all other fuel-gas-burning *appliances* within the same room so they will operate at their full inputs. Follow lighting instructions for each *appliance*.

13. Repeat Steps 10 and 11 on the *appliance* being inspected.

14. Return doors, windows, exhaust fans, *fireplace dampers* and any other fuel-gas-burning *appliance* to their previous conditions of use.

15. **Furnace installations:** Check both the limit *control* and the fan *control* for proper operation. Limit *control* operation can be checked by blocking the circulating air inlet or temporarily disconnecting the electrical supply to the blower motor and determining that the limit *control* acts to shut off the *main burner* gas.

16. **Boiler installations:** Verify that the water pumps are in operating condition. Test low water cutoffs, automatic feed *controls*, pressure and temperature limit *controls*, and *relief valves* in accordance with the manufacturer's recommendations to determine that they are in operating condition.

APPENDIX E

MANUFACTURED HOUSING USED AS DWELLINGS

(The provisions contained in this appendix are not mandatory unless specifically referenced in the adopting ordinance.)

SECTION AE101
SCOPE

AE101.1 General. These provisions shall be applicable only to a *manufactured home* used as a single *dwelling unit* installed on privately owned (nonrental) lots and shall apply to the following:

1. Construction, *alteration* and repair of any foundation system which is necessary to provide for the installation of a *manufactured home* unit.

2. Construction, installation, *addition*, *alteration*, repair or maintenance of the building service *equipment* which is necessary for connecting *manufactured homes* to water, fuel, or power supplies and sewage systems.

3. *Alterations*, *additions* or repairs to existing *manufactured homes*. The construction, *alteration*, moving, demolition, repair and use of accessory buildings and structures and their building service *equipment* shall comply with the requirements of the codes adopted by this *jurisdiction*.

These provisions shall not be applicable to the design and construction of *manufactured homes* and shall not be deemed to authorize either modifications or *additions* to *manufactured homes* where otherwise prohibited.

Exception: In addition to these provisions, new and replacement *manufactured homes* to be located in flood hazard areas as established in Table R301.2(1) of the *International Residential Code* shall meet the applicable requirements of Section R322 of the *International Residential Code*.

SECTION AE102
APPLICATION TO EXISTING MANUFACTURED HOMES AND BUILDING SERVICE EQUIPMENT

AE102.1 General. *Manufactured homes* and their building service *equipment* to which *additions*, *alterations* or repairs are made shall comply with all the requirements of these provisions for new facilities, except as specifically provided in this section.

AE102.2 Additions, alterations or repairs. *Additions* made to a *manufactured home* shall conform to one of the following:

1. Be certified under the National Manufactured Housing Construction and Safety Standards Act of 1974 (42 U.S.C. Section 5401, et seq.).

2. Be designed and constructed to conform with the applicable provisions of the National Manufactured Housing Construction and Safety Standards Act of 1974 (42 U.S.C. Section 5401, et seq.).

3. Be designed and constructed in conformance with the code adopted by this *jurisdiction*.

Additions shall be structurally separated from the *manufactured home*.

Exception: A structural separation need not be provided when structural calculations are provided to justify the omission of such separation.

Alterations or repairs may be made to any *manufactured home* or to its building service *equipment* without requiring the existing *manufactured home* or its building service *equipment* to comply with all the requirements of these provisions, provided the *alteration* or repair conforms to that required for new construction, and provided further that no hazard to life, health or safety will be created by such *additions*, *alterations* or repairs.

Alterations or repairs to an existing *manufactured home* which are nonstructural and do not adversely affect any structural member or any part of the building or structure having required fire protection may be made with materials equivalent to those of which the *manufactured home* structure is constructed, subject to approval by the *building official*.

Exception: The installation or replacement of glass shall be required for new installations.

Minor *additions*, *alterations* and repairs to existing building service *equipment* installations may be made in accordance with the codes in effect at the time the original installation was made subject to approval of the *building official*, and provided such *additions*, *alterations* and repairs will not cause the existing building service *equipment* to become unsafe, insanitary or overloaded.

AE102.3 Existing installations. Building service *equipment* lawfully in existence at the time of the adoption of the applicable codes may have their use, maintenance or repair continued if the use, maintenance or repair is in accordance with the original design and no hazard to life, health or property has been created by such building service *equipment*.

AE102.4 Existing occupancy. *Manufactured homes* which are in existence at the time of the adoption of these provisions may have their existing use or occupancy continued if such use or occupancy was legal at the time of the adoption of these provisions, provided such continued use is not dangerous to life, health and safety.

The use or occupancy of any existing *manufactured home* shall not be changed unless evidence satisfactory to the *building official* is provided to show compliance with all applicable provisions of the codes adopted by this *jurisdiction*. Upon any change in use or occupancy, the *manufactured home* shall cease to be classified as such within the intent of these provisions.

AE102.5 Maintenance. All *manufactured homes* and their building service *equipment*, existing and new, and all parts thereof shall be maintained in a safe and sanitary condition. All device or safeguards which are required by applicable codes or by the *Manufactured Home* Standards shall be maintained in conformance with the code or standard under which it was installed. The owner or the owner's designated agent shall be responsible for the maintenance of *manufactured homes*, accessory buildings, structures and their building service *equipment*. To determine compliance with this subsection, the *building official* may cause any *manufactured home*, accessory building or structure to be reinspected.

AE102.6 Relocation. *Manufactured homes* which are to be relocated within this *jurisdiction* shall comply with these provisions.

SECTION AE201
DEFINITIONS

AE201.1 General. For the purpose of these provisions, certain abbreviations, terms, phrases, words and their derivatives shall be construed as defined or specified herein.

ACCESSORY BUILDING. Any building or structure, or portion thereto, located on the same property as a *manufactured home* which does not qualify as a *manufactured home* as defined herein.

BUILDING SERVICE EQUIPMENT. Refers to the plumbing, mechanical and electrical *equipment* including piping, wiring, fixtures and other accessories which provide sanitation, lighting, heating ventilation, cooling, fire protection and facilities essential for the habitable occupancy of a *manufactured home* or accessory building or structure for its designated use and occupancy.

MANUFACTURED HOME. A structure transportable in one or more sections which, in the traveling mode, is 8 body feet (2438 body mm) or more in width or 40 body feet (12 192 body mm) or more in length or, when erected on site, is 320 or more square feet (30 m²), and which is built on a permanent chassis and designed to be used as a *dwelling* with or without a permanent foundation when connected to the required utilities, and includes the plumbing, heating, air-conditioning and electrical systems contained therein; except that such term shall include any structure which meets all the requirements of this paragraph except the size requirements and with respect to which the manufacturer voluntarily files a certification required by the secretary (HUD) and complies with the standards established under this title.

For mobile homes built prior to June 15, 1976, a *label* certifying compliance to the Standard for Mobile Homes, NFPA 501, ANSI 119.1, in effect at the time of manufacture is required. For the purpose of these provisions, a mobile home shall be considered a *manufactured home*.

MANUFACTURED HOME INSTALLATION. Construction which is required for the installation of a *manufactured home*, including the construction of the foundation system, required structural connections thereto and the installation of on-site water, gas, electrical and sewer systems and connections thereto which are necessary for the normal operation of the *manufactured home*.

MANUFACTURED HOME STANDARDS. The *Manufactured Home* Construction and Safety Standards as promulgated by the United States Department of Housing and Urban Development.

PRIVATELY OWNED (NONRENTAL) LOT. A parcel of real estate outside of a *manufactured home* rental community (park) where the land and the *manufactured home* to be installed thereon are held in common ownership.

SECTION AE301
PERMITS

AE301.1 Initial installation. A *manufactured home* shall not be installed on a foundation system, reinstalled or altered without first obtaining a *permit* from the *building official*. A separate *permit* shall be required for each *manufactured home* installation. When *approved* by the *building official*, such *permit* may include accessory buildings and structures and their building service *equipment* when the accessory buildings or structures will be constructed in conjunction with the *manufactured home* installation.

AE301.2 Additions, alterations and repairs to a manufactured home. A *permit* shall be obtained to alter, remodel, repair or add accessory buildings or structures to a *manufactured home* subsequent to its initial installation. *Permit* issuance and fees therefor shall be in conformance with the codes applicable to the type of work involved.

An *addition* made to a *manufactured home* as defined in these provisions shall comply with these provisions.

AE301.3 Accessory buildings. Except as provided in Section AE301.1, *permits* shall be required for all accessory buildings and structures and their building service *equipment*. *Permit* issuance and fees therefor shall be in conformance with the codes applicable to the types of work involved.

AE301.4 Exempted work. A *permit* shall not be required for the types of work specifically exempted by the applicable codes. Exemption from the *permit* requirements of any of said codes shall not be deemed to grant authorization for any work to be done in violation of the provisions of said codes or any other laws or ordinances of this *jurisdiction*.

SECTION AE302
APPLICATION FOR PERMIT

AE302.1 Application. To obtain a *manufactured home* installation *permit*, the applicant shall first file an application in writing on a form furnished by the *building official* for that purpose. At the option of the *building official*, every such application shall:

1. Identify and describe the work to be covered by the *permit* for which application is made.

2. Describe the land on which the proposed work is to be done by legal description, street address or similar description that will readily identify and definitely locate the proposed building or work.

3. Indicate the use or occupancy for which the proposed work is intended.

4. Be accompanied by plans, diagrams, computations and specifications and other data as required in Section AE302.2.

5. Be accompanied by a soil investigation when required by Section AE502.2.

6. State the valuation of any new building or structure or any *addition*, remodeling or *alteration* to an existing building.

7. Be signed by permittee, or permittee's authorized agent, who may be required to submit evidence to indicate such authority.

8. Give such other data and information as may be required by the *building official*.

AE302.2 Plans and specifications. Plans, engineering calculations, diagrams and other data as required by the *building official* shall be submitted in not less than two sets with each application for a *permit*. The *building official* may require plans, computations and specifications to be prepared and designed by an engineer or architect licensed by the state to practice as such.

Where no unusual site conditions exist, the *building official* may accept *approved* standard foundation plans and details in conjunction with the manufacturer's *approved* installation instructions without requiring the submittal of engineering calculations.

AE302.3 Information on plans and specifications. Plans and specifications shall be drawn to scale on substantial paper or cloth and shall be of sufficient clarity to indicate the location, nature and extent of the work proposed and shown in detail that it will conform to the provisions of these provisions and all relevant laws, ordinances, rules and regulations. The *building official* shall determine what information is required on plans and specifications to ensure compliance.

SECTION AE303
PERMITS ISSUANCE

AE303.1 Issuance. The application, plans and specifications and other data filed by an applicant for *permit* shall be reviewed by the *building official*. Such plans may be reviewed by other departments of this *jurisdiction* to verify compliance with any applicable laws under their *jurisdiction*. If the *building official* finds that the work described in an application for a *permit* and the plans, specifications and other data filed therewith conform to the requirements of these provisions and other data filed therewith conform to the requirements of these provisions and other pertinent codes, laws and ordinances, and that the fees specified in Section AE304 have been paid, the *building official* shall issue a *permit* therefor to the applicant.

When the *building official* issues the *permit* where plans are required, the *building official* shall endorse in writing or stamp the plans and specifications *APPROVED*. Such *approved* plans and specifications shall not be changed, modified or altered without authorization from the *building official*, and all work shall be done in accordance with the *approved* plans.

AE303.2 Retention of plans. One set of *approved* plans and specifications shall be returned to the applicant and shall be kept on the site of the building or work at all times during which the work authorized thereby is in progress. One set of *approved* plans, specification and computations shall be retained by the *building official* until final approval of the work.

AE303.3 Validity of permit. The issuance of a *permit* or approval of plans and specifications shall not be construed to be a *permit* for, or an approval of, any violation of any of the provisions of these provisions or other pertinent codes of any other ordinance of the *jurisdiction*. No *permit* presuming to give authority to violate or cancel these provisions shall be valid.

The issuance of a *permit* based on plans, specifications and other data shall not prevent the *building official* from thereafter requiring the correction of errors in said plans, specifications and other data, or from preventing building operations being carried on thereunder when in violation of these provisions or of any other ordinances of this *jurisdiction*.

AE303.4 Expiration. Every *permit* issued by the *building official* under these provisions shall expire by limitation and become null and void if the work authorized by such *permit* is not commenced within 180 days from the date of such *permit*, or if the work authorized by such *permit* is suspended or abandoned at any time after the work is commenced for a period of 180 days. Before such work can be recommenced, a new *permit* shall be first obtained, and the fee therefor shall be one-half the amount required for a new *permit* for such work, provided no changes have been made or will be made in the original plans and specifications for such work, and provided further that such suspension or abandonment has not exceeded one year. In order to renew action on a *permit* after expiration, the permittee shall pay a new full *permit* fee.

Any permittee holding an unexpired *permit* may apply for an extension of the time within which work may commence under that *permit* when the permittee is unable to commence work within the time required by this section for good and satisfactory reasons. The *building official* may extend the time for action by the permittee for a period not exceeding 180 days upon written request by the permittee showing that circumstances beyond the control of the permittee have prevented action from being taken. No *permit* shall be extended more than once.

AE303.5 Suspension or revocation. The *building official* may, in writing, suspend or revoke a *permit* issued under these provisions whenever the *permit* is issued in error or on the basis of incorrect information supplied, or in violation of any ordinance or regulation or any of these provisions.

SECTION AE304
FEES

AE304.1 Permit fees. The fee for each *manufactured home* installation *permit* shall be established by the *building official*.

When *permit* fees are to be based on the value or valuation of the work to be performed, the determination of value or valuation under these provisions shall be made by the *building official*. The value to be used shall be the total value of all work required for the *manufactured home* installation plus the total value of all work required for the construction of accessory buildings and structures for which the *permit* is issued as well as all finish work, painting, roofing, electrical, plumbing, heating, air conditioning, elevators, fire-extinguishing systems and any other permanent *equipment* which is a part of the accessory building or structure. The value of the *manufactured home* itself shall not be included.

AE304.2 Plan review fees. When a plan or other data are required to be submitted by Section AE302.2, a plan review fee shall be paid at the time of submitting plans and specifications for review. Said plan review fee shall be as established by the *building official*. Where plans are incomplete or changed so as to require additional plan review, an additional plan review fee shall be charged at a rate as established by the *building official*.

AE304.3 Other provisions.

AE304.3.1 Expiration of plan review. Applications for which no *permit* is issued within 180 days following the date of application shall expire by limitation, and plans and other data submitted for review may thereafter be returned to the applicant or destroyed by the *building official*. The *building official* may extend the time for action by the applicant for a period not exceeding 180 days upon request by the applicant showing that circumstances beyond the control of the applicant have prevented action from being taken. No application shall be extended more than once. In order to renew action on an application after expiration, the applicant shall resubmit plans and pay a new plan review fee.

AE304.3.2 Investigation fees: work without a permit.

AE304.3.2.1 Investigation. Whenever any work for which a *permit* is required by these provisions has been commenced without first obtaining said *permit*, a special investigation shall be made before a *permit* may be issued for such work.

AE304.3.2.2 Fee. An investigation fee, in addition to the *permit* fee, shall be collected whether or not a *permit* is then or subsequently issued. The investigation fee shall be equal to the amount of the *permit* fee required. The minimum investigation fee shall be the same as the minimum fee established by the *building official*. The payment of such investigation fee shall not exempt any person from compliance with all other provisions of either these provisions or other pertinent codes or from any penalty prescribed by law.

E304.3.3 Fee refunds.

AE304.3.3.1 Permit fee erroneously paid or collected. The *building official* may authorize the refunding of any fee paid hereunder which was erroneously paid or collected.

AE304.3.3.2 Permit fee paid when no work done. The *building official* may authorize the refunding of not more than 80 percent of the *permit* fee paid when no work has been done under a *permit* issued in accordance with these provisions.

AE304.3.3.3 Plan review fee. The *building official* may authorize the refunding of not more than 80 percent of the plan review fee paid when an application for a *permit*

for which a plan review fee has been paid is withdrawn or canceled before any plan reviewing is done.

The *building official* shall not authorize the refunding of any fee paid except upon written application by the original permittee not later than 180 days after the date of the fee payment.

SECTION AE305
INSPECTIONS

AE305.1 General. All construction or work for which a *manufactured home* installation *permit* is required shall be subject to inspection by the *building official*, and certain types of construction shall have continuous inspection by special inspectors as specified in Section AE306. A survey of the *lot* may be required by the *building official* to verify that the structure is located in accordance with the *approved* plans.

It shall be the duty of the *permit* applicant to cause the work to be accessible and exposed for inspection purposes. Neither the *building official* nor this *jurisdiction* shall be liable for expense entailed in the removal or replacement of any material required to allow inspection.

AE305.2 Inspection requests. It shall be the duty of the person doing the work authorized by a *manufactured home* installation *permit* to notify the *building official* that such work is ready for inspection. The *building official* may require that every request for inspection be filed at least one working day before such inspection is desired. Such request may be in writing or by telephone at the option of the *building official*.

It shall be the duty of the person requesting any inspections required either by these provisions or other applicable codes to provide access to and means for proper inspection of such work.

AE305.3 Inspection record card. Work requiring a *manufactured home* installation *permit* shall not be commenced until the *permit* holder or the *permit* holder's agent shall have posted an inspection record card in a conspicuous place on the premises and in such position as to allow the *building official* conveniently to make the required entries thereon regarding inspection of the work. This card shall be maintained in such position by the *permit* holder until final approval has been issued by the *building official*.

AE305.4 Approval required. Work shall not be done on any part of the *manufactured home* installation beyond the point indicated in each successive inspection without first obtaining the approval of the *building official*. Such approval shall be given only after an inspection has been made of each successive step in the construction as indicated by each of the inspections required in Section AE305.5. There shall be a final inspection and approval of the *manufactured home* installation, including connections to its building service *equipment*, when completed and ready for occupancy or use.

AE305.5 Required inspections.

AE305.5.1 Structural inspections for the manufactured home installation. Reinforcing steel or structural framework of any part of any *manufactured home* foundation system shall not be covered or concealed without first obtaining the approval of the *building official*. The *building official*, upon notification from the *permit* holder or the *permit* holder's agent, shall make the following inspections and shall either approve that portion of the construction as completed or shall notify the *permit* holder or the *permit* holder's agent wherein the same fails to comply with these provisions or other applicable codes:

1. Foundation inspection: To be made after excavations for footings are completed and any required reinforcing steel is in place. For concrete foundations, any required forms shall be in place prior to inspection. All materials for the foundation shall be on the job, except where concrete from a central mixing plant (commonly termed "transit mixed") is to be used, the concrete materials need not be on the job. Where the foundation is to be constructed of *approved* treated wood, additional framing inspections as required by the building official may be required.

2. Concrete slab or under-floor inspection: To be made after all in-slab or underfloor building service *equipment*, conduit, piping accessories and other ancillary *equipment* items are in place but before any concrete is poured or the *manufactured home* is installed.

3. Anchorage inspection: To be made after the *manufactured home* has been installed and permanently anchored.

AE305.5.2 Structural inspections for accessory building and structures. Inspections for accessory buildings and structures shall be made as set forth in this code.

AE305.5.3 Building service equipment inspections. All building service *equipment* which is required as a part of a *manufactured home* installation, including accessory buildings and structures authorized by the same *permit*, shall be inspected by the building official. Building service *equipment* shall be inspected and tested as required by the applicable codes. Such inspections and testing shall be limited to site construction and shall not include building service *equipment* which is a part of the *manufactured home* itself. No portion of any building service *equipment* intended to be concealed by any permanent portion of the construction shall be concealed until inspected and *approved*. Building service *equipment* shall not be connected to the water, fuel or power supply or sewer system until authorized by the building official.

AE305.5.4 Final inspection. When finish grading and the *manufactured home* installation, including the installation of all required building service *equipment*, is completed and the *manufactured home* is ready for occupancy, a final inspection shall be made.

AE305.6 Other inspections. In addition to the called inspections specified above, the building official may make or require other inspections of any construction work to as certain compliance with these provisions or other codes and laws which are enforced by the code enforcement agency.

SECTION AE306
SPECIAL INSPECTIONS

AE306.1 General. In addition to the inspections required by Section AE305, the building official may require the owner to employ a special inspector during construction of specific types of work as described in this code.

SECTION AE307
UTILITY SERVICE

AE307.1 General. Utility service shall not be provided to any building service *equipment* which is regulated by these provisions or other applicable codes and for which a *manufactured home* installation *permit* is required by these provisions until *approved* by the building official.

SECTION AE401
OCCUPANCY CLASSIFICATION

AE401.1 Manufactured homes. A *manufactured home* shall be limited in use to use as a single *dwelling unit*.

AE401.2 Accessory buildings. Accessory buildings shall be classified as to occupancy by the building official as set forth in this code.

SECTION AE402
LOCATION ON PROPERTY

AE402.1 General. *Manufactured homes* and accessory buildings shall be located on the property in accordance with applicable codes and ordinances of this *jurisdiction*.

SECTION AE501
DESIGN

AE501.1 General. A *manufactured home* shall be installed on a foundation system which is designed and constructed to sustain within the stress limitations specified in this code and all loads specified in this code.

> **Exception:** When specifically authorized by the building official, foundation and anchorage systems which are constructed in accordance with the methods specified in Section AE600 of these provisions, or in the United States Department of Housing and Urban Development Handbook, *Permanent Foundations for Manufactured Housing,* 1984 Edition, Draft, shall be deemed to meet the requirements of this Appendix E.

AE501.2 Manufacturer's installation instructions. The installation instructions as provided by the manufacturer of the *manufactured home* shall be used to determine permissible points of support for vertical loads and points of attachment for anchorage systems used to resist horizontal and uplift forces.

AE501.3 Rationality. Any system or method of construction to be used shall admit to a rational analysis in accordance with well-established principles of mechanics.

SECTION AE502
FOUNDATION SYSTEMS

AE502.1 General. Foundation systems designed and constructed in accordance with this section may be considered as a permanent installation.

AE502.2 Soil classification. The classification of the soil at each *manufactured home* site shall be determined when required by the *building official*. The *building official* may require that the determination be made by an engineer or architect licensed by the state to conduct soil investigations.

The classification shall be based on observation and any necessary tests of the materials disclosed by borings or excavations made in appropriate locations. Additional studies may be necessary to evaluate soil strength, the effect of moisture variation on soil-bearing capacity, compressibility and expansiveness.

When required by the *building official*, the soil classification design bearing capacity and lateral pressure shall be shown on the plans.

AE502.3 Footings and foundations. Footings and foundations, unless otherwise specifically provided, shall be constructed of materials specified by this code for the intended use and in all cases shall extend below the frost line. Footings of concrete and masonry shall be of solid material. Foundations supporting untreated wood shall extend at least 8 inches (203 mm) above the adjacent finish *grade*. Footings shall have a minimum depth below finished *grade* of 12 inches (305 mm) unless a greater depth is recommended by a foundation investigation.

Piers and bearing walls shall be supported on masonry or concrete foundations or piles, or other *approved* foundation systems which shall be of sufficient capacity to support all loads.

AE502.4 Foundation design. When a design is provided, the foundation system shall be designed in accordance with the applicable structural provisions of this code and shall be designed to minimize differential settlement. Where a design is not provided, the minimum foundation requirements shall be as set forth in this code.

AE502.5 Drainage. Provisions shall be made for the control and drainage of surface water away from the *manufactured home*.

AE502.6 Under-floor clearances—ventilation and access. A minimum clearance of 12 inches (305 mm) shall be maintained beneath the lowest member of the floor support framing system. Clearances from the bottom of wood floor joists or perimeter joists shall be as specified in this code.

Under-floor spaces shall be ventilated with openings as specified in this code. If combustion air for one or more heat-producing *appliances* is taken from within the under-floor spaces, ventilation shall be adequate for proper *appliance* operation.

Under-floor access openings shall be provided. Such openings shall be not less than 18 inches (457 mm) in any dimension and not less than 3 square feet (0.279 m²) in area and shall be located so that any water supply and sewer drain connections located under the *manufactured home* are accessible.

SECTION AE503
SKIRTING AND PERIMETER ENCLOSURES

AE503.1 Skirting and permanent perimeter enclosures. Skirting and permanent perimeter enclosures shall be installed only where specifically required by other laws or ordinances. Skirting, when installed, shall be of material suitable for exterior exposure and contact with the ground. Permanent perimeter enclosures shall be constructed of materials as required by this code for regular foundation construction.

Skirting shall be installed in accordance with the skirting manufacturer's installation instructions. Skirting shall be adequately secured to assure stability, to minimize vibration and susceptibility to wind damage, and to compensate for possible frost heave.

AE503.2 Retaining walls. Where retaining walls are used as a permanent perimeter enclosure, they shall resist the lateral displacements of soil or other materials and shall conform to this code as specified for foundation walls. Retaining walls and foundation walls shall be constructed of *approved* treated wood, concrete, masonry or other *approved* materials or combination of materials as for foundations as specified in this code. Siding materials shall extend below the top of the exterior of the retaining or foundation wall or the joint between siding and enclosure wall shall be flashed in accordance with this code.

SECTION AE504
STRUCTURAL ADDITIONS

AE504.1 General. Accessory buildings shall not be structurally supported by or attached to a *manufactured home* unless engineering calculations are submitted to substantiate any proposed structural connection.

> **Exception:** The *building official* may waive the submission of engineering calculations if it is found that the nature of the work applied for is such that engineering calculations are not necessary to show conformance to these provisions.

SECTION AE505
BUILDING SERVICE EQUIPMENT

AE505.1 General. The installation, *alteration*, repair, replacement, *addition* to or maintenance of the building service *equipment* within the *manufactured home* shall conform to regulations set forth in the *Manufactured Home* Standards. Such work which is located outside the *manufactured home* shall comply with the applicable codes adopted by this *jurisdiction*.

SECTION AE506
EXITS

AE506.1 Site development. Exterior stairways and ramps which provide egress to the public way shall comply with applicable provisions of this code.

AE506.2 Accessory buildings. Every accessory building or portion thereof shall be provided with exits as required by this code.

SECTION AE507
OCCUPANCY, FIRE SAFETY AND ENERGY CONSERVATION STANDARDS

AE507.1 General. *Alterations* made to a *manufactured home* subsequent to its initial installation shall conform to the occupancy, fire-safety and energy conservation requirements set forth in the *Manufactured Home* Standards.

SECTION AE600
SPECIAL REQUIREMENTS FOR FOUNDATION SYSTEMS

AE600.1 General. Section AE600 is applicable only when specifically authorized by the *building official*.

SECTION AE601
FOOTINGS AND FOUNDATIONS

AE601.1 General. The capacity of individual load-bearing piers and their footings shall be sufficient to sustain all loads specified in this code within the stress limitations specified in this code. Footings, unless otherwise *approved* by the *building official*, shall be placed level on firm, undisturbed soil or an engineered fill which is free of organic material, such as weeds and grasses. Where used, an engineered fill shall provide a minimum load-bearing capacity of not less than 1,000 psf (48 kN/m²). Continuous footings shall conform to the requirements of this code. Section AE502 of these provisions shall apply to footings and foundations constructed under the provisions of this section.

SECTION AE602
PIER CONSTRUCTION

AE602.1 General. Piers shall be designed and constructed to distribute loads evenly. Multiple section homes may have concentrated roof loads which will require special consideration. Load-bearing piers may be constructed utilizing one of the methods listed below. Such piers shall be considered to resist only vertical forces acting in a downward direction. They shall not be considered as providing any resistance to horizontal loads induced by wind or earthquake forces.

1. A prefabricated load-bearing device that is listed and *labeled* for the intended use.

2. Mortar shall comply with ASTM C 270 Type M, S or N; this may consist of one part portland cement, one-half part hydrated lime and four parts sand by volume. Lime shall not be used with plastic or waterproof cement.

3. A cast-in-place concrete pier with concrete having specified compressive strength at 28 days of 2,500 psi (17 225 kPa).

Alternate materials and methods of construction may be used for piers which have been designed by an engineer or architect licensed by the state to practice as such.

Caps and leveling spacers may be used for leveling of the *manufactured home*. Spacing of piers shall be as specified in the manufacturer's installation instructions, if available, or by an *approved* designer.

SECTION AE603
HEIGHT OF PIERS

AE603.1 General. Piers constructed as indicated in Section AE602 may have heights as follows:

1. Except for corner piers, piers 36 inches (914 mm) or less in height may be constructed of masonry units, placed with cores or cells vertically. Piers shall be installed with their long dimension at right angles to the main frame member they support and shall have a minimum cross-sectional area of 128 square inches (82 560 mm²). Piers shall be capped with minimum 4-inch (102 mm) *solid masonry* units or equivalent.

2. Piers between 36 and 80 inches (914 mm and 2032 mm) in height and all corner piers over 24 inches (610 mm) in height shall be at least 16 inches by 16 inches (406 mm by 406 mm) consisting of interlocking masonry units and shall be fully capped with minimum 4-inch (102 mm) *solid masonry* units or equivalent.

3. Piers over 80 inches (2032 mm) in height may be constructed in accordance with the provisions of Item 2 above, provided the piers shall be filled solid with grout and reinforced with four continuous No. 5 bars. One bar shall be placed in each corner cell of hollow masonry unit piers or in each corner of the grouted space of piers constructed of *solid masonry* units.

4. Cast-in-place concrete piers meeting the same size and height limitations of Items 1, 2 and 3 above may be substituted for piers constructed of masonry units.

SECTION AE604
ANCHORAGE INSTALLATIONS

AE604.1 Ground anchors. Ground anchors shall be designed and installed to transfer the anchoring loads to the ground. The load-carrying portion of the ground anchors shall be installed to the full depth called for by the manufacturer's installation directions and shall extend below the established frost line into undisturbed soil.

Manufactured ground anchors shall be listed and installed in accordance with the terms of their listing and the anchor manufacturer's instructions and shall include means of attachment of ties meeting the requirements of Section AE605. Ground anchor manufacturer's installation instructions shall include the amount of preload required and load capacity in various types of soil. These instructions shall include tensioning adjustments which may be needed to prevent damage to the *manufactured home*, particularly damage that can be caused by frost heave. Each ground anchor shall be marked with the manufacturer's identification and listed model identification number which shall be visible after installation. Instructions shall accompany each listed ground anchor specifying the types of soil for which the anchor is suitable under the requirements of this section.

Each *approved* ground anchor, when installed, shall be capable of resisting an allowable working load at least equal to 3,150 pounds (14 kN) in the direction of the tie plus a 50 percent overload [4,725 pounds (21 kN) total] without failure. Failure shall be considered to have occurred when the anchor moves more than 2 inches (51 mm) at a load of 4,725 pounds (21 kN) in the direction of the tie installation. Those ground anchors which are designed to be installed so that loads on the anchor are other than direct withdrawal shall be designed and installed to resist an applied design load of 3,150 pounds (14 kN) at 40 to 50 degrees from vertical or within the angle limitations specified by the home manufacturer without displacing the tie end of the anchor more than 4 inches (102 mm) horizontally. Anchors designed for connection of multiple ties shall be capable of resisting the combined working load and overload consistent with the intent expressed herein.

When it is proposed to use ground anchors and the *building official* has reason to believe that the soil characteristics at a given site are such as to render the use of ground anchors advisable, or when there is doubt regarding the ability of the ground anchors to obtain their listed capacity, the *building official* may require that a representative field installation be made at the site in question and tested to demonstrate ground anchor capacity. The *building official* shall approve the test procedures.

AE604.2 Anchoring equipment. Anchoring *equipment*, when installed as a permanent installation, shall be capable of resisting all loads as specified within these provisions. When the stabilizing system is designed by an engineer or architect licensed by the state to practice as such, alternative designs may be used, providing the anchoring *equipment* to be used is capable of withstanding a load equal to 1.5 times the calculated load. All anchoring *equipment* shall be listed and *labeled* as being capable of meeting the requirements of these provisions. Anchors as specified in this code may be attached to the main frame of the *manufactured home* by an *approved* $^3/_{16}$-inch-thick (4.76 mm) slotted steel plate anchoring device. Other anchoring devices or methods meeting the requirements of these provisions may be permitted when *approved* by the *building official*.

Anchoring systems shall be so installed as to be permanent. Anchoring *equipment* shall be so designed to prevent self-disconnection with no hook ends used.

AE604.3 Resistance to weather deterioration. All anchoring *equipment*, tension devices and ties shall have a resistance to deterioration as required by this code.

AE604.4 Tensioning devices. Tensioning devices, such as turnbuckles or yoke-type fasteners, shall be ended with clevis or welded eyes.

SECTION AE605
TIES, MATERIALS AND INSTALLATION

AE605.1 General. Steel strapping, cable, chain or other *approved* materials shall be used for ties. All ties shall be fastened to ground anchors and drawn tight with turnbuckles or other adjustable tensioning devices or devices supplied with the ground anchor. Tie materials shall be capable of resisting an allowable working load of 3,150 pounds (14 kN) with no more than 2 percent elongation and shall withstand a 50 percent overload [4,750 pounds (21 kN)]. Ties shall comply with the weathering requirements of Section AE604.3. Ties shall connect the ground anchor and the main structural frame. Ties shall not connect to steel outrigger beams which fasten to and intersect the main structural frame unless specifically stated in the manufacturer's installation instructions. Connection of cable ties to main frame members shall be $^5/_8$-inch (15.9 mm) closed-eye bolts affixed to the frame member in an *approved* manner. Cable ends shall be secured with at least two U-bolt cable clamps with the "U" portion of the clamp installed on the short (dead) end of the cable to assure strength equal to that required by this section.

Wood floor support systems shall be fixed to perimeter foundation walls in accordance with provisions of this code. The minimum number of ties required per side shall be sufficient to resist the wind load stated in this code. Ties shall be evenly spaced as practicable along the length of the *manufactured home* with the distance from each end of the home and the tie nearest that end not exceeding 8 feet (2438 mm). When continuous straps are provided as vertical ties, such ties shall be positioned at rafters and studs. Where a vertical tie and diagonal tie are located at the same place, both ties may be connected to a single anchor, provided the anchor used is capable of carrying both loadings. Multisection *manufactured homes* require diagonal ties only. Diagonal ties shall be installed on the exterior main frame and slope to the exterior at an angle of 40 to 50 degrees from the vertical or within the angle limitations specified by the home manufacturer. Vertical ties which are not continuous over the top of the *manufactured home* shall be attached to the main frame.

SECTION AE606
REFERENCED STANDARDS

ASTMC 270-04 Specification for Mortar
for Unit Masonry AE602

NFPA 501-03 Standard on Manufactured
Housing AE201

RADON CONTROL METHODS

(The provisions contained in this appendix are not mandatory unless specifically referenced in the adopting ordinance.)

SECTION AF101
SCOPE

AF101.1 General. This appendix contains requirements for new construction in *jurisdictions* where radon-resistant construction is required.

Inclusion of this appendix by *jurisdictions* shall be determined through the use of locally available data or determination of Zone 1 designation in Figure AF101.

SECTION AF102
DEFINITIONS

AF102.1 General. For the purpose of these requirements, the terms used shall be defined as follows:

SUBSLAB DEPRESSURIZATION SYSTEM (Passive). A system designed to achieve lower sub-slab air pressure relative to indoor air pressure by use of a vent pipe routed through the *conditioned space* of a building and connecting the sub-slab area with outdoor air, thereby relying on the convective flow of air upward in the vent to draw air from beneath the slab.

SUBSLAB DEPRESSURIZATION SYSTEM (Active). A system designed to achieve lower sub-slab air pressure relative to indoor air pressure by use of a fan-powered vent drawing air from beneath the slab.

DRAIN TILE LOOP. A continuous length of drain tile or perforated pipe extending around all or part of the internal or external perimeter of a *basement* or crawl space footing.

RADON GAS. A naturally-occurring, chemically inert, radioactive gas that is not detectable by human senses. As a gas, it can move readily through particles of soil and rock and can accumulate under the slabs and foundations of homes where it can easily enter into the living space through construction cracks and openings.

SOIL-GAS-RETARDER. A continuous membrane of 6-mil (0.15 mm) polyethylene or other equivalent material used to retard the flow of soil gases into a building.

SUBMEMBRANE DEPRESSURIZATION SYSTEM. A system designed to achieve lower-sub-membrane air pressure relative to crawl space air pressure by use of a vent drawing air from beneath the soil-gas-retarder membrane.

SECTION AF103
REQUIREMENTS

AF103.1 General. The following construction techniques are intended to resist radon entry and prepare the building for post-construction radon mitigation, if necessary (see Figure AF102). These techniques are required in areas where designated by the *jurisdiction*.

AF103.2 Subfloor preparation. A layer of gas-permeable material shall be placed under all concrete slabs and other floor systems that directly contact the ground and are within the walls of the living spaces of the building, to facilitate future installation of a sub-slab depressurization system, if needed. The gas-permeable layer shall consist of one of the following:

1. A uniform layer of clean aggregate, a minimum of 4 inches (102 mm) thick. The aggregate shall consist of material that will pass through a 2-inch (51 mm) sieve and be retained by a $^{1}/_{4}$-inch (6.4 mm) sieve.

2. A uniform layer of sand (native or fill), a minimum of 4 inches (102 mm) thick, overlain by a layer or strips of geotextile drainage matting designed to allow the lateral flow of soil gases.

3. Other materials, systems or floor designs with demonstrated capability to permit depressurization across the entire sub-floor area.

AF103.3 Soil-gas-retarder. A minimum 6-mil (0.15 mm) [or 3-mil (0.075 mm) cross-laminated] polyethylene or equivalent flexible sheeting material shall be placed on top of the gas-permeable layer prior to casting the slab or placing the floor assembly to serve as a soil-gas-retarder by bridging any cracks that develop in the slab or floor assembly and to prevent concrete from entering the void spaces in the aggregate base material. The sheeting shall cover the entire floor area with separate sections of sheeting lapped at least 12 inches (305 mm). The sheeting shall fit closely around any pipe, wire or other penetrations of the material. All punctures or tears in the material shall be sealed or covered with additional sheeting.

AF103.4 Entry routes. Potential radon entry routes shall be closed in accordance with Sections AF103.4.1 through AF103.4.10.

AF103.4.1 Floor openings. Openings around bathtubs, showers, water closets, pipes, wires or other objects that penetrate concrete slabs or other floor assemblies shall be filled with a polyurethane caulk or equivalent sealant applied in accordance with the manufacturer's recommendations.

AF103.4.2 Concrete joints. All control joints, isolation joints, construction joints and any other joints in concrete slabs or between slabs and foundation walls shall be sealed with a caulk or sealant. Gaps and joints shall be cleared of loose material and filled with polyurethane caulk or other elastomeric sealant applied in accordance with the manufacturer's recommendations.

AF103.4.3 Condensate drains. Condensate drains shall be trapped or routed through nonperforated pipe to daylight.

AF103.4.4 Sumps. Sump pits open to soil or serving as the termination point for sub-slab or exterior drain tile loops shall be covered with a gasketed or otherwise sealed lid. Sumps used as the suction point in a sub-slab depressurization system shall have a lid designed to accommodate the vent pipe. Sumps used as a floor drain shall have a lid equipped with a trapped inlet.

AF103.4.5 Foundation walls. Hollow block masonry foundation walls shall be constructed with either a continuous course of *solid masonry*, one course of masonry grouted solid, or a solid concrete beam at or above finished ground surface to prevent passage of air from the interior of the wall into the living space. Where a brick veneer or other masonry ledge is installed, the course immediately below that ledge shall be sealed. Joints, cracks or other openings around all penetrations of both exterior and interior surfaces of masonry block or wood foundation walls below the ground surface shall be filled with polyurethane caulk or equivalent sealant. Penetrations of concrete walls shall be filled.

AF103.4.6 Dampproofing. The exterior surfaces of portions of concrete and masonry block walls below the ground surface shall be dampproofed in accordance with Section R406 of this code.

AF103.4.7 Air-handling units. Air-handling units in crawl spaces shall be sealed to prevent air from being drawn into the unit.

> **Exception:** Units with gasketed seams or units that are otherwise sealed by the manufacturer to prevent leakage.

AF103.4.8 Ducts. Ductwork passing through or beneath a slab shall be of seamless material unless the air-handling system is designed to maintain continuous positive pressure within such ducting. Joints in such ductwork shall be sealed to prevent air leakage.

Ductwork located in crawl spaces shall have all seams and joints sealed by closure systems in accordance with Section M1601.4.1.

AF103.4.9 Crawl space floors. Openings around all penetrations through floors above crawl spaces shall be caulked or otherwise filled to prevent air leakage.

AF103.4.10 Crawl space access. Access doors and other openings or penetrations between *basements* and adjoining crawl spaces shall be closed, gasketed or otherwise filled to prevent air leakage.

AF103.5 Passive submembrane depressurization system. In buildings with crawl space foundations, the following components of a passive sub-membrane depressurization system shall be installed during construction.

> **Exception:** Buildings in which an *approved* mechanical crawl space ventilation system or other equivalent system is installed.

AF103.5.1 Ventilation. Crawl spaces shall be provided with vents to the exterior of the building. The minimum net area of ventilation openings shall comply with Section R408.1 of this code.

AF103.5.2 Soil-gas-retarder. The soil in crawl spaces shall be covered with a continuous layer of minimum 6-mil (0.15 mm) polyethylene soil-gas-retarder. The ground cover shall be lapped a minimum of 12 inches (305 mm) at joints and

shall extend to all foundation walls enclosing the crawl space area.

AF103.5.3 Vent pipe. A plumbing tee or other *approved* connection shall be inserted horizontally beneath the sheeting and connected to a 3- or 4-inch-diameter (76 mm or 102 mm) fitting with a vertical vent pipe installed through the sheeting. The vent pipe shall be extended up through the building floors, terminate at least 12 inches (305 mm) above the roof in a location at least 10 feet (3048 mm) away from any window or other opening into the *conditioned spaces* of the building that is less than 2 feet (610 mm) below the exhaust point, and 10 feet (3048 mm) from any window or other opening in adjoining or adjacent buildings.

AF103.6 Passive subslab depressurization system. In *basement* or slab-on-grade buildings, the following components of a passive sub-slab depressurization system shall be installed during construction.

AF103.6.1 Vent pipe. A minimum 3-inch-diameter (76 mm) ABS, PVC or equivalent gas-tight pipe shall be embedded vertically into the sub-slab aggregate or other permeable material before the slab is cast. A "T" fitting or equivalent method shall be used to ensure that the pipe opening remains within the sub-slab permeable material. Alternatively, the 3-inch (76 mm) pipe shall be inserted directly into an interior perimeter drain tile loop or through a sealed sump cover where the sump is exposed to the sub-slab aggregate or connected to it through a drainage system.

The pipe shall be extended up through the building floors, terminate at least 12 inches (305 mm) above the surface of the roof in a location at least 10 feet (3048 mm) away from any window or other opening into the *conditioned spaces* of the building that is less than 2 feet (610 mm) below the exhaust point, and 10 feet (3048 mm) from any window or other opening in adjoining or adjacent buildings.

AF103.6.2 Multiple vent pipes. In buildings where interior footings or other barriers separate the sub-slab aggregate or other gas-permeable material, each area shall be fitted with an individual vent pipe. Vent pipes shall connect to a single vent that terminates above the roof or each individual vent pipe shall terminate separately above the roof.

AF103.7 Vent pipe drainage. All components of the radon vent pipe system shall be installed to provide positive drainage to the ground beneath the slab or soil-gas-retarder.

AF103.8 Vent pipe accessibility. Radon vent pipes shall be accessible for future fan installation through an *attic* or other area outside the *habitable space*.

> **Exception:** The radon vent pipe need not be accessible in an *attic* space where an *approved* roof-top electrical supply is provided for future use.

AF103.9 Vent pipe identification. All exposed and visible interior radon vent pipes shall be identified with at least one *label* on each floor and in accessible *attics*. The *label* shall read: "Radon Reduction System."

AF103.10 Combination foundations. Combination *basement*/crawl space or slab-on-grade/crawl space foundations shall have separate radon vent pipes installed in each type of foundation area. Each radon vent pipe shall terminate above the roof or shall be connected to a single vent that terminates above the roof.

AF103.11 Building depressurization. Joints in air ducts and plenums in un*conditioned spaces* shall meet the requirements of Section M1601. Thermal envelope air infiltration requirements shall comply with the energy conservation provisions in Chapter 11. Firestopping shall meet the requirements contained in Section R602.8.

AF103.12 Power source. To provide for future installation of an active sub-membrane or sub-slab depressurization system, an electrical circuit terminated in an *approved* box shall be installed during construction in the *attic* or other anticipated location of vent pipe fans. An electrical supply shall also be accessible in anticipated locations of system failure alarms.

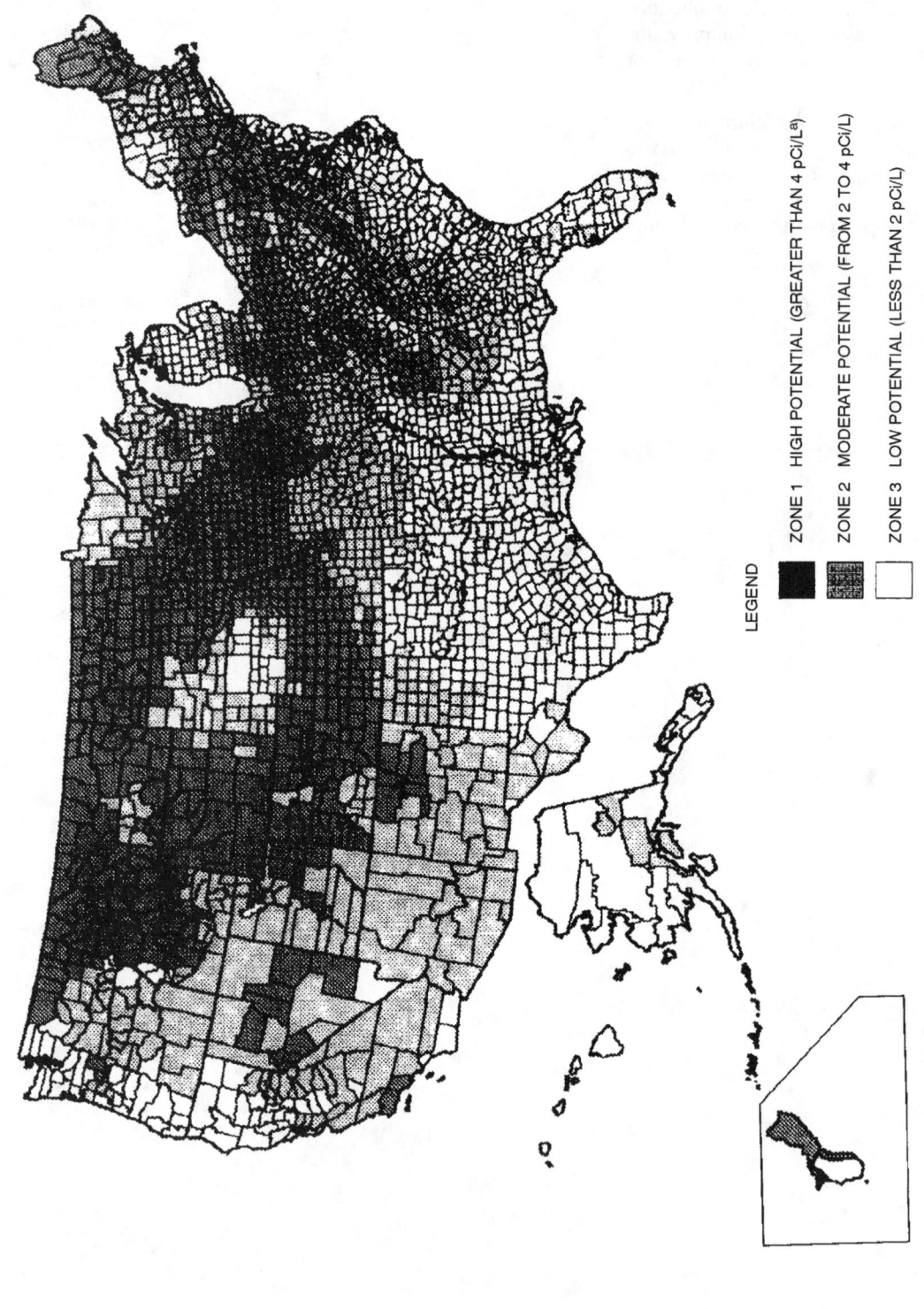

a. pCi/L standard for picocuries per liter of radon gas. EPA recommends that all homes that measure 4 pCi/L and greater be mitigated.

The United States Environmental Protection Agency and the United States Geological Survey have evaluated the radon potential in the United States and have developed a map of radon zones designed to assist building officials in deciding whether radon-resistant features are applicable in new construction.

The map assigns each of the 3,141 counties in the United States to one of three zones based on radon potential. Each zone designation reflects the average short-term radon measurement that can be expected to be measured in a building without the implementation of radon control methods. The radon zone designation of highest priority is Zone 1. Table AF101 of this appendix lists the Zone 1 counties illustrated on the map. More detailed information can be obtained from state-specific booklets (EPA-402-R-93-021 through 070) available through State Radon Offices or from U.S. EPA Regional Offices.

FIGURE AF101
EPA MAP OF RADON ZONES

LEGEND

ZONE 1   HIGH POTENTIAL (GREATER THAN 4 pCi/L[a])

ZONE 2   MODERATE POTENTIAL (FROM 2 TO 4 pCi/L)

ZONE 3   LOW POTENTIAL (LESS THAN 2 pCi/L)

2009 INTERNATIONAL RESIDENTIAL CODE®

TABLE AF101(1)
HIGH RADON POTENTIAL (ZONE 1) COUNTIES[a]

ALABAMA
Calhoun
Clay
Cleburne
Colbert
Coosa
Franklin
Jackson
Lauderdale
Lawrence
Limestone
Madison
Morgan
Talladega

CALIFORNIA
Santa Barbara
Ventura

COLORADO
Adams
Arapahoe
Baca
Bent
Boulder
Chaffee
Cheyenne
Clear Creek
Crowley
Custer
Delta
Denver
Dolores
Douglas
El Paso
Elbert
Fremont
Garfield
Gilpin
Grand
Gunnison
Huerfano
Jackson
Jefferson
Kiowa
Kit Carson
Lake
Larimer
Las Animas
Lincoln
Logan
Mesa
Moffat
Montezuma
Montrose
Morgan
Otero
Ouray
Park
Phillips
Pitkin
Prowers
Pueblo
Rio Blanco
San Miguel
Summit
Teller
Washington
Weld
Yuma

CONNECTICUT
Fairfield
Middlesex
New Haven
New London

GEORGIA
Cobb
De Kalb
Fulton
Gwinnett

IDAHO
Benewah
Blaine
Boise
Bonner
Boundary
Butte
Camas
Clark
Clearwater
Custer
Elmore
Fremont
Gooding
Idaho
Kootenai
Latah
Lemhi
Shoshone
Valley

ILLINOIS
Adams
Boone
Brown
Bureau
Calhoun
Carroll
Cass
Champaign
Coles
De Kalb
De Witt
Douglas
Edgar
Ford
Fulton
Greene
Grundy
Hancock
Henderson
Henry
Iroquois
Jersey
Jo Daviess
Kane
Kendall
Knox
La Salle
Lee
Livingston
Logan
Macon
Marshall
Mason
McDonough
McLean
Menard
Mercer

Morgan
Moultrie
Ogle
Peoria
Piatt
Pike
Putnam
Rock Island
Sangamon
Schuyler
Scott
Stark
Stephenson
Tazewell
Vermilion
Warren
Whiteside
Winnebago
Woodford

INDIANA
Adams
Allen
Bartholomew
Benton
Blackford
Boone
Carroll
Cass
Clark
Clinton
De Kalb
Decatur
Delaware
Elkhart
Fayette
Fountain
Fulton
Grant
Hamilton
Hancock
Harrison
Hendricks
Henry
Howard
Huntington
Jay
Jennings
Johnson
Kosciusko
Lagrange
Lawrence
Madison
Marion
Marshall
Miami
Monroe
Montgomery
Noble
Orange
Putnam
Randolph
Rush
Scott
Shelby
Steuben
St. Joseph
Tippecanoe
Tipton
Union
Vermillion

Wabash
Warren
Washington
Wayne
Wells
White
Whitley

IOWA
All Counties

KANSAS
Atchison
Barton
Brown
Cheyenne
Clay
Cloud
Decatur
Dickinson
Douglas
Ellis
Ellsworth
Finney
Ford
Geary
Gove
Graham
Grant
Gray
Greeley
Hamilton
Haskell
Hodgeman
Jackson
Jewell
Johnson
Kearny
Kingman
Kiowa
Lane
Leavenworth
Lincoln
Logan
Marion
Marshall
McPherson
Meade
Mitchell
Nemaha
Ness
Norton
Osborne
Ottawa
Pawnee
Phillips
Pottawatomie
Pratt
Rawlins
Republic
Rice
Riley
Rooks
Rush
Russell
Saline
Scott
Sheridan
Sherman
Smith
Stanton

Thomas
Trego
Wallace
Washington
Wichita
Wyandotte

KENTUCKY
Adair
Allen
Barren
Bourbon
Boyle
Bullitt
Casey
Clark
Cumberland
Fayette
Franklin
Green
Harrison
Hart
Jefferson
Jessamine
Lincoln
Marion
Mercer
Metcalfe
Monroe
Nelson
Pendleton
Pulaski
Robertson
Russell
Scott
Taylor
Warren
Woodford

MAINE
Androscoggin
Aroostook
Cumberland
Franklin
Hancock
Kennebec
Lincoln
Oxford
Penobscot
Piscataquis
Somerset
York

MARYLAND
Baltimore
Calvert
Carroll
Frederick
Harford
Howard
Montgomery
Washington

MASS.
Essex
Middlesex
Worcester

MICHIGAN
Branch
Calhoun

Cass
Hillsdale
Jackson
Kalamazoo
Lenawee
St. Joseph
Washtenaw

MINNESOTA
Becker
Big Stone
Blue Earth
Brown
Carver
Chippewa
Clay
Cottonwood
Dakota
Dodge
Douglas
Faribault
Fillmore
Freeborn
Goodhue
Grant
Hennepin
Houston
Hubbard
Jackson
Kanabec
Kandiyohi
Kittson
Lac Qui Parle
Le Sueur
Lincoln
Lyon
Mahnomen
Marshall
Martin
McLeod
Meeker
Mower
Murray
Nicollet
Nobles
Norman
Olmsted
Otter Tail
Pennington
Pipestone
Polk
Pope
Ramsey
Red Lake
Redwood
Renville
Rice
Rock
Roseau
Scott
Sherburne
Sibley
Stearns
Steele
Stevens
Swift
Todd
Traverse
Wabasha
Wadena
Waseca

Washington
Watonwan
Wilkin
Winona
Wright
Yellow Medicine

MISSOURI
Andrew
Atchison
Buchanan
Cass
Clay
Clinton
Holt
Iron
Jackson
Nodaway
Platte

MONTANA
Beaverhead
Big Horn
Blaine
Broadwater
Carbon
Carter
Cascade
Chouteau
Custer
Daniels
Dawson
Deer Lodge
Fallon
Fergus
Flathead
Gallatin
Garfield
Glacier
Granite
Hill
Jefferson
Judith Basin
Lake
Lewis and Clark
Liberty
Lincoln
Madison
McCone
Meagher
Mineral
Missoula
Park
Phillips
Pondera
Powder River
Powell
Prairie
Ravalli
Richland
Roosevelt
Rosebud
Sanders
Sheridan
Silver Bow
Stillwater
Teton
Toole
Valley
Wibaux

a. EPA recommends that this county listing be supplemented with other available State and local data to further understand the radon potential of Zone 1 area.

(continued)

TABLE AF101(1)—continued
HIGH RADON POTENTIAL (ZONE 1) COUNTIES[a]

Yellowstone National Park

NEBRASKA
Adams
Boone
Boyd
Burt
Butler
Cass
Cedar
Clay
Colfax
Cuming
Dakota
Dixon
Dodge
Douglas
Fillmore
Franklin
Frontier
Furnas
Gage
Gosper
Greeley
Hamilton
Harlan
Hayes
Hitchcock
Hurston
Jefferson
Johnson
Kearney
Knox
Lancaster
Madison
Nance
Nemaha
Nuckolls
Otoe
Pawnee
Phelps
Pierce
Platte
Polk
Red Willow
Richardson
Saline
Sarpy
Saunders
Seward
Stanton
Thayer
Washington
Wayne
Webster
York

NEVADA
Carson City
Douglas
Eureka
Lander
Lincoln
Lyon
Mineral
Pershing
White Pine

NEW HAMPSHIRE
Carroll

NEW JERSEY
Hunterdon
Mercer
Monmouth
Morris
Somerset
Sussex
Warren

NEW MEXICO
Bernalillo
Colfax
Mora
Rio Arriba
San Miguel
Santa Fe
Taos

NEW YORK
Albany
Allegany
Broome
Cattaraugus
Cayuga
Chautauqua
Chemung
Chenango
Columbia
Cortland
Delaware
Dutchess
Erie
Genesee
Greene
Livingston
Madison
Onondaga
Ontario
Orange
Otsego
Putnam
Rensselaer
Schoharie
Schuyler
Seneca
Steuben
Sullivan
Tioga
Tompkins
Ulster
Washington
Wyoming
Yates

N. CAROLINA
Alleghany
Buncombe
Cherokee
Henderson
Mitchell
Rockingham
Transylvania
Watauga

N. DAKOTA
All Counties

OHIO
Adams
Allen
Ashland

Auglaize
Belmont
Butler
Carroll
Champaign
Clark
Clinton
Columbiana
Coshocton
Crawford
Darke
Delaware
Fairfield
Fayette
Franklin
Greene
Guernsey
Hamilton
Hancock
Hardin
Harrison
Holmes
Huron
Jefferson
Knox
Licking
Logan
Madison
Marion
Mercer
Miami
Montgomery
Morrow
Muskingum
Perry
Pickaway
Pike
Preble
Richland
Ross
Seneca
Shelby
Stark
Summit
Tuscarawas
Union
Van Wert
Warren
Wayne
Wyandot

PENNSYLVANIA
Adams
Allegheny
Armstrong
Beaver
Bedford
Berks
Blair
Bradford
Bucks
Butler
Cameron
Carbon
Centre
Chester
Clarion
Clearfield
Clinton
Columbia
Cumberland
Dauphin

Delaware
Franklin
Fulton
Huntingdon
Indiana
Juniata
Lackawanna
Lancaster
Lebanon
Lehigh
Luzerne
Lycoming
Mifflin
Monroe
Montgomery
Montour
Northampton
Northumberland
Perry
Schuylkill
Snyder
Sullivan
Susquehanna
Tioga
Union
Venango
Westmoreland
Wyoming
York

RHODE ISLAND
Kent
Washington

S. CAROLINA
Greenville

S. DAKOTA
Aurora
Beadle
Bon Homme
Brookings
Brown
Brule
Buffalo
Campbell
Charles Mix
Clark
Clay
Codington
Corson
Davison
Day
Deuel
Douglas
Edmunds
Faulk
Grant
Hamlin
Hand
Hanson
Hughes
Hutchinson
Hyde
Jerauld
Kingsbury
Lake
Lincoln
Lyman
Marshall
McCook
McPherson

Miner
Minnehaha
Moody
Perkins
Potter
Roberts
Sanborn
Spink
Stanley
Sully
Turner
Union
Walworth
Yankton

TENNESSEE
Anderson
Bedford
Blount
Bradley
Claiborne
Davidson
Giles
Grainger
Greene
Hamblen
Hancock
Hawkins
Hickman
Humphreys
Jackson
Jefferson
Knox
Lawrence
Lewis
Lincoln
Loudon
Marshall
Maury
McMinn
Meigs
Monroe
Moore
Perry
Roane
Rutherford
Smith
Sullivan
Trousdale
Union
Washington
Wayne
Williamson
Wilson

UTAH
Carbon
Duchesne
Grand
Piute
Sanpete
Sevier
Uintah

VIRGINIA
Alleghany
Amelia
Appomattox
Augusta
Bath
Bland
Botetourt

Bristol
Brunswick
Buckingham
Buena Vista
Campbell
Chesterfield
Clarke
Clifton Forge
Covington
Craig
Cumberland
Danville
Dinwiddie
Fairfax
Falls Church
Fluvanna
Frederick
Fredericksburg
Giles
Goochland
Harrisonburg
Henry
Highland
Lee
Lexington
Louisa
Martinsville
Montgomery
Nottoway
Orange
Page
Patrick
Pittsylvania
Powhatan
Pulaski
Radford
Roanoke
Rockbridge
Rockingham
Russell
Salem
Scott
Shenandoah
Smyth
Spotsylvania
Stafford
Staunton
Tazewell
Warren
Washington
Waynesboro
Winchester
Wythe

WASHINGTON
Clark
Ferry
Okanogan
Pend Oreille
Skamania
Spokane
Stevens

W. VIRGINIA
Berkeley
Brooke
Grant
Greenbrier
Hampshire
Hancock
Hardy
Jefferson

Marshall
Mercer
Mineral
Monongalia
Monroe
Morgan
Ohio
Pendleton
Pocahontas
Preston
Summers
Wetzel

WISCONSIN
Buffalo
Crawford
Dane
Dodge
Door
Fond du Lac
Grant
Green
Green Lake
Iowa
Jefferson
Lafayette
Langlade
Marathon
Menominee
Pepin
Pierce
Portage
Richland
Rock
Shawano
St. Croix
Vernon
Walworth
Washington
Waukesha
Waupaca
Wood

WYOMING
Albany
Big Horn
Campbell
Carbon
Converse
Crook
Fremont
Goshen
Hot Springs
Johnson
Laramie
Lincoln
Natrona
Niobrara
Park
Sheridan
Sublette
Sweetwater
Teton
Uinta
Washakie

a. EPA recommends that this county listing be supplemented with other available State and local data to further understand the radon potential of Zone 1 area.

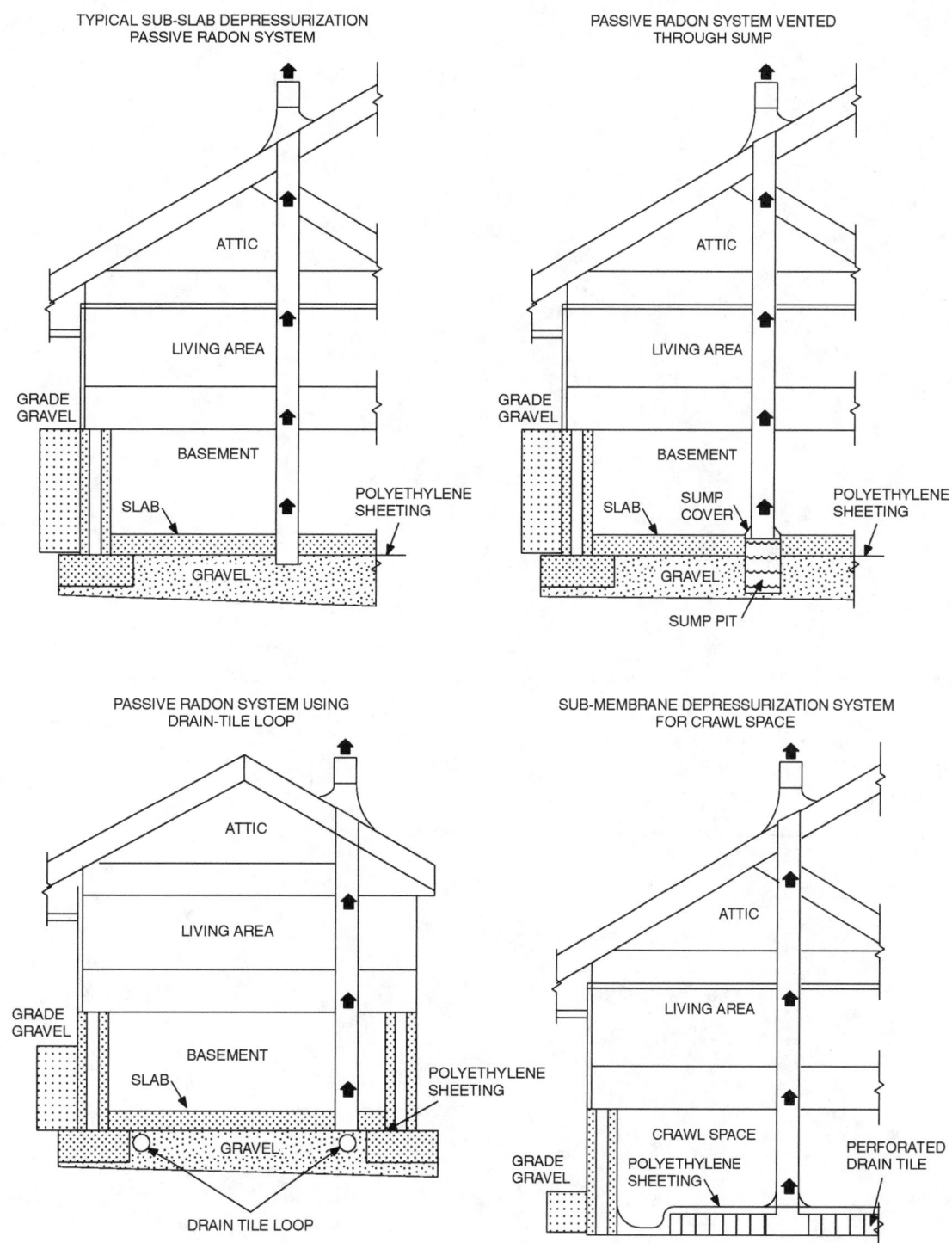

FIGURE AF102
RADON-RESISTANT CONSTRUCTION DETAILS FOR FOUR FOUNDATION TYPES

APPENDIX G

SWIMMING POOLS, SPAS AND HOT TUBS

(The provisions contained in this appendix are not mandatory unless specifically referenced in the adopting ordinance.)

SECTION AG101
GENERAL

AG101.1 General. The provisions of this appendix shall control the design and construction of swimming pools, spas and hot tubs installed in or on the *lot* of a one- or two-family dwelling.

AG101.2 Pools in flood hazard areas. Pools that are located in flood hazard areas established by Table R301.2(1), including above-ground pools, on-ground pools and in-ground pools that involve placement of fill, shall comply with Sections AG101.2.1 or AG101.2.2.

> **Exception:** Pools located in riverine flood hazard areas which are outside of designated floodways.

AG101.2.1 Pools located in designated floodways. Where pools are located in designated floodways, documentation shall be submitted to the *building official*, which demonstrates that the construction of the pool will not increase the design flood elevation at any point within the *jurisdiction*.

AG101.2.2 Pools located where floodways have not been designated. Where pools are located where design flood elevations are specified but floodways have not been designated, the applicant shall provide a floodway analysis that demonstrates that the proposed pool will not increase the design flood elevation more than 1 foot (305 mm) at any point within the *jurisdiction*.

SECTION AG102
DEFINITIONS

AG102.1 General. For the purposes of these requirements, the terms used shall be defined as follows and as set forth in Chapter 2.

ABOVE-GROUND/ON-GROUND POOL. See "Swimming pool."

BARRIER. A fence, wall, building wall or combination thereof which completely surrounds the swimming pool and obstructs access to the swimming pool.

HOT TUB. See "Swimming pool."

IN-GROUND POOL. See "Swimming pool."

RESIDENTIAL. That which is situated on the premises of a detached one- or two-family dwelling or a one-family *townhouse* not more than three stories in height.

SPA, NONPORTABLE. See "Swimming pool."

SPA, PORTABLE. A nonpermanent structure intended for recreational bathing, in which all controls, water-heating and water-circulating *equipment* are an integral part of the product.

SWIMMING POOL. Any structure intended for swimming or recreational bathing that contains water over 24 inches (610 mm) deep. This includes in-ground, above-ground and on-ground swimming pools, hot tubs and spas.

SWIMMING POOL, INDOOR. A swimming pool which is totally contained within a structure and surrounded on all four sides by the walls of the enclosing structure.

SWIMMING POOL, OUTDOOR. Any swimming pool which is not an indoor pool.

SECTION AG103
SWIMMING POOLS

AG103.1 In-ground pools. In-ground pools shall be designed and constructed in conformance with ANSI/NSPI-5 as listed in Section AG108.

AG103.2 Above-ground and on-ground pools. Above-ground and on-ground pools shall be designed and constructed in conformance with ANSI/NSPI-4 as listed in Section AG108.

AG103.3 Pools in flood hazard areas. In flood hazard areas established by Table R301.2(1), pools in coastal high hazard areas shall be designed and constructed in conformance with ASCE 24.

SECTION AG104
SPAS AND HOT TUBS

AG104.1 Permanently installed spas and hot tubs. Permanently installed spas and hot tubs shall be designed and constructed in conformance with ANSI/NSPI-3 as listed in Section AG108.

AG104.2 Portable spas and hot tubs. Portable spas and hot tubs shall be designed and constructed in conformance with ANSI/NSPI-6 as listed in Section AG108.

SECTION AG105
BARRIER REQUIREMENTS

AG105.1 Application. The provisions of this chapter shall control the design of barriers for residential swimming pools, spas and hot tubs. These design controls are intended to provide protection against potential drownings and near-drownings by restricting access to swimming pools, spas and hot tubs.

AG105.2 Outdoor swimming pool. An outdoor swimming pool, including an in-ground, above-ground or on-ground pool, hot tub or spa shall be surrounded by a barrier which shall comply with the following:

1. The top of the barrier shall be at least 48 inches (1219 mm) above *grade* measured on the side of the barrier which faces away from the swimming pool. The maximum vertical clearance between grade and the bottom of

the barrier shall be 2 inches (51 mm) measured on the side of the barrier which faces away from the swimming pool. Where the top of the pool structure is above grade, such as an above-ground pool, the barrier may be at ground level, such as the pool structure, or mounted on top of the pool structure. Where the barrier is mounted on top of the pool structure, the maximum vertical clearance between the top of the pool structure and the bottom of the barrier shall be 4 inches (102 mm).

2. Openings in the barrier shall not allow passage of a 4-inch-diameter (102 mm) sphere.

3. Solid barriers which do not have openings, such as a masonry or stone wall, shall not contain indentations or protrusions except for normal construction tolerances and tooled masonry joints.

4. Where the barrier is composed of horizontal and vertical members and the distance between the tops of the horizontal members is less than 45 inches (1143 mm), the horizontal members shall be located on the swimming pool side of the fence. Spacing between vertical members shall not exceed $1^3/_4$ inches (44 mm) in width. Where there are decorative cutouts within vertical members, spacing within the cutouts shall not exceed $1^3/_4$ inches (44 mm) in width.

5. Where the barrier is composed of horizontal and vertical members and the distance between the tops of the horizontal members is 45 inches (1143 mm) or more, spacing between vertical members shall not exceed 4 inches (102 mm). Where there are decorative cutouts within vertical members, spacing within the cutouts shall not exceed $1^3/_4$ inches (44 mm) in width.

6. Maximum mesh size for chain link fences shall be a $2^1/_4$-inch (57 mm) square unless the fence has slats fastened at the top or the bottom which reduce the openings to not more than $1^3/_4$ inches (44 mm).

7. Where the barrier is composed of diagonal members, such as a lattice fence, the maximum opening formed by the diagonal members shall be not more than $1^3/_4$ inches (44 mm).

8. Access gates shall comply with the requirements of Section AG105.2, Items 1 through 7, and shall be equipped to accommodate a locking device. Pedestrian access gates shall open outward away from the pool and shall be self-closing and have a self-latching device. Gates other than pedestrian access gates shall have a self-latching device. Where the release mechanism of the self-latching device is located less than 54 inches (1372 mm) from the bottom of the gate, the release mechanism and openings shall comply with the following:

    8.1. The release mechanism shall be located on the pool side of the gate at least 3 inches (76 mm) below the top of the gate; and

    8.2. The gate and barrier shall have no opening larger than $1/_2$ inch (12.7 mm) within 18 inches (457 mm) of the release mechanism.

9. Where a wall of a *dwelling* serves as part of the barrier, one of the following conditions shall be met:

    9.1. The pool shall be equipped with a powered safety cover in compliance with ASTM F 1346; or

    9.2. Doors with direct access to the pool through that wall shall be equipped with an alarm which produces an audible warning when the door and/or its screen, if present, are opened. The alarm shall be listed and *labeled* in accordance with UL 2017. The deactivation switch(es) shall be located at least 54 inches (1372 mm) above the threshold of the door; or

    9.3. Other means of protection, such as self-closing doors with self-latching devices, which are *approved* by the governing body, shall be acceptable as long as the degree of protection afforded is not less than the protection afforded by Item 9.1 or 9.2 described above.

10. Where an above-ground pool structure is used as a barrier or where the barrier is mounted on top of the pool structure, and the means of access is a ladder or steps:

    10.1. The ladder or steps shall be capable of being secured, locked or removed to prevent access; or

    10.2. The ladder or steps shall be surrounded by a barrier which meets the requirements of Section AG105.2, Items 1 through 9. When the ladder or steps are secured, locked or removed, any opening created shall not allow the passage of a 4-inch-diameter (102 mm) sphere.

AG105.3 Indoor swimming pool. Walls surrounding an indoor swimming pool shall comply with Section AG105.2, Item 9.

AG105.4 Prohibited locations. Barriers shall be located to prohibit permanent structures, *equipment* or similar objects from being used to climb them.

AG105.5 Barrier exceptions. Spas or hot tubs with a safety cover which complies with ASTM F 1346, as listed in Section AG107, shall be exempt from the provisions of this appendix.

SECTION AG106
ENTRAPMENT PROTECTION FOR SWIMMING POOL AND SPA SUCTION OUTLETS

AG106.1 General. Suction outlets shall be designed and installed in accordance with ANSI/APSP-7.

SECTION AG107
ABBREVIATIONS

AG107.1 General.

ANSI—American National Standards Institute
11 West 42nd Street
New York, NY 10036

APSP—Association of Pool and Spa Professionals
NSPI—National Spa and Pool Institute
2111 Eisenhower Avenue
Alexandria, VA 22314

ASCE—American Society of Civil Engineers
1801 Alexander Bell Drive
Reston, VA 98411-0700

ASTM—ASTM International
100 Barr Harbor Drive,
West Conshohocken, PA 19428

UL—Underwriters Laboratories, Inc.
333 Pfingsten Road
Northbrook, IL 60062-2096

SECTION AG108
STANDARDS

AG108.1 General.

ANSI/NSPI

ANSI/NSPI-3-99 Standard for
Permanently Installed Residential Spas AG104.1

ANSI/NSPI-4-99 Standard for Above-ground/
On-ground Residential Swimming Pools AG103.2

ANSI/NSPI-5-2003 Standard for
Residential In-ground Swimming Pools. AG103.1

ANSI/NSPI-6-99 Standard for
Residential Portable Spas AG104.2

ANSI/APSP

ANSI/APSP-7-06 Standard for Suction Entrapment
avoidance in Swimming Pools, Wading Pools, Spas,
Hot Tubs and Catch Basins. AG106.1

ASCE

ASCE/SEI-24-05 Flood Resistant
Design and Construction. AG103.3

ASTM

ASTM F 1346-91 (2003) Performance
Specification for Safety Covers and Labeling
Requirements for All Covers for Swimming Pools,
Spas and Hot Tubs AG105.2, AG105.5

UL

UL 2017-2000 Standard for General-purpose
Signaling Devices and Systems—with Revisions
through June 2004. . . . . AG105.2

APPENDIX H

PATIO COVERS

(The provisions contained in this appendix are not mandatory unless specifically referenced in the adopting ordinance.)

SECTION AH101
GENERAL

AH101.1 Scope. Patio covers shall conform to the requirements of this appendix chapter.

SECTION AH102
DEFINITION

Patio covers. One-story structures not exceeding 12 feet (3657 mm) in height. Enclosure walls shall be permitted to be of any configuration, provided the open or glazed area of the longer wall and one additional wall is equal to at least 65 percent of the area below a minimum of 6 feet 8 inches (2032 mm) of each wall, measured from the floor. Openings shall be permitted to be enclosed with (1) insect screening, (2) *approved* translucent or transparent plastic not more than 0.125 inch (3.2 mm) in thickness, (3) glass conforming to the provisions of Section R308, or (4) any combination of the foregoing.

SECTION AH103
PERMITTED USES

AH103.1 General. Patio covers shall be permitted to be detached from or attached to *dwelling units*. Patio covers shall be used only for recreational, outdoor living purposes and not as carports, garages, storage rooms or habitable rooms.

SECTION AH104
DESIGN LOADS

AH104.1 General. Patio covers shall be designed and constructed to sustain, within the stress limits of this code, all dead loads plus a minimum vertical live load of 10 pounds per square foot (0.48 kN/m^2) except that snow loads shall be used where such snow loads exceed this minimum. Such covers shall be designed to resist the minimum wind loads set forth in Table R301.2(1).

SECTION AH105
LIGHT AND VENTILATION/EMERGENCY EGRESS

AH105.1 General. Exterior openings required for light and ventilation shall be permitted to open into a patio structure con-forming to Section AH101, provided that the patio structure shall be unenclosed if such openings are serving as emergency egress or rescue openings from sleeping rooms. Where such exterior openings serve as an exit from the *dwelling unit*, the patio structure, unless unenclosed, shall be provided with exits conforming to the provisions of Section R310 of this code.

SECTION AH106
FOOTINGS

AH106.1 General. In areas with a frostline depth of zero as specified in Table R301.2(1), a patio cover shall be permitted to be supported on a slab on *grade* without footings, provided the slab conforms to the provisions of Section R506 of this code, is not less than 3.5 inches (89 mm) thick and the columns do not support live and dead loads in excess of 750 pounds (3.34 kN) per column.

SECTION AH107
SPECIAL PROVISIONS FOR ALUMINUM SCREEN ENCLOSURES IN HURRICANE-PRONE REGIONS

AH107.1 General. Screen enclosures in *hurricane-prone regions* shall be in accordance with the provisions of this Section.

AH107.1.1 Habitable spaces. Screen enclosures shall not be considered *habitable spaces*.

AH107.1.2 Minimum ceiling height. Screen enclosures shall have a ceiling height of not less than 7 feet (2134 mm).

AH107.2 Definitions.

SCREEN ENCLOSURE. A building or part thereof, in whole or in part self-supporting, and having walls of insect screening and a roof of insect screening, plastic, aluminum, or similar lightweight material.

AH107.3 Screen enclosures.

AH107.3.1 Thickness. Actual wall thickness of extruded aluminum members shall be not less than 0.040 inches (1.02 mm).

AH107.3.2 Density. Screen density shall be a maximum of 20 threads per inch by 20 threads per inch mesh.

AH107.4 Design.

AH107.4.1 Wind load. Structural members supporting screen enclosures shall be designed to support minimum wind loads given in Table AH107.4(1) and AH107.4(2). Where any value is less than 10 psf (0.479 kN/m^2) use 10 psf (0.479 kN/m^2).

AH107.4.2 Deflection limit. For members supporting screen surfaces only, the total load deflection shall not exceed *l/60*. Screen surfaces shall be permitted to include a maximum of 25 percent solid flexible finishes.

AH107.4.3 Importance factor. The wind factor for screen enclosures shall be 0.77 in accordance with Section 6.5.5 of ASCE 7.

AH107.4.4 Roof live load. The minimum roof live load shall be 10 psf (0.479 kN/m²).

AH107.5 Footings. In areas with a frost line is zero, a screen enclosure shall be permitted to be supported on a concrete slab on *grade* without footings, provided the slab conforms to the provisions of Section R506, is not less than 3¹/₂ inches (89 mm) thick, and the columns do not support loads in excess of 750 pounds (3.36 kN) per column.

TABLE AH107.4(1)
DESIGN WIND PRESSURES FOR ALUMINUM SCREEN ENCLOSURE FRAMING
WITH AN IMPORTANCE FACTOR OF 0.77[a, b, c]

LOAD CASE	WALL	Basic Wind Speed (mph)											
		100		110		120		130		140		150	
		Exposure Category Design Pressure (psf)											
		C	B	C	B	C	B	C	B	C	B	C	B
A[d]	Windward and leeward walls (flow thru) and windward wall (non-flow thru) L/W = 0-1	12	8	14	10	17	12	19	14	23	16	26	18
A[d]	Windward and leeward walls (flow thru) and windward wall (non-flow thru) L/W = 2	13	9	16	11	19	14	22	16	26	18	30	21
B[e]	Windward: Non-gable roof	16	12	20	14	24	17	28	20	32	23	37	26
B[e]	Windward: Gable roof	22	16	27	19	32	23	38	27	44	31	50	36
	ROOF												
All[f]	Roof-screen	4	3	5	4	6	4	7	5	8	6	9	7
All[f]	Roof-solid	12	9	15	11	18	13	21	15	24	17	28	20

For SI: 1 mile per hour = 0.44 m/s, 1 pound per square foot = 0.0479 kPa, 1 foot = 304.8 mm.

a. Values have been reduced for 0.77 Importance Factor in accordance with Section AH107.4.3.

b. Minimum design pressure shall be 10 psf in accordance with Section AH107.4.1.

c. Loads are applicable to screen enclosures with a mean roof height of 30 feet or less. For screen enclosures of different heights the pressures given shall be adjusted by multiplying the table pressure by the adjustment factor given in Table AH107.4(2).

d. For Load Case A flow thru condition the pressure given shall be applied simultaneously to both the upwind and downwind screen walls acting in the same direction as the wind. The structure shall also be analyzed for wind coming from the opposite direction. For the non-flow thru condition the screen enclosure wall shall be analyzed for the load applied acting toward the interior of the enclosure.

e. For Load Case B the table pressure multiplied by the projected frontal area of the screen enclosure is the total drag force, including drag on screen surfaces parallel to the wind, which must be transmitted to the ground. Use Load Case A for members directly supporting the screen surface perpendicular to the wind. Load Case B loads shall be applied only to structural members which carry wind loads from more than one surface.

f. The roof structure shall be analyzed for the pressure given occurring both upward and downward.

TABLE AH107.4(2)
HEIGHT ADJUSTMENT FACTORS

MEAN	EXPOSURE	
Roof Height (ft)	B	C
15	1	0.86
20	1	0.92
25	1	0.96
30	1	1.00
35	1.05	1.03
40	1.09	1.06
45	1.12	1.09
50	1.16	1.11
55	1.19	1.14
60	1.22	1.16

For SI: 1 foot = 304.8 mm.

APPENDIX I

PRIVATE SEWAGE DISPOSAL

(The provisions contained in this appendix are not mandatory unless specifically referenced in the adopting ordinance.)

SECTION AI101
GENERAL

AI101.1 Scope. Private sewage disposal systems shall conform to the *International Private Sewage Disposal Code.*

APPENDIX J

EXISTING BUILDINGS AND STRUCTURES

(The provisions contained in this appendix are not mandatory unless specifically referenced in the adopting ordinance.)

SECTION AJ101
PURPOSE AND INTENT

AJ101.1 General. The purpose of these provisions is to encourage the continued use or reuse of legally existing buildings and structures. These provisions are intended to permit work in existing buildings that is consistent with the purpose of the *International Residential Code*. Compliance with these provisions shall be deemed to meet the requirements of the *International Residential Code*.

AJ101.2 Classification of work. For purposes of this appendix, all work in existing buildings shall be classified into the categories of repair, renovation, *alteration* and reconstruction. Specific requirements are established for each category of work in these provisions.

AJ101.3 Multiple categories of work. Work of more than one category may be part of a single work project. All related work permitted within a 12-month period shall be considered a single work project. Where a project includes one category of work in one building area and another category of work in a separate and unrelated area of the building, each project area shall comply with the requirements of the respective category of work. Where a project with more than one category of work is performed in the same area or in related areas of the building, the project shall comply with the requirements of the more stringent category of work.

SECTION AJ102
COMPLIANCE

AJ102.1 General. Regardless of the category of work being performed, the work shall not cause the structure to become unsafe or adversely affect the performance of the building; shall not cause an existing mechanical or plumbing system to become unsafe, hazardous, insanitary or overloaded; and unless expressly permitted by these provisions, shall not make the building any less conforming to this code or to any previously *approved* alternative arrangements than it was before the work was undertaken.

AJ102.2 Requirements by category of work. Repairs shall conform to the requirements of Section AJ301. Renovations shall conform to the requirements of Section AJ401. *Alterations* shall conform to the requirements of Section AJ501 and the requirements for renovations. Reconstructions shall conform to the requirements of Section AJ601 and the requirements for *alterations* and renovations.

AJ102.3 Smoke detectors. Regardless of the category of work, smoke detectors shall be provided where required by Section R314.3.1.

AJ102.4 Replacement windows. Regardless of the category of work, when an existing window, including sash and glazed portion is replaced, the replacement window shall comply with the requirements of Chapter 11.

AJ102.5 Flood hazard areas. Work performed in existing buildings located in a flood hazard area as established by Table R301.2(1) shall be subject to the provisions of Section R105.3.1.1.

AJ102.6 Equivalent alternatives. These provisions are not intended to prevent the use of any alternate material, alternate design or alternate method of construction not specifically prescribed herein, provided any alternate has been deemed to be equivalent and its use authorized by the *building official*.

AJ102.7 Other alternatives. Where compliance with these provisions or with this code as required by these provisions is technically infeasible or would impose disproportionate costs because of structural, construction or dimensional difficulties, other alternatives may be accepted by the *building official*. These alternatives may include materials, design features and/or operational features.

AJ102.8 More restrictive requirements. Buildings or systems in compliance with the requirements of this code for new construction shall not be required to comply with any more restrictive requirement of these provisions.

AJ102.9 Features exceeding *International Residential Code* requirements. Elements, components and systems of existing buildings with features that exceed the requirements of this code for new construction, and are not otherwise required as part of *approved* alternative arrangements or deemed by the *building official* to be required to balance other building elements not complying with this code for new construction, shall not be prevented by these provisions from being modified as long as they remain in compliance with the applicable requirements for new construction.

SECTION AJ103
PRELIMINARY MEETING

AJ103.1 General. If a building *permit* is required at the request of the prospective *permit* applicant, the *building official* or his designee shall meet with the prospective applicant to discuss plans for any proposed work under these provisions prior to the application for the *permit*. The purpose of this preliminary meeting is for the *building official* to gain an understanding of the prospective applicant's intentions for the proposed work, and to determine, together with the prospective applicant, the specific applicability of these provisions.

SECTION AJ104
EVALUATION OF AN EXISTING BUILDING

AJ104.1 General. The *building official* may require an existing building to be investigated and evaluated by a registered design professional in the case of proposed reconstruction of any portion of a building. The evaluation shall determine the existence of any potential nonconformities with these provisions, and shall provide a basis for determining the impact of the proposed changes on the performance of the building. The evaluation shall use the following sources of information, as applicable:

1. Available documentation of the existing building.

    1.1. Field surveys.

    1.2. Tests (nondestructive and destructive).

    1.3. Laboratory analysis.

Exception: Detached one- or two-family dwellings that are not irregular buildings under Section R301.2.2.2.5 and are not undergoing an extensive reconstruction shall not be required to be evaluated.

SECTION AJ105
PERMIT

AJ105.1 Identification of work area. The work area shall be clearly identified on all *permits* issued under these provisions.

SECTION AJ201
DEFINITIONS

AJ201.1 General. For purposes of this appendix, the terms used are defined as follows.

ALTERATION. The reconfiguration of any space, the *addition* or elimination of any door or window, the reconfiguration or extension of any system, or the installation of any additional *equipment*.

CATEGORIES OF WORK. The nature and extent of construction work undertaken in an existing building. The categories of work covered in this Appendix, listed in increasing order of stringency of requirements, are repair, renovation, *alteration* and reconstruction.

DANGEROUS. Where the stresses in any member; the condition of the building, or any of its components or elements or attachments; or other condition that results in an overload exceeding 150 percent of the stress allowed for the member or material in this code.

EQUIPMENT OR FIXTURE. Any plumbing, heating, electrical, ventilating, air conditioning, refrigerating and fire protection *equipment*, and elevators, dumb waiters, boilers, pressure vessels, and other mechanical facilities or installations that are related to building services.

LOAD-BEARING ELEMENT. Any column, girder, beam, joist, truss, rafter, wall, floor or roof sheathing that supports any vertical load in addition to its own weight, and/or any lateral load.

MATERIALS AND METHODS REQUIREMENTS. Those requirements in this code that specify material standards; details of installation and connection; joints; penetrations; and continuity of any element, component or system in the building. The required quantity, fire resistance, flame spread, acoustic or ther-mal performance, or other performance attribute is specifically excluded from materials and methods requirements.

RECONSTRUCTION. The reconfiguration of a space that affects an exit, a renovation and/or *alteration* when the work area is not permitted to be occupied because existing means of egress and fire protection systems, or their equivalent, are not in place or continuously maintained; and/or there are extensive *alterations* as defined in Section AJ501.3.

REHABILITATION. Any repair, renovation, *alteration* or reconstruction work undertaken in an existing building.

RENOVATION. The change, strengthening or *addition* of load-bearing elements; and/or the refinishing, replacement, bracing, strengthening, upgrading or extensive repair of existing materials, elements, components, *equipment* and/or fixtures. Renovation involves no reconfiguration of spaces. Interior and exterior painting are not considered refinishing for purposes of this definition, and are not renovation.

REPAIR. The patching, restoration and/or minor replacement of materials, elements, components, *equipment* and/or fixtures for the purposes of maintaining those materials, elements, components, *equipment* and/or fixtures in good or sound condition.

WORK AREA. That portion of a building affected by any renovation, *alteration* or reconstruction work as initially intended by the owner and indicated as such in the *permit*. Work area excludes other portions of the building where incidental work entailed by the intended work must be performed, and portions of the building where work not initially intended by the owner is specifically required by these provisions for a renovation, *alteration* or reconstruction.

SECTION AJ301
REPAIRS

AJ301.1 Materials. Except as otherwise required herein, work shall be done using like materials or materials permitted by this code for new construction.

    AJ301.1.1 Hazardous materials. Hazardous materials no longer permitted, such as asbestos and lead-based paint, shall not be used.

    AJ301.1.2 Plumbing materials and supplies. The following plumbing materials and supplies shall not be used:

        1. All-purpose solvent cement, unless listed for the specific application;

        2. Flexible traps and tailpieces, unless listed for the specific application; and

        3. Solder having more than 0.2 percent lead in the repair of potable water systems.

AJ301.2 Water closets. When any water closet is replaced with a newly manufactured water closet, the replacement water closet shall comply with the requirements of Section P2903.2.

AJ301.3 Safety glazing. Replacement glazing in hazardous locations shall comply with the safety glazing requirements of Section R308.1.

AJ301.4 Electrical. Repair or replacement of existing electrical wiring and *equipment* undergoing repair with like material shall be permitted.

Exceptions:

1. Replacement of electrical receptacles shall comply with the requirements of Chapters 34 through 43.

2. Plug fuses of the Edison-base type shall be used for replacements only where there is no evidence of overfusing or tampering per the applicable requirements of Chapters 34 through 43.

3. For replacement of nongrounding-type receptacles with grounding-type receptacles and for branch circuits that do not have an *equipment* grounding conductor in the branch circuitry, the grounding conductor of a grounding type receptacle outlet shall be permitted to be grounded to any accessible point on the grounding electrode system, or to any accessible point on the grounding electrode conductor, as allowed and described in Chapters 34 through 43.

SECTION AJ401
RENOVATIONS

AJ401.1 Materials and methods. The work shall comply with the materials and methods requirements of this code.

AJ401.2 Door and window dimensions. Minor reductions in the clear opening dimensions of replacement doors and windows that result from the use of different materials shall be allowed, whether or not they are permitted by this code.

AJ401.3 Interior finish. Wood paneling and textile wall coverings used as an interior finish shall comply with the flame spread requirements of Section R302.9.

AJ401.4 Structural. Unreinforced masonry buildings located in Seismic Design Category D_2 or E shall have parapet bracing and wall anchors installed at the roofline whenever a reroofing *permit* is issued. Such parapet bracing and wall anchors shall be of an *approved* design.

SECTION AJ501
ALTERATIONS

AJ501.1 Newly constructed elements. Newly constructed elements, components and systems shall comply with the requirements of this code.

Exceptions:

1. Openable windows may be added without requiring compliance with the light and ventilation requirements of Section R303.

2. Newly installed electrical *equipment* shall comply with the requirements of Section AJ501.5.

AJ501.2 Nonconformities. The work shall not increase the extent of noncompliance with the requirements of Section AJ601, or create nonconformity with those requirements which did not previously exist.

AJ501.3 Extensive alterations. When the total area of all the work areas included in an *alteration* exceeds 50 percent of the area of the *dwelling unit*, the work shall be considered as a reconstruction and shall comply with the requirements of these provisions for reconstruction work.

Exception: Work areas in which the *alteration* work is exclusively plumbing, mechanical or electrical shall not be included in the computation of total area of all work areas.

AJ501.4 Structural. The minimum design loads for the structure shall be the loads applicable at the time the building was constructed, provided that no dangerous condition is created. Structural elements that are uncovered during the course of the *alteration* and that are found to be unsound or dangerous shall be made to comply with the applicable requirements of this code.

AJ501.5 Electrical equipment and wiring.

AJ501.5.1 Materials and methods. Newly installed electrical *equipment* and wiring relating to work done in any work area shall comply with the materials and methods requirements of Chapters 34 through 43.

Exception: Electrical *equipment* and wiring in newly installed partitions and ceilings shall comply with all applicable requirements of Chapters 34 through 43.

AJ501.5.2 Electrical service. Service to the *dwelling unit* shall be a minimum of 100 ampere, three-wire capacity and service *equipment* shall be dead front having no live parts exposed that could allow accidental contact. Type "S" fuses shall be installed when fused *equipment* is used.

Exception: Existing service of 60 ampere, three-wire capacity, and feeders of 30 ampere or larger two- or three-wire capacity shall be accepted if adequate for the electrical load being served.

AJ501.5.3 Additional electrical requirements. When the work area includes any of the following areas within a *dwelling unit*, the requirements of Sections AJ501.5.3.1 through AJ501.5.3.5 shall apply.

AJ501.5.3.1 Enclosed areas. Enclosed areas other than closets, kitchens, *basements*, garages, hallways, laundry areas and bathrooms shall have a minimum of two duplex receptacle outlets, or one duplex receptacle outlet and one ceiling or wall type lighting outlet.

AJ501.5.3.2 Kitchen and laundry areas. Kitchen areas shall have a minimum of two duplex receptacle outlets. Laundry areas shall have a minimum of one duplex receptacle outlet located near the laundry *equipment* and installed on an independent circuit.

AJ501.5.3.3 Ground-fault circuit-interruption. Ground fault circuit interruption shall be provided on newly installed receptacle outlets if required by Chapters 34 through 43.

AJ501.5.3.4 Lighting outlets. At least one lighting outlet shall be provided in every bathroom, hallway, stairway, attached garage and detached garage with electric power to illuminate outdoor entrances and exits, and in utility rooms and *basements* where these spaces are used for storage or contain *equipment* requiring service.

AJ501.5.3.5 Clearance. Clearance for electrical service *equipment* shall be provided in accordance with Chapters 34 through 43.

AJ501.6 Ventilation. All reconfigured spaces intended for occupancy and all spaces converted to habitable or occupiable space in any work area shall be provided with ventilation in accordance with Section R303.

AJ501.7 Ceiling height. *Habitable spaces* created in existing *basements* shall have ceiling heights of not less than 6 feet 8 inches (2032 mm). Obstructions may project to within 6 feet 4 inches (1930 mm) of the *basement* floor. Existing finished ceiling heights in nonhabitable spaces in *basements* shall not be reduced.

AJ501.8 Stairs.

AJ501.8.1 Stair width. Existing *basement* stairs and handrails not otherwise being altered or modified shall be permitted to maintain their current clear width at, above, and below existing handrails.

AJ501.8.2 Stair headroom. Headroom height on existing *basement* stairs being altered or modified shall not be reduced below the existing stairway finished headroom. Existing *basement* stairs not otherwise being altered shall be permitted to maintain the current finished headroom.

AJ501.8.3 Stair landing. Landings serving existing *basement* stairs being altered or modified shall not be reduced below the existing stairway landing depth and width. Existing *basement* stairs not otherwise being altered shall be permitted to maintain the current landing depth and width.

SECTION AJ601
RECONSTRUCTION

AJ601.1 Stairways, handrails and guards.

AJ601.1.1 Stairways. Stairways within the work area shall be provided with illumination in accordance with Section R303.6.

AJ601.1.2 Handrails. Every required exit stairway that has four or more risers, is part of the means of egress for any work area, and is not provided with at least one handrail, or in which the existing handrails are judged to be in danger of collapsing, shall be provided with handrails designed and installed in accordance with Section R311 for the full length of the run of steps on at least one side.

AJ601.1.3 Guards. Every open portion of a stair, landing or balcony that is more than 30 inches (762 mm) above the floor or *grade* below, is part of the egress path for any work area, and does not have guards or in which the existing guards are judged to be in danger of collapsing, shall be provided with guards designed and installed in accordance with Section R312.

AJ601.2 Wall and ceiling finish. The interior finish of walls and ceilings in any work area shall comply with the requirements of Section R302.9. Existing interior finish materials that do not comply with those requirements shall be removed or

shall be treated with an *approved* fire-retardant coating in accordance with the manufacturer's instructions to secure compliance with the requirements of this section.

AJ601.3 Separation walls. Where the work area is in an attached *dwelling unit*, walls separating *dwelling units* that are not continuous from the foundation to the underside of the roof sheathing shall be constructed to provide a continuous fire separation using construction materials consistent with the existing wall or complying with the requirements for new structures. Performance of work shall be required only on the side of the wall of the *dwelling unit* that is part of the work area.

AJ601.4 Ceiling height. *Habitable spaces* created in existing *basements* shall be permitted to have ceiling heights of not less than 6 feet 8 inches (2032 mm). Obstructions may project to within 6 feet 4 inches (1930 mm) of the *basement* floor. Existing finished ceiling heights in nonhabitable spaces in *basements* shall not be reduced.

APPENDIX K

SOUND TRANSMISSION

(The provisions contained in this appendix are not mandatory unless specifically referenced in the adopting ordinance.)

SECTION AK101
GENERAL

AK101.1 General. Wall and floor-ceiling assemblies separating *dwelling units* including those separating adjacent *townhouse* units shall provide air-borne sound insulation for walls, and both air-borne and impact sound insulation for floor-ceiling assemblies.

SECTION AK102
AIR-BORNE SOUND

AK102.1 General. Air-borne sound insulation for wall and floor-ceiling assemblies shall meet a Sound Transmission Class (STC) rating of 45 when tested in accordance with ASTM E 90. Penetrations or openings in construction assemblies for piping; electrical devices; recessed cabinets; bathtubs; soffits; or heating, ventilating or exhaust ducts shall be sealed, lined, insulated or otherwise treated to maintain the required ratings. *Dwelling unit* entrance doors, which share a common space, shall be tight fitting to the frame and sill.

AK102.1.1 Masonry. The sound transmission class of concrete masonry and clay masonry assemblies shall be calculated in accordance with TMS 0302 or determined through testing in accordance with ASTM E 90.

SECTION AK103
STRUCTURAL-BORNE SOUND

AK103.1 General. Floor/ceiling assemblies between *dwelling units* or between a *dwelling unit* and a public or service area within a structure shall have an Impact Insulation Class (IIC) rating of not less than 45 when tested in accordance with ASTM E 492.

SECTION AK104
REFERENCED STANDARDS

ASTM E 90-04 Test Method for Laboratory
Measurement of Airborne Sound Transmission
Loss of Building Partitions and Elements AK102

ASTM E 492-04 Specification for
Laboratory Measurement of Impact Sound
Transmission through Floor-ceiling Assemblies
Using the Tapping Machine AK103

The Masonry Society

TMS 0302-07 Standard for Determining
the Sound Transmission Class Rating
for Masonry Walls. AK102.1.1

APPENDIX L

PERMIT FEES

(The provisions contained in this appendix are not mandatory unless specifically referenced in the adopting ordinance.)

TOTAL VALUATION	FEE
$1 to $ 500	$24
$501 to $2,000	$24 for the first $500; plus $3 for each additional $ 100 or fraction thereof, to and including $2,000
$2,001 to $40,000	$69 for the first $2,000; plus $11 for each additional $1,000 or fraction thereof, to and including $40,000
$40,001 to $100,000	$487 for the first $40,000; plus $9 for each additional $1,000 or fraction thereof, to and including $100,000
$100,001 to $500,000	$1,027 for the first $100,000; plus $7 for each additional $1,000 or fraction thereof, to and including $500,000
$500,001 to $1,000,000	$3,827 for the first $500,000; plus $5 for each additional $1,000 or fraction thereof, to and including $1,000,000
$1,000,001 to $5,000,000	$6,327 for the first $1,000,000; plus $3 for each additional $1,000 or fraction thereof, to and including $5,000,000
$5,000,001 and over	$18,327 for the first $ 5,000,000; plus $1 for each additional $1,000 or fraction thereof

APPENDIX M

HOME DAY CARE—R-3 OCCUPANCY

(The provisions contained in this appendix are not mandatory unless specifically referenced in the adopting ordinance.)

SECTION AM101
GENERAL

AM101.1 General. This appendix shall apply to a home day care operated within a *dwelling*. It is to include buildings and structures occupied by persons of any age who receive custodial care for less than 24 hours by individuals other than parents or guardians or relatives by blood, marriage, or adoption, and in a place other than the home of the person cared for.

SECTION AM102
DEFINITIONS

EXIT ACCESS. That portion of a means of egress system that leads from any occupied point in a building or structure to an exit.

SECTION AM103
MEANS OF EGRESS

AM103.1 Exits required. If the occupant load of the residence is more than nine, including those who are residents, during the time of operation of the day care, two exits are required from the ground-level *story*. Two exits are required from a home day care operated in a *manufactured home* regardless of the occupant load. Exits shall comply with Section R311.

AM103.1.1 Exit access prohibited. An exit access from the area of day-care operation shall not pass through bathrooms, bedrooms, closets, garages, fenced rear *yards* or similar areas.

> **Exception:** An exit may discharge into a fenced *yard* if the gate or gates remain unlocked during day-care hours. The gates may be locked if there is an area of refuge located within the fenced *yard* and more than 50 feet (15 240 mm) from the *dwelling*. The area of refuge shall be large enough to allow 5 square feet (0.5 m²) per occupant.

AM103.1.2 Basements. If the *basement* of a *dwelling* is to be used in the day-care operation, two exits are required from the *basement* regardless of the occupant load. One of the exits may pass through the *dwelling* and the other must lead directly to the exterior of the *dwelling*.

> **Exception:** An emergency and escape window complying with Section R310 and which does not conflict with Section AM103.1.1 may be used as the second means of egress from a *basement*.

AM103.1.3 Yards. If the *yard* is to be used as part of the day-care operation it shall be fenced.

AM103.1.3.1 Type of fence and hardware. The fence shall be of durable materials and be at least 6 feet (1529 mm) tall completely enclosing the area used for the day-care operations. Each opening shall be a gate or door equipped with a self-closing and self-latching device to be installed at a minimum of 5 feet (1528 mm) above the ground.

> **Exception:** The door of any *dwelling* which forms part of the enclosure need not be equipped with self-closing and self-latching devices.

AM103.1.3.2 Construction of fence. Openings in the fence, wall or enclosure required by this section shall have intermediate rails or an ornamental pattern that do not allow a sphere 4 inches (102 mm) in diameter to pass through. In addition, the following criteria must be met:

1. The maximum vertical clearance between *grade* and the bottom of the fence, wall or enclosure shall be 2 inches (51 mm).

2. Solid walls or enclosures that do not have openings, such as masonry or stone walls, shall not contain indentations or protrusions except for tooled masonry joints.

3. Maximum mesh size for chain link fences shall be $1^1/_4$-inches (32 mm) square unless the fence has slats at the top or bottom which reduce the opening to no more than $1^3/_4$ inches (44 mm). The wire shall not be less than 9 gage [(0.148 in.) (3.8 mm)].

AM103.1.3.3 Decks. Decks that are more than 12 inches (305 mm) above *grade* shall have a guard in compliance with Section R312.

AM103.2 Width and height of an exit. The minimum width of a required exit is 36 inches (914 mm) with a net clear width of 32 inches (813 mm). The minimum height of a required exit is 6 feet 8 inches (2032 mm).

AM103.3 Type of lock and latches for exits. Regardless of the occupant load served, exit doors shall be openable from the inside without the use of a key or any special knowledge or effort. When the occupant load is 10 or less, a night latch, dead bolt or security chain may be used, provided such devices are openable from the inside without the use of a key or tool and mounted at a height not to exceed 48 inches (1219 mm) above the finished floor.

AM103.4 Landings. Landings for stairways and doors shall comply with Section R311 except that landings shall be required for the exterior side of a sliding door when a home day-care is being operated in a Group R-3 Occupancy.

SECTION AM104
SMOKE DETECTION

AM104.1 General. Smoke detectors shall be installed in *dwelling* units used for home day-care operations. Detectors shall be installed in accordance with the approved manufacturer's instructions. If the current smoke detection system in the *dwelling* is not in compliance with the currently adopted code for smoke detection, it shall be upgraded to meet the currently adopted code requirements and Section AM103 before daycare operations commence.

AM104.2 Power source. Required smoke detectors shall receive their primary power from the building wiring when that wiring is served from a commercial source and shall be equipped with a battery backup. The detector shall emit a signal when the batteries are low. Wiring shall be permanent and without a disconnecting switch other than those required for over-current protection. Required smoke detectors shall be interconnected so if one detector is activated, all detectors are activated.

AM104.3 Location. A detector shall be located in each bedroom and any room that is to be used as a sleeping room and centrally located in the corridor, hallway or area giving access to each separate sleeping area. When the *dwelling* unit has more than one *story*, and in *dwellings* with *basements*, a detector shall be installed on each *story* and in the *basement*. In *dwelling* units where a *story* or *basement* is split into two or more levels, the smoke detector shall be installed on the upper level, except that when the lower level contains a sleeping area, a detector shall be installed on each level. When sleeping rooms are on the upper level, the detector shall be placed at the ceiling of the upper level in close proximity to the stairway. In *dwelling* units where the ceiling height of a room open to the hallway serving the bedrooms or sleeping areas exceeds that of the hallway by 24 inches (610 mm) or more, smoke detectors shall be installed in the hallway and in the adjacent room. Detectors shall sound an alarm audible in all sleeping areas of the *dwelling* unit in which they are located.

APPENDIX N

VENTING METHODS

(This appendix is informative and is not part of the code.
This appendix provides examples of various of venting methods.)

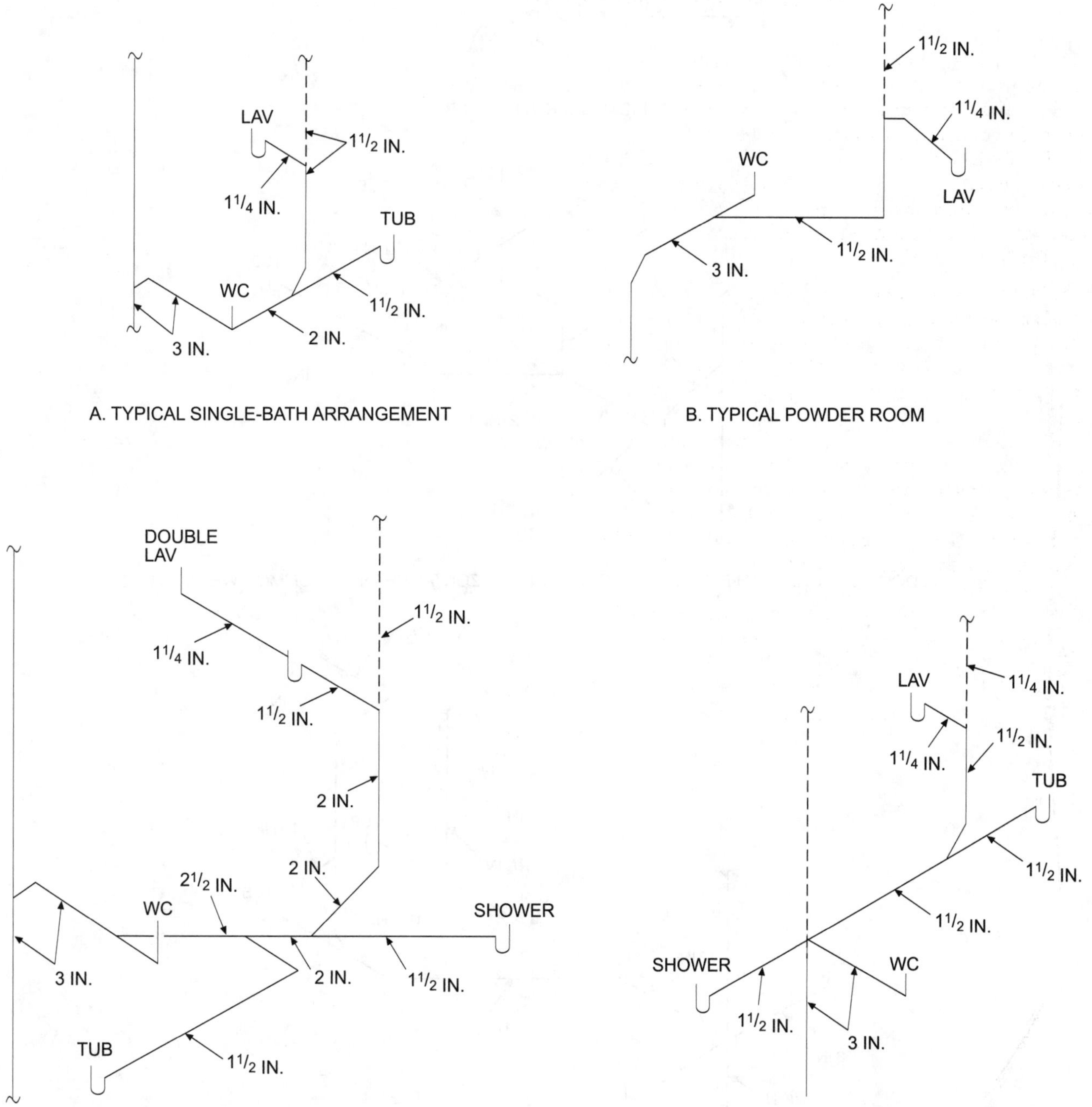

A. TYPICAL SINGLE-BATH ARRANGEMENT

B. TYPICAL POWDER ROOM

C. MORE ELABORATE SINGLE-BATH
ARRANGEMENT

D. COMBINATION WET- AND STACK-VENTING
WITH STACK FITTING

For SI: 1 inch = 25.4 mm.

FIGURE N1
TYPICAL SINGLE-BATH WET-VENT ARRANGEMENTS

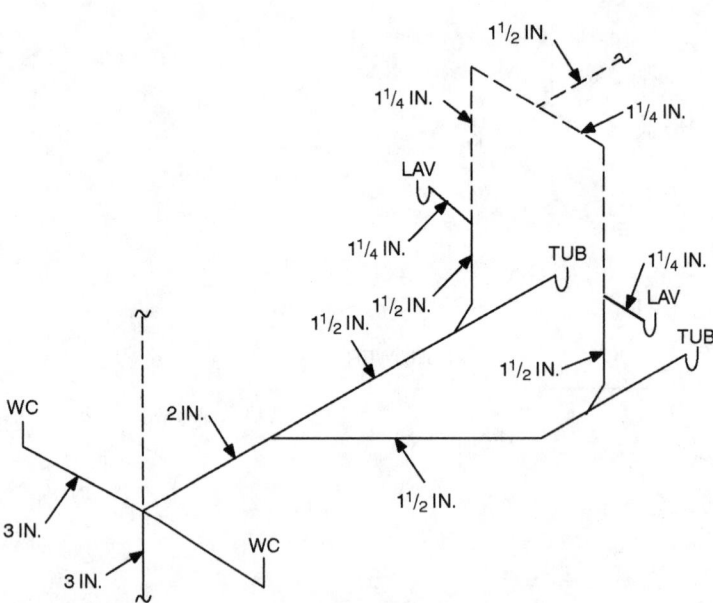

A. TYPICAL BACK-TO-BACK BATHS

B. DOUBLE BATHS WITH FIXTURES ON COMMON HORIZONTAL BRANCH, COMMON WET VENT

C. DOUBLE BATHS WITH WASTE FIXTURES ON COMMON HORIZONTAL BRANCH, INDIVIDUAL WET VENTS

For SI: 1 inch = 25.4 mm.

FIGURE N2
TYPICAL DOUBLE-BATH WET-VENT ARRANGEMENTS

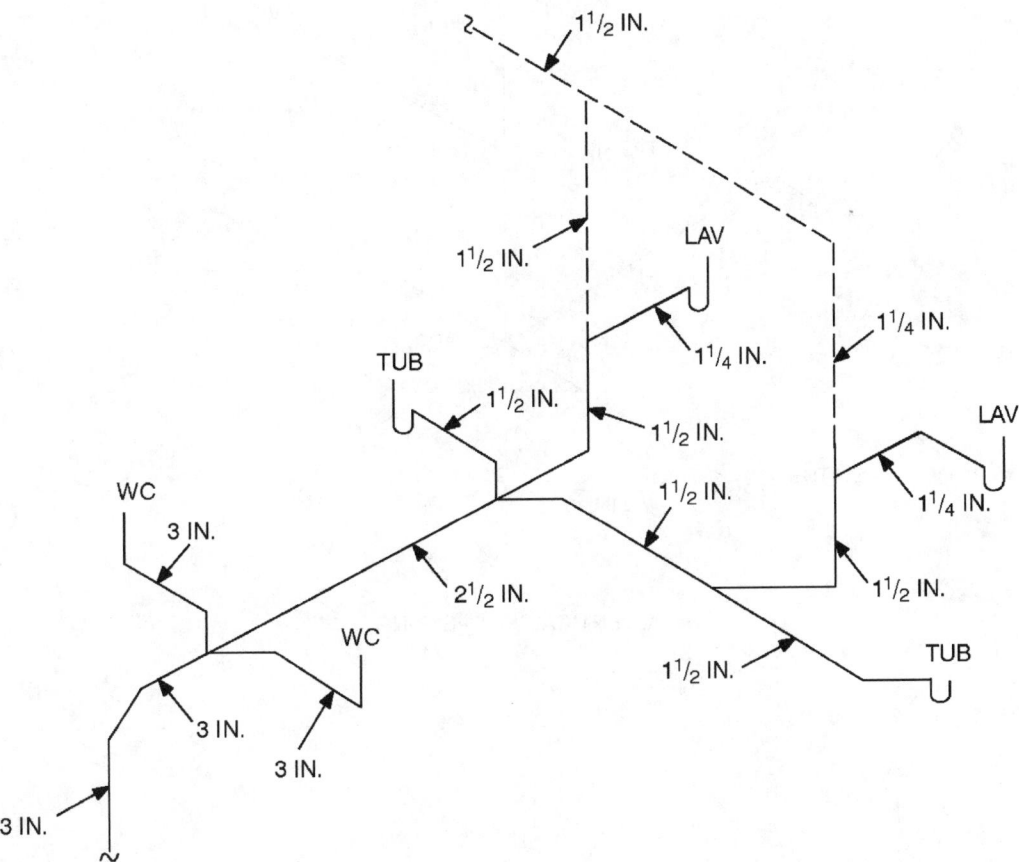

For SI: 1 inch = 25.4 mm.

FIGURE N3
TYPICAL HORIZONTAL WET VENTING

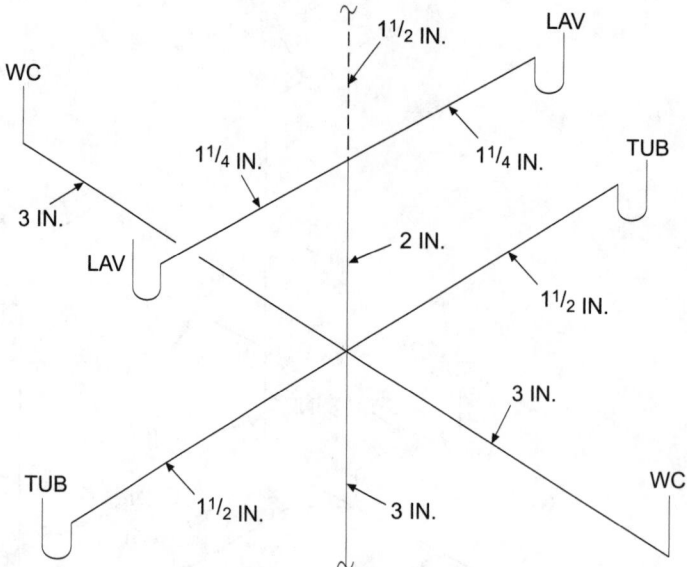

A. VERTICAL WET VENTING

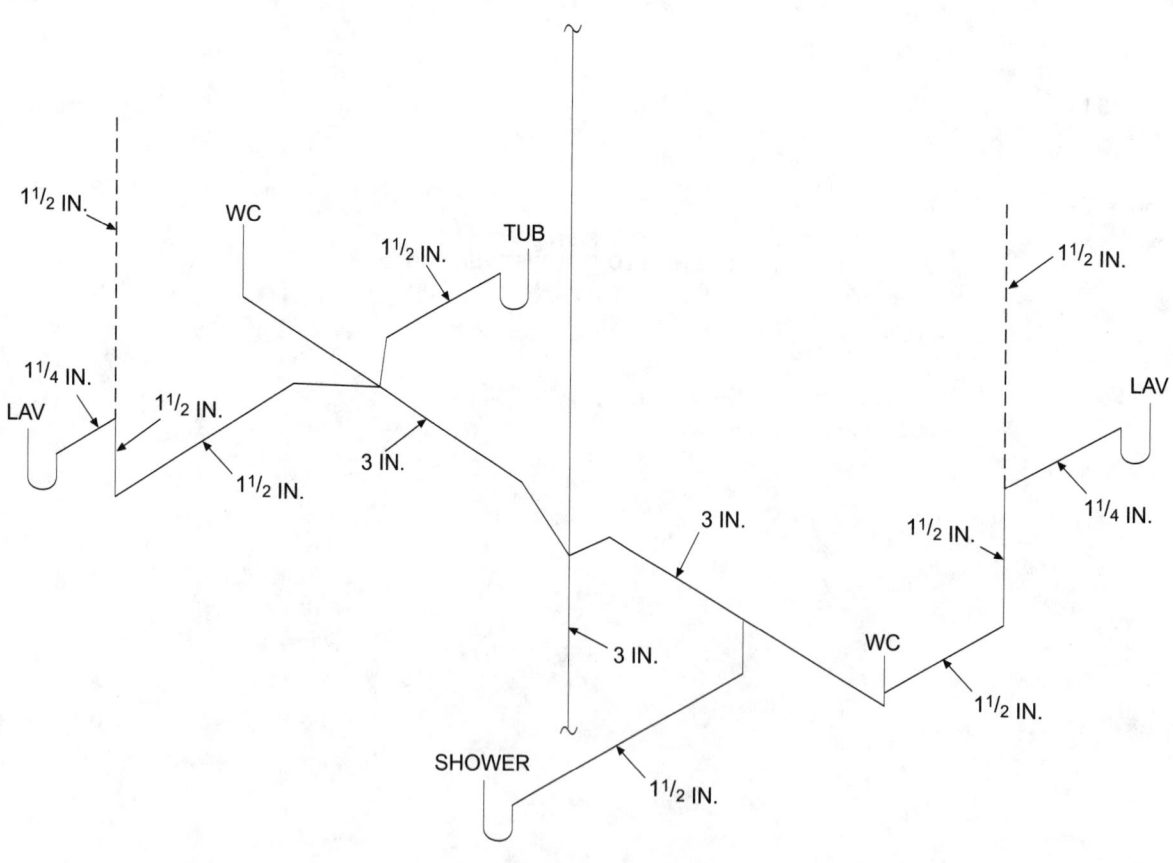

B. HORIZONTAL WET VENTING

For SI: 1 inch = 25.4 mm.

FIGURE N4
TYPICAL METHODS OF WET VENTING

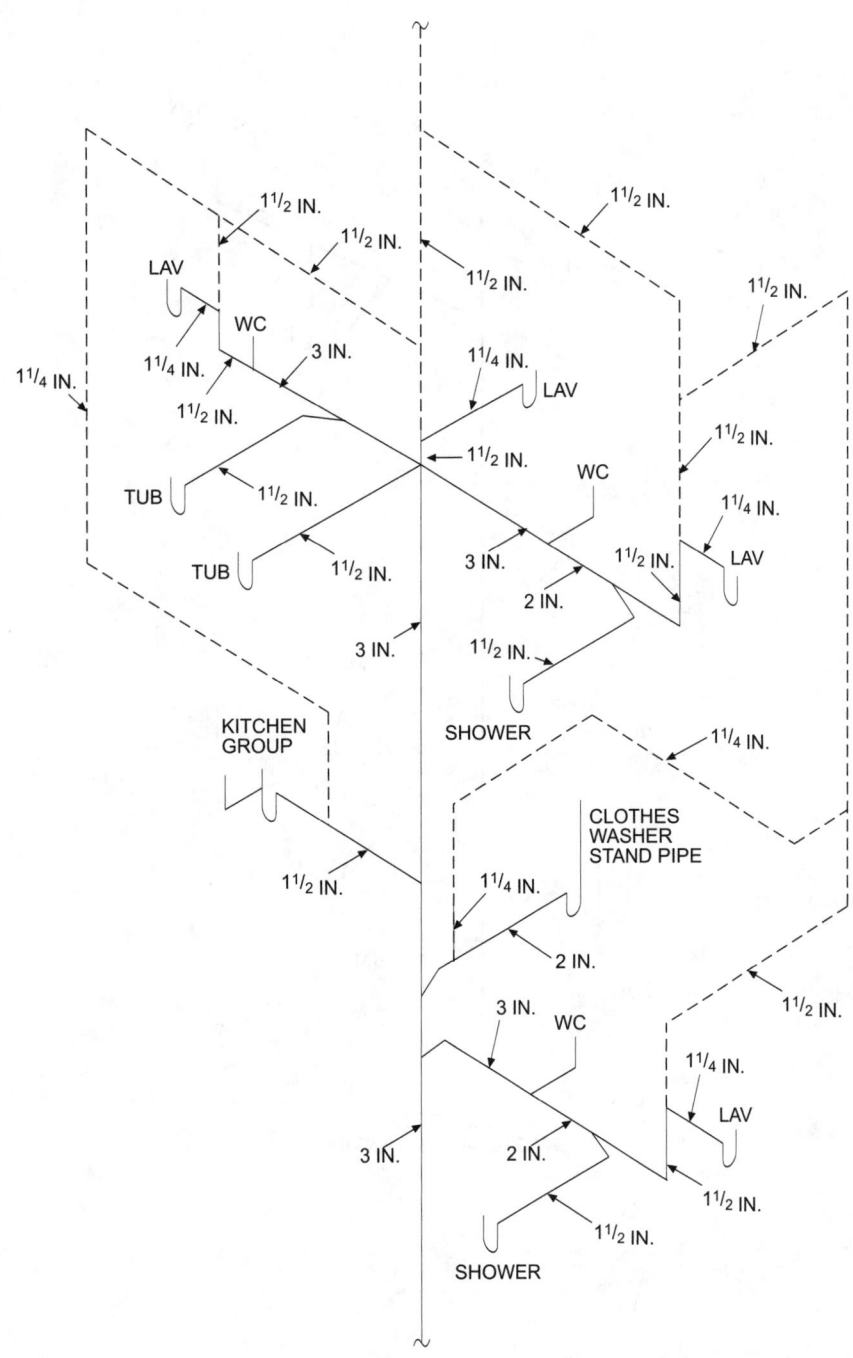

For SI: 1 inch = 25.4 mm.

FIGURE N5
SINGLE STACK SYSTEM FOR A TWO-STORY DWELLING

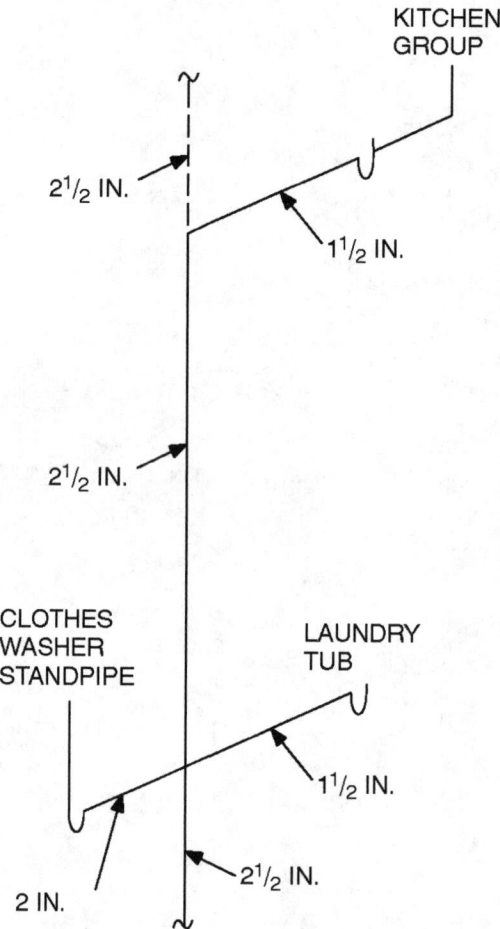

KITCHEN
GROUP

$2^1/_2$ IN.

$1^1/_2$ IN.

$2^1/_2$ IN.

CLOTHES
WASHER
STANDPIPE

LAUNDRY
TUB

$1^1/_2$ IN.

$2^1/_2$ IN.

2 IN.

For SI: 1 inch = 25.4 mm.

FIGURE N6
WASTE STACK VENTING

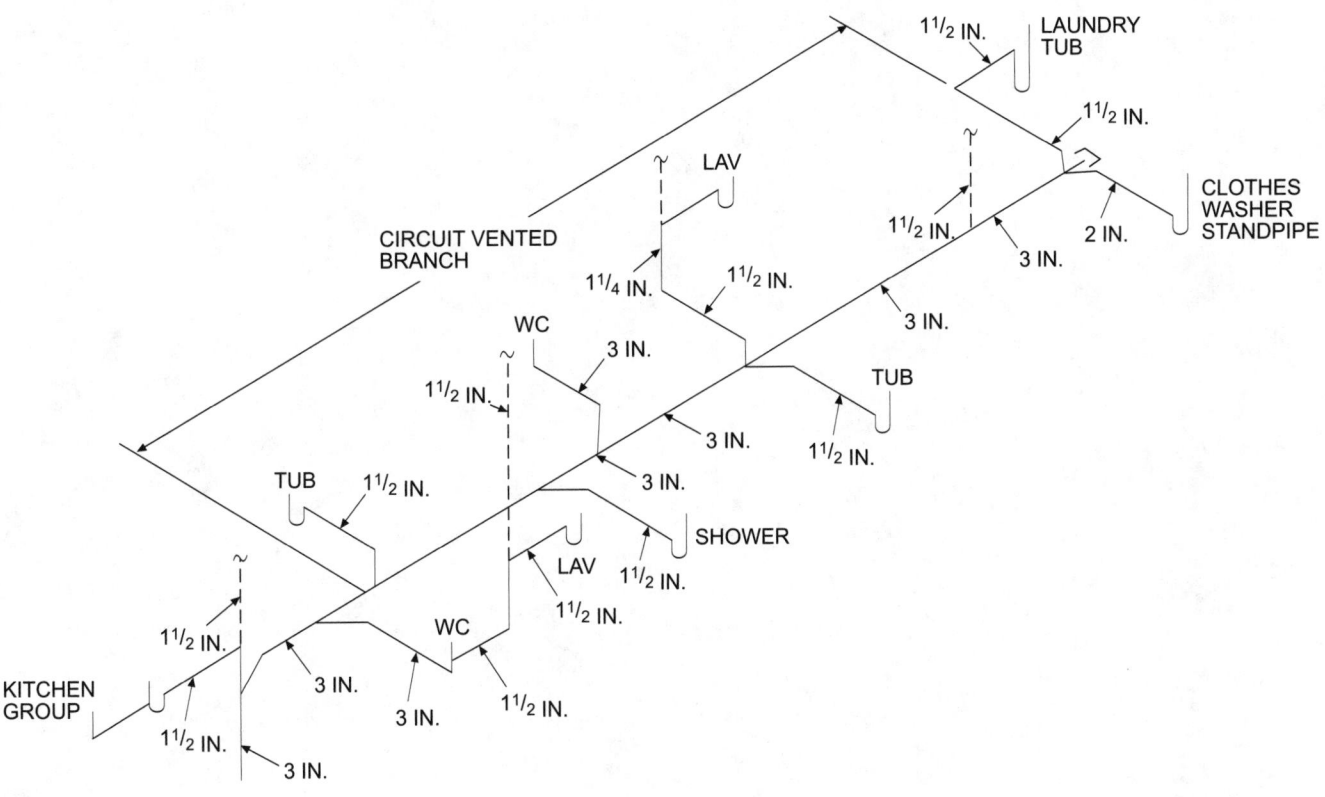

For SI: 1 inch = 25.4 mm.

FIGURE N7
CIRCUIT VENT WITH ADDITIONAL NONCIRCUIT VENTED BRANCH

GRAY WATER RECYCLING SYSTEMS

(The provisions contained in this appendix are not mandatory unless specifically referenced in the adopting ordinance.)

Note: *Section P2601.2 of the* International Residential Code *requires all plumbing fixtures that receive water or waste to discharge to the sanitary drainage system of the structure. To allow for the use of a gray water recycling system, Section P2601.2 of the* International Residential Code *should be revised to read as follows:*

P2601.2 Connections. Plumbing fixtures, drains and appliances used to receive or discharge liquid wastes or sewage shall be directly connected to the sanitary drainage system of the building or premises, in accordance with the requirements of this code. This section shall not be construed to prevent indirect waste systems.

Exception: Bathtubs, showers, lavatories, clothes washers and laundry trays are not required to discharge to the sanitary drainage system where those fixtures discharge to an *approved* gray water recycling system.

SECTION AO101
GENERAL

AO101.1 Scope. The provisions of this appendix shall govern the materials, design, construction and installation of gray water systems for flushing of water closets and urinals and for subsurface landscape irrigation [see Figures AO101.1(1) and AO101.1(2)].

AO101.2 Definition. The following term shall have the meaning shown herein.

GRAY WATER. Waste discharged from lavatories, bathtubs, showers, clothes washers and laundry trays.

AO101.3 Permits. Permits shall be required in accordance with Section R105 of the *International Residential Code.*

AO101.4 Installation. In addition to the provisions of Section AO101, systems for flushing of water closets and urinals shall comply with Section AO102 and systems for subsurface landscape irrigation shall comply with Section AO103. Except as provided for in Appendix O, all systems shall comply with the provisions of the *International Residential Code.*

AO101.5 Materials. Above-ground drain, waste and vent piping for gray water systems shall conform to one of the standards listed in Table P3002.1(1) of the *International Residential Code.* Gray water underground *building drainage* and vent pipe shall conform to one of the standards listed in Table P3002.1(2) of the *International Residential Code.*

AO101.6 Tests. Drain, waste and vent piping for gray water systems shall be tested in accordance with Section P2503 of the *International Residential Code.*

AO101.7 Inspections. Gray water systems shall be inspected in accordance with Section P2503 of the *International Residential Code.*

AO101.8 Potable water connections. Only connections in accordance with Section AO102.3 shall be made between a gray water recycling system and a potable water system.

AO101.9 Waste water connections. Gray water recycling systems shall receive the waste discharge only of bathtubs, showers, lavatories, clothes washers and laundry trays.

AO101.10 Filtration. Gray water entering the reservoir shall pass through an *approved* filter such as a media, sand or diatomaceous earth filter.

AO101.10.1 Required valve. A full-open valve shall be installed downstream of the last fixture connection to the gray water discharge pipe before entering the required filter.

AO101.11 Collection reservoir. Gray water shall be collected in an *approved* reservoir constructed of durable, nonabsorbent and corrosion-resistant materials. The reservoir shall be a closed and gas-tight vessel. Access openings shall be provided to allow inspection and cleaning of the reservoir interior.

AO101.12 Overflow. The collection reservoir shall be equipped with an overflow pipe of the same diameter as, or larger than, the influent pipe for the gray water. The overflow pipe shall be trapped and shall be indirectly connected to the sanitary drainage system.

AO101.13 Drain. A drain shall be located at the lowest point of the collection reservoir and shall be indirectly connected to the sanitary drainage system. The drain shall be the same diameter as the overflow pipe required in Section AO101.12.

AO101.14 Vent required. The reservoir shall be provided with a vent sized in accordance with Chapter 31 of the *International Residential Code* and based on the diameter of the reservoir influent pipe.

SECTION AO102
SYSTEMS FOR FLUSHING WATER
CLOSETS AND URINALS

AO102.1 Collection reservoir. The holding capacity of the reservoir shall be a minimum of twice the volume of water required to meet the daily flushing requirements of the fixtures supplied with gray water, but not less than 50 gallons (189 L). The reservoir shall be sized to limit the retention time of gray water to a maximum of 72 hours.

AO102.2 Disinfection. Gray water shall be disinfected by an *approved* method that uses one or more disinfectants such as chlorine, iodine or ozone that are recommended for use with the pipes, fittings and equipment by the manufacturer of the pipes, fittings and equipment.

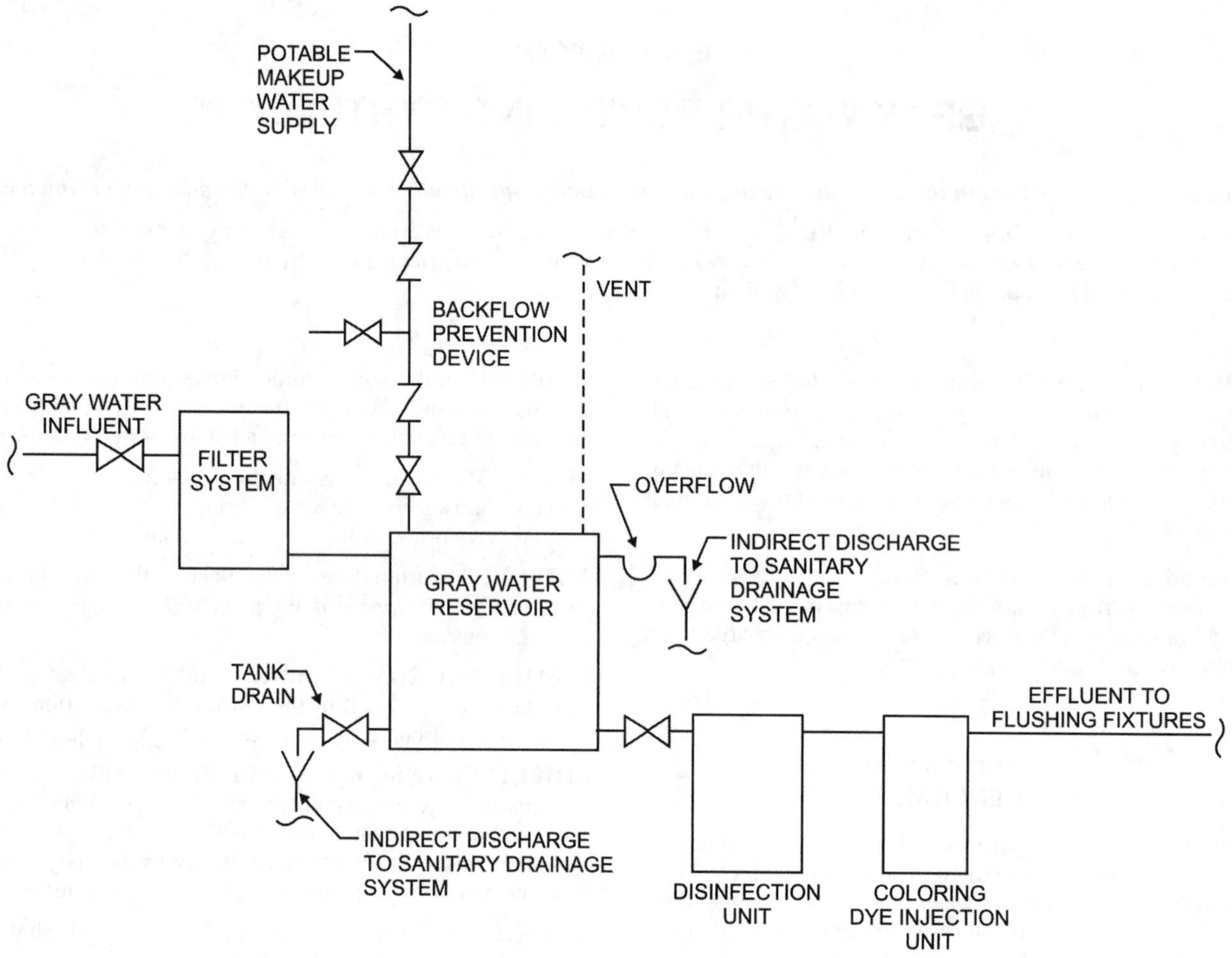

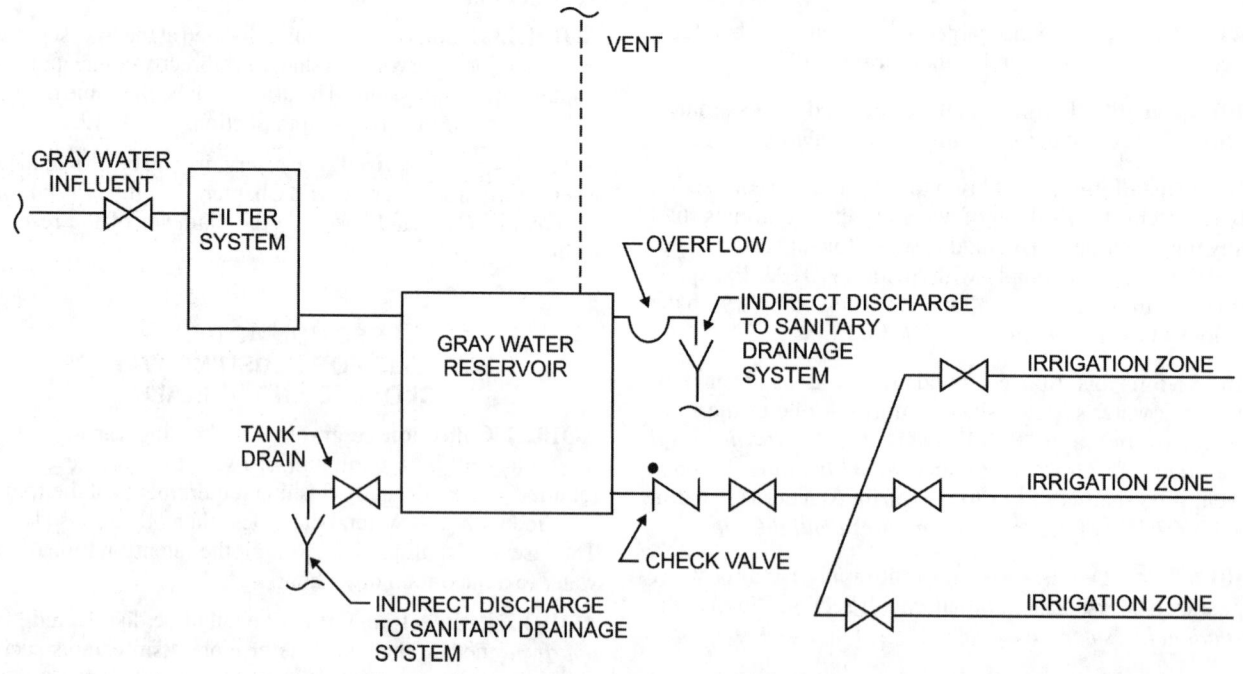

FIGURE AO101.1(1)
GRAY WATER RECYCLING SYSTEM FOR FLUSHING WATER CLOSETS AND URINALS

FIGURE AO101.1(2)
GRAY WATER RECYCLING SYSTEM FOR SUBSURFACE LANDSCAPE IRRIGATION

AO102.3 Makeup water. Potable water shall be supplied as a source of makeup water for the gray water system. The potable water supply shall be protected against backflow in accordance with Section P2902 of the *International Residential Code*. A full-open valve shall be located on the makeup water supply line to the collection reservoir.

AO102.4 Coloring. The gray water shall be dyed blue or green with a food grade vegetable dye before such water is supplied to the fixtures.

AO102.5 Materials. Distribution piping shall conform to one of the standards listed in Table P2905.4 of the *International Residential Code*.

AO102.6 Identification. Distribution piping and reservoirs shall be identified as containing nonpotable water. Piping identification shall be in accordance with Section 608.8 of the *International Plumbing Code®*.

SECTION AO103
SUBSURFACE LANDSCAPE
IRRIGATION SYSTEMS

AO103.1 Collection reservoir. Reservoirs shall be sized to limit the retention time of gray water to a maximum of 24 hours.

AO103.1.1 Identification. The reservoir shall be identified as containing nonpotable water.

AO103.2 Valves required. A check valve, and a full-open valve located on the discharge side of the check valve, shall be installed on the effluent pipe of the collection reservoir.

AO103.3 Makeup water. Makeup water shall not be required for subsurface landscape irrigation systems. Where makeup water is supplied, the installation shall be in accordance with Section AO102.3.

AO103.4 Disinfection. Disinfection shall not be required for gray water used for subsurface landscape irrigation systems.

AO103.5 Coloring. Gray water used for subsurface landscape irrigation systems shall not be required to be dyed.

AO103.6 Estimating gray water discharge. The system shall be sized in accordance with the demands per day per occupant based on the type of fixtures connected to the gray water system. The discharge shall be calculated by the following equation:

$$C = A \times B \qquad \text{(Equation AO-1)}$$

A = Number of occupants:

Number of occupants shall be determined by the actual number of occupants but not less than two occupants for 1 bedroom and one occupant for each additional bedroom.

B = Estimated flow demands for each occupant:

25 gallons per day (95 Lpd) per occupant for showers, bathtubs and lavatories and 15 gallons per day (57 Lpd) per occupant for clothes washers or laundry trays.

C = Estimated gray water discharge based on the total number of occupants.

AO103.7 Percolation tests. The permeability of the soil in the proposed absorption system shall be determined by percolation tests or permeability evaluation.

AO103.7.1 Percolation tests and procedures. At least three percolation tests shall be conducted in each system area. The holes shall be spaced uniformly in relation to the bottom depth of the proposed absorption system. More percolation tests shall be made where necessary, depending on system design.

AO103.7.1.1 Percolation test hole. The test hole shall be dug or bored. The test hole shall have vertical sides and a horizontal dimension of 4 inches to 8 inches (102 mm to 203 mm). The bottom and sides of the hole shall be scratched with a sharp-pointed instrument to expose the natural soil. All loose material shall be removed from the hole and the bottom shall be covered with 2 inches (51 mm) of gravel or coarse sand.

AO103.7.1.2 Test procedure, sandy soils. The hole shall be filled with clear water to a minimum of 12 inches (305 mm) above the bottom of the hole for tests in sandy soils. The time for this amount of water to seep away shall be determined and this procedure shall be repeated if the water from the second filling of the hole seeps away in 10 minutes or less. The test shall proceed as follows: Water shall be added to a point not more than 6 inches (152 mm) above the gravel or coarse sand. Thereupon, from a fixed reference point, water levels shall be measured at 10-minute intervals for a period of 1 hour. Where 6 inches (152 mm) of water seeps away in less than 10 minutes, a shorter interval between measurements shall be used, but in no case shall the water depth exceed 6 inches (152 mm). Where 6 inches (152 mm) of water seeps away in less than 2 minutes, the test shall be stopped and a rate of less than 3 minutes per inch (7 s/mm) shall be reported. The final water level drop shall be used to calculate the percolation rate. Soils not meeting the requirements of this section shall be tested in accordance with Section AO103.7.1.3.

AO103.7.1.3 Test procedure, other soils. The hole shall be filled with clear water, and a minimum water depth of 12 inches (305 mm) shall be maintained above the bottom of the hole for a 4-hour period by refilling whenever necessary or by use of an automatic siphon. Water remaining in the hole after 4 hours shall not be removed. Thereafter, the soil shall be allowed to swell not less than 16 hours or more than 30 hours. Immediately after the soil swelling period, the measurements for determining the percolation rate shall be made as follows: Any soil sloughed into the hole shall be removed, and the water level shall be adjusted to 6 inches (152 mm) above the gravel or coarse sand. Thereupon, from a fixed reference point, the water level shall be measured at 30-minute intervals for a period of 4 hours, unless two successive water level drops do not vary by more than 0.62 inch (16 mm). At least three water level drops shall be observed and recorded. The hole shall be filled with clear water to a point not more than 6 inches (152 mm) above the gravel or coarse sand whenever it becomes nearly empty. The water level shall not be adjusted during the three measurement periods except to the limits of the last measured water level drop. When the first 6 inches (152 mm) of water seeps away in less than 30 minutes, the time interval between measurements shall be 10 minutes and the test run for 1 hour. The water depth shall not exceed 5 inches (127 mm) at any time during the measurement period. The drop that occurs during the final measurement period shall be used in calculating the percolation rate.

AO103.7.1.4 Mechanical test equipment. Mechanical percolation test equipment shall be of an *approved* type.

AO103.7.2 Permeability evaluation. Soil shall be evaluated for estimated percolation based on structure and texture in accordance with accepted soil evaluation practices. Borings shall be made in accordance with Section AO103.7.1 for evaluating the soil.

AO103.8 Subsurface landscape irrigation site location. The surface grade of all soil absorption systems shall be located at a point lower than the surface grade of any water well or reservoir on the same or adjoining property. Where this is not possible, the site shall be located so surface water drainage from the site is not directed toward a well or reservoir. The soil absorption system shall be located with a minimum horizontal distance between various elements as indicated in Table AO103.8. Private sewage disposal systems in compacted areas, such as parking lots and driveways, are prohibited. Surface water shall be diverted away from any soil absorption site on the same or neighboring lots.

TABLE AO103.8
LOCATION OF GRAY WATER SYSTEM

ELEMENT	MINIMUM HORIZONTAL DISTANCE	
	HOLDING TANK (feet)	IRRIGATION DISPOSAL FIELD (feet)
Buildings	5	2
Property line adjoining private property	5	5
Public water main	10	10
Seepage pits	5	5
Septic tanks	0	5
Streams and lakes	50	50
Water service	5	5
Water wells	50	100

For SI: 1 foot = 304.8 mm.

AO103.9 Installation. Absorption systems shall be installed in accordance with Sections AO103.9.1 through AO103.9.5 to provide landscape irrigation without surfacing of gray water.

AO103.9.1 Absorption area. The total absorption area required shall be computed from the estimated daily gray water discharge and the design-loading rate based on the percolation rate for the site. The required absorption area equals the estimated gray water discharge divided by the design-loading rate from Table AO103.9.1.

TABLE AO103.9.1
DESIGN LOADING RATE

PERCOLATION RATE (minutes per inch)	DESIGN LOAD FACTOR (gallons per square foot per day)
0 to less than 10	1.2
10 to less than 30	0.8
30 to less than 45	0.72
45 to 60	0.4

For SI: 1 minute per inch = 2.362 s/mm;
1 gallon per square foot = 40.743 L/m².

AO103.9.2 Seepage trench excavations. Seepage trench excavations shall be a minimum of 1 foot (305 mm) to a maximum of 5 feet (1524 mm) wide. Trench excavations shall be spaced a minimum of 2 feet (610 mm) apart. The soil absorption area of a seepage trench shall be computed by using the bottom of the trench area (width) multiplied by the length of pipe. Individual seepage trenches shall be a maximum of 100 feet (30 480 mm) in *developed length*.

AO103.9.3 Seepage bed excavations. Seepage bed excavations shall be a minimum of 5 feet (1524 mm) wide and have more than one distribution pipe. The absorption area of a seepage bed shall be computed by using the bottom of the trench area. Distribution piping in a seepage bed shall be uniformly spaced a maximum of 5 feet (1524 mm) and a minimum of 3 feet (914 mm) apart, and a maximum of 3 feet (914 mm) and a minimum of 1 foot (305 mm) from the sidewall or headwall.

AO103.9.4 Excavation and construction. The bottom of a trench or bed excavation shall be level. Seepage trenches or beds shall not be excavated where the soil is so wet that such material rolled between the hands forms a soil wire. All smeared or compacted soil surfaces in the sidewalls or bottom of seepage trench or bed excavations shall be scarified to the depth of smearing or compaction and the loose material removed. Where rain falls on an open excavation, the soil shall be left until sufficiently dry so a soil wire will not form when soil from the excavation bottom is rolled between the hands. The bottom area shall then be scarified and loose material removed.

AO103.9.5 Aggregate and backfill. A minimum of 6 inches (152 mm) of aggregate ranging in size from $^1/_2$ to $2^1/_2$ inches (13 mm to 64 mm) shall be laid into the trench below the distribution piping elevation. The aggregate shall be evenly distributed a minimum of 2 inches (51 mm) over the top of the distribution pipe. The aggregate shall be covered with *approved* synthetic materials or 9 inches (229 mm) of uncompacted marsh hay or straw. Building paper shall not be used to cover the aggregate. A minimum of 9 inches (229 mm) of soil backfill shall be laid above the covering.

AO103.10 Distribution piping. Distribution piping shall be not less than 3 inches (76 mm) in diameter. Materials shall comply with Table AO103.10. The top of the distribution pipe shall be not less than 8 inches (203 mm) below the original surface. The slope of the distribution pipes shall be a minimum of

2 inches (51 mm) and a maximum of 4 inches (102 mm) per 100 feet (30 480 mm).

AO103.11 Joints. Distribution pipe shall be joined in accordance with Section P3003 of the *International Residential Code*.

TABLE AO103.10
DISTRIBUTION PIPE

MATERIAL	STANDARD
Polyethylene (PE) plastic pipe	ASTM F 405
Polyvinyl chloride (PVC) plastic pipe	ASTM D 2729
Polyvinyl chloride (PVC) plastic pipe with pipe stiffness of PS 35 and PS 50	ASTM F 1488

SIZING OF WATER PIPING SYSTEM

(The provisions contained in this appendix are not mandatory unless specifically referenced in the adopting ordinance.)

SECTION AP101
GENERAL

AP101.1 Scope.

AP101.1.1 This appendix outlines two procedures for sizing a water piping system (see Sections AP103.3 and AP201.1). The design procedures are based on the minimum static pressure available from the supply source, the head charges in the system caused by friction and elevation, and the rates of flow necessary for operation of various fixtures.

AP101.1.2 Because of the variable conditions encountered in hydraulic design, it is impractical to specify definite and detailed rules for sizing of the water piping system. Accordingly, other sizing or design methods conforming to good engineering practice standards are acceptable alternatives to those presented herein.

SECTION AP102
INFORMATION REQUIRED

AP102.1 Preliminary. Obtain the necessary information regarding the minimum daily static service pressure in the area where the building is to be located. If the building supply is to be metered, obtain information regarding friction loss relative to the rate of flow for meters in the range of sizes likely to be used. Friction loss data can be obtained from most manufacturers of water meters.

AP102.2 Demand load.

AP102.2.1 Estimate the supply demand of the building main and the principal branches and risers of the system by totaling the corresponding demand from the applicable part of Table AP103.3(3).

AP102.2.2 Estimate continuous supply demands in gallons per minute (L/m) for lawn sprinklers, air conditioners, etc., and add the sum to the total demand for fixtures. The result is the estimated supply demand for the building supply.

SECTION AP103
SELECTION OF PIPE SIZE

AP103.1 General. Decide from Table P2903.1 what is the desirable minimum residual pressure that should be maintained at the highest fixture in the supply system. If the highest group of fixtures contains flush valves, the pressure for the group should not be less than 15 pounds per square inch (psi) (103.4 kPa) flowing. For flush tank supplies, the available pressure should not be less than 8 psi (55.2 kPa) flowing, except blowout action fixtures must not be less than 25 psi (172.4 kPa) flowing.

AP103.2 Pipe sizing.

AP103.2.1 Pipe sizes can be selected according to the following procedure or by other design methods conforming to acceptable engineering practice and *approved* by the administrative authority. The sizes selected must not be less than the minimum required by this code.

AP103.2.2 Water pipe sizing procedures are based on a system of pressure requirements and losses, the sum of which must not exceed the minimum pressure available at the supply source. These pressures are as follows:

1. Pressure required at fixture to produce required flow. See Sections P2903.1 of this code and Section 604.5 of the *International Plumbing Code*.

2. Static pressure loss or gain (due to head) is computed at 0.433 psi per foot (9.8 kPa/m) of elevation change.

   Example: Assume that the highest fixture supply outlet is 20 feet (6096 mm) above or below the supply source. This produces a static pressure differential of 8.66 psi (59.8 kPa) loss [20 feet by 0.433 psi/foot (2096 mm by 9.8 kPa/m)].

3. Loss through water meter. The friction or pressure loss can be obtained from meter manufacturers.

4. Loss through taps in water main.

5. Losses through special devices such as filters, softeners, backflow prevention devices and pressure regulators. These values must be obtained from the manufacturers.

6. Loss through valves and fittings. Losses for these items are calculated by converting to *equivalent length* of piping and adding to the total pipe length.

7. Loss caused by pipe friction can be calculated when the pipe size, the pipe length and the flow through the pipe are known. With these three items, the friction loss can be determined. For piping flow charts not included, use manufacturers' tables and velocity recommendations.

Note: For all examples, the following metric conversions are applicable:

1 cubic foot per minute = 0.4719 L/s

1 square foot = 0.0929 m²

1 degree = 0.0175 rad

1 pound per square inch = 6.895 kPa

1 inch = 25.4 mm

1 foot = 304.8 mm

1 gallon per minute = 3.785 L/m

AP103.3 Segmented loss method. The size of water service mains, branch mains and risers by the segmented loss method, must be determined according to water supply demand [gpm (L/m)], available water pressure [psi (kPa)] and friction loss caused by the water meter and *developed length* of pipe [feet (m)], including *equivalent length* of fittings. This design procedure is based on the following parameters:

- The calculated friction loss through each length of the pipe.

- A system of pressure losses, the sum of which must not exceed the minimum pressure available at the street main or other source of supply.

- Pipe sizing based on estimated peak demand, total pressure losses caused by difference in elevation, equipment, *developed length* and pressure required at the most remote fixture, loss through taps in water main, losses through fittings, filters, backflow prevention devices, valves and pipe friction.

Because of the variable conditions encountered in hydraulic design, it is impractical to specify definite and detailed rules for sizing of the water piping system. Current sizing methods do not address the differences in the probability of use and flow characteristics of fixtures between types of occupancies. Creating an exact model of predicting the demand for a building is impossible and final studies assessing the impact of water conservation on demand are not yet complete. The following steps are necessary for the segmented loss method.

1. **Preliminary.** Obtain the necessary information regarding the minimum daily static service pressure in the area where the building is to be located. If the building supply is to be metered, obtain information regarding friction loss relative to the rate of flow for meters in the range of sizes to be used. Friction loss data can be obtained from manufacturers of water meters. Enough pressure must be available to overcome all system losses caused by friction and elevation so that plumbing fixtures operate properly. Section 604.6 of the *International Plumbing Code* requires that the water distribution system be designed for the minimum pressure available taking into consideration pressure fluctuations. The lowest pressure must be selected to guarantee a continuous, adequate supply of water. The lowest pressure in the public main usually occurs in the summer because of lawn sprinkling and supplying water for air-conditioning cooling towers. Future demands placed on the public main as a result of large growth or expansion should also be considered. The available pressure will decrease as additional loads are placed on the public system.

2. **Demand load.** Estimate the supply demand of the building main and the principal branches and risers of the system by totaling the corresponding demand from the applicable part of Table AP103.3(3). When estimating peak demand, sizing methods typically use water supply fixture units (w.s.f.u.) [see Table AP103.3(2)]. This numerical factor measures the load-producing effect of a single plumbing fixture of a given kind. The use of fixture units can be applied to a single basic probability curve (or table), found in the various sizing methods

[Table AP103.3(3)]. The fixture units are then converted into gallons per minute (L/m) flow rate for estimating demand.

    2.1. Estimate continuous supply demand in gallons per minute (L/m) for lawn sprinklers, air conditioners, etc., and add the sum to the total demand for fixtures. The result is the estimated supply demand for the building supply. Fixture units cannot be applied to constant-use fixtures such as hose bibbs, lawn sprinklers and air conditioners. These types of fixtures must be assigned the gallon per minute (L/m) value.

3. **Selection of pipe size.** This water pipe sizing procedure is based on a system of pressure requirements and losses, the sum of which must not exceed the minimum pressure available at the supply source. These pressures are as follows:

    3.1. Pressure required at the fixture to produce required flow. See Section P2903.1 of this code and Section 604.5 of the *International Plumbing Code.*

    3.2. Static pressure loss or gain (because of head) is computed at 0.433 psi per foot (9.8 kPa/m) of elevation change.

    3.3. Loss through a water meter. The friction or pressure loss can be obtained from the manufacturer.

    3.4. Loss through taps in water main [see Table AP103.3(4)].

    3.5. Losses through special devices such as filters, softeners, backflow prevention devices and pressure regulators. These values must be obtained from the manufacturers.

    3.6. Loss through valves and fittings [see Tables AP103.3(5) and AP103.3(6)]. Losses for these items are calculated by converting to *equivalent length* of piping and adding to the total pipe length.

    3.7. Loss caused by pipe friction can be calculated when the pipe size, the pipe length and the flow through the pipe are known. With these three items, the friction loss can be determined using Figures AP103.3(2) through AP103.3(7). When using charts, use pipe inside diameters. For piping flow charts not included, use manufacturers' tables and velocity recommendations. Before attempting to size any water supply system, it is necessary to gather preliminary information which includes available pressure, piping material, select design velocity, elevation differences and *developed length* to most remote fixture. The water supply system is divided into sections at major changes in elevation or where branches lead to fixture groups. The peak demand must be determined in each part of the hot and cold water supply system which includes the corresponding water supply fixture unit and conversion to gallons per minute (L/m) flow rate to be expected through each section. Sizing methods require determination of the "most hydraulically remote" fixture to compute the pressure loss caused by pipe and fittings. The hydraulically remote fixture represents the most downstream fixture along the circuit of piping requiring the most available pressure to operate properly. Consideration must be given to all pressure demands and losses, such as friction caused by pipe, fittings and equipment; elevation; and the residual pressure required by Table P2903.1. The two most common and frequent complaints about water supply system operation are lack of adequate pressure and noise.

Problem: What size Type L copper water pipe, service and distribution will be required to serve a two-story factory building having on each floor, back-to-back, two toilet rooms each equipped with hot and cold water? The highest fixture is 21 feet (6401 mm) above the street main, which is tapped with a 2-inch (51 mm) corporation cock at which point the minimum pressure is 55 psi (379.2 kPa). In the building basement, a 2-inch (51 mm) meter with a maximum pressure drop of 11 psi (75.8 kPa) and 3-inch (76 mm) reduced pressure principle backflow preventer with a maximum pressure drop of 9 psi (62.1 kPa) are to be installed. The system is shown by Figure AP103.3(1). To be determined are the pipe sizes for the service main and the cold and hot water distribution pipes.

Solution: A tabular arrangement such as shown in Table AP103.3(1) should first be constructed. The steps to be followed are indicated by the tabular arrangement itself as they are in sequence, columns 1 through 10 and lines A through L.

Step 1

Columns 1 and 2: Divide the system into sections breaking at major changes in elevation or where branches lead to fixture groups. After point B [see Figure AP103.3(1)], separate consideration will be given to the hot and cold water piping. Enter the sections to be considered in the service and cold water piping in Column 1 of the tabular arrangement. Column 1 of Table AP103.3(1) provides a line-by-line recommended tabular arrangement for use in solving pipe sizing.

The objective in designing the water supply system is to ensure an adequate water supply and pressure to all fixtures and equipment. Column 2 provides the pounds per square inch (psi) to be considered separately from the minimum pressure available at the main. Losses to take into consideration are the following: the differences in elevations between the water supply source and the highest water supply outlet, meter pressure losses, the tap in main loss, special fixture devices such as water softeners and backflow prevention devices and the pressure required at the most remote fixture outlet.

The difference in elevation can result in an increase or decrease in available pressure at the main. Where the water supply outlet is located above the source, this results in a loss in the available pressure and is subtracted from the pressure at the water source. Where the highest water supply outlet is located below the water supply source, there will be an increase in pressure that is added to the available pressure of the water source.

Column 3: According to Table AP103.3(3), determine the gpm (L/m) of flow to be expected in each section of the system. These flows range from 28.6 to 108 gpm. Load values for fixtures must be determined as water supply fixture units and then converted to a gallon-per-minute (gpm) rating to determine peak demand. When calculating peak demands, the water supply fixture units are added and then converted to the gallon-per-minute rating. For continuous flow fixtures such as hose bibbs and lawn sprinkler systems, add the gallon-per-minute demand to the intermittent demand of fixtures. For example, a total of 120 water supply fixture units is converted to a demand of 48 gallons per minute. Two hose bibbs × 5 gpm demand = 10 gpm. Total gpm rating = 48.0 gpm + 10 gpm = 58.0 gpm demand.

Step 2

Line A: Enter the minimum pressure available at the main source of supply in Column 2. This is 55 psi (379.2 kPa). The local water authorities generally keep records of pressures at different times of day and year. The available pressure can also be checked from nearby buildings or from fire department hydrant checks.

Line B: Determine from Table P2903.1 the highest pressure required for the fixtures on the system, which is 15 psi (103.4 kPa), to operate a flushometer valve. The most remote fixture outlet is necessary to compute the pressure loss caused by pipe and fittings, and represents the most downstream fixture along the circuit of piping requiring the available pressure to operate properly as indicated by Table P2903.1.

Line C: Determine the pressure loss for the meter size given or assumed. The total water flow from the main through the service as determined in Step 1 will serve to aid in the meter selected. There are three common types of water meters; the pressure losses are determined by the American Water Works Association Standards for displacement type, compound type and turbine type. The maximum pressure loss of such devices takes into consideration the meter size, safe operating capacity (gpm) and maximum rates for continuous operations (gpm). Typically, equipment imparts greater pressure losses than piping.

Line D: Select from Table AP103.3(4) and enter the pressure loss for the tap size given or assumed. The loss of pressure through taps and tees in pounds per square inch (psi) is based on the total gallon-per-minute flow rate and size of the tap.

Line E: Determine the difference in elevation between the main and source of supply and the highest fixture on the system. Multiply this figure, expressed in feet, by 0.43 psi (2.9 kPa). Enter the resulting psi loss on Line E. The difference in elevation between the water supply source and the highest water supply outlet has a significant impact on the sizing of the water supply system. The difference in elevation usually results in a loss in the available pressure because the water supply outlet is generally located above the water supply source. The loss is caused by the pressure required to lift the water to the outlet. The pressure loss is subtracted from the pressure at the water source. Where the highest water supply outlet is located below the water source, there will be an increase in pressure which is added to the available pressure of the water source.

Lines F, G and H: The pressure losses through filters, backflow prevention devices or other special fixtures must be obtained from the manufacturer or estimated and entered on these lines. Equipment such as backflow prevention devices, check valves, water softeners, instantaneous or tankless water heaters, filters and strainers can impart a much greater pressure loss than the piping. The pressure losses can range from 8 psi to 30 psi.

Step 3

Line I: The sum of the pressure requirements and losses that affect the overall system (Lines B through H) is entered on this line. Summarizing the steps, all of the system losses are subtracted from the minimum water pressure. The remainder is the pressure available for friction, defined as the energy available to push the water through the pipes to each fixture. This force can be used as an average pressure loss, as long as the pressure available for friction is not exceeded. Saving a certain amount for available water supply pressures as an area incurs growth, or because of aging of the pipe or equipment added to the system is recommended.

Step 4

Line J: Subtract Line I from Line A. This gives the pressure that remains available from overcoming friction losses in the system. This figure is a guide to the pipe size that is chosen for each section, incorporating the total friction losses to the most remote outlet (measured length is called *developed length*).

> **Exception:** When the main is above the highest fixture, the resulting psi must be considered a pressure gain (static head gain) and omitted from the sums of Lines B through H and added to Line J.

The maximum friction head loss that can be tolerated in the system during peak demand is the difference between the static pressure at the highest and most remote outlet at no-flow conditions and the minimum flow pressure required at that outlet. If the losses are within the required limits, every run of pipe will also be within the required friction head loss. Static pressure loss is at the most remote outlet in feet × 0.433 = loss in psi caused by elevation differences.

Step 5

Column 4: Enter the length of each section from the main to the most remote outlet (at Point E). Divide the water supply system into sections breaking at major changes in elevation or where branches lead to fixture groups.

Step 6

Column 5: When selecting a trial pipe size, the length from the water service or meter to the most remote fixture outlet must be measured to determine the *developed length*. However, in systems having a flush valve or temperature controlled shower at the topmost floors the *developed length* would be from the water meter to the most remote flush valve on the system. A rule of thumb is that size will become progressively smaller as the system extends farther from the main source of supply. Trial pipe size may be arrived at by the following formula:

Line J: (Pressure available to overcome pipe friction) × 100/*equivalent length* of run total *developed length* to most remote fixture × percentage factor of 1.5 (note: a percentage factor is used only as an estimate for friction losses imposed for fittings for initial trial pipe size) = psi (average pressure drop per 100 feet of pipe).

For trial pipe size see Figure AP103.3(3) (Type L copper) based on 2.77 psi and 108 gpm = $2^1/_2$ inches. To determine the *equivalent length* of run to the most remote outlet, the *developed length* is determined and added to the friction losses for fittings and valves. The *developed lengths* of the designated pipe sections are as follows:

A - B	54 ft
B - C	8 ft
C - D	13 ft
D - E	150 ft

Total *developed length* = 225 ft

The *equivalent length* of the friction loss in fittings and valves must be added to the *developed length* (most remote outlet). Where the size of fittings and valves is not known, the added friction loss should be approximated. A general rule that has been used is to add 50 percent of the *developed length* to allow for fittings and valves. For example, the *equivalent length* of run equals the *developed length* of run (225 ft × 1.5 = 338 ft). The total *equivalent length* of run for determining a trial pipe size is 338 feet.

> **Example:** 9.36 (pressure available to overcome pipe friction) × 100/ 338 (*equivalent length* of run = 225 × 1.5) = 2.77 psi (average pressure drop per 100 feet of pipe).

Step 7

Column 6: Select from Table AP103.3(6) the *equivalent lengths* for the trial pipe size of fittings and valves on each pipe section. Enter the sum for each section in Column 6. (The number of fittings to be used in this example must be an estimate.) The *equivalent length* of piping is the *developed length* plus the *equivalent lengths* of pipe corresponding to friction head losses for fittings and valves. Where the size of fittings and valves is not known, the added friction head losses must be approximated. An estimate for this example is found in Table AP.1.

Step 8

Column 7: Add the figures from Column 4 and Column 6, and enter in Column 7. Express the sum in hundreds of feet.

Step 9

Column 8: Select from Figure AP103.3(3) the friction loss per 100 feet (30 480 mm) of pipe for the gallon-per-minute flow in a section (Column 3) and trial pipe size (Column 5). Maximum friction head loss per 100 feet is determined on the basis of total pressure available for friction head loss and the longest *equivalent length* of run. The selection is based on the gallon-per-minute demand, the uniform friction head loss, and the maximum design velocity. Where the size indicated by the hydraulic table indicates a velocity in excess of the selected velocity, a size must be selected which produces the required velocity.

Step 10

Column 9: Multiply the figures in Columns 7 and 8 for each section and enter in Column 9.

Total friction loss is determined by multiplying the friction loss per 100 feet (30 480 mm) for each pipe section in the total *developed length* by the pressure loss in fittings expressed as *equivalent length* in feet. Note: Section C-F should be considered in the total pipe friction losses only if greater loss occurs in Section C-F than in pipe Section D-E. Section C-F is not considered in the total *developed length*. Total friction loss in *equivalent length* is determined in Table AP.2.

Step 11

Line K: Enter the sum of the values in Column 9. The value is the total friction loss in *equivalent length* for each designated pipe section.

Step 12

Line L: Subtract Line J from Line K and enter in Column 10.

The result should always be a positive or plus figure. If it is not, repeat the operation using Columns 5, 6, 8 and 9 until a balance or near balance is obtained. If the difference between Lines J and K is a high positive number, it is an indication that the pipe sizes are too large and should be reduced, thus saving materials. In such a case, the operations using Columns 5, 6, 8 and 9 should be repeated.

The total friction losses are determined and subtracted from the pressure available to overcome pipe friction for trial pipe size. This number is critical because it provides a guide to whether the pipe size selected is too large and the process should be repeated to obtain an economically designed system.

Answer: The final figures entered in Column 5 become the design pipe size for the respective sections. Repeating this operation a second time using the same sketch but considering the demand for hot water, it is possible to size the hot water distribution piping. This has been worked up as a part of the overall problem in the tabular arrangement used for sizing the service and water distribution piping. Note that consideration must be given to the pressure losses from the street main to the water heater (Section A-B) in determining the hot water pipe sizes.

TABLE AP.1

COLD WATER PIPE SECTION	FITTINGS/VALVES	PRESSURE LOSS EXPRESSED AS EQUIVALENT LENGTH OF TUBE (feet)	HOT WATER PIPE SECTION	FITTINGS/VALVES	PRESSURE LOSS EXPRESSED AS EQUIVALENT OF TUBE (feet)
A-B	3-2^1/$_2$″ Gate valves	3	A-B	3-2^1/$_2$″ Gate valves	3
	1-2^1/$_2$″ Side branch tee	12	—	1-2^1/$_2$″ Side branch tee	12
B-C	1-2^1/$_2$″ Straight run tee	0.5	B-C	1-2″ Straight run tee	7
	—	—	—	1-2″ 90-degree ell	0.5
C-F	1-2^1/$_2$″ Side branch tee	12	C-F	1-1^1/$_2$″ Side branch tee	7
C-D	1-2^1/$_2$″ 90-degree ell	7	C-D	1-1^1/$_2$″ 90-degree ell	4
D-E	1-2^1/$_2$″ Side branch tee	12	D-E	1-1^1/$_2$″ Side branch tee	7

TABLE AP.2

PIPE SECTIONS	FRICTION LOSS EQUIVALENT LENGTH (feet)	
	Cold Water	Hot Water
A-B	0.69 × 3.2 = 2.21	0.69 × 3.2 = 2.21
B-C	0.085 × 3.1 = 0.26	0.16 × 1.4 = 0.22
C-D	0.20 × 1.9 = 0.38	0.17 × 3.2 = 0.54
D-E	1.62 × 1.9 = 3.08	1.57 × 3.2 = 5.02
Total pipe friction losses (Line K)	5.93	7.99

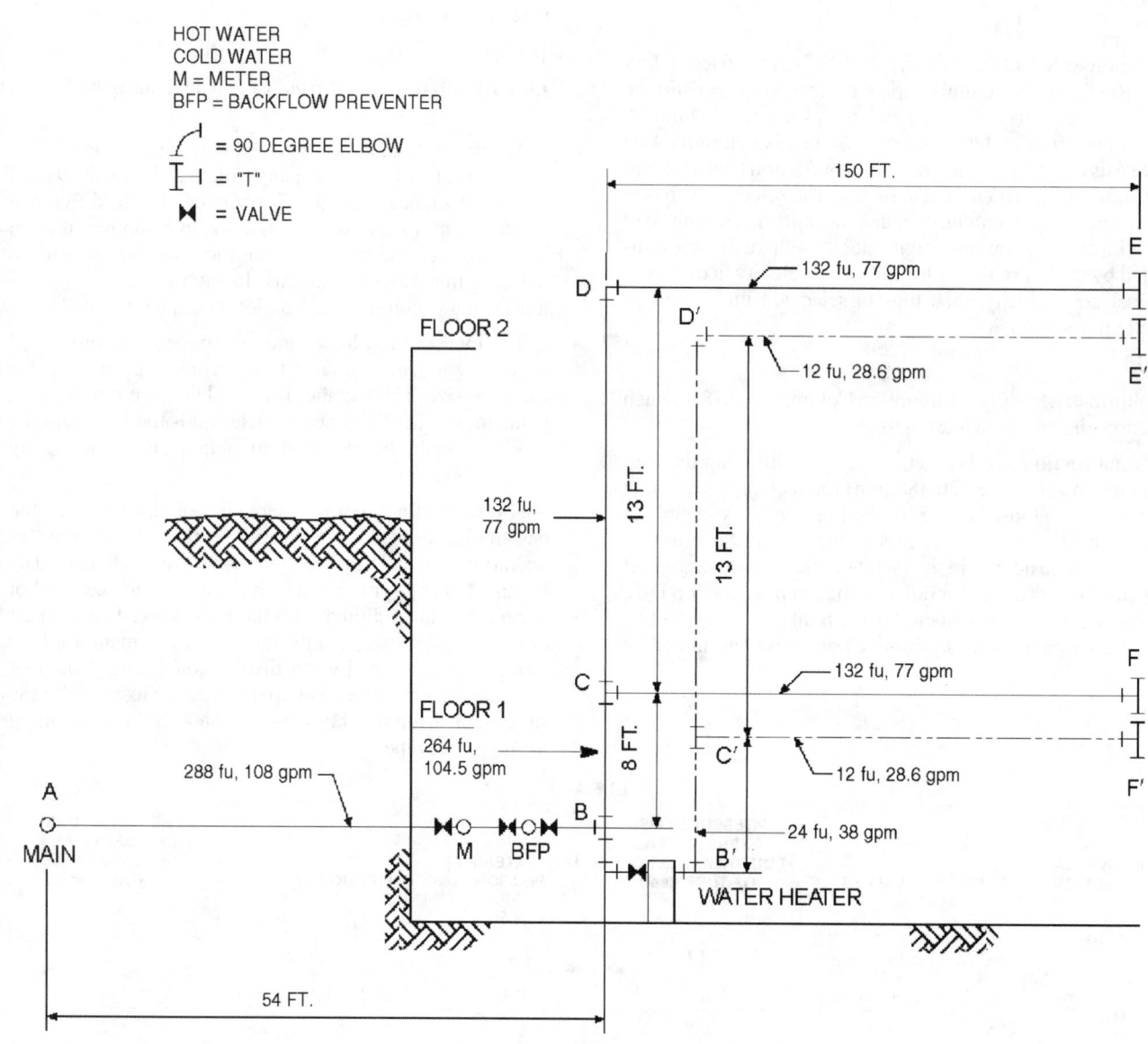

HOT WATER
COLD WATER
M = METER
BFP = BACKFLOW PREVENTER

⌐ = 90 DEGREE ELBOW

⊥ = "T"

▶◀ = VALVE

150 FT.

E

132 fu, 77 gpm

D

FLOOR 2

D'

12 fu, 28.6 gpm

E'

13 FT.

132 fu,
77 gpm

13 FT.

F

132 fu, 77 gpm

C

FLOOR 1

264 fu,
104.5 gpm

8 FT.

C'

12 fu, 28.6 gpm

F'

288 fu, 108 gpm

A

B

24 fu, 38 gpm

MAIN

M   BFP

B'

WATER HEATER

54 FT.

For SI: 1 foot = 304.8 mm, 1 gpm = 3.785 L/m.

FIGURE AP103.3(1)
EXAMPLE-SIZING

TABLE AP103.3(1)
RECOMMENDED TABULAR ARRANGEMENT FOR USE IN SOLVING PIPE SIZING PROBLEMS

COLUMN		1	2	3	4	5	6	7	8	9	10
Line		Description	Lb per square inch (psi)	Gal. per min through section	Length of section (feet)	Trial pipe size (inches)	Equivalent length of fittings and valves (feet)	Total equivalent length col. 4 and col. 6 (100 feet)	Friction loss per 100 feet of trial size pipe (psi)	Friction loss in equivalent length col. 8 x col. 7 (psi)	Excess pressure over friction losses (psi)
A	Service and cold water distribution piping[a]	Minimum pressure available at main . . 55.00									
B		Highest pressure required at a fixture (Table P2903.1) 15.00									
C		Meter loss 2″ meter 11.00									
D		Tap in main loss 2″ tap [Table AP103.3(4)] . 1.61									
E		Static head loss 21 ft × 0.43 psi/ft. 9.03									
F		Special fixture loss backflow preventer 9.00									
G		Special fixture loss—Filter 0.00									
H		Special fixture loss—Other 0.00									
I		Total overall losses and requirements (Sum of Lines B through H) 45.64									
J		Pressure available to overcome pipe friction (Line A minus Line I) 9.36									
	DESIGNATION Pipe section (from diagram) Cold water Distribution piping	FU AB 288	108.0	54	$2^1/_2$	15.00	0.69	3.2	2.21	—
		BC 264	104.5	8	$2^1/_2$	0.5	0.85	3.1	0.26	—
		CD 132	77.0	13	$2^1/_2$	7.00	0.20	1.9	0.38	—
		CF[b] 132	77.0	150	$2^1/_2$	12.00	1.62	1.9	3.08	—
		DE[b] 132	77.0	150	$2^1/_2$	12.00	1.62	1.9	3.08	—
K	Total pipe friction losses (cold)		—	—	—	—	—	—	—	5.93	—
L	Difference (Line J minus Line K)		—	—	—	—	—	—	—	—	3.43
	Pipe section (from diagram) Diagram Hot water Distribution Piping	A′B′ 288	108.0	54	$2^1/_2$	12.00	0.69	3.3	2.21	—
		B′C′ 24	38.0	8	2	7.5	0.16	1.4	0.22	—
		C′D′ 12	28.6	13	$1^1/_2$	4.0	0.17	3.2	0.54	—
		C′F′[b] 12	28.6	150	$1^1/_2$	7.00	1.57	3.2	5.02	—
		D′E′[b] 12	28.6	150	$1^1/_2$	7.00	1.57	3.2	5.02	—
K	Total pipe friction losses (hot)		—	—	—	—	—	—	—	7.99	—
L	Difference (Line J minus Line K)		—	—	—	—	—	—	—	—	1.37

For SI: 1 inch = 25.4 mm, 1 foot = 304.8 mm, 1 psi = 6.895 kPa, 1 gpm = 3.785 L/m.

a. To be considered as pressure gain for fixtures below main (to consider separately, omit from "I" and add to "J").

b. To consider separately, in K use C-F only if greater loss than above.

TABLE AP103.3(2)
LOAD VALUES ASSIGNED TO FIXTURES[a]

FIXTURE	OCCUPANCY	TYPE OF SUPPLY CONTROL	LOAD VALUES, IN WATER SUPPLY FIXTURE UNITS (wsfu)		
			Cold	Hot	Total
Bathroom group	Private	Flush tank	2.7	1.5	3.6
Bathroom group	Private	Flush valve	6.0	3.0	8.0
Bathtub	Private	Faucet	1.0	1.0	1.4
Bathtub	Public	Faucet	3.0	3.0	4.0
Bidet	Private	Faucet	1.5	1.5	2.0
Combination fixture	Private	Faucet	2.25	2.25	3.0
Dishwashing machine	Private	Automatic	—	1.4	1.4
Drinking fountain	Offices, etc.	$^3/_8''$ valve	0.25	—	0.25
Kitchen sink	Private	Faucet	1.0	1.0	1.4
Kitchen sink	Hotel, restaurant	Faucet	3.0	3.0	4.0
Laundry trays (1 to 3)	Private	Faucet	1.0	1.0	1.4
Lavatory	Private	Faucet	0.5	0.5	0.7
Lavatory	Public	Faucet	1.5	1.5	2.0
Service sink	Offices, etc.	Faucet	2.25	2.25	3.0
Shower head	Public	Mixing valve	3.0	3.0	4.0
Shower head	Private	Mixing valve	1.0	1.0	1.4
Urinal	Public	1″ flush valve	10.0	—	10.0
Urinal	Public	$^3/_4''$ flush valve	5.0	—	5.0
Urinal	Public	Flush tank	3.0	—	3.0
Washing machine (8 lb)	Private	Automatic	1.0	1.0	1.4
Washing machine (8 lb)	Public	Automatic	2.25	2.25	3.0
Washing machine (15 lb)	Public	Automatic	3.0	3.0	4.0
Water closet	Private	Flush valve	6.0	—	6.0
Water closet	Private	Flush tank	2.2	—	2.2
Water closet	Public	Flush valve	10.0	—	10.0
Water closet	Public	Flush tank	5.0	—	5.0
Water closet	Public or private	Flushometer tank	2.0	—	2.0

For SI: 1 inch = 25.4 mm, 1 pound = 0.454 kg.

a. For fixtures not listed , loads should be assumed by comparing the fixture to one listed using water in similar quantities and at similar rates. The assigned loads for fixtures with both hot and cold water supplies are given for separate hot and cold water loads and for total load. The separate hot and cold water loads being three-fourths of the total load for the fixture in each case.

TABLE AP103.3(3)
TABLE FOR ESTIMATING DEMAND

SUPPLY SYSTEMS PREDOMINANTLY FOR FLUSH TANKS			SUPPLY SYSTEMS PREDOMINANTLY FOR FLUSH VALVES		
Load	Demand		Load	Demand	
(Water supply fixture units)	(Gallons per minute)	(Cubic feet per minute)	(Water supply fixture units)	(Gallons per minute)	(Cubic feet per minute)
1	3.0	0.04104	—	—	—
2	5.0	0.0684	—	—	—
3	6.5	0.86892	—	—	—
4	8.0	1.06944	—	—	—
5	9.4	1.256592	5	15.0	2.0052
6	10.7	1.430376	6	17.4	2.326032
7	11.8	1.577424	7	19.8	2.646364
8	12.8	1.711104	8	22.2	2.967696
9	13.7	1.831416	9	24.6	3.288528
10	14.6	1.951728	10	27.0	3.60936
11	15.4	2.058672	11	27.8	3.716304
12	16.0	2.13888	12	28.6	3.823248
13	16.5	2.20572	13	29.4	3.930192
14	17.0	2.27256	14	30.2	4.037136
15	17.5	2.3394	15	31.0	4.14408
16	18.0	2.90624	16	31.8	4.241024
17	18.4	2.459712	17	32.6	4.357968
18	18.8	2.513184	18	33.4	4.464912
19	19.2	2.566656	19	34.2	4.571856
20	19.6	2.620128	20	35.0	4.6788
25	21.5	2.87412	25	38.0	5.07984
30	23.3	3.114744	30	42.0	5.61356
35	24.9	3.328632	35	44.0	5.88192
40	26.3	3.515784	40	46.0	6.14928
45	27.7	3.702936	45	48.0	6.41664
50	29.1	3.890088	50	50.0	6.684
60	32.0	4.27776	60	54.0	7.21872
70	35.0	4.6788	70	58.0	7.75344
80	38.0	5.07984	80	61.2	8.181216
90	41.0	5.48088	90	64.3	8.595624
100	43.5	5.81508	100	67.5	9.0234
120	48.0	6.41664	120	73.0	9.75864
140	52.5	7.0182	140	77.0	10.29336
160	57.0	7.61976	160	81.0	10.82808
180	61.0	8.15448	180	85.5	11.42964
200	65.0	8.6892	200	90.0	12.0312
225	70.0	9.3576	225	95.5	12.76644
250	75.0	10.026	250	101.0	13.50168

(continued)

TABLE AP103.3(3)—continued
TABLE FOR ESTIMATING DEMAND

SUPPLY SYSTEMS PREDOMINANTLY FOR FLUSH TANKS			SUPPLY SYSTEMS PREDOMINANTLY FOR FLUSH VALVES		
Load	Demand		Load	Demand	
(Water supply fixture units)	(Gallons per minute)	(Cubic feet per minute)	(Water supply fixture units)	(Gallons per minute)	(Cubic feet per minute)
275	80.0	10.6944	275	104.5	13.96956
300	85.0	11.3628	300	108.0	14.43744
400	105.0	14.0364	400	127.0	16.97736
500	124.0	16.57632	500	143.0	19.11624
750	170.0	22.7256	750	177.0	23.66136
1,000	208.0	27.80544	1,000	208.0	27.80544
1,250	239.0	31.94952	1,250	239.0	31.94952
1,500	269.0	35.95992	1,500	269.0	35.95992
1,750	297.0	39.70296	1,750	297.0	39.70296
2,000	325.0	43.446	2,000	325.0	43.446
2,500	380.0	50.7984	2,500	380.0	50.7984
3,000	433.0	57.88344	3,000	433.0	57.88344
4,000	535.0	70.182	4,000	525.0	70.182
5,000	593.0	79.27224	5,000	593.0	79.27224

TABLE AP103.3(4)
LOSS OF PRESSURE THROUGH TAPS AND TEES IN POUNDS PER SQUARE INCH (psi)

GALLONS PER MINUTE	SIZE OF TAP OR TEE (inches)						
	$5/_8$	$3/_4$	1	$1^1/_4$	$1^1/_2$	2	3
10	1.35	0.64	0.18	0.08	—	—	—
20	5.38	2.54	0.77	0.31	0.14	—	—
30	12.10	5.72	1.62	0.69	0.33	0.10	—
40	—	10.20	3.07	1.23	0.58	0.18	—
50	—	15.90	4.49	1.92	0.91	0.28	—
60	—	—	6.46	2.76	1.31	0.40	—
70	—	—	8.79	3.76	1.78	0.55	0.10
80	—	—	11.50	4.90	2.32	0.72	0.13
90	—	—	14.50	6.21	2.94	0.91	0.16
100	—	—	17.94	7.67	3.63	1.12	0.21
120	—	—	25.80	11.00	5.23	1.61	0.30
140	—	—	35.20	15.00	7.12	2.20	0.41
150	—	—	—	17.20	8.16	2.52	0.47
160	—	—	—	19.60	9.30	2.92	0.54
180	—	—	—	24.80	11.80	3.62	0.68
200	—	—	—	30.70	14.50	4.48	0.84
225	—	—	—	38.80	18.40	5.60	1.06
250	—	—	—	47.90	22.70	7.00	1.31
275	—	—	—	—	27.40	7.70	1.59
300	—	—	—	—	32.60	10.10	1.88

For SI: 1 inch = 25.4 mm, 1 pound per square inch = 6.895 kPa, 1 gallon per minute = 3.785 L/m.

TABLE AP103.3(5)
ALLOWANCE IN EQUIVALENT LENGTHS OF PIPE FOR FRICTION LOSS IN VALVES AND THREADED FITTINGS (feet)

FITTING OR VALVE	PIPE SIZE (inches)							
	$\frac{1}{2}$	$\frac{3}{4}$	1	$1\frac{1}{4}$	$1\frac{1}{2}$	2	$2\frac{1}{2}$	3
45-degree elbow	1.2	1.5	1.8	2.4	3.0	4.0	5.0	6.0
90-degree elbow	2.0	2.5	3.0	4.0	5.0	7.0	8.0	10.0
Tee, run	0.6	0.8	0.9	1.2	1.5	2.0	2.5	3.0
Tee, branch	3.0	4.0	5.0	6.0	7.0	10.0	12.0	15.0
Gate valve	0.4	0.5	0.6	0.8	1.0	1.3	1.6	2.0
Balancing valve	0.8	1.1	1.5	1.9	2.2	3.0	3.7	4.5
Plug-type cock	0.8	1.1	1.5	1.9	2.2	3.0	3.7	4.5
Check valve, swing	5.6	8.4	11.2	14.0	16.8	22.4	28.0	33.6
Globe valve	15.0	20.0	25.0	35.0	45.0	55.0	65.0	80.0
Angle valve	8.0	12.0	15.0	18.0	22.0	28.0	34.0	40.0

For SI: 1 inch = 25.4 mm, 1 foot = 304.8 mm, 1 degree = 0.0175 rad.

TABLE AP103.3(6)
PRESSURE LOSS IN FITTINGS AND VALVES EXPRESSED AS EQUIVALENT LENGTH OF TUBE[a] (feet)

NOMINAL OR STANDARD SIZE (inches)	FITTINGS					VALVES			
	Standard Ell		90-Degree Tee						
	90 Degree	45 Degree	Side Branch	Straight Run	Coupling	Ball	Gate	Butterfly	Check
$\frac{3}{8}$	0.5	—	1.5	—	—	—	—	—	1.5
$\frac{1}{2}$	1	0.5	2	—	—	—	—	—	2
$\frac{5}{8}$	1.5	0.5	2	—	—	—	—	—	2.5
$\frac{3}{4}$	2	0.5	3	—	—	—	—	—	3
1	2.5	1	4.5	—	—	0.5	—	—	4.5
$1\frac{1}{4}$	3	1	5.5	0.5	0.5	0.5	—	—	5.5
$1\frac{1}{2}$	4	1.5	7	0.5	0.5	0.5	—	—	6.5
2	5.5	2	9	0.5	0.5	0.5	0.5	7.5	9
$2\frac{1}{2}$	7	2.5	12	0.5	0.5	—	1	10	11.5
3	9	3.5	15	1	1	—	1.5	15.5	14.5
$3\frac{1}{2}$	9	3.5	14	1	1	—	2	—	12.5
4	12.5	5	21	1	1	—	2	16	18.5
5	16	6	27	1.5	1.5	—	3	11.5	23.5
6	19	7	34	2	2	—	3.5	13.5	26.5
8	29	11	50	3	3	—	5	12.5	39

For SI: 1 inch = 25.4 mm, 1 foot = 304.8 mm, 1 degree = 0.01745 rad.

a. Allowances are for streamlined soldered fittings and recessed threaded fittings. For threaded fittings, double the allowances shown in the table. The equivalent lengths presented above are based on a C factor of 150 in the Hazen-Williams friction loss formula. The lengths shown are rounded to the nearest half-foot.

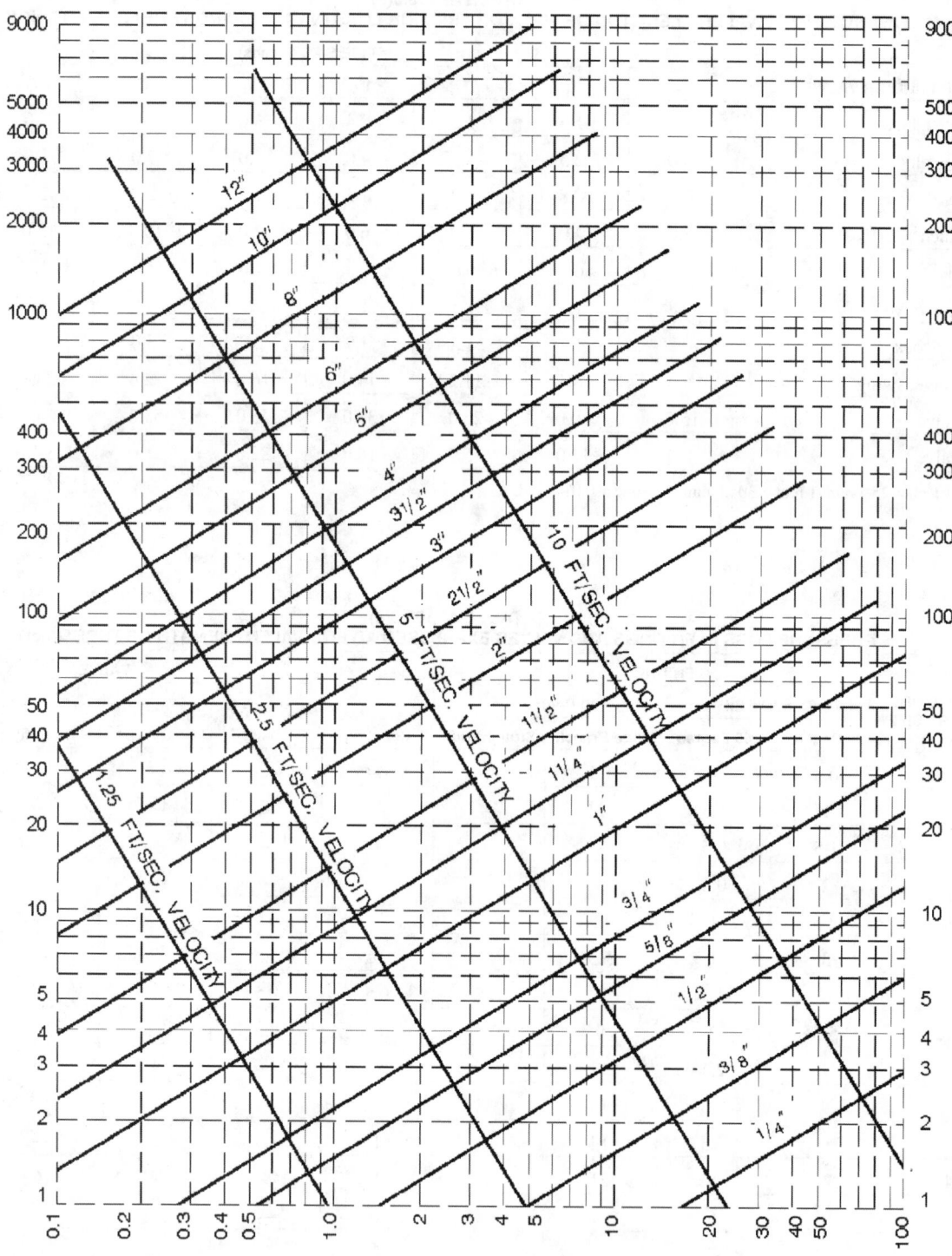

WATER FLOW RATE, GALLONS PER MINUTE

PRESSURE DROP PER 100 FEET OF TUBE, POUNDS PER SQUARE INCH

Note: Fluid velocities in excess of 5 to 8 feet/second are not usually recommended.

FIGURE AP103.3(2)
FRICTION LOSS IN SMOOTH PIPE[a] (TYPE K, ASTM B 88 COPPER TUBING)

For SI: 1 inch = 25.4 mm, 1 foot = 304.8 mm, 1 gpm = 3.785 L/m, 1 psi = 6.895 kPa, 1 foot per second = 0.305 m/s.
a. This chart applies to smooth new copper tubing with recessed (streamline) soldered joints and to the actual sizes of types indicated on the diagram.

Note: Fluid velocities in excess of 5 to 8 feet/second are not usually recommended.

FIGURE AP103.3(3)
FRICTION LOSS IN SMOOTH PIPE[a] (TYPE L, ASTM B 88 COPPER TUBING)

For SI: 1 inch = 25.4 mm, 1 foot = 304.8 mm, 1 gpm = 3.785 L/m, 1 psi = 6.895 kPa, 1 foot per second = 0.305 m/s.

a. This chart applies to smooth new copper tubing with recessed (streamline) soldered joints and to the actual sizes of types indicated on the diagram.

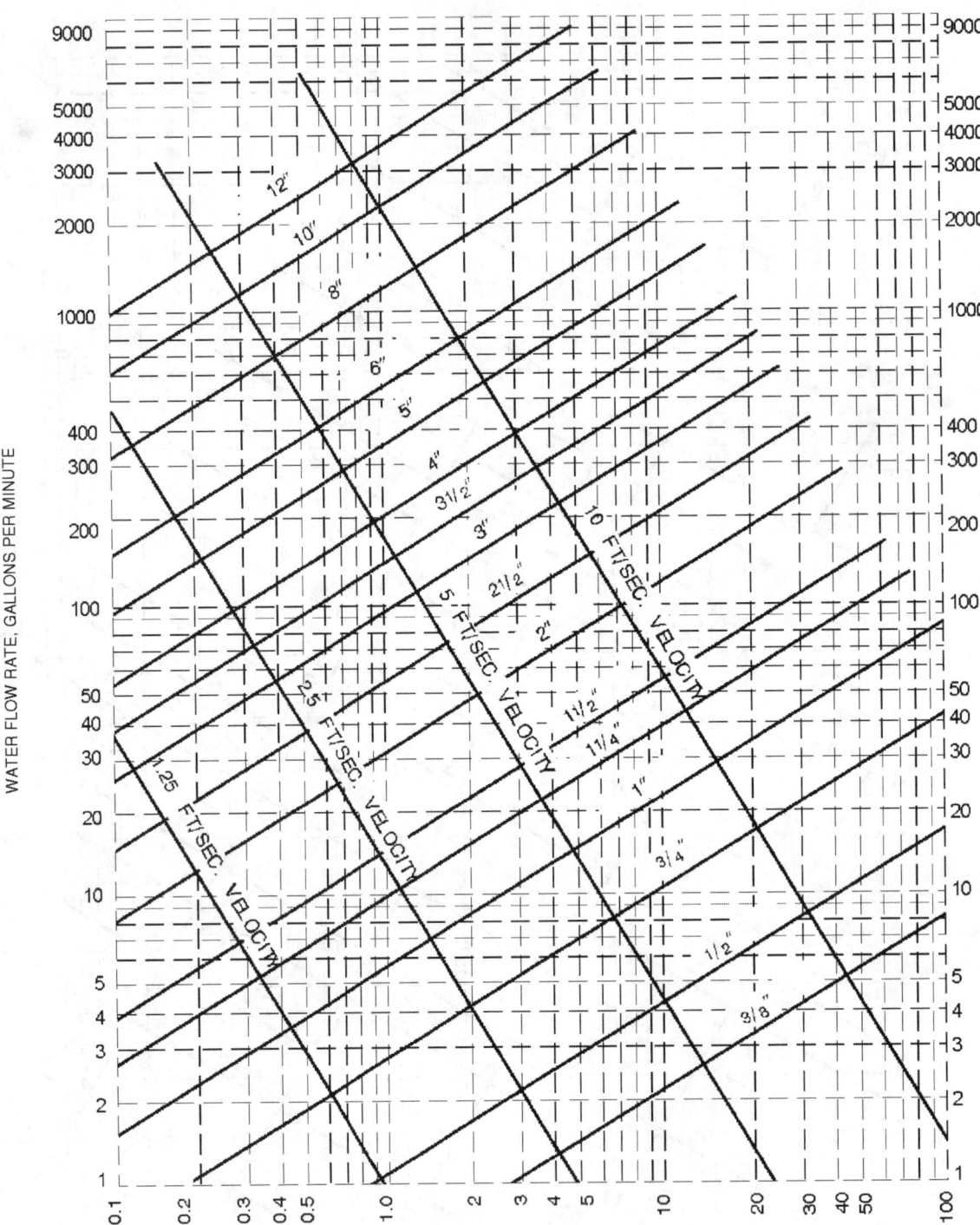

WATER FLOW RATE, GALLONS PER MINUTE

PRESSURE DROP PER 100 FEET OF TUBE, POUNDS PER SQUARE INCH

Note: Fluid velocities in excess of 5 to 8 feet/second are not usually recommended.

FIGURE AP103.3(4)
FRICTION LOSS IN SMOOTH PIPE[a] (TYPE M, ASTM B 88 COPPER TUBING)

For SI: 1 inch = 25.4 mm, 1 foot = 304.8 mm, 1 gpm = 3.785 L/m, 1 psi = 6.895 kPa, 1 foot per second = 0.305 m/s.
a. This chart applies to smooth new copper tubing with recessed (streamline) soldered joints and to the actual sizes of types indicated on the diagram.

2009 INTERNATIONAL RESIDENTIAL CODE®

FRICTION LOSS POUNDS PER SQUARE INCH HEAD PER 100 FEET LENGTH

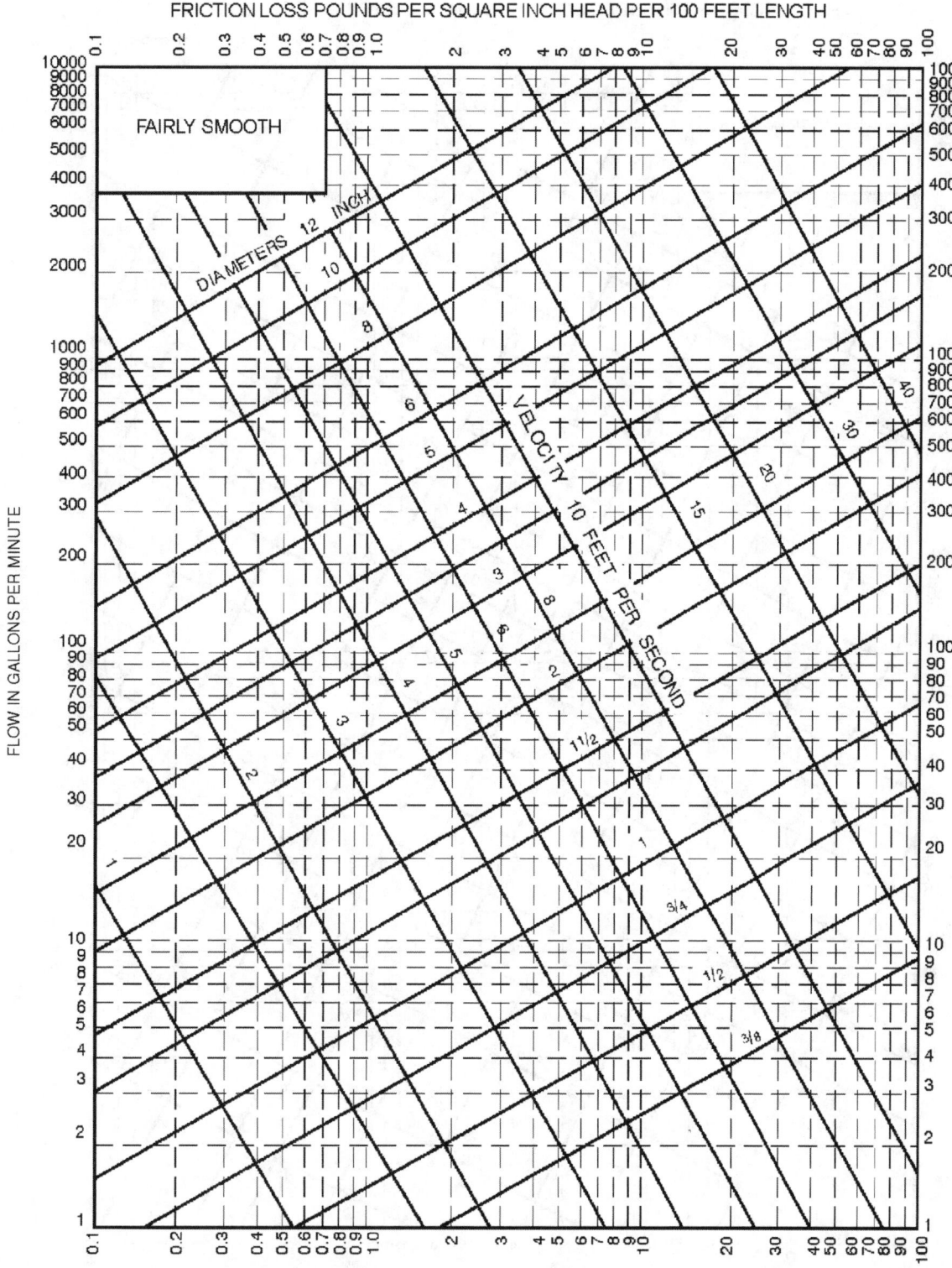

FRICTION LOSS POUNDS PER SQUARE INCH HEAD PER 100 FEET LENGTH

FIGURE AP103.3(5)
FRICTION LOSS IN FAIRLY SMOOTH PIPE[a]

For SI: 1 inch = 25.4 mm, 1 foot = 304.8 mm, 1 gpm = 3.785 L/m, 1 psi = 6.895 kPa, 1 foot per second = 0.305 m/s.

a.   This chart applies to smooth new steel (fairly smooth) pipe and to actual diameters of standard-weight pipe.

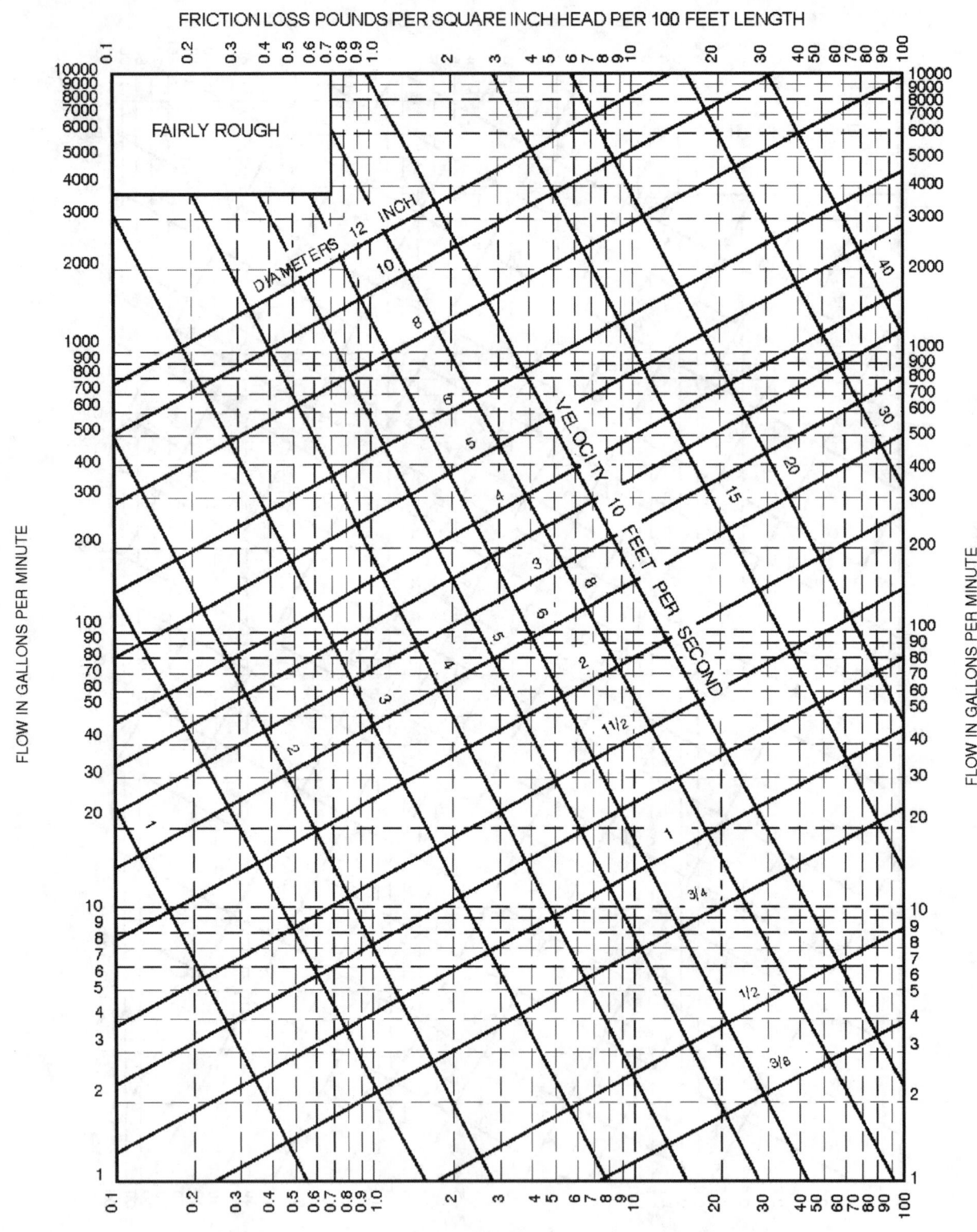

FIGURE AP103.3(6)
FRICTION LOSS IN FAIRLY ROUGH PIPE[a]

For SI: 1 inch = 25.4 mm, 1 foot = 304.8 mm, 1 gpm = 3.785 L/m, 1 psi = 6.895 kPa, 1 foot per second = 0.305 m/s.
a. This chart applies to fairly rough pipe and to actual diameters which in general will be less than the actual diameters of the new pipe of the same kind.

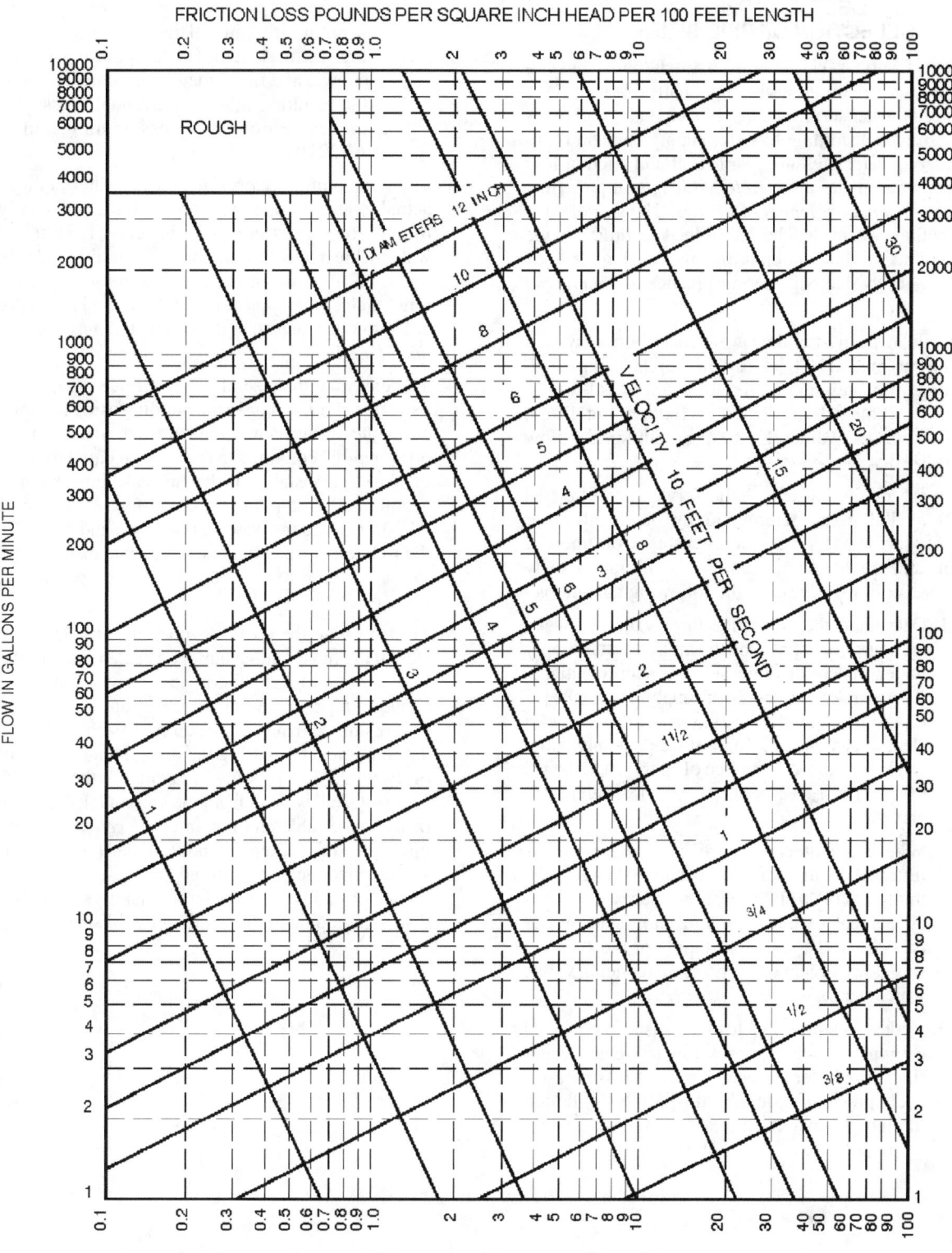

FRICTION LOSS POUNDS PER SQUARE INCH HEAD PER 100 FEET LENGTH

FIGURE AP103.3(7)
FRICTION LOSS IN FAIRLY ROUGH PIPE[a]

For SI: 1 inch = 25.4 mm, 1 foot = 304.8 mm, 1 gpm = 3.785 L/m, 1 psi = 6.895 kPa, 1 foot per second = 0.305 m/s.

a. This chart applies to very rough pipe and existing pipe and to their actual diameters.

SECTION AP201
SELECTION OF PIPE SIZE

AP201.1 Size of water-service mains, branch mains and risers. The minimum size water service pipe shall be $^3/_4$ inch (19.1 mm). The size of water service mains, branch mains and risers shall be determined according to water supply demand [gpm (L/m)], available water pressure [psi (kPa)] and friction loss caused by the water meter and *developed length* of pipe [feet (m)], including *equivalent length* of fittings. The size of each water distribution system shall be determined according to the procedure outlined in this section or by other design methods conforming to acceptable engineering practice and *approved* by the code official:

1. Supply load in the building water-distribution system shall be determined by total load on the pipe being sized, in terms of water-supply fixture units (w.s.f.u.), as shown in Table AP103.3(2). For fixtures not listed, choose a w.s.f.u. value of a fixture with similar flow characteristics.

2. Obtain the minimum daily static service pressure [psi (kPa)] available (as determined by the local water authority) at the water meter or other source of supply at the installation location. Adjust this minimum daily static pressure [psi (kPa)] for the following conditions:

   2.1. Determine the difference in elevation between the source of supply and the highest water supply outlet. Where the highest water supply outlet is located above the source of supply, deduct 0.5 psi (3.4 kPa) for each foot (0.3 m) of difference in elevation. Where the highest water supply outlet is located below the source of supply, add 0.5 psi (3.4 kPa) for each foot (0.3 m) of difference in elevation.

   2.2. Where a water pressure reducing valve is installed in the water distribution system, the minimum daily static water pressure available is 80 percent of the minimum daily static water pressure at the source of supply or the set pressure downstream of the pressure reducing valve, whichever is smaller.

   2.3. Deduct all pressure losses caused by special equipment such as a backflow preventer, water filter and water softener. Pressure loss data for each piece of equipment shall be obtained through the manufacturer of the device.

   2.4. Deduct the pressure in excess of 8 psi (55 kPa) resulting from installation of the special plumbing fixture, such as temperature-controlled shower and flushometer tank water closet. Using the resulting minimum available pressure, find the corresponding pressure range in Table AP201.1.

3. The maximum *developed length* for water piping is the actual length of pipe between the source of supply and the most remote fixture, including either hot (through the water heater) or cold water branches multiplied by a factor of 1.2 to compensate for pressure loss through fittings. Select the appropriate column in Table AP201.1 equal to or greater than the calculated maximum *developed length*.

4. To determine the size of water service pipe, meter and main distribution pipe to the building using the appropriate table, follow down the selected "maximum *developed length*" column to a fixture unit equal to or greater than the total installation demand calculated by using the "combined" water supply fixture unit column of Table AP201.1. Read the water service pipe and meter sizes in the first left-hand column and the main distribution pipe to the building in the second left-hand column on the same row.

5. To determine the size of each water distribution pipe, start at the most remote outlet on each branch (either hot or cold branch) and, working back toward the main distribution pipe to the building, add up the water supply fixture unit demand passing through each segment of the distribution system using the related hot or cold column of Table AP201.1. Knowing demand, the size of each segment shall be read from the second left-hand column of the same table and maximum *developed length* column selected in Steps 1 and 2, under the same or next smaller size meter row. In no case does the size of any branch or main need to be larger that the size of the main distribution pipe to the building established in Step 4.

TABLE AP201.1
MINIMUM SIZE OF WATER METERS, MAINS AND DISTRIBUTION PIPING
BASED ON WATER SUPPLY FIXTURE UNIT VALUES (w.s.f.u.)

METER AND SERVICE PIPE (inches)	DISTRIBUTION PIPE (inches)	MAXIMUM DEVELOPMENT LENGTH (feet)									
Pressure Range 30 to 39 psi		40	60	80	100	150	200	250	300	400	500
$^3/_4$	$^1/_2$ [a]	2.5	2	1.5	1.5	1	1	0.5	0.5	0	0
$^3/_4$	$^3/_4$	9.5	7.5	6	5.5	4	3.5	3	2.5	2	1.5
$^3/_4$	1	32	25	20	16.5	11	9	7.8	6.5	5.5	4.5
1	1	32	32	27	21	13.5	10	8	7	5.5	5
$^3/_4$	$1^1/_4$	32	32	32	32	30	24	20	17	13	10.5
1	$1^1/_4$	80	80	70	61	45	34	27	22	16	12
$1^1/_2$	$1^1/_4$	80	80	80	75	54	40	31	25	17.5	13
1	$1^1/_2$	87	87	87	87	84	73	64	56	45	36
$1^1/_2$	$1^1/_2$	151	151	151	151	117	92	79	69	54	43
2	$1^1/_2$	151	151	151	151	128	99	83	72	56	45
1	2	87	87	87	87	87	87	87	87	87	86
$1^1/_2$	2	275	275	275	275	258	223	196	174	144	122
2	2	365	365	365	365	318	266	229	201	160	134
2	$2^1/_2$	533	533	533	533	533	495	448	409	353	311

METER AND SERVICE PIPE (inches)	DISTRIBUTION PIPE (inches)	MAXIMUM DEVELOPMENT LENGTH (feet)									
Pressure Range 40 to 49 psi		40	60	80	100	150	200	250	300	400	500
$^3/_4$	$^1/_2$ [a]	3	2.5	2	1.5	1.5	1	1	0.5	0.5	0.5
$^3/_4$	$^3/_4$	9.5	9.5	8.5	7	5.5	4.5	3.5	3	2.5	2
$^3/_4$	1	32	32	32	26	18	13.5	10.5	9	7.5	6
1	1	32	32	32	32	21	15	11.5	9.5	7.5	6.5
$^3/_4$	$1^1/_4$	32	32	32	32	32	32	32	27	21	16.5
1	$1^1/_4$	80	80	80	80	65	52	42	35	26	20
$1^1/_2$	$1^1/_4$	80	80	80	80	75	59	48	39	28	21
1	$1^1/_2$	87	87	87	87	87	87	87	78	65	55
$1^1/_2$	$1^1/_2$	151	151	151	151	151	130	109	93	75	63
2	$1^1/_2$	151	151	151	151	151	139	115	98	77	64
1	2	87	87	87	87	87	87	87	87	87	87
$1^1/_2$	2	275	275	275	275	275	275	264	238	198	169
2	2	365	365	365	365	365	349	304	270	220	185
2	$2^1/_2$	533	533	533	533	533	533	533	528	456	403

(continued)

TABLE AP201.1—continued
MINIMUM SIZE OF WATER METERS, MAINS AND DISTRIBUTION PIPING
BASED ON WATER SUPPLY FIXTURE UNIT VALUES (w.s.f.u.)

METER AND SERVICE PIPE (inches)	DISTRIBUTION PIPE (inches)	MAXIMUM DEVELOPMENT LENGTH (feet)									
Pressure Range 50 to 60 psi		40	60	80	100	150	200	250	300	400	500
$^3/_4$	$^1/_2$ a	3	3	2.5	2	1.5	1	1	1	0.5	0.5
$^3/_4$	$^3/_4$	9.5	9.5	9.5	8.5	6.5	5	4.5	4	3	2.5
$^3/_4$	1	32	32	32	32	25	18.5	14.5	12	9.5	8
1	1	32	32	32	32	30	22	16.5	13	10	8
$^3/_4$	$1^1/_4$	32	32	32	32	32	32	32	32	29	24
1	$1^1/_4$	80	80	80	80	80	68	57	48	35	28
$1^1/_2$	$1^1/_4$	80	80	80	80	80	75	63	53	39	29
1	$1^1/_2$	87	87	87	87	87	87	87	87	82	70
$1^1/_2$	$1^1/_2$	151	151	151	151	151	151	139	120	94	79
2	$1^1/_2$	151	151	151	151	151	151	146	126	97	81
1	2	87	87	87	87	87	87	87	87	87	87
$1^1/_2$	2	275	275	275	275	275	275	275	275	247	213
2	2	365	365	365	365	365	365	365	329	272	232
2	$2^1/_2$	533	533	533	533	533	533	533	533	353	486

METER AND SERVICE PIPE (inches)	DISTRIBUTION PIPE (inches)	MAXIMUM DEVELOPMENT LENGTH (feet)									
Pressure Range Over 60		40	60	80	100	150	200	250	300	400	500
$^3/_4$	$^1/_2$ a	3	3	3	2.5	2	1.5	1.5	1	1	0.5
$^3/_4$	$^3/_4$	9.5	9.5	9.5	9.5	7.5	6	5	4.5	3.5	3
$^3/_4$	1	32	32	32	32	32	24	19.5	15.5	11.5	9.5
1	1	32	32	32	32	32	28	28	17	12	9.5
$^3/_4$	$1^1/_4$	32	32	32	32	32	32	32	32	32	30
1	$1^1/_4$	80	80	80	80	80	80	69	60	46	36
$1^1/_2$	$1^1/_4$	80	80	80	80	80	80	76	65	50	38
1	$1^1/_2$	87	87	87	87	87	87	87	87	87	84
$1^1/_2$	$1^1/_2$	151	151	151	151	151	151	151	144	114	94
2	$1^1/_2$	151	151	151	151	151	151	151	151	118	97
1	2	87	87	87	87	87	87	87	87	87	87
$1^1/_2$	2	275	275	275	275	275	275	275	275	275	252
2	2	365	368	368	368	368	368	368	368	318	273
2	$2^1/_2$	533	533	533	533	533	533	533	533	533	533

For SI: 1 inch = 25.4, 1 foot = 304.8 mm.
a. Minimum size for building supply is $^3/_4$-inch pipe.

ICC INTERNATIONAL RESIDENTIAL CODE ELECTRICAL PROVISIONS/NATIONAL ELECTRICAL CODE CROSS-REFERENCE

(This appendix is informative and is not part of the code. This table is a cross-reference of the
International Residential Code, Chapters 34 through 43, and the 2008 *National Electrical Code,* NFPA 70).

INDEX

T

U

V

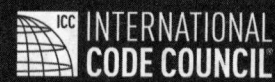
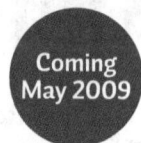
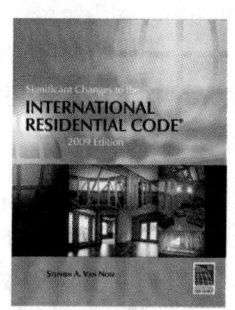
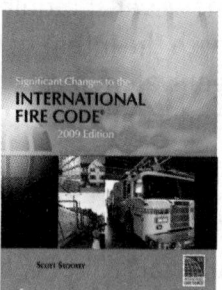
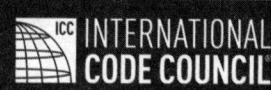

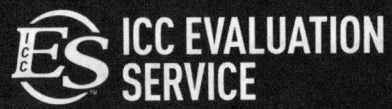

Innovative Building Products:

The Code Requirement

The International Building Code® Section 104.11 allows for the use of alternate building products. However, it requires building officials to verify that the proposed design is satisfactory and complies with the intent of the code. Specifically, the material, method or work offered must be at least the equivalent of that prescribed in the code in quality, strength, effectiveness, fire resistance, durability and safety.

What's in an ICC-ES Evaluation Report

Evaluation reports from ICC Evaluation Service® are the most preferred resource used by code officials to verify that new and innovative building products comply with code requirements. The evaluation reports provide information about what code requirements or acceptance criteria were used to evaluate the product, how the product should be installed to meet the requirements, how to identify the product, and much more. ES Reports are divided into eleven major areas.

1 **CSI Division Number**—ICC-ES Evaluation Reports, and the building products represented in them, are organized according to the Construction Specifications Institute's (CSI) Masterformat system.

2 **Report Holder**—The name and address of the company or organization that has applied for the Evaluation Report.

3 **Evaluation Subject**—The specific product(s) covered by the report.

4 **Evaluation Scope**—The code(s) that were used to evaluate the product.

5 **Properties Evaluated**—A brief description of the properties the product was evaluated against such as fire resistance and wind resistance. This section also shows if the product can be used for structural purposes.

6 **Uses**—Identifies the scope of the Evaluation Report and relates the product evaluated to code provisions.

7 **Description**—Provides a general description of the product and its features, such as length, thickness, etc.

8 **Installation**—Identifies general and often specific requirements to help the inspector ensure the product is installed properly according to the code requirements or acceptance criteria.

9 **Conditions of Use**—Statement that the product, as described in the Evaluation Report, complies with or is a suitable alternative to the requirements of the applicable code and a list of conditions under which the report is issued.

10 **Evidence Submitted**—Data (i.e. test reports, calculations, installation instructions) that was used in evaluating the product.

11 **Identification**—Information that can be used to identify the product, including the manufacturer's name, product code, Evaluation Report number, etc.

8-61804-64

Make sure they are up to code with ICC-ES Evaluation Reports

The ICC-ES Solution

ICC Evaluation Service® (ICC-ES®), a subsidiary of ICC®, was created to assist code officials and industry professionals in verifying that new and innovative building products meet code requirements. This is done through a comprehensive evaluation process that results in the publication of ICC-ES Evaluation Reports for those products that comply with requirements in the code or acceptance critiera. Today, more code officials prefer using ICC-ES Evaluation Reports over any other resource to verify products comply with codes.

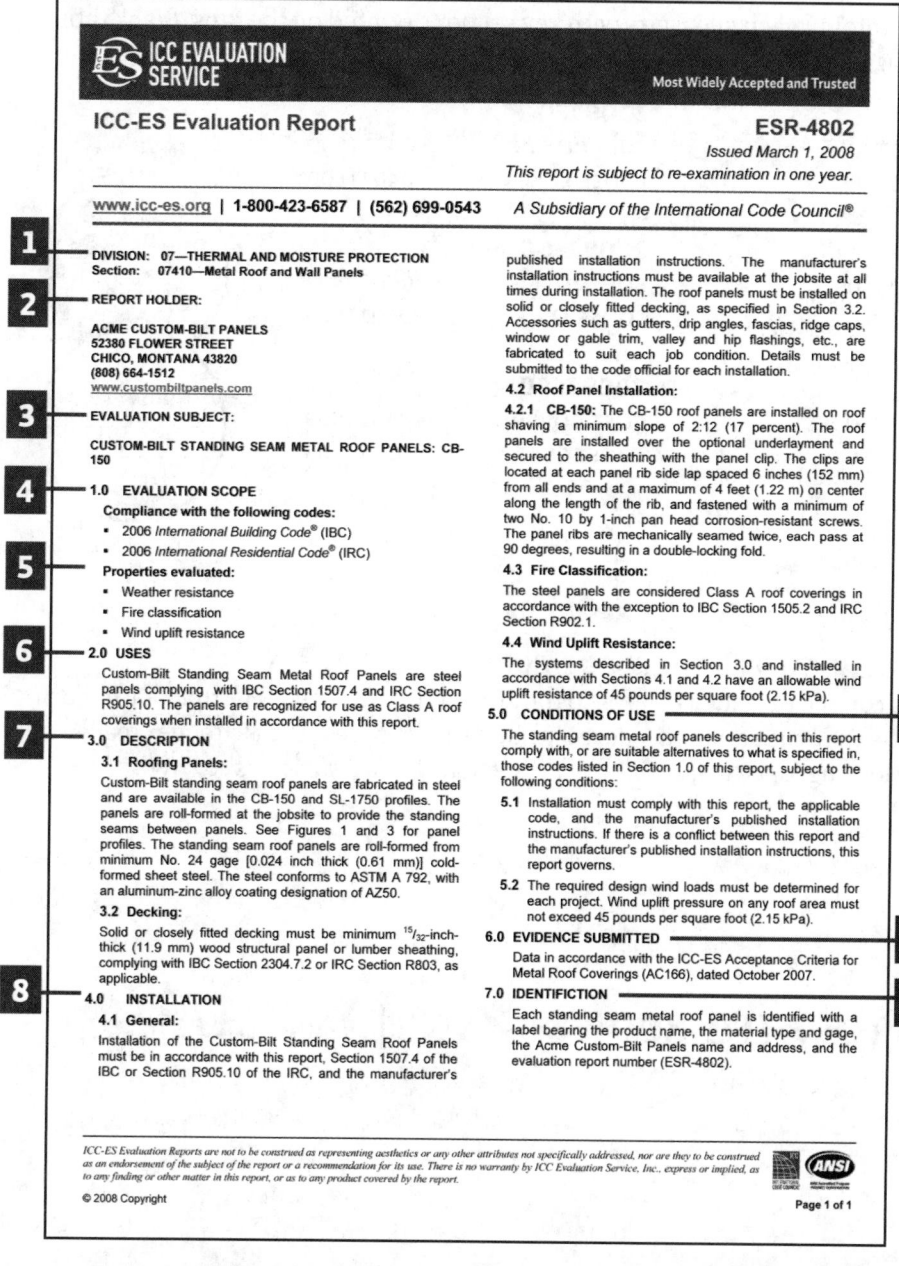

FREE Access to ICC-ES Evaluation Reports!

VIEW ONLINE NOW!
www.icc-es.org

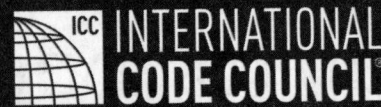

INTERNATIONAL CODE COUNCIL®

People Helping People Build a Safer World™

Cruise Through Your New I-Code

Tools that help you navigate the new codes

TURBO TABS

Find I-Code sections quickly using Turbo Tabs. With the most commonly-used sections of the code printed on each Tab, you can flip through the code and find frequently used sections fast!

Turbo Tabs are available for both soft cover and loose leaf codes. The soft cover versions contain clear plastic, self-adhesive tabs with key sections of the codes printed in an easy-to-read format. The loose leaf versions contain full-page inserts with key sections printed on the tabs. Blank tabs are now included allowing you to customize your tabs.

2009 IBC		**2009 IFC**	
SOFT COVER	#0001TS09	SOFT COVER	#0401TS09
LOOSE LEAF	#0001TL09	LOOSE LEAF	#0401TL09

2009 IRC		**2009 IFGC**	
SOFT COVER	#0101TS09	SOFT COVER	#0601TS09
LOOSE LEAF	#0101TL09	LOOSE LEAF	#0601TL09

2009 IPC		**2009 IEBC**	
SOFT COVER	#0201TS09	SOFT COVER	#0551TS09
LOOSE LEAF	#0201TL09	LOOSE LEAF	#0551TL09

2009 IMC	
SOFT COVER	#0301TS09
LOOSE LEAF	#0301TL09

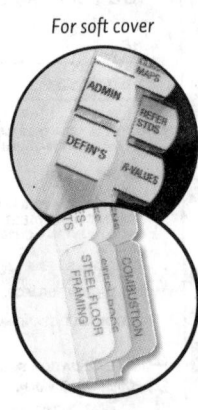

For soft cover

For loose leaf

EXTENDEX: EXTENDED INDEXES TO THE 2009 I-CODES®

These helpful references contain extended indexes to the 2009 IBC®, IRC®, and IFC® that reach much deeper into subject matter than the standard indexes included in the codes. Each Extendex makes it easy to find what you're looking for by listing the specific section where a subject is covered.

2009 IBC EXTENDEX	#4009S09
2009 IRC EXTENDEX	#4103S09
2009 IFC EXTENDEX	#4402S09

ORDER YOURS TODAY! 1-800-786-4452 | www.iccsafe.org

08-01106